# The Cleveland Clinic Intensive Review of Internal Medicine

**FOURTH EDITION**

**EDITORS**

■ **JAMES K. STOLLER, MD, MS**

Professor of Medicine, Cleveland Clinic Lerner College
of Medicine of Case Western Reserve University
Vice Chairman, Division of Medicine
Department of Pulmonary and Critical Care Medicine
Associate Chief of Staff
The Cleveland Clinic Foundation
Cleveland, Ohio

■ **FRANKLIN A. MICHOTA, Jr., MD**

Head, Section of Hospital Medicine
Department of General Internal Medicine
The Cleveland Clinic Foundation
Cleveland, Ohio

■ **BRIAN F. MANDELL, MD, PhD**

Vice Chairman, Division of Medicine for Education
Department of Rheumatic and Immunologic Disease
Deputy Editor
The Cleveland Clinic Journal of Medicine
The Cleveland Clinic Foundation
Cleveland, Ohio

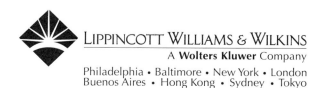

**LIPPINCOTT WILLIAMS & WILKINS**
A **Wolters Kluwer** Company

Philadelphia • Baltimore • New York • London
Buenos Aires • Hong Kong • Sydney • Tokyo

*Acquisitions Editor*: Sonya Seigafuse
*Developmental Editor*: Mary Choi
*Project Manager*: Nicole Walz
*Senior Manufacturing Manager*: Ben Rivera
*Senior Marketing Manager*: Kathy Neely
*Design Coordinator*: Holly McLaughlin
*Cover Designer*: Becky Baxendell
*Compositor*: TechBooks
*Printer*: Quebecor World–Taunton

© 2005 by LIPPINCOTT WILLIAMS & WILKINS
© 2002, 2000, and 1998 by Lippincott Williams & Wilkins
530 Walnut Street
Philadelphia, PA 19106 USA
LWW.com

**Library of Congress Cataloging-in-Publication Data**

The Cleveland Clinic intensive review of internal medicine / editors, James K. Stoller, Franklin A. Michota, Jr., Brian F. Mandell.— 4th ed.
      p. ; cm
   Includes bibliographical references and index.
   ISBN 0-7817-5733-9 (pbk.)
   1.   Internal medicine—Outlines, syllabi, etc. 2.   Internal medicine—Study guides. I. Stoller, James K. II. Michota, Franklin A. III. Mandell, Brian F., 1951– IV. Cleveland Clinic Foundation. V. Title: Intensive review of internal medicine.   [DNLM:
   1.   Internal Medicine—Examination Questions.   WB 18.2 C635 2005]
RC46.C548 2005 616'.0076—dc22

                                                              2005003223

Care has been taken to confirm the accuracy of the information presented and to describe generally accepted practices. However, the authors, editors, and publisher are not responsible for errors or omissions or for any consequences from application of the information in this book and make no warranty, expressed or implied, with respect to the currency, completeness, or accuracy of the contents of the publication. Application of this information in a particular situation remains the professional responsibility of the practitioner.

The authors, editors, and publisher have exerted every effort to ensure that drug selection and dosage set forth in this text are in accordance with current recommendations and practice at the time of publication. However, in view of ongoing research, changes in government regulations, and the constant flow of information relating to drug therapy and drug reactions, the reader is urged to check the package insert for each drug for any change in indications and dosage and for added warnings and precautions. This is particularly important when the recommended agent is a new or infrequently employed drug.

Some drugs and medical devices presented in this publication have Food and Drug Administration (FDA) clearance for limited use in restricted research settings. It is the responsibility of health care providers to ascertain the FDA status of each drug or device planned for use in their clinical practice.

10 9 8 7 6 5 4 3 2 1

To Terry and Jake, whose love and support have made this possible.

J.K.S.


To my wife and children for their ongoing support of a career that focuses my attention as much outside the home as it does inside.

F.A.M.


This textbook began several editions ago as a labor of love and commitment to life-long professional education by Jamie Stoller and David Longworth, the first course directors. The annual Internal Medicine Review course, and this text's existence as a vibrant experience, would be impossible without the dedication and clinical expertise of the many Cleveland Clinic physician educators noted within these pages. On a personal note, I gratefully acknowledge the patience and support of my family during this enterprise of late night editing sessions.

B.F.M.

# Contents

## SECTION X: MOCK BOARD SIMULATION  893

# Contributing Authors

**LOUTFI S. ABOUSSOUAN, MD**  Department of Pulmonary, Allergy, and Critical Care Medicine, The Cleveland Clinic Foundation, Cleveland, Ohio

**DAVID J. ADELSTEIN, MD**  Department of Hematology and Medical Oncology, The Cleveland Clinic Foundation, Cleveland, Ohio

**AMJAD ALMAHAMEED, MD**  Department of Cardiovascular Medicine, The Cleveland Clinic Foundation, Cleveland, Ohio

**JOHN ANDREFSKY, MD**  Northeast Ohio College of Medicine, Akron General Medical Center, Akron, Ohio

**STEVEN ANDRESEN, DO**  Department of Hematology and Medical Oncology, The Cleveland Clinic Foundation, Cleveland, Ohio

**GERALD B. APPEL, MD**  Professor of Clinical Medicine, Columbia University College of Physicians and Surgeons, New York, New York, and Director of Clinical Nephrology, Department of Medicine, Columbia-Presbyterian Hospital, New York, New York

**WENDY ARMSTRONG, MD**  Department of Infectious Diseases, The Cleveland Clinic Foundation, Cleveland, Ohio

**ALEJANDRO C. ARROLIGA, MD**  Professor of Medicine, Cleveland Clinic Lerner College of Medicine of Case Western Reserve University; Head, Section of Critical Care Medicine, Department of Pulmonary, Allergy, and Critical Care Medicine, The Cleveland Clinic Foundation, Cleveland, Ohio

**PELIN BATUR, MD**  Department of General Internal Medicine, The Cleveland Clinic Foundation, Cleveland, Ohio

**GERALD J. BECK, PhD**  Department of Biostatistics and Epidemiology, The Cleveland Clinic Foundation, Cleveland, Ohio

**DAVID E. BLUMENTHAL, MD**  Division of Rheumatology, Metro Health Medical Center, Cleveland, Ohio

**BRIAN J. BOLWELL, MD**  Professor of Medicine, Cleveland Clinic Lerner College of Medicine of Case Western Reserve University; Director, Bone Marrow Transplant Program, Department of Hematology and Medical Oncology, The Cleveland Clinic Foundation, Cleveland, Ohio

**JULIA BREYER-LEWIS, MD**  Professor, Department of Medicine, Division of Nephrology, Vanderbilt University School of Medicine, Nashville, Tennessee

**DAVID L. BRONSON, MD**  Chairman, Regional Medical Practice, The Cleveland Clinic Foundation, Cleveland, Ohio

**AARON BRZEZINSKI, MD**  Center for Inflammatory Bowel Disease, Department of Gastroenterology and Hepatology, The Cleveland Clinic Foundation, Cleveland, Ohio

**MARIE M. BUDEV, DO, MPH**  Assistant Medical Director, Lung Transplant Program, Department of Pulmonary, Allergy, and Critical Care Medicine, The Cleveland Clinic Foundation, Cleveland, Ohio

**CAROL A. BURKE, MD, FACP, FACG**  Director, Center for Colon Polyps and Cancer, Department of Gastroenterology, The Cleveland Clinic Foundation, Cleveland, Ohio

**LEONARD H. CALABRESE, DO**  Professor of Medicine, Cleveland Clinic Lerner College of Medicine of Case Western Reserve University; R. J. Fasenmyer Chair of Clinical Immunology, Department of Rheumatic and Immunologic Disease, The Cleveland Clinic Foundation, Cleveland, Ohio

**WILLIAM D. CAREY, MD**  Professor of Medicine, Cleveland Clinic Lerner College of Medicine of Case Western Reserve University; Director, Center for Continuing Education, Division of Hepatology, Department of Gastroenterology and Hepatology, The Cleveland Clinic Foundation, Cleveland, Ohio

**JEFFREY T. CHAPMAN, MD**  Department of Pulmonary, Allergy, and Critical Care Medicine, The Cleveland Clinic Foundation, Cleveland, Ohio

**MINA K. CHUNG, MD**  Department of Cardiovascular Medicine, The Cleveland Clinic Foundation, Cleveland, Ohio

**DARWIN L. CONWELL, MD**  Department of Gastroenterology and Hepatology, The Cleveland Clinic Foundation, Cleveland, Ohio

**AMANDA CURNOCK, MD**  Practice, Lafayette, Indiana

**ROSSANA D. DANESE, MD**  Division of Endocrinology, University Hospitals of Cleveland, Cleveland, Ohio

**STEVEN R. DEITCHER, MD**   Vice President, Medical Affairs, Nuvelo, Sunnyvale, California

**JOHN A. DUMOT, DO**   Section Head, Department of Gastroenterology and Hepatology, The Cleveland Clinic Foundation, Cleveland, Ohio

**RAED A. DWEIK, MD**   Associate Professor of Medicine, Cleveland Clinic Lerner College of Medicine of Case Western Reserve University; Department of Pulmonary, Allergy, and Critical Care Medicine, The Cleveland Clinic Foundation, Cleveland, Ohio

**CHARLES FAIMAN, MD**   Department of Endocrinology, Diabetes, and Metabolism, The Cleveland Clinic Foundation, Cleveland, Ohio

**GARY W. FALK, MD**   Director, Center for Swallowing and Esophageal Disorders, Department of Gastroenterology and Hepatology, The Cleveland Clinic Foundation, Cleveland, Ohio

**RICHARD A. FATICA, MD**   Department of Hypertension and Nephrology, The Cleveland Clinic Foundation, Cleveland, Ohio

**ANDREW J. FISHLEDER, MD**   Professor of Pathology, Cleveland Clinic Lerner College of Medicine of Case Western Reserve University; Chairman, Division of Education, The Cleveland Clinic Foundation, Cleveland, Ohio

**KATHLEEN S. N. FRANCO-BRONSON, MD, MS**   Director, Consultation-Liaison Psychiatry, Department of Psychiatry and Psychology, The Cleveland Clinic Foundation, Cleveland, Ohio

**SASAN GHAFFARI, MD**   Pacific Cardiovascular Associates, Costa Mesa, California

**BRIAN P. GRIFFIN, MD**   Vice Chairman, Department of Cardiovascular Medicine, The Cleveland Clinic Foundation, Cleveland, Ohio

**RICHARD A. GRIMM, DO**   Section of Cardiac Imaging, Department of Cardiovascular Medicine, The Cleveland Clinic Foundation, Cleveland, Ohio

**AMIR H. HAMRAHIAN, MD**   Adjunct Assistant Professor of Medicine, Cleveland Clinic Lerner College of Medicine of Case Western Reserve University; Department of Endocrinology, Diabetes, and Metabolism, The Cleveland Clinic Foundation, Cleveland, Ohio

**ROBERT E. HOBBS, MD**   Department of Cardiovascular Medicine, The Cleveland Clinic Foundation, Cleveland, Ohio

**GARY S. HOFFMAN, MD**   Professor of Medicine, Cleveland Clinic Lerner College of Medicine of Case Western Reserve University; Harold C. Schott Chair and Chairman, Department of Rheumatic and Immunologic Disease, and Director, Center for Vasculitis Care and Research, The Cleveland Clinic Foundation, Cleveland, Ohio

**EDWARD P. HORVATH, MD, MPH**   Department of Veterans Affairs Medical Center, Cleveland, Ohio

**MOHAMAD A. HUSSEIN, MD**   Department of Hematology and Medical Oncology, The Cleveland Clinic Foundation, Cleveland, Ohio

**CARLOS M. ISADA, MD**   Fellowship Program Director, Department of Infectious Diseases, The Cleveland Clinic Foundation, Cleveland, Ohio

**AMIR K. JAFFER, MD**   Medical Director, Impact Center and the Anticoagulation Clinic, Department of General Internal Medicine, The Cleveland Clinic Foudation, Cleveland, Ohio

**ANIL K. JAIN, MD**   Department of General Internal Medicine, The Cleveland Clinic Foundation, Cleveland, Ohio

**HANI JNEID, MD**   Cardiology Fellow, Division of Cardiology, University of Louisville, Louisville, Kentucky

**VIDYASAGAR KALAHASTI, MD**   Fellow in Training, Department of Cardiovascular Medicine, The Cleveland Clinic Foundation, Cleveland, Ohio

**MATT KALAYCIO, MD**   Director, Leukemia Program, Department of Hematology and Medical Oncology, The Cleveland Clinic Foundation, Cleveland, Ohio

**SAMIR R. KAPADIA, MD**   Department of Cardiovascular Medicine, The Cleveland Clinic Foundation, Cleveland, Ohio

**MANI S. KAVURU, MD**   Director, Pulmonary Function Laboratory, Department of Pulmonary, Allergy, and Critical Care Medicine, The Cleveland Clinic Foundation, Cleveland, Ohio

**THOMAS F. KEYS, MD**   Associate Professor of Medicine, Cleveland Clinic Lerner College of Medicine of Case Western Reserve University; Department of Infectious Diseases, The Cleveland Clinic Foundation, Cleveland, Ohio

**RICHARD S. LANG, MD, MPH**   Chairman, Department of General Internal Medicine, The Cleveland Clinic Foundation, Cleveland, Ohio

**SUSAN B. LEGRAND, MD, FACP**   Director of Education, The Cleveland Clinic Taussig Cancer Center, The Cleveland Clinic Foundation, Cleveland, Ohio

**DAVID S. LEVER, MD**   Department of Gastroenterology and Hepatology, The Cleveland Clinic Foundation, Cleveland, Ohio

**ANGELO A. LICATA, MD, PhD**   Clinical Assistant Professor of Medicine, Cleveland Clinic Lerner College of Medicine of Case Western Reserve University; Department of

Endocrinology, Diabetes, and Metabolism, The Cleveland Clinic Foundation, Cleveland, Ohio

**ALAN E. LICHTIN, MD**   Associate Professor of Medicine, Cleveland Clinic Lerner College of Medicine of Case Western Reserve University; Department of Hematology and Medical Oncology, The Cleveland Clinic Foundation, Cleveland, Ohio

**A. MICHAEL LINCOFF, MD**   Professor of Medicine, Cleveland Clinic Lerner College of Medicine of Case Western Reserve University; Department of Cardiovascular Medicine, The Cleveland Clinic Foundation, Cleveland, Ohio

**DAVID L. LONGWORTH, MD**   Chairman, Department of Medicine, Baystate Medical Center, Springfield, Massachusetts, and Deputy Chairman, Department of Medicine, Tufts University School of Medicine, Boston, Massachusetts

**CAREEN Y. LOWDER, MD, PhD**   Division of Ophthalmology, Cole Eye Institute, The Cleveland Clinic Foundation, Cleveland, Ohio

**BRIAN F. MANDELL, MD, PhD**   Professor of Medicine, Cleveland Clinic Lerner College of Medicine of Case Western Reserve University; Chairman, Division of Medicine (for Education), Department of Rhematic and Immunologic Disease, and Deputy Editor, Cleveland Clinic Journal of Medicine, The Cleveland Clinic Foundation, Cleveland, Ohio

**MAURIE MARKMAN, MD**   Vice President for Clinical Research, and Professor of Medicine, Department of Gynecologic Medical Oncology, University of Texas MD Anderson Cancer Center, Houston, Texas

**THOMAS H. MARWICK, MD, PhD**   Head, Section of Medicine, and Professor of Medicine, University of Queensland, Princess Alexandra Hospital Campus, Brisbane, Australia, and Director of Echocardiography, Princess Alexandra Hospital, Brisbane, Australia

**STEVEN D. MAWHORTER, MD**   Director, Travel Clinic, Department of Infectious Diseases, The Cleveland Clinic Foundation, Cleveland, Ohio

**PETER MAZZONE, MD, MPH**   Department of Pulmonary, Allergy, and Critical Care Medicine, The Cleveland Clinic Foundation, Cleveland, Ohio

**ADI E. MEHTA, MD**   Department of Endocrinology, Diabetes, and Metabolism, The Cleveland Clinic Foundation, Cleveland, Ohio

**ATUL C. MEHTA, MB, BS**   Vice Chairman, Department of Pulmonary, Allergy, and Critical Care Medicine, The Cleveland Clinic Foundation, Cleveland, Ohio

**TAREK MEKHAIL, MD, MSC**   Director, Lung Cancer Medical Oncology Program, The Cleveland Clinic Taussig Cancer Center, The Cleveland Clinic Foundation, Cleveland, Ohio

**FRANKLIN A. MICHOTA, JR., MD**   Head, Section of Hospital Medicine, Department of General Internal Medicine, The Cleveland Clinic Foundation, Cleveland, Ohio

**DOUGLAS S. MOODIE, MD, MS**   Chairman, Department of Pediatrics, Ochsner Clinic, New Orleans, Louisiana

**HALLE C. F. MOORE, MD**   Department of Hematology and Medical Oncology, The Cleveland Clinic Foundation, Cleveland, Ohio

**DARIUS M. MOSHFEGHI, MD**   Assistant Professor, Department of Ophthalmology, and Head, Opthalmic Oncology, Stanford University, Palo Alto, California

**SHERIF B. MOSSAD, MD**   Department of Infectious Diseases, The Cleveland Clinic Foundation, Cleveland, Ohio

**JOSEPH V. NALLY, JR., MD**   Department of Nephrology and Hypertension, The Cleveland Clinic Foundation, Cleveland, Ohio

**CRAIG NIELSEN, MD**   Program Director, Internal Medicine Residency Program, The Cleveland Clinic Foundation, Cleveland, Ohio

**ROBERT M. PALMER, MD, MPH**   Head, Section of Geriatric Medicine, Department of General Internal Medicine, The Cleveland Clinic Foundation, Cleveland, Ohio

**DAVID PEEREBOOM, MD**   Department of Hematology and Medical Oncology, The Cleveland Clinic Foundation, Cleveland, Ohio

**ROBERT J. PELLEY, MD**   Department of Hematology and Medical Oncology, The Cleveland Clinic Foundation, Cleveland, Ohio

**VICTOR PEREZ, MD**   Division of Ophthalmology, Cole Eye Institute, The Cleveland Clinic Foundation, Cleveland, Ohio

**MELISSA PECK PILIANG, MD**   Department of Dermatology, The Cleveland Clinic Foundation, Cleveland, Ohio

**MARC A. POHL, MD**   Ray W. Gifford Jr. Endowed Chair in Hypertension, Department of Nephrology and Hypertension, and Section Head, Clinical Hypertension and Nephrology, The Cleveland Clinic Foundation, Cleveland, Ohio

**BRAD L. POHLMAN, MD**   Department of Hematology and Medical Oncology, The Cleveland Clinic Foundation, Cleveland, Ohio

**VAKESH RAJANI, MD**   Practice, Clearwater, Florida

**S. SETHU K. REDDY, MD, MBA**   Chairman and Program Director, Department of Endocrinology, Diabetes, and Metabolism, The Cleveland Clinic Foundation, Cleveland, Ohio

**KAREN E. RENDT, MD**   Education Program Co-Director, Department of Rheumatic and Immunologic Disease, The Cleveland Clinic Foundation, Cleveland, Ohio

**JOEL E. RICHTER, MD**    Professor of Medicine, and Chair, Department of Medicine, Temple University, School of Medicine, Philadelphia, Pennsylvania

**CURTIS M. RIMMERMAN, MD, MBA**    Gus P. Karos Chair in Clinical Cardiovascular Medicine, Department of Cardiovascular Medicine, The Cleveland Clinic Foundation, Cleveland, Ohio

**ELISA K. ROSS, MD**    Department of Obstetrics and Gynecology, The Cleveland Clinic Foundation, Cleveland, Ohio

**MARTIN A. SAMUELS, MD**    Chairman, Department of Neurology, Brigham and Women's Hospital, Boston, Massachusetts, and Professor of Neurology, Harvard Medical School, Boston, Massachusetts

**RAYMOND J. SCHEETZ, JR., MD**    Department of Rheumatic and Immunologic Disease, The Cleveland Clinic Foundation, Cleveland, Ohio

**STEVEN K. SCHMITT, MD**    Department of Infectious Diseases, The Cleveland Clinic Foundation, Cleveland, Ohio

**MARTIN J. SCHREIBER, JR., MD**    Department of Nephrology and Hypertension, The Cleveland Clinic Foundation, Cleveland, Ohio

**EDY E. SOFFER, MD**    GI Motility Program, Cedars-Sinai Medical Center, Los Angeles, California; Department of Gastroenterology and Hepatology, The Cleveland Clinic Foundation, Cleveland, Ohio

**DENNIS L. SPRECHER, MD**    Adjunct Professor, Division of Cardiology, University of Pennsylvania, Philadelphia, Pennsylvania, and Director, Dyslipidemia, Discovery Medicine, GlaxoSmithKline, Philadelphia, Pennsylvania

**JAMES K. STOLLER, MD, MS**    Professor of Medicine, Cleveland Clinic Lerner College of Medicine of Case Western Reserve University; Vice Chairman, Division of Medicine, Head, Section of Respiratory Therapy, Department of Pulmonary, Allergy, and Critical Care Medicine, and Associate Chief of Staff, The Cleveland Clinic Foundation, Cleveland, Ohio

**ALAN J. TAEGE, MD**    Department of Infectious Diseases, The Cleveland Clinic Foundation, Cleveland, Ohio

**HOLLY L. THACKER, MD**    Head, Section of Women's Health, Departments of General Internal Medicine and Gynecology and Obstetrics, The Cleveland Clinic Foundation, Cleveland, Ohio

**KENNETH J. TOMECKI, MD**    Department of Dermatology, The Cleveland Clinic Foundation, Cleveland, Ohio

**J. WALTON TOMFORD, MD**    Department of Infectious Diseases, The Cleveland Clinic Foundation, Cleveland, Ohio

**DONALD A. UNDERWOOD, MD**    Head, Section of Electrocardiography, Department of Cardiovascular Medicine, The Cleveland Clinic Foundation, Cleveland, Ohio

**JOHN J. VARGO II, MD**    Director, Fellowship Training Program, Department of Gastroenterology and Hepatology, The Cleveland Clinic Foundation, Cleveland, Ohio

**DONALD G. VIDT, MD**    Department of Nephrology and Hypertension, The Cleveland Clinic Foundation, Cleveland, Ohio

**ROBERT S. ZIMMERMAN, MD**    Department of Endocrinology, Diabetes, and Metabolism, The Cleveland Clinic Foundation, Cleveland, Ohio

# Preface

This fourth edition of *The Cleveland Clinic Intensive Review of Internal Medicine* reflects our ongoing fascination with how physicians learn best and our continued passion for clinical medicine, medical education, and scholarship—values that define the culture of The Cleveland Clinic Foundation. This book has its origin in the Foundation's Intensive Review of Internal Medicine Symposium, a 6-day course offered annually since 1989, that is designed for physicians preparing for the certification and recertification examinations in internal medicine, and for those wishing for a comprehensive, state-of-the-art review of the field. The symposium celebrates its seventeenth offering in the United States in June 2005, and it has been presented four times internationally.

We continue to be humbled and gratified by the success of the Symposium and of the first three editions of this book. Experience has taught us that practicing physicians learn best when using a case-driven format, and that factual knowledge and new developments in the field are best integrated into clinical practice through a discussion of case management. Never meant to be a comprehensive textbook of internal medicine, the fourth edition builds on this concept and continues to use bulleted points, clinical vignettes, and review exercises to convey important "clinical pearls."

Each chapter in the fourth edition has been reviewed and carefully updated where necessary, and many chapters have been substantially revised or rewritten. Several chapters are new since the third edition, reflecting input from our readers and attendees of the Intensive Review of Internal Medicine Symposium. Updated references have been provided in the suggested readings at the end of each chapter. The mock Board examination has been revised and now includes 205 multiple-choice questions, with an explanation and discussion of the correct and incorrect answers.

This book serves as the syllabus for both domestic and international offerings of the Intensive Review of Internal Medicine Symposium. It also provides an independent study guide for preparing for the certification and recertification examinations in internal medicine.

We remain extraordinarily grateful to our colleagues and contributors who have supported the Symposium and this book over the years. They represent the best and brightest among clinician scholars and educators, adept at teaching the art and science of medicine and facile in distilling their clinical wisdom into a concise and practical document. In addition, we are indebted to our students, residents, fellows, and colleagues, who have taught us so much over the years about clinical medicine and about how physicians learn best. Finally, there are several people without whom this book would not have come to fruition. We are indebted to David Longworth, MD, our friend and former editor, now Chair of Medicine at Baystate Medical Center in Springfield, Massachusetts. As one of the founding editors of the book, his wisdom and organizational skills are still evident in the fourth edition. We are grateful to Danette Somers and to Sonya Seigafuse of Lippincott Williams & Wilkins (LWW) for their ongoing support, both editorial and intellectual, in building on past editions. Mary Choi of LWW provided superb developmental editorial help. We also thank Beth Dobish, our administrative assistant, who contributed energy and craftsmanship in shepherding each chapter through editorial revision, completion, and submission to the publisher. Finally, we are grateful to our families, who tolerated and supported the many hours we devoted to this book.

As editors, we take pride in this book's content, and we accept sole responsibility for its shortcomings. We hope that this book deepens your own passion for clinical medicine and medical education, just as it has continued to fuel our own.

*James K. Stoller, MD, MS*
*Franklin A. Michota, Jr, MD*
*Brian A. Mandell, MD, PhD*

# Multidisciplinary Skills for the Internist

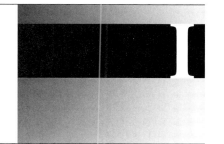

# Health Screening and Adult Immunizations

*Craig Nielsen    Richard S. Lang*

Conceptually, preventive medicine involves four tasks for the clinician: screening, counseling, immunization, and prophylaxis. Preventive interventions have been categorized as primary, secondary, and tertiary. *Primary prevention* is the reduction of risk factors before a disease or condition has occurred. Examples are immunization, use of safety equipment, dietary management, and smoking cessation. Primary prevention aims to reduce the incidence of a disease or condition. *Incidence* is the number of persons developing a condition or disease in a specific period of time. *Secondary prevention* is the detection of a condition or disease to reverse or slow the condition or disease and thereby improve prognosis. Examples of secondary prevention are mammography and Papanicolaou (Pap) smears. Secondary prevention ideally detects and intervenes in a condition before that condition is clinically apparent. Secondary prevention therefore aims to reduce the prevalence of a disease. *Prevalence* is the total number of individuals who have a condition or disease at a particular time. *Tertiary prevention* is the minimizing of the future negative health effects of a disease or condition. An example of tertiary prevention is the aggressive treatment of cholesterol in a patient with a known history of coronary artery disease.

The considerations in screening for a disease or condition should include the following questions:

- Is the disease or condition an important problem? (What are the morbidity and mortality of the condition?)
- Is the disease or condition a common problem? (What are its prevalence and incidence?)
- Is the screening test accurate? (What are its sensitivity, specificity, and predictive value?)
- Does the screening determine prevalence or incidence?
- What is the cost of the screening procedure? (Consider both financial and health risks.)
- What are the available follow-up diagnostic procedures?
- What is the available treatment for the disease or condition?
- How acceptable to patients is the screening procedure?
- What are the circumstances for the screening? (What is the context—for example, health maintenance, occupational, preoperative screening?)
- What are the current recommendations for screening and the medical evidence to support these recommendations?

The ideal screening situation uses an inexpensive, noninvasive test with a high level of sensitivity and specificity to detect a common problem that can be treated but, if left untreated, leads to significant morbidity and mortality.

*Sensitivity* is the ability of a test to correctly identify those who have a condition or disease.

*Specificity* is the ability of a test to correctly identify those who do not have the disease or condition in question. The *predictive values* for a screening test are the proportions of people correctly labeled as having the condition or disease (positive predictive value) and those not having the condition or disease (negative predictive value). Table 1.1 illustrates these terms. This 2 $\times$ 2 table is a common method for viewing the application of a screening test in a population.

## LEADING CAUSES OF MORTALITY

The optimal use of screening requires a basic understanding of the common causes of mortality. Table 1.2 outlines the most common causes of mortality for adult age groups, and Table 1.3 shows the average life expectancy of males and females at different ages.

Accidents, homicide, and suicide are common causes of mortality in young adults. Motor vehicle injuries account for more than 25% of the deaths in persons 15 to 24 years of age. The use of seat belts, a form of primary prevention, can reduce crash mortality by as much as 50%. Homicide is the leading cause of death of black males in the 15- to 24-year-old age group. Counseling regarding handgun safety is therefore an important intervention for this population. Suicide is another common cause of death in the young age group and is more common in those infected with the human immunodeficiency virus (HIV). Surveillance and counseling for suicide in this patient population are therefore important. HIV infection continues as an important cause of morbidity in the younger age groups. Preventive efforts related to sexual practices and to use of intravenous drugs are important interventions.

Heart disease and cancer are the leading causes of mortality in adults older than 45 years. Preventive efforts therefore should be directed to these conditions. Projections indicate that cancer will become the leading cause of adult mortality

|                | Disease | No Disease | Total |
|----------------|---------|------------|-------|
| Test positive  | True (+)[a] | False (+) | All (+) |
| Test negative  | False (−) | True (−) | All (−) |
| Total          | All with disease | All without disease | Total patients |

[a] Sensitivity = True (+) | [True (+) + False (−)] = how well the test correctly detects those with disease. Specificity = True (−) | [True (−) + False (+)] = how well the test identifies those without disease. Positive predictive value = True (+) | [True (+) + False (+)] = when a test is positive, the proportion of those with the disease. Negative predictive value = True (−) | [True (−) + False (−)] = when a test is negative, the proportion of those without the disease.

**TABLE 1.3**
**AVERAGE LIFE EXPECTANCY (UNITED STATES 2001)**

| Gender and Age | Years of Survival Life | Expectancy |
|----------------|------------------------|------------|
| Males |  |  |
| 65 | 16.4 | 81.4 |
| 70 | 13.1 | 83.1 |
| 75 | 10.2 | 85.2 |
| Females |  |  |
| 65 | 19.4 | 84.4 |
| 70 | 15.7 | 85.7 |
| 75 | 12.4 | 87.4 |
| 85 | 6.9 | 91.9 |

in the near future. The lifetime probability of developing cancer is estimated to be 45% in males and 38% in females. Common cancer sites in women are the breast, lung, colon/rectum, uterus, and ovary (Fig. 1.1). Leading cancer sites in men are the prostate, lung, colon/rectum, and bladder. Common causes of cancer death in women are lung, breast, and colon/rectum cancers; in men, lung, prostate, and colon/rectum cancers. Screening and prevention efforts are therefore targeted at the most common cancers as well as those most often leading to death—lung, colon/rectum, breast, and prostate cancers (Fig. 1.1).

## SCREENING TESTS BY ORGAN SYSTEM AND DISEASE

### Cardiovascular System

For preventive purposes, atherosclerotic heart disease, stroke, and peripheral vascular disease are grouped together because of their similar risk factors:

- Previous atherosclerotic vascular disease
- Family history of premature vascular disease
- Smoking
- Hypertension

- Diabetes
- Hyperlipidemia
- Age older than 45 years in men and older than 55 years in women
- Premature menopause in women without estrogen replacement therapy

A high-density lipoprotein (HDL) cholesterol level greater than 60 mg/dL is thought to be a negative risk factor, or "protective" factor, for the development of coronary vascular disease. Low-density lipoprotein (LDL) cholesterol reduction has been proved to result in cardiovascular disease benefits in the setting of both primary and secondary prevention. The U.S. Preventive Services Task Force recommends the measurement of total serum cholesterol level and HDL cholesterol level in a nonfasting state in "asymptomatic" adults, generally every 5 years beginning at age 35 in men, at age 45 in women, and at younger ages (20 to 35 in men and 20 to 45 in women) in those with additional cardiovascular risk factors. In persons of high risk, more frequent and earlier screening is suggested. The National Cholesterol Education Program (NCEP) recommends screening beginning at age 20 with a fasting lipid profile. An age to stop screening is not established, nor is there clear evidence to support the measurement of triglycerides as a routine screening test.

**TABLE 1.2**
**LEADING CAUSES OF DEATH (UNITED STATES 2001)**

| Rank | Overall Population | Aged 25–34 | Aged 35–64 | Aged 65–74 | Aged 75–84 |
|------|--------------------|-----------|-----------|-----------|-----------|
| 1 | Heart disease | Accidents | Cancer | Cancer | Heart |
| 2 | Cancer | Suicide | Heart | Heart | Cancer |
| 3 | Stroke | Homicide | Accidents | COPD | Stroke |
| 4 | COPD[a] | Cancer | Cirrhosis | Stroke | COPD |
| 5 | Accidents | Heart | Suicide | Diabetes | Diabetes |
| 6 | Diabetes | Diabetes | Stroke | Accidents | Influenza and pneumonia |

[a] COPD, chronic obstructive pulmonary disease

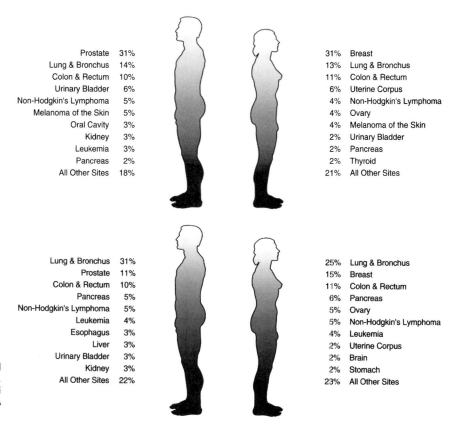

Estimated New Cases*

| Prostate | 31% | | 31% | Breast |
| Lung & Bronchus | 14% | | 13% | Lung & Bronchus |
| Colon & Rectum | 10% | | 11% | Colon & Rectum |
| Urinary Bladder | 6% | | 6% | Uterine Corpus |
| Non-Hodgkin's Lymphoma | 5% | | 4% | Non-Hodgkin's Lymphoma |
| Melanoma of the Skin | 5% | | 4% | Ovary |
| Oral Cavity | 3% | | 4% | Melanoma of the Skin |
| Kidney | 3% | | 2% | Urinary Bladder |
| Leukemia | 3% | | 2% | Pancreas |
| Pancreas | 2% | | 2% | Thyroid |
| All Other Sites | 18% | | 21% | All Other Sites |

Estimated Deaths

| Lung & Bronchus | 31% | | 25% | Lung & Bronchus |
| Prostate | 11% | | 15% | Breast |
| Colon & Rectum | 10% | | 11% | Colon & Rectum |
| Pancreas | 5% | | 6% | Pancreas |
| Non-Hodgkin's Lymphoma | 5% | | 5% | Ovary |
| Leukemia | 4% | | 5% | Non-Hodgkin's Lymphoma |
| Esophagus | 3% | | 4% | Leukemia |
| Liver | 3% | | 2% | Uterine Corpus |
| Urinary Bladder | 3% | | 2% | Brain |
| Kidney | 3% | | 2% | Stomach |
| All Other Sites | 22% | | 23% | All Other Sites |

**Figure 1.1** Estimated new cancer cases and cancer deaths: ten leading sites by gender, United States, 2004. [From Jemal A, Tiwari RC, Murray T, et al. Cancer Statistics, 2004. *CA Cancer J Clin* 2004;54:8–29.]

Most authorities advise measuring the blood pressure in normotensive persons at least every 2 years, particularly in those with prior diastolic readings of 85 to 89 mm Hg, prior systolic readings of 135 to 139 mm Hg, or those who are obese or who have a first-degree relative with hypertension. The current recommended classification of blood pressure, based on the Seventh Report of the Joint National Committee on Prevention, Detection, Evaluation, and Treatment of High Blood Pressure (JNC 7), is as follows:

- Normal BP          S BP <120          D BP <80
- Prehypertension    S BP 120–139       D BP 80–89
- Stage 1 HTN        S BP 140–159       D BP 90–99
- Stage 2 HTN        S BP >160          D BP >100

Lifestyle modifications are appropriate for all stages of hypertension, including prehypertension. These modifications include optimizing weight; limiting alcohol; participating in regular aerobic exercise; reducing sodium intake; and maintaining an adequate intake of dietary potassium, calcium, and magnesium. Drug therapy is indicated for Stage 1 and Stage 2 hypertension.

Low-dose aspirin therapy should be considered for the primary prevention of ischemic heart disease in men older than age 40 who are at high risk. The optimal preventive aspirin dosage is not clearly established and ranges from 81 to 325 mg daily. The side effects and potential complications of chronic aspirin usage should be considered carefully.

The electrocardiogram is not a sensitive screening test for coronary artery disease in asymptomatic patients and therefore is not generally advised as a screening test. Considerations for obtaining a preoperative electrocardiogram include the patient's age, procedure planned, anesthesia to be used, cardiovascular risk factors, and the presence of other systemic disease. Exercise treadmill testing has limited sensitivity (approximately 65%) and specificity (approximately 75% to 85%) for detecting coronary artery disease. Stress testing is most useful when coronary artery disease is suspected or likely to be present. Therefore, treadmill testing is most effectively used for those with multiple risk factors. Stress testing also should be considered for those engaging in occupations that demand physical exertion or that may impact on public safety. Otherwise, exercise treadmill testing should not be used routinely in asymptomatic persons.

Similarly, the use of noninvasive vascular evaluation of the carotid arteries should be reserved for patients in whom disease is suspected, based either on symptoms or the presence of carotid bruits. The prevalence of carotid bruits in the adult population is approximately 4% to 5%. Ultrasonographic screening of the abdominal aorta for aortic aneurysm should be reserved for men older than 50 years with a family history of aortic aneurysm and vascular disease risk factors, especially hypertensive males who smoke tobacco products.

In summary, risk factors for the development of vascular disease should be assessed in all patients; modifiable risk factors should be addressed; blood pressure and cholesterol should be monitored and treated appropriately; and stress testing and assessment of carotid arteries and abdominal aorta are best undertaken in patients in whom coronary artery disease, carotid atherosclerosis, or aortic aneurysm are most likely to be present.

## LUNG CANCER

The numbers of new cancer cases and cancer deaths for specific types of cancers are shown in Figure 1.1. Lung cancer is the most common cause of cancer death in the United States. Cigarette smoking is the most important risk factor for the development of lung cancer. Generally, smokers are 10 times more likely to die of lung cancer than nonsmokers. The risk for developing lung cancer depends on the number of cigarettes smoked, the age when smoking began, and the degree of inhalation. The risk for lung cancer decreases after smoking is stopped, particularly after 5 years or more. Therefore, the most important preventive interventions for lung cancer are avoidance and cessation of smoking. Other risk factors for the development of lung cancer are occupational exposures (asbestos, arsenic, chloromethyl ethers, chromium, polycyclic aromatic compounds, nickel, and vinyl chloride), chronic obstructive lung disease, previous lung cancer, previous head and neck cancer, and radon exposure.

Generally, screening for lung cancer in asymptomatic patients has not been advised, because large-scale studies have not demonstrated a reduction in mortality when screening interventions such as serial chest x-rays and frequent sputum cytology were applied to high-risk populations. Therefore, routine screening chest radiography should be reserved for situations in which clinical evidence suggests the presence of disease. More recently, computerized tomographic (CT) scanning techniques of the chest have shown promise as a screening modality in high-risk patients. This type of testing is under continued study and is still not currently advocated as a general screening test.

## BREAST CANCER

Risk factors for breast cancer are:

■ Family history of breast cancer
■ BRCA-1 and BRCA-2 genes
■ Previous breast cancer
■ Menarche before age 13
■ Late menopause (after age 50)
■ Late first pregnancy (after age 35)
■ Previous lobular carcinoma *in situ* of the breast
■ Previous cancer of the uterus, ovary, or salivary gland

A family history of breast cancer is a particularly important risk factor when diagnosed in a premenopausal first-degree relative or bilaterally in any first-degree relative. A

woman with a premenopausal first-degree relative who had breast cancer has a threefold risk of developing breast cancer herself. An estimated 80% of women diagnosed with breast cancer do not have a positive family history, however. High socioeconomic status, nulliparity, hormone replacement therapy, and prior exposure to high-dose radiation also convey modestly increased risk.

Screening for breast cancer includes breast self-examination, clinical breast examination by a physician or nurse, and mammography. A large number of breast cancers are found by palpation. Breast self-examination has low sensitivity and unknown specificity. Appropriate teaching is required for effective breast self-examination. Many advisory groups now list self breast-examination as an optional test because of lack of evidence regarding its effectiveness. Annual clinical breast examination by a physician or healthcare professional is recommended by the major advisory panels for women older than age 40. Mammography has a variable but good sensitivity for detecting breast cancer, in the range of 74% to 93%. Specificity is also relatively good, at approximately 90% to 95%. The positive predictive value of an abnormal mammogram is approximately 10% to 20%. A normal mammogram has a negative predictive value of approximately 99%. All major authoritative groups recommend routine mammography screening after age 50. Studies have shown that mammography screening in women 50 to 69 years of age leads to a reduction of approximately 30% in breast cancer mortality. The benefits of mammography for women of normal risk younger than age 50 have been uncertain, and much debate has taken place regarding screening for this age group. More recent data suggest a positive benefit from screening in the age group of 40 to 50 years, leading most authorities to recommend mammography screening for women in this age group. Evidence is lacking as to the efficacy of screening mammography in women older than age 70, but because of the high risk for breast cancer in this age group, many have recommended a continuation of screening. Life expectancy of the individual woman is a major factor to consider for screening in this age group. If life expectancy is greater than 10 years, mammogram screening may be reasonable to consider. In general, clinical breast examinations should be instituted in women at around the age of 40, and mammography screening should be started between the ages of 40 and 50. Risk assessment tools have been developed, such as the Gail model, which helps to stratify risk for an individual. Women with the greatest risk should be considered for screening at an earlier age. Screening women in a higher risk category beginning at age 40 and screening women of no increased risk at 45 to 50 appears to be a reasonable approach. Mammography frequency depends on the individual's risk factors. Less frequent screenings for low-risk women can be undertaken, but generally screening is done yearly. Screening should be continued into the later years until less frequent screening in that age group is supported by clinical studies.

## COLON AND RECTAL CANCER

Risk factors for colon cancer are:

- Prior colon cancer
- Familial polyposis
- Family history of hereditary nonpolyposis colorectal cancer
- Inflammatory bowel disease
- Family history of colorectal cancer
- History of endometrial, ovarian, or breast cancer
- History of adenomatous polyps of the colon
- Lifestyle factors: tobacco use, obesity, excessive alcohol use

The overall lifetime risk for colon cancer in the U.S. population is approximately 6%. The younger the age of a first-degree relative encountering colon cancer, and the more numerous the number of family members having had colon cancer, the greater the risk to the patient. Screening for colon cancer is best conducted by determining whether a patient has normal or high risk. The testing type and frequency can then be selected based on that risk stratification. Screening strategies for colon cancer vary somewhat between different advisory groups, but all agree that some form of screening is very important.

Fecal occult blood testing is a cheap screening test but often involves poor patient compliance, has a limited sensitivity of approximately 50% to 65% for colon cancer, and has a positive predictive value for cancer of approximately 10% to 15%. It is estimated that yearly fecal occult blood testing lowers colon cancer mortality in an individual by approximately 30%, however. In those of normal risk older than age 50, most authoritative groups have advised yearly fecal occult blood testing. This test can be falsely positive due to diet or medications and, for accuracy, should be combined with other screening tests.

Sigmoidoscopy has a relatively low sensitivity for detecting cancer of the colon, approximately 40% to 60%. Sigmoidoscopy is limited by examiner technique and the length of colon examined. In those of average risk, screening sigmoidoscopy is generally advised every 5 years beginning at approximately age 50.

Colonoscopy conveys a sensitivity for colon cancer of approximately 80% to 90%. Colonoscopy has the advantage of examining the whole colon and is believed by many to be the preferred method for screening (every 10 years). Cost, bowel preparation, the potential need for sedation, the advanced training needed for the endoscopist, and limited data regarding its effect on colon cancer mortality must be factored in the screening decision-making process, however. In high-risk patients, most authoritative groups have advised screening starting at an earlier age, usually around age 40 or even 10 years earlier. The advised type of screening varies. Most authoritative groups have suggested periodic colonoscopy at a frequency of approximately once every 5 years.

An air-contrast barium enema also has a high sensitivity for colon cancer, approximately 90% or greater. The air-contrast barium enema is generally cheaper than colonoscopy, has a lower complication rate, and can provide a better view of the cecum, but it does not allow for biopsy or removal of polyps, as can be done during colonoscopy. Many advisor groups no longer recommend air-contrast barium enema for routine screening, but in some patients, air-contrast barium enema may still be used because of patient preference. Both CT colonography (*virtual colonoscopy*) and fecal DNA mutation testing are promising new screening modalities, but these are currently not recommended until further studies are completed.

In summary, the risk for future development of colon cancer should be assessed in each patient. In those of low or average risk, screening should consist of fecal occult blood testing yearly and sigmoidoscopy every 5 years after the age of 50 or by colonoscopy every 10 years. In patients with a family history of colon cancer, the risk depends on the number of relatives affected. For patients with a family history that includes one first-degree relative or two second-degree relatives with colon cancer, fecal occult blood testing and sigmoidoscopy can be initiated at around the age of 40, with consideration given to screening with colonoscopy. For patients with a family history that includes two or more first-degree relatives or one first-degree relative with cancer or adenomatous polyp before the age of 40, a colonoscopy should be performed every 5 years after the age of 40 or 10 years younger than the youngest affected family member. Those in a very high-risk group (e.g., familial polyposis, inflammatory bowel disease) should generally be referred to a specialty center for more aggressive screening and monitoring.

## PROSTATE CANCER

Risk factors for prostate cancer are:

- Advanced age
- African American race
- Family history of prostate cancer
- Smoking

With the advent of widespread screening for prostate cancer, the lifetime risk of a man being diagnosed with prostate cancer is approximately 15%, but the risk of death from prostate cancer is only around 3%. Digital rectal examination has a sensitivity of approximately 33% to 70% and a specificity of 50% to 95% for detecting prostate cancer. Digital rectal examination has not been shown to decrease mortality from prostate cancer. Prostate-specific antigen (PSA) has been used to screen for prostate cancer. A PSA level of greater than 4 ng/mL has a sensitivity of approximately 71%, specificity of approximately 75%, positive predictive value of approximately 35% to 40%, and negative predictive value of approximately 90% for prostate cancer.

PSA levels increase in both benign and malignant prostate disease. Variations on PSA testing, such as age-specific PSA, PSA density, PSA velocity, and free PSA levels, have sought to improve the sensitivity and specificity of the test but are currently not recommended by most advisory groups for routine screening. To date, no clear evidence has shown that the early detection and treatment of prostate cancer decreases mortality. Randomized clinical trials are currently in progress to try to answer these questions. Likewise, when prostate cancer is found at an early stage, presently no simple method exists for distinguishing clinically significant cancer from an indolent form. Screening for prostate cancer can lead to morbidity in those who may never have been affected by the disease and is costly when follow-up diagnostic studies are considered. The use of digital rectal examination and PSA to screen for prostate cancer is therefore at this juncture controversial and not advocated based on evidence. The American Cancer Society has recommended offering annual digital rectal examination and PSA testing to men older than age 50 whose life expectancy is at least 10 years and screening men in a high-risk group yearly beginning at age 45. Other groups have not recommended the use of PSA as a screening test for prostate cancer based on current evidence. When considering prostate cancer screening, a discussion with the patient regarding the pros and cons of screening should take place.

## CERVICAL CANCER

Risk factors for the development of cervical cancer are:

- Multiple sexual partners
- History of sexually transmitted disease (especially human papilloma virus and HIV)
- Previously abnormal Pap smear or cervical dysplasia
- First coitus at an early age
- Smoking
- Low socioeconomic status

The use of the cervical Pap smear has been shown to decrease mortality from invasive cervical cancer. The positive benefit of cervical Pap smear screening occurs because the natural history of the disease is known; the disease progresses relatively slowly; and screening via Pap smear is relatively accurate, inexpensive, and safe. A Pap smear has a low sensitivity of approximately 30% to 40%, but a high specificity greater than 90%. Liquid-based Pap smears have a higher sensitivity. Most advisory groups suggest Pap screening be initiated with the onset of sexual activity or at age 21, whichever occurs first. Thereafter, most advisory groups recommend annual Pap smears (or once every 2 years using liquid-based tests) in patients younger than 30 years of age. Above age 30, Pap smears can be performed every 3 years if patients have undergone regular screening previously and are not considered high risk. Some advisory groups recommend human papilloma virus (HPV) testing

be combined with Pap smear screening every 3 years in patients over the age of 30. Beyond age 65, screening should be continued based on risk; in women who have been adequately screened at a younger age whose tests have been consistently negative, screening may be discontinued. Screening also may be discontinued in women who have undergone hysterectomy (with removal of the cervix) for benign gynecologic disease.

## OTHER CANCERS

Insufficient evidence exists to recommend routine screening for testicular cancer by physician examination or patient self-examination. Similarly, the effectiveness of routine screening of women for ovarian cancer by pelvic examination, vaginal or abdominal ultrasound, or serologic testing (carcinoembryonic antigen CA-125) is not established. The screening of high-risk patients (for testicular cancer, those males aged 13 to 39 with history of cryptorchidism, orchiopexy, or testicular atrophy; for ovarian cancer, those women with family history of ovarian cancer, familial breast-ovarian cancer syndrome, familial cancer syndrome, or BRCA-1 mutation carriers) should be considered. Lysophosphatidic acid (LPA), a tumor marker for ovarian cancer, is being evaluated as a possible screening test.

An increase in melanoma incidence has occurred in the past few decades. Those with a high risk for melanoma (familial melanoma syndrome, or with first-degree relatives with melanoma) should be referred to and screened by a dermatologist. The benefit of screening average-risk patients for melanoma is currently not supported by medical evidence.

## GENERAL PHYSICAL EXAMINATION

Over time, the use of the general physical examination as a screening tool has changed significantly. The general physical examination is now usually used to establish a baseline. Thereafter, only blood pressure, weight, breast examination, and pelvic examination are advised by most advocacy groups for the screening of asymptomatic adults. The intervals to perform these examinations are not generally agreed on. Other components of the physical examination are not generally advised in truly asymptomatic persons. A more cost-effective approach for healthcare providers is to instead spend time and resources counseling patients about:

- Smoking
- Diet
- Exercise
- Mental health
- Sexual practices
- Alcohol use
- Drug abuse
- Use of seat belts

## OTHER TESTS

Hearing testing is advised in all adults when hearing loss is suspected. In patients exposed to excess noise on a regular basis, audiograms should be performed periodically.

No general consensus exists for visual acuity testing. Some authorities have recommended screening in adults older than age 65.

Tonometry is generally not recommended because of the lack of a good screening test. Schiotz tonometry has a specificity of 10% to 30% and a sensitivity of 50% to 70%. Patients at high risk for glaucoma should instead be referred to an ophthalmologist for evaluation. Glaucoma prevalence is significantly higher in African Americans; the risk steadily increases with age. Neither hematocrit/hemoglobin nor leukocyte determinations have been shown to be useful in screening asymptomatic patients. Chemistry profile panels are similarly not recommended for screening asymptomatic healthy adults. Fasting plasma glucose levels should be measured every 3 years in patients at a high risk for diabetes because of a family history of diabetes, in obese persons older than age 40, and in women with a personal history of gestational diabetes. Native Americans, Hispanics, and African Americans have a higher risk for development of diabetes mellitus. The American Diabetes Association considers a fasting plasma glucose level of greater than 126 mg/dL diagnostic of type II diabetes.

Urinalysis also is not advised for screening asymptomatic patients. Population-based studies have shown low rates for detecting serious and treatable urinary tract disorders in asymptomatic adults with either hemoglobin or protein present on dipstick urinalysis. All major authorities do recommend screening urinalysis in the prenatal care of pregnant women. Some groups have advised urinalysis for asymptomatic bacteriuria in diabetic patients and elderly patients older than age 65.

Generally, laboratory tests such as chemistry profiles, blood count, urinalysis, and other similar tests should be used for targeted select patients based on increased risk and likelihood of disease. Routine screening of asymptomatic healthy adults via these methods is not advised or supported by the current medical literature.

## ADULT IMMUNIZATIONS

### Influenza

Influenza vaccine is made from an inactivated virus grown in eggs. It contains three viruses—two A-type and one B-type virus. The vaccine is given yearly in the fall, optimally in October or November. It is 65% to 80% effective. Side effects include local skin reaction, fever, myalgia, and malaise, which, if they occur, begin soon after the vaccination and last 1 to 2 days. Patients may mistake these side effects for influenza symptoms, which may create a barrier for their future use of the vaccine. The vaccine is made from an inactivated virus and does not cause influenza. Hypersensitivity reactions are rare. The vaccine should be avoided in those with a history of hypersensitivity reactions to eggs or to a previous dose of influenza vaccine and in those with a febrile illness. The vaccination can be given safely to pregnant women. Recommended recipients of the vaccine include:

- Those older than age 50
- Those with chronic illness such as diabetes, chronic lung disease, asthma, congestive heart failure, kidney disease, cirrhosis, or hemoglobinopathy
- Nursing home patients
- Medical personnel
- Those with weakened immune systems, such as persons on long-term corticosteroid treatment or patients receiving cancer treatment with radiation or chemotherapy
- Those infected with HIV
- Those younger than age 18 on long-term aspirin therapy (to prevent Reye's syndrome)
- Persons frequently exposed to or living with persons at high risk
- Those who perform essential community service
- Pregnant women past 13 weeks gestation

The vaccine, particularly in the elderly, is less protective for the recipient contracting the illness but does reduce the severity of the illness. The greatest percentage of deaths due to influenza occurs in those older than age 65. Consequently, vaccination in this age group is particularly important. Also, the vaccine has been shown to be cost effective in healthy working adults between the ages of 18 to 64 years old (through fewer missed work days).

### Pneumococcus

The current 23-valent vaccine was established in 1983. The vaccine is approximately 60% effective for establishing immunity and covers approximately 88% of bloodstream isolates of pneumococcal infections in the United States. High-risk patients include those 65 years of age and older and those younger than age 65 with the following conditions:

- Chronic cardiac or pulmonary conditions
- Anatomic or functional asplenia
- Chronic liver disease
- Alcoholism
- Diabetes
- Immunocompromise
- Chronic renal disease
- Residents of long-term care facilities

Patients with chronic renal disease, Hodgkin's disease, or multiple myeloma; those who have undergone organ transplantation; and those receiving hemodialysis or chemotherapy for cancer may have a diminished response to the vaccine. Adverse reactions to the vaccine are rare. Minor local side effects, such as pain and redness, are common. For those adults who are most at risk for serious pneumococcal infection, one-time revaccination after 5 years is recommended. This is particularly important in patients with functional or anatomic asplenia and in those who are likely to have diminishing antibody levels (e.g., patients on dialysis, those with nephrotic syndrome, those having had organ transplantation). Revaccination for healthy adults is advised for those who received the vaccine before age 65 and more than 5 years have elapsed. Revaccination is generally safe and well-tolerated. An Arthus-type reaction can occur. Pregnancy is not a contraindication to the use of this vaccine.

## Hepatitis B

Hepatitis B vaccination is a three-part procedure presently given at 0, 1 to 2, and 4 to 6 months. The vaccination is 85% to 95% effective and is administered in the deltoid muscle. A decreased antibody response is seen in the presence of renal failure, diabetes, chronic liver disease, HIV infection, smoking, and advanced age. The vaccination series is advised for all adolescents, for young adults aged 20 to 39 years who have not been previously immunized, and for adults at high risk, including:

- Healthcare workers
- Dentists
- Hemodialysis patients
- Intravenous drug users
- Institutionalized persons
- Homosexuals and bisexuals
- Public safety personnel
- International travelers to areas of high risk
- Immigrants from countries where hepatitis B is endemic

Vaccination also is recommended for contacts of hepatitis B virus carriers, those positive for anti-Hepatitis C virus, heterosexuals with multiple partners, and those with recent sexually transmitted disease. The vaccine is contraindicated for those with yeast hypersensitivity (the vaccine is yeast recombinant). The vaccine is safe, producing in some patient's only mild soreness at the injection site that may last 1 to 2 days. Rarely, constitutional symptoms have been experienced. Postvaccination serologic testing to demonstrate immunity is advised in those with high occupational risk (e.g., healthcare workers) and in patients on hemodialysis. When antibodies to the hepatitis B surface antigen are not present, revaccination should use the three-dose series. After one dose, 20% of nonresponders will produce antibodies. Between 30% and 50% will respond after three additional doses. After six doses, further attempts to immunize the patient are not likely to be fruitful. The need for booster vaccinations to provide clinical protection is unproven. In patients receiving hemodialysis, and whose immunity declines rapidly, annual serologic testing is recommended and booster vaccination may be administered to those whose antibody level falls below 10 mIU/mL. The vaccine is safe to give to pregnant women.

## Tetanus/Diphtheria

The primary tetanus/diphtheria toxoid vaccination should be given to all adults who have not received the primary series previously. The general recommendation for booster dosing has been every 10 years throughout life. One usually gets a last childhood booster at the age of 15. If a patient presents with a contaminated wound, a booster should be given if the last Td vaccine was given more than 5 years earlier. Local reactions of tenderness and erythema are common after tetanus/diphtheria injections. Severe reactions to the vaccine are rare. Hypersensitivity occurs most commonly in those receiving multiple booster vaccinations; therefore, those who have received the vaccination within 5 years should not be revaccinated. The vaccine is not contraindicated in pregnancy.

## Rubella

The rubella vaccine is a live attenuated virus vaccine. It is available alone or in combination with measles and mumps. Rubella vaccine is recommended for all adults, particularly women. Infection in pregnant women during the first trimester usually results in congenital rubella syndrome, and vaccination attempts to prevent this disease. Susceptible women of childbearing age who do not have acceptable evidence of rubella immunity or vaccination should be vaccinated. Women of childbearing age should receive the vaccine only if they say they are not pregnant. They should be counseled not to become pregnant for at least 4 weeks after receiving the vaccination. If a pregnant woman is found to be rubella susceptible (no serologic evidence of immunity), she should be vaccinated as early in the postpartum period as possible. Adverse reactions occur only in susceptible persons. Those already immune to rubella, who are receiving a second vaccination, are not at risk for developing side effects. Side effects have included joint pain and inflammation, which have been persistent in some. Hospital workers who have the potential to transmit rubella to pregnant women should have their immunity checked and be vaccinated appropriately.

## Measles

The measles vaccine is a live attenuated vaccine. Those born before 1957 are likely to have had the virus and need not be vaccinated. Adults born after 1957, not previously vaccinated, and without demonstrated immunity to measles should receive the vaccine. A second dose is recommended in adults recently exposed to measles, healthcare workers, patients vaccinated between years 1963 and 1967 with an inactivated virus vaccine, students entering college, and persons who plan to travel internationally. Reactions to the vaccine are local redness, sometimes accompanied by a low-grade fever. Higher fevers developing 5 to 12 days after the vaccination and lasting 1 to 2 days occur in 5% to 15% of recipients.

## Mumps

The mumps vaccine should be administered to adolescent boys who previously have not had mumps or been given the vaccine because of the possibility of mumps orchitis complicating mumps infection. The vaccine also should be given to adults not previously immunized and without immunity to mumps. The vaccine should be avoided when hypersensitivity to eggs is present. The mumps vaccine is a live attenuated virus vaccine and contains trace amounts of neomycin. Therefore, contraindications include pregnancy, anaphylaxis to neomycin, and the presence of immunosuppressive conditions. Asymptomatic HIV-positive patients can receive the vaccine. Side effects include fever and rash 5 to 14 days after the vaccination, arthralgia or arthritis when given with the rubella vaccine, and local pain.

## Hepatitis A

Preexposure immunization with the hepatitis A vaccine is advised for the following groups:

- Adults traveling to or working in countries in which hepatitis A is endemic
- Homosexual men
- Users of illicit drugs
- Those with chronic liver disease
- Those residing in an institutional setting where hepatitis A is an ongoing problem
- Those with an occupational risk for developing the disease
- Those with clotting factor disorders, such as hemophilia
- Food handlers, when health authorities determine the vaccination to be cost effective

The intramuscular injection is given as a primary vaccination followed in 6 to 12 months by a booster vaccination. Postexposure management of hepatitis A should employ immune globulin. Side effects of the vaccine include soreness at the injection site, headache, and malaise. Generally, the vaccine has a good safety profile.

## Varicella

Those with a history of having varicella are assumed to be immune and need not be considered for vaccination. Many other adults without a reliable history of varicella infection often carry immunity to varicella. Therefore, serologic testing before vaccination should be considered. Persons for whom the varicella vaccination should be considered include the following groups:

- Healthcare workers
- Household contacts of immunocompromised patients
- Those living or working in high-risk environments for varicella transmission, such as schools and daycare centers
- College students
- Military personnel

- Nonpregnant women of childbearing age
- International travelers
- Those without a history of the disease

The vaccine is given subcutaneously in two doses 4 to 8 weeks apart. The vaccine is a live attenuated virus and therefore is contraindicated in immunocompromised individuals. The vaccine is also contraindicated in those who have anaphylaxis to neomycin or untreated active tuberculosis, and in recent recipients of blood products or in pregnant women. Side effects may include pain and erythema at the injection site or a varicella-like rash.

## Lyme Disease

The Lyme disease vaccination is a noninfectious genetically engineered vaccine advised for those at significant risk for contracting Lyme disease: those who reside, work, or recreate in endemic areas and are thereby exposed frequently to vector ticks. The vaccine is given in three parts at 0, 1, and 12 months. The vaccine is generally well tolerated.

## Meningococcus

College students, particularly freshmen living in dormitories, are at moderately increased risk for meningococcal disease and are advised to consider receiving the meningococcal vaccination to prevent meningococcal meningitis. Adults with functional or anatomic asplenia or terminal complement component deficiency should receive the meningococcal vaccination. Travelers to certain areas of the world (e.g., sub-Saharan Africa and Mecca, Saudi Arabia) should also be vaccinated. This single-dose polysaccharide vaccination has few side effects, principally localized erythema.

## REVIEW EXERCISES

### QUESTIONS

**1.** The optimal timing for the administration of the pneumococcal vaccination includes all of the following *except*
a) Before a planned splenectomy
b) After 5 years in a patient with chronic renal failure who received the vaccination previously
c) Before administration of chemotherapy in a patient with lymphoma
d) When a person is found to be HIV-positive
e) After immunosuppressive therapy in a patient undergoing organ transplantation

**2.** All of the following statements regarding influenza vaccination are true *except*
a) It can be given at the same time as the pneumococcal vaccination.

b) It is 60% to 80% effective.
c) It often causes an influenza-like illness.
d) It is contraindicated in the presence of allergy to eggs.
e) It should be postponed in the setting of a febrile illness.

3. A 35-year-old man presents to office for the first time requesting a "routine physical." He is on no medications, has no significant past medical or family history, and his review of systems is negative. Which of the following screening tests would be considered to be most appropriate?
a) Blood pressure, lipid panel, urinalysis, complete blood count
b) Blood pressure, lipid panel, glucose
c) Blood pressure, glucose
d) Blood pressure, lipid panel
e) Blood pressure, lipids, EKG

4. All of the following are incorrect, *except*
a) Varicella vaccination is contraindicated in pregnant patients.
b) PSA and digital rectal exams are proven screening methods to reduce prostate cancer mortality.
c) Measles vaccine is recommended in individuals born before 1957.
d) Self-breast exam is a proven screening method to reduce breast cancer mortality.
e) Hepatitis B vaccination is contraindicated in pregnant patients.

5. A 35-year-old woman presents to you for a new patient evaluation. She is here for her "annual physical." Her current medications include an oral contraceptive and ibuprofen as needed. Her mother has a history of hypertension. She is married and works as a legal secretary. Her review of systems is negative. Her previous records report that she had a normal liquid-based Pap smear and an HPV screen 2 years ago. She doesn't remember any recent lab work and thinks her last immunizations were when she was a teenager. Which of the following screening tests are most appropriate for this patient?
a) Pap smear, lipid panel
b) Tetanus (Td) vaccination, lipid panel
c) Pap smear, Td
d) Td
e) Pap smear, HPV testing, lipid panel, Td

6. All of the following are correct, *except*
a) Fecal occult blood testing (FOBT) has been proven by a randomized clinical trial to decrease colon cancer mortality.
b) Lung cancer is the leading cause of cancer deaths in the United States.
c) Complete blood count, EKG, and urinalysis testing are not recommended in asymptomatic healthy adults.

d) Colonoscopy has been proven by a randomized clinical trial to decrease colon cancer mortality.
e) A meningococcal vaccination should be offered to incoming college freshman.

## ANSWERS

**1. e.**
Generally, the pneumococcal vaccination should be given to immunosuppressed patients before their immunosuppression occurs or becomes advanced. Therefore, the vaccination should be given before a planned splenectomy, the administration of chemotherapy, or immunosuppressant therapy, and when HIV infection is first detected. The correct answer therefore is e. Because of waning immunity, the vaccination should be given after 5 years in a patient with chronic renal failure who received the vaccination previously.

**2. c.**
A common misconception among patients is that the influenza vaccination causes influenza infection. The vaccine may cause local skin reaction, fever, myalgia, and malaise, side effects that the patient may mistake for influenza symptoms. The vaccine does not cause influenza because the vaccine is made from an inactivated virus. The vaccine is contraindicated in those allergic to eggs because the vaccine is made from inactivated virus grown in eggs. It should be postponed in those with a febrile illness. It is 60% to 80% effective and can be given safely at the same time as the pneumococcal vaccination. The correct answer is therefore c.

**3. d.**
In asymptomatic patients, routine EKGs and screening lab tests, such as urinalysis, complete blood counts, chemistry panels, and liver function tests are generally not recommended. All major advisory groups recommend blood pressure screening and lipid panel testing by the age of 35. Therefore, d is the correct answer.

**4. a.**
All of the statements are false except for a. Varicella is a live attenuated viral vaccine and is contraindicated in pregnancy.

**5. b.**
With both a normal Pap smear and negative HPV screen done 2 years ago, this patient doesn't need another Pap smear until next year (a 3-year interval). A Pap smear could be done sooner if this patient were considered to be at high risk for cervical cancer. A tetanus booster immunization should be administered every 10 years after the primary series is completed, and almost all major advisory groups recommend cholesterol screening in asymptomatic patients by the age of 35. Therefore b is the correct answer.

## 6. d.

All the listed statements are correct except d. To date, a randomized clinical trial has not been done to demonstrate the effectiveness of colonoscopy in reducing colon cancer mortality. FOBT screening is supported by several randomized clinical trials, and flexible sigmoidoscopy screening is supported by the results of case-control studies.

## SUGGESTED READINGS

### General

Jemal A, Tiwari RC, Murray T, et al. Cancer statistics, 2004. *CA Cancer J Clin* 2004;54:8–29.

Lang RS, Hensrud DD, eds. *Clinical Preventive Medicine*, 2nd ed. Chicago: AMA Press, 2004.

The Third U.S. Preventive Services Task Force: background, methods, and first recommendations. *Am J Prev Med* 2001;20:35.

U.S. Preventive Services Task Force Report. *Guide to Clinical Prevention Services*, 2nd ed. Alexandria, VA: International Medical Publishing, 1996.

U.S. Preventive Services Task Force Web site: http://www.preventiveservices.ahrq.gov

### Screening

American Cancer Society. Update of early detection guidelines for prostate, colorectal, and endometrial cancers. *CA Cancer J Clin* 2001;51:38–75.

American Cancer Society guideline for the early detection of cervical neoplasia and cancer. *CA Cancer J Clin* 2002;52:342–362.

American College of Physicians. Guidelines for using cholesterol, HDL cholesterol, and triglyceride levels as screening tests for preventing coronary artery disease in adults. *Ann Intern Med* 1996;124:515–517.

Amin SH, Kuhle CL, Fitzpatrick LA. Comprehensive evaluation of the older woman. *Mayo Clin Proc* 2003;78:1157–1185.

Antman K, Shea S. Screening mammography under age 50. *JAMA* 1999;281:1470–1472.

Barry MJ. Prostate specific-antigen testing for early diagnosis of prostate cancer. *N Engl J Med* 2001;344:1373–1377.

Coley CM, Barry MJ, Mulley AG. Screening for prostate cancer. *Ann Intern Med* 1997;126:480–484.

Chobanian AV, Bakris GL, Black HR, et al. The seventh report of the Joint National Committee on Prevention, Evaluation, and Treatment of High Blood Pressure. *JAMA* 2003;289:2560–2572.

Expert Panel on Detection, Evaluation, and Treatment of High Blood Cholesterol in Adults. Executive summary of the third report of the National Cholesterol Education Program (NCEP) Expert Panel on Detection, Evaluation, and Treatment of High Blood Cholesterol in Adults (Adult Treatment Panel III). *JAMA* 2001;285:2486–2497.

Giovannucci E. Modifiable risk factors for colon cancer. *Gastroenterol Clin North Am* 2002;31:935–943.

Imperiale TF, Wagner DR, Lin CY, et al. Results of screening colonoscopy among persons 40 to 49 years of age. *NEJM* 2002;346:1781–1785.

Jin XW, Nielsen C, Brainard J, Yen-Lieberman B. New advances transform the management of women with abnormal Pap tests. *Clev Clin J of Med* 2003;70:641–648.

Mahadevia PF, Fleisher LA, Frick KD, et al. Lung cancer screening with helical computed tomography in older adult smoker. A decision and cost-effective analysis. *JAMA* 2003;289:313–322.

Marcus PM, Fagerstrom RM, Prorok C, et al. Screening for lung cancer with helical CT scanning. *Clin Pulm Med* 2002;9:323–329.

Oboler SK, La Force FM. The periodic physical examination in asymptomatic adults. *Ann Intern Med* 1989;110:214–226.

Olsen O, Gotzche PC. Cochrane review on screening for breast cancer with mammography. *Lancet* 2001;358:1340–1342.

Rex DK, Johnson DA, Lieberman DA, et al. *ACG Recommendations on Colorectal Cancer Screening for Average and Higher Risk Patients in Clinical Practice*. Arlington, VA: American College of Gastroenterology, 2001.

Sawaya GF, Brown AD, Washington AE, et al. Current approaches to cervical cancer screening. *N Engl J Med* 2001;344:1603–1607.

Schlant RC, Blomqvist CG, Brandenburg RO, et al. Report of the Joint American College of Cardiology and American Heart Association Task Force on Assessment of Cardiovascular Procedure. Guidelines for exercise testing. *Circulation* 1986;74:653A–667A.

Smith RA, Cokkinides V, Eyre HJ. American Cancer Society guidelines for the early detection of cancer, 2004. *CA Cancer J Clin* 2004; 54:41–52.

Spitzer WO (chairman). Canadian Task Force on the Periodic Health Examination. The periodic health examination. *Can Med Assoc J* 1979;121:1193–1254; 1984;130:1278–1285; 1986;134:721 (see also yearly updates).

Takahashi PY, Okhravi HR, Lim LS, Kasten MJ. Preventive health care in elderly population: a guide for practicing physicians. *Mayo Clin Proc* 2004;79:416–427.

U.S. Preventive Services Task Force. Screening adults for lipid disorders: recommendations and rationale. *Am J Prev Med* 2001;20: 77–89.

U.S. Preventive Services Task Force. Screening for colorectal cancer: recommendations and rationale. *Ann Intern Med* 2002;137: 132–141.

U.S. Preventive Services Task Force. Screening for breast cancer: recommendations and rationale. *Ann Intern Med* 2002;137:344–346.

U.S. Preventive Services Task Force. Screening for prostate cancer: recommendations and rationale. *Ann Intern Med* 2002;137:915–916.

U.S. Preventive Services Task Force. Screening for high blood pressure: recommendations and rationale. *Am J Prev Med* 2003;25:159–164.

U.S. Preventive Services Task Force. Screening for coronary heart disease: recommendation statement. *Ann Intern Med* 2004;140: 569–572.

U.S. Preventive Services Task Force. Screening for lung cancer: recommendations and rationale. *Ann Intern Med* 2004;140:740–753.

Walsh JME. Controversies in cancer prevention and screening. *Adv Stud Med* 2003;3:316–325.

Winawer S, Fletcher R, Rex D, et al. Colorectal cancer screening and surveillance: clinical guidelines and rationale—update based on new evidence. *Gastroenterology* 2003;124:544–560.

### Immunizations

Advisory Committee on Immunization Practices (ACIP) recommendations and statements: http://www.cdc.gov/nip/publications/ACIP-list.htm.

Canadian Medical Association National Advisory Committee on Immunizations. *Canadian Immunization Guide*, 5th ed. Minister of Public Works and Government Services Ottawa, Ontario, Canada, 1998.

Centers for Disease Control and Prevention. Prevention of pneumococcal disease: recommendations of the Advisory Committee on Immunization Practices. *MMWR Morb Mortal Wkly Rep* 1997;46: 1–24.

Immunization Action Coalition (IAC) Web site: http://www.immunize.org.

World Health Organization—immunizations: http://www.who.int/vaccines.

# Women's Hormonal Health Issues

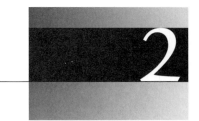

*Pelin Batur, MD*    *Marie M. Budev DO, MPH*
*Holly L. Thacker, MD, FACP*

With the increasing interest in women's health and gender-based biology, physicians are now more than ever being asked to have a greater understanding of gender-specific healthcare issues. In an effort to understand these issues effectively, it is helpful to divide a woman's life into the different hormonal phases—the reproductive phase, the menopausal phase, and the postmenopausal state. Understanding the changes in hormonal states during each of these phases depends on a keen understanding of the hypothalamic/pituitary/ovarian/endometrial axis. Any changes within this axis can lead to certain physiologic and metabolic consequences. This chapter provides an overview of the three major hormonal phases in a woman's life, concentrating on the pathobiology, medical treatment, and management of these conditions.

## ANATOMY AND HORMONES

### Ovary

The ovary is composed of stroma and germ cells (oocytes). The greatest number of oocytes is present at the fifth month of gestation. Through atresia, a great number are reduced. At birth, 1 to 2 million oocytes exist, with only 400,000 existing by menarche; only a few hundred to a few thousand exist before menopause. The ovary is primarily responsible for synthesizing estrogen, progesterone, androgens, and peptides such as inhibin.

### Estrogen

There are three human estrogens: estradiol ($E_2$), estrone ($E_1$), and estriol ($E_3$). Over 200 estrogenic substances (from plant, animal, and synthetic sources), however, interact with the estrogen receptors (ERα and ERβ) and substances that affect estrogen metabolism. 17β-estradiol ($E_2$) is the most potent human estrogen.

During reproductive years, the main source of estrogen, 17β-estradiol ($E_2$), is produced by the dominant ovarian follicle (Fig. 2.1). $E_1$, the second major estrogen, is derived principally from the metabolism of $E_2$ and from the arom-atization of androstenedione in peripheral adipose tissue. Only a small quantity of $E_1$ is secreted by the ovary and the adrenal glands.

In the postmenopausal state, estrogen production ceases, and the $E_1$ peripheral aromatication of androstenedione becomes the dominant form of estrogen. An increase in androstenedione conversion to $E_1$ occurs as a woman's weight increases, which results in increased overall estrogen levels.

The peripheral aromatization of testosterone to $E_2$ and $E_1$ has only a minimal contribution to overall $E_1$ and $E_2$ levels in the postmenopausal state. $E_2$ can also be converted to $E_1$ and vice versa through a reversible conversion that occurs in the liver. Another source of $E_1$ is from the reversible metabolism of estrone ($E_1$)-3 sulfate.

The liver plays an important role in the metabolism and excretion of estrogens and is influenced directly by estrogen status. The first-pass effect of estrogens absorbed from the gastrointestinal tract and subsequent reabsorption of estrogens secreted in bile affect liver metabolism. The liver is also the primary conversion site of $E_1$ to $E_2$ as well as for the conjugation of estrogens.

All estrogens circulating in the body are either protein-bound or free. Estrogen is bound tightly to sex hormone–binding globulin (SHBG) and more loosely bound to serum albumin. Alterations in SHBG change the concentration of unbound $E_2$, altering its bioavailability. Estrogen therapy, pregnancy, and hyperthyroidism increase SHBG, whereas hypothyroidism, androgen excess, insulin, and obesity lower SHBG.

The biologic activity of each estrogen depends on (i) its ability to cross the cell membrane, (ii) its binding ability to a specific receptor protein and activation of the receptor, and (iii) subsequent DNA synthesis. $E_2$ has the highest binding affinity of the estrogens. Two identified estrogen receptors (ERα and ERβ) are located throughout the body, in different proportions.

### Progesterone

Progestogens are divided into two classes: natural and synthetic. Progesterone is the sole naturally occurring progestogen. Synthetic progestins include 17-hydroxyprogesterone

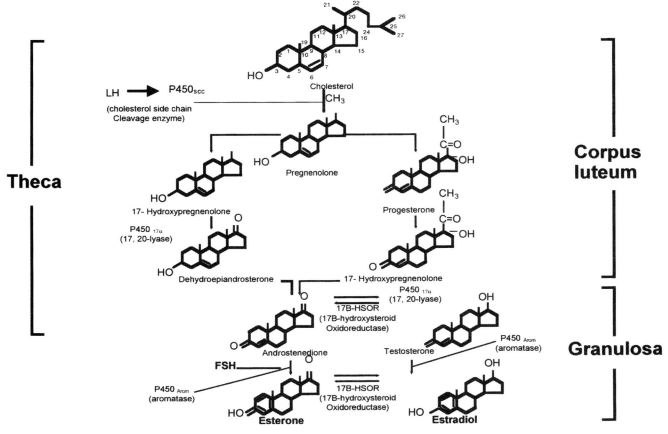

**Figure 2.1** Steroid hormone biosynthesis in the ovary.

acetate, megestrol acetate, and compounds related to testosterone, including norethindrone and levonorgestrel and its derivatives. Naturally occurring progesterone is produced by the corpus luteum, and it prepares a secretory endometrium to accept a fertilized ovum. During anovulation no corpus luteum develops, thus estrogen is unopposed. This unopposed estrogen causes endometrial proliferation, leading to an endometrial lining that is unstable and subsequently sheds, leading to dysfunctional uterine bleeding. Therefore, progestins are prescribed to oppose the continuous effect of estrogen on the endometrium.

## Androgen

In a premenopausal woman, androgens are produced by the adrenal gland and ovary. The ovarian androgens produced are androstenedione (which can be peripherally converted to $E_1$ in adipose tissue) and testosterone. Surgically induced menopause reduces not only a woman's level of estrogen and progesterone but also of total testosterone. Even with estrogen therapy (ET) many women may experience the effects of sexual dysfunction related to the relative androgen deficiency.

## Inhibin

Inhibin is produced by the granulocytes of the ovary and inhibits pituitary gonadotropin production, specifically of follicular-stimulating hormone (FSH). When inhibin is at its highest level, FSH is suppressed. In the postmenopausal state, when inhibin in no longer produced, FSH levels remain elevated even in the face of estrogen therapy.

## MENSTRUAL CYCLE

The menstrual cycle begins with the onset of menarche, usually around 12 years of age, with a monthly cycle eventually occurring every 21 to 42 days. When menses occur at less than 21-day periods or more than 42-day periods, it is deemed to be irregular and likely anovulatory in etiology. It is important to note that the menstrual cycle is irregular usually at the extremes of reproductive life due to anovulatory cycles, during the perimenarcheal and perimenopausal time frame. Other common causes for a change in the usual menstrual cycle include changes in body mass index, changes in exercise patterns, parturition, and significant psychosocial distress (Tables 2.1 and 2.2). The menstrual

## TABLE 2.1
### CAUSES OF CHRONIC ANOVULATION

Chronic anovulation because of inappropriate pituitary feedback
   (e.g., in polycystic ovary syndrome)
Excessive extraglandular estrogen (as in obesity)
Functional androgen excess from adrenal or ovarian cause
Neoplasms that produce either androgens or estrogens
Neoplasms producing chorionic gonadotropin
Abnormal sex hormone–binding globulin (including liver disease)
Chronic anovulation because of endocrine or metabolic disorders
Thyroid dysfunction, either hyper- or hypothyroidism
Prolactin and/or growth hormone excess
Pituitary micro- or macroadenomas
Hypothalamic dysfunction
Drug-induced hyperprolactinemia
Malnutrition
Adrenal hyperfunction (Cushing's disease)
Congenital adrenal hyperplasia
Chronic anovulation of hypothalamic pituitary origin
Hypothalamic chronic anovulation
Psychogenic
Exercise induced
Associated malnutrition, weight loss, or systemic illness
Eating disorder (anorexia nervosa and/or bulimia)
Isolated gonadotropin deficiency (Kallmann's syndrome)
Hypothalamic pituitary damage
After surgery, trauma, radiation, or infection
Empty sella syndrome
After infarction (postdelivery Sheehan's syndrome)
Pituitary and para-pituitary tumors
Idiopathic hypopituitarism

## TABLE 2.2
### CAUSES OF SECONDARY AMENORRHEA

Pregnancy
Ovarian failure—menopause
Chronic anovulation
Endometrial atrophy (e.g., from continuous progestin use)
Traumatic amenorrhea (Asherman's syndrome)
Adrenal and/or thyroid dysfunction
Pituitary prolactinoma
Gestational trophic disease

cycle is divided into three phases: *follicular, ovulatory*, and *luteal*.

### Follicular Phase

The first day of menstrual bleeding marks the beginning of the follicular phase (Fig. 2.2). During this time, one dominant follicle produces high levels of $E_2$. At this time, the other ovarian follicles become atretic. In response to the high levels of estrogen produced by the dominant follicle, the endometrium begins to proliferate. In response to high estrogen levels, the pituitary gland and hypothalamus decrease the production of FSH through negative feedback. An increase in luteinizing hormone (LH) release causes ovulation (the LH surge).

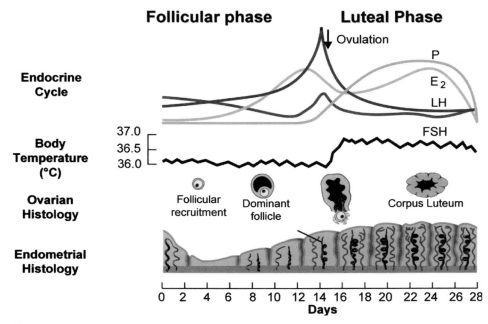

**Figure 2.2**   Follicular and luteal phases. $E_2$, estradiol; FSH, follicular-stimulating hormone; LH, luteinizing hormone; P, progesterone.

## Ovulatory Phase

When LH reaches its peak, ovarian estrogen is temporarily inhibited and estrogen levels dip before ovulation, while progesterone levels continue to increase. Ovulation occurs due to the rupture of the dominant follicle and release of the mature oocyte into the peritoneal cavity. Often, with the release of the oocyte, women note symptoms of lower abdominal pain, termed *mittelschmerz*, which may be due to the release of follicular fluid and bleeding with the mature oocyte.

## Luteal Phase

The luteal phase begins after the dominant follicle ruptures and then convolutes, forming the corpus luteum (Fig. 2.2). The term *corpus luteum* is used due to its yellow appearance as a result of the uptake of lipids and lutein pigment by the granulosa cells of the follicular walls. Once formed, the corpus luteum begins to secrete estrogen, progesterone, and androgens. The progesterone and the estrogens secreted by the corpus luteum begin the secretory phase, characterized by a coiling of the endometrial glands, resulting in a highly vascularized endothelium. If pregnancy does not occur, autolysis occurs, and the levels of progesterone and estrogen fall, owing to the absence of placenta human chorionic gonadotropin. With the fall in both estrogen and progesterone, the endometrium undergoes shedding.

## PREMATURE MENOPAUSE/PREMATURE OVARIAN INSUFFICIENCY

Premature menopause is better termed *premature ovarian insufficiency* (POI); this is said to occur before the age of 40 years and occurs in less than 1% of all women. POI before the age of 40 years usually occurs owing to premature cessation of ovarian function rather than depletion of the ovarian follicles. This is often termed *hypergonadotropic amenorrhea* (Table 2.3). The diseases associated with premature ovarian failure include sex chromosome abnormalities. POI has been linked to both familial and nonfamilial X chromosome abnormalities such as Turner's syndrome or XO chromosome and fragile X syndrome.

Women with POI should be offered testing for fragile X syndrome using *FMR-1* gene testing, particularly if any mental retardation exists in the family. Autoimmune disorders such as Addison's disease, myasthenia gravis, rheumatoid arthritis, systemic lupus erythematosus, and thyroid and parathyroid disease have been associated in women with POI. Physical insults to the ovary, including surgery, radiation, or chemotherapy (especially cyclophosphamide), or infection such as tuberculosis or mumps *in utero* can destroy ovarian follicles.

Other rare causes of premature ovarian failure and accelerated follicular atresia include isolated ovarian antibodies,

## TABLE 2.3

**DIFFERENTIAL DIAGNOSIS OF HYPERGONADOTROPIC AMENORRHEA (FOLLICLE-STIMULATING HORMONE >20–40 IU/L)**

Natural menopause (age range of 40–56 yr. with mean of 51.3 yr.)
Physical causes
Surgical removal (castration)
Gonadal irradiation
Chemotherapy (especially alkylating agents)
Autoimmune disorders
Polyglandular failure involving the ovaries
Isolated ovarian failure associated with ovarian antibodies
Chromosomal abnormalities
Inherited tendencies producing premature ovarian failure
Genetically reduced cell endowment
Accelerated atresia
Gonadotropin receptor and/or postreceptor defects causing resistant ovary syndrome

interstitial diseases, and reduced follicular cell endowment. In rare cases, gonadotropic receptor defects leading to resistant ovarian syndrome can account for premature ovarian failure. Hormonal contraceptives (HCs) (pills, patches, vaginal rings) do not suppress rare instances of ovulation in women with hypergonadotropic amenorrhea because contraceptive doses of hormones were developed to suppress ovulation in eugonadotropic women.

## MENOPAUSE TRANSITION

Perimenopause or "menopause transition" is the time before and after the last period when hormone fluctuations occur, yielding some of the early symptoms of menopause. Symptoms during this time vary depending on the production of $E_2$, androgens, and progesterone levels. Diagnosis is made clinically, and no method of serologic testing can predict the time of menopause. A persistent elevation in FSH (and LH) can signal that menopause is imminent.

## MENOPAUSE

*Menopause* is defined as the permanent cessation of menses. This is diagnosed retrospectively after the absence of periods for 1 year. *Postmenopause* is the term used to refer to the time after menopause. The median age of menopause is 51 years of age. It has been noted that the average age of menopause is lowered in certain groups, such as smokers and women with chronic illness. Menopause occurs when the ovary no longer has active follicles producing $E_2$. The main symptoms of menopause are manifested by estrogen deficiency expressed by estrogen target tissues that are rich in estrogen

---

**TABLE 2.4**

**EFFECTS OF ESTROGEN LOSS**

| | |
|---|---|
| Symptoms (early onset) | Hot flashes/vasomotor symptoms |
| | Mood disturbances |
| | Sleep disturbances |
| | Irritability |
| | Urogenital symptoms |
| Physical signs (intermediate onset) | Vaginal atrophy |
| | Cervical atrophy |
| | Skin/dermal thinning |
| | Hair thinning |
| Diseases (later onset) | Osteoporosis |

---

receptors, including the urogenital system, breast, bone, the cardiovascular system (including the vascular endothelium), the central nervous system, and the gastrointestinal tract (Table 2.4).

Fluctuations in $E_2$ levels can trigger vasomotor symptoms such as hot flashes or flushes, the most commonly reported symptoms of menopausal transition and post-menopausal women. Other conditions can mimic vasomotor symptoms (Table 2.5).

## MENOPAUSAL SYMPTOMS

*Hot flashes* are the sensation of warmth to extreme heat in the upper body, arms, and face. Usually hot flashes are followed by a hot flush (visible erythema), which is characterized by the vasodilation of blood vessels and a noticeable

---

**TABLE 2.5**

**DIFFERENTIAL DIAGNOSIS OF HOT FLASH/FLUSH**

| | |
|---|---|
| Psychiatric manifestations | Panic attacks |
| | Anxiety |
| Medications | Nitroglycerin |
| | Niacin |
| | Nifedipine |
| | Calcitonin |
| | Clomiphene citrate |
| | Danazol |
| | Gonadotropin-releasing hormone analogs |
| Endocrine | Thyrotoxicosis |
| | Carcinoid |
| | Diabetic insulin reaction |
| | Pheochromocytoma |
| | Insulinoma |
| | Autonomic dysfunction |
| Substances | Monosodium glutamate |
| Other | Lymphoma |
| | Tuberculosis |

---

blush to the skin. A prodromal aura may occur, consisting of head pressure, headache, and nausea, present with or without diaphoresis. The severity and resultant debilitating effects of these symptoms on each woman vary. This may be due to various hypothalamic receptors and dietary factors that are specific to an individual woman. Although the vasomotor phenomenon is not life threatening, it can frequently disrupt sleep and lead to chronic sleep deprivation, which can then lead to fatigue and mood changes, including depression. The pathobiology of hot flushes has yet to be clearly defined but is suggestive of a triggering response in the thermal regulatory centers in the hypothalamus. Hot flashes usually resolve with age, with a mean duration lasting 2 to 5 years after onset, although a small percentage of women continue to have these symptoms for greater than 15 years.

Women who have induced menopause experience the most intense hot flash symptoms, but not all women with induced menopause experience vasomotor symptoms. Other vasomotor symptoms may include palpitations, dizziness, and, rarely, skin crawling sensations.

*Psychiatric diseases* such as major depression and panic disorder do not appear to occur at an increased rate in postmenopausal women. But women who have suffered from affective disorders after a reproductive event (depression, premenstrual dysphoric disorder, and postpartum depression) are at an increased risk for reoccurrence related to changes in their reproductive hormonal status. Vasomotor symptoms can exacerbate panic disorders, depression, and anxiety. Estrogen therapy (ET) does have a role in ameliorating vasomotor symptoms, but standard psychiatric treatment and pharmacologic as well as psychological therapy should be recommended in these instances. In postmenopausal women without psychiatric disorders, mild mood changes can improve with ET.

Although epidemiologic data seem to indicate that ET reduces senile dementia of Alzheimer's type, recent placebo-controlled trials in patients with senile dementia of Alzheimer's type failed to show any delay in disease progression. Furthermore, the Women's Health Initiative (WHI), a large preventive trial, estrogen-progestin study in late postmenopausal women suggested an increased risk of dementia in older women. The timing of use of HT may explain the disparate findings between observation studies and randomized controlled trials in both dementia and cardiovascular disease.

### Integument

Decrease or loss of $E_2$ decreases the mitotic activity of the dermis and epidermis and leads to a reduction in the synthesis of collagen and elastin fibers. Hair thinning may occur in an androgenic pattern in predisposed women. Also, excessive facial hair may occur with the change of the estrogen–androgen ratio. ET reverses some of these changes and may improve skin texture.

## Genitourinary System

*Multiple vulvar changes* occur, including atrophy of the labia majora and the labia minora, atrophy of urethra, overall dryness, and sparser pubic hair owing to lack of estrogen and androgen. Reduced estrogen levels lead to a decrease in the vaginal rugae, with pale, dry vaginal mucosa noted on speculum examination. Atrophic vaginitis develops, which can lead to pain with routine pelvic examination and during intercourse. There may be an increase in urinary symptoms and urinary tract infections owing to a reduction in vaginal lactobacilli populations.

*Cervical atrophy*, which may cause the cervix to become flush with the vaginal wall, and uterine shrinkage may occur with decreased estrogen levels. Uterine fibroids generally shrink, and the ovaries also reduce in size and should not be palpable on routine examination within 1 to 2 years after menopause.

*Urodynamic changes* occur with the reduction in local estrogen levels as well, with changes in the epithelium of the urethra and a reduced closing pressure of the urethral sphincter. Frequently, urethral syndromes during menopause mimic symptoms of urinary tract infections, including urgency, frequency, dysuria, and suprapubic pain, which may occur without evidence of infection on routine dipstick examination.

*Stress incontinence* may develop during pelvic stress maneuvers such as coughing, sneezing, or lifting. Other types of incontinence include urge, overflow, function, and mixed (stress and urge) and can occur in combination in the postmenopausal period. Risk factors for stress incontinence include a history of obstetric trauma, weakness of pelvic floor muscles, and chronic cough. Kegel or pelvic floor exercises can be used for mild stress incontinence to strengthen the voluntary muscles of the pelvic floor and urethral sphincter. ET locally may help reconstitute the integrity of the vaginal and urethral mucosa. Bladder retraining and biofeedback may be helpful in treating mild cases of female incontinence.

*Urge incontinence* is associated with a strong urge to urinate but the inability to get to the bathroom before the onset of urination. The physiology of urge incontinence includes an uninhibited bladder contraction that is significant enough to overcome baseline urethral sphincter tone. Estrogen deficiency may further exacerbate bladder irritability owing to atrophy of the trigone of the bladder, thus worsening urge incontinence. Other substances that can worsen urge incontinence include caffeine, spices, and citrus products. Treatment for urge incontinence includes local estrogen treatment and medications such as tolterodine tartrate (Detrol) or oxybutynin chloride (Ditropan) along with bladder behavioral therapy.

The endopelvic fascia may also weaken with menopause, aging, weight gain, and trauma from childbirth, and this can lead to cystocele, rectocele, and cystourethrocele or frank prolapse at the vaginal introitus, leading to irritation, incontinence, and frequent infections.

## Bone Mass and Osteoporosis

Bone mass in a woman depends on multiple factors, including genetics, estrogen exposure, dietary calcium with vitamin D intake, and exercise. A rapid increase in bone mass occurs in puberty, with peak bone mass being reached by age 30. Bone mass declines starting in a woman's 30s and is accelerated during the menopausal transition period and early postmenopausal time. When menopause occurs and estrogen levels fall, the most rapid decline in bone mass is in the trabecular spine. Estrogen acts as an antiresorptive agent and inhibits bone loss. Evidence also suggests that progesterone plays a role in protecting bone mass, but overall it is primarily estrogen that preserves bone mass. The protection offered by estrogen-progestin therapy (named hormone therapy or HT) is greatest if therapy is continuous. If therapy stops, typical menopausal bone loss will commence. Women who have used long-term HT for osteoporosis (OP) prophylaxis should have a bone density assessment periodically because a small percentage of these women on long-term therapy are considered bone nonresponders. Women using HT solely for bone benefits should consider other bone-specific options.

### Alternatives to HT in the Prevention and Treatment of OP

Bisphosphonates such as alendronate (Fosamax) 5 mg or 10 mg daily, respectively, or 35 mg or 70 mg weekly, respectively, and risedronate (Actonel), 5 mg daily, or 35 mg weekly, is approved for both the treatment and prevention of OP. For many women, another alternative to HT is the use of selective estrogen receptor modulators (SERMs). Raloxifene (Evista) is the first SERM that was approved for both the prevention and treatment of OP. The SERMs act similarly to estrogen on certain tissues. Raloxifene also has some positive lipid effects and effects on vascular reactivity, although overall these effects seem to be less potent than those of estrogen. Raloxifene is currently being evaluated in the Raloxifene Use for the Heart (RUTH) trial, a large, randomized, prospective trial examining the use of raloxifene in cardiovascular outcomes. In addition, early data from the clinical trials Multiple Outcomes of Raloxifene Evaluation (MORE) and Continuing Outcomes Relevant to Evista (CORE) have generated evidence that raloxifene may reduce the risk of breast cancer in certain women.

The Study of Tamoxifen and Raloxifene (STAR) trial currently under way compares raloxifene and tamoxifen for breast cancer protection outcomes (the latter of which is currently the only drug approved by the U.S. Food and Drug Administration [FDA] to reduce breast cancer diagnosis in high-risk women). One significant clinical difference that exists in comparing raloxifene and tamoxifen is the estrogenic effect on the uterus by tamoxifen, which can lead to endometrial hyperplasia, thus increasing the risk of endometrial cancer. Raloxifene appears to have no endometrial effects. The use of raloxifene and tamoxifen has been found to cause a slight increase in the risk of thromboembolism, similar to that of ET. Raloxifene does not treat any menopausal symptoms of hot flashes or vaginal atrophy and has not been shown to specifically reduce hip fracture, but it has been shown to reduce vertebral fractures.

Osteoprotegerin is a naturally occurring protein that is a regulator of osteoclast formation. A small, randomized, double-blinded study showed an 80% reduction in bone turnover markers in postmenopausal women who received daily injections of osteoprotegerin. Larger trials looking at these results are currently under way. Injectable Forteo (ter-aperatide) is FDA-approved for the treatment of osteoporosis and has osteoblastic bone building effects. Women with Paget's disease or bone irradiation are not candidates due to the concern of osteosarcoma (seen in rats given very high doses).

## Cardiovascular System

Despite significant advances in cardiovascular medicine over the decade, cardiovascular disease is still the leading killer of women in the United States and in the majority of developed countries. In the United States alone, over 0.5 million women die yearly due to cardiovascular disease, thus exceeding the number of deaths in men. Risk factors for cardiovascular disease in women are similar to those in men including dyslipidemia, hypertension, diabetes mellitus, and smoking, but some gender-specific differences do exist. Selected studies have indicated that women are less likely than men to achieve risk factor goal therapies. Overall the awareness of cardiovascular disease has increased in women, but a significant gap still exists in women's perceived and actual risk of cardiovascular disease.

Hypertension is more common in older women than older men. Early observational studies have suggested that ET can reduce the risk of coronary artery disease (CAD) up to 50% with estrogen alone and 34% with HT. The Heart and Estrogen/Progestin Replacement Study (HERS), the first large, randomized, placebo-controlled trial of estrogen for secondary prevention of CAD in postmenopausal women with established coronary artery disease showed no clinical benefit in HT users compared to placebo on overall cardiovascular events, despite favorable effects on the lipid profile. In fact, the HERS trial indicated a three-fold hazard for venous thromboembolic events in HT users, particularly during early use. Based on the HERS findings, the American Heart Association (AHA) recommended that HT not be initiated solely for the purpose of secondary prevention of CAD. In 2002, the Women's Health Initiative (WHI) Randomized Controlled Trial, the first primary prevention trial of HT in postmenopausal women, failed to demonstrate any benefit of estrogen plus progestin in the prevention of CAD or stroke after 5.2 years of follow-up. In addition, the WHI study demonstrated a

twofold hazard of pulmonary embolism. It was concluded that HT should not be initiated or continued for the primary prevention of CAD.

Recently, the unopposed estrogen arm of the WHI, involving women without an intact uterus, showed no benefit and no risk of ET for the primary prevention of CAD. In the wake of the results from these major clinical trials, the AHA issued a set of collaborative evidence-based guidelines for the prevention of CAD in women, depending on clinical diagnosis and scenarios that group women into categories of high, intermediate, and lower risk.

In addition, the new guidelines show risk groups as defined by their absolute probability of having a coronary event in 10 years, according to the Framingham Risk Score for women. The new guidelines stress lifestyle interventions, including smoking cessation, encouraging physical activity every day of the week, cardiac rehabilitation after any recent cardiac event, heart-healthy diet including omega-3 fatty acids and folic acid supplementation in high-risk women, weight maintenance and reduction, and evaluation for depression. Major risk factor interventions include encouragement to achieve a new optimal blood pressure of <120/80 mm Hg through lifestyle approaches. In addition, optimal levels of lipoproteins in women including a LDL-C of <100 mg/dL, HDL-C of >50 mg/dL, and triglycerides of <150 mg/dL are described in the new guidelines. The guidelines stress the initiation of pharmacotherapy in high-risk women with an LDL-C of >100 mg/dL or in moderate-risk women with an LDL-C of >130 mg/dL to lower LDL-C with a statin simultaneously with lifestyle therapy. Statin agents, such as atorvastatin (Lipitor), lovastatin (Mevacor), pravastatin (Pravachol), rosuvastatin (Crestor), and simvastatin (Zocor), are recommended as initial first-line therapy. ET appears to have complementary effects on the lipid profile when combined with statin therapy, particularly in women with elevated levels of lipoprotein(a) [Lp(a)], although it is not used specifically for cardiovascular risk reduction, only for treatment of menopausal symptoms.

Preventative measures, including aspirin therapy, are highly recommended in high- and intermediate-risk women, but should not be used in low-risk women. The AHA guidelines do not support the initiation or continuation of estrogen plus progestin HT to prevent cardiovascular disease in postmenopausal women. In addition, the guidelines do not support the use of antioxidant vitamin supplements in the prevention of cardiovascular disease, and the new guidelines recommend against the preventive use of aspirin in women at low risk for cardiovascular disease.

## Breast Tissue

In the postmenopausal period, involution of the ductal and glandular breast tissue occurs with a reduction in estrogen and progesterone levels. For most women, the breast shrinks and becomes replaced with adipose tissue. The Gail Model Breast Cancer Risk Assessment Tool, a seven-question logistical mathematical regression model, computes an individual woman's 5-year risk and lifetime risk of breast cancer diagnosis. If a woman has a high Gail Model assessment percentage (lifetime risk of 30% or more), she should be further counseled regarding breast cancer risk assessment and be referred to a breast center for breast cancer chemoprevention study, tamoxifen therapy, or breast ductal lavage for further risk assessment.

Increased exposure to estrogen modestly raises the risk of breast cancer. Early menarche (before age 12) and/or late menopause (after age 55), both markers of increased estrogen exposure, confer some increased risk. The WHI showed a 26% increased risk of breast cancer at 5.2 years in women who use combination estrogen and progestin in the form of Prempro. When this same data is interpreted in the form of absolute risk, it is evident that the risk of breast cancer diagnosis to the individual woman is low. In the WHI, 38 cases of breast cancer occurred in HT users per year, compared with 30 cases in women not using HT—an absolute difference of 8 cases. In contrast, women in the estrogen-only arm of this trial, using Premarin, had no increased risk of breast cancer. The Million Women Study in the United Kingdom is the largest nonrandomized study of hormone use. This study concluded that all types of hormone use, including estrogen-only forms, increased the risk of breast cancer compared with women receiving no hormone therapy.

# DIAGNOSIS OF MENOPAUSE

The diagnosis of menopause is officially made retrospectively after the cessation of menses for 1 year. Pregnancy, however, should be considered as the number one cause of secondary amenorrhea in all women. If secondary amenorrhea remains suspected, and pregnancy is ruled out, considerations in the differential diagnosis should include polycystic ovarian disease (most common ovarian cause), chronic anovulation, structural changes such as cervical stenosis or Asherman's syndrome (endometrial scarring), adrenal or thyroid dysfunction, endometrial atrophy (i.e., continuous progesterone use), pituitary prolactinoma, gestational trophoblastic disease, and nutritional disorders.

## Clinical Diagnosis

The history and physical examination should focus on the skin, the bone, and the genitourinary structures, and the cardiovascular system. Key questions to ask about menopause include symptoms of estrogen deficiency, including hot flashes or hot flushes, sleep disturbances, palpitations, changes in skin texture, history of irritable bladder or incontinence, and history of painful intercourse. It is also pertinent to ask about symptoms of

androgen deficiency, which may present as hypoactive sexual desire and a decreased ability to reach sexual climax, because this may represent a true female androgenic deficiency syndrome in a minority of postmenopausal women. Symptoms of progesterone deficiency in perimenopause present as heavy irregular menses (owing to unopposed estrogen).

The height, weight, and blood pressure should be recorded and compared with prior values. Thyroid examination; breast examination in sitting and supine position; skin examination; cardiovascular examination; and abdominal, pelvic, and rectal examinations should be performed. The clinician should note signs of genitourinary atrophy, including a thin, pale, atrophic vaginal mucosa, which may present with petechia or may be atrophic diffusely or in patches. The periurethral tissue is the most estrogen-sensitive tissue and usually shows initial signs of estrogen deficiency. Examples of severe vaginal estrogen deficiency include a stenotic introitus, varying degrees of urethral caruncle, and the presence of a small cervical os or possible stenotic os. In severe cases, the cervix may actually be flush with the vaginal walls and may be very difficult to distinguish from this surrounding vaginal tissue. A screening Papanicolaou (Pap) smear should be obtained of the ectocervix and the endocervix using a spatula and a cytobrush to screen for cervical cancer, with HPV testing in women over 30 or women with abnormal Paps. A Gail Model assessment of breast cancer risk should be considered to further define an individual woman's risk for breast cancer, and a Framingham Score should be used to assess for low, moderate, or high risk for cardiovascular disease.

## Laboratory Studies

In most cases, FSH and $E_2$ levels are not needed to diagnose the menopausal state. In a woman who has had a simple hysterectomy (ovaries remaining), ovarian function may be present after the hysterectomy, and FSH and $E_2$ levels may aid the clinician in the decision to initiate ET. If a woman has been on hormone contraceptives (HCs)—pills, patch, ring, injection, or implants or hormonal intra-uterine systems) up to the time of menopause—measuring hormonal levels after several months of being off HCs (while a woman uses a barrier method) may also be helpful in determining whether menopause has occurred. Measuring these values in a menopausal transition female are not as clinically useful because these levels may fluctuate widely through the menopausal transition state. Again, this emphasizes that the diagnosis of menopause is always retrospective.

The American College of Physicians recommends screening of thyroid-stimulating hormone in all women older than age 50, whereas the American College of Clinical Endocrinology recommends screening by age 35. Women receiving thyroxine, who may be clinically euthyroid, may actually be biochemically hyperthyroid and, therefore, at an increased risk for bone loss. Perimenopausal women who present with menopause-like symptoms and menstrual disorders may actually have hypo- or hyperthyroidism.

Standard screening mammograms and examinations of the breasts by a healthcare provider should be performed yearly, beginning at the age of 40 for all women. Women with a strong family history of breast cancer (and/or those who have Gail Model–calculated lifetime risk of breast cancer of 30% or more) should be referred to a breast center. One randomized, double-blinded, placebo-controlled trial (Postmenopausal Estrogen/Progestin Interventions Trial) actually showed an increased breast density in some HT users, which in theory may make mammographic breast cancer detection more difficult. In women with dense breasts, the clinician may consider stopping hormonal therapy 2 to 3 weeks prior to annual mammography.

The National Osteoporosis Foundation (NOF) recommends that all women be screened for OP by the age of 65 or earlier if one or more risk factors (including natural and surgically induced menopause, maternal or personal history of hip fracture, a weight of less than 128 lb, and smoking) are present. The NOF guidelines suggest that all women who have been on long-term HT have a bone density assessment because a small subset of women are bone nonresponders, even though they have been on long-term treatment. For a healthy postmenopausal woman who is contemplating initiating any therapy for bone protection reasons, a dual X-ray absorptometry (DXA) scan may assist her in the decision to institute therapy. Any woman with a history of vertebral compression fractures or skeletal deformity should have a DXA performed initially at baseline. DXA scans also serve as screening for OP prevention in women with POI and for other persons with risk factors for OP (glucocorticoid use, eating disorders, anticonversant therapy, height loss, a history of prolonged amenorrhea).

Along with body mass index calculations (weight in kilograms over height in meters), waist to hip ratios (waist circumference should be <35 inches in women and <40 inches in men), blood pressure, smoking history, diabetes, and lipids stratify a woman's cardiovascular risk. Several large studies indicate that ultrasensitive C-reactive protein (US CRP) screening, in addition to standard lipid screening, provided further information in identifying women who were at high risk for future cardiovascular events. These results may influence clinicians to more aggressively treat with statin agents in this subset of patients with elevated US CRP levels.

## MANAGEMENT OF MENOPAUSE

The key to managing menopause and its associated symptoms is to tailor therapy to the individual woman. The minimum effective dose of replacement therapy should be used to treat the symptoms of menopause (vasomotor symptoms, genitourinary symptoms). The benefits and risks should be discussed with patients regarding standard HT with the lowest effective dose used. Options should be provided regarding other bone therapy options with SERMs or bisphosphonates. Dietary, exercise, and lifestyle advice is paramount. A woman's individual medical history, family history, current menopausal symptoms, and her response to HT should periodically be reassessed.

## Risks and Benefits of HT

### Benefits
- Relief of vasomotor symptoms
- Prevention of postmenopausal OP, fractures, and dental loss
- Curing of genitourinary atrophy
- Reduction in colon cancer and colon polyps in HT users
- Possible benefit in reducing age-related macular degeneration
- Probable improvement in mood and energy level and a sense of well-being in symptomatic women
- Possible reduction in cataract formation, knee osteoarthritis, and obstructive sleep apnea syndrome

### Risks
- Five- to tenfold increase in endometrial cancer risk if ET is unopposed
- Slight increase in breast cancer diagnosis in women on estrogen-progestin HT for several years
- Increase in the relative risk of thromboembolic events of two- to threefold in HT users
- Increased stroke risk
- Increased incidence of gallbladder disease, which may necessitate cholecystectomy
- Premenstrual-like side effects on a combination (estrogen/progestin) therapy
- Withdrawal menstrual bleeding on a cycled HT regimen
- Elevations of triglyceride levels on oral ET in susceptible women

If a woman has had a hysterectomy, ET alone is prescribed, but if a woman has an endometrium and uterus, *both* estrogen and progestin therapy should be given to avoid unopposed estrogen that can lead to endometrial hyperplasia and thus increase the risk of endometrial cancer.

If a woman is still using contraception before menopause, she should continue with contraception use 1 year after initiating HT therapy because the level of hormones in postmenopausal therapy is not high enough to inhibit the hypothalamic-pituitary-ovarian axis, which is needed for contraceptive protection.

## Estrogen Therapy

### Conjugated Equine Estrogens
A blend of multiple equine estrogens, Premarin, has been available the longest and studied the most extensively of all ET. Esterified estrogen preparations (Estratab and

## TABLE 2.6
### ORAL ESTROGEN DOSAGES

| Trade Name | Ultra-Low Dose (mg) | Low Dose (mg) | Medium Dose (mg) | Intermediate Dose (mg) | Higher Dose (mg) | Highest Dose (mg) |
|---|---|---|---|---|---|---|
| Premarin (CEEs) | 0.3 | 0.45 | 0.625 | 0.9 | 1.25 | 2.5 |
| Estrace (micronized estradiol) | 0.5 | | 1.000 | | 2.00 | |
| Ogen (estrone) | | | 0.625 | | 1.25 | 2.5 |
| Ortho-Est (estrone) | | | 0.625 | | 1.25 | |
| Estratab (esterified estrogen preparation) | 0.3 | | 0.625 | | 1.25 | 2.5 |
| Menest (esterified estrogen preparation) | 0.3 | | 0.625 | | 1.25 | 2.5 |
| Cenestin (synthetic CEE)[a] | | | 0.625 | | 0.9 | |
| Estrasorb (lotion) | | | 0.625 (Apply one dose daily) | | | |
| Femring every 3 months | | | 0.05 | | | |

[a] CEE=conjugated equine estrogen.

Menest) contain $E_1$ and equilin sulfate, but are not exact biochemical equivalents to conjugated equine estrogen (CEE). Cenestin is a synthetic conjugated estrogen formulation. Micronized 17β-estradiol ($E_2$) (Estrace) can be given orally and is well absorbed by the gastrointestinal tract, but has a short half-life, necessitating a twice-daily dosage. Estropipate ($E_1$) is available as Ogen and Ortho-Est and is dosed daily. Dosages for oral estrogen therapy are shown in Table 2.6.

The $E_2$ transdermal patch offers an alternative to women who prefer the convenience of dosing (most patches are changed every 3.5 days or once a week), who experienced nausea or drug-induced hypertension on oral preparations (Table 2.7), or who want to use "bio-identical" estradiol. In women who have elevated triglycerides, the patch preparation is also preferred. The patch preparation avoids enterohepatic metabolism. In women with a history of deep venous thrombosis, theoretically, transdermal ET may be advantageous; however, no evidence suggests that transdermal or "bio-identical" HT is any safer than other regimens.

Overall, the side effects of estrogen include nausea, bloating, and breast tenderness, but they are lower with ET preparations in comparison with standard HC because the overall estrogenic doses are 4 to 5 times lower in comparison with low-dose HC. Lower doses of estrogen with CEE at 0.45 or 0.3 mg are recommended as starting doses, or patches may be used (0.025, 0.0375, or 0.045 mg). In general, women who have undergone surgical- or chemotherapy-induced menopause may need higher doses of estrogen to control vasomotor symptoms. Higher doses of CEE of 0.625, 0.9, or 1.25 mg daily, either by the oral route or the transdermal $E_2$ patches of 0.05, 0.075, 0.100 mg may be needed. Several weeks should elapse before dosages are increased. If women are on standard oral ET and continue to have genitourinary symptoms, vaginal preparations, in addition to systemic therapy, may be beneficial (Table 2.8). An example of this is Estrace or Premarin vaginal cream, 2 g daily for 2 weeks and then 1 g one to three times per week, given intravaginally. Some systemic absorption of estrogen cream in preparation occurs through the vaginal mucosa, but once

## TABLE 2.7
### ESTRADIOL PATCH DOSAGES

| Trade Name | Ultra-Low & Low Dose (mg) | Medium Dose (mg) | Intermediate Dose (mg) | Higher Dose (mg) | Change Patch |
|---|---|---|---|---|---|
| Estraderm | | 0.05 | | 0.10 | Every 3.5 days |
| Vivelle | 0.025 0.0375 | 0.05 | 0.075 | 0.10 | Every 3.5 days |
| Alora | | 0.05 | 0.075 | 0.10 | Every 3.5 days |
| Climara | 0.025 | 0.05 | 0.075 | 0.10 | Weekly |
| CombiPatch | Contains 0.05 mg of estradiol with either 0.14 mg or 0.25 mg of norethindrone acetate (NA) | | | | |
| ClimaraPro | Contains 0.045 mg of estradiol with NA—weekly 0.015 of levonorgestrel | | | | |

## TABLE 2.8

### OPTIONS FOR GENITOURINARY MENOPAUSAL SYMPTOMS

| | |
|---|---|
| Premarin cream/Estrace cream/Ogen cream | 2 g daily intravaginally for 2 weeks, then 1 g intravaginally 1–3 times weekly |
| Vagifem tablets (estradiol hemihydrate) | Insert 1 tablet in vagina each night for 2 weeks, then 1 tablet 2 times weekly for maintenance |
| Estring (estradiol ring) | Place ring intravaginally, change every 3 months |

the mucosal integrity is restored with local therapy, systemic absorption is minimal. If a woman prefers not to use vaginal cream preparations due to variability, absorbability, and application, other options have become available for urogenital symptoms of estrogen deficiency. A silicone vaginal ring (Estring) impregnated with $E_2$ can be inserted in the vagina by the woman every 3 months for relief of urogenital symptoms. Little systemic absorption of estrogen has been noted with the vaginal ring, thus making it a possible therapeutic option in women who want to avoid systemic estrogen treatment.

In addition, the Vagifem intravaginal tablet [17β-estradiol $(E_2)$] is another option for women who need local vaginal therapy and who have continued urogenital symptoms, or for women who currently are not on systemic therapy and continue to have urogenital symptoms. One tablet is inserted into the lower third of the vagina every night for 2 weeks, then twice a week thereafter for the relief of urogenital symptoms. An approximate 5% rate of systemic absorption of $E_2$ occurs using this treatment, unlike the vaginal ring, so endometrial stimulation is possible. Other kinds of estrogen systemic therapy include the Femring vaginal ring, changed every 3 weeks, which provides local and systemic estrogen, and Estrasorb estrogen lotion, which is rubbed on the arms and legs and provides systemic estrogen to treat hot flashes.

Women who have low free testosterone levels may benefit from preparations containing esterified estrogen, 1.25 mg or 0.625 mg, combined with methyltestosterone, 2.5 mg or 1.25 mg (Estratest or Estratest HS). Side effects of androgen therapy include acne, hirsutism, and other virilization effects. It is important to note that any oral androgen may cause an elevation in transaminases and potential liver damage. Therefore, it is recommended that periodic monitoring of transaminases, lipid levels, and $E_2$ free testosterone levels be performed in a women taking oral androgens. Compounded testosterone preparations are not routinely recommended because of a variability in absorption and lack of standardization. Although testosterone patches are available (for male hypogonadism),

the doses are generally too high for women. The FDA is expected to approve a testosterone patch, called Intrinsa, for women in 2005.

Tibolone, available in Europe, is a synthetic steroid analog that has estrogenic, androgenic, and progestin activity without endometrial stimulation. After metabolism, the progestogenic metabolite predominates, producing an atrophic endometrium. Tibolone may prove to be a useful alternative in women wanting to avoid uterine bleeding or in women with endometriosis; however, in the Million Women Study, tibolone was shown to increase the risk of breast cancer. Tibolone may reduce bone reabsorption and decrease total cholesterol, Lp(a), and triglyceride levels but also has been noted to decrease high density lipoprotein levels as well.

### Progestins

Combined estrogen/progestin therapy is mandatory in a woman with an endometrium to avoid stimulation of the endometrial lining, which may lead to the endometrial hyperplasia associated with unopposed estrogen use. In a hysterectomized patient, progestins are not recommended unless a residual endometriosis exists. The side effects of progestins include premenstrual-like symptoms, which often cause women the discomfort that is associated initially with starting combined estrogen/progestin therapy. Progestins may have androgenic effects, depending on the type of agent used, dosage, and route of delivery. Current epidemiologic studies do not recommend adding progestins to estrogen to prevent OP.

Cycled progestins are taken for the first 12 days of every calendar month. This *cyclic regimen* is associated with withdrawal bleeding in most women. If progestins are taken on a daily basis with estrogen, this is termed *continuous therapy*, and usually induces amenorrhea in most menopausal women within a 6- to 9-month period.

Provera, Cycrin, and Amen (medroxyprogesterone acetate, 5 to 10 mg) are examples of progestins that are given on days 1 through 12 of each calendar month for a cycled regimen (Table 2.9). Micronized progesterone (Prometrium, 100 mg continuous regimen or 200 mg cycled regimen, days 1 through 12) is centrally metabolized and may have sedative-hypnotic effects (Table 2.9). This may be an option for women who suffer from sleep disturbances secondary to menopause. Prometrium is micronized with peanut oil, therefore, women with peanut allergies must have progesterone compounded with another oil. Prochieve vaginal gel (4%–8%) is available for women intolerant of Prometrium use and is a vaginal progesterone.

A woman should expect mild to moderate bleeding during cycled therapy, usually occurring mid month between days 10 through 15. As long as the cervical os is not stenosed, the absence of withdrawal bleeding indicates the endometrial lining may simply be atrophic. Any abnormal bleeding occurring outside of the day 10 to day 15 period must be further investigated with an endometrial biopsy,

## TABLE 2.9

### MEDROXYPROGESTERONE ACETATE (MPA) AND COMBINATION CONTINUOUS REGIMENS

| Brand Name | Dosage |
|---|---|
| MPA regimens | |
| Provera | MPA 5–10 mg on days 1–12, or 2.5 mg daily |
| Cycrin | MPA 5–10 mg on days 1–12, or 2.5 mg daily |
| Amen | MPA 10 mg on days 1–12 (tablet is scored) |
| Combination continuous regimens | |
| Prempro (2.5 or 5.0) | MPA, 2.5 or 5.0 mg daily, and CEE[a] 0.625 mg daily (28-day pill pack), or new starting dose ultra-low-dose Premarin (CEE), 0.45 mg/1.5 mg of MPA or 0.3 mg/1.5 mg |
| Premphase | MPA, 5 mg/day for 14 days, with CEE, 0.625 mg daily (28-day pill pack) |
| Prometrium | Micronized progesterone, 200 mg for 14 days or 100 mg for 28 days in addition to ET, to be taken with food to improve absorption and in the evening due to sedative side effect |
| FemHRT | Norethindrone acetate, 1 mg with 5 μg EE daily (28-day pill pack) |
| Activella | Norethindrone acetate, 0.5 mg with 1 mg EE daily (28-day pill pack) |
| Prefest | Norgestimate, 0.09 mg with 1 mg estradiol daily (28-day pill pack); daily estrogen with *intermittent* norgestimate |

[a] CEE=conjugated equine estrogens; EE=ethinyl estradiol; ET=estrogen therapy.

hysteroscopy, or saline-infused sonogram to detect endometrial abnormalities.

If HT is given to relieve postmenopausal symptoms, therapy can be tapered off gradually while still monitoring for bone loss with periodic DXA scanning. The key to HT is to tailor the therapy based on an individual woman's risks and benefits and re-evaluate the need for HT periodically based on treatment goals using the lowest effective dose.

## Contraindications to Hormone Therapy

Absolute contraindications to HT include pregnancy and undiagnosed vaginal bleeding. Any postmenopausal vaginal bleeding must be investigated with an endometrial biopsy, owing to a 5% to 10% incidence of simple or complex hyperplasia (with or without atypia), adenomatous endometrial hyperplasia, or frank endometrial cancers. The majority of women with postmenopausal bleeding have a proliferative endometrium (because of a lack of progesterone), endometrial polyps, cervical or vulvar lesions, submucosal fibroids, or simple bleeding from an atrophic vagina or atrophic endometrium.

Once uterine cancer is cured either by surgical excision of low-grade, early-stage cancer or by lack of occurrence after 5 years from initial surgical treatment, ET is an option. Ovarian cancers are not usually thought to be estrogen-dependent and therefore do not constitute a contraindication to HT.

A remote history of deep venous thrombosis (DVT) is not an absolute contraindication to HT. Any patient with a history of recurrent DVT or a family history of thromboembolic events, however, should be evaluated for the presence of a hypercoagulable state. Migraine headaches that have a hormonal pattern may improve or worsen at menopause. Postmenopausal women with a history of migraines usually benefit from continuous replacement therapy rather than cyclical therapy, thereby avoiding the variation in hormone levels that may actually exacerbate migraines.

A rare side effect of HT is an idiosyncratic elevation of blood pressure in a small percentage of women. Also, women with hepatic disease or gallbladder disease may have worsening of the disease state on oral HT and may want to consider transdermal HT as an alternative (Climara-Propatch or CombiPatch).

## Alternative Options for Treatment of Menopausal Symptoms

Over-the-counter vaginal lubricants offer some temporary relief of symptoms of vaginal dryness but do not revive the atrophic vaginal mucosa. For the treatment of hot flashes, some of the selective serotonin reuptake inhibitors (SSRIs) and the norepinephrine serotonin reuptake inhibitor (NSRI) venlafaxine have been shown to be reduce hot flashes. Vitamin E, 400 IU per day, may also alleviate some vasomotor symptoms by reducing LH levels. In women with breast cancer, megestrol acetate (Megace) has also been used to treat vasomotor instability.

*Alternative therapies* such as black cohosh or red clover leaf have potential estrogen-like effects and may help in reducing vasomotor symptoms, but it is advisable to caution patients that these are not regulated substances in the United States; therefore, purity and strength can vary from product to product. Recently, soy products containing soy proteins and isoflavones (if ingested in amounts greater than 25 mg per day) have been shown in studies to reduce total cholesterol levels. The resolution of vasomotor symptoms with soy has not been as consistent in studies. In a recent study, isoflavones in comparison with placebo were found to be no better in controlling vasomotor symptoms. In a recent placebo-controlled trial, dong quai was found to be no better than placebo in controlling hot flashes as well. In advising women regarding "natural remedies," it is important to stress that most herbal supplements have not been studied in large, controlled, prospective trials, and, therefore, the risk associated with these therapies remains questionable.

## Diet and Exercise during Menopause

It is important to counsel patients that aging and menopause are risks for weight gain. During the menopausal transition period, women can gain on average 2 to 5 lb or more. Also, a hormonally driven shift in fat distribution occurs, making central obesity more prevalent. A diet rich in fruits, vegetables, whole grains, nuts, and low-fat dairy products and low in saturated animal fats should be recommended. Trans-fat ("partial hydrogenated oils") should be avoided and essential fatty acids, like omega-3 oils, should be consumed regularly.

Adequate calcium and vitamin D intake is important for OP prevention in women, as well as possibly reducing the risk of colon cancer and decreasing PMS symptoms. Three major sources for calcium exist: foods, calcium-fortified foods, and supplements. Dietary foods are the preferred means of obtaining adequate calcium intake. Dairy products have a high calcium content, have high calcium bioavailability, and are affordable. However, 25% of the U.S. population exhibits some degree of lactase nonpersistence (lactose intolerance) and have poor dairy intake. Calcium supplements should be considered if lactose intolerance or dietary preferences limit dietary dairy intake. The National Institutes of Health recommend the following daily elemental calcium intakes in women:

- Premenopausal women 25 to 50 years: 1,000 to 1,200 mg per day in divided doses
- Postmenopausal women younger than 65 years using ET: 1,200 mg per day total in divided doses
- Postmenopausal women not using ET: 1,500 mg per day total in divided doses
- All women older than age 65 years: 1,500 mg per day total in divided doses

The use of higher calcium intakes produces no currently recognized health benefits and may expose the individual to further side effects. Vitamin D is essential for the intestinal absorption of calcium. The National Osteoporosis Foundation recommends up to 800 IU per day of vitamin D for women at risk of deficiency because of poor sunlight exposure, advanced age, chronic illness, being homebound, and living in northern latitudes. Daily requirements can usually be met with a multivitamin supplement (usually containing 400 IU of vitamin D) and with brief sun exposure of the skin.

Aerobic exercise and weight training are also beneficial for postmenopausal women and have been shown to increase bone mineral density, reduce OP fracture risks, and reduce the overall risk for fatal and nonfatal myocardial events, as well as to reduce breast and colon cancer risks.

## Treatment of the Menopausal Transition State

Some women may experience only vasomotor symptoms while they are still menstruating regularly. Very low-dose ET may be a treatment option in this population. In the menopausal transition state, the failing ovary responds inconsistently to elevated levels of stimulating gonadotropins with estrogen surges. The endometrium may subsequently become thickened owing to this unopposed estrogen. Periodic monitoring (endometrial biopsy) of the endometrium is imperative to assess for hyperplasia if an unopposed estrogen state is suspected. Some women during the perimenopausal period may produce adequate amounts of estrogen from the ovaries and adrenal glands but may have evidence of progesterone deficiency because of a lack of production from the corpus luteum. These women may exhibit symptoms of mood irritability and menstrual disturbances, usually with heavy bleeding being the most common manifestation. The use of oral micronized progesterone in the form of Prometrium or the use of synthetic progestins may regulate menstrual flow in these women.

### Hormonal Contraception (HC)

In the perimenopausal woman who is a *nonsmoker* and in general good health, HC can be continued up to the ages of 50 to 55. HC controls the irregular cycles associated with the menopausal transition state and can control vasomotor symptoms and provide contraceptive protection as well. Once the woman becomes menopausal, if symptomatic, HC can be converted to progestin/estrogen therapy [e.g., FemHRT, which is 5 µg ethinyl estradiol ($E_2$) and 1.0 mg norethindrone acetate]. Progestin/estrogen menopausal therapy *does not* provide contraceptive protection.

HC provides 4 to 5 times more estrogenic activity than is needed during the menopausal state. Low-dose HC [30 to 35 µg of ethinyl estradiol ($E_2$)] does not increase the risk of breast cancer or diabetes and has little effect on carbohydrate metabolism. For women who experience nausea, bloating, and other estrogenic side effects, very low-dose HC, such as 20 µg of ethinyl estradiol ($E_2$, Loestrin, Alesse, Mircette, Levlite) are options. All these preparations should preserve bone mass, alleviate dysmenorrhea, and reduce menstrual blood flow (alleviating iron deficiency anemia). In women with a history of ovarian cysts, higher doses of estrogen-containing HC are needed to suppress ovulation. HC is also beneficial in the treatment of acne and hirsutism by reducing absolute free testosterone levels via ovarian steroidogenesis suppression and reduced adrenal androgen production.

### Newer HC: Yasmin, Ortho Evra, NuvaRing

*Yasmin* is a monophasic, low-dose oral contraceptive pill that contains $E_2$ and drospirenone, a progestin analogue of spironolactone. Drospirenone is the only progestin with both antimineralocorticoid and antiandrogenic properties. Yasmin's 99% efficacy is similar to most other HC. Yasmin helps to improve acne, seborrhea, and hirsutism while providing good weight stability due to its antiandrogenic, diuretic properties. As a result, it is a good choice in those with severe premenstrual symptoms such as bloating. Each Yasmin pill contains 3 mg of drospirenone, the equivalent to 25 mg of spironolactone, a potassium-sparing diuretic. Therefore, the serum potassium level should be monitored during the first month of therapy. Yasmin should be used with caution in women taking medications that predispose to hyperkalemia, such as other potassium-sparing diuretics, angiotensin-converting enzyme (ACE) inhibitors, aldosterone antagonists, and nonsteroidal anti-inflammatory medications. Yasmin is contraindicated in women with renal, hepatic, or adrenal insufficiency.

Data from the Nurses Health Study indicate no increased risk exists for CAD, stroke, or other cardiovascular complications in healthy HC users. A risk for cardiovascular complications does exist in women, older than age 35 years, who *continue to smoke* while on HC. In a woman who is generally healthy, is a nonsmoker, and is without hypertension and with well-controlled cholesterol levels, HC can be continued well beyond the age of 40 years.

*Ortho Evra* is the first transdermal contraceptive patch that releases 20 µg E2 and 150 µg norelgestromin per 24 hours. Norelgestromin is a metabolite of norgestimate, the progestin in the third-generation pills Ortho-Cyclen and Ortho Tri-Cyclen. A new patch is applied weekly, on the same day each week, for 3 weeks. Week four is patch free and withdrawal bleeding is expected during this time. When compared to daily HC, the patch is equally safe, with similar contraceptive efficacy and menstrual cycle control, but has the benefit of improved compliance. Experience with more than 70,000 Ortho Evra patches worn showed that 4.7% of patches were replaced because they either fell off (1.8%) or were partly detached (2.9%). If detached, a new patch should be applied immediately. Packages of single replacement patches are available; supplemental adhesives or wraps should never be used. The patient should be encouraged to enjoy her usual physical activities (i.e., sauna, whirlpool, swimming). Used patches still contain active hormones, and they should be carefully folded in half before being discarded.

In clinical trials, most unintended pregnancies were among women weighing more than 198 lb. (90 kg), therefore, Ortho Evra should be used with caution in these women. The most common side effects reported are (in decreasing order): breast tenderness, headache, skin irritation, and nausea. Because Ortho Evra avoids first-pass metabolism, it is unknown if the risk of venous thromboembolism while using Ortho Evra is different from that of other HC.

*NuvaRing* is a contraceptive vaginal ring that releases 120 µg of $E_2$ daily. The vaginal ring is colorless, odorless, 2 inches in diameter, and easily inserted vaginally by most women. The ring is left in place for 3 weeks, with withdrawal bleed occurring during the fourth, ring-free week. Although not recommended if a cystocele, rectocele, or uterine prolapse is present, NuvaRing is an excellent, convenient choice for most women.

A study comparing NuvaRing to standard HC containing 30 µg of $E_2$ showed that NuvaRing users had less frequency of irregular bleeding and better cycle control. NuvaRing may cause a higher incidence of vaginal discomfort and vaginitis, however. Also, the ring may be accidentally expelled from the vagina, and if the ring is left out for more than 3 hours, efficacy is significantly reduced. To maintain the highest contraceptive efficacy, NuvaRing should be rinsed with warm water and reinserted in the vagina.

The other potential noncontraceptive health benefits of HC include:

- Protection against endometrial and ovarian cancer (because of the suppression of chronic ovulation)
- Reduction of the risk of colon cancer (by induction of favorable changes in bile synthesis and reduction of bile acid in the colon)
- Reduction in incidence and severity of dysmenorrhea and *mittelschmerz* (ovulatory mid-cycle pain)
- Resolution of menstrual irregularity related to hormonal fluxes
- Stabilization of bone mineral density (which is advantageous in the female athlete with amenorrhea)
- Decrease in iron deficiency anemia (because of the decrease in the length and flow of the menses)
- Reduction in ovarian cyst formation (higher doses of estrogen HC may be needed for the suppression of large cysts)
- Lower incidence of endometriosis
- Reduction in the risk for developing uterine fibroids
- A reduced risk of benign breast disease
- Decrease in the risk of ectopic pregnancy
- Decreased risk of salpingitis/pelvic inflammatory disease
- Reduced risk of rheumatoid arthritis
- Possible improvement in menstrual exacerbations of porphyria and asthma

Since the introduction of HC in the last 40 years, the overall dose of estrogen has been decreased by 90% and the dose of progestin by 80%. Third-generation progestins such as desogestrel (Desogen, Ortho-Cept) and norgestimate (Ortho-Cyclen, Ortho Tri-Cyclen) have been developed to decrease some of the androgenic side effects that were present in higher-dose progestin-containing HC. Studies from Europe, however, have indicated that the risk of nonfatal thromboembolic events associated with third-generation HC (containing desogestrel or gestodene) seems to be higher than for the second-generation HC (which contain levonorgestrel or norethindrone). In a woman with an increased risk of thromboembolic disease or with risk factors such as obesity or varicosities, these third-generation HC should be generally avoided as first choice.

HCs have a mild favorable effect on lipid profiles, including a 5% to 10% increase in high-density lipoprotein

(HDL) cholesterol levels and a mild decrease of 5% in low-density lipoprotein (LDL) cholesterol levels. Factor V Leiden mutation testing is *not* recommended before starting HC in a patient who has no family history of thromboembolic events or no personal history of thromboembolic disease.

The first-generation oral HCs contain 50 μg or more of ethinyl estradiol ($E_2$) and are indicated only for use in women with recurrent ovarian cysts needing ovarian suppression or in women with a seizure disorder on anticonvulsant therapy who may metabolize contraceptives at a faster rate.

*Medroxyprogesterone acetate* suspension (Depo-Provera) is an injectable hormone contraceptive that acts primarily by preventing ovulation by inhibiting the secretion of gonadotropins. The chief advantage of Depo-Provera is the avoidance of estrogenic side effects and the reduction of menstrual bleeding. By the end of the first year of use, approximately 50% of users will develop amenorrhea. The contraceptive protection of Depo-Provera lasts for approximately 12 to 14 weeks. The ideal time to initiate Depo-Provera is within 5 days after the onset of menses, and it is given by intramuscular injection (150 mg) in the upper outer quadrant of the gluteal region. The efficacy of Depo-Provera is high, with failure rates between 0.0% to 0.7%. Depo-Provera may be more desirable over HC in certain disease states and in terms of compliance to therapy. Disease states such as hypertension exacerbated by synthetic estrogens, renal hepatic disease, vascular disease, thromboembolic disease, hemoglobinopathies, and seizure disorders, and the postpartum lactating state are examples of medical conditions that make the use of Depo-Provera more desirable over HC.

Contraindications to Depo-Provera use include pregnancy, undiagnosed bleeding, history of suspected malignancy or known malignancy of the breast, active thrombophlebitis, active liver disease, or known hypersensitivity to medroxyprogesterone acetate. The most common side effect of Depo-Provera is spotting bleeding (which makes it a poor choice of birth control in women whom further investigation of vaginal spotting would be deemed appropriate, such as older women). Other side effects include weight gain (approximately 2-kg weight gain in the first year), exacerbation of headaches or migraines, abdominal pain, dizziness, and fatigue. If a woman has complete amenorrhea with ovarian suppression for prolonged periods of time, osteopenia is a concern and assessment of the bone mineral density should be considered.

*Lunelle* is the first monthly combination contraceptive injection containing both medroxyprogesterone acetate (25 mg) and $E_2$ (5 mg) available in the United States. Intramuscular injections should be given every 28 to 30 days. The failure rate has been reported to be from 0.1% to 1.0%. The most common side effect noted is weight gain within the first year of use. Contraindications for use are similar to those of HC.

*Implanon* is a progestin-only contraceptive implant that is effective against pregnancy for 3 years. It consists of a single plastic rod measuring 40 mm in length and 2 mm in diameter (about the size of a matchstick). The rod is inserted just under the skin on the inside of the upper arm, is very flexible, and not likely to be visible. The hormone etonogestrel is released slowly from the device into the bloodstream over 3 years. This is the active metabolite of desogestrel, one of the third-generation progestins commonly used in HC. In clinical trials involving over 2,300 women, no pregnancies have been reported after approximately 73,000 monthly cycles. This product is expected to be available in the United States after 2005.

*Postcoital contraception* can be offered to women in the form of steroidal and nonsteroidal estrogens alone or in combination with progestin. Success rates are up to 75% if given within the first 72 hours after sexual exposure. Of note is that the earlier the administration of the first dose of postcoital contraception, the lower the failure rate. One example of postcoital contraception is the Yuzpe regimen, which consists of norgestrel and 100 μg ethinyl estradiol ($E_2$) (Ovral, two pills, or Lo/Ovral, four pills) followed by a repeat dose 12 hours later. Major side effects with postcoital contraception include nausea (25% to 66%) and vomiting (5% to 24%). Preven Kit (estrogen and progestin) and Plan B (progestin only) are approved by the FDA for emergency contraception.

Plan B is associated with less nausea compared with the Preven and may be the agent of first choice. It has FDA approval for over-the-counter availability.

*Intrauterine contraceptive devices (IUDs)* are an option still for parous, monogamous women. The copper IUD provides effective contraception for 7 to 10 years. Mirena-IUS (levonorgestrel-IUS) may be a treatment option to reduce bleeding in women with menorrhagia, and in a recent study, it is a cost-effective alternative to hysterectomy to reduce heavy vaginal bleeding. The levonorgestrel IUS (Mirena) is therapeutic for 5 to 7 years. Women older than 35 years (particularly if they smoke, thus making HC unacceptable) are excellent candidates for IUDs, assuming they have no history of pelvic inflammatory disease, ectopic pregnancy, leukemia, sickle cell disease, or valvular heart disease. IUDs are not the first choice for a young nulliparous woman due to the potential for dysmenorrhea and the high risk of sexually transmitted diseases.

*Sterilization* remains the most popular form of contraception in the United States either by tubal ligation or vasectomy, which are both considered irreversible procedures. Other options include *barrier methods*, such as latex condoms for men (or polyurethane condoms if either partner has a latex allergy). Several new female barriers have been developed in Europe, in addition to the Femdom (the female condom), including the Oves cap, Femcaps, and Lea's Shield (diaphragms), which require concomitant spermicidal use, as well as the contraceptive sponge, which is back on the market. All of the above caps come with user kits to promote correct and consistent use. Only a few clinical trials exist using these methods of contraception, thus limiting the availability of contraceptive efficacy data.

## CONCLUSION

The various hormonal phases in a woman's life are periods of potential positive change that provide the patient and the physician a unique opportunity to address specific healthcare issues and health maintenance activities. Each life cycle hormonal phase requires the clinician to understand the physiology of gonadal hormones, pharmacology of the hormonal agent prescribed, and the importance of lifestyle modifications to individualize a woman's health regimen. The current approach to menstrual disorders management, contraceptive management, and menopausal care provides the potential for improved quality of life for women. Menopausal risk assessment and treatment provide the potential for improved quality of life for women and may include: HT for symptoms, bone specific agents for bone protection, and statin use for women at increased cardiovascular risk, with periodic re-evaluation.

## REVIEW EXERCISES

### QUESTIONS

**1.** A 54-year-old woman presents to your office with the chief complaint of vaginal dryness. She became post-menopausal spontaneously at 52 years of age and has had occasional nondescriptive hot flashes since then. She reports having at least two urinary tract infections in the last year, has noted that sexual intercourse has become more painful over the last year, and has experienced some stress urinary incontinence. Otherwise, she is healthy, has no history of breast or endometrial cancer, and has had a normal Pap smear and screening mammogram. She is not interested in systemic HT at this time. Your best recommendations at this time are which of the following?
**a)** Vaginal over-the-counter moisturizers and lubricants during intercourse
**b)** Estring vaginal ring
**c)** OCP therapy
**d)** Assessment of bone status
**e)** a, b, and d

**2.** A 55-year-old Hispanic female who became menopausal 3 years ago presents to your office for routine physical examination. She is currently on CEEs and medroxyprogesterone acetate (Prempro), 0.625 mg/2.5 mg daily, and denies any vasomotor symptoms, sleep disturbances, or change in libido. She does report some

"vaginal spotting" twice over the last 3 months. You would recommend which of the following?
**a)** Bleeding calendar to mark her days of bleeding
**b)** Hysterectomy
**c)** Increasing the progestin portion to Prempro, 0.625 mg/5 mg by mouth every day
**d)** Endometrial biopsy and consider Prempro-low dose

**3.** A 53-year-old white woman with a history of total abdominal hysterectomy, bilateral salpingo-oophorectomy for fibroids, and seizure disorder presents to your office with the chief complaint of having "hot flashes." She has been on CEEs (Premarin), 0.625 mg, since her hysterectomy. She is also taking phenytoin and folic acid in addition to Premarin. She also has an isolated elevation of her triglyceride levels to 250 mg/dL. You would recommend which of the following?
**a)** Adding progestin, 5 mg daily
**b)** Increasing her oral Premarin dose to 1.25 mg daily
**c)** Recommend adding isoflavones to her diet and then stopping Premarin
**d)** Changing her ET to a transdermal patch therapy such as weekly Climara

**4.** A 48-year-old African American woman with a history of total abdominal hysterectomy and bilateral salpingo-oophorectomy 4 years ago for benign reasons comes to your office complaining of low sexual interest and an inability to reach sexual climax. She is currently on esterified estrogen (Menest), 0.625 mg every day, and denies other symptoms. You check her total serum $E_2$ level, which is 50 pg/mL. She has a normal vaginal and pelvic examination. You recommend which of the following?
**a)** Sertraline (Zoloft), 25 mg by mouth every day and sex therapy
**b)** Vaginal lubrication
**c)** Changing to esterified estrogens, 0.625 mg, plus methyltestosterone, 1.25 mg (Estratest HS) by mouth every day
**d)** Increasing her dose of Premarin to 1.25 mg by mouth every day

**5.** A 56-year-old white woman who has been post-menopausal for 6 years comes to you for a routine examination. She has intermittent symptoms of gastro-esophageal reflux disease and has a past medical history of esophagitis. She also had a recent DXA scan of her spine and hip that showed a T score of −2.5 standard deviations below young normal. She states her mother was diagnosed with breast cancer, and she is not interested in HT. She has no personal or family history of DVT. You recommend which of the following?
**a)** Medroxyprogesterone acetate (Depo-Provera) injections every 3 months
**b)** Raloxifene, 60 mg by mouth every day
**c)** Alendronate, 70 mg by mouth every week

**d)** Calcium supplementation to a total of 1,500 mg daily with vitamin D, 400 IU to 800 IU daily

**e)** Both b and d

**6.** A 36-year-old obese smoker presents to you for contraceptive counseling. She is married with two children and has no history of sexually transmitted diseases, pelvic inflammatory disease, or DVT. She has normal periods with no heavy bleeding or clots. You recommend which of the following?

**a)** IUD or IUS-Mirena

**b)** Second-generation birth control pill

**c)** Medroxyprogesterone acetate (Depo-Provera) injection

**d)** Estratest

**7.** A 54-year-old G2P2 white female has tried multiple nonhormonal therapies for menopausal symptoms. None have provided her relief. She stopped menstruating for 13 months at age 52, but subsequently had 2 days of spotting, which resolved on its own. She has a past medical history of DVT in her 30s. This occurred while she was involved in a significant motor vehicle accident. She has an aunt and sister with breast cancer. Her father had an myocardial infarction at age 48, subsequently developed a stroke a year later, and died.

You discuss the risks, benefits, alternatives of HT with her, but advise her against HT due to the following absolute contraindication:

**a)** Personal history of remote thromboembolism

**b)** Undiagnosed uterine bleeding

**c)** Strong family history of breast cancer

**d)** Early family history of CV disease and stroke

**e)** a and c

**f)** All of the above.

**8.** A 49-year-old white woman presents with symptoms of hot flashes, difficulty sleeping, decreased libido, fatigue, and feeling irritable and depressed. These symptoms started a few years ago, but have now significantly worsened over the last 6 to 8 months. Her past medical history is significant for hyperlipidemia (LDL 164). She is classified as pre-hypertensive by the new JNCVII criteria. No known heart disease. Her past surgical history is significant for an appendectomy. She is G4P4, s/p total abdominal hysterectomy at age 48 for a history of fibroids. Family history shows breast cancer in sister (age 63), osteoporosis in mother, and stroke in grandmother. She now asks you for advice, you tell her:

**a)** To have her FSH levels checked to determine if she is in menopause.

**b)** To combine over-the-counter soy formulations until she gets symptom relief, since these products have a better safety profile than ET

**c)** That ET is discouraged in her case due to the pre-hypertension, elevated cholesterol, and a family history of breast cancer

**d)** That ET will help symptoms, but there is an increased risk of stroke, breast cancer, heart attack, and cholecystitis

**e)** That she may try using off-label antidepressants to treat vasomotor signs and mood symptoms

## ANSWERS

**1. e.**

The use of the Estring vaginal ring would be an option for local ET in a patient with vaginal atrophy and genitourinary symptoms. The estrogen ring provides local estrogen to the vaginal mucosa to help alleviate symptoms of vaginal dryness. The use of nonhormonal over-the-counter vaginal moisturizers and lubricants, including Silk-E or KY Jelly, may provide some relief during sexual intercourse. In a woman *not* on systemic HT, it is important to establish her bone mineral density status because this might affect her decision to initiate HT, or select alternative therapy with a bisphosphonate (Actonel or Fosamax) or SERM such as raloxifene (Evista).

**2. d.**

The presence of abnormal vaginal bleeding or spotting in any postmenopausal woman on continuous combined HT should alert the physician to the possibility of endometrial hyperplasia or endometrial cancer. Other causes of spotting include endometrial polyps and uterine fibroids. The next step for therapy would be an endometrial biopsy to further evaluate the endometrial lining for changes. If the endometrial biopsy is benign, consideration should be given to a different hormonal therapy such as $E_2$/ norgestimate (Prefest), $E_2$/norethindrone acetate (Activella), or FermHRT (ethinylestradiol/NA), or low dose Prempro (0.45/1.5 or 0.3/1.5) (which may offer this patient a better chance of amenorrhea).

**3. d.**

Because of her history of using phenytoin for her seizure disorder, this patient probably metabolizes estrogen at a faster rate than normal. By changing her ET to a transdermal patch, consistent estrogen levels can be maintained, which should alleviate her symptoms. Adding isoflavones and other plant-based estrogens in addition to her ET may or may not also help her symptoms. Other causes for her hot flashes should also be excluded, including checking for thyroid-stimulating hormone (TSH) and a fasting blood sugar level. The patient will also benefit from transdermal patch therapy instead of oral ET due to her elevated triglyceride level. Fasting lipid levels should be periodically monitored.

**4. c.**

This patient's symptoms seem to correlate with a female androgen deficiency (FAD) syndrome requiring therapy.

Because she is already on adequate estrogen replacement, the only method currently available for androgen therapy is oral Estratest HS (1.25 methyltestosterone and 0.625 mg of esterified estrogen). At present, no agent is FDA approved for FAD, however, the testosterone patch for women is expected soon. She should have periodic monitoring of her triglycerides, cholesterol profile, and free and total testosterone level before and after therapy is initiated [a transdermal testosterone patch, Intrinsa, for hypoactive sexual desire disorder (HSDD) is expected soon].

### 5. e.

This patient has OP on DXA, which is of concern and must be treated. Although calcium supplementation at 1.5 g plus vitamin D, 800 IU per day, is necessary but not sufficient to treat OP, she needs additional treatment to prevent further bone loss. The best option for treatment in this patient is a SERM such as raloxifene. Raloxifene will not only prevent further bone loss but may also offer her the possibility of breast cancer reduction as well as a decrease in total cholesterol without an increase in US CRP. Because of this patient's past medical history of esophagitis and gastroesophageal reflux disease, Fosamax or Actonel would not be the best option for treatment. Injectable Forteo, a bone building agent, could be considered.

### 6. a.

Because she is a smoker and older than age 35, this patient is at risk for thromboembolic disease if placed on birth control pills. The best choice in this married, monogamous female with no risk factors for pelvic inflammatory disease would be the IUD or IUS. Depo-Provera may cause a weight gain in this already obese patient.

### 7. b.

Absolute contraindications to HT include pregnancy and undiagnosed vaginal bleeding. Any postmenopausal vaginal bleeding must be investigated with an endometrial biopsy, owing to a 5% to 10% incidence of simple or complex hyperplasia (with or without atypia), adenomatous endometrial hyperplasia, or frank endometrial cancers. A remote history of DVT is not an absolute contraindication to HT. Although a strong family history of breast cancer or cardiovascular disease is an important consideration when advising women on HT, these factors do not make the decision for or against starting HT.

### 8. e.

Hormone levels such as FSH do not contribute to the diagnosis of menopause, which is made clinically. ET can be started at any time symptoms occur; therefore, an FSH level fluctuation would not change management in this case. The long term safety of the over-the-counter menopausal supplements is not yet clear. Although ET remains the gold standard for vasomotor symptom relief, the SSRIs (fluoxetine, paroxetine) and NSRI inhibitor (Effexor) have been shown to reduce hot flashes when compared with placebo. Patient preferences and individualized assessment will dictate which therapy is initiated first. ET is clearly the most effective and only FDA-approved therapy for menopausal hot flashes. A family history of breast cancer or risk factors for VTE is an important consideration when advising women on ET, but do not preclude the use of ET in women who need it. ET did not increase the risk of breast cancer or heart attacks in the WHI trial, which makes choice d incorrect.

## SUGGESTED READINGS

Anderson GL, Limacher M, Assaf AR, et al. Effects of conjugated equine estrogen in postmenopausal women with hysterectomy: the Women's Health Initiative randomized controlled trial. *JAMA* 2004; 291:1701–1712.

Batur P, Elder J, Mayer M. Update on contraception: benefits and risks of the new formulations. *Cleve Clin J Med* 2003;70:681–668.

Estrogen and progestogen use in peri- and postmenopausal women: September 2003 position statement of the North American Menopause Society. *Menopause* 2003;10:497–506.

Hulley S, Grady D, Bush T, et al. Randomized trial of estrogen plus progestin for secondary prevention of coronary heart disease in postmenopausal women. Heart and estrogen/progestin replacement study (HERS) research group. *JAMA* 1998;280: 605–613.

Kubba A, Guillebaud J, Anderson RA, et al. Contraception. *Lancet* 2000;356:1913–1919.

Ridker PM, Hennekens CH, Buring JE, et al. C-reactive protein and other markers of inflammation in the prediction of cardiovascular disease in women. *N Engl J Med* 2000;342:836–843.

Treatment of menopause-associated vasomotor symptoms: position statement of the North American Menopause Society. *Menopause* 2004;11(1):11–33.

Utian W, Shoupe D, Bachmann G, et al. Relief of vasomotor symptoms and vaginal atrophy with lower doses of conjugated equine estrogens and medroxyprogesterone acetate. *Fertil Steril* 2001;75: 1065–1075.

Writing group for the WHI investigators. Risks and benefits of estrogen plus progestin in healthy postmenopausal women: principal results from the Women's Health Initiative randomized controlled trial. *JAMA* 2002;288:321–333.

http://www.menopause.org (Web site of the North American Menopause Society; contains comprehensive information about menopause).

http://www.nof.org (Web site of the National Osteoporosis Foundation; contains guidelines for osteoporosis screening and management).

# Medical Diseases in Pregnancy

**3**

*Elisa K. Ross*

Chronic disease has an effect on pregnancy, and pregnancy has an effect on chronic disease. When considering the interactions of chronic medical disease and pregnancy, the general principles are as follows:

- The healthier the mother, the healthier the child.
- Although no drug is guaranteed to be absolutely safe in pregnancy, the risks of not treating a condition may outweigh the potential risks of treatment.
- The lowest effective dose should be used.
- Half of all pregnancies are unplanned.

## PRECONCEPTION CARE

Primary care providers are in a unique position to practice preventive medicine for the not-yet-conceived patient (the fetus). Some women will consult with a provider before conception, but because up to half of all pregnancies are unplanned, and birth control methods are known to fail, it seems prudent to touch on these four points—preconception counseling in a nutshell—with all women of childbearing age, even those who "can't get pregnant":

- Recommend folic acid supplementation (0.4 mg/day), found in most multivitamins, to prevent neural tube defects (NTDs).
- Confirm immunities. A history of vaccination is not predictive of rubella immunity; delay pregnancy 1 month after vaccination. Check for varicella immunity; if no history of the disease is present, check blood titers; vaccinations are available. Check for hepatitis B in susceptible patients, because most vertical transmission (mother to fetus) occurs in chronic carriers.
- Consider family and genetic history and offer consultation as needed.
- Consider medical history and the optimization of chronic disease—one-third of pregnancy complications are related to pre-existing conditions. "Tuning up" the treatment of chronic disease and a realistic risk assessment are helpful.

## REVIEW OF FOOD AND DRUG ADMINISTRATION (FDA) PREGNANCY CATEGORIES

Many medications are rated according to their potential risk to a developing fetus. These ratings are requested by the manufacturing companies themselves. For liability reasons, many manufacturers do not want their drugs used during pregnancy. To this end, some will provide no information concerning drug use during pregnancy, and some will stipulate contraindications not borne out in the literature (e.g., terbutaline, pitocin). Other medications receive category B ratings even in their first years of general use. Because certain risk profiles may be acceptable to one patients but not to another, the following letter risk category designations of the U.S. FDA do not tell the whole story, but rather give general guidance:

- A  Controlled human studies show no adverse effect.
- B  Animal studies show no risk, and no anecdotal human evidence suggests otherwise; or animal studies have shown risk, but human studies have not.
- C  Animal studies have shown risk, and there are no human studies.
- D  Evidence exists for human fetal risk, but benefits may outweigh risk.
- X  Evidence exists of human risk, and no benefit appears to outweigh it.

Ninety-five percent of the 200 most-prescribed drugs appear to be safe for use during pregnancy. Currently, most medications used in pregnancy are category B or C. These categories may change soon to a descriptive system based on the strength of the evidence and the severity of the potential fetal effect.

Few drugs are rated category A because it is difficult to recruit pregnant patients for randomized, controlled, double-blind studies. A potential participant may be reluctant to forego a believed beneficial treatment, or conversely, may not be eager to expose her fetus to an unknown substance. Not all teratogens are category X. This applies only to those for which the indication for using the drug does not appear to outweigh the potential risk. Other known teratogens may be category C or D.

Most teratogens increase the relative rate of malformation from the background rate two- to threefold. Because the background rate of each particular malformation is usually less than 1%, the absolute incidence of any effect will be small, usually 2% to 3% at most. Even the most teratogenic substances known (e.g., thalidomide, isotretinoin) will affect only approximately 30% of exposed fetuses, leaving 70% unaffected. The factors involved are dose, timing of exposure, and the cytogenetic makeup of the individual.

So, in the face of exposure to a teratogen, the mother must be counseled that it is more likely that her fetus will show no effect. It is nevertheless preferable to use the safest-rated medications during pregnancy in all potentially fertile women.

Examples of category X drugs and their potential effects:

- Live attenuated vaccines for measles, mumps, rubella, and varicella—Congenital viral syndromes.
- Danazol—Ambiguous genitalia.
- Warfarin—Warfarin embryopathy: hypoplastic nose, epiphyseal stippling, optic atrophy, microcephaly, and growth restriction (despite this, it is used in certain uniquely risky situations).
- Diethylstilbestrol—Vaginal adenosis and clear cell carcinoma in offspring.
- Vitamin A—More than 25,000 U/day is unsafe; tripled risk of renal and facial anomalies exists. Beta carotene is not implicated.
- Isotretinoin—Isotretinoin syndrome; etretinate has been detected in maternal serum 7 years after the cessation of use; topical retinoin is not implicated.
- Triazolam—Cleft palate.
- Lovastatin—Weak evidence for bone malformation.
- Thalidomide—Limb-shortening defects.
- Ribavirin—A purine analog, embryocidal; an occupational hazard exists where aerosolized.
- Occupational agents such as lead, methyl mercury, polychlorinated biphenyls (PCBs), polybrominated biphenyls, and organic solvents—Assorted mental, physical, and metabolic effects.
- Ionizing radiation—An all-or-none effect is believed to occur in early gestation, causing miscarriage rather than birth defect. Most radiographic studies expose the mother to less than 1 rad, and the fetus to far less; 5 rads is considered acceptable fetal exposure. Patients who work near radiation should wear their detection badge near their pelvis to approximate the fetal exposure. When counseling a patient about the need for imaging, it is sometimes useful to remember that if the fetus was born, even prematurely, he or she would be radiographed as necessary for care.

Known teratogens that have some usefulness in pregnancy (category D):

- Angiotensin-converting enzyme (ACE) inhibitors—Unsafe after the first trimester; renal failure and death in neonate can occur.
- Anticholinergic drugs—Neonatal meconium ileus.
- Antithyroid drugs—Neonatal goiter and hypothyroidism, aplasia cutis (methimazole).
- Carbamazepine—NTDs.
- Lithium—Ebstein's anomaly.
- Nonsteroidal anti-inflammatory drugs (NSAIDs)—Constriction of the ductus arteriosus in third trimester.
- Phenytoin (Dilantin)—Fetal hydantoin syndrome.
- Psychoactive drugs—Fetal withdrawal syndrome.
- Tetracycline—Tooth discoloration, bone malformation.
- Valproic acid—NTDs.

Some commonly avoided medications that have been shown to be *not* teratogenic, as once thought:

- Bendectin (doxylamine and pyridoxine)
- Diazepam (although some withdrawal syndrome occurs if used in the third trimester)
- Metronidazole
- Oral contraceptives
- Salicylates
- Spermicides

Updated information may be found at http://www.motherisk.org, http://www.cdc.gov, or http://orpheus.ucsd.edu/ctis/.

## GENERAL ASPECTS OF CARE DURING PREGNANCY

The rest of this chapter is organized roughly from head to toe, emphasizing those aspects of care that might be different from the expected. The following are basic maternal physiologic changes that occur during pregnancy and that may have a bearing on each disease process:

- Increased cardiac output
- Decreased systemic vascular resistance
- Increased intravascular volume and volume of distribution
- Increased minute ventilation
- Increased renal flow and excretion
- Slowed gastrointestinal functioning
- Hypercoagulability
- Increased binding globulins affecting drug metabolism
- Immune suppression

## HEAD

### Headache

Headache is common in pregnancy, and workup and treatment are the same as for the nonpregnant patient.

Preeclampsia must be ruled out as a cause of headache. Acetaminophen and narcotics are first-line treatment choices. Ergot alkaloids are contraindicated, as are NSAIDs in the last trimester. Imitrex can be used for refractory migraines (pregnancy category C), as can propranolol. A post-epidural headache is treated with caffeine and narcotics, and, if needed, an injection of blood into the epidural space—blood patch.

## Cerebrovascular Accident

Pregnancy is a hypercoagulable state. Occlusive disease is rare but increases fivefold during pregnancy, with the most common site being the middle cerebral artery. Atherosclerosis is not a major cause of occlusive disease during pregnancy. The diagnosis is made by computerized tomography (CT), magnetic resonance imaging (MRI), or cerebral arteriography. The potential benefit of making the diagnosis outweighs the minimal risk of fetal radiation exposure. Therapeutic heparin may be used if no evidence of intracranial bleeding is present. Heparin is too large and positively charged a molecule to cross the placenta. In these cases, vaginal delivery is preferable to cesarean section.

Subarachnoid hemorrhage accounts for 10% of maternal deaths. Arteriovascular malformations are the most common cause in those younger than age 25. Berry aneurysms in the circle of Willis are a more common cause in those older than age 25. The most common symptom is unrelenting headache. The diagnosis should be made via CT, lumbar puncture, or cerebral arteriography, as usual. Surgical repair is strongly recommended because rebleeding is common in pregnancy and often fatal. After repair, vaginal delivery is preferred. If the lesion is not completely repaired, performing a cesarean section will minimize Valsalva maneuvers and the risk of repeat subarachnoid hemorrhage.

Pseudotumor cerebri is managed in the usual way.

## Epilepsy

Forty percent of epileptics experience increased seizure activity, and 50% remain unchanged. Medications are indicated to prevent seizures because status epilepticus may be associated with a maternal mortality rate of 25% and a fetal mortality rate of 50%.

Among the offspring of epileptics on medication, an increased risk (up to 10%) of congenital anomalies is present. It is unclear if this is from medication use or from cytogenetic causes, but current studies point toward the medications. An increased risk of seizure disorders in offspring is also present, up to 9% if the mother is the affected parent and 2% if the father (the background rate is less than 1%). Low birth weight, neonatal death, stillbirth, lower Apgar scores, and prematurity are also increased. Despite these findings, most babies born to epileptic mothers will be healthy.

The general principles of medication use in pregnant epileptics are:

- Single-agent treatment is preferred, if possible.
- Frequent dosing is advised to avoid high peak concentrations.
- Doses of all medications are frequently increased, based on monthly serum levels and clinical status.
- Seizure control is most important, regardless of how much and what medications are required.
- If there has been no seizure activity in the last two years, or if the diagnosis is suspect, it may be worthwhile to re-evaluate and/or withdraw medications prior to conception.

All seizure medications have the potential to cause birth defects but do so at a rate of 5% to 10%, depending on timing and dose of exposure. If the patient has a choice of agents, she should choose the risk profile most acceptable to her. Carbamazepine (Tegretol) is the most widely used antiepileptic agent. Phenobarbital is next, despite a risk of cleft palate. Phenytoin is associated with fetal hydantoin syndrome: microcephaly, facial clefts and dysmorphism, limb defects, and distal phalangeal and nail hypoplasia. Valproic acid (Depakote) is associated with NTDs. Carbamazepine also is associated with NTDs, but to a lesser extent.

Supplemental superdose folate (4 g/day) is added in early pregnancy and preconceptually to help neutralize the increased risk of NTDs. Maintenance folate during the rest of an epileptic's pregnancy is 1 g/day. Oral vitamin K may be added at some time toward the end of the pregnancy (20 mg/day) and during labor to avoid neonatal bleeding. The fetus is always given 1 mg vitamin K intramuscularly at birth.

If seizures occur in the third trimester, fetal monitoring is useful. Seizures can be stopped using lorazepam and/or phenytoin. Eclampsia is treated with magnesium, but epileptic seizures are not.

Postpartum, the dose of antiepileptic medications should go back to the prepregnancy regimen. Breastfeeding is not contraindicated. The mother should be advised of the importance of adequate sleep and of taking precautions for protecting the baby in the case of maternal seizure—such precautions may include changing the diaper on the floor and having someone else present during the bathing of the baby.

## Prolactinoma

Prolactin levels are normally elevated in pregnancy and lactation. If a patient with hyperprolactinemia is on bromocriptine to enhance the chance of conception, the medication can be discontinued for the remainder of the pregnancy. If a prolactinoma enlarges during pregnancy, bromocriptine may be safely given to reduce tumor size.

## Depression

Depression is common and underdiagnosed. Selective serotonin reuptake inhibitors (SSRIs) and tricyclics are used in pregnancy. In severe cases, electroconvulsive therapy is considered safe. Postpartum exacerbation is common, affecting 10% of all mothers. Selective serotonin reuptake inhibitors are safe for use during breastfeeding. For bipolar depression, valproic acid or lithium may be used, although both are associated with anomalies if used in the first trimester.

## Eye

It is common to have temporary refractive changes that resolve after pregnancy. Diabetics need a retinal examination every trimester to guard against undiagnosed proliferative retinopathy. Scotomata may be a sign of preeclampsia.

## Nose

Nosebleeds are common and benign, although some may require cautery.

The incidence of rhinitis is increased because of progesterone vasodilation. Oxymetazoline spray and pseudoephedrine can be used for 5 days in symptomatic patients. Intranasal cromolyn, intranasal beclomethasone, oral tripelennamine, or chlorpheniramine also may be tried, in that order.

The incidence and severity of colds and upper respiratory infections is unchanged during pregnancy, but sinusitis is reported to be six times more prevalent in pregnant women. Sinusitis can trigger asthma. Acetaminophen, guaifenesin with or without dextromethorphan, pseudoephedrine, diphenhydramine, and loratadine are often used to treat sinus and asthma symptoms. Azithromycin, ampicillin-clavulanate, and ampicillin are preferred for sinusitis. A 3-week course is recommended because of difficulty with relapse and the increased chance of sepsis in treatment failure.

## Dentition

Pyogenic granuloma occurs in the papilla between the teeth, and this condition is commonly seen in pregnancy. Gingivitis of pregnancy is common.

Dental care can be provided as usual. Local anesthetics without epinephrine, narcotics, acetaminophen, and beta-lactams are used regularly. Nitrous oxide is best avoided. Shielded radiography is not contraindicated.

## Substance Abuse

Smoking is associated with decreased fertility and decreased birth weight, as well as an increased risk of miscarriage, ectopic pregnancy, preterm delivery, abruptio placentae, sudden infant death syndrome, and developmental problems. Nicotine patches are preferable to smoking.

Alcohol use of as little as 3 oz/day is associated with fetal alcohol syndrome (FAS), the most common cause of mental retardation besides genetic causes. No safe amount of alcohol use in pregnancy has been documented, and expression of FAS is variable.

Cocaine use is associated with maternal hypertension, abruption, fetal loss, prematurity, growth restriction, congenital somatic defects, and behavior problems in the child.

Neither marijuana nor hallucinogens have shown any definite, reproducible effect. Nevertheless, they cannot be recommended.

Opiates are associated with stillbirth, growth restriction, prematurity, and potentially fatal neonatal withdrawal syndrome. Maternal methadone improves outcomes, but infants still withdraw.

## Bell's Palsy

Bell's palsy is common after delivery and requires no treatment. Symptoms often resolve spontaneously.

## Ptyalism

Excessive salivation is common and refractory to treatment. It usually resolves promptly after delivery.

## NECK

### Thyroid

Thyroid function generally remains normal throughout pregnancy. The presence of increased binding proteins may confound the usual measurements of thyroid function, so determining the free thyroxine level is the best way to measure function. The level of thyroid-stimulating hormone remains the same during pregnancy.

#### Hyperthyroidism

Hyperthyroidism is found in 0.2% of pregnancies; 85% of these patients have Graves' disease. One must also consider acute and subacute thyroiditis, chronic lymphocytic (Hashimoto's disease) thyroiditis, toxic nodular goiter, hydatidiform mole, and choriocarcinoma.

Hyperthyroidism is treated with propylthiouracil in pregnancy, which has less placental transfer than methimazole. The patient need not be made completely euthyroid. Suppression adequate to allow good growth of the baby is sufficient. The neonate may be transiently hypothyroid after delivery. Propylthiouracil is not transferred to breast milk, but methimazole is transferred. Radioactive iodine is contraindicated in pregnancy.

The postpartum period is a time of relatively increased risk for autoimmune thyroiditis. Two-thirds of cases are a reactivation of Graves' disease, in which the radioactive iodine uptake is normal or high, and one-third of cases are "silent" thyroiditis, in which radioactive iodine uptake is low. Spontaneous resolution usually occurs over months. Hypothyroidism follows in 25% of cases. Postpartum thyroiditis is histologically similar to Hashimoto's thyroiditis with lymphocytic infiltration. The rate is increased in patients who were previously type I diabetics (30%) or have had Hashimoto's thyroiditis previously (75%).

Thyroid storm can be precipitated by terbutaline (often used for preterm labor) if the hyperthyroidism is uncontrolled. Propranolol is used to counteract symptoms.

### Hypothyroidism

Hypothyroidism is rarely diagnosed during pregnancy because it often disrupts fertility. Treated hypothyroidism is common, however, and there appears to be no adverse effects of medication use during pregnancy. In cases in which hypothyroidism is inadequately treated, one report finds a decrease in fetal intelligence may be possible. Free thyroxine or thyroid-stimulating hormone levels must be monitored every trimester as the binding protein concentration increases, and the dose of thyroxine may need to be adjusted.

## BONE MARROW

### Anemia

Anemia is a common finding in pregnancy, occurring because of an average 1,000-mL increase in plasma volume but only a 300-mL increase in red cell mass. Therefore, some dilutional decrease in hemoglobin and hematocrit is normal. Anemia in pregnancy is defined as a hematocrit level of less than 30% and a hemoglobin level of less than 10 g/dL. Besides dilutional factors, iron deficiency is the most common cause of anemia (90%). A trial of iron therapy is reasonable as a first step. Craving ice, starch, or dirt (pica) is a sign of iron deficiency. Folate deficiency is the second most common cause and is seen in multiple gestations and with drug therapy involving phenytoin, nitrofurantoin, pyrimethamine, or trimethoprim or with large ethanol consumption. Thalassemias may present with microcytic, hypochromic anemia, and this has genetic implications for the offspring. Sickle cell or sickle-C disease may cause vasoocclusive episodes (crises) that may lead to uteroplacental insufficiency, fetal growth restriction, and prematurity. Sickle trait carriers are at higher risk for urinary tract infections and should be screened regularly.

Pregnant and postpartum women can tolerate much lower hemoglobin levels than others. No mortality or cardiac failure has been reported in patients with hemoglobin of greater than 4.5 mg/dL as their only complicating factor. If transfusion is necessary for any pregnant patient, cytomegalovirus-negative blood is preferred to decrease the chance of devastating fetal infection. This precaution is not necessary postpartum.

## Thrombocytopenia

In pregnancy, thrombocytopenia is defined as fewer than 100,000 platelets/μL, but serious bleeding rarely occurs if counts are greater than 20,000/μL. The various causes are similar to those in nonpregnant women, in addition to HELLP syndrome (hemolysis, elevated liver enzymes, and low platelet count) and disseminated intravascular coagulopathy (DIC). Gestational thrombocytopenia is seen in up to 8% of normal women.

In immune thrombocytopenic purpura, immunoglobulin G (IgG) class antiplatelet antibody crosses the placenta. The delivery route depends on an estimation of fetal platelets. A variation on this is IgG directed against the fetal platelets. Systemic lupus erythematosus (SLE) can be associated with thrombocytopenia.

Some medications cause thrombocytopenia. Thrombotic thrombocytopenic purpura is not unusual, mostly occurring during the first two trimesters. Hemolytic-uremic syndrome is seen mostly in postpartum renal failure.

HELLP syndrome is associated with preeclampsia. DIC is seen with retained dead fetus syndrome, preeclampsia, abruption, amniotic fluid embolism, and hemorrhage, in addition to the usual causes.

## White Blood Cells

The normal white blood cell count in pregnancy can be as high as 16,000/μL.

## Clotting Disorders

Von Willebrand's disease is common in pregnancy, but because of increases in various factors, it is difficult to diagnose during pregnancy. The most accurate way to diagnose von Willebrand's disease is to measure bleeding time at 36 weeks. Most patients do not bleed clinically despite abnormal tests. The mechanism of hemostasis after delivery has more to do with contraction of the uterus than the clotting cascade. Delayed bleeding is not uncommon. Desmopressin, von Willebrand's factor concentrate, or both may be needed to alleviate excess bleeding.

## EXTREMITIES

Carpal tunnel syndrome is a common complaint of pregnant women, especially on awakening. It is caused by the normal fluid retention present in later pregnancy. Braces worn at night help, and symptoms usually resolve after delivery.

Joints are prone to injury because of ligament softening secondary to progesterone, and because of increased weight and change in posture. Patients most often complain about their hip, pubic bone, and sacroiliac joints. Back pain tends to be more muscular in nature.

Swelling of the lower extremities is common and is treated with elevation, after preeclampsia and deep venous thrombosis (DVT) have been ruled unlikely.

## LUNGS

In normal pregnancy, pulmonary function changes: Oxygen consumption goes up 20%, tidal volume goes up 40%, minute ventilation increases 50%, but vital capacity shows no change. All other parameters decrease.

### Infectious Diseases

Pneumonia is uncommon but is a leading cause of nonobstetric death. The most common causes are *Streptococcus pneumoniae*, *Mycoplasma pneumoniae*, *Haemophilus influenzae*, fungi, varicella, and aspiration. Varicella can cause florid pneumonitis and death. Coccidioidomycosis can cause cavitary lesions and dissemination in pregnancy. Aspiration pneumonia is increased because of decreased esophageal sphincter tone and delayed gastric emptying.

Tuberculosis is common in high prevalence areas. Inactive disease is often treated by oral isoniazid, 300 mg/day for 1 year. Active disease is treated with oral isoniazid, 5 mg/kg/day, plus rifampin, 10 mg/kg/day, plus pyridoxine.

### Asthma

Asthma is seen in 1% of pregnant patients, of whom 15% have a severe attack. The course is unpredictable. One-third get better, one-third get worse, and one-third stay the same. Most pregnancies proceed uneventfully, but an increased risk of prematurity and growth restriction is present among asthmatics.

The general principles of management in asthma patients include continuing prepregnancy treatment and minimizing triggers. The routine use of a flow meter can detect onset before an attack becomes severe. Most asthma medications are safely used in pregnancy, including antibiotics and steroids, because minimizing the known risks of maternal hypoxia is preferred to minimizing the theoretical risk to the fetus from the medications. Inhaled medications minimize fetal exposure. Systemic theophylline levels must be reassessed every trimester and postpartum because binding globulins increase for two trimesters, then clearance decreases. Allergy shots may be continued in pregnancy but are rarely initiated. Terbutaline is preferred to epinephrine, which may constrict uterine blood flow.

During a severe attack, fetal monitoring may be indicated. Oxygen pressure of less than 60 mm Hg correlates with fetal compromise. An aggressive attention to the patient's acid-base status, including early intubation, will optimize fetal health. Carbon dioxide pressure ($P_{CO_2}$) of greater than 38 mm Hg or a pH level of less than 7.35 is highly abnormal for pregnancy and may represent retention and need for intubation.

### Embolic States

Amniotic fluid embolism manifests as sudden a cardiovascular collapse, followed by DIC, seizures, left ventricular dysfunction, and acute respiratory distress syndrome. It carries a 50% mortality rate. The mechanism is unknown, but is possibly a response to a bolus of fetal antigen, pulmonary artery spasm, or mechanical blockage by fetal cells. The best treatment is also unknown but is usually supportive, inotropic medications, and fresh frozen plasma.

Pulmonary embolus is covered in detail in the thrombosis section; however, the vital point is to treat immediately with full heparin anticoagulation when pulmonary embolus is suspected and then get diagnostic tests. A delay in treatment can be dangerous.

Pulmonary edema is seen in the usual situations, as well as in association with tocolytic (terbutaline and magnesium sulfate) use. It is more likely in multiple gestations (twins, triplets). Careful diuresis and oxygen are used to treat edematous conditions.

## HEART

Cardiac output increases 40% during pregnancy, thus leading to a potentially serious compromise of mother and fetus, depending on the nature of the maternal cardiac defect. Common signs of cardiovascular compromise, such as shortness of breath, palpitations, and tachycardia, are also found in normal pregnancies. The signs that may indicate the presence of actual cardiac disease include a progressive limitation of physical activity secondary to worsening dyspnea, chest pain, and syncope preceded by palpitations. The cardiovascular changes seen in normal pregnancy may confound the interpretation of diagnostic studies: The chest radiograph shows cardiomegaly and venous congestion, and the electrocardiogram in normal pregnancy may include ST-T depression and flattening of T waves. Therefore, echocardiography is the preferred technique to evaluate cardiovascular disease in pregnancy.

When trying to predict the effect of pregnancy on any given cardiac condition, keep in mind the following five principles:

■ A 50% increase in intravascular volume and cardiac output occurs by the third trimester. Thus, if cardiac output is limited by defective valves or general dysfunction, an increased chance of congestive failure or the formation or dissection of an aneurysm exists.
■ Systemic vascular resistance decreases during pregnancy. This may worsen left-to-right shunts.
■ Pregnancy is a hypercoagulable state, so dysfunctional valves and atrial fibrillation may need meticulous anticoagulation.

- Cardiac fluctuations occur during labor and delivery.
- Cardiac output increases by a further 50% during labor.

Fluid shifts at delivery could go either way: Blood loss or epidural-induced pooling can decrease effective volume, and redistribution from the contracted uterus or relief of caval obstruction may cause sudden increases in blood pooling. These fluid shifts affect both patients with preload-dependent cardiac output (pulmonary hypertension) and those with fixed cardiac output (stenosis). Tachycardia also worsens cardiac output in stenosis. To avoid complications, patients with venous return dysfunction should avoid pushing and Valsalva maneuvers, which compromise venous return.

Cardiac output peaks at 24 to 28 weeks gestation, even during bed rest, and decreases somewhat during the last 10 weeks of pregnancy. Therefore, the most severe effects of cardiac disease are seen before the fetus is viable, thus making management difficult.

A 50% maternal mortality rate has been associated with the following lesions:

- Marfan's syndrome with aortic root dilation
- Eisenmenger's syndrome (pulmonary hypertension from shunting)
- Primary pulmonary hypertension
- Uncorrected tetralogy of Fallot

A significant morbidity rate also is associated with dilated cardiomyopathy and severe mitral or aortic stenosis.

Good outcomes are expected from the following:

- New York Heart Association functional classes I and II
- Mitral valve prolapse
- Mild mitral and aortic disorders
- Septal defects
- Patent ductus arteriosus
- Repaired tetralogy of Fallot
- American Heart Association endocarditis prophylaxis

Endocarditis prophylaxis is of limited value for vaginal delivery or elective cesarean section because of the low risk of bacteremia in these situations. For low- or moderate-risk lesions, antibiotics are *not* recommended; they are considered optional for high-risk cardiac lesions. Nevertheless, most practitioners treat endocarditis because of possible intrapartum infection or the need for intrapartum cesarean section. The standard regimens for both high- and low-risk lesions are followed in the usual way in pregnancy.

A cesarean section after a long labor should be given prophylactic antibiotics. Aggressive antibiotics are used for frank infection. Patients with mitral valve prolapse without regurgitation are not given prophylactic antibiotics.

The offspring of patients with congenital heart disease are at increased risk over the general population for cardiac anomalies (up to 5%) but not necessarily the same ones as their parents have. If a sibling is affected too, the risk increases to 10%. The fetus of a functionally impaired car-

diac patient may exhibit growth restriction or premature delivery.

The careful management of preload and afterload is necessary for the severely affected patient. Most pregnancy-related cardiac deaths occur after delivery, probably exacerbated by the large fluid shifts that accompany delivery. Most cardioactive medications are safe for use during pregnancy, falling with FDA categories B or C (e.g., digitalis, loop diuretics, thiazides, hydralazine, isosorbide, propranolol, metoprolol, nifedipine, and verapamil).

Peripartum cardiomyopathy can occur in the last month of pregnancy or the first 6 months after delivery. It is treated similarly to other cardiomyopathies. Prognosis is related to cardiac size 6 months after delivery. Recurrence is likely, and death is a real possibility during the next pregnancy if the heart remains enlarged.

Maternal cardiac arrhythmias are treated as needed. Clinically significant arrhythmias are rare. Premature ventricular contractions and atrial contractions are common, as is paroxysmal supraventricular tachycardia. Wolff-Parkinson-White syndrome is managed with medication. Catheter ablation is not generally performed in pregnancy because of the fluoroscopy risk to the fetus. The most commonly used medications to treat Wolff-Parkinson-White syndrome are atenolol, quinidine, and procainamide. Larger doses than expected are often needed. Also used are the pregnancy category C drugs diltiazem, verapamil, disopyramide, flecainide, propafenone, sotalol, adenosine, and digoxin. Seldom-used drugs include amiodarone, lidocaine, and mexiletine.

Rheumatic heart disease predisposes to congestive failure, pulmonary edema, subacute bacterial endocarditis, thromboembolic disease, and fetal loss. Symptomatic aortic or mitral valve stenosis can be treated with balloon commissurotomy or other procedures if necessary.

Women with mechanical valve prostheses need anticoagulation. Heparin is preferred in the first trimester to avoid fetal anomalies (warfarin syndrome). It is also preferred in the third trimester because of easy reversibility. Warfarin is sometimes used in the middle trimester because heparin can induce osteoporosis and thrombocytopenia in the mother. Low-molecular-weight heparin is used increasingly to avoid these side effects. Women with valvular bioprostheses do not need to be anticoagulated, but their chance of needing a replacement valve increases with each pregnancy.

## BREASTS

Stage for stage, breast cancer is unaffected by pregnancy. The termination of a pregnancy has no proven effect for localized disease, although disseminated cancer is responsive to hormonal ablation. Theoretically, then, termination or early delivery could be beneficial. Chemotherapy can be given in the second and third trimesters, if necessary.

Survivors (>5 yrs tumor free) need not be discouraged from conceiving if they are disease-free for an additional 6 months or more.

Breast masses in pregnant women should be examined as usual, via unilateral shielded mammography or needle or open biopsy. The differential diagnosis includes adenoma, blocked duct, cyst, and mastitis. Cancer is sometimes found in this situation, however, so a complete workup is always appropriate.

## LIVER

Jaundice in pregnancy can be caused by obstruction of the bile duct or by several other major disease processes.

*Hepatitis* is the major cause of jaundice, having the same distribution of types as in the nonpregnant population. Pregnancy does not affect the course of any type of hepatitis, except for occasional worsening of hepatitis E (up to 10% maternal mortality). Hepatitis A does not cross the placenta.

Hepatitis B accounts for 80% of cases of hepatitis during pregnancy. It is diagnosed through the characteristic elevations of aminotransferases and a history of appropriate exposure. Vertical transmission to the fetus at birth is the major risk. Most infected infants become chronic carriers. Universal screening of mothers is the norm, and infants receive hepatitis B immune globulin and vaccination if exposed.

Intrahepatic cholestasis of pregnancy, also called *pruritus gravidarum*, is the second most common cause of jaundice in pregnancy. Bile acids are increased to 10 to 100 times normal, the alkaline phosphatase level is elevated, and the bilirubin level can be as high as 5 mg/mL, with a mild elevation of aminotransferases and cholestasis. The main symptom is intractable itching. Cholestasis of pregnancy is treated by delivery at term because an increase in fetal demise is reported if early induction is attempted. Diphenhydramine (Benadryl), hydroxyzine, calamine lotion, and cholestyramine are first-line therapy for symptomatic relief. Phenobarbital is used in severe cases. Pruritis gravidarium usually presents in late pregnancy, and recurrence in future pregnancies and with oral contraceptive use is likely.

*HELLP syndrome* is associated with preeclampsia and thus is usually found during the second half of pregnancy. Hypertension and proteinuria are often seen, but these are not required for the diagnosis. Jaundice is mild, and aminotransferase levels are moderately elevated. HELLP syndrome is caused by a disruption in the vascular endothelium. Liver infarction and rupture can occur. DIC may follow. Delivery is the treatment of choice, even remote from term. HELLP syndrome rarely recurs.

*Acute fatty liver of pregnancy* carries a mortality rate of 30%. It is usually seen during the last trimester in primigravidas. Symptoms include gastrointestinal dysfunction, epigastric pain, jaundice, confusion, coma, or coagulopathy. Bilirubin and transaminase levels are only moderately elevated, and biopsy shows small-droplet steatosis. A high index of suspicion and timely delivery decrease mortality.

*Cholelithiasis* has the same incidence as in the nonpregnant population. Symptomatic stones are treated in the usual way with nasogastric suction, intravenous hydration, pain medication, and antibiotics as needed. Failure of the above or the development of pancreatitis is an indication for cholecystectomy. Laparoscopic surgery is preferred in any trimester. All surgeries are safest in the second trimester.

## PANCREAS

Diabetes mellitus, both preexisting and of gestational onset, affects 2% of pregnancies. Gestational diabetes mellitus is diagnosed during pregnancy and typically resolves after delivery. The proper preconception care of diabetics, types I and II, presents a unique opportunity for the internist to prevent birth defects. The incidence of malformations and miscarriages correlates with the quality of blood glucose level control. Even in well-controlled diabetes, a threefold increase in congenital anomalies is possible over the usual 2% baseline risk. Defects of the heart and neural tube are most common. The mermaid syndrome, or caudal regression (sacral agenesis), is seen only in diabetics.

Glucose is difficult to control during pregnancy because the fetus is a constant energy sink, causing glucose values to dip when they otherwise would not have. Conversely, placental hormones, such as human placental lactogen, act as an antiinsulin agent and cause relative hyperglycemia. This effect intensifies as the pregnancy progresses and the placenta grows larger. The altered eating habits of early and late gestation further complicate the picture.

Incredibly tight control is desired of all diabetics (a fasting serum glucose level of less than 100 mg/dL and a 2-hour postprandial level of less than 120 mg/dL). Blood glucose is typically measured four times a day until a stable pattern emerges. Insulin is administered in two or three divided doses. Hemoglobin A1c is periodically measured for assessment of long-term control. Oral hypoglycemics are currently not used for fear of fetal effects, but this practice is currently under reconsideration. Oral hypoglycemic medication does cross the placenta; insulin does not cross the placenta, but glucose does.

Measurement of urine glucose has no value in the management of the pregnant diabetic because urine glucose does not correlate with serum levels during pregnancy. Glucosuria is common in any pregnancy and more so in patients with diabetes mellitus. Increased renal flow increases the diffusion of glucose into the urine beyond the capability of tubular reabsorption, thus resulting in the normal glucosuria of pregnancy of approximately 300 mg/day.

The pregnant woman with diabetes is at higher risk for pregnancy-induced hypertension, proliferative retinopathy, urinary tract infection, postpartum hemorrhage, and cesarean delivery. Diabetic ketoacidosis occurs more often as well. Retinopathy progresses in 15% of diabetic pregnant women, so an ophthalmologic examination is needed every 3 months.

The neonatal consequences seen with increased frequency in gestational and preexisting diabetes include macrosomia, respiratory distress syndrome, polyhydramnios, hypoglycemia, hypocalcemia, hyperbilirubinemia, and shoulder dystocia with resultant Erb's palsy. Neonatal death and intrauterine growth restriction are seen in brittle diabetics or those with preexisting end-organ compromise.

Gestational diabetes mellitus is diagnosed during pregnancy. Universal screening is done with a 50-g, 1-hour screening glucola test during the second trimester. If the results of the 1-hour screen are abnormal, a diagnostic 3-hour test is indicated. The diagnosis is made with at least two abnormal values on a 100-g, 3-hour glucola test. Earlier screening is recommended for higher-risk patients (obese, hypertensive, carrying multiple fetuses, glucosuria, history of a large baby, history of unexplained fetal death, strong family history diabetes mellitus, or multiple miscarriages). The screen is repeated in the third trimester if the first result is negative. Fifteen percent of all gravidas will have an abnormal screen result, 15% of these will be diagnosed with gestational diabetes mellitus, and most of these patients will have diet-controlled diabetes.

Postpartum, the gestational diabetic rarely needs insulin; types I and II diabetics also experience a brief honeymoon period postpartum.

Glucose screening is advised 4 months after delivery and periodically thereafter (usually every 1 or 2 years) for any woman who had gestational diabetes because of an increased rate of regular diabetes later in life in these patients, particularly in women of Hispanic and Native American origins.

Oral hypoglycemic agents are now under investigation for use in pregnancy, and their continued use seems likely at this writing. Metformin is often used for women diagnosed prepregnancy as having metabolic syndrome or polycystic ovarian syndrome. Some studies have found metformin to help weight loss, regulation of menstruation, and in delaying the onset of type 2 diabetes. If a patient conceives while using metformin, current practice continues the metformin throughout the pregnancy. Metformin use confers a decreased chance of miscarriage and gestational diabetes.

The continuation of glyburide therapy during pregnancy for some diabetics, and the initiation of glyburide therapy for some gestational diabetics, is not yet the standard of care. Insulin therapy remains the safest approach.

# KIDNEYS

A 50% increase in glomerular filtration rate is seen in normal pregnancies, with a corresponding decrease in serum creatinine (to 0.6 mg/dL) and blood urea nitrogen (to 9 mg/dL). Pregnancy often has no adverse effect on those chronic renal disease patients with preconception creatinine levels of less than 1.4 mg/dL. Proteinuria occurs in half of all pregnancies and, in the absence of hypertension, is not a cause for concern. Patients with preconception serum creatinine levels of 1.5 to 2.5 mg/dL may have some worsening of renal function during and after the pregnancy. Poor fetal outcome is increased when creatinine levels are greater than 2.5.

Hypertension in addition to any chronic renal process, either before or during the pregnancy, drastically complicates the picture and increases the chance of poor outcomes for the pregnancy and the course of the underlying renal disease.

The prognosis for pregnancy after renal transplantation is fairly good if 2 years have passed since transplantation and no sign of impairment or rejection is present. Growth restriction, prematurity, and preeclampsia are more common in this group, but outcomes are generally good for mother and baby.

## Hypertension

When hypertension occurs in pregnancy, four distinct syndromes may be in play: chronic hypertension, preeclampsia, preeclampsia superimposed on chronic hypertension, and gestational hypertension.

### Chronic Hypertension
Chronic hypertension exists, by definition, before pregnancy or appears during the first 20 weeks of pregnancy. Consistent pressures of 140/90 mm Hg qualify as hypertension; medication use is not part of the definition. Chronic hypertension during pregnancy can be masked by the vasodilation that occurs in the first two trimesters. Methyldopa, hydralazine, and labetalol are antihypertensives with long-term track records of not adversely affecting fetal outcome. Nifedipine is a relative newcomer and has been used with good results.

Chronic hypertensives who are contemplating pregnancy are best started on medications that can be safely given during pregnancy. If a patient is stable on another medication, however, it is usual to wait until pregnancy actually occurs before changing it. Diuretics should not be started during pregnancy because they may change fluid dynamics. They may be continued, however, if the patient has been stable while using them before pregnancy. Diuretics are most useful in left ventricular hypertrophy or salt-sensitive hypertension. They should be discontinued if growth restriction or preeclampsia develops. ACE inhibitors are contraindicated in pregnancy; these agents are associated with fetal growth restriction, neonatal renal failure, and death. Most of these effects are seen with ACE inhibitor exposure later in pregnancy, thus it is prudent to change the medication upon diagnosis of pregnancy. Atenolol has been associated with uteroplacental hemodynamic changes; if used, fetal monitoring toward term is recommended.

Poor maternal and fetal outcome is seen with diastolic pressures of greater than 110 mm Hg. Treatment of mild hypertension in pregnancy is not of proven benefit.

### Preeclampsia or Pregnancy-Induced Hypertension

Pregnancy-induced hypertension is a multiorgan disease that involves much more than elevated blood pressure. It is a disease of vascular endothelial cell damage (mechanism unknown) and volume contraction. Delivery of the placenta seems to remove the thus far unidentified precipitating agent, so delivery is the only "cure" for this condition. Maternal seizures are unpredictable but happen mostly within 24 hours before or after delivery. Magnesium is given intravenously as seizure prophylaxis. Neither phenobarbital nor phenytoin is as effective as magnesium in preeclamptic seizure control.

The subsets of pregnancy-induced hypertension are recognized depending on end-organ effects:

- Preeclampsia (renal)
- Proteinuria, edema, hypertension, decreased renal function
- Eclampsia (neurologic)
- Convulsions
- HELLP syndrome (hepatic microvascular)
- Hemolysis, elevated liver enzymes, low platelets, possible liver rupture

In the basic pathophysiology of pregnancy-induced hypertension, peripheral resistance is increased. Patients are volume constricted, not hypovolemic. Thus, they are not underfilled but rather constricted by the increased sensitivity of the arterioles to endogenous pressor substances, with a consequent increase in hematocrit in the early stages. Later, a decrease in hematocrit can occur from microangiopathic hemolytic anemia, a consequence of endothelial damage resulting from arteriolar spasm. Placental perfusion is decreased, as is perfusion of some end organs such as kidneys. Diuretics and antihypertensive agents do not improve uterine blood flow, but may decrease plasma volume even further and decrease uterine perfusion.

Mild preeclampsia is diagnosed by a sustained blood pressure of at least 140/90 mm Hg, 300 mg protein/24-hour urine, or nondependent edema. Some experts believe that an increase of 30 mm Hg systolic or 15 mm Hg diastolic over screening values represents significant hypertension, but this is currently a controversial point. The treatment of mild preeclampsia is to temporize with bed rest until fetal maturity or until the syndrome becomes severe. Delivery is the only "cure," and the syndrome resolves fairly promptly after delivery. Vaginal delivery is preferred, with cesarean section reserved for the usual obstetric indications. Intravenous magnesium is used during labor and 12 to 24 hours afterward to prevent seizures.

Severe preeclampsia is diagnosed with any of the following symptoms:

- Blood pressure greater than 160/110 mm Hg
- Nephrotic-range proteinuria (5 g protein/24 hours)
- Oliguria (less than 25 mL/hour)
- Eclampsia
- HELLP syndrome, DIC
- Fetal distress

In these cases, prompt delivery is required, despite prematurity. Again, induction of labor is undertaken, hoping for a vaginal delivery. Magnesium is given intravenously during labor and for 24 hours after delivery to prevent seizures. Neither low-dose aspirin nor high-dose calcium has actually been proved to reduce the 30% risk of preeclampsia in subsequent pregnancies.

Preeclampsia superimposed on chronic hypertension carries the worst prognosis for both mother and child. Chronic hypertensives are at increased risk for preeclampsia. Proteinuria and increased serum uric acid are the first signs of preeclampsia in these patients, besides worsening hypertension.

Gestational hypertension that develops late in pregnancy with no signs of preeclampsia usually resolves after delivery.

## Urinary Tract Infections

Asymptomatic bacteriuria is common (8%) in pregnancy. Twenty-five percent of patients left untreated will progress to symptomatic urinary tract infections or pyelonephritis. The most common organisms implicated are *Escherichia coli* and *Klebsiella*. Pyelonephritis is the most common medical complication of pregnancy requiring hospitalization. Twenty percent of pyelonephritis patients will have premature contractions; 10% will have positive blood cultures.

Treatment of asymptomatic bacteriuria or urinary tract infection requires 3 days of antibiotics. Typical antibiotics include oral ampicillin, 500 mg four times daily; oral amoxicillin, 500 mg three times daily; oral cephalexin, 500 mg four times daily; oral nitrofurantoin, 100 mg twice daily; and oral sulfisoxazole, 1 g four times daily. Sulfas and nitrofurantoin are avoided in the last month because they may theoretically displace bilirubin from the carrier proteins or cause hemolysis in a glucose-6-phosphate dehydrogenase–deficient neonate, respectively. The usual treatment for pyelonephritis is intravenous ampicillin and gentamicin, with prolonged oral therapy after resolution of pain. Gentamicin has been shown to be nephrotoxic in the neonate but not in the fetus. If intravenous therapy with appropriate antibiotics does not resolve pyelonephritis in 72 hours, obstruction needs to be ruled out using ultrasonography or a "single-shot" intravenous pyelogram.

## INFECTIOUS DISEASE

Antibiotics commonly used in pregnancy include:

- Penicillins—All
- Cephalosporins—All
- Nitrofurantoin—Some question of fetal risk in the third trimester if glucose-6-phosphate dehydrogenase–deficiency is present in fetus
- Erythromycin—Avoid estolate
- Clindamycin—Oral, intravenous, and topical
- Metronidazole—Studies show no risk despite commonly held beliefs to the contrary
- Spectinomycin—Alternative gonorrhea treatment
- Azithromycin—Preferred agent because of long duration of action
- Gentamicin—No fetal effects, despite causing neonatal renal failure
- Vancomycin—Only used if necessary
- Quinolones—Associated with cartilage problems in animals but no human evidence
- Trimethoprim-sulfamethoxazole—Not generally used in first trimester because trimethoprim is a folate antagonist; theoretical problems near delivery are suspected because the sulfa portion can displace bilirubin from binding proteins in the newborn and cause kernicterus

The following antibiotics are contraindicated during pregnancy:

- Chloramphenicol—"Gray baby" syndrome
- Tetracycline and derivatives—Tooth discoloration from second and third trimester use
- Kanamycin, streptomycin—Eighth nerve deafness
- For current recommendations on antibiotic use, the reader is referred to http://www.cdc.gov.

### Human Immunodeficiency Virus

The universal screening of all pregnant women for HIV is recommended. Reproductive-age women represent an increasing percentage of the HIV-infected people in the United States. The majority of pediatric HIV infection occurs because of vertical transmission from mother to fetus. Up to 33% of infants born to untreated mothers are infected. With treatment, rates of transmission are decreased to less than 7%. Antiviral medication is given orally to the mother from 14 weeks' gestation to delivery, intravenously during labor, and orally to the infant for 6 weeks at least. If resources are tight, intrapartum ZVD alone conveys most of the benefit. A triple-drug regimine is usually recommended, however, to reduce the development of resistance. Breastfeeding is discouraged when sterile formula is available.

The preferred route of delivery is an ongoing controversy, but currently, planned cesarean section is favored to decrease the baby's exposure to maternal fluids.

Viral titers are correlated with transmission rates; thus if the viral load is undetectable, perinatal transmission rates approach zero. Bactrim or aerosolized pentamidine are used for *Pneumocystis carinii* pneumonia (PCP) prophylaxis when indicated. HIV has no effect on the obstetric course when social factors are controlled. Pregnancy has no effect on the progression of HIV disease. If multiple drugs are used to control disease, they should be continued during the first trimester. If newly discovered, the start of medications should be delayed to the second trimester.

### Bacterial Vaginosis

Bacterial vaginosis was formerly known as *Gardnerella vaginalis vaginitis*, *Haemophilus vaginalis vaginitis*, and *nonspecific vaginitis*. It is not sexually transmitted. Bacterial vaginosis represents an overgrowth of the anaerobic flora. The fishy odor comes from amines, activated when pH is basic (such as the day after intercourse). Bacterial vaginosis is associated with an increased incidence of preterm delivery, preterm rupture of membranes, amnionitis, postpartum endometritis, pelvic inflammatory disease, posthysterectomy cellulitis, and postabortal infection. No change in treatment is needed because of pregnancy. Typical treatments include oral metronidazole (Flagyl), 500 mg twice daily for 7 days; metronidazole vaginal gel 0.75%, one applicator daily for 5 days; or clindamycin cream 2%, one applicator daily for 5 days. Theoretical concern exists for the folate-inhibiting potential of metronidazole, but multiple retrospective studies have confirmed its safety.

### Group B Beta-Hemolytic Streptococcus

Group B beta-hemolytic streptococcus colonizes 20% to 30% of women. The reservoir is the gastrointestinal tract, so the rectum is cultured in addition to the vagina. Approximately 0.1% of infants contract B streptococcus meningitis or sepsis. Prevention of this disease is a hot topic with obstetricians and pediatricians. Currently, patients with risk factors are treated using intrapartum penicillin to decrease the colonization of the infant and subsequent infection. The risk factors for neonatal disease are prematurity, rupture of membranes for longer than 18 hours, maternal fever, previously affected infant, and B streptococcus urinary tract infection at any time during the pregnancy, which is thought to represent heavy colonization in the mother. Some practitioners culture all patients and treat the carriers during labor, even in the absence of risk factors. No regimen is 100% protective.

## Chlamydia

Chlamydia in pregnancy is treated with 1 g of azithromycin or a 10-day course of erythromycin. Ampicillin also may be effective in a prolonged course. Tetracycline and doxycycline are not used because of tooth discoloration in the fetus.

## Cytomegalovirus

Cytomegalovirus causes primary or recurrent infections in 1% of fetuses, with varying degrees of effects. Ten percent have anomalies such as hepatosplenomegaly, growth restriction, microcephaly, and intracranial calcifications. These are worse with primary infection but also occur in recurrent infections. No adequate screening method exists and no treatment is available. Even asymptomatic infants can develop hearing loss, chorioretinitis, and neurologic or dental defects.

## Gonorrhea

Screening for gonorrhea is routinely performed in pregnancy. The treatment is the same as for nonpregnant patients, but quinolones are avoided. Ceftriaxone or azithromycin are best practice. Neonatal ophthalmia can be prevented at birth with the application opthalmalic erythromycin ointment. Presumed coincident chlamydia is always treated with azithromycin, erythromycin, ampicillin, or clindamycin. Tetracycline derivatives are avoided if possible.

## Herpes Simplex Virus

Herpes simplex virus is prevalent in the general population. Primary infection poses the greatest risk to the fetus because the IgG that forms with recurrent infection crosses the placenta and has a fetoprotective effect. Cesarean delivery is indicated if visible vulvar/vaginal lesions are present at labor. Cultures are not useful to predict shedding. Famcyclovir and valcyclovir are pregnancy category B drugs and are used if clearly needed for symptomatic relief. These medications do not exert a definite effect on neonatal disease nor on asymptomatic shedding.

## Malaria

Mefloquine is an FDA pregnancy category C drug and should be used with caution. Chloroquine may be used, but is not FDA rated.

## Lyme Disease

Early localized disease is treated with amoxicillin, 500 mg three times daily for 21 days. With asymptomatic seropositivity, no treatment is necessary.

## Rubella (German or Three-Day Measles)

Fifteen percent of reproductive-age women may lack immunity. A history of vaccination or infection is unreliable, so serum status is routinely checked during each pregnancy. Infection in the first trimester may lead to mental retardation, deafness, cataracts, and heart defects. The earlier the exposure, the worse outcome for the fetus. IgM may be used to make the diagnosis, but immunoglobulin does not have a protective effect. Conception should be avoided for 3 months after infection or vaccination with the live virus on theoretical grounds.

## Syphilis

Screening for syphilis is routinely performed once or twice during each pregnancy. Syphilis is caused by *Treponema pallidum*, which crosses the placenta. Abortion, stillbirth, and neonatal death are common. The classic stigmata of neonatal syphilitic syndrome are maculopapular rash, snuffles, mucous patches of the oral pharynx, hepatosplenomegaly, jaundice, lymphadenopathy, and chorioretinitis. Mulberry molars, Hutchinson's teeth, saddle nose, and saber shins may develop later. The diagnosis is made through blood screening tests. Because penicillin is the only effective antibiotic that crosses the placenta, treatment must use benzathine penicillin. In patients with penicillin allergies, desensitization may be needed before initiating treatment.

## Toxoplasmosis

Toxoplasmosis develops as a result of exposure to undercooked meat from an infected animal or the infected feces of outdoor cats. Presently, in the United States, serial titers are not routinely determined in pregnant women. Infection is usually asymptomatic in the mother, but potential fetal effects are more severe the earlier in pregnancy the infection occurs. Maternal-fetal transmission rates, however, are increased later in pregnancy. Fetal effects include mental retardation, chorioretinitis, blindness, epilepsy, intracranial calcifications, and hydrocephalus. Treatment uses sulfadiazine and pyrimethamine.

## Varicella

Varicella exposure during pregnancy rarely results in adverse neonatal outcomes, although a neonatal varicella syndrome that includes microcephaly and skin cicatrices has been described. Varicella pneumonia is more common in pregnant patients and is often fatal; acyclovir is used in this context. Presumed exposures are treated with varicella-zoster immune globulin if the patient is not immune. A history of disease is predictive of immunity. Half of those without a positive history are also immune. Conception should be delayed for 3 months after live attenuated vaccination. No cases of neonatal syndrome from a fetus exposed to vaccine have been reported.

## ABDOMEN

### Abdominal Surgery

Appendicitis is the most common surgical emergency during pregnancy. The maternal mortality rate in the first and second trimesters is 2%; mortality rises to almost 10% in the third trimester (compared with 0.25% for nonpregnant individuals). A delay in diagnosis and a doubling of the perforation rate are responsible for this increase, usually because the position of the appendix is thought to migrate toward the right upper quadrant as pregnancy progresses, thus making diagnosis more difficult.

It is essential to thoroughly evaluate all pregnant women presenting with unusual abdominal pain for any potentially life-threatening conditions. Fetal risk from radiographic or invasive studies is low.

### Abdominal Trauma

Trauma is most commonly seen with automobile accidents, falls, and interpersonal violence (up to 10% of pregnant women are subject to violence). The possibility of abruptio placentae must be kept in mind in all cases of direct abdominal trauma or sudden deceleration events (as occurs in automobile accidents). Bleeding caused by abruption may be concealed or may present vaginally. Serial hematocrits and coagulation studies will aid in the diagnosis, as will fetal hemoglobin titers (Kleihauer-Betke test) and ultrasonography. A normal ultrasonographic result, however, does not rule out abruption. In cases of suspected abruption, $Rh_0(D)$ immune globulin should be given to Rh-negative patients.

In cases of penetrating trauma, surgical exploration is usually warranted.

### Inflammatory Bowel Disease

Ulcerative colitis is not exacerbated by pregnancy, but patients with ulcerative colitis have higher rates of miscarriage and preterm labor. Sulfasalazine, diphenoxylate, and steroids can be used safely during pregnancy. Regional enteritis is unaffected by pregnancy.

### Pregnancy After Gastrointestinal Bypass

Late complications of gastrointestinal bypass can include diarrhea; decreased levels of vitamins, including folic acid and vitamin $B_{12}$; nephrolithiasis; cholelithiasis; and chronic liver dysfunction. Normal metabolism is found in most pregnant women who have undergone gastrointestinal bypass surgery. Screening for diabetes should be performed during pregnancy, and water-soluble emulsions of fat-soluble vitamins should be prescribed.

## NEUROLOGIC DISEASE

### Spinal Cord Injury

Spinal cord injured patients can complete a successful pregnancy, although in patients with lesions higher than T-10, self-palpation is needed to detect labor and forceps delivery is required at the end of the birthing process because patients cannot push. If the lesion is above T-6, autonomic hyperreflexia can be life threatening during labor. Ironically, epidural anesthesia can help prevent this, even though it is not needed for pain management.

### Multiple Sclerosis

The severity of multiple sclerosis is often reduced during pregnancy, although postpartum relapses are common. No increase in fetal anomalies is reported. An increased incidence (up to a 5% lifetime risk vs. 0.1% in the general population) of multiple sclerosis in offspring is noted. Disease progression is not affected by pregnancies.

### Myasthenia Gravis

Pregnancy has no significant effect on the course of the disease. Labor and delivery are critical because of the increased work requirement and risk of anesthesia. Oral anticholinesterase drugs produce no fetal effects. A pyridostigmine parenteral preparation may be ordered during labor. Edrophonium also may be used safely during labor and delivery. Patients with myasthenia gravis are sensitive to narcotics, thus their use must be carefully montiored. Magnesium should not be used. Neonatal myasthenia gravis occurs in 10% of neonates and is often transient.

## THROMBOEMBOLIC CONDITIONS

### Deep Vein Thrombosis

The risk of thrombosis increases during pregnancy and postpartum. Venous stasis, relaxed vasculature, occlusion by the gravid uterus, and hypercoagulability are contributing factors. Other factors, such as bed rest, pelvic surgery (cesarean section), obesity, increasing parity, and preexisting coagulation disorders can exacerbate the risk. Deep venous thrombosis (DVT) has an estimated incidence of up to 3%. The left leg is most often involved. Doppler screening of the lower extremity is helpful, but because venography presents minimal risk to the fetus, it can be used to confirm the diagnosis of DVT. Treatment of DVT consists of heparin anticoagulation. Coumadin is relatively contraindicated because of teratogenesis in the first trimester and risk of bleeding at delivery later in pregnancy.

Pulmonary embolism (PE) and DVT are more difficult to diagnose in pregnancy because many signs and symptoms of both are found in normal pregnancies. A false-positive Doppler test result may be caused by the uterus interfering with venous return. An arterial oxygen pressure of less than 80 mm Hg may suggest PE. Diagnostic spiral CT and angiography present little radiation risk to the fetus. Ventilation-perfusion scans may also be used. Most of the radiation exposure to the fetus in this test is from collection of radiographic contrast agents in the bladder; therefore, hydration and a Foley catheter for drainage further decreases fetal exposure. Prompt anticoagulation reduces the mortality from PE. If PE is suspected, it is wise to heparinize the patient even before diagnostic tests are done. Low-molecular-weight heparin is the best choice in pregnancy, but a switch to regular heparin should occur before delivery for easy reversibility. Vena cava ligation or placement of a filter is acceptable during pregnancy if needed.

Sixty percent of women with venous thromboembolism in pregnancy also have activated protein C resistance. Others may have anticardiolipin antibody, lupus anticoagulant, or protein C, S, or antithrombin III deficiency. A diagnosis of protein S deficiency should not be made near term or postpartum because levels are normally low at that time.

## Autoimmune-Associated Thrombosis

Lupus anticoagulant (LAC) and anticardiolipin antibodies are collectively known as *antiphospholipid antibodies* and may be found in up to 50% of SLE patients and 4% of normal pregnant patients. The term *LAC* is a misnomer because in vitro this substance acts as an anticoagulant, but in vivo it promotes coagulation. The activated partial thromboplastin time is a good stand-in assay for LAC levels. Low-titer anticardiolipin antibodies in asymptomatic women are not worrisome because not all patients with antibodies have antiphospholipid antibody syndrome. Features of the antiphospholipid antibody syndrome include:

- Recurrent thrombosis
- Recurrent pregnancy loss
- Thrombocytopenia
- High-titer anticardiolipin antibodies, especially IgG
- Growth restriction, early-onset pregnancy-induced hypertension, severe pregnancy-induced hypertension, prematurity

Treatment is controversial, with minidose aspirin, heparin, or steroids used, depending on the seriousness of the history of thrombosis.

## ARTHRITIS AND AUTOIMMUNE DISEASES

### Systemic Lupus Erythematosus

SLE is exacerbated in approximately half of all pregnancies. It is difficult to tell a lupus flare from preeclampsia (hypertension, proteinuria, thrombocytopenia, and edema). The flare, but not preeclampsia, will respond to steroids.

The course of SLE in pregnancy usually mimics recent activity. The best time for pregnancy is when there are no recent flares, the disease is controlled on less than 10 mg/day of prednisone, and no renal compromise is present. Active SLE increases the risk to the fetus, with a 50% miscarriage rate.

Many patients have antiphospholipid antibodies. LAC and anticardiolipin antibodies are associated with intrauterine death, growth restriction, and prematurity, even in the absence of SLE. Neonatal lupus syndrome is associated with anti-Ro (SSa) and anti-La (SSb). Neonatal heart block, dermatitis, hemolytic anemia, thrombocytopenia, and hepatitis can be seen in severe cases. These resolve when the mother's IgG antibodies are cleared from the infant's circulation, usually within 3 to 6 months postpartum. The exception to this clearance time occurs with the heart block, which is often fatal, but otherwise requires a pacemaker. Common SLE medications used in pregnancy include aspirin, prednisone, azathioprine, and NSAIDs (first trimester only). Contraindicated medications include hydroxychloroquine sulfate, cyclophosphamide, warfarin, gold, and penicillamine.

### Rheumatoid Arthritis

Most arthritides improve during pregnancy, but flare during postpartum. Methotrexate is a known teratogen and must be avoided; NSAIDs in the third trimester can close the ductus arteriosus so should be used with extreme caution. Aspirin and steroids may be safely used throughout pregnancy.

### Scleroderma

In patients with scleroderma, perinatal loss is increased, especially if the disease presents with renal involvement. Esophageal dysfunction is worsened during pregnancy.

## LIFESTYLE ISSUES

For the pregnant or soon-to-become pregnant patient, here are the answers to a few common lifestyle questions ("Is it safe . . . ?"):

- Hair dyeing—Yes.
- Caffeine—Limit intake to three cups of coffee or tea per day.

- Aspartame—Yes.
- Exercise—Use perceived exertion as a guide and protect joints.
- Scuba diving below 30 feet—No.
- Sky diving or mountain climbing above 10,000 feet—No.
- Physically hazardous job—If desired, the patient has a legal right to keep any job, although restricted duty is often appropriate. Time-honored restrictions are no lifting of more than 20 pounds, no pushing of more than 50 pounds, no standing for more than 4 hours without a break, and no exposure to known toxins, although these restrictions have not been proved to improve outcome in uncomplicated pregnancies.
- Flying—Flying in commercial airlines should be no problem at any gestational age, unless the cervix has started to dilate.

## REVIEW EXERCISES

### QUESTIONS

**1.** If a woman presents for preconception counseling (or even if she doesn't), you should include all *except*:
a) Folic acid supplementation (0.4mg/day)
b) Rubella and varicella immunity
c) Family and genetic history
d) Baseline CXR, EKG, and U/A
e) Medical history and optimization of chronic disease

**2.** Which of the following are *not* rated pregnancy-category X?
a) Vaccines: measles, mumps, rubella, varicella
b) Lovastatin (Mevacor)
c) Retin-A
d) DES
e) Thalidomide

**3.** Which of the following medications are absolutely safe (category A) for use in pregnancy?
a) Tylenol (acetaminophen)
b) Ampicillin
c) Synthroid (L-thyroxine)
d) Sudafed (pseudoephedrine)
e) Maalox (magnesium/aluminum hydroxides)

**4.** Your patient asks if there are any absolute contraindications to pregnancy. You say:
a) Not really
b) Marfan's syndrome with aortic root dilation
c) Primary pulmonary hypertension
d) Eisenmenger's pulmonary hypertension
e) Uncorrected tetralogy of Fallot

**5.** A young woman presents with dilated cardiomyopathy and a left ventricular (LV) ejection fraction of 30%.

The expected change of pregnancy most likely to cause trouble is:
a) Decreased systemic resistance
b) Increased heart rate
c) Increased intravascular volume
d) Decreased pulmonary vascular resistance
e) Iron-deficiency anemia

**6.** A 25-year-old woman presents for urinary frequency and dysuria. She is 20 weeks pregnant. The urinalysis shows many leukocytes per high-power field and numerous bacteria. You diagnose UTI.
The patient has no allergies. What would you recommend?
a) No treatment until the culture is returned from the lab
b) Single dose trimethoprim-sulfamethoxazole
c) Chronic suppression with nitrofurantoin
d) Three-day course of amoxicillin
e) Seven-day course of ciprofloxacin

**7.** A patient with sickle cell trait was found to have >100,000 colonies/mL of *E. coli* on routine urine culture at her 8-week prenatal visit. Treatment should include the following:
a) Do nothing in the absence of symptoms
b) Advise cranberry juice TID and reculture at next visit
c) Minimize fetal drug exposure with a single dose of amoxicillin, 2 gm
d) Give a three-day course of cephalexin
e) Get a catheter-collected urine specimen to confirm the diagnosis

**8.** A pregnant woman is found to have HIV on routine screening. Which of the following is true?
a) The confirmatory Western blot test may be falsely positive in pregnancy
b) Untreated, perinatal transmission approaches 60%
c) Perinatal antiviral treatment will decrease the transmission rate to under 7%
d) PCP prophylaxis should be started
e) Termination of the pregnancy will offer some protection against progression of her disease

**9.** A patient with known HIV becomes pregnant. Treatment should include:
a) Recommendation for amniocentesis
b) Cessation of medications until 14 weeks gestation, when organogenesis is complete
c) Encouragement of breastfeeding
d) Deference of evaluation of abnormal Pap test
e) Increase in surveillance for sexually transmitted diseases (STDs)

**10.** A pregnant asthmatic comes to the ER in severe respiratory distress. She stopped all medications because of

concerns for the fetus. Appropriate therapy might include all *but*:
a) Subcutaneous epinephrine
b) Inhaled metaproterenol
c) Oxygen by mask
d) Inhaled albuterol
e) Intravenous steroids

**11.** Your junior residents don't know how to manage a pregnant asthmatic in respiratory distress. You remind them that:
a) The dosing of IV steroids must be altered because of altered protein binding.
b) Epinephrine may be used in repeated doses before exposing the fetus to the risk of other drugs.
c) Fetal monitoring is not needed until the hypoxia has been corrected.
d) Sinusitis as a trigger should be treated with 10 days of Ciprofloxacin.
e) An ABG with $Pco_2$ in the normal range means intubation may be necessary.

**12.** A 32-year-old woman with epilepsy presents for preconception counseling. She is currently seizure-free on phenytoin (Dilantin). You tell her:
a) Epilepsy is a contraindication to pregnancy
b) All epilepsy medications carry some increased risk to the fetus
d) Valproic acid is the drug of choice
e) She should maintain the same dose throughout her pregnancy
f) Her offspring have a 50% chance of also having epilepsy

**13.** An epileptic patient's seizures are well controlled on valproic acid and phenobarbital. She discovers that she is already 12 weeks pregnant and calls you in a panic. You:
a) Berate her for not taking her oral contraceptive properly
b) Berate yourself for not documenting that you advised her to take folic acid 0.4 mg daily "just in case"
c) Discontinue one of her medications immediately
d) Recommend a detailed fetal ultrasound
e) Prescribe folic acid 4 mg/day

**14.** All of the following have been associated with poor glycemic control in diabetic women who become pregnant, *except*:
a) Increased first trimester miscarriages
b) Increased NTDs
c) Increased birth weight
d) Increased neonatal glucose levels
e) Increased neonatal respiratory distress syndrome

**15.** Which of the following medications is contraindicated for the treatment of hypertension in pregnancy?

a) Propranolol
b) Methyldopa
c) Hydralazine
d) Enalapril
e) Labetalol

**16.** A 40-year-old in her eighth month of pregnancy notes increasing edema and scotomata. BP is 145/95 resting on her left side. Abnormal laboratory values are BUN 30 mg/dL, creatinine 2.1 mg/dL, serum uric acid 8.6, new-onset 4+ proteinuria. What is your first step?
a) Observation on left-sided bed rest
b) Phenytoin to prevent seizures
c) Immediate cesarean delivery
d) Magnesium sulfate intravenously
e) Furosemide to mobilize fluid

**17.** A patient with SLE contemplating pregnancy should consider all of the following *except*:
a) Decreased fertility
b) Increased miscarriage rate
c) Disease exacerbation
d) Neonatal heart block
e) Low birth weight infant

**18.** Which one of the following autoantibodies is associated with thromboses and recurrent miscarriages?
a) Anti-Sm
b) Anti-Ro/SSA
c) Anti-centromere
d) Anti-cardiolipin
e) Anti-Scl-70

**19.** A woman in her seventh month of pregnancy presents to the emergency department with hypoxia and left leg swelling. You give oxygen and arrange for:
a) Doppler study of leg, then IV heparin if positive
b) Spiral CT, then heparin if indicated
c) V/Q scan, then heparin if positive
d) IV heparin while awaiting radiology
e) Doppler leg study and vena cava filter to prevent PE

**20.** A 32-year-old in her eighth month of pregnancy presents with intense itching, but no rash, and mild jaundice. AST is 85 u/L and total bilirubin is 4.0 mg/dL. CBC is normal, as is the PT and aPTT. Which do you suspect?
a) Acute viral hepatitis
b) Intrahepatic cholestasis of pregnancy
c) HELLP syndrome
d) Acute fatty liver of pregnancy
e) Choledocolithiasis

**21.** A 32-year-old in her eighth month of pregnancy presents with nausea, anorexia, somnolence, and jaundice. You are not surprised when your obstetric consultant recommends:

a) NG suction, IV hydration, and antibiotics
b) Stat c-section and ICU admission
c) IV magnesium and induction of labor
d) HBIG for all household contacts
e) Benadryl and observation

## ANSWERS

### 1. d.

Preconception counseling with baseline values of CXR, EKG, and U/A are not cost-effective in the preconceptual situation in an otherwise healthy woman. A U/A would be obtained if this were her first prenatal visit. The other choices are examples of good preventive care for the as yet unconceived patient—the fetus. Folic acid at this dose is found in most multivitamins and prevents NTDs in children born to average-risk women. Vaccinations should be brought up to date; a varicella vaccine is available for the nonimmune, and rubella vaccination should be considered because rubella immunity may wear off despite childhood vaccination. Genetic counseling can be offered if there is family or ethnic-group risk. Optimizing chronic disease care will optimize the healthiness of the baby and mother.

### 2. c.

All are FDA drug category X treatments except Retin-A, which is a topical vitamin A analog. Accutane (isotretinoin), the oral form of retinoin causes, birth defects in the children of some users. Live, attenuated vaccines are thought to pose theoretical risk to the fetus, but no actual viral syndromes have been reported in this context (of inadvertant exposure). The other category X medications are thought to convey no worthwhile benefit to the mother to justify their use in pregnancy. Other known teratogens that may have benefit to the mother (antiepileptics are prime examples) are rated category D.

### 3. c.

All these medications are commonly used in pregnancy, but only one, L-thyroxine, has been the subject of a prospective, controlled study and submitted for approval of the FDA. It is difficult to recruit pregnant women for such studies, and politics and liability are issues when the FDA assigns a rating. The literature may be a better source of information about the true risks of a medication, rather than the current FDA rating system.

### 4. a.

Although each of these cardiac lesions carries with it a possible 50% maternal mortality rate, the decision to proceed with pregnancy is ultimately a personal one, and as long as the risks and potential outcomes are described to the patient and her partner, any decision should be honored.

### 5. c.

Several of these normal physiologic changes in pregnancy may be less than optimal for her, but the possible fluid overload in the mid-trimester may prove most difficult to manage.

### 6. d.

Prompt treatment is prudent, given the high chance of progression to pyelonephritis. More than a 1-day course of treatment is necessary because of the physiologic changes of pregnancy. Penicillins, cephalosporins, nitrofurantoin, and erythromycin derivatives are the most widely used antibiotics in pregnancy. Seven days of ciprofloxacin is too long and too strong; the organism is likely to respond to a narrower-spectrum medication.

### 7. d.

Asymptomatic bacteriuria is more common is patients with sickle trait. Despite the lack of symptoms, she should be treated as if she has a UTI because of the risk of progression.

### 8. c.

Perinatal antiviral medication reduces transmission rates to near 7%. Up to 33% of infants born to untreated mothers are infected. Either trimethoprim-sulfamethoxazole or aerosolized pentamidine is used for PCP prophylaxis, only if indicated. Pregnancy does not affect the progression of disease.

### 9. e.

HIV is often sexually transmitted. High-risk behavior may continue during the pregnancy. Repeat screening for sexually transmitted diseases is reasonable. Abnormal cervical cytology can progress to cancer more quickly in HIV-positive patients. Amniocentesis can increase the chance that the fetus will be exposed to maternal fluids. Any drug regimen that is controlling the disease well should not be changed or temporarily discontinued because the theoretic risk for transmission due to increasing viral load outweighs the theoretical risk of fetal exposure to the medications. Discontinuation may also select for a resistant strain of the virus. Breastfeeding is known to increase the chance of transmission. Pregnancy does not further immunosuppress the patient, so the usual parameters of starting PCP prophylaxis apply and the usual medications are used.

### 10. a.

Minimizing the known risks of maternal hypoxia to the fetus is preferred to minimizing the theoretical risks of medications. Therefore, encouraging compliance with medications is important. Almost all asthma medications are used safely during pregnancy. The exception is epinephrine, which can decrease uterine perfusion. A better choice is terbutaline, 0.25 mg subcutaneously, which often is used also to treat preterm labor.

**11. e.**

Steroids are given in the usual doses based on body weight. Sinusitis requires 3 weeks of treatment in pregnancy. Aminophylline, if used, will probably need to be given in a larger than usual dose because clearance is increased and volume expanded. Epinephrine is contraindicated in pregnancy because it may restrict uterine blood flow. A normal pregnant woman has a decreased $P_{CO_2}$. Therefore, a "normal" $P_{CO_2}$ represents carbon dioxide retention and prompts intubation.

**12. b.**

Most epileptics can successfully complete pregnancy. Each commonly used medication has its own risk profile, and no one preferred medication exists. It is most important to keep the seizure activity to a minimum by frequently checking drug levels. Up to 10% of the offspring of epileptics develop epilepsy.

**13. d.**

Phenobarbital may well have interfered with the effectiveness of her oral contraceptive, no matter how conscientious she was. The 0.4-mg folate dose should be recommended to every woman in the reproductive years. A higher dose, 4 mg, is used for those at risk for a NTDs, such as valproic acid users and those with a family or personal history of NTDs. The weaning of medications must be done cautiously, if at all. Because organogenesis is complete and the period for birth defects has already passed, it is unlikely that ultrasonography would identify a NTD or cleft palate; most exposed fetuses will not have these anomalies, so automatic termination of the pregnancy is not reasonable. It is too late in the pregnancy for the larger dose of folate to exert a protective effect against NTDs. Berating yourself or your patient is usually counterproductive.

**14. e.**

Insulin does not cross the placenta, but glucose does. The fetus will make its own insulin to respond to high glucose levels. This leads to hypoglycemia after the umbilical cord is cut, which abruptly ends the glucose supply. Both large-for-gestational-age and growth-restricted babies are born to diabetics, depending on the effect on the placenta, which is also an end-organ, like kidneys and eyes. Larger babies tend to have less mature lungs; the mechanism for this is unknown. Miscarriages and birth defects are more common in preexisting diabetics, as opposed to gestational diabetics.

**15. d.**

Angiotensin-converting enzyme (ACE) inhibitors are associated with fetal compromise and death when exposure occurs during the second and third trimesters. The other medications listed are commonly used.

**16. d.**

This patient has classic severe preeclampsia. Although the blood pressure may be treated with labetalol, the process of endothelial damage goes on. Therefore, emergent delivery is indicated. Vaginal delivery is preferred if possible, so labor is induced, blood pressure is controlled to prevent stroke, and magnesium is started to prevent seizures. A decreased dose will reach therapeutic levels in this patient with decreased clearance. Toxicity is a danger. Magnesium is preferred to phenytoin (Dilantin) and phenobarbital for seizure prevention in preeclampsia. Diuretics may cause catastrophic volume depletion. Although the patient has edema and decreased urine output, she is not volume overloaded.

**17. a.**

Patients with lupus usually have no problem conceiving, but do have trouble maintaining a healthy pregnancy. Patients with lupus conceive at the normal rate, as long as their kidneys are not affected. They do, however, have an increased chance of miscarriage, low birth weight infant, neonatal heart block, and symptom flare.

**18. d.**

Anti-Ro/SSa is associated with neonatal heart block. Anti-cardiolipin and LAC, the antiphospholipid antibodies, are associated with recurrent thrombosis and miscarriage. The listed antibodies have no specific application to obstetrics.

**19. d.**

Early anticoagulation with heparin decreases mortality. DVT and PE are increased during pregnancy. Heparin does not cross the placenta and is easily reversed, so immediate anticoagulation carries little risk. Once that is done, do not hesitate to make the definitive diagnosis. Fetal risk from radiation is minimal compared with risk the of untreated DVT or PE or of unindicated treatment. Ventilation-perfusion scanning, spiral CT, angiography, and venography are all worth the risk. Long-term full anticoagulation with heparin or low-molecular-weight heparin is preferred to warfarin. A filter is indicated only if anticoagulation cannot be safely accomplished.

**20. b.**

The degree of jaundice and of liver function test elevation may help differentiate these causes of jaundice in pregnancy, but look for these clues: for hepatitis, appropriate exposure; for cholestasis, pruritus; for

HELLP syndrome, preeclampsia; for acute fatty liver, encephalopathy; for stones, pain. The treatment of each differs: for hepatitis B, hepatitis B immune globulin and vaccine for infant on delivery; for cholestasis, benadryl, cholestyramine, delivery at term; for HELLP syndrome, magnesium and immediate delivery, even if preterm; for fatty liver, immediate delivery because of a 30% maternal mortality rate; for stones, supportive measures, antibiotics, then surgery if all else fails.

**21. b.**
See answer for item 20.

## SUGGESTED READINGS

Coleman MT, Rund DA. Nonobstetric conditions causing hypoxia during pregnancy: asthma and epilepsy. *Am J Obstet Gynecol* 1997;177:1–7.

Coleman MT, Trianfo VA, Rund DA. Nonobstetric emergencies in pregnancy: trauma and surgical conditions. *Am J Obstet Gynecol* 1997;177:497–502.

Koren G, Pastuszak A, Ito S. Drugs in pregnancy. *N Engl J Med* 1998;338:1128–1137.

Medical and surgical complications of pregnancy. In: Beckman CRB, Ling FW, Herbert WN, et al, eds. *Obstetrics and Gynecology*, 3rd ed. Baltimore: Williams & Wilkins, 1998:196–246.

Rayburn WF. Chronic medical disorders during pregnancy, guidelines for prescribing drugs. *J Reprod Med* 1997;42:1–24.

Sibai BM. Treatment of hypertension in pregnant women. *N Engl J Med* 1996;335:257–265.

# Biostatistics in Clinical Medicine: Diagnostic Tests

**4**

*Gerald J. Beck*

When determining the presence of a disease in a patient, physicians use the results of diagnostic tests (e.g., laboratory, radiologic, physical symptoms) to modify their pretest impression of the likelihood of the disease being present. Therefore, it is important that clinicians understand how diagnostic tests are used in reaching clinical decisions and how the accuracy of the diagnostic test can impact their conclusions. This chapter defines and illustrates the concepts of the sensitivity, specificity, and predictive value of a diagnostic test. A good general reference to the interpretation and use of diagnostic tests is given by Griner et al. (1).

A diagnostic test is used as a decision-making tool in that the results of the test are used to predict whether a disease is present or absent. The relationship between a dichotomous test result (i.e., positive or negative) and the true diagnosis of disease can be summarized using a standard $2 \times 2$ table with four cells (A to D, as in Table 4.1). This table shows that the test may provide the clinician with the correct answer [true positive (A) or true negative (D)] or may result in the wrong conclusion [false positive (B) or false negative (C)].

To quantify the accuracy of the test in making a correct decision, several diagnostic summary values can be calculated. To illustrate this, Table 4.2 gives some hypothetical data on the relationship of a screening test using prostate-specific antigen (PSA) in diagnosing prostate cancer. In this group of 400 men having both the PSA test and the definitive biopsy(gold standard test in this disease), 160 men were correctly identified as having prostate cancer and 120 were correctly identified as not having prostate cancer. However, 120 men were misdiagnosed as either false positives (n = 80) or false negatives (n = 40). The accuracy of the PSA test can be summarized by (i) the proportion of truly diseased patients who test positive, called the *sensitivity of the test* (160 of 200, or 0.80, or 80% in the example), and (ii) the proportion of truly nondiseased patients who test negative, called the *specificity of the test* (120 of 200, or 0.60, or 60% in the example). Similarly, the false-positive rate (1 − specificity) would be 80 of 200, or 40%, and the false-negative rate (1 − sensitivity) would be 40 of 200, or 20%.

The quantities of sensitivity and specificity can be determined for a diagnostic test, in general, when the result of the diagnostic test and the true disease status is known for a group of persons and tabulated, as shown in Table 4.1. Cells A, B, C, and D represent the frequencies of the various combinations of test and disease status. The sensitivity of the diagnostic test is $A/(A + C)$ and the specificity is $B/(B + D)$.

As in the PSA example, many diagnostic tests are based on a continuous measurement. The accuracy of the test is

## TABLE 4.1

**RELATIONSHIP BETWEEN A DICHOTOMOUS DIAGNOSTIC TEST RESULT AND THE OCCURRENCE OF DISEASE: THE 2 × 2 TABLE**

|  | True Disease Status | | |
|---|---|---|---|
|  | **Disease Present** | **Disease Absent** | **Total** |
| Test Result |  |  |  |
| Positive | True positive (A) | False-positive (B) | A + B |
| Negative | False-negative (C) | True negative (D) | C + D |
| Total | A + C | B + D |  |

## TABLE 4.2

**RELATIONSHIP BETWEEN PROSTATE-SPECIFIC ANTIGEN TEST AND OCCURRENCE OF PROSTATE CANCER (HYPOTHETICAL DATA)**

|  | True Disease Status | | |
|---|---|---|---|
|  | **Prostate Cancer** | **No Prostate Cancer** | **Total** |
| Prostate-specific antigen test |  |  |  |
| Positive ($\geq$4 $\mu$g/L) | 160 | 80 | 240 |
| Negative (<4 $\mu$g/L) | 40 | 120 | 160 |
| Total | 200 | 200 | 400 |

then specific to a given cut-point value of the test that distinguishes between a positive and negative test. As shown in Figure 4.1, the choice of a cut-point will change the sensitivity, specificity, and false-positive and false-negative rates. The two curves in the figure represent the frequency distribution of the test value in the "disease absent" and "disease present" populations. Overlap usually occurs in these curves because no test perfectly discriminates between the "disease absent" and "disease present" groups. The different areas under the curves give the proportions of persons who are correctly or incorrectly classified in the "disease absent" and "disease present" groups. Therefore, moving the cut-point affects all the different areas. Moving the cut-point to the left (lower test value) increases the sensitivity but decreases the specificity (assuming a larger test value indicates the presence of disease). Hence, changing the cut-point cannot simultaneously increase both the sensitivity and specificity or simultaneously decrease the false-positive and false-negative rates. The choice of an optimal cut-point is beyond the scope of this chapter, but it can be determined using receiver operating characteristic curves (2). The cut-point choice also depends on the purpose of the diagnostic test. For example, when screening donated blood for human immunodeficiency virus (HIV), one should choose a cut-point that would reduce the false-negative rate as much as possible. If one uses the HIV blood test to identify infected

individuals, however, one should reduce the false-positive rate as much as possible to avoid falsely alarming individuals about the presence of disease. Of course, in practice, repeating the test or using a second type of test to confirm the diagnosis is often done.

Of main interest to the physician (and patient) is the probability of having the disease given that the test was positive. This is easily seen in the PSA example in Table 4.2, in which out of the 240 men with a positive test, 160 actually have prostate cancer. That is, the test gave the correct diagnosis 0.667, or 66.7%, of the time (number of times the test was positive and the disease was present out of the total number of positive tests). This quantity is called the *positive predictive value* and is calculated by A/(A + B) using the general frequencies in Table 4.1. Similarly, the negative predictive value is the proportion of patients who have a negative test result and actually have no disease, out of the total number with a negative test result. In the example, this is 120 of 160 = 0.75, or 75%, or D/(C + D). In practice, the clinician only knows the result of the diagnostic test and is trying to determine the true disease status of the patient without having knowledge of the frequencies in Table 4.1.

The pretest probability of disease in a given individual is based on the physician's personal experience with patients who have characteristics similar to the patient being diagnosed and/or on the prevalence of disease in

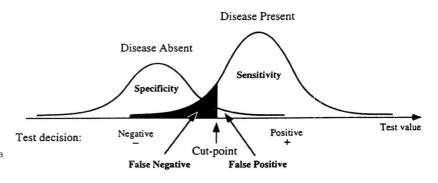

**Figure 4.1** Diagnostic test terms when there is a continuous outcome for the test.

such patients, as reported in the published literature. The key point is that the person's probability of having the disease is modified from the pretest probability to the posttest probability (positive predictive value) by incorporating the information on the accuracy of the test. In the PSA example, the pretest probability of disease was 0.50 because 200 of the 400 men represented in Table 4.2 had prostate cancer, but this is not likely the case in practice.

Therefore, a general way of calculating the positive and negative predictive values is needed.

The positive and negative predictive values are calculated, in general, using the two equations below, which are derived from Bayes' theorem.

Positive predictive value =

$$\frac{(\text{Prevalence})(\text{Sensitivity})}{(\text{Prevalence})(\text{Sensitivity}) + (1 - \text{Prevalence})(1 - \text{Specificity})}$$

Negative predictive value =

$$\frac{(1 - \text{Prevalence})(\text{Specificity})}{(1 - \text{Prevalence})(\text{Specificity}) + (\text{Prevalence})(1 - \text{Sensitivity})}$$

In the PSA example, the sensitivity was 0.80 and the specificity was 0.60. So, if the prevalence is 0.5 (as assumed above), the positive predictive value is $(0.5)(0.80)/[(0.5)(0.80) + (1 - 0.5)(1 - 0.60)]$, which equals 0.667, the same (160/240) as previously determined from Table 4.2. Likewise, the negative predictive value is $(1 - 0.5)(0.60)/[(1 - 0.5)(0.60) + (0.5)(1 - 0.80)]$, which equals 0.75, as before (120/160 in Table 4.2).

Suppose now that the prevalence (pretest probability) is 0.1 instead of 0.5. Applying the above equations would give a positive predictive value of 0.182 and a negative predictive value of 0.964, quite a bit different from the previous values, in which the prevalence was 0.5. Table 4.3 shows these values and also gives the predictive values assuming

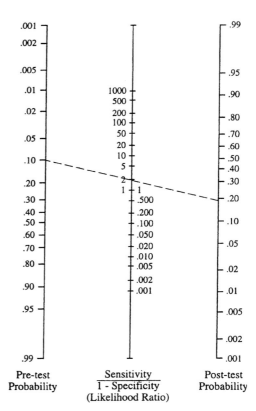

**Figure 4.2**   Fagan's nomogram to determine the posttest probability from the pretest probability, sensitivity, and specificity of a diagnostic test.

other values of disease prevalence. This table dramatically shows that the positive and negative predictive values depend on the prevalence of the disease and that, as the prevalence increases, the positive predictive value increases while the negative predictive value decreases. This occurs even if the diagnostic test has very high sensitivity and specificity. Also, as can be seen from the equations above, the positive predictive value can be increased by increasing the specificity of the test, and the negative predictive value can be increased by increasing the sensitivity of the test. It is important that the clinician understand these interrelationships when interpreting a diagnostic test or beginning a screening program. For example, if the general population, with low prevalence of HIV infection, is screened for HIV, the positive predictive value may be very low despite a very high sensitivity and specificity of the test. Also, this situation could lead to many more false-positive results than the number of true cases identified (3).

It is also important to understand how the diagnostic test result will modify the pretest probability (prevalence) values into the posttest probability. That is, a positive test will give a posttest probability (positive predictive value) larger than the pretest probability, whereas a negative test will give a posttest probability smaller (equal to 1 − the negative predictive probability) than the pretest probability. For example (as seen in Table 4.3), with a pretest

**TABLE 4.3**

**INFLUENCE OF PREVALENCE OF DISEASE ON THE POSITIVE AND NEGATIVE PREDICTIVE PROBABILITIES (HYPOTHETICAL DATA, ASSUMING 80% SENSITIVITY AND 60% SPECIFICITY)**

| Prevalence | Positive Predictive Value | Negative Predictive Value |
|---|---|---|
| 0.10 | 0.182 | 0.964 |
| 0.30 | 0.462 | 0.875 |
| 0.50 | 0.667 | 0.750 |
| 0.70 | 0.926 | 0.562 |
| 0.90 | 0.947 | 0.250 |

probability of disease equal to 0.1, if the diagnostic test is positive, the posttest probability of disease is increased to 0.182; whereas, if the test is negative, the probability of disease is decreased to $1 - 0.964$, or 0.036.

Without having to use the equations based on Bayes' theorem for determining the positive and negative predictive probabilities from the sensitivity, specificity, and prevalence of the disease (in the group setting of the individual being tested), one can use the simple nomogram of Fagan (4) to go from the pretest to the posttest probability. This nomogram (Fig. 4.2) uses the ratio of the sensitivity and the false-positive rate (or $1 -$ specificity) as a way of incorporating both the sensitivity and specificity. This ratio also is called the *likelihood ratio*, and it is the ratio of obtaining a positive test result given the disease is present versus given the disease is absent. As in the PSA example, if the sensitivity is 80% and the specificity is 60%, the likelihood ratio is $0.80/(1.0 - 0.60) = 2.0$. Then, if the pretest probability is 0.10, the posttest probability can be obtained using the nomogram in Figure 4.2 by drawing a straight line between the pretest value and the likelihood ratio and extending it to the posttest probability scale to reach a value. In this example, the posttest probability value read from Figure 4.2 is approximately 0.18 (very close to the exact value of 0.182 previously calculated). Selecting other pretest probabilities yields different posttest probabilities. Also, changing the sensitivity or specificity of the test gives different results. If the likelihood ratio is above (or below) 1, the posttest probability will be larger (or smaller) than the pretest probability.

In summary, diagnostic tests are commonplace in the practice of medicine. Understanding the interpretation of these tests is important and includes knowing the concepts of sensitivity, specificity, and positive and negative predictive value, the relationships among these, and the influence of the setting in which the test is applied—that is, the prevalence (or pretest probability) of the disease. Other biases can occur when using diagnostic tests; these have not been covered (5) but should be considered, to gain a better understanding of diagnostic testing. These biases

## TABLE 4.4
### DIAGNOSTIC VALUE OF X-OMETRY FOR DISEASE X

| | Disease X | | |
| | Present | Absent | Total |
|---|---|---|---|
| X-ometry Positive Negative | | | |
| Total | 20 | 80 | 100 |

Population prevalence = 20/100 (20%).

## TABLE 4.5
### DIAGNOSTIC VALUE OF X-OMETRY FOR DISEASE X

| | Disease X | | |
| | Present | Absent | Total |
|---|---|---|---|
| X-ometry Positive Negative | | | 40 60 |
| Total | 20 | 80 | 100 |

Population prevalence = 20%.
Positive X-ometry in 40/100 (40%).

include referral or verification bias, the use of an imperfect gold standard, the handling of uninterpretable results, and the influence of the case-mix or spectrum of patients to which the test is being applied.

## REVIEW EXERCISES

### QUESTIONS

**1.** Assume that 20% of patients truly have disease X. Using a new test (X-ometry) to test 100 patients in your office for disease X, a total of 40 of these 100 patients are found to have positive X-ometry. The specificity of X-ometry is known to be 60%. What is the positive predictive value of positive X-ometry under these conditions?

**2.** Suppose that a screening mammography test for breast cancer has both high sensitivity and specificity, say 95% each. What are the positive and negative predictive values of the test when applied to
**a)** Women with a 1% prevalence of breast cancer?
**b)** Women with a 10% prevalence of breast cancer (e.g., those with a self-diagnosed lump in a breast)?

### ANSWERS

**1.** Tables 4.4 to 4.6 use the partial information provided about a diagnostic test to complete the $2 \times 2$ table and then calculate the positive predictive value.

Step 1. The example specifies a population prevalence of disease X of 20%. Thus, of 100 patients who are tested, 20 are expected to have the condition disease X—that is, the frequencies A and C add to 20 (Table 4.4).

Step 2. The problem specifies that 40 of the 100 patients tested have a positive test, so $A + B$ is 40, and the other marginal values of the table can be determined by subtracting the known values from 100, which is the total number of patients examined in this example (Table 4.5).

**TABLE 4.6**

## DIAGNOSTIC VALUE OF X-OMETRY FOR DISEASE X

| | Disease X | | |
| | Present | Absent | Total |
| --- | --- | --- | --- |
| X-ometry | | | |
| Positive | 8 | 32 | 40 |
| Negative | 12 | 48 | 60 |
| Total | 20 | 80 | 100 |

Population prevalence = 20%.
Positive X-ometry = 40%.
Specificity X-ometry = 60%.

Step 3. The specificity of the test is designated to be 60%, so that 60% of the 80 patients without disease X in this example have a negative X-ometry test result: Frequency D is thus 60% of 80, or 48. The frequency in each of the other cells in this 2 × 2 table can then be specified (Table 4.6).

Step 4. Once the cells are all filled in, it is possible to calculate the value of the positive predictive value of X-ometry in this example by calculating cell A (= 8) divided by the sum of cells A + B (= 8 + 32, or 40). The correct answer for the positive predictive value is therefore 8 of 40, or 20% in this example.

**2.** Apply Bayes' theorem to calculate the positive and negative predictive values given the specified values of sensitivity, specificity, and prevalence.

**a)** The prevalence is 0.01, so the positive predictive value is $(0.01)(0.95)/[(0.01)(0.95) + (1 - 0.01)(1 - 0.95)]$, which equals $0.0095/(0.0095 + 0.0495)$, or 0.161. Likewise, the negative predictive value is $(1 - 0.01)(0.95)/[(1 - 0.01)(0.95) + (0.01)(1 - 0.95)]$, which equals $0.9405/(0.9405 + 0.0005)$, or 0.999.

**b)** The prevalence is 0.10, so the positive predictive value is $(0.10)(0.95)/[(0.10)(0.95) + (1 - 0.10)(1 - 0.95)]$, which equals $0.095/(0.095 + 0.045)$, or 0.679. Likewise, the negative predictive value is $(1 - 0.10)(0.95)/[(1 - 0.10)(0.95) + (0.10)(1 - 0.95)]$, which equals $0.855/(0.855 + 0.005)$, or 0.994.

Think about how the positive and negative predictive values changed when the prevalence increased from part a to part b.

Using Fagan's nomogram (Fig. 4.2), the positive and negative predictive values can be approximated. Calculate the likelihood ratio, which is sensitivity/$(1 - $ specificity). This equals $0.95/(1 - 0.95)$, or 19. Then, drawing a straight line from the pretest probability (prevalence) of 0.01 in part a, or 0.10 in part b, through the likelihood ratio of 19, one can read off the posttest probability (positive predictive value). These values are very close to those calculated above by Bayes' theorem.

## REFERENCES

1. Griner PF, Mayewski RJ, Mushlin AI, et al. Selection and interpretation of diagnostic tests and procedures: principles and applications. *Ann Intern Med* 1981;94:553–600.
2. Metz CE. Basic principles of ROC analysis. *Semin Nucl Med* 1978; 8:283–298.
3. Meyer KB, Pauker SG. Screening for HIV: can we afford the false positive rate? *N Engl J Med* 1987;317:238–241.
4. Fagan TJ. Nomogram for Bayes theorem [Letter]. *N Engl J Med* 1975;293:257.
5. Begg CB. Biases in the assessment of diagnostic tests. *Stat Med* 1987;6:411–423.

# 5

# Ocular Manifestations of Systemic Disease

*Darius M. Moshfeghi*     *Careen Y. Lowder*     *Victor L. Perez*

The ability of the physician to directly visualize ocular structures is unique to the eye as an organ system. The physician is able to make an immediate assessment of many systemic diseases, such as diabetes and hypertension, using ocular manifestations. In systemic diseases with ocular manifestations, close collaboration between the ophthalmologist and the internist is required to provide the best medical care to the patient. The main goal of this chapter is to provide internists a comprehensive and simplified journey through the eye that will make for better communication between our specialties.

## EYE EXAMINATION

The first step in the evaluation of any suspected ophthalmic disorder is a complete eight-part eye examination, which can be performed at the bedside in the following order:

- Vision
- Ocular motility
- Pupil examination
- Visual fields
- External examination
- Anterior segment examination (conjunctiva, sclera, cornea, anterior chamber, iris, and lens)
- Intraocular pressure examination
- Dilated fundus examination

Vision should always be documented first, even if it means noting simply that the patient withdraws from light, which is the vital sign of the eye. The most common system is the Snellen notation, ranging from 20/20 (normal) to approximately 20/800. This is easily performed using a near card at the appropriate testing distance (check the card). Remember, the vision is checked for each eye separately while the fellow eye is occluded, and then with both eyes open. In the emergency room setting or at bedside, lower visual acuities are usually denoted as counting fingers at a specified distance (CF6′ is counting fingers at 6 ft), followed by the ability to see hand motions (HM12″ is hand motions at 12 in), light perception and no light perception. The most common error in vision testing is not completely occluding the fellow eye, leading to better vision recorded than is actually the case in an eye with poor vision.

Ocular motility testing is assessed by measuring version and ductions. *Versions* are the movements of both eyes together while they are simultaneously viewing the object of regard, whereas *ductions* are the movements of one eye while the other eye is occluded. These can be quickly evaluated by having the patient track the examiner's finger as it is moved through the 12 clock hours for both eyes together and then for each eye alone. Similarly, the patient is then asked to look in the six cardinal directions of gaze (up and right, right, down and right, up and left, left, and down and left), as well as up, down, and straight ahead for both eyes together and then for each eye alone. The evaluation of ocular movements may reveal cranial nerve palsies and mechanical restrictions of the muscles (thyroid eye disease, orbital inflammatory syndrome, and trauma).

Pupil responses are a very important part of the ophthalmic exam. These responses should be tested by using a bright light source (muscle lamp or penlight). Pupillary testing may demonstrate a tonic pupil (Adie's syndrome, pharmacologic), relative afferent pupillary defect (asymmetric optic nerve damage; i.e., aneurysm), light-near dissociation (midbrain tumors), and Argyll-Robertson pupils (syphilis, chronic diabetes mellitus). Foremost, no drops should be placed in the patient's eyes before evaluation. The patient is then asked to focus on a distant object (at least 6 m away) and maintain that focus throughout the examination. The light is shone into the right eye and the pupillary response is noted. This is the direct response. A normal pupil should constrict immediately and briskly to a smaller circumference, followed by a small redilation to a level midway between the pre-light stimulus and the maximal light stimulus. At this point (approximately 3 s), the light is swung to stimulate the left pupil (hence the name *swinging flashlight test*). The pupillary response of the left eye should be documented; this is called the *consensual response*. The normal consensual response is a pupil that may minimally dilate or stay constricted at the midlevel of the direct response. This is because the pupillary fibers cross in the optic chiasm, contributing approximately equal amounts of response to both sides. An abnormal pupillary response would be a redilation of the left eye to a size equal to or greater than the prelight stimulus. This would indicate that the left eye's optic nerve is not perceiving as much light stimulus. Another abnormal pupillary response would be a significant constriction of the left pupil, indicating that it is perceiving more light stimulus than the right eye. The light is then returned rapidly to the right eye after 3 s, and this process is repeated several times until the abnormality, if any, is determined. The patient is then allowed to recover, and the process is repeated starting with the left eye. Pupillary testing should be done in both dim and bright lighting conditions. One important point to remember is that if both optic nerves are equally damaged, no evidence of a relative afferent pupillary defect will present because there is no difference in the amount of light each optic nerve perceives it is receiving. Common errors to avoid are not having the patient focus on the light source (this induces the near response with subsequent pupillary constriction) and not shining the light directly into the pupil (obliquely holding light in front of one pupil, but not the other, can simulate a relative afferent pupillary defect).

Confrontation visual field testing is easy, quickly performed, and reveals important information about the integrity of the visual system. While facing the patient at approximately arm's length, ask the patient to look directly and only at your nose. Have the patient cover his or her left eye while you occlude your right eye so that you should both have similar fields of view (this only works if the examiner does not have a visual field defect). At this point, the examiner holds up the left hand at a distance midway between the examiner and the patient, extending fingers in the various fields of gaze (see previous discussion) so that the patient also can see them. Then the patient is asked to say how many fingers are present. Repeat the process for the other eye, reversing the eyes that are occluded for both the patient and the examiner, and the hand that is being used to count fingers. Visual field testing can reveal the presence of pituitary masses, orbital masses, retinal detachments, advanced glaucoma, and intraocular lesions. Common errors of visual field testing include the patient not focusing on the examiner's nose (looks at the fingers), the examiner not occluding his or her own eye (could test outside the patient's field), and not having the patient wear his or her corrective lenses (the patient may not be able to see without them).

The external examination may reveal exophthalmos (anterior displacement of the globe), enophthalmos (posterior displacement of the globe), ptosis (lid droop), lid lesions, erythema, and edema. Palpation of the bony orbit may reveal discontinuities (orbital fractures) or masses (tumors, foreign body). Care should be taken to evaluate for the presence of a preauricular lymph node (common in viral conjunctivitis).

The anterior segment examination is best performed using a slit-lamp biomicroscope; however, a direct ophthalmoscope is just as useful at the bedside. A systematic approach is most useful: (i) lashes, lids, lacrimal system; (ii) conjunctiva and sclera; (iii) cornea; (iv) iris; (v) anterior chamber; (vi) lens; and (vii) anterior vitreous. Conjunctival and scleral examination can demonstrate jaundice, paleness of the tarsal conjunctiva (anemia), subconjunctival hemorrhages (bleeding diatheses), or conjunctival edema (chemosis). Vascular congestion is common in conjunctivitis, and chemosis is typical of an allergic response. Ciliary flush or redness associated with severe iritis and light sensitivity (photophobia) should be taken seriously because these represent signs of severe inflammation of the anterior segment of the eye. The anterior chamber is assessed for depth, presence of cell (absent is normal), and flare (absent is normal).

The measurement of intraocular pressure (IOP) is also very important. The normal range is 10 to 21 mm Hg, with a skewing toward the higher numbers. IOP should be assessed before dilation to minimize the possibility of worsening an attack of angle-closure glaucoma. Acute increases in IOP can mimic a systemic illness with the presence of headache, severe eye pain, nausea, vomiting, fatigue, loss of appetite, and abdominal pain.

The important structures of the posterior segment, such as the optic nerve, macula, and the major arcades and some of their branches, are easily visualized using the direct ophthalmoscope. The nerve is assessed for color (pale or pink), edema (crisp margins or blurred), hemorrhage, and the ratio of cup to disc. Symmetry between the nerves is noted. The presence of a foveal reflex should be noted. Narrowing and tortuosity of the arteries, arteriolar sclerosis, congestion and tortuosity of the veins, and arteriovenous (AV) crossing changes reflect disease processes such as hypertension, anemia, diabetes mellitus, and vasculopathies, among others. None of these finding is pathognomic of a specific disease; they only represent the limited number of ways that the retina can respond to injury.

## RETINAL NONSPECIFIC SIGNS

Cotton-wool spots, hard exudates, and intraretinal hemorrhages are the most common nonspecific manifestations of retinopathy. All these findings can be seen in disease processes such as diabetes mellitus, hypertension, hypotension, venous stasis, collagen vascular disease, and radiation damage to the orbit.

Cotton-wool spots represent infarcts that result from the closure of the precapillary arterioles within the nerve fiber layer (NFL) of the retina. The subsequent edema results in the classic appearance of small fluffy white lesions that may obscure the retinal blood vessels (Fig. 5.1). These lesions will characteristically disappear within 6 to 8 weeks.

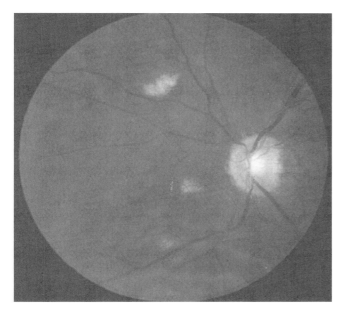

**Figure 5.1** Cotton-wool spots. (See Color Fig. 5.1.)

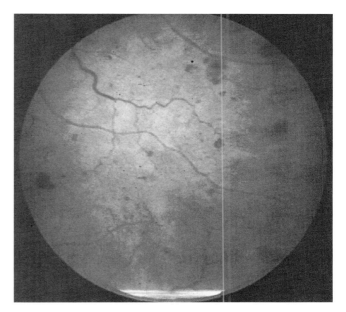

**Figure 5.3** Intraretinal hemorrhages. (See Color Fig. 5.3.)

Hard exudates are visualized as punctate yellowish spots that result from conditions that produce leaky blood vessels (Fig. 5.2).

Hemorrhages may be intraretinal or extraretinal extravasations of blood. Intraretinal hemorrhages may be flame-shaped when present in the nerve fiber layer or dot shaped if in the outer plexiform layer (Fig. 5.3).

Neovascularization of the retina is characterized by the appearance of either loop or capillary structures that proliferate along the retinal surface and extend into the vitreous cavity. The new vessels demonstrate abnormal growth out of the retina, bleed easily, are prone to leaking exudate, and may involute. Retinal neovascularization is best associated with diabetes mellitus, but is also seen in numerous entities including carotid artery disease, retinopathy of prematurity, inflammatory processes, and sickle cell disease. The vascular proliferation in diabetes mellitus typically appears on the optic nerve head (neovascularization of the disc, or NVD; Fig. 5.4) or may be present elsewhere (neovascularization elsewhere, or NVE; Fig. 5.5), but it is usually seen along blood vessels in the posterior pole.

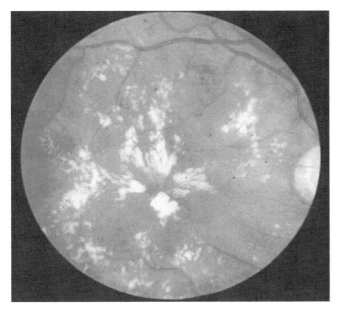

**Figure 5.2** Hard exudates. (See Color Fig. 5.2.)

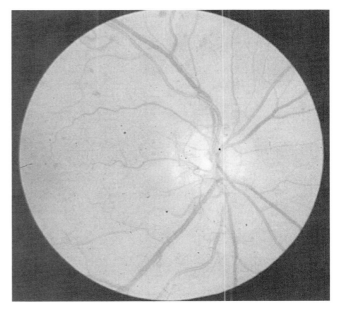

**Figure 5.4** Neovascularization of the disc. (See Color Fig. 5.4.)

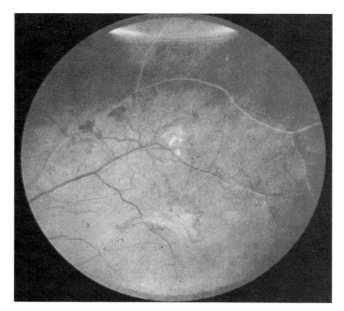

**Figure 5.5** Neovascularization elsewhere. (See Color Fig. 5.5.)

Papilledema refers to swelling of the optic nerve head in patients with increased intracranial pressure. Disk edema refers to swelling of the optic nerve head from any other cause. These swellings are associated with stasis rather than inflammation. Swelling of the optic nerve associated with inflammation is called papillitis and is differentiated from papilledema by a reduction in vision. Papilledema usually does not cause reduction in visual acuity unless it is long-standing.

## OPHTHALMIC SIGNS OF SPECIFIC CONDITIONS

### Giant Cell Arteritis and Temporal Arteritis

Giant cell arteritis (GCA) is a systemic vasculitis that affects people over 60 years of age, with an increasing prevalence in each subsequent decade. No case has been documented histologically in a patient younger than 50 years of age. Histologically, the arteritis consists of cellular infiltration of the arterial wall by multinucleated giant cells and a breakdown of the internal elastic lamina.

Giant cell arteritis may present with the onset of sudden loss of visual acuity in one or both eyes and diplopia. Patients may have systemic symptoms such as headache, arthralgias, myalgias, fever, weight loss, anemia, scalp tingling, jaw claudication, and depression prior to loss of vision. The diminished visual acuity is attributed to the occlusion of the posterior ciliary blood vessels that supply the optic nerve head. This results in an anterior ischemic optic neuropathy. Examination of the optic nerve head demonstrates typical pallid edema (Fig. 5.6). The diagnosis is based upon a high degree of clinical suspicion in a

patient population of the appropriate age having the symptoms outlined above. Two useful tests are the erythrocyte sedimentation rate and the c-reactive protein level check, which will generally both be elevated in the presence of giant cell arteritis. These tests are nonspecific, however, and can be elevated normally in the typical age-range of patients with this disease. Diagnosis can only be confirmed by a histologic demonstration of multinucleated giant cells within the muscular lining of the arterial wall and an accompanying breakdown of the internal elastic lamina, following biopsy of the superficial temporalis artery. In the appropriate clinical setting, the initiation of high-dose oral corticosteroid should be instituted immediately (prednisone 60–100 mg daily), even pending temporal artery biopsy. Patients can rapidly progress to no light perception vision in both eyes in the absence of treatment. A temporal artery biopsy should be scheduled, but it should not delay treatment. Several studies have demonstrated that the biopsy remains positive for at least 3 weeks, even with intravenous corticosteroid treatment, and there have been anecdotal reports of positive biopsies several months after continuous corticosteroid use. The absence of a positive temporal artery biopsy does not ensure absence of disease. In the setting of high clinical suspicion and a negative biopsy, a biopsy of the uninvolved side is warranted. It has been reported that up to 10% of patients with giant cell arteritis have a negative temporal artery biopsy. The response to therapy and a tapering of corticosteroids are guided by the erythrocyte sedimentation rate, which should be kept below 30 mm/h. Therapy may need to be continued for over a year.

### Hypertension

Hypertensive retinopathy may develop through several stages, but in severe hypertension these stages may not be

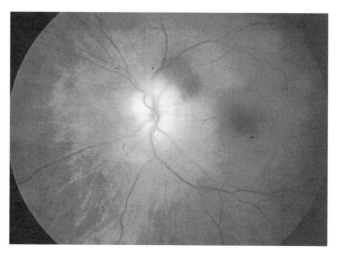

**Figure 5.6** Pallid optic nerve edema in giant cell arteritis. (See Color Fig. 5.6.)

detected because of the accelerated nature of the hypertensive retinopathy. The stages of hypertensive retinopathy are:

1. Vasoconstrictive phase
2. Sclerotic phase
3. Exudative phase
4. Complications of the sclerotic phase

In the vasoconstrictive phase, elevated blood pressure causes the retinal arteries to increase their tone through autoregulation, resulting in arterial narrowing and tortuosity. The primary site of vasoconstriction is the precapillary arteriole, occurring most frequently in the second-order and third-order arteries. A persistent elevation in blood pressure results in the hyalinization of the blood vessels, leading to a change in the light reflex of the vessel wall; AV crossing changes develop, and the arteries become more tortuous. In the exudative phase, flame-shaped hemorrhages develop from damaged blood vessel walls; cotton-wool spots or microinfarcts develop from closure of the pre-capillary arterioles.

## Malignant Hypertension

Malignant hypertension is characterized ophthalmologically by papilledema and numerous flame-shaped hemorrhages and cotton-wool spots in the peripapillary area and posterior pole (Fig. 5.7). Malignant hypertension is a medical emergency, but care must be taken not to decrease the systemic blood pressure too rapidly because this may lead to infarction of the optic nerve.

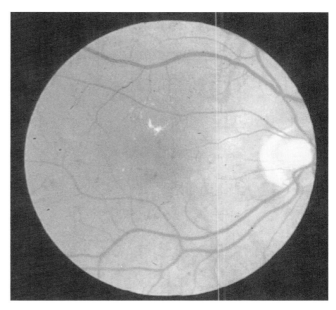

**Figure 5.8** Background diabetic retinopathy consisting of dot hemorrhages and hard exudates. (See Color Fig. 5.8.)

## Diabetic Retinopathy

In the Western Hemisphere, diabetic retinopathy is the leading cause of blindness in patients under 65 years of age. The onset of diabetic retinopathy varies with the type of diabetes mellitus present. In type I diabetes (insulin-dependent diabetes mellitus, IDDM), there is a delay of approximately 5 years between the diagnosis of diabetes and the onset of retinopathy. In type II diabetes (non–insulin-dependent diabetes mellitus, NIDDM), the retinopathy may be present at the time of diagnosis. Patients with diabetes mellitus should be referred to an ophthalmologist for proper evaluation and care.

Most patients with diabetes mellitus develop characteristic abnormalities of the retinal blood vessels. Retinal hemorrhages and hard exudates are not peculiar to diabetes mellitus, but their distribution and relative proportions lead to the highly characteristic and essentially pathognomonic appearance of the eye in patients with diabetes mellitus (Fig. 5.8). The hemorrhages and exudates are usually confined to the posterior pole, bounded by the superior and inferior temporal vessels. The leading cause of irreversible vision loss in patients with diabetes is macular edema. One test that is useful in the evaluation of diabetic retinopathy is intravenous fluorescein angiography (IVFA). Fluorescein angiography is not needed to diagnose clinically significant macular edema (CSME) or proliferative diabetic retinopathy, but it is necessary to identify areas of precapillary closure and capillary nonperfusion (Fig. 5.9). Clinically, areas of capillary nonperfusion may have overlying cotton-wool spots. Patients with extensive capillary closure are at high risk for the development of proliferative diabetic retinopathy. Patients with diabetes mellitus who

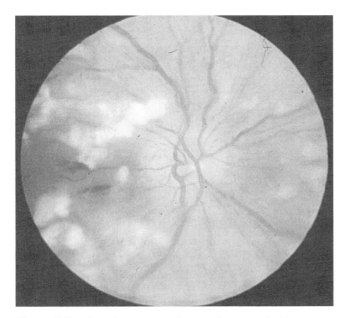

**Figure 5.7** The edematous optic nerve is surrounded by cotton-wool spots and intraretinal hemorrhages in malignant hypertension. (See Color Fig. 5.7.)

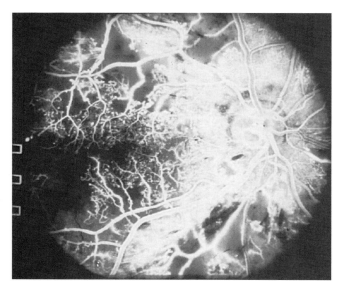

**Figure 5.9** Fluorescein angiogram reveals areas of capillary nonperfusion.

are noted to have cotton-wool spots should be monitored closely for the development of neovascularization or proliferative diabetic retinopathy. Neovascularization of the disc or of blood vessels elsewhere in the posterior pole characterize the proliferative stage. Panretinal laser photocoagulation is indicated in these patients.

After the ophthalmologic examination, and according to the results from either the eye examinations or from the angiographic study, the patient is classified into one of nine different categories that will guide the treatment and follow-up care.

Depending on the presence or absence of retinopathy, the management of diabetic retinopathy will be as follows:

- *Normal or minimal nonproliferative retinopathy.* Fundus photographs, angiography, and laser treatment are not necessary. These patients should be examined once a year.
- *Nonproliferative retinopathy without macular edema.* These patients occasionally present with hard exudates and dot and blot hemorrhages, and fundus photographs may be taken to be used as baseline. Follow-up visits should be scheduled within 6 to 12 months.
- *Nonproliferative retinopathy with nonsignificant macular edema.* Nonsignificant macular edema does not involve the center of the fovea nor does it reduce visual acuity. Fluorescein angiography and color fundus photography occasionally may be indicated for these patients. Follow-up visits should be scheduled within 4 to 6 months because these patients are at risk of developing CSME.
- *Nonproliferative retinopathy with CSME.* CSME has been defined as the presence of macular thickening, with 500 microns of the center of the fovea, hard exudates at or within 500 microns of the center of the fovea if associated with an area of adjacent retinal thickening, or an area of

thickening 1 disc area or larger, any part of which is located within 1 disc diameter of the center of the fovea. These patients should be considered for fluorescein angiography and focal laser photocoagulation. Referral to an endocrinologist should be considered. Follow-up visits should take place within 1 to 3 months.
- *Severe nonproliferative (preproliferative) retinopathy.* Nonproliferative retinopathy is characterized by the presence of four quadrants of hemorrhage and microaneurysm, two quadrants of venous beading, or one quadrant of intraretinal microvascular abnormalities. Depending on the extent of pathology, 10% to 50% of these patients will develop proliferative diabetic retinopathy within 1 year. Color fundus photography as well as fluorescein angiography are indicated. Follow-up visits should occur every 3 to 4 months.
- *Non–high-risk proliferative retinopathy.* Non–high-risk proliferative retinopathy refers to patients who have not developed NVD and vitreous hemorrhage. Fluorescein angiography may help to assess the extent of these areas of retinal nonperfusion and areas of retinal neovascularization. Laser surgery may occasionally be indicated for these patients, depending on their reliability to follow-up and the status of their fellow eye. Follow-up visits should occur within 3 to 4 months.
- *Non–high-risk proliferative diabetic retinopathy with CSME.* Fluorescein angiography should be considered in these patients. Focal macular laser surgery is indicated for these patients. Follow-up visits should occur within 1 to 3 months.
- *High-risk proliferative diabetic retinopathy.* High-risk proliferative retinopathy refers to patients who have developed NVD alone (greater than one-third to one-fourth of the surface disc area) or in association with vitreous hemorrhage. Panretinal photocoagulation is indicated for these patients. Some of them are candidates for early vitrectomy. Follow-up visits should occur every 3 to 4 months.
- *High-risk proliferative diabetic retinopathy not amenable to photocoagulation.* High-risk proliferative retinopathy not amenable to photocoagulation refers to patients who have developed severe vitreous hemorrhage or to patients with active proliferative retinopathy in spite of laser treatment. Vitreous surgery may be indicated in these patients because it may be impossible to perform laser photocoagulation due to the vitreous hemorrhage. Follow-up visits should occur every 4 to 6 weeks.

## Retinal Artery Occlusion

Patients with central retinal artery occlusion have sudden loss of vision. Examination will reveal markedly narrow arteries with boxcar segmentation. The retina is opacified, with a cherry-red spot in the macular area (Fig. 5.10). Central retinal artery occlusion (CRAO) is a true ophthalmic emergency. The usual site of obstruction is at the lamina cribrosa, the sieve-like membrane at the optic nerve

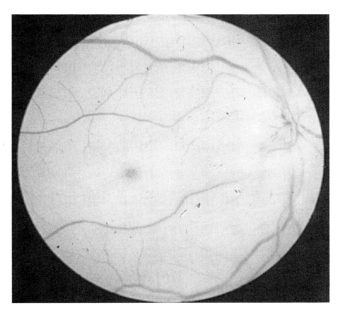

**Figure 5.10** The retina is edematous, and there is a cherry-red spot in the macula of a patient with central retinal artery occlusion. (See Color Fig. 5.10.)

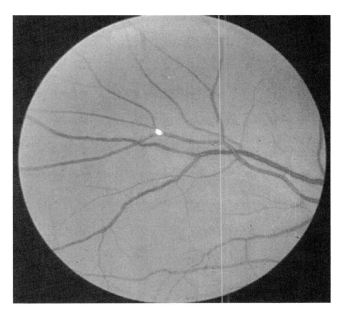

**Figure 5.11** Hollenhorst's plaque. (See Color Fig. 5.11.)

head. This is the location where the periarterial fibrous membrane becomes a mechanical barrier to the expansion of the artery. Digital massage over closed lids after instillation of antihypertensive drops such as a beta blocker (timolol 0.5%) or an alpha-adrenergic agonist (alphagan) can be performed immediately to decrease the intraocular pressure in the setting of acute CRAO. Systemic medications such as a carbonic anhydrase inhibitor also may be given to the patient. Alternatively, an anterior chamber paracentesis can be performed to acutely lower the intraocular pressure. Lowering the intraocular pressure may dislodge emboli and improve circulation. All reports of improvement following intervention are anecdotal in nature, and no intervention has ever been demonstrated to be effective over observation in restoring vision. Visual loss is permanent if the circulation is not restored within 90 minutes.

Atheromata and emboli are the most common causes of artery obstruction. The emboli may consist of calcific vegetations that originate from valvular disease of the heart, or they may be particles from atheromatous plaques found in the carotid artery or aorta. Calcific emboli are matte white and nonscintillating, in contrast to lipid emboli, which appear yellowish and scintillating (Fig. 5.11). Lipid emboli usually originate in an atheroma of a stenotic carotid artery. Usually, multiple lipid emboli are seen clinically, and they tend to lodge at the bifurcations of the retinal arteries. These emboli are responsible for transient ischemic attacks. Platelet-fibrin emboli cause transient blindness and usually occur after myocardial infarction. Platelet-fibrin emboli are abolished with aspirin intake. Whenever a patient presents with CRAO, consider the possibility of giant cell arteritis, which can rapidly progress to involve the fellow eye.

## Wegener's Granulomatosis

Wegener's granulomatosis is a necrotizing vasculitis of the small arteries and veins and is associated with granuloma formation. About 95% of patients have respiratory tract disease; 85% may have renal disease. Eye, adnexal, and orbital involvement are present in 50% of patients. Virtually any vascularized part of the eye may be involved. Orbital disease is the most common ophthalmic manifestation of Wegener's granulomatosis and is usually secondary to nasal or paranasal sinus disease (Fig. 5.12).

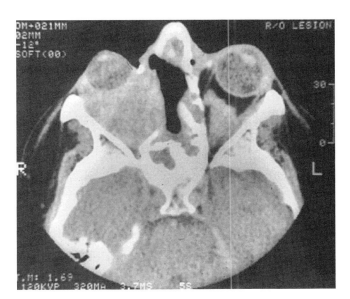

**Figure 5.12** Computed tomography reveals involvement of the paranasal sinuses and orbits in a patient with Wegener's granulomatosis.

Orbital disease presents with pain, tenderness, limited extraocular movement, and proptosis. Optic nerve compression is the usual cause of blindness.

## Rheumatoid Arthritis

The most common ocular problem in patients with rheumatoid arthritis is keratoconjunctivitis sicca or secondary Sjögren's syndrome associated with connective tissue disease. Dry eyes occur in 11% to 13% of patients. The lacrimal and salivary glands are infiltrated by lymphocytes, leading to glandular destruction with loss of tear and saliva production. Dry eyes should be treated with the frequent instillation of tears or bland ointment to prevent corneal opacification and melting.

Scleritis is the second most common ocular finding, occurring in 1% to 6% of patients with rheumatoid arthritis. The scleritis may be anterior, posterior, or necrotizing. Necrotizing scleritis has a poor prognosis, because it is usually associated with systemic vasculitis (Fig. 5.13). Scleritis requires systemic treatment with nonsteroidal anti-inflammatory agents (NSAIDs), in addition to topical corticosteroids. In severe cases, systemic corticosteroids and immunosuppressive drugs may be necessary.

Posterior segment lesions due to rheumatoid arthritis are rare. Probably the most common reason for a dilated eye examination in patients with rheumatoid arthritis is to screen for antimalarial drug toxicity. Hydroxychloroquine is accumulated in pigmented tissues, such as the retinal pigment epithelium, and may cause a bull's-eye pigmentary maculopathy (Fig. 5.14). The retinopathy may be reversible if discovered early, but it is irreversible and even progressive despite discontinuation of the drug if not detected early. The frequency of retinopathy is less than 1% when dosages of less than 6.5 mg/kg/day of hydroxychloroquine are used (<400 mg/day) for a duration of less than 10 years.

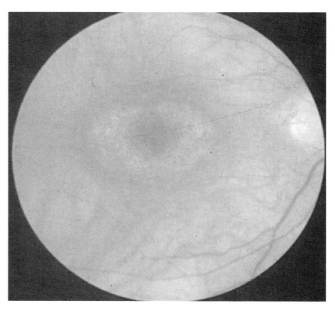

**Figure 5.14** Bull's-eye of hydroxychloroquine pigmentary maculopathy. (See Color Fig. 5.14.)

## HLA-B27–Associated Uveitis

Over 50% of acute anterior uveitis (iritis or iridocyclitis) is associated with the HLA-B27 antigen. In patients who have recurrent, unilateral, or acute attacks of iritis that alternate between the eyes, almost 90% of patients have the HLA-B27 antigen. The iritis is characterized by severe pain, redness, and photophobia. Clinically, a marked conjunctival injection and ciliary flush is present (Fig. 5.15). The cornea may be hazy. Fibrinous exudates or a hypopyon may be present. The anterior lens surface may be obscured by fibrin (Fig. 5.16). All of these findings may be visualized using a direct ophthalmoscope. Both men and women may be affected, and approximately 50% of patients have an

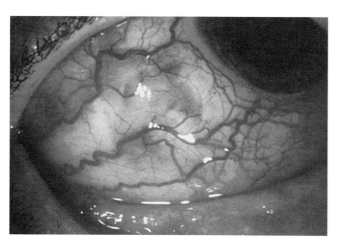

**Figure 5.13** Avascularity of the sclera leads to scleromalacia in a patient with rheumatoid arthritis. (See Color Fig. 5.13.)

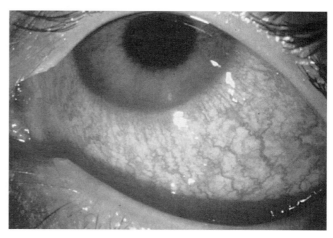

**Figure 5.15** Marked conjunctival injection and ciliary flush in acute iritis. (See Color Fig. 5.15.)

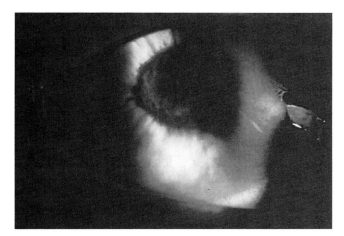

**Figure 5.16** The anterior lens capsule is covered by a fibrinous exudate in a patient with HLA-B27–associated acute iritis. (See Color Fig. 5.16.)

associated seronegative spondyloarthropathy. The most commonly associated systemic diseases are ankylosing spondylitis, Reiter's syndrome, psoriatic arthritis, and inflammatory bowel disease.

## Thyroid Eye Disease

Thyroid-related immune orbitopathy (Graves' orbitopathy, dysthyroid ophthalmopathy, thyroid eye disease) is the most common cause of unilateral and bilateral proptosis in adults. Thyroid eye disease usually occurs between the ages of 25 and 50 years. Findings include proptosis, eyelid retraction and lagophthalmos, and restriction of the extraocular muscles, resulting in diplopia. The signs may occur alone or all at the same time. The compression of the optic nerve results from extraocular muscle enlargement and is sight threatening (Fig. 5.17). Formal visual field tests will reveal scotomas in patients with thyroid optic neuropathy. The clinical course of thyroid eye disease does not usually follow a linear progression in severity. Patients may have acute episodes characterized by edema and swelling of the tissues, followed by resolution and scarring. Swelling of the extraocular muscles causes diplopia. The patient, however, should not have corrective strabismus surgery until the inflammatory process has subsided and stabilized and scarring has developed.

## Leukemia

The ocular involvement in leukemia varies in different series from a prevalence of 28% to 82%, the latter figure in an autopsy series. Leukemic infiltrates may be seen in the iris, retina, choroid, and optic nerve. Leukemic cells invading the anterior chamber mimic iritis, and in the vitreous, vitritis.

Leukemic retinopathy refers to the ocular findings in patients with leukemia who are suffering with anemia, thrombocytopenia, or increased blood viscosity. Hemorrhages may present as blots, dots, and flame shapes with

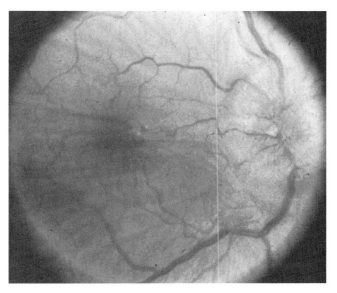

**Figure 5.17** Fundus photograph show a swollen optic nerve and choroidal folds secondary to compression by enlarged muscles in a patient with thyroid optic neuropathy. (See Color Fig. 5.17.)

or without white centers. The hemorrhage may spill into the vitreous. Cotton-wool spots also are commonly seen. Hyperviscosity of the blood may lead to vein occlusions, microaneurysms, retinal hemorrhages, and neovascularization (Fig. 5.18).

## Acquired Immunodeficiency Syndrome

The most common ocular manifestation in AIDS is the cotton-wool spot, a nonspecific finding seen in many other diseases. Infections of every ocular structure by unusual

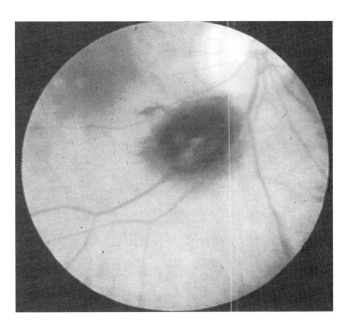

**Figure 5.18** Leukemic retinopathy characterized by intraretinal and preretinal hemorrhages. (See Color Fig. 5.18.)

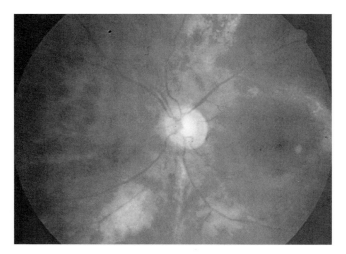

**Figure 5.19**    CMV retinitis in a patient with AIDS.

organisms have been reported in patients with AIDS. The most common and sight-threatening ocular infection is cytomegalovirus (CMV) retinitis (Fig. 5.19), which in the pre-highly active antiretroviral therapy (HAART) era affected 20% to 35% of patients with AIDS and 30% to 40% of patients with a CD4$^+$ cell count under 50/$\mu$L. The treatment of CMV retinitis with currently available antiviral agents such as ganciclovir, foscarnet, and cidofovir requires close collaboration between the ophthalmologist and the internist.

## OPHTHALMIC CONDITION OF RELEVANCE TO THE INTERNIST

### Glaucoma

Glaucoma is a condition in which the pressure caused by the fluid in the eye is abnormally high. Elevated pressure within the eye can damage the cells of the retina (the lining of the eye) and the optic nerve (Fig. 5.20). The eye is like a ball that does not increase in size with more pressure: As the pressure increases, the walls of the ball become constricted and damage occurs to the structures lining the ball (eye). Damage to the inner structures of the eye, because of eye pressure, leads to loss of visual field.

The risk of developing glaucoma increases with age. It usually occurs in people over 45 years of age. According to the National Society for the Prevention of Blindness, 1 in 50 Americans over the age of 35, and 3 out of 100 over the age of 65 have glaucoma.

People at greatest risk are those who have diabetes or who have relatives with glaucoma.

There are different types of glaucoma:

- *Open-angle glaucoma*—About 90% of cases; progresses slowly and is often unnoticed for months or years. Therapy is usually antiglaucomatous drops. This type of glaucoma is chronic and slowly progressive if untreated. Untreated open-angle glaucoma leads to loss of peripheral vision, which may be unnoticed by the patient because of its slow progression. It ultimately leads to blindness.
- *Angle-closure glaucoma*—This is very different from open-angle glaucoma in that patients develop a sudden, drastic increase in pressure, severe pain, blurred vision, halos around light, and vomiting. Laser iridotomy is the treatment indicated. (See the following section on Laser Surgery.) Unlike open-angle glaucoma, an attack of angle closure is a medical emergency and must be treated immediately. If pressure is not relieved within several hours, the patient may develop permanent loss of vision.
- *Secondary glaucoma*—This increased intraocular pressure is caused by other conditions such as uveitis, corticosteroid treatment, trauma, and other factors. The increased intraocular pressure must be treated and monitored by an ophthalmologist.
- *Congenital glaucoma*—Present at birth. The infant may have cloudy corneas, corneas that appear larger than normal, protruding eyes, tearing, and light sensitivity. The intraocular pressure must be relieved as soon as possible by means of a surgical procedure called goniotomy or trabeculotomy, where the outflow or anterior chamber angle is incised to improve the flow of fluid out of the eye.

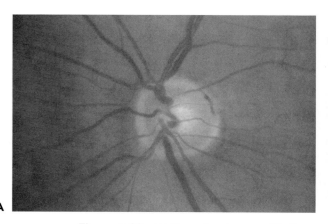

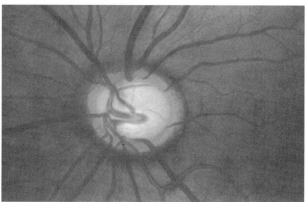

A                                                                                                    B

**Figure 5.20**    **(A)** Normal optic nerve. **(B)** Glaucomatous optic nerve. (See Color Fig. 5.20.)

### Treatment

#### Medical

Patients who have glaucoma need to have their intraocular pressures monitored and medications (drops) prescribed according to the intraocular pressure. Medications decrease eye pressure by either slowing the production of fluid in the eye or by improving drainage of fluid from the eye. For the medications to work, the patient must take them regularly and continuously. Even skipping one or two times can cause the pressure to go up. These topical medications can have systemic side effects, and these should be considered by internists in their assessment of patients with glaucoma (Table 5.1).

## TABLE 5.1
### SYSTEMIC SIDE EFFECTS OF TOPICAL GLAUCOMA MEDICATIONS

| Class Compound | Brand Name | Method of Action | Side Effects Systemic |
|---|---|---|---|
| **Beta-adrenergic antagonists (beta blockers)** | | | |
| Timolol maleate | Timoptic XE Timoptic Ocudose Timolol gel | Decrease aqueous production | Bradycardia, heart block, bronchospasm, decreased libido, CNS depression, mood swings |
| Betaxolol | Betoptic (S) | Same as above | Fewer pulmonary complications |
| **Adrenergic agonists** | | | |
| Epinephrine | Epifrin | Improve aqueous outflow | Hypertension, headaches, extra systoles |
| **Alpha-adrenergic agonists** | | | |
| Apraclonidine HCl | Iopidine | Decrease aqueous production, decrease episcleral venous pressure | Hypotension, vasovagal attack, dry mouth and nose, fatigue |
| Brimonidine tartrate | Alphagan | Decrease aqueous production, increase uveoscleral outflow | Headache, fatigue, hypotension, insomnia, depression, syncope, dizziness, anxiety |
| **Parasympathomimetic (miotic) agents** | | | |
| Pilocarpine HCl | Isopto Carpine Pilocar | Increase trabecular outflow | Increased salivation, increased secretion (gastric), abdominal cramps |
| Echothiophate iodide | Phospholine Iodide | | Same as pilocarpine, more gastrointestinal difficulties |
| **Prostaglandin analogues** | | | |
| Lantanoprost | Xalatan | Increase uveoscleral outflow | Flu-like symptoms, joint/muscle pain |
| **Hyperosmotic agents** | | | |
| Mannitol (parenteral) | Osmitrol | Osmotic gradient dehydrates vitreous | Urinary retention, headache, congestive heart failure, expansion of blood volume, diabetic complications, nausea, vomiting, diarrhea, electrolyte disturbance, renal failure |
| Glycerin (oral) | Osmoglyn | | Can cause problems in diabetic patients; similar to above |
| Isosorbide (oral)[†] | Ismotic | | Similar to mannitol |
| **Carbonic anhydrase inhibitors ORAL** | | | |
| Acetazolamide | Diamox | Decrease aqueous production | Poor tolerance of carbonated beverages, acidosis, depression, malaise, hirsutism, flatulence, paresthesias, numbness, lethargy, blood dyscrasias, diarrhea, weight loss, renal stones, loss of libido, bone marrow depression, hypokalemia, cramps, anorexia, taste, increased serum urate, enuresis |
| Methazolamide | Neptazane | | Same as above |
| **TOPICAL** | | | |
| Dorzolamide | Trusopt | | Less likely to induce systemic effects of CA1, but may occur; bitter taste |

[†] Adapted from Basic and Clinical Science Course 2002. American Academy of Ophthalmology.

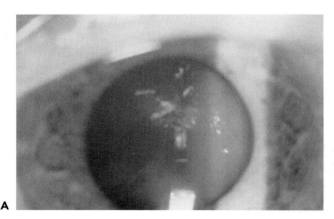

A

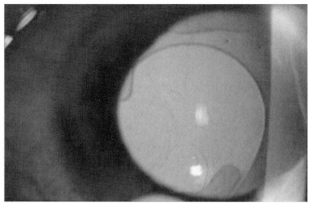

B

**Figure 5.21** **(A)** Cataract. **(B)** Intraocular lens implant. (See Color Fig. 5.21.)

### Laser Surgery

Laser surgery for glaucoma depends on the type of glaucoma.

In *open-angle glaucoma*, the drain itself is treated. Laser is used to increase fluid flow through the drain in a procedure called laser trabeculoplasty.

In *angle-closure glaucoma*, in which there is no room in the anterior chamber, the laser creates a hole in the iris (the colored portion of the eye). The procedure is called laser iridotomy, and the fluid behind the iris flows into the anterior chamber through the hole made by the laser, into the drain.

### Surgery or Trabeculectomy

When a patient's intraocular pressures cannot be controlled with medications and/or laser treatment, the surgeon must make an opening in the eye to allow the fluid to leave the eye. The fluid exits the eye through the opening and filters underneath a "bleb" or bubble covered by the conjunctiva, the covering of the sclera.

*Untreated glaucoma or increased intraocular pressure can lead to blindness.*

## CATARACT AND CATARACT SURGERY

A cataract is a clouding of the normal clear lens of the eye (Fig. 5.21A) that results in decreased vision, which may be described as:

- Blurred vision
- Fogged vision
- Glare
- Double vision
- Needing brighter light to read
- Frequent prescription changes
- Can't see colors well

Cataracts are usually a result of aging, but may also develop because of medicines taken by the patient (such as steroids), ocular trauma, long-term exposure to bright lights, or medical conditions such as diabetes.

### Treatment

Cataract surgery or the removal of the cloudy lens is the only way to clear the vision. An ophthalmologist must determine whether the patient can have improvement in vision by examining the eye thoroughly to exclude any other causes of decreased vision. Cataract surgery, if recommended, is an elective procedure, meaning a patient should only have surgery if the patient would like to have an improvement in vision because the decreased vision is interfering with the normal daily activities.

Currently, the procedure is *phacoemusification* (removal of the cataract by ultrasound to dissolve the cataract) and placement of a lens implant (a plastic lens, previously calculated to give good vision, to replace the biologic lens; Fig. 5.21B). The surgery is performed as an outpatient procedure and under local anesthesia. Patients must have a preoperative evaluation (physical examination and laboratory tests including blood, chest X-ray, and EKG) to ascertain that they are able to have the procedure. Because sedation is used, patients must have someone to take

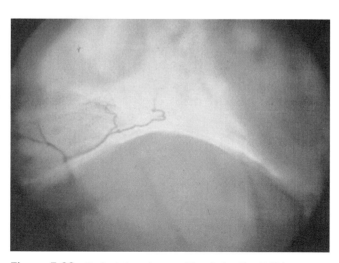

**Figure 5.22** Retinal detachment. (See Color Fig. 5.22.)

them home after surgery; the eye is patched overnight, and the patch is removed on the first postoperative visit.

## RETINAL DETACHMENT

The retina is the lining of the eye, and it is responsible for vision. The eye works in a way similar to that of a camera: The light passes through the lens and is focused on the film (the retina is the film of the eye). The images on the film or retina are transmitted to the brain via nerve fibers.

Retinal detachment occurs when the lining of the eye comes off, thus causing loss of vision. Causes of retinal detachment include ocular trauma, posterior vitreous detachment, traction from an inflamed vitreous, long eyeballs (as in very nearsighted people), family predisposition, degenerative changes in the retina, complications from diabetes, and as a complication of intraocular surgery, including cataract surgery. A retinal detachment can be caused by a retinal tear or by scar tissue pulling the retina away from the wall of the eye. If the tear is not sealed (by laser), the liquid in the vitreous—the gel-like substance

## TABLE 5.2
## OPHTHALMIC EMERGENCIES

| Disease | Symptoms | Signs | Urgent (Ophthalmologist in 12 Hours) | Emergent (Immediate ER) | Treatment (Internist) |
|---|---|---|---|---|---|
| Trauma | Pain, photophobia, blurred vision or loss of vision | Laceration of the globe, redness, limitation of eye movements | | X | Protective eye shield without underlying patch |
| Acute angle closure glaucoma | Pain, halos around lights, nausea, vomiting | Severe redness, corneal opacification | | X | IV medication (mannitol) |
| Foreign body | Foreign body sensation, tearing, pain | Redness, discharge | X | | Protective eye shield without underlying patch |
| Foreign body sensation in contact lens wearers | Tearing, severe pain | Redness, discharge, contact lens | | X | Immediate removal of the contact lens, eye shield |
| Retinal detachment | Sudden loss of vision or field of vision, floaters, flashes of light | None | X | | Bilateral eye patching, bed rest |
| Sudden crossed eyes (adults) | Double vision | Crossed eyes | | X | Glucose, head CT |
| Uveitis | Blurred vision, pain, tearing, floaters, photophobia | Hyperemia, anterior chamber cells, redness, vitritis, retinitis | X | | |
| Scleritis | Severe pain with eye movements, photophobia | Diffuse or localized severe scleral injection, watery discharge | X | | Oral NSAIDs, oral corticosteroid |
| Optic neuritis | Sudden loss of vision, severe pain | Papillitis, afferent pupillary defect | | X | IV (pulse) corticosteroid |
| Chemical burn | Severe pain, photophobia | Epithelial defect, chemosis, redness, whitening of the cornea or conjunctiva | | X | Copious irrigation with saline solution, patch with antibiotic ointment |

in the eye—goes through the tear and gets under the retina, detaching it from the underlying tissues (Fig. 5.22). Vision is lost wherever the retina is detached.

## Symptoms

The patient may notice loss of side and/or central vision, or a dark shadow, a veil, and—with total detachment—loss of vision.

## Treatment

### Retinal Tear

Laser treatment or cryotherapy or both may be used to seal a retinal tear to prevent a retinal detachment from occurring. The laser beam is directed through a special contact lens. Cryotherapy freezes that part of the retina requiring treatment.

### Retinal Detachment

If the retinal detachment is too large for laser treatment or cryotherapy alone, surgery becomes necessary to reattach the retina. The goal of treatment is reattachment of the retina. Successful reattachment of the retina does not mean a return of good vision; vision depends on the length of time the macular area of the retina was detached prior to reattachment. Once the macula is detached, vision rarely returns to normal. An improvement in vision may require several months. Various procedures are available, and only the ophthalmologist can determine which procedure is most applicable after examining the patient and evaluating the type and extent of detachment.

## OPHTHALMIC EMERGENCIES

Some ophthalmic emergencies (Table 5.2) occur that, for better visual outcome, the internist must identify and either treat or send immediately to an ophthalmologist.

## REVIEW EXERCISES

### QUESTIONS

**1.** The most common cause of visual decline in a patient with diabetes mellitus is
a) Macular edema
b) Proliferative diabetic retinopathy
c) Diabetic papillopathy
d) Tractional retinal detachment

**2.** The most appropriate initial intervention for a patient with a corneal ulcer is
a) No treatment
b) Corneal cultures and sensitivities
c) Oral antibiotics
d) Broad-spectrum topical antibiotics four times a day

**3.** The most common ocular manifestation in patients with rheumatoid arthritis is
a) Uveitis
b) Keratoconjunctivitis sicca
c) Conjunctivitis
d) Keratitis

**4.** In the Western Hemisphere, the leading cause of irreversible blindness in patients over 60 is
a) Cataract
b) Diabetic retinopathy
c) Glaucoma
d) Age-related macular degeneration

### ANSWERS

1. a.

2. b.

3. b.

4. d.

## SUGGESTED READINGS

Early Treatment Diabetic Retinopathy Study Research Group. Photocoagulation for diabetic macular edema. Early Treatment Diabetic Retinopathy Study Report Number 1. *Arch Ophthalmol* 1985;103:1796–1806.

The Diabetic Retinopathy Study Research Group. Four risk factors for severe visual loss in diabetic retinopathy. The third report from the Diabetic Retinopathy Study. *Arch Ophthalmol* 1979;97:654–555.

Ernst BB, Lowder CY, Meisler DM, Gutman FA. Posterior segment manifestations of inflammatory bowel disease. *Ophthalmology* 1991;98:1272–1280.

Fauci AS, Haynes BF, Katz P, et al. Wegener's granulomatosis: prospective clinical and therapeutic experience with 85 patients for 21 years. *Ann Intern Med* 1983;98:76–85.

Foster RE, Lowder CY, Meisler DM, et al. *Pneumocystis carinii* choroiditis. *Ophthalmology* 1991;98:1360–1365.

Freeman WR, Friedberg DN, Berry C, et al. Risks factors for development of rhegmatogenous retinal detachment in patients with CMV retinitis. *Am J Ophthalmol* 1993;116:713–720.

Holland GN, Levinson RD, Jacobson MA, AIDS Clinical Trials Group. Dose-related difference in progression rates of CMV retinopathy during foscarnet maintenance therapy. *Am J Ophthalmol* 1995;119:576–586.

Holland GN, Engstrom REJ, Glasgow BJ, et al. Ocular toxoplasmosis in patients with AIDS. *Am J Ophthalmol* 1988;106:653–657.

Pepose J, Wilhelmus K, Holland GN, eds. *Ocular Infection and Immunity.* St. Louis: Mosby-Yearbook, 1995.

Johnson MW, Vine AK. Hydroxychloroquine therapy in massive total doses without retinal toxicity. *Am J Ophthalmol* 1987;104: 139–144.

Keltner JL. Giant cell arteritis; signs and symptoms. *Ophthalmology* 1982;89:1101–1110.

Kishi S, Tso MO, Hayreh SS. Fundus lesions in malignant hypertension. *Arch Ophthalmol* 1985;103:1198–1206.

Laties AM. Central retinal artery innervation; absence of adrenergic innervation to the intraocular branches. *Arch Ophthalmol* 1967; 77:405–409.

Lowder CY, Meisler DM, McMahon JT, et al. Microsporidia infection of the cornea in a man seropositive for human immunodeficiency virus. *Am J Ophthalmol* 1990;109:242–244.

Lowder CY, Butler CP, Dodds EM, et al. CD8⁺ T-lymphocytes and CMV retinitis in patients with AIDS. *Am J Ophthalmol* 1995;120: 283–290.

Margolis TP, Lowder CY, Holland G, et al. Varicella zoster virus retinitis in patients with the acquired immunodeficiency syndrome. *Am J Ophthalmol* 1991;112:119–131.

Mizen TR. Giant cell arteritis: diagnostic and therapeutic considerations. *Ophthalmol Clin North Am* 1991;4:547–556.

Moss SE, Klein R, Klein BE. Ocular factors in the incidence and progression of diabetic retinopathy. *Ophthalmology* 1994;101: 77–83.

Studies of the Ocular Complications of AIDS Group. Foscarnet-ganciclovir cytomegalovirus retinitis trial: 4. Visual outcomes. *Ophthalmology* 1994;101:1250–1261.

Tay-Kearney ML, Schwam BL, Lowder C, et al. Clinical features and associated systemic diseases of HLA-B27 uveitis. *Am J Ophthalmol* 1996;121:47–56.

Tso MO, Jampol LM. Pathophysiology of hypertensive retinopathy. *Ophthalmology* 1982;89:1132–1145.

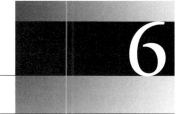

# Preoperative Evaluation and Management Before Major Noncardiac Surgery

*Amir K. Jaffer, MD    David L. Bronson, MD, FACP*

Each year, over 36 million procedures are performed in the United States, with approximately a third performed on patients over the age of 65 (1). This group of patients is the fastest growing subset of the population and estimated to double from 35 million to 70 million people by 2030 (2). A recent prospective cohort study done at a major academic center showed that elderly patients have a higher rate of major perioperative complications and mortality after noncardiac surgery compared with their younger counterparts (3). Complications occur frequently, and cardiovascular events are the leading cause of perioperative death. The cost of perioperative cardiovascular morbidity alone is approximately $20 billion in the United States (4). Therefore, a preoperative evaluation designed to reduce risk is especially needed in the elderly and in younger patients with existing medical problems. This evaluation should be geared toward risk assessment and the implementation of risk reduction therapies that may help decrease perioperative morbidity and mortality, thereby improving patient outcomes and decreasing associated costs. Effective preoperative medical consultation depends on the internist's understanding of the issues faced by anesthesiologists and surgeons in planning and performing a surgical procedure and on communicating clear strategies to optimize the patient's medical status.

Perioperative risks fall into four major categories: *patient-specific, procedure-specific, anesthesia-specific,* and *provider-specific risks.* Patient-specific risks refer to a patient's characteristics (e.g., age, gender, race, level of fitness, etc.) and underlying medical conditions (e.g., diabetes, hypertension, coronary artery disease, etc.). Optimizing these underlying conditions and identifying new risk factors or medical conditions that can be modified are some of the goals of the medical consultant.

The risk of a specific surgical procedure (procedure-specific risk) is proportional to the physiologic stress associated with the procedure, as outlined in Table 6.1. Procedures associated with major blood loss or those that involve cross-clamping of the aorta cause the patient to experience the highest level of physiological stress and carry a cardiac event risk of >5%. Patients undergoing surgery in which the blood loss is intermediate (e.g., major joint replacement) have an intermediate level of cardiac event risk of 1 to 5%. The lowest level of risk, <1% (5), occurs in minor procedures associated with minimal blood loss and physiologic stress (e.g., breast biopsy).

In a review of over 100,000 surgical procedures performed under anesthesia, patient-specific and surgical-specific risk factors were much more important in predicting seven-day mortality than the anesthesia factors studied (6). Modern anesthesia is generally safe, but anesthesia-specific risks exist that involve the direct and indirect effects of anesthetic agents in the context of the physiologic responses to surgically induced hypotension, blood loss, anemia, and postoperative pain. During anesthesia induction, tachycardia and hypertension occur in response to anxiety and the mechanical effects of tracheal manipulation with intubation. Ten percent of cardiac events occur during this time.

**TABLE 6.1**

## CARDIAC RISK (NONFATAL MYOCARDIAL INFARCTION OR DEATH) STRATIFICATION FOR NONCARDIAC SURGICAL PROCEDURES*

**High (reported cardiac risk often >5%)**
Emergent major operations, particularly in the elderly
Aortic and other major vascular surgery
Peripheral vascular surgery
Anticipated prolonged surgical procedures associated with large
    fluid shifts or blood loss
Intermediate (reported cardiac risk generally 1%–5%)
Carotid endarterectomy
Head and neck surgery
Intraperitoneal and intrathoracic surgery
Orthopedic surgery
Prostate surgery (other than TURP)

**Low (reported cardiac risk generally <1%)**
Endoscopic procedures
Superficial procedure
Cataract surgery
Breast biopsy
TURP (based on most studies, but not included by ACC/AHA)

(* Reproduced with permission from Eagle et al. *Circulation* 2002;
105(10):1257–1267.)

Later hypotension may occur as a result of the vasodilation and myocardial depression associated with anesthetic agents, intermittent positive pressure ventilation, hemorrhage, or infection. Balanced anesthetic techniques using opiates, sedative hypnotics, neuromuscular blockers, and inhalation agents cause fewer cardiovascular effects than anesthesia using inhalation agents alone. Most anesthetic deaths are due to failure to ventilate adequately, unsuspected hypoxia, or anesthetic agent overdose (7). No one best anesthetic technique exists to reduce cardiac risk. A meta-analysis of 141 trials involving 9,559 patients found that epidural or spinal anesthesia significantly reduced the risk of mortality, thromboembolic complications, myocar-

dial infarction (MI), transfusion requirements, pneumonia, and respiratory depression compared with general anesthesia (8). The authors commented that the inconsistency of their findings versus other smaller clinical trials potentially resulted from insufficient statistical power. It is probably safe to conclude at this time that epidural anesthesia, both with or without opioid analgesia, has similar if not improved morbidity when compared with general anesthesia with or without opioid, patient-controlled analgesia. The American Society of Anesthesiologists (ASA) Classification of Preoperative Risk (Table 6.2) roughly classifies patients into groups correlated with overall and anesthesia-specific risks. This scale is a useful tool for quickly defining a patient's risk, but it does not consider procedure-specific issues. The anesthesia-associated death rate of healthy patients in class I and II is 1 in 200,000. In emergency surgery, anesthetic and surgical mortality doubles for classes I, II, and III. Provider-specific risk is related to the experience of the surgeon and the surgical team and may vary according to the volume of surgeries performed and their expertise with a particular procedure. The medical consultant cannot modify this risk.

## MANAGING CARDIOVASCULAR RISK

The overall risk of postoperative cardiac death or major cardiac complications is less than 6% in patients over the age of 40 undergoing major noncardiac surgeries (9). Approximately 8 million individuals undergoing surgical procedures each year have known coronary artery disease (CAD) or coronary risk factors (10), however, and approximately 1 million individuals will have some perioperative cardiac complication. The most common cardiovascular complications are:

■ Perioperative acute ischemia and MI
■ Congestive heart failure (CHF)

**TABLE 6.2**

## AMERICAN SOCIETY OF ANESTHESIOLOGISTS (ASA) CLASSIFICATION OF PREOPERATIVE RISK*

| ASA Class Definition | | Mortality (%) |
|---|---|---|
| I | Healthy patient with no disease outside of the surgical process | <0.03 |
| II | Mild to moderate systemic disturbance caused by the surgical condition or by other pathological processes, medically well-controlled | 0.2 |
| III | Severe systemic disturbance which limits activity but not necessarily life threatening | 1.2 |
| IV | Severe systemic disturbance that is life threatening | 8 |
| V | Moribund with little chance of survival at 24 hours with or without operation | 34 |

(* Adapted from Cohen, MM et al. Does anesthesia contribute to operative mortality? *JAMA* 1998;260;2859.)

- Arrhythmias
- Hypotension
- Hypertension

In the early postoperative period, pain, hypotension, and increased catecholamine release with associated tachycardia may lead to cardiovascular stress by increasing myocardial oxygen demand and coronary vascular tone. The catecholamine effects also may increase plaque instability and, with enhanced platelet aggregation and hypercoagulability owing to tissue injury, elevate the risk of coronary thrombosis. A limited cardiovascular reserve, particularly in elderly patients, increases the risk of a cardiac event. The incidence of MI peaks on the third postoperative day, and increased risk persists for up to 6 months after the surgery. The greatest risk for acute pulmonary edema is in patients with known CHF; this risk occurs especially in the first few hours after anesthesia, when anesthesia-induced hypotension abates and fluid resorption is most vigorous.

The critical first step in the cardiac evaluation of a patient having noncardiac surgery is identifying the patient's clinical features, including the presence of unstable symptoms. Evidence suggests that decompensated CHF, significant arrhythmia, severe valvular disease, or unstable angina (USA) are associated with increased perioperative cardiac morbidity. A high index of suspicion may also identify individuals with occult symptoms. For example, dyspnea may be the only manifestation of underlying CAD. The identification and management of uncontrolled symptoms before elective surgery will greatly reduce postoperative cardiac morbidity.

In an attempt to quantify the preoperative risk in patients with known or suspected cardiac disease, several multivariate indices of risk have been developed. Some of the more well-known and studied indices include the Goldman Cardiac Risk Index (Table 6.3), Detsky Modified Risk Index (Table 6.4), and the revised Goldman Cardiac Risk Index—also called the Lee Risk Index (Table 6.5). The role of risk indices is to assist physicians in identifying patients at low-, intermediate-, and high-risk for postoperative cardiac complications. Indices developed by Eagle (11) (Table 6.6) and Vanzetto (12) support the usefulness of preoperative dipyridamole-thallium imaging (DTI) and clinical variables in predicting ischemic events after vascular surgery.

In 1977, Goldman and colleagues published a landmark article evaluating 1,001 patients undergoing noncardiac surgery (9). Nine independent correlates of perioperative fatal or major nonfatal cardiac events were identified and assigned a certain number of points. Patients were then placed in four classes, depending on the total number of points. In Class IV (highest risk category), 78% of patients had a major cardiac event compared with less than 1% of patients in Class 1 (lowest risk category) group. The Cardiac Risk Index (CRI) developed from this study (Table 6.3) divides patients into high- and low-risk categories; for the large group of patients in the intermediate risk category, a 9% chance of major perioperative cardiac event still exists. Other limitations of this index include: (i) relatively few vascular surgery patients were included in the study; (ii) it was developed in the mid-1970s and does not take into account advances in medical, anesthetic, or surgical care; and (iii) the data was collected only at one institution.

## TABLE 6.4
### MODIFIED MULTIFACTORIAL INDEX*

| Clinical Feature | Points |
| --- | --- |
| MI <6 months | 10 |
| MI >6 months | 5 |
| Angina–Class 3 unstable | 10 |
| Angina–Class 4 | 20 |
| Pulmonary edema | |
| Within 1 week | 10 |
| Ever | 5 |
| Critical aortic stenosis | 20 |
| Nonsinus rhythms, PACs, or >5 PVCs | 5 |
| Age >70 | 5 |
| Emergency operation | 10 |
| Poor general medical condition | 5 |

(* Adapted with permission from Detsky et al. Cardiac assessment for patients undergoing noncardiac surgery. A multifactorial clinical risk index. *Arch Intern Med* 1986;146:2131–2134.)

## TABLE 6.3
### CARDIAC RISK INDEX*

| Indicator | Points |
| --- | --- |
| Age >70 years | 5 |
| MI <6 months | 10 |
| $S_3$ gallop or JVD | 11 |
| Important valvular aortic stenosis | 3 |
| Nonsinus rhythm, PACs or >5 PVCs/min | 7 |
| $PO_2$ <60 or $Pco_2$ >50 mm Hg, K <3.0 or $HCO_3$ <20 mEg/L, BUN >50 or Cr >3.0 mg/dL abnormal SGOT, signs of chronic liver disease, or patients bedridden from noncardiac cause | 3 |
| Intraperitoneal, intrathoracic, or aortic operation | 3 |
| Emergency operation | 4 |

**Risk Assessment**

| Class | Points | Risk |
| --- | --- | --- |
| I | 0–5 | 0.7% Complication 0.2% Death |
| II | 6–12 | 5.0% Complication 2.0% Death |
| III | 13–25 | 11% Complication 2.0% Death |
| IV | 26+ | 22% Complication 56% Death |

(* Adapted with permission from Goldman et al. Multifactorial index of cardiac risk in noncardiac surgical procedures. *N Engl J Med* 1977;297:845–850.)

## TABLE 6.5

### REVISED CARDIAC RISK INDEX (LEE RISK INDEX)*

**Risk Factors**

High-risk type of surgery: intraperitoneal, intrathoracic, or suprainguinal vascular procedure

History of ischemic heart disease: history of MI, positive exercise stress test, current complaint of ischemic chest pain or use of nitrate therapy, or electrocardiogram with Q waves. Patients with prior CABG or percutaneous transluminal coronary angioplasty were included only if they had current complaints of chest pain presumed due to ischemia

History of CHF, PE, or paroxysmal nocturnal dyspnea, physical examination with bilateral rales or $S_3$, or chest radiograph showing pulmonary vascular redistribution

History of cerebrovascular disease

Diabetes mellitus treated with insulin

Preoperative serum creatinine >2.0 mg/dL

| Revised Cardiac Risk Class | Number of Risk Factors | Major Cardiac Events | Rate (%) |
|---|---|---|---|
| I | 0 | 5/1,071 | 0.5 |
| II | 1 | 14/1,106 | 1.3 |
| III | 2 | 18/506 | 3.6 |
| IV | >3 | 19/210 | 9.1 |

(* Adapted from Lee TH, Marcantonio ER, Mangione CM, et al. Derivation and prospective validation of a simple index for prediction of cardiac risk of major noncardiac surgery. *Circulation* 2001;100:1043–1049.)

The Modified Multifactorial Index by Detsky and coworkers (13) (Table 6.4) modified the Goldman Index by assigning a higher score to emergency surgery and recent MI (<6 months) and included angina and pulmonary edema in the index. Like the Goldman Index, however, Detsky may also underestimate the cardiac risk in vascular patients. The Detsky modification of the Goldman Index is the starting point of the American College of Physicians (ACP) guidelines for preoperative testing for CAD (14). These guidelines are discussed in more detail in the section on Guidelines for Assessing Perioperative Cardiac Risk.

The revised Goldman Cardiac Risk Index (Table 6.5), also referred to as the Lee Risk Index (15), seeks to simplify the original criteria. In a prospective study of 4,315 patients ≥50 years of age undergoing elective major noncardiac surgeries, Lee et al. identified six independent predictors of perioperative complications:

- High-risk type of surgery
- History of ischemic heart disease
- History of CHF
- History of stroke or transient ischemic attack (TIA)
- Diabetes on insulin
- Preoperative serum creatinine of >2 mg/dL

Each predictor was assigned one point. Table 6.5 shows the rate of complication in each risk category during this study. This index appears to be more accurate than older indices in predicting major postoperative cardiac complications (16).

The second step during the preoperative evaluation is to determine the patient's functional class. Self-reported exercise tolerance is the key for cardiovascular risk stratification and is an independent predictor for postoperative cardiovascular complications (17). The Duke Activity Status Index (18) (Table 6.7) is one way of dividing patients into four functional classes (I–IV), based on their activity level, that can help generate an estimate of their metabolic equivalents (METs). The ability to perform >4 METs of activity has been associated with a lower cardiovascular risk (17).

The third step is to determine the patient's surgery-specific risk; Table 6.1 groups surgical procedures into three different categories labeled as high risk (reported cardiac risk >5%), intermediate risk (reported cardiac risk 1–5%), and low risk (cardiac risk <1%).

The first three evaluation steps determine the need for noninvasive testing (step 4). Patients who are at low risk based on clinical features, functional status, and proposed low-risk surgery do not generally require any further evaluation. Conversely, those patients deemed high risk, using the clinical features developed by Lee (15) (Table 6.5)—often termed as the "intermediate clinical predictors" per the American College of Cardiology and American Heart Association (ACC/AHA) guidelines (Fig. 6.1)—may benefit from further noninvasive evaluation if they have either a poor functional class or are undergoing a high-risk procedure. In addition, patients with unreliable histories and poor functional status from vascular or orthopedic disease may make the assessment of angina difficult. In such patients, noninvasive cardiac testing may also be useful.

## TABLE 6.6

### DIPYRIDAMOLE-THALLIUM IMAGING TO PREDICT POSTOPERATIVE CARDIAC ISCHEMIA[†]

| Clinical Group* | Postoperative Event** | |
|---|---|---|
| 0 Factors | 2/64 | (3%) |
| 1–2 Factors and − Thallium | 2/62 | (3%) |
| 1–2 Factors and + Thallium | 16/54 | (30%) |
| 3+ Factors | 10/24 | (50%) |

* Factors including age >70, history of angina, history of VEA requiring treatment, DM on therapy, Q-wave on EKG
** Cardiac death, MI, ischemic pulmonary edema, unstable angina
([†] Adapted with permission from Eagle et al., Combining clinical and thallium data optimizes preoperative assessment of cardiac risk before major vascular surgery. *Ann Intern Med* 1989;110:859.)

## TABLE 6.7
## EVALUATION OF FUNCTIONAL STATUS USING SPECIFIC ACTIVITIES: THE DUKE ACTIVITY STATUS INDEX*

| Activity | Estimated Metabolic Cost of Each Activity (MET Units) |
|---|---|
| **Can You:** | |
| Walk indoors, such as around your house? | 1.75 |
| Do light work around the house, such as dusting or washing dishes? | 2.70 |
| Take care of yourself, that is, eating, dressing, bathing, using the toilet? | 2.75 |
| Walk a block or two on level ground? | 2.75 |
| Do moderate work around the house such as vacuuming, sweeping floors, or carrying in groceries? | 3.50 |
| Do yard work such as raking leaves, weeding, or pushing a power mower? | 4.50 |
| Have sexual relations? | 5.25 |
| Climb a flight of stairs or walk up a hill? | 5.50 |
| Participate in moderate recreational activities, such as golf, bowling, dancing, doubles tennis, or throwing a baseball or football? | 6.00 |
| Participate in strenuous sports, such as swimming, singles tennis, football, basketball, or skiing? | 7.50 |
| Do heavy work around the house, such as scrubbing floors or lifting or moving heavy furniture? | 8.00 |
| Run a short distance? | 8.00 |

(* Reproduced with permission from Hlatky MA, et al. *Am J Cardiol* 1989;64(10):651–654.)

The ACC/AHA guidelines favor the use of noninvasive testing for patients with two or more of the following indicators:

- Undergoing high-risk procedures
- Poor functional capacity (i.e., performing less than 4 METs in activity)
- Intermediate clinical predictors (i.e., angina, prior MI, compensated or prior CHF, chronic renal insufficiency with a creatinine of 2 mg/dL or more, or diabetes mellitus)

In patients who can exercise, exercise stress testing can accurately stratify cardiovascular risk in major vascular surgery. Patients who achieve 75% of maximally predicted heart rate (HR) without EKG changes are at low risk for cardiac complications (10). Dipyridamole-thallium imaging (DTI) can accurately predict cardiac complications in selected patients undergoing vascular surgery. In patients with one or two risk factors (intermediate risk), a positive test is associated with a high cardiac complication rate and a negative test is associated with a substantially lower rate (Table 6.6) (11). Data are limited in nonvascular surgery patients, but it is likely that DTI may be useful in intermediate-risk patients, as defined by the ACC/AHA guidelines.

Dobutamine stress echocardiography (DSE) may be useful in both intermediate- and high-risk patients, as defined by the ACC/AHA guidelines. In the largest study of preoperative DSE in patients undergoing vascular surgery, a normal test was associated with a very low cardiac compli-

cation rate (19). In a meta-analysis of six noninvasive tests, DSE showed a positive trend toward better diagnostic performance than other tests, but this was only significant in the comparison with myocardial perfusion scintigraph (20). DSE should be avoided in patients with significant arrhythmias, very high or low blood pressures, and critical aortic stenosis.

The fifth step is to decide when to refer patients for preoperative coronary angiography. In general, the indications are similar to those for nonoperative settings—that is, those who are at high risk based on findings from a noninvasive test, who have angina unresponsive to medical therapy or USA, and those scheduled for intermediate- or high-risk surgery after an equivocal noninvasive study.

The sixth step is to optimize medical therapy preoperatively. This includes, but is not limited to, titrating medications to better control blood pressure and initiating beta-blocker (β-blocker) therapy on those patients who would benefit from this therapy. Details regarding β-blocker therapy are discussed in the section on this topic.

Two well-written and often cited guidelines have been developed, one by the ACC/AHA (Figure 6.1) and the other by the American College of Physicians (ACP) (21,22). Our own preference and practice is to use the ACC/AHA guidelines outlined in Figure 6.1, which were first published in 1996 and updated in 2002 (5). These guidelines integrate clinical risk factors, exercise capacity, and type of surgery into the preoperative decision process.

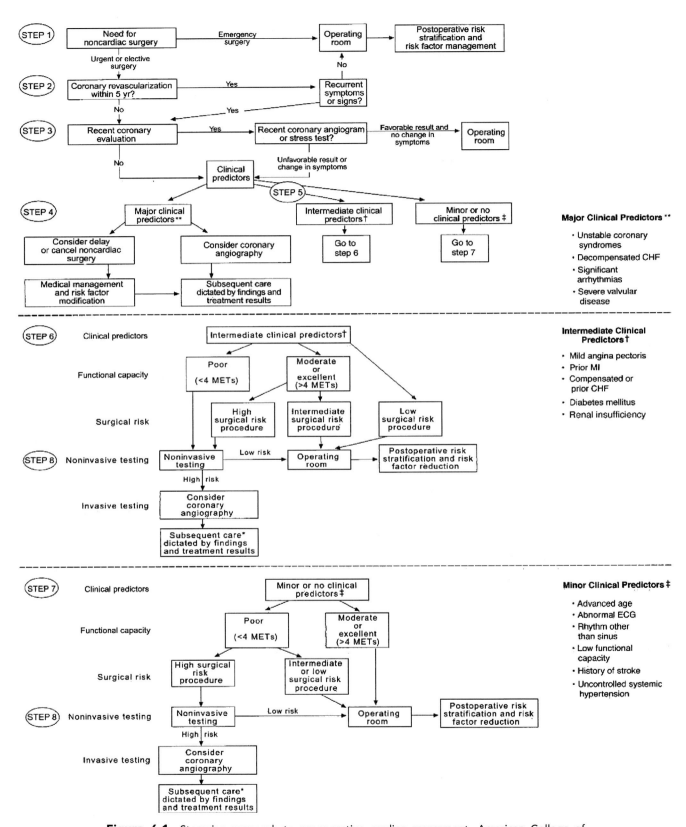

**Figure 6.1** Stepwise approach to preoperative cardiac assessment. American College of Cardiology/American Heart Association Guidelines. (Reprinted with permission from Eagle et al. ACC/AHA guideline update for perioperative cardiovascular evaluation for noncardiac surgery–executive summary a report of the American College of Cardiology/American Heart Association Task Force on Practice Guidelines. Committee to Update the 1996 Guidelines on Perioperative Cardiovascular Evaluation for Noncardiac Surgery. *Circulation* 2002;105(10):1257–1267.)

The ACC/AHA guidelines are based on both evidence and expert opinion and suggest that first the urgency of the surgery be evaluated, then a determination be made if the patient has had previous coronary revascularization or coronary evaluation. Next, any patient with unstable coronary syndromes should be stabilized prior to surgery, and the decision for further testing should be based on a combination of clinical risk factors, surgery-specific risk, and functional capacity. Patients with minor or no clinical predictors generally require no further testing unless they have poor functional capacity and are undergoing high-risk procedures. Of importance, no preoperative testing should be performed if the results will not change perioperative management (21).

The ACP guidelines (22) use the Detsky modification of the Goldman CRI as the initial evaluation point. Patients who have multiple markers for cardiovascular disease and are undergoing major vascular surgery are candidates for further testing. The ACP guidelines are purely evidence-based and suggest that not enough evidence exists for further testing in patients undergoing nonvascular surgery or for using exercise tolerance in evaluating the need for further preoperative testing. Strict adherence to these guidelines would result in fewer stress tests, but they may be overly conservative.

A recent MI carries a significant risk of perioperative infarction, although contemporary post-MI risk stratification and anesthetic techniques have lowered this risk considerably. In the patient without post-MI ischemia and good functional capacity on stress testing, elective surgical procedures usually should be delayed for 3 months; if needed clinically, surgery can often be performed as soon as 6 weeks after the cardiac event. In the patient needing more urgent surgery after an uncomplicated MI and satisfactory post-MI risk stratification, the use of β-blockers and invasive monitoring should be considered to minimize cardiovascular instability, depending on the planned procedure and the individual patient's risk (5).

## MANAGEMENT OF NONISCHEMIC CARDIAC DISEASE

### Hypertension

Patients with hypertension have a higher incidence of silent CAD and previous MI than the general population. Traditionally, surgery was delayed for patients presenting with a diastolic blood pressure (DBP) of >110 mm Hg, but review of the literature shows that these patients may be at increased risk for hemodynamic lability but not necessarily for MI. Chronic antihypertensive medications can be continued in the perioperative period, with some exceptions for the morning of surgery (discussed in a following paragraph). Preoperatively, a systolic blood pressure (SBP)

of >180 mm Hg and a DBP of >110m Hg are definite indications for preoperative intervention.

### Congestive Heart Failure

Compensated CHF patients have a 5% to 7% incidence of perioperative cardiac complications in comparison with the 20% to 30% in patients with decompensated CHF (5). In addition to stabilizing CHF prior to surgery and delaying surgery if necessary, the etiology of CHF must be determined—if not known already—because perioperative monitoring will differ depending on the etiology. Optimizing the medical management of patients with CHF is critical prior to elective surgeries and, if the surgery is emergent, invasive monitoring may be useful.

### Cardiac Murmurs

When a murmur is detected on physical examination as part of the preoperative evaluation, an effort should be made to ascertain the chronicity of the murmur and to determine whether the murmur is functional or structural. If the murmur is believed to be functional, then a search for anemia, thyroid disorders, and other causes should be initiated. Evaluation by echocardiography is recommended for all diagnosed murmurs, if none has been performed previously. Echocardiography can help determine the severity of the lesion and appropriate medical management as needed. Aortic stenosis increases the risk of perioperative mortality (23) and nonfatal MI by fivefold regardless of the presence of other revised cardiac risk index criteria. The need for bacterial endocarditis prophylaxis should be kept in mind for individuals undergoing most major procedures. Cardiac conditions and surgical procedures, along with recommended prophylactic antibiotic regimens, are outlined in Table 6.8 (24).

## BETA-BLOCKERS AND REDUCTION OF CARDIAC EVENTS

Several trials examine the use of β-blockers to reduce perioperative cardiac morbidity and mortality. Auerbach and Goldman (25) reviewed six publications, including five randomized trials studying the effectiveness of β-blockade in reducing perioperative myocardial ischemia and cardiac or all-cause mortality. The studies used different agents and dosing schedules, but they all administered a β-blocker before the induction of anesthesia and continued β-blockade throughout the intraoperative and postoperative period. All studies except one titrated the dose to a target heart rate of less than 80 bpm. The number of patients needed to treat to prevent cardiac death or nonfatal MI with β-blocker therapy were very favorable, ranging from 2.5 to 8.3 for up to 2 years of follow-up (25). Despite the evidence

**TABLE 6.8**

**RECOMMENDED PROPHYLACTIC ANTIBIOTIC REGIMENS***

| Patient | Regimen |
|---|---|
| Standard | Amoxicillin 2.0 g orally 1 h before procedure or |
| | Ampicillin 2.0 g IM or IV within 30 min before procedure |
| Patients allergic to penicillin | Clindamycin 600 mg orally 1 h before procedure or |
| | Cephalexin or cefadroxil 2.0 g orally 1 h before procedure or |
| | Azithromycin or clarithromycin 500 mg orally 1 h before procedure or |
| | Clindamycin 600 mg IV within 30 min before procedure or |
| | Cefazolin 1.0 g within 30 min before procedure |
| High-risk patients | Ampicillin 2.0 g IM or IV plus gentamicin 1.5 mg/kg IV or IM patients to exceed 120 mg) within 30 min of starting procedure and |
| | Ampicillin 1.0 g IM or IV or amoxicillin 1 g orally 6 h later |
| High-risk patients allergic to penicillin | Vancomycin 1.0 g IV over 1–2 h plus gentamicin 1.5 mg/kg (not to exceed 120 mg) IV or IM; complete injection/infusion within 30 min of starting procedure |
| Moderate-risk patients | Amoxicillin 2.0 g orally 1 h before procedure or |
| | Ampicillin 2.0 g IM or IV within 30 min of starting procedure |
| Moderate-risk patients allergic to penicillin | Vancomycin 1.0 g IV over 1–2 h; complete infusion within 30 min of starting procedure |

**Cardiac Conditions and Surgical Procedures in Which Endocarditis Prophylaxis Is Recommended**

| Cardiac Conditions | Surgical Procedures |
|---|---|
| High risk | Respiratory tract |
| Prosthetic heart valves | Tonsillectomy or adenoidectomy |
| Previous bacterial endocarditis | Rigid bronchoscopy |
| Complex cyanotic congenital heart disease | Surgical operations involving the respiratory mucosa |
| Surgically constructed pulmonary shunts or conduits | Gastrointestinal tract |
| | Sclerotherapy |
| Moderate risk | Esophageal stricture dilation |
| Other congenital heart lesions | Endoscopic retrograde cholangiography with biliary obstruction |
| Acquired valvular dysfunction | Surgical operations involving the intestinal mucosa |
| Hypertrophic cardiomyopathy | Biliary-tract surgery |
| Mitral-valve prolapse with regurgitation or thickened leaflets | Genitourinary tract |
| | Prostate surgery |
| | Cystoscopy |
| | Urethral dilation |

(* Adapted with permission from Dajani AS, et al. Prevention of bacterial endocarditis. Recommendations by the American Heart Association. *JAMA* 1997;277:1797.)

supporting the beneficial effects, some physicians remain concerned about the side-effects of β-blockers and underutilize these drugs in the perioperative setting. All the studies used β–1 selective agents; no evidence shows an advantage of one selective agent over another, thereby suggesting that the efficacy of β-blockade is a class effect and not drug dependent. Table 6.9 shows which patients are candidates for β-blockade; we believe all patients who fit these criteria should receive β-blockade perioperatively, unless they have an absolute contraindication.

## POSTOPERATIVE PULMONARY COMPLICATIONS

Postoperative pulmonary complications (PPC) may include atelectasis, infection (tracheobronchitis or pneumonia), acute respiratory failure requiring mechanical ventilation, acute exacerbation of underlying lung disease, and bronchospasm. The frequency of these complications is higher than that of cardiovascular complications. Risk factors for PPC include smoking, poor exercise tolerance, chronic obstructive pulmonary disease (COPD), surgical site (the risk of PPC increases as the incision approaches the diaphragm), surgery duration greater than 3 hours, general anesthesia, and intraoperative pancuronium use (26). Most pulmonary complications are the result of an alteration of normal pulmonary physiology. Postoperative pain may cause splinting, and the residual effects of anesthesia and narcotics may impair cough and the mucociliary clearance of respiratory secretions. In addition, altered pulmonary mechanics and altered pattern of breathing postoperatively may lead to a PPC.

Preoperative pulmonary risk-reduction strategies (26) include:

■ Encouraging patients to stop smoking for at least 8 weeks before surgery. Practically, this may not be

**TABLE 6.9**

**ELIGIBILITY CRITERIA FOR USE OF PERIOPERATIVE β-BLOCKERS***

Minor Clinical Criteria [Adapted from Mangano et al. (45).]
Use β-blockers in patients meeting any two of the following criteria:
- Aged 65 years or older
- Hypertension
- Current smoker
- Serum cholesterol concentration at least 240 mg/dL
- Diabetes mellitus not requiring insulin therapy

*or*

Major Clinical Criteria [Adapted from Lee et al. (15).]
Use β-blockers in patients meeting any one of the following criteria:
- High risk surgery
- Ischemic heart disease
- Cerebrovascular disease
- Diabetes mellitus on insulin therapy
- Chronic renal insufficiency with Cr >2.0 mg/dL

(* Adapted with permission from Auerbach, et al. Beta-blockers and reduction of cardiac events in noncardiac surgery: clinical applications beta-blockers and reduction of cardiac events in noncardiac surgery: scientific review [comment]. *JAMA* 2002;287(11):1435–1444.)

possible because patients undergo a preoperative evaluation only a few weeks prior to surgery.
- Treating airflow obstruction with β-agonists and steroids in patients with COPD or asthma.
- Using antibiotics and delaying surgery for about 6 weeks if upper respiratory or pulmonary infection is present.
- Educating patients preoperatively regarding lung-expansion exercises.
- Educating patients postoperatively regarding the techniques and use of incentive spirometry.

## PREOPERATIVE PULMONARY TESTING

In general, no single test or combination of tests will predict pulmonary complications reliably. A preoperative history should focus on exercise tolerance, chronic cough, or unexplained dyspnea. Preoperative pulmonary function tests (PFTs) are not useful for noncardiothoracic surgery except in cases where there is a significant smoking history, unexplained dyspnea, or uncharacterized lung disease, in which case preoperative PFTs may help provide a diagnosis or evaluate the degree of impairment. Forced expiratory volume vital capacity in 1 second ($FEV_1$) remains a good indicator of surgical risk. If the $FEV_1$ is greater than 2 L, the risk of complications is low. An $FEV_1$ less than 1 L is associated with a high risk of pulmonary complications or prolonged ventilation, whereas patients with an $FEV_1$ between 1 and 2 L have a moderately elevated risk that must be weighed against the need for the procedure.

The following are the ACP guidelines for situations in which preoperative spirometry is indicated (27):

- Lung resection
- Coronary artery bypass surgery (CABG) and smoking history or dyspnea
- Upper abdominal surgery and smoking history or dyspnea
- Lower abdominal surgery and uncharacterized pulmonary disease, particularly if the surgery will be prolonged or extensive
- Other surgery and uncharacterized pulmonary disease, particularly in those who might require strenuous postoperative rehabilitation programs

Arterial blood gases are generally not indicated preoperatively except perhaps in patients planned for lung resection or in patients with underlying lung disease or risk for lung disease who have dyspnea. Small case series have asserted that a partial pressure of carbon dioxide ($PaCO_2$) greater than 45 mm Hg suggests a limited pulmonary reserve and an increased risk for postoperative pulmonary complications. Clinicians should not use arterial blood gas analyses to delay surgery (26), however.

Perhaps the most comprehensive risk index is that developed by Arozullah et al. (28). This multifactorial risk index for postoperative respiratory failure was derived and validated from a large Veterans Affairs (VA) database. The factors in this index are listed in Table 6.10. The total points are added to develop a risk score, and patients are assigned to Classes 1 through 5. Patients in Class 1 are at significantly lower risk for respiratory failure than patients in Class 5. The type of surgery, emergency surgery, and metabolic factors play a large role in predicting postoperative respiratory failure. In addition to developing an index to assess the risk of postoperative respiratory failure, Arozullah has also developed a similar index to assess the risk for postoperative pneumonia. The type of surgery, age, and functional status appear to be the most predictive factors for postoperative pneumonia.

In general, a careful history and physical examination is key in identifying potential postoperative pulmonary complications. Lung expansion maneuvers, including deep breathing and incentive spirometry, are the mainstays in the postoperative prevention of pulmonary complications. Medical optimization of COPD and asthma will reduce the risk of postoperative complications significantly.

## DIABETES MELLITUS

Advances in surgical management mean that patients have shorter preoperative and postoperative hospital stays, thus increasing the challenge of the perioperative management of patients with diabetes mellitus. The patient with diabetes carries a cardiac event risk that is equivalent to the nondiabetic patient with known ischemic heart disease. An evaluation of the patient with diabetes must include the careful assessment of long-term complications, particularly those renal, cardiovascular, and neuropathic complications that

**TABLE 6.10**
**RESPIRATORY FAILURE RISK INDEX***

| Preoperative Predictor | Point Value |
| --- | --- |
| Type of surgery | |
| Abdominal aortic aneurysm | 27 |
| Thoracic | 21 |
| Neurosurgery, upper abdominal, or peripheral vascular | 14 |
| Neck | 11 |
| Emergency surgery | 11 |
| Albumin 3 mg/dL | 9 |
| Blood urea nitrogen >30 mg/dL | 8 |
| Partially or fully dependent functional status | 7 |
| History of chronic obstructive pulmonary disease | 6 |
| Age years | |
| >70 | 6 |
| 60–69 | 4 |

| Class | Points | N (%) | Rate of Respiratory Failure (%) |
| --- | --- | --- | --- |
| 1 | ≤10 | 48% | 0.5 |
| 2 | 11–19 | 23% | 2.1 |
| 3 | 20–27 | 17% | 5.3 |
| 4 | 28–40 | 10% | 11.9 |
| 5 | >40 | 2% | 30.9 |

(* Adapted with permission from Arozullah, et al. Multifactorial risk index for predicting postoperative respiratory failure in men after major noncardiac surgery. *Am Surg* 2000;232:242.)

add to overall risk. A key factor in planning the preoperative and intraoperative care of patients with diabetes is a careful coordination of the management with the anesthesiologist. The stress of anesthesia and surgery generally promotes hyperglycemia by increasing the counterregulatory hormones epinephrine, cortisol, glucagon, and growth hormone. It is desirable to maintain intraoperative glucoses in the range of 150 to 200 mg/dL to avoid both hypoglycemia and hyperglycemia. Hyperglycemia above 250 to 300 mg/dL is associated with osmotic diuresis and increased vascular instability. Preoperative glucose levels >300 mg/dL cause an osmotic diuresis, thus complicating volume management. Therefore, surgery usually should be delayed until the fasting glucose is <200 mg/dL. In type 2 diabetes mellitus treated with diet alone, supplemental short-acting insulin is used to maintain glucoses in the therapeutic range if needed. For patients with type 2 diabetes mellitus treated with oral agents, these medications are taken the day before surgery, but held on the morning of surgery. Short-acting intravenous (IV) insulin may be used intraoperatively and in the postoperative period, especially with major surgery or in poorly controlled diabetics on oral therapy. Renal function should be monitored in those patients receiving contrast media or having borderline renal insufficiency before restarting metformin after surgery. In those patients with type 1 or type 2 diabetes mellitus using insulin, the timing and expected duration of the procedure and the usual insulin regimen must be considered when planning therapy. For early morning minor procedures, delaying the usual daily therapy until after surgery may be appropriate. If the patient uses insulin, then one-third to one-half of the usual dose is given before the planned surgery for minor procedures. For patients undergoing major surgery, the anesthesiologist monitors glucose control intraoperatively and uses IV insulin (29). Increasing evidence shows the benefit of tight blood sugar control in the postoperative period in reducing complications.

## THYROID DISORDERS

Patients with preexisting hypothyroidism should be questioned as to recent changes in therapy, symptoms of hypothyroidism or hyperthyroidism, and the results of any recent thyroid tests. Newly diagnosed hypothyroid patients do not need to be treated before surgery unless signs of severe hypothyroidism or myxedema are present. It is not essential for patients to take their thyroid replacement on the morning of surgery.

Patients currently under treatment for hyperthyroidism should take their antithyroid drugs on the day of surgery and resume therapy as soon as possible postsurgery because these drugs have a short half-life. Elective surgery should be postponed until hyperthyroid patients become euthyroid because of the mortality associated with "thyroid storm." Patients with hyperthyroidism or severe hypothyroidism

**TABLE 6.11**

## RECOMMENDED PERIOPERATIVE HYDROCORTISONE DOSAGE FOR PATIENTS ON LONG-TERM STEROID THERAPY[†]

| Surgery Type | Stress Dose | Duration* |
|---|---|---|
| Minor (e.g., inguinal herniorrhaphy) | 25 mg/day | 1 day |
| Moderate (e.g., total joint replacement) | 50–75 mg/day | 1–2 days |
| Major (e.g., cardiopulmonary bypass) | 100–150 mg/day | 2–3 days |

* In the absence of complications.
([†] Reproduced with permission from Shaw, M. When is perioperative steroid coverage necessary? *Cleveland Clin J Med* 2002;69(1):9–11.)

should be managed in conjunction with an endocrinologist preoperatively and perhaps perioperatively.

## CHRONIC STEROID USE

Patients receiving ≥5 mg of prednisone or its equivalent daily for more than 2 weeks over the last year are at risk for adrenal insufficiency during stress after cessation of steroid therapy. Given the degree of morbidity and mortality associated with adrenal insufficiency, prophylactic glucocorticoid administration is outlined in Table 6.11.

## DELIRIUM RISK

The incidence of postoperative delirium is in the range of 10% to 15% and is associated with higher mortality and poor functional recovery. The costs of care increase substantially when an acute confusional state complicates postoperative recovery. Marcantonio and colleagues (30) developed and validated a clinical prediction rule for the postoperative development of delirium. The findings were confirmed and slightly modified by Litaker et al. (31). Independent correlates of delirium risk included age over 70 years; preexisting cognitive impairment; previous episodes of delirium; self-reported alcohol use; poor functional status; markedly abnormal serum sodium, potassium, or glucose level; noncardiac chest surgery; and aortic abdominal surgery. Assessing risk allows for potential interventions to reduce delirium incidence. In addition to correcting preoperative metabolic abnormalities, the best preventive intervention is to avoid psychotropic drug use and hypoxia perioperatively, and pay careful attention to managing perioperative metabolic abnormalities, particularly in those patients identified as high risk.

## PREOPERATIVE LABORATORY STUDIES

The goals of preoperative testing are to identify and minimize the risk factors for surgery. Potential reasons for ordering preoperative laboratory tests are:

- To detect unsuspected abnormalities that might influence the risk of perioperative morbidity or mortality
- To establish a baseline value for a test that will be monitored or altered after the surgery is complete

Existing literature suggests that 30% to 60% of abnormalities discovered on routine preoperative tests are ignored (32). Given this fact, routine preoperative testing without documentation of abnormalities may actually lead to more medico-legal risk. In general, it is safe to use test results that were performed within the last 4 months and that gave normal results, given that no change has occurred in the patient's clinical status. Macpherson et al. reported that only 0.4% of such tests repeated at the time of surgery were abnormal and could have been predicted by the patient's history (33). Table 6.12 provides some evidence-based recommendations for laboratory testing before elective surgery.

## MANAGEMENT OF MEDICATIONS

Few controlled trials have been performed on the safety of drugs in the perioperative period. Therefore, the recommendations on which medications to stop or continue during this time are based on expert consensus, case reports, in vitro studies, manufacturer's recommendations in the package insert, and on known information such as the drug's pharmacokinetics, known effects, known perioperative risks, and possible interactions with anesthetic agents (34). In addition, it is key to take a detailed history to include not only prescribed medications but over-the-counter medications, vitamins, and herbal supplements. A recent review found that one-third of the presurgical population took a herbal medication and concluded that physicians should explicitly elicit and document a history of herbal medication and be aware of the potentially serious perioperative problems associated with the continued use of herbals (35). The potentially harmful perioperative effects of some herbs include excessive bleeding, sedation, and even hypoglycemia. As a general rule, we recommend that all herbal remedies and vitamins be stopped 14 days prior to surgery.

Aspirin irreversibly inhibits platelet cyclooxygenase and should be discontinued 7 to 10 days before surgery to allow the replacement of the circulating platelet pool. In patients undergoing CABG, a prospective study showed that continuing aspirin leads to increased postoperative bleeding (36).

Nonsteroidal anti-inflammatory drugs (NSAIDs) reversibly inhibit platelet cyclooxygenase. Most NSAIDs can be stopped 3 to 5 days before surgery, except for some

| TABLE 6.12 |
|---|

## RECOMMENDATIONS FOR LABORATORY TESTING BEFORE ELECTIVE SURGERY

| Test | Incidence of Abnormalities Influencing Management | Indications |
|---|---|---|
| Hemoglobin | 0.1 % | Anticipated major blood loss or symptoms of anemia |
| White blood cell count | 0.0 % | Symptoms suggest infection, myeloproliferative disorder, or myelotoxic medications |
| Platelet count | 0.0 % | History of bleeding diathesis, myeloproliferative disorder, or myelotoxic medications |
| Prothrombin time | 0.0 % | History of bleeding diathesis, chronic liver disease, malnutrition, recent or long-term antibiotic use |
| Partial thromboplastin time | 0.1 % | History of bleeding diathesis |
| Electrolytes | 1.8 % | Known renal insufficiency, congestive heart failure, medications that affect electrolytes |
| Renal function | 2.6 % | Age >50 years, hypertension, cardiac disease, major surgery, medications that may affect renal function |
| Glucose | 0.5 % | Obesity or known diabetes |
| Liver function tests | 0.1 % | No indication. Consider albumin measurement for major surgery or chronic illness |
| Urinalysis | 1.4 % | No indication |
| Electrocardiogram | 2.6 % | Men >40 years, women >50 years, known CAD, diabetes, or hypertension |
| Chest radiograph | 3.0 % | Age >50 years, known cardiac or pulmonary disease, symptoms or examination suggest cardiac or pulmonary disease |

(Adapted with permission from Smetana, GW, et al. The case against routine preoperative laboratory testing. *Med Clin North Am* 2003;87(1):7–40.)
CAD=coronary artery disease.

long-acting drugs such as piroxicam and oxaprozin, which must be stopped 14 days prior to surgery. In vitro studies show no increased risk of bleeding associated with cyclooxygenase-2 inhibitors (COX-2) therefore, theoretically, these can be continued perioperatively. Because all NSAIDs can inhibit renal prostaglandin synthesis, however, they can induce renal failure in combination with other drugs and hypotension. Therefore, it may be best to stop all NSAIDs in patients with underlying renal insufficiency.

Clopidogrel causes irreversible antiplatelet effect by inhibiting the adenosine diphosphate-induced stimulation of platelets. Therefore, it should be discontinued at least 7 days before surgery.

Hormone replacement therapy (HRT) use is associated with a 2.7-fold increased risk of venous thromboembolism (VTE) compared with nonusers (37). The perioperative management of HRT is still controversial, however. Some still recommend stopping HRT about 4 weeks before surgery; however, we recently completed a case-control study that found no association between perioperative HRT use and postoperative VTE in patients undergoing major orthopedic surgery as long as they were receiving pharmacological prophylaxis with either enoxaparin or warfarin postoperatively (38).

Among cardiovascular medications, all forms of nitrates, digoxin, β-blockers, calcium channel blockers, statins and antiarrhythmics can be safely continued, including on the morning of surgery. Diuretics, angiotensin converting enzyme (ACE) inhibitors, and angiotensin receptor antago-

nists (ARBs), however, should be held on the morning of surgery (39,40) due to reports of refractory hypotension.

Pulmonary medications such as theophylline, inhaled β-agonists, ipratropium, and corticosteroids can be continued safely perioperatively. In addition, all antiseizure medications, H2-blockers, and proton pump inhibitors should also be continued perioperatively.

Among the antidepressants, selective serotonin reuptake inhibitors (SSRIs) are safe perioperatively. Monoamine oxidase inhibitors (MAO-I) have a large number of drug interactions and the potential for hypertensive crisis. Tricyclic antidepressants (TCAs) may enhance the action of sympathomimetics. Patients on these last two classes of medications usually have more severe depression, and the potential exists for these patients to have a severe recurrence of depressive symptoms postoperatively, with a concurrent increased risk for suicide. Therefore, in our own practice, we tend to continue all antidepressants but alert anesthesiologists to these medications so that potentially interacting sedatives and or anesthetics can be avoided.

Warfarin is a commonly used anticoagulant. Most patients needing major surgery or invasive procedures require discontinuation of warfarin. It takes approximately 5 days for the antithrombotic effect of warfarin to wear off (41). Therefore, in many patients with preoperative INRs between 2 and 3, warfarin can be discontinued 5 days before surgery. During this time, patients may be at increased risk of thromboembolism. In addition, the discontinuation of oral anticoagulation may be associated with a rebound hypercoagulable state, which has been described but not validated in clinical practice. Surgery also poses an increased risk for the development of VTE. To minimize the risk of thromboembolism, some higher risk patients may require treatment with intravenous (IV) unfractionated heparin (UFH) in the hospital, or as outpatients with subcutaneous (SQ) low-molecular-weight heparin (LMWH) as a bridge to surgery. Patients undergoing minor surgery can be managed using a normogram that adjusts the perioperative dose of warfarin and minimizes the time the patient has a subtherapeutic INR (42). Certain procedures, such as cataract surgery and minor dermatologic and dental procedures, can be performed without stopping or adjusting warfarin dosing. For further reading on this topic of perioperative management of anticoagulation, we refer you to a recent comprehensive review (43).

## VENOUS THROMBOEMBOLISM PREVENTION

The risk of VTE is determined by several factors including the type of surgery, the patient's clinical risk factors for VTE, and the period of perioperative immobilization. The clinical risk factors for VTE include:

- Increasing age
- Prior VTE
- Obesity
- Stroke
- Immobility
- Paralysis
- CHF
- Cancer
- Trauma
- Varicose veins
- Pregnancy

### TABLE 6.13

**CATEGORIES OF RISK FOR VENOUS THROMBOEMBOLISM IN SURGICAL PATIENTS[†]**

Low risk:
Minor surgery in patients <40 years of age with no additional risk factors present*
Moderate risk:
Minor surgery in patients with additional risk factor present*, or non-major surgery in patients aged 40–60 with no additional risk factor, or major surgery in patients <40 with no additional risk factors
High Risk:
Non-major surgery in patients >60 or with additional risk factor present*, or major surgery in patients >40, or with additional risk factor
Highest risk:
Major surgery in patients >40 with additional risk factor present*, or hip or knee arthroplasty, hip fracture surgery, or major trauma, spinal cord injury

---

* Additional risk factors include one or more of the following: advanced age, prior venous thromboembolism, obesity, heart failure, paralysis, or presence of a molecular hypercoagulable state (e.g., protein C deficiency, factor V Leiden).
([†] Adapted with permission from Geerts, WH, et al. Prevention of venous thromboembolism. *Chest* 2001;119:132S.)

- Estrogen use
- Hypercoagulable state (e.g., protein C deficiency, Factor V Leiden)

Table 6.13 outlines a risk stratification scheme put forth for surgical patients by the American College of Chest Physicians (ACCP). The risk categories range from low risk to highest risk. The approximate prevalence of calf deep vein thrombosis (DVT), proximal DVT, and clinical pulmonary embolism (PE) in the absence of prophylaxis is listed for each category of risk in Table 6.14 along with the

### TABLE 6.14

**LEVELS OF VENOUS THROMBOEMBOLISM RISK AND RECOMMENDATIONS FOR PROPHYLAXIS[†]**

| Level of Risk | Calf DVT % | Proximal DVT % | Clinical PE % | Fatal PE % | Prevention Strategies |
|---|---|---|---|---|---|
| Low risk | 2 | 0.4 | 0.2 | 0.002 | No specific measures<br>Aggressive mobilization |
| Moderate risk | 10–20 | 2–4 | 1–2 | 0.1–0.4 | LDUH q12h or LMWH, or ES or IPC |
| High risk | 20–40 | 4–8 | 2–4 | 0.4–1.0 | LDUH q8h or LMWH or IPC |
| Very high risk | 40–80 | 10–20 | 4–10 | 0.2–5 | LMWH or OA,<br>IPC/ES + LDUH/LMWH, or ADH. Consider pharmacologic prophylaxis for extended duration (i.e., up to 30 days) |

LDUH = low dose unfractionated heparin (e.g., UH 5,000 U SQ q12)
LMWH = low molecular weight heparin (e.g., Enoxaparin 40 mg sq qd, Dalteparin 5000 IV/d)
ES = Elastic stocking
IPC = Intermittent pneumatic compression level
OA = Oral anticoagulant (e.g., warfarin with target INR = 2–3)
ADH = Adjusted dose heparin
([†] Adapted with permission from Geerts, WH, et al. Prevention of venous thromboembolism. *Chest* 2001;119:132S.)

suggested prevention strategies. A more detailed discussion is covered in a recent review (44).

# CONCLUSION

Many medical considerations are part of the preoperative evaluation and perioperative management of patients undergoing major noncardiac surgery. Careful attention to risk assessment during the history and examination, optimization of the preoperative medical conditions, institution of evidence-based risk-reduction therapies, and excellent communication with other members of the healthcare team can assist the anesthesiologist and surgeon in delivering the best care to the patient.

# REVIEW EXERCISES

## QUESTIONS

**1.** You are asked to see a 54-year-old man with a 15-year history of non–insulin-dependent diabetes mellitus and hypertension. His medications include glyburide, metformin, and lisinopril. He has mild retinopathy and 300 mg/d of proteinuria. His last laboratory studies 2 weeks ago showed a creatinine of 1.4 mg/dL, total cholesterol of 216 mg/dL, high-density lipoprotein cholesterol 39 mg/dL, low-density lipoprotein cholesterol of 122 mg/dL, triglycerides of 210 mg/dL, and glycosylated hemoglobin of 7.2%. He has no past history of cardiovascular disease and denies current chest pain, palpitations, or dyspnea of exertion. For the past year, he has had limited physical activity due to progressive osteoarthritis of the hip and is scheduled for a total hip replacement in 3 weeks. The surgeon has asked you for advice regarding his perioperative management. On examination, his weight is 220 lb with a body mass index of 32, his BP is 132/84, and his pulse is 84. His funduscopic examination shows mild background retinopathy. His cardiac and pulmonary examinations are normal, while the remainder of his examination is otherwise unremarkable except for mildly diminished dorsalis pedis pulses, and decreased position sense in his toes. His ECG shows nonspecific ST-T wave changes.
As part of his evaluation, you recommend:
a) Ultrasound vascular evaluation of the lower extremities
b) Dipyridamole thallium imaging or dobutamine stress echocardiography
c) No further cardiac testing and proceed with surgery
d) Cardiac catheterization

**2.** As part of his perioperative management, you also recommend:

a) Holding his oral diabetes medications on the day of surgery
b) Maintaining his intraoperative glucose between 150 and 200 mg/dL with regular insulin if necessary
c) Atenolol preoperatively, intraoperatively, and in the postoperative period
d) All of the above

**3.** You are asked to evaluate a 73-year-old man with stable class II angina treated with nitrates and atenolol and no previous MI or CHF. He has mild hypertension controlled on lisinopril and has no history of diabetes. He had moderate exercise capacity (5 MTEs) until he injured his ankle 2 weeks ago. At that time, he was found to have a 5.2-cm abdominal aortic aneurysm. His examination is unremarkable, and his BP is 154/86. His ECG is normal. He is scheduled to undergo abdominal aortic aneurysm repair. You recommend which of the following?
a) Exercise stress test
b) DSE or DTI
c) No further cardiac testing and proceed with surgery
d) Cardiac catheterization

**4.** A 63-year-old man with a past history of angina and three-vessel disease underwent successful CABG surgery 3 years ago. He is now asymptomatic and presents for preoperative evaluation before total knee replacement for severe osteoarthritis. His current medications are simvastatin for controlled hyperlipidemia and one aspirin daily. He does not have diabetes mellitus or a history of MI or CHF. His examination is unremarkable except for knee arthritis, and his BP is 142/85. His ECG shows unchanged chronic, nonspecific ST-T wave changes. You recommend which of the following?
a) Cardiac catheterization
b) DSE or DTI
c) A standard exercise ECG stress test
d) No further testing; proceed with surgery

**5.** You are asked to evaluate a 73-year-old man before planned transurethral resection prostate surgery for benign prostatic hyperplasia. He had an uncomplicated inferior wall MI 4 years ago and has had mild angina only with extreme physical activity. He exercises regularly and takes aspirin daily and rarely uses nitroglycerin. He does not have diabetes and has no history of CHF. A recent ECG stress test was normal until his heart rate reached 150 at peak exercise and 1 mm of ST depression occurred. His examination is normal, and his BP is 160/92. You recommend which of the following?
a) Start intravenous nitroglycerin at the onset of surgery
b) Cancel the surgery and obtain a cardiac catheterization
c) Start atenolol before surgery
d) No further testing; proceed with surgery

**6.** A 48-year-old woman is referred for preoperative evaluation before planned elective laparoscopic chole-cystectomy. She has no prior cardiac history but has had asthma since age 16 years. Her current medications are oral theophylline and inhaled albuterol. She does not smoke and notes no dyspnea on moderate exertion. On examination, her weight is 97 kg (213.4 lb), her height is 163 cm (5 ft, 4 in.), her BP is 144/78, and her pulse is 76 and regular. Her lungs reveal moderate wheezing that does not clear with cough. Her heart is normal, and other than obesity, the remainder of her examination is normal. You recommend which of the following?
a) Add inhaled salbutamol before surgery
b) Add inhaled betamethasone before surgery
c) Reassure her that her risk is low because of the planned laparoscopic approach
d) Cancel the surgery and optimize antiasthma treatment regimen before rescheduling

**7.** A 35-year-old man is referred to you for a preoperative evaluation prior to inguinal hernia repair. He has no prior cardiac history and does not smoke or drink. On exam, he weighs 80 kg (176 lbs), his BP is 140/80, and his pulse is 80. His heart, lungs, and remainder of his examination are normal. You recommend which of the following?
a) Complete metabolic profile (CMP)
b) Complete blood count (CBC)
c) Urine analysis (UA)
d) All of the above
e) None of the above

**8.** A 50-year-old woman with a history of rheumatoid arthritis for about 20 years is scheduled for spine surgery. Her medications include prednisone 10 mg orally per day for the last year, vitamin E, gingko biloba, garlic, and aspirin. Her functional class is limited but she can still climb a flight of stairs with her groceries (>4 METs). She denies history of chest pain, shortness of breath, and prior cardiac problems. Her exam reveals a weight of 60 kg and height of 5 ft 5 inches; her BP is 120/70 mm Hg, and her heart rate is 80. Heart and lung examination are normal. Her neck exam reveals decreased range of motion; extremities reveal deformities consistent with rheumatoid arthritis. You recommend which of the following:
1. Continue Vitamin E, gingko biloba, and garlic because they are natural products
2. Discontinue aspirin 10 days before surgery
3. C-spine films
4. Hydrocortisone 100 mg IV q8h on call to the OR
Select the correct answer:
a) All of the above
b) 2, 3, and 4
c) Only 4
d) 2 and 4

**ANSWERS**

**1. b.**
Using the ACC/AHA guidelines, this patient has intermediate risk predictors (h/o type 2 DM) and is scheduled for an intermediate risk surgery. Because his functional class is poor, with activity at <4 METs, he should undergo further risk stratification with noninvasive testing.

**2. d.**
Stopping oral agents on the day of surgery usually is sufficient to protect against hypoglycemia. The anesthesiologist must monitor glucoses intraoperatively and supplement with short-acting subcutaneous insulin to maintain glucoses in the stated therapeutic range or use intraoperative intravenous insulin for longer procedures. Several studies show that β-blockers decrease the risk of perioperative ischemia and infarct and therefore should be prescribed whenever possible as outlined in Table 6.8.

**3. b.**
Applying the ACC/AHA guidelines to this patient with chronic stable class II angina (intermediate risk predictor) before a high-risk vascular procedure would require that he undergo further risk stratification with a stress test. Exercise ECG is impractical because of his recent ankle injury. Pharmacologic stress testing is the best approach to assess ischemic risk. Even with a negative test result, perioperative β-blockade is recommended.

**4. d.**
His past history of successful CABG 3 years ago and the absence of symptoms keep this patient in the low-risk category. The Coronary Artery Surgery Study showed that successful coronary revascularization returns cardiac risk to near normal levels for several years.

**5. c.**
In similar patients, β-blockers have been shown in randomized clinical trials to reduce the risk of cardiac morbidity and mortality perioperatively and for up to 2 years following surgery in similar patients. The indications for cardiac catheterization are the same as in the nonsurgical population.

**6. d.**
The presence of active wheezing places this patient at greater risk for postoperative pulmonary complications as well as increased bronchospasm during anesthesia induction. The patient should delay surgery until her asthma treatment is optimized. The laparoscopic approach may reduce the risk of pulmonary complications compared with open cholecystectomy, but a level of risk remains because of gaseous peritoneal distention and postoperative pain.

**7. e.**

This patient is completely healthy, and evidence would suggest that ordering routine preoperative blood work would be both unnecessary and costly and not indicated. Table 6.12 reviews in detail the indications for various tests. A screening urine analysis is never indicated unless symptoms suggest that the patient may have an underlying infection.

**8. b.**

Current evidence and consensus would support discontinuing vitamin E, ginkgo biloba, and garlic about 2 weeks prior to surgery because they all increase the risk of bleeding. Aspirin irreversibly inhibits platelet cyclooxygenase and should be stopped 7 to 10 days before surgery. Cervical spine films are indicated in patients with rheumatoid arthritis before they undergo general anesthesia because the presence of severe atlantoaxial disease can cause compromise of the cervical cord during manipulation of the neck during intubation.

## REFERENCES

1. National Center for Health Statistics: Advance Data No. 301, August 31, 1998.
2. Centers for Disease Control and Prevention: CDC Fact Book, 2001–2002.
3. Polanczyk CA, Marcantonio E, Goldman L, et al. Impact of age on perioperative complications and length of stay in patients undergoing noncardiac surgery. *Ann Intern Med* 2001;134:637–643.
4. Wallace A, Layug B, Tateo I, et al. Prophylactic atenolol reduces postoperative myocardial ischemia. McSPI Research Group. *Anesthesiology* 1998;88:7–17.
5. Eagle KA, Berger PB, Calkins H, et al. ACC/AHA guideline update for perioperative cardiovascular evaluation for noncardiac surgery—executive summary. A report of the American College of Cardiology/American Heart Association Task Force on Practice Guidelines. Committee to Update the 1996 Guidelines on Perioperative Cardiovascular Evaluation for Noncardiac Surgery. *Circulation* 2002;105:1257–1267.
6. Cohen MM, Duncan PG, Tate RB. Does anesthesia contribute to operative mortality?[See comment.] *JAMA* 1988;260:2859–2863.
7. Kroenke K. Preoperative evaluation: the assessment and management of surgical risk. *J Gen Intern Med* 1987;2:257–269.
8. Rodgers A, Walker N, Schug S, et al. Reduction of postoperative mortality and morbidity with epidural or spinal anaesthesia: results from overview of randomised trials. *BMJ* 2000;321:1493.
9. Goldman L, Caldera DL, Nussbaum SR, et al. Multifactorial index of cardiac risk in noncardiac surgical procedures. *N Engl J Med* 1977;297:845–850.
10. Mangano DT, Goldman L. Preoperative assessment of patients with known or suspected coronary disease. *N Engl J Med* 1995; 333:1750–1756.
11. Eagle KA, Coley CM, Newell JB, et al. Combining clinical and thallium data optimizes preoperative assessment of cardiac risk before major vascular surgery. *Ann Intern Med* 1989;110:859–866.
12. Vanzetto G, Machecourt J, Blendea D, et al. Additive value of thallium single-photon emission computed tomography myocardial imaging for prediction of perioperative events in clinically selected high cardiac risk patients having abdominal aortic surgery. *Am J Cardiol* 1996;77:143–148.
13. Detsky AS, Abrams HB, Forbath N, et al. Cardiac assessment for patients undergoing noncardiac surgery. A multifactorial clinical risk index. *Arch Intern Med* 1986;146:2131–2134.
14. Palda VA, Detsky AS. Perioperative assessment and management of risk from coronary artery disease. *Ann Intern Med* 1997;127: 313–328.
15. Lee TH, Marcantonio ER, Mangione CM, et al. Derivation and prospective validation of a simple index for prediction of cardiac risk of major noncardiac surgery. *Circulation* 1999;100:1043–1049.
16. Gilbert K, Larocgue BJ, Patrick LT. Prospective evaluation of cardiac risk indices for patients undergoing noncardiac surgery. [comment]. *Annals of Internal Med* 2000;133:356–359.
17. Reilly DF, McNeely MJ, Doerner D, et al. Self-reported exercise tolerance and the risk of serious perioperative complications. *Arch Intern Med* 1999;159:2185–2192.
18. Hlatky MA, Boineau RE, Higginbotham MB, et al. A brief self-administered questionnaire to determine functional capacity (the Duke Activity Status Index). *Am J Cardiol* 1989;64:651–654.
19. Poldermans D, Arnese M, Fioretti PM, et al. Improved cardiac risk stratification in major vascular surgery with dobutamine-atropine stress echocardiography. *J Am Coll Cardiol* 1995;26: 648–653.
20. Kertai MD, Boersma E, Bax JJ, et al. A meta-analysis comparing the prognostic accuracy of six diagnostic tests for predicting perioperative cardiac risk in patients undergoing major vascular surgery. *Heart* 2003;89:1327–1334.
21. Eagle KA. ACC/AHA guideline update for perioperative cardiovascular evaluation for noncardiac surgery—executive summary. A report of the American College of Cardiology/American Heart Association Task Force on Practice Guidelines. Committee to Update the 1996 Guidelines on Perioperative Cardiovascular Evaluation for Noncardiac Surgery [comment]. *Anesth Analg* 2002; 94:1378–1379.
22. Palda VA, Detsky AS. Perioperative assessment and management of risk from coronary artery disease. *Ann Intern Med* 1997;127: 313–328.
23. Kertai MD, Bountioukos M, Boersma E, et al. Aortic stenosis: an underestimated risk factor for perioperative complications in patients undergoing noncardiac surgery. *Am J Med* 2004;116: 8–13.
24. Dajani AS, Taubert KA, Wilson W, et al. Prevention of bacterial endocarditis. Recommendations by the American Heart Association. *JAMA* 1997;277:1794–1801.
25. Auerbach AD, Goldman L. Beta-Blockers and reduction of cardiac events in noncardiac surgery: scientific review [comment]. *JAMA* 2002;287:1435–1444.
26. Smetana GW. Preoperative pulmonary evaluation. *N Engl J Med* 1999;340:937–944.
27. American College of Physicians. Preoperative pulmonary function testing. *Ann Intern Med* 1990;112:793–794.
28. Arozullah AM, Daly J, Henderson WG, Kituri SF. Multifactorial risk index for predicting postoperative respiratory failure in men after major noncardiac surgery. *Annals of Surgery* 2000; 232:242–253.
29. Schiff RL, Welsh GA. Perioperative evaluation and management of the patient with endocrine dysfunction. *Med Clin North Am* 2003; 87:175–192.
30. Marcantonio ER, Goldman L, Mangione CM, et al. A clinical prediction rule for delirium after elective noncardiac surgery. *JAMA* 1994;271:134–139.
31. Litaker D, Locala J, Franco K, et al. Preoperative risk factors for postoperative delirium. *Gen Hosp Psychiatry* 2001; 23:84–89.
32. Roizen MF. More preoperative assessment by physicians and less by laboratory tests. *N Engl J Med* 2000;342:204–205.
33. Macpherson DS, Litaker D. Preoperative screening. *Med Clin North Am* 2003;87:7–40.
34. Spell NO, 3rd. Stopping and restarting medications in the perioperative period. *Med Clin North Am* 2001;85:1117–1128.
35. Ang-Lee MK, Moss J, Yuan CS. Herbal medicines and perioperative care. *JAMA* 2001;286:208–216.
36. Taggart DP, Siddiqui A, Wheatley DJ. Low-dose preoperative aspirin therapy, postoperative blood loss, and transfusion requirements. *Ann Thorac Surg* 1990;50:424–428.
37. Grady D, Wenger NK, Herrington D, et al. Postmenopausal hormone therapy increases risk for venous thromboembolic disease. The Heart and Estrogen/Progestin Replacement Study. *Ann Intern Med* 2000;132:689–696.

38. Hurbanek JG, Jaffer A, Morra N, Brotman DJ. Postmenopausal hormone replacement therapy and venous thromboembolism following orthopedic surgery. *Thromb Haemost* 2004;92:337–343.

39. Brabant SM, Bertrand M, Eyraud D, et al. The hemodynamic effects of anesthetic induction in vascular surgical patients chronically treated with angiotensin II receptor antagonists. *Anesth Analg* 1999;89:1388–1392.

40. Coriat P, Richer C, Douraki T, et al. Influence of chronic angiotensin-converting enzyme inhibition on anesthetic induction. *Anesthesiology* 1994;81:299–307.

41. White RH, McKittrick T, Hutchinson R, Twitchell J. Temporary discontinuation of warfarin therapy: changes in the international normalized ratio. *Ann Intern Med* 1995;122:40–42.

42. Marietta M, Bertesi M, Simoni L, et al. A simple and safe nomogram for the management of oral anticoagulation prior to minor surgery. *Clin Lab Haematol* 2003;25:127–130.

43. Jaffer AK, Brotman DJ, Chukwumerije N. When patients on warfarin need surgery. *Cleve Clin J Med* 2003;70:973–984.

44. Kaboli P, Henderson MC, White RH. DVT prophylaxis and anticoagulation in the surgical patient. *Med Clin North Am* 2003;87:viii, 77–110.

## SUGGESTED READINGS

Arozullah AM, Daly J, Henderson WG, Kituri SF. Multifactorial risk index for predicting postoperative respiratory failure in men after major noncardiac surgery. *Annals of Surgery* 2000;232: 242–253.

Auerbach AD, Goldman L. Beta-blockers and reduction of cardiac events in noncardiac surgery: scientific review [comment]. *JAMA* 2002;287:1435–1444.

Cohn SL. The role of the medical consultant. *Med Clin North Am* 2003;87:1–6.

Dajani AS, Taubert KA, Wilson W, et al. Prevention of bacterial endocarditis. Recommendations by the American Heart Association. *JAMA* 1997;277:1794–1801.

Eagle KA, Berger PB, Calkins H, et al. ACC/AHA guideline update for perioperative cardiovascular evaluation for noncardiac surgery—executive summary. A report of the American College of Cardiology/American Heart Association Task Force on Practice Guidelines. Committee to Update the 1996 Guidelines on Perioperative Cardiovascular Evaluation for Noncardiac Surgery. *Circulation* 2002;105:1257–1267.

Hlatky MA, Boineau RE, Higginbotham MB, et al. A brief self-administered questionnaire to determine functional capacity (the Duke Activity Status Index). *Am J Cardiol* 1989;64:651–654.

Jaffer AK, Brotman DJ, Chukwumerije N. When patients on warfarin need surgery. *Cleve Clin J Med* 2003;70:973–984.

Kaboli P, Henderson MC, White RH. DVT prophylaxis and anticoagulation in the surgical patient. *Med Clin North Am* 2003;87:viii, 77–110.

Kertai MD, Boersma E, Bax JJ, et al. A meta-analysis comparing the prognostic accuracy of six diagnostic tests for predicting perioperative cardiac risk in patients undergoing major vascular surgery. *Heart* 2003;89:1327–1334.

Kroenke K. Preoperative evaluation: the assessment and management of surgical risk. *J Gen Intern Med* 1987;2:257–269.

Lee TH, Marcantonio ER, Mangione CM, et al. Derivation and prospective validation of a simple index for prediction of cardiac risk of major noncardiac surgery. *Circulation* 1999;100:1043–1049.

Mangano DT, Layug EL, Wallace A, Tateo I. Effect of atenolol on mortality and cardiovascular morbidity after noncardiac surgery. Multicenter Study of Perioperative Ischemia Research Group. *N Engl J Med* 1996;335:1713–1720.

Mukherjee D, Eagle KA. Perioperative cardiac assessment for noncardiac surgery: eight steps to the best possible outcome. *Circulation* 2003;107:2771–2774.

Palda VA, Detsky AS. Perioperative assessment and management of risk from coronary artery disease. *Ann Intern Med* 1997;127:313–328.

Schiff RL, Welsh GA. Perioperative evaluation and management of the patient with endocrine dysfunction. *Med Clin North Am* 2003;87: 175–192.

Smetana GW, Macpherson DS. The case against routine preoperative laboratory testing. *Med Clin North Am* 2003; 87:7–40.

Smetana GW. Preoperative pulmonary evaluation. *N Engl J Med* 1999; 340:937–944.

Spell NO, 3rd. Stopping and restarting medications in the perioperative period. *Med Clin North Am* 2001;85:1117–1128.

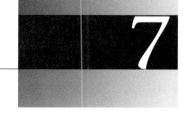

# Geriatric Medicine

*Robert M. Palmer*

The aging process predisposes elderly patients to homeostatic failure, chronic disease, and functional decline (i.e., a loss of independence in performing daily activities). Illness often manifests as a *geriatric syndrome*, a clinical problem with a wide array of etiologies and complex pathophysiology. Included among these geriatric syndromes are cognitive dysfunction (altered mental status), falls, and urinary incontinence.

These syndromes, which increase in frequency and importance in advanced age (older than 75 years), are frequently encountered by internists in ambulatory, hospital, and long-term care settings. These common problems often are left undiagnosed or untreated, resulting in a loss of quality of life for older patients. Through careful assessment, however, internists can detect, prevent, and manage effectively these common problems of old age.

## COGNITIVE DYSFUNCTION: DELIRIUM

The common causes of cognitive dysfunction in elderly patients are dementia, delirium, and depression. (Dementia and depression are discussed in Chapter 10, but key points are included here.) Delirium (acute confusion) is an organic mental syndrome characterized by:

- A reduced ability to maintain or shift attention
- Disorganized thinking
- An altered level of consciousness
- Perceptual disturbances
- Increased or decreased psychomotor activity
- Disturbances of the sleep–wake cycle
- Disorientation to time, place, or person
- Memory impairments

Typically, the disturbance in cognition develops over a short period (hours to days) and fluctuates throughout the day. Delirium occurring in hospitalized elderly patients often goes undetected or is misdiagnosed as dementia, depression, functional psychosis, or personality disorder. The sequelae of delirium include prolonged length of hospitalization, higher costs of care, and a greater risk of institutionalization and mortality, all underscoring the importance of early detection, a search for likely etiologies, and appropriate therapeutic interventions designed to prevent or rapidly resolve the syndrome of delirium.

## Etiology

Virtually any acute physical stress can precipitate delirium in vulnerable patients. Delirium is most commonly associated with:

- Infection (e.g., urosepsis or pneumonia)
- Hypoxemia
- Hypotension
- Psychoactive medications (e.g., narcotics or benzodiazepines)
- Anticholinergic medications

Other causes of delirium include:

- Alcohol withdrawal or intoxication
- Partial complex seizures
- Stroke
- Uremia
- Electrolyte disorders (e.g., hyponatremia)

Drugs are common, but preventable, causes of delirium. Many antiarrhythmics, tricyclic antidepressants, neuroleptics, analgesics, and gastrointestinal medications can induce delirium in elderly patients. One common characteristic of many of these agents is their central anticholinergic effect. Some medications to avoid prescribing to elderly patients, and their alternatives, are shown in Table 7.1.

## Epidemiology

Delirium occurs primarily in patients who are acutely ill or hospitalized. Among medically ill hospitalized elderly

### TABLE 7.1
### MEDICATIONS TO AVOID IN ELDERLY PATIENTS: REASONS, EXAMPLES, AND ALTERNATIVES

**Antihistamines**

Reasons: Confusion (delirium), oversedation, orthostatic hypotension, falls, constipation, and urinary retention due to anticholinergic effects

Examples: diphenhydramine; hydroxyzine

Alternatives: *Hypnotics*: temazepam 7.5 mg hs; zolpidem 5 mg hs; trazodone 50 mg hs
*Nonsedating antihistamines*: loratadine 10 mg daily; fexofenadine 60 mg daily or bid

**Benzodiazepines**

Reasons: Confusion, sedation, and falls

Examples: diazepam; chlordiazepoxide

Alternatives: *Anxiety or withdrawal*: lorazepam 0.5–1 mg q6h prn; oxazepam 10 mg q6h prn
*Agitation/psychosis*: haloperidol 0.5–2 mg bid or tid; risperidone 0.5 mg bid

**Tricyclic Antidepressants**

Reasons: Confusion, oversedation, orthostatic hypotension, falls, constipation, and urinary retention due to anticholinergic effects

Examples: amitriptyline; imipramine; doxepin

Alternatives: *Neuropathic pain*: desipramine 10–20 mg daily; nortriptyline 10–25 mg daily

**Antiemetics**

Reasons: Confusion, oversedation, orthostatic hypotension, falls, constipation, and urinary retention due to anticholinergic effects

Examples: trimethobenzamide (a low potency antiemetic, highly anticholinergic)

Alternatives: promethazine 12.5 mg q6h prn; prochlorperazine 5 mg q6h prn

**Narcotic Analgesics**

Reasons: Meperidine—confusion, oversedation, orthostatic hypotension, falls, constipation, and urinary retention due to anticholinergic effects; metabolite may produce agitation and seizures; short duration of analgesia. Propoxyphene—poor analgesic effect with usual opioid anticholinergic effects

Examples: meperidine; propoxyphene

Alternatives: Acetaminophen—provides analgesia equivalent to propoxyphene; add codeine or oxycodone if pain relief is inadequate; oxycodone 2.5 mg q4–6h; morphine—initially low doses (e.g., 2–4 mg q3–4h) suffice

patients, the prevalence of delirium at admission is 10% to 15%; the incidence is 10% to 15% during hospitalization. Postoperative delirium occurs in 10% to 15% of general surgical patients and in 30% to 50% of patients admitted to the hospital with hip fractures or to undergo knee surgery.

The risk factors for incident delirium were elucidated in prospective cohort studies. Independent risk factors for delirium in elderly patients admitted to the hospital include:

- Dementia
- Fever
- Use of psychoactive drugs
- Azotemia
- Fracture
- Abnormal serum sodium (dehydration)

Dementia is the major risk factor for delirium, increasing the risk nearly threefold. Other medical conditions that are often associated with delirium include prolonged sleep deprivation, sensory impairments (vision and hearing), and changes in environment.

Delirium that occurs in the hospital in high-risk patients is precipitated by factors that are potentially amenable to medical interventions or change in therapies. In one study, five independent precipitating or antecedent factors for delirium in the hospital were identified:

- Use of physical restraints
- Malnutrition
- More than three added medications
- Use of a bladder catheter
- Any iatrogenic event (e.g., unintentional injury or pressure ulcer)
- Pathophysiology

The pathophysiology of delirium remains poorly understood. Patients with risk factors for delirium are regarded as vulnerable, based on the hypothetical assumption of limited homeostatic (brain) reserves. For a high-risk patient, even a minor insult such as fever can precipitate delirium. A metabolic derangement with disturbances in neurotransmitter activity likely accounts for the cognitive features of delirium. For example, delirium can be induced by centrally acting anticholinergic drugs. In hepatic encephalopathy, the presence of delirium correlates with the accumulation of toxic metabolites (e.g., ammonia). In other patients, lymphokines, interleukin-1 and interleukin-2, are associated with delirium.

## Clinical Presentation

An acute change in mental status with disturbed consciousness, impaired cognition, and fluctuating course is characteristic of delirium. A reduced ability to focus, sustain, or shift attention is evident and accounts for the behavioral manifestations of incoherent or tangential speech and disorganized or erratic thought processes. Perceptual disturbances (misperceptions), illusions, or delusions and hallucinations are common, particularly in patients with increased psychomotor activity. Most often, delirium presents as a "quiet confusion" in acutely ill patients, although extremes in behavior and cognition may occur throughout the day. Delirium is often the initial symptom or a common presentation of many acute illnesses.

## Diagnosis

The diagnostic evaluation of a patient with detected delirium is driven by a search for the most probable etiologies and the need to exclude life-threatening diseases. In many cases, the etiology seems obvious (e.g., urosepsis), but vigilance is needed to exclude other possible causes (e.g., hypoxemia) that may contribute to the delirium.

Rarely is an extensive laboratory evaluation needed. Because infection is so frequently the precipitant of delirium, a complete blood count and blood chemistry panel is usually obtained. In select cases (e.g., fever, hypotension), blood and urine cultures are warranted; likewise, chest films, electrocardiography, arterial blood gases, lumbar puncture, head neuroimaging, or electroencephalography may be useful.

## Screening

Even subtle cases of delirium can be detected through careful observation of the patient (e.g., change in cognition, reasoning, or alertness) and the use of screening instruments, such as the digit span test and the confusion assessment method. With the digit span test, patients are asked to repeat a random list of numbers that are stated in a monotone at 1-second intervals. Typically, healthy patients can correctly repeat five or more of these numbers in correct order, whereas delirious patients repeat fewer than five numbers. With the confusion assessment method, a diagnosis of delirium can be achieved with greater than 90% sensitivity and specificity by documenting a change in mental status characterized by inattention, an acute onset and fluctuating course, and either or both disorganized thinking or an altered level of consciousness. Instruments to measure cognitive function (e.g., Mini-Mental State Examination) are often used to quantify the degree of dysfunction or to monitor the patient's response to treatment.

## Differential Diagnoses

Delirium should be distinguished from functional psychosis, depression, and dementia as follows:

- Functional psychosis (e.g., late-onset schizophrenia) is not characterized by impaired attention or fluctuating mental status.
- Depression is suspected in patients who give variable responses or many "I don't know" answers to questions during a mental status examination. A dysphoric mood, irritability, and a withdrawn appearance further suggest the diagnosis. Depressed patients are alert and attentive, although their ability to concentrate may be limited, especially if they are anxious or agitated.
- Although delirium occurs more often in demented patients, clinical features help to distinguish these conditions (Table 7.2).

**TABLE 7.2**
**DELIRIUM VERSUS DEMENTIA**

| Feature | Delirium | Dementia |
|---|---|---|
| Onset | Rapid, often at night | Usually insidious, as in Alzheimer's disease |
| Duration | Hours to weeks (usually transient) | Months to years (persistent) |
| Consciousness | Depressed | Normal |
| Awareness | Always impaired | Usually normal |
| Alertness | Reduced or increased (fluctuates) | Usually normal |
| Attention span | Decreased (less than four digits) | Usually normal (in mild to moderate states) |

## Treatment

### Prevention

Delirium can be prevented in hospitalized elderly patients. A clinical trial of intervention protocols targeted at risk factors for delirium resulted in a 40% reduction in the incidence of delirium. The protocols served to optimize cognitive function (reorientation, therapeutic activities), prevent sleep deprivation (relaxation, noise reduction), avoid immobility (ambulation, exercises), improve vision (visual aids, illumination), improve hearing (hearing devices), and treat dehydration (volume repletion).

### Management

The management of delirium begins with the treatment of the underlying etiologies. Effective nursing and environmental interventions include:

- Continuity of nursing care
- Alternatives to physical restraints (restraints can paradoxically increase patient agitation)
- Correction of sensory impairments (visual and hearing)
- Placement of the patient in a room near the nurses' station for closer observation and greater socialization
- Social visits with a family member, caregiver, or hired sitter
- Promotion of normal sleep cycles through noise control, dim lighting at night, and reality orientation

### Pharmacologic Treatment

No medication has an indication for treating delirium. Medications are considered for treatment of symptoms that disturb the patient or behaviors that threaten to disrupt life-maintaining therapies. Antipsychotic agents (neuroleptics) are considered for the treatment of hallucinations, delusions, or frightening illusions. Haloperidol, 0.5 to 1.0 mg, can be given orally or intramuscularly every 6 to 8 hours as necessary. Higher doses or more frequent intervals are often used in critically ill patients whose heart rhythm and vital signs are continuously monitored, but the long-term safety of high doses of haloperidol is unknown. Anxious or frightened patients and those with drug or alcohol withdrawal should be considered for treatment with lorazepam, 0.5 to

1.0 mg given orally or parenterally every 4 to 6 hours as necessary. Delirious patients in severe pain can be treated with morphine sulfate, 4 to 6 mg (lower doses in very old or frail patients). Repeated doses of meperidine should be avoided because of the neurotoxic effect of its metabolite. Psychotropic medications, however, should be used judiciously and for the shortest time necessary because they can cause paradoxic confusion and increase the risk of falls. Likewise, physical restraints should be avoided in most cases because they can increase patient agitation and the risks of pressure ulcer and physical deconditioning.

## Prognosis

Most episodes of delirium improve rapidly, usually within days of appropriate therapy. Functional and cognitive deficits often persist after discharge from the hospital, however, probably related to the underlying etiology or risk factors for delirium, especially dementia. The patient's mental status should be reevaluated after hospital discharge, and the patient should be monitored for possible dementia.

## FALLS

Accidental falls, defined as "unintentionally coming to rest on the ground, floor, or other lower level," are common and potentially preventable causes of morbidity and mortality in the elderly. Falls account for many serious injuries, including hip fractures and soft tissue trauma. A loss of mobility and fear of falling again are common consequences of a fall and contribute to the patient's inability to live independently. Falls are often attributed to either host (intrinsic) or environmental (extrinsic) predisposing or situational risk factors.

## Etiology

### Epidemiology

The incidence of falls and related injuries increases with advancing age. Falls occur in approximately one-third of community-residing persons 65 years of age and older and in approximately 50% of persons 80 years of age and older. Approximately 5% of falls by community-residing elderly persons result in a fracture. Falling increases the probability of hospitalization, nursing home placement, and death. Approximately 90% of hip fractures in elderly people result from falls.

In prospective studies, significant independent risk factors for falls are sedative use (benzodiazepines), cognitive impairment, disability of the lower extremities, abnormalities of balance and gait, and foot problems. In a cohort study of women over age 65, hip fractures were more common in women with multiple risk factors for falling, a prior history of falls, poor performance on tests of neuromuscular function (e.g., gait speed), and low bone mineral density.

### Clinical Causes

Accidental falls stem from the combination of environmental hazards and the increased susceptibility to falls related to aging or diseases. Accidents, simple slips, or trips are the most common cause of falls occurring in the community-dwelling elderly population, and these occur more often in the presence of environmental hazards. Lower extremity weakness from deconditioning, stroke, and chronic diseases is the second most common cause of gait impairment leading to falls. Syncope accounts for fewer than 3% of falls. Dizziness, vertigo, delirium, postural hypotension, and visual disorders are less frequent causes of falls.

## Pathophysiology

The maintenance of normal balance and gait requires the successful integration of sensory (afferent), central (brain and spinal cord), and musculoskeletal systems. A disturbance in sensory input (e.g., peripheral neuropathy), central nervous system functioning (e.g., dementia), or motor function (e.g., arthritis, muscle weakness) predisposes elderly patients to falls. Weakness of the lower extremity muscles, which is often associated with deconditioning, impairs gait and predisposes the patient to falling in the face of a minor perturbation. The aging process may also predispose patients to falls by increasing postural sway and reducing adaptive reflexes.

## Diagnosis

Patients at risk for falls can be identified with a medical history, brief physical examination, and basic laboratory studies. A review of risk factors, medications (vasodilators, adrenergic blockers, psychotropic agents), and screening instruments (vision, mental status, balance, and gait) helps to identify patients at risk. Observation of the patient's balance and gait identifies patients at risk of falling. The Timed Up and Go (TUG) test is quickly performed and predictive of falling. This test requires a patient to stand up, walk 10 feet, turn, walk back, and sit down. Older adults at risk of falls require longer than 20 seconds to complete this task. As the patient performs this task, postural instability, lower extremity weakness, reduced steppage, increased lateral sway, stride variability, and ataxia can be readily identified and further diagnostic evaluation can be pursued. Further diagnostic assessment is invaluable for patients who have a prolonged TUG or risk factors for recurrent falls. Examination of the patient's vision, gait and balance, lower extremity strength and function, mental status and basic neurological examination are advisable. Often this assessment is completed with the assistance of other health professionals, such as physical therapists. Routinely, elderly patients should be asked about the occurrence of falls since their last office visit.

The diagnostic evaluation of a patient who has fallen is based on the circumstances surrounding the fall. Syncopal falls are evaluated differently from nonsyncopal falls. An ambulatory cardiac monitor is indicated for the patient with syncope, unexplained lightheadedness, or palpitations preceding the fall. With an acute fall, an acute illness should be suspected, as a fall is often the sentinel symptom of underlying disease. A basic chemistry panel could reveal evidence of dehydration or electrolyte disorders; a complete blood count might indicate anemia or an elevated white blood count, implying the presence of an infection. A head computed tomography (CT) scan is indicated if there is evidence from the history or physical examination of head trauma or an acute change in mental status associated with the fall.

## Treatment

The specific causes of falls are easily treated (e.g., syncope owing to complete heart block). More often, however, the intervention to reduce the risk of falls is multifactorial, directed at optimizing the patient's sensory, central, and musculoskeletal systems (Table 7.3).

Clinical trials support the effectiveness of multifactorial interventions. In a trial of community-residing persons 70 years of age and older who had risk factors for falling, a multicomponent intervention reduced the incidence of falls. The intervention included an adjustment of medications, behavioral instructions, and an exercise program (balance exercises, gait training, low-intensity resistive exercises). The patients receiving the intervention had a significant reduction in the numbers of falls in the subsequent year compared with controls. In another clinical trial, an exercise program conducted in home visits by a physiotherapist led to a nearly 50% reduction in the 1-year incidence of falls in women 80 years of age and older. Similar results were seen in a clinical trial involving elderly patients who had sustained a recent fall. A home visit by an occupational therapist (home safety evaluation) resulted in a 39% reduction in the 1-year incidence of recurrent falls. Balance exercises also lower the rate of falls. Tai chi exercises to enhance balance and body awareness reduce the rate of falls in elderly healthy people.

**TABLE 7.3**

**INTERVENTION TO DECREASE THE RISK OF FALLS**

| Risk Factor | Intervention |
|---|---|
| Polypharmacy medication review | Reduce or discontinue doses of psychotropic agents, vasodilators, and adrenergic blockers |
| Lower-extremity weakness, deconditioning | Low-intensity resistive exercises, high-intensity resistance exercises under therapist supervision, tai chi exercises, water-walking exercises, and assistive devices (e.g., cane, walker) |
| Hearing and visual impairment | Hearing aid and corrective lenses |
| Postural hypotension | Reconditioning exercises, graded compression stockings, salt repletion, and medication changes (diuretics, vasodilators) |
| Environmental hazards | Home safety evaluation (rugs, lighting, stairs, handrails, assistive devices) |

The effectiveness of both low-intensity and progressive high-intensity resistive exercise in improving lower extremity strength is well established. Bands, tubes, pulleys, and weight machines have been used under therapist supervision in these studies. Resistance exercises increase the patient's muscle strength and mass.

Other approaches to the prevention of fractures due to falls are effective. The treatment of osteoporosis (calcium and vitamin D supplementation, bisphosphonates) reduces the risk of hip fractures. Hip protectors have been found in some studies to reduce the risk of hip fracture in nursing home patients and in ambulatory frail elderly patients. Compliance with hip protectors is problematic.

The benefit of supplemental vitamin D on falls risk is uncertain. A recent review found that vitamin D supplementation appears to reduce the risk of falls by more than 20% among ambulatory or institutionalized older individuals with stable health.

# URINARY INCONTINENCE

Urinary incontinence is the involuntary loss of urine of sufficient severity to be a social or health problem. Incontinence impairs the quality of life of older patients, is costly to treat, and is a risk factor for institutionalization. Never a consequence of normal aging, urinary incontinence is always treatable and often curable.

## Epidemiology

The prevalence of urinary incontinence in community-residing elderly people increases with advancing age from 5% to 15% in women 65 years of age to more than 25% in men and women 85 years of age and older, and nearly 50% in nursing home residents. Urinary incontinence is strongly associated with impaired cognition and physical function. Medications, fecal impaction, environmental barriers (e.g., lack of bathrooms in close reach), estrogen depletion in women, and pelvic muscle weakness increase the risk of incontinence. The adverse consequences of urinary incontinence include the placement of indwelling urinary catheters, impaired healing of perineal pressure ulcers, and rashes.

## Pathophysiology

Urinary incontinence results from neurologic or anatomic defects that interfere with normal urinary micturition. The urinary bladder is responsible for the storage and emptying of urine. Lesions that interfere with bladder contraction and emptying (e.g., sensory neuropathy) predispose patients to incontinence. Parasympathetic stimulation by the sacral nerves (S2–S4) produces detrusor muscle contractions; disruption of these nerves results in an acontractile bladder. As the bladder fills, the parasympathetic system is inhibited. When intravesical pressure increases (typically with bladder volumes of greater than 250 mL), inhibitory pathways from the frontal lobe are overcome and detrusor contraction is able to exceed urethral resistance to allow urinary flow from the bladder.

The contraction of the detrusor muscle at low bladder-filling volumes (detrusor instability or overactivity) occurs in patients with central nervous system disease (e.g., stroke) or increased sensory stimulation from the bladder (e.g., urinary tract infection, prostatic hyperplasia). Loss of detrusor contractility or bladder outlet obstruction results in a distended bladder; intravesical pressure exceeds urethral resistance and results in incontinence. Incompetence of the internal urethral sphincter (e.g., secondary to pelvic relaxation) allows urine to leak from the bladder during increases in intraabdominal pressure).

## Clinical Presentations

Four basic types of urinary incontinence occur in elderly patients (Table 7.4):

- Stress incontinence
- Urge incontinence
- Overflow incontinence
- Functional incontinence

Stress incontinence is the most common type in women younger than 75 years of age, whereas urge incontinence is the most common type in patients older than 75 years. Stress incontinence results from sphincteric incompetence; urge incontinence results from detrusor overactivity. Overflow incontinence is seen in patients with an acontractile bladder or bladder outlet obstruction. Functional

### TABLE 7.4
### TYPES, CHARACTERISTICS, AND TREATMENT OF URINARY INCONTINENCE

| Type | Characteristics | Cause | Treatment |
|------|-----------------|-------|-----------|
| Stress | Urinary leakage with an increase in intraabdominal pressure (cough, sneeze, physical exertion) | Sphincteric incompetence | Medical: pelvic-muscle exercises, scheduled toileting, α-adrenergic agonists (pseudoephedrine), estrogen (oral, or topical)<br>Surgical: bladder-neck suspension, vaginal sling, and periurethral injections |
| Urge | Urinary urgency and frequency, usually with small to moderate volume of urine | Detrusor overactivity | Bladder retraining (scheduled or prompted voiding) and anticholinergics/bladder relaxants:<br>Oxybutynin, 5–15 mg in divided doses or extended-release form once daily<br>Tolterodine, 2–4 mg divided in two doses or long-acting form once daily |
| Overflow | Incomplete or unsuccessful voiding or continuous dribbling | Outlet obstruction or inability to toilet | Acontractile bladder: intermittent or chronic catheter drainage<br>Obstructed outlet: surgical relief of obstruction |
| Functional | Inability or unwillingness to get to toilet | Physical or cognitive disability | Change treatments (e.g., loop diuretics, restraints), bedside commode or urinal, prompted voiding, and absorbent pads and garments |

incontinence occurs as a consequence of cognitive, physical, psychological, or environmental barriers to urination (e.g., delirious patient in physical restraint). Often two or more clinical types, commonly stress and urge, are present in elderly patients. Patients with polyuric states (e.g., uncontrolled diabetes), gait impairments, and cognitive impairments are particularly likely to have a functional component of incontinence.

## Diagnosis

Urinary incontinence may present as either an acute (*transient*) or chronic (*established*) condition. Acute incontinence typically has a sudden onset and is associated with an acute illness (e.g., infection, delirium) or iatrogenic event (e.g., polypharmacy, restricted mobility). Incontinence may occur in hospitalized patients as a result of delirium, excessive infusions of intravenous fluids, and metabolic disorders such as hyperglycemia with glucosuria. Incontinence is also associated with functional impairments, including cognitive dysfunction and an inability to toilet in time.

The clinical type and most likely cause of established urinary incontinence are often determined by a careful medical history, a brief physical examination, and a few laboratory studies (urinalysis, blood chemistries). The medical history is key to the diagnosis (Table 7.4). Elderly patients should be asked about symptoms of incontinence (e.g., "How often do you lose urine when you don't want to?"). The physical examination identifies pelvic conditions such as vaginal prolapse, genital atrophy, or urethral leakage in women and abnormal prostate glands in men; and rectal or abdominal masses due to bladder distention or fecal impaction in both men and women. A postvoid residual urine obtained by straight catheterization of the bladder or estimated by a bladder scan can exclude urinary retention resulting from either an acontractile bladder or bladder outlet obstruction. A residual of greater than 150 mL is abnormal and indicates the need for further urologic evaluation.

Surgical referral should be considered for patients with complicated urinary tract infections (e.g., when upper urinary tract obstruction or stones are suspected), severe pelvic prolapse (prominent cystocele with observed leakage of urine), severe symptoms of prostatism, hematuria, and poor response to behavioral and medical treatments. When the pathophysiologic mechanism of incontinence is unclear, office cystometry is useful to determine bladder-filling capacity, detrusor compliance and contractility, and postvoid residual urine. A detailed urodynamic evaluation is needed in cases of incontinence refractory to medical treatments, and particularly before surgical treatments. These studies can identify a definitive cause of overflow incontinence due to an acontractile bladder or outlet obstruction, secure the diagnosis of detrusor hyperactivity with impaired contractility, and determine whether stress incontinence is due to urethral hypermobility or intrinsic sphincter deficiency (ISD).

## Treatment

Therapeutic strategies for the management of urinary incontinence include behavioral techniques, medications, patient and caregiver education, surgical procedures, and catheters and incontinence supplies. Behavioral interventions including bladder training, biofeedback, and pelvic muscle exercises are recommended as a first line of treatment in the management of stress and urge incontinence in motivated women. Pelvic muscle exercise is assumed to enhance urethral resistance by increasing the strength and endurance of the periurethral and perivaginal muscles and by improving the anatomic support to the bladder neck and proximal urethra.

Intravaginal, oral, or transdermal estrogen replacement therapy have modest effects on stress incontinence in elderly patients, but concerns regarding their long-term adverse effects limit their use in practice. Likewise, α-adrenergic agonists improve stress incontinence in some women, but their usefulness is limited by potentially serious adverse effects. Surgical options for stress incontinence include bladder neck suspension for women with urethral hypermobility that fails to respond to conservative measures, a vaginal sling for women with findings of both urethral hypermobility and sphincteric incompetence, and periurethral injections of collagen for women with ISD, which is commonly associated with multiple incontinence surgical procedures or hypoestrogenism.

Urge incontinence resulting from detrusor instability (overactive bladder) often responds to scheduled toileting and bladder retraining, scheduled toileting (e.g., every 2 hours), or prompted voiding. Bladder relaxant medications, with anticholinergic properties, are the most effective drug therapies for urge incontinence. Oxybutynin and tolterodine are the most commonly prescribed agents. These medications are moderately effective but can produce significant side effects of constipation, dry mouth, blurred vision, and occasionally confusion in vulnerable patients. Long-acting preparations of oxybutynin (XL) and tolterodine (LA) are available, are similar in efficacy, and may enhance compliance compared to the shorter-acting preparations.

Acute overflow incontinence, which may have been precipitated by medications (e.g., anticholinergic drugs), anesthesia, or urethral manipulation may be treated with intermittent urethral catheterization until the acute precipitating event subsides. Overflow incontinence resulting from bladder outlet obstruction (e.g., urethral stricture, prostatic hyperplasia) needs either surgical correction or intermittent catheterization. Some patients with urge symptoms and outlet obstruction resulting from prostatic hyperplasia may respond to α-adrenergic antagonists (e.g., terazosin, tamsulosin, doxazosin) that reduce internal sphincter tone. Intermittent self-catheterization is warranted for patients with atonic or neurogenic bladders. Chronic indwelling urinary catheterization usually is reserved for patients who cannot be catheterized intermittently because of discomfort or terminal illness. External (condom) catheters for men often fail and can lead to local skin infection. The condom catheter is most useful in mobility-impaired patients with either functional or urge incontinence at night.

Functional incontinence responds to improved caregiving, frequent toileting, and treatment of underlying causes. When incontinence is incurable, incontinence aids such as absorbent pads or external catheters are helpful.

## REVIEW EXERCISES

### QUESTIONS

**1.** A previously well 78-year-old man is admitted to the hospital for treatment of community-acquired pneumonia. The nurses report that he is sometimes hard to arouse, quiet, and withdrawn and other times agitated, disoriented, and accusatory and behaves inappropriately. Physical examination is unremarkable except for findings of pneumonia. Which of the following is the most accurate statement about his mental status?
a) He has dementia with "sundowning"
b) The symptoms are potentially preventable
c) A head computed tomographic scan is needed
d) He has the "pseudodementia" of depression

**2.** A 77-year-old man has a 6-month history of frequent falling. He loses his balance while walking. He is walking less and has a fear of falling. He takes a diuretic for hypertension and a nitrate for angina pectoris. On physical examination, he takes small, short steps and has postural instability and decreased steppage. Routine blood test results are normal. The treatment most likely to reduce this patient's risk of falling is
a) Change in medications
b) Gait training
c) Low-intensity resistive exercises
d) All of the above
e) None of the above

**3.** An 82-year-old woman presents with a 2-year history of urinary frequency and leakage of small amounts of urine after coughing, sneezing, or straining. She has a past history of a vaginal hysterectomy and takes no daily medications. Physical examination shows that she has a small cystocele and slight urinary leakage. A postvoid residual urine is 20 mL. Her chemistry panel and urinalysis are normal. The treatment most likely to improve this patient's symptoms is
a) Anticholinergic drugs (oxybutynin)
b) Vaginal estrogen
c) Intermittent catheterization
d) Periurethral injections (collagen)
e) Cholinergic drugs (bethanechol)

**4.** An 84-year-old man is recovering from abdominal surgery in the hospital. Four days after surgery, he attempts to get out of bed for the first time. He feels lightheaded and unsteady and falls without an injury. He is now afraid to walk. Before the operation, he walked normally. He is taking a cardioselective β-blocker, a statin, and acetaminophen. Physical examination reveals normal cognition and vital signs and generalized weakness. He appears worried. Laboratory studies are unremarkable. Which of the following is most likely to improve his symptoms?

a) A beta blocker with intrinsic sympathomimetic activity rather than the cardioselective agent
b) Low-intensity resistive exercises for his lower extremities
c) A low dose of a psychostimulant (e.g., methylphenidate)
d) A four-prong cane
e) A benzodiazepine (e.g., lorazepam) to treat anxiety

**5.** A 79-year-old man is admitted to the hospital for treatment of congestive heart failure (left ventricular ejection fraction is 30%). His past medical history includes mild Alzheimer's disease, osteoarthritis, and reflux gastroesophageal disease (GERD). He is restless, attempts to get out of bed, and remains awake at night. He is given medications for heart failure, sleep, GERD, and arthritis pain. Which of the following medications is most likely to cause symptoms of delirium in this man?
a) Omeprazole
b) Diphenhydramine
c) Acetaminophen
d) Atenolol
e) Lisinopril

**6.** A 71-year-old woman presents with an 8-month history of urinary urgency, frequency and nocturia, and daily urinary incontinence. Her past medical history is significant for occasional "stress incontinence" (with sneezing, coughing, straining) for 12 years. She takes no daily medications. Physical examination reveals slight anterior vaginal prolapse and no visible leakage or pelvic mass. A screening urinalysis and basic metabolic panel are normal. Which of the following is most likely to relieve her urinary incontinence?
a) Bladder relaxant (oxybutynin)
b) Topical (vaginal) estrogen
c) α-agonist (pseudoephedrine)
d) Behavioral therapies
e) Periurethral injections (collagen)

**7.** A 72-year-old man is admitted to the hospital with "dehydration." He has a past medical history of benign prostatic hyperplasia, gait impairment due to lumbar canal stenosis, hypertension, and glucose intolerance. He reports constant dribbling of urine that is worse when he stands, strains, or coughs. He has no dysuria or sensation of urinary urgency. Laboratory studies done in the office show normal renal function and urine analysis. Which of the following is the most appropriate treatment of his urinary incontinence?
a) Bladder relaxant
b) Urethral catheterization
c) α-agonist (pseudoephedrine)
d) Behavioral therapies
e) α-blocker (tamsulosin)

## ANSWERS

**1. b.**
The acute onset of change in mental status, the fluctuating course, and the altered level of consciousness are diagnostic of delirium. Although cognitive dysfunction at night in a new environment (sundowning) can occur in patients with either dementia or delirium, the patient does not have a history of dementia, in which symptoms usually progress over a duration of months to years, and attention and level of consciousness are normal. A head CT scan is rarely useful in the diagnostic evaluation of a patient with delirium and is reserved for patients with new or focal neurologic signs or suspected head trauma. Patients with major depressive disorder often have cognitive dysfunction ("pseudodementia") but are alert and attentive and do not have a fluctuating course. A clinical trial of hospitalized elderly patients demonstrated a 40% decrease in the incidence of delirium with an intervention that targeted risk factors for delirium (cognitive impairment, sleep deprivation, immobility, visual and hearing impairment, dehydration); total days of delirium also were reduced by the intervention.

**2. d.**
Recurrent falls occur in patients with disorders of balance and gait, lower extremity weakness (often from muscular deconditioning or atrophy), polypharmacy, and a fear of falling. Drugs with cardiovascular (e.g., α-blockers, vasodilators) or central nervous system (e.g., benzodiazepines) effects may worsen postural stability or balance, increasing the risk of a fall. Clinical trials provide strong evidence that balance and gait training, low-intensity resistive exercise (e.g., with weights, bands, or tubes), walking, or tai chi exercises can reduce the incidence of falls.

**3. d.**
Leakage of urine with stress maneuvers and small residual volumes is characteristic of stress incontinence resulting from either urethral hypermobility or ISD. Her advanced age, prior hysterectomy, and frequency of urinary leakage are consistent with ISD, although urodynamic studies are needed to confirm that diagnosis. Although estrogen (oral or vaginal) may be considered an adjunctive pharmacologic agent for postmenopausal women with stress or mixed (urge and stress) incontinence, guidelines recommend sling procedures for women who have ISD with coexisting hypermobility or periurethral bulking injections for women with ISD who do not have coexisting hypermobility. Oxybutynin and tolterodine have both anticholinergic and direct smooth muscle relaxant properties; they are moderately effective in the treatment of urge incontinence resulting from detrusor instability, but they have no role in treating pure stress incontinence. Bethanechol is a cholinergic

agent that is used rarely in the treatment of overflow incontinence attributable to a hypocontractile bladder.

### 4. b.

The patient probably has deconditioning associated with major surgery and prolonged immobility. With prolonged bed rest, generalized weakness of the extensor and flexor muscles of the knees and hips is common. Low-intensity exercises, active resistance against flexion or extension, and therapeutic bands or tubes increase muscle strength and lessen the chance of a fall. A β-blocker with intrinsic sympathomimetic activity could cause orthostatic hypotension and more lightheadedness. A psychostimulant might be considered for a patient with depression and delayed recovery from surgery but will not increase muscle strength. A four-prong cane is helpful when patients have weakness in one extremity, but is not indicated for a patient with generalized weakness due to deconditioning. An anxiolytic could cause gait impairment and increase the risk of a fall.

### 5. b.

The patient has delirium. Drugs with psychoactive or anticholinergic effects and opiates are among the most common medications associated with delirium, especially in hospitalized patients. The antihistamine, diphenhydramine, has strong anticholinergic properties. In a case-controlled study of 426 elderly patients admitted to a medical service, cognitive decline and symptoms of delirium occurred more commonly in patients treated with diphenhydramine compared with controls not given this medication. The patient is at risk of delirium due to the Alzheimer's disease. He is likely to be more sensitive to the adverse central nervous system effects of anticholinergic drugs. Although most classes of medications have cognitive effects at high doses, the other medications taken by the patient are not known to have adverse effects on cognition at usual therapeutic doses.

### 6. d.

The patient has mixed stress and urge incontinence. The stress incontinence is most likely a result of urethral hypermobility whereas the urge incontinence likely represents an overactive bladder. Although bladder relaxants alone reduce the frequency of incontinent episodes due to urge incontinence, they have little or no effect on stress incontinence. Behavioral therapies (training) including pelvic floor exercise, pelvic floor stimulation, and biofeedback are more effective than placebo or bladder muscle relaxants for mixed forms of incontinence. In one study, biofeedback to teach pelvic floor muscle control, verbal feedback based on vaginal palpation, and a self-help booklet in a first-line behavioral training program all achieved comparable improvements in urge

incontinence in community-dwelling older women. Periurethral injections with bulking agents (collagen) are indicated for ISD and have no effect on urge incontinence. The α-agonists and vaginal estrogen are of questionable value in the treatment of stress incontinence and have no proven effect in women with ISD.

### 7. b.

The patient has overflow incontinence. Symptoms can be confused with those of stress incontinence, thus underscoring the need to exclude overflow as the cause of incontinence in every patient. The two common causes of overflow incontinence are bladder outlet obstruction and acontractile (atonic or "neurogenic") bladder. Outlet obstruction in men most often results from benign prostatic hyperplasia, and less often from urethral stricture or tumor. An acontractile bladder is seen after prolonged outlet obstruction, autonomic neuropathy (for example in diabetics), and with medications that depress detrusor muscle contractility (e.g., anticholinergics). Although prostatectomy might eventually cure bladder outlet obstruction, the patient first needs further evaluation to determine the type of overflow incontinence. Surgery will not be helpful and could even worsen incontinence if he has an acontractile bladder. An α-agonist has no effect on bladder contractility and will not reduce the symptoms of a bladder outlet obstruction. An α-blocker might be helpful in preventing urinary retention and overflow incontinence if his symptoms are due to benign prostatic hyperplasia, but will not relieve his symptoms as promptly as urethral catheterization.

## SUGGESTED READINGS

Agostini JV, Leo-Summers L, Inouye SK. Cognitive and other adverse effects of diphenhydramine use in hospitalized older patients. *Arch Intern Med* 2001;161:2091–2097.

American Geriatrics Society, British Geriatrics Society, American Academy of Orthopaedic Surgeons Panel on Falls Prevention. Guideline for the prevention of falls in older persons. *J Am Geriatr Soc* 2001;49:664–672.

American Psychiatric Association. Practice guideline for the treatment of patients with delirium. *Am J Psychiatry* 1999;156[5 Suppl]:1–20.

Bischoff-Ferrari HA, Dawson-Hughes B, Willett WC, et al. *JAMA* 2004; 291:1999–2006.

Burgio KL, Locher JL, Goode PS, et al. Behavioral vs. drug treatment for urge incontinence in older women: a randomized controlled trial. *JAMA* 1998;280:1995–2000.

Burgio KL, Goode PS, Locher JL, et al. Behavioral training with and without biofeedback in the treatment of urge incontinence in older women: a controlled trial. *JAMA* 2002;288:2293–2299.

Campbell AJ, Robertson MC, Gardner MM, et al. Randomised controlled trial of a general practice program of home-based exercise to prevent falls in elderly women. *BMJ* 1997;315:1065–1069.

Close J, Elis M, Hooper R, et al. Prevention of falls in the elderly trial (PROFET): a randomised controlled trial. *Lancet* 1999;353:93–97.

Dargent-Molina P, Favier F, Grandjean H, et al. Fall-related factors and risk of hip fracture: the EPIDOS prospective study. *Lancet* 1996;348:145–149.

Fantl JA, Newman DK, Cooling J, et al. Urinary incontinence in adults: acute and chronic management. Clinical Practice Guideline no. 2. In: *AHCPR Publication 96-0682, March 1996*. Rockville, MD: U.S. Department of Health and Human Services, Public Health Services, Agency for Health Care Policy and Research.

Gillespie LD, Gillespie WJ, Robertson MC, et al. Interventions for preventing falls in elderly people. *Cochrane Database Syst Rev* 3: 2003.

Goode PS, Burgio KL, Lochner JL, et al. Effect of behavioral training with or without pelvic floor electrical stimulation on stress incontinence in women: a randomized controlled trial. *JAMA* 2003;290:345–352.

Inouye SK, Bogardus ST, Charpentier PA, et al. Multicomponent intervention to prevent delirium in hospitalized older patients. *N Engl J Med* 1999;340:669–676.

Inouye SK, Charpentier PA. Precipitating factors for delirium in hospitalized elderly persons. *JAMA* 1996;275:852–857.

Kannus P, Pakkari J, Niemi S, et al. Prevention of hip fracture in elderly people with use of a hip protector. *N Engl J Med* 2000;343:1506–1513.

Marcantonio ER, Flacker JM, Wright RJ, et al. Reducing delirium after hip fracture: a randomized trial. *J Amer Geriatr Soc* 2001;49:516–522.

McCusker J, Cole M, Abrahamowicz M, et al. Delirium predicts 12-month mortality. *Arch Intern Med* 2002;162:457–463.

Ouslander JG, Schnelle JF. Incontinence in the nursing home. *Ann Intern Med* 1995;122:438–449.

Tinetti ME, Baker DI, McAvay G, et al. A multifactorial intervention to reduce the risk of falling among elderly people living in the community. *N Engl J Med* 1994;331:821–827.

Tinetti ME. Clinical practice. Preventing falls in elderly persons. *N Engl J Med* 2003;348:42–49.

Van Schoor NM, Smit JH, Twisk JW, et al. Prevention of hip fractures by external hip protectors: a randomized controlled trial. *JAMA* 2003;289:1957–1962.

Winters JC, Chiverton A, Scarpero HM, et al. Collagen injection therapy in elderly women: long-term results and patient satisfaction. *Urology* 2000;55:856–861.

Wu G. Evaluation of the effectiveness of Tai Chi for improving balance and preventing falls in the older population—a review. *J Am Geriatr Soc* 2002;50:746–754.

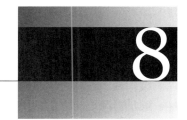

# Dermatology for the Internist

*Melissa Peck Piliang     Kenneth J. Tomecki*

The skin is often a window to systemic disease. An awareness and appreciation of the cutaneous manifestations of systemic diseases helps to guide the internist in determining the diagnosis, therapy, or need for referral to a dermatologist. This chapter provides a broad overview of skin diseases that are clinically germane and relevant to internists and medical subspecialists.

## GENERAL DERMATOLOGY

### Common Benign Cutaneous Disorders

*Acne vulgaris* is an inflammatory disorder of the pilosebaceous follicle, characterized by comedones, papules, pustules, and nodules, occasionally with scars, on the face, neck, chest, and back. Disease typically affects youngsters and young adults. Concomitant hyperandrogenism may occur in women with acne, hirsutism, and irregular menses.

*Rosacea*, or adult acne, is an inflammatory disease of the midface characterized by erythema, telangiectasia, papules, and pustules. Rhinophyma is an uncommon complication.

*Seborrheic dermatitis* is a common inflammatory disease that favors hair-bearing areas such as the scalp, face, ears, and central chest. Seborrheic dermatitis is characterized by erythematous plaques with greasy, yellow scale. Scalp pruritus is a common symptom. Disease can affect infants and adults and tends to be common and extensive in patients with neurologic disorders such as Parkinson's disease and human immunodeficiency virus (HIV) infection.

*Seborrheic keratoses* are warty, age-related plaques. Although common and benign, they may indicate an underlying adenocarcinoma of the gastrointestinal tract if they appear suddenly in great numbers (sign of Leser-Trélat).

*Urticaria*, or hives, is most frequently caused by medication (antibiotics, aspirin), food (shellfish, nuts, chocolate), or infection (chronic sinusitis). Affected patients have pruritic, edematous, evanescent wheals that usually resolve within 24 hours. Acute urticaria may last 4 to 6 weeks.

*Pruritus* may be a symptom of a primary dermatosis, eczema, internal disorder [e.g., hepatic or renal disease, hematologic malignancy (especially lymphoma)], iron deficiency, psychiatric disease, or endocrinologic disorders. Aquagenic pruritus is unique to polycythemia vera.

*Drug eruptions* (Fig. 8.1) occur in approximately 2% of all hospitalized patients. The most common type of reaction is *exanthematous* or *morbilliform*, which can resemble a viral exanthem; common causes are penicillin, sulfonamides, and blood products. *Urticarial reactions*, characterized by transient wheals and edematous plaques, may occur with systemic anaphylaxis; the most common causes are aspirin, penicillin, and blood products. Phototoxic and photoallergic reactions are two types of drug-induced

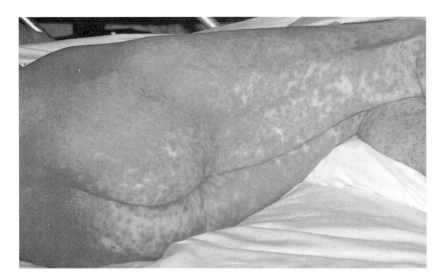

**Figure 8.1** Drug eruption: exanthematous type caused by vancomycin.

photosensitivity. *Phototoxic reactions*, essentially exaggerated sunburn responses, may occur in anyone; tetracycline is a common cause. In contrast, *photoallergic reactions* are immunologic responses that occur only in previously sensitized individuals; they occur on sun-exposed areas and may spread to unexposed areas. Drugs that cause photoallergic reactions include sulfonamides, thiazides, griseofulvin, and phenothiazines.

*Erythema multiforme* (Fig. 8.2) is a hypersensitivity reaction of the skin and mucosal surfaces characterized by macules, papules, plaques, vesicles, or bullae, often with a targetoid appearance. The most common cause of erythema multiforme is recurrent herpes simplex virus infection; less common causes are other infections such as mycoplasma pneumonia and hypersensitivity to medications such as sulfonamides, barbiturates, and antibiotics.

*Psoriasis* (Fig. 8.3) is a common disease that affects 1% to 2% of the population. The characteristic silvery-white scaly papules and plaques commonly occur on the scalp, elbows, and knees. Often, nail dystrophy such as onycholysis, pitting, and oil spots are seen. Disease often begins in the third decade, and about 50% of patients have an affected family member. Approximately 5% of patients develop psoriatic arthritis (see Psoriasis and Psoriatic Arthritis, later in this chapter).

*Vitiligo,* characterized by depigmented macules, affects approximately 1% of the population. The disease can be localized, usually to bony prominences or orifices, or it can be generalized. Associated autoimmune diseases include thyroid disease (30% of all patients), alopecia areata, type I diabetes mellitus, pernicious anemia, or Addison's disease.

*Erythema nodosum* (Fig. 8.4) is a hypersensitivity panniculitis characterized by painful reddened nodules on the shins and less so on the thighs and forearms. The most common cause of erythema nodosum is a streptococcal pharyngitis, closely followed by drug sensitivity (e.g., sulfonamides, oral contraceptives), and a variety of illnesses, primarily inflammatory bowel disease and sarcoidosis.

## Autoimmune Bullous Diseases

Autoimmune bullous diseases are characterized by the deposition of immunoglobulin within the epidermis (pemphigus) or at the dermal–epidermal junction (dermatitis herpetiformis, bullous pemphigoid, epidermolysis bullosa). *Pemphigus vulgaris* is a chronic, debilitating, blistering disease characterized by painful mucosal erosions and flaccid, often eroded blisters. Immunologically, deposition of immunoglobulin G (IgG) occurs within the epidermis. Even

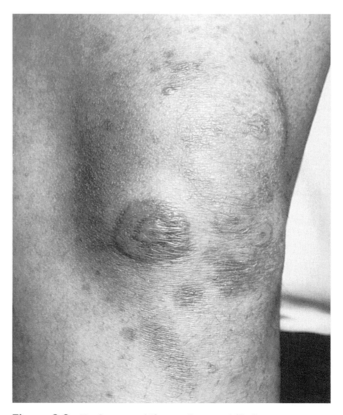

**Figure 8.2** Erythema multiforme: "targetoid" plaques.

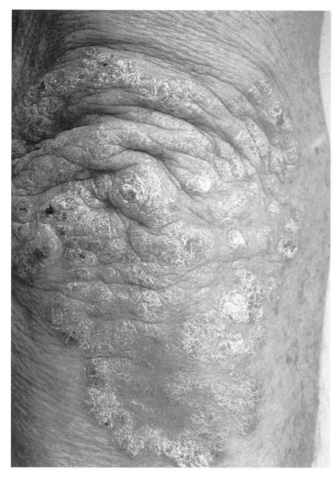

**Figure 8.3**   Psoriasis: scaly plaques.

with treatment using systemic corticosteroids and immuno-suppressives, morbidity and mortality are appreciable. *Bullous pemphigoid* is the most common autoimmune bullous disease. It almost invariably affects the elderly, usually with large, tense blisters and urticarial plaques. Pruritus may

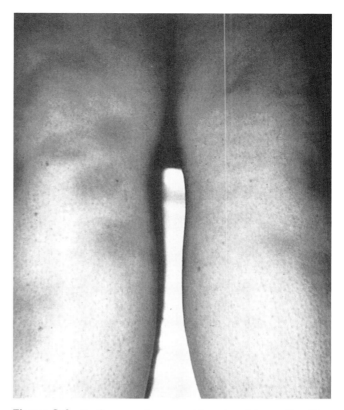

**Figure 8.4**   Erythema nodosum: reddened nodules on the shins.

be severe. Mucosal disease is rare. Immunologically, a deposition of IgG at the dermal–epidermal junction occurs. With treatment, affected patients have a good prognosis.

*Dermatitis herpetiformis* (Fig. 8.5) is a chronic, intensely pruritic, papulovesicular disease characterized by the deposition of IgA at the dermal–epidermal junction. Affected patients have symmetric groups of vesicles, papules, and wheals that appear on the elbows, knees, scalp, and buttocks. Most patients have an asymptomatic gluten-sensitive

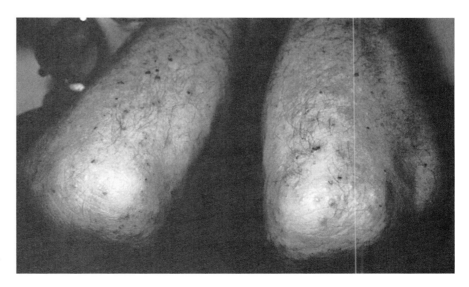

**Figure 8.5**   Dermatitis herpetiformis: excoriated papules and vesicles.

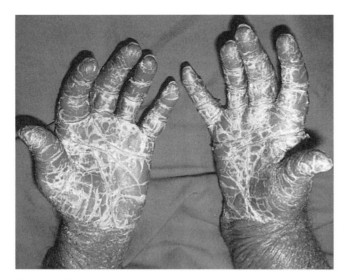

**Figure 8.6** Exfoliative dermatitis: eczematous, scaly plaques.

enteropathy; about 35% have thyroid disease. *Epidermolysis bullosa acquisita* is a bullous disease characterized by skin fragility, milia, scarring alopecia, and nail dystrophy. Skin disease typically follows trauma. Immunologically, IgG deposition occurs at the dermal–epidermal junction (similar to bullous pemphigoid).

## Exfoliative Dermatitis

*Exfoliative dermatitis* (Fig. 8.6) is an uncommon itchy eczematous disease that is usually generalized and insidious in nature. The most common causes are a preexisting skin disease (e.g., psoriasis, atopic eczema) and drug hypersensitivity (drug rash). A less common but important etiology is early, evolving a cutaneous lymphoma (T cell type).

## PRIMARY SKIN CANCER

*Basal cell carcinoma* (BCC) (Fig. 8.7) and *squamous cell carcinoma* (SCC) (Fig. 8.8) are the most common types of skin cancer. Together, they account for more than 1 million skin cancers each year. At a 5:1 ratio, BCCs are more common. BCCs are usually a "pearly" papule, plaque, or nodule with a telangiectatic surface and a rolled border. The vast majority occur on the head and neck. The tumor can be locally aggressive, although its ability to metastasize is limited (less than 0.1%). Tumors near the nose, eye, or ear may invade the eye or brain.

*Squamous cell carcinoma* is typically an ill-defined indurated papule, plaque, or nodule with central ulceration and a hyperkeratotic edge, most commonly found on the face, ears, dorsal hands, and forearms. SCCs can metastasize in 3% to 4% of cases. Lesions on the head and neck have the

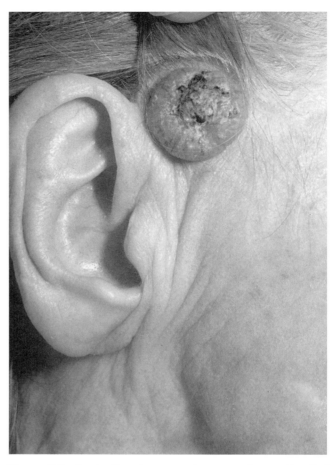

**Figure 8.7** Basal cell carcinoma: erythematous plaque with rolled border.

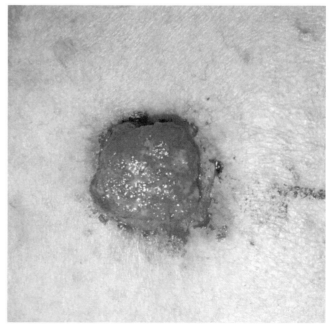

**Figure 8.8** Squamous cell carcinoma: indurated, erythematous papule.

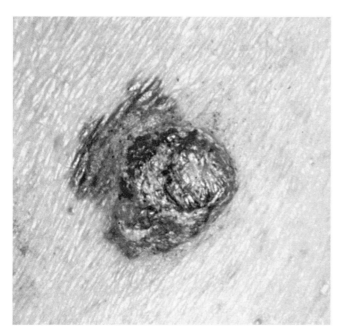

**Figure 8.9** Melanoma: asymmetric plaque with an irregular bor-der, uneven brown-black color, and large diameter (greater than 6 mm), the "ABCD" signs of melanoma.

highest metastatic potential and require more aggressive treatment.

*Melanoma* (Fig. 8.9) affects approximately 60,000 peo-ple each year in the United States. The lifetime risk in fair-skinned individuals is 1 in 75 (approximately 1%). Approximately 30% of melanomas arise in a preexisting melanocytic nevus; the remainder arise de novo. Most melanomas have *a*symmetry, an irregular *b*order, uneven

color, and a large *d*iameter (greater than 6 mm), all of which constitute the "ABCD" signs of melanoma. Most occur on the head, neck, upper extremities, back, chest, and legs. Common sites for metastases are the skin, lungs, liver, bone, and brain. The most important prognostic indi-cator is the histologic depth of invasion (Breslow depth). Thinner melanomas (<0.75 mm) have an excellent prog-nosis (greater than 95% 5-year survival), but thicker melanomas (>3.5 mm) carry a much graver prognosis (35–40% 5-year survival).

## SKIN DISEASE AND INTERNAL CANCER

### Cutaneous Metastases

*Cutaneous metastases* (Fig. 8.10) occur in 3% to 5% of patients with cancer, and most commonly are seen on the head, neck, and trunk, often in close proximity to the underlying tumor. Metastases typically reflect the more common types of cancer in the general population (e.g., cancers of the breast, lung, or gastrointestinal tract). Clinically, cutaneous metastases may be nondescript, but often are juicy red to violaceous nodules.

### Paget's Disease of the Breast

*Paget's disease of the breast* (Fig. 8.11), a unilateral, eczema-tous plaque of the nipple and areola, invariably implies an underlying intraductal carcinoma of the breast. *Extramam-mary Paget's disease* (Fig. 8.12), typically a persistent, eczematous plaque on the perineum, often indicates the presence of an underlying adnexal (apocrine) carcinoma or an underlying cancer of the genitourinary tract or distal

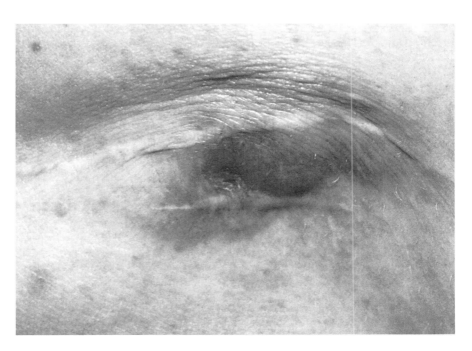

**Figure 8.10** Metastatic breast cancer: thoracic nodule.

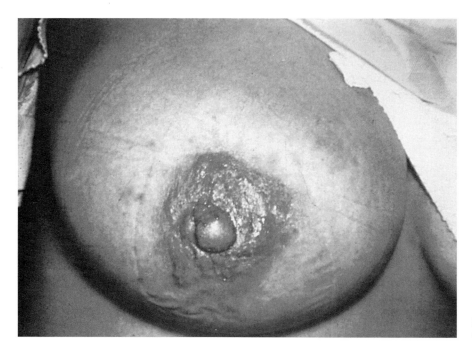

**Figure 8.11**   Paget's disease: unilateral eczematous plaque on areola.

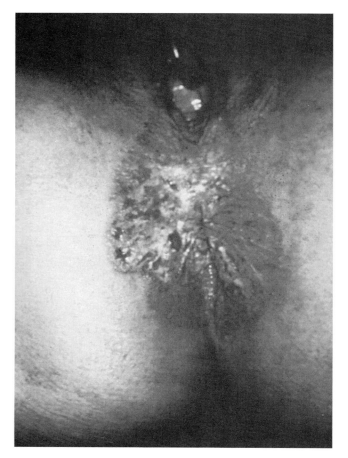

**Figure 8.12**   Extramammary Paget's disease: eczematous plaque on perineum.

gastrointestinal tract. Approximately 50% of affected patients have an underlying malignancy.

## Acanthosis Nigricans

*Acanthosis nigricans* (Fig. 8.13), smooth, velvet-like, hyperkeratotic plaques of intertriginous areas, may indicate an underlying adenocarcinoma of the gastrointestinal tract, usually the stomach. The most common causes of acanthosis nigricans are obesity and type II diabetes. Occasionally, disease occurs with certain medications, such as systemic corticosteroids, nicotinic acid, diethylstilbestrol, and isoniazid.

## Acquired Ichthyosis

*Acquired ichthyosis* (Fig. 8.14), a scaly platelike thickening of the skin, is a relatively specific marker for lymphoma when it appears de novo in an adult.

## Glucagonoma Syndrome

The *glucagonoma syndrome* (Fig. 8.15), characterized by a distinctive necrolytic migratory erythema (erosive, crusted plaques usually on the perineum, sometimes on the face and trunk), implies the presence of an islet cell (glucagon-secreting) tumor of the pancreas. Skin disease without glucagonoma may occasionally occur with malabsorption (e.g., zinc deficiency). Affected patients usually have weight loss, diarrhea, stomatitis, glossitis, and anemia. An elevated serum glucagon level confirms the diagnosis.

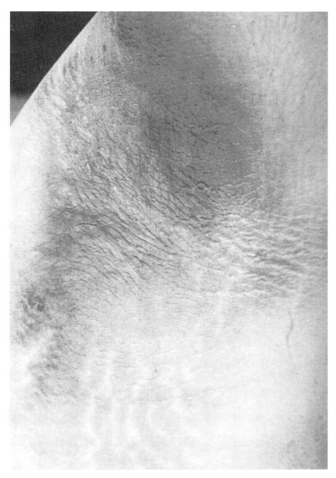

**Figure 8.13** Acanthosis nigricans: velvety hyperpigmented axillary plaques.

## Carcinoid Syndrome

The triad of flushing, secretory diarrhea, and valvular heart disease characterizes *carcinoid tumor*. Other manifestations include telangectasia, wheezing, and paroxysmal hypotension. Carcinoid tumors most commonly secrete serotonin. Affected patients have elevated levels of urinary 5-hydroxyindolaceticacid (5-HIAA), a byproduct of serotonin metabolism.

## Gardner's Syndrome

*Gardner's syndrome* (Fig. 8.16) is an autosomal dominant cancer syndrome, characterized by colonic polyposis; osteomas of the maxilla, mandible, and skull; scoliosis; epidermoid cysts; and soft tissue tumors such fibromas, desmoids, and lipomas. Approximately 60% of affected patients will develop adenocarcinoma of the colon by age 40, secondary to a malignant transformation of the gastrointestinal polyps.

## Torre's Syndrome

*Torre's syndrome* is an uncommon autosomal dominant cancer syndrome characterized by at least one sebaceous gland tumor (sebaceous adenoma, epithelioma, carcinoma) and one or more internal malignancies, usually colorectal, genitourinary, or lymphoma. The sebaceous gland tumors generally appear on the face and trunk.

## Cowden's Syndrome

*Cowden's syndrome* (a.k.a. multiple hamartoma syndrome) is a rare autosomal dominant cancer syndrome characterized

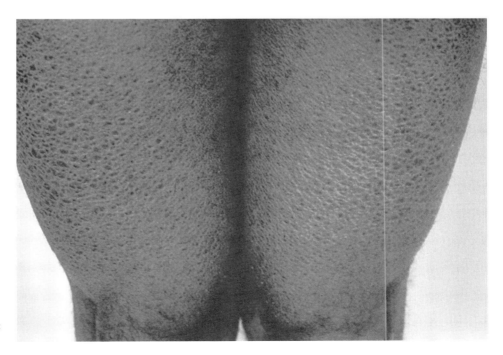

**Figure 8.14** Acquired ichthyosis: plate-like, scaly plaques.

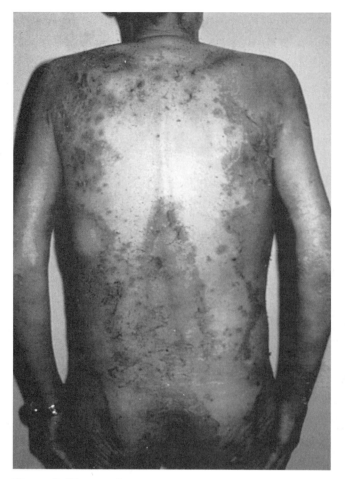

**Figure 8.15**  Necrolytic migratory erythema (glucagonoma syndrome): erosive, necrolytic plaques.

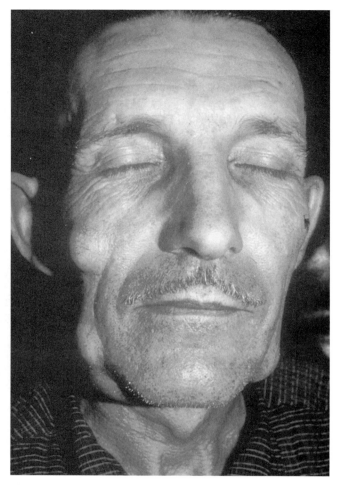

**Figure 8.16**  Gardner's syndrome: facial cysts.

by multiple tricholemmomas (which resemble warts) on the nose and ears, and periorally. A high incidence of breast and thyroid cancer appears in affected individuals.

### Hirsutism

*Hirsutism* (Fig. 8.17), the presence of coarse male-type hair in a woman, may indicate androgen excess, with or without an adrenal or ovarian tumor.

### Sweet's Syndrome

*Sweet's syndrome* (Fig. 8.18), or acute febrile neutrophilic dermatosis, is characterized by the presence of painful, reddened plaques on the face, extremities, and trunk. The syndrome is associated with acute leukemia in about 20% of patients, either myelocytic or myelomonocytic. Sweet's may be induced by medications that stimulate neutrophil production, such as G-CSF. A flu-like illness and arthralgias often accompany the symptoms of Sweet's syndrome. The syndrome primarily affects women.

### Multiple Mucosal Neuromas Syndrome

*Multiple mucosal neuroma syndrome,* characterized by numerous fibromas of the skin and mucosa, is associated with multiple endocrine neoplasia II, which includes medullary thyroid carcinoma, pheochromocytoma, and parathyroid adenoma.

### Dermatomyositis

*Dermatomyositis* (Fig. 8.19) is a connective tissue disease characterized by symmetric proximal muscle weakness (myositis); pathonomonic papules and plaques on the hands, elbows, and knees (Gottron's papules); and periorbital edema with a violaceous hue (heliotrope). Other features include poikiloderma (hypopigmented/hyperpigmented, telangiectatic, atrophic macules) on the face, neck, trunk, and extremities; malar erythema; and nail abnormalities (periungual telangiectasiae and cuticular hypertrophy). Accurate diagnosis requires a muscle biopsy, electromyelogram, and muscle enzyme tests. Adult dermatomyositis has a strong association with

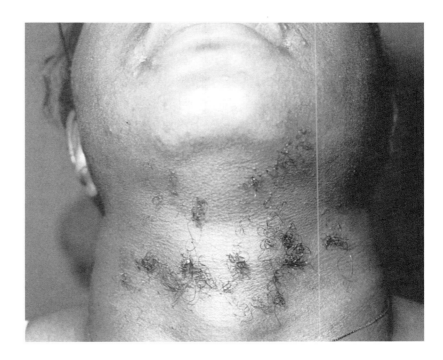

**Figure 8.17**  Hirsutism: coarse, male-type hair.

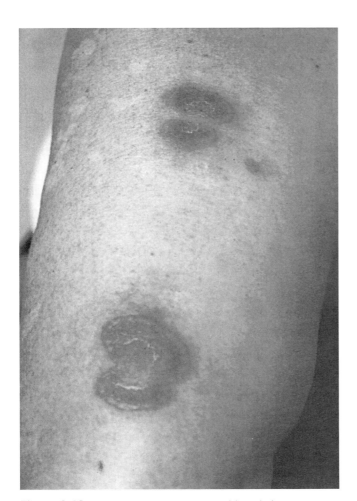

**Figure 8.18**  Sweet's syndrome: juicy, reddened plaques.

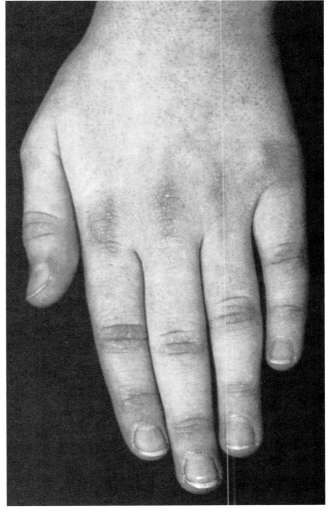

**Figure 8.19**  Dermatomyositis: Gottron's papules and plaques.

malignancy, usually adenocarcinoma of the breast, ovary, gastrointestinal tract, or lung.

## Amyloidosis of the Skin

*Amyloidosis* of the skin, typically expressed as waxy papules of the orbits and midface that become purpuric with pressure or rubbing, may be a sign of multiple myeloma. Other features include macroglossia, "pinch purpura" after trauma, and alopecia.

## Autoimmune Bullous Diseases and Cancer

Some autoimmune bullous diseases (see the preceding section on Autoimmune Bullous Diseases) may occur as a paraneoplastic phenomenon. *Paraneoplastic pemphigus*, which clinically and histologically resembles pemphigus vulgaris, bullous pemphigoid, and erythema multiforme has a strong association with leukemia and lymphoma. Dermatitis herpetiformis has rarely preceded an intestinal lymphoma, and epidermolysis bullosa acquisita has a weak association with multiple myeloma.

## Erythema Gyratum Repens

*Erythema gyratum repens* is a rare but distinctive skin disease characterized by reddened concentric bands in a whorled pattern; it has a strong association with breast cancer.

# SKIN DISEASE AND CARDIOVASCULAR DISEASE

## Multiple Lentigines

Multiple lentigines and cardiac abnormalities occur with *LEOPARD syndrome* (a.k.a. Moynahan syndrome), which includes *l*entigines *e*lectrocardiographic changes, *o*cular telorism, *p*ulmonary stenosis, *a*bnormal genitalia, *r*etarded growth, and *d*eafness. Variants of LEOPARD syndrome include *LAMB syndrome* (*l*entigines, *a*trial myxoma, *m*ucocutaneous myxomas, and *b*lue nevi), and *NAME syndrome* (*n*evi, *a*trial myxoma, *m*yxoid neurofibromas, and *e*phelides).

## Pseudoxanthoma Elasticum

*Pseudoxanthoma elasticum* (Fig. 8.20) is an inherited disease (either autosomal dominant or recessive) characterized by yellowed, pebbled skin on the neck, abdomen, and intertriginous areas. The disease represents a defect in elastic fibers, which become brittle and calcified. Associated internal manifestations include hypertension, peripheral vascular and coronary artery disease, and retinal and gastrointestinal hemorrhage. Funduscopic examination reveals angioid streaks in Bruch's membrane.

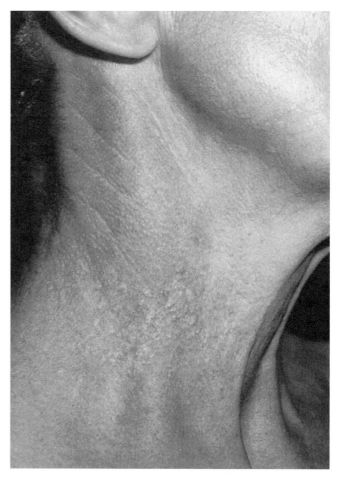

**Figure 8.20**   Pseudoxanthoma elasticum: pebbled skin on the neck.

## Ehlers-Danlos Syndrome

*Ehlers-Danlos syndrome*, characterized by hyperextensible and hypermobile joints, fragile skin, and "fish-mouth" scars, represents an abnormality in collagen biosynthesis. Several variants exist, and associated features include angina, gastrointestinal bleeding (perforation), poor wound healing, hernias, and peripheral vascular disease.

## Marfan's Syndrome

*Marfan's syndrome* is an autosomal dominant connective tissue disease affecting the skin, cardiovascular, musculoskeletal, and ocular systems. Patients are generally thin, with long, spindly extremities. Complications include striae distensae, elastosis perforans serpiginosa, aortic aneurysms, mitral valve prolapse, and displacement of the lens.

## Fabry's Disease

*Fabry's disease* is an X-linked abnormality of glycosphingolipid metabolism caused by a deficiency of α-galactosidase A, characterized by angiokeratoma corporis diffusum (blue-black nonblanchable papules in a bathing trunk distribution). Associated cardiovascular abnormalities include mitral valve prolapse, angina, myocardial infarction, congestive heart failure, and hypertension. Other features are painful neuropathy, renal failure, and stroke.

## SKIN DISEASE AND PULMONARY DISEASE

### Sarcoidosis

*Sarcoidosis* (Fig. 8.21) is a chronic, often multisystem, granulomatous disease. Of affected patients, 30% to 35% have skin disease, which can have a variety of presentations on the skin, including nasal edema, midfacial papules, annular plaques, scaly plaques, or nodules. Lupus pernio is sarcoidosis of the central face and upper airway tract. Skin disease occurs in approximately one-third of patients with sarcoidosis. Erythema nodosum, an acute painful panniculitis that commonly affects the shins, may accompany acute sarcoidosis.

## SKIN DISEASE AND RHEUMATIC DISEASE

### Psoriasis and Psoriatic Arthritis

*Psoriatic arthritis* (Fig. 8.22) is an uncommon, asymmetric, seronegative spondyloarthropathy characterized by fusiform swelling of the distal and proximal interphalangeal joints. It affects 5% to 6% of psoriatic patients. The most common presentation is asymmetric oligoarthritis, which is characterized by "sausage" digits and the involvement of a few large joints.

### Reiter's Syndrome

*Reiter's syndrome* (Fig. 8.23) is an inflammatory disorder with three features: urethritis, conjunctivitis, and arthritis. Reiter's invariably affects young men, and most patients have skin disease that resembles psoriasis: erythematous scaly plaques on the penis (circinate balanitis) and palms and soles (keratoderma blenorrhagicum). Most patients have the HLA-B27 antigen.

### Acrosclerosis

*Acrosclerosis* (Fig. 8.24), a thickened tapering of the skin, often with secondary ulceration, may occur with angiitis, chilblains, cryopathies, and scleroderma, or may follow exposure to polyvinyl chlorides.

### Erythema Chronicum Migrans

*Erythema chronicum migrans* (Fig. 8.25) is an annular erythematous plaque that follows and surrounds the site of a tick bite. Lyme disease is a multisystem illness that includes fever, arthralgia, and myalgia and may also include meningoencephalitis, myocarditis, and peripheral neuropathy. The causative agent in the United States is usually *Ixodes scapularis* or *I. pacificus*, whose bite transmits the spirochete *Borrelia burgdorferi*. Primary endemic areas are New England, the upper Midwest, and Pacific Northwest.

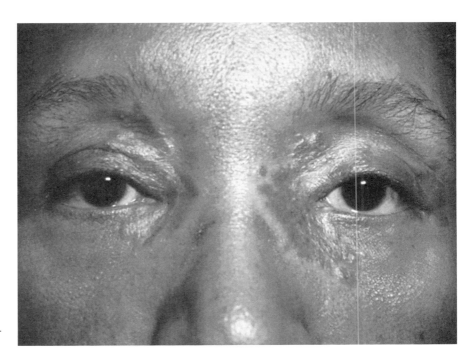

**Figure 8.21** Cutaneous sarcoidosis: annular facial plaques.

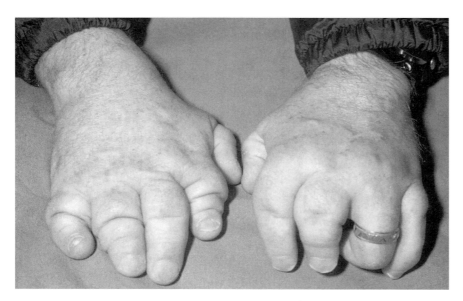

**Figure 8.22**   Psoriatic arthritis: "sausage" digits.

# SKIN DISEASE AND GASTROINTESTINAL DISEASE

## Aphthae

*Aphthae* are common painful superficial ulcerations of the mucosa. They may occur with Crohn's disease, gluten-sensitive enteropathy or HIV infection.

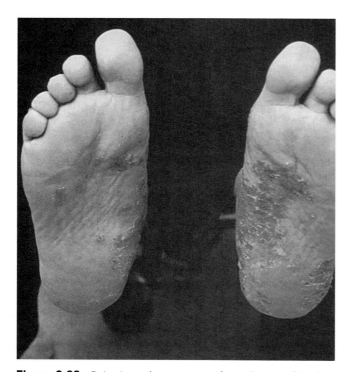

**Figure 8.23**   Reiter's syndrome: psoriasiform plaques of the feet (keratoderma blenorrhagicum).

## Acrodermatitis Enteropathica

*Acrodermatitis enteropathica* is an inflammatory disease, either inherited or acquired, characterized by a deficiency of zinc, diarrhea, alopecia, and erosive plaques in the perineum and on the face, hands, and feet. Affected individuals have a zinc deficiency.

## Hepatitis C Infection

*Hepatitis C infection* is a common cause of chronic liver disease and hepatoma. It can induce cryoglobulinemia with vasculitis, porphyria cutanea tarda, chronic arthropathy, and lichen planus.

## Hereditary Hemorrhagic Telangiectasia

*Hereditary hemorrhagic telangiectasia* (Osler-Weber-Rendu syndrome) (Fig. 8.26) is an autosomal dominant disease characterized by cutaneous (typically on the palms, but elsewhere as well) and mucosal (lips, nose, and tongue) telangiectasiae that may bleed. Affected patients typically have frequent nosebleeds (epistaxis) and occasionally gastrointestinal bleeding. Pulmonary arteriovenous fistulae and central nervous system vascular malformations may occur; aortic aneurysms are rare.

## Peutz-Jeghers Syndrome

*Peutz-Jeghers syndrome* (Fig. 8.27) is an autosomal dominant disease characterized by perioral, mucosal, and acral lentigines and gastrointestinal polyps, usually hamartomas, in the small intestine. The malignant potential of the polyps is low, but affected patients do have a higher risk of colon cancer than the general population.

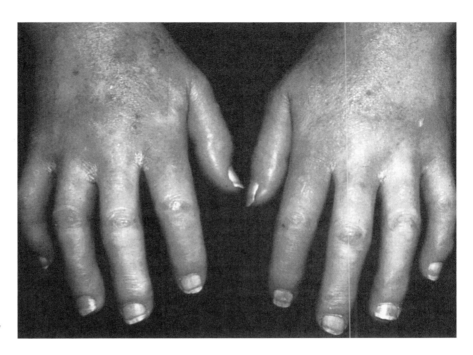

**Figure 8.24** Acrosclerosis: thickened, sclerotic digits.

## Pyoderma Gangrenosum

*Pyoderma gangrenosum* (Fig. 8.28) is an inflammatory ulcerative skin disease with a distinctive morphology: inflammatory ulcers with undermined edges and a border of gray or purple pigmentation. The legs are most commonly affected. The ulcers typically follow trauma. Most patients have either inflammatory bowel disease (usually ulcerative colitis) or rheumatoid arthritis. Some may have paraproteinemia, usually an IgA gammopathy. Bullous pyoderma gangrenosum occurs with leukemia.

## SKIN DISEASE AND ENDOCRINE OR METABOLIC DISEASE

### Skin Disease with Diabetes

Approximately one-third to one-half of all patients with diabetes have skin disease, most commonly diabetic dermopathy (shin spots), thickened skin, acanthosis nigricans, yellowed nails and skin, or cutaneous infections (fungal or yeast, or bacterial most commonly).

*Shin spots* (diabetic dermopathy) are small, discrete, scarlike plaques on the legs. They are a common, though nonspecific, occurrence in diabetic patients.

*Thickened skin*, which may vary from pebbling to sclerodermalike changes, is another common finding. *Scleredema*, a chronic thickening of the skin on the upper back and shoulders, usually affects men with long-standing uncontrolled diabetes. *Stiff hand syndrome*, a waxy thickening of the skin combined with restricted mobility, occurs in young patients with insulin-dependent juvenile diabetes; renal and retinal vascular disease often follows the syndrome.

Acanthosis nigricans (see earlier section) commonly occurs with obesity and other insulin-resistant disorders, primarily diabetes.

*Yellowed nails and skin* occur in approximately 50% of patients with diabetes, primarily on the palms and soles,

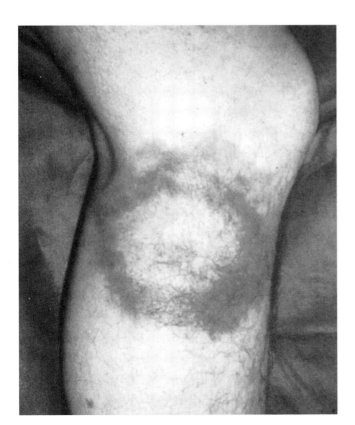

**Figure 8.25** Erythema chronicum migrans (Lyme disease): annular, reddened plaque.

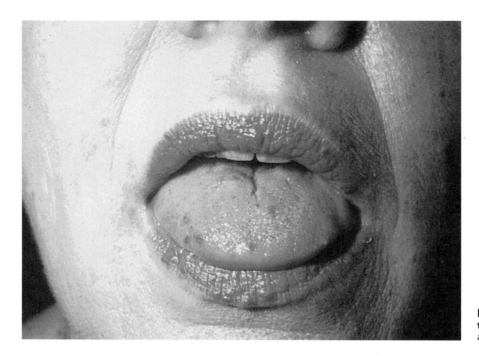

**Figure 8.26** Hereditary hemorrhagic telangiectasia: telangiectasiae of the skin and mucosa.

probably secondary to either carotenemia or protein glycosylation. The significance is unknown.

Less common concerns include perforating disorders, calciphylaxis, and perhaps granuloma annulare.

*Acquired perforating disorders* primarily affect patients with diabetes mellitus and renal failure, especially those on hemodialysis. Patients have pruritic hyperkeratotic papules in a generalized distribution, especially on the legs.

*Calciphylaxis* is characterized by painful, inflammatory necrotic plaques that primarily affect adults with end-stage renal disease, diabetes mellitus, and secondary hyperparathyroidism. It is caused by calcium deposits, within the cutaneous vasculature, which lead to necrosis.

*Granuloma annulare,* characterized by reddened annular papules and plaques, usually on the hands and feet, may occur with or without diabetes.

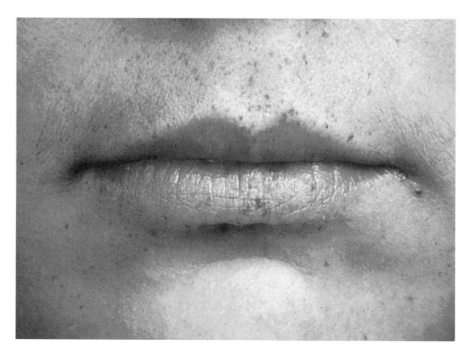

**Figure 8.27** Peutz-Jeghers syndrome: hyperpigmented macules (lentigines) on the skin and mucosa.

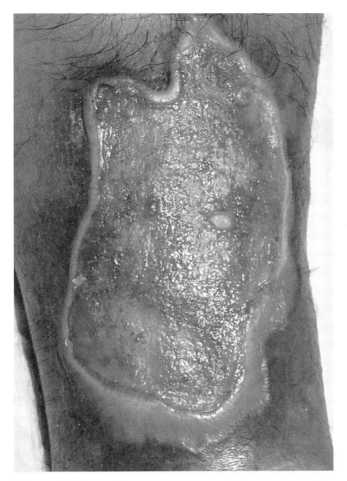

**Figure 8.28** Pyoderma gangrenosum: inflammatory, undermined ulcer.

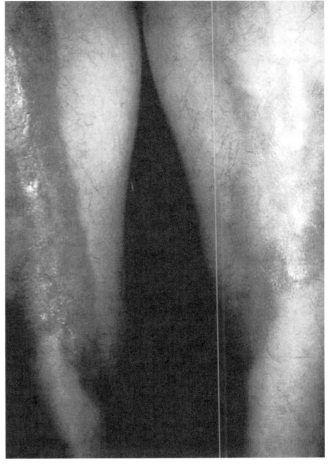

**Figure 8.29** Necrobiosis lipoidica diabeticorum: shiny atrophic plaques.

Uncommon but specific concerns include necrobiosis lipoidica diabeticorum, diabetic bullae (bullous diabeticorum), and eruptive xanthoma.

*Necrobiosis lipoidica diabeticorum* (Fig. 8.29)—yellowed, atrophic plaques usually on the shins that may ulcerate—is uncommon but highly specific for diabetes.

*Diabetic bullae* are also very uncommon. Bullae erupt and resolve spontaneously and heal without scarring. They occur mainly in male patients with type II diabetes mellitus.

*Eruptive xanthomas,* characterized by discrete yellow papules on the extremities and buttocks, occur in patients with diabetes and hyperlipidemia (elevated triglycerides). Pruritus can be significant. Xanthomas resolve with treatment of the hyperlipidemia.

## Porphyrias

Porphyrias are a group of disorders of heme biosynthesis that may be erythropoietic, hepatic, or mixed; each type, whether inherited or acquired, has a specific enzyme defect. Porphyria cutanea tarda (Fig. 8.30), the most common porphyria, is a hepatic porphyria that may be inherited or acquired. Affected patients lack uroporphyrinogen decarboxylase, which converts uroporphyrin to coproporphyrin; as such, uroporphyrins accumulate in the urine. Precipitating factors include hepatitis C infection, alcohol ingestion, estrogens, and toxins such as hexachlorobenzene. Skin disease typically includes photosensitivity, skin fragility, vesicles, bullae, and erosions, usually on the hands, forearms, and face. Hyperpigmentation and hypertrichosis (excess hair growth) may occur, usually on the face.

*Pseudoporphyria* resembles porphyria cutanea tarda but without the enzyme defect; plasma and urinary porphyrins are normal. Common causes are hemodialysis and certain medications, such as nonsteroidal anti-inflammatory drugs (NSAIDs), furosemide, nalidixic acid, and tetracycline.

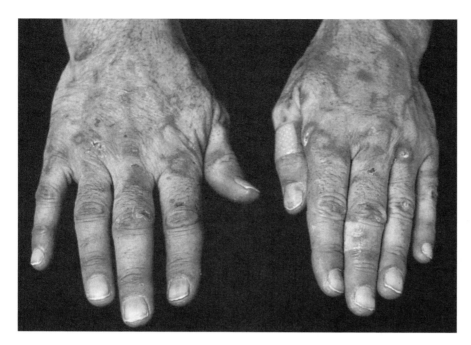

**Figure 8.30**  Porphyria cutanea tarda: vesicles and erosions.

# REVIEW EXERCISES

## QUESTIONS

**1.** Acute urticaria in a healthy young woman commonly follows all the following *except*
a) Crash dieting
b) Chocolate ingestion
c) Pregnancy
d) Alcohol ingestion

**2a.** A 35-year-old woman developed several painful, reddened plaques on the face, arms, legs, and trunk associated with fever, arthralgia, and myalgia. The most likely diagnosis is
a) Lyme disease
b) Sweet's syndrome
c) Dermatomyositis
d) Sarcoidosis
e) Erythema multiforme

**2b.** Affected patients often develop which of the following?
a) Adenocarcinoma of the breast
b) Adenocarcinoma of the gastrointestinal tract
c) Pulmonary disease
d) Myocarditis
e) Leukemia

**3.** Which is the most common type of drug eruption?
a) Exanthematous or morbilliform
b) Urticarial
c) Phototoxic
d) Photoallergic
e) None of the above

**4.** Which is the most important prognostic indicator for melanoma?
a) Lymph node involvement
b) Site of the tumor
c) Histologic depth of invasion (Breslow depth)
d) Age and sex of the patient
e) Tumor size

**5.** A 30-year-old man with ulcerative colitis developed an inflammatory undermined ulcer on his left leg. The most likely diagnosis is
a) Necrobiosis lipoidica diabeticorum
b) Stasis ulcer
c) Gangrene
d) Pyoderma gangrenosum
e) Kaposi's sarcoma

**6.** An elderly woman with tense bullae on the extremities most likely has
a) Bullous pemphigoid
b) Pemphigus vulgaris
c) Dermatitis herpetiformis
d) Erythema multiforme

**7.** Dermatitis herpetiformis is strongly associated with
a) Recurrent herpes virus infection
b) Atopic dermatitis
c) Gluten-sensitive enteropathy
d) Nonsteroidal anti-inflammatory drug (NSAID) use

**8.** A 35-year-old woman has tender targetoid plaques on her hands and oral erosions. What is the most likely cause?
**a)** Toxic shock syndrome
**b)** Herpes simplex virus infection
**c)** Diabetes mellitus
**d)** Pemphigus vulgaris

**9.** Lupus pernio is the central face and airway involvement of
**a)** Tuberculosis
**b)** Systemic lupus erythematosus
**c)** Psoriasis
**d)** Sarcoidosis
**e)** Granuloma annulare

## ANSWERS

**1. c.**
The most common causes of acute urticaria are medications, food, and infection.

**2a. b.**
Sweet's syndrome, characterized by painful, reddened plaques on the face, extremities, and trunk, typically affects women, often in association with a flu-like illness.

**2b. e.**
Sweet's syndrome is strongly associated with myelocytic or myelomonocytic leukemia.

**3. a.**
The most common type of drug eruption is the exanthematous reaction.

**4. c.**
The histologic depth of invasion is the most important prognostic indicator for melanoma.

**5. d.**
Pyoderma gangrenosum is an inflammatory ulcerative disease of the legs. Ulcers have undermined edges and gray or purple borders. Approximately 50% of affected patients have inflammatory bowel disease, usually ulcerative colitis or rheumatoid arthritis.

**6. a.**
Bullous pemphigoid is an uncommon blistering disease of the elderly, characterized by tense bullae, most commonly on the extremities. Mucosal involvement is rare.

**7. c.**
Most patients with dermatitis herpetiformis have an asymptomatic gluten-sensitive enteropathy; some have thyroid disease.

**8. b.**
Erythema multiforme is most commonly associated with recurrent oral herpes simplex virus infection.

**9. d.**
Sarcoidal involvement of the central face and upper respiratory tract characterizes lupus pernio.

## SUGGESTED READINGS

Callen JP. Pyoderma gangrenosum. *Lancet* 1998;351:581.
Callen JP. Neutrophillic dermatoses. *Dermatol Clinics* 2002;20:409.
Giuffrida TJ, Kerdel FA. Sarcoidosis. *Dermatol Clinics* 2002;20:435.
Kahn LE, Russo G, Millikan LE. Genetic and acquired cutaneous disorders associated with internal malignancy. *Int J Dermatol* 1995;34: 749.
McDonnell JK. Cardiac disease and the skin. *Dermatol Clinics* 2002; 20:503.
Perez MI, Kohn SR. Cutaneous manifestations of diabetes mellitus. *J Am Acad Dermatol* 1994;30:519.
Poole S, Fenske NF. Cutaneous markers of internal malignancy. I, II. *J Am Acad Dermatol* 1993;28:147.
Rivers JK. Melanoma. *Lancet* 1996;347:803.
Scott JE, Ahmed AR. The blistering diseases. *Med Clin North Am* 1998; 82:1239.

# Occupational Medicine

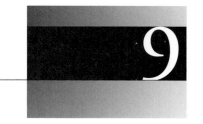

*Peter J. Mazzone    Edward P. Horvath Jr.*

General internists are called upon to manage many occupational health–related issues. Services commonly provided include preplacement examinations, injury care, and return-to-work evaluations. In addition, the internist must be knowledgeable about the evaluation and management of toxicity related to exposures in the environment and the workplace.

This chapter provides information that will help the internist recognize and manage three common chemical exposures, three common pneumoconioses, and occupational asthma. The suggested readings expand on these and other topics.

## CHEMICAL EXPOSURES

Chemical exposures can result from occupational exposure, industrial accidents, natural disasters, recreational contact, chemical warfare, or acts of terrorism. Here we discuss three common exposures—the asphyxiant carbon monoxide, cholinesterase inhibitors such as organophosphate insecticides, and heavy metal exposure to lead.

### Asphyxiants–Carbon Monoxide

Asphyxiants are chemicals that lead to tissue hypoxia after exposure. Cardiovascular and neurologic symptoms predominate. Simple asphyxiants (e.g., methane, propane, nitrogen, carbon dioxide) cause tissue hypoxia by displacing oxygen in inspired air. Chemical asphyxiants (e.g., carbon monoxide, cyanide, hydrogen sulfide) cause tissue hypoxia by interfering with oxygen transport and/ or cellular respiration in the body. Carbon monoxide is the most commonly encountered chemical asphyxiant.

Carbon monoxide poisoning is one of the most common forms of poisoning in both occupational and nonoccupational settings. As a by-product of incomplete combustion, it is present in virtually every workplace and home environment, particularly during the heating season. As an odorless, colorless, and tasteless gas, it gives no warning of its presence. Additionally, the typical early symptoms of exposure—nausea, headache, and dizziness—occur frequently with common disorders, such as viral illness. Practicing physicians must be aware of the possibility of carbon monoxide poisoning, particularly among certain workers, and during

the heating season. A measurement of blood carboxyhemoglobin always should be obtained in such circumstances.

#### Occupational Exposure

Certain employees are recognized as being at particular risk for carbon monoxide poisoning, including firefighters, coal miners, coke oven and smelter workers, mechanics, and drivers. Exhaust from the operation of vehicles indoors, such as propane-powered forklift trucks, is a frequently overlooked source of exposure. Overexposure is particularly likely to occur during winter months, when the ventilation of the work environment may be decreased to lower the costs of heating. Methylene chloride, a solvent widely used as a paint stripper, produces a unique form of carbon monoxide poisoning by being metabolized to carbon monoxide in the body.

#### Environmental Exposure

Carbon monoxide is also a significant cause of poisoning in nonoccupational environments. Despite widespread recognition of this hazard, fatalities occur each year from prolonged exposure to automobile exhaust in enclosed spaces. Deaths of entire families from carbon monoxide poisoning caused by malfunctioning furnaces or space heaters are disturbingly common. Deliberate personal exposure from cigarette or cigar smoke can produce blood carboxyhemoglobin levels from 2% to 10% and sometimes as high as 18%. Nonexposed persons have an average level of 1% or less from endogenous hemoglobin metabolism.

#### Clinical Effects

Carbon monoxide has an affinity for hemoglobin of approximately 200 to 300 times that of oxygen; however, the formation of carboxyhemoglobin is not the only way in which carbon monoxide exerts adverse physiologic effects. It also shifts the oxygen–hemoglobin dissociation curve and binds to both myoglobin and cytochrome oxidase. The central nervous system and myocardium are sensitive to the tissue hypoxia produced by carbon monoxide. The clinical effects in a given patient depend on the intensity and duration of clinical exposure and the presence of any preexisting conditions, such as atherosclerosis. Blood carboxyhemoglobin levels of 10% or less rarely produce symptoms. At levels of 10% to 30%, patients may complain of headache, nausea, weakness, and dizziness. Mentation begins to be impaired at 30% to 35%, and levels of 35% to 40% may result in coma. Death can occur with levels exceeding 50%. As with many chemical exposures, considerable individual variation occurs. Death has occurred from blood levels of 36% to 38% in circumstances of prolonged exposure, presumably from the longer time available for the cytochromes to be inhibited. Although many patients with carbon monoxide poisoning recover completely, others exhibit delayed neurologic and neuropsychiatric manifestations thought to be due to diffuse demyelination. These complications can include a parkinsonian movement disorder, cranial nerve dysfunction, peripheral motor or sensory loss, and disorders of cognition and affect.

### Laboratory Studies

A person who has been overcome by carbon monoxide and brought to the emergency room from a typical exposure environment (e.g., a running vehicle in a closed garage) seldom poses a diagnostic problem. In some instances, however, exposure to carbon monoxide may not be readily apparent, and the patient's symptoms may be nonspecific. A key diagnostic clue is the presence of discordance between the oxygen saturation as measured by pulse oximetry and that measured by an arterial blood gas (by co-oximetry). The oxygen saturation measured by pulse oximetry is usually falsely normal. Arterial blood gases show a normal partial pressure of oxygen, but the oxygen saturation is decreased. Electrolytes may show hypokalemia. In the presence of tissue damage, creatine kinase and lactate dehydrogenase are elevated. The electrocardiogram may show ischemic changes. The measurement of the carboxyhemoglobin level confirms the diagnosis.

### Treatment

The objectives of treatment are to increase tissue oxygenation and speed the elimination of carbon monoxide. Administration of 100% oxygen by a tightly fitting face mask reduces the half-life from 5.5 hours to approximately 1.5 hours. Hospitalization should be considered if evidence of end-organ dysfunction is present (e.g., an abnormal electrocardiogram or neurologic findings) or carbon monoxide levels are greater than 25%. Assisted ventilation is required for patients in respiratory distress. Treatment with hyperbaric oxygen at 2 to 3 atm should be considered for severely affected patients with coma or seizures or for those in whom neurologic and cardiovascular dysfunction does not resolve with other forms of oxygen therapy. Oxygen at 3 atm not only reduces the half-life for carbon monoxide elimination to 23 minutes, but it also results in enough available oxygen dissolved in the plasma to support metabolism, even in the absence of functioning hemoglobin. The prompt use of hyperbaric oxygen also may reduce the risk of delayed neurologic symptoms.

## Cholinesterase Inhibitors–Organophosphate Insecticides

Chemicals that inhibit the enzyme acetylcholinesterase include organic phosphorus pesticides, carbamate pesticides, and organophosphorus "nerve agents" (e.g., sarin, VX). The result of exposure is overstimulation of the cholinergic system, with both muscarinic and nicotinic effects. Exposure may result from inhalation, ingestion, or absorption through the skin. Antidotes include atropine, pralidoxime, and benzodiazepines (for seizure control). Here we focus on organophosphate insecticides.

Internists occasionally encounter patients either acutely poisoned by pesticides or fearful of potential the long-term effects from past exposure. Although a large number of different pesticides are in commercial use, physicians are most likely to encounter clinical problems caused by the organophosphate insecticides. The toxicity of organophosphate insecticides varies widely. One of the least toxic, malathion, commonly results in home-use exposures. Poisoning from more toxic agents, such as parathion, is rare except in agricultural regions or in a pesticide manufacturing or formulating facility.

### Occupational Exposure

In occupational settings, exposures occur during the manufacturing, formulation, transportation, and application of pesticides. Firefighters and hazardous waste workers may encounter these substances in their work. Organophosphate insecticides are readily absorbed by inhalation, through intact skin, and by ingestion.

### Environmental Exposure

Exposures may occur among families of field workers or farmers who come in contact with contaminated clothing. Haphazard aerial spraying also can result in exposure in rural families. The general public often expresses concern about pesticide contamination of food or water, although actual clinical toxicity in such circumstances is rare. Organophosphate poisoning from accidental ingestion by children remains regrettably common, particularly when unused pesticide is stored in an inappropriate container, such as a pop bottle or can.

### Clinical Effects

Anticholinesterase compounds produce their clinical effects through the phosphorylation of the acetylcholinesterase enzyme at nerve endings. The resultant accumulation of the neurotransmitter acetylcholine at these nerve endings produces overstimulation and then paralysis of nerve transmission. Both nicotinic (ganglionic and neuromuscular) and muscarinic (parasympathetic) effects are observed. Various mnemonics have been devised to assist clinicians in remembering the clinical signs and symptoms of cholinesterase inhibition. A common one, *STUMBLED*, stands for *sal*ivation, *t*remors, *u*rination, *m*iosis, *b*radycardia, *l*acrimation, emesis, and diarrhea. The developmental sequence of systemic effects and the time of onset after exposure can vary. Acute toxicity is usually rapid in onset, although symptoms may be delayed up to 12 hours after exposure. In cases of inhalation, respiratory and ocular symptoms may appear first. In cases of ingestion, gastrointestinal effects may be the initial manifestation. Occupational exposures insufficient to produce symptoms following a single event can result in symptoms after continued daily exposure. Depending on treatment, a complete symptomatic recovery usually occurs within a week; however, increased susceptibility to the effects of anticholinesterase agents may persist for several weeks after a single exposure.

A delayed peripheral neuropathy has been reported after poisoning by some organophosphates. This condition, organophosphate-induced delayed neuropathy, is thought to be due to the phosphorylation and inhibition of the enzyme neurotoxic esterase, followed by degradation of the phosphoryl-enzyme complex. This predominantly motor polyneuropathy occurs 2 to 3 weeks after acute poisoning, usually by intentional ingestion. An "intermediate syndrome" after acute poisoning also has been reported. It consists of a paralytic syndrome involving primarily proximal limb muscles, neck flexors, certain cranial motor nerves, and the muscles of respiration, which occurs 24 to 96 hours after heavy exposure. Neuropsychiatric or cognitive complaints, such as irritability, depression, anxiety, fatigue, difficulty in concentration, and short-term memory impairment, are commonly reported after acute exposures. In the assessment of individual cases, however, it is often difficult to distinguish organically based neurobehavioral symptoms from the psychologic reactions likely to occur after exposure events.

### Laboratory Studies

The diagnosis of organophosphate poisoning depends on a history of exposure, the presence of typical signs and symptoms, and laboratory documentation of cholinesterase inhibition. Two types of cholinesterase levels can be measured: plasma cholinesterase (pseudocholinesterase) and red cell cholinesterase (true acetylcholinesterase). Plasma cholinesterase, which is synthesized by the liver, declines sooner but regenerates faster than does red cell cholinesterase. Typical regeneration time is days to a few weeks. Depressed plasma cholinesterase levels also are seen in genetic pseudocholinesterase deficiency and in chronic liver disease. Red cell cholinesterase more accurately reflects the degree of actual enzyme inactivation at neuroeffector sites; however, it is depressed more slowly and for longer periods than plasma cholinesterase. Typical regeneration time is 1 to 3 months. Cholinesterase levels are of greater clinical utility when they can be compared with a preexposure baseline. Unfortunately, such data are rarely available except in pesticide-exposed workers in whom prior medical surveillance testing has been conducted. A cholinesterase depression of 25% or more, compared with the pre-exposure baseline, is regarded as evidence of excessive absorption. A reduction of greater than 50% is usually seen with frank poisoning.

### Treatment

For relatively mild cases, treatment may consist only of removal from further exposure and decontamination of clothing and skin. Healthcare personnel must avoid direct cutaneous contact with obviously contaminated clothing inasmuch as organophosphate compounds are readily absorbed through intact skin. Gastric lavage is indicated in cases of pesticide ingestion. Anticonvulsant medication may be necessary (benzodiazepines are the agents of choice). In severe cases, a patent airway must be established, both for removal of excess secretions and to institute ventilatory support. In the absence of cyanosis, atropine sulphate should be administered intravenously in high doses, typically 1 to 4 mg. This is repeated every 15 minutes until signs of atropinization appear: a dry, flushed skin; tachycardia as high as 140 beats per minute; and a pupillary dilatation. A mild degree of atropinization should be maintained for at least 24 hours. Pralidoxime chloride (Protopam) reactivates the enzyme cholinesterase by breaking the acetylcholinesterase–phosphate complex; 1 to 2 g are given as an intravenous infusion and can be repeated 1 to 2 hours later if muscle weakness has not improved. Additional doses can be given at 10- to 12-hour intervals. Treatment with pralidoxime chloride is most effective if initiated within 24 hours after exposure. In addition to an assessment of clinical response, red cell cholinesterase levels should be monitored.

## Heavy Metals–Lead Intoxication

Lead has been used extensively since antiquity. Considerable information regarding the cause, clinical effects, prevention, and treatment of lead poisoning has been compiled. Despite a reduction in clinical cases arising in industrialized settings, lead poisoning continues to occur in both occupational and nonoccupational environments, providing a challenge to both internists and pediatricians.

### Occupational Exposure

Although many industrial workers still regularly come in contact with lead-containing compounds, modern control measures, such as those found in the Occupational Safety and Health Administration's (OSHA) lead standard, have reduced the incidence of overt cases of clinical poisoning in high-risk operations, such as battery manufacturing, brass and bronze foundry work, and lead smelting and refining. Cases continue to be reported in occupations in which lead exposure is less well appreciated, however. Bridge reconstruction workers are exposed to airborne lead arising from lead-painted surfaces that are subjected to abrasive blasting or oxyacetylene torch cutting or welding.

Avid marksmen, particularly those frequently engaged in shooting competitions, may develop symptoms from exposures in inadequately ventilated indoor firing ranges. The risk of clinical toxicity is generally low in occupations such as soldering and lead glass manufacturing.

### Environmental Exposure

Exposure to leaded paint continues to be a serious hazard to both children and adults. Youngsters, particularly those in inner cities, regularly ingest paint chips from deteriorating interior surfaces. Adults are exposed to lead-containing dust generated by the abrasion of painted surfaces during building renovation. Although lead water pipes and storage tanks are no longer used in homes, some pipes still contain lead solder. Lead can enter domestic water supplies under certain conditions, particularly if the water is slightly acidic and has been in contact with a leaded surface for a prolonged time.

The declining use of alkyl lead compounds as antiknock agents in gasoline has decreased the risk from this source of exposure. Improperly manufactured lead-glazed earthenware can be an unusual source of lead poisoning, particularly with acidic foods and beverages, which may dissolve lead from the glaze. The risk is low with commercially manufactured stoneware, which is fired at a sufficiently high temperature. Although improvements in canning technology have decreased the lead content of canned foods substantially, folk remedies and "health foods" are generally unregulated and may be a source of unsuspected exposure.

### Clinical Effects

Inorganic lead can enter the body by inhalation or ingestion. The former is more common in occupational exposures and the latter in environmental settings. After absorption, it is distributed to the erythrocytes, liver, and kidneys. Over time, lead is redistributed to the bones, following a metabolic pathway similar to that of calcium. Through its ability to interact with sulfhydryl groups, lead exerts toxic effects on a number of organ systems, resulting in a wide range of clinical effects.

Classic lead colic, which is due to the spasmodic contraction of intestinal smooth muscle, is now encountered only rarely. More common are its insidious gastrointestinal symptoms, including vague abdominal discomfort, anorexia, and constipation. Because lead interferes with hemoglobin synthesis, anemia is a frequent clinical finding. This condition has been described as microcytic, hypochromic and normocytic, or normochromic anemia. Lead also shortens erythrocyte life span through a poorly understood mechanism. The resulting increased erythropoiesis in the bone marrow leads to the additional findings of reticulocytosis and basophilic stippling of red cells. Heavy, persistent exposure lasting 10 years or longer may result in a lead nephropathy, characterized by progressive renal impairment and hypertension. Tubular dysfunction may be sufficiently severe as to result in a Fanconi-like syndrome with aminoaciduria, glucosuria, and hyperphosphaturia. Lead interferes with the excretion of urates. The resulting hyperuricemia can lead to a form of gout referred to as *saturnine*, an old term for lead poisoning.

Severe involvement of the peripheral nervous system, leading to paralysis of the extensor muscles of the wrist (wrist drop) or ankles (foot drop), is now uncommon. Likewise, occupationally induced lead encephalopathy is rare; however, acute encephalopathy remains a regrettably frequent and serious complication of childhood lead poisoning. Although chelation treatment has reduced the mortality substantially, approximately 25% of survivors exhibit permanent brain damage. Some cases of mild poisoning in adults may present with vague neuropsychiatric complaints such as headache, poor concentration, and memory loss. Because these symptoms are relatively common, nonspecific complaints in clinical practice, the diagnosis of lead poisoning may not be suspected without obtaining a thorough occupational history. Reproductive effects in both men and women have been described, including increased rates of miscarriages and stillbirths, prematurity, reduced birth weights, and decreased sperm counts and motility.

### Laboratory Studies

The diagnosis of lead poisoning, like that of all occupational and environmental disorders, is an exercise in clinical judgment requiring a full consideration of the medical and occupational history, the physical examination, and the relevant laboratory studies. The measurement of blood lead is the single most useful diagnostic test. It is also the preferred test for the biologic monitoring of exposed workers. It reflects recent exposure and is less variable than urinary lead measurements; however, the mere elevation of blood lead slightly above the upper limits of laboratory "normal" should not necessarily lead to a diagnosis of lead poisoning. Clinical symptoms (e.g., abdominal complaints) or organ-system effects (e.g., anemia) should be present before the diagnosis is made. Concentrations greater than 40 μg/dL, but less than 60 μg/dL, indicate increased absorption, but they may or may not be accompanied by clinical symptoms. Patients with blood lead levels greater than 80 μg/dL usually have clinical manifestations of lead toxicity and detectable anemia. Although an approximate dose–response relationship exists between blood lead levels and clinical effects, differences occur in individual susceptibility and in the interpretation of test results.

The measurement of free erythrocyte protoporphyrin or zinc protoporphyrin relates to lead's effect on heme synthetase. Free erythrocyte protoporphyrin and zinc protoporphyrin levels begin to increase when the blood lead level exceeds 40 μg/dL. These levels stay elevated longer than blood lead and are therefore better indicators of chronic intoxication; however, they are less specific than blood lead and also may be elevated in patients with iron deficiency anemia. Other laboratory studies that should be ordered in the initial assessment of any lead-exposed patient include a complete blood count with peripheral smear, blood urea nitrogen, creatinine, and urinalysis.

The assessment of a causal role for remote lead exposure in a chronic disorder, such as nephropathy, can be difficult. The usual measures of recent exposure, such as the blood lead level, are generally normal. Over time, most of the body burden is redistributed to the kidneys, liver, and especially bone. A lead-mobilization test using edetate calcium disodium (CaEDTA) has been advocated. A newer technique using radiographic fluorescence and bone densitometry also can measure accumulated lead.

### Treatment

The initial treatment of lead poisoning is a removal of the patient from further exposure. In adults with mild symptoms and only slight anemia, this may be all that is necessary. In patients with higher blood levels, more striking clinical symptoms, and significant anemia, chelation therapy is indicated. CaEDTA is the parenteral agent of choice and is usually given in cases of acute or severe poisoning. An orally administered agent, 2,3-dimercaptosuccinic acid (Succimer), has gained acceptance for lead poisoning in both children and adults. The prophylactic use of chelating agents to prevent elevated blood lead levels in workers who have been occupationally exposed is expressly prohibited by OSHA's lead standard.

## PNEUMOCONIOSES

The term *pneumoconiosis* is derived from Greek and simply means "dusty lungs." The term is used to describe the permanent alteration of lung structure caused by the inhalation of a mineral dust and the reaction of the lung tissue to this dust. The reactions that occur within the lungs vary with the size of the dust particle and its biologic activity. Some dusts (like barium, tin, and iron) do not result in a fibrogenic reaction in the lungs. Others can evoke a variety of tissue responses. Nodular fibrosis may occur with exposure to crystalline silica, diffuse fibrosis with exposure to asbestos, and macule formation with focal emphysema after exposure to coal. Still others, such as beryllium, can evoke a systemic response and induce a granulomatous reaction in the lungs. Treatment is supportive because specific therapies do not exist. This section contains a discussion of the traditional dust exposures (asbestos, silica, coal) and the illnesses they produce.

### Asbestos

Exposure to asbestos can lead to a variety of manifestations in the lungs. Pleural disease, parenchymal disease (asbestosis), and asbestos as a carcinogen are discussed in the next three sections.

### Exposure

Exposure to asbestos occurs during its mining, milling, and transport, as well as during the manufacture and application of asbestos-containing products. Plumbers, pipefitters, insulators, and electricians working in the construction and shipbuilding industries are most commonly exposed. Manifestations of the various associated lung diseases typically occur many years after the initial exposure. A careful occupational history is often needed to identify the exposure.

### Clinical Manifestations
Pleural Diseases
Four forms of pleural disease related to asbestos exposure have been described: pleural plaques, benign asbestos pleural effusions, pleural fibrosis, and malignant mesotheliomas.

*Pleural plaques* are the most common manifestation of asbestos exposure. They are smooth, white, raised, irregular lesions found on the parietal pleura. Most commonly located in the lateral and posterior midzones or over the diaphragms, the plaques are typically asymptomatic, recognized only on chest imaging. Macroscopic calcification is common. Plaques are not associated with the development of a malignant mesothelioma. They are, however, markers of asbestos exposure, and thus individuals with pleural plaques are at risk of developing parenchymal disease, mesothelioma, and lung cancer.

*Benign asbestos pleural effusions* may be silent or present with pain, fever, and shortness of breath. They are an early manifestation of asbestos exposure, occurring within 15 years after initial exposure. The diagnosis of this condition is one of exclusion. It requires known asbestos exposure; the finding of an exudative, bloodstained, lymphocyte-predominant effusion; the lack of tumor development over a 3-year follow-up; and no evidence of another cause of the effusion. Frequently, a thoracoscopy with biopsy is performed to exclude other causes. A benign asbestos pleural effusion is usually transient but requires close follow-up. No specific therapy is required. Benign asbestos pleural effusions are not associated with the development of a malignant mesothelioma.

*Pleural fibrosis* typically occurs in individuals who have had a remote exposure to asbestos (more than 20 years earlier) that was short-lived and heavy in intensity. Individuals may be asymptomatic or present with progressive shortness of breath and restriction on pulmonary function testing depending on the degree of fibrosis. The fibrosis can occur as a focal or diffuse process. The fibrosed pleura may surround the lung, leading to a trapped lung, or fold in on itself, encasing a portion of the parenchyma. The masslike lesion that results is known as *rounded atelectasis*. All degrees of pleural fibrosis are difficult to distinguish from malignancy and frequently require biopsies to ensure benignity. Pleural stripping ("decortication") is a treatment option for those who are symptomatic with a trapped lung and otherwise well enough to tolerate the procedure. The presence of pleural fibrosis indicates an increased risk of parenchymal disease.

Asbestos exposure is responsible for most cases of *malignant mesothelioma*. The presentation is typically the insidious onset of nonpleuritic chest wall pain, 20 to 40 years after the initial exposure. The pain can radiate to the upper abdomen or shoulder and is often associated with dyspnea and systemic symptoms. The mass typically involves both the parietal and visceral pleura. Local invasion is common, with symptoms stemming from the organs invaded. Chest imaging frequently reveals an effusion ipsilateral to the pleural disease and may show pleural plaques in the contralateral hemithorax. Open biopsy is required for the diagnosis. Treatment options are unsatisfactory. For local disease in an otherwise healthy individual, extrapleural pneumonectomy with adjuvant chemotherapy +/− local radiation therapy is recommended. For unresectable disease, a platinum-containing chemotherapy regimen is used. No synergy exists between smoking and asbestos exposure for the development of a malignant mesothelioma.

### Asbestosis

The term *asbestosis* refers to pulmonary fibrosis secondary to asbestos exposure. Risk factors for the development of asbestosis include increased levels and duration of exposure, younger age at initial exposure, and exposure to the amphibole fiber type. It is not associated with smoking. Common symptoms include progressive shortness of breath and a nonproductive cough. Chest pain may be reported. On examination, inspiratory crackles on lung auscultation and digital clubbing are present with variable frequency.

The parenchymal fibrotic changes are most prominent in the lower lobes and subpleural areas. Pulmonary function testing reveals restrictive lung disease with a decreased diffusing capacity for carbon monoxide. These radiographic and physiologic findings can be indistinguishable from those of other causes of pulmonary fibrosis. The presence of concomitant pleural disease and the finding of asbestos or ferruginous bodies in pathologic samples help to support the diagnosis.

Asbestosis may appear and progress long after exposure has ceased. It may remain static or advance over time. No known effective therapy is available. The number of reported deaths from asbestosis has increased over time, related to the time-delayed use of asbestos. The age-adjusted mortality rate from asbestosis is 5.0 per million population from 1985 to 1999.

### Asbestos as a Carcinogen

Asbestos is classified as a class I carcinogen (carcinogenic to humans) by the International Agency for Research on Cancer (IARC). Lung cancer and mesothelioma have been consistently linked with asbestos exposure, whereas the evidence for laryngeal and gastrointestinal malignancies is more variable.

The risk of developing lung cancer in an individual exposed to asbestos is enhanced in a multiplicative fashion by concomitant cigarette smoking. Lung cancer more commonly occurs in individuals who also have asbestosis. All cell types are associated with exposure. The lag time to the development of lung cancer is usually more than 20 years. Treatment follows the principles of lung cancer therapy in individuals without prior asbestos exposure (see Chapter 36). Comorbid lung disease may limit the treatment options.

## Silica

### Exposure

Exposure to crystalline silica occurs when silica-containing rock and sand are encountered. This most commonly occurs in occupations associated with construction, mining, quarrying, drilling, and foundry work. A variety of conditions have been associated with the inhalation of crystalline silica, including silicosis, tuberculosis, obstructive lung disease, and lung cancer.

### Clinical Manifestations

#### Silicosis

The inhalation of crystalline silica can lead to a fibronodular parenchymal lung disease known as silicosis. This most commonly occurs in a form known as chronic or simple silicosis. Individuals with chronic silicosis typically have had more than 20 years of silica exposure. They are frequently without symptoms, although shortness of breath and cough can develop. Their disease is thus recognized radiographically as multiple small nodules with an upper lobe predominance. Hilar adenopathy with "eggshell" calcification can be seen. Pulmonary function abnormalities do not invariably occur. Pathologically, the nodules are recognized as silicotic nodules.

The pulmonary nodules seen with chronic silicosis can become progressive. They may be seen to conglomerate and be accompanied by fibrosis, which has been termed *conglomerate silicosis* and *progressive massive fibrosis*. Shortness of breath and cough can become debilitating. Pulmonary function testing often shows a mixed obstructive and restrictive defect, with a reduction in the diffusing capacity. Death due to silicosis continues to occur. The age adjusted mortality rate was 1.4 per million population from 1985 to 1999.

Acute and accelerated forms of silicosis are more rapidly progressive, typically associated with intense exposure to silica. Acute silicosis can develop within months of exposure. The exposed individual may develop progressive shortness of breath and coughing. The radiographic picture is compatible with acute airspace disease. Pathology mimics alveolar proteinosis, with proteinaceous material in the alveoli, but interstitial involvement and early nodule formation can be seen. A rapid progression to acute respiratory failure is common. Accelerated silicosis occurs after 5 to 15 years of exposure. Patients are usually symptomatic and often progress to respiratory failure and death. They are recognized by the development of upper zone nodules and fibrosis on radiographs and numerous nodules with interstitial fibrosis on pathology.

### Mycobacterial Disease

Mycobacterial disease is known to occur with increased frequency in individuals with silicosis. Individuals with chronic silicosis have an incidence of mycobacterial tuberculosis that is three times greater than that of age-matched controls. Those with acute and accelerated silicosis have the highest incidence of mycobacterial disease. Others exposed to silica but without silicosis may have an excess risk of developing tuberculosis. It is recommended that individuals with silicosis (or long-term exposure to crystalline silica) should receive a tuberculin skin test. If the reaction is 10 mm or greater, and no evidence of active tuberculosis is present, standard treatment for latent tuberculosis should be administered. If symptoms or radiographic changes suggest the possibility of active mycobacterial disease, routine or induced sputum should be obtained. If active tuberculosis is confirmed, standard tuberculosis therapy, with a regimen containing rifampin, should be administered. Similarly, if a nontuberculous mycobacterium is identified, standard therapy for that organism should be administered.

### Obstructive Lung Disease and Lung Cancer

Exposure to crystalline silica has been associated with the development of obstructive lung disease, chronic bronchitis, and emphysema. These associations are more prominent in those with silicosis. The intensity of dust exposure appears to affect the development of obstructive lung diseases. Tobacco smoking may cause an additive effect.

According to the IARC, sufficient evidence exists to classify silica as carcinogenic in humans. Available studies are complicated by multiple confounders and selection biases. Despite this, the bulk of the evidence supports an increased risk for lung cancer in tobacco smokers with silicosis. The relationship is less clear for never-smokers and for individuals exposed to silica who do not have silicosis.

### Other Associations

Evidence suggests a relationship between appreciable silica exposure and the development of scleroderma. Less evidence is available to support an association with rheumatoid arthritis or systemic lupus erythematosus. Similarly, reports of renal disease associated with silica exposure require further evidence to confirm a link.

## Coal Dust

The deposition of coal dust in the lungs can lead to lung disease. In addition to coal worker's pneumoconiosis (CWP), coal dust exposure is also related to the development of airflow limitation, chronic bronchitis, and emphysema. Silica exposure frequently occurs in combination with coal dust exposure; thus, the above-described silica-related illnesses may also be seen.

### Exposure

Coal mining is the major source of exposure. The tissue reaction to coal dust inhalation is the development of a *coal macule*. Over the course of years to decades, focal emphysema may form around the macule. This combination is termed a *coal nodule* and is the characteristic lesion of simple CWP.

### Clinical Manifestations

#### Coal Worker's Pneumoconiosis

Most individuals with CWP are asymptomatic. This presentation is termed *simple CWP*. Given the frequent absence of symptoms, simple CWP is often a radiographic diagnosis. Chest imaging reveals small nodules with upper and posterior zone predominance. Hilar lymph node enlargement is not uncommon, although eggshell calcification does not generally occur. Simple CWP tends to have little effect on lung function.

The presence of shortness of breath or a productive cough in an individual with simple CWP is often related to the coexistence of chronic bronchitis or airflow obstruction. Progressive massive fibrosis (PMF) can occur, more frequently when there has also been exposure to silica. Symptoms advance as the PMF worsens. When PMF occurs, the small nodules seen in simple CWP coalesce, forming opacities larger than 1 cm. These lesions are odd-shaped, usually bilateral, progressive, and may cavitate or become calcified. Care must be taken since lesions diagnosed radiographically as PMF are often shown later to have been tumors, tuberculosis scars, or Caplan's nodules (see following paragraph). Airflow limitation, restriction, and a reduction in diffusing capacity can all be seen when PMF develops. Pulmonary hypertension may develop in advanced disease. Deaths from CWP continue to occur.

The complications of CWP include a higher incidence of mycobacterial disease (although not as high as with silicosis), scleroderma, and an increased risk of stomach cancer. Tuberculin skin testing, chemoprophylaxis, and the treatment of active tuberculosis are recommended, as in silicosis. *Caplan's syndrome* is a nodular form of CWP seen in individuals with rheumatoid arthritis. The nodules are multiple, tend to be larger than typical coal nodules, develop over short periods of time, and more frequently cavitate. These findings usually occur concomitantly with the joint manifestations, active arthritis, and the presence of circulating rheumatoid factor.

## OCCUPATIONAL ASTHMA

Occupational asthma now represents 5% to 15% of new asthma in working adults.

## Exposures

Over 250 exposures are known to cause occupational asthma. Individuals may be exposed to sensitizing agents in a repeated fashion or have had a single exposure to a potent respiratory irritant. Latex exposure is the leading cause of occupational asthma in healthcare workers. Isocyanates found in auto body shops or spray painters are also common. Many others exist, including wood products, textiles, and grains as sensitizing exposures, and chlorine gas, bleach, and strong acids as respiratory irritants.

## Clinical Manifestations

The symptoms of occupational asthma are the same as those for nonoccupational asthma (see Chapter 37). The additional feature is a work-related pattern to these symptoms. The work-related pattern of illness can mean that the asthma symptoms began after a new workplace exposure, or that preexisting asthma was made worse by the exposure. The asthma can be *work aggravated*, producing an exacerbation of asthma that was previously subclinical or in remission; *asthma with latency*, producing new onset asthma caused by a sensitizing exposure; or *asthma without latency*, producing asthma resulting from a single heavy exposure to a potent respiratory irritant. Symptoms are made worse by continuing exposure. This is manifest by increased asthma symptoms in the workplace, which diminish when away from work.

To diagnose occupational asthma the physician must confirm the presence of asthma, confirm an exposure, and confirm a work-related pattern. Asthma may be confirmed by the classic symptoms and signs—shortness of breath, cough, and wheeze. An exposure can be confirmed from a detailed history, including review of Material Safety Data Sheets from the workplace. When the diagnosis is not clear, further testing is necessary.

## Diagnostic Testing

Testing to confirm the presence of asthma includes spirometry, which looks for obstruction with a bronchodilator response. If this is not present, then a methacholine challenge test may be useful. Testing to confirm a sensitizing exposure may include skin or RAST testing, which demonstrates antigen-specific antibodies. Testing to confirm a work-related pattern of the asthma manifestations may include peak flow recordings at work and away from work. Peak flows that fall while the exposure is occurring can objectify the work-related pattern of illness. This is complicated in that some substances (e.g., isocyanates) produce a delayed onset of symptoms (6–8 hrs).

## Treatment

Treatment follows the principles of asthma management for nonoccupational asthma. This includes a patient-centered approach, including education about the illness and active monitoring of symptoms and peak flows. Inhaled corticosteroids and bronchodilators are the mainstays of medical therapy (see Chapter 37). Avoidance of the incriminated exposure must be highlighted.

## REVIEW EXERCISES

### QUESTIONS

**1.** During a preplacement examination for a bridge reconstruction job, a 32-year-old woman was found to have a blood lead level of 4.0 μg/dL (normal, 0.0 to 11.0 μg/dL) and a zinc protoporphyrin of 104 μg/dL (normal, 0.0 to 70.0 μg/dL). She is asymptomatic, and her physical examination is normal. Her medical history is unremarkable except for four pregnancies. The most likely explanation for these laboratory results is
a) Unrecognized environmental lead exposure
b) Iron deficiency anemia
c) Erythropoietic protoporphyria
d) Laboratory error
e) Thalassemia minor

**2.** In the proper medical management of lead toxicity, all the following are true, except
a) Removal from exposure is mandatory.
b) Symptomatic patients with high lead levels should undergo chelation therapy.
c) All patients with elevated blood lead levels should be chelated even if asymptomatic.
d) CaEDTA is the preferred parenteral agent.
e) 2,3-Dimercaptosuccinic acid (Succimer) is the oral agent of choice.

**3.** The appropriate management of a patient poisoned by organophosphate cholinesterase-inhibiting agents includes all the following, except
a) Atropine
b) Sodium nitrite
c) Pralidoxime chloride (Protopam)
d) Maintenance of airway
e) Decontamination

**4.** Acute poisoning from organophosphate insecticides can result in which of the following delayed neurologic effects?
a) Cerebellar degeneration
b) Dementia
c) Bell's palsy
d) Motor polyneuropathy
e) Seizure disorder

**5.** A 52-year-old male employee of a local warehouse operation is seen at an urgent care center complaining of gradual onset of headache, nausea, and dizziness. He relates experiencing similar symptoms over the past few days, which tend to occur near the end of his workshift and resolve overnight. During this time, all windows in his warehouse have remained closed to reduce heating costs. None of his family members is ill, but he claims other employees in his work area are experiencing similar complaints. He has been in good health, in spite of having smoked one-half pack of cigarettes daily for the past 30 years. Physical examination is unremarkable. A blood carboxyhemoglobin level is 20%. An electrocardiogram and cardiac enzymes are normal. Proper medical management of this patient would entail which of the following

a) Nothing, except removal from exposure
b) Administration of 100% oxygen by face mask
c) Assisted ventilation
d) Hospitalization overnight for observation
e) Hyperbaric oxygen at 2 to 3 atm

**6.** The most likely source of carbon monoxide poisoning in a warehouse operation is
a) Malfunctioning central heating unit
b) Indoor vehicular exhaust
c) Employee smoking
d) Ambient (outside) air pollution
e) Methylene chloride

**7.** A 67-year-old man presents to your office concerned about his health. Two of his friends have developed lung disease from dusts they inhaled in their workplace. He wonders if his lungs are all right because he had worked in several dusty places—the shipyards for 20 years, followed by foundry work for another 20 years. He is a prior smoker who is currently asymptomatic. Which of the following statements about the pneumoconioses is most correct?
a) Because he is asymptomatic, he does not have a pneumoconiosis.
b) The most common manifestation of asbestos exposure is a benign asbestos pleural effusion.
c) The risk of developing asbestosis is increased by smoking.
d) Complications of silicosis include mycobacterial infections and an increased risk of lung cancer.
e) Individuals with coal workers' pneumoconiosis never develop progressive massive fibrosis.

**8.** A 36-year-old woman presents to your office with complaints of intermittent shortness of breath, cough, and wheeze of 6 months duration. She notes her symptoms are worse during the week than on the weekend and were relieved during a recent vacation. She is a nonsmoker, with no prior illnesses, who works as a spray-painter in an autobody shop. Which of the following statements about her condition is most true?

a) Very few exposures are known to cause this condition.
b) Diagnosis can only be established by challenge testing.
c) Exposure to latex is the leading cause in healthcare workers.
d) Exposure can be allowed to continue as long as treatment is provided.
e) An individual must have a preexisting condition to be affected.

## ANSWERS

**1. b**
An elevated zinc protoporphyrin with a normal blood lead level is most often due to iron deficiency anemia, particularly in a woman of reproductive age. Because these studies were obtained during the preplacement evaluation, the patient has not yet encountered lead exposure in the workplace. The physician always should inquire about possible environmental or household exposures, such as the use of glazed ceramic ware, folk remedies, or lead-soldered water pipes. A completely normal lead level excludes recent or ongoing lead exposure from any source.

Erythropoietic protoporphyria is a rare disorder that results in significant symptoms, including photosensitivity. Thalassemia minor and laboratory error are theoretically possible, but highly unlikely, explanations for these results.

**2. c.**
The first step in the management of lead toxicity is removal from exposure, and in some cases, this may be all that is necessary. Chelation therapy in adults should be reserved for patients with significant signs or symptoms (e.g., encephalopathy or renal injury). Commonly used chelators have potential side effects (e.g., CaEDTA can cause acute tubular necrosis) and should not be used routinely in asymptomatic patients. The indications for chelation therapy in children are more liberal. The Centers for Disease Control and Prevention recommend that children with blood levels of 45 µg/dL be referred for therapy, and some practitioners routinely treat children having levels between 25 and 44 µg/dL.

Although several chelators have been used in the treatment of lead poisoning, CaEDTA is the drug of choice when a parenteral agent is needed. When an oral agent is preferred (e.g., in children), Succimer is used.

**3. b.**
Atropine blocks the muscarinic effects of organophosphates and should be administered promptly. Pralidoxime chloride (Protopam) reactivates the enzyme cholinesterase by breaking the acetylcholinesterase–phosphate complex. Its advantages over atropine include its ability to reverse muscle paralysis and possible central nervous system depression.

Decontamination procedures may include removal of contaminated clothing, washing of skin and hair, and, if indicated by route of exposure, emptying the stomach. In severe cases, a patent airway must be established for the removal of excess secretions and institution of ventilatory support.

Sodium nitrite is used in cyanide poisoning. It has no role in the management of organophosphate toxicity.

## 4. d.

Acute poisoning with organophosphate insecticides can result in a variety of central nervous system manifestations. A small percentage of patients may exhibit neuropsychiatric or cognitive complaints, such as irritability, depression, anxiety, and short-term memory impairment, weeks to months after initial intoxication. It is often difficult, however, to distinguish organically based neurobehavioral symptoms from the psychological or emotional responses likely to occur after acute chemical exposures.

A delayed peripheral neuropathy has been reported after poisoning by some organophosphates. This condition, organophosphate-induced delayed neuropathy, is a predominantly motor polyneuropathy that occurs 2 to 3 weeks after acute poisoning.

## 5. b.

Removal from further exposure is usually the first step in the management of any toxic event. This has already been accomplished in this case, at least for the time being. The treating physician, however, does have an obligation to promptly report the diagnosis of work-related carbon monoxide poisoning to the employer to ensure appropriate corrective measures are undertaken to lower further employee exposure below permissible limits.

Although this patient would ultimately recover without specific therapy, administration of 100% oxygen by face mask would reduce the half-life from 5.5 to 1.5 hours and hasten the patient's symptomatic improvement.

Assisted ventilation, hospitalization, or hyperbaric oxygen are indicated only for those more severely affected than this patient.

## 6. b.

Although the central heating unit always should be inspected in any episode of carbon monoxide poisoning occurring within a building, propane-powered vehicles, such as forklift trucks, are a more likely source of this problem in a warehouse.

Exposure to environmental tobacco smoke and ambient air pollution, although undesirable, are unlikely to result in clinically significant carbon monoxide poisoning under usual exposure circumstances.

Methylene chloride is metabolized to carbon monoxide, but poisoning from this agent occurs during its use

as a paint stripper, an unlikely operation to be routinely conducted in a warehouse.

## 7. d.

Individuals with silicosis are known to have a higher incidence of mycobacterial infections. All patients with silicosis should receive a standardized intradermal tuberculin skin test. If positive (>10 mm) and no sign of active infection exists, then treatment for latent tuberculosis should be administered. If evidence of active tuberculosis is present, then a standard treatment regimen including rifampin should be administered. Treatment for nontuberculosis mycobacteria is no different in for those with silicosis.

Many individuals with silicosis and CWP are asymptomatic. The most common manifestation of asbestos exposure is a pleural plaque. No increased risk exists of developing asbestosis in smokers. Individuals with CWP may develop progressive massive fibrosis. This more commonly occurs where there may be concomitant exposure to silica.

## 8. c.

Exposure to latex can act as a sensitizer that leads to occupational asthma. It is the most common cause of occupational asthma in healthcare workers. Over 250 exposures are known to cause occupational asthma. The diagnosis requires the presence of asthma (symptoms, pulmonary function testing), the recognition of an exposure (history, skin testing, RAST testing), and a work-related pattern to the symptoms. The cornerstone of therapy is avoidance of the exposure. Preexisting asthma may be made worse by the exposure, or asthma can be of new onset and related to the exposure of concern.

## SUGGESTED READINGS

Agency for Toxic Substances and Disease Registry (ATSDR). *Case studies in environmental medicine.* Washington, DC: U.S. Department of Health and Human Services, 1990–2000.

Asbestos Standard for the Construction Industry. OSHA 3096, U.S. Department of Labor, 2002 (Revised).

Beckett W, Abraham J, Becklake M, et al. Adverse effects of crystalline silica exposure. Official statement of the American Thoracic Society Committee of the Scientific Assembly on Environmental and Occupational Health. *Am J Respir Crit Care Med* 1997;155:761–768.

Beckett WS. Occupational respiratory diseases. *N Engl J Med* 2000; 342:406–413.

Bowler RM, Cone JE. *Occupational Medicine Secrets.* Philadelphia: Hanley & Belfus, 1999.

Brooks SM, Gochfeld M, Herzstein J, et al., eds. *Environmental Medicine.* St. Louis: Mosby, 1995.

Ernst A, Zibrak JD. Carbon monoxide poisoning. *N Engl J Med* 1998; 339:1603–1608.

Harbison RD. *Hamilton and Hardy's Industrial Toxicology,* 5th ed. St. Louis: Mosby, 1998.

Hathaway G, Proctor NH, Hughes JP. *Proctor and Hughes' Chemical Hazards of the Workplace*, 4th ed. New York: John Wiley and Sons, 1996.

http://monographs.iarc.fr/monoeval/crthgr01.html.

Kales SN, Christiani DC. Acute chemical emergencies. *N Engl J Med* 2004;350:800–808.

LaDou J, ed. *Occupational and Environmental Medicine*, 2nd ed. Stamford, CT: Appleton & Lange, 1997.

McCunney RH, ed. *A Practical Approach to Occupational and Environmental Medicine*, 2nd ed. Philadelphia: Lippincott Williams & Wilkins, 1994.

NIOSH Hazard Review. Health Effects of Occupational Exposure to Respirable Crystalline Silica. DHHS (NIOSH) publication no. 2002-129, April 2002.

Rom WN. *Environmental and Occupational Medicine*, 3rd ed. Boston: Little, Brown and Company, 1998.

Rosenstock L, Cullen MR, eds. *Textbook of Clinical Occupational and Environmental Medicine*. Philadelphia: WB Saunders, 1994.

Sullivan JB, Krieger GR. *Clinical Environmental Health and Toxicology*, 2nd ed. Baltimore: Williams & Wilkins, 2001.

Wagner GR. Asbestosis and silicosis. *Lancet* 1997;349:1311–1315.

Work-Related Lung Disease Surveillance Report, 1999. USDHHS, CDC, Division of Respiratory Disease Studies; DHHS (NIOSH) publication no. 2003-111.

www-cie.iarc.fr/htdocs/monographs/vol68/silica.htm.

Zenz C, Dickerson OB, Horvath EP, eds. *Occupational Medicine*, 3rd ed. St. Louis: Mosby, 1994.

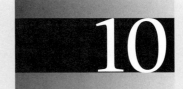

# BOARD SIMULATION: Psychiatric Disorders in Medical Practice

*Kathleen S. N. Franco-Bronson*

Primary care physicians can find almost any psychiatric presentation in their practices, but some are more frequent and require that diagnostic and treatment skills be kept up to date. Most depressed patients present to their primary care physician rather than to a psychiatrist and have physical complaints rather than opening with emotional concerns. Major depression can be a life-threatening illness requiring a rapid assessment of suicide risk and expedient, safe therapy. Somatoform disorders can lead to expensive, unnecessary testing or risky procedures if medical mimics have not been considered. The same can be said for panic disorders, which if accompanied by depression, can carry the highest suicide risk. Patients with generalized anxiety disorder frequently seek medical attention and pharmacologic relief. Hospitalized patients, particularly elderly patients, are at risk for delirium or acute confusional states. As a greater number of people survive into later years, primary care physicians find themselves providing for not only the physical needs but also the cognitive and emotional needs of patients with dementia.

This chapter explores the initial assessment and treatment for commonly seen psychiatric disorders and provides selected real-life cases for more in-depth exploration.

## DEPRESSION

### Case 1

A 76-year-old woman complained of epigastric pain, constipation, and a secondary loss of appetite for longer than

1 month. The pain awakens her at night, which she believes is the cause of daytime fatigue. Various gastrointestinal medications have been tried without success. The results of the upper and lower gastrointestinal series ordered by your partner for this patient were normal. Although the chart indicates that her husband died 3 months ago, she states that she does not believe this event is holding her back and would not describe herself as depressed. She has been devoted to her church throughout her life, but she believes her physical symptoms have kept her from going to services the past few months. She moved out of her home a month ago and into a senior's apartment to live near a female friend. Her friend was admitted to the hospital 2 weeks earlier and has been diagnosed with cancer. The patient has never been treated for a psychiatric disorder, and there is no family history for this. The patient has a 10-lb weight loss since her last visit 6 weeks ago. She has a history of partially controlled hypertension. On an electrocardiogram, her heart rate is 82, PR 0.120 sec, QRS 0.100 sec, and QT 0.430/0.465 sec. She has a 15-mm Hg orthostatic blood pressure drop, but she does not complain of dizziness. Her electrolytes, blood urea nitrogen, creatinine, and physical examination indicate dehydration. Her total protein is slightly low, as are her hemoglobin and hematocrit. Her liver function tests and urine analysis are normal. Her physical examination and chest x-ray do not reveal any additional information.

The best course of action is

a) This is probably normal grief response; just let it run its course.

**b)** Admit her to the hospital for a full workup.

**c)** Give her a 2-week prescription for alprazolam (Xanax); have her return for a follow-up visit

**d)** Order a thyroid stimulating hormone (TSH) test, and call her daughter for additional information; consider prescribing a selective serotonin reuptake inhibitor (SSRI)

**e)** Refer her to a gastroenterologist

Bereavement generally occurs within the first 2 to 3 months after the death of a loved one. Subjects with depression at 2 months are much more likely to be depressed at 2 years, are less likely to engage in new relationships, and are more likely to experience worse generalized health than before their loss. Admitting her to the hospital does not seem necessary at this stage, although we would want to do some basic laboratory studies, including a TSH. It would be unlikely that referral to a gastroenterologist is necessary with two normal gastrointestinal series. The weight loss, insomnia, fatigue, and discontinuation of normal activities are quite possibly symptoms of depression. Starting an anxiolytic is not advisable and likely would slow recognition and treatment of major depression. Additional information and observations by family are always helpful. The best answer is d.

As you talk to her longer, you learn that she believes she must have done something wrong for her husband to die, and now she is losing her best friend. She talks about her daughters, one who is a nun and has much responsibility and the other who lives in a distant state with her husband and the patient's only grandchildren.

She admits to withdrawal from others. She says, "I should be stronger. My daughters have important things to do. As for other friends, if I get close, they'll just be taken away from me." The patient acknowledges that she thinks about these things a great deal and also wonders whether her body is developing cancer. She does not drink alcohol or smoke cigarettes, and she has no suicidal thoughts.

Which do you think most closely identifies her situation?

**a)** Generalized anxiety disorder

**b)** Occult affective disorder (major depression without psychosis, single episode)

**c)** Hypochondriasis

**d)** Psychotic delusional disorder

**e)** Posttraumatic stress disorder

The patient has many of the criteria for major depressive disorder and few of those for the other diagnoses (see criteria for Major Depressive Episode in *Diagnostic and Statistical Manual of Mental Disorders*, Fourth Edition). Prior to her husband's death, the patient had no history of free floating or pervasive anxiety. She did not have a "track record" for believing she had serious, life-threatening illness in the absence of any findings. No hallucinations, delusions, or evidence that she is out of touch with reality are present. There is also no evidence of flashbacks, nightmares, or intrusive thoughts of an extremely horrific event that would never be expected to occur. The correct answer is b.

The mnemonic SIGECAPS is helpful in remembering the common signs and symptoms of depression. To meet criteria for major depression, the patient should have been depressed or dysphoric most of the day for 2 or more weeks, with difficulties in social interactions or at work and problems with at least four of the following:

**S** Sleep is poor with early morning awakening and a fragmented pattern or excessive

**I** Interest in normal activities is diminished

**G** Guilt is excessive or inappropriate

**E** Energy is lower than normal

**C** Concentration is poor

**A** Appetite is reduced or increased, with a consistent weight change

**P** Psychomotor retardation, slowed speech, and physical involvement or agitation is present

**S** Suicidal thoughts or thoughts of death are reported

Because patients who have physical illness alone may have disturbances of sleep, appetite, and energy, it is wise to further explore psychological symptoms.

In the medically ill patient with depression, we also consider the mnemonic WART; H/H:

**W** Withdrawal from others

**A** Anhedonia

**R** Ruminating thoughts

**T** Tearfulness

**H/H** Helplessness/Hopelessness

Listen for the emotional aspects. Patients may not identify themselves as depressed and may continue stoically despite their losses. It may take some additional questions to find the psychologic aspects of their condition. Ruminating on negative thoughts, excessive guilt, or belief of punishment and a lack of interest and pleasure in former activities are key symptoms. Physical symptoms of weight loss and insomnia may be associated with a variety of conditions and can be explored further, but depression should be treated when the criteria exist. Treat patients who meet the criteria for major depression whether a comorbid physical illness or any "good reason to be depressed" exists.

### Effective Treatment

Which of the following is an effective, appropriate, and safe treatment to begin today?

**a)** Escitalopram 10 mg daily

**b)** Electroconvulsive therapy (ECT)

**c)** Amitriptyline, 75 mg twice daily

**d)** Doxepin, 150 mg at bedtime

**e)** Psychoanalytic psychotherapy

The best answer is a. In this case, avoiding additional orthostasis, cardiac conduction delay (quinidine-like), and anticholinergic effects would recommend against a tricyclic.

A rapid, safe first-line choice would be a selective serotonin reuptake inhibitor (SSRI), such as escitalopram. Psychoanalytic psychotherapy is a lengthy procedure and would not be recommended as a stand-alone treatment in this case. Electroconvulsive therapy would be a later option if two or more antidepressants were not effective or if the patient were acutely suicidal.

During any given week, approximately 60% to 80% of the general public has a physical complaint, and physicians may be unable to identify an organic cause in 20% to 80% of patients bringing these symptoms to the office visit. Patients with a diagnosis of major depression more often present with physical symptoms to their primary care physician.

## Case 2

A 52-year-old woman reports that she "just doesn't feel well." You also hear in her history that she has had poor appetite, with an 8-lb weight loss over the last 2 months. She has gradually withdrawn from her family and friends because she is just "too tired." Her interests in her church and grandchildren have deteriorated. She feels guilty about this but cannot seem to energize herself. Although she sometimes wishes she were dead, she convinces you that she would never do anything to hurt herself and has no plan or intent to commit suicide. Your patient is significantly overweight, demonstrates psychomotor retardation, and has marked orthostasis (170/90 mm Hg sitting, 140/80 mm Hg standing, pulse 85). Her evaluation includes a TSH testing of 5.5 and cholesterol of 240. On her electrocardiogram, she has a normal sinus rhythm and ventricular rate of 80, PR of 0.150 sec, QRS of 0.100 sec, and QT/QTc of 0.420/0.468 sec. She had one earlier episode of depression at age 25 and responded to amitriptyline.

Which medication would likely have a greater safety and tolerability for this patient?

a) Amitriptyline (Elavil)
b) Venlafaxine (Effexor)
c) Trazodone (Desyrel)
d) Mirtazapine (Remeron)
e) Sertraline (Zoloft)

Although she responded to amitriptyline in the past, her current QTc, orthostasis, and weight would advise against that. With her preexisting hypertension, venlafaxine would not be the first choice. Her orthostasis, psychomotor retardation, and no indication of anxiety or insomnia would direct away from trazodone. Weight gain, orthostasis, and hypercholesterolemia could be more problematic with mirtazapine. Of these choices, sertraline would be the best choice. The answer is e.

After 2 weeks of 50 mg of sertraline and a partial response, you increase the dose to 100 mg. The patient tells you she has started to have rapid-onset sweating that occasionally occurs during the day and awakens her about five nights out of seven. She wonders whether this is a side effect of sertraline (she read the package insert). You gather more information about her irregular menses. In fact, she has had periods only twice in the past 12 months. As you question her, she remembers her mother going through menopause at about this age.

If augmentation were to be considered, which has been reported to be helpful?

a) Low-dose levothyroxine ($T_4$)
b) Light therapy
c) Estrogen (hormone replacement therapy)
d) Buspirone
e) Any of these

The sweating could be secondary to an SSRI, but it is more likely to be hot flashes heralding the onset of menopause. Some patients will respond to an antidepressant medication only after $T_4$ has been added. Her TSH is toward high normal, so it is worth monitoring and is a consideration. Light therapy may help if it is winter and she is living in an area with few hours of sunlight.

Although initially we would use an antidepressant in this patient, who had an earlier episode of major depression, women in the perimenopausal age group often respond well to hormone replacement therapy (e.g., 0.625 mg estrogen and 2.5 mg progesterone).

Buspirone augments diverse serotonin receptor sites and has been used to improve response to various SSRIs with or without anxiety being present. Certainly, we would not try all these agents at once, but any of these choices has the potential to be helpful to this patient, as would an increase in sertraline. The correct answer is e.

## Case 3

A 76-year-old man presents with a poor appetite, weight loss, and sleep disturbance and is generally apathetic. He is not tearful or suicidal. The patient does not report any significant loss during the past year but is aware that his interest in nearby family, friends, neighbors, and hobbies (gardening, local community groups) has diminished. He feels little energy and finds concentrating on the newspaper too great a challenge. He has a distant history of "hepatitis" in his 20s. You have ordered baseline laboratory tests, including liver function studies, and are ready to order an antidepressant when you notice that his TSH is undetectable and $T_4$ is elevated. You decide to try radioactive iodine to treat his hyperthyroidism first. Although he makes some physical improvements, symptoms of depression continue. He feels more hopeless and withdrawn from others. He ruminates on the time he has lost and wonders whether life is worthwhile at his age. He takes one aspirin a day and astemizole (Hismanal) for a respiratory allergy. He also has a history of coronary artery disease and acute myocardial infarction (MI) 5 years ago. Today his vitals are: temperature 37.1 C, pulse 105, BP 130/85, respirations 16, $O_2$ saturation 95%.

You decide to do which of the following?

a) Wait
b) Start him on citalopram (Celexa)
c) Place him in assisted living several states away where his brother lives
d) Try him on trazodone (Desyrel) to improve his sleep disturbance as well as his depression
e) Begin methylphenidate to activate him

The risk of not treating a major depression in this patient can have more serious consequences than the risk of treatment side effects. Current research confirms that when all else is held constant, depressed patients have a two- to four-fold greater risk for an MI. Many choices are safe for this patient, such as an SSRI (e.g., citalopram). This class of medications is considered a first-line option. Although trazodone might be a good choice for another patient, it is unlikely to be an adequate antidepressant alone and can increase the risk of orthostasis. Methylphenidate is used for some medically ill and depressed patients; however, the potential for tachycardia in this case makes it a less preferable choice. The best answer is b.

While educating our patient and his family about the vascular effects of depression and his new medication (an SSRI), we explain which of the following?

a) SSRI reuptake inhibitors reduce platelet aggregation.
b) Depression increases bleeding time.
c) Depression increases the number of platelets.
d) Depression reduces platelet aggregation.

Research demonstrates that depression increases platelet aggregation and that SSRIs reduce platelet aggregation, with or without depression being present. No evidence suggests that depression increases platelets, and it certainly would not increase bleeding time. SSRIs can also compete with warfarin through the P450 cytochrome 2C9. Although generally not a problem clinically, if acute bleeding occurs, the SSRI should be stopped. The correct answer is a.

## Case 4

In the next examination room, you encounter another elderly man who had an MI 2 weeks ago and is back for follow-up as an outpatient. His hypertension has been treated with the same beta blocker for 5 years. You find he meets criteria now for his first major depression and recommend an antidepressant. His daughter says, "Isn't this a normal reaction, and can we just wait it out?"

You reflect on her comment and respond as follows:

a) "Sure, it's probably only an adjustment reaction. Let's just wait."
b) "He has a tenfold risk of dying within the year, but we can decide at any point before the end of the first 6 months, and he will be fine."
c) "Although I would also hope not to add another medication, it is better that we begin treatment now

since patients after myocardial infarction experiencing depression have a three- to fivefold greater cardiac mortality at 6 months."
d) "We should admit him to the hospital today. His condition is too fragile to treat him as an outpatient."
e) "You're probably right, but I also think if we just stop his antihypertensive now, his depression will disappear."

The correct answer for this question is c. The patient should be started on antidepressant medication, such as an SSRI. The risk of cardiovascular mortality is high (three- to fivefold), and the benefit is significant in patients who have had a recent MI. If he has been on the same beta blocker for 5 years, it is unlikely to contribute to new onset apathy.

Evidenced-based medicine has *not* proven that for patients like this treatment with antidepressants will accomplish which of the following?

a) Improve his rehabilitation effort
b) Reduce depression
c) Increase his survival
d) Enhance quality of life

The answer is c. Although the impact may be more significant in patients who have had prior depressions, no evidence suggests that the patient with his first depression will survive longer if he is treated. Evidence supports, however, that rehabilitation effort, mood, and quality of life will improve.

## Case 5

A 32-year-old woman reports more frequent headaches extending from both temples to the back of her head and down her neck. As you explore her history further and complete your physical examination, you find adequate criteria to merit a diagnosis of major depressive disorder, recurrent. Although she is willing to try an antidepressant medication because her symptoms responded in the past, she admits she discontinued the antidepressant early because she experienced side effects. She wants to discuss the pros and cons of various options before the two of you make a selection.

Patients on which antidepressants are most likely to complain of sexual dysfunction?

a) Trazodone (Desyrel)
b) Bupropion (Wellbutrin)
c) Paroxetine (Paxil)
d) Lithium
e) Mirtazapine (Remeron)

Patients taking SSRIs (fluoxetine, sertraline, paroxetine, fluvoxamine) are more likely to report sexual dysfunction than those taking the other agents listed. The correct answer is c. Trazodone, however, can induce priapism in rare cases if increased too rapidly.

Taking which antidepressant is most likely to lead to weight gain?

a) Mirtazapine (Remeron)
b) Fluoxetine (Prozac)
c) Venlafaxine (Effexor)
d) Trazodone (Desyrel)
e) Sertraline (Zoloft)

Although it is of great benefit in many cases, the agent mirtazapine is associated with more weight gain than the other options offered. The correct answer is a.

Akathesia is most common with which drug?

a) Venlafaxine (Effexor)
b) Mirtazapine (Remeron)
c) Fluoxetine (Prozac)
d) Trazodone (Desyrel)

Again, the traditional SSRIs (e.g., fluoxetine) are more likely to induce this side effect than the other agents listed, although there can be some weight gain with other choices, particularly if the patient has Parkinson's disorder. The correct answer is d.

Insomnia would most likely be a side effect of which antidepressant?

a) Imipramine (Tofranil)
b) Sertraline (Zoloft)
c) Trazodone (Desyrel)
d) Mirtazapine (Remeron)

Although only a minority of patients will report insomnia, this side effect is more prominent in patients taking traditional SSRIs (e.g., sertraline). The others listed tend to be more sedating. Mirtazapine is unique in that lower doses are sedating, but above 30 mg, it is more activating. The correct answer is b.

Board review questions about patients with psychiatric disorders draw on your knowledge of psychopharmacology. To assist with learning how medications differ, tables are included throughout of this chapter. The pharmacologic information for common psychiatric medications is summarized in Tables 10.1 through 10.3; side effects are reviewed in Tables 10.4, 10.5, and 10.7; and drug interactions are listed in Table 10.6. The relative use of different compounds is summarized in Table 10.8. Mood stabilizers are listed in Table 10.9.

## TABLE 10.1
### ANTIDEPRESSANT THERAPY

| Drug | Starting Single Dose (mg) for Elderly or Frail Medically Ill Patients | Average Total Daily Dose (mg) for Many Patients | Important Considerations |
|---|---|---|---|
| Amitriptyline (Elavil) | 10–25 | 75–150 | Highly sedating; anticholinergic, orthostasis, EKG changes |
| Amoxapine | 25 | 75–150 | Antipsychotic properties with EPS |
| Bupropion (Wellbutrin) | 75–150 | 300 | Less weight gain, watch BP ↑, less sexual side effects |
| Citalopram[a] (Celexa) | 10–20 | 20 | Less drug interaction |
| Clomipramine (Anafranil) | 25 | 75–150 | For obsessive-compulsive disorder; ↑ orthostasis and anticholinergic |
| Desipramine[a] (Norpramin) | 25 | 75–150 | More ODs associated with death |
| Doxepin (Sinequam) | 25 | 75–150 | Weight gain, sedating |
| Escitalopram[a] (Lexapro) | 5–10 | 10–20 | Less drug interactions |
| Fluvoxamine | 25–50 | 100–150 | For obsessive-compulsive disorder |
| Fluoxetine[a] (Prozac) | 10–20 | 20 | Longest half-life, self-tapers |
| Imipramine (Tofranil) | 10–25 | 75–150 | Orthostasis, ↑ EKG changes, anticholinergic |
| Maprotiline | 25 | 75 | Side effects similar to other TCAs |
| Mirtazapine[a] (Remeron) | 7.5–15.0 | 15–30 | Less sexual side effects; sedating at low doses activating at higher doses, weight gain |
| Nortriptyline[a] (Pamelor) | 10–25 | 50–100 | Less orthostasis, some EKG changes |
| Paroxetine[a] (Paxil) | 10–20 | 20 | Constipation on higher doses and more sedation; must taper; more withdrawal symptoms |
| Protriptyline (Vivactyl) | 5–10 (a.m.) | 20 (10 mg, a.m. and noon) | Activating, but very anticholinergic |
| Sertraline[a] (Zoloft) | 25–50 | 50–100 (a.m.) | Loose stools, less drug interaction at lowest levels |
| Trazodone[a] (Desyrel) | 50 | 150–300 | Sedating, orthostasis, priapism with rapid increase |
| Trimipramine (Surmontil) | 10–25 | 50–100 (a.m.) | Very anticholinergic, sedating and increased EKG cardiac changes |
| Venlafaxine[a] (Effexor) | 25 | 100–150 | Reduces pain, ↑ BP at higher doses |

[a] Used in elderly patients.

## TABLE 10.2

**ANTIPSYCHOTIC MEDICATIONS: DOSAGE FOR MEDICALLY ILL PATIENTS WITH PROMINENT CHARACTERISTICS**

| Agent | Starting Oral Dose (mg)[a] | Comments and Characteristics |
|---|---|---|
| **Phenothiazines** | | |
| Chlorpromazine (Thorazine) | 10–25 | Significant hypotension risk, lowers seizure threshold, highly sedating, anticholinergic |
| Thioridazine (Mellaril) | 10–25 | Similar to chlorpromazine but more likely to alter ECG (prolongs QT more than others), not available IM |
| Mesoridazine (Serentil) | 10–25 | Similar to chlorpromazine and thioridazine |
| Perphenazine (Trilafon) | 4 | Moderate sedation and hypotension than haloperidol, but less than chlorpromazine |
| Trifluoperazine (Stelazine) | 2 | High frequency of EPS (acute dystonias, akasthesias, pseudoparkinsonian syndrome, tardive dyskinesia) |
| Fluphenazine (Prolixin) | 2 | High frequency of EPS similar to trifluoperazine |
| Prochlorperazine (Compazine) | 5–10 | Weak antipsychotic, used more as an antiemetic, but can produce EPS |
| Pimozide (Orap) | 2 | Has been used for monodelusional disorder, Tourette's syndrome, and during anesthesia |
| **Other traditional or classic antipsychotics** | | |
| Haloperidol (Haldol) | 0.5–2.0 | High frequency of EPS except when given IV (twice as potent when given IV) |
| Thiothixene (Navane) | 1–2 | High frequency of EPS similar to trifluoperazine |
| Loxapine (Loxitane) | 10 | Moderate in most side effects noted above |
| Molindone (Moban) | 5–10 | Less weight gain, but blurring of vision frequently |
| Atypical antipsychotics | | |
| Aripiprazole (Abilify) | 10 mg q.d. | Takes longer to act, watch for hypomania in some, weight gain |
| Clozapine (Clozaril) | 25 q.d. | Recommended for patients who have treatment-resistant or chronic schizophrenia or evidence of tardive dyskinesia; 5-HT blockade may be helpful with patients with Parkinson's disorder (very few EPS), weight gain, orthostasis |
| Risperidone (Risperdal) | 0.5–1.0 q.d. or b.i.d. | At low dose, few EPS, but more than clozapine; IM for two week dose, helpful with "negative" symptoms of psychosis, occasional headache, increased TIAs and strokes over age 85 reported |
| Olanzapine (Zyprexa) | 2.5–5.0 | Sedation, orthostasis, weight gain, increased diabetes mellitus reported, very few EPS, helpful in Parkinson's disorder, increased pancreatitis, strokes and TIAs reported |
| Ziprasidone (Geodon) | 20 b.i.d. | Few EPS, less sedating, less weight gain, do not use if ↑ QTc on ECG, oral must be b.i.d, available IM for acute use |

ECG, electrocardiogram; EPS, extrapyramidal side effects (akasthesia, pseudoparkinsonian syndrome, acute dystonias, tardive dyskinesthesia); 5-HT, 5-hydroxytryptamine (serotonin).

## SOMATOFORM DISORDERS

### Case 1

A 45-year-old woman presents to your office complaining of intermittent chest pain for the past month. She initially noticed it walking up the stairs from her basement with a basket of laundry. Since then, she has been aware of the pain on several occasions: once at the office while working on a complex project for her boss, another time when rushing to the school performance of her youngest child, and, most recently, during a phone call with her mother. She believes the pain is growing in intensity and is taking longer before it passes.

What would be your first step?

a) Reassure her and have her call back if the pain continues to occur over the next 2 weeks.
b) Schedule her for a stress echocardiogram.
c) Gather additional past and family history.
d) Prescribe an anxiolytic, such as alprazolam.
e) Prescribe an SSRI, such as sertraline.

The information provided suggests that some or all these episodes occur when the patient is fatigued or potentially under duress. Rather than jumping in to order costly tests or prescribe unnecessarily, the optimal choice is to gather further history. The answer is c.

The patient confirms that her demands at work are increasing and that it is difficult to get everything done on time, both at work and at home. Past history from the patient includes irregular menses, double vision, pelvic pain, fatigue, headaches, nausea and vomiting, joint symptoms, insomnia, bouts of diarrhea, and frequent upper respiratory infections and urinary tract infections, among a variety of other symptoms. As you peruse the archival record, you notice your predecessor has done extensive

## TABLE 10.3

### ANTIANXIETY AGENTS AND NIGHTTIME SEDATIVES[a]

| Agent | Half-Life (h) | Onset | Starting Dose (mg)[b] | |
|---|---|---|---|---|
| **Benzodiazepines** | | | | |
| Triazolam (Halcion) | 1.5–3.5 | Rapid | 0.125 q.h.s. | More frequent amnesia and hallucinations, rarely used |
| Oxazepam (Serax)[a] | 8–20 | Moderate | 10 t.i.d. | More gradual onset |
| Lorazepam (Ativan)[a] | 10–20 | Rapid | 0.5 t.i.d. | IV, IM, or PO preferably short-term use |
| Temazepam (Restoril)[a] | 12–24 | Rapid | 15 q.h.s. | Bedtime only |
| Alprazolam (Xanax) | 12–24 | Moderate | 0.25 t.i.d. | Higher risk for dependency |
| Chlordiazepoxide (Librium) | 12–48 | Moderate | 10 b.i.d. or t.i.d. | Taper, used for benzodiazepine or alcohol withdrawal at higher doses |
| Clonazepam (Klonopin) | 20–30 | Rapid | 0.5 b.i.d. | Long half-life, may be used for withdrawal taper |
| Diazepam (Valium) | 20–90 | Rapid | 2–5 b.i.d. | Rapid onset, increased dependency may be used for withdrawal taper, IV, PO, or IM |
| Clorazepate (Tranxene) | 20–100 | Rapid | 7.5 b.i.d. | Significant dependency risk, rarely used |
| Flurazepam (Dalmane) | 20–100 | Rapid | 15 q.h.s. | Rebound insomnia when stopped, long half-life, rarely used |
| **Nonbenzodiazepines** | | | | |
| Zolpidem tartrate (Ambien) | 2.6 | Rapid | 5 q.h.s. | Short half-life, sleep may not last through the night |
| Zaleplon (Sonata)[c] | 1.0 | Rapid | 5 q.h.s. | Similar to zolpidem, very mild depression at higher doses |

Other:
For generalized anxiety disorder Buspirone (BuSpar). Slow; takes 2 weeks 5 mg t.i.d. and increase; may need 45 or even 60 mg/24 hours. Elderly or extremely debilitated patients should be given lower doses. Caution should be used when prescribing long-acting sedating medications because they have been associated with a high incidence of falls and hip fractures.

[a] Preferred for elderly patients, one pass through liver. a) Gluconidation or conjugation only in lorazepam, oxazepam, and temazepam. (All others additionally require oxidation and should be given in lower doses to avoid accumulation, increasing risk for falls and fractures.)
Note: i) Antidepressants (for panic disorder): May use lower doses than for depression; for example, an imipramine starting dose of 10 mg t.i.d. ii) Beta blockers (for autonomic symptom control): Performance anxiety but not panic disorder. Propranolol (Inderal) 10–20 mg t.i.d. iii) Antipsychotics (for anxiety associated with delirium or psychosis). iv) Antihistamines: May be safer in some cases when dependency is a concern, but not advisable in the elderly or anyone prone to delirium. Diphenhydramine (Benadryl), 25 mg; starting doses b.i.d.; hydroxyzine (Vistaril), 25–50 mg; starting doses t.i.d.

workup on this patient on a variety of occasions and found little. Talking to her further, she tells you that her 75-year-old father died of an MI several months ago. She describes her mother as one who frequently requests others to take her to the doctor for a variety of concerns. Her mother is now quite distraught and needs or requests more visits with her doctors and more time from her daughter. The rest of the family history is unremarkable. Sleeping and eating patterns, concentration, and general interest level are all good at this time. The physical examination on the patient is completely normal.

### Diagnostic Criteria for Somatoform Disorder (from Diagnostic and Statistical Manual of Mental Disorders, Fourth Edition)

The DSMMD criteria include finding a history of many physical complaints beginning before age 30 years that occur over a period of several years and result in treatment being sought or significant impairment in social, occupational, or other area of functioning. These criteria include:

- Four pain symptoms at different sites or functions
- Two gastrointestinal symptoms other than pain
- One sexual symptom
- One pseudoneurologic symptom
- After appropriate investigation, symptoms not fully explained by a known medical condition or effects of a substance
- When a related general medical condition exists, physical complaints or resulting social or occupational impairment are in excess of what would be expected

Watch closely the patient's affect and behavior while questioning about how easy or difficult daily life has been and how upsetting recent social changes have been. These responses can add clues to a psychosocial connection when there is a lack of support from physical findings.

## TABLE 10.4
### ANTIPSYCHOTICS—SIDE EFFECTS MORE FREQUENT WITH INCREASING Ts

| | Aripiprazole (Abilify) | Haloperidol (Haldol) | Thioridazine (Mellaril) | Clozapine (Clozaril) | Risperidone (Risperdal) | Olanzapine (Zyprexa) | Quetiapine (Seroquel) | Ziprasidone (Geodon) |
|---|---|---|---|---|---|---|---|---|
| Anticholinergic | | + | ++ | ++ | | + | + | |
| Sedating | | | ++ | ++ | + | ++ | + | + |
| Extrapyramidal | | ++ | + | | + | | | |
| Orthostatic hypotension | | | ++ | ++ | + | + | + | |
| Weight gain | + | | ++ | ++ | ++ | ++ | + | |
| Weekly CBC required (agranulocytosis) | | | | + | | | | |
| Reduces apathy and other negative symptoms | + | | | + | + | + | + | + |
| Intravenous use | | + | | | | | | |
| Intramuscular use | | + | | | + q 2 weeks | | | + |
| Can prolong conduction | | | ++ PR, QRS, QTc | | | | | + QTc |
| CBC weekly or biweekly | | | | + | | | | |

Reviewing medical records and emergency room visits are also a must.

### Evaluating for Somatoform Disorders

In evaluating patients for somatoform disorders, key questions to ask include the following:

- In general, how stressful or difficult is this patient's daily life?
- Have there been newer or recent changes in the life of the patient or his loved ones, moves, job loss or switch, financial problems, disagreements with family members, or other concerns?
- Are there anniversary responses to past loss around this time of year?
- Is there a time connection with physical symptom(s)?
- Could symptom(s) serve to distract from emotional conflict?

## TABLE 10.5
### SELECTIVE SEROTONIN REUPTAKE INHIBITORS—SIDE EFFECTS

1. Anticholinergic: very few side effects. (Paroxetine has some; still lower than tricyclic antidepressant.)
2. Arrhythmias: very few side effects; occasional bradycardia.
3. Sedation: very little, but some patients respond in paradoxical fashion; can increase with dose. Paroxetine most, fluoxetine least.
4. Seizure threshold is of very little concern.
5. Gastrointestinal side effects: sertraline provokes more diarrhea; paroxetine provokes constipation at higher doses.
6. Sexual dysfunction.
7. Toxicity in overdose: little to none.
8. Extrapyramidal symptoms: tremor and akasthesia.
9. Headache.
10. Hyponatremia occasional.
11. Reduced platelet aggregation; prolongs bleeding time, especially with higher doses of antidepressant, presence of warfarin, preexisting bleeding.

## TABLE 10.6
### SELECTED SSRI DRUG INTERACTIONS

1. Antiarrhythmic (propafenone, flecainide); increased plasma level of antiarrhythmic due to inhibited metabolism.
2. Beta blockers (propranolol, metoprolol); decreased heart rate (addictive effect) reported with fluoxetine. Increased side effects, lethargy, bradycardia with fluoxetine due to decreased metabolism. Up to fivefold increase in propranolol level has been reported with fluvoxamine.
3. Calcium channel blockers (nifedipine, verapamil); increased side effects (headache, flushing, edema) resulting from inhibited clearance of blocker with fluoxetine.
4. Digoxin; decreased level (area under curve) of digoxin by 18% reported with paroxetine.
5. Warfarin can displace warfarin through p450 2C9/19 and secondarily increase risk of bleeding.

## TABLE 10.7
### CYCLIC ANTIDEPRESSANTS

1. Anticholinergics
   Most: amitriptyline, imipramine
   Less: desipramine
2. Quinidinelike
   Most: amitriptyline, imipramine
   Less: protriptyline
3. Sedation
   Most: amitriptyline, doxepin
   Less: desipramine, nortriptyline
4. Seizures
   Most: clomipramine (TCA/SSRI), maprotiline (tetracyclic), amoxapine (TCA/antipsychotic)
   Less: desipramine
5. Weight gain
   Most: doxepine, amitriptyline
   Less: desipramine
6. Orthostatic
   Most: amitriptyline, imipramine
   Less: nortriptyline
7. Gastrointestinal
   Most: clomipramine (TCA/SSRI)
   Less: desipramine
8. Sexual dysfunction
   Most: "toss up" may be slightly better than SSRIs
9. Toxicity in overdose
   Most: "toss up" (more deaths reported with desipramine)

SSRI, selective serotonin reuptake inhibitor; TCA, tricyclic antidepressant.

■ Are there any potential gains or benefits from others having the symptom(s)?

Treating the patient with short but regularly scheduled visits; reassurance; referral to a psychoeducational group, if available, to enhance optimal health; ordering only "necessary" testing; and treating comorbid psychiatric disorders, such as depression if it arises, are the cornerstones of managing these cases.

Somatoform disorders respond better when intervention is early, without reinforcement by the excessive ordering of tests and evaluations and when patients are told that the symptoms are "real" but not life threatening and that you want to see them again for a scheduled return visit.

## Case 2

A 24-year-old female student in allied health is admitted to the hospital 1 month after a motor vehicle accident. She complains of severe pain, edema, and skin temperature and coloration changes. Your anesthesiology colleagues performed three separate nerve blocks to reduce symptoms of reflex sympathetic dystrophy. The pain was relieved for only a few hours each time. They have discovered that she had two earlier admissions to your hospital 3 years ago. The patient was admitted at that time for red cells in her urine in close proximity to the appearance of a "butterfly" rash on her cheeks. The workup for systemic lupus erythematosus and other autoimmune disorders was negative, as well as negative for urinary tract conditions. Your colleagues want to know whether the current symptoms have anything to do with those identified during the two prior hospitalizations.

As you talk to the patient, you realize there are many stressors and concerns in her life in addition to the physical symptoms limiting her ability to do her part-time work and studies.

Which is the best plan?

a) Pursue repeat autoimmune testing, and if the results are normal, sign off the case.
b) Confront the patient that you think she is malingering and recommend she be discharged.
c) Wait until she is out of the room and search her possessions.
d) Be certain that all appropriate testing has been ordered and reviewed while requesting a psychiatric consultation.
e) Pursue all of the above.

The correct response is d. It is important that all appropriate, but not excessive, testing be ordered and reviewed to provide quality healthcare for the patient. It is critical to listen closely, while being open with her about concerns that stress, depression, and anxiety can greatly impact both emotional and physical well-being. Patients can be directly or indirectly causing harm to themselves without their physician being aware. This patient met criteria for both major depressive disorder recurrent and factitious disorder. Included in the criteria for factitious disorder is the intentional production or feigning of physical or psychologic symptoms. Symptoms of factitious disorder are motivated by psychological gain, as when a person wishes to be in a sick role, either physically or emotionally. Alternatively, malingering would have been diagnosed if the patient was attempting to avoid financial or legal responsibility or otherwise "better" her current situation. Working closely with mental health professionals, the internist in this case was able to treat the patient successfully. After the depression was treated and adequate individual and group psychotherapy provided, the self-destructive behavior ended (rubber band tourniquets, scratching with razor blades), and the patient returned to regular activities. Although patients like this are at risk during periods of great stress, reentry into therapy as early as possible is of great advantage.

## PANIC DISORDER

### Case 1

A 20-year-old man presents to the office and states that last week, during his examination at the university, he had two episodes of choking. They came on unexpectedly and made it difficult for him to finish the test. On another occasion,

## TABLE 10.8
### COMORBIDITY TABLE: PSYCHOTROPICS EFFECTIVE WITH AFFECTIVE AND RELATED DISORDERS

| Psychotropic | MDD | PMDD | ADD | OCD | Panic | Eating Disorder | GAD | Bipolar | Chronic Benign Pain |
|---|---|---|---|---|---|---|---|---|---|
| Clomipramine (Anafranil) | T | T | | T | T | | T | a | ? |
| Fluoxetine (Prozac) | T | T | T | T | T | T | T | a | T |
| Sertraline (Zoloft) | T | T | T | T | T | T | T | a | T |
| Paroxetine (Paxil) | T | T | T | T | T | T | T | a | T |
| Fluvoxamine (Luvox) | T | T | T | T | T | T | T | a | ? |
| Citalopram (Celexa) | T | T | T | T | T | T | T | a | ? |
| Mirtazapine (Remeron) | T | ? | | | | T | ? | T | a |
| Trazodone (Desyrel) | T | | | | | | T | a | ? |
| Venlafaxine (Effexor) | T | ? | | | T | ? | T | a | T |
| Amitriptyline (Elavil) | T | | | | T | | T | a | T |
| Imipramine (Tofranil) | T | | | | T | | T | a | T |
| Bupropion (Wellbutrin) | T | | | | | | | a | |
| Alprazolam (Xanax) | | | | | T | | T | | |
| Buspirone (BuSpar) | T | | T | | | | | | |
| Methylphenidate (Ritalin)[b] | IM | | T | | | | | | |
| Lithium (Eskalith) | M | | | | | | | T | |
| Atomoxetine (Strattera) | | | | | | | | | |
| Carbamazepine (Tegretol) | M | | | | | | | T | |
| Valproate (Depakote) | M | | | | | | | T | |
| Gabapentin (Neurontin) | | | | | | | ? | ? | T |
| Topiramate (Topamax) | | | | | | | | ? | |
| Lamotrigine (Lamictal) | | | | | | | | T | |
| Oxcarbazepine (Trileptal) | | | | | | | | ? | |
| Tiagabine (Gabitril) | | | | | | | | ? | |
| Levetiracetam (Keppra) | | | | | | | | | |

ADD, attention deficit disorder; GAD, generalized anxiety disorder; IM, alternative for medically ill patient with depression; M, may be used to augment an antidepressant; MDD, major depressive disorder; OCD, obsessive compulsive disorder; PMDD, premenstrual dysphoric disorder; T, effective treatment; ?, possibly effective or partially effective due to mechanism of action, but currently inadequate evidence-based data.
[a] Okay if depressed and on a mood stabilizer.
[b] Psychomotor retarded, medically ill.

## TABLE 10.9
### MOOD STABILIZERS

| Medication | Starting Dose | Maximum Dose (mg) | Common Drug Interactions or Concerns |
|---|---|---|---|
| Lithium | 300 mg q.h.s. | 900–1,200 | (Will ↑ Li level), ACE inhibitors, NSAIDS, thiorazide diuretics |
| Carbamazepine | 100 mg | 300–600 | Divalproate and many others |
| Divalproate | 125–250 mg | 500–750 | Carbamazepine, lamotrigene, and many others |
| Gabapentin | 100 mg | 300–600 | ↓ level if creatinine is ↑; helpful for pain |
| Lamotrigine | 25 mg<br>Increase slowly q 1–2 weeks; if need to taper off must be over 4 weeks | 500–700 | Valproate can ↑ lamotrigine |
| Oxcarbazepine | 150 mg<br>Increase q 3 days | 900–1,800 | Like carbamazepine, can ↓ sodium |
| Topiramate | 25 mg<br>Increase q week | 400–1,000 | Can ↓ new learning |
| Tiagabine | 2 mg<br>Increase q week | 32 | |

he was watching television in his room. The patient is concerned that these episodes will return and is fearful of going anywhere alone that would make it difficult for him to get to medical care. As you begin to question him further, he answers that he did feel short of breath, as though he might pass out for some minutes. The patient remembers feeling dizzy and sweaty toward the end of the episode. He does not recall chest pain, headache, or abdominal pain.

Past history indicates some complaints of dizziness 2 years earlier that did not occur on more than a few occasions and then disappeared. He stated that he was told once that he might have mitral valve prolapse. Although he states that he never visited a mental health professional, his parents had planned to take him during elementary school because he did not want to leave them to attend class. A 35-year-old aunt had a history of chest pain and a rapid heart rate off and on; she has been taking fluoxetine for several years.

### Criteria for Panic Attack (from Diagnostic and Statistical Manual of Mental Disorders, Fourth Edition)

The criteria include a discrete period of intense fear or discomfort in which four (or more) of the following symptoms develop abruptly and reach a peak within 10 minutes:

- Palpitations, pounding heart, or accelerated heart rate
- Sweating
- Trembling or shaking
- Sensations of shortness of breath or smothering
- Feeling of choking
- Chest pain or discomfort
- Nausea or abdominal distress
- Feeling dizzy, unsteady, lightheaded, faint
- Derealization (feelings of unreality) or depersonalization (being detached from oneself)
- Fear of losing control or going crazy
- Fear of dying
- Paresthesias (numbness or tingling sensation)
- Chills or hot flashes

### Panic Disorder (from Diagnostic and Statistical Manual of Mental Disorders, Fourth Edition)

To establish a diagnosis of panic disorder, both 1 and 2 must be present:

1. Recurrent unexpected panic attacks
2. At least one of the attacks has been followed by 1 month (or longer) of one (or more) of the following:

   a) Persistent concern about having additional attacks
   b) Worry about the implications of the attack or its consequences
   c) Significant change in behavior related to attacks

In addition, one should determine if comorbid agoraphobia is present.

A frequently chosen treatment option is low-dose antidepressants. To avoid precipitating an attack, panic patients require tiny increments of antidepressant until they are able to tolerate a therapeutic amount with good control of symptoms. A small amount of benzodiazepine can be added for any breakthrough panic attacks occurring during the first 2 weeks.

Your impression is that this patient

a) Probably plans to request a medical note to allow him to drop two classes
b) May have panic disorder and requires further assessment
c) Should be referred to your ear, nose, and throat colleague
d) Needs a bronchoscopy
e) Should take a semester off and will be fine

The correct answer is b, because the patient has had panic attacks and now has increased concern about future ones. He is also at risk for agoraphobia, considering that he is starting to alter where he will go for fear of an attack. Any medical concerns (e.g., thyroid, cardiac or respiratory and substance issues) should be explored.

It is reported that patients with panic disorder often have six medical visits or more before the diagnosis is entertained. Past history of separation anxiety or school phobia during childhood may be an important clue, as is a positive family history. After basic laboratory studies, a chest film, and the electrocardiogram are determined to be normal, the patient can be reassured and educated about panic disorder. A stress test may be recommended for some, as reports indicate a reduced heart rate variability in some patients with panic disorder as well as those with depression and schizophrenia.

A wide range of therapeutic options for panic disorder is available, including antidepressants, anxiolytics, and cognitive or other behavioral therapies. Often low-dose antidepressants are prescribed to avoid the frequent side effects that panic patients experience. A small amount of benzodiazepine can be prescribed for the first 2 to 3 weeks while the antidepressant is slowly increased. An appropriate rate of increase for the antidepressant would be, for example, 12.5 mg of sertraline or 5 mg of paroxetine or citalopram added every 2 to 3 days until the typical therapeutic dosage is reached.

## Case 2

On your rounds at the extended-care facility, you are asked to see a new resident. She is 60 years old and suffers from late-stage Huntington's disease. During her 20s and 30s, she suffered from recurrent major depression and obsessive-compulsive disorder. Her daughter took care of her at home until a few years ago, at which time her son took her to live in a facility near his home. Over the last few years, her medication was changed from haloperidol to risperidone. In addition, she was "out of control" at times. The onset of these episodes was sudden, with loud vocalizations and pounding on her chest. They were infrequent 1 year ago, and the 0.5 mg of lorazepam twice daily seemed to control them well. Later, the dose was increased to three times a day, but eventually the symptoms recurred and led to 1.0 mg three times daily dosing. Now on the new ward, her nurse tells you she thinks the patient awakens with these attacks, but once they get "medication into her she begins to calm down." Although the patient has limited detail in her spontaneous communication, she is able to indicate "yes" and "no" appropriately. She acknowledges her heart beating rapidly and feeling short of breath when the events occur. During the day, the patient does not fall asleep while taking lorazepam. She communicates great distress when her chest pain begins, and she worries that the episodes are coming more often. You order a dipyridamole thallium stress test, and it returns normal. Although the patient never drank alcohol, her father and brother were alcoholics. Her mother and aunts were treated for depression.

Besides her prior psychiatric diagnosis, you believe she may also have which of the following?

a) Dissociative disorder
b) Psychotic paranoid condition
c) Delirium
d) Somatoform disorder
e) Panic disorder

It is difficult for her to communicate, but the symptoms seem likely to be those of panic disorder. Her yes and no responses are consistent and indicate no hallucinations or delusions. She does not have fluctuations in her attention or a long history of somatic complaints without physical findings. She does not meet criteria for the other disorders. As she became tolerant of lorazepam, breakthrough panic occurred nearly every morning, when blood level was lowest. Before discounting other conditions, it is important to rule out hypoxia and various endocrinopathies.

When comorbid psychiatric disorders exist, medication adjustments are more important. For example, if panic disorder exists with depression, doses must start low, with gentle titration upward (e.g., fluoxetine, 2 to 5 mg, taken orally each day for several days before increasing by another 2 to 5 mg daily). It may take 2 to 3 weeks to titrate up to the maintenance level (e.g., 20 mg fluoxetine). If obsessive-compulsive disorder exists along with major depression, it is not unusual for the patient eventually to need higher doses of SSRI (e.g., paroxetine, 40 to 80 mg daily).

## Delirium

A 51-year-old male patient in the intensive care unit presents with acute onset of confusion 36 hours postoperatively, after a successful coronary artery bypass graft. The patient is taking several medications, including insulin, atenolol, promethazine, metoclopramide, levothyroxine, and others. The patient has no respiratory distress and has good arterial blood gases. His electrolytes, blood sugar, electrocardiogram, creatinine, and liver function tests are within normal range at present. A TSH is ordered, and oral haloperidol (5 mg) is given to reduce symptoms of delirium. The patient does not improve; in fact, the nurses report his behavior has further deteriorated, and his arms and legs have become somewhat rigid.

What would you do?

a) Reconfirm that the patient has not used alcohol or benzodiazepines daily.
b) Consider the possibility of anticholinergic activity causing his agitation.
c) Try a dose of lorazepam (1 to 2 mg).
d) Monitor vitals and cogwheeling, hold the haloperidol; consider checking creatinine phosphokinase, iron, and white blood cell count if temperature increases or stiffness occurs.
e) All of the above.

The correct answer is e. Drug–drug interactions are frequent delirium inducers. It is wise to avoid multiple anticholinergic drugs that may cause delirium, including antipsychotic agents, antiemetic agents, antiparkinsonian agents, tricyclic antidepressants, and antihistamines. Using multiple agents that block dopamine (e.g., haloperidol, promethazine, metoclopramide) may affect multiple dopamine receptors, producing a paradoxical response and severe hypotension. If this occurs, a nondopaminergic pressor agent can be used.

If the patient's QTc had been long, it would have been quite important to avoid medications that might further lengthen that interval: tricyclic antidepressants; carbamazepine; antipsychotics, including pimozide; and antiarrhythmics including lidocaine, propafenone, and quinidine. Even haloperidol can increase the QTc interval in patients with a history of Torsade de Pointes or alcoholic cardiomyopathy.

The prolonged metabolism of some QTc-increasing drugs can occur with fluoxetine, fluvoxamine, grapefruit juice, sertraline, ketoconazole, and astemizole via the P450 3A4 isoenzyme.

Numerous reasons may exist for this patient's acute confusional state. Medication-induced delirium (anticholinergic), thyroid disease, alcohol or benzodiazepine withdrawal, and other conditions should be ruled out. It is less likely that he is developing neuroleptic malignant syndrome, but this is still a possibility. It is more likely that the metoclopramide and oral haloperidol may have increased his extrapyramidal side effects. A close monitoring of vital signs, laboratory studies, and patient responses will further direct treatment.

## Mania

A 50-year-old female who is followed by your partner drops in to ask if she can start a medicine she "saw on TV for smoking cessation." The two of you determine that she is probably talking about bupropion (Zyban or Wellbutrin).

As you assess her smoking dependency, you also consider contraindications to the medication.

The contraindications might include all of the following, except

a) Bulimia nervosa and being overweight
b) Anorexia nervosa and being underweight
c) Epilepsy
d) Coronary artery disease
e) Recent closed-head injury

Patients who have epilepsy or who have brain pathology may have an increased risk for seizures while using this medication. Being overweight alone is not a contraindication, and in fact, this antidepressant is more effective in allowing patients who follow a healthy diet and exercise to lose weight. Patients with either anorexia or bulimia nervosa, however, are at higher risk for seizures when taking buproprion. Patients with cardiac disease can be treated safely, unless their blood pressure increases, which can sometimes occur at higher doses. The correct answer is d.

After 3 days, the patient's husband calls you on the phone stating that "there's something wrong with her." He says she hasn't been able to sleep, and he wants you to prescribe a sleeping pill. As you are in a hurry, you start to ask where he wants you to call in the prescription, but then reconsider and ask to speak with his wife, the patient. When you ask her how she is doing, she responds "terrific" and goes on to tell you all the many, many activities she's planning.

Now, your thoughts are

a) Oh my goodness, I forgot to ask about past and family history for any hypomanic or manic symptoms.
b) Is she really talking that fast?
c) Can she ever have that much energy, money, and time for all those projects?
d) I better stop the bupropion and get her in to see a psychiatrist as soon as possible.
e) All of the above.

The answer is e, all of the above. The symptoms of a classic hypomanic/manic phase include pressured speech, racing thoughts, little to no sleep, boundless energy, euphoric mood, grandiose plans, and inappropriate judgment. Manic symptoms can develop quickly, although this patient's course is rapid.

The psychiatrist wants to begin lithium carbonate and asks you to order the following. You agree to order all except which one?

a) TSH
b) Complete blood cell count
c) Electrocardiogram
d) Creatinine
e) Liver function tests

Over 10% of patients on lithium develop hypothyroidism, so you would like to know the level of her TSH before starting lithium. Likewise, her white blood count may rise with lithium, and ST elevation can occur. If we have baseline values before initiating the drug, we can better assess possible side effects. If her creatinine is elevated, she is unlikely to clear lithium adequately and would be at greater risk for toxicity. Lithium has renal clearance and is not hepatically metabolized, so we would not agree to spend the extra money on liver function tests at this point. The answer is e. As part of our responsibility, we thoughtfully consider drug interactions that increase lithium levels and remember that it will rise in combination with which of the following?

a) Lisinopril and other angiotensin-converting enzyme inhibitors
b) Nonsteroidal anti-inflammatory drugs (NSAIDs)
c) Hydrochlorothiazide
d) All of the above
e) None of the above

Some drugs can lead to significant increases in lithium to the point of toxicity in only several days. All of these listed are able to do this, thus the answer is d.

Others that also increase serum lithium levels (morning trough) include which of the following?

a) Theophylline
b) Osmotic diuretics
c) Steroids
d) All of the above
e) None of the above

The answer is e, none of the above, as all the drugs in this list reduce lithium level. When any of these are added to the regimen of a patient stable on lithium, the level may fall, and the patient's mood may switch into depression or mania.

### Dementia

A 72-year-old man is brought to see you for "agitation" secondary to dementia. He has diabetes mellitus, is significantly overweight, and has hyperlipidemia. His EKG was read as normal with QT350, QTc 400. The family would like to avoid placing him in a nursing home. They say he has tantrums when he cannot find his wallet, glasses, or other personal possessions. Lists, color coding possessions, reminder signs, and other behavioral techniques have been tried, but to no avail. The family asks if a medicine could help.

Your first choice might be which of the following?

a) Antianxiety agent
b) Antidepressant
c) Anticholinesterase medication
d) Antipsychotic
e) Anticonvulsant

The answer is c. Although these drugs have all been used for agitation in dementia, the etiology of the symptom, the intensity or nature of the behavior, and the side effects should be considered. In this case, the patient is likely forgetting where he placed his possessions, and if an anticholinesterase agent helps improve his recall, it would be the optimal choice with which to start.

Donepezil is successful for several years until paranoid delusions about his neighbors stealing from him are heard. He insists that they send criminals into his home to remove his favorite shoes and gloves. He even saw them in his living room, although when the family arrived, they found no evidence anyone had been there.

At this point in his care, you would

a) Add rivastigmine, 3 mg b.i.d., to the 10 mg of donepezil he is already taking.
b) Suggest thioridazine (Mellaril) to reduce the symptoms and improve his sleep.
c) Try olanzapine (Zyprexa) nightly to reduce the symptoms and improve his sleep.
d) Try ziprasidone (Geodon) to reduce hallucinations and delusions.
e) Select haloperidol because it is inexpensive. He has little risk for tardive dyskinesia, having used it only for 3 months 2 years ago after the onset of postoperative delirium.

The answer is d. It would be risky and of no advantage to add a second cholinesterase inhibitor. More gastrointestinal side effects and drug complications with little return would make no sense. Because he has visual hallucinations and paranoid delusions, an antipsychotic is in order. If the patient had used a traditional antipsychotic agent for more than 30 days in the past and would now start a traditional antipsychotic, at the end of 1 year, the risk for tardive dyskinesia would be approximately 37%. A newer agent with less risk for tardive dyskinesia and orthostatic and anticholinergic effects is preferable. Of the two options remaining, ziprasidone is less likely to increase appetite, weight gain, or lipids.

### Psychotropics in the Medically Ill
Several psychotropic medications have been implicated in association with the onset of diabetes mellitus.

Which of the following has been reported during this transition?

a) Insulin resistance
b) Hypoinsulinemia
c) Reduced leptin
d) Weight loss
e) None of the above

The answer is a, insulin resistance. Hyperinsulinemia, increased leptin, and weight gain are also described. The weight gain, however, is not necessarily a cause or believed to be the sole reason for the development of diabetes.

Before starting various psychiatric medications in the elderly patient with multisystem disease, it is wise to assess all *except* which of the following?

a) Blood pressure—venlafaxine (Effexor), bupropion (Wellbutrin)
b) Renal clearance—gabapentin (Neurontin)
c) Electrocardiogram for QTc—nortriptyline, ziprasidone (Geodon), haloperidol
d) Lipid profile, blood sugar—mirtazapine (Remeron), olanzapine (Zyprexa)
e) Red blood count—clozapine (Clozaril)

White blood count is most closely monitored for clozapine to avoid agranulocytosis, so the answer is e. Blood is drawn weekly for the first 6 months and biweekly from that time until the medication is discontinued. All the other drugs are paired with areas where alterations or side effects can occur. It is important to evaluate for underlying medical problems before prescribing these agents.

Withdrawal syndromes occur when which of these drugs is abruptly discontinued?

a) Clozapine—cholinergic rebound (extreme nausea, vomiting, headache)
b) Paroxetine—flu-like symptoms and dizziness
c) Fluoxetine—diarrhea
d) a and b
e) a, b, and c
f) None of the above

Fluoxetine, with its long half-life, self-tapers. Abrupt cessation of clozapine and paroxetine lead to the symptoms listed, so the correct response is d.

## Case 3

A 50-year-old male has been in the hospital for over 6 weeks after developing multiple complications post coronary artery bypass graft. This unfortunate gentleman experienced acute respiratory distress syndrome, acute renal failure, and sepsis.

His past medical history includes congestive heart failure and chronic obstructive pulmonary disease from many years of smoking tobacco. He has no other substance abuse history (alcohol, benzodiazepines, analgesics or illicit drugs). His father and older brother died of complications of alcoholic cirrhosis, however. His mother's early demise at age 50 was secondary to a myocardial infarction.

The patient's archival includes a year-old stress test indicating reduced heart rate variability and heart rate recovery and increased blood pressure variability. A note states that the patient requested refills for the fluoxetine that he took for his anxiety disorder. His wife confirms her husband's anxiety and has been worried that his nothing by mouth (NPO) status did not allow him to take his medication. She wonders if he could take his old medication (amitriptyline) if he can't have fluoxetine now. He has been getting lorazepam IV q 4 to 6 hours. Initially, it was 1 mg, but now the dose is 2 mg and still doesn't seem to keep him calm. He seems to awaken feeling acute discomfort at the upper midline of his chest with a choking sensation.

What is unusual about this case of panic disorder?

a) The patient's atypical chest pain
b) The patient's reduced heart variability
c) The patient's reduced increased blood pressure variability
d) The patient's history of self-reported anxiety
e) The patient's age and gender

The answer is e. Atypical chest pain, reduced heart rate variability, increased blood pressure variability, and self-reported anxiety is frequently associated with panic disorder. Although it is unclear when his anxiety actually began, younger females are more typical of panic disorder patients than middle-aged or older men.

## Case 4

A 29-year-old female presents to your office with concerns about her weight (250 pounds). You saw this woman 4 months ago and treated her for major depression. Initially, you started buproprion because she didn't want to add extra pounds, but a day later she reported extreme agitation, and you switched her to fluoxetine. She has done quite well, but still wants to lose some weight. Her first question is "can I stop the fluoxetine?" Your reply would be

a) "Even if this is your first episode, you should continue for 2 years."
b) "Fluoxetine will definitely help you lose weight the longer you're on it."
c) "You should continue it for 6 to 12 months before tapering, but 12 months is safer."
d) "Let's switch back to buproprion; you are unlikely to have the same side-effect and you would likely lose 20 pounds."
e) "I know you've been walking 1.5 miles per day, but that is far too little to lose weight."

The answer is c. A patient has roughly an 80% chance of relapse if she stops her medication prior to 6 months, even if it this is her first episode of depression. The recommended continuation is 6 to 12 months, with more literature supporting a full year. Patients on fluoxetine are most likely to lose weight during the first 3 months, but may have some increase in appetite later, although possibly less with fluoxetine than some other SSRIs. Buproprion's dopaminergic action can lead to agitation. The average weight loss with buproprion is 6 pounds.

Topamax has been used to help patients get started with weight loss, but poorer cognitive performance and a tendency toward mania in some bipolar patients limit its use. Orlistat could reduce lipid absorption. Sibutramine might induce potentially lethal serotonin syndrome if combined with fluoxetine.

## SUGGESTED READINGS

Alarcon FJ, Isaacson JH, Franco-Bronson K. Diagnosing and treating depression in primary care patients: looking beyond physical complaints. *Cleve Clin J Med* 1998;65:251–260.

Bakish D. The patient with comorbid depression and anxiety: the unmet need. *J Clin Psychiatry* 1999;60[Suppl 6]:20–24.

Beliles K, Stoudemier A. Psychopharmacologic treatment of depression in the medically ill. *Psychosomatics* 1998;39[Suppl]:2–19.

Ferketich AK, Schwartzbaum JA, Frid DJ, Moeschberger ML. Depression as an antecedent to heart disease among women and men in the NHANES1 Study. National Health and Nutrition Examination Survey. *Arch Intern Med* 2000;160:1261–1268.

Fleet RP, Marchand A, Dupuis G, et al. Comparing emergency department and psychiatry setting patients with panic disorder. *Psychosomatics* 1998;39:512–519.

Franco-Bronson K, Williams K. Emotional and psychiatric problems in patients with cancer. In: Skeel R, ed. *Handbook of Cancer Chemotherapy*. New York: Lippincott Williams & Wilkins, 1999.

Garre-Olmo J, Lopez-Pousa S, Vilalta-Franch J, et al. Evolution of depressive symptoms in Alzheimer disease—one year follow-up. *Alzheimer Dis Assoc Disord* 2003;17:77–85.

Glassman AH, Shapiro PA. Depression and the course of coronary artery disease. *Am J Psychiatry* 1998;155:4–11.

Inouye SH, Bogardus ST, Charpentier PA, et al. A multicomponent intervention to prevent delirium in hospitalized older patients. *N Engl J Med* 1999;340:669–676.

Jorge RE, Robinson RG, Tateno A. Repetitive transcranial magnetic stimulation as treatment of poststroke depression: a preliminary study. *Biol Psychiatry* 2004;55:398–405.

Kashner TM, Rost K, Cohens B, et al. Enhancing the health of somatization disorder patients. *Psychosomatics* 1995;36:462–470.

Kroenke K, Spitzer RL, DeGruny FV, et al. A somatoform checklist to screen for somatoform disorders in primary care. *Psychosomatics* 1998;39:263–272.

Lavretsky H. Late-life depression: risk factors, treatment and sex difference. *Clin Geriatr Med* 1998;6:13–24.

Lee HB, Lyketsos CG. Depression in Alzheimer's disease: heterogeneity and related issues. *Biol Psychiatry* 2003;54:353–362.

Perez V, Soler J, Puigdemont D, et al. A double blind, randomized, placebo controlled trial of pindolol augmentation in depressive patients resistant to serotonin reuptake inhibitors. *Arch Gen Psychiatry* 1999;56:375–379.

Pozuelo L, Franco K, Palmer R. Agitated dementia: drug vs. nondrug treatment. *Cleve Clin J Med* 1998;5:191–199.

Preskorn SH. Clinically relevant pharmacology of selective serotonin reuptake inhibitors. *Clin Pharmacokinet* 1997;32[Suppl 1]:1–21.

Preskorn SH. Comparison of the tolerability of bupropion, fluoxetine, imipramine, nefazodone, paroxetine, sertraline, venlafaxine. *J Clin Psychiatry* 1995;56:12–21.

Robinson RG. Poststroke depression: Prevalence, diagnosis, treatment and disease progression. *Biol Psychiatry* 2003;54:376–387.

Rosenzweig A, Prizerson H, Miller MD, et al. Bereavement and late-life depression: grief and its complications in the elderly. *Annu Rev Med* 1997;48:421–428.

Sauer WH, Berlin JA, Kimmel SE. Effect of antidepressants and their relative affinity for the serotonin transporter on the risk of myocardial infarction. *Circulation* 2003;108:32–36.

Sephton S, Spiegel D. Circadian disruption in cancer: a neuroendocrine–immune pathway from stress to disease? *Brain Behav Immun* 2003;17:321–328.

Stahl SM. Basic pharmacology of antidepressants, part 2: estrogen as an adjunct to antidepressant treatment. *J Clin Psychiatry* 1998;59:15–23.

Stahl SM. Selecting an antidepressant by using mechanism of action to enhance efficacy and avoid side effects. *J Clin Psychiatry* 1998;59[Suppl 18]:23–29.

Stahl S. *Essential Psychopharmacology*, 2nd ed. Cambridge, MA: Cambridge University Press, 2000.

Stoudemire A. Expanding psychopharmacologic treatment options for the depressed medical patient. *Psychosomatics* 1995;36:S19–S26.

Stoudemire A, Fogel B, Greenbert D. *Psychiatric Care of the Medical Patient*, 2nd ed. New York: Oxford Press, 2000.

Strik JJ, Denoller J, Lousberg R, Honig A. Comparing symptoms of depression and anxiety as predictors of cardiac events and increased health care consumption after myocardial infraction. *J Am Coll Cardiol* 2003;42:1801–1807.

Stunkard AJ, Faith MS, Allison KC. Depression and obesity. *Biol Psychiatry* 2003;54:330–337.

Tan RS, Brown J. Cognitive and estrogens in the elderly woman. *Clin Geriatr Med* 1998;6:10–19.

Thase ME. Redefining antidepressant efficacy toward long-term recovery. *J Clin Psychiatry* 1999;60[Suppl 6]:15–19.

Workgroup on Delirium. Practice guideline for the treatment of patients with delirium. *Am J Psychiatry* 1999;56[Suppl 5]: 1–20.

Writing Committee for ENRICHD investigations. Effects of treating depression and low perceived social support on clinical events after myocardial infarction. *JAMA* 2003;289:3106–3116.

Yonkers KA. The association between premenstrual dysphoric disorder and other mood disorders. *J Clin Psychiatry* 1997;58:19–25.

# BOARD SIMULATION: Genetic Diseases in Internal Medicine

**11**

*Franklin A. Michota, Jr.*

## GENETIC DISEASES

Most diseases encountered in the practice of medicine have genetic components in both cause and pathogenesis. The following cases illustrate several genetic diseases that internists may see.

## Case 1

A 44-year-old man reports intermittent gross hematuria. He is very concerned about his health following the recent death of his younger brother from a subarachnoid hemorrhage. Family history is remarkable for kidney disease. On examination, he is hypertensive with a mitral regurgitation murmur. No rash or skin lesions are found. Urinalysis shows more than 25 red blood cells (RBCs) but no white blood cells, casts, protein, or stones. Blood urea nitrogen is 31 mg/dL, and creatinine is 2 mg/dL.

Of the following tests, which is most likely to be helpful in diagnosis?

a) 24-hour urine collection for protein
b) Plasma immunoglobulin A levels
c) Renal ultrasound
d) Total and C3 complement levels
e) Renal biopsy

The answer is c. This case involves a middle-aged man with a family history of renal disease. He has hematuria without casts, valvular heart disease, hypertension, elevated creatinine, and a recent death of a sibling from subarachnoid hemorrhage. Closer physical examination might reveal hepatomegaly or palpable kidneys. He most likely has adult polycystic kidney disease (PKD).

Adult PKD is the most common hereditary renal disease and represents 10% of all cases of renal failure that reach end-stage disease. Inheritance is autosomal dominant, with wide phenotypic variability. Adult PKD is caused by mutations in two different genes, *PKD1* on chromosome 16 (85%–90% of cases) and *PKD2* on chromosome 4 (10%–15% of cases). The two types of adult PKD have similar pathologic and physiologic features, but *PKD2* patients have a later onset of symptoms, a slower rate of progression to renal failure, and a longer life expectancy (69 years) compared with *PKD1* patients (53 years). The PKD genes encode integral membrane proteins, polycystin-1 and polycystin-2, which occur on renal tubular epithelia. Polycystin-1 is a membrane receptor capable of binding and interacting with many proteins, carbohydrates, and lipids and eliciting intracellular responses through phosphorylation pathways, whereas polycystin-2 is thought to act as a calcium-permeable channel. No ethnic predominance is noted, and the prevalence of PKD is 1 in 1,000 persons. From birth, thin-walled spherical cysts develop in the cortex and medulla of both kidneys. The cysts range from millimeters to centimeters in diameter and are usually visible on ultrasonography or computerized tomography by 25 years of age. Other cysts can be found in the liver, spleen, pancreas, and brain (arachnoid cysts) and occasionally in the esophagus, ovaries, uterus, and seminal vesicles. Liver cysts are common, with a higher prevalence in women. Pregnancy is a risk factor for massive hepatic cystic involvement, thought to be related to estrogens.

Overall, symptoms typically develop in the third to fourth decades, with flank pain and hematuria. Urinary tract infections are common and must be treated using lipophilic antibiotics (flouroquinolones, sulfonamides) that penetrate the cysts. Other manifestations include nocturia, kidney stones, and hypertension. Left ventricular hypertrophy is a common early complication of adult PKD, with cardiovascular disease representing the leading cause of death. PKD is also associated with cardiac valve myxomatous degeneration, diverticulosis, and intracranial aneurysms. Subarachnoid hemorrhage from an intracranial aneurysm causes death or neurologic injury in approximately 10% of patients. Hematocrit may be increased secondary to elevated erythropoietin levels or decreased from excessive hematuria and blood loss.

Acute renal failure can result from infection, ureteral obstruction due to clots or stone, or sudden angulation of a ureter by a nearby cyst. Azotemia progresses slowly in the absence of these complications. In contrast to other renal conditions, angiotensin-converting enzyme (ACE) inhibitors are not superior to other drugs in slowing progression to renal failure. Patients with PKD and chronic renal failure tend to have higher hematocrits than their counterparts with other renal diseases. Fluid overload is infrequent because of a tendency for renal salt wasting. On hemodialysis, 5-year survival is 10% to 15% greater in PKD than in non-PKD patients.

Renal ultrasound is the diagnostic method of choice for screening individuals at risk. Sensitivity is greater than 85% in those from 20 to 30 years of age. Although proteinuria is common in PKD, it rarely exceeds 2 g/d. Immunoglobulin A nephropathy may present with hematuria but is usually associated with erythrocyte casts and glomerulonephritis. Complement levels are normal in PKD and have no role in the diagnosis of this disorder.

## Case 2

A 56-year-old white man with a history of pseudogout and diabetes mellitus type II complains of fatigue and weight loss. His family history is significant for diabetes, liver cancer, and arthritis. On examination, a mildly enlarged liver is noted, together with palmar erythema and bilateral knee effusions. Blood chemistry reveals mildly elevated alanine transaminase and aspartate transaminase values; total bilirubin is 2.0 mg/dL, international normalized ratio (INR) is 1.95, and ferritin is 2,500 ng/mL (normal range, 10 to 200 ng/mL).

The treatment most likely to decrease this patient's risk for hepatocellular carcinoma is which of the following?

a) Ursodeoxycholic acid (ursodiol)
b) Repeated phlebotomy
c) Penicillamine
d) Deferoxamine
e) None of the above

The answer is e. This case illustrates the clinical presentation of symptomatic hereditary hemochromatosis (HHC), one of the most common autosomal recessive disorders. The principal determinant for HHC has been identified as the *HFE* gene on chromosome 6, with two mutations (C282Y and H63D) representing the majority (>90%) of the world cases. Recently, an autosomal dominant form of HHC has been described and associated with a mutation in the *SLC11A3* gene, thus establishing a non-*HFE* linked hereditary hemochromatosis. Among people of Northern European descent, the prevalence of HHC is 1 in 500 persons, with a carrier frequency as high as 1 in 8. HHC is a disorder of iron storage, whereby an inappropriate increase in intestinal iron absorption results in deposition of excessive quantities of iron in parenchymal cells, with eventual tissue damage and functional impairment. The most commonly affected organs include the liver, pancreas, heart, and pituitary gland. Clinical expression of HHC is modified by several factors, including blood loss in menstruating women. HHC is expressed five to ten times more frequently in men.

Symptoms develop in most untreated patients between the fourth and sixth decades. HHC is rarely clinically evident before age 20 years. Early symptoms include weakness, weight loss, change in skin color, abdominal pain, loss of libido, and symptoms related to the onset of diabetes mellitus. More established disease presents with hepatomegaly, skin pigmentation, spider angiomas, palmar erythema, splenomegaly, ascites, loss of body hair, testicular atrophy, arthropathy, cardiac arrhythmias, congestive heart failure, and jaundice.

The liver is usually the first affected organ. Hepatomegaly develops and, when hepatic iron concentration reaches a threshold of 400 micromol/g dry weight, cirrhosis is common. The iron threshold is lower in patients with other risk factors for liver diseases, such as heavy alcohol consumption or chronic hepatitis. Splenomegaly develops in 50% of symptomatic patients. Manifestations of portal hypertension and esophageal varices occur less commonly than in alcoholic cirrhosis. Hepatocellular carcinoma develops in 30% of those with cirrhosis and is the most common cause of death among treated patients.

Arthropathy most commonly occurs after age 50 years, but may occur at any time in the course of the disease. The small joints of the hands, especially the second and third metacarpophalangeal joints, are the first joints to be involved. A progressive polyarthritis of the wrists, hips, ankles, and knees may follow. Deposition of calcium pyrophosphate may be seen following acute brief attacks of synovitis, especially in the knees.

A fasting transferrin saturation is the best screening test for asymptomatic individuals. Population screening of adults has been advocated, but has yet to become accepted public policy. Genetic testing for the missense mutation (C282Y) of the *HFE* gene is available and provides a potentially powerful noninvasive method of disease susceptibility. Clinical HHC is only present in the setting of iron overload, however, and the standard for diagnosis still requires a liver biopsy with histologic evaluation and biochemical quantification of hepatic iron concentration. The serum ferritin level defines the point at which hemochromatosis is expressing iron overload and treatment should be initiated. Treatment involves removal of mobilizable iron stores. Weekly phlebotomy is usually required for 2 to 3 years. When the transferrin saturation and ferritin level become normal, phlebotomy is performed at the time intervals required to maintain levels in the normal range. Chelating agents, such as deferoxamine, are more expensive and less effective than phlebotomy, but may play a role in HHC when anemia or hypoproteinemia are severe enough to preclude further blood removal. When treatment is initiated before the development of hepatic cirrhosis or diabetes, patients with HHC appear to have a normal life expectancy. In the case example, elevations in INR, bilirubin, and transaminases suggest that liver damage and cirrhosis have already occurred. Once hepatic cirrhosis develops, however, no treatment is available to alter the risk of hepatocellular carcinoma.

## Case 3

A 19-year-old African American man presents to the emergency department with severe abdominal pain and jaundice. His past medical history is unremarkable, although his mother reports "growing pains" as a child. Further questioning reveals the patient is adopted. He is febrile and tachycardic. The abdomen is diffusely tender. No rebound is present, and bowel sounds are present throughout. A small skin ulcer is noted on his left lower extremity. Complete blood cell count shows white blood cells at 17 K/μL, hemoglobin (Hgb) at 6.3 g/dL, and mean corpuscular volume at 89 μm³. Aspartate transaminase and alanine transaminase values are normal. Indirect bilirubin is 3.6 mg/dL. A peripheral smear was performed (Fig. 11.1) and displays the crescent-shaped (sickle) RBCs of sickle cell disease.

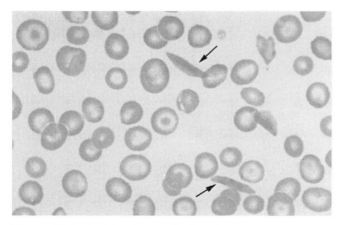

**Figure 11.1** Peripheral smear for Case 3.

Which of the following statements regarding this patient's condition is true?

a) Sepsis is the most common cause of death in adults.
b) In the United States, few patients survive beyond the fifth decade.
c) A selective advantage against *Plasmodium vivax* malaria is present.
d) Transmission is autosomal dominant with variable penetrance.
e) Symptoms do not develop until the patient is older than 6 months.

The answer is e. Given this finding and the clinical presentation, this patient most likely has sickle cell anemia (SSA), the most common heritable hematologic disease affecting humans. Inheritance is autosomal recessive, and among African American adults, SSA has a prevalence of 1 in 500, with 10% being carriers of the sickle trait. Patients have an electrophoretically abnormal hemoglobin (HgbS) that differs from HgbA by substitution of valine for glutamic acid at the sixth position of the β chain. On deoxygenation, HgbS begins to polymerize and changes the RBC from a biconcave disk to an elongated sickle shape. Patients with SSA have a selective advantage against *Plasmodium falciparum* malaria, with preferential sickling of parasitized cells. The rate of polymerization depends on the concentration of HgbS and the extent of deoxygenation. The sickling may be irreversible if enough cell damage occurs. Fetal hemoglobin (HgbF) is protective against polymerization and varies in its distribution among RBCs in patients with SSA. Signs and symptoms of the disease do not usually appear until the sixth month of life, at which time most HgbF has been replaced by HgbS.

The elongated sickle shape of RBCs is responsible for the vaso-occlusive phenomena seen in patients with SSA. Microinfarcts develop, leading to painful bone crises, and macroinfarcts cause chronic organ damage. SSA leads to impaired growth and development, and recurrent splenic infarction results in an increased susceptibility to serious infections, particularly pneumococcal infections. Patients with SSA typically have severe hemolytic anemia, with an RBC life span of only 2 weeks. Infection or folate deficiency may suppress erythropoiesis enough to cause aplastic crisis. Chronic anemia often causes congestive heart failure, and progressive renal insufficiency typically develops, with most patients suffering from hyposthenuria. Other clinical findings include chronic skin ulcers, retinal infarcts and ocular disease, seizures, neurologic thrombosis with an increased risk for subarachnoid hemorrhage, avascular necrosis of bone, and increased risk of gallstones. The most common cause of death in adult patients with SSA is from acute chest syndrome. In a multicenter study, 45% of all acute chest syndrome cases had an unknown etiology. Its cardinal features are fever, pleuritic chest pain, referred abdominal pain, cough, lung infiltrates, and hypoxia. Approximately 30% were due to infections with atypical organisms and 9% from fat embolism secondary to long-bone infarction.

The treatment for sickle cell disease is evolving. Patients should be well hydrated and receive folate supplementation and vaccination against the pneumococcus. Hydroxyurea may increase HgbF concentration and decrease the number of painful crises. Its use should be reserved for patients with frequent episodes of pain, a history of the acute chest syndrome, other severe vaso-occlusive complications, or severe symptomatic anemia. Blood counts should be monitored every 2 weeks until a stable dose is achieved. Mean corpuscular volume parallels the rise in HgbF concentrations and is an inexpensive surrogate for HgbF concentration during therapy. Blood transfusions are only indicated in acute chest syndrome with hypoxia, symptomatic episodes of acute anemia, surgery with general anesthesia, or severe symptomatic chronic anemia. Transfusions may be useful in complicated obstetric problems, refractory leg ulcers, acute severe priapism, and refractory and protracted painful episodes. Straight transfusion, when the patient is given additional units of blood without removal of sickle blood, is best used when the hemoglobin concentration is lower than 8 or 9 g/dL. Exchange transfusion is better when the hemoglobin concentration is high, thus reducing the complications from increased viscosity. All transfused blood should be matched for minor blood group antigens, screened negative for sickle cells by sickle-dex, and undergo leukoreduction. Bone marrow transplantation offers the potential for cure. Children and adolescents younger than 16 years of age who have severe complications and a human leukocyte antigen–matched donor available are the best candidates. Only 1% of all patients with SSA meet these requirements. If successful, hematopoietic stem cell transplantation may obviate the need for bone marrow transplantation in SSA.

Worldwide, approximately 120,000 babies with SSA are born each year, but less than 2% survive to the age of 5. In the United States and other developed countries, SSA patients often survive into their fifth or sixth decade.

## Case 4

A thin, 21-year-old white woman presents to the emergency department with acute-onset shortness of breath. Examination is consistent with pneumothorax. Chest radiography confirms this finding, along with evidence of mild hyperinflation and ring shadows in the upper lobes. She states that she was a "sickly" child with many episodes of sinusitis and bronchitis and that lately she cannot get rid of a productive cough. Cystic fibrosis (CF) is suspected.

Which of the following statements regarding this patient's condition is false?

a) Adults make up approximately 40% of patients with this disease.

b) Pneumothorax and female sex are poor prognostic indicators.

c) *Pseudomonas aeruginosa* is associated with rapid deterioration in lung function.

d) Two-year survival for lung transplantation patients exceeds 50%.

e) Allergic bronchopulmonary aspergillosis has been noted in 10% of patients.

The answer is c. This case concerns a young woman with spontaneous pneumothorax, chest radiologic abnormalities consistent with bronchiectasis, and a personal history of chronic respiratory infections. She most likely has cystic fibrosis (CF).

In white populations, CF, which occurs in approximately 1 in 2,500 live births, is the most common lethal autosomal recessive genetic disorder, with a carrier frequency of 1 in 25 persons. During the past three decades, however, the number of adults with CF has increased dramatically, attributable in large part to a significant improvement in survival. For patients born in the 1990s, the median survival is now predicted to be greater than 40 years. Over one-third of the patients in the Cystic Fibrosis Foundation Registry are now older than 30 years.

CF is a monogenetic disorder caused by mutation in the CF transmembrane conductance regulator (*CFTR*) gene on chromosome 7. The clinical manifestations are due primarily to the dysfunction of exocrine glands, producing viscid dehydrated secretions. Diagnosis is based on one or more typical clinical features, a history of CF in a sibling, and laboratory evidence of a *CFTR* abnormality, such as elevated sweat chloride values. Approximately 3% to 4% of patients with CF are diagnosed as adults. This group usually presents with chronic respiratory problems and, in contrast to CF patients diagnosed as children, they have milder lung disease, less pseudomonal infection, and are more likely to be pancreatic sufficient.

Clinically, CF is characterized by chronic airway infection leading to bronchiectasis and bronchiolectasis, exocrine pancreatic deficiency, abnormal sweat glands, and urogenital dysfunction. Patients typically have chronic sinusitis as children, with eventual lower respiratory tract involvement represented by cough. The cough is progressive and productive, ultimately leading to frequent exacerbations with decrements in pulmonary function. Advanced lung disease ensues, leading to digital clubbing, respiratory failure, and cor pulmonale. Other respiratory complications include pneumothorax and hemoptysis, both of which are poor prognostic indicators. The earliest chest radiographic change in CF lungs is hyperinflation. Later, evidence of luminal mucous impaction, bronchial cuffing, and bronchiectasis is noted. The right upper lobes display the earliest and most severe changes.

Patients with CF exhibit characteristic sputum microbiology, with *Haemophilus influenzae* and *Staphylococcus aureus* often the first organisms recovered from lung samples in patients newly diagnosed with CF. After multiple clinical exacerbations and antibiotic exposures, *P. aeruginosa* becomes the predominant organism recovered. Almost 50%

of patients have *Aspergillus fumigatus* in their sputum, with up to 10% exhibiting the syndrome of allergic bronchopulmonary aspergillosis. Infection with *Burkholderia cepacia* species is pathogenic and causes rapid clinical deterioration, often with fulminating pneumonia, bacteremia, and death (cepacia syndrome).

More than 85% of patients with CF demonstrate some degree of exocrine pancreas deficiency, but most adults remain asymptomatic. Insufficient pancreatic enzyme release, however, yields the typical pattern of protein and fat malabsorption with frequent, bulky, and foul-smelling stools. Young adults may present with distal intestinal instruction, which may be confused with appendicitis. Late onset of puberty in CF is common in both sexes, with almost all men being azoospermic. The delayed maturational pattern is likely secondary to the effects of chronic lung disease and inadequate nutrition on reproductive endocrine function.

The major objective of treatment is to promote clearance of secretions and control infection in the lung, improve nutritional status, and encourage a reasonable quality of life. More than 95% of patients with CF die from complications resulting from lung infections. Approaches to the prevention of pulmonary deterioration must be individualized, but they usually include aggressive antibiotic therapy for established infection, airway clearance techniques, a mucoactive agent, regular exercise, and treatment of airway reactivity. Prophylaxis with nebulized antipseudomonal antibiotics has also been shown to improve lung function and reduce the frequency of lung infections. Currently, the only effective treatment for respiratory failure in CF is lung transplantation. Bilateral transplantation is the procedure of choice. More recent results indicate a 70% survival at 1 year, 62% at 2 years, and 53% at 3 years after transplantation. Phase I human gene therapy studies using adenovirus and liposomal vectors for the *CFTR* gene suggest that gene transfer is safe, but not clinically efficacious. Current research is now focusing more on the barriers faced by delivery agents, with the aim that more efficient gene delivery will lead to a gene therapeutic for CF.

## Case 5

A 43-year-old man undergoes a preoperative evaluation for inguinal hernia repair. He is a tall, thin man without previous medical problems. Examination reveals normal vital signs, pectus excavatum, mild kyphoscoliosis, and a mitral regurgitation murmur. Subsequent echocardiography demonstrates normal left ventricular function, 2+ mitral regurgitation, and mild ascending aortic aneurysm. Further workup reveals a negative urine cyanide-nitroprusside test result and a slit-lamp examination consistent with ectopia lentis.

Which of the following is the most likely diagnosis?

a) Ehlers-Danlos syndrome type IV
b) Homocystinuria
c) Marfan syndrome
d) Familial aortic aneurysm
e) Ehlers-Danlos syndrome type VI

The answer is c. This case illustrates the clinical presentation of Marfan syndrome. Marfan syndrome is inherited as an autosomal dominant disorder with a wide phenotypic range both within affected families and between families. The common mutations producing Marfan syndrome involve the fibrillin gene (*FBN1*) on chromosome 15. Fibrillin is a glycoprotein that is a vital component of elastin-associated microfibrils. The prevalence has been reported as high as 1 in 2,000 persons, with an incidence of 1 in 10,000 in most racial and ethnic groups. Approximately 25% to 30% of patients do not have affected parents and most likely represent spontaneous mutations.

Severe Marfan syndrome is characterized by a triad of features: (i) long, thin extremities frequently associated with other skeletal changes, (ii) reduced vision as the result of dislocations of the lenses (ectopia lentis), and (iii) aortic aneurysm that typically begins at the base of the aorta. Other skeletal abnormalities include severe chest deformities, scoliosis, kyphosis, and pes planus. Joint hypermobility may be seen, although not commonly. Cardiovascular abnormalities are the major source of morbidity and mortality. The rate of aortic dilatation is unpredictable, but dilatation can cause aortic regurgitation, dissection, and rupture. Dilatation is probably accelerated by physical and emotional stress, particularly pregnancy. Mitral valve prolapse is common and progresses to regurgitation in 25% of patients. Other clinical manifestations include spontaneous pneumothorax and inguinal and incisional hernias.

Marfan syndrome shares clinical characteristics with other syndromes, and in the absence of classic features, diagnosis may be difficult. Patients with homocystinuria may have tall stature, pectus deformities, scoliosis, pes planus, and progressive lens dislocation. Homocystinuria may be detected by a positive urinary nitroprusside test result or elevated urinary homocystine by amino acid chromatography. Ehlers-Danlos syndrome type IV (vascular type) presents with aortic aneurysms and rupture, joint hypermobility, mitral valve prolapse, and spontaneous pneumothorax. Ehlers-Danlos syndrome type VI (ocular type) may exhibit characteristics similar to those of type IV, with the addition of retinal detachment and ocular symptoms. Ectopia lentis is not a feature of Ehlers-Danlos syndrome. Diagnostic criteria for Marfan syndrome are based on the presence of an affected first-degree relative or major clinical manifestations.

No established treatment exists for Marfan syndrome, but most investigators recommend the use of β-adrenergic blocking agents to delay or prevent aortic dilatation. Surgical replacement of the aorta, aortic valve, and mitral valve has been successful in some patients, and all patients should be followed carefully with echocardiography. Patients should be advised of the risks of pregnancy and should avoid contact sports and other strenuous exercise.

# REVIEW EXERCISES

## QUESTIONS

For each condition, select the appropriate sign and symptom:

| Sign | Disease |
|---|---|
| 1. Fabry disease | a) Acroparesthesia |
| 2. Von Recklinghausen disease | b) Café-au-lait macules |
| 3. Stickler syndrome | c) Degenerative joint disease |
| 4. Kartagener syndrome | d) Recurrent pneumonia |
| 5. Gaucher disease | e) Splenomegaly |
| 6. Charcot-Marie-Tooth disease | f) Telangiectasia |
| | g) Deafness |

For each condition, select the appropriate laboratory value:

| Disorder | Laboratory Value |
|---|---|
| 7. Alport syndrome | a) Hgb = 8.2 mg/dL |
| 8. Von Hippel–Lindau disease | b) Glucose = 280 mg/dL |
| 9. Osler-Weber-Rendu disease | c) Calcium = 11.4 mg/dL |
| 10. Friedreich ataxia | d) Urinalysis with RBC casts |
| 11. Becker muscular dystrophy | e) Hgb = 18.1 mg/dL |
| | f) Glucose = 45 mg/dL |
| | g) Creatine kinase = 8,500 U/L |

## ANSWERS

### 1. a and f.

Fabry disease is a lysosomal storage disease resulting from a deficiency of α-galactosidase A. The inheritance pattern is X-linked recessive. Onset is usually in childhood or adolescence. Clinical signs include telangiectatic angiokeratomas of skin and mucous membranes; acroparesthesia; corneal opacities and cataracts; infiltrative cardiac disease with left ventricular hypertrophy, arrhythmias, and occasionally a short PR interval on electrocardiography; and renal disease with hypertension. The most frequent cause of death is renal failure, followed by cardiac or cerebrovascular disease.

### 2. b.

Von Recklinghausen disease, or neurofibromatosis type 1, is the first of two genetically distinct types of neurofibromatosis, both autosomal dominant disorders. Type 1 is associated with café-au-lait macules, axillary and inguinal freckling, Lisch nodules of the iris, neurofibromas, and occasionally pheochromocytomas and scoliosis. Type 2 is characterized by bilateral vestibular schwannomas with associated symptoms of tinnitus, hearing loss, and balance dysfunction, other nervous system gliomas, and cataracts.

### 3. c and g.

Stickler syndrome is an autosomal dominant disorder of type II collagen. The four most affected systems are craniofacial, skeletal, ocular, and auditory. Clinical associations include severe myopia, vitreal degeneration, retinal detachment, conductive and sensorineural hearing loss, midfacial underdevelopment, cleft palate, epiphyseal dysplasia, and premature osteoarthritis.

### 4. d.

Kartagener syndrome is an autosomal recessive disorder of ciliary ultrastructure with absent or reduced ciliary motility. Patients have recurrent pneumonia, sinusitis, bronchitis, and bronchiectasis. Kartagener syndrome is clinically distinct from other ciliary dyskinesias by the presence of situs inversus and dextrocardia. Female patients are fertile. Male patients have immotile spermatozoa, and in the absence of micromanipulation, they are functionally infertile.

### 5. e and c.

Gaucher disease is an autosomal recessive, lysosomal storage disorder caused by a deficiency of the enzyme β-glucocerebrosidase. Lipid storage is found in the spleen, liver, bone marrow, and other organs. Gaucher disease encompasses a continuum of clinical findings from a perinatal lethal form to an asymptomatic form or one that is initially diagnosed in the elderly. Five clinical subtypes have been identified. Type 1 is the most common and is characterized by the absence of central nervous system disease; it occurs most frequently in Ashkenazi Jews (1 in 1,000) and responds well to enzyme replacement treatment. Hepatomegaly, splenomegaly, anemia, thrombocytopenia, and degenerative bone disease (osteopenia, focal or sclerotic lesions, osteonecrosis) may develop in untreated patients. Types 2 and 3 are characterized by the presence of primary neurologic disease, with expected life spans ranging from childhood to the third and fourth decades.

### 6. g.

Charcot-Marie-Tooth disease is a hereditary neuropathy categorized by mode of inheritance and causative gene or chromosomal locus. Charcot-Marie-Tooth disease is the most common genetic cause of neuropathy and is characterized by chronic motor and sensory nerve symptoms. The typical patient has distal muscle weakness and atrophy often associated with mild to moderate sensory loss, depressed tendon reflexes, and high-arched feet. Charcot-Marie-Tooth disease is genetically heterogeneous and may be inherited through autosomal dominant, autosomal recessive, and X-linked patterns. *CMT1* is autosomal dominant, represents the most common of the subtypes, and is associated with hearing loss.

## 7. a and d.

Alport syndrome is a genetically heterogeneous disorder characterized by hereditary nephritis, sensorineural hearing loss, and eye abnormalities. It is caused by mutations in several different genes encoding isoforms of type IV collagen, a major component of basement membranes. X-linked dominant and autosomal recessive forms have been described. The renal disease presents with hematuria, proteinuria, and nephrosis, with end-stage renal disease by 16 to 30 years of age.

## 8. a and e.

Von Hippel-Lindau disease is an autosomal dominant disorder characterized by retinal, spinal cord, and cerebellar hemangioblastomas; cysts of the kidneys, pancreas, and epididymis; pheochromocytoma and renal cell cancers; and endolymphatic sac tumors. Cerebellar hemangioblastomas may be associated with headache, vomiting, gait disturbances, or ataxia. Retinal hemangioblastomas may be the initial manifestation of von Hippel-Lindau syndrome and can cause vision loss. Renal cell carcinoma occurs in 40% of patients and is the most common cause of death. If renal cell carcinoma occurs, hematuria and anemia are typical, but erythrocytosis may be seen in up to 5% of patients.

Endolymphatic sac tumors can cause hearing loss of varying severity, which can be a presenting symptom.

## 9. a.

Osler-Weber-Rendu disease, or hereditary hemorrhagic telangiectasia, is an autosomal dominant condition in which occult or overt gastrointestinal bleeding is often present. Telangiectases of the skin and mucous membranes are seen, and approximately 20% of patients have pulmonary arteriovenous malformations.

## 10. b.

Friedreich ataxia is an autosomal recessive disorder characterized by slowly progressive ataxia with onset usually before the age of 25 years, typically associated with depressed tendon reflexes, dysarthria, Babinski responses, loss of position and vibration senses, and cardiomyopathy. Approximately 25% of cases have an atypical presentation with later onset (after age 25 years), retained tendon reflexes, or unusually gradual progression of disease. Almost all Friedreich ataxia patients have identifiable mutations in the *X25/FRDA* gene on chromosome 6. Other clinical associations include diabetes mellitus (10%), optic atrophy (25%), dementia, and respiratory dysfunction due to kyphoscoliosis. Death is often related to cardiomyopathy and diabetes. The mean age of loss of ambulation is 25 years.

## 11. g.

Duchenne and Becker muscular dystrophies are caused by mutations in the dystrophin gene located on chromosome 21. Inheritance is X-linked recessive, with one third of cases arising by spontaneous mutation. Progressive skeletal weakness occurs, with the clinical diagnosis being supported by markedly increased creatine kinase levels. Duchenne muscular dystrophy is rapidly progressive, with affected children being wheelchair bound by the age of 12 years. Cardiomyopathy occurs in all patients after the age of 18, and few survive beyond the third decade. Becker muscular dystrophy has later onset muscular weakness, with patients remaining ambulatory into their 20s. Despite the milder skeletal muscle involvement, heart failure from dilated cardiomyopathy is a common cause of morbidity and the most common cause of death. Mean age of death for Becker muscular dystrophy is in the mid-40s.

## SUGGESTED READINGS

Alton E, Kitson C. Gene therapy for cystic fibrosis. *Expert Opin Investig Drugs* 2000;9:1523–1535.

Burke W, Thomson E, Khoury M, et al. Hereditary hemochromatosis: gene discovery and its implications for population-based screening. *JAMA* 1998;280:172–178.

Charrow J, Esplin JA, Gribble TJ, et al. Gaucher disease: recommendations on diagnosis, evaluation, and monitoring. *Arch Intern Med* 1998;158:1754–1760.

Claster S, Vichinsky EP. Managing sickle cell disease. *BMJ* 2003;327: 1151–1155.

Davidson DJ, Porteous DJ. Genetics and pulmonary medicine: the genetics of cystic fibrosis lung disease. *Thorax* 1998;53:389–397.

Gray JR, Davies SJ. Marfan syndrome. *J Med Genet* 1996;33:403–408.

Griffiths W, Cox T. Hemochromatosis: novel gene discovery and the molecular pathophysiology of iron metabolism. *Hum Mol Genet* 2000;9:2377–2382.

Maher ER, Kaelin WG. Von Hippel-Lindau disease. *Medicine* 1997;76: 381–391.

McCarthy GM, McCarthy CJ, Kenny D, et al. Hereditary hemochromatosis: a common, often unrecognized genetic disease. *Clev Clin J Med* 2002;69:224–242.

Motulsky AG, Beutler E. Population screening in hereditary hemochromatosis. *Ann Rev Public Health* 2000;21:65–79.

Pietrangelo A. Hemachromatosis. *Gut* 2003;52(Supp):23–30.

Powell LW, George KD, McDonnel SM, et al. Diagnosis of hemochromatosis. *Ann Intern Med* 1998;129:925–931.

Rosenstein BJ, Zeitlin PL. Cystic fibrosis. *Lancet* 1998;351:277–282.

Ryan G, Mukhopadhyay S, Singh M. Nebulized anti-pseudomonal antibiotics for cystic fibrosis. *Cochrane Database Syst Rev* 2000; (2):CD001021.

Steinberg MH. Drug therapy: management of sickle cell disease. *N Engl J Med* 1999;340:1021–1030.

Wilson PD. Mechanisms of disease: polycystic kidney disease. *N Engl J Med* 2004;350:151–164.

Wu G, Somlo S. Molecular genetics and mechanism of autosomal dominant polycystic kidney disease. *Mol Genet Metab* 2000; 69:1–15.

Yankaskas JR, Mallory GB. Lung transplantation in cystic fibrosis: consensus conference statement. *Chest* 1998;113:217–226.

Yankaskas JR, Marshall, BC, Sufian BJD, et al. Cystic fibrosis adult care: consensus conference statement. *Chest* 2004;125(Supp):1S–39S.

## SUGGESTED WEB SITES

GeneClinics: http://www.geneclinics.org
OMIM (Mendelian Inheritance in Man, Online): http:// www.ncbi.nlm.nih.gov/Omim

## 12

# Neurology

*Martin A. Samuels*    *John C. Andrefsky*

Neurologic medicine is an enormous field that contains its own core information and, in addition, borders on a number of other fields of medicine, including internal medicine, pediatrics, neurosurgery, neuroimaging, neurophysiology, psychiatry, physiatry, geriatrics, and neuropathology. This chapter focuses on the major subjects in clinical neurology. It is divided into two major sections: neurologic symptoms and neurologic disorders.

## NEUROLOGIC SYMPTOMS

### Disorders of Consciousness

Consciousness is difficult to define, but in neurologic terms, it consists of two components: (i) arousal or wakefulness and (ii) awareness. Each of these two components has its own functional neuroanatomic basis. *Arousal* or *wakefulness*, defined simply as whether a person will open her eyes either spontaneously or in response to a stimulus, is mediated by a diffuse system of neurons, dendrites, and axons, which occupy the core of the brainstem from about the level of the midpons rostrally. This system is known as the *ascending reticular activating system* (ARAS), and it forms a component of the reticular formation, a system of neurons and their connections that ascend from high in the cervical spinal cord to the thalamus. The ARAS gains much of its input from structures in the midpons, the most important of which is the locus ceruleus, a noradrenergic nucleus that supplies much or all of the norepinephrine for the entire central nervous system (CNS).

The ARAS terminates in the midline, nonspecific nuclei of the thalamus. Taken together, the ARAS and the nonspecific nuclei of the thalamus are sometimes referred to as the *centrencephalon*, meaning the center of the head. This system sets the normal sleep and wake cycle. The second component of consciousness is known as *awareness*, and it refers to a person's ability to have an understanding of himself and the environment. This function requires the sum of many cortical functions that reside throughout the cerebral cortex. Awareness is therefore generated by the total action of the cerebral cortex. The nonspecific nuclei of the thalamus project to the dendrites of the neurons of the cerebral cortex responsible for the function of awareness. Therefore, in summary, arousal or wakefulness is mediated by the ascending reticular activating system and nonspecific thalamic nuclei, and awareness is mediated by the nonspecific thalamic nuclei and the cerebral cortex. This discussion underlines the fulcrum function of the nonspecific thalamic nuclei in mediating consciousness because these nuclei belong to both the awareness and the arousal subsystems.

Disorders of consciousness are divided into two categories: those caused by an abnormality in arousal and those attributable to an abnormality in awareness. Arousal disorders are a group of abnormalities in consciousness on a spectrum that ranges from alertness to deep coma, which in many respects resembles sleep. Names have been assigned to the different depths of arousal disorders so that clinicians can communicate with each other easily using brief descriptions of the patient's state. Four major depths of disordered arousal are recognized. The mildest disorder is characterized by an inability to maintain a coherent stream of thought or action, an attentional disorder known as *confusion* or the *confusional state*.

Patients in a confused state have their eyes open but are unable to carry out tasks that require a coherent stream of thought or action, such as serial or digit span testing. Some confused patients also show hyperactivity of the sympathetic limb of the autonomic nervous system. Such patients have dilated pupils and are diaphoretic, tremulous, and tachycardic. This latter state is known as *delirium*. Delirium and confusion are the mildest disorders of arousal and are often due to a diffuse abnormality of the nervous system caused by metabolic or toxic encephalopathy. Evidence does point, however, to an attentional system lateralized to the right cerebral hemisphere in a way analogous to language, which is usually lateralized to the left cerebral hemisphere. Thus, right cerebral hemisphere disorders sometimes may cause a patient to become confused or delirious. In general, delirium is caused by metabolic and toxic disorders characterized by increased levels of circulating catecholamines in the blood, such as sedative drug withdrawal, alcohol withdrawal, high fever, or the use of stimulant medications such as amphetamines.

The next deepest level of disordered arousal is known as *drowsiness*, which is defined as a state of *apparent sleep*, which can be overcome by a verbal command. The next deepest level of disordered arousal is known as *stupor* and is characterized by an apparent sleep state that can be overcome only by a noxious stimulus, not by a simple verbal command. The deepest state of disordered arousal is known as *coma*, from which the patient cannot be aroused even with a noxious stimulus.

*Awareness disorders* refer to states during which the patient may be awake or asleep, often at different times during the day, but has an abnormality of interaction with the environment even when apparently awake. This category has five major disorders: *abulia* is defined as a state of reduced effervescence and spontaneity. It is often caused by bilateral prefrontal disease such as hydrocephalus, anterior cerebral artery distribution infarctions, or tumors infiltrating the frontal lobe. *Catatonia* refers to a state of waxy rigidity caused by a psychologic conflict, which ordinarily can be revealed using a barbiturate interview. *Conversion disorder* refers to the use of body language to express a psychologic conflict. *A dissociative state* or trance-like state is a hypnotic condition in which the patient dissociates various components of the personality, one from the other; it often is induced by stress. *Nonconvulsive seizures* refer to epileptic seizures rendering the patient unaware but not disabling the arousal mechanisms. Telltale clues often are present, such as small-amplitude repetitive motor movements (e.g., blinking).

The examination of the patient with an abnormality of consciousness is carried out in the same order as the general neurologic examination and consists of an assessment of a level of consciousness, a detailed eye examination to assess brainstem function, a motor and sensory examination, and an evaluation of the reflexes.

The patient's level of consciousness is assessed according to these definitions (i.e., alert, confused, delirious, stuporous, or comatose). Examination of the eyes is extremely useful in the patient with abnormal consciousness because eye-movement control centers use pathways that are closely related to the ARAS of the brainstem, which mediates arousal. Neurologic forms of unconsciousness virtually always show some abnormality in the eye-movement examination.

Examining the eyes is done in three steps. The first step is to examine the fundi using an ophthalmoscope. Clues to the unconscious state may be found, such as papilledema or subhyaloid hemorrhages, which are indicative of increased intracranial pressure and subarachnoid hemorrhage, respectively. The pupils then are measured, and their reaction to light, both direct and consensually, is recorded. Eye movements are tested by observing spontaneous eye movements and then inducing eye movements using the vestibulo-ocular reflex. In unconscious patients arriving in an emergency department, it may be unsafe to turn the head passively because a neck injury may have occurred. It is wiser and more revealing to elicit the vestibulo-ocular reflex using caloric techniques. In the emergency department, the simplest method for carrying out a caloric examination is to infuse 25 to 50 mL of ice water into the external auditory canal and observe the eye movements over the next 30 to 60 seconds. Normally, the eyes will turn conjugately toward the side of the ice water infusion,

followed by a jerking corrective movement away from the side of the ice water infusion. The slow movement of this nystagmus is generated by the vestibulo-ocular pathways in the brainstem extending from the vestibular nuclei in the pons and medulla to the oculomotor nuclei in the midbrain. This slow movement would not be normal in a patient with significant lesions in the ascending reticular activating system of the brainstem. The rapid correction phase is generated from the frontal eye fields in the frontal lobe, which transmit the signal through the white matter of the hemispheres to the pontine gaze centers near the abducens nuclei and from there up the brainstem through the medial longitudinal fasciculus to the oculomotor nuclei. Thus, the fast phase of the nystagmus induced by ice water is a test of cerebral hemisphere function, at least in part.

The motor examination consists of observing for spontaneous movement and seizures, which maybe subtle and found only around the eyes and mouth. Painful stimulation of the stuporous or comatose patient will allow the clinician to observe purposeful movements that indicate patterns of weakness such as hemiparesis, paraparesis, tetraparesis, or monoparesis. Antigravity reflexes also are observed either with spontaneous movement or on noxious stimulation. *Decerebration* consists of extension and internal rotation of all four extremities, often reflecting a disorder in the midportions of the brainstem. *Decortication* is characterized by extension and internal rotation of the lower extremities and flexion and adduction of the upper extremities, often reflecting a disease in the diencephalon. The sensory examination is difficult to perform in detail, but sometimes the patient's face can be observed for wincing reactions when noxious stimuli are applied to various parts of the body. It is sometimes possible to recognize a hemisensory loss or a sensory level on the trunk, as would be seen in a spinal cord injury even in a relatively unarousable patient. Three categories of reflexes are tested in the unconscious patient. Proprioceptive reflexes are also known as the *tendon jerks*. Five such reflexes are present: the biceps, triceps, and brachioradialis reflexes in the upper extremities and the quadriceps and gastrocnemius reflexes in the lower extremities. Nociceptive reflexes are elicited by stimulating the skin with a noxious stimulus. The two nociceptive reflexes regularly elicited in unconscious patients are the *plantar response* (Babinski reflex) and the *corneal response*. Release reflexes, such as sucking, rooting, and grasping, are not particularly useful in this setting.

*Death by brain criteria* is defined as a state of absent arousal and awareness with absent brainstem reflexes and apnea despite an adequate $P_{CO_2}$ (>60 mm Hg) to stimulate breathing in the absence of drugs, toxins, and hypothermia. The *vegetative state* is defined as a state of absent awareness despite preservation of some brain functions, often those involving brainstem centers for cardiovascular and autonomic control. The management of the acutely unconscious patient can be done using an algorithmic method shown in Figure 12.1.

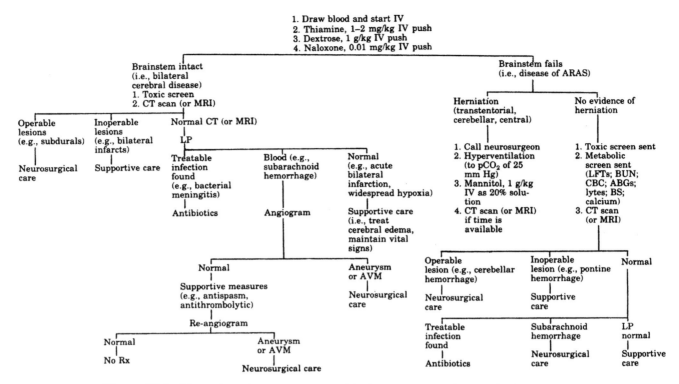

**Figure 12.1** Diagnosis and treatment protocol in the comatose patient. *LP*, lumbar puncture; *LFT*, liver function test; *ABGs*, arterial blood gases; *BS*, blood sugar; *AVM*, arteriovenous malformation. (Reprinted with permission from Samuels MA, ed. *Manual of Neurologic Therapeutics*, 6th ed. Philadelphia: Lippincott Williams & Williams, 1999.)

## Headache

Headache is one of the most common complaints for which people seek medical attention. To understand this problem, it is useful to review the neuroanatomic basis of head pain. Not all structures within the head are pain sensitive. In fact, nociceptors are present only in the dura mater and closely related structures, in proximal portions of the cerebral arteries, and in the scalp and its vessels. The brain itself is not invested with proprioceptive fibers and therefore is not pain sensitive. Two main pathways exist for the transmission of nociceptive information from the head and neck, both of which converge in the CNS. From most of the head to the vertex of the skull and to a location just behind the ear, nociceptors are carried in divisions of the fifth (trigeminal) cranial nerve. The cell bodies responsible for the dendrites carrying this nociceptive information lie in the gasserian ganglion just outside the pons. The nociceptive structures behind the ear and posterior to the vertex of the head use an analogous structure, the dorsal root ganglion for the second cervical spinal cord segment (C-2). For the gasserian ganglion, the axon carrying nociception enters the pons and descends in the spinal tract of the trigeminal and then synapses in the spinal nucleus of the trigeminal in the upper cervical region. The analog of this system for C-2 is the substantia gelatinosa, located in the

spinal cord at C-2. Fibers leave the substantia gelatinosa and the spinal nucleus of V, cross and ascend together as the spinothalamic tract and the quintothalamic tract, respectively, to the lateral thalamus. The ventral posterolateral nucleus of the thalamus is specialized for this purpose. Fibers arising in the ventral posterolateral nucleus of the thalamus then project through the white matter to the parietal cortex.

Superimposed on this ascending pain transmission system is a descending pain modulation pathway for the endogenous control of nociceptive information. Fibers in this system arise in the limbic brain and descend to the gray matter around the aqueduct of Sylvius in the midbrain (the periaquductal gray). Fibers from the periaquductal gray descend in the dorsal lateral funiculus of the spinal cord and provide presynaptic inhibition on the cells in the spinal nucleus of V and the substantia gelatinosa, probably by releasing endogenous opiate-like substances.

It is useful clinically to distinguish among nociception, pain, and suffering. *Nociception* refers to the transmission of potentially tissue-damaging stimuli. *Pain* refers to the unpleasant quality of the nociceptive information that reaches the thalamus. *Suffering* refers to the behavioral effect of many unpleasant experiences, one of which is pain. In general, the pathways for nociception are limited to the peripheral nervous system, brainstem, and spinal cord. Pain is mediated by the thalamus and suffering by the cerebral cortex, probably primarily the limbic cortex.

With this background in neuroanatomy, it is possible to generate three major theories for head pain. The *vascular theory* of head pain is based on the concept that the pain is related primarily to vasodilation and the stimulation of nociceptive fibers by this process. Supporting this theory is the fact that serotonin receptors are known to exist on blood vessels, and medications that affect these serotonin receptors, such as the triptan drugs [5-hydroxytryptamine (5-HT1d) agonists], are known to improve head pain. The older theory that migraine was due to a biphasic phenomenon of vasoconstriction followed by vasodilation is probably incorrect. The second theory is the *neurologic theory*, which argues that head pain is an entirely neurologic phenomenon caused by abnormalities in the way the brain handles nociception. The effect of drugs that act on catecholamines (e.g., tricyclic antidepressive drugs) in pain syndromes supports the neurologic theory of head pain. The current leading theory for the cause of head pain is the *neurovascular theory*, which provides a unifying hypothesis arguing that some aspects of head pain are generated from peripheral mechanisms on blood vessels and other aspects are mediated by the CNS processing of these signals. The neurovascular theory also argues that head pain actually may be related to neurogenic inflammation caused by the release of inflammatory substances from synaptic terminals into blood vessels and related tissues in the periphery.

Regardless of the cause, several major headache syndromes are recognizable clinically and can be managed by syndrome recognition. The *migraine syndrome* is probably the most common of all the headache syndromes. Ordinarily, a family history is present. The syndrome is sex influenced, usually expressing itself more commonly and severely in women than in men. People with migraine often have a characteristic personal life history that includes colic in infancy, motion sickness in childhood, episodic abdominal pain in childhood, catamenial headaches at the time of menarche, and food-induced headaches, particularly for such foods as red wine, aged cheeses, peanuts, and chocolate. Other associated headache syndromes during life include caffeine-withdrawal headaches, exercise-induced headaches, ice-cream headaches, jabs and jolts, ice-pick pains, sex headaches, and hangovers. Finally, among elderly patients, transient global amnesia may be a migraine equivalent. Neurologic phenomena (*auras*) sometimes accompany migraines. These tend to be positive phenomena, such as lights and tingling, as opposed to the negative phenomena, such as hemiparesis, which are seen in transient ischemic attacks (TIAs). The auras of migraine tend to migrate in a rather leisurely fashion over an approximately 20-minute period, moving from one part of the body to the other. This may be due to an electric phenomenon in the brain known as the *spreading depression*, which is possibly the electric cause of the neurologic auras of migraine. People with migraine have a slight increase in the risk of stroke,

either because of vasospasm or because of the platelet aggregation and hypercoagulability associated with the phenomenon. An overlap also exists in families and in individual patients between epileptic seizures and migraine, and often both disorders respond to similar classes of medication, such as valproic acid (valproate). The current view of managing migraine is to use abortive treatments unless the headaches are so frequent that they interfere with daily life, in which case prophylactic treatment can be used.

*Cluster headaches* refer to nonpulsating eye pains and usually are seen in men without a personal or family history, similar to the migraine syndrome. Headaches of this kind last for hours and are associated with autonomic abnormalities, such as ptosis and Horner syndrome. Twenty-minute eye pains are called *hemicrania*.

*Tension-type headache* is a nonpulsating head pain that feels as though a band is being tightened around the head. Synonyms for tension-type headache are muscle contraction headache and psychogenic headache.

*Chronic daily headache* refers to headaches that occur more than 5 days a week. It is believed that most chronic daily headache is related to analgesic withdrawal. This syndrome is the final common pathway for any chronic headache problem that is characterized by excessive analgesic use.

*Thunderclap headache* refers to a headache that is maximal at onset. In such circumstances, subarachnoid hemorrhage should be ruled out by using noncontrast computed tomography (CT) and a lumbar puncture if the CT scan is normal. Most thunderclap headaches are benign headaches seen in people with migraine.

Headaches in elderly persons are a special problem. If no prior history of headache is elicited, arteritis should be excluded, but many of these headaches actually are related to cervical spondylosis and other neck problems. Most patients with temporal arteritis have an extremely elevated erythrocyte sedimentation rate, but only a biopsy can make the diagnosis with certainty. If the syndrome is quite suggestive of arteritis, these patients should be treated with steroids until the results of the biopsy are available.

Headaches attributable to increased intracranial pressure tend to be worse in the morning because of relative hypoventilation during the night, combined with a reduction in venous return from the head while the patient is in the supine or prone positions. *Pseudotumor cerebri* or *idiopathic intracranial hypertension* is a syndrome characterized by diffuse headaches, transient visual obscurations, visual field defects, and 6th nerve palsies usually found in obese females.

Headaches caused by cervical radiculopathy and cervical spondylosis tend to be worse posteriorly and are more common as people age.

Headaches from eye disease are almost never seen unless the eye is red. If the eye is quiet, the headache should not be attributed to eye problems, including refractive errors.

Headaches from acute paranasal sinus disease usually are associated with fever and a nasal discharge. Chronic sinusitis does not cause headaches.

Headaches from intracranial masses occur only when the mass involves pain-sensitive structures such as the meninges and the proximal portions of the cerebral arteries. Parenchymal brain tumors, which do not disturb pain-sensitive structures, will not cause head pain unless increased intracranial pressure is present.

The treatment of the common primary headache disorders is based on a clear understanding of the anatomy and neuropharmacology of head pain. Therapy for migraine is based on the frequency of headaches that the patient experiences. For patients with infrequent headaches (one per week), nonoral abortive treatment is best because the stomach rarely empties normally during a migraine, even if no nausea occurs. Currently available nonoral treatments include subcutaneous sumatriptan, sumatriptan nasal spray, rizatriptan sublingual wafer, indomethacin per rectum, ergotamine and caffeine (Cafergot) per rectum, dihydroergotamine nasal spray or intravenously, and antiemetics such as metoclopramide or prochlorperazine, either intravenously or intramuscularly. If oral abortive treatment is tried, an antiemetic such as metoclopramide probably should be administered first so that the oral medication is absorbed. Once the stomach is empty, any oral medication can be used, including any of the triptans and any of the nonsteroidal anti-inflammatory drugs (NSAIDs). Although caffeine is helpful, it is not recommended because caffeine-withdrawal headaches are a common problem and may contribute to the syndrome of chronic daily headache. For refractory headaches, dihydroergotamine 0.75 to 1.5 mg administered intravenously after an antiemetic usually provides excellent headache relief. Isometheptene, the active ingredient in Midrin, is safe, but a fairly weak medication; steroids may be used for short courses to abort recurrent migraines.

Prophylactic treatment for migraine is usually considered when patients experience two or more headaches per week. Three classes of drugs commonly are used: the β-blockers, the antiepileptic drugs, and the polycyclic antidepressants. Among the β-blockers, propranolol appears to be the best, probably because it penetrates the blood–brain barrier most effectively. Other β-blockers also may work. Among the antiepileptic drugs, valproic acid is probably the most effective, but the side effects of hair loss and its lack of safety in pregnancy make it difficult to use in the patient population susceptible to migraine, which includes a large number of young women. Gabapentin is another useful anticonvulsant that is not metabolized by the liver and has a minimal side effect profile. Among the polycyclic antidepressants, amitriptyline has been shown to be most effective, but it also has the most side effects in the form of dry mouth, constipation, and blurred vision as well some degree of confusion and drowsiness.

Treating migraine during pregnancy is a particular problem. In general, no medication is completely safe for the fetus. It is generally believed, however, that acetaminophen is relatively safe. Short courses of steroids can be used. Opiates are probably safe if given occasionally, and promethazine also may be useful for occasional use, when administered per rectum to abort a migraine during pregnancy.

The treatment of acute Horton (cluster) headache is 100% oxygen by face mask to abort the attacks. Prophylactic treatment involves the use of lithium carbonate or verapamil, a calcium channel blocker.

Hemicrania is responsive to indomethacin, which can be given per rectum to abort attacks and orally for prophylaxis. Calcium channel blockers, such as verapamil, sometimes work prophylactically.

Muscle-contraction headache is generally treated using nonpharmacologic techniques such as exercise, biofeedback, and relaxation techniques. If possible, the underlying cause also can be treated, for example, depression, anxiety, or neck pain. Recently, clinicians have used the spasticity drug tizanidine (Zanaflex) for its muscle relaxant properties. Botulinum toxin (Botox) injections of the frontalis muscle are also used for muscle-contraction headaches.

Chronic daily headache is best avoided by not using analgesics more than 3 days a week, whether prescription or over-the-counter analgesics. Treatment requires withdrawing the analgesics, often giving the patient steroids if necessary during this period.

## Dementia

Dementia is one of a group of disorders characterized by intellectual dysfunction. It is important when evaluating dementia to define the three major abnormalities in intellectual dysfunction. *Dementia* is a usually progressive loss of previously acquired intellectual ability. *Mental retardation* is subnormal intellectual capacity. *Pseudodementia* comprises intellectual problems caused by disorders in affect, mood, or thought. When a patient, or more likely the family of a patient, complains of an abnormality in intellectual function, any one of a number of abbreviated screening examinations may be carried out, including the Folstein mini-mental status examination and the Solomon 7-minute mental status battery. The neurologic examination itself involves a careful evaluation of the mental status screening for the four major spheres of mental functioning: level of consciousness, memory, language, and visual–spatial skills. The level of consciousness is tested using specific tests of attention, such as the digit span or the serial seven test. If the patient is confused or delirious, a careful search should be done for a metabolic or toxic cause or a right-hemisphere problem, such as stroke or tumor. Short-term memory is tested by discussing current events with which the patient should have some knowledge with sports, hobbies, politics, and music all useful subjects that can be discussed. Long-term memory is quite difficult to test in the office and is best relegated to a formal neuropsychologic evaluation, if necessary. Language is assessed by analyzing fluency, comprehension, and repetition. Visual–spatial skills are evaluated by having the patient write his or her name and address and a sentence about the weather, followed by a large rendition of a clock face with the hands put on the clock at an arbitrary location. This four-part mental status examination should be kept in the record for future reference. The rest of the elemental neurologic examination is done with the aim of uncovering visual field defects, weakness, sensory loss, or incoordination. The laboratory evaluation for a demented patient will vary depending on the history and the findings but always should include some form of brain imaging, preferably magnetic resonance imaging (MRI), at some point during an evaluation. Ancillary testing, depending on the history, would include metabolic and toxic screens; serological test for syphilis and human immunodeficiency virus (HIV); thyroid function tests; vitamin B12 and folate level tests; homocysteine and methylmalonic acid level tests; a lumbar puncture for measurements of pressure, cellularity, opportunistic infection, and the clinical response to lowering the spinal fluid pressure; and formal psychological tests done by a neuropsychologist. At present, specific genetic tests have no role in the clinical evaluation.

The most important dementing illness in terms of its prevalence and conceptual importance is Alzheimer's disease, which is probably a cerebral amyloidosis caused by an accumulation of a neurotoxic amyloid $\beta$-protein (A-$\beta$), which is cleaved from a normally occurring amyloid precursor protein (APP) by a $\gamma$-secretase enzyme. The neurotoxicity may be mediated in part by an inflammatory reaction to the amyloid and preferentially may affect cholinergic systems that are important for memory. Oxidative stress and excitotoxicity also may contribute to neuronal death.

Many routes to this final common pathway exist; these include (i) having a third copy of chromosome 21 (Down's syndrome) that contains the gene for APP, thus having 50% too much APP; (ii) having a mutation in the genes that code for the $\gamma$-secretase enzyme such as occurs in the two known presenillin mutations on chromosomes 1 and 14; (iii) having an abnormal isotype of the transport protein apoprotein E (APO E4) coded on chromosome 19, which may lead to increased amounts of the neurotoxic form of A-$\beta$ in neurons; and (iv) having a reduced amount of estrogen (as in men and postmenopausal women), which normally partially protects neurons against the neurotoxic effects of A-$\beta$.

At present, the treatment of Alzheimer's disease is not particularly satisfactory. It includes the use of so-called cholinergic therapy with centrally acting anticholinesterase drugs. Donepezil (Aricept), rivastigmine (Exelon), and galantamine (Reminyl) are available and have been demonstrated to have a modest beneficial effect on the natural history of Alzheimer's disease. Memantine (Namenda), an N-methyl D aspartate (NMDA) receptor antagonist, has recently been approved by the FDA for use in patients with moderate to severe dementia. *Ginko biloba*, an over-the-

counter complementary medication, may contain a weak anticholinesterase drug. Estrogen replacement therapy also may delay and or slow the progression of the disease, as do NSAIDs. Antioxidants such as vitamin E also may delay the onset or slow the progression of the disease in susceptible persons. Currently, most therapies involve the use of symptomatic therapy for behavioral problems and include the use of benzodiazepines and phenothiazine drugs when necessary. $\gamma$-Secretase-inhibiting drugs and drugs that interfere with the amyloid fibril self-assembly are presently under development but are not currently clinically available. *Vascular dementia* refers to patients who become demented because of multiple cerebral infarcts or because of chronic cerebral ischemia (*Binswanger's disease*). No specific treatment for the disorder is available, but stroke prevention and maintaining reasonably good blood pressure throughout life should decrease the incidence.

*Hydrocephalus* is divided into two types, *noncommunicating* and *communicating*, depending on whether the ventricles of the brain are openly communicating with each other. Most dementias caused by hydrocephalus are of the communicating type. Normal-pressure hydrocephalus is a disorder in which patients present with dementia, gait abnormalities, and urinary incontinence. Imaging studies often suggest the diagnosis because the ventricles are large and the cerebral sulci are not particularly deep. A lumbar puncture or subarachnoid drainage is the best predictive test as to whether a shunt procedure will help.

Many multisystem neurodegenerative diseases cause dementia as part of a larger syndrome. The most common of these diseases are Parkinson's disease, diffuse Lewy body disease, progressive supranuclear palsy, cortical basal ganglionic degeneration, multisystem atrophy (Shy-Drager syndrome), fronto-temporal dementia (Pick disease), and olivopontocerebellar atrophy.

Several infectious diseases can cause dementia. The most important among these are syphilis, HIV, toxoplasmosis (most commonly seen in immunocompromised persons), and various diseases caused by prions, such as Creutzfeldt-Jacob disease, fatal familial insomnia, Gerstmann-Straussler disease, and bovine spongioform encephalopathy (mad cow disease).

Several nutritional diseases are known to cause dementia. The most important of these is cobalamin (vitamin B12) deficiency, thiamine deficiency (Wernicke-Korsakoff), and nicotinamide (niacin deficiency), otherwise known as pellagra.

Demyelinating disease may cause dementia when the number of white-matter lesions becomes enormous. The most important of these diseases is multiple sclerosis (MS), but progressive multifocal leukoencephalopathy and osmotic demyelination (formerly known as *central pontine myelinolysis*) are also in this category.

Several chronic metabolic insults may result in dementia, such as hypoglycemia, hypoxemia, uremia, and hepatic failure with portosystemic shunting.

Among the endocrine disorders, only thyroid disorders cause dementia as a prominent component of the disease. These disorders include both adult hypothyroidism and cretinism in children. Autoimmune thyroid disease is associated with a rapidly progressive dementing illness (Hashimoto's encephalopathy) that clinically may resemble a prion disease.

Intracranial space-occupying lesions also may cause dementia. These include primary brain tumors such as gliomas, metastases, and brain abscesses, often in patients who have had oral surgery or ear infections or are known to be immunocompromised.

Brain trauma is also an important cause of dementia. The combination of neurotrauma and carrying two copies of the APO E4 genotype greatly increases the risk of dementia.

## Dizziness

Dizziness is an extremely common problem for which people seek medical attention. *Dizziness* is a layperson's term that generally refers to one or more of four common sensations: vertigo, near syncope, disequilibrium, and ill-defined lightheadedness.

*Vertigo* is defined as an illusion of movement and always reflects a disorder of the vestibular system. To understand vertigo, one must review the functional anatomy of the vestibular system, which is a proprioceptive apparatus meant to record angular acceleration of the head and linear acceleration attributable to gravity. For this purpose, three semicircular ducts containing endolymph and surrounded by perilymph, are embedded in the temporal bone in structures known as *semicircular canals*. The three semicircular ducts record angular acceleration of the head. A utricle and saccule, also containing endolymph and surrounded by perilymph, record linear acceleration particularly and, most importantly, acceleration due to gravity. The vestibular nerves travel through the internal auditory meatus with the cochlear and facial nerves to synapse in the medullary vestibular nuclei. The vestibular nuclei then project up the brainstem to the temporal lobe for conscious appreciation of vestibular sensations. The vestibular nuclei also coordinate various vestibularly generated eye movements (the vestibular ocular reflex), antigravity reflexes via the spinal cord, and arousal mechanisms in the reticular formation. Vertigo emanating from the peripheral nervous system may also involve the cochlear apparatus, thereby causing hearing loss or tinnitus and producing violent torsional vertigo; this vertigo often is associated with rotatory nystagmus.

Vertigo emanating from the CNS tends to spare hearing, to produce less torsional vertigo, and to be associated with other brainstem symptoms and signs, such as double vision, dysarthria, and ataxia. Common causes of peripheral vertigo are benign paroxysmal positional vertigo (BPPV) resulting from the escape of otoliths from the utricle and saccule into the posterior semicircular duct, thus rendering that duct gravity sensitive and producing violent spinning vertigo when the affected ear is turned down in the supine position. This vertigo is transient (i.e., lasting less than 60 seconds), fatigues with repeated movements into the "bad" position, reverses direction on sitting up, spares hearing, and is associated with rotatory nystagmus.

*Vestibular neuronitis* and *labyrinthitis* are postviral, probably inflammatory, disorders that follow viral illnesses. In labyrinthitis, hearing is affected, whereas in vestibular neuronitis it is spared.

*Labyrinthine concussion* refers to nystagmus and vertigo after head trauma and should be distinguished from the so-called postconcussion syndrome, a vague and poorly defined syndrome occurring after relatively minor head injury and associated with the various signs and symptoms of depression.

Labyrinthotoxic drugs such as quinine, aspirin, and aminoglycoside antibiotics also can affect the labyrinthine system and produce vertigo.

Vestibular schwannoma, a benign nerve-sheath tumor, almost always produces hearing loss by compressing the cochlear nerve. It also can produce vertigo. The term *acoustic neuroma* is incorrect and should be avoided.

Common causes of vertigo emanating from the CNS are vertebrobasilar insufficiency, demyelinating disease, and centrally acting vestibulotoxic drugs, such as antiepileptic drugs, barbiturates, and benzodiazepines.

Treatment of vertigo depends on the cause. For BPPV, the best treatment is to reposition the otoliths by moving them from the posterior semicircular duct back into the utricle and saccule, from whence they came. This treatment can be done using a physical therapy maneuver originally invented by John Epley and therefore called the *Epley maneuver* (Fig. 12.2). Other repositioning maneuvers are also possible but are not used as commonly. If the Epley maneuver fails, the labyrinth can be reconditioned by placing the head in the "bad" position over and over again each day. This treatment is unpleasant and less than satisfactory. Vestibular sedatives also can be used. These drugs have in common the fact that they are all anticholinergic and act in the CNS. Many are available over the counter, including meclizine (Bonine, Antivert), diphenhydrinate (Dramamine), diphenhydramine (Benadryl). Promethazine (Phenergan) and scopolamine (Scope Trans-Derm) are prescription drugs. An acoustic or vestibular schwannoma usually can be excised by neurosurgeons and otologic surgeons often working as a team. In patients with vertebrobasilar insufficiency, the blood pressure should be raised slightly and aspirin or other antiplatelet drugs used because surgical procedures are usually not helpful to this kind of problem. Demyelinating disease can be treated, if necessary, and all known vestibulotoxic drugs should be discontinued, if possible.

*Near syncope* refers to a sensation of near faint caused by inadequate cerebral perfusion pressure. This usually occurs in the upright position and represents a failure of the

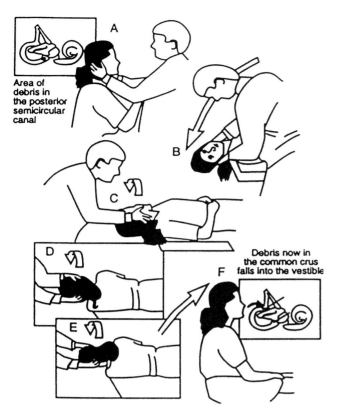

Area of debris in the posterior semicircular canal

Debris now in the common crus falls into the vestibe

**Figure 12.2** The otololith repositioning maneuver of Epley.

nervous system's autonomic response to the upright posture. In clinical practice, it is often associated with the use of medications that cause vasodilation, volume depletion, or both. Drugs that interfere with the ability of the heart to respond to low blood pressure, such as β-blockers, which prevent tachycardia, also can aggravate the symptoms of this type of dizziness. A careful cardiac evaluation should be performed to ensure that the patient is not suffering from a serious cardiac condition, such as left ventricular outflow obstruction, as seen in aortic stenosis, asymmetric septal hypertrophy, or coronary artery disease. Most causes of near syncope are benign and often are related to volume depletion and vasodilation; these problems can be managed by reducing the medications that cause these adverse effects.

*Disequilibrium* refers to a sensation of dizziness caused by gait disorder. In clinical practice, the common gait disorders that cause dizziness include cerebellar ataxia, spasticity, and proprioceptive difficulties such as those commonly seen in cervical spondylosis. Vitamin B12 deficiency has the tendency to produce stiff, weak legs and poor proprioception. An extrapyramidal disorder such as Parkinson's disease also may cause a gait disorder that patients call dizziness. Treatment of the gait disorder often improves the sensation of dizziness.

*Ill-defined lightheadedness* refers to a sensation caused by anxiety, which many patients call dizziness. In some of these patients, episodes of severe dizziness are caused by

hyperventilation attacks, but in many others the sensation is simply a chronic feeling of dysphoria in which the word *dizziness* is used metaphorically to mean anxious or depressed. Such patients are best treated without medications or, if necessary, with medications aimed specifically at the anxiety and depression.

## Back and Neck Pain

Back and neck pains are among the most common complaints for which people seek medical attention and that disable patients so that they cannot work or enjoy their leisure time. For clinical purposes, it is useful to divide these patients into two major categories: those suffering from low back and leg pain and those suffering from neck and arm pain.

Most lower back and leg pain is due to degenerative disease of the lumbar spine or intervertebral disc disease. Nondiscogenic pain should be suspected when the pain is worse at night or at rest, when severe local tenderness is present, or when systemic symptoms or signs of an underlying disease are present. In most patients, the pain is localized to the lower back without much local tenderness or radiation to one or the other leg. Using proprioceptive reflexes, it is usually possible to ascertain the level of the greatest nerve root compression. Table 12.1 demonstrates how it is possible to do this using the reflexes and the sensory and the motor examination. Conservative therapy consists of bed rest for 72 hours, NSAIDs, and muscle relaxants. Patients with pain that is refractory to conservative measures may benefit from epidural steroid injections into the affected lumbar roots. Surgical therapy is reserved for patients who fail all medical and pain management therapies.

Most neck and arm pain is due to degenerative changes in the cervical spine or intervertebral disk disease. *Cervical spondylosis* refers to degenerative change in the cervical spine resulting from degeneration of the intervertebral discs and their intermittent protrusions and calcifications, which lead to nerve root or spinal cord compression. Unlike intervertebral disc disease in the lumbosacral spine, disk disease in the neck can be dangerous in that it can compress the spinal cord, producing a myelopathy.

Fortunately, most cervical spondylosis produces radiculopathy, with its consequent pain in the shoulder, arm, and hand. This disease has a natural history that is characterized by waxing and waning symptoms, but no significant long-term disability result. The vast majority of patients can be treated medically with episodic use of a collar, anti-inflammatory and antispasmodic drugs, and time. Table 12.2 demonstrates how it is possible using proprioceptive reflexes and motor and sensory examination to determine the level of the intervertebral disc that is most likely to be responsible. Patients who fail medical treatment using immobilization and analgesia may benefit from epidural steroid injections into the affected cervical roots. For patients who fail conservative and epidural

**TABLE 12.1**

**SYMPTOMS AND SIGNS OF LATERAL RUPTURE OF LUMBAR DISK**

| Disk | Root | Pain and Parasthesias | Sensory Loss | Motor Loss | Reflex Loss |
|------|------|----------------------|--------------|------------|-------------|
| L3−4 | L4 | Anterior surface of thigh, inner surface of shin | Anteromedial surface of thigh, extending down along shin to inner side of foot | Quadriceps | Knee jerk |
| L4−5 | L5 | Radiating down outer side of back of thigh and outer side of calf, and across dorsum of foot to great toe | Usually involves outer side of calf and the great toe | Extensor hallucis longus; less commonly, muscles of dorsiflexion and eversion of foot | None |
| L5−1 | S1 | Radiating down back of thigh and outer side and back of calf, to foot and the lesser toes | Almost always involves outer side of calf, outer border of foot, and the lesser toes; less commonly, the back of the thigh | Gastrocnemius and occasionally muscles of eversion of foot | Ankle jerk |

Reproduced with permission from Samuels MA, ed. *Manual of Neurologic Therapeutics*, 6th ed. Philadelphia: Lippincott Williams & Wilkins, 1999; Table 5-1, p. 89.

therapies, surgical approaches are available using both the anterior and posterior approaches, depending on the specific location of the disk protrusion.

## Seizures and Epilepsy

An epileptic seizure (usually an abbreviated seizure) is any stereotypical experience or activity arising from hypersynchronous discharge in the cerebral cortex and perhaps some subcortical structures. *Epilepsy* is a disorder characterized by recurrent seizures that are not due to a demonstrable metabolic insult. *Status epilepticus* is the term used to describe seizures lasting for longer than 30 minutes or repeated seizures lasting a total of 30 minutes from which the patient does not recover between episodes. A *nonepileptic* seizure (or *pseudoseizure*) refers to episodic neuropsychiatric phenomena that cannot be demonstrated to be due to hypersynchronous discharges (such as psychogenic seizures). Epileptic seizures are divided into four

major categories: *primary generalized* (centencephalic seizures), *secondary generalized* (beginning partial), *partial* (formerly called *focal*), and *neonatal* (occurring in the first 30 days of life). Primary generalized seizures are subdivided further into *tonic* or *clonic seizures*, formerly known as *grand mal seizures*, and *absence seizures*, formally known as *petit mal seizures*. Partial seizures also are subdivided further into *complex partial seizures*, which affect consciousness, and *simple partial seizures*, which do not affect consciousness.

In evaluating a presumed seizure, it is important to obtain a careful history that includes a birth and developmental history and any history of remote neurotrauma or neurologic infectious disease. An examination, in addition to a standard neurologic examination, should include a careful evaluation of the head and the skin, giving particular attention to body asymmetries because these may reflect early-life brain disease. Ancillary tests include the use of imaging, which in a case of seizures almost always should be MRI, unless this is completely impossible.

**TABLE 12.2**

**SYMPTOMS AND SIGNS OF LATERAL RUPTURE OF CERVICAL DISK**

| Disk | Root | Pain and Parasthesias | Sensory Loss | Motor Loss | Reflex Loss |
|------|------|----------------------|--------------|------------|-------------|
| C4−5 | C5 | Neck, shoulder, upper arm | Shoulder | Deltoid, biceps | Biceps |
| C5−6 | C6 | Neck, shoulder, lateral aspect of arm, and radial aspect of forearm to thumb and forefinger | Thumb, forefinger, radial aspect of forearm, lateral aspect of arm | Biceps | Biceps, supinator |
| C6−7 | C7 | Neck, lateral aspect of arm, and ring and index fingers | Forefinger, middle finger, radial aspect of forearm | Triceps, extensor carpi ulnaris | Triceps, supinator |
| C7−T1 | C8 | Ulnar aspect of forearm and hand | Ulnar half of ring finger, little finger | Intrinsic muscles of the hand, wrist extensors | None |

Reproduced with permission from Samuels MA, ed. *Manual of Neurologic Therapeutics*, 6th ed. Philadelphia: Lippincott Williams & Wilkins, 1999; Table 5-2, p. 93.

Electroencephalography (EEG) is often useful in determining the nature of the seizure and its localization. A spinal fluid analysis may be performed to look for the cause of the seizure, and a metabolic and toxic screen should be done because many seizures are due to metabolic or toxic insults. Common causes of seizures in adults include cerebral infarction, trauma, infection, and alcohol and drug withdrawal.

The general principles for the treatment of seizures are quite straightforward. Treatment should aim to treat only epilepsy (not seizures), except in specific life-threatening circumstances, such as toxemia of pregnancy. Otherwise, the antiepileptic medication will have greater toxicity than benefits. When using antiepileptic drugs (AEDs), monotherapy is preferred. It is now possible to obtain drug levels at the *trough* (i.e., just before the next dose of medication), which often helps to keep the medications to a minimum. The choice of AEDs is becoming quite straightforward. For generalized seizures, valproic acid is the first choice, with phenytoin as backup (Fig. 12.3). For partial seizures, carbamazepine is the drug of choice, with valproate as backup. For certain seizure types, individual drugs have been known to be particularly effective. Those include ethosuximide for typical absence seizures, valproic acid for juvenile myoclonic epilepsy, and magnesium sulfate for toxemia of pregnancy. In general, it is best to avoid newer medications such as gabapentin, lamotrigene, topiramate, felbamate, and tiagabine until more time has been allowed to ascertain the long-term toxic effects. These drugs are best used by experts in epileptology rather than by general neurologists or general physicians. Over time, some of them will enter the armamentarium of the generalist.

Surgical treatment of epilepsy is reserved for a small number of patients and should be done only in specialized centers where it is possible to document medical intractability carefully and to perform a detailed neuropsychological, physiological, and anatomic mapping study before the surgery is performed. Available procedures include removal of the focus, callosotomy, lobectomy, and hemispherectomy. Vagal nerve stimulation also may help certain patients who have intractable seizures, although the mechanism of action is unknown.

Epilepsy in pregnancy is particularly challenging. All AEDs are potentially teratogenic, so the general rule is to keep AEDs to an absolute minimum, especially during first trimester organogenesis. All female seizure patients of child-bearing years should be maintained on folate to minimize the risk of neural tube defects. Severe seizures are probably worse for the fetus than any AED because of the potential for anoxic injury to the fetus. The risks versus the benefits must be weighed for each patient and then treatment individualized. The rules for stopping AEDs have been learned from experience. A long seizure-free period (about 4 years) is recommended. A normal EEG at the time AEDs are discontinued and a normal MRI predict a better long-term outcome. Nonetheless, the risk of seizure recurrence in the "best" group of patients is still about 30%.

Epilepsy and seizures cause a sudden loss of consciousness in many circumstances and therefore may interfere with the activities of daily living; thus, they can be quite

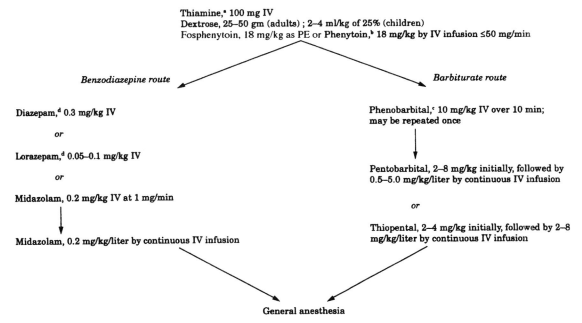

**Figure 12.3** Treatment of generalized tonic-clonic status epilepticus. (A) Thiamine is given when alcoholism or malnutrition is suspected. (B) Never dilute in glucose-containing fluids. (C) Drug of first choice in neonates. (D) In children, usually diazepam or lorezepam is the initial drug, followed by phenytoin.

dangerous. In general, patients should not drive unless the seizures are under control. Each state within the United States, as well as other countries, has specific rules about what is meant by the phrase *seizure free for a long enough period*. Generally, this period ranges from 6 to 12 months without seizure and on an appropriate AED regimen. Some states require that the physician or patient must report such cases to the Registry of Motor Vehicles; in other states, this is not necessary. Familiarity with local laws on this subject is advised. Other activities such as swimming usually are not regulated specifically but also can be quite dangerous.

It is known that epileptics have an increased risk of sudden death. Many causes are possible; most deaths are due to an autonomic storm with consequent cardiac arrhythmias.

# NEUROLOGIC DISEASES

## Stroke

A *stroke* is the sudden or rapid onset of a neurologic deficit in a vascular territory caused by an underlying cerebrovascular disease lasting longer than 24 hours. A TIA is the same, but it lasts less than 24 hours. The major contributing cerebrovascular diseases include atherosclerosis, lipohyalinosis (arteriolar sclerosis), cerebral embolism, arterial dissection, fibromuscular dysplasia, berry aneurysm, vascular malformations, and vasculitis. Hypercoagulable states that may predispose to stroke include both prethrombotic and thrombosis-prone conditions.

All strokes are divided into two subtypes: *ischemic* and *embolic* strokes. Ischemic strokes themselves are subdivided into two types: *thrombotic* and *embolic*. Thrombotic stroke is subdivided into those caused by large-vessel disease and those caused by small-vessel disease. The large vessels that tend to cause thrombotic stroke are the *carotid arteries*, otherwise known as the *anterior circulation*, and the *vertebral* and *basilar arteries*, otherwise known as the *posterior circulation*. Small vessels also can thrombose, leading to small infarcts deep in the brain, known as *lacunes*. Embolic stroke is divided into *cardiac-* and *arterial-source emboli*. Cardiac-source emboli are generally larger and more likely to produce serious stroke deficits. Embolism tends to affect midsized cerebral vessels, as in middle cerebral artery syndrome, anterior cerebral artery syndrome, and posterior cerebral artery syndrome.

*Hypercoagulable states* are subdivided into two types: *primary* and *secondary*. The primary hypercoagulable state are disorders in known endogenous anticoagulant mechanisms and include protein S and protein C deficiency, antithrombin III deficiency, and various fibrinolytic disorders. Secondary hypercoagulable states include antiphospholipid antibody syndrome, paraneoplastic (Trousseau's) syndrome, and various rheologic problems, such as those caused by immobility, obesity, and pressure from artificial surfaces.

*Hemorrhagic strokes* are divided into two types: those in which bleeding occurs into the substance of the brain, known as *intracerebral hemorrhages (ICH)*, and those bleeding into the subarachnoid space, known as *subarachnoid hemorrhages (SAH)*. ICH tend to be due to hypertensive vascular disease, in which case they occur deep in the brain, particularly in the putamen, thalamus, pons, and cerebellum. ICH caused by a rupture of fragile arteries affected by amyloid (congophilic angiopathy) tend to be lobar and closer to the surface of the brain where the affected pial vessels are plentiful. SAH most commonly is produced by a rupture of a congenital (berry) aneurysm or of an abnormal vascular malformation, such as an arteriovenous malformation (AVM), capillary malformation, or venous malformation.

The diagnosis of stroke or TIA is largely a clinical one. The clinical picture for each of the major cerebral territories is fairly characteristic. When the ophthalmic artery is involved, patients complain of transient or permanent episodes of monocular blindness. Anterior cerebral artery ischemia produces contralateral leg weakness, sparing the arm and face. The middle cerebral syndrome consists of hemiparesis that is worse in the face and hand, sparing the leg. Vertebral artery occlusions tend to cause infarction in the cerebellum and lateral medulla, producing ipsilateral ataxia, facial numbness, Horner's syndrome, hoarseness, and vertigo with contralateral body numbness. This syndrome, when it affects the lateral medulla, is known as *Wallenberg's stroke*. Basilar artery disease is divided into main-stem basilar disease and basilar-branch disease. Main-stem basilar disease tends to produce episodes of progressive tetraparesis, dysarthria, dysphagia, ataxia, and eye-movement abnormalities as well as changes in the level of consciousness. Basilar-branch disease tends to produce episodic or progressive contralateral hemiparesis with ipsilateral cranial nerve findings. The top of the basilar syndrome is a characteristic cerebral embolism syndrome in which a sudden loss of consciousness occurs. If the patient awakens, he manifests a major abnormality in vision, such as blindness, with denial of deficit (Anton's syndrome) or a visual agnosia, such as Balint's syndrome, often with a major visual field cut, such as a hemianopsia.

Various noninvasive studies are available for evaluating cerebral vascular disease, including ultrasound evaluation of the carotid, transcranial Doppler for the vertebral and middle cerebral intracranial arteries, magnetic resonance angiography, CT angiography, nuclear flow studies, functional imaging such as positron emission tomography (PET), single-photon emission CT, and functional MR. Stroke centers are commonly using MR diffusion and perfusion imaging in the assessment of acute stroke. MR diffusion indicates infarcted tissue, whereas MR perfusion indicates areas of the brain that are not adequately perfused. In combination, MR diffusion and perfusion can assess the extent of the penumbra. The penumbra is brain tissue that is not adequately perfused but which remains viable if blood flow can be quickly reestablished. CT perfusion and angiography may be used to delineate those areas of brain tissue having poor flow and that are at risk for infarction. Conventional angiography remains the gold standard for assessment of embolus localization in acute stroke, investigation to exclude an aneurysm or AVM, and as a screening tool to exclude vasculitis. Urgent angiography is only performed if an interventional procedure to remove an embolus is being considered. When cerebral embolism is suspected, a cardiac ultrasound evaluation is considered to be routine. Transesophageal echocardiography has been demonstrated to be superior to transthoracic studies for demonstrating a potential cardiac source for a cerebral embolism.

The treatment of acute stroke involves the maintenance of euvolemia and a minimization of fluids that contain free water, to avoid cerebral edema; nothing by mouth for a day or two to avoid aspiration; and moderation in the control of blood pressure. Sudden drops in blood pressure from hypovolemia or drug therapy during stroke may make the patients deteriorate if cerebral blood flow is impaired through extracranial or intracranial stenosis. Steroids are not only ineffective, but probably dangerous in the context of stroke.

Intravenous thrombolytic therapy is becoming more popular in small- to medium-sized vessel disease. Intravenous tissue plasminogen activator (IV-tPA) has been shown to be beneficial when given in the first 3 hours after a stroke. Patients must meet strict inclusion and exclusion criteria (see Table 12.3) to be eligible for IV-tPA. Symptomatic hemorrhages after IV-tPA usually occur within the first 24 hours after treatment and are associated with protocol violations. Intra-arterial thrombolysis using urokinase, prourokinase, or tPA is probably also effective, particularly in larger vessel disease. Only one randomized trial has shown benefit using intra-arterial prourokinase. It can only be utilized in specialized centers where the technical capability to use intra-arterial therapy is present. Other experimental therapies, such as the use of hemodilution to improve cerebral perfusion, hypothermia, angioplasty, stents, cerebral bypass surgery, laser lysis of clots, and cellular protection protocols using glutamate receptor blockers, free radical scavengers, and calcium entry blockers are all under investigation, but not generally available at this time. Multiple devices for the mechanical removal of clots are currently being investigated for use in the 0- to 6-hour time window. Newer MR and CT imaging techniques are being investigated to expand the available time window for thrombolysis and mechanical clot removal.

Carotid endarterectomy is considered for patients with symptomatic and asymptomatic stenosis of 60% to 99%. Patients who are symptomatic and have higher degrees of stenosis benefit more than those who are asymptomatic with less stenosis. Carotid angioplasty and stenting with distal emboli protection for high-risk patients will probably be approved by the FDA by the end of 2005. Catheter-guided techniques allow interventionalists to treat lesions not amenable to surgery.

Neurologists use antiplatelet therapy for patients with acute stroke unless a high-risk condition such as atrial fibrillation exists. If a high-risk condition exists, heparin for the prevention of further acute strokes may be considered depending on the size of the infarction and other comorbid conditions. Most neurologists use heparin in nonhemorrhagic strokes that are progressing, even though no good evidence-based data support this use. Warfarin, aiming for an international normalized ratio (INR) of 2 to 3, is used in patients with known significant risk factors for cerebral embolism, such as atrial fibrillation, patent foramen ovale, myocardial infarction with a dyskinetic left ventricular wall, and cardiomyopathy. Warfarin is relatively contraindicated in unreliable or alcoholic patients, in persons who have active infective endocarditis or a known blood dyscrasia, and in patients who tend to fall frequently. High-intensity warfarin with an INR greater than 3 is indicated in patients having antiphospholipid antibody syndrome and mechanical heart valves.

Antiplatelet therapy using aspirin appears to be effective in reducing the risk of stroke and death in patients with threatened stroke, in the form of either subtotal stroke or past TIAs. The exact most effective dose of aspirin is still not known. The lowest proved effective dose is 30 mg a day, but most neurologists prescribe either 81 or 325 mg a day. For patients who are aspirin failures, a combination of dipyridamole and aspirin (Aggrenox) or clopidogrel (Plavix) may be used for stroke prevention. Coumadin has not been shown to reduce the risk of recurrent stroke with

## TABLE 12.3

### INCLUSION AND EXCLUSION CRITERIA FOR THE ADMINISTRATION OF IV-tPA

| Inclusion Criteria | Exclusion Criteria |
|---|---|
| Onset of symptoms <3 hours | Systolic BP >185, diastolic BP |
| Screening NIH[a] stroke scale | <110 |
| CT scan of brain without | Rapidly resolving symptoms |
| hemorrhage and early | Seizure at onset |
| infarction less than | Stroke within 3 months |
| 1/3 MCA[b] territory | Head trauma within 3 months |
| | GI of urinary tract hemorrhage |
| | within 3 months |
| | Noncompressible arterial |
| | puncture within 7 days |
| | Anticoagulants or heparin within |
| | 48 hours |
| | Elevated PTT or PT >15 |
| | Platelet count <100,000 |
| | Glucose <50 or >400 |

[a] NIH, National Institutes of Health Stroke Scale;
[b] MCA, Middle Cerebral Artery
Reproduced with permission from The National Institute of Neurological Disorders and Stroke rt-PA Stroke Study Group. Tissue plasminogen activator for acute ischemic stroke. *N Engl J Med* 1995;333;1581–1587.

an unknown etiology. The combination of dipyridamole and aspirin has demonstrated a significant difference in reducing the risk of stroke compared to both placebo and aspirin therapy. Clopidogrel, an inhibitor of ADP-induced platelet aggregation that binds directly to the ADP receptor, is as effective as its analog ticlopidine, roughly the same price, and is probably slightly less toxic.

The treatment of subarachnoid hemorrhage is surgical clipping or intra-arterial coiling of the aneurysm at the earliest possible time to prevent another SAH. The use of antithrombolytic therapy to prevent rebleeding is uncommon because of its tendency to produce thrombosis throughout the body, including pulmonary embolism. Antispasm therapy consists of hydration, blood pressure augmentation, and hemodilution and is usually not initiated until the aneurysm has been treated. If medical therapy fails, interventional procedures such as angioplasty and the intra-arterial administration of papavarine may be tried to open the vasospastic artery. Hydrocephalus and seizures are other complications of SAH that may be life-threatening and need to be urgently treated. In general, cerebral edema is not treated unless the patient clearly has a major problem of cerebral tissue shifts and increased intracranial pressure that may progress to uncal herniation.

## Peripheral Neuropathy

To understand the common problems of peripheral neuropathy, it is necessary to review the functional neuroanatomy. The ordinary peripheral nerve is a mixed nerve that contains at least two major types of afferent fibers and two major types of efferent fibers. The afferent fibers include small-diameter unmyelinated fibers carrying nociceptive sensations, such as pain and temperature information, and large-diameter myelinated fibers carrying nonnociceptive information, such as proprioception, vibration sense, position sense, and touch to the spinal cord or brainstem. The efferent fibers consist of small-diameter unmyelinated fibers carrying autonomic information and large-diameter myelinated fibers carrying motor information to muscles. Neuropathy is a disorder of the nerve and can include all or some of the four major fiber types, including effects on the myelin sheaths of the large-diameter fibers, both efferent and afferent. In general, diseases of the roots, known as *radiculopathies*, are "lumped together" with neuropathies in the same category of illness.

The pathology of peripheral neuropathy consists of three major categories: infarction or compression of the nerve, which produces mononeuropathy; axonal degeneration, which produces polyneuropathy; and segmental demyelination, which produces polyneuropathy or mononeuropathy.

In taking a history from a patient with tingling, numbness, weakness, or autonomic change, the possibility of a peripheral neuropathy should be considered. The rate of onset and progression of the illness is extremely important because some neuropathies progress rapidly and are life

threatening, whereas others are slow or nonprogressive. Because the peripheral nerve is predictably susceptible to toxic metabolic insults, a careful history of any known toxins, such as metals, solvents, and glue, also is important. Drugs are often toxic to peripheral nerves; therefore, in taking a history, inquiry should be made about the use of quinine derivatives, phenytoin, glutethimide, gold, hydralazine, isoniazid, nitrofurantoin, and vincristine. This list is not complete, however, and any drug is potentially neurotoxic. A history of recent immunizations, such as those against influenza, rabies, typhoid, or smallpox, also may be responsible for some of the immune-mediated demyelinating neuropathies. Recent infections, particularly gastrointestinal infections that might be due to *Campylobacter*, are particularly important because immune reactions against this organism are known to cause certain kinds of neuropathy. The history of underlying malignancy is also important because a number of paraneoplastic and nutritional neuropathies exist, and a family history is particularly important because about a third of patients with chronic neuropathy of unknown cause eventually are found to have a familial form of the syndrome.

The clinical picture is generally divided into the major categories of the syndrome of mononeuropathy and the syndrome of polyneuropathy. Mononeuropathy involves the loss of motor or sensory function in the distribution of one nerve or asymmetrically in multiple nerves (in which case it is known as *mononeuropathy multiplex*) associated with pain and a loss of appropriate reflexes. The pain and loss of reflexes may or may not be present, depending on the nerve that is affected. In polyneuropathy, a loss of motor or sensory function occurs symmetrically, in a distribution that usually affects the longest nerves first. This so-called dying-back phenomenon is extremely accurate and helpful in distinguishing axonal polyneuropathy from mononeuropathy or demyelinating diseases. In axonal polyneuropathy, the loss of reflexes affects the longest nerves first, and pain is variable, depending on the cause and nature of the neuropathic disease.

Among the neuropathies, one of the most common forms is compression or entrapment neuropathy. Sometimes these neuropathies are related to amyloid, acromegaly, or hypothyroidism, but usually they are associated with recurrent trauma or are completely cryptogenic. Any nerve that is susceptible to such an injury could suffer this kind of problem, but the most common are carpal tunnel syndrome of the median nerve at the wrist, the peroneal nerve at the knee, the radial nerve in the arm, the ulnar nerve at the elbow, and the lateral femoral cutaneous nerve (meralgia paresthetica) in the inguinal ligament. Mononeuritis and mononeuritis multiplex commonly are seen in systemic vasculitis diseases, such as periarteritis; in various vasculopathy syndromes, such as diabetes mellitus; in some hyperviscosity circumstances, such as Waldenstrom's syndrome, multiple myeloma, and polycythemia; in certain toxic circumstances, particularly those caused by lead; in some infectious diseases, particularly those caused by herpes zoster or leprosy; and sometimes cryptogenically or postinfectious, such as Bell's palsy.

Among the polyneuropathies, segmental demyelination is seen in the postinfectious or postimmunization syndrome of Guillain-Barré, now known as *acute inflammatory demyelinating polyneuropathy (AIDP)*. A chronic form also exists, known as chronic IDP (CIDP). Metachromatic leukodystrophy and Krabbe's disease are inherited forms of segmental demyelinating polyneuropathy having central nervous system myelin involvement as well. Genetically, the most common form is known as Charcot-Marie-Tooth disease. Axonal degeneration-type polyneuropathy is the most common of all. It can be associated with vitamin deficiencies sometimes associated with alcohol, such as thiamine, vitamin B6, and folate. It is seen in diabetes mellitus, hepatic failure, renal failure, paraneoplastic syndromes, diphtheria, amyloidosis, porphyria, and in exposures to large numbers of toxins. It can also be genetically determined. It may be immune mediated, as when it is associated with monoclonal gammopathy of unknown significance and in the so-called POEMS syndrome (*p*olyneuropathy, *o*rganomegaly, *e*ndocrinopathy, *m*onoclonal gammopathy, and *s*kin changes) seen in osteosclerotic myeloma. Lastly, axonal degeneration may be completely cryptogenic, as in many motor neuron diseases.

The treatment of neuropathy depends a great deal on the underlying cause. The best protocol is to treat the underlying condition, such as repleting vitamin deficiency, treating diabetes mellitus, discontinuing intoxications, or treating an underlying malignancy. Steroids can be beneficial in certain categories of neuropathy, such as Bell's palsy and CIDP. Plasmapheresis has been demonstrated to be useful in AIDP, CIDP, and possibly in certain paraneoplastic neuropathies. Intravenous immunoglobulin also may be effective for AIDP, CIDP, and paraneoplastic neuropathies. Hospitalization for respiratory support is often necessary for patients with severe AIDP; therefore, plasmapheresis can be used frequently during that period. Lastly, genetic counseling often is useful for patients with a known genetically determined neuropathy.

## Movement Disorders

Disorders of movement are divided into two major categories: those characterized by too little movement and those characterized by too much movement. Movement disorders characterized by too little movement fall into three major syndromes: paralysis, rigidity, and akinesia. *Paralysis* (or paresis when incomplete) refers to the inability to use a limb voluntarily. Paralysis is divided into two subtypes: upper motor neuron (or supranuclear) and lower motor neuron (or infranuclear). *Supranuclear paralysis* means a weakness of voluntary effort in a limb that will move under other circumstances, such as part of a tendon reflex or as a result of automatic movement, such as yawning. Lower motor neuron or infranuclear weakness refers to the inability of the limb to move under any circumstance, with associated trophic change and wasting of the muscle. Diseases that affect both upper and lower motor neurons simultaneously are known as *motor neuron diseases*, the most common of which is amyotrophic lateral sclerosis (ALS). The second movement disorder characterized by too little movement is *rigidity*, meaning an abnormal stiffness in a muscle. Rigidity falls into three subtypes: spasticity, lead-pipe stiffness, and paratonic rigidity. *Spasticity* is a velocity-dependent stiffness seen in persons who have upper motor neuron disease. *Lead-pipe stiffness* is not velocity dependent and is seen in extrapyramidal disorders such as parkinsonism. *Paratonic stiffness* varies in severity and is seen in frontal-lobe disease, such as hydrocephalus, or in degenerative diseases of the nervous system, such as Alzheimer's disease. The third category of movement disorder characterized by too little movement is akinesia and bradykinesia. *Akinesia* refers to a delay between the beginning of the effort to make a movement and the beginning of the movement itself. *Bradykinesia* refers to slowness of movement. Akinesia and bradykinesia often occur together; when they do, they are often referred to generically as parkinsonism. This tendency not to move produces a rigid appearance of the face and body, as though the patient were wearing a mask. Such patients blink less often than normally and, when walking, have fewer than normal associated movements, such as swinging of the arms.

Many movement disorders are characterized by too much movement. *Tremor* is the most common movement disorder characterized by too much movement; it refers to an oscillating involuntary movement around some fulcrum. Tremors may be proximal or distal, fast or slow, and are generated by synchronous or asynchronous activity at a joint. It is useful from a clinical perspective to divide all tremors into two categories: those that are obvious in repose, known as *repose* or *resting tremor*, and those present on action (known as *intention tremor*). Among the tremors in repose, one group improves on action and one group worsens and changes in character on action. A tremor in repose that is relieved by action is most likely due to parkinsonism. The tremor is slow and alternating at about three or four cycles per second in repose. On action, the tremor reduces in amplitude and frequency. Patients are often aware of the fact that their tremor is better on action. A tremor in repose that is exaggerated on action is known as a *rubral* or *cerebellar outflow tremor* and often is due to a disease in the white matter superior cerebellar peduncle as it crosses the midbrain on its way to the lateral thalamus. Patients with MS and head trauma are particularly susceptible to the rubral tremor. Among the action tremors, some are present only on goal-directed action, such as pointing at a particular goal. This intention tremor is due to cerebellar disease either in the cerebellum itself or in fibers going to or coming from the cerebellum. Action tremors that are activated simply by a particular position (e.g., the antigravity posture) are known as *postural action tremors*. The *physiological* (normal) tremor is an example of a postural action tremor. This type of tremor can be exaggerated by the use of medication that activates β-receptors in muscle or that leads to increased amounts of circulating catecholamines in the blood. Thus, caffeine, theophylline, asthma medications, and catecholamine reuptake inhibitors all exaggerate physiologic tremor and make it a symptom. A somewhat slower tremor that occurs on postural action is known as *essential tremor*. It tends to run in families, beginning asymmetrically and progressing slowly over many years.

A *fibrillation* is the smallest possible movement disorder. It consists of the firing of one muscle fiber within a muscle belly occurring without command. It is always pathologic and represents denervation supersensitivity. It can be seen only by carrying out electrophysiologic studies, which is performed by placing recording electrodes into muscles to observe the electromyogram. A fibrillation usually reflects neuropathic diseases.

A *fasciculation* is the firing of all muscle fibers connected to one motor neuron (a *motor unit*). A fasciculation is often visible but is usually not large enough to move a joint unless the joint is small, such as in the fingers. Fasciculations are commonly normal and may be exacerbated by anxiety and various metabolic disturbances, in particular, hyperventilation and hypomagnesemia. If fasciculations are associated with both upper and lower motor neuron signs, the clinician needs to consider the diagnoses of ALS or cervical myelopathy with multiple cervical radiculopathies. In the absence of wasting and weakness, fasciculations have no pathologic importance; occasionally, they may be treated with magnesium or membrane-stabilizing drugs, such as AEDs and quinine.

*Myoclonus* refers to the sudden contraction of all the muscles at a given joint, producing a quick movement of that joint. Sudden interruptions of muscular contraction at the same joint produces inverse myoclonus or *asterixis*. Myoclonus and asterixis are commonly seen in metabolic encephalopathies, such as in the circumstances of renal and hepatic failure, pulmonary disease, or the use of opiates. Myoclonus and asterixis also can be seen in various neurologic conditions, particularly the prion diseases; in such cases, the clinical picture is dominated by dementia and movement disorders of other sorts, not by the myoclonus and asterixis alone. In a general hospital, myoclonus and asterixis usually means metabolic encephalopathy.

*Chorea* refers to a quick movement involving more than one joint. It tends to have a semi-involuntary appearance, but it is, in fact, completely involuntary. It was originally noted in rheumatic fever, where it was called *Sydenham chorea* (or *St. Vitus' dance*). *Huntington disease* is another illness that produces chorea; however, most chorea is seen as the result of the chronic use of those neuroleptic drugs that block dopamine receptors in the CNS. This chorea probably occurs because of denervation supersensitivity and is known as *tardive chorea*. This is only one of the many tardive movement disorders (*tardive dyskinesias*) seen with the use of

neuroleptic drugs, but it is probably the most common among them. Chorea may involve proximal structures, such as the mouth and lips, in which case it is called *oral* or *buccolingual chorea*, or it can be quite distal in the limbs. It is seen in pregnancy (*chorea gravidarum*), with the use of oral contraceptives in patients with lupus, and in some otherwise normal elderly people (*senile chorea*).

*Dystonia* refers to an abnormal posture or a movement into an abnormal posture. Dystonia may be focal, segmental, or generalized. An example of a focal dystonia is writer's cramp or various musicians' and occupational dystonias brought about by particular repetitive movements in a highly skilled action. Segmental dystonias include torticollis, blepharospasm, and Meige syndrome. Generalized dystonias (formerly known as *dystonia musculorum deformans*) are genetically determined diseases characterized by progressive torsion dystonia. Several genes have been identified to explain many of the known dystonia syndromes. A few of the dystonias are dopamine responsive. These dystonias are recognizable when patients feel better in the morning, but worse as the day goes on.

*Athetosis* refers to the slow, writhing movement from one dystonic posture to another dystonic posture. It can be thought of as a moving dystonia. Athetosis has no meaning in its own right beyond that of dystonia.

*Ballismus* refers to the sudden flinging movements of a limb. If one side of the body is involved, it is called *hemiballismus*; it may affect all four limbs or only one of the four limbs. It generally is due to a small infarction in the subthalamic nucleus resulting from a stroke in the distribution of the mesencephalic artery, a branch of the posterior circulation of the brain.

*Akathisia* refers to the inability to hold still. It is part of the Ekbom syndrome and represents a spectrum from a simple feeling of wanting to move, sometimes called the restless leg syndrome, to actually moving. It may be a form of tardive dyskinesia and may occur completely randomly and for no apparent cause. It is known to be associated with certain metabolic diseases that produce neuropathy and also with iron deficiency anemia.

A *tic* is a semi-voluntary movement that often affects muscles derived from branchial arches. A tic is otherwise known as a *habit*. The tic relieves an inner tension, which then builds up again and leads to another tic. Tic is associated with and may be a neurologic example of obsessive-compulsive disorder, and it responds to the same treatments to which obsessive-compulsive disorder responds in other circumstances, such as polycyclic antidepressants, specific serotonin reuptake inhibitors, or clonidine, a centrally active α-receptor agonist.

Among the many movement disorders, particular syndromes are common in clinical practice. The most common of these is parkinsonism syndrome, referring to the triad of akinesia, lead-pipe stiffness or rigidity, and a tremor in repose that improves with action. The differential diagnosis for parkinsonism includes (i) Parkinson's disease, a cryptogenic loss of cells in the substantia nigra with the subsequent loss of dopamine in the striatum; and (ii) postencephalic parkinsonism, an epidemic disease occurring in North America until about 1920, with occasional sporadic cases still occurring. In postencephalic parkinsonism, a neurotrophic virus apparently produces a mesencephalic encephalitis with drowsiness, followed by parkinsonism; it formerly was known as *sleeping sickness*.

Parkinsonism may be induced by drugs that block dopamine receptors in the CNS, particularly those neuroleptic drugs used in psychiatric circumstances. Parkinsonism often is associated with other degenerative diseases of the nervous system, such as progressive supranuclear palsy and multisystem atrophy, strionigral degeneration, and olivopontocerebellar atrophy. Occasionally, it occurs in endemic areas, such as in Guam, in the Parkinson dementia complex. Parkinsonism is sometimes familial, but it is usually a sporadic illness. Parkinsonism can be seen in association with the deposition of certain minerals in the basal ganglia, as in the case of Wilson's disease (copper), Fahr's disease (calcium and magnesium), Hallervorden-Spatz disease (iron), and miner's parkinsonism (manganese). Parkinsonism may be toxic, as occurs with intoxication with N-methl-phenyl-1,2,3,6-tetrahydropydropyridine and even may be metabolic, as in subacute necrotizing encephalomyelopathy of Leigh and other mitochondrial diseases.

The treatment of parkinsonism has undergone significant changes over the past 5 years. Patients with early or mild parkinsonian symptoms are now treated using central dopamine agonists instead of using dopamine replacement with carbidopa. Newer agents such as pramipexole (Mirapex) and ropinirole (Requip), and older agents such as bromocriptine (Parlodel) and pergolide (Permax), are dopamine agonists that improve early parkinsonian symptoms as well as levadopa does. The early initiation of these agents significantly delays the need for levadopa for years and decreases the number of patients who develop dyskinesias, as compared with levadopa. Levadopa is used in the later stages of the disease or if patients fail dopamine agonists. Catechol-O-methyltransferase (COMT) inhibitors decrease the peripheral metabolism of levadopa by the gut and liver, thereby increasing the amount available for the CNS; these are used as adjunctive therapy to levadopa. Stalevo, a combination of levodopa, carbidopa, and entacopone (Comtan), has been shown to be effective in patient's with advanced Parkinson's disease. In patients having predominately tremor, anticholinergics such as trihexyphenidyl (Artane) or benztropine (Cogentin) may be used. Amantadine (Symmetrel) improves central dopamine release and may be used alone or in combination with the anticholinergics or levadopa. Selegiline (Eldepryl) is used in patients younger than 65 years old and in those with mild parkinsonian features. It delays the progression of parkinsonian symptoms and prolongs the symptomatic benefit of levadopa. Given the high incidence of intolerance to parkinsonism medication, all drugs should be initiated slowly and titrated to the lowest possible effective dose. In patients with psychiatric manifestations of parkinsonism (in particular, hallucinations), clozapine (Clozaril) is the best drug choice because it produces little parkinsonism itself.

The deep brain stimulation of areas involved in the pathophysiology of parkinsonism is usually reserved for patients who fail conventional therapy. Recent advancements in stereotactic techniques have made the placement of electrodes into deep regions of the brain more beneficial and less risky for patients. The stimulation of the subthalamic nucleus (STN) and the globus pallidus (GP) are both efficacious, with the STN being an easier target and the GP slightly more effective. The advantages of electrical stimulation include and improvement of all parkinsonian symptoms, doubled "on" time, no dyskinesias, and the potential of neuroprotection.

The transplantation of dopamine-producing fetal cells from the carotid body or adrenal medulla into the striatum of patients has been tried for refractory patients. Stereotactically placed destructive lesions in the thalamus are mainly used to treat tremor, whereas lesions in the GP improve all symptoms.

Treatment of chorea is difficult unless levels of the offending drug, such as hormonal birth control, can be reduced. Antidopamine therapy using a central dopamine receptor antagonist, such as haloperidol (Haldol), is sometimes useful, but haloperidol often produces parkinsonism and other side effects. Cholinergic therapy using a centrally acting acetylcholine precursor, such as choline or lecithin or a cholinergic agonist such as deanol (Deaner), or anticholinesterase therapy using physostigmine or donepezil are occasionally beneficial.

Myoclonus is treated using serotonergic agonists, such as 5-hydroxytryptophan and carbidopa, or with centrally acting serotonin reuptake inhibitors, such as fluoxetine (Prozac).

Dystonia is difficult to treat unless it happens to be a dopamine-responsive dystonia. Otherwise, the injection of the affected muscles with small doses of botulinum toxin is often helpful. Tardive dyskinesia, whether it be dystonia, athetosis, chorea, or akathisia, is often best treated by discontinuing the offending drug, even though to do so may transiently increase the movement disorder. Sometimes a small benefit can be obtained by using a centrally acting catecholamine-depleting drug, such as reserpine or tetrabenazine.

Tics are best ignored and not treated at all unless they are particularly bothersome. Developmental tics will disappear spontaneously. Severe tic disorder can be treated in a manner similar to the treatment of obsessive-compulsive disorders or sometimes with haloperidol or clonidine.

## Diseases of Myelin

Myelin is a lipoprotein that allows underlying axons to conduct impulses at a much more rapid rate than otherwise because of saltatory (jumping) conduction. Peripheral myelin is made by Schwann cells, and central myelin is made by oligodendrocytes. In both cases, myelin is a lipoprotein composed of 70% lipid and 30% protein. The major proteins in myelin are proteolipid protein and basic protein. The lipids are mainly galactose-containing glycolipids, such as cerebroside and sulfatide. The myelin sheath is in fact a modified plasma membrane. *Demyelination* refers to an acquired illness that causes a loss of myelin while other elements of the nervous system are relatively intact. The most common CNS demyelinating disease is MS. Other CNS demyelinating diseases are optic neuropathy, transverse myelitis, acute disseminated encephalomyelitis, neuromyelitis optica (Devic's disease), and progressive multifocal leukoencephalopathy. MS is a disease of CNS myelin that is manifested by attacks separated in both time and space: lesions must occur in more than one location, and the lesions must have occurred at more than one time. The disease has an interesting epidemiology in that it most tends to affect populations that are farthest from the equator. Initially, this was thought to be due to a possible infectious etiology of the disease, but it appears more probably because of a genetic predisposition for what is probably an autoimmune demyelinating process. The pathology consists of perivenular inflammation, with demyelination limited completely to the CNS. The current view is that MS is probably an immune-mediated illness for which a genetic predisposition exists to some triggers in the environment, such as otherwise benign viral illness. The diagnosis is based on the clinical history of multiple lesions in space and time. No single diagnostic test for MS exists at this time. The spinal fluid is abnormal in 90% of patients, an elevated γ-globulin level is found in about 75% of cases, and more than five lymphocytes per cubic millimeter are found in about 50% of cases. MRI is the most useful and diagnostic study, but even it is not perfectly sensitive and specific for the diagnosis of MS. Patients with MS may have one attack and never have any trouble again, or they may have multiple attacks from which they relatively recover, or the disease may progress unremittingly. The treatment of relapsing-remitting MS has been studied in the greatest detail because this is the most common form of the disease. It is generally believed that intravenous methylprednisolone should be given for acute attacks at a dose of about 1 g per day for 5 days. Strong evidence now suggests that β-interferon reduces the attack rate in the relapsing-remitting form of the disease by about 20%. Three forms of β-interferon are presently available: β-interferon 1A (Avonex) is given intramuscularly once a week, β-interferon 1A (Rebif) is given subcutaneously three times per week, and β-interferon 1B (Betaseron) is given subcutaneously every other day. Another medication, glatiramer acetate (Copaxone), is a synthetic polypeptide that is administered daily subcutaneously; it is roughly as effective as the interferons.

Symptomatic therapy to control spasticity includes baclofen, both orally and intrathecally. Limb weights, thalamic surgery, and thalamic stimulation may be used to help control ataxia. Carbamazepine, amitriptyline, gabapentin, and narcotics are used to treat pain associated with MS. Oxybutynin is used for bladder spasticity, and cholinomimetics are used for hypotonicity of the bladder. The serotonin reuptake inhibitors and polycyclic drugs are used to treat the depression associated with the disease, and amantadine is used to treat fatigue. Treating underlying infections, such as urinary tract infections, is also extremely useful in reducing the severity and number of attacks. Several experimental treatments, including use of oral myelin, oral interferons, oral glatiramer, and other immune system modulators, are under investigation, but they are not clinically available for general use at this time. In severely resistant patients with progressive disease, more radical immune modulation includes the use of cyclophosphamide, azathioprine, and methotrexate.

Optic neuropathy is a demyelinating disease of the optic nerve and may or may not be part of the general syndrome of MS. Patients present with pain in the eye, loss of visual acuity with particularly severe loss of the ability to see red (*red desaturation*), and a reduction in the reaction of pupils to direct light, which is best compared with a reaction to consensual light (the *Marcus-Gunn deafferented pupil*).

In managing a patient who shows signs of this syndrome, the possibility of temporal arteritis, tumor in the optic nerve, toxic amblyopia from cyanide exposure or vitamin deficiency, and Leber hereditary optic neuropathy (a mitochondrial disease) should be excluded. A relationship exists between optic neuropathy and MS, but it is not a 1:1 relationship. About 20% of patients with optic neuropathy eventually develop MS, and this percentage is probably greater in women. About 40% of MS patients have had clinical optic neuritis, and more than 80% have had subclinical optic neuritis, as judged by visual evoked responses. The treatment is intravenous methylprednisolone; about one-third of the patients recover completely, about one-third recover partially, and one-third do not recover.

*Transverse myelitis* is another acute demyelinating illness that affects the spinal cord. It is treated with a short course of intravenous methylprednisolone. It has about the same relationship to MS as does optic neuritis.

*Acute disseminated encephalomyelitis* is an acute demyelinating disease that sometimes involves hemorrhage and necrosis (*Weston-Hurst disease*). This monophasic illness can be severe and even fatal following a viral illness or immunization. If the patient recovers, he may do well, and the illness may never recur.

*Neuromyelitis optica* (*Devic's disease*) is a demyelinating disease that affects the optic nerves and the spinal cord. It can be an extremely aggressive illness. It is treated with intravenous immunoglobulin and intravenous steroids. This form of MS is seen in certain parts of the world more commonly than others, in particular, parts of Africa.

*Progressive multifocal leukoencephalopathy* is caused by an infection of the oligodendrocyte with the papovavirus JC. The virus itself is probably ubiquitous and usually innocuous, but it becomes pathogenic in persons who are immunocompromised, such as those with lymphoma or leukemia, those who have undergone organ transplantation, patients with a history of chronic use of immunosuppression, or patients with HIV. The disease has no known effective treatment and is usually lethal in a matter of months.

*Peripheral nervous system demyelinating diseases* are divided into two categories according to their course. AIDP is a postinfectious inflammatory demyelinating disease that can be life threatening. Its course is shortened by the use of plasmapheresis or intravenous immunoglobulin. Many patients require some period of respiratory support, but 95% of patients will recover more than 95% of their original neurologic state. CIPD, formerly thought to be a chronic form of the AIDP syndrome, is probably a different immune-mediated disease. It is slowly progressive or episodic and never affects respiratory musculature. It is ordinarily treated with immunosuppression using steroids or the episodic use of intravenous immunoglobulin. It is sometimes secondary to an underlying malignancy or plasma cell dyscrasia. When it is not, it is a chronic illness that often requires treatment for many years.

## Sleep Disorders

Sleep is a natural, reversible, and universal phenomenon found throughout the animal kingdom. Human beings sleep at night and are awake during the day based on a circadian rhythm. The amount of sleep necessary for a typical adult varies from 5 to 10 hours per day and changes with advancing age. The exact function of sleep is unknown and has been debated for centuries by both philosophers and scientists. Sleep is thought to allow for body restoration and energy conservation, the consolidation of learning and memories, adaptation to a broader range of environments, thermoregulation, and brain development. Human sleep is divided into two main stages, non–rapid eye movement (NREM) and rapid eye movement (REM) sleep, based on the observation and electroencephalographic analysis of sleeping patients. Normal subjects pass through stages 1, 2, 3, and 4 of NREM sleep in about 80 to 90 minutes and 10 to 15 minutes of REM sleep. Depending on the total sleep time, about four to six cycles of alternating NREM–REM continue throughout the night, with a period of about 100 minutes in which the amount of stages 3 and 4 decreases and REM increases as the night progresses.

Complaints of excessive daytime sleepiness (EDS) are common in general medical practice and may indicate the presence of serious medical or sleep hygiene problems. Fatigue, EDS, and snoring are symptoms of *obstructive sleep apnea (OSA)*, which is characterized by frequent apneas and hypopneas. The consequent oxygen desaturation causes awakenings during sleep to maintain airway patency. Risk factors for OSA include obesity, craniofacial abnormalities, structural airway abnormalities, and neurologic diseases

that cause airway weakness. Bed partners frequently complain that OSA patients exhibit loud snoring, restless sleeping, and cessation of breathing for varying amounts of time. Patients with OSA have a significantly increased risk of essential hypertension, TIA, cerebral infarction, and cardiac dysfunction. The evaluation of patients with suspected OSA consists of a complete history and physical and a polysomnogram (PSG) that measures multiple physiologic parameters such as EEG, electromyography (EMG), EKG, eye movements, oxygen saturation, airflow, and respiratory effort. The PSG documents the frequency and severity of physiologic abnormalities in OSA patients as well as their response to treatment. The treatment of mild OSA for most patients consists of weight loss if obesity is a problem and positional therapy, where patients avoid sleeping in a position that worsens the sleep apnea. A dental consult for the custom construction of an oral appliance is an alternate form of therapy. For patients with more severe sleep apnea, continuous positive airway pressure (CPAP) to prevent airway collapse during sleep is indicated. Bilevel positive airway pressure (BiPAP) is a method of delivering positive pressure in which patients exhale against a lower pressure. All symptoms of OSA respond well to CPAP if patients comply with the treatment. If patients cannot tolerate CPAP or BiPAP, various surgical techniques are available.

EDS is caused by other sleep disorders including *jet lag syndrome, shift-work sleep disorder, narcolepsy*, and *periodic limb movement disorder (PLMD)*. Jet lag syndrome and shift-work sleep disorder can be managed with improvements in sleep hygiene. Narcolepsy is characterized by EDS and sleep attacks, which are brief episodes of sleep that occur anytime during the day. *Cataplexy*, which is present in about two-thirds of narcoleptics, is an episode of bilateral weakness associated with excitement or emotion without a change in the level of consciousness. Diagnosis is supported by a multiple sleep latency test, which demonstrates decreased time to sleep and early onset REM. The treatments of choice for narcolepsy are CNS stimulants such as modafinil (Provigil), methyphenidate (Ritalin), pemoline (Cylert), and dextroamphetamine (Dexedrine). Patients with PLMD present with EDS, frequent awakenings, difficulty falling asleep, and bed partners who complain about excessive partner movement during the night. A polysomnogram is indicated to confirm the presence and assess the severity of the movements and sleep disruption. The treatments of choice are dopaminergic parkinsonism medicines such as pramipexole (Mirapex), ropinirole (Requip), levodopa (Sinemet).

## REVIEW EXERCISES

### Case 1: Headaches

A 50-year-old woman complains of headaches. She has never had headaches before and has no history of neurologic or psychiatric disease. The headaches began about

6 weeks before and are not severe, but they seem to be getting worse and are beginning to worry her. They wax and wane throughout the day without any particular pattern. They respond well to aspirin but seem to return when the aspirin wears off. They do not wake her from sleep, nor do they cause nausea or vomiting. No neurologic prodrome is present, and she cannot think of anything that exacerbates the pain. It is difficult to localize the headache, and it is not pulsating in character. The pain sometimes improves when her husband massages her neck. No significant past medical, family, or social history is taken. She takes no drugs and does not drink alcohol or smoke. General physical examination is normal, as is the mental status and cranial nerve examination. Motor examination shows a slight but definite pronation of the left arm on extension of upper limbs. Careful sensory examination shows some extinction to double simultaneous stimulation on the left. Coordination is normal. Reflexes are symmetric and of average amplitude. Both plantars are flexor.

What is the diagnosis?

Are any diagnostic studies indicated?

### Discussion

This case raises many important issues encountered in the management of a patient complaining of headache. In this particular case, the history itself is worrisome and is enough to warrant further testing. Although the headaches are mild, they are different for this patient than her usual pattern. This is probably the most important part of the history in a headache patient. Headaches that have changed in quality are more worrisome than severe headaches that are the same as always. The fact that the headaches respond to mild analgesic medication or to massage should not be reassuring to the physician. Pains of all sort respond to analgesic medication, and this in and of itself does not mean that the cause of the headache is benign. Of the greatest importance is the abnormality in the neurologic examination. A slight but definite pronation of the left arm on extension of the upper limbs indicates a mild left hemiparesis. A positive neurologic examination in the presence of headache should always lead to further evaluation. Furthermore, this patient showed some extinction to double simultaneous stimulation on the left side. That is, when sensory stimuli were given to both sides of her body, she sometimes ignored the left side. This is a right parietal lobe sign and is further indication of something wrong over the right hemisphere. In such a circumstance, when the history is worrisome, and in particular when the examination is abnormal, it is absolutely required that a CT scan be done. In some centers, it may be possible to do an MRI, but CT scanning is a more widespread and available technology. For this patient, there is really no reason to obtain skull radiographs or any other noninvasive evaluation other than a CT scan. The CT scan may be done without contrast, at which time a lesion may be found. If nothing is found, a decision about injecting contrast can be made later. It should be recalled that the only real risk of a CT scan in a conscious, alert patient is the injection of the iodinated contrast medium. In summary, this patient's history and examination are worrisome and point to a process in the right hemisphere that should lead the physician to carry out a CT scan. In this case, the CT scan showed a right-hemisphere cerebral convexity meningioma.

## Case 2: Movement Disorder

A 68-year-old man is complaining that his handwriting is deteriorating and that his hands shake when he tries to drink from a glass or coffee cup. He has no significant past medical history and no family history of neurologic or psychiatric disease. He does not drink alcohol or smoke. His only medication is Sinemet 10/100 four times a day given to him by a physician whom he saw once while on vacation in Florida 2 years before. A physician friend of the patient has been rewriting the prescription since then. His general examination is normal. On motor examination, he is noted to have a rather expressionless face and sits rigidly in his chair with arms flexed, bent slightly forward. Tone is diffusely increased with "cogwheeling." Power is normal. There is a 2- to 3-second alternating tremor noted in both hands while he is seated. When asked to extend his hands, this tremor becomes finer but more rapid. On finger-nose-finger testing, the tremor intensifies, but no dysmetria is noted. When he attempts to write, the tremor becomes severe, leading to illegible script. Sensory examination is intact. Reflexes are average and symmetric. Both plantars are extensor. His gait is shuffling but with a narrow base. He has difficulty getting started, but, once he is going, he walks quite well although slightly bent forward.

What is the diagnosis?

What therapy would you recommend?

### Discussion

This case demonstrates some of the salient features in the diagnosis and management of various movement disorders. This 68-year-old man has two separate, unrelated problems. The first is a tendency not to move, known as *akinesia* or *bradykinesia*. This gives him the expressionless face and accounts for his sitting rigidly in a chair with his arms flexed and bent slightly forward. This akinesia is sometimes referred to as *parkinsonism*. In addition to the akinesia, he shows the classic tremor of parkinsonism, which is characterized as a slow alternating tremor with a frequency of about three cycles per second. This tremor is most prominent in the position of repose and improves when the limb moves into action. It is therefore clear, based on his akinesia and tremor in repose, that he does in fact have parkinsonism. When a tremor is superimposed on rigidity, the phenomenon of cogwheeling develops.

Cogwheeling is not essential to parkinsonism but may be present, as in this patient. Parkinsonism has multiple etiologies. The common causes include idiopathic Parkinson's disease, postencephalitic parkinsonism, and drug-induced parkinsonism. Rare causes include toxic parkinsonism and parkinsonism in the context of other neurodegenerative diseases, such as progressive supranuclear palsy, olivopontocerebellar atrophy, and Shy-Drager syndrome. In this case, it is most likely that this man suffers from idiopathic Parkinson's disease. There is no history of any exposure to neuroleptic drugs, which induce parkinsonism, and there is no history of an episode of childhood encephalitis. No evidence is seen of any other neurodegenerative disease. The patient's second problem is that of a tremor. *Tremor* is defined as an alternating movement around some fulcrum. Tremors may be proximal or distal, rapid or slow, synchronous or alternating. They may be greatest in the position of repose or on action. A simple classification of tremor that works clinically is based on dividing all tremors into two major categories. The first is tremors that are prominent in the position of repose, and the second is tremors that are prominent on action. Tremors that are prominent in repose are themselves subdivided into two categories. The first type is characterized by tremor in repose that improves on action. This patient, in fact, had that form of tremor, known as *parkinsonian tremor*, which is present in most forms of parkinsonism. The second subtype of tremor changes on action into a cerebellar tremor. This type of tremor is known as a *rubral* or *cerebellar outflow tremor*. It is commonly seen in demyelinating diseases such as MS or in head trauma patients. The second large category of tremor is the *action tremors*, which are subdivided into two types. The first type is the *goal-directed action tremor*, which is present only when the patient attempts to make a projected precise movement. When attempting to carry out such a movement, a side-to-side, alternating low-frequency tremor at about three cycles per second develops. This tremor is known in some circles as *cerebellar tremor*, and it is due to disease in the cerebellum or its connections. The second subcategory of action tremors is the category characterized by tremor that occurs when the affected limb attains an antigravity posture, such as raising the hand. This tremor is not prominent in repose, and it does not require a goal-directed movement; rather, it requires simply an antigravity movement of any sort. These are known as the *postural action tremors*, of which there are two major types. *Physiologic tremor* is a rapid (approximately nine cycles per second), synchronous action tremor that occurs on attaining an antigravity posture. It is often most prominent in the extremities distally and interferes with carrying out fine motor activity, such as writing. It also can be seen, however, in axial structures, such as the head, and is known by some as *titubation*. The physiologic tremor is a normal phenomenon and is present to some extent in everyone. It is caused by the peripheral action of catecholemines or their agonists on receptors in muscle. It is usually not symptomatic, but it may become symptomatic when it is exaggerated, in which case it is called *exaggerated physiologic tremor*. Such patients may complain of the tremor, and it may interfere with their carrying out fine motor activities. Physiologic tremor is ordinarily exaggerated by situations that increase the sensitivity of peripheral catecholemine receptors or increase the amount of circulating catecholemines. Such circumstances include anxiety, hyperthyroidism, or the use of drugs that functionally raise the circulating catecholemine levels, such as antiasthma medications, lithium carbonate, theophylline, and caffeine. This tremor is treated best by reducing the exacerbating factors or, if necessary, with a small dose of β-blocker. Alcohol is also effective against this tremor, but it is not recommended as a therapy. The second form of postural tremor is known as *essential tremor*. It is also rapid and synchronous, usually slightly slower than the physiologic tremor, averaging about seven cycles per second. It is also present in the extremities most commonly, but it can be seen in the head and other axial structures. This tremor may occur in families, in which case it is called *familial essential tremor*; it may develop only in older people, in which case it is called *senile essential tremor*. Sound evidence suggests that this tremor is at least partially centrally mediated; it does not respond as well or as quickly to the oral administration of β-blockers. It also responds well and rapidly to alcohol, but alcohol is not a recommended therapy.

The treatment of essential tremors, including familial and senile tremor, consists of either β-blockade or use of the antiepileptic drug primidone (Mysoline). The mechanism of action of these drugs on essential tremor remains obscure. This patient has two related problems. The first problem is parkinsonism, probably due to idiopathic Parkinson's disease, including akinesia and rigidity and tremor. The tremor of his Parkinson's disease is probably not bothering him because it is present only in repose and improves on action. His major complaint concerned deterioration of handwriting. In fact, he is complaining about a second tremor, some form of postural tremor, which could be either an essential tremor or an exaggerated physiologic tremor. Evidence suggests that the incidence of essential tremor is higher in patients with parkinsonism than in age-matched controls; that is, it may be true that action tremor is part of Parkinson's disease. It is also possible that this man has an exaggerated physiologic tremor, possibly caused by the peripheral metabolism of Sinemet to norephinephrine, which then acts on receptors in the muscle. A tremor study done in an experienced neurophysiology laboratory might be helpful in distinguishing these two types of tremor, but a therapeutic trial of reduction in Sinemet may work just as well. In this case, discontinuation of Sinemet resulted in reduction in the action tremor, leading to the conclusion that the action component of this patient's tremor is an enhanced physiologic tremor resulting from the catecholamine metabolites of Sinemet.

## Case 3: TIA and Stroke

A 65-year-old man arrived at the hospital after awakening with right-sided weakness. His family says that for about a year he has complained of brief episodes of blurred vision in his left eye. On the evening before admission he had a short period of word-finding difficulty, which cleared after about 5 minutes, and he seemed to be normal when he retired for the night. On examination, his blood pressure is 160/100. The neurologic examination shows a mild degree of naming difficulty and mild pronation of the right arm on extension of the limb. Circumduction of the right leg occurs when walking, and mild deficits to all sensory modalities can be discerned on the right side. Reflexes are 2+ on the left and 1+ on the right, and a right-sided Babinski's sign is present. Carotid pulses are faint but palpable bilaterally without bruits. Flow in the external carotid branches on the face cannot be estimated clinically. You decide to admit this patient to the hospital. While having his chest radiograph, he has a 5-minute episode of dense right hemiplegia and mutism, from which he recovers and returns to his baseline state as described.

What is the likely diagnosis?
What therapy is indicated?

### Discussion

This case raises some important issues in the management of a patient with a TIA and involves some of the most controversial issues in the field of neurology. A great deal of disagreement arises about the best management of patients of this kind. One issue is unequivocal. This patient is complaining of episodes of TIAs. A TIA is defined as the sudden onset of a neurologic deficit that fits a vascular territory and lasts less than 24 hours. This

patient's spell fits a disorder in the distribution of a left middle cerebral artery. The initial thought that this represented a carpal tunnel syndrome is incorrect because the patient has numbness in the right corner of the mouth as well as the right hand. Although the spells seem mild and completely disappear between attacks, one should not feel comfortable that this does not foreshadow a serious subsequent stroke. There is no way to predict, based on the severity of the attack or its quality, whether a patient will go on to develop a stroke and whether this stroke will be severe or mild. It is unequivocal that this patient is suffering from TIAs in the territory of the left carotid. The physical examination yields little information about the severity of carotid disease. In particular, the presence or absence of a cervical bruit is nearly useless, although bruits often represent vascular disease; but the bruit may be on the wrong side (as in this patient) or not present at all if flow through a tight stenosis is slowed sufficiently. Dynamic palpations of facial pulses is a way of evaluating the direction of flow in the external carotid branches in the face. With a tight stenosis or occlusion of the internal carotid distal to the takeoff of the external carotid, it is often possible to demonstrate reversed flow in the branches of the external carotid artery of the face. In this patient, this test was positive, indicating a tight stenosis or an occlusion of the left internal carotid. This test, however, does not distinguish between a tight stenosis and an occlusion, an important distinction because surgical intervention is possible only in a case of tight stenosis, not in a case of total occlusion. Once it is recognized that this patient is undergoing TIAs in the distribution of the left carotid, the most difficult decision will involve which maneuver should be carried out next. Some experienced physicians would not investigate such a patient any further but would simply give the patient aspirin. Most experienced neurologists and neurosurgeons probably would carry out some form of neurodiagnostic study to evaluate the carotid. Some would obtain a battery of noninvasive tests. The difficulty with these studies is that significant numbers of false-positives and false-negatives occur. If a test is positive, it will probably be necessary to carry out a more invasive study to give the vascular surgeon or neurosurgeon enough data with which to consider operating. If the noninvasive studies are negative, but the history still strongly suggests TIAs, it will probably still be necessary to go on with a more invasive study. It is rare that noninvasive studies yield enough information to preclude the use of a more "dangerous" study. The most difficult question is to determine which of the invasive studies to order in such a patient. The simplest test, which gives the most information, is a magnetic resonance angiogram (MRA). This obtains a reasonably good angiogram at the lowest risk.

The advantage of such a study is that no contrast infusion is used. Some experienced physicians would order a CT angiogram (CTA), which often can be done in an emergency department with only CT technology available, but this test requires the use of intravenous contrast material. The gold standard for cerebral vascular disease remains the arteriogram done using a femoral catheterization with individual catheterizations of the major cerebral vessels. In good hands, such a study has an approximately 1% morbidity rate. Most of the neurologic complications are reversible. Nonetheless, it requires an injection of contrast through an arterial catheterization, including individual catheterizations of cerebral vessels. This is risky but often necessary to make a final decision about whether carotid endarterectomy is feasible. In summary, this patient has a definite left carotid distribution TIA history. This patient probably should undergo either a MRA, CTA, or an ordinary carotid arteriogram. If a tight carotid stenosis is found, most experienced neurologists would recommend a carotid endarterectomy done by an experienced neurosurgeon or vascular surgeon. If the carotid is occluded, most physicians would recommend the use of aspirin in an attempt to prevent further TIAs, which may be due to platelet emboli from the distal stump of the occlusion. If no carotid disease is found, a careful evaluation of the heart would follow, including transesophageal echocardiography, a set of blood cultures, and a careful cardiac examination, probably including a Holter monitor study. It is possible that these TIAs actually represent cardiac-source emboli. In this case, this is unlikely because the TIAs always seem to involve the left hemisphere. If no carotid disease is found, one must consider this possibility. If a cardiac source, such as intermittent atrial fibrillation, is found, warfarin therapy probably would be the treatment of choice.

## SUGGESTED READINGS

Adams RD, Victor M, Ropper AH. *Principles of Neurology.* New York: McGraw-Hill, 1997.

Aldrich MS. *Sleep Medicine.* New York: Oxford Press, 1999.

Samuels MA. *Manual of Neurologic Therapeutics,* 7th ed. Philadelphia: Lippincott Williams & Wilkins, 2004.

Samuels MA, Feske S. *Office Practice of Neurology,* 2nd ed. Philadelphia: WB Saunders, 2004.

Samuels MA. *Video Textbook of Neurology for the Practicing Physician.* Boston: Butterworth-Heinemann, 1997.

Samuels MA. *Hospitalist Neurology.* Boston: Butterworth-Heinemann, 1999.

Samuels MA. Neurologic disorders. In: Stein JH, ed. *Internal Medicine,* 5th ed. St. Louis: Mosby, 1998.

Samuels MA. *Journal Watch Neurology.* Boston: Massachusetts Medical Society, 1999.

The National Institute of Neurological Disorders and Stroke rt-PA Stroke Study Group.

Tissue plasminogen activator for acute ischemic stroke. *N Engl J Med* 1995;333;1581–1587.

# Infectious Disease

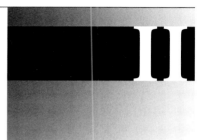

# Sexually Transmitted Diseases

### 13

## Carlos M. Isada  David L. Longworth

Sexually transmitted diseases (STDs) remain among the most common problems encountered in the practice of general internal medicine. Despite their ubiquity, STDs remain a diagnostic and therapeutic challenge. This chapter focuses on the clinical manifestations, diagnosis, and treatment of the classic STDs, with emphasis on common clinical syndromes and their differential diagnoses. The topics of vaginitis and genital warts also are discussed. Treatment recommendations are based on the 2002 guidelines from the Centers for Disease Control and Prevention (CDC).

## URETHRITIS AND CERVICITIS

### Urethritis

In sexually active men, urethritis is characterized by dysuria and discharge of purulent material from the urethra. It is traditionally divided into two types: gonococcal and nongonococcal. Diagnostic testing to identify the offending pathogen is presently recommended because (i) both infections are reportable to state health departments, (ii) treatment compliance may be better with a specific diagnosis, and (iii) partner notification and treatment may be improved. The CDC recommends that if the diagnostic means are not available, patients should be treated for both gonococcal and chlamydial infections, although establishing a specific microbiologic diagnosis is preferred.

### Nongonococcal Urethritis

#### Etiology and Clinical Manifestations

*Chlamydia trachomatis* is the most common cause of nongonococcal urethritis (NGU), accounting for approximately 50% of cases, although the frequency is variable depending on the case series. In males who have NGU but test negative for *C. trachomatis*, establishing an etiology is often difficult. *Ureaplasma urealyticum*, *Trichomonas vaginalis*, and herpes simplex virus (HSV) account for approximately 15% of cases. No etiologic diagnosis is found in up to 35% of cases.

NGU tends to have a more indolent presentation compared with gonococcal urethritis. The incubation period of NGU is 1 to 3 weeks. A mucoid or watery discharge from the urethra is the typical clinical presentation, although up

to 25% of infected men may be asymptomatic. Fevers and chills are unusual, and symptoms of urinary tract infection are usually absent; patients may have some dysuria or itching, but hematuria, urinary frequency, or pelvic pain are unusual.

Complications arising from NGU include epididymitis and Reiter's syndrome. Partner notification is important because female sexual partners are at high risk for chlamydial infection and its complications.

#### Laboratory Diagnosis

It is important to objectively confirm the presence of urethritis in all suspected cases, particularly since some patients may present with vague or nonspecific genital symptoms. Urethritis can be diagnosed on clinical grounds alone when a purulent urethral discharge is found on physical examination, either on initial inspection or by milking the penis from the base to the glans. In less clear cases, however, urethritis also can be diagnosed by either of the following:

- Presence of five or more polymorphonuclear leukocytes per oil immersion field on a smear of a urethral swab specimen, or
- A positive leukocyte esterase test from a first-void urine specimen or first-void urine with greater than or equal to 10 white blood cells (WBCs) per high power field.

Although the leukocyte esterase test is convenient, a positive test result should be confirmed with a Gram-stained smear of a urethral swab specimen.

NGU is confirmed when a male meets one or more of the above criteria and shows no evidence of Gram-negative intracellular diplococci on Gram's stain. Urethra specimens should be submitted routinely for detection of *N. gonorrhoeae* and *C. trachomatis*. A number of different nucleic acid amplification systems are available that are more sensitive than traditional culture techniques, particularly for *C. trachomatis*. Persons who present with nonspecific genitourethral symptoms and who fail to meet objective criteria for urethritis should still be tested for *C. trachomatis* and *N. gonorrhoeae* because if infection is minimally symptomatic, antibiotic treatment is generally deferred. In some instances, the empiric treatment of urethral symptoms in the absence of documented urethritis may be considered if the patient is unlikely to return for follow-up if contacted.

### Therapy

Regimens presently recommended by the CDC for the treatment of NGU include:

- Doxycycline, 100 mg orally twice daily for 7 days, or
- Azithromycin, 1 g orally (single dose)

  Alternative regimens include:

- Erythromycin base, 500 mg orally four times daily for 7 days, or
- Erythromycin ethylsuccinate, 800 mg orally four times daily for 7 days, or
- Ofloxacin (Floxin), 300 mg orally twice daily for 7 days, or
- Levofloxacin, 500 mg orally once daily for 7 days

## Mucopurulent Cervicitis

### Etiology and Clinical Manifestations

The major infectious causes of mucopurulent cervicitis (MPC) include *C. trachomatis, N. gonorrhoeae,* and HSV. In many women, however, no organism is isolated. The CDC recommends that patients with MPC have cervical specimens tested for *C. trachomatis* and *N. gonorrhoeae.*

In sexually active women, MPC is the counterpart to urethritis in men. It is characterized by a yellow endocervical exudate that can be seen in the endocervical canal or on a swab of cervical secretions. In many women, the infection is minimally symptomatic or completely asymptomatic; others may have abnormal vaginal bleeding after intercourse. Serious complications of MPC include pelvic inflammatory disease (PID), tubal infertility, ectopic pregnancy, and chronic pelvic pain.

### Laboratory Diagnosis

The diagnosis of MPC is supported by the visualization of yellow or green endocervical mucopus on a white swab (positive swab test result). The utility of the Gram's stain of an endocervical swab specimen for confirming MPC is somewhat controversial. The presence of ten or more polymorphonuclear leukocytes per high-powered field of a Gram-stained specimen of endocervical mucopus correlates with the presence of recognized infectious causes of MPC. This test has a number of limitations, however, including a poor positive predictive value; it is not as clinically useful as the Gram's stain of urethral exudates in males with urethritis. It is important to emphasize that most women with *C. trachomatis* or *N. gonorrhoeae* infection *do not* have active MPC.

### Therapy

The therapy of MPC should be guided by the results of specific testing for *C. trachomatis* or *N. gonorrhoeae.* In

patients unlikely to return for follow-up, treatment for both pathogens should be initiated. Treatment should cover both organisms if the likelihood of infection with either organism is high in a particular population. Current population-specific treatment recommendations from the CDC include the following:

- If there is a high prevalence of both *C. trachomatis* and *N. gonorrhoeae* (as in many STD clinics), treat for both agents.
- If the incidence of *N. gonorrhoeae* is low in the population and the likelihood of *C. trachomatis* is high, treat for chlamydial infection only.
- If both infections are uncommon, and if the likelihood of compliance for a return visit is good, await test results to guide specific therapy.

## Chlamydia trachomatis Infection

### Epidemiology and Clinical Manifestations

*C. trachomatis* is the most common bacterial sexually transmitted disease in the United States. Approximately 2.8 million Americans are infected with this organism each year. The majority of these infections are asymptomatic, with asymptomatic infection in three-fourths of women with documented infection and about one-half of males. Teenage girls and young women are particularly predisposed to infection because the cervix has not fully matured. In women, the organism first infects the cervix and/or urethra. *C. trachomatis* may produce a variety of clinical syndromes, including urethritis, cervicitis, and proctocolitis in men who have sex with men (MSM). Approximately 40% of untreated infections in women progress from the cervix to involve the fallopian tubes or the uterus. *C. trachomatis* is a major contributing pathogen in women with PID, particularly in those with multiple reinfections. A number of women with PID suffer long-term complications, such as chronic pelvic pain, ectopic pregnancy, and infertility (about one-fifth). In addition, women with chlamydial infection are five times more likely to develop HIV if they become exposed. For these reasons, the CDC has expanded its recommendations for chlamydia screening among women. The CDC recommends routine annual screening for *C. trachomatis* in all sexually active adolescents (19 years old and under) and sexually active women 20 to 25 years of age, including those who are asymptomatic. Annual screening also is recommended for older women with risk factors for infection, such as a new sexual partner or multiple partners. Because many of these infections are asymptomatic, the CDC recommends aggressive treatment for patients with *C. trachomatis* infection, as well as for their partners, even if asymptomatic, particularly those who have new or multiple sexual partners or who do not consistently use barrier contraceptives. Some women with apparently uncomplicated cervical *C. trachomatis* infections are likely to have subclinical upper reproductive tract involvement and are thus at high risk for PID, ectopic pregnancy, and infertility. The treatment of such cervical infections likely reduces these sequelae.

### Therapy

Current recommendations from the CDC for the treatment of uncomplicated chlamydial infection include the following regimens:

- Doxycycline, 100 mg orally twice daily for 7 days, or
- Azithromycin, 1 g orally (one dose)

The efficacy of doxycycline and azithromycin is comparable, provided the patient is adherent to the 7-day regimen of doxycycline. Azithromycin has the advantage of single-dose administration, which is particularly attractive in noncompliant patients. Doxycycline has a longer history of safety, efficacy, and use, however, and is much less expensive. Azithromycin should not be used in persons under the age of 15 years because its safety and efficacy in this group has not yet been established.

Alternative regimens for the treatment of chlamydial infection include:

- Ofloxacin, 300 mg orally twice daily for 7 days, or
- Erythromycin base, 500 mg orally four times daily for 7 days, or
- Erythromycin ethylsuccinate, 800 mg orally four times daily for 7 days, or
- Levofloxacin, 500 mg orally for 7 days.

Ofloxacin has proven efficacy against *C. trachomatis*, but clinical trials have shown no advantage in efficacy compared with doxycycline. Ofloxacin is expensive and also has no dosing advantages over doxycycline. Levofloxacin is a new recommendation by the CDC in 2002. No clinical trial data examine the efficacy of levofloxacin for treatment of *C. trachomatis*, but the in vitro activity of levofloxacin is similar to ofloxacin, and levofloxacin has the advantage of once-daily dosing. Other fluoroquinolones are not as yet recommended.

A routine test of cure for chlamydia soon after treatment with doxycycline or azithromycin (less than 3 weeks) is not recommended; the value of early retesting has not been proven and some of the nucleic acid–based tests for *C. trachomatis* may remain positive at 3 weeks despite microbiologic eradication by traditional culture methods. In contrast, it is now recommended by the CDC that women with documented chlamydial infections undergo routine rescreening 3 to 4 months after the completion of treatment. This guideline was issued due to the high prevalence of chlamydia found in women who had been diagnosed and treated in the preceding months, presumably from reinfection rather than failure of the initial antibiotic course.

The sexual partners of patients with chlamydial infection should be referred for evaluation and treatment. All partners of symptomatic patients with chlamydial infection should be treated if the last sexual contact with the index patient occurred within 30 days from the onset of the index patient's symptoms. If the index patient is asymptomatic, all sexual partners whose last sexual contact with the index patient occurred within 60 days of diagnosis should be evaluated and treated. In partners of index patients who fulfill neither of these criteria, the most recent sexual partner of the index patient should be treated even if the last sexual contact occurred beyond these time intervals.

For pregnant women with chlamydial infection, the CDC recommends the following regimen:

- Erythromycin base, 500 mg orally four times daily for 7 days, or
- Amoxicillin, 500 mg orally three times daily for 7 days

An alternative regimen includes:

- Erythromycin base, 250 mg orally four times a day for 14 days, or
- Erythromycin ethylsuccinate, 800 mg orally four times a day for 7 days, or
- Erythromycin ethylsuccinate, 400 mg orally four times a day for 14 days, or
- Azithromycin, 1 gram orally as a single dose.

Retesting at 3 weeks after completion of the treatment regimen is recommended in pregnancy. Doxycycline, ofloxacin, and erythromycin estolate are contraindicated during pregnancy.

## GONOCOCCAL INFECTION

### Gonorrhea

Gonorrhea remains endemic in the United States, despite public health measures to track and eradicate the infection. It is estimated that more than 700,000 new cases occur annually in this country. In men, gonococcal infection is usually sufficiently symptomatic for patients to seek medical care. In women, gonococcal infections are often asymptomatic, and a significant proportion of symptoms are nonspecific and may be confused with common vaginal or bladder infections. Women are at risk for complications such as PID, infertility, and ectopic pregnancy. Because of this, the CDC recommends screening high-risk women for gonorrhea, even if asymptomatic.

### Therapy

Several factors influence the therapy of patients with suspected or confirmed gonococcal infection. Over the past 20 years, resistant strains of *N. gonorrhoeae* have become increasingly common. These include penicillinase-producing and tetracycline-resistant organisms, as well as strains with chromosomally mediated resistance to multiple antimicrobial agents. In recent years, an increasing spread of quinolone resistant *N. gonorrhoeae* has occurred, to an extent that alters empiric quinolone use in some areas of the country. In addition, patients with gonococcal infection are frequently coinfected with *C. trachomatis*, thus making empiric therapy for this infection mandatory for most individuals. This strategy of dual therapy is usually accompanied by specific laboratory testing for *C. trachomatis*, but in some situations, testing for chlamydia in persons with gonococcal infection may be deferred because of financial constraints; if 10% to 30% of gonococcal infections in a given area are coinfected with *C. trachomatis*, dual therapy without specific testing for *C. trachomatis* might be cost-effective. In most circumstances, however, it is recommended that persons with gonococcal infection be treated and tested for chlamydia.

The current CDC treatment recommendations for uncomplicated urethral, endocervical, and rectal gonorrhea are as follows:

- Ceftriaxone, 125 mg intramuscularly (single dose, 99.1% cure), or
- Cefixime (Suprax), 400 mg orally (single dose, 97.1% cure), or
- Ciprofloxacin, 500 mg orally (single dose), or
- Ofloxacin, 400 mg orally (single dose), or
- Levofloxacin, 250 mg orally in a single dose.

Each of these regimens should be given with an agent active against *C. trachomatis*, such as doxycycline, 100 mg orally twice daily for 7 days, or azithromycin, 1 g orally as a single dose. The 2002 CDC guidelines included cefixime as a recommended regimen, but this agent is no longer available in most areas.

In recent years, the CDC has reported a significant increase in quinolone-resistant *N. gonorrhoeae* (QRNG). In 2002, the CDC recommended that fluoroquinolones should be avoided in patients whose gonorrhea was acquired in Asia, Hawaii, other Pacific islands, California, and some other areas of the world such as England and Wales. In 2004, the CDC noted that local and national data showed a 5% prevalence of QRNG in MSM. This led to the 2004 recommendation that fluoroquinolones not be used to treat known or suspected gonorrhea in MSM, unless susceptibility testing or tests of cure are available. This is a somewhat complicated situation because many STD clinics use nucleic acid–based testing for *N. gonorrhoeae*, and susceptibility testing requires culture media and additional laboratory expense. Empiric therapy for gonorrhea in geographic areas with high rates of QRNG or MSM patients is with ceftriaxone, cefixime (currently not available in the United States), or spectinomycin.

Alternative regimens for uncomplicated gonococcal infection include:

- Spectinomycin (Trobicin), 2 g intramuscularly (single dose), or
- An injectable cephalosporin: ceftizoxime (Cefizox), cefotaxime (Claforan), cefotetan (Cefotan), or cefoxitin (Mefoxin), or
- Cefuroxime (Ceftin), 1 g orally (single dose), or

- Other quinolones: gatifloxacin, 400 mg orally (single dose), lomefloxacin (Maxaquin), 400 mg by mouth (single dose), or norfloxacin (Noroxin), 800 mg orally (single dose).

Each of these regimens should be given with an agent active against *C. trachomatis*, such as doxycycline, 100 mg orally twice daily for 7 days, or azithromycin, 1 g orally as a single dose.

### Management of Sexual Partners

All sexual partners of symptomatic individuals with gonococcal infection should be evaluated and treated for both gonorrhea and chlamydial infection if their last sexual contact with the index patient was within 30 days of the onset of the patient's symptoms. If the index patient has no symptoms, sexual partners whose last sexual contact with the index patient was less than 60 days from the diagnosis should be evaluated and treated. In circumstances in which no partners fulfill these criteria, the most recent sexual partner should be treated, even if the last sexual contact took place beyond these time periods.

## Disseminated Gonococcal Infection

### Etiology and Clinical Manifestations

In the past, disseminated gonococcal infection (DGI) was invariably produced by penicillin-susceptible strains of *N. gonorrhoeae*. In more recent years, however, documented cases of DGI due to penicillinase-producing strains have been described. In this unique clinical syndrome, patients may exhibit a number of clinical manifestations, as summarized in Table 13.1.

The differential diagnosis of patients with suspected DGI includes infections such as meningococcemia, endocarditis, septic arthritis, infectious tenosynovitis, and other bacteremias; seronegative arthritides such as Reiter's syndrome, ankylosing spondylitis, psoriatic arthritis, and dermal vasculitis; and collagen vascular diseases such as systemic lupus erythematosus (SLE).

**TABLE 13.1**

**CLINICAL MANIFESTATIONS OF DISSEMINATED GONOCOCCAL INFECTION**

| Common | Unusual | Rare |
|---|---|---|
| Fever | Endocarditis | Pneumonia |
| Leukocytosis | Meningitis | Adult respiratory distress syndrome |
| Skin lesions | Perihepatitis | |
| Tenosynovitis | | Osteomyelitis |
| Polyarthralgia | | |
| Oligoarthritis | | |
| Hepatitis | | |
| Myopericarditis | | |

## TABLE 13.2
### DISSEMINATED GONOCOCCAL INFECTION: DIAGNOSIS

**Patients with Positive Test Results (%)**

| Site | Culture | Gram's Stain | Immunofluo-rescence |
|------|---------|--------------|---------------------|
| Skin lesions | 10 | 10 | 60 |
| Joint fluid | 20–30 | 10–30 | 25 |
| Blood | 10–30 | — | — |
| Mucosal (pharynx, urethra, cervix, rectum) | 80–90 | — | — |

### Diagnosis

The diagnosis of DGI should be suspected in individuals with the classic hemorrhagic pustules and symptoms of tenosynovitis or oligoarthritis. Skin lesions may be relatively asymptomatic and should be carefully sought. Usually, fewer than ten lesions are evident. In those with suspected DGI, cultures for *N. gonorrhoeae* should be obtained from skin lesions, joint fluid, blood, and mucosal surfaces such as the urethra, cervix, rectum, and pharynx. The diagnostic sensitivity of culture, Gram's stain, and immunofluorescent testing are summarized in Table 13.2.

### Therapy

The treatment for DGI should be initiated in the hospital with the administration of ceftriaxone 1 g intramuscularly or intravenously every 24 hours, based on CDC recommendations in 2002. Alternative regimens include cefotaxime, 1 g intravenously every 8 hours, or ceftizoxime, 1 g intravenously every 8 hours. For patients allergic to β-lactam agents, acceptable alternative regimens include ciprofloxacin, 400 mg intravenously every 12 hours, ofloxacin, 400 mg intravenously every 12 hours, levofloxacin, 250 mg intravenously daily, or spectinomycin. Twenty-four to 48 hours after improvement, the patient can be switched to an oral regimen such as cefixime, 400 mg twice a day, ciprofloxacin, 500 mg twice a day, ofloxacin, 400 mg twice a day, or levofloxacin 500 mg daily to complete a 7-day course of therapy.

## GENITAL ULCERATION WITH REGIONAL LYMPHADENOPATHY

The syndrome of genital ulceration with regional lymphadenopathy is characteristic of five of the six classic STDs: primary syphilis, primary genital HSV infection, chancroid, lymphogranuloma venereum (LGV), and granuloma inguinale (donovanosis) (Table 13.3). Of note, gonorrhea is not a cause of this syndrome. Genital ulcers are frequently misdiagnosed as to cause when the history and physical examination are used alone; thus, laboratory

## TABLE 13.3
### GENITAL ULCERATION WITH REGIONAL LYMPHADENOPATHY: SUMMARY OF CLINICAL MANIFESTATIONS

| Genital Lesions | Incubation (d) | Type | Pain | Number | Duration |
|-----------------|----------------|------|------|--------|----------|
| Primary syphilis | 3–90 | Clean ulcer, raised | No | Usually single | 3–6 wk |
| Primary herpes simplex virus | 1–26 | Grouped papules, vesicles, pustules, ulcers | Yes | Often multiple | 1–3 wk |
| Chancroid | 1–21 | Purulent ulcer, shaggy border | Yes | Single in men, multiple in women | Progressive |
| Lymphogranuloma venereum | 3–21 | Papule, vesicle, ulcer | No | Usually single | Few days |
| Granuloma inguinale | 8–80 | Nodules, coalescing granulomatous ulcers | No | Single or multiple | Progressive |

| Inguinal Adenopathy | Onset | Pain | Type | Frequency | Constitutional Symptoms |
|---------------------|-------|------|------|-----------|-------------------------|
| Primary syphilis | Same time | No | Firm | 80%, 70% bilateral | Absent |
| Primary herpes simplex virus | Same time | Yes | Firm | 80%, usually bilateral | Common |
| Chancroid | Same time | Yes | Fluctuant, may fistulize | 50–65%, usually unilateral | Uncommon |
| Lymphogranuloma venereum | 26 wk later | Yes | Indurated, fluctuant, may fistulize | Unilateral, one-third bilateral | Common |
| Granuloma inguinale | Variable | | Suppurating pseudobubo | 10% | 15% |

**TABLE 13.4**

**GENITAL ULCERS: RECOMMENDED
DIAGNOSTIC EVALUATION**

Serologic test for syphilis
Dark-field examination or direct immunofluorescence test for
  *Treponema pallidum*
Culture or antigen test for herpes simplex virus
**In selected cases**
Culture for *Haemophilus ducreyi*
Lymphogranuloma venereum titers
Biopsy for Donovan's bodies

---

tests are important to confirm the clinical suspicion. An increased risk of human immunodeficiency virus (HIV) infection is associated with each of these infections. HIV testing should be performed in the management of patients who have genital ulcers caused by *Treponema pallidum* or *Haemophilus ducreyi*, and it should be considered in those who have ulcers caused by HSV.

Genital HSV infection is the most common cause of the syndrome of genital ulceration with regional lymphadenopathy in the United States. Based on serologic studies, it is estimated that approximately 50 million individuals in the United States are infected with HSV-2. The second most common cause of this syndrome in the United States is primary syphilis. Other infectious causes (the so-called minor venereal diseases), although common in other parts of the world, are relatively uncommon in the United States, although outbreaks have been reported. The diagnostic evaluation of patients with genital ulceration and regional lymphadenopathy is summarized in Table 13.4.

## Primary Herpes Simplex Virus Infection

### Etiology and Clinical Manifestations

Genital herpes may be produced by either HSV type 1 or type 2. In the United States, herpes simplex type 2 accounts for the majority of cases of genital HSV, although in some groups (particularly teenage populations), almost 30% of cases may be from HSV type 1. In other parts of the world, such as Japan, herpes simplex type 1 produces the majority of cases. The presence of HSV-2 antibody indicates prior anogenital infection (symptomatic or not) because HSV-2 is a very rare cause of oral herpes infections. In contrast, the presence of HSV-1 antibodies is very common in the general population due to prior oral herpes infections, thus, it is not useful in distinguishing orolabial from anogenital herpes.

The incubation period after exposure for primary genital HSV infection is 1 to 26 days, with an average of 1 week. Before lesions appear, patients may complain of burning or pruritus. The initial lesions are grouped papules, which are often painful. They progress to vesicles and pustules

and then form small, clean-based ulcerations. Inguinal lymphadenopathy, usually bilateral, is apparent at the same time as the genital lesions in approximately 80% of patients. The nodes are firm and painful.

Primary genital HSV infection may be a systemic illness, and constitutional symptoms are common. Patients frequently complain of low-grade fever, malaise, headache, and fatigue. In severe cases, patients with primary HSV infection may present with aseptic meningitis, pelvic radiculomyelitis, flank pain simulating pyelonephritis, or abdominal pain resembling a surgical abdomen.

Based on recent studies using newer techniques for serologic testing, it is estimated that 20% to 25% of the adult U.S. population is infected with genital herpes. Many infections go unrecognized by both physicians and patients. The majority of genital herpes cases do not present in a "classic" manner. About 10% to 20% of persons with genital herpes will have genital ulcers, 10% to 20% will be asymptomatic, and 60% will have atypical symptoms such as genital itching, back pain, leg pain, vaginal discharge, and other nonspecific symptoms.

### Diagnosis

Although the presence of grouped vesicles in the genital region is nearly pathognomonic for HSV infection, many patients present later in the course of the infection, when vesicles have already ulcerated. Thus, laboratory confirmation is important in many instances. Several methods are available for confirming the presence of HSV in genital ulcerations. The *Tzanck smear* is an established, rapid, and reasonably accurate method for presumptively diagnosing HSV infection. Definitive diagnosis is still established by the isolation of HSV in tissue culture, a technique available in most laboratories. In most cases, the turnaround time to isolation of the virus is short (relative to other viruses, such as varicella-zoster virus or cytomegalovirus) because HSV grows rapidly and well in tissue culture systems. The introduction of the shell vial for primary viral isolation has further shortened the time to identification of HSV, to 48 hours in many cases. Alternative methods for HSV detection include several enzyme immunoassays that identify HSV-1 and HSV-2 antigen directly in clinical specimens. HSV also can be detected using the polymerase chain reaction (PCR) technique. It should be noted that a number of patients with primary HSV-2 or HSV-1 genital infection will be culture negative, particularly if the lesions have already crusted. False negative cultures are even more common with recurrent genital HSV.

Serologic studies may be useful in certain patients with culture-negative primary infections. The detection of specific HSV immunoglobulin M strongly suggests recent infection. Immunoglobulin M (IgM) antibody also may be detectable in some individuals during recurrent episodes of genital HSV infection, however. A fourfold rise in HSV immunoglobulin G (IgG) between the acute and convalescent periods also is diagnostic of a primary HSV episode.

Recently, newer serologic tests with high specificity for the detection of HSV-2 and HSV-1 antibody have been made commercially available. Older serologic tests for HSV-2 and HSV-1 lacked specificity and had limited clinical utility. Newer tests are based on the detection of the HSV-specific glycoprotein G2 for HSV-2 infection and glycoprotein G1 for HSV 1 infection; the sensitivity is in the range of 80% to 98%, and specificity is about 96%. These glycoprotein-based tests are useful in diagnosing culture-negative HSV-2 infections. Type-specific serologic tests also can be used to identify persons with atypical symptoms and to evaluate the sex partners of persons with genital herpes infections. Screening of the general population is not recommended.

### Therapy

#### First Episode of Herpes Simplex Virus Infection

The first episode of HSV infection should be treated for 7 to 10 days with one of the following regimens:

- Acyclovir (Zovirax), 400 mg three times daily, or
- Acyclovir (Zovirax), 200 mg five times daily, or
- Famciclovir (Famvir), 250 mg orally three times daily, or
- Valacyclovir (Valtrex), 1 g orally twice daily.

Longer treatment courses may be necessary in some cases. Patients with severe disease or with complications of primary HSV infection such as pneumonitis, encephalitis, or hepatitis may be treated with acyclovir, 5 mg/kg intravenously every 8 hours for 5 to 7 days. Acyclovir shortens the course of primary HSV infection and accelerates viral clearance and healing of ulcers. It has no effect, however, on the rate of subsequent recurrences. The drug is active only against replicating virus and does not target latent HSV. Topical acyclovir is less effective than acyclovir given orally.

The safety of acyclovir in pregnancy has not been definitively established. The U.S. Public Health Service recommends that pregnant women should only be treated if a life-threatening maternal primary HSV infection is present.

#### Recurrent Episodes

Recurrences of genital HSV infection are common and problematic. Recurrent attacks are less frequently associated with regional lymphadenopathy and constitutional symptoms than primary HSV infection. In addition, genital lesions associated with recurrent episodes heal more quickly than do those of primary HSV infection. False-negative cultures for HSV are more common than with primary infection, and it is estimated that, on the average, only 20% of cultures are positive during a recurrence.

In addition to recurrent ulcers, persons with genital herpes frequently demonstrate asymptomatic shedding of the virus, which is potentially transmissible to a susceptible partner. Over 90% of persons with genital HSV-2 shed live virus at some point after the primary infection. In the first few years after primary infection, it is estimated that

virus is shed on 10% to 20% of days in the absence of visible lesions.

The number of recurrences is highly variable. Recurrences are much more common with genital infection from HSV-2 than HSV-1. On the average, persons with genital HSV-2 experience four outbreaks in the first year following primary infection, which subsequently decreases by 0.5 outbreaks per year for subsequent years; however, this is only an average rate and the actual number in an individual person is difficult to predict.

The optimal therapy for recurrent attacks remains controversial. Data from large studies suggest that acyclovir is of limited benefit when recurrent episodes are treated individually, shortening the duration of viral shedding and the time to crusting of lesions by less than 1 day. No beneficial effect is seen on the rate of recurrences. In severe recurrent disease, some individuals start acyclovir at the start of the prodrome and continue therapy for 5 days. Possible regimens include oral acyclovir, 200 mg five times daily, 400 mg three times daily, or 800 mg twice daily. Famciclovir, 125 mg orally twice daily, or valacyclovir, 500 mg orally twice daily, are alternative regimens.

#### Daily Suppressive Therapy

Another approach for patients with frequent severe recurrences is daily suppressive acyclovir therapy. Studies have shown that individuals with frequent recurrences of HSV infection, defined as six or more outbreaks per year, may have a 75% reduction in the number of recurrences using daily suppressive therapy. Chronic suppression using acyclovir appears to be safe for up to 6 years, and for 1 year with famciclovir and valacyclovir; however, the U.S. Public Health Service recommends a 1-year course followed by reassessment of the need for daily therapy. Acyclovir-resistant HSV has been isolated from patients on suppressive therapy, but this has not been clearly associated with treatment failure. One limitation of daily suppressive therapy is its lack of long-term benefit; the frequency of outbreaks often returns to baseline once acyclovir is discontinued.

Recommended regimens for daily suppressive therapy include:

- Acyclovir, 400 mg orally twice daily, or
- Famciclovir, 250 mg orally twice daily, or
- Valacyclovir, 500 mg orally daily, or 1 g orally daily.

Because the safety of acyclovir in pregnancy has not been established, daily suppressive acyclovir should not be used for recurrent genital HSV infections in pregnant women, nor should recurrent episodes be treated individually unless life threatening.

#### Genital Herpes Treatment in AIDS

Severe progressive HSV infections were commonly seen in individuals with acquired immunodeficiency syndrome (AIDS) in the era before highly active antiretroviral therapy. Fortunately, these infections are less common with the advent of highly active antiretroviral therapy. Progressive genital and perianal ulcers with proctocolitis may be due to either HSV-1 or HSV-2 in persons with HIV. When HSV proctitis occurs, it may be quite debilitating, with anorectal pain, bloody stools, and fever. In patients with advanced immunodeficiency and HSV proctitis, recurrences are common. Such patients with AIDS are often placed on chronic suppressive acyclovir therapy. This has led to reports of the emergence of acyclovir-resistant HSV mutants. Recurrent episodes are often suppressed using daily acyclovir, especially if severe or associated with HSV proctitis. The dosage of acyclovir in this setting is controversial. In 2002, the CDC recommended acyclovir, 400 mg orally two to three times daily, famciclovir, 500 mg orally twice a day, or valacyclovir, 500 mg orally twice a day. For episodic treatment of genital herpes in HIV, several regimens may be used for 5 to 10 days, including:

- Acyclovir, 400 mg orally three times daily, or
- Acyclovir, 200 mg orally five times daily, or
- Famciclovir, 500 mg orally twice daily, or
- Valacyclovir, 1 gram orally twice daily.

If lesions fail to heal while on appropriate therapy, the possibility of a drug-resistant HSV isolate should be considered. Acyclovir-resistant HSV isolates also usually are cross resistant to famciclovir and valacyclovir and generally require alternative treatments such as foscarnet and cidofovir. This problem seems to have decreased with the advent of antiretroviral therapy.

# CHANCROID

## Etiology and Clinical Manifestations

Chancroid is caused by *Haemophilus ducreyi*, a Gram-negative coccobacillus. Although uncommon in the United States, its worldwide incidence may exceed that of syphilis. From 1971 to 1980, the number of cases of chancroid in the United States was less than 900 annually. In the 1980s, the incidence of chancroid increased markedly, with 3,418 cases reported in 1986. Chancroid is a known cofactor for HIV transmission, and an estimated 10% of patients who have chancroid could be coinfected with *T. pallidum* or HSV. Chancroid is endemic in many areas of the United States; from 1981 to 1987, nine major outbreaks were reported, primarily in Florida, New York City, California, Boston, and Dallas. Chancroid was seen mainly in Hispanic and black heterosexual men who patronized prostitutes. In Florida, chancroid was seen in highly sexually active men without clear prostitute exposure. In Boston, the outbreak may have been related to individuals who had originally been infected in foreign countries where the disease is endemic, such as Haiti and the Dominican Republic.

After exposure, the incubation period for chancroid is 1 to 21 days, with an average of 7 days. Chancroid ulcers are painful, deep, shaggy, and friable, and their borders are undermined. Ulcers are commonly single in men but multiple in women.

Regional adenopathy occurs simultaneously with the ulcer and is seen in 50% to 65% of patients. The nodes are quite tender and tend to be unilateral. In addition, they tend to become fluctuant and can easily fistulize. The combination of a painful ulcer with suppurative inguinal lymphadenopathy is almost diagnostic of chancroid. Constitutional symptoms are uncommon.

## Diagnosis

The isolation of *H. ducreyi* from an active genital ulcer is the only definitive means of confirming the diagnosis of chancroid. Special media and culture techniques are required to isolate this fastidious organism. Gram's stain of an ulcer specimen may be misleading because of the presence of polymicrobial flora colonizing genital ulcers, and culture confirmation remains the gold standard. The sensitivity of culture isolation of *H. ducreyi* from active genital ulcers is variable, ranging from 50% to 80%, depending on the culture medium employed. It is important to note that *H. ducreyi* is almost never isolated from aspiration of inguinal buboes. Alternatives to culture confirmation have been described but are investigational.

A probable diagnosis of chancroid can be made if the following criteria are met:

- One or more painful genital lesions
- No evidence of syphilis (a negative dark-field examination or negative rapid plasma reagin test result more than 7 days after onset of the ulcer)
- No evidence of HSV (clinically or by testing)

## Therapy

Regimens recommended by the CDC for the treatment of chancroid include:

- Azithromycin (Zithromax), 1 g orally (single dose), or
- Ceftriaxone (Rocephin), 250 mg intramuscularly (single dose), or
- Ciprofloxacin (Cipro), 500 mg orally twice daily for 3 days, or
- Erythromycin, 500 mg orally four times daily for 7 days.

For individuals with chancroid who are coinfected with HIV, some experts recommend the erythromycin regimen; close follow-up is necessary.

# LYMPHOGRANULOMA VENEREUM

## Etiology and Clinical Manifestations

LGV is caused by *Chlamydia trachomatis*, serovars L1, L2, or L3. The incubation period for LGV is variable, ranging from 3 to 21 days. The genital lesion is not striking and may be missed by both patients and physicians. It is usually single and painless and may be a papule, vesicle, or ulcer. It resolves within several days.

The key to the diagnosis of LGV is the nature of the regional adenopathy, not the genital lesion. Inguinal lymphadenopathy in LGV develops 2 to 6 weeks after the primary lesion, but in rare cases, the genital lesion may still be present. The nodes are matted, fluctuant, and large. Typically, they are painful. Adenopathy is unilateral in two thirds of patients and bilateral in the remainder. Fistulas have been described, especially after diagnostic needle aspiration. Constitutional symptoms such as fever, headache, myalgia, and malaise are often prominent.

## Diagnosis

Serologic titers for LGV may be useful in selected cases. The complement fixation test result is positive in most patients with active LGV at titers of 1:64 or higher. Titers become positive between 1 and 3 weeks after infection. Occasionally, high complement fixation titers have been found in individuals with other chlamydial infections and in asymptomatic individuals. Titers less than 1:64 are suggestive but not diagnostic of LGV. It is difficult to demonstrate a classic fourfold rise in specific antibody titer in LGV because of the late presentation in many patients.

## Therapy

Doxycycline, 100 mg orally twice daily for 21 days, is the treatment of choice for LGV. An alternative regimen is erythromycin, 500 mg orally four times daily for 21 days. Treatment is the same in HIV-infected patients.

## GRANULOMA INGUINALE (DONOVANOSIS)

### Etiology and Clinical Manifestations

Granuloma inguinale, also termed *donovanosis*, is caused by the Gram-negative bacillus *Calymmatobacterium granulomatis*. It is quite rare in the United States, but in many developing countries, it is one of the most prevalent STDs. Granuloma inguinale is common in India, the Caribbean islands, and Africa. In 1984, an outbreak of 20 cases was recognized in Texas. The epidemiology and pathogenesis of donovanosis in the United States (and endemic countries as well) are poorly characterized. The precise role of sexual transmission is unclear, but repeated anal intercourse appears to be a risk factor for rectal and penile lesions in homosexual couples. Available data suggest that the infection is only mildly contagious.

The incubation period varies from 8 to 80 days. The lesion or lesions initially appear as subcutaneous nodules that later erode. Ulcerations forming above the nodules are

painless, clean, and granulomatous. Granulation tissue often appears "beefy-red" and with occasional contact bleeding. The lesions are most common on the glans or prepuce in men and on the labial area in women. The ulcers progressively enlarge in a chronic destructive fashion. They may be misidentified as carcinoma of the penis, chancroid, condyloma latum of secondary syphilis (when perianal lesions are present), and other causes of genital ulceration. Constitutional symptoms are usually absent.

Infection with *C. granulomatis* does not produce true regional lymphadenopathy. Instead, the granulomatous process in the genitals may extend into the inguinal region, causing further fibrosis and granulation tissue (pseudobuboes). These pseudobuboes are present in only 10% of patients with donovanosis and are variably painful.

## Diagnosis

The diagnosis of granuloma inguinale can be confirmed by finding the characteristic *Donovan's bodies* in a crush preparation of fresh granulation tissue from a genital ulcer, which is spread over a clean microscope slide, air-dried, and stained with Wright's or Giemsa's stain. Donovan's bodies are multiple, darkly staining intracytoplasmic bacteria (*C. granulomatis*) found within the vacuoles of large mononuclear cells. They also can be identified in formal biopsy specimens with the use of standard light microscopy.

## Therapy

Granuloma inguinale responds well to the following first-line oral antibiotics used singly, as recommended by the CDC:

- Doxycycline, 100 mg orally twice daily, or
- Trimethoprim-sulfamethoxazole, double-strength (160 mg trimethoprim/800 mg sulfamethoxazole) tablet orally twice daily

Antibiotics are continued until the lesions are completely healed, usually 21 days or more. Alternative regimens include ciprofloxacin, 750 mg orally twice daily, or erythromycin base, 500 mg orally four times daily. In pregnancy, erythromycin is recommended. HIV-infected individuals with granuloma inguinale are treated in the same manner as otherwise healthy individuals.

## SYPHILIS

### Primary Syphilis

#### Etiology and Clinical Manifestations

Syphilis is caused by the spirochete *Treponema pallidum*. The incubation period ranges from 3 to 90 days (mean, 21 days). The syphilitic chancre is typically a single, painless ulcer with raised and indurated borders. The base of the ulcer is clean and usually without purulence. Up to one-third of syphilitic ulcers, however, may be mildly painful. Development of the ulcer is usually slow. In the absence of treatment, chancres persist for up to 6 weeks. Constitutional symptoms are usually absent.

Inguinal lymphadenopathy is present in approximately 80% of patients with primary syphilis. The onset of lymphadenopathy usually occurs at the same time as the genital lesion. Characteristically, the adenopathy is painless (like the chancre), and the nodes are firm. In 70% of patients, the adenopathy is bilateral.

### Diagnosis

The definitive methods of diagnosing early syphilis are dark-field examination and direct fluorescent antibody tests on active lesions or tissue biopsies. Serologic tests for syphilis, commonly used, are not diagnostic. A presumptive diagnosis of active syphilis can be made with one of various serologic tests, which are classified as nontreponemal and treponemal. Nontreponemal tests include the Venereal Disease Research Laboratory (VDRL) and Rapid Plasma Reagin (RPR) tests. Treponemal tests include the fluorescent treponemal antibody absorption test, the micro-hemagglutination assay for antibody to *T. pallidum*, and the *T. pallidum* immobilization test.

Both positive treponemal and nontreponemal test results are necessary to presumptively diagnose syphilis, in the absence of direct tests on primary lesions. As a rule, treponemal test results stay positive for life after the initial infection, whether appropriate therapy has been administered. Because treponemal test results do not correlate with disease activity, they are usually reported as either positive or negative. In contrast, nontreponemal test results do correlate with disease activity, reaching high titers with primary infection or recent reinfection and decreasing over time after appropriate therapy. Nontreponemal test results are reported as quantitative titers. The adequacy of therapy can be determined using serial RPR (or VDRL) tests; ideally, the same test in the same laboratory should be followed sequentially.

In primary syphilis, the VDRL test result is positive in approximately 70% of patients, and the RPR test result is positive in approximately 80%. Thus, it is important to realize that a substantial number of patients with a typical syphilitic chancre may have a negative nontreponemal test result. Treponemal test results also may be negative early on in primary syphilis. The percentage of positive test results for the fluorescent treponemal antibody absorption test is 85%, for the microhemagglutination assay for antibody to *T. pallidum* 65%, and for the *T. pallidum* immobilization test 50%. Thus, the diagnosis of primary syphilis should be considered in patients with lesions compatible with a chancre, even if nontreponemal and treponemal tests are negative.

All patients with syphilis, regardless of stage, should be tested for HIV according to the CDC recommendations.

### TABLE 13.5

#### CLINICAL MANIFESTATIONS OF SECONDARY SYPHILIS

| Manifestation | Cases (%) |
|---|---|
| Skin | 90 |
| Mouth and throat | 35 |
| Genital lesions | 20 |
| Constitutional symptoms | 70 |
| Central nervous system | |
|     Asymptomatic | 8–40 |
|     Symptomatic | 1–2 |

Modified and used with permission from Mandell GL, Bennett JE, Dolin R, eds. *Mandell, Douglas and Bennett's Principles and Practice of Infectious Diseases*, 5th ed. Philadelphia: Churchill Livingstone, 1999.

## Secondary and Tertiary Syphilis

### Clinical Manifestations and Laboratory Diagnosis

In the absence of specific therapy, clinical manifestations may develop, in addition to genital ulceration with regional adenopathy. Secondary syphilis may present up to 2 years after the initial infection. Common clinical manifestations of secondary syphilis are summarized in Table 13.5. The most common manifestation is rash, and clinicians must consider secondary syphilis in all patients with unexplained rash, especially if accompanied by a risk history to suggest the diagnosis. The rash may be protean in its appearance, but involvement of the palms of the hands and soles of the feet should suggest the diagnosis.

Patients with syphilis and clinical signs suggesting either meningitis or uveitis should be fully evaluated for neurosyphilis or luetic uveitis, with testing including lumbar puncture and slit-lamp examination. During primary or secondary syphilis, invasion of the cerebrospinal fluid (CSF) by *T. pallidum* is common; abnormalities in the CSF often can be demonstrated. If primary or secondary syphilis is treated appropriately, however, neurosyphilis develops in only a small percentage of patients. The CDC does not recommend routine lumbar puncture in patients with primary or secondary syphilis, unless signs or symptoms of neurologic or ophthalmic involvement are present.

The natural history of untreated secondary syphilis is spontaneous resolution after 3 to 12 weeks, although viable organisms persist. VDRL, RPR, and treponemal test results are positive in nearly 100% of patients with secondary syphilis. In the absence of specific treatment, patients enter a stage of asymptomatic infection termed *latency*. They are classified as having *early-latent* disease if they are asymptomatic and have acquired infection within the past year. Those without symptoms and with infection of greater than 1 year's duration are said to have *late-latent* syphilis. In asymptomatic patients with a positive serology, it may be difficult to distinguish early- from late-latent disease.

Tertiary syphilis may produce cardiac or neurologic disease, as well as a variety of less common manifestations. The most common cardiac manifestation is aortitis. Neurologic manifestations of tertiary syphilis may include meningovascular syphilis, tabes dorsalis, and generalized paresis. *Gummatous syphilis* is a rare manifestation of late syphilis in which granulomatous lesions present as space-occupying lesions in a variety of organs such as liver, bone, central nervous system, respiratory tract, and bowel.

### Therapy

Primary, secondary, and early-latent syphilis is treated with a single dose of benzathine penicillin G, 2.4 million U intramuscularly. For penicillin-allergic patients, the alternative is doxycycline, 100 mg orally twice daily for 2 weeks, or tetracycline, 500 mg orally four times daily for 2 weeks. Later stages of syphilis require more prolonged therapy. Current treatment recommendations for the respective stages of syphilis are summarized in Table 13.6.

## Syphilis and HIV Infection

In HIV-infected individuals, syphilis can be highly aggressive. Patients may progress from primary to tertiary disease over the course of several years rather than several decades, as occurs in non–HIV-infected individuals. Several important caveats regarding syphilis in HIV-infected patients are summarized in Table 13.7. All individuals who present with syphilis should be offered HIV testing. In younger individuals who present with unexplained stroke, meningovascular syphilis in the setting of unrecognized HIV infection should

| TABLE 13.7 |
| --- |

### SYPHILIS IN HUMAN IMMUNODEFICIENCY VIRUS (HIV)-INFECTED PATIENTS: CAVEATS

Progression to tertiary syphilis may occur rapidly (several years).

Neurosyphilis should always be considered in HIV-infected patients with neurologic disease.

When findings suggest syphilis at any stage but serologic test results are negative, diagnosis with biopsy, dark-field examination, or direct fluorescent antibody staining should be pursued.

**Treatment**

Use penicillin.

No changes in therapy for early syphilis.

Consider cerebrospinal fluid examination in all patients with clues and HIV infection.

Follow-up with VDRL or rapid plasma reagin test at 3, 6, 9, 12, and 24 months; if titers fail to decrease fourfold after 6 months, treat again and perform lumbar puncture.

be considered in the differential diagnosis, along with infective endocarditis and more common causes of stroke.

## VAGINAL INFECTIONS

## Etiology and Clinical Manifestations

Vaginal discharge is a common complaint in primary care practice, accounting for approximately 10 million office visits annually in the United States. Vaginal signs and symptoms are nonspecific, however, and more serious conditions such as cervical neoplasia, MPC, and PID may mimic

| TABLE 13.6 |
| --- |

### TREATMENT RECOMMENDATIONS FOR THE DIFFERENT STAGES OF SYPHILIS

| Stage | Recommended | Alternative |
| --- | --- | --- |
| Primary | Benzathine PCN G, 2.4 million units i.m. for 1 wk | Doxycycline, 100 mg p.o. b.i.d., or tetracycline,[a] 500 mg p.o. q.i.d. for 2 wk |
| Secondary Early latent (<1 yr) Late latent (>1 yr) | Benzathine PCN G, 2.4 million units i.m. weekly for 3 wk | Doxycycline, 100 mg p.o. b.i.d., or tetracycline,[a] 500 mg p.o. q.i.d. for 4 wk |
| Gummas Cardiovascular Neurosyphilis | Aqueous PCN G, 18–24 million units i.v. daily for 10–14 days | Procaine PCN G, 2.4 million units i.m. daily; probenecid, 500 mg q.i.d. for 10–14 days |

PCN, penicillin.
[a] Avoid tetracycline during pregnancy.

## TABLE 13.8
### VAGINAL INFECTIONS: CLINICAL MANIFESTATIONS

|  | Normal Vagina | Yeast Vaginitis | Trichomoniasis | Bacterial Vaginosis |
|---|---|---|---|---|
| Etiology | — | *Candida albicans*, other yeasts | Trichomonas vaginalis | *Gardnerella vaginalis*, mycoplasmas, anaerobes |
| Symptoms | — | Itching, irritation, discharge | Malodorous discharge, often profuse | Malodorous discharge |
| **Discharge** |  |  |  |  |
| Color | Clear or white | White | Yellow | White or gray |
| Consistency | Nonhomogeneous, floccular | Clumped, adherent plaques | Thin, homogeneous, frothy | Homogenous, coats vaginal mucosa |
| Inflammation of vulva/introitus | — | Vaginal erythema, vulvar dermatitis | Vaginal erythema, strawberry cervix | None |

Modified and reproduced with permission from Paavonen J, Stamm WE. Sexually transmitted diseases: lower genital tract infections in women. *Infect Dis Clin North Am* 1987;1:179–198.

vaginitis. The most common causes of vaginitis include bacterial vaginosis (BV, i.e., nonspecific vaginitis), *Trichomonas vaginalis* vaginitis, and yeast vulvovaginitis due to *Candida albicans* and other yeasts.

The symptoms of vaginitis are rarely specific enough to suggest a precise etiologic diagnosis. Nevertheless, the common clinical manifestations of the respective causes of vaginitis are summarized in Table 13.8.

## Diagnosis

The diagnostic evaluation of patients with suspected vaginitis should include the microscopic examination of vaginal secretions, testing of secretions for pH, and application of 10% potassium hydroxide to secretions to elicit a fishy odor (whiff test). The results of these tests may distinguish the respective causes, as summarized in Table 13.9.

BV may be caused by *Gardnerella vaginalis*, mycoplasmas, and occasionally anaerobic bacteria. Criteria for the

clinical diagnosis of BV include the following:

- Gray homogeneous discharge adherent to the vaginal epithelium and cervix
- Fishy odor
- pH 4.5
- Clue cells
- Positive whiff test

## Therapy

The sexual partners of individuals with BV do not require treatment. Recommended regimens for the therapy of BV include the following antibiotics:

- Metronidazole, 500 mg orally twice daily for 7 days, or
- Clindamycin 2% cream (Cleocin), 5 g intravaginally at bedtime for 7 days, or
- Metronidazole, 0.75% gel, 5 g intravaginally twice daily for 5 days.

## TABLE 13.9
### VAGINAL INFECTIONS: DIAGNOSIS

|  | Normal Vagina | Yeast Vaginitis | Trichomoniasis | Bacterial Vaginosis |
|---|---|---|---|---|
| pH | <4.5 | <4.5 | ≥4.5 | ≥4.5 |
| Ammonia odor with 10% potassium hydroxide | None | None | Usually present | Present |
| Microscopy | Epithelial cells, lactobacilli | Leukocytes, epithelial cells; yeast, mycelia, pseudomycelia in up to 80% | Leukocytes, motile trichomonads in 80%–90% | Clue cells, few leukocytes, profuse mixed flora |

Modified and reproduced with permission from Paavonen J, Stamm WE. Sexually transmitted diseases: lower genital tract infections in women. *Infect Dis Clin North Am* 1987;1:179–198.

Alternative regimens include:

- Metronidazole, 2 g orally (single dose), or
- Clindamycin, 300 mg orally twice daily for 7 days
- Clindamycin ovules, 100 g intravaginally once at bedtime for 3 days.

A number of controversies arise regarding bacterial vaginosis in pregnancy, including the optimal regimens, screening of asymptomatic pregnant women, and safety of various antibiotics. Metronidazole has remained somewhat controversial, although studies on the safety of this antibiotic in pregnancy have failed to show a definite association with adverse pregnancy outcomes. Bacterial vaginosis has been linked with a number of pregnancy complications including chorioamnionitis, preterm birth, and others. Recent studies have shown an increase in adverse events associated with clindamycin cream, and this is no longer recommended. The CDC has recommended against the use of topical agents during pregnancy for BV. The recommendations for the treatment for BV during pregnancy is as follows:

- Metronidazole, 250 mg orally three times daily for 7 days, or
- Clindamycin, 300 mg orally twice daily for 7 days.

For the treatment of trichomonas infection, metronidazole, 2 g orally (single dose), is recommended for the treatment of trichomoniasis. An alternative regimen is metronidazole, 500 mg orally twice daily for 7 days. Metronidazole gel is not recommended for trichomonas due to poor efficacy, although it is approved for BV. Sexual partners also should be treated.

Trichomonas infection in pregnancy has been associated with a variety of adverse outcomes. It is not clear, however, whether treatment of asymptomatic trichomoniasis in pregnancy decreases adverse outcomes. The recommended regimen in pregnancy is 2 g of metronidazole given as a single dose; the CDC feels that no clear teratogenic effect of metronidazole has been shown.

The recommended regimens for the treatment of vulvovaginal candidiasis include the following agents:

- Butoconazole 2% cream (Femstat), 5 g intravaginally for 3 days, or
- Clotrimazole 1% cream, 5 g intravaginally for 7 to 14 days, or
- Clotrimazole, 100-mg vaginal tablet for 7 days, or
- Clotrimazole, 100-mg vaginal tablet, two tablets for 3 days, or
- Clotrimazole, 500-mg vaginal tablet, one tablet in a single application, or
- Miconazole (Monistat) 2% cream, 5 g intravaginally for 7 days, or
- Miconazole, 200-mg vaginal suppository for 3 days, or
- Miconazole, 100-mg vaginal suppository for 7 days, or
- Terconazole (Terazol) 0.4% cream, 5 g intravaginally for 7 days, or

- Terconazole 0.8% cream, 5 g intravaginally for 3 days, or
- Terconazole, 80-mg suppository for 3 days, or
- Tioconazole 6.5% ointment (Vagistat-1), 5 g intravaginally in a single application, or Fluconazole (Diflucan), 150 mg orally as a single dose.

Sexual partners do not require treatment (unless balanitis is present). Pregnant women are treated in the same manner as nonpregnant women.

# GENITAL WARTS

## Etiology and Clinical Manifestations

Over 100 strains or types of human papillomavirus (HPV) exist, and over 30 types can infect the genital tract. They have been broadly classified into low-risk (e.g., HPV-6 and HPV-11) and high-risk (e.g., HPV-16, 18, 31, 33, 35) types on the basis of their association with cancer. HPV-6 and 11 are the most common types found in external genital warts. Most visible genital warts are associated with low-risk HPV types. Occasionally, visible warts are associated with the high-risk types, but this is much less common.

External genital warts are one of the most commonly diagnosed STDs in the United States, with an estimated prevalence of 20 million cases and an incidence of 6 million new infections annually. About 50% of sexually active persons in the United States will acquire genital HPV infection at some point. Genital warts accounted for more than one-third of the total cost for STDs in the United States in 1995. The sexual and behavioral risk factors associated with genital HPV infections include multiple sexual partners, sex with a person with warts, or anoreceptive intercourse (for intra-anal but not perianal warts). Condoms do not completely protect against HPV transmission, especially in women.

Most HPV infections are subclinical and asymptomatic, but lesions that do occur usually appear between 3 weeks and 8 months after infection of genital tract cells. Genital warts affect a variety of sites including the penis, scrotum, vulva, perineal and perianal areas, pubic area, and crural folds. HPV types that cause external genital warts also can cause warts in the vagina or cervix and inside the urethra or anus. Persons who practice anal receptive intercourse are at risk for developing intra-anal warts; this is in contrast to perianal warts, which can develop as an extension of genital warts, unrelated to anal intercourse. Intraurethral warts may cause terminal hematuria or intermittent spotting. Genital warts may occur as discrete lesions or may coalesce into confluent plaques. Four morphologic types exist:

- Condyloma acuminatum: cauliflower-shaped, usually on moist surfaces
- Smooth papular: dome-shaped, usually on dry surfaces
- Keratotic: thick horny layer, possibly resembling a common wart or seborrheic keratosis, usually on dry surfaces

■ Flat to slightly raised flat-topped papular: on any mucosal or cutaneous surface

A strong association exists between infection with certain types of HPV and anogenital cancer. Bowenoid papulosis, almost always associated with HPV-16 or HPV-18, is characterized by dome-shaped or flat papules 1 to 5 mm in size that may be hyperpigmented or bluish hued. Histologic examination of these papules shows high-grade squamous intraepithelial lesions. Buschke-Löwenstein tumor, a form of verrucous squamous cell carcinoma, is perhaps the only neoplastic lesion associated with low-risk HPV types. Cervical, vulvar, and perianal intraepithelial neoplasia and carcinomas of the vulva, cervix, anus, and penis have all been associated with HPV, mostly types 16 and 18.

## Diagnosis

Clinical trials have demonstrated that diagnosis based on clinical examination is reliable and consistent with histologic diagnosis. Bright light and magnification may assist in the diagnosis of flat or small warts. The application of a 3% to 5% acetic acid solution to genital tissues for 5 to 10 minutes (acetowhite test) before examination may be useful in populations with a high prevalence of warts and for the identification of flat-topped warts that may be particularly difficult to visualize. This test is not recommended for routine screening, however. An examination of the cervix using colposcopy after the acetowhite test is sensitive but not specific and should not be employed as a diagnostic tool. Biopsy is not routinely required but should be considered when:

■ One or more lesions are indurated, ulcerated, or fixed to underlying structures.
■ An individual lesion is larger than 10 mm.
■ The diagnosis is in doubt.
■ Lesions are unresponsive to standard therapy.
■ Lesions are pigmented.
■ The condition worsens during therapy.
■ The patient is immunocompromised.

The detection of HPV DNA in genital tissue is used in studies of the epidemiology and pathogenesis of HPV infection. Although assays for HPV DNA are commercially available, type-specific HPV DNA assays are not indicated for the routine management of visible genital warts. DNA detection assays may be useful in confirming infection in patients with equivocal Papanicolaou (Pap) smears. Viral cultures for HPV detection are not widely available, and currently no useful serologic tests for HPV are available.

Although HPV typing has no proven benefit in the management of external genital warts because the prevalence of high-risk types is low in this circumstance, typing may be valuable in providing prognostic information for patients with cervical intraepithelial neoplasia. Women with exophytic cervical warts require an evaluation for high-grade squamous intraepithelial lesions. Subclinical genital HPV infection, however, is much more common than visible cervical warts. Subclinical genital infection is usually suspected on the basis of an abnormal Pap smear, colposcopy, or abnormal skin or mucous membrane areas after acetic acid testing. In women, subclinical HPV infection is commonly diagnosed on Pap testing, which shows squamous intraepithelial lesions (SIL). Some cases of HPV on Pap smear are probably false positive tests, however, with no HPV DNA detectable. HPV infection can be diagnosed definitively by the detection of HPV nucleic acid, and type-specific testing may be useful in evaluating women with atypical squamous cells of undetermined significance (ASCUS) but less useful in other types of abnormal cytologies. The routine screening of skin or normal genital tissue for subclinical HPV using DNA or RNA tests is not advised.

Patients with genital warts and their partners should be screened for other STDs. Because women with external genital warts have a greater probability of exposure to high-risk oncogenic HPV types, these women and the female partners of men with warts should be screened annually for cervical cancer using a Pap smear until receiving three negative test results. Subsequent screening should be considered. There are no guidelines for anal cancer screening, but patients with perianal warts, HIV-infected patients, and patients with a history of anoreceptive intercourse should be asked about symptoms of melena or hematochezia and should be tested for occult blood; possibly, anal cytology also should be considered.

## Therapy

External genital warts are usually asymptomatic, but depending on their size, number, and location, they may be painful, friable, or pruritic and may interfere with normal function. In addition, they may be socially stigmatizing and emotionally distressing. Although unpredictable, some warts may resolve spontaneously, but regression is often followed by disease recurrence later. In most patients, however, warts either remain unchanged or increase in size and number, especially during pregnancy and immune deficiency. Currently available therapies may eliminate the warts but not the infection and may not decrease infectivity. No simple, routinely effective therapies are available, and this often makes the treatment of genital warts a frustrating experience for both patients and clinicians. Most treatment modalities have similar efficacy. The size, location, number, and character of the warts affect treatment decisions, as do coexisting medical conditions (e.g., pregnancy or immune deficiency).

Patient-controlled therapies are best suited for patients who desire more control over their care; they are usually less invasive and require patient education. Their safety and efficacy have not been established in pediatric patients and pregnant women. One commonly used agent is 0.5% podofilox solution or gel (Condylox), which should be applied twice daily for 3 consecutive days. This cycle is repeated weekly until the warts are gone, but no longer than 4 weeks. Another agent is 5% imiquimod (Aldara) cream applied at bedtime on 3 alternating days per week until the lesions clear or for 16 weeks. The cream is washed off 6 to 10 hours after application.

Physician-applied therapies include:

- Trichloroacetic acid or bichloracetic acid applied every 1 to 2 weeks, or
- Podophyllin resin (10% to 25%) in tincture of benzoin applied one to two times weekly for six treatments, or
- 5-Fluorouracil (5%) cream one to three times weekly for several weeks, or
- Cryotherapy with liquid nitrogen applied by cryoprobe, spray, or loosely wound cotton on a wooden applicator (this requires training for proper administration), or
- Office surgery, including curettage, electrosurgery, and fine-scissor or tangential shave excision (these require equipment and significant training)

Complex destructive modalities include laser or intralesional interferon. These require in-depth training and are not recommended for first-line treatment. Systemic interferon is not efficacious. Treatment should be changed or the patient should be referred when:

- Three treatment sessions have resulted in no improvement.
- Complete clearance has not occurred after six treatment sessions.
- Continued treatment would extend beyond the manufacturer's recommendations for patient-applied therapies.

Immune compromise decreases the likelihood of spontaneous regression and responsiveness to conventional therapies and increases the likelihood of relapse. In HIV-infected patients, the ulcerations caused by therapy increase the risk of transmission of HIV and other STDs to sexual partners.

An integral component of therapy for patients with genital warts is counseling. Many patients respond to the appearance of warts with a strong mix of emotions, ranging from embarrassment to anger to fear. Genital warts can damage a patient's feelings of self-esteem and interactions with sexual partners. Worry about the possibility of cancer or transmission of the disease to sexual partners or to a newborn during delivery also can cause anguish. Clinicians can be sensitive to these concerns by addressing them with both verbal reassurance and written information. A nonjudgmental attitude is critical to the success of counseling, which is aimed at preventing or alleviating the significant emotional, psychological, and social sequelae that may result from the disease.

## REVIEW EXERCISES

### QUESTIONS

**1.** A 19-year-old man has a low-grade fever, tender inguinal adenopathy, and grouped vesicles on his penis. He has never had an STD before, and he has a new female partner. How should this patient be managed?
a) Acyclovir cream applied to the lesions three times daily until resolution
b) No therapy because trials have failed to demonstrate efficacy in this setting
c) Acyclovir, 400 mg orally three times daily; famciclovir, 250 mg orally three times daily; or valacyclovir, 1 g orally twice daily for 7 days
d) Acyclovir, 5 mg/kg intravenously every 8 hours
e) None of the above

**2.** A 26-year-old man has a several-week-old penile lesion with new inguinal adenopathy. On examination, a single nontender ulcer is present. Bilateral palpable inguinal nodes are present, which also are nontender. RPR test results are negative. The most likely diagnosis is:
a) Lymphogranuloma venereum
b) Chancroid
c) Primary syphilis
b) Variant HSV infection
e) Granuloma inguinale

**3.** A 44-year-old man has had a painful penile ulcer for several weeks. He is HIV-negative, but has frequent prostitute exposure. He has tender inguinal lymph nodes on the right, which appeared at the same time as the genital ulcer. He has seen several physicians, apparently without a diagnosis. On examination, the node is fluctuant and has a fistula with pus. Which of the following would be effective treatment?
a) Azithromycin, 1 g orally twice daily for 7 days
b) Ceftriaxone, 250 mg intramuscularly once
c) Ciprofloxacin, 500 mg orally once
d) All of the above
e) None of the above

**4.** A 27-year-old woman comes to the office because her boyfriend was recently diagnosed with genital herpes. She is sexually active without condoms, but is asymptomatic. Pelvic examination is normal. She is requesting some type of evaluation for herpes. What is the most appropriate next step?
a) Begin oral acyclovir for 7 to 10 days
b) Tzanck smear of the cervix
c) Glycoprotein G-based HSV serologies
d) HSV nucleic acid testing from blood and cervix

**5.** A 60-year-old woman is seen on referral for a positive VDRL test result. She is asymptomatic, except for mild memory loss. She recalls having had syphilis as a teenager but was never treated. CSF examination shows no white blood cells, normal protein, and normal glucose; the CSF VDRL is nonreactive. How should she be managed next?

a) Erythromycin, 250 mg orally four times daily for 2 weeks
b) Hospitalization and treatment with aqueous crystalline penicillin G at 12 million U intravenously daily for 14 days
c) Benzathine penicillin G, 2.4 million U intramuscularly once
d) Benzathine penicillin G, 2.4 million U intramuscularly each week for 3 weeks

**6.** Which of the following statements about secondary syphilis is false?

a) Rash is the most common clinical manifestation.
b) Erythromycin is the treatment of choice in penicillin-allergic patients.
c) Up to 20% of patients have a genital lesion evident.
d) Nontreponemal test results are almost always positive.

**7.** A 19-year-old sexually active man (HIV-negative) has dysuria and a urethral discharge. He has a new partner. Gram stain of the discharge shows >10 WBCs per oil immersion field. Which of the following statements is false?

a) He should be specifically tested for *C. trachomatis*.
b) He should be specifically tested for *N. gonorrhoeae*.
c) If the patient is unreliable for follow-up, he should be treated with antibiotics empirically.
d) This condition could be caused by HSV.
e) Asymptomatic infection is rare.

**8.** A 19-year-old man presents with a painful urethral discharge. He denies any history of prior STDs. Gram's stain of the discharge shows WBCs with intracellular Gram-negative diplococci. The next step is:

a) No treatment until cultures of the discharge are finalized
b) Ciprofloxacin, 500 mg orally once
c) Ceftriaxone, 125 mg intramuscularly once
d) Ceftriaxone, 250 mg intramuscularly once
e) None of the above

**9.** A 37-year-old man comes to clinic for a urethral discharge. He has recently returned from a vacation in Hawaii, where he had unprotected intercourse with a new female partner. He has a purulent urethral exudate and staining shows Gram-negative intracellular diplococci. He has no antibiotic allergies. A swab of the urethral exudate is submitted for nucleic acid testing for *N. gonorrhoeae* and *C. trachomatis*. Which of the following is *not* appropriate empiric therapy?

a) Ceftriaxone and doxycycline
b) Ofloxacin and doxycycline
c) Cefixime and doxycycline
d) Ceftriaxone and azithromycin

**10.** Which of the following statements is false regarding HPV infection?

a) HPV-6 is the most common type associated with external genital warts.
b) External genital warts are one of the most commonly diagnosed STDs in the United States.
c) Condoms completely protect against HPV transmission.
d) Screening for cervical cancer is recommended in patients with genital warts.

**11.** A 35-year-old woman complains of a several-day history of malodorous vaginal discharge. On pelvic examination, a gray homogeneous discharge is present. Examination of the discharge reveals a pH of 6. Gram's stain shows clue cells. The most likely diagnosis is:

a) Trichomoniasis
b) *C. trachomatis* infection
c) Bacterial vaginosis
d) Yeast vulvovaginitis
e) None of the above

## ANSWERS

**1. c.**

The patient has primary HSV infection. Topical agents have no role in therapy, and intravenous therapy is reserved for patients who experience complications of primary HIV infection, such as pneumonitis, encephalitis, or hepatitis. The patient should receive some form of treatment because therapy partially relieves symptoms and accelerates healing. Newer antivirals are now available as alternatives to acyclovir.

**2. c.**

RPR test results are positive in primary syphilis in only 70% of patients. Thus, a negative RPR result does not rule out the diagnosis. The five options listed constitute the differential possibilities for the syndrome of genital ulcers with regional adenopathy. The three most common etiologies in the United States are HIV, syphilis, and chancroid.

**3. b.**

The correct diagnosis is chancroid. One intramuscular dose of ceftriaxone is a recommended regimen. Azithromycin is another option, but a single dose is sufficient, rather than a 7-day course of therapy. Ciprofloxacin is effective but needs to be given twice daily for 3 days. Finally, erythromycin can be used at a dose of 500 mg orally four times daily for 7 days.

**4. c.**

The CDC has recently advocated the use of type-specific glycoprotein G-based serologic tests for the diagnosis of genital herpes in certain circumstances, particularly in suspected cases that are culture negative. A positive HSV-2 antibody test is indicative of infection with anogenital herpes at some time in the past. The antibody test may be useful in partner evaluation, although pretest counseling is important. The test is not recommended for routine screening in the population but should be available to anyone requesting testing.

**5. d.**

The patient has late-latent syphilis. The recommended therapy is 3 weekly intramuscular doses of benzathine penicillin G. In penicillin-allergic patients, doxycycline or tetracycline should be given for 4 weeks.

**6. b.**

Doxycycline, not erythromycin, is the treatment of choice for secondary syphilis in penicillin-allergic patients. All the other statements are correct. Of note, the presence of the primary chancre should not divert from the diagnosis. The rash can manifest in many different ways, but by the time it is present, nontreponemal test results are positive almost 100% of the time, making the diagnosis relatively easy, if considered.

**7. e.**

Many men and women with urethritis/MPC are minimally symptomatic or asymptomatic. Causative agents include *N. gonorrhoeae*, *C. trachomatis*, HSV, *T. vaginalis*, and *U. urealyticum*. If a patient is unreliable, he should be treated empirically to help prevent further spread of the infection to other sexual partners.

**8. e.**

The patient has gonorrhea. Gram's stain is diagnostic, so there is no need to await culture results. All three listed regimens would work, although the lower dose of ceftriaxone is sufficient. None of the answers is correct as stated, however, because empiric therapy for chlamydial infection should always be used concurrently with antigonococcal therapy.

**9. b.**

This patient has gonococcal urethritis that was likely acquired in Hawaii. Because of an increasing prevalence of quinolone resistant *N. gonorrheoae* in some areas, including Hawaii and California, empiric therapy with ofloxacin or other quinolone is not recommended. The patient should receive ceftriaxone and an agent active against chlamydia.

**10. c.**

Condoms do not completely protect against HPV transmission. Genital warts are one of the most common STDs in the United States. HPV-6 and HPV-11 are considered low-risk and HPV-16 and HPV-18 high-risk for cervical cancer. Thus, all female patients with genital warts should be screened.

**11. c.**

Gram's stain shows clue cells, which are characteristic of BV. Trichomoniasis also can cause an increased vaginal pH, but does not demonstrate clue cells on the wet-mount preparation. Neither of these findings is present in vaginal yeast infections or chlamydial cervicitis.

## SUGGESTED READINGS

### General

Brown TJ, Yen-Moore A, Tyring SK. An overview of sexually transmitted diseases. Part I. *J Am Acad Dermatol* 1999;41:511–532.

Brown TJ, Yen-Moore A, Tyring SK. An overview of sexually transmitted diseases. Part II. *J Am Acad Dermatol* 1999;41:661–677.

Cates W, Jr. Estimates of the incidence and prevalence of sexually transmitted diseases in the United States. American Social Health Association panel. *Sex Trans Dis* 1999;26[Suppl 4]:S2–S7.

Centers for Disease Control and Prevention. Sexually transmitted diseases treatment guidelines. *Morb Mortal Wkly Rep* 2002;51 (RR-6):1–80.

Centers for Disease Control and Prevention. Increases in fluoroquinolone-resistant *Neisseria gonorrhoeae* among men who have sex with men; United States, 2003, and revised recommendations for gonorrhea treatment, 2004. *MMWR* 2004;53(16):335–338.

Czelusta A, Yen-Moore A, Van der Straten M, et al. An overview of sexually transmitted diseases. Part III. Sexually transmitted diseases in HIV-infected patients. *J Am Acad Dermatol* 2000;43:409–432.

### Drugs for Sexually Transmitted Diseases

IDCP guidelines: sexually transmitted diseases, part I. *Infect Dis Clin Pract* 1995;4:407–418.

IDCP guidelines: sexually transmitted diseases, part II. *Infect Dis Clin Pract* 1996;5:6–11.

IDCP guidelines: sexually transmitted diseases, part III. *Infect Dis Clin Pract* 1996;5:85–93.

### Genital Ulcer Disease

DiCarlo RP, Martin DH. The clinical diagnosis of genital ulcer disease in men. *Clin Infect Dis* 1997;25:292–298.

Dillon SM, Cummings M, Rajagopalan S, et al. Prospective analysis of genital ulcer disease in Brooklyn, New York. *Clin Infect Dis* 1997; 24:945–950.

### Herpes Simplex Virus Infection

Diaz-Mitoma F, Sibbald RG, Shafran SD, et al. Oral famciclovir for the suppression of recurrent genital herpes: a randomized, controlled trial. *JAMA* 1998;280:887–892.

Leung DT, Sacks SL. Current recommendations for the treatment of genital herpes. *Drugs* 2000;60:1329–1352.

Marques AR, Straus SE. Herpes simplex type 2 infections—an update. *Adv Intern Med* 2000;45:175–208.

Mertz GJ, Loveless MO, Levin MJ, et al. Oral famciclovir for suppression of recurrent genital herpes simplex virus infection in women: a multicenter, double-blind, placebo-controlled trial. *Arch Intern Med* 1997;157:343–349.

Reitano M, Tyring S, Lang W, et al. Valacyclovir for the suppression of recurrent genital herpes simplex virus infection: a large-scale dose range-finding study. *J Infect Dis* 1998;178:603–610.

Sacks SL, Aoki FY, Diaz-Mitoma F, et al. Patient-initiated, twice daily oral famciclovir for early recurrent genital herpes: a randomized, double-blind multicenter trial. *JAMA* 1996;276:44–49.

Tetrault I, Boivin G. Recent advances in management of genital herpes. *Can Fam Physician* 2000;46:1622–1629.

Wald A. New therapies and prevention strategies for genital herpes. *Clin Infect Dis* 1999;28[Suppl 1]:S4–S13.

Whitley RJ, Kimberlin DW, Roizman B. Herpes simplex viruses. *Clin Infect Dis* 1998;26:541–545.

## Chancroid

Lewis DA. Diagnostic tests for chancroid. *Sex Trans Infect* 2000; 76:137–141.

Mertz KJ, Weiss JB, Webb RM, et al. An investigation of genital ulcers in Jackson, Mississippi, with use of a multiplex polymerase chain reaction assay: high prevalence of chancroid and human immunodeficiency virus infection. *J Infect Dis* 1998; 178:1060–1066.

Schmid GP. Treatment of chancroid, 1997. *Clin Infect Dis* 1999; 28[Suppl 1]:S14–S20.

## Lymphogranuloma Venereum

Heaton ND, Yates-Bell A. Thirty-year follow-up of lymphogranuloma venereum. *Br J Urol* 1992;70:693–694.

## Donovanosis

Hart G. Donovanosis. *Clin Infect Dis* 1997;25:24–32.

## Syphilis

Augenbraun MH, Rolfs R. Treatment of syphilis, 1998: nonpregnant adults. *Clin Infect Dis* 1999;28[Suppl 1]:S21–S28.

Blocker ME, Levine WC, St. Louis ME. HIV prevalence in patients with syphilis, United States. *Sex Trans Dis* 2000;27:53–59.

Clyne B, Jerrard DA. Syphilis testing. *J Emerg Med* 2000;18:361–367.

Genc M, Ledger WJ. Syphilis in pregnancy. *Sex Trans Infect* 2000; 76:73–79.

Larsen SA, Steiner BM, Rudolph AH. Laboratory diagnosis and interpretation of tests for syphilis. *Clin Microbiol Rev* 1995;8:1–21.

Singh AE, Romanowski B. Syphilis: review with emphasis on clinical, epidemiologic, and some biologic features. *Clin Microbiol Rev* 1999;12:187–209.

## Urethritis and Cervicitis

Burstein GR, Zenilman JM. Nongonococcal urethritis: a new paradigm. *Clin Infect Dis* 1999;28[Suppl 1]:S66–S73.

Molodysky E. Urethritis and cervicitis. *Aust Fam Physician* 1999;28: 333–338.

## Chlamydia Infection

Burstein GR, Gaydos CA, Diener-West M, et al. Incident *Chlamydia trachomatis* infections among inner-city adolescent females. *JAMA* 1998;280:521–526.

Fenton KA. Screening men for *Chlamydia trachomatis* infection: have we fully explored the possibilities? *Commun Dis Public Health* 2000;3:86–89.

Howell MR, Quinn TC, Gaydos CA. Screening for *Chlamydia trachomatis* in asymptomatic women attending family planning clinics: a cost-effectiveness analysis of three strategies. *Ann Intern Med* 1998;128:277–284.

Magid D, Douglas JM Jr, Schwartz JS. Doxycycline compared with azithromycin for treating women with genital *Chlamydia trachomatis* infections: an incremental cost-effectiveness analysis. *Ann Intern Med* 1996;12:389–399.

Weber JT, Johnson RE. New treatments for *Chlamydia trachomatis* genital infection. *Clin Infect Dis* 1995;20[Suppl 1]:S66–S71.

## Gonorrhea

Emmert DH, Kirchner JT. Sexually transmitted diseases in women. Gonorrhea and syphilis. *Postgrad Med* 2000;107:189–190,193–197.

Moran JS, Levine WC. Drugs of choice for the treatment of uncomplicated gonococcal infections. *Clin Infect Dis* 1995; 20[Suppl 1]: S47–S65.

Robinson AJ, Ridgway GL. Concurrent gonococcal and chlamydial infection: how best to treat. *Drugs* 2000;59:801–813.

## Human Papillomavirus Infection

Alexander KA, Phelps WC. Recent advances in diagnosis and therapy of human papillomaviruses. *Expert Opinion Invest Drugs* 2000;9: 1753–1765.

Beutner KR, Reitano MV, Richwald GA, et al. External genital warts: report of the American Medical Association consensus conference. *Clin Infect Dis* 1998;27:796–806.

Beutner KR, Wiley DJ, Douglas JM, et al. Genital warts and their treatment. *Clin Infect Dis* 1999;28[Suppl 1]:S37–S56.

Palefsky JM. Human papillomavirus-related tumors. *AIDS* 2000; 14[Suppl 3]:S189–S195.

Severson J, Evans TY, Lee P, et al. Human papillomavirus infections: epidemiology, pathogenesis, and therapy. *J Cutan Med Surg* 2001; 5:43–60.

## Vaginal Infections

Egan ME, Lipsky MS. Diagnosis of vaginitis. *Am Fam Physician* 2000;62:1095–1104.

Haefner HK. Current evaluation and management of vulvovaginitis. *Clin Obstet Gynecol* 1999;42:184–195.

Joesoef MR, Schmid GP, Hillier SL. Bacterial vaginosis: review of treatment options and potential clinical indications for therapy. *Clin Infect Dis* 1999;28[Suppl 1]:S57–S65.

Petrin D, Delgaty K, Bhatt R, et al. Clinical and microbiological aspects of *Trichomonas vaginalis*. *Clin Microbiol Rev* 1998;11: 300–317.

Reef SE, Levine WC, McNeil MM, et al. Treatment options for vulvovaginal candidiasis, 1993. *Clin Infect Dis* 1995;20[Suppl 1]: S80–S90.

Sobel JD. Vaginitis. *N Engl J Med* 1997;337:1896–1903.

Sobel JD. Bacterial vaginosis. *Annu Rev Med* 2000;51:349–346.

# Human Immunodeficiency Virus Infections and Acquired Immunodeficiency Syndrome

# 14

*Wendy S. Armstrong    Alan J. Taege*

The acquired immunodeficiency syndrome (AIDS) is caused by the human immunodeficiency virus (HIV). HIV is a double-stranded RNA retrovirus from the lentivirus family. It primarily targets CD4+ T-helper lymphocytes, thus depleting the immune system and leading to a state of immunodeficiency. As the immune system deteriorates and the CD4+ count approaches 200 cells/mm$^3$, opportunistic infections often occur.

The clinical syndrome of AIDS was first described in 1981, when a cluster of cases of *Pneumocystis carinii* pneumonia (PCP) was noted in a group of homosexual men (1). The causative agent, HIV, was identified in 1984. By 1987, the first medication to treat HIV, azidothymidine (AZT, Retrovir) became available. Currently, 20 medications are available to be utilized in combination cocktails of three or more drugs (highly active antiretroviral therapy, HAART).

Two genetic types of HIV have been identified, HIV-1 and HIV-2. HIV-1 is the predominant type throughout the world. HIV-2 appears to be concentrated in West Africa, with small numbers of cases noted in France, Portugal, Angola, and Mozambique. HIV-2 appears to be less easily transmitted, results in disease that progresses more slowly, and is believed to be less virulent (2,3).

HIV-1 is divided into three subtypes (also referred to as *clades*), designated group M (composed of subtypes A–K), N, and O. HIV-1 in the United States is 98% subtype B (2,3).

## EPIDEMIOLOGY

It is estimated that 40 million people worldwide have been infected with HIV through the end of 2003 (4). The adult population accounts for over 37 million cases, whereas more than 2.5 million are children younger than 15 years of age. The epidemic has claimed nearly 22 million lives since its onset in 1981, of which 4.5 million were children. An estimated 14 million children are orphans because of the epidemic.

Sub-Saharan Africa has borne a disproportionate number of cases of HIV/AIDS, in part attributable to poverty, low educational levels, and social upheaval, which results in medical care that is either unavailable or severely fragmented. This region may have as many as 28 million people living with HIV/AIDS. The epidemic has begun to unfold in China and the former Soviet Union, where the number of active cases is beginning to be realized.

Globally, the most common means of acquiring HIV is through heterosexual contact. All age groups are affected, with the largest number of cases occurring between the ages of 20 and 50 years, the most productive years of life.

Over 900,000 cases of AIDS have been diagnosed in the United States. The vast majority of cases are in adults, whereas less than 10,000 cases have occurred in children. Males comprise 82% of cases; females account for 18%. Over 500,000 people have died of AIDS in the United States. The most common mode of transmission in the United States is male-to-male sexual contact (46%), followed by injection drug use (25%), then heterosexual contact (11%). Mother-to-child transmission (which occurs prenatally, during birth, or postnatally via breast feeding) makes up a small group of cases in the United States. Rare cases occur through transfusion of blood products (5).

Although African Americans constitute slightly more than 12% of the U.S. population, nearly 40% of all cases of HIV/AIDS have occurred in this group (6). In the most recently available statistics, African Americans accounted for 50% of new cases in 2002. From 1999 to 2002, African American females represented 72% of the new cases in the female population (6). Hispanics represent 19% of HIV/AIDS cases. Caucasians account for ~40% of the total. See Tables 14.1–3 for a summary of the statistics.

The age group between 25 and 45 years account for nearly two-thirds of all cases in the United States. A recent alarming trend demonstrates increasing numbers of infections in the 15- to 25-year age group. The majority of cases are clustered along the coastal areas, with major metropolitan areas having the largest numbers of cases. New York, California, Florida, and Texas have 49% of all cases. The

## TABLE 14.1
### HIV INFECTION: GENDER

| | |
|---|---|
| Male | 82% |
| Female | 18% |

## TABLE 14.3
### HIV INFECTION: MODE OF TRANSMISSION

| | |
|---|---|
| MSM | 48% |
| IDU | 27% |
| Heterosexual | 15% |
| MSM/IDU | 7% |
| Other | 3% |

epidemic has steadily infiltrated all areas of the country, however, urban and rural.

## PATHOPHYSIOLOGY

The HIV viruses belong to the lentivirus subfamily of the RNA retroviruses. Like most retroviruses, the HIV genome consists of three structural genes: *gag, pol,* and *env.* The *gag* gene codes for viral capsid proteins, *env* for the viral envelope proteins, and *pol* for the proteins responsible for viral replication, including the RNA-dependent DNA polymerase known as reverse transcriptase. In addition, several other regulatory genes are present, including *nef, rev,* and *tat.*

Most commonly, transmission of the virus occurs after a breach in the integument or mucous membranes. HIV infection occurs when the envelope subunit gp120 binds the human CD4 T-cell receptor, found primarily on lymphocytes and monocyte-derived macrophages. In addition, binding also requires the presence on the host cell of the chemokine receptor CCR5 or CXCR4. The viral envelope then fuses with the host cell, allowing the release of the viral core into the host cell. Viral DNA is synthesized by reverse transcriptase and incorporated into the host genome by the protein integrase. Once the viral gene products are transcribed and assembled, the HIV protease mediates the packaging of new virions for release into serum, thus propagating the infection (7).

Over time, infected persons have a progressive loss of CD4+ lymphocytes, although in the early stages of infection, this is not associated with increased immunosuppression. The rate of CD4+ cell loss is variable and depends on viral and host factors. On average, infected persons lose 40 to 80 cells/mm$^3$ per year (8). A subset of individuals will progress rapidly; however, 5% of infected persons, known as long-term nonprogressors, will have little or no progression of clinical disease or decline in CD4 counts over 10 years, even without antiretroviral therapy (9).

## TABLE 14.2
### HIV INFECTION: ETHNICITY

| | |
|---|---|
| White | 42% |
| African American | 40% |
| Hispanic | 18% |

Transmission of the virus occurs via exposure to infected body fluids. These include blood, semen, and vaginal fluid. The most common modes of transmission are sexual contact (male–male or heterosexual sex), parenteral exposure to blood and blood products, and vertical transmission during pregnancy. The magnitude of risk depends on the exposure. For example, the risk of HIV transmission from a known HIV-positive source from receptive anal intercourse is 0.1% to 0.3%, whereas receptive vaginal intercourse carries a risk per episode of 0.08% to 0.2%. A percutaneous exposure through a needlestick injury or intravenous drug use results in transmission 0.4% or 0.67% of the time respectively (10). The risk of vertical transmission from mother to fetus without any preventive therapy is approximately 25% (11). The efficiency of transmission increases with greater degrees of viremia in the source patient and the presence of concurrent sexually transmitted diseases.

## SIGNS AND SYMPTOMS

### Acute HIV Infection

In an estimated 40% to 90% of individuals, HIV seroconversion is associated with a clinical syndrome known as acute/primary HIV infection or acute retroviral syndrome. In one prospective study, among those with symptoms at the time of seroconversion, 95% sought medical care. Nevertheless, acute HIV infection is rarely diagnosed, partly because the symptoms are protean. The onset of illness is between 2 and 6 weeks after viral transmission and is thought to correlate with peak viremia, often in excess of 1 million viral copies/mL. Fever (mean 38.9° C), rash, lymphadenopathy, and nonexudative pharyngitis are each present in more than 70% of individuals (Table 14.4). Most often, the rash is reminiscent of a viral exanthem, with erythematous maculopapular lesions on the face and trunk, although many types of lesions have been described. Headache with or without cerebrospinal fluid (CSF) pleocytosis, myalgias, and gastrointestinal symptoms are also common. Although present in only 5% to 20% of patients, oral or genital ulcers can be an important diagnostic clue. Laboratory abnormalities, specifically leukopenia, thrombocytopenia, and elevated transaminases are not uncommon. Opportunistic infections, such as mucocutaneous

### TABLE 14.4
#### ACUTE HIV INFECTION: FREQUENCY OF ASSOCIATED SIGNS AND SYMPTOMS

| | |
|---|---|
| Fever – 96% | Headache – 32% |
| Lymphadenopathy – 74% | Nausea and Vomiting – 27% |
| Pharyngitis – 70% | Hepatosplenomegaly – 14% |
| Rash – 70% | Weight Loss – 13% |
| Myalgia or Arthralgia – 54% | Thrush – 12% |
| Diarrhea – 32% | Neurologic Symptoms – 12% |

Adapted with permission from the DHHS Guidelines for the Use of Antiretroviral Agents in HIV-infected Adults and Adolescents, March 23, 2004.

### TABLE 14.5
#### AIDS INDICATOR DISEASES

| | |
|---|---|
| Candidiasis, invasive | Lymphoma: primary CNS, Non-Hodgkin's lymphoma |
| Cervical cancer, invasive | Mycobacterial disease, disseminated or extrapulmonary |
| Coccidioidomycosis, extrapulmonary | |
| Cryptococcosis, extrapulmonary | *Mycobacterium tuberculosis* infection |
| Cryptosporidiosis of >1 mo duration | Nocardiosis |
| Cytomegalovirus disease outside lymphoreticular system | *Pneumocystis carinii* pneumonia |
| Dementia, HIV | Pneumonia, recurrent (>1 episode in 1 yr) |
| Encephalopathy, HIV-related | Progressive multifocal leukoencephalopathy |
| Herpes simplex infection of >1 mo duration or visceral | Strongyloidiasis, extraintestinal |
| *Salmonella* bacteremia, recurrent | Toxoplasmosis, cerebral |
| Histoplasmosis, extrapulmonary | Wasting syndrome due to HIV |
| Isosporiasis of >1 mo duration | |
| Kaposi's sarcoma | |

candidiasis and PCP, may present during acute HIV infection as a result of transient but dramatic CD4 cell count depletion due to the high level of viremia.

The symptoms of acute HIV infection are self-limited and most likely correlate with viremia. After reaching high levels, the viral load declines to a steady state or set point, and the CD4 count recovers. HIV-1–specific cytotoxic T lymphocytes are present in high titer and appear to play an important role in controlling viral replication. The magnitude of the viral set point and the severity of initial symptoms predict disease progression. Some experts advocate early antiretroviral treatment, which may alter the viral set point and slow the progression of disease. Patients treated acutely appear to have a more robust HIV-specific cell-mediated immune response. Recognition of this syndrome has obvious implications for public health but may also impact the individual's disease course (12).

### Chronic HIV Infection

A variety of historical details, findings on physical examination, and laboratory abnormalities should prompt testing to identify individuals with established HIV infection. As expected, these findings are more prominent in patients with more advanced disease. Frequently, the initial diagnosis of HIV infection is made when the patient develops an AIDS-indicator condition (Table 14.5) (13). The astute clinician, however, can often detect signs and symptoms of HIV infection earlier in the course of disease, thus allowing access to appropriate therapy and prophylaxis prior to the development of significant illness.

Physicians must conduct a thorough, nonjudgmental assessment of risk factors for HIV infection. Testing should be offered to individuals with a history of intravenous drug use, sexually transmitted diseases including human papillomavirus (HPV), hemophilia, and receipt of blood products between 1977 and 1985. Men who have had sex with men, sex workers, and heterosexual persons with multiple partners are also at high risk, as are the sexual partners of high-risk or HIV-infected individuals. Mental illness and incarceration may serve as markers for high-risk behavior,

as does a history of hepatitis B or C infection. Persons who consider themselves at risk should receive testing even if risk behaviors are not disclosed.

A history of certain illnesses can also be suggestive of HIV infection (Table 14.5). Infections such as active tuberculosis, recurrent community-acquired pneumonia, esophageal candidiasis, and either multidermatomal herpes zoster or zoster in younger adults should lead to HIV testing. Neoplastic diseases such as B-cell lymphoma, severe anal or cervical dysplasia, or invasive carcinoma and Kaposi's sarcoma are indications for HIV testing, as is idiopathic dilated cardiomyopathy. The evaluation of fever of unknown origin or unexplained weight loss should always include an HIV test, even in elderly patients without identified risk factors.

Various findings on physical examination may suggest coexisting HIV infection. An examination of the skin can be particularly revealing. Seborrheic dermatitis or molluscum contagiosum are common in early disease, as is psoriasis. Oral candidiasis and oral hairy leukoplakia can be seen, typically with CD4 counts less than 500 cells/mm$^3$. Generalized lymphadenopathy is common. Recurrent or severe lesions of HSV may be indicative of underlying HIV infection. Neurologic findings such as unexplained peripheral neuropathy or dementia are suggestive.

On laboratory evaluation, idiopathic thrombocytopenia (ITP), unexplained anemia, neutropenia, and/or leukopenia are frequent early clues to underlying HIV infection.

## DIAGNOSIS

Multiple tests have been developed for the serologic diagnosis of HIV-1 and -2. Samples of blood, urine, and oral secretions have been utilized for testing. The standard approach employs a two-step process using the enzyme linked immunosorbent assay (ELISA or EIA) and the Western blot (WB) (14). Both are designed to detect antibodies to HIV. The EIA is a highly sensitive screening test, which when positive is repeated for verification. A positive EIA is only presumptive evidence of infection by HIV and should never be accepted as a diagnostic confirmation by itself. It must be followed and confirmed by a WB. Most individuals develop a positive EIA approximately 2 weeks after infection, with the vast majority seroconverting in 4 weeks. Currently available rapid screening tests (OraQuick, OraSure, Recombigold, and Reveal) are also EIAs and require WB confirmation. False-positive EIAs occur as a result of cross-reacting antibodies (common HLA antigens), chronic renal failure, malignancies, severe liver disease, vaccination, or autoreactive antibodies (i.e., ANA).

The WB is an immunoblot electrophoretic assay that measures antibodies to the HIV gene products of *env, pol,* and *gag* (including the p24 antigen). A positive study is defined as one in which bands to two of the following three proteins are present: the envelope proteins gp41 and gp120/160 and the viral capsid protein p24. A negative Western blot has no positive bands, but a study with any positive bands that do not meet the above criteria is considered indeterminate. Indeterminate assays are usually caused by nonspecific cross-reacting proteins, HIV-2 infection, pregnancy, transfusions, malignancy, autoimmune diseases, or connective tissue diseases. Indeterminate assays, however, also are seen in early seroconversion. A repeat assay should be performed within 2 to 4 weeks to evaluate the progression or regression of the test result. Repeated indeterminate tests are common. In a low-risk population, these results are usually of no clinical consequence. When in doubt, an expert in the field of HIV disease should be consulted (15).

## INITIAL EVALUATION

The last decade of advances in therapy and care have allowed us to view HIV as a chronic condition. As such, the initial encounter should be an important data gathering session but also an opportunity to establish a long-term relationship with the patient. The initial evaluation should include a very detailed comprehensive history and physical examination, coupled with appropriate lab and x-ray tests.

The history should include all the basics of any thorough medical history. In addition, focus should be directed to common HIV-related symptoms of unexplained fevers, night sweats, weight loss, skin rashes and lesions, diarrhea, weight loss, oral or vaginal candida, oral ulcers, shingles, neurologic symptoms (i.e., neuropathy), changes in mental status, or symptoms of depression.

A nonjudgmental careful sexual history is necessary and includes sexual practices, number and type of partners, use of condoms, and previous or current sexually transmitted

diseases. It is also important to know if the patient's sexual partners have been notified. This information may provide an important avenue for the education of the patient, partner, and family of the patient.

Intravenous drug users should be asked about needle sharing and their sexual partners. Appropriate education, counseling, and rehabilitation should be offered.

Travel and residential history may be pertinent. Those living in endemic geographic locales may be at risk for various infections (histoplasmosis in the Ohio and Mississippi River valleys or coccidiodomycosis in the southwest United States).

A routine vaccination history should be recorded. Previous testing for hepatitis A, B, or C or the administration of hepatitis vaccines should be noted. Knowledge of previous chickenpox or vaccination status is also important when considering the risk of varicella or herpes zoster.

Previous PPD testing and tuberculosis exposure or treatment should be included in the record. Because of the increased risk of acquisition and reactivation, annual PPD skin tests are recommended. A positive test in an HIV-infected individual is ≥5 mm.

Throughout the interview, the knowledge base of the patient should be noted and educational needs assessed, with subsequent planning to address these needs.

The physical examination also must be thorough. Specific HIV-related findings should be sought. The skin examination may reveal seborrheic dermatitis, Kaposi's sarcoma (KS), psoriasis, or extensive folliculitis. Evidence of cytomegalovirus retinitis on fundoscopic examination suggests advanced disease. If the examiner does not feel adept at fundoscopy, referral to an ophthalmologist is appropriate. Oral findings may include thrush, KS, aphthous ulcers, or oral hairy leukoplakia (OHL). Dental hygiene and dental health should be noted, with appropriate care or referral planned. The size and location of enlarged lymph nodes are important because varying degrees of generalized lymphadenopathy are common in HIV. Focal lymphadenopathy that persists or enlarges, however, may require further evaluation. Pelvic and rectal examination should be directed toward evidence of candidiasis, sexually transmitted diseases, or malignancy. All women should have PAP tests performed because there exists a higher rate of cervical dysplasia, carcinoma in situ, and frank cervical carcinoma than in the general population. Two normal PAP tests should be obtained 6 months apart, then annual testing is routine. All abnormalities should be pursued aggressively.

Laboratory testing is an important aspect of the evaluation of an HIV-positive patient. Table 14.6 lists those baseline tests that are recommended. If the patient presents with an anonymous HIV test result, it may be appropriate to repeat and confirm the serology.

The CBC may reveal the typical lymphocytopenia of HIV but may also disclose HIV-related leukopenia, thrombocytopenia, or anemia. All are common. Nutritional status

## TABLE 14.6

### THE INITIAL EVALUATION: LABORATORY TESTING

| | |
|---|---|
| CBC with diff | CD4+ count |
| Chemistry | HIV viral load |
| RPR | HIV genotype |
| Urinalysis | CMV IgG |
| Hepatitis A,B,C serologies | Toxoplasma IgG |
| G-6-PD* | Lipid profile |

* When indicated.

(albumin) or evidence of hepatitis (AST/ALT) may be noted on the chemistry panel. Underlying renal insufficiency may be evident and influence subsequent drug therapy and evaluation.

RPR and hepatitis serologies (A, B, and C) are necessary because syphilis and hepatitis are more common in this population. If the RPR or VDRL is positive, an FTA-Abs should be performed. If active syphilis is diagnosed, the administration of appropriate therapy should follow. Evidence of active hepatitis may require therapy for hepatitis B or C. If no evidence exists for hepatitis A or B, vaccination is recommended.

Baseline lipid profiles are important because HIV disease should be viewed as a long-term condition, and lipid screening is a routine aspect of healthcare and maintenance. In addition, certain HIV medications are associated with lipid elevations, often requiring dietary intervention and medical therapy for control.

A knowledge of the CD4+ count and HIV viral load are important prognostic indicators. Patients with high viral loads (typically >100,000 copies/mm$^3$) and low CD4+ counts experience a more rapid progression of their disease and more frequent complications. The CD4+ count is also used for staging purposes (Table 14.7). The numerical aspect of staging is determined by the CD4+ cell count (1: CD4 ≥500, 2: CD4 = 200–499 and 3: CD4 <200), whereas the letter designations of A, B, or C refer to symptoms associated with HIV disease or indicator illnesses. Category A patients are asymptomatic, whereas category C patients have experi-

enced an AIDS indicator condition (Table 14.5). Most, but not all, AIDS indicator conditions occur when the CD4+ count drops below 200 cells/mm$^3$. By definition, a CD4+ count of 200/mm$^3$ is an AIDS indicator event. Category B patients are symptomatic but have not experienced an AIDS indicator condition. Category B patients may have herpes zoster, persistent or recurrent thrush, persistent or recurrent vaginal candidiasis, constitutional symptoms, prolonged unexplained diarrhea (>1 month), ITP, OHL, cervical dysplasia, or neuropathy. Some degree of variation may be noted in CD4+ counts and viral loads between testing sessions, as well as between laboratories. It is important to establish a trend with respect to counts and to attempt to utilize the same laboratory for testing.

Newly infected patients are increasingly acquiring drug-resistant virus. Currently, a baseline HIV genotype is recommended to evaluate for the presence of drug resistance mutations in all newly diagnosed patients in whom recent infection is suspected. This information may be used to guide current or future drug therapy.

## THERAPY

The appropriate treatment of the HIV-infected individual requires much more than a consideration of antiretroviral therapy. Preventive care is essential to treating the HIV-infected patient. Some infections can be minimized by avoiding uncooked and undercooked foods such as seafood, eggs, and meats, abstaining from drinking lake and river water, avoiding contact with animals with diarrhea and litter boxes, and the institution of careful handwashing. All patients should receive the pneumococcal vaccine, updated every 3 to 6 years. The influenza vaccine is recommended, as is hepatitis B vaccination if the patient is seronegative. Although hepatitis A vaccination is indicated if the patient has existing hepatitis B or C, most practitioners favor vaccinating all seronegative individuals. Tetanus boosters are indicated every 10 years. At present, live vaccines are not recommended in patients with advanced disease. The safety of these vaccines, which include varicella, measles-mumps-rubella (MMR), and yellow fever, early in disease is unknown and can be considered individually. The inactivated vaccines for typhoid (Typhim Vi CPS) and polio (IPV) should be administered when required, rather than the live vaccines (16).

The identification of a durable power of attorney and a discussion of advanced directives is valuable early in disease. Annual ophthalmologic and dental visits are recommended. Consultation with a nutritionist experienced in HIV care and a social worker are beneficial.

Patients with advanced HIV disease require prophylaxis to prevent opportunistic infections (Table 14.8). At CD4 counts less than 200 cells/mm$^3$ or CD4+ <14, *P. carinii* prophylaxis should be initiated promptly because the incidence

## TABLE 14.7

### CDC HIV CLINICAL STAGING

| CD4+ Count (mm$^3$) | Asymptomatic | Symptomatic | AIDS Indicator |
|---|---|---|---|
| ≥500 | A1 | B1 | C1 |
| 200–499 | A2 | B2 | C2 |
| <200 | A3 | B3 | C3 |

## TABLE 14.8
### PRIMARY PROPHYLAXIS AGAINST OPPORTUNISTIC INFECTIONS

| Pathogen | Indication | Drug of Choice | Alternatives |
|---|---|---|---|
| Pneumocystis carinii | CD4 count <200/μL or oropharyngeal candidiasis | TMP-SMZ, 1 SS, or DS tablet daily | Dapsone, pyrimethamine, leucovorin, aerosol pentamidine, atovaquone, TMP-SMZ 3 × week |
| Mycobacterium tuberculosis[a,b] | TST positive (5 mm) or prior positive TST without treatment or contact with active case | INH, 300 mg daily, plus pyridoxine, 50 mg daily, for 9 mo; INH, 900 mg, plus pyridoxine, 100 mg 2 × week for 9 mo; or rifampin, 600 mg, plus pyrazinamide, 15–20 mg/kg, daily for 2 mo[c] | Rifabutin, 300 mg, plus pyrazinamide, 15–20 mg/kg, daily for 2 mo; or rifampin, 600 mg daily, for 4 mo |
| INH-resistant M. tuberculosis | Same as above; high probability of exposure to INH-resistant tuberculosis | Rifampin, 600 mg, plus pyrazinamide, 20 mg/kg, daily for 2 mo[c] | Rifabutin plus pyrazinamide daily for 2 mo; or rifampin or rifabutin daily for 4 mo |
| Toxoplasma gondii | CD4 count <100/μL and IgG antibodies to Toxoplasma | TMP-SMZ, 1 DS tablet, daily | Low-dose TMP-SMZ; dapsone plus pyrimethamine plus leucovorin; atovaquone pyrimethamine plus leucovorin daily |
| Mycobacterium avium complex[b] | CD4 count <50/μL | Clarithromycin, 500 mg b.i.d., or azithromycin, 1,200 mg, weekly | Rifabutin daily or azithromycin weekly plus rifabutin daily |
| Varicella zoster virus | Significant exposure in seronegative patient or patient with no history of chickenpox or shingles | VZIG, 5 vials IM, .96 h after exposure | None |

INH, isoniazid; TMP-SMZ, trimethoprim-sulfamethoxazole; TST, tuberculin skin test; VZIG, varicella-zoster immunoglobulin.

[a] Consult USPHS/IDSA document for recommendations on prophylaxis of INH-resistant or multidrug-resistant M. tuberculosis. Modified with permission from Centers for Disease Control and Prevention.

[b] Pharmacokinetic interactions may occur when rifampin, rifabutin, or clarithromycin are administered concurrently with protease inhibitors or non-nucleoside reverse transcriptase inhibitors.

[c] Because of potential liver injury, the 9-month daily INH regimen is preferred unless the patient has been exposed to an INH-resistant strain or is unlikely to complete the course of therapy. Use the 2-month regimen with caution, especially in patients taking other medications associated with liver injury and those with alcoholism.

Modified with permission from Draft 2001 USPHS/IDSA guidelines for the prevention of opportunistic infections in persons infected with human immunodeficiency virus. http://www.aidsinfo.nih.gov/guidelines/op_infections/OI_112801.pdf, accessed 9/13/04. Dosing modifications may be indicated for individuals with renal or hepatic dysfunction.

of disease approaches 20% per year. The first-line agent is trimethoprim-sulfamethoxazole (TMP-SMX), one double-strength tablet daily. Dapsone (100 mg/day) is recommended for patients who are TMP-SMX intolerant and not G6PD deficient. When the CD4 count falls below 100 cells/mm³, patients with positive T. gondii IgG serologies require prophylaxis to prevent reactivation. Daily TMP-SMX is again the drug of choice. Patients on dapsone require the addition of pyrimethamine. Although Mycobacterium avium complex (MAC) prophylaxis is recommended at CD4 counts below 50 cells/mm³, initiation is never emergent and active MAC disease should be ruled out prior to starting prophylaxis if the patient has any suggestive symptoms. The most common regimen is azithromycin 1,200 mg/week. More detailed information can be obtained from the USPHS/IDSA guidelines for the prevention of opportunistic infections (16).

## ANTIRETROVIRAL THERAPY

During the past decade, the selection of highly active antiretroviral therapy (HAART) has become increasingly complex. The ideal time to start HAART therapy remains undefined. Many studies confirm that poorer outcomes are seen when antiretroviral therapy is initiated after the CD4+ T-cell count falls below 200 cells/mm³. The appropriate time to initiate therapy prior to this, however, remains in doubt. All patients with symptomatic HIV disease should be offered HAART. Current DHHS recommendations (2004) suggest that treatment should be offered to asymptomatic individuals with CD4+ T cells between 200 cells/mm³ and 350 cells/ mm³, regardless of viral load but acknowledge that this remains controversial. They also note that some experienced clinicians recommend initiating therapy in those with CD4+ T-cell counts above 350 cells/mm³ and with viral loads above 55,000 copies/cc. In general, recent guidelines suggest initiating HAART later than previously recommended, due to the emerging problems of drug resistance and medication side effects, coupled with uncertain benefit. Most importantly, the decision to start HAART must be individualized in every case. Factors including the rate of CD4 T cell decline or viral load increase and the readiness of the patient to initiate therapy are critical. Often, the decision to start therapy should be delayed in those with untreated depression or substance abuse. Because the guidelines and expert opinion change regularly based on ongoing studies, interested individuals should review the most current set of guidelines (17).

Currently four different antiretroviral drug classes are licensed: nucleoside/nucleotide reverse transcriptase inhibitors (NRTIs), non-nucleoside reverse transcriptase inhibitors (NNRTIs), protease inhibitors (PIs), and a single fusion inhibitor (Table 14.9). The NRTIs are nucleoside/nucleotide analogues and act as chain terminators that impair the process of reverse transcription of viral

## TABLE 14.9
### CURRENTLY AVAILABLE ANTIRETROVIRAL AGENTS (2004)

**Nucleoside Reverse Transcriptase Inhibitors**
Zidovudine (AZT, Retrovir)
Didanosine (ddI, Videx)
Zalcitabine (ddC, Hivid)
Lamivudine (3TC, Epivir)
Stavudine (d4T, Zerit)
Abacavir (ABC, Ziagen)
Emtricitabine (FTC, Emtriva)

**Nucleotide Reverse Transcriptase Inhibitors**
Tenofovir (TDF, Viread)

**Non-Nucleoside Reverse Transcriptase Inhibitors (NNRTI)**
Nevirapine (Viramune)
Delavirdine (Rescriptor)
Efavirenz (Sustiva)

**Protease Inhibitors**
Ritonavir (Norvir)
Indinavir (Crixivan)
Saquinavir (Invirase, Fortovase)
Nelfinavir (Viracept)
Amprenavir (Agenerase)
Fosamprenavir (Lexiva)
Atazanavir (Reyataz)
Lopinavir/ritonavir (Kaletra)

**Fusion Inhibitor**
Enfuvirtide (T20, Fuzeon)

**Combination Pills**
Combivir (zidovudine/lamivudine)
Trizivir (zidovudine/lamivudine/abacavir)
Epzicom (abacavir/lamivudine)
Truvada (tenofovir/emtricitabine)

RNA into DNA. The NNRTIs inhibit reverse transcriptase by binding the RT enzyme-preventing function. The PIs impair the packaging of viral particles into a mature virion capable of budding from the cell and productively infecting additional T lymphocytes. Finally, the fusion inhibitor impairs membrane fusion of the HIV virion to the T cell, thus preventing initial infection of the lymphocyte. Agents in additional classes are in development, including chemokine receptor antagonists and other entry inhibitors as well as integrase inhibitors. Initial therapy should always include a minimum of three agents, and no single regimen is appropriate for all patients. Recommended first-line regimens include two NRTIs and either an NNRTI or a PI. Regimens containing triple NRTIs have been shown to have higher rates of virologic failure and therefore are not recommended as first-line therapy, except in the rare instances when an NNRTI- or PI-containing regimen cannot or should not be used. The DHHS guidelines currently indicate that the preferred NNRTI-containing regimen is efavirenz + lamivudine + zidovudine (or tenofovir or stavudine), except in those who are or may become pregnant. The preferred PI-based regimen is lopinavir/ritonavir + lamivudine + zidovudine or stavudine. Many other regimens are acceptable alternatives. Currently available protease inhibitors, with the exception of nelfinavir, are frequently prescribed in combination with low-dose ritonavir, a technique known as *boosting*. Ritonavir is a potent inhibitor of the CYP3A4 isoenzyme that is part of the cytochrome P450 system of hepatic metabolism. All PIs are substrates of this enzyme. As a result, low-dose ritonavir increases the trough and prolongs the half-life of the coadministered PI, thus enhancing the drug exposure and allowing for less frequent dosing. Many experts now believe that all first-line PI-containing regimens should now utilize ritonavir boosted PIs (17,18).

The response to therapy should be carefully monitored. Patients on initial regimens should achieve undetectable viral loads 16 to 24 weeks after initiating therapy. Viral loads should be followed every 4 to 8 weeks immediately after starting the regimen, however. Failure to achieve an undetectable viral load or a rebound in plasma viremia after reaching this goal should lead to a careful assessment of the reasons for virologic failure. These considerations should include nonadherence, decreased drug absorption, drug-drug interactions altering drug metabolism, and the development of resistance. Resistance testing should be performed if alternative reasons for virologic failure are not apparent. The most critical and modifiable factor affecting success is patient adherence. Only 45% of patients taking 90% to 95% of their prescribed doses of antiretroviral medications will achieve viral suppression (<400 copies/cc) compared to 78% in those taking more than 95% of their doses (19). Incomplete viral suppression leads to the development of drug resistance. Adherence to the antiviral regimen should be addressed at every visit with every physician

| TABLE 14.10 | | | |
|---|---|---|---|
| **SELECTED COMMON ADVERSE EVENTS (AEs) DUE TO ANTIRETROVIRAL AGENTS, INCLUDING AEs UNIQUE TO SELECTED AGENTS AND AEs COMMON ACROSS MEMBERS OF THE CLASS** | | | |
| Nucleoside and Nucleotide Reverse Transcriptase Inhibitors (NRTIs) | Zidovudine (AZT,ZDV) | Anemia, neutropenia | Lactic acidosis with hepatic steatosis, lipodystrophy* |
| | Didanosine (ddI) | Peripheral neuropathy, pancreatitis | |
| | Zalcitabine (ddC) | Peripheral neuropathy | |
| | Stavudine (d4T) | Peripheral neuropathy | |
| | Lamivudine (3TC) | | |
| | Abacavir (ABC) | Hypersensitivity syndrome | |
| | Tenofovir (TDF) | | |
| | Emtricitabine (FTC) | | |
| Non-Nucleoside Reverse Transcriptase Inhibitors (NNRTIs) | Nevirapine | Hepatitis | Rash |
| | Delavirdine | | |
| | Efavirenz | CNS symptoms | |
| Protease Inhibitors (PIs) | Indinavir | Nephrolithiasis | Lipodystrophy*, GI intolerance, hyperglycemia, lipid abnormalities |
| | Ritonavir | | |
| | Nelfinavir | | |
| | Saquinavir | | |
| | Amprenavir | | |
| | Fosamprenavir | | |
| | Atazanavir** | | |
| | Lopinavir/Ritonavir | | |

* The role of various antiretroviral agents in the development of lipodystrophy is not fully understood.
** Lipid abnormalities appear to be less prominent with this agent.
Adapted with permission from the DHHS Guidelines for the Use of Antiretroviral Agents in HIV-infected Adults and Adolescents, March 23, 2004.

in a detailed fashion, and the importance of careful adherence should be stressed.

The clinician must also be aware of side effects and toxicities that may occur due to the prescribed antiretroviral medications (Table 14.10). The most common and potentially serious include:

- Cytopenias, with the use of zidovudine
- Pancreatitis, with the use of didanosine
- Peripheral neuropathy, with the use of didanosine and stavudine
- Hypersensitivity including rash, fever, and risk of death with re-exposure to abacavir
- Rash, with the use of all NNRTIs
- Hepatitis, with the use of nevirapine
- Nephrolithiasis, with the use of indinivir
- GI toxicity, including diarrhea and nausea, with the use of all protease inhibitors

More recently appreciated are the metabolic abnormalities that can occur in patients taking HAART. Hyperglycemia, hypercholesterolemia, and hypertriglyceridemia should be carefully monitored and treated (with attention to interactions between the protease inhibitors and many HMG CoA reductase inhibitors). Fat distribution abnormalities (lipodystrophy) are frequently noted, including wasting of the limbs and face (lipoatrophy) and enlargement of the dorsocervical fat pad and central obesity (fat accumulation). An increased risk of osteopenia and aseptic joint necrosis has been noted. Nucleoside analogues, again notably stavudine, didanosine, and zidovudine, can lead to mitochondrial dysfunction due to the inhibition of mitochondrial $\gamma$-DNA polymerase. Likely the etiology of lipoatrophy and other effects, mitochondrial dysfunction can also lead to potentially fatal lactic acidosis with hepatic steatosis. Early symptoms of this syndrome are protean and include fatigue, abdominal pain and bloating, nausea and vomiting, tachypnea, and parasthesias. Elevated lactate levels establish the diagnosis; however, transaminase elevations may be suggestive. Treatment requires the discontinuation of the inciting drugs. In addition, significant drug interactions can occur between antiretroviral agents and commonly prescribed drugs; these interactions can lead either to drug toxicities or a reduction in levels of the drug or the antiretroviral agent, thus rendering them ineffective. For a complete listing of adverse effects, toxicities, and medication interactions, please refer to the DHHS Adult/Adolescent Guidelines (17).

## SPECIAL CIRCUMSTANCES: PREGNANCY

Pregnant women who are HIV-infected pose special treatment challenges. The risks of antiretroviral medications to the fetus are not fully known for all available agents. Most experts believe that, with a few exceptions as noted below, the benefits of therapy to the mother and the reduction in the risk of vertical transmission to the infant outweigh the risks of antiretroviral therapy. Currently, antiretroviral medications that are avoided in pregnancy include efavirenz (due to the occurrence of birth defects in monkeys) and the combination of stavudine and didanosine (increased risks of mitochondrial toxicity in pregnancy). Recent data suggest that there may be an increased risk of hepatotoxicity or Stevens-Johnson syndrome in pregnant women with preserved CD4 cell counts. The greatest amount of data in pregnancy exists for zidovudine, and it should be included as part of the treatment regimen when feasible.

Delivery by cesarean section at 38 weeks is recommended for women if the plasma viral load late in pregnancy exceeds 1,000 copies/cc. Current data suggest that women with viral loads below this level appear to have equivalent risks of mother-to-child transmission regardless of mode of delivery; that rate is <1%. All HIV-infected women should receive intravenous zidovudine during labor (or as a continuous infusion, beginning with a loading dose prior to planned cesarean section), and the infant should receive zidovudine for 6 weeks after birth. Women declining HAART in the second and third trimester should be encouraged to take zidovudine at a minimum, although single-drug therapy does increase the risk of developing resistant virus in the mother and potentially transmitting resistant virus to the infant. When used alone, this three-part zidovudine regimen has been shown to reduce the risk of mother-to-child transmission from 23% to 8% (20).

## SPECIAL CIRCUMSTANCES: POSTEXPOSURE PROPHYLAXIS

Limited data suggest that treatment with antiretroviral medications immediately after exposure to potentially infectious material from an HIV-infected source may reduce the risk of seroconversion in the exposed individual. The data largely is derived from a single retrospective cohort study of zidovudine prophylaxis after occupational exposures. In this study, however, the risk of transmission was reduced by 81%. Animal data, scientific theory, and mother-to-child transmission studies all support the concept that antiretroviral therapy may be beneficial. Currently established guidelines have been established for occupational exposures, and extrapolation of these concepts to nonoccupational exposures is left to the treating physicians.

Exposures are evaluated based on risk of the exposure. Percutaneous exposures carry a greater risk of transmission than mucus membrane exposures. Exposures resulting from a deep injury, from a device on which blood was either visible, or from a device that had been in the source patient's artery or vein also carry a greater risk of seroconversion. Fluids from source patients with advanced disease, as measured by disease activity or viremia, place the exposed worker at greater risk than those from lower-risk individuals.

Based on these criteria, the exposure is rated as either a more or less severe percutaneous or mucus membrane exposure from a higher- or lower-risk source patient. Individuals sustaining percutaneous exposures or high-volume mucus membrane exposures from high-risk patients or severe percutaneous exposures from lower-risk patients are offered a three-drug prophylaxis regimen. Those with less severe percutaneous exposures or high-volume mucus membrane exposures from lower-risk patients or small-volume mucus membrane exposures from high-risk patients are offered two-drug prophylactic regimens. Individuals with small-volume mucus membrane exposures from low-risk patients can consider a two-drug regimen. The most common two-drug regimen offered is zidovudine + lamivudine. The expanded three-drug regimen may include a PI or efavirenz. The regimen should be initiated as soon as possible, ideally within 1 hour of the exposure, and continued for 28 days. Baseline HIV serologic tests should be obtained. Follow-up testing at 6 weeks, 3 months, and 6 months is recommended. Expert consultation should be sought if the source patient is known to have drug-resistant virus (21).

## VACCINES

Vaccines have been one of the most effective means of combating and controlling infectious diseases. An extensive effort is under way to find such a treatment for HIV. Despite several vaccine trials evaluating both therapeutic and preventative vaccines, none has been found effective to date. Critical to this effort are ongoing attempts to seek an understanding of the basic immune correlates of protection from HIV. In addition, methods must be developed to deal with the marked genetic variability between different strains of HIV. Vaccines appear to hold the most promise for the world as a whole in conquering the HIV epidemic. Unfortunately, none appears to be on the horizon at this time.

## OPPORTUNISTIC INFECTIONS (OIs)

Many uncommon infections may occur in HIV patients as the disease progresses and cell-mediated immunity deteriorates. Table 14.11 lists the more common OIs. As noted, toxoplasmosis, MAC, and PCP are targeted for primary prophylaxis (no evidence of active disease, but the patient is at risk). Secondary prophylaxis (ongoing treatment after acute infection has been diagnosed and treated) is indicated for PCP, toxoplasmosis, MAC, cryptococcosis, CMV, histoplasmosis, and coccidiodomycosis. Although various OIs have

## TABLE 14.11
### COMMON OPPORTUNISTIC INFECTIONS

| | |
|---|---|
| PCP | CMV |
| Candida | MAC |
| HSV | *Cryptococcus neoformans* |
| HHV-8 | *Histoplasma capsulatum* |
| *Toxoplasma gondii* | JC virus |

## TABLE 14.12
### CD4+ CELL COUNT AND OPPORTUNISTIC INFECTIONS

| CD4+/mm$^3$ | Infection/complication |
|---|---|
| <500 | VZV, oral candida, tuberculosis, HSV, KS (HHV-8) |
| <200 | PCP, severe mucocutaneous HSV |
| <100 | Toxoplasmosis, cryptococcosis, MAC, CMV, microsporidiosis |
| <50 | PML, cryptosporidiosis |

occurred at higher CD4+ counts, most begin when the CD4 count approaches 200 cells/mm$^3$. Table 14.12 lists OIs and the typical level of CD4+ count at which they are known to occur with increased frequency. With the arrival of HAART and subsequent improvement of the immune system through control of the virus (immune reconstitution), it has become possible to discontinue the use of primary and secondary prophylactic medications. Table 14.13 reviews the UPHS/IDSA guidelines for starting and stopping primary and secondary prophylaxis (16).

A detailed discussion of all OIs is beyond the intent of this chapter. A brief overview of the salient aspects of the presentation and diagnosis of PCP, toxoplasmosis, MAC, and cryptococcosis follows.

## PNEUMOCYSTIS CARINII PNEUMONIA (PCP)

PCP is the most common pulmonary infection in HIV patients, typically occurring when the CD4+ T cell count approaches 200 cells/mm$^3$ or less. Although the organism exists in cyst, tachyzoite, and sporozoite forms, it is taxonomically most closely associated with the fungi. Symptoms are nonspecific, insidious in onset, and include shortness of breath, dyspnea, nonproductive cough, fever, chest tightness, fatigue, and weight loss. The chest radiograph most commonly demonstrates interstitial infiltrates, although it may be normal in 20% of cases (22). Spontaneous pneumothoraces may occur. Laboratory tests are of little assistance in the diagnosis. The serum lactate dehydrogenase (LDH) may be elevated but is nonspecific. An exercise desaturation test may reveal exercise-induced hypoxia, which may aid in the diagnosis of PCP. The diagnosis is based upon clinical suspicion and the demonstration of the organisms on silver stain or by other means in the laboratory. Open-lung biopsy has been the gold standard, but more commonly bronchoscopy and bronchoalveolar lavage (BAL) are utilized, with yields of nearly 100% (23). Expectorated or induced sputum samples generally have variable yields that are inferior to BAL. Treatment is trimethoprim-sulfamethoxazole for 3 weeks. If the PO$_2$ is less than 70 mm Hg, a tapering dose of prednisone is recommended, starting at 40 mg twice daily. Alternate therapies include pentamidine and dapsone or trimethoprim. When acute therapy has been completed, secondary prophylaxis should be initiated.

## TABLE 14.13
### INITIATION AND DISCONTINUATION OF PRIMARY PROPHYLAXIS

| Pathogen | Criteria for Initiation | Criteria for Discontinuation | Criteria for Restarting |
|---|---|---|---|
| *Pneumocystis carinii* pneumonia | CD4+ <200 cells/μL or oropharyngeal candidiasis | CD4+ >200 cells/μL for ≥3 months | CD4+ <200 cells/μL |
| Toxoplasmosis | CD4 count <100/μL or IgG antibody to toxoplasma | CD4+ >200 cells/μL for ≥3 months | CD4 <100–200 cells/μL |
| Disseminated *Mycobacterium avium* complex | CD4 count <50/μL | CD4+ >100 cells/μL for ≥3 months | CD4 <100–200 cells/μL |

Modified with permission from Draft 2001USPHS/IDSA guidelines for the prevention of opportunistic infections in persons infected with human immunodeficiency virus. http://www.aidsinfo.nih.gov/guidelines/op_infections/OI_112801.pdf. Accessed September 13, 2004.

## TOXOPLASMA ENCEPHALITIS

*Toxoplasma gondii* is an obligate intracellular parasite. The cat is the definitive host, whereas humans and other animals are secondary hosts. It is the most common cause of intracerebral lesions in HIV patients (24) and usually presents as encephalitis.

The clinical presentation is subacute and may include subtle progressive changes in mental status or neuropsychiatric function, focal motor weakness, coma, and seizures. Neuroimaging is very important in the diagnosis and characteristically reveals multiple intracranial ring-enhancing lesions with surrounding edema. The lesions have a predilection for the basal ganglia. The differential diagnosis of toxoplasmosis includes CNS lymphoma, histoplasmoma, cryptococcoma, tuberculoma, bacterial abscesses, or metastatic carcinoma. A lumbar puncture often yields a nonspecific elevation of protein, minimal change in glucose, and mild mononuclear pleocytosis. Nearly all patients have a positive toxoplasma IgG serology, indicating prior exposure and subsequent risk for reactivation. Where available, PCR of the CSF for toxoplasma may be helpful. The demonstration of organisms on brain biopsy makes a definitive diagnosis, but biopsy is reserved for those cases that do not appear to respond to treatment or that have a negative baseline toxoplasma serology. First-line therapy of toxoplasmic encephalitis is pyrimethamine, sulfadiazine, and folinic acid. Alternative therapies include TMP-SMX, clindamycin, or other macrolides combined with pyrimethamine. Initial treatment for 3 to 6 weeks is followed by secondary prophylaxis.

## CRYPTOCOCCOSIS

*Cryptococcus neoformans* is an encapsulated dimorphic fungus that is ubiquitous in nature, found in the soil and in high concentrations in pigeon feces. It is the most common cause of meningitis in HIV patients. Cryptococcal infections occur as CD4+ counts approach $\leq$100 cells/mm$^3$.

The clinical presentation is often subtle, with fever and headache. Meningoencephalitis may occur with altered mental status, headache, and fever. Despite a high burden of organisms, the inflammatory response is muted or absent. The CSF will usually have elevated protein, decreased glucose, and a pleocytosis that seems minor for the degree of disease present. The serum and CSF cryptococcal antigen and fungal culture are the best diagnostic tools. The CSF antigen will be present in >90% of cases of meningitis, and the serum antigen will be present in 94% to 100% of cases (25).

Treatment for 10 weeks starting with amphotericin B 0.7 mg/kg/day for 2 weeks, followed by fluconazole 400 mg daily is recommended (26). Flucytosine may be added to the first 2 weeks of therapy. Initial therapy is followed by fluconazole prophylaxis. Alternatively, fluconazole may be used for the entire course of therapy.

## MYCOBACTERIUM AVIUM COMPLEX (MAC)

MAC is a rapid-growing mycobacterium that presents as a disseminated disease in advanced HIV, typically at CD4+ counts of <100/mm$^3$. The clinical syndrome is nonspecific, with a combination of several symptoms and findings that may include wasting, fever, night sweats, anorexia, diarrhea, enlarged liver and spleen, central and peripheral lymph node enlargement, or anemia. The organism may be cultured from blood, bone marrow, stool, lymph nodes, or liver biopsy. Although an elevated serum alkaline phosphatase is a nonspecific laboratory finding, it is frequently noted with MAC infection. The burden of organisms in the various tissues is usually massive. Prolonged therapy is necessary and includes at a minimum clarithromycin or azithromycin with ethambutol.

## NATIONAL GUIDELINES

The following guidelines are all available at http://AIDSinfo.nih.gov/guidelines:

■ DHHS Guidelines for the Use of Antiretroviral Agents in HIV-infected Adults and Adolescents, March 23, 2004.
■ Public Health Service Task Force Recommendations for the Use of Antiretroviral Drugs in Pregnant HIV-1 Infected Women for Maternal Health and Interventions to Reduce Perinatal HIV-1 Transmission in the United States, June 23, 2004.
■ NPHRC/HRSA/NIH Guidelines for the Use of Antiretroviral Agents in Pediatric HIV Infection, January 20, 2004.
■ 2001 USPHS/IDSA Guidelines for the Prevention of Opportunistic Infections in Persons Infected with Human Immunodeficiency Virus, U.S. Public Health Service and Infectious Diseases Society of America, November 28, 2001.
■ Updated U.S. Public Health Guidelines for Management of Occupational Exposure to HBV, HCV, and HIV and Recommendations for Postexposure Prophylaxis, June 29, 2001.

## REFERENCES

1. Pneumocystis pneumonia—Los Angeles. *MMWR* 1981;30:250–252.
2. Markovitz DM. Infections with human immunodeficiency virus type 2. *Ann Intern Med* 1993;118:211–218.
3. Weidle PJ, Ganea CE, Irwin KL, et al. Presence of human immunodeficiency (HIV) type 1, group M, non-B subtypes, Bronx, New York: a sentinel site for monitoring HIV genetic diversity in the United States. *J Infect Dis* 2000;181:470–475.
4. World HIV and AID Statistics 2003. http://www.avert.org/worldstats.htm. April 2004.
5. CDC Divisions of HIV/AIDS Prevention. http://www.cdc.govt/hiv/stats.htm. May 2004.
6. HIV/AIDS among African Americans. CDC Divisions of HIV/AIDS Prevention. http://www.cdc.gov/hiv/pubs/facts/afam.htm. April 2004.

7. Geleziunas R, Greene WC. Molecular insights into HIV-1 infection and pathogenesis. In: Sande MA, Volberding PA, eds. *The Medical Management of AIDS*, 6th ed. Philadelphia: WB Saunders Co., 1999;23–39.

8. Mellors JW, Muñoz A, Giorgi JV, et al. Plasma viral load and CD4+ lymphocytes as prognostic markers of HIV-1 infection. *Ann Intern Med* 1997;126:946–954.

9. Cao Y, Qin L, Zhang L, et al. Virologic and immunologic characterization of long-term survivors of human immunodeficiency virus type 1 infection. *N Engl J Med* 1995;332:201–208.

10. Centers for Disease Control and Prevention. Management of possible sexual, injecting-drug-use, or other nonoccupational exposure to HIV, including considerations related to antiretroviral therapy. Public Health Service Statement. *MMWR* 1998;47(No. RR-17): 1–14.

11. Sperling RS, Shapiro DE, Coombs RW, et al. Maternal viral load, zidovudine treatment, and the risk of transmission of human immunodeficiency virus type 1 from mother to infant. *N Engl J Med* 1996;335:1621–1629.

12. Kahn JO, Walker BD. Current concepts: acute human immunodeficiency virus type 1 infection. *N Engl J Med* 1998;339:33.

13. 1993 Revised classification system for HIV infection and expanded surveillance case definition for AIDS among adolescents and adults. *MMWR* 1992;41(RR-17).

14. Mylonakis E, Paliou M, Lally M, et al. Laboratory testing for infection with the human immunodeficiency virus: established and novel approaches. *Am J Med* 2000;109:568–576.

15. CDC. Interpretation and use of the Western blot assay for serodiagnosis of human immunodeficiency virus type 1 infections. *MMWR* 1989;38:7.

16. USPHS/IDSA Prevention of Opportunistic Infections Working Group. USPHS/IDSA guidelines for the prevention of opportunistic infections in persons infected with human immunodeficiency virus. http://www.aidsinfo.nih.gov/guidelines/op_infections/OI_112801.pdf. Nov. 28, 2001.

17. Panel on Clinical Practices for Treatment of HIV infection. DHHS Guidelines for the Use of Antiretroviral Agents in HIV-infected Adults and Adolescents. http://www.aidsinfo.nih.gov/guidelines/adult/AA_032304.pdf. March 23, 2004.

18. Yeni PG, Hammer SM, Hirsch MS, et al. Treatment for adult HIV infection: 2004 recommendations of the International AIDS Society–USA Panel. *JAMA* 2004;292:251–265.

19. Paterson DL, Swindells S, Mohr J, et al. Adherence to protease inhibitor therapy and outcomes in patients with HIV infection. *Ann Intern Med* 2000;133:21–30.

20. Perinatal HIV Working Group. Public Health Service Task Force Recommendations for the Use of Antiretroviral Drugs in Pregnant HIV-1 Infected Women for Maternal Health and Interventions to Reduce Perinatal HIV-1 Transmission in the United States, http://www.aidsinfo.nih.gov/guidelines/perinatal/PER_062304.pdf. June 23, 2004.

21. Centers for Disease Control and Prevention. Updated U.S. public health guidelines for management of occupational exposure to HBV, HCV, and HIV and recommendations for postexposure prophylaxis. *MMWR* 2001;50(No. RR-11). June 29, 2001.

22. Brenner M, Ognibene FP, Lack EE, et al. Prognostic factors and life expectancy of patients with acquired immunodeficiency syndrome and *Pneumocystis carinii* pneumonia. *Am Rev Respir Dis* 1987;136:1199.

23. Broaddus V, Dake M, Stulbarg M, et al. Bronchoalveolar lavage and transbronchial biopsy for the diagnosis for pulmonary infections in patients with the acquired immunodeficiency syndrome. *Ann Int Med* 1985;102:747.

24. Luft B, Remington J. Toxoplasmic encephalitis in AIDS. *Clin Infect Dis* 1992;15:211.

25. Chuck S, Sande M. Infections with *Cryptococcus neoformans* in the acquired immunodeficiency syndrome. *N Engl J Med* 1989;321: 794.

26. Saag MS, Graybill RJ, Larsen RA, et al. Practice guidelines for the management of cryptococcal disease. *Clin Infect Dis* 2000;30.

# Infective Endocarditis    15

*Thomas F. Keys*

Infective endocarditis remains a challenge to American medicine. The incidence has remained stable during the antibiotic era: an estimated 1 case per 1,000 hospital admissions or approximately 8,000 cases per year. The most appropriate medical and surgical management for infective endocarditis is a challenge in this era of great technology, but increasing restraints from third-party payers. Its prevention is a challenge because of the threat of nosocomial bacteremia from intravascular catheters or surgical wounds, which often is caused by antibiotic-resistant microorganisms. And its medical treatment remains a challenge because of the relative lack of new or innovative antimicrobial agents that are needed to confront those enterococci and staphylococci that have become absolutely or relatively insensitive to vancomycin. This chapter discusses the epidemiology of infective endocarditis, current diagnostic methods, pharmacologic and surgical treatments, persistent fever during therapy, neurologic complications, and preventive strategies.

## EPIDEMIOLOGY

In the preantibiotic era, survival was rare after an attack of infective endocarditis. With the introduction of effective chemotherapy, beginning in the early 1940s, and surgical intervention beginning in the late 1960s, the outcome of infective endocarditis was no longer bleak (Table 15.1). Despite these striking advances, however, mortality remains around 20%. In part, this is because more patients are living longer with prosthetic heart valves, and intravenous drug abuse (IVDA) continues to be a problem. Furthermore, our technically complex healthcare system often exposes patients

## TABLE 15.1

### DECLINING INCIDENCE OF DEATH FROM INFECTIVE ENDOCARDITIS

| Series | Years | Patients | Deaths (%) |
|---|---|---|---|
| Cates and Christie | 1945–1949 | 442 | 44 |
| Lerner and Weinstein | 1939–1959 | 100 | 37 |
| Pelletier and Petersdorf | 1963–1972 | 125 | 37 |
| Keys et al. | 1981–1982 | 90 | 21 |
| Sandre and Shafron | 1985–1993 | 135 | 19 |

Data adapted with permission from Cates JE, Christie RV. Subacute bacterial endocarditis: a review of 442 patients treated in 14 centers appointed by the Penicillin Trials Committee of the Medical Research Council. *QJM* 1951;20:93; Keys TF, Schaber D, Lever H, et al. Treatment of infective endocarditis. *Proceedings of the 14th International Congress on Chemotherapy, Kyoto, Japan.* Tokyo: University of Tokyo Press, June 25, 1985:1981–1982; Lerner PI, Weinstein L. Infective endocarditis in the antibiotic era. *N Engl J Med* 1966;274:199; Pelletier LL Jr, Petersdorf RG. Infective endocarditis: a review of 125 cases from the University of Washington Hospitals, 1963–1972. *Me Med* 1977;56:287–313; Sandre RM, Shafran SD. Infective endocarditis: review of 135 cases over 9 years. *Clin Infect Dis* 1996;22:276–286.

to nosocomial blood stream infections that may result in endocarditis. In the modern era, death usually is not due to uncontrolled infection but more commonly to congestive heart failure (CHF) and mechanical failure of heart valves.

Although rheumatic valvulitis was historically considered a frequent predisposing disease to infective endocarditis, times have changed (Table 15.2). Mitral valve prolapse, aortic sclerosis, and even bicuspid aortic valvular heart disease are more frequent factors. Prosthetic valvular heart disease accounts for approximately one third of all cases of infective endocarditis and is seen in 1% to 3% of patients undergoing valvular heart surgery. Twenty years ago, early-onset (within 1 year of surgery) prosthetic valve endocarditis (PVE) was often fatal; surgeons were reluctant to operate on patients who had active endocarditis involving freshly implanted heart valves. Mortality was reported at 90% in one series. Infection most often resulted from intraoperative contamination by nosocomial bacteria, especially *Staphylococcus epidermidis*, as well as by inexperience with surgical techniques. Despite advancing surgical

## TABLE 15.2

### UNDERLYING HEART DISEASE IN 60 PATIENTS WITH NATIVE VALVE ENDOCARDITIS

| Lesion | Patients (n) | Prevalence (%) |
|---|---|---|
| Mitral valve prolapse | 14 | 23 |
| Aortic sclerosis | 12 | 20 |
| Bicuspid aortic valve | 6 | 10 |
| Miscellaneous | 6 | 10 |
| Rheumatic | 5 | 8 |
| Unknown | 17 | 28 |

## TABLE 15.3

### FREQUENCY OF SOURCES RESPONSIBLE FOR ENDOCARDITIS DUE TO *STAPHYLOCOCCUS AUREUS*

| | Cases (n) | |
|---|---|---|
| Presumed Source | Hospital | Community |
| Intravenous catheter | 12 | 11 |
| Hemodialysis fistula | 2 | 5 |
| Surgical wound | 12 | 2 |
| Other | 1 | 1 |
| None | 0 | 13 |

expertise and standard antibiotic prophylaxis against staphylococci, early-onset PVE continues to be a problem, although mortality is now around 25% because of more aggressive surgical intervention combined with antibiotic therapy. In addition to valve replacement, preferably with homograft tissue, surgeons are successfully debriding and repairing native valves without replacement.

Late-onset PVE (at least 1 year after surgery) is much more frequent because more patients with prosthetic heart valves survive longer. Fortunately, these cases are usually caused by the same organisms as native valve endocarditis (NVE). Cure rates are nearly as good, and reoperation may not be necessary.

Pacemaker endocarditis, another complication of advancing technology, is usually caused by skin bacteria from a battery pack that migrate from a pocket infection or erosion through the skin. Early cases are usually caused by *Staphylococcus aureus* and late cases by *S. epidermidis*. Pacemaker leads may encapsulate into the ventricle, making explantation tedious and difficult.

A recent study demonstrated a high frequency of *S. aureus* endocarditis secondary to preventable sources. Of 59 cases reported from Duke University, 23 were caused by infected intravascular catheters and 14 from surgical wounds (Table 15.3). It has been estimated that 25% of vascular catheter–associated bacteremias caused by *S. aureus* result in endocarditis.

A significant risk factor for endocarditis is IVDA. Patients who use injection drugs tend to be younger and may be coinfected with human immunodeficiency virus. IVDA-associated endocarditis is usually quite responsive to antibiotic therapy. The quoted overall mortality is around 10%.

## PATHOGENESIS

Infective endocarditis usually follows endothelial trauma, as might occur from regurgitant blood flow or a high pressure gradient. Microorganisms with adherence factors are preferentially attracted to these lesions and proliferate within a fibrin meshwork, resulting in a vegetation. Adherence is promoted by dextran-producing streptococci. For example, *Streptococcus mutans* produces large concentrations of dextran and is commonly associated with endocarditis, whereas this is rarely caused by non–dextran-secreting organisms such as group A β-hemolytic streptococci.

## MICROBIOLOGY

Viridans and other streptococci, including *S. bovis* and *Enterococcus faecalis*, are responsible for the largest percentage of endocarditis cases (Table 15.4). *S. mitis* is nutritionally deficient and requires vitamin B6 and thio compounds for growth. It accounts for 10% all cases of viridans endocarditis and tends to be less responsive to penicillin therapy. Occasionally, cases of group B streptococcal endocarditis occur, and they often present with major embolic events from vegetations. Rarely, *S. pneumoniae* may cause endocarditis. This has been reported in alcoholic men, who may present with the Osler triad of pneumonia, meningitis, and endocarditis; mortality is high.

Endocarditis due to *S. aureus* may result in a sepsis syndrome with a fulminating coagulopathy. Metastatic foci of infection occur in the brain, lungs, liver, and kidneys. Overall, this infection has the highest mortality when cases related to IVDA are excluded. *S. aureus* is also a common cause of early-onset PVE, although not as frequently as *S. epidermidis* (Table 15.5). Although historically related to intraoperative contamination from skin bacteria, infections of vascular catheters and surgical wounds are now more important sources of infection. Endocarditis due to *Staphylococcus lugdunensis* has recently been emphasized in the literature. This organism, first described in 1988, is coagulase-negative, but may be confused with *S. aureus* in the laboratory. Although usually very susceptible to penicillin, isolates appear highly virulent. Cases present acutely, and infection is associated with a very high mortality rate. In one series, death was certain unless patients

### TABLE 15.4
**NATIVE VALVE ENDOCARDITIS MICROBIOLOGY**

| Organism | Cases (%) |
| --- | --- |
| *Streptococcus viridans* | 30–40 |
| *Enterococcus* species | 5–10 |
| Other streptococci | 10–25 |
| *Staphylococcus aureus* | 10–27 |
| Coagulase-negative staphylococci | 1–3 |
| Gram-negative bacilli | 2–13 |
| Fungi | 2–4 |
| Other | 5 |
| "Culture negative" | 5–24 |

### TABLE 15.5
**EARLY-ONSET PROSTHETIC VALVE ENDOCARDITIS MICROBIOLOGY**

| Organism | Cases (%) |
| --- | --- |
| *Staphylococcus epidermidis* | 35 |
| *Staphylococcus aureus* | 17 |
| Streptococcal species | 8 |
| Diphtheroids | 10 |
| Gram-negative bacilli | 16 |
| Fungi | 11 |
| Other | 3 |

underwent emergency valve replacement. *S. epidermidis*, the most frequent cause of early onset PVE, is almost always resistant to methicillin (Staphcillin) or oxacillin, but has a more favorable prognosis.

The HACEK group of fastidious Gram-negative microorganisms occasionally cause endocarditis. HACEK is an all-inclusive term for endocarditis due to *Haemophilus*, *Actinobacillus*, *Cardiobacterium*, *Eikenella*, and *Kingella* species of bacteria. Clinically, these cases are characterized by a subacute or chronic course and often present with embolic lesions from large vegetations.

Most cases of fungal endocarditis occur in patients who are receiving prolonged antibiotics or parenteral nutrition through central vascular catheters. Such patients may also be immunocompromised. The most common species is *Candida albicans*, followed by *C. parapsilosis*. Endocarditis due to *Histoplasma capsulatum* or *Aspergillus* species is rare.

Finally, unusual cases of endocarditis should be considered when standard microbiologic techniques fail to provide a diagnosis. Q fever endocarditis, due to *Coxiella burnetii*, usually has an atypical presentation. Patients may not have fever but frequently have underlying valvular heart disease and are on immunosuppressive therapy. Vegetations are rarely detected on echocardiogram. Routine blood cultures are negative. Serologic studies are reasonably specific, and an alerted microbiology laboratory may recover the organism from buffy-coat cultures. *Bartonella henselae* may also cause endocarditis. This infection, often of the homeless and alcoholic population, is difficult to diagnose. Blood cultures are negative, but serology may be helpful. Studies using the polymerase chain reaction (PCR) technique on resected valve tissue may provide the diagnosis if the technology is available.

## DIAGNOSIS

The diagnostic clues noted by Sir William Osler in 1908 remain true today: remittent fever with a valvular heart lesion, embolic findings, skin lesions, and progressive cardiac changes. In 1981, Von Reyn and colleagues reported the benefit of strict definitions for managing cases and comparing outcomes. The use of echocardiography improved the specificity of diagnosis, and, in 1984, Durack and colleagues from Duke University, proposed updated criteria that have now been accepted for diagnosis:

- Positive valve culture or histology
- Two major criteria: typical organism, persistent bacteremia, positive echocardiogram for vegetations, abscess, or valve dehiscence
- Five of six minor criteria: predisposing lesions or IVDA, temperature greater than 38°C, vasculitis, skin lesions, suggestive echocardiogram, microbiology
- One major and three minor criteria

Transesophageal echocardiography is more sensitive and specific than transthoracic echocardiography for detecting vegetations and other lesions, such as ring abscesses and valve dehiscence (Table 15.6).

The clinical features of patients with PVE are not much different from those with NVE (Table 15.7). Fever, skin lesions, a newly appreciated heart murmur, and splenomegaly occur with equal frequency. Weight loss may be more common in NVE, however, presumably because patients are sicker longer before they seek medical attention.

The most important laboratory study to confirm a clinical diagnosis of endocarditis is the blood culture. In a landmark study reported by Werner and colleagues (1967), a clear majority of patients with suspected bacterial endocarditis had positive blood cultures within a period of 2 days, provided that they had not been on antibiotics

## TABLE 15.6

### ECHOCARDIOGRAM DETECTION OF VEGETATIONS IN PATIENTS WITH INFECTIVE ENDOCARDITIS

| | | | Sensitivity (%) | |
|---|---|---|---|---|
| Study | Year | Patients | TTE[a] | TEE[b] |
| Daniel et al. | 1987 | 69 | 78 | 94 |
| Mugge et al. | 1989 | 91 | 58 | 90 |
| Shively et al. | 1991 | 16 | 44 | 94 |
| Birmingham et al. | 1992 | 31 | 30 | 88 |

[a] TTE, transthoracic echocardiography; [b] TEE, transesophageal echocardiography.
Data adapted with permission from Birmingham GD, Rahko PS, Ballantyne F III. Improved detection of infective endocarditis with transesophageal echocardiography. *Am Heart J* 1992;123:774–781; Daniel WG, Mugge A, Grote J, et al. Comparison of transthoracic and transesophageal echocardiography for detection of abnormalities of prosthetic and bioprosthetic valves in the mitral and aortic positions. *Am J Cardiol* 1993;71:210–215; Mugge A, Danile WG, Frank G, et al. Echocardiography in infective endocarditis: reassessment of the prognostic implications of vegetation size determined by the transthoracic and transesophageal approach. *J Am Coll Cardiol* 1989;14:631–638; Shively BK, Gurule FT, Roldan CA, et al. Diagnostic value of transesophageal compared with transthoracic echocardiography in infective endocarditis. *J Am Coll Cardiol* 1991;18:391–397.

## TABLE 15.7

### CLINICAL FINDINGS IN 90 PATIENTS WITH INFECTIVE ENDOCARDITIS

| Symptom | NVE[a] (%) (n = 60) | PVE[b] (%) (n = 30) |
|---|---|---|
| Fever | 75 | 87 |
| Weight loss | 52 | 20 |
| Skin lesions | 51 | 47 |
| New murmur | 33 | 33 |
| Splenomegaly | 20 | 20 |

[a] NVE, native valve endocarditis; [b] PVE, prosthetic valve endocarditis.

recently. Therefore, one need not collect more than three blood cultures during a 24-hour period unless antibiotics are already on board. More sophisticated blood culture techniques have also improved the recovery of organisms: BACTEC system (Johnston Laboratories Inc., Towson, MD) for staphylococcal species and the ISOLATER system (E.I. du Pont de Nemours and Company, Wilmington, DE) for Gram-negative bacilli and yeasts. Other laboratory features, although nonspecific, may suggest the diagnosis. These include an elevated erythrocyte sedimentation rate, a positive rheumatoid factor, proteinuria, and circulating immune complexes.

## TREATMENT

### Pharmacologic Treatment

In the preantibiotic era, infective endocarditis was a fatal disease. Now, penicillin, often in combination with gentamicin, remains a cornerstone of therapy for endocarditis caused by susceptible streptococci (Table 15.8). For penicillin-allergic patients, vancomycin is substituted. Intravenous ceftriaxone (Rocephin), given once a day for 4 weeks, has been reported to cure penicillin-sensitive streptococcal endocarditis. More recently, ceftriaxone in combination with gentamicin has proved successful with only 2 weeks of therapy. This is not recommended, however, for

## TABLE 15.8

### THERAPY OF NATIVE VALVE ENDOCARDITIS: PENICILLIN-SENSITIVE STREPTOCOCCI

| Antibiotic | Regimen | Duration (wk) |
|---|---|---|
| Penicillin G | 12–18 MU i.v. daily | 4 |
| Ceftriaxone | 2 g i.v. daily | 4 |
| Ceftriaxone + gentamicin | 2 g i.v. daily 3 mg/kg i.v. daily | 2 |
| Vancomycin | 1 g i.v. every 12 h | 4 |

MU, million units.
Doses assume normal renal function. Minimum inhibitory concentration ≤0.1 μg/mL.

### TABLE 15.9

**THERAPY OF NATIVE VALVE ENDOCARDITIS FOR PENICILLIN-INSENSITIVE STREPTOCOCCI[a] OR ENTEROCOCCI[b]**

| Antibiotic | Regimen | Duration (wk) |
|---|---|---|
| Penicillin G | 18 MU i.v. daily | 4–6[c] |
| + Gentamicin | 1 mg/kg i.v./i.m. every 8 h | 2–6[c] |
| Vancomycin | 1 g i.v. every 12 h | 4–6 |
| + Gentamicin[d] | 1 mg/kg i.v./i.m. every 8 h | 4–6 |

MU, million units.
Doses assume normal renal function.
[a] Minimum inhibitory concentration = 0.10.5 μg/mL.
[b] Minimum inhibitory concentration > 0.5 μg/mL.
[c] Prolonged therapy for enterococci.
[d] Gentamicin with vancomycin only for enterococci.

patients who have PVE, major embolic complications, or symptoms lasting longer than 2 months. In one series reported from the Mayo Clinic, 24% of all patients required valvular heart surgery within 5 to 36 days after beginning treatment. Therefore, careful follow-up is essential, especially if patients are discharged from the hospital to complete antibiotic therapy at home.

For streptococci that are relatively insensitive to penicillin (minimum inhibitory concentration 0.1 to 0.5 μg/mL), penicillin dosage is increased and the antibiotic continued for 4 weeks (Table 15.9). Gentamicin is given for the first 2 weeks. The treatment of enterococcal endocarditis is longer, using penicillin with gentamicin for 6 weeks. Vancomycin may be substituted for penicillin, provided that the isolate is susceptible. For vancomycin-resistant enterococci, anecdotal success has been reported using quinupristin-dalfopristin or linezolid.

The therapy for NVE caused by methicillin-susceptible staphylococci is oxacillin or cefazolin for 4 to 6 weeks. If the organism is methicillin-resistant, vancomycin is substituted. Gentamicin can be added for the first 3 to 5 days. Although this may shorten the duration of bacteremia, it

### TABLE 15.11

**THERAPY OF ENDOCARDITIS DUE TO HACEK[a] MICROORGANISMS**

| Antibiotic | Regimen | Duration (wk) |
|---|---|---|
| Ceftriaxone | 2 g i.v. every 24 h | 4 |
| Ampicillin | 2 g i.v. every 4 h | 4 |
| + Gentamicin | 1 mg/kg i.v./i.m. every 8 h | 4 |

[a] HACEK, *Haemophilus, Actinobacillus, Cardiobacterium, Eikenella,* and *Kingella* species of bacteria.
Doses assume normal renal function.

does not improve the cure rate and, if continued longer, may cause renal toxicity.

Antibiotic therapy for staphylococcal PVE must be more aggressive because of the greater likelihood of treatment failure or relapse (Table 15.10). Oxacillin is prescribed for 6 weeks, with gentamicin for the first 2 weeks. If the isolate is methicillin-resistant, vancomycin is substituted for oxacillin. Rifampin is added, providing the organism is susceptible.

Endocarditis caused by *S. aureus* associated with IVDA is generally more responsive to short-course antibiotic therapy. In one study, a cure rate of 89% was reported using a 2-week course of intravenous cloxacillin alone.

The current recommended treatment for the HACEK group of Gram-negative bacteria is ceftriaxone alone or ampicillin plus gentamicin for 4 weeks (Table 15.11). Patients with late-onset PVE often may be cured medically without valve surgery.

Patients with fungal endocarditis generally have a poor prognosis. In one study, only 30% of patients survived despite aggressive antifungal therapy, often in combination with surgery. My colleagues and I recently reported a 67% survival rate in treating cases of fungal PVE. The mainstay of therapy was aggressive surgery accompanied by intravenous amphotericin B (Fungizone) and followed by life-long suppression with oral azole compounds such as fluconazole (Diflucan) or itraconazole (Sporanox).

### TABLE 15.10

**THERAPY OF PROSTHETIC VALVE STAPHYLOCOCCAL ENDOCARDITIS**

| Isolate | Antibiotic | Regimen | Duration (wk) |
|---|---|---|---|
| MSSA or MSSE | Oxacillin | 2 g i.v. every 4 h | ≥6 |
| | + Gentamicin | 1 mg/kg i.v./i.m. every 8 h | First 2 |
| | + Rifampin | 300 mg p.o. every 8 h | ≥6 |
| MRSA or MRSE | Vancomycin | 1 g i.v. every 12 h | ≥6 |
| | + Gentamicin | 1 mg/kg i.v./i.m. every 8 h | First 2 |
| | + Rifampin | 300 mg p.o. every 8 h | ≥6 |

MRSA, methicillin-resistant *Staphylococcus aureus*; MRSE, methicillin-resistant *Staphylococcus epidermidis*; MSSA, methicillin-sensitive *Staphylococcus aureus*; MSSE, methicillin-sensitive *Staphylococcus epidermidis*.
Doses assume normal renal function.

Approximately 10% of patients with clinically suspected endocarditis will have negative blood cultures. A trial of empiric therapy can be considered using ampicillin plus gentamicin for NVE or vancomycin plus ampicillin and gentamicin for PVE. Approximately 50% of these patients respond, as the typical organisms may not be recovered from the blood but may still be within vegetations. A common reason is that prior antibiotic treatment has suppressed growth in blood cultures. If a patient remains ill despite empiric therapy, however, one must look for an unusual organism or a noninfectious cause of endocarditis.

## Surgical Treatment

Death from infective endocarditis is usually due to CHF, often accompanied by valve dysfunction. In the last quarter century, aggressive surgery has been the most important advance in therapy. Surgery during acute infection does not increase mortality; in fact, restoration of a failing pump improves function and outcome. Valve dysfunction causing moderate to severe CHF (New York Heart Association class III or IV) is a strong indication for urgent surgery, as are endocardial abscesses. These frequently involve the aortic root, a valve ring, or the ventricular septum. Other conditions favoring surgery include vegetations larger than 1 cm in diameter and failure or relapse of medical therapy due to organisms such as *S. aureus, Pseudomonas aeruginosa,* or *Candida* species.

Even if surgery is not required during the period of antimicrobial therapy, it may be required later, when heart failure develops because of valve damage from endocarditis. In one study, 47% of patients required surgery, usually within 2 years after completing medical therapy.

## Complications of Treatment

A significant number of patients will have persistent fever during treatment (Table 15.12). Annular or ring abscesses may cause fever and are a strong indication for surgery. Other causes of prolonged fever during therapy include myocarditis, pulmonary and systemic emboli, drug hypersensitivity, and intravenous site infections.

## TABLE 15.12

**PERSISTENT FEVERS DURING TREATMENT OF INFECTIVE ENDOCARDITIS**

| Reason | Patients | % |
| --- | --- | --- |
| Annular abscesses | 11 | 26 |
| Pulmonary or systemic emboli | 7 | 17 |
| Drug hypersensitivity | 7 | 17 |
| Myocarditis | 3 | 7 |
| Intravenous site infection | 2 | 5 |
| Other | 6 | 14 |
| Unknown | 6 | 14 |

## TABLE 15.13

**NEUROLOGIC COMPLICATIONS IN NATIVE (NVE) AND PROSTHETIC VALVE ENDOCARDITIS (PVE)**

| Complication | NVE[a] (%) (n = 13) | PVE[b] (%) (n = 62) |
| --- | --- | --- |
| Stroke | 15 | 21 |
| Encephalopathy | 9 | 8 |
| Retinal emboli | 3 | 3 |
| Headache | 4 | 3 |
| Mycotic aneurysm | 3 | — |
| Abscess | 1 | 2 |
| Meningitis | 1 | 2 |
| Seizures | 1 | — |
| Total | 37 | 39 |

[a] NVE, native valve endocarditis; [b] PVE, prosthetic valve endocarditis.

Major neurologic complications from endocarditis are fortunately rare (Table 15.13). They can present difficult and sometimes vexing management dilemmas, however. Leading causes are stroke, encephalopathy, and retinal emboli. Brain abscess and mycotic aneurysms are relatively infrequent. As a general rule, anticoagulation should be avoided because of the increased risk of intracranial bleeding. One may elect to continue anticoagulation in patients with mechanical heart valves, but dosing should be in the low therapeutic range to minimize the risk of bleeding. Fortunately, most cases of mycotic aneurysm do not require surgery and resolve after appropriate medical therapy.

## PREVENTION

The need for and adequacy of antibiotic prophylaxis to prevent infective endocarditis continues to be debated. In 1986, Bayliss and colleagues observed that a presumed dental portal of entry was recognized less than 20% of the time. In two-thirds of cases, no portal of entry could be determined. Further controversy was stimulated by a recently published case-control study from the greater Philadelphia area (Table 15.14). Controls were matched for age, sex, and neighborhood. Information was collected through structured telephone interviews and outside medical and dental records. Patients with cases of endocarditis were no more likely than controls to have had recent dental procedures, with a procedure rate of around 20% (similar to the finding in the Bayliss study). One interesting caveat was present: Six cases of endocarditis were preceded by dental extraction, although none was noted in the control group. More important, however, cardiac risk factors dominated endocarditis cases. Mitral valve prolapse, congenital heart disease, rheumatic valvular heart disease, previous cardiac surgery, a history of infective endocarditis, and a known heart murmur were

## TABLE 15.14
### DENTAL AND CARDIAC RISK FACTORS FOR INFECTIVE ENDOCARDITIS

| Risk Factor | Cases (*n* = 273) | Controls (*n* = 273) |
|---|---|---|
| Dental prophylaxis | 24 | 23 |
| Extractions | 6 | 0 |
| Gingival surgery | 1 | 0 |
| History of endocarditis | 17 | 1 |
| Cardiac valvular surgery | 37 | 2 |
| Mitral valve prolapse | 52 | 6 |

nearly six times more frequent in endocarditis patients than in the control group.

The 1997 American Heart Association prophylaxis guidelines may be too liberal (Table 15.15). An accompanying editorial suggested that appropriate prophylaxis for dental procedures might include only patients undergoing dental extractions or gingival surgery who have prosthetic valvular heart disease or a history of endocarditis.

The compliance with the current guidelines is not known, but it is likely that antibiotics are overprescribed and may not be timely for the procedure intended. Furthermore, the risk of side effects is probably greater than the benefit of preventing endocarditis in patients at relatively low risk. Nevertheless, prophylaxis remains accepted, standard practice.

In the 1997 American Heart Association guidelines, indications for prophylaxis were stratified into high- and moderate-risk categories, completely excluding a negligible-risk category (Table 15.16). Examples of patients at high risk include those with prosthetic heart valves and previous endocarditis; moderate-risk patients are those with acquired valvular heart disease and mitral valve prolapse with regurgitation.

## TABLE 15.15
### EXAMPLES OF AMERICAN HEART ASSOCIATION RECOMMENDATIONS FOR PROPHYLAXIS DURING PROCEDURES

| Yes | No |
|---|---|
| Dental extractions | Dental restoration |
| Periodontal procedures | Adjustment of braces |
| Dental implants | Flexible bronchoscopy |
| Prophylactic cleaning | Gastrointestinal endoscopy |
| Tonsillectomy | Cesarean section deliveries |
| Esophageal dilatation | Cardiac catheterization |
| Sclerotherapy | Urethral catheterization[a] |
| Cystoscopy | |
| Urethral dilatation | |

[a] When urine is sterile.

## TABLE 15.16
### PREVENTION OF BACTERIAL ENDOCARDITIS: DISEASES AT RISK FOR INFECTIVE ENDOCARDITIS

High risk
   Prosthetic heart valves
   Previous bacterial endocarditis
   Complex cyanotic congenital heart disease
   Surgically constructed pulmonary shunts
Moderate risk
   Acquired valvular dysfunction
   Hypertrophic cardiomyopathy
   Mitral valve prolapse with regurgitation
Negligible risk
   Isolated atrial septal defect
   Surgical repair of atrial septal defect, ventricular septal defect, or patent ductus arteriosus
   Previous coronary artery bypass grafting
   Mitral valve prolapse without regurgitation
   Cardiac pacemakers

For high- and moderate-risk patients undergoing dental, oral, respiratory tract, or esophageal procedures, amoxicillin, 2 g orally, is recommended 1 hour before the procedure. For penicillin-allergic patients, clindamycin (Cleocin), 600 mg orally; cephalexin, 2 g orally; or azithromycin (Zithromax), 500 mg orally, may be substituted. No postprocedure dose is needed (Table 15.17).

For high-risk patients undergoing genitourinary and gastrointestinal procedures, ampicillin, 2.0 g intramuscularly or intravenously, plus gentamicin, 1.5 mg/kg (not to exceed 120 mg), should be given within 30 minutes of the procedure and a single dose of amoxicillin, 1 g orally, 6 hours later (Table 15.18). For penicillin-allergic patients, vancomycin, 1 g intravenously, is substituted for ampicillin. A second dose is not needed. For moderate-risk patients, amoxicillin, 2 g orally, should be given 1 hour before the procedure or ampicillin, 2 g intramuscularly or intravenously, within 30 minutes of the procedure. Vancomycin, 1 g intravenously, is substituted in penicillin-allergic patients.

## TABLE 15.17
### PROPHYLACTIC REGIMENS FOR DENTAL, ORAL, RESPIRATORY, AND ESOPHAGEAL PROCEDURES

| Situation | Agent | Regimen |
|---|---|---|
| Standard | Amoxicillin | 2 g p.o. 1 h before |
| Unable to take p.o. | Ampicillin | 2 g i.m./i.v. 30 min before |
| Penicillin allergy | Clindamycin | 600 mg p.o. 1 h before |
| | Cephalexin | 2 g p.o. 1 h before |
| | Azithromycin | 500 mg p.o. 1 h before |

## TABLE 15.18

**PROPHYLACTIC REGIMENS FOR GENITOURINARY AND GASTROINTESTINAL PROCEDURES**

| Category | Regimen |
| --- | --- |
| High risk | Ampicillin,[a] 2 g i.m./i.v., 30 min before + Gentamicin, 1.5 mg/kg, 30 min before |
| Moderate risk | Amoxicillin, 2 g p.o., 1 h before or ampicillin, 2 g i.m./i.v., 30 min before |

[a] For penicillin allergy, substitute vancomycin, 1 g i.v.; infuse over 12 h and complete 30 min before procedure.

For patients undergoing cardiac valve surgery, perioperative prophylaxis with a first- or second-generation cephalosporin is recommended. The antibiotic infusion should be completed within 30 minutes of the skin incision and need not be continued longer than 24 hours afterward. If surgery is longer than 4 hours, another dose should be given intraoperatively before closure. Hospitals with a high prevalence of methicillin-resistant staphylococci (*S. aureus* and *S. epidermidis*) should use vancomycin rather than a cephalosporin.

## REVIEW EXERCISES

### QUESTIONS

**1.** Probable infective endocarditis by the Duke Criteria Diagnosis:
**a.** Typical organism
**b.** Persistent bacteremia
**c.** Classic skin/mucosal lesions
**(1)** a, b
**(2)** a, c
**(3)** b, c
**(4)** a, b, c

**2.** Predictable organisms causing early-onset prosthetic valve endocarditis:
**a.** *Staphylococcus epidermidis*
**b.** *Staphylococcus aureus*
**c.** Vancomycin-resistant *Enterococcus species*
**(1)** a
**(2)** a, b
**(3)** a, c
**(4)** a, b, c

**3.** Unusual causes of endocarditis: diagnosis by PCR
**a.** *Coxiella burnetii*
**b.** *Whippeli trophyeryma*
**c.** *Bartonella species*
**(1)** a, b

**(2)** a, c
**(3)** b, c
**(4)** a, b, c

**4.** Presumptive therapy of late-onset prosthetic valve endocarditis
**a.** Penicillin + gentamicin
**b.** Penicillin + vancomycin
**c.** Penicillin + vancomycin + gentamicin
**d.** Vancomycin + gentamicin
**(1)** a
**(2)** b
**(3)** c
**(4)** d

**5.** Infective endocarditis: indication(s) for surgery
**a.** Congestive heart failure
**b.** Vegetations on ECHO
**c.** Ring abscesses
**(1)** a
**(2)** a, b
**(3)** c
**(4)** a, b, c

**6.** Infective endocarditis: indications for prophylaxis
**a.** Probable mitral valve prolapse
**b.** Prosthetic valvular heart disease
**c.** History of infective endocarditis
**(1)** a
**(2)** a, b
**(3)** b, c
**(4)** a, b, c

**7.** History of penicillin allergy: alternatives for dental prophylaxis
**a.** Vancomycin
**b.** Cephalexin
**c.** Clindamycin
**d.** Azithromycin
**(1)** a, b
**(2)** c, d
**(3)** b, c, d
**(4)** a, b, c, d

### ANSWERS

**1.** (1)

**2.** (2)

**3.** (4)

**4.** (3)

**5.** (3)

**6.** (3)

**7.** (3)

## SUGGESTED READINGS

Bayliss R, Clarke C, Oakley CM, et al. Incidence, mortality and prevention of infective endocarditis. *J R Coll Physicians Lond* 1986; 20:15–20.

Dajani AS, Taubert KA, Wilson W, et al. Prevention of bacterial endocarditis: recommendations by the American Heart Association. *JAMA* 1997;277:1794–1801.

Douglas A, Moore-Gillon J, Eykyn S. Fever during treatment of infective endocarditis. *Lancet* 1986;1:1341–1343.

Durack DT, Lukes AS, Bright KD, et al. New criteria for diagnosis of infective endocarditis: utilization of specific echocardiographic findings. *Am J Med* 1994;96:200–209.

Fowler VG, Sanders LL, Kong LK, et al. Infective endocarditis due to *Staphylococcus aureus. Clin Infect Dis* 1994;28:106–114.

Hoesley CJ, Cobbs CG. Endocarditis at the millennium. *J Infect Dis* 1999;179[Suppl 2]:S360–S365.

Melgar GR, Nasser RM, Gordon SM, et al. Fungal prosthetic valve endocarditis in 16 patients. *Medicine* 1997;76:1–10.

Murray HW, Roberts RB. *Streptococcus bovis* bacteremia and underlying gastrointestinal disease. *Arch Intern Med* 1978;138:1097–1099.

Sexton DJ, Tenenbaum MJ, Wilson WR, et al. Ceftriaxone once daily for 4 weeks compared with ceftriaxone plus gentamicin once daily for 2 weeks for treatment of endocarditis due to penicillin-susceptible streptococci. *Clin Infect Dis* 1998;27:1470–1474.

Strom BL, Abrutyn E, Berlin JA, et al. Dental and cardiac risk factors for infective endocarditis. *Ann Intern Med* 1998;129:761–769.

Von Reyn CF, Levy BS, Arbeit RD, et al. Infective endocarditis: an analysis based on strict case definitions. *Ann Intern Med* 1981;94: 505–518.

Werner AS, Cobbs CG, Kaye D, et al. Studies on the bacteremia of bacterial endocarditis. *JAMA* 1967;202:127–131.

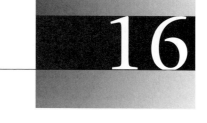

# Pneumonias

*Steven K. Schmitt*

Sir William Osler described pneumonia as the "captain of the men of death" (1). Although the advent of the antimicrobial age has somewhat reduced this rank, pneumonia remains the sixth leading cause of death in the United States. In 2001, the age-adjusted death rate due to pneumonia was 22.0 per 100,000 persons. Estimates of the incidence of pneumonia range from 4 to 5 million cases per year, with about 25% requiring hospitalization. Because pneumonia crosses the boundaries of all internal medicine subspecialties, a discussion of difficult issues regarding diagnosis, antimicrobial selection, treatment setting, and prevention is appropriate.

## ETIOLOGY OF PNEUMONIA

### Pathogenesis

Six mechanisms have been identified in the pathogenesis of pneumonia in immunocompetent adults:

- Inhalation of infectious particles
- Aspiration of oropharyngeal or gastric contents
- Hematogenous deposition
- Invasion from infection in contiguous structures
- Direct inoculation
- Reactivation

The inhalation of infectious particles is probably the most important pathogenic mechanism in the community. It is thought to be particularly contributory in pneumonia due to *Legionella* species and *Mycobacterium tuberculosis.*

The aspiration of oropharyngeal or gastric contents is by far the most prevalent pathogenetic mechanism in cases of nosocomial pneumonia, with a variety of factors contributing to this risk. Swallowing and epiglottic closure may be impaired by neuromuscular diseases or stroke. States of altered consciousness, such as in chemical sedation, delirium, coma, or seizures, can also depress swallowing, the gag reflex, and closure of the epiglottis. In addition, endotracheal and nasogastric tubes may interfere with these anatomic defenses. Finally, impaired lower esophageal sphincter function and nasogastric and gastrostomy tubes increase the risk of the regurgitation of gastric contents. Fortunately, aspiration rarely leads to overt bacterial pneumonitis. It is probable that the nature of the resident flora, the size of the inoculum, and underlying diseases may determine which aspirations result in lung infection.

Direct inoculation rarely occurs as a result of surgery or bronchoscopy but may play a role in the development of pneumonia in patients supported with mechanical ventilation. The hematogenous deposition of bacteria in the lung is also uncommon but is responsible for some cases of pneumonia due to *Staphylococcus aureus, Pseudomonas aeruginosa,* and *Escherichia coli.* The reactivation of latent infection likely plays an important role in the development of pneumonia due to cytomegalovirus and *Mycobacterium tuberculosis.* The direct extension of infection to the lung from contiguous areas such as the pleural or subdiaphragmatic spaces is rare.

Once bacteria reach the tracheobronchial tree, infectivity may be enhanced by defects in local pulmonary defenses. The cough reflex can be impaired by stroke, neuromuscular disease, sedatives, or poor nutrition. Mucociliary transport is depressed with the aging process, dehydration, morphine, atropine, prior infection with influenza virus, tobacco smoking, and chronic bronchitis. Anatomic derangements, including emphysema, bronchiectasis, and obstructive mass lesions, also can hinder clearance of organisms. Proteolytic enzymes, such as neutrophil elastase, are released by inflammatory cells recruited to infected areas of the pulmonary tree, thus altering the bronchial epithelium and ciliary clearance mechanisms as well as stimulating excess mucus production.

Bacteria in the tracheobronchial tree may encounter a blunted cellular and humoral immune response, thus increasing the risk of pneumonia. For example, granulocyte chemotaxis is reduced with aging, diabetes mellitus, malnutrition, hypothermia, hypophosphatemia, and corticosteroid administration. Absolute granulocytopenia may be caused by cytotoxic chemotherapy. Alveolar macrophages may be rendered dysfunctional by corticosteroids, cytokines, viral illnesses, and malnutrition. Diminished antibody production or function can be the sequelae of hematologic malignancies, such as multiple myeloma or chronic lymphocytic leukemia.

## Pathologic Agents

Despite the emergence of several newer pathogens as causes of community-acquired pneumonia, *Streptococcus pneumoniae* remains the most commonly identified pathogen. A variety of other pathogens have been reported to cause pneumonia in the community, with their order of importance dependent on the location and population studied. These include long-recognized pathogens such as *Haemophilus influenzae, Mycoplasma pneumoniae,* and influenza A, along with newer pathogens such as *Legionella* species and *Chlamydophila pneumoniae.* Other common causes in the immunocompetent patient include *Moraxella catarrhalis, Mycobacterium tuberculosis,* and aspiration pneumonia.

The following organisms are the causative agents in the 50% to 70% of cases for which a cause is identified (2):

- *S. pneumoniae,* 20% to 60%
- *H. influenzae,* 3% to 10%
- *S. aureus,* 3% to 5%
- Gram-negative bacilli, 3% to 10%
- *Legionella* species, 2% to 8%
- *M. pneumoniae,* 1% to 6%
- *C. pneumoniae,* 4% to 6%
- Viruses, 2% to 15%
- Aspiration, 6% to 10%
- Others, 3% to 5%

Whereas pneumonias arising in the nursing home can be caused by community-acquired pathogens, higher percentages are caused by pathogens seen with relatively low frequency in the community. *S. aureus* should be sought in the setting of aspiration or as a result of influenza in the nursing home. Gram-negative organisms are also more prominent.

Because of the different pathogenetic mechanisms leading to its development, nosocomial pneumonia is caused by a group of microorganisms quite different from those causing community-acquired pneumonia. Organisms known to colonize the respiratory tree of hospitalized patients, such as *S. aureus* and enteric Gram-negative organisms of the genuses *Pseudomonas, Enterobacter, Citrobacter, Serratia, Acinetobacter,* and *Stenotrophomonas,* are commonly isolated. Outbreaks of *Legionella* pneumonia and tuberculosis also have occurred in nursing homes and hospitals.

# DIAGNOSIS OF PNEUMONIA

Because the clinical syndromes characterizing pneumonic infections caused by various agents frequently overlap with each other and with many noninfectious processes, the diagnosis of pneumonia can be challenging. The diligent clinician can narrow the differential diagnosis, however, by considering the place of acquisition and patient characteristics along with diagnostic tests.

## Place of Acquisition

The differential diagnosis of pneumonia acquired in the community is quite different from that acquired in the nursing home or hospital.

A residence and travel history can help focus the differential diagnosis of pneumonia. Coccidioidomycosis should be considered in patients developing pneumonia upon return from the southwestern United States. A patient developing pneumonia after a trip to Southeast Asia may have melioidosis or tuberculosis. A patient infected with human immunodeficiency virus (HIV) living in New York City with cough, fever, and night sweats may have multidrug-resistant tuberculosis. Residents of the desert southwestern United States with pneumonia and exposure to rodent excreta should be evaluated for the hantavirus pulmonary syndrome. A person returning from an area with an active outbreak of severe acute respiratory syndrome (SARS) should be tested for SARS coronavirus.

## Clinical Presentation

Typical bacterial pathogens such as *S. pneumoniae, H. influenzae,* and the enteric Gram-negative organisms usually present acutely with high fever, chills, tachypnea, tachycardia, productive cough, and examination findings localized to a specific lung zone. In contrast, atypical pathogens such as *Mycoplasma, Chlamydophila,* and viruses can present in a subacute fashion with low-grade fever, nonproductive cough, constitutional symptoms, and absent or diffuse findings on lung examination. Rapid progression of disease can be seen in severe pneumococcal or *Legionella* pneumonia. The overlap between the presentations of typical and atypical pathogens, however, weakens the specificity of these categorizations considerably.

Certain extrapulmonary physical findings can provide clues to the diagnosis. Poor dentition and foul-smelling sputum may indicate the presence of a polymicrobial lung abscess. Bullous myringitis can accompany infection with *M. pneumoniae.* An absent gag reflex or altered sensorium raises the question of aspiration. Encephalitis can complicate pneumonia with *M. pneumoniae* or *Legionella pneumophila.* Cutaneous manifestations of infection can include erythema multiforme (*M. pneumoniae*), erythema nodosum (*C. pneumoniae* and *M. tuberculosis*), or ecthyma gangrenosum (*P. aeruginosa*).

## Patient Characteristics

The age of the patient can play an important role in disease etiology and presentation. Older patients often have humoral and cellular immunodeficiency as a result of underlying diseases, immunosuppressive medications, and aging. They are more frequently institutionalized with anatomic problems that inhibit the pulmonary clearance of pathogens. The presentation is often more subtle than in younger adults, with more advanced disease and sepsis despite minimal fever and sputum production. More prolonged antimicrobial therapy is often required.

The occupation and hobbies of the patient can provide important clinical clues. For example, exposure to construction sites or old buildings with accumulations of bat or bird droppings can predispose to pneumonias due to *Histoplasma capsulatum* or *Cryptococcus neoformans.* Hunters who skin their own rabbits may be exposed to *Francisella tularensis.* Farmers working with stored hay may be exposed to *Aspergillus* species, as may patients who smoke marijuana. Laboratory workers handling the SARS-coronavirus can develop disease with this pathogen.

Underlying diseases are a critical part of the history of the patient with pneumonia. Risk factors for HIV infection should be sought in the clinical history. HIV increases the risk for pneumonias due to common bacterial pathogens, as well as opportunistic pathogens such as *Pneumocystis carinii,* cytomegalovirus, and *Mycobacterium avium-intracellulare.* Fungal pneumonias caused by *H. capsulatum, Coccidioides immitis,* and *C. neoformans* have been seen in HIV-infected patients in appropriate epidemiologic settings and can have especially severe courses. Neutropenic patients are especially prone to fungal pneumonias, such as those caused by *Aspergillus* species. Patients treated with prolonged courses of immunosuppressive medications, such as corticosteroids, are at risk for pulmonary infections with various viral, fun-

gal, and mycobacterial agents. Alcoholism predisposes individuals to aspiration pneumonia, with mixed Gram-positive and Gram-negative aerobic and anaerobic flora, as well as to tuberculosis. *M. catarrhalis, H. influenzae,* and *S. pneumoniae* are more likely in those with chronic obstructive pulmonary disease. Diabetic patients are more prone to staphylococcal infections. Patients with functional or surgical asplenia are prone to infection with encapsulated organisms such as *S. pneumoniae* and *H. influenzae.*

## Radiography

A cornerstone of diagnosis is the chest radiograph, which usually reveals an infiltrate at presentation. This finding, however, may be absent in the dehydrated patient during the first 24 to 48 hours of rehydration. Also, the radiographic manifestations of chronic diseases such as congestive heart failure, chronic obstructive pulmonary disease (COPD), and malignancy may obscure the infiltrate of pneumonia.

Although radiographic patterns are usually nonspecific, they can suggest a microbiologic differential diagnosis. Lobar consolidation or a large pleural effusion suggests a bacterial pathogen. Cavitation may be found in bacterial abscesses, as well as mycobacterial, fungal, or nocardial infections. Pneumonias caused by *S. pneumoniae* may present as a lobar or bronchopneumonia. Gram-negative and staphylococcal pneumonias can cause consolidation and cavitation. The infiltrate that progresses rapidly from a single lobe to multiple lobes should raise suspicion of *L. pneumophila.*

Although aspiration more commonly affects the right lung because of tracheobronchial anatomy, both lungs can be affected simultaneously. The affected site may depend on position at the time of aspiration. Aspiration while recumbent will commonly lead to clinical and radiographic pneumonia in the posterior segments of the upper lobes and superior segments of the lower lobes. Upright aspiration usually affects the lung bases.

When diffuse interstitial infiltrates predominate in the absence of clinical evidence of fluid overload, pneumonias caused by viruses or *P. carinii* should be considered in the differential diagnosis.

## Cultures

A Gram-stained sputum specimen also can provide critical information in choosing empiric therapy. Unfortunately, sputum is frequently difficult to obtain from elderly patients because of a weak cough, obtundation, and dehydration. Inhaled nebulized saline may help mobilize secretions. Nasotracheal suctioning can sample the lower respiratory tract directly, but this technique risks oropharyngeal contamination and is therefore of lesser value. A sputum specimen is thought to reflect lower respiratory secretions when more than 25 white blood cells (WBCs) and less than 10 epithelial cells are seen in a low-powered microscopic field. When such a specimen also shows a predominant organism, it lends a high positive predictive value for the choice of appropriate antimicrobial therapy. Other stains, such as the acid-fast stain for mycobacteria, modified acid-fast stain for *Nocardia,* or the toluidine blue and Gomori methenamine silver stains for *P. carinii,* may prove useful when historically indicated. The direct fluorescent antibody staining of sputum, bronchoalveolar lavage fluid, or pleural fluid may help identify *Legionella* species.

The sputum culture remains a controversial tool but is still recommended to help tailor therapy. It may prove particularly helpful in identifying resistant nosocomial bacterial pathogens. Expectorated morning sputum specimens also can be sent for mycobacterial culture when a compatible clinical syndrome is noted.

When a patient is hospitalized with pneumonia, blood cultures drawn within 8 hours may improve clinical outcome.

When these procedures fail to yield a microbiologic diagnosis, and when the patient fails to respond to empiric antibiotic therapy, more invasive diagnostic techniques may be indicated. Fiberoptic bronchoscopy allows the use of several techniques in the diagnosis of pneumonia. Bronchoalveolar lavage with saline can obtain deep respiratory specimens for the gamut of stains and cultures mentioned above. A transbronchial biopsy of infiltrated lung parenchyma can reveal alveolar or interstitial pneumonitis, viral inclusion bodies, and invading fungal or mycobacterial organisms. The protected brush catheter is used to quantitatively distinguish between tracheobronchial colonizers and pneumonic pathogens. When recovered secretions contain $10^3$ colony-forming units (cfu)/mL of a bacterial pathogen, lower respiratory infection should be suspected.

In some centers, mini-bronchoalveolar lavage is another method used in the diagnosis of nosocomial pneumonia. This procedure is performed through the nonbronchoscopic passage of a telescoping catheter through the endotracheal tube. Several recent articles have suggested a high culture concordance between this method and the bronchoscopic protected-brush catheter technique.

A more substantial amount of lung tissue may be obtained for culture and histologic examination using thoracoscopic or open-lung biopsy. Because these procedures can carry considerable morbidity, their timing in the diagnostic algorithm is controversial. They are usually reserved for the deteriorating patient with a pneumonia that defies diagnosis by less invasive techniques.

## Serologic Testing

Serologic testing for such pathogens as *Legionella* species, *Mycoplasma* species, and *C. pneumoniae* should include sera drawn in both the acute and convalescent phases for comparison. A fourfold increase in the immunoglobulin G (IgG) titer is suggestive of recent infection with these organisms.

IgM assays are prone to false positives, but can provide evidence of acute infection. A single IgM titer of $\geq$1:16 is judged to be diagnostic of acute infection with *C. pneumoniae.*

A sensitive enzyme immunoassay has been developed for the detection of *L. pneumophila* antigen in urine. Because the antigen persists for prolonged periods after infection, it is difficult to differentiate between past and current infections when using this assay. A similar urine antigen test has been developed for the detection of *Streptococcus pneumoniae,* and it may be used to augment standard techniques of culture and Gram staining.

A urinary assay for the detection of *H. capsulatum* antigen is also available and can be a useful diagnostic adjunct to traditional fungal complement fixation and immunodiffusion test batteries.

## Molecular Techniques

Powerful molecular techniques are being applied to the early diagnosis of pneumonia. DNA probes have been used for the detection of *Legionella* species, *M. pneumoniae,* and *M. tuberculosis* in sputum. These probes have excellent sensitivity and specificity, but can produce some false-positive results. The polymerase chain reaction (PCR) has been shown to be a sensitive tool for the early detection of *M. tuberculosis* in sputum specimens. Given the large percentage of pneumonia cases for which no microbial etiology is identified, it is likely that molecular tools will eventually be applied to the identification and antimicrobial susceptibility testing of nearly all agents of pneumonia.

## TREATMENT OF PNEUMONIA

### Hospitalization

Healthcare budgetary constraints have given rise to a number of studies addressing the issue of hospitalization in community-acquired pneumonia. A recent study (3) validated a risk scale for mortality in community-acquired pneumonia. Patients less than 50 years of age without significant coexisting diseases or vital sign abnormalities were assigned to risk group I. All others were grouped in classes II ($\leq$70 points), III (71–90 points), IV (91–130 points), and V (>130 points) using a system assigning points for age, residence, coexisting diseases, physical examination findings, and laboratory abnormalities:

- Age: Males, 1 point per year; females, 1 point per year minus 10
- Nursing home resident, 10 points
- Coexisting illnesses: Neoplastic disease, 30 points; chronic renal disease, 10 points; congestive heart failure, 10 points; chronic liver disease, 20 points; cerebrovascular disease, 10 points
- Physical findings: Respiratory rate 30 breaths/min, 20 points; systolic blood pressure <90 mm Hg, 20 points;

pulse 125 beats/min, 10 points; temperature 40°C or <35°C, 15 points; altered mental status, 20 points
■ Diagnostic tests: $PaO_2$ <60 mm Hg, 10 points; hematocrit <30%, 10 points; blood urea nitrogen >30 mg/dL, 20 points; pleural effusion on chest radiograph, 10 points; sodium <130 mM, 20 points; glucose >250 mg/dL, 10 points; arterial pH <7.35, 30 points

Patients in the first three risk classes had less than 1% mortality, with steep increases to 9.3% in class IV and 27.0% in class V. Fewer than 6% of patients in the first three groups treated as inpatients required intensive care unit admission, and fewer than 10% of patients in the first two groups treated as outpatients were subsequently hospitalized. Although these data can help in patient assessment, the decision to admit must ultimately be individualized to each patient encounter.

## Pharmacologic Treatment

With concerns about antimicrobial overuse, healthcare costs, and bacterial resistance increasing, pharmacologic therapy should always follow the confirmation of the diagnosis of pneumonia and should always be accompanied by a diligent effort to identify an etiologic agent. When the history, chest radiograph, and a Gram-stained sputum fail to suggest a specific cause for pneumonia, a trial of empiric antibiotics is warranted. Antibiotic therapy is best initiated after obtaining appropriate specimens for culture, when appropriate. The choice of antimicrobial is dictated by severity of illness, treatment setting, and comorbid diseases. Table 16.1 provides a framework for the initial therapy of community-acquired pneumonia, based on the recommendations of the Infectious Disease Society of America (IDSA) (4,5). Expert panels from several groups, including the American Thoracic Society (ATS) (6), have also rendered guidelines with similar treatment recommendations.

In the outpatient treatment of pneumonia, the IDSA recommends the use of an oral macrolide, tetracycline, or newer fluoroquinolone (i.e., levofloxacin, gatifloxacin, or moxifloxacin). Of note, ATS guidelines limit the use of fluoroquinolones in the outpatient setting to patients with comorbid diseases or risks for resistant pathogens. The use of the newer fluoroquinolones as first-line agents for pneumonia remains controversial and should be considered in the context of evolving, significant data regarding the side effect profiles of and emerging resistance to these agents. If HIV infection is a suspected comorbidity, then strong consideration should be given to the inclusion of trimethoprim-sulfamethoxazole in the treatment regimen.

When patients with community-acquired pneumonia require hospitalization but are not critically ill, intravenous therapy with cefotaxime, ceftriaxone, or a β-lactam/β-lactamase inhibitor combination plus a macrolide is warranted. Newer fluoroquinolones provide a monotherapeutic option, although this recommendation remains con-

troversial. When the pneumonia is severe, empiric intravenous therapy should include cefotaxime, ceftriaxone, or a β-lactam/β-lactamase inhibitor combination (the latter is preferred if resistant Gram-negative pathogens are suspected) plus either high-dose erythromycin, azithromycin, or a newer fluoroquinolone. Intravenous antibiotics may be switched to oral antibiotics when the patient is stable and afebrile, provided that the patient can adhere to the selected regimen and has adequate swallowing and gastrointestinal function.

Because Gram-negative organisms predominate in pneumonia acquired in hospital settings, an agent possessing antipseudomonal activity (such as an antipseudomonal cephalosporin or penicillin, β-lactam/β-lactamase inhibitor, imipenem, or a fluoroquinolone) and an aminoglycoside are usually used. When nosocomial pneumonia is severe, and the institution has a significant percentage of methicillin-resistant staphylococci, consideration should be given to the empiric addition of vancomycin until culture data excluding the presence of these pathogens can be obtained. If the hospitalized patient is also neutropenic, and the response to antibacterials is suboptimal, some consideration should be given to the early addition of antifungal therapy.

Clindamycin is preferred over penicillin for the treatment of community-acquired aspiration pneumonia because of its superiority in the treatment of oral anaerobes such as *Bacteroides melaninogenicus*. Amoxicillin/clavulanic acid also provides excellent coverage in this setting. When large-volume aspiration is documented in the hospital, a β-lactam/β-lactamase inhibitor combination or the combination of clindamycin and an antipseudomonal agent should be used.

When the diagnostic techniques described above yield a specific causative agent for the pneumonia, special effort should be made to narrow the spectrum of activity used as early as possible. Overuse of broad-spectrum agents encourages the development of resistance and should be avoided whenever possible.

Despite a lack of controlled data specifically addressing length of therapy, many cases of community-acquired pneumonia are adequately treated with 10 to 14 days of therapy. Certain organisms, however (e.g., *Legionella, S. aureus, Pseudomonas*, or *C. pneumoniae*), may require longer courses. Similarly, patients with comorbidities that compromise local (COPD) or systemic (hematologic malignancy) immunity may take longer to clear their illness.

With concern for healthcare costs on the rise, much attention has been given to the oral treatment of pneumonia. Fully oral and intravenous-to-oral "switch" therapies offer potential reductions in length of stay, antibiotic administration costs, complications of venous access, and disruption of families and careers. Many antibiotics are well-absorbed from the gastrointestinal tract, lending further credence to the notion of effective oral treatment. Because well-controlled, risk-stratified data comparing oral

**TABLE 16.1**

**ANTIBIOTIC THERAPY FOR COMMUNITY-ACQUIRED PNEUMONIA IN IMMUNOCOMPETENT ADULTS**

| Setting | Patient | Common Pathogens | Empiric Therapy |
|---|---|---|---|
| Outpatient | No comorbid diseases; no recent prior antibiotic therapy | *S. pneumoniae* <br> *M. pneumoniae* <br> *C. pneumoniae* <br> Viruses <br> *H. influenzae* | A macrolide or doxycycline |
| | No cormorbid diseases; recent prior antibiotic therapy | *S. pneumoniae* <br> *M. pneumoniae* <br> *C. pneumoniae* <br> Viruses <br> *H. influenzae* | Fluoroquinolone alone; newer macrolide plus high-dose amoxicillin or amoxicillin/ clavulanate |
| | Having comorbid disease; no recent prior antibiotic therapy | *S. pneumoniae* <br> Viruses <br> *H. influenzae* <br> Gram-negative bacilli[b] <br> *S. aureus*[b] | Newer macrolide or a fluoroquinolone[a] |
| | Having comorbid disease; recent prior antibiotic therapy | *S. pneumoniae* <br> Viruses <br> *H. influenzae* <br> Gram-negative bacilli[b] <br> *S. aureus*[b] | Fluoroquinolone alone or a newer macrolide plus a β-lactam[c] |
| Inpatient | Not severely ill | *S. pneumoniae* <br> *H. influenzae* <br> Polymicrobial <br> Anaerobes <br> *S. aureus* <br> *C. pneumoniae* <br> Viruses | A macrolide and cefotaxime or ceftriaxone or a β-lactam/β-lactamase inhibitor[f]; a fluoroquinolone[d] alone |
| | Severely ill | *S. pneumoniae*[e] <br> *Legionella* <br> Gram-negative bacilli <br> *M. pneumoniae* <br> Viruses <br> *S. aureus* | Erythromycin, azithromycin, or a fluoroquinolone[c] and cefotaxime, ceftriaxone, or a β-lactam/β-lactamase inhibitor[f] |

[a] In the outpatient setting, many authorities prefer to reserve fluoroquinolones (levofloxacin, gatifloxacin, moxifloxacin) for patients with comorbid diseases/risk factors.
[b] In most cases, patients with pneumonias due to these organisms should be hospitalized.
[c] High-dose amoxicillin, high-dose amoxicillin-clavulanate, cefpodoxime, cefprozil, or cefuroxime.
[d] Levofloxacin, gatifloxacin, moxifloxacin.
[e] Critically ill patients in areas with significant rates of high-level pneumococcal resistance and a suggestive sputum Gram stain should receive vancomycin or a newer quinolone pending microbiologic diagnosis.
[f] Piperacillin-tazobactam or ampicillin-sulbactam.
Modified with permission from Mandell LA, Bartlett JG, Dowell SF, et al. Update of practice guidelines for the management of community-acquired pneumonia in immunocompetent adults. *Clin Infect Dis* 2003;37:1405–1433.

and intravenous therapies are few, appropriate patient populations and treatment settings for oral therapy are yet to be fully defined. Better data exist for the use of switch therapies for the stabilized patient who has good gastrointestinal and swallowing function and adequate social support, and such regimens have gained wide acceptance.

## SPECIFIC PATHOGENS

Certain emerging pathogens have been the subject of considerable research in recent years. Given their importance, they are worthy of special attention.

### *Streptococcus pneumoniae*

Although the pneumococcus is a familiar enemy, it has become even more formidable in recent years. The exact incidence of pneumococcal pneumonia is unknown, but it has been estimated at 1 to 2 per 1,000 persons per year in the United States. It is more common in the elderly, with incidence estimates ranging from 14 to 46 per 1,000 persons per year. Untreated mortality has been estimated at about 30%.

Although pneumococci have traditionally been exquisitely sensitive to penicillin, strains of the organism possessing low- or high-level resistance to penicillin have established a foothold in many communities. The Centers for Disease Control and Prevention (CDC) states that 5% to 15% of pneumococcal isolates in many areas of the United States exhibit high-level penicillin resistance, with several areas reporting 35% of isolates with at least intermediate resistance. Some of these strains are multiply resistant, with resistance to multiple cephalosporins, erythromycin, tetracyclines, and trimethoprim-sulfamethoxazole. No strains resistant to vancomycin have been isolated. This has led to the recommendation by several authorities that empiric therapy for life-threatening disease suspected or proven to be due to pneumococci include vancomycin or a newer fluoroquinolone (in nonmeningitic disease) until susceptibility patterns are known. Because peak penicillin levels in high-dose intravenous therapy reach 50 to 60 μg/mL, many authorities feel that pneumonia due to pneumococci that are inhibited by a minimum concentration (MIC) of 0.12 to 2.0 μg/mL of penicillin can be treated with high-dose penicillin (150,000–200,000 U/kg/day in divided doses). Ceftriaxone or cefotaxime may be used for strains with reduced susceptibility to penicillin (MIC >0.1 μg/mL), providing the MIC for these agents is <2 μg/mL. If the penicillin MIC is more than 2.0 μg/mL (penicillin-resistant *S. pneumoniae*) and the cephalosporin MIC is also elevated, then vancomycin and the newer fluoroquinolones are the treatments of choice. Whenever possible, vancomycin should be changed to β-lactam therapy, because of both improved efficacy and the continuing emergence of vancomycin resistance among Gram-positive pathogens such as enterococci and staphylococci.

### Legionella Species

Although difficult to visualize on sputum Gram's stain and slow to grow even on specialized culture media, members of the *Legionella* genus frequently leave several epidemiologic clues helpful to the diagnosis of Legionnaire's disease. Most frequently occurring in the spring or summer months, Legionnaire's disease can occur sporadically or in epidemics in settings with recirculated air, such as hotels, airplanes, and hospitals. It can occur in adults of all ages but is more common in middle-aged and elderly persons. A prodrome of malaise, myalgia, and headache frequently is present, sometimes accompanied by gastrointestinal symptoms such as watery diarrhea, nausea, or abdominal pain. The pneumonia is often explosive, with nonproductive cough, high fever, shaking chills, tachycardia, and tachypnea. Focal findings on lung examination and chest radiograph (initially patchy areas of bronchopneumonia) can progress within hours to a multilobe process. Confusion and disorientation can be present.

Laboratory evaluation can also yield information useful in the diagnosis. Left-shifted leukocytosis may be present on the complete blood count. Elevated liver function tests, azotemia, hypophosphatemia, hyponatremia, and hypoxemia may be seen, but none of these findings are pathognomonic for legionellosis. Urinalysis may reveal hematuria.

The sputum Gram's stain in *Legionella* pneumonia usually reveals many WBCs but no predominant organism. Culture is best attempted with charcoal-yeast extract agar, but sensitivities of 50% to 70% are common. Therefore, a variety of alternative tests have been developed to support the diagnosis. Serology is 70% to 96% sensitive and more than 95% specific, but results may not be available for several days. Sputum-direct fluorescent antibody testing is likewise highly specific, but quite technique-dependent, with sensitivities of 25% to 80% reported. DNA probing of sputum specimens is expensive, available only in a few laboratories, and relatively insensitive (50%–65%). Urinary antigen testing is sensitive (75%–90%), uniformly specific, and may turn positive as early as 72 hours into the illness. It only detects *L. pneumophila* type 1, however, which accounts for 80% of cases of legionellosis. The test fails to distinguish acute from remote infection because antigenuria may be present for up to a year after infection. The IDSA recommends culture and urinary antigen testing as the primary diagnostic modalities for *Legionella* pneumonia. Empiric therapy for legionellosis may still be warranted, however, when the clinical setting is appropriate, despite extensive negative testing.

Standard therapy has traditionally consisted of a macrolide, typically erythromycin, intravenously at a high dose (1 g intravenously every 6 hours). Many authorities advocate the addition of rifampin, which also offers good intracellular penetration. A lengthy course (at least 3 weeks) may be required for cure. More recently, clinical preference has drifted toward the use of azithromycin or quinolones; the IDSA panel prefers the use of azithromycin, doxycycline, ofloxacin, levofloxacin, or ciprofloxacin over erythromycin for severe legionellosis.

### Chlamydophila pneumoniae

Only recognized as a cause of respiratory infection in 1986, this obligate intracellular pathogen was originally designated as the TWAR agent from the laboratory numbers of the first two strains isolated. Predicted over 40 years ago by epidemiologic studies of psittacosis-like infections with no exposure to birds, *C. pneumoniae* is now classified as a pathogen distinct from *C. psittaci*, and having person-to-person respiratory transmission. Current seroepidemiology suggests that *C. pneumoniae* accounts for about 10% of all cases of community-acquired pneumonia, with a seroprevalance in the United States of about 50%. Data indicate that most adults are exposed during the teenage years, outside the home. Outbreaks have been reported to spread somewhat more slowly than influenza through closed populations such as military recruits and college students.

The clinical presentation of respiratory infections due to *C. pneumoniae* is frequently nonspecific. Cough (productive or nonproductive) and sore throat are common, occurring in more than 80% of patients. A clinical clue present in only 30% of cases is hoarseness, which is present in less than 5% of patients with mycoplasmal or viral infections. Mild fever and leukocytosis are common. The presentation on lung examination and chest radiography is usually that of a localized infiltrate. The illness is usually indolent, although severe pneumonias can occur in elderly and immunocompromised adults.

Culture diagnosis is uncommon because the organism is difficult to cultivate. The diagnosis is made more commonly by serology, with IgM titers ≥1:16 or a fourfold titer increase considered diagnostic.

Both tetracyclines and macrolides have been shown to have excellent in vitro activity against *C. pneumoniae* and are considered the treatment agents of choice despite a relative paucity of clinical data. Alternatives to these agents may include quinolones such as levofloxacin, gatifloxacin, and moxifloxacin.

### *Mycoplasma pneumoniae*

Like *C. pneumoniae*, *M. pneumoniae* accounts for 5% to 20% of community-acquired pneumonia, with slow spread through closed populations. It produces a syndrome of low-grade fever, nonproductive cough, and pharyngitis. Headache and otalgia also are frequently reported. The most common respiratory syndrome is bronchitis, with up to one-fourth of these patients proceeding to pneumonia. Radiographic presentations range from single to multilobe, with patchy infiltrates. Uncommon but sometimes severe extrapulmonary manifestations can include hemolytic anemia, myocarditis, pericarditis, meningoencephalitis, monoarthritis or polyarthritis, and erythema multiforme.

The culture of *M. pneumoniae* requires broth medium and a 7- to 10-day span of time, so it usually is not performed. Diagnosis is serologic, with specific IgM positivity, IgG titers ≥1:256, or a fourfold increase in IgG titer considered diagnostic. The cold agglutinin test is nonspecific but supports the diagnosis of mycoplasmal infection when a high titer (≥1:128) is present.

Therapy consists of the administration of a macrolide, tetracycline, or fluoroquinolone for at least 14 days.

### Influenza and Other Viruses

In some series of community-acquired pneumonia, no etiologic agent was established in 40% to 50% of cases. It is likely that a portion of these is due to viral agents, which are an underdiagnosed cause of pneumonia. Among immunocompetent adults, influenza viruses (especially influenza A) are the most common causes of viral pneumonia. Mainly occurring between October and March, influenza pneumonia is characterized by nonproductive cough, wheezing, myalgia, sore throat, and fever. Chest radiographs may show localized or diffuse patchy infiltrates. The diagnosis is established by serology or by swab collection of nasopharyngeal cells for culture or rapid antigen detection, such as direct immunofluorescent staining. Rapid methods, which can provide an answer in minutes to hours, are perhaps most useful when treatment is contemplated. The standard treatment of influenza A pneumonia has been amantidine or the less toxic rimantidine. Two newer agents, zanamivir and oseltamivir, have activity against both influenza A and B. If given soon after the onset of symptoms, these drugs can shorten the duration of symptoms and viral shedding by 1 to 2 days.

When the patient with suspected or documented influenza develops a secondary, more acute phase of illness with high fever and productive cough, bacterial superinfection must be considered. *S. aureus*, *S. pneumoniae*, and *H. influenzae* are the most common causes of pneumonia in this setting.

Adenoviruses have been demonstrated to cause pneumonia in military recruits. Along with adenoviruses, respiratory syncytial virus, influenza virus, and parainfluenza virus can cause viral pneumonia in immunocompromised patients. Direct immunofluorescent staining of the nasopharyngeal cells provides the most rapid diagnostic method.

### Hantavirus Pulmonary Syndrome

In 1993, a cluster of 24 patients living in the Four Corners area of New Mexico, Arizona, Colorado, and Utah developed acute respiratory failure following an influenza-like illness. Twelve of these patients died, sparking an epidemiologic investigation that led to the isolation of a new pathogen in the hantavirus family, the Sin Nombre virus. Subsequent characterization of the illness caused by this agent suggests that it is transmitted to humans by exposure to the excreta of the deer mouse (*Peromyscus maniculatus*). The epidemiologic range of this disease has grown steadily since its characterization, and cases have been noted in several regions of the United States.

Fever, myalgia, nausea, vomiting, and abdominal pain mark the prodromal phase of the disease, lasting 3 to 6 days. Upper respiratory symptoms are uncommon. The cardiopulmonary phase is heralded by progressive cough and dyspnea, with tachypnea, tachycardia, fever, and severe hypotension. Laboratory evaluation reveals thrombocytopenia, abnormal coagulation parameters, and leukocytosis, sometimes with atypical lymphocytosis. Renal failure is rare, but ventilatory failure is common, with 88% of patients requiring mechanical ventilation. The chest radiograph progresses rapidly to diffuse interstitial edema. Lung pathology reveals evidence of vascular permeability without parenchymal necrosis.

The diagnosis is serologic, with demonstration of IgM or a fourfold increase in IgG antibodies. Treatment is largely supportive. Ribavirin, either in the intravenous or aerosolized form, has been proposed by some as a potential therapy, but controlled data to support the use of this toxic drug are lacking.

## Severe Acute Respiratory Syndrome (SARS)

An outbreak of severe respiratory disease spread from southern China worldwide within several weeks of first reports in early 2003. A novel virus, SARS-coronavirus, was quickly identified and diagnostic tests were developed. The outbreak was aggressively controlled by quarantine methods.

The CDC case definition of SARS requires an epidemiologic exposure to the virus, either by travel, close contact, or occupation, within 10 days of developing the prodromal symptoms of headache, chills, myalgias, and malaise. The more severe syndrome of high fever, cough, dyspnea, and radiographic abnormalities follows in some cases. The diagnosis involves the exclusion of and empiric therapy for severe CAP while awaiting the results of diagnostic testing by serology and PCR of blood, respiratory, or stool specimens. Specific treatment has not yet been defined and is currently supportive in nature.

## PREVENTION OF PNEUMONIA

Given the increased resistance among pneumococci and the undiminished importance of influenza as a respiratory pathogen, emphasis on immunization against these agents should be intensified. Immunization can play a critical role in the prevention of pneumonia, particularly in immunocompromised and older adults. The influenza vaccine is formulated and administered annually. Given the risk of postinfluenza bacterial superinfection in elderly and immunocompromised individuals, this vaccine should be given to all patients in these groups, except those allergic to eggs.

The pneumococcal vaccine, containing polysaccharide antigens of the 23 strains responsible for 88% of cases of bacteremic pneumococcal disease, has been shown to be 60% to 70% effective in immunocompetent patients. Side effects are rarely serious and consist of local pain and erythema, which occur in up to 50% of recipients. Patients who are immunosuppressed and those with severely debilitating cardiovascular, pulmonary, renal, hepatic, or diabetic disease may not have sustained titers of protective antibody and should be considered for revaccination after 6 years.

Selective digestive decontamination uses a combination of antibacterial and antifungal agents in an attempt to reduce gastrointestinal and oropharyngeal colonization with microorganisms. The simultaneous administration of these agents as an oral paste and a nasogastric suspension has been shown to reduce the incidence of nosocomial pneumonia in some studies but without a convincing improvement in morbidity, mortality, or length of intensive care unit stay.

Nosocomial pneumonia is frequently preventable, and recent guidelines from the CDC address strategies to reduce the incidence of this entity. Hand washing and bar-

rier precautions are stressed as strategies to reduce patient-to-patient transmission of respiratory pathogens by healthcare workers in the intensive care unit. Many hospitals now employ teams to evaluate swallowing function and aspiration risk. The modified barium swallow can help establish the types of liquid and solid foodstuffs likely to be aspirated. Elevation of the upper airway to above the level of the stomach and the use of jejunostomy (rather than gastrostomy) tubes for enteral feeding can help diminish aspiration risk in patients with incompetent lower esophageal sphincters. Finally, careful attention to pulmonary toilet can assist debilitated persons in clearing tracheobronchial secretions.

## REVIEW EXERCISES

### QUESTIONS

1. A 58-year-old woman presents with a 3-week history of nonproductive cough and hoarseness. She reports a temperature of 100.4°F. She is not short of breath and has no chills or sweats. She has a smoking history of 20-packs per year but quit 20 years ago. She lives at home with her husband, who is asymptomatic. She has had several antibiotics in the past week, of which she comments, "I felt a little better after the clarithromycin, but not much, so my doctor changed me to cefuroxime, and I felt worse." On examination, she appears healthy. She has a low-grade fever at 38.0°C, but her vital signs are otherwise normal. The physical examination is unremarkable. Laboratory evaluation is notable only for a normal WBC count with a mild left shift. Chest radiograph reveals a subtle right-sided infiltrate. The most appropriate next step in the care of this patient would be:
   a) Admission for high-dose intravenous erythromycin
   b) Outpatient therapy with oral doxycycline
   c) Admission for intravenous ceftriaxone
   d) Outpatient therapy with oral ciprofloxacin
   e) Home intravenous antibiotic therapy with piperacillin/tazobactam

2. A 23-year-old college student presents in late December with a 5-day history of nonproductive cough and shortness of breath. He notes that a number of fellow students have had respiratory illnesses over the past 2 months. He has recently tested HIV negative. Physical examination shows he is in good physical condition. His temperature is 38.3°C, his heart rate is 120/min, his respiratory rate is 22 breaths/min, and his blood pressure is 90/60 mm Hg. The examination otherwise is remarkable only for a few scattered rales at the lung bases. On laboratory evaluation, he is hypoxemic with a $PO_2$ of 76. The WBC count is 14,000/mm$^3$, with a marked left shift. His hemoglobin is 8.3 g/dL, and his peripheral smear shows

red cell fragments. Chest radiograph reveals bilateral patchy lower lobe infiltrates.

The patient deteriorates soon after admission, requiring mechanical ventilation and pressors. Chest radiography reveals a progression of the infiltrates to involve all five lung lobes. A Swan-Ganz catheter is placed, revealing a high systemic vascular resistance but a low cardiac output.

The most appropriate empiric antimicrobial therapy for this patient is:

a) Trimethoprim-sulfamethoxazole 5 mg/kg intravenously every 6 hours
b) Doxycycline 100 mg intravenously every 12 hours
c) Piperacillin/tazobactam 3.375 g intravenously every 6 hours
d) Azithromycin 500 mg intravenously every day plus ceftriaxone 1 g intravenously every day
e) Clindamycin 900 mg intravenously every 8 hours plus ceftazidime 1 g intravenously every 8 hours

3. A 66-year-old man with a history of non-Hodgkin's lymphoma presents with a 2-week history of dry cough and low-grade fever in January. He has a pet parakeet and a grandchild has a respiratory illness. His lung exam is remarkable for a few rales at the lung bases. His CXR initially reveals a faint infiltrate in both lung bases.

The patient is admitted to the hospital and levofloxacin is administered intravenously. Despite this therapy, the patient's respiratory status worsens over the first 48 hours of hospitalization. He is admitted to the intensive care unit and requires mechanical ventilation. A repeat CXR shows reticulonodular infiltrates throughout both lung fields.

Which of the following are causes of failure to respond to therapy in community-acquired pneumonia?

a) Wrong diagnosis
b) Empyema
c) Poor adherence to medical regimen.
d) a and c
e) a, b, and c

## ANSWERS

### 1. b.

The patient presents with a subacute, indolent illness and radiographic evidence of community-acquired pneumonia. No risk factors for mortality are present, and admission is probably not warranted. Piperacillin/tazobactam has no activity against common atypical bacterial organisms. Ciprofloxacin has poor activity against Gram-positive organisms and should not be used in this setting. Correct therapeutic options include oral tetracyclines, macrolides, levofloxacin, gatifloxacin, or moxifloxacin. In this case, the symptom of hoarseness and partial response to clarithromycin raise suspicion for *C. pneumoniae* as a pathogen. Doxycycline is preferred in this setting.

### 2. d.

The patient is acutely and severely ill with a community-acquired process. By IDSA guidelines, appropriate therapy consists of a macrolide or fluoroquinolone and ceftriaxone, cefotaxime, or a β-lactam/β-lactamase inhibitor combination. Because he is HIV negative and acutely ill, trimethoprim-sulfamethoxazole would not provide adequate coverage for either atypical or serious Gram-negative pathogens. Likewise, neither piperacillin-tazobactam or the combination of clindamycin and ceftazidime would cover atypical pathogens. Intravenous doxycycline alone would not cover all likely typical bacterial pathogens. Of the provided answers, only the combination of azithromycin and ceftriaxone would treat severe pneumonia due to both *Legionella* and typical bacterial pathogens.

This patient presents with several clinical clues to the correct diagnosis. He presents with a nonproductive cough and low-grade fever, suggesting an atypical pathogen. His sputum Gram's stain shows no predominant organism, despite a fulminant process. He has evidence of hemolytic anemia and cardiac dysfunction. His *Mycoplasma* IgM titer was strongly positive, illustrating the potentially severe complications of this ordinarily indolent pathogen.

### 3. e.

Several factors can contribute to failure to respond to initial antibiotic therapy in community-acquired pneumonia. First, one should consider the correctness of the diagnosis. A number of diagnoses may lead to pulmonary infiltrates, including noninfectious diseases such as heart failure. Host factors such as empyema, immunodeficiency, and bronchial tree obstruction may slow the response to antibiotics. It is also important to consider difficulties with the regimen itself: Is this the wrong drug or dose? Is the patient adhering to the regimen? The clinician must also place less common microbial pathogens in the differential diagnosis, as some pathogens do not respond to standard antibiotic regimens. Finally, certain pathogens, such as *Legionella* species and *Streptococcus pneumoniae*, may cause overwhelming infection that may not immediately respond to antibiotics.

In this circumstance, the patient is immunocompromised by virtue of his lymphoma. He has a pet parakeet and might have pneumonia caused by an unusual pathogen, such as *C. psittaci*. He has a granddaughter with a respiratory illness and it is January, raising the question of viral pathogens such as influenza, respiratory syncytial virus, adenovirus, parainfluenza virus, and others. Given his rapid decline, bronchoscopy is likely indicated to obtain a specimen for staining and culture for a broad range of pathogens. Serology may be useful to help diagnose chlamydial infection and other atypical pathogens, such as *Legionella* and *Mycoplasma* species.

## REFERENCES

1. Osler W. *Principles and Practice of Medicine.* New York: Appleton, 1892.
2. Bartlett JG, Mundy LM. Community-acquired pneumonia. *N Engl J Med* 1995;333:1618–1624.
3. Fine MJ, Auble TE, Yealy DM, et al. A prediction rule to identify low-risk patients with community-acquired pneumonia. *N Engl J Med* 1997;336:243–250.
4. Bartlett JG, Dowell SF, Mandell LA, et al. Practice guidelines for the management of community-acquired pneumonia in adults. *Clin Infect Dis* 2000;31:347–382.
5. Mandell LA, Bartlett JG, Dowell SF, et al. Update of practice guidelines for the management of community-acquired pneumonia in immunocompetent adults. *Clin Infect Dis* 2003;37:1405–1433.
6. American Thoracic Society. Guidelines for the management of adults with community-acquired pneumonia in adults: diagnosis, assessment of severity, antimicrobial therapy, and prevention. *Am J Resp Crit Care Med* 2001;163:1730–1754.

## SUGGESTED READINGS

Ailani RK, Agastya G, Mukunda BN, et al. Doxycycline is a cost-effective therapy for hospitalized patients with community-acquired pneumonia. *Arch Intern Med* 1999;159:266–270.
Butler JC, Peters CJ. Hantaviruses and hantavirus pulmonary syndrome. *Clin Infect Dis* 1994;19:387–395.

Cassiere HA, Fein AM. Duration and route of antibiotic therapy in community-acquired pneumonia: switch and step-down therapy. *Semin Respir Infect* 1998;13:36–42.
Centers for Disease Control and Prevention. Guidelines for prevention of nosocomial pneumonia. *MMWR* 1997;46:1–85.
Friedland IR, McCracken GH. Management of infections caused by antibiotic-resistant *Streptococcus pneumoniae*. *N Engl J Med* 1994; 331:377–382.
Grayston JT, Campbell LA, Kuo CC, et al. A new respiratory tract pathogen: *Chlamydia pneumoniae* strain TWAR. *J Infect Dis* 1990;161:618–625.
Marrie TJ. Community-acquired pneumonia. *Clin Infect Dis* 1994;18: 501–513.
Marrie TJ. *Mycoplasma pneumoniae* pneumonia requiring hospitalization, with emphasis on infection in the elderly. *Arch Intern Med* 1993;153:488–494.
McEachern R, Campbell GD. Hospital-acquired pneumonia: epidemiology, etiology, and treatment. *Infect Dis Clin North Am* 1998;12: 761–769.
Meeker DP, Longworth DL. Community-acquired pneumonia: an update. *Cleve Clin J Med* 1996;63:16–30.
Murray HW, Masur H, Senterfit LB, Roberts RB. The protean manifestations of *Mycoplasma pneumoniae* infection in adults. *Am J Med* 1975;58:229–242.
Rello J, Quintana E, Ausina V, et al. Incidence, etiology, and outcome of nosocomial pneumonia in mechanically ventilated patients. *Chest* 1991;100:439–444.
Scheld WM, Mandell GL. Nosocomial pneumonia: pathogenesis and recent advances in diagnosis and therapy. *Rev Infect Dis* 1991; 13(suppl):743–751.
Stout JE, Yu VL. Legionellosis. *N Engl J Med* 1997;337:682–687.

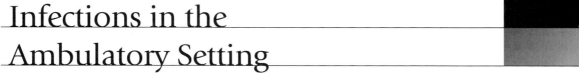

# Infections in the Ambulatory Setting

# 17

*Sherif B. Mossad*

Several other important topics on infections in the ambulatory setting, such as community-acquired pneumonia, sexually transmitted diseases, hepatitis, and tuberculosis, are discussed in other chapters of this book.

## ACUTE INFECTIOUS DIARRHEA

Acute diarrhea is defined as having more than three liquid stools (more than 200 grams) per day for a period of less than 14 days. Acute infectious diarrhea (AID) is second only to the common cold in frequency of healthcare-related visits. AID is more common during the winter months, with an average incidence of 1.4 episodes per person a year. AID results in about 900,000 hospitalizations and 6,000 deaths annually in the United States. The mortality rate is much higher in the developing world, particularly among infants.

Viruses, such as noroviruses, rotaviruses, and norwalk-like viruses cause most cases of AID. In the United States, bacterial causes of AID in adults, in order of frequency, are *Campylobacter*, *Salmonella*, *Shigella*, and *Escherichia coli* O157:H7 [Shigella toxin producing *E. coli* (STEC)].

The most important step in evaluating a patient with AID is to differentiate between inflammatory and noninflammatory causes. Symptoms suggestive of inflammatory AID include fever, presence of blood in stools, and tenesmus. Because most cases of AID are self-limited, laboratory investigation is not indicated for patients presenting within 24 hours of illness, unless they have one of the above symptoms. Testing for fecal leukocytes using microscopy or an immunoassay for lactoferrin may be used if the history is

## TABLE 17.1

### INCUBATION PERIOD FOR VARIOUS CAUSES OF ACUTE INFECTIOUS DIARRHEA

| Less than 6 Hours | 6 to 24 Hours | 16 to 72 Hours |
|---|---|---|
| Staphylococcus aureus<br>Bacillus cereus | Clostridium perfringens<br>Bacillus cereus | Noroviruses, enterotoxigenic<br>E. coli, Vibrio, Salmonella, Shigella,<br>Campylobacter, Yersinia, STEC, Giardia,<br>Cyclospora, Cryptosporidium |

equivocal. Stool cultures are grossly overused, making the cost per positive result greater than $1,000. The incubation period between exposure to the presumed culprit food and the onset of illness may offer some clues for specific etiologic diagnoses (Table 17.1), but significant overlap occurs, thus making this an inaccurate measure. Epidemiologic clues, such as the type of food consumed, recent hospitalization, recent travel, regional outbreaks, and daycare exposure can be very helpful in narrowing down the differential diagnosis. Similarly, clinical clues, such as fever, bloody stools, and dysentery, as well as host-related defenses and immune defects should offer further clues to the etiologic diagnosis.

Rehydration is the most important measure in the management of AID. Ample evidence refutes the misconception that the bowels need to rest in AID. Oral rehydration suffices in most cases, using home remedies such as soups and Gatorade. Glucose-containing electrolyte solutions are preferred over hyperosmolar fluids. A standard oral rehydration formulation is recommended by the World Health Organization, particularly in resource-poor areas. Bismuth subsalicylate and kaolin-pectin are effective antidiarrheal agents. The antimotility agents, loperamide and diphenoxylate should be avoided in cases of bloody diarrhea, particularly those proven to be due to STEC. Antimicrobial agents are effective in the treatment of traveler's diarrhea, shigellosis, Clostridium difficile–associated diarrhea, and when given early, in cases of campylobacteriosis. A concern exists for prolonged fecal shedding in cases of salmonellosis treated with antibiotics. Antimicrobial therapy is contraindicated in cases of STEC infection because some studies have shown that this increases the risk of serious complications. Trimethoprim-sulfamethoxazole (TMP-SMX), or fluoroquinolones, such as ciprofloxacin are appropriate empiric options, when indicated. Macrolides should be used when quinolone-resistant campylobacteriosis is suspected, such as in travelers returning from Southeast Asia. Oral metronidazole and stopping of systemic antibiotics are the treatment for C. difficile colitis. Healthy adults should be treated for 3 days (10 days for the latter infection) in most cases, but immunocompromised patients usually require a longer duration of therapy. Advising travelers about appropriate eating and drinking habits is crucial in preventing travelers' diarrhea. Prophylactic bismuth subsalicylate decreases the incidence of travelers' diarrhea, but causes blackening of the tongue and stools. Self-treatment with empiric antibiotics is recommended for travelers with AID, but not prophylactic antibiotics.

## URINARY TRACT INFECTIONS

Urinary tract infection (UTI) results in 7 million visits to outpatient clinics and 100,000 hospitalizations annually, with an estimated cost to the healthcare system of $1.6 billion. UTI may be classified into four categories: acute cystitis, acute pyelonephritis, catheter-related, and prostatitis. E. coli is the most common causative organism in all these categories, but the distribution of other causative agents varies (Table 17.2).

### Acute Cystitis

The first step in the management of acute cystitis is to differentiate this from cervicitis, vaginitis, and urethritis. If symptoms of cystitis (frequency, dysuria, urgency) are most prominent, one should ask about other symptoms suggestive of upper UTI, such as fever, chills, and flank pain. Next, risk factors for having complicated cystitis should be evaluated. These include having symptoms for >14 days, most UTI in men, diabetics, renal transplant recipients, other immunosuppressed individuals, and during pregnancy. In addition, patients with history of urinary stones, and those with anatomic genitourinary abnormalities, should also be considered to have a potentially complicated UTI.

The detection of pyuria by leukocyte esterase test or urine microscopy, and the detection of bacteriuria by nitrite test or urine Gram staining, have low sensitivity and positive predictive value, and high specificity and negative predictive value for the diagnosis of UTI. Both of these tests have their limitations and perform better when used together. Routine urine culture is not indicated for the management of simple cystitis, and empiric therapy is appropriate. The first line of therapy remains TMP-SMX or trimethoprim alone, with fluoroquinolones, nitrofurantoin, and fosfomycin considered as second-line agents. Due to the high rate of antimicrobial resistance in the pathogens causing UTI to penicillins and cephalosporins, these agents are not recommended for empiric therapy.

**TABLE 17.2**

**CLASSIFICATION AND MICROBIOLOGY OF URINARY TRACT INFECTIONS**

| Acute Cystitis and Acute Pyelonephritis | Catheter-related UTI | Prostatitis |
|---|---|---|
| *E. coli* (80%) | *E. coli* | *E. coli* |
| *Staphylococcus saprophyticus* (10%) | Proteus | Proteus |
| Klebsiella | Candida | Providencia |
| Enterobacter | Enterococcus | Klebsiella |
| Proteus | Pseudomonas | Enterobacter |
| Enterococcus | Klebsiella | Pseudomonas |
| | Enterobacter | Citrobacter |
| | *Staphylococcus aureus* | Enterococcus |
| | | *Staphylococcus aureus* and *S. epidermidis* |

The following factors increase the risk of antimicrobial resistance to TMP-SMX:

- Local resistance pattern to TMP-SMX of >20%
- Recent use of TMP-SMX
- Current use of any antimicrobial agents
- Recent hospitalization
- Recurrent UTI
- Estrogen exposure for contraception or hormone replacement
- Diabetes mellitus

Single-dose therapy has been advocated for women, but a high failure rate may be seen with associated occult upper urinary tract infection or with certain organisms such as *Staphylococcus saprophyticus*. Treatment for 3 days is appropriate for most women. Treatment for 7 to 10 days is recommended for most men, diabetics, and renal transplant recipients; during pregnancy; in patients older than 65 years; in women who concomitantly use cervical diaphragms; in patients with symptoms lasting more than 7 days and who have known antimicrobial resistance. Options for recurrent cystitis in women are continuous prophylaxis, postcoital prophylaxis, or self-initiated therapy. The latter option has been well-studied and proven reliable.

## Acute Pyelonephritis

The differential diagnosis for acute pyelonephritis includes renal calculi and renal infarction. The majority of patients with acute pyelonephritis have more than $10^5$ colony-forming units/mL of organisms on urine culture; however 20% may have $10^2$ to $10^5$ colony-forming units/mL. Blood cultures are positive in 15% to 20% of patients ill enough to require hospitalization. Discordance between blood and urine cultures occurs in less than 3% of cases, however. Empiric outpatient antibiotic therapy includes either oral fluoroquinolones or TMP-SMX for 7 to 14 days. Hospitalization and initial parenteral antimicrobial therapy

is advised in patients presenting with nausea and vomiting, and in diabetic and immunosuppressed individuals.

Empiric parenteral antibiotic choices include ampicillin in conjunction with gentamicin, fluoroquinolones, and third-generation cephalosporins. A change to oral antimicrobial therapy can be done as soon as oral intake is restored. Extending antimicrobial therapy beyond 2 weeks will not benefit uncomplicated cases of pyelonephritis, even in bacteremic patients. The persistence of symptoms despite appropriate antimicrobial therapy for more than 48 to 72 hours warrants an imaging study, such as ultrasonography or computerized tomography (Fig. 17.1) to look for intrarenal abscess or evidence of obstruction. Antimicrobial resistance may be seen with any urinary pathogen, particularly *Pseudomonas aeruginosa* and enterococci. The latter organisms may need combination antimicrobial agents or

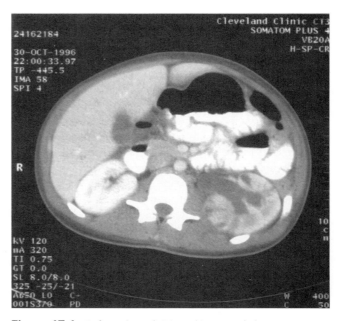

**Figure 17.1**  Left pyelonephritis and intrarenal abscess.

longer-duration therapy. If no anatomic defect that could be corrected is detected, a "test of cure" urine culture is recommended 1 to 2 weeks after the completion of therapy.

### Catheter-Related UTI

Catheter-related UTI is the most common nosocomial infection, accounting for 1 million cases per year. Pyuria is strongly associated with catheter-related UTI due to Gram-negative bacilli, but not Gram-positive cocci or yeast. In addition, bacteriuria with as few as 100 cfu/mL may be indicative of infection in catheterized patients. Because most patients with catheter-related UTI do not have urinary symptoms, one should obtain urine culture and consider empiric therapy for UTI if a catheterized patient develops signs of sepsis that cannot be otherwise explained. In general, however, the treatment of asymptomatic bacteriuria is not recommended.

Antimicrobial prophylaxis should be considered in renal transplant recipients and in patients undergoing transurethral resection of the prostate. Measures to prevent catheter-related UTI include avoiding catheterization in the first place, following strict aseptic insertion techniques, using a closed drainage system, using silver-coated catheters, discontinuing catheterization as soon as the indication resolves, or using alternatives such as condom or suprapubic catheters.

## ACUTE BACTERIAL PROSTATITIS

About one-fourth of men are diagnosed with prostatitis during their lifetime. Patients with acute bacterial prostatitis present with symptoms suggestive of cystitis, associated with deep pelvic pain and constitutional symptoms. In such cases, the prostate gland is swollen and extremely tender on digital rectal exam. Prostate massage should be avoided in these patients because it may precipitate bacteremia; urine culture suffices. An infection is not present in most patients with chronic symptoms. The "four-cup" localization culture test should be utilized in these patients to differentiate between chronic bacterial prostatitis, chronic nonbacterial prostatitis, or chronic pelvic pain syndrome. Similar to acute cystitis, empiric therapy for bacterial prostatitis includes TMP-SMX or fluoroquinolones; however, the recommended duration of therapy is 4 weeks for acute cases, and 6 to 12 weeks for chronic cases.

## UPPER RESPIRATORY TRACT INFECTIONS

Antibiotic prescriptions for upper respiratory tract infection (URI) account for 75% of all antibiotics prescribed for adults, with a total annual cost of $726 million. Fortunately, after years of extensive educational interventions to both physicians and the public, recent surveys have shown a downward trend in the proportion of patients diagnosed with the common cold or bronchitis who are prescribed antibiotics. The use of broad-spectrum antimicrobial agents in these patients has increased by threefold, however. Several symptoms predictive of physicians' behavior to prescribe antibiotics for URI, such as production of yellow sputum, sore throat, fever, and colored nasal discharge, actually have poor predictive evidence in the literature for the efficacy of the prescribed antibiotics. Several studies have shown the importance of a personal explanation of the lack of efficacy and the potential adverse effects of antibiotics to patients presenting with nonspecific URI. In addition, counseling patients about the cost of antibiotics, the false sense of security created by taking them, and the increasing problem of antimicrobial resistance resulting from selective pressure and elimination of normal flora is also very important.

### Infectious Mononucleosis Syndrome

Epstein-Barr virus (EBV) is the most common cause of a "monolike" illness, consisting of the triad of fever, sore throat, and lymphadenopathy. Several other infectious agents can produce a similar illness, however, including cytomegalovirus, human immunodeficiency virus (HIV), human herpesvirus 6 (HPV-6), parvovirus B-19, toxoplasmosis, and group A β-*hemolytic streptococcus* (GABHS) pharyngitis. Patients with EBV infection may also present with fatigue, which can last for 3 weeks or more, headache, and myalgia. Physical examination findings include generalized lymphadenopathy in 95% of cases, pharyngitis in 80%, splenomegaly in 50%, and hepatomegaly and jaundice in 10%. A maculopapular rash is noted on presentation in 5% to 10% of cases, and this rash is more likely to develop in patients who receive ampicillin or amoxicillin for presumed GABHS pharyngitis. Large, lobulated "atypical" lymphocytes often are seen on peripheral blood smear. Mild to moderate leukopenia, thrombocytopenia, and hemolytic anemia may also be seen during the acute illness. Liver function abnormalities occur in up to 80% of patients, particularly in older adults. Monospot test detects heterophile antibodies in 70% to 90% of cases within 1 to 5 weeks of the onset of illness. Specific EBV immunoglobulin M (IgM) is positive with acute infection and usually wanes within 3 months, whereas EBV immunoglobulin G (IgG) remains positive, often for life.

This is a self-limited illness, so treatment is only supportive. Treatment with antiviral agents or corticosteroids is not recommended. A confirmed association exists between EBV and oral hairy leukoplakia and certain types of lymphoma. More recently, a relation between EBV and multiple sclerosis has been suggested by epidemiologic studies.

### Influenza

In the United States, yearly influenza epidemics result in 25 million healthcare visits, with 140,000 resultant hospitalizations and 40,000 to 60,000 deaths at an average of

$12 million. Epidemics in the Northern Hemisphere occur between the months of September and March, usually start in schoolchildren, then spread to the rest of the community. Transmission occurs by small-particle aerosol from infected persons. Viral shedding peaks within 2 to 3 days of infection but may last for 1 week or more. Yearly minor antigenic changes, or *antigenic drift*, in the viral glycoprotein hemagglutinin allow for the viral evasion of any immunological protection built up from influenza infections or immunizations in preceding seasons, thus resulting in annual epidemics. Major changes in viral antigenic composition, or *antigenic shift*, on the other hand, result in pandemics.

Patients present with sudden diffuse or throbbing headache, high fever, severe myalgia, and dry cough. Sore throat and rhinorrhea may occur, but the systemic symptoms are much more prominent. Patients with underlying chronic medical problems such as obstructive lung disease and congestive heart failure are at risk for developing serious complications, through exacerbation of their underlying illness or bacterial superinfection. Bacterial pneumonia after influenza is caused by *Streptococcus pneumoniae*, *Haemophilus influenzae*, or *Staphylococcus aureus* and usually develops several days or weeks later. During epidemics, clinical diagnosis in those presenting with typical symptoms is 80% accurate. The gold standard to confirm the diagnosis for epidemiologic purposes is either viral culture or acute and convalescent serology. Because these measures are not practical for clinical use, several rapid diagnostic tests have been developed, including direct fluorescent antigen detection, enzyme immunoassay, and optical immunoassay.

The therapeutic agents amantadine and rimantadine have been available for several years, and more recently, the neuraminidase inhibitors zanamivir and oseltamivir have become available. The main advantages of these newer agents are their activity against both influenza A and B, better tolerability, and lower incidence of developing viral resistance. They are considerably more expensive, however. For maximum benefit, all influenza antiviral agents should be started within 1 to 2 days of the onset of illness. When used early in the course of influenza, studies have shown these anitviral agents to shorten the duration of illness by 1 to 2 days and to significantly decrease the severity of symptoms. These benefits are more evident in patients presenting with severe illness.

Vaccination remains the primary preventive measure against influenza. The trivalent, inactivated, intramuscular vaccine is recommended for children aged 6 to 23 months, adults aged >50 years, patients with chronic medical problems and their household members, and healthcare providers. Several large studies have shown that influenza vaccine is both efficacious and cost effective. It is well-tolerated and, contrary to false belief, it cannot cause influenza. Vaccination rates in the United States have improved during the last decade but are still less than opti-

mal. In June 2003, the live-attenuated, cold-adapted, intranasal influenza vaccine became available in the United States. It is as effective as the inactivated vaccine, and may be more appealing for those who would like to avoid an injection. It is only approved for healthy persons aged 5 to 49 years, however. In addition, because shedding of live-attenuated virus occurs after receiving this vaccine, healthcare providers and the household contacts of immunocompromised patients should receive the inactivated vaccine to avoid the theoretical risk of virus transmission causing disease. Although all the approved antiviral agents have been shown to be effective in preventing influenza during outbreaks, they should not be regarded as a substitute to the vaccine.

## Acute Rhinosinusitis

Patients are considered to have acute rhinosinusitis if their symptoms last less than 4 weeks. Subacute sinusitis is defined as symptoms lasting 4 to 12 weeks, and chronic sinusitis is present if symptoms last more than 12 weeks. *S. pneumoniae*, *H. influenzae*, *Moraxella catarrhalis*, *S. aureus*, and GABHS are the major causative agents, with viruses causing approximately 5% to 15% of cases. Paranasal sinus ostial blockade due to mucosal edema is the main precipitating factor for the development of sinusitis. This is most commonly predisposed to by an antecedent viral infection or "common cold," but may also be associated with nasal allergies; anatomic abnormalities, such as deviated nasal septum, concha bullosum, and ciliary dysfunction; or immune deficiency, such as hypogammaglobulinemia and HIV infection. Other, less common predisposing factors include diving and cocaine abuse.

Characteristic clinical findings include maxillary toothache, unilateral facial pain, purulent nasal and postnasal discharge, lack of response to decongestants, and decreased transillumination. Computed tomography (CT) is more informative and priced comparably to plain radiography and should be done to define the anatomy before an anticipated corrective surgery. However, neither CT, sinus endoscopy, nor sinus aspiration is recommended before the treatment of an initial episode of acute sinusitis. Most cases of mild sinusitis improve with topical intranasal steroids and topical or systemic nasal decongestants, without the need for antimicrobial therapy.

Because the microbiology of acute sinusitis is somewhat predictable, empiric treatment for moderate and severe cases with amoxicillin, TMP-SMX, or doxycycline as first-line agents is recommended. Alternatives include cefpodoxime, cefuroxime, cefdinir, and macrolides. Broader-spectrum penicillins, such as amoxicillin-clavulanate, and "respiratory" fluoroquinolones, such as levofloxacin, gatifloxacin, and moxifloxacin, should be reserved as second-line agents in situations such as (i) lack of response to first-line agents, (ii) multiple prior antibiotic courses, and (iii) a high incidence of β-lactamase–producing organisms in the community.

## Streptococcal (Tonsillo) Pharyngitis

The differential diagnosis for someone presenting with sore throat includes pharyngitis, epiglottitis, Ludwig's angina, thyroiditis, and gastroesophageal reflux disease. The most important question to answer in a patient presenting with pharyngitis is whether it is caused by GABHS, a readily treatable infection, which may prevent suppurative and immunological complications. Common cold viruses, such as rhinovirus and coronavirus, cause the majority of cases of pharyngitis, and other bacteria, including group C β-hemolytic streptococci, *Corynebacterium diphtheriae*, *Neisseria gonorrhoeae*, *Arcanobacterium haemolyticum*, *Chlamydia pneumoniae*, and *Mycoplasma pneumoniae* each cause a small percentage of cases. The Centor clinical criteria increase the diagnostic likelihood of GABHS infection; these criteria include fever, tonsillar exudate, tender anterior cervical lymphadenopathy, the absence of cough, and exposure within 2 weeks to someone with strep throat. In adults, streptococcal rapid antigen detection test is 80% to 90% sensitive and 95% specific, whereas culture is 90% to 95% sensitive and 95% specific.

Oral penicillin for 10 days is the treatment of choice. Alternatives include intramuscular penicillin, oral first-generation cephalosporins, and oral macrolides.

## Acute Tracheobronchitis

This illness is characterized by cough, with or without sputum production, lasting 1 to 3 weeks. Other commonly associated symptoms include wheezing, coryza, and constitutional symptoms. Viruses, such as influenza A and B, parainfluenza, respiratory syncytial virus, rhinovirus, coronavirus, and adenovirus cause the majority of cases. Fewer than 10% of cases are caused by *Bordetella pertussis*, *B. parapertussis*, *M. pneumoniae*, and *C. pneumoniae* (TWAR). In otherwise healthy patients presenting with cough, pneumonia can be reasonably excluded if the vital signs are normal and if clinical signs of consolidation, such as rales and egophony, are absent. Purulence of sputum is a poor predictor of bacterial infection. Chest radiography should be reserved for patients with comorbid conditions, those with abnormal vital signs or signs of consolidation, or those with persistent symptoms for more than 3 weeks. A normal C-reactive protein can reasonably exclude pneumonia, but may be elevated in the presence of several other infectious and noninfectious conditions. If cough lasts more than weeks, postnasal drip, asthma, and gastroesophageal reflux disease account for the majority of causes. Treating acute tracheobronchitis with antibiotics is not recommended. Most cases resolve spontaneously. Selective β-agonist bronchodilators and antitussive agents may offer symptomatic relief. Other measures used to treat

nonspecific URI, such as vaporizers, and acetaminophen may also be used.

## SOFT TISSUE INFECTIONS

### Cellulitis

Cellulitis is infection involving the subcutaneous tissues. Risk factors include diabetes mellitus, arterial or venous insufficiency, and tinea pedis. Patients whose saphenous veins have been harvested for coronary artery bypass surgery, and those who undergo mastectomy and axillary lymph node dissection for breast cancer are at increased risk of recurrent cellulitis due to lymphatic disruption and lymphedema. Differentiating staphylococcal from streptococcal cellulitis is not possible on clinical grounds alone, so empiric antimicrobial coverage should include an agent active against both types of organisms, such as oral dicloxacillin or intravenous oxacillin, and oral or intravenous first-generation cephalosporins, depending on the severity of illness. The generally accepted course of therapy is 7 to 14 days. Elevation and rest of the involved limb is necessary to reduce edema. Patients with chronic limb edema and lymphedema are advised to use elastic support stockings after cellulitis resolves to avoid recurrence. Interdigital epidermophytosis should be treated with topical antifungal agents. Cellulitis surrounding a decubitus ulcer or a diabetic foot ulcer is likely to be polymicrobial, so a broad-spectrum antimicrobial agent such as ampicillin-sulbactam is appropriate. Pain, tenderness, or crepitus extending outside the area of erythema should raise suspicion for necrotizing fasciitis, which warrants immediate surgical consultation. *H. influenzae* commonly causes buccal cellulitis, so treatment with a third-generation cephalosporin is appropriate. Confirmed Group A streptococcal cellulitis is best treated using penicillin combined with clindamycin to overcome the inoculum effect, which is a stationary microorganism growth phase that makes penicillin less effective. Clindamycin is a logical choice because it acts by inhibiting protein and bacterial toxin synthesis. Rapidly progressive cellulitis in immunocompromised patients, particularly cirrhotics, who are exposed to saltwater or who eat raw oysters should raise the suspicion for *Vibrio vulnificus* as the etiologic agent. Hemorrhagic bullae are characteristically seen in infections by this organism. Bacteremic cases are fatal in 30% to 50% of cases. Doxycycline is the treatment of choice, and thorough cooking of seafood remains the only effective preventive measure.

Cellulitis due to *Aeromonas hydrophila* is another serious form of cellulitis, similarly seen more frequently in cirrhotics and cancer patients who are exposed to fresh water. Some reports linking this infection to medicinal leeches have been published. Other manifestations of infection by this organism include gastroenteritis and spontaneous bacterial peritonitis. Ciprofloxacin is the treatment of choice.

Erysipeloid, caused by *Erysipelothrix rhusiopathiae*, is usually an occupational infection that occurs in healthy people handling meat products or saltwater fish. A violaceous lesion that spreads peripherally and has a raised border and central clearing is characteristic. Ulceration usually does not develop, and this infection is almost always localized to the site of inoculation. It responds well to penicillin therapy. Several mimics of cellulitis exist, including insect bites, acute gout, deep venous thrombosis, fixed drug eruption, pyoderma gangrenosa, and Sweet's syndrome.

## Erysipelas

Erysipelas is infection involving the superficial skin and cutaneous lymphatics. Older literature indicated the face to be the most common site of occurrence, but more recent studies show the lower extremities to account for 80% of cases. Those classic features of erysipelas that distinguish it from cellulitis are the sharp demarcating edge and palpable induration "peau d'orange." Sometimes, however, it is not possible to distinguish both clinically; this is important from the management point because almost all cases of erysipelas are caused by GABHS and are treatable with penicillin, whereas cellulitis, as noted earlier, should be treated with antimicrobial agents that are β-lactamase–resistant. Blood culture and surface culture are rarely positive in erysipelas, and aspirating the leading edge for culture is likewise of low yield. A rising antistreptolysin O titer may be helpful in confirming the diagnosis. Patients with lymphedema are at risk for recurrent erysipelas in up to 30% of cases.

## Bites

Almost one-half of all Americans will be bitten at some point during their lifetime by an animal or by another person. Humans are most frequently bitten by, in order, dogs, cats, wild animals, and other humans. When it comes to potential complications of bites, however, this order is reversed. When bite wounds get infected, *Pasteurella multocida* is the organism seen most frequently in cat bites, α-hemolytic streptococci in dog bites, and *Eikenella corrodens* in human bites. In addition, *S. aureus* and mixed anaerobic organisms are seen in approximately 30% of infected bites. In fact, the bacteriologic analysis of infected dog and cat bites yields a median of five bacterial isolates per culture.

Radiographic studies should be considered when fracture or an impacted foreign body, such as a tooth fragment, is suspected, or if the bite is close to a joint. If the bite is less than 8 hours old and does not appear to be clinically infected, culture from the wound is not recommended. Most bite wounds should be left open with delayed closure. Irrigation, debridement, elevation, and immobilization are important steps in managing any bite wound. A tetanus booster is recommended if the patient has not received one within the preceding 10 years. Rabies vaccine is not recommended for dog or cat bites occurring in the United States, but should be considered for rodent or wild animal bites. The antimicrobial agent of choice in infected bites is amoxicillin-clavulanic acid; for penicillin-allergic individuals, tetracyclines or a combination of a quinolone and clindamycin are reasonable alternatives.

Prophylactic antibiotics in clinically uninfected wounds are not recommended except in those involving severe crush injuries, involving joints or bones, near prosthetic joints, or on the hands. In addition, any bite in immunocompromised patients who are at risk for developing more serious infections should be treated with antibiotics. Prompt surgical intervention is imperative for any deep hand or facial bite that becomes infected.

## Herpetic Whitlow

Autoinnoculation by herpes simplex virus (HSV) type 1 as a complication of oral herpes, or by HSV type 2 as a complication of genital herpes, may result in herpetic whitlow, particularly with an antecedent trauma to the nail cuticle. Exposure may also occur during manual sexual contact, or in healthcare workers exposed to oral secretions. The pain associated with this condition is severe and out of proportion to the physical findings. Systemic symptoms and regional lymphadenopathy are common. Lesions may mimic bacterial infections, such as paronychia, which is an infection of the epidermis bordering the nail, and felon, which is an infection of the distal phalanx pad. Treatment with antiviral agents, such as acyclovir, may shorten illness if started within 48 hours of the onset. Contrary to paronychia or felon, incision and drainage is contraindicated for herpetic whitlow because this may result in viremia or secondary bacterial infection. To avoid occupational exposure, respiratory therapists and dental hygienists should wear gloves when exposed to oral secretions. Unfortunately, recurrence occurs in up to 30% of patients, so either suppressive therapy or treatment during the prodromal stage may be beneficial.

## Onychomycosis

A fungal infection of fingernails and toenails is a very common condition, accounting for approximately half of all nail problems. The distal subungual form is more common than the proximal subungual, superficial, or total dystrophic forms. Most cases are caused by either *Trichophyton rubrum* or *T. mentagrophytes*. Risk factors include increasing age, familial predisposition, diabetes mellitus, peripheral arterial occlusive disease, and HIV infection, as well as other immunosuppressive conditions. Concomitant tinea pedis is present in almost half the patients with onychomycosis. Even though this infection is frequently perceived as a cosmetic problem, it may have psychologic, social, and medical consequences, the direst of which is diabetic foot infection, which may lead

## TABLE 17.3

### INFECTIONS IN THE AMBULATORY SETTING: SUMMARY

| Condition | Etiology | Treatment |
|---|---|---|
| Acute infectious diarrhea | Viral | Rehydration |
| | Bacterial | Quinolone or TMP–SMX |
| Acute cystitis | *E. coli* | TMP–SMX |
| Acute pyelonephritis | *E. coli* | Quinolone or TMP–SMX |
| Catheter–related UTI | *E. coli* | Quinolone or TMP–SMX |
| Acute prostatitis | *E. coli* | Quinolone or TMP–SMX |
| Infectious mononucleosis | EBV | Symptomatic |
| Influenza | Influenza A and B | Amantadine, rimantadine, zanamivir, or oseltamivir |
| Acute rhinosinusitis | *Streptococcus pneumoniae* | Amoxicillin |
| Acute (tonsillo) pharyngitis | GABHS | Penicillin |
| Acute bronchitis | Viral | Beta agonists |
| Cellulitis | *Staphylococcus aureus* and streptococci | Penicillinase-resistant penicillin or first-generation cephalosporin |
| Erysipelas | GABHS | Penicillin |
| Herpetic whitlow | HSV types 1 and 2 | Acyclovir |
| Onychomycosis | *Tricophyton rubrum* | Terbinafine or itraconazole |

to amputation. Other conditions, such as psoriasis, may resemble onychomycosis. This, together with the fact that treatment is both lengthy and costly, has led most health insurance companies to require mycologic confirmation of the diagnosis before reimbursing the cost of treatment. This confirmation may be accomplished by using either a potassium hydroxide preparation of the nail bed scrapings or by fungal culture. Systemic antifungal treatment is generally much more effective than topical therapies, such as ciclopirox nail varnish. Older antifungal agents, such as griseofulvin and ketoconazole, have been largely replaced by safer and more effective options, such as itraconazole and terbinafine. The duration of therapy is several weeks, longer for toenails than fingernails. Intermittent "pulse" therapy with itraconazole for 1 week per month has been shown to be both efficacious and cost effective. Patients should be reminded that continued improvement is expected for several weeks after completing the course of therapy. Unfortunately, relapse may occur in approximately 15% of cases.

## SUMMARY

Table 17.3 summarizes the signs and symptoms and treatment of the infectious diseases presented in this chapter.

## REVIEW EXERCISES

### QUESTIONS

**1.** A 30-year-old healthy woman presents with non-bloody diarrhea that has persisted for less than 24 hours. She has nausea and abdominal cramping, but no fever or tenesmus. No recent travel is noted, and her exam is normal. You should:

a) Ask her if other family members are affected.
b) Check fecal leukocytes by microscopy or lactoferrin.
c) Collect stools for bacterial culture and rotavirus PCR.
d) Tell her to avoid antidiarrheal agents, such as loperamide.
e) Start empiric ciprofloxacin.

**2.** A 22-year-old woman presents with dysuria and foul-smelling urine for 24 hours. No fever or suprapubic or flank pain is present. She had four similar episodes in the past year. She uses spermicide-coated condoms and diaphragms for contraception. Her exam is normal. You should:

a) Collect urine for culture.
b) Order ultrasound of the urinary bladder and kidneys.
c) Prescribe trimethoprim-sulfamethoxazole for 7 days.
d) Advise her to avoid vaginal spermicides.
e) Advise against future self-treatment or prophylaxis.

**3.** A 20-year-old college student presents with fever, sore throat, myalgia, splenomegaly, and generalized lymphadenopathy. Which of the following is true?

a) HIV testing should be considered. Treatment is symptomatic.
b) A vaccine could have prevented this illness. Specific therapy is indicated if presenting within 48 hours.
c) *S. pneumoniae* and *H. influenzae* are likely causes. Amoxicillin remains the first-line agent.
d) Fever, tonsillar exudate, and palatal petechiae increase the likelihood of group A β-hemolytic streptococcus (GABHS) infection.

**e)** Rhinovirus is the most common cause. No diagnostic tests are needed.

**4.** An 80-year-old diabetic woman with varicose veins has fever, pain, and ill-defined redness surrounding an erosion over her tibia. Which of the following is true?

**a)** Blood cultures are rarely positive. Penicillin is the drug of choice.

**b)** Herpes simplex is in the differential diagnosis. Ask about sexual practices.

**c)** Hospital admission for IV antibiotics and surgical consultation is warranted.

**d)** Initiate antimicrobial coverage for streptococci and penicillinase-producing staphylococci.

**e)** Antifungal therapy is needed.

## ANSWERS

**1. a.**

If AID can be linked to the ingestion of a certain meal, such as in a family outbreak setting, the incubation period can be helpful for diagnosis (see Table 17.1). Certain foods are also linked to particular infections; for example, undercooked poultry and campylobacteriosis, undercooked hamburger and STEC, seafood and *Vibrio* species, improperly refrigerated fried rice and *Bacillus cereus*, fresh soft cheeses and *Listeria monocytogenes*, contaminated eggs and *Salmonella* species, unrefrigerated potato salad and *S. aureus* (preformed enterotoxin), and undercooked pork and *Yersinia enterocolytica*. The most likely cause in this case is a viral infection.

Because this illness is less than 24 hours in duration, and is not associated with inflammatory features, the detection of fecal leukocytes and stool cultures are not indicated at this time. Rotavirus PCR should not be used in routine clinical care. Oral rehydration is the appropriate management here. Antimotility agents, such as loperamide and diphenoxylate may be used here if needed, because the diarrhea is not bloody. Empiric antimicrobials are indicated for moderate to severe travelers' diarrhea, and febrile, community-acquired, inflammatory diarrhea, particularly in immunocompromised patients, unless STEC is suspected on epidemiologic grounds. Severe nosocomial diarrhea in patients receiving systemic antibiotics or chemotherapeutic agents should also be treated empirically with metronidazole, pending the results of a *C. difficile* toxin assay. Persistent diarrhea for more than 10 days should raise the concern of protozoal pathogens, such as Giardia and Cryptosporidium; empiric therapy with metronidazole, pending stool microscopy or immunoassay, is reasonable in this setting.

**2. d.**

The microbiology of acute uncomplicated cystitis in women is predictable, so empiric antimicrobial therapy would be appropriate. Collecting urine for culture should be considered if empiric therapy fails. Ultrasound of the urinary bladder may be useful in cases with persistent symptoms to rule out the presence of stone or diverticulum. Renal ultrasound should be considered if a clinical suspicion for upper UTI is present. Treatment with TMP-SMX for 3 days is appropriate in most women; extending therapy for 7 days may be considered in patients with persistent symptoms. The use of vaginal spermicides is a known risk factor for UTI; women with recurrent UTI should be advised to use another form of contraception. Once the diagnosis is established, antimicrobial self-treatment at the onset of dysuria and post-coital prophylaxis are reasonable options for this young woman with recurrent cystitis.

**3. a.**

In the appropriate setting, patients presenting with mononucleosis-type illness should be questioned about their sexual practices because the acute retroviral syndrome has a similar presentation. HIV antibody test is usually negative during the acute illness and may require several weeks or months to become positive. An accurate diagnosis requires a plasma HIV RNA test or HIV p24 antigen detection. This has clear clinical and public health implications. The statement in (b) refers to a patient with influenza; an illness that, unlike infectious mononucleosis, may be preventable with a vaccine and is treatable with specific antiviral agents. The statement in (c) refers to a patient with acute sinusitis, which is not associated with splenomegaly or generalized lymphadenopathy. The statement in (d) refers to a patient with "strep throat," a form of pharyngitis more common in children than adults, and associated with certain clinical features which do not include splenomegaly or generalized lymphadenopathy. The statement in (e) could apply to a patient with nonspecific upper respiratory tract infection (common cold) or bronchitis; these illnesses are gradual in onset and, again, not associated with splenomegaly or generalized lymphadenopathy.

**4. d.**

Risk factors for soft tissue infection in this elderly woman include diabetes and varicose veins. The portal of entry for the causative organism is likely the erosion overlying her tibia. The ill-defined redness is more consistent with cellulitis than erysipelas. It is true that blood cultures are usually not positive in most cases of cellulitis, but treatment with penicillin would only be appropriate for erysipelas. Herpes simplex virus infection is not a consideration here, and sexual activity is not a risk factor for cellulitis. Even though one might consider admission to the hospital to initiate intravenous antimicrobial therapy and observe clinical improvement in this elderly patient, surgical consultation would only be warranted for this case if necrotizing fasciitis is clinically suspected. Topical antifungal therapy may be considered here only if tinea pedis is present.

## SUGGESTED READINGS

Mossad S. Common infections in clinical practice: dealing with the daily uncertainties. *Cleve Clin J Med* 2004;71:129–143.

### Acute Infectious Diarrhea

Aranda-Michel J, Giannella RA. Acute diarrhea: a practical review. *Am J Med* 1999;106:670–676.
Centers for Disease Control and Prevention. Diagnosis and management of foodborne illness. A primer for physicians and other health care professionals. *MMWR* 2004;53(No. RR-4).
Guerrant RL, Van Gilder T, Steiner TS, et al. Practice guidelines for the management of infectious diarrhea. *Clin Infect Dis* 2001;32:331–350.
Thielman NM, Guerrant RL. Acute infectious diarrhea. *N Engl J Med* 2004;350:38–47.

### Urinary Tract Infections

Estathiou SP, Pefanis AV, Tsioulos DI, et al. Acute pyelonephritis in adults. Prediction of mortality and failure of treatment. *Arch Intern Med* 2003;163:1206–1212.
Fihn SD. Acute uncomplicated urinary tract infection in women. *N Engl J Med* 2003;349:259–266.
Gupta K, Hooton TM, Stamm WE. Increasing antimicrobial resistance and the management of uncomplicated community-acquired urinary tract infections. *Ann Intern Med* 2001;135:41–50.
Hooton TM, Besser R, Foxman B, et al. Acute uncomplicated cystitis in an era of increasing antibiotic resistance: a proposed approach to empirical therapy. *Clin Infect Dis* 2004;39:75–80.
Lipsky BA. Prostatitis and urinary tract infection in men: What's new, what's true? *Am J Med* 1999;106:327–334.
Saint S, Lipsky BA. Preventing catheter-related bacteriuria. Should we? Can we? How? *Arch Intern Med* 1999;159:800–808.
Tambyah PA, Maki DG. The relationship between pyuria and infection in patients with indwelling urinary catheters. A prospective study of 761 patients. *Arch Intern Med* 2000;160:673–677.
Warren JW, Abrutyn E, Hebel R, et al. Guidelines for antimicrobial treatment of uncomplicated acute bacterial cystitis and acute pyelonephritis in women. *Clin Infect Dis* 1999;29:745–758.
Wilson ML, Gaido L. Laboratory diagnosis of urinary tract infections in adult patients. *Clin Infect Dis* 2004;38:1150–1158.

### Upper Respiratory Tract Infections

Auwaerter PG. Infectious mononucleosis in middle age. *JAMA* 1999;281:454–459.
Bisno AL, Gerber MA, Gwaltney Jr JM, et al. Practice guidelines for the diagnosis and management of group A streptococcal pharyngitis. *Clin Infect Dis* 2002;35:113–125.
Bisno AL, Peter GS, Kaplan EL. Diagnosis of strep throat in adult: are clinical criteria really good enough? *Clin Infect Dis* 2003;35:126–129.
Bisno AL. Acute pharyngitis. *N Engl J Med* 2001;344:205–211.
Centers for Disease Control and Prevention. Prevention and control of influenza. Recommendations of the advisory committee on immunization practices (ACIP). *MMWR* 2004;53:1–40.

Cohen JI. Epstein-Barr virus infection. *N Engl J Med* 2000;343:481–92.
Couch RB. Influenza: prospects for control. *Ann Intern Med* 2000;133:992–998.
Ebell MH, Smith MA, Barry HC, et al. Does this patient have strep throat? *JAMA* 2000;284:2912–2918.
Gonzales R, Sande MA. Uncomplicated acute bronchitis. *Ann Intern Med* 2000;133:981–991.
Gonzales R. A 65-year-old woman with acute cough illness and an important engagement. *JAMA* 2003;289:2701–2708.
Levin LI, Munger KL, Rubertone MV, et al. Multiple sclerosis and Epstein-Barr virus. *JAMA* 2003;289:1533–1536.
McIsaac WJ, Kellner JD, Aufricht P, et al. Epirical validation of guidelines for the management of pharyngitis in children and adults. *JAMA* 2004;291:1587–1595.
Neuner JM, Hamel M, Phillips RS, et al. Diagnosis and management of adults with pharyngitis. A cost effectiveness analysis. *Ann Intern Med* 2003;139:113–122.
Poole MD. A focus on acute sinusitis in adults: changes in disease management. *Am J Med* 1999;106:38S–47S.
Rothberg MB, Bellantonio S, Rose DN. Management of influenza in adults older than 65 years of age: Cost-effectiveness of rapid testing and antiviral therapy. *Ann Intern Med* 2003;139:321–329.
Sinus and Allergy Health Partnership. Antimicrobial treatment guidelines for acute bacterial rhinosinusitis. *Otolaryngol Head Neck Surg* 2004;130:S1–S45.
Snow V, Mottur-Pilson C, Cooper RJ, Hoffman JR, for the American College of Physicians-American Society of Internal Medicine. Principles of appropriate antibiotic use for acute pharyngitis in adults. *Ann Intern Med* 2001;134:506–508.
Snow V, Mottur-Pilson C, Gonzales R, for the American College of Physicians-American Society of Internal Medicine. *Ann Intern Med* 2001;134:518–520.
Snow V, Mottur-Pilson C, Hickner JM, for the American College of Physicians–American Society of Internal Medicine. Principles of appropriate antibiotic use for acute sinusitis in adults. *Ann Intern Med* 2001;134:495–497.
Steinman MA, Gonzales R, Linder JA, Landefeld CS. Changing use of antibiotics in community-based outpatient practice, 1991–1999. *Ann Intern Med* 2003;138:525–533.
Straus SE, Cohen JI, Tosato G, et al. NIH conference. Epstein-Barr virus infections: biology, pathogenesis, and management. *Ann Intern Med* 1993;118:45–58.
Thorley-Lawson DA, Gross A. Persistence of the Epstein-Barr virus and the origins of associated lymphomas. *N Engl J Med* 2004;350:1328–1337.
Weintrob AC, Giner J, Menezes P, et al. Infrequent diagnosis of primary human immunodeficiency virus infection. Missed opportunities in acute care settings. *Arch Intern Med* 2003;163:2097–2100.
Williams JW, Simel DL, Roberts L, et al. Clinical evaluation for sinusitis. Making the diagnosis by history and physical examination. *Ann Intern Med* 1992;117:705–710.

### Soft Tissue Infections

Bisno AL, Stevens DL. Streptococcal infections of skin and soft tissues. *N Engl J Med* 1996;334:240–245.
Clark DC. Common acute hand infections. *Am Fam Physician* 2003;68:2167–2176.
Elewski BE. Onychomycosis. Treatment, quality of life, and economic issues. *Am J Clin Dermatol* 2000;1:19–26.
Faergemann J, Baran R. Epidemiology, clinical presentation and diagnosis of onychomycosis. *Br J Dermatol* 2003;149 (S 65):1–4.
Goldstein EJC. Bite wounds and infection. *Clin Infect Dis* 1992;14:633–640.
Swartz MN. Cellulitis. *N Engl J Med* 2004;350:940–912.
Talan D, Citron DM, Abrahamian FM, et al., for the Emergency Medicine Animal Bite Infection Study Group. Bacteriologic analysis of infected dog and cat bites. *N Engl J Med* 1999:340:85–92.

## 18

# BOARD SIMULATION:
## Infectious Diseases

*Alan J. Taege    Steven D. Mawhorter    J. Walton Tomford*

This board simulation chapter on infectious diseases is not meant to be a comprehensive review of the questions likely to be encountered on the certifying examination in internal medicine. Rather, it is designed to supplement the material presented elsewhere in the text, both in the Infectious Disease section and in other subspecialty sections. Entire chapters have been devoted to the important topics of sexually transmitted diseases, endocarditis, pneumonia, human immunodeficiency virus (HIV) infection, and new and emerging infections, which are favorite areas for the boards.

This chapter is divided into several segments: first, a discussion of mycobacterial disease; second, a series of case scenarios with questions addressing different methods of diagnosis and management in different areas of infectious diseases; and finally, a series of short matching and multiple-choice questions.

## MYCOBACTERIAL INFECTIONS

Mycobacterial infections have been important causes of morbidity and mortality for thousands of years. From a clinical microbiologic perspective, mycobacteria can be divided into three major types: *Mycobacterium leprae*, nontuberculous mycobacteria, and *Mycobacterium tuberculosis*. Rare infections due to the therapeutic use of bacille Calmette-Guérin (BCG) vaccination will not be covered.

Leprosy is occasionally seen in the United States in patients from Asia, Africa, and other parts of the world. Nontuberculous mycobacterial infections have increased in the United States due, in part, to better recognition, the HIV epidemic, increased use of immunosuppression, and greater numbers of organ transplants. Leprosy and diseases due to nontuberculous mycobacteria are serious clinical disorders with complex diagnostic and therapeutic aspects. This chapter, however, only emphasizes tuberculosis (TB). The important aspects of diagnosis and therapy are covered for both active disease and latent TB infection (LTBI). The latter was termed *TB prophylaxis*. The Centers for Disease Control (CDC) has issued new, simpler guidelines for the interpretation of TB skin testing (TST) and for the treatment and monitoring of patients with LTBI. These new recommendations are emphasized.

TB remains one of the major microbial "killers" worldwide, with an estimated 2 to 3 million deaths per year. Approximately one-third of the world is infected with *M. tuberculosis*; a considerable number of these individuals will at some point develop tuberculous disease, with its attendant morbidity and potential mortality. Although the upsurge of TB in the early 1990s prompted renewed attention of the disease in the United States, case rates have been progressively declining for the last 7 years, with less than 17,000 cases in the United States for 2000. Additional demographic information includes the observation that foreign-born persons now comprise almost half the patients with TB in the United States. Despite the decline of TB cases in the United States, the disease is still a frequent cause of morbidity and even occasional mortality. Reports continue to surface of delayed or even missed diagnoses, with disastrous infection control situations, not to mention direct patient care issues. Thus, a review of TB, with emphasis on diagnosis, therapy of active cases, and preventative therapy, seems an appropriate topic for a comprehensive review of internal medicine.

The pathophysiology of TB is important in helping to understand the rationale behind treatment of LTBI, and to comprehend the various forms of extrapulmonary TB. The near universal portal of entry for TB is the inhalation of droplet nuclei from the lungs of another human infected with TB. These infectious particles settle in the lower-lung zones and develop into a primary pulmonary infection. The vast majority of the time, a containment of this process occurs with the development of delayed-type hypersensitivity to tuberculin protein manifested by skin testing reactivity to the purified protein derivative (PPD). A silent lymphohematogenous spread usually occurs, however, throughout the rest of the body. Disease becomes manifest when *M. tuberculosis* is not contained during the initial infection or a later reactivation of the microbe occurs, with clinical symptoms in the lungs or in extrapulmonary areas such as pleura, lymph nodes, bone, joints, kidney, peritoneum, pericardium, central nervous system, and even miliary spread.

*M. tuberculosis* is an acid-fast bacillus that usually results in granulomatous inflammation. To not miss the diagnosis of this treatable contagious disease, TB should always be in the differential of any inflammatory disorder, especially when granulomas are present. Although most cases are pulmonary, extrapulmonary forms account for 15% to 20% of cases. TB outside the lung tends to be paucibacillary; acid-fast bacillus (AFB) stains are commonly negative, so that the clinician has to rely on a culture analysis of body fluids or biopsy material. TB can mimic carcinoma and can present with emergent problems such as miliary spread, tuberculous meningitis, endobronchial spread, hemoptysis, or fever of unknown origin. Thus, the clinician should always entertain TB in the differential diagnosis of any inflammatory disorder.

A positive Mantoux five-unit PPD should heighten the suspicion but does not have infallible diagnostic sensitivity. A significant rate of false-positive and false-negative skin tests, the confusion potentially produced by prior BCG, and the booster phenomenon created by frequent TST make for difficulty in interpretation of PPD skin testing. The laboratory can be of great help in confirming the clinician's suspicion of TB through microscopic and culture techniques, provided good quality body fluids and tissue, where appropriate, are sent for AFB culture and smear. Although great promise was placed on the development and practical use of molecular techniques such as polymerase chain reaction (PCR) and ribotyping, these expensive modalities have not proven better than experienced microbiology labs. With recent improvement in culture techniques and the application of molecular probes once the culture has turned positive, the clinician is usually aware of the growth of acid-fast bacilli by 3 weeks. Molecular probes used in this manner can distinguish between *M. tuberculosis, Mycobacterium avium-intracellulare, Mycobacterium kansasii,* and *Mycobacterium gordonae* with a very high rate of sensitivity and specificity. When the molecular techniques are used in this manner, information becomes available to guide correct microbiologic diagnosis and has a direct influence on infection control measures as well as therapeutic decisions. Once appropriate specimens have been sent, however, therapy should not be delayed until cultural confirmation in the case of suspected pulmonary parenchymal disease, tuberculous meningitis, or miliary TB.

The therapy of active disease includes the use of multiple medications from the list of first-line and—in the case of resistance or intolerable side effects—from the second-line medications. The first-line antituberculous medications include isoniazid (INH), rifampin, pyrazinamide (PZA), ethambutol, and streptomycin. Second-line drugs include other aminoglycosides, certain quinolones, ethionamide, rifabutin, rifapentine, cycloserine, and para-aminosalicylic acid. In starting these medications, the clinician should be aware of their major but infrequent side effects, including toxicities to the liver, eyes, ears, and gait. Drug–drug

interactions occur with INH and especially rifampin. In a case of TB in an HIV-infected patient, rifampin adversely affects the blood levels of many antiretrovirals in the non-nucleoside reverse-transcriptase inhibitor and protease inhibitor classes. In these situations, rifampin should be changed to rifabutin, and HIV medications still need to be chosen with skill. Other issues to consider in standard TB therapy include the chance of primary versus secondary drug resistance and the careful use of adjunctive steroids in certain select situations. The length of therapy is for many months, and directly observed therapy via the public health department is very important. To violate the basic tenets of therapy using multiple medications and directly supervised therapy is to invite a clinical and public health disaster if the patient's TB strain develops multidrug resistance. Thus, the clinician has an obligation to make the correct diagnosis, begin carefully chosen multidrug therapy, and to ensure vigorous outpatient follow-up, monitoring, and assurance of clinical improvement, as well as notification of the local public health authorities.

The therapy of latent tuberculous infection is founded on the absolute necessity of exclusion of active disease and, as in treatment of active disease, patient adherence. In hopes of further elimination of TB in the United States, the CDC has published recent guidelines for tuberculin skin testing to be used in the treatment of LTBI. In this scenario, TST should be targeted to those groups of patients with an increased incidence of TB infection, as well as those with an increased risk for the progression from latent infection to active disease (Tables 18.1 and 18.2).

In addition, TST should be performed on all patients, including those receiving organ transplants and others who are being considered for the administration of 15 mg/day or greater of prednisone for more than 1 month. This caveat also includes patients who are being started on the monoclonal antibody infliximab. To clarify a former point of great confusion, when serial PPD testing is applied, as it commonly is in the employee infection-control programs of most U.S. hospitals, a PPD conversion is considered to have occurred when there is a 10-mm or greater increase in the amount of induration at the PPD site.

Before discussing the size interpretation of a positive PPD for particular populations, new guidelines for the treatment of LTBI should be mentioned. HIV-negative

## TABLE 18.1

### GROUPS AT HIGH RISK OF TUBERCULOSIS INFECTION

Close contacts of patients with active pulmonary tuberculosis
Persons from Asia, Africa, Latin America
Medically underserved groups: African Americans, Hispanics, Native Americans
Residents of prisons, nursing homes, institutions
Healthcare workers in high-incidence jobs or institutions

## TABLE 18.2

### GROUPS AT HIGH RISK OF PROGRESSION FROM LATENT INFECTION TO ACTIVE DISEASE

Human immunodeficiency virus
Corticosteroid use (prolonged use at high dose)
Diabetes mellitus
Silicosis
Gastrectomy
Disorder requiring chronic immunosuppression (including organ transplants)
Chest radiograph suggestive of old tuberculosis
Malignancy, especially in lung cancer, head and neck carcinoma, and lymphoma
Chronic renal failure
Intravenous drug abuse
Infliximab use

patients should be given INH/vitamin B6 for 9 months, as should HIV-positive patients and those with lung fibrotic scars larger than 2 cm, compatible with old TB. HIV-positive or HIV-negative patients may be candidates for a shorter course with rifampin plus PZA for 2 months, but very recent reports of severe hepatitis using this dual regimen has led to recommendations for closer monitoring of these patients. Finally, HIV-positive or HIV-negative patients may be treated with rifampin alone for 4 months. Recommendations for monitoring patients while on LTBI have been simplified, but the reports of hepatitis when rifampin plus PZA is used for 2 months may complicate matters. Otherwise, on INH monotherapy, baseline liver function tests are only suggested for patients with HIV positivity, pregnancy, postpartum state, chronic liver disease, or heavy alcohol intake. The most important aspect of monitoring to prevent drug toxicity is an emphasis on adherence, yet education on potential side effects and availability for rapid assessment in the clinic.

Tables 18.3, 18.4, and 18.5 list the guidelines for the interpretation of a positive tuberculin skin test at measurement of induration of 5 mm, 10 mm, and 15 mm, respectively. These three tables formulate those medical situations in which a strong consideration of treatment for LTBI should be present, with the previously mentioned caveats concerning the regimen chosen and the monitoring needed during treatment.

## TABLE 18.3

### TUBERCULOSIS (TB) SKIN TESTING POSITIVITY—RISK GROUPS 5 MM

Human immunodeficiency virus–positive
Recent contacts—active pulmonary TB
Changes on chest radiograph compatible with old TB
Immunosuppressed patients on 15 mg prednisone daily for more than 1 mo
Patients being started on infliximab

## TABLE 18.4

### TUBERCULOSIS SKIN TESTING POSITIVITY— RISK GROUPS 10 MM

Immigration within 5 yr from an area of incidence
Intravenous drug abuse
Residents of jails and nursing homes; the homeless
Hospital clinical personnel or acid-fast bacillus lab employees
Patients with conditions with increased risk of reactivation (i.e., silicosis, etc; see Table 18.2)
Children <4 yr old; infants, children, adolescents exposed to adults in high-risk categories

## CASE 1

A 60-year-old African-American man originally from Alabama is transferred from his home in southern Ohio to a Cleveland hospital. He had been a foundry worker for many years and had never had a tuberculin skin test. He has chronic obstructive pulmonary disease (COPD) for which he has received steroids for the last 6 months. He was admitted to the outside hospital 1 week ago for worsening respiratory failure and pneumonia requiring mechanical ventilation. One week later, he has not improved and, in fact, has worsened on broad-spectrum antibiotics for Gram-negative bacilli that grew from the sputum. He is transferred to a tertiary care facility for "weaning." His chest radiograph is shown in Figure 18.1.

### Questions

**1.** To confirm the most likely diagnosis, endotracheal tube sputum should be sent for:
**a)** Giemsa stain
**b)** Wright's stain
**c)** PCR
**d)** Ziehl-Neelsen stain
**e)** Papanicolaou's stain

**2.** If results of the above stain were positive for many beaded red-staining organisms, what would be the correct treatment plan?
**a)** INH, vitamin B6, rifampin, PZA, and ethambutol
**b)** Ethionamide, cycloserine, streptomycin, and ethambutol

## TABLE 18.5

### TUBERCULOSIS SKIN TESTING POSITIVITY— RISK GROUPS 15 MM

All others (minimal risk of tuberculosis) regardless of age
Those at start of employment in healthcare facility with no other risk or incidence factors

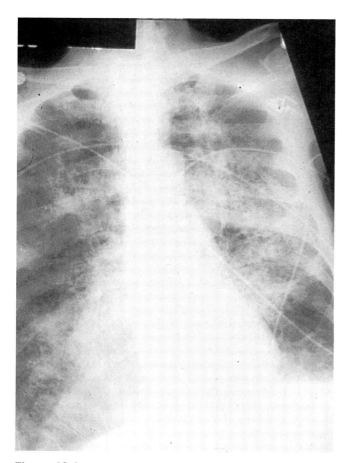

**Figure 18.1**   Chest radiograph of patient in Case 1.

c) INH and vitamin $B_6$
d) Wait for cultures
e) Ciprofloxacin

## Discussion

This case illustrates the importance of considering mycobacteria, especially *M. tuberculosis*, in any case of pneumonia that fails to respond to antibacterial therapy. Corticosteroid therapy for COPD has been associated with a variety of infectious complications. The patient's silica exposure in a foundry should have prompted a baseline tuberculin skin test years earlier, certainly before the initiation of steroids for COPD.

The presence of Gram-negative rods in the sputum analysis does not necessarily indicate a true Gram-negative pneumonia: Clinical judgment, knowledge of the Gram's stain result, and additional laboratory data are necessary to distinguish colonization from true infection. AFBs are sometimes weakly Gram-positive, but Gram's stain is not a reliable way to exclude TB.

Once AFBs are found on the sputum smear, one has to decide the likelihood of *M. tuberculosis* versus nontuberculous mycobacteria (also referred to as atypical mycobac-

teria, environmental mycobacteria, or mycobacteria other than TB). In a clinically serious situation such as this, *M. tuberculosis* must be at the top of the list, although *M. kansasii*, *M. avium-intracellulare*, and rapidly growing mycobacteria, such as *Mycobacterium chelonae*, can also produce serious acute pulmonary disease.

The decision to treat this pulmonary process as TB is a wise one. Therapy should begin promptly using a very aggressive multidrug regimen. In regions of the United States in which the incidence of multidrug-resistant TB is less than 5%, a three-drug regimen of INH, rifampin, and PZA is probably adequate, but it is probably safer to include ethambutol as well until sensitivities can be obtained. Vitamin B6 in a dose of 50 to 100 mg orally per day should be given to prevent INH peripheral neuropathy.

## Answers and Explanations

**1. d.**
A Giemsa stain is not usually requested for sputum. It is useful in detecting malarial parasites or *Babesia*. Wright's stain of the sputum would detect eosinophils suggestive of asthma or allergic bronchopulmonary aspergillosis. At present, molecular methods for direct detection of *M. tuberculosis* in sum are available but much more costly and, practically speaking, not necessarily more sensitive than conventional methods of TB microscopy. The use of the Ziehl-Neelsen stain, which is properly decolorized on a carefully collected and handled endotracheal sputum specimen, would be strongly indicated in this patient receiving steroids. The results would likely be positive and clinically suggestive of severe infection from *M. tuberculosis*. Papanicolaou's staining on sputum might be useful if one were looking for malignant cells. In addition, an alerted cytologist can sometimes recognize certain fungal organisms such as *Blastomyces dermatitidis* or *Histoplasma capsulatum*, two organisms that are epidemiologically possible causes of pneumonia in this case and could be especially virulent in the presence of steroids. Fungi are best seen using a potassium hydroxide–prepared fluorescence stain.

**2. a.**
The regimen in answer choice b includes two second-line drugs, ethionamide and cycloserine, which are toxic and often poorly tolerated. Therapy with INH and vitamin B6 alone would be foolish in the presence of obvious active disease and would lead to the development of secondary resistance. To withhold therapy pending cultures in a patient with severe illness and positive sputum smears would be inappropriate. Monotherapy with ciprofloxacin may be appropriate in selected patients with certain types of Gram-negative pneumonia but would be inappropriate in someone with suspected or proven TB. Quinolones are sometimes used with other medications for TB and certain types of nontuberculous mycobacteria.

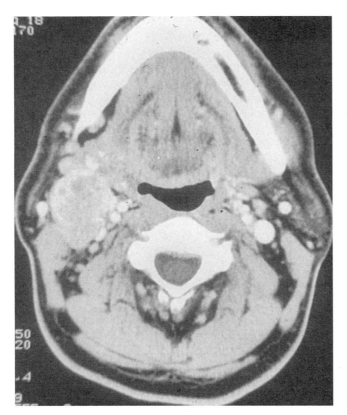

**Figure 18.2** Computerized tomography scan of neck of patient in Case 2.

## CASE 2

A 50-year-old Indian physician presents with a right neck mass. The patient received BCG as a child. Results of a tuberculin skin test were strongly positive 10 years ago on immigration to the United States. A computerized tomography (CT) scan of the neck is shown in Figure 18.2. Two major surgical procedures and a prolonged course of expensive medications were required to produce a successful clinical and cosmetic result.

### Question

3. In retrospect, what should have been done a decade ago?
a) Offered INH/vitamin B6 for 9 months.
b) Offered INH/PZA/streptomycin for 1 year.
c) Excluded active disease.
d) Observation, especially because the patient has a history of being hepatitis B surface antigen positive
e) a and c

### Discussion

This case illustrates the importance of understanding the concepts of treatment for LTBI. Updated American Thoracic Society and CDC guidelines address issues regarding BCG vaccination and skin test conversions. It is always important to first exclude active disease because monotherapy with INH quickly produces resistance in such situations. In fact, when in doubt, treat as if active disease is present. If this is a possibility, one needs to start at least two new drugs to which the patient's mycobacteria have not been previously exposed.

Remote BCG vaccination is not necessarily a contraindication to INH prophylaxis, nor is it a reason not to offer INH prophylaxis in appropriate clinical situations, as outlined in the text discussion, tables, and clinical vignette.

### Answer and Explanation

3. e.
The exclusion of active disease by history, compulsive physical examination, and routine laboratory studies, such as a complete blood cell count, chest radiography, and urinalysis to exclude silent sterile pyuria, is the first order of business. The presence of active disease would require multidrug therapy, as outlined earlier. Once active disease is excluded, the need for the treatment of LTBI is determined by the size of the PPD reaction, as well as the presence of risk factors for a high incidence of TB infection or risk factors for progression of LTBI to active disease.

In most circumstances, INH plus vitamin B6 is the recommended regimen, although shorter alternative regimens have been proposed, with certain caveats owing to recent reports of increased hepatitis from shorter courses of therapy. If the contact person has drug-resistant TB, then recommendations are different and include the use of combinations of rifampin, PZA, ethambutol, and ciprofloxacin, depending on the susceptibility profile of the organism from the contact source. In this case, answer b would be inappropriate because drug-resistant disease is not a concern. Hepatitis from INH and rifampin is not generally predictable, although the risk does increase with age, so close education, outpatient follow-up, and compliance are of great importance.

## CASE 3

A 35-year-old construction worker from southern Ohio is transferred to your hospital for meningitis. The patient was sick with fever and malaise for 3 weeks before admission and received an empiric course of therapy with trimethoprim-sulfamethoxazole for possible sinusitis. The patient is known to be HIV negative. A lumbar puncture is performed on admission to the patient's local hospital, which shows 85 white blood cells (WBCs)/mm³ with 95% polymorphonuclear cells (PMNs), glucose 45 mg/dL, and protein 180 mg/dL. The patient's condition worsens despite therapy with vancomycin and ceftriaxone.

Cryptococcal antigen in the cerebrospinal fluid (CSF) is negative on the initial and follow-up spinal taps. A head CT scan shows hydrocephalus, meningeal enhancement, and a basal ganglia infarct. The patient is transferred to your hospital and dies shortly after arrival. A postmortem examination shows chronic meningitis with caseating granulomas.

## Question

**4.** Which of the following two diseases would be likely causes for this patient's death?
a) *M. tuberculosis* or *Cryptococcus neoformans*
b) *M. kansasii* or *Brucella* species
c) *M. tuberculosis* or *H. capsulatum*
d) *M. avium-intracellulare* or sarcoidosis

## Discussion

This case illustrates the varied presentations of TB. This patient's presentation was not typical for tuberculous meningitis, which can occur alone or as a manifestation of miliary disease. In a suspected case, even if the smear is negative, empiric therapy should not be withheld pending culture and may be lifesaving if initiated in a timely fashion. The PMN predominance in this patient's CSF is not uncommon in tuberculous meningitis—it occurs in 20% to 30% of cases in the early stages of the disease. This patient's CT findings are characteristics of TB involving the meninges. Basilar meningitis can lead to obstructive hydrocephalus and inflammatory vasculitis, which results in infarcts. The pathologic finding of granulomas should always make one think of mycobacteria, especially TB. Although caseation is often said to be almost pathognomonic for TB, it can be seen in histoplasmosis, blastomycosis, cryptococcosis, coccidioidomycosis, and certain other infections. Sarcoidosis is rarely associated with caseation necrosis. In patients with chronic or basilar meningitis, however, the distinction between TB and sarcoidosis can be difficult. In addition, TB and the other fungal infections discussed earlier can occasionally coexist with or complicate sarcoidosis and its treatment.

## Answer and Explanation

**4. c.**
The CSF cryptococcal antigen is very sensitive and is positive in more than 95% of patients with cryptococcal meningitis. Although *C. neoformans* can produce caseating granulomatous necrosis, the spinal fluid usually tests positive for antigen. Brucellosis would be an unlikely consideration in this setting, given the absence of any history of travel, animal exposure, or unusual food ingestion. Most mycobacteria, other than *M. tuberculosis*, do not disseminate to the meninges, even in the presence of HIV infection. Although sarcoidosis is possible, it is rarely this fulminant. Histoplasmosis, next to TB, is the most likely organism to explain this particular patient's problem.

## CASE 4

A 25-year-old fisherman from the Gulf Coast of Florida presents to your office with a 1-day history of erythema of the hand, fever to 39°C, and shaking chills. No lymphangitis is present. History is notable for chronic hepatitis C.

## Question

**5.** Choose the least likely agent for the cellulitis.
a) *Aeromonas hydrophila*
b) *Vibrio vulnificus*
c) *Streptococcus pyogenes*
d) *Mycobacterium marinum*
e) *Erysipelothrix rhusiopathiae*

## Discussion

This case involves the differential diagnosis of cellulitis acquired in a marine environment. Although most organisms on the skin are Gram-positive cocci, most organisms in water are Gram-negative bacilli. *Aeromonas* and *Vibrio* cellulitis occur after skin trauma in individuals who are exposed to water contaminated with these organisms. Secondary bacteremia is common with both organisms, and *Vibrio* infections have a propensity for individuals with underlying liver disease. *Erysipelothrix* cellulitis occurs in meat handlers and fisherman after minor skin trauma. The localized cutaneous form tends to be subacute and classically has a serpiginous purple-red appearance. Fever may be absent. Diffuse cellulitis is less common and may evolve from erysipeloid. In cases presenting with diffuse cellulitis, fever is common. *M. marinum* produces a chronic cellulitis, often with nodular lymphangitis, and is usually seen in fishermen or owners of aquaria. Fever is uncommon. Salient facts regarding waterborne cellulitis are summarized in Table 18.2.

## Answer and Explanation

**5. d.**
Although *M. marinum* can produce cellulitis in fishermen, it produces a chronic cellulitis. The patient described has an acute rather than a chronic cellulitis. All the other organisms would be common causes of acute cellulitis in this setting.

## CASE 5

A 63-year-old married, white, retired natural gas company serviceman from Ohio presents with a 3-day history of progressive tingling in his fingers and toes, clumsiness of his hands, and unsteadiness on his feet. He notes coughing and choking when he attempts to eat or drink. Although his speech is slightly slurred, he has not been confused. He has no fever, chills, sweats, or headache. Two or 3 weeks before, he had a diarrheal illness lasting approximately 4 days. Blood was noted in multiple stools. His wife recently removed a tick from his hair. He has also been spraying his apple trees with an insecticide. He eats deli meats but no raw meats. A history of chronic lymphocytic leukemia with a Richter's transformation is present, which required chemotherapy with fludarabine, radiation, and Campath (a monoclonal antibody) 3 months ago. Examination discloses no rash, clear mentation, minimal dysarthria, a weak gag reflex, areflexia, ataxia, and diffuse symmetric weakness, which progresses over the next 24 hours and results in intubation 48 hours after admission.

## Questions

6. The differential diagnosis should include all of the following, *except*
a) Botulism
b) Organophosphate poisoning
c) Paraneoplastic syndrome
d) Tickborne encephalitis
e) Guillain-Barré syndrome (GBS)
f) Tickborne paralysis
g) Listeria meningitis

A lumbar puncture is performed that discloses two WBCs, no red blood cells (RBCs), glucose 65 mg/dL (serum glucose 107 mg/dL), and protein 88 mg/dL. Gram's, fungal, and AFB stains are negative.

7. Additional appropriate tests could include all of the following, *except*
a) Blood cultures
b) CSF PCR for TB
c) Nerve conduction studies
d) Stool culture for enteric pathogens
e) MRI of the brain and brainstem
f) Blood and CSF PCR for cytomegalovirus (CMV)

8. The nerve conduction study reveals an acute inflammatory demyelinating polyneuropathy. Appropriate therapeutic interventions could include all of the following, *except*
a) High-dose corticosteroids
b) Plasmapheresis
c) Supportive care
d) Immunoglobulin therapy
e) Moving the patient to an intensive care unit

## Discussion

This case represents the Miller-Fisher variant of GBS, which is characterized by ataxia, cranial nerve involvement, areflexia, and progressive muscle weakness. The typical case of GBS is characterized by a progressive ascending weakness, areflexia, and sensory sparing but not cranial nerve involvement. It is an immune-mediated, acute inflammatory demyelinating polyneuropathy. Preceding infections are associated with approximately two-thirds of cases such as CMV, Epstein-Barr virus, Varicella-zoster virus, *Campylobacter*, *Mycoplasma*, Lyme borreliosis, and HIV. Other systemic conditions, such as Hodgkin's disease, systemic lupus erythematosus, and sarcoidosis, are also linked to the Miller-Fisher variant of GBS. The association with vaccines is not well supported as a major factor in this syndrome.

## Answers and Explanations

### 6. d.

Although a tick was removed, the patient's sensorium is normal and therefore does not suggest encephalitis. The numerous pieces of history and physical findings allow for the other possibilities. Botulism is a possibility. He demonstrates cranial nerve deficits but lacks ophthalmoplegia. Most cases are foodborne, however, and no other family members are ill. Organophosphate poisoning should be considered. He was spraying his apple trees with insecticides; however, the onset of his syndrome is too slow, and he lacks the gastrointestinal symptoms and muscarinic manifestations. His history of chronic lymphocytic leukemia with transformation makes a paraneoplastic syndrome possible. Manifestations may vary depending on the anatomic location of injury.

GBS could occur in association with his underlying malignancy. The history of bloody diarrhea preceding this presentation, however, should alert the clinician to the possibility of foodborne infectious etiologies. Further questioning of family members revealed at least three other members with a concurrent diarrheal illness, probably related to eating chicken salad. This would make *Campylobacter*—the most commonly identified foodborne bacterial pathogen—a very likely suspect. Tickborne paralysis is a possibility. Once the tick is removed, however, the symptoms should resolve, not progress.

His immunocompromised state and consumption of deli meats raise the question of listeriosis, which typically affects the very young, immunocompromised, pregnant, or elderly. It has the highest mortality and hospitalization rates of any foodborne illnesses. It may present as a rhomboencephalitis with asymmetric cranial nerve palsies, cerebellar signs, weakness, and altered consciousness.

### 7. b.

No history of exposure to TB is present, and the CSF formula did not suggest tuberculous meningitis. Blood cultures may recover *Listeria* or other bacterial pathogens. Because CMV has been associated with GBS, appropriate investigations are warranted. Electrophysiologic studies could be very beneficial, as the demonstration of an acute demyelinating polyneuropathy would be highly suggestive of GBS in this clinical setting. These are considered the most sensitive and specific diagnostic tests.

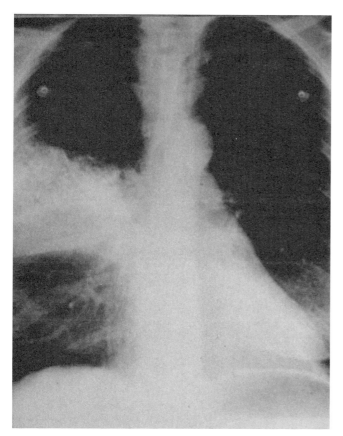

**Figure 18.3**   Chest radiograph of patient in Case 6. (See Color Fig. 18.3.)

Stool cultures for enteric pathogens are indicated because of the history of bloody diarrhea. Be sure the lab routinely cultures for *Campylobacter* or other pathogens in your differential diagnosis. The pathogens are not often isolated, however, as the initial infection has frequently resolved before the onset of GBS.

MRI of the brain and brainstem may reveal space-occupying lesions, inflammation, or demyelination.

**8. a.**

Steroids have not been shown to benefit GBS. Plasmapheresis and immunoglobulin therapy have demonstrated efficacy. Supportive care is critical to avoid aspiration. Patients should be monitored for autonomic instability, which develops in up to 50%, and for dysrhythmias. Ventilatory support may be necessary in up to one-third of affected patients. Eighty percent make a near total recovery.

This patient has two immediate adverse prognostic factors—age more than 60 years and rapidly progressive disease. Additional factors associated with a less favorable outcome are underlying pulmonary disease, prolonged ventilation (more than 1 month), or persistent severe abnormal electrophysiologic studies. Mortality is 3% to 8%.

## CASE 6

A 61-year-old white male resident of Cleveland presents to the emergency room complaining of the acute onset of fever (39°C), chills, productive cough of yellow-rusty sputum, and pleuritic right chest pain over the past 12 to 18 hours. He is an unemployed alcoholic smoker who is cachectic and toxic appearing. His WBC is 16,000/mm$^3$, and an arterial blood gas demonstrates a PaO$_2$ of 49 mm Hg on room air. His chest radiograph is shown in Figure 18.3.

### Questions

**9.** The most likely etiology of his pneumonia is
a) Aspiration
b) Legionella
c) *Streptococcus pneumoniae*
d) Mycoplasma
e) Influenza

He is admitted to your hospital intensive care unit service. Sputum Gram's stain is shown in Figure 18.4.

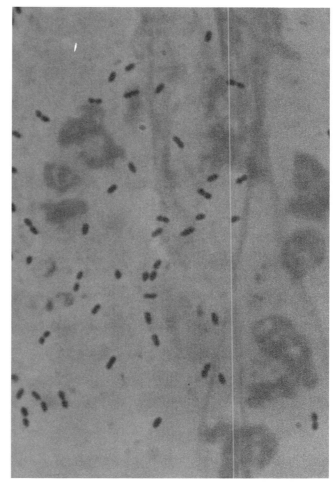

**Figure 18.4**   Sputum Gram's stain of patient in Case 6. (See Color Fig. 18.4.)

**10.** The most appropriate antibiotic coverage would be (may include more than one answer)
a) Penicillin G
b) Azithromycin
c) Clindamycin
d) Oseltamivir
e) Ceftriaxone

At 24 hours, his blood cultures are growing Gram-positive cocci in pairs. Because of his poor nutritional status and poor oral intake, TPN is initiated. He appears to be improving. On the fifth hospital day, he has recurrent fever to 38.9°C. A repeat chest radiograph shows his previous lobar pneumonia with a small effusion, not amenable to thoracentesis. His respiratory status deteriorates, and he requires intubation. Blood cultures are repeated.

**11.** At this time, antibiotic coverage should be changed to
a) Levofloxacin
b) Ceftazidime
c) Cefotaxime
d) Vancomycin and piperacillin/tazobactam
e) Imipenem and azithromycin

On day 6, he develops an erythematous, nonblanching, nonpruritic, macronodular rash (Fig. 18.5), and his fever persists despite the change in antibiotic regimen.

**12.** The most appropriate next step in management is to
a) Discontinue his antibiotic regimen, assuming a drug reaction, and start of an unrelated class of antipneumococcal antibiotics.
b) Add fluconazole and remove his central line.
c) Apply steroid cream and moisturizers to the rash.
d) Treat his scabies with lindane.
e) Ask dermatology to evaluate and biopsy the rash.

## Discussion

This is a case of pneumococcal pneumonia with bloodstream infection in a debilitated, malnourished alcoholic patient. The sudden onset with chills, pleurisy, and lobar consolidation all point toward pneumococcus as a likely etiology.

## Answers and Explanations

### 9. c.

All the etiologic agents listed should be considered, although no history of blackouts or vomiting is present to make one suspicious of aspiration. *Legionella* tends to have a more insidious onset, less sputum production, and may have gastrointestinal symptoms as a clue to assist in the diagnosis. *Mycoplasma*, another cause of atypical pneumonia (along with *Chlamydia* and *Legionella*), also has an insidious onset, nonproductive cough, and an overall less toxic-appearing presentation, hence the term *walking pneumonia*. Influenza generally presents with

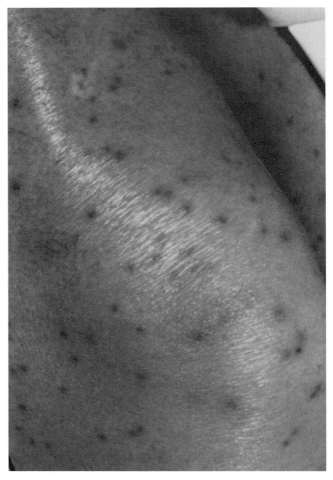

**Figure 18.5** Erythematous, nonblanching, nonpruritic, macronodular rash of patient in Case 6. (See Color Fig. 18.5.)

coryza, arthralgia and myalgia, a nonproductive cough, and high fever, often in a seasonal epidemic setting.

Many risk factors are associated with pneumococcal pneumonia including age older than 60 years, smoking, COPD, cancer, HIV, diabetes, congestive heart failure, alcohol abuse, and liver disease; however, alcohol use was the single most commonly associated condition from one study.

### 10. b, e.

Azithromycin affords coverage of atypical organisms, many Gram-positive bacteria, and some *Haemophilus influenzae*. Ceftriaxone provides coverage for Gram-negative bacteria and many of the penicillin-resistant organisms. Penicillin resistance has become a significant issue in the treatment of pneumococcal pneumonia. The incidence of penicillin resistance among *S. pneumoniae* varies between 15% and 35% in various parts of the United States (see Chapter 16). Therefore, penicillin would not be a good choice. Clindamycin may cover many *S. pneumoniae* and is appropriate for aspiration but lacks atypical and Gram-negative coverage. Oseltamivir

## TABLE 18.6
### RISK FACTORS FOR DISSEMINATED CANDIDIASIS

| | |
|---|---|
| Diabetes | Malignancy |
| Alcoholism | Neutropenia |
| Catheters | Total parenteral nutrition |
| Abdominal surgery | Intensive care unit length of stay |
| Hemodialysis | Colonization |
| Antibiotics | Neonates |
| Burn patient | Transplantation |
| Steroids | |

would be appropriate for influenza, but this is an unlikely diagnosis in our patient.

### 11. d.

We now must consider the possibility of a mixed population of *S. pneumoniae*, some of which may have had high-level penicillin or ceftriaxone resistance, as well as hospital-acquired infections, such as methicillin-resistant *Staphylococcus aureus* from the line, intensive care unit Gram-negative organisms (which will vary at each hospital), drug reactions, empyema, deep vein thrombosis, aspiration, or possibly fungal infections.

Vancomycin would cover all *S. pneumoniae*, methicillin-resistant *S. aureus*, and other potential Gram-positive organisms. Piperacillin-tazobactam would provide good Gram-negative and anaerobic coverage. You must be aware of your institution's endemic antimicrobial resistance patterns, which vary from one hospital to another, to ascertain the best empiric coverage. Levofloxacin, ceftazidime, cefotaxime, imipenem, and azithromycin do not provide methicillin-resistant *S. aureus* coverage. If the *S. pneumoniae* were resistant to ceftriaxone, it is also likely to be resistant to ceftazidime and cefotaxime.

### 12. b.

The rash is consistent with disseminated candidiasis, which is the fourth-leading cause of nosocomial bloodstream infection. His blood cultures eventually grow *Candida albicans*. Our patient has several risk factors for candidemia (Table 18.6). Most infections are caused by *C. albicans*; however, increasing numbers of other non-*albicans* species of *Candida* exist, which produce bloodstream infection. This is important because non-*albicans* *Candida* are not uniformly susceptible to the azoles (Table 18.7).

## CASE 7

A 23-year-old healthy single white man from south-central Missouri presents in early December with a 3-week history of a sudden onset of fever to 39°C, chills, and headache. His symptoms wax and wane. Associated fatigue, weakness, sweats, and a 5- to 8-lb weight loss is also present. He lives alone, works as a cabinetmaker in a factory, smokes, and drinks socially. He was treated empirically with amoxicillin without improvement. He had tender lymph nodes at the right epitrochlear and axillary regions. Biopsy of one reveals caseating granulomas and a negative routine culture at an outside hospital. Subsequent oral cephalexin therapy had no effect on the illness. Your history reveals no travel, exposures to illness, or substance abuse. He is an avid outdoorsman who hunts year round. The week before the onset of his illness, he shot several rabbits and an eight-point whitetail buck. Physical examination reveals an ill but nontoxic-appearing young man with a temperature of 38.8°C. He has numerous abrasions on his hands from work and tender right epitrochlear and axillary nodes measuring 2 to 3 cm. No rash or hepatosplenomegaly is noted. Lab results reveal a hemoglobin of 14.7 g/dL, WBC 11,200/mm³, platelet 300 K/μL, and normal liver enzymes and creatinine.

### Questions

**13.** Your differential diagnosis should include all of the following, *except*
**a)** Rocky Mountain spotted fever (RMSF)
**b)** Lyme disease
**c)** Ehrlichiosis
**d)** Tularemia
**e)** TB
**f)** Babesiosis

## TABLE 18.7
### SUSCEPTIBILITY

| | Fluconazole | Itraconazole | Amphotericin |
|---|---|---|---|
| *Candida albicans* | S | S | S |
| *Candida parapsilosis* | S | S | S |
| *Candida tropicalis* | S-DD | S | S |
| *Candida glabrata* | S-DD | S-DD | S |
| *Candida krusei* | R | S-DD | S |
| *Candida lusitanae* | S | S-DD | R |

R, resistant; S, sensitive; S-DD, sensitive, dose-dependent.

**14.** Appropriate diagnostic tests would include all of the following, *except*
a) Blood cultures on cysteine-enriched media
b) Wright's stain of blood smear for morulae
c) Thick and thin blood smears
d) Paired serology for RMSF
e) Weil-Felix agglutination test

The blood cultures grow a Gram-negative pleomorphic rod.

**15.** Appropriate treatment would be
a) Doxycycline
b) Augmentin
c) Cefuroxime
d) Ampicillin
e) Acyclovir

## Discussion

Although the symptoms are nonspecific, several clues suggest the diagnosis of tularemia, caused by *Francisella tularensis*, a somewhat fastidious intracellular Gram-negative coccobacillus.

## Answers and Explanations

### 13. e.

The sudden onset within 1 week of hunting deer and rabbits suggests an exposure or perhaps vector-borne disease. Tularemia can occur as a result of tick, deerfly, or mosquito bites or contact with infected blood and animal carcasses through breaks in the skin, such as the numerous cuts and abrasions on his hands. Tender regional adenopathy is representative of the glandular clinical syndrome of tularemia (Table 18.8). Also typical are the waxing and waning fevers with the lack of response to penicillin and first-generation cephalosporins. This zoonotic clinical picture would include in the differential diagnosis RMSF, ehrlichiosis, babesiosis, and perhaps Lyme disease. This would be an unusual presentation for TB, and, therefore, this is the answer.

### 14. e.

The Weil-Felix agglutination is a nonspecific test with several potential cross reactions; it is obsolete with today's technology. Cysteine-enriched blood cultures are helpful in culturing *F. tularensis*. If suspected, you should notify the lab of your suspicions, as it is highly contagious. The infective inoculum is 10 organisms by contact or 15 by aerosol. Morulae are found in the cytoplasm of WBCs

| TABLE 18.8 |
|---|
| **TULAREMIA CLINICAL SYNDROMES** |

| | |
|---|---|
| Ulceroglandular | Typhoidal |
| Glandular | Oropharyngeal |
| Oculoglandular | Pneumonic |

during *Ehrlichia* infections but require a trained microscopist to make the diagnosis. Thick and thin blood smears are used to search for *Babesia*. PCR is also available. Paired sera are used for the diagnosis of RMSF, but, obviously, the diagnosis must be made earlier, either clinically or by direct fluorescent antibody of a biopsy of the skin rash because successful treatment is at least partially dependent on the early initiation of appropriate therapy.

### 15. a.

Doxycycline is an appropriate therapy for tularemia but requires a longer course of treatment than streptomycin, the drug of choice. *F. tularensis* is also susceptible to other aminoglycosides, rifampin, chloramphenicol, erythromycin, third-generation cephalosporins, and probably most quinolones. It is resistant to penicillin and first-generation cephalosporins.

## CASE 8

A 23-year-old man undergoes bilateral lung transplantation for cystic fibrosis; the donor and recipient are CMV seropositive. He receives postoperative cyclosporine A and prednisone. A history of exposure during childhood to a brother with active pulmonary TB is noted. The results of a pretransplant tuberculin skin test were negative.

On day 5 postoperatively, fever develops to 39°C. On physical examination, the patient appears ill. The incision is clean. A few rales are present along the right parasternal border. The WBC count is 18,000/mm³, with 90% granulocytes. A chest radiograph discloses a subtle right basilar infiltrate.

## Questions

**16.** Which of the following is the least likely consideration?
a) CMV pneumonia
b) Anastomotic leak from the right mainstem bronchus
c) Mediastinitis
d) *Pseudomonas cepacia* pneumonia
e) Acute rejection
f) *Haemophilus parainfluenzae* pneumonia from the donor

The patient undergoes bronchoscopy and is found to have *H. parainfluenzae* pneumonia and responds to a course of parenteral antibiotics. Ganciclovir is given for 4 weeks postoperatively according to standard preventive prophylactic protocol. The patient is compliant with trimethoprim-sulfamethoxazole prophylaxis maintenance. At 5 months posttransplant, the patient presents with fever and a left-upper infiltrate.

**17.** On a statistical basis, what is the most likely diagnosis?
a) *Pneumocystis carinii* pneumonia
b) CMV pneumonia
c) TB
d) Bacterial pneumonia
e) Cryptococcal pneumonia

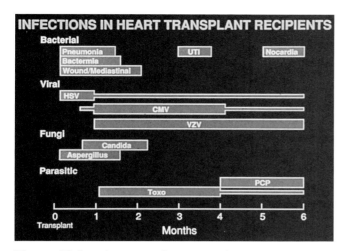

**Figure 18.6** Infections in heart transplant recipients. CMV, cytomegalovirus; HSV, herpes simplex virus; PCP, *Pneumocystis carinii* pneumonia; Toxo, toxoplasmosis; UTI, urinary tract infection; VZV, varicella-zoster virus.

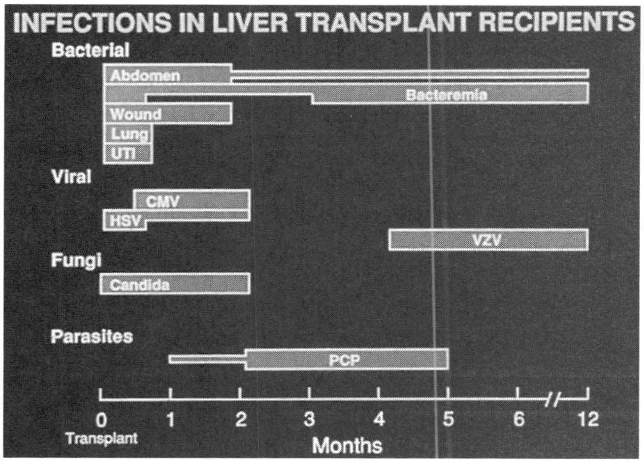

**Figure 18.7** Infections in liver transplant recipients. CMV, cytomegalovirus; HSV, herpes simplex virus; PCP, *Pneumocystis carinii* pneumonia; UTI, urinary tract infection; VZV, varicella-zoster virus.

## Discussion

This case deals with the differential diagnosis of fever in patients undergoing solid organ transplantation. In approaching such patients, several important considerations directly affect the differential diagnosis:

- Type of organ transplanted
- Timing of fever relative to transplantation
- CMV donor-recipient status
- Prior and current epidemiologic exposures

In general, infectious complications occurring within the first month are most often attributable to postoperative bacterial infections involving the allograft (or surrounding structures), wound infections, or nosocomial bacterial infections (e.g., intravascular lines, urinary tract infections from Foley catheters, etc.). CMV disease most often presents during months 1 to 4 posttransplantation and is especially problematic in originally CMV-seronegative patients who have received organs from CMV-seropositive donors. Infectious complications beyond month 4 are often attributable to pathogens associated with impaired cellular immunity, which occur in the setting of chronic immunosuppression. An exception to this occurs in lung transplant recipients: Bacterial pneumonia is the most common infectious complication, regardless of posttransplantation time. The common infectious complications and their temporal onset after transplantation are summarized by the organ transplants in Figures 18.6 through 18.8.

## Answers and Explanations

### 16. a.

Although at risk for CMV pneumonia, day +5 would be very early in the course for this to occur. Most patients with CMV pneumonia present 1 to 4 months posttrans-

plantation. Mediastinitis, anastomotic leak at the bronchial anastomosis, and acute rejection would all be major concerns. In addition, cystic fibrosis patients may seed their new lungs with organisms that continue to colonize their native trachea and sinuses, such as *P. cepacia*, *Pseudomonas aeruginosa*, and *S. aureus*. Finally, some studies have shown that colonizing organisms in the donor bronchus may produce postoperative pneumonia in the transplanted lung, as occurred in this patient.

### 17. d.

As noted earlier, bacterial pneumonia is the correct answer and is the leading cause of infection in lung transplant recipients during all posttransplantation time periods. All the other answers, however, would be appropriate concerns at 5 months, in view of the cellular immunodeficiency from chronic immunosuppression.

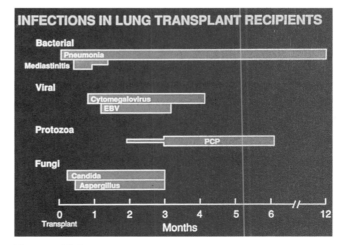

**Figure 18.8** Infections in lung transplant recipients. EBV, Epstein-Barr virus; PCP, *Pneumocystis carinii* pneumonia.

## CASE 9

A 23-year-old woman undergoes allogeneic bone marrow transplantation for acute myelogenous leukemia. The donor was seropositive for CMV, whereas the recipient was seronegative. The patient presented 1 year ago with fever, petechiae, and gingival bleeding and was found to have acute myelogenous leukemia. Induction therapy with high-dose cytosine arabinoside and daunorubicin achieved remission. Treatment was complicated by *Escherichia coli* bacteremia during neutropenia. No source for the bacteremia was found. Six months later, the patient relapsed and underwent reinduction with the same regimen. This time, treatment during neutropenia was complicated by transient candidemia, for which 1 g of amphotericin B was given. Remission was achieved, and a Hickman catheter was placed in preparation for allogeneic bone marrow transplantation.

The patient is admitted and receives a preparative regimen of busulfan, cyclophosphamide (Cytoxan), and etoposide, which produces considerable vomiting. Prophylaxis with oral ciprofloxacin is begun on day 0 at the time of allogeneic transplantation. She is treated with granulocyte colony–stimulating factor, cyclosporine, and prednisone. She becomes absolutely neutropenic on day +2.

On day +3 she develops fever to 39.4°C. On examination, she appears chronically but not acutely ill and is vomiting. There is mild oral mucositis. The remainder of the physical examination is normal. The WBC count is 100 cells/mm³, and the alkaline phosphatase is elevated at 235 IU/mL. A chest radiograph raises the question of a vague right-middle lobe infiltrate.

### Questions

18. Which is the least likely diagnosis?
a) CMV pneumonia
b) Aspiration pneumonia
c) Hickman-related bacteremia
d) Fever from mucositis
e) Gram-negative bacteremia with early adult respiratory distress syndrome

Therapy with vancomycin, piperacillin, and tobramycin is begun. Blood cultures grow *Streptococcus viridans* in one set of peripheral cultures. Blood cultures obtained via the Hickman catheter are negative. The chest radiograph does not evolve. She promptly defervesces but is slow to engraft. On day 15, she spikes to 40°C. She has diarrhea, and the physical examination is normal. The WBC count is 250 cells/mm³ with 5% PMNs. The alkaline phosphatase is 600 IU/mL, aspartate aminotransaminase 42 IU/mL; alanine aminotransferase 55 IU/mL, and bilirubin 1.5 mg%. A CT scan of the abdomen discloses ill-defined areas of mottling in the liver.

19. Which is the most likely diagnosis?
a) Graft-versus-host disease
b) Veno-occlusive disease
c) Hepatic candidiasis
d) Liver abscess from prior bacteremia
e) *Clostridium difficile* colitis

Blood cultures grow *C. albicans*, and amphotericin B is given. The patient engrafts at day 20 and is discharged to complete 100 days of outpatient ganciclovir and 2.5 g of amphotericin B. Trimethoprim-sulfamethoxazole is begun, and the patient is maintained on cyclosporine A and prednisone, 30 mg/day; she does well until day +120, when a fever that spikes at 38.5°C and a dry cough develop. A chest radiograph discloses a large left-upper lobe cavity. The patient has forgotten to take trimethoprim-sulfamethoxazole for the past month and has returned to work as a supervisor on construction sites. The patient also recalled that an uncle with whom she had lived as a child died of TB.

20. Which is the least likely diagnosis?
a) *Nocardia* pneumonia
b) *P. carinii* pneumonia
c) CMV pneumonia
d) Pulmonary TB
e) Cryptococcal pneumonia

Bronchoscopy is performed. For each potential finding shown in Figures 18.9 through 18.12, choose the best therapy.

21. For the pathogen in Figure 18.9

22. For the pathogen in Figure 18.10

23. For the pathogen in Figure 18.11

24. For the pathogen in Figure 18.12
a) Trimethoprim-sulfamethoxazole
b) Amphotericin B plus flucytosine

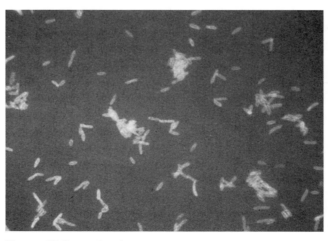

**Figure 18.9**   Finding for Case 9. (See Color Fig. 18.9.)

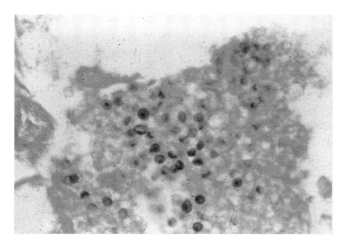

**Figure 18.10**   Finding for Case 9.  (See Color Fig. 18.10.)

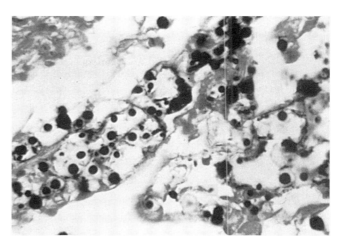

**Figure 18.12**   Finding for Case 9.  (See Color Fig. 18.12.)

c)  INH plus rifampin plus PZA plus ethambutol
d)  Amphotericin B at 1 mg/kg/day
e)  Erythromycin

## Discussion

This case deals with the differential diagnosis of fever in the bone marrow transplant recipient. The differential diagnosis of fever in such patients is invariably broad, but several important considerations are helpful in approaching a microbial differential diagnosis:

■  Time of onset relative to transplantation
■  Presence or absence of neutropenia
■  CMV donor-recipient status
■  Prior infections or exposures
■  Autologous versus allogeneic transplant
■  Immunosuppressive regimen
■  Presence of graft-versus-host disease
■  Prophylactic regimens

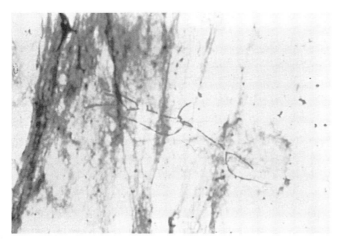

**Figure 18.11**   Finding for Case 9.  (See Color Fig. 18.11.)

The temporal onset of infectious complications after allogeneic bone marrow transplantation is summarized in Table 18.9.

In general, the first month after transplantation is the period associated with neutropenia and thus with invasive bacterial infections such as bacteremias, line-related infections, *C. difficile* colitis (given the use of empiric antimicrobials), and bacterial pneumonias. Oral herpes simplex virus infections and fungal infections, such as candidiasis or aspergillosis, may also be encountered. The use of growth factors has shortened the duration of neutropenia and, thus, the incidence of these infectious complications.

During months 1 to 4, CMV becomes a diagnostic consideration in patients with unexplained fever, cytopenia, or pneumonia, especially in those with concomitant graft-versus-host disease. In all solid organ and autologous bone marrow transplant settings, patients who are originally CMV negative and receive organs from CMV-positive donors are at highest risk of subsequent CMV disease. After allogeneic bone marrow transplantation, the immune system is comprised of donor cells with potential reservoirs of CMV residing in patients' organs, such that the highest risk is found when the donor bone marrow is CMV negative and the recipient is CMV positive. CMV disease is rare in autologous bone marrow transplant recipients who do not require long-term immunosuppression. Beyond month 4, allogeneic recipients are at risk of infectious complications associated with chronic immunosuppression, such as *P. carinii* pneumonia, herpes zoster, cryptococcosis, and reactivation TB.

## Answers and Explanations

**18. a.**
CMV is the least likely diagnosis, given that the patient is only at day +3, posttransplantation.

**19. c.**
Hepatic candidiasis is the best answer. Clues to this diagnosis in the history include the prior candidemia, the

## TABLE 18.9

### TIMING OF COMPLICATIONS IN PATIENTS UNDERGOING ALLOGENEIC BONE MARROW TRANSPLANTATION

| Risk Factor | Neutropenia | Acute GVHD | Chronic GVHD |
|---|---|---|---|
| Immunosuppression | Immunosuppression | Chronic immunosuppression | Chronic immunosuppression |
| Bacterial infections | Mucositis | Mucositis | Encapsulated organisms |
| | Bacteremias | Bacteremias | |
| | Intravenous line infections | Intravenous line infections | |
| | *Candida difficile* | *C. difficile* | |
| Fungal | *Candida* and *Aspergillus* | *Candida* and *Aspergillus* | *Candida* and *Aspergillus* |
| Viral | Herpes simplex virus | CMV and adenovirus | Varicella-zoster virus |
| Pneumonia | Bacterial | CMV | Tuberculosis |
| | | | *Nocardia* |
| | | | Encapsulated bacteria |
| Interstitial | | PCP | PCP |
| Months | 1 | 4 | 12 |

CMV, cytomegalovirus; GVHD, graft-versus-host disease; PCP, *Pneumocystis carinii* pneumonia.

abnormalities on CT scan of the abdomen, and the elevated alkaline phosphatase out of proportion to the transaminases, which is characteristic of hepatic candidiasis. Graft-versus-host disease often produces diarrhea when it involves the gut but occurs after engraftment and rarely produces fever. Veno-occlusive disease may occur early but is usually associated with jaundice. Antibiotic-associated colitis is a reasonable concern but does not account for the liver function abnormalities. Bacteremic seeding of the liver occurs but is rare; thus, this is not the best answer.

### 20. c.

CMV is the correct answer because CMV pneumonia, although not unexpected at day +120, does not cavitate. All the other choices can produce cavitary pneumonia in the immunocompromised patient and might occur at this point after allogeneic bone marrow transplantation.

### 21–24.

Transbronchial biopsy might conceivably show one of several pathogens depicted in Figures 18.9 to 18.12, which could produce a cavity. Figure 18.9 shows *Legionella* species, for which erythromycin would be appropriate therapy. Although not a common pathogen in allogeneic bone marrow transplant recipients, the construction site exposure and cavitary infiltrate necessitate its inclusion in the differential diagnosis. Figure 18.10 shows *P. carinii*, which rarely may cavitate, although generally with small rather than large cavities. The patient stopped taking prescribed trimethoprim-sulfamethoxazole, making this a concern. Trimethoprim-sulfamethoxazole would be the best therapy of the choices offered for *P. carinii* pneumonia. Figure 18.11 shows the weakly acid-fast branching filamentous bacilli typical of *Nocardia asteroides*, for which trimethoprim-sulfamethoxazole is the best choice. Figure 18.12 shows *C. neoformans*, for which amphotericin B and flucytosine would be appropriate. Some may

have chosen amphotericin B alone (choice d), concerned about the bone marrow–suppressive side effects of flucytosine. Given the severity of the patient's immunosuppression, it is best to take advantage of the additive effects of both antifungal agents (choice b).

## CASE 10

A 42-year-old HIV-positive businessman consults you for periumbilical crampy abdominal pain and nonbloody, watery diarrhea. He has recently returned from a 2-week trip to Moscow and St. Petersburg. His CD4 count is 560/mm$^3$, and his history is otherwise unremarkable.

### Questions

**25.** All of the following would be likely causes of diarrhea, *except*
a) Enteropathogenic *E. coli*
b) Giardiasis
c) Cryptosporidiosis
d) Microsporidiosis
e) Amebiasis

Stool examinations for ova and parasites demonstrate several organisms. Select the appropriate therapy for each pathogen shown in Figures 18.13 through 18.15.

**26.** For the pathogen in Fig. 18.13

**27.** For the pathogen in Fig. 18.14

**28.** For the pathogen in Fig. 18.15
a) No therapy
b) Paromomycin, 500 mg orally twice daily for 1 week
c) Metronidazole, 250 mg orally three times daily for 7 days

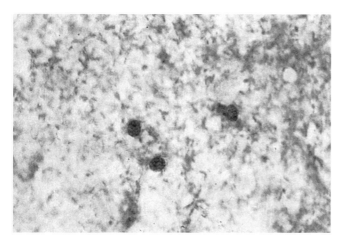

**Figure 18.13** Pathogen in Case 10. (See Color Fig. 18.13.)

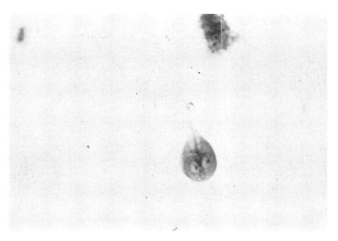

**Figure 18.15** Pathogen in Case 10. (See Color Fig. 18.15.)

d) Metronidazole, 750 mg orally three times daily for 5 to 10 days plus diloxanide furoate, 500 mg orally three times daily for 10 days

## Discussion

This case involves the differential diagnosis of diarrhea in an HIV-positive traveler. The most important consideration in the differential diagnosis is the patient's CD4 count, which is normal. Opportunistic pathogens such as *M. avium intracellulare*, microsporidiosis, and CMV would not be considerations in an individual with a normal CD4 count. These infections are usually seen in patients with advanced immunodeficiency and CD4 counts of less than 100 cells/ mm$^3$. In this patient, all the common causes of nonbloody traveler's diarrhea would be appropriate concerns, including enterotoxigenic *E. coli*, giardiasis, cryptosporidiosis (a self-limited disease in immunocompetent individuals), and amebiasis (although in most homosex-

ual men, entamoebas detected in stool usually represent the nonpathogenic zymodeme *Entamoeba dispar*).

## Answers and Explanations

### 25. d.
As described previously, microsporidiosis would not be a concern in an HIV-positive individual with a normal CD4 count.

### 26. a.
Figure 18.13 demonstrates acid-fast organisms of *Cryptosporidium*. Although paromomycin has been beneficial in some HIV-infected patients with advanced immunodeficiency and chronic cryptosporidiosis, its usefulness in the therapy of acute cryptosporidiosis in immunocompetent individuals and HIV-infected individuals with normal CD4 counts has not been proven. Quinacrine and metronidazole are not effective in cryptosporidiosis.

### 27 and 28. c.
Figures 18.14 and 18.15 show a cyst and trophozoite of *Giardia lamblia*. Metronidazole, 250 mg orally three times daily for 1 week, would be appropriate. High-dose metronidazole and diloxanide furoate are the recommended treatment for intestinal amebiasis. A trophozoite and cyst form of *Entamoeba histolytica* are depicted in Figures 18.16 and 18.17, respectively.

Salient facts concerning cryptosporidiosis, giardiasis, microsporidiosis, and amebiasis are summarized in Tables 18.10 through 18.17.

## CASE 11

You are a general internist in a small community in Oklahoma. A family, long-time patients in your practice,

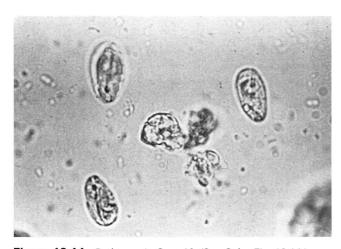

**Figure 18.14** Pathogen in Case 10. (See Color Fig. 18.14.)

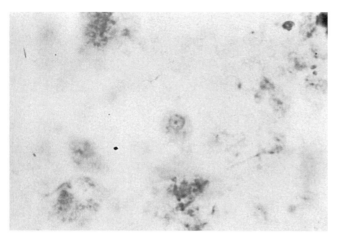

**Figure 18.16** *Entamoeba histolytica* trophozoite. (See Color Fig. 18.16.)

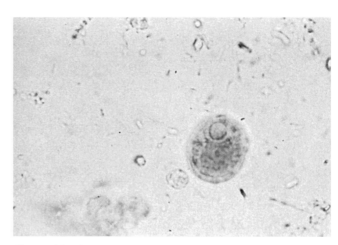

**Figure 18.17** *Entamoeba histolytica* cyst. (See Color Fig. 18.17.)

presents to your office again with febrile illnesses. They have recently returned from another extended exotic vacation. Six weeks earlier, they traveled to the Amazon basin in central Brazil, where they worked for 3 weeks in a rural missionary hospital. Three weeks earlier, they returned to the United States and spent 1 week vacationing at their private home on Nantucket. While there, they cared for a neighbor's infant daughter who had an unexplained febrile illness. Two weeks ago, they returned to their ranch in Oklahoma, where they spent several days working with their dogs herding cattle. Several family members recall removing ticks from the dogs.

Patient 1 is a healthy 52-year-old male business executive. The patient developed falciparal malaria last year after a trip to Nigeria. Ten days ago, he complained of the gradual onset of fever, shaking chills, headache, lethargy, and cough. These symptoms have waxed and waned but persist. Physical examination is notable for a temperature of 39.0°C, heart rate of 78 beats/min, mild diaphoresis, hepatosplenomegaly, and a faint cluster of pink macules on the abdomen. The WBC count is 3,000/mm³.

Patient 2 is a 48-year-old female schoolteacher, previously healthy except for a bout of babesiosis acquired on Martha's Vineyard. Two days ago, she noted gradual onset of fever that spiked at 38.7°C, arthralgias, anorexia, chills, fatigue, and headache. Physical examination is notable for a temperature of 38.7°C, a heart rate of 104 beats/min, tender nonswollen joints of the hands, cervical lymphadenopathy, and a faint reticular rash on the trunk and limbs. The WBC count is 3,500/mm³.

Patient 3 is an 18-year-old male college freshman who was healthy previously, except for a bout of ehrlichiosis last year. The patient presents with a 3-day history of fever that spiked to 38.5°C, headache, diarrhea, myalgia, and arthralgia. At physical examination his temperature is 38.4°C and other findings are normal.

Patient 4 is a 16-year-old male junior in high school who was previously healthy as well, except for a football injury last year that led to a splenectomy. Five days ago, the patient complained of fever, chills, myalgia, and headache. Physical examination is notable for a temperature of 38.7°C and a healed left-upper quadrant scar.

**TABLE 18.10**
**CRYPTOSPORIDIOSIS**

|  | Immunocompetent Individuals | Immunocompromised Individuals |
|---|---|---|
| High-risk | Travelers, daycare workers, veterinarians, homosexual men, healthcare workers, household contacts | Acquired immunodeficiency syndrome, congenital immunodeficiency, immunosuppression |
| Incubation period | 1–12 d (mean = 7 d) | Same |
| Clinical | Self-limited gastroenteritis | Intractable secretory diarrhea, weight loss, malabsorption, bronchial and biliary |
| Duration | 2–26 d (mean = 12 d) | Prolonged |

## TABLE 18.11
### CRYPTOSPORIDIOSIS: DIAGNOSIS

Conventional stool examination unreliable
Special techniques
Sugar-coverslip flotation
Kinyoun or Giemsa stains
Phase contrast microscopy
Small bowel biopsy

## TABLE 18.12
### CRYPTOSPORIDIOSIS: THERAPY

| Immunocompetent Individuals | Immunocompromised Individuals |
| --- | --- |
| Supportive | Supportive |
| Hydrate, sometimes total parenteral nutrition | Reverse immunosuppression |
| Antimotility agents | |
| Paromomycin | |

## TABLE 18.13
### GIARDIASIS: TRANSMISSION

Known reservoirs include humans, dogs, and beavers
Transmission via person-to-person spread, food, or water
Groups at high risk
Travelers to areas with poor sanitation
Campers who drink from streams
Male homosexuals
Children in day care centers
Institutionalized patients
Communities with inadequate or faulty water purification systems
Hypogammaglobulinemia or achlorhydria

## TABLE 18.14
### GIARDIASIS: CLINICAL MANIFESTATIONS

| Illness | Manifestations |
| --- | --- |
| Asymptomatic | Passes organisms |
| Acute illness | Incubation period 1–3 wk |
| | Watery nonbloody diarrhea |
| | Anorexia, nausea, distention, flatulence |
| | Sulfur burps, crampy pain |
| | Duration more than 1 wk |
| Chronic illness | Evolves from acute illness or insidiously alternating diarrhea and constipation |
| | Distention, belching, flatulence common |
| | Malabsorption and weight loss on occasion |

## TABLE 18.15
### GIARDIASIS: DIAGNOSIS

| Test | Sensitivity (%) | Comment |
| --- | --- | --- |
| Stool ova and parasites | 40–80 | — |
| Upper gastrointestinal sampling | 80–100 | — |
| Stool antigen | 90–95 | — |
| String test | — | — |
| Aspirate | — | — |
| Small bowel biopsy | — | — |
| Serology | >95 | Not widely available |
| Enzyme-linked immunoassay (serum and stool) | — | — |
| Immunofluorescent antibody (serum) | — | — |
| Upper gastrointestinal series | Poor | Nonspecific |

Patient 5 is a 14-year-old male foreign exchange student from Scotland spending the year with the family. The patient presents with a 4-day history of fever that spiked to 38.8°C, headache, myalgia, and arthralgia. At physical examination, his temperature is 38.6°C, and other findings are normal. The patient's WBC count is 3,900/mm$^3$ (65% PMNs, 30% lymphocytes, and 5% monocytes), platelet count is 105,000/mm$^3$, and aminotransaminase and alanine aminotransferase are 115 U/L and 135 U/L, respectively.

Because of the extensive travel history, you obtain peripheral thick and thin smears on the family, which are shown in Figures 18.18 through 18.22.

### Questions

Based on the history, findings, laboratory studies, and blood smear results, choose the best therapy for each of the patients.

**29.** Patient 1

**30.** Patient 2

**31.** Patient 3

**32.** Patient 4

**33.** Patient 5

a) Chloroquine phosphate, 1 g followed by 500 mg in 6 hours, then 500 mg/day for 2 days

b) Clindamycin, 600 mg orally three times daily and quinine sulfate, 650 mg orally three times daily for 7 to 10 days

c) Ciprofloxacin, 500 mg orally twice daily

d) Tetracycline, 500 mg orally four times daily

e) Quinine sulfate, 650 mg orally three times daily for 3 to 7 days, and pyrimethamine-sulfadoxine, three tablets at once on last day of quinine therapy

f) No therapy

## TABLE 18.16
### GIARDIASIS: THERAPY

| Agent | Regimen | Efficacy (%) | Comment |
|---|---|---|---|
| Quinacrine | 100 mg t.i.d. × 5 d | ~90 | Side effects: toxic psychosis, liver necrosis, dermatitis; contraindicated in psoriasis; limited availability, not in United States |
| Metronidazole | 250 mg t.i.d. × 5 d | 80–100 | Antabuse effect |
| Furazolidone | 100 mg q.i.d. × 7–10 d | 90–95 | Elixir available; brown urine, rash, disulfiram (Antabuse) effect, gastrointestinal, hemolysis in glucose-6-phosphate dehydrogenase deficiency |
| Tinidazole | 1.5–2.0 g × 1 d | 90 | Not available in the United States; lactose-free diet |

## Discussion

The patients present with acute febrile illnesses in the setting of extensive travel to the Amazon basin, Nantucket, and, subsequently, home to Oklahoma where several of them recall tick bites. The patients also recall exposure to an infant with an unexplained febrile illness. This places them at risk for a number of acute infectious diseases.

## Answers and Explanations

### 29. c.
*Patient 1.* This illness could be mistaken for a viral illness, especially given the leukopenia. Malaria and ehrlichiosis are major concerns; blood smear results (Fig. 18.18) are normal, however, and the presence of hepatosplenomegaly

## TABLE 18.17
### CLINICAL FEATURES OF MICROSPORIDIOSIS IN HUMAN IMMUNODEFICIENCY VIRUS–INFECTED PATIENTS

Enterocytozoon
CD4 counts <100
Chronic diarrhea, anorexia, weight loss most common
Cholecystitis, cholangitis, sinusitis, bronchitis rare
Encephalitozoon
CD4 counts <100
Keratoconjunctivitis, bronchiolitis, pneumonitis
Sinusitis, nephritis, cystitis, ureteritis
*Septata intestinalis*
Enteritis, cholecystitis
Diagnosis
Microscopic visualization in tissues or body fluids using Gram's, Weber's, and Giemsa stains
Reliable serodiagnostic tests lacking
Therapy
Albendazole may be effective for *S. intestinalis*, encephalitozoon, and enterocytozoon gastrointestinal illness
Fumagillin or propamidine for ocular encephalitozoon

and rose spots should suggest the diagnosis of typhoid fever, which is endemic in the tropics. Of the offered choices, the correct treatment for patient 1 is ciprofloxacin. In the past, chloramphenicol has been the treatment of choice, but resistance to this drug, as well as to ampicillin and trimethoprim-sulfamethoxazole, has emerged in some parts of the world. Third-generation cephalosporins, such as ceftriaxone, and quinolones, such as ciprofloxacin, have excellent activity against *Salmonella typhi*.

### 30. f.
*Patient 2.* Results of the peripheral blood smear (Fig. 18.19) are normal, arguing against a diagnosis of malaria. Rash, cervical lymphadenopathy, and tender joints should suggest a diagnosis of parvovirus B19, likely acquired from the infant on Nantucket. No therapy is available for this illness.

### 31. e.
*Patient 3.* This patient's illness could easily be confused with acute gastroenteritis, a viral illness, or typhoid fever. His peripheral smear, however, shows the typical banana

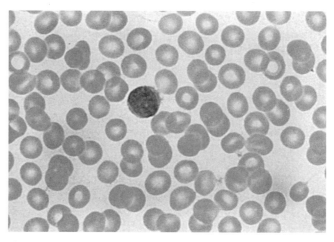

**Figure 18.18** Smear for patient 1. (See Color Fig. 18.18.)

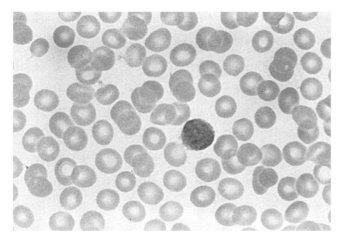

**Figure 18.19**    Smear for patient 2. (See Color Fig. 18.19.)

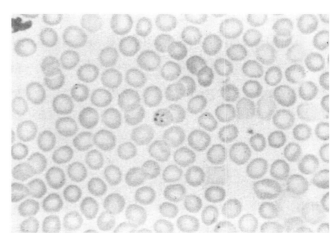

**Figure 18.21**    Smear for patient 4. (See Color Fig. 18.21.)

gametocyte of *Plasmodium falciparum* (Fig. 18.20). His illness is a medical emergency. It is imperative to consider the diagnosis of malaria in all patients with an acute febrile illness returning from a malaria-endemic part of the world, even if they have taken prophylaxis. Malaria may be accompanied by diarrhea, which should not dissuade one from considering the diagnosis. Chloroquine resistance occurs throughout South America. The correct treatment for the patient is therefore a combination of quinine sulfate and pyrimethamine-sulfadoxine.

### 32. b.
*Patient 4.* Peripheral smear demonstrates the tetrad of *Babesia microti* (Fig. 18.21), which was likely acquired during his sojourn on Nantucket. Clinically severe babesiosis occurs more commonly in splenectomized individuals. Appropriate therapy consists of clindamycin plus quinine sulfate. Compared to this combination, recent tests of azithromycin plus atovaquone showed a

greatly reduced side effect profile at 15% versus 72% (azithromycin plus atovaquone vs. clindamycin plus quinine sulfate). Symptom resolution was similar at 65% versus 73% (azithromycin plus atovaquone vs. clindamycin plus quinine sulfate). In severe cases, exchange transfusion may be necessary.

### 33. d.
*Patient 5.* This patient has a febrile, flu-like illness, a normal peripheral smear (Fig. 18.22), leukopenia, thrombocytopenia, and mild hepatitis. These findings are nonspecific and raise numerous possibilities. In someone residing in Oklahoma, with a history of tick exposure, however, this should suggest the diagnosis of ehrlichiosis or RMSF, for which doxycycline, tetracycline, or chloramphenicol would be appropriate therapy.

Key points concerning typhoid fever, parvovirus B19, malaria, babesiosis, ehrlichiosis, and RMSF are summarized in Tables 18.18 through 18.28.

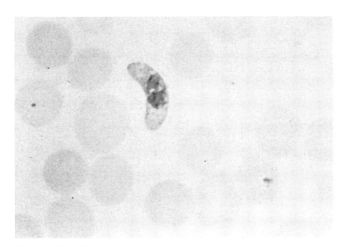

**Figure 18.20**    Smear for patient 3. (See Color Fig. 18.20.)

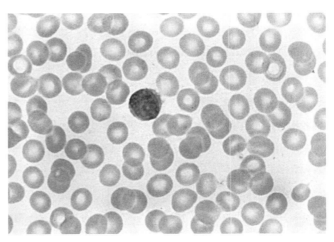

**Figure 18.22**    Smear for patient 5. (See Color Fig. 18.22.)

## TABLE 18.18
### BABESIOSIS

Epidemiology
Etiology in North America is usually *Babesia microti*
Transmission occurs via ixodid ticks and, rarely, transfusion
Most cases contracted on Nantucket, Martha's Vineyard, Long
   Island, Shelter Island
Clinical manifestations
Incubation period 1–4 wk
Many do not recall a tick bite
Spectrum of illness ranges from asymptomatic to prolonged
   severe illness
Splenectomy predisposes to more severe illness with higher levels
   of parasitemia
Diagnosis
Thick and thin smears stained with Giemsa
Serology
Therapy
Clindamycin, 1.2 g i.v. b.i.d. or 600 mg p.o. t.i.d. × 7 d *plus*
   quinine sulfate 650 mg p.o. t.i.d. × 7 d
Azithromycin, 500 mg p.o. q.d. × 1 d; 250 mg p.o. × 6 d *plus*
   atovaquone 750 mg p.o. b.i.d. × 7 d
Consider exchange transfusion in critically ill patient

## CASE 12

A 42-year-old male insulin-dependent diabetic archaeologist presents to your office with a 6-week history of intermittent fever, dry cough, a 10-lb weight loss, and night sweats. In the past 6 months, the patient has worked on various digs at Native American burial sites in New Mexico, Wisconsin, and southern Ohio. In addition, the patient traveled to rural Thailand 4 months earlier for a 2-week holiday.

At physical examination his temperature is 38°C and other findings are normal. A chest radiograph discloses a

## TABLE 18.20
### FEATURES SUGGESTING *PLASMODIUM FALCIPARUM*

Banana gametocytes
High-grade parasitemia
Double-applique forms
Multiply parasitized red blood cells
Absence of trophozoites or schizonts in periphery

left-upper lobe cavitary lesion with surrounding infiltrate. A bronchoscopy is performed.

For each potential finding shown in Figures 18.23 through 18.25, choose which answer is incorrect regarding the associated disease.

### Questions

**34.** Choose the incorrect statement for Figure 18.23.
a) This disease is produced by *Pseudomonas pseudomallei*.
b) Amoxicillin-clavulanate, 1 g three times daily would be an appropriate antibiotic in this setting.
c) This disease can produce acute, subacute, and chronic illness and may mimic pulmonary TB.
d) No therapy is indicated.
e) Prolonged therapy for several months is indicated.

**35.** Choose the incorrect statement for Figure 18.24.
a) Diabetics and those with compromised immunity are at higher risk of developing this form of the disease.
b) Surgical removal of cavitary disease is indicated for persistent, severe, or recurrent hemoptysis; rupture into the pleura; or enlargement of the cavity despite therapy.
c) The skin test result will likely be positive and is helpful in confirming the diagnosis.
d) Therapy is indicated.

## TABLE 18.19
### BIOLOGIC AND CLINICAL CHARACTERISTICS OF HUMAN MALARIA

|  | Falciparum | Vivax | Ovale | Malariae |
|---|---|---|---|---|
| Prevalence | Common | Common | Uncommon | Uncommon |
| Incubation (d) | 7–27 | 10–40 | 12–26 | 18–76 |
| Red blood cell cycle (h) | 48 | 48 | 48 | 72 |
| Hepatic relapse | No | Yes | Yes | No |
| Persistence (yr) | <3 | <3 | <3 | Many |
| Parasitemia | Up to 60% | <1% | <1% | <1% |
| Morbidity | Hemolysis | Hemolysis | — | Nephrosis |
|  | Acute tubular necrosis | Splenic rupture | — | — |
|  | Pulmonary edema | — | — | — |
|  | Central nervous system | — | — | — |
| Mortality | Common without therapy | Uncommon | Rare | Rare |
| Chloroquine resistance | Widespread | Rare | No | No |

## TABLE 18.21

### THERAPY OF MALARIA: ALL FORMS EXCEPT CHLOROQUINE-RESISTANT *PLASMODIUM FALCIPARUM*

| Route | Drug | Adult Dosage | Pediatric Dosage |
|---|---|---|---|
| Oral | Chloroquine phosphate | 600-mg base (1 g), then 300-mg base (0.5 g) at 6, 24, and 48 h | 10 mg base/kg (maximum 600 mg), then 5 mg base/kg at 6, 24, and 48 h |
| Parenteral | Quinidine gluconate | 10 mg/kg loading dose (maximum 600 mg) in normal saline over 1 h, followed by continuous infusion 0.02 mg/kg/min × 3 d maximum | Same as adult |
| | or Quinine dihydrochloride | 20 mg salt/kg loading dose in 10 mL/kg dextrose 5% in water over 4 h, then 10 mg salt/kg over 2–4 h every 8 h (maximum 1,800 mg/d) until oral therapy | Same as adult |

e) Triazole may be efficacious, and therapy should be continued at least 6 months beyond resolution of disease activity.

**36.** Choose the incorrect statement for Figure 18.25.

a) A careful examination for subcutaneous nodules and skin lesions should be performed because these are commonly seen.

b) Genitourinary disease is common in men, and urine culture may yield the organism after prostatic massage.

c) A complement fixation test may help confirm the diagnosis.

d) Ketoconazole or itraconazole is appropriate for patients with mild to moderate pulmonary disease.

e) Amphotericin B is indicated for those with life-threatening disease or central nervous system disease, and for those who are immunocompromised.

## Discussion

This question examines the differential diagnosis of a subacute respiratory illness together with a cavitary infiltrate in a diabetic archaeologist with an extensive travel history.

## Answers and Explanations

### 34. d.

Figure 18.23 shows Gram-negative bacilli. The travel history to Thailand should suggest the diagnosis of melioidosis, produced by the Gram-negative bacillus *P. pseudomallei*. Melioidosis may produce a variety of syndromes, including subacute pulmonary disease mimicking TB, acute pneumonitis, septicemia, chronic localized suppurative infection involving a variety of organs (including the lung), and acute localized suppurative infection. In patients with localized disease who are not toxic, amoxicillin-clavulanate, trimethoprim-sulfamethoxazole, chloramphenicol, or tetracycline has been shown to be effective. For septicemic patients, trimethoprim-sulfamethoxazole plus ceftazidime is recommended. Melioidosis is not endemic in the United States. Therapy is definitely indicated.

## TABLE 18.22

### THERAPY OF MALARIA: CHLOROQUINE-RESISTANT *PLASMODIUM FALCIPARUM*

| Route | Drug | Adult Dosage | Pediatric Dosage |
|---|---|---|---|
| Oral | Quinine SO$_4$ | 650 mg p.o. t.i.d. × 3–7 d | 25 mg/kg/d in 3 doses × 3 d <1 yr, |
| | Pyrimethamine-sulfadoxine | 3 tabs × 1 d, last day of quinine SO$_4$ | ¼ tab; 1–3 yr, ½ tab; 4–8 yr, 1 tab; 9–14 yr, 2 tabs |
| | or Tetracycline | 250 mg q.i.d. × 7 d[a] | 20 mg/kg/d every 6 h × 7 d |
| | or Clindamycin | 900 mg t.i.d. × 3 d | 20–40 mg/kg/d every 8 h × 3 d |
| Oral alternatives | Mefloquine | 1,250 mg × 1 d | 25 mg/kg once |
| | Halofantrine | 500 mg every 6 h × 3 doses | 8 mg/kg every 6 h × 3 doses |
| Parenteral | Quinidine gluconate | As before | As before |
| | Quinine dihydrochloride | As before | As before |

[a] Avoid in children younger than 8 years.

## TABLE 18.23

### PREVENTION OF MALARIA RELAPSES: *PLASMODIUM VIVAX* AND *PLASMODIUM OVALE*

| Adult Dosage | Pediatric Dosage |
| --- | --- |
| Primaquine phosphate, 15-mg base (26.3 mg)/d × 14 d or 45-mg base (79 mg)/wk × 8 wk | 0.3-mg base/kg/d × 14 d |

**35. c.**

Figure 18.24 shows a spherule of *Coccidioides immitis*. This illness is consistent with acute pulmonary coccidioidomycosis evolving into chronic cavitary disease. Diabetics and immunocompromised hosts are at increased risk of developing chronic pulmonary disease. The diagnosis is based on visualization of spherules in sputum, bronchoscopy specimens, or other tissue or fluid samples, as well as on culture isolation. Serum immunoglobulin M (IgM) precipitins are present in 75% of individuals 1 to 3 weeks into the acute illness. Complement-fixing immunoglobulin G (IgG) antibodies are present in 50% to 90% of patients with symptomatic primary coccidioidomycosis by 3 months. Elevated complement fixation titers are characteristic of disseminated disease. The results of skin tests with coccidioidal antigens are positive in most individuals by 1 month, but skin tests alone do not confirm the diagnosis in the absence of serologic or microbiologic evidence of infection. Therapy is indicated for those with severe primary infection, high complement fixation antibody titers, symptoms persisting beyond 6 weeks, pregnancy, progressive pulmonary disease, or significant underlying diseases (diabetes, immunosuppression, asthma, etc.). Amphotericin B is indicated in patients with extrapulmonary disease, and the triazoles can be used in those with nonmeningeal disease.

## TABLE 18.24

### MALARIA CHEMOPROPHYLAXIS: CHLOROQUINE-SENSITIVE AREAS

| Drug | Adult Dosage | Pediatric Dosage |
| --- | --- | --- |
| Chloroquine phosphate | 300-mg base (500 mg salt) p.o. every wk, beginning 1 wk before and continuing 4 wk after last exposure | 5 mg/kg base (8.3 mg/kg salt) every wk, up to adult dose |

Prolonged therapy is indicated for at least 6 months beyond resolution of a clinically apparent disease.

**36. c.**

Figure 18.25 shows the broad-based yeast form of *B. dermatitidis*. All the answer choices except (c) are true statements about North American blastomycosis. Complement fixation tests are neither sensitive nor specific for serologic diagnosis.

## CASE 13

An 18-year-old young woman with type 1 (insulin-requiring) diabetes who provides childcare for a toddler after school develops chickenpox. She has a typical illness for 5 days, with a maximum temperature of 38°C. After showing slight improvement for 2 days, she has an abrupt spiking temperature to 39.2°C; blood pressure, 142/85 mm Hg; pulse, 120 bpm and regular; and respiration, 14 per minute and easy. She presents to the emergency department with a 0.5-cm crusted papule with 2 cm of surrounding erythema. Minimal edema is present and no subcutaneous crepitance. She describes the area as having "12 out of 10 pain." A radiograph is negative for fracture or foreign body.

She is treated with a nonsteroidal anti-inflammatory drug and released. The next day she returns to the emergency room with temperature of 38.6°C and spreading erythema, warmth, and tenderness. She complains of a tingling and burning in her hand. The center of the lesion has progressed to a violaceous bulla.

### Questions

**37.** The most likely diagnosis is
a) Pyomyositis
b) Diabetic myonecrosis
c) Cellulitis
d) Necrotizing fasciitis
e) Traumatic hematoma

**38.** The definitive diagnostic modality is
a) Muscle biopsy with frozen section
b) Blood cultures
c) Bullae fluid culture
d) Serum creatine phosphokinase with isoenzymes
e) Radiograph to look for tissue gas

**39.** In addition to surgery, treatment consists of all the following, *except*
a) Extended spectrum, penicillin, β-lactamase inhibitor combination
b) Clindamycin
c) Tetanus toxoid
d) Ceftazidime
e) Intravenous immune globulin

## TABLE 18.25
### MALARIA CHEMOPROPHYLAXIS: CHLOROQUINE-RESISTANT AREAS

| Drug | Adult Dosage | Pediatric Dosage | Days before/Days after Malarious Exposure | Common Side Effects |
|---|---|---|---|---|
| Mefloquine | 250 mg p.o. weekly | 15–19 kg, ¼ tab weekly; 20–30 kg, ½ tab weekly; 31–45 kg, ¾ tab weekly; >45 kg, 1 tab weekly | Begin 1–2 wk before End 4 wk after | Vivid dreams |
| Doxycycline | 100 mg daily | >8 yr old, 2 mg/kg/d up to adult dose | Begin 1–2 d before End 4 wk after | Sunburn Vaginal yeast |
| Malarone (atovaquone/ proguanil HCL) | 250 mg atovaquone/ 100 mg proguanil HCL daily | Pediatric tab = 62.5 mg atovaquone (25 mg proguanil HCL) daily; 2–11 kg, 1 tab; 21–30 kg, 2 tabs daily; 31–40 kg, 3 tabs daily | Begin 1–2 d before End 7 d after leaving endemic area | Gastrointestinal upset |

HCL, hydrochloride.

## Discussion

Chickenpox is usually a moderate to severe viral illness with self-limited and characteristic progression. The overall disease process can be somewhat more severe in adolescence; however, it typically resolves from an early severe illness over several days. This case is a good reminder of the role of varicella vaccine in adolescents who have not had chickenpox previously. Vaccination before her exposure could likely have prevented this illness.

The presentation of a new abrupt fever and cellulitis spreading around a classic vesicular or crusted lesion should raise the possibility of secondary infection. In particular, case reports have indicated the presence of a severe group A streptococcal cellulitis on the heels of the original viral infection.

## Answers and Explanations

**37. d.**

The extremely rapid progression with extreme pain and distal neuropathy in a host with diabetes should increase the consideration of necrotizing fasciitis over simple cellulitis. Although the other diagnoses are possible, they are less likely and less ominous.

**38. a.**

It is appropriate to do blood cultures in patients with this degree of fever. A culture of the bullae fluid is most often sterile. Serum creatine phosphokinase and radiographs

## TABLE 18.26
### HUMAN EHRLICHIOSIS VERSUS ROCKY MOUNTAIN SPOTTED FEVER

| | Ehrlichiosis | Rocky Mountain Spotted Fever |
|---|---|---|
| Vector | Amblyomma americanum, Dermacentor variabilis | D. variabilis |
| Organism | Ehrlichia chaffeensis | Rickettsia rickettsii |
| Seasonality | Late spring, summer | Same |
| Geography | Oklahoma, Arkansas, Missouri, Georgia, Carolinas | Same plus South Atlantic |
| Peak age | Adults | Children |
| Symptoms | Fever, headache, myalgias | Same |
| Rash | <35% | >90% |
| Leukopenia | Common | Rare |
| Thrombopenia | Common | Occasional |
| Hepatitis | Common | Common |
| Therapy | Tetracycline, doxycycline | Same |

## TABLE 18.27
### TYPHOID FEVER

Incubation Period 5–21 d
Onset may be insidious
Fever, constitutional symptoms typical; diarrhea in only 20%–40%, neuropsychiatric symptoms in 10%
Signs include relative bradycardia (50%), rose spots (30%), hepatosplenomegaly (50%)
Anemia and leukopenia common
Blood cultures positive in 50%–70%
Blood, bone marrow, or stool cultures positive in more than 90%
Serologic tests unreliable
Resistance to chloramphenicol, ampicillin, and trimethoprim-sulfamethoxazole increasingly common
Third-generation cephalosporin or quinolone are drugs of choice

### TABLE 18.28
### CLINICAL SYNDROMES OF PARVOVIRUS B19

| Host | Disease |
| --- | --- |
| Children, adults | Erythema infectiosum |
| Adults, children | Arthritis |
| Chronic hemolysis | Aplastic crisis |
| Immunocompromised | Chronic anemia |
| Fetuses | Hydrops fetalis, fetal death |
| Various | Isolated reports of cardiac, neurologic, vasculitic disease |

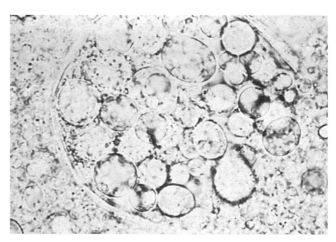

**Figure 18.24** Pathogen in Case 12. (See Color Fig. 18.24.)

are both insensitive means to evaluate for muscle- or tissue-necrotizing infection. A deep muscle biopsy with frozen section is the most definitive way to diagnose this condition. Surgical intervention is so essential to the resolution of this infection that surgical consultation must be sought immediately. Wide debridement and even multiple debridements are often necessary to effect a full cure, even with the rapid initiation of powerful broad-spectrum antibiotic therapy.

Necrotizing fasciitis may follow minor and even non-penetrating trauma or illnesses such as chickenpox. Pain out of proportion to the surface examination is something of a hallmark of this diagnosis. Bullae are often present and rapidly "mature" from clear fluid to a maroon or violaceous color. Cutaneous gangrene and an extension of inflammation appears along the planes, resulting in cutaneous anesthesia as the surface nerve areas undergo necrosis. The cutaneous anesthesia may proceed or follow the cutaneous gangrene.

### 39. d.

Although surgery is the most necessary intervention, extended-spectrum penicillins provide excellent spectrum for the organisms most often involved in necrotiz-ing fasciitis. Clindamycin is also very effective and will provide additional antitoxin effects. Tetanus toxoid is important to consider because many cases are preceded by trauma. Up to 70% of adults are not up to date in their tetanus toxoid immunization. With a recommendation of a once-a-decade vaccination after completion of the childhood series at approximately 5 years of age, this 18-year-old patient would likely be at her immune nadir for tetanus. Some centers have published small series indicating a beneficial effect of intravenous immune globulin, especially in cases of streptococcus group, a severe infection. Ceftazidime is an excellent antibiotic, but does not cover any of the anaerobic bacteria, which are often involved in this condition.

When selecting empiric antibiotics, one must first consider the likely flora associated. Table 18.29 provides a condensed summary of antibiotic selections based on general principles of antimicrobial coverage.

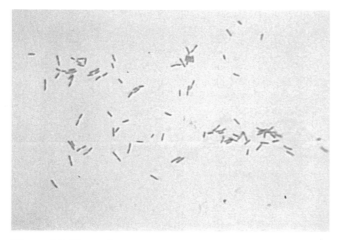

**Figure 18.23** Pathogen in Case 12. (See Color Fig. 18.23.)

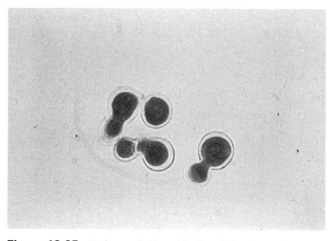

**Figure 18.25** Pathogen in Case 12. (See Color Fig. 18.25.)

**TABLE 18.29**
## EMPIRIC ANTIBIOTICS SELECTION SUMMARY

| Antimicrobial Agents | Example | Gram-Positive | | Gram-Negative | Anaerobes (Gram-Positive and Gram-Negative) |
|---|---|---|---|---|---|
| | | MSSA | MRSA | | |
| Glycopeptide | Vancomycin | +++ | +++ | −− | + (Gram-positive only) |
| Extended spectrum penicillin +β-lactamase inhibitor | Zosyn or Timentin | +++ | −− | +++ | +++ |
| Third-generation cephalosporin | Ceftazidime or ceftriaxone | −− | −− | +++ | −− |
| Quinolone | Ciprofloxacin | −− | −− | +++ | −− |
| First-generation cephalosporin | Cefazolin | +++ | −− | + | −− |

+, weak activity against listed organisms; +++, strong activity against listed organisms; −, no efficacy; MSSA, methicillin-susceptible *Staphylococcus aureus*; MRSA, methicillin-resistant *Staphylococcus aureus*.

## GENERAL KNOWLEDGE: MATCHING AND MULTIPLE CHOICE QUESTIONS

40. Match the most likely side effect profile with the antivirals listed. More than one answer may be correct for each drug.

**Drug**
40. Ritonavir
41. Stavudine
42. Abacavir
43. Indinavir
44. Zidovudine
45. Didanosine
46. Nelfinavir
47. Efavirenz
48. Amprenavir

**Side Effects**
a) Potentially fatal hypersensitivity reaction with rechallenge
b) Peripheral neuropathy
c) Crystalluria, dysuria, nephrolithiasis
d) Nausea, vomiting, diarrhea
e) Malaise, anemia, headache
f) Oral paresthesia
g) Pancreatitis
h) Dizziness, vivid dreams, depersonalization, and false-positive cannabinoid test

### Answers
40. d, f.
41. b, g.
42. a.
43. c.
44. e.
45. b, g.
46. d.
47. h.
48. f, d.

49. All of the following can cause a bloody foodborne diarrhea, *except*
a) Salmonella
b) Campylobacter
c) *E. coli* O157:H7
d) Cyclospora
e) Shigella

### Answer
49. d.

For questions 50 to 54, choose the most typical CSF formula for each clinical scenario.

50. A healthy 25-year-old man with fever, headache, and photophobia after a summer diarrheal illness

51. A 50-year-old splenectomized man with sudden-onset fever, headache, and obtundation who presents with nuchal rigidity and hypotension

52. A 40-year-old woman with onset of fever and confusion over 24 hours; she presents with a seizure and demonstrates enhancement and hemorrhage in the right temporal lobe on magnetic resonance imaging

53. A 60-year-old man with fever and headache 1 week after frontal sinus surgery; he demonstrates a right frontal subdural collection on CT

54. A 65-year-old woman with stage 4 non-Hodgkin's lymphoma; she presents with subacute onset of headache and right facial weakness
a) WBC count 3,000/mm$^3$ (98% PMNs, 2% lymphocytes), RBC count 10/mm$^3$, glucose 10 mg/dL, and protein 125 mg/dL
b) WBC count 75/mm$^3$ (85% lymphocytes, 15% PMNs), RBC count 325/mm$^3$, glucose 65 mg/dL, and protein 55 mg/dL

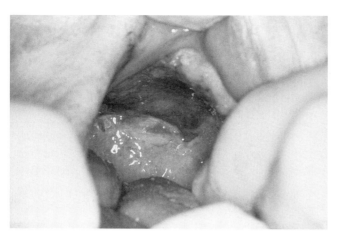

**Figure 18.26** Palatal lesion of patient in Question 54. (See Color Fig. 18.26.)

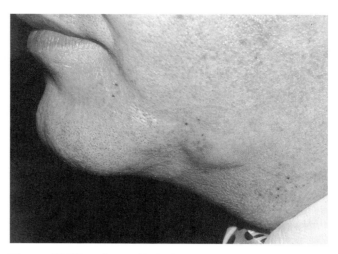

**Figure 18.28** Left mandibular lesion of patient in Question 58. (See Color Fig. 18.28.)

c) WBC count 35/mm$^3$ (50% lymphocytes, 50% PMNs), RBC count 5/mm$^3$, glucose 75 mg/dL, and protein 125 mg/dL

d) WBC count 125/mm$^3$ (90% lymphocytes, 10% PMNs), RBC count 0, glucose 65 mg/dL, and protein 55 mg/dL

e) WBC count 50/mm$^3$ (90% lymphocytes, 10% reactive cells), RBC count 0, glucose 0 mg/dL, and protein 85 mg/dL

For each clinical scenario in questions 55 to 58, choose the best therapy.

**55.** A 70-year-old previously healthy woman presents with confusion, right eye proptosis, a blood sugar of 450 mg/dL, and the palatal lesion shown in Figure 18.26.

**56.** A 30-year-old healthy female gardener presents with findings involving the left arm shown in Figure 18.27. She is otherwise asymptomatic. Biopsy of a nodule discloses cigar-shaped yeast forms.

**57.** The 33-year-old husband of the patient in question 56 presents with similar lesions to those shown in Figure 18.27. He is previously healthy and has an aquarium that he regularly tends. A biopsy of a nodule discloses AFBs.

**58.** A 37-year-old male attorney presents with painless swelling of the left mandible (Fig. 18.28). He reports temperature sensitivity of several months' duration involving a left lower molar. Gram's smear of discharge from the lesion discloses Gram-positive filamentous bacilli.
a) Rifampin plus ethambutol
b) Saturated solution of potassium iodide
c) Penicillin
d) Amphotericin B and surgical debridement

## Answers and Explanations

**50. d.**
This patient has enteroviral meningitis, which is usually characterized by a lymphocytic pleocytosis and normal (or mildly depressed) CSF glucose. In the first 12 hours of the illness, however, the pleocytosis may be polymorphonuclear.

**51. a.**
This patient has bacterial meningitis until proven otherwise, most likely pneumococcal, given the prior splenectomy and the acute, fulminant illness. A marked polymorphonuclear pleocytosis and profound hypoglycorrhachia would be consistent with this presentation.

**52. b.**
This case scenario suggests the diagnosis of herpes simplex encephalitis, and the hemorrhagic lymphocytic pleocytosis would be most characteristic of this diagnosis.

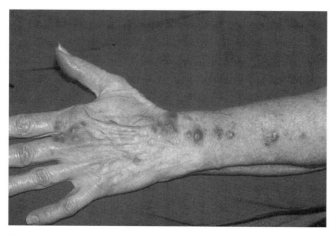

**Figure 18.27** Left arm lesions of patients in Questions 56 and 57. (See Color Fig. 18.27.)

**53. c.**

This patient has a parameningeal focus of infection that is often accompanied by a mixed polymorphonuclear and lymphocytic pleocytosis, an elevated protein, and a normal CSF glucose.

**54. e.**

This patient has lymphomatous meningitis. In patients with carcinomatous or lymphomatous meningitis, the clues in the formula are the reactive cells and the undetectable CSF glucose.

**55. d.**

This patient presents with previously unrecognized diabetes mellitus, proptosis, and a necrotic palatal lesion. This constellation of clinical findings suggests mucormycosis (zygomycosis). Medical therapy alone is rarely curative, and the combination of aggressive surgical debridement combined with antifungal therapy with high-dose amphotericin B is indicated.

**56. b.**

This woman has cutaneous sporotrichosis caused by *Sporothrix schenckii,* for which saturated solution of potassium iodide is appropriate therapy. Sporotrichosis is an important consideration in patients with nodular lymphangitis.

**57. a.**

Her husband also has nodular lymphangitis, but in this case it is caused by *M. marinum.* This diagnosis is suggested by his fish tank exposure and the finding of AFBs on biopsy of a nodule. Other nontuberculous mycobacteria can produce a similar clinical syndrome. Rifampin plus ethambutol is one of several regimens appropriate in patients with *M. marinum* infection producing this syndrome.

**58. c.**

This patient has cervicofacial actinomycosis, for which penicillin is appropriate therapy. Such patients often present with unrecognized dental disease. Several months of therapy are typically required. Actinomycosis also may present with chronic empyema occasionally draining to the skin, enteric fistulas mimicking Crohn's disease, and endometritis in the setting of an indwelling intrauterine device.

## SUGGESTED READINGS

ATS/CDC Statement Committee on Latent Tuberculosis Infection. Targeted tuberculin testing and treatment of latent tuberculosis infection. *MMWR* 2000;49(RR06):1–54.

Blumberg H, Jarvis W, Soucie M, et al. Risk factors for candidal bloodstream infections in surgical intensive care unit patients: the NEMIS Prospective Multicenter Study. *Clin Inf Dis* 2001; 33:177.

Hahn A. The Guillian-Barré syndrome. *Lancet* 1998;352:635.

Iseman MD. *A Clinician's Guide to Tuberculosis.* Philadelphia: Lippincott Williams & Wilkins, 2000.

Jacobs B, Rothbart P, van der Meche F, et al. The spectrum of antecedent infections in Guillian-Barré syndrome: a case-control study. *Neurology* 1998;51:1110.

Musher D, Alexandrake I, Graviss EA, et al. Bacteremic and nonbacteremic pneumonococcal pneumonia: a prospective study. *Medicine* 2000;79(4):210.

Pfaller M, Jones R, Doern G, et al. Bloodstream infections due to *Candida* species: SENTRY antimicrobial surveillance program in North America and Latin America, 1997–1998. *Antimicr Agents Chemother* 2000;44:747.

Rees J, Soudain S, Gregson N, et al. *Campylobacter jejuni* infection and Guillain-Barré syndrome. *N Engl J Med* 1995;333;1374.

Rex J, Walsh T, Sobel J, et al. Practice guidelines for the treatment of candidiasis. *Clin Inf Dis* 2000;30:62.

Roper A. The Guillain-Barré Syndrome. *N Engl J Med* 1992;326:1130.

Small PM, Fujiwara PI. Medical progress: management of tuberculosis in the United States. *N Engl J Med* 2001;345:189–200.

Wenzel R. Nosocomial candidemia: risk factors and attributable mortality. *Clin Inf Dis* 1995;20:1531.

# Hematology and
# Medical Oncology

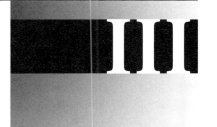

# Oncologic Emergencies

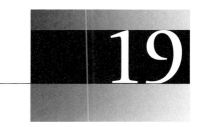

*Tarek Mekhail    David J. Adelstein*

Malignancies can produce medical emergencies from both local and metastatic disease. This discussion focuses on some of the common structural problems associated with cancer.

A number of malignancy-related metabolic and endocrinologic conditions also are emergencies, including hyponatremia, hypoglycemia, acute renal failure, and ectopic hormone production. Hematologic emergencies include both leukopenia and hyperleukocytosis, thrombocytopenia and thrombocytosis, as well as polycythemia, hyperviscosity, and disseminated intravascular coagulation. These syndromes are not addressed in this chapter.

## SUPERIOR VENA CAVA SYNDROME

The superior vena cava is a thin-walled, low-pressured, vascular structure rigidly confined in the mediastinum and surrounded by lymph nodes. It is readily occluded or thrombosed by any distortion of the normal architecture. Fortunately, an extensive collateral network exists, allowing for decompression and venous return. Patients with superior cava obstruction usually present with complaints of neck and facial swelling, dyspnea, and cough. Physical examination is notable for distended jugular veins; prominent superficial venous collaterals; and edema of the face, shoulders, and arms.

The diagnosis is usually made at the bedside. Chest radiography may reveal mediastinal widening or a right hilar mass. Further delineation of the anatomic abnormality can be obtained via computerized tomography (CT), contrast venography, or ultrasonography. The differential diagnosis should include congestive heart failure, pericardial tamponade/constriction, and pulmonary hypertension.

Although the clinical presentation of superior vena cava syndrome is often dramatic, death from superior vena cava obstruction alone is not well described. Overall, the prognosis of patients with this syndrome depends entirely on the prognosis of their underlying disease.

Symptomatic measures, such as diuretics and elevation of the head of the bed, are usually sufficient and allow time for an accurate etiologic diagnosis.

The etiology of superior vena cava syndrome includes the following:

- Malignancy
- Small cell and non-small cell lung cancer
- Lymphoma
- Thrombosis
- Fibrosis
- Substernal goiter
- Syphilitic aneurysm

Most patients with superior vena cava obstruction have malignancy. Lung cancer, particularly small cell carcinoma, is the cause in most of these cases. Malignant lymphoma is also commonly responsible. Many patients now develop superior vena cava syndrome as a result of the more frequent use of central venous catheters.

An accurate etiologic diagnosis is crucial, and tissue confirmation is required to verify the presence of malignancy. Despite fears to the contrary, invasive diagnostic procedures carry little additional risk in these patients. Although it was recommended in the past, radiation therapy before the histologic confirmation of malignancy is inappropriate and may confound accurate histologic diagnosis. Several cancers commonly implicated are potentially curable with appropriate treatment, thus justifying an aggressive diagnostic and therapeutic approach.

Clinical improvement occurs in most patients, although this improvement may largely result from the development of adequate collateral circulation. Anticoagulation has not been used extensively, except when thrombosis has resulted from a central venous catheter. The treatment plan generally should be based on the tumor histology and disease extent, not just on the presence of superior vena cava obstruction. Radiation therapy is most appropriate in those patients with non-small cell lung cancer or other neoplasms unresponsive to chemotherapy. Patients with small cell lung cancer or lymphoma, however, can be treated primarily with chemotherapy, with the expectation of a rapid response.

Although clinical improvement can be expected in 70% to 95% of patients, radiologic evidence of recannulation and patency of the superior vena cava at autopsy is much less frequent. It is the development of adequate collateral circulation that allows for this symptomatic resolution, despite continued superior vena caval obstruction.

## SPINAL CORD COMPRESSION

Neoplastic epidural spinal cord compression (ESCC) is a common complication of cancer that causes pain and sometimes irreversible loss of neurologic function. In adults, the tip of the spinal cord usually lies at the L1 vertebral level; below this level, the lumbosacral nerve roots form the cauda equina, which floats in cerebrospinal fluid (CSF). Because the pathophysiology of compression of the thecal sac at the level of the cauda equina does not differ significantly from that of more rostral compression, compression of the cauda equina is still generally referred to by the slightly inaccurate name of ESCC.

Spinal cord compression resulting from malignancy usually occurs in patients with incurable disease and is responsible for serious morbidity. Indeed, treatment success is usually measured by whether a patient remains ambulatory and continent. The diagnosis of spinal cord compression must be anticipated: Once neurologic dysfunction develops, it is rarely reversible.

Most often, spinal cord compression arises from a metastasis that involves the vertebral body and extends to produce an anterior epidural cord compression. Hematologic neoplasms, however, such as lymphoma and myeloma, may produce epidural cord compression by direct extension from a paravertebral mass without bone involvement. The thoracic spine represents the most common site of cord compression, and the lesions are often multiple.

### Etiology

The most common tumors responsible include:

- Lung cancer
- Breast cancer
- Prostate cancer
- Myeloma
- Lymphoma

The gastrointestinal tumors metastasize to bone less frequently and are therefore relatively less likely to cause this syndrome.

### Pathophysiology

The pathophysiology of spinal cord compression is shown in Figure 19.1.

### Clinical Picture

The symptomatic hallmark of spinal cord compression is back pain. Although a common symptom, its presence in association with known spinal metastases mandates further evaluation. The presence of a symptomatic radiculopathy or myelopathy in a patient with malignancy is also a clear indication for further evaluation. Although epidural

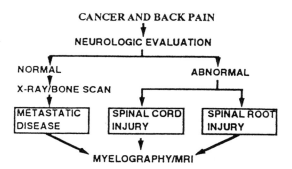

**Figure 19.1** Cancer and back pain neurologic evaluation. MRI, magnetic resonance imaging.

cord compression is the most common cause of myelopathic symptomatology in a patient with malignancy, the following etiologies must also be considered:

- Intradural or intramedullary tumor
- Carcinomatous meningitis
- Radiation myolpathy
- Paraneoplastic syndrome

Diagnostic options include:

- Neurologic examination
- Plain films
- Bone scan
- Complete myelogram
- CT
- Magnetic resonance imaging (MRI); MRI with contrast is required if intramedullar tumor is suspected

The results of neurologic examination are often normal in these patients. If abnormal, however, the findings may be useful in localizing the level of cord disease. Either an MRI scan or complete myelography is required for diagnosis. Although most patients with spinal metastases and a radiculopathy or myelopathy will have evidence of epidural lesions, cord compression will also be found in a significant number of patients with spinal metastases and back pain alone.

### Treatment

Once myelopathic signs have developed, the treatment of spinal cord compression is imperfect. Nonambulatory patients rarely recover the ability to ambulate. When diagnosed early, however, the preservation of neurologic function is the rule. Steroids should be initiated, and radiation and surgical consultation should be obtained as soon as possible.

Corticosteroids appear to have a short-term benefit. Guidelines for their use include:

- Prevent secondary pathologic changes
- Dexamathasone 10 mg followed by 4 mg q 6h
- High-dose steroids may help for quick pain control

Radiation is indicated in most patients. Radiation can shrink the tumor within days.

Recently, a randomized study indicated that surgery might be more effective than radiation therapy, resulting in more ambulatory patients at the end of treatment. Surgical decompression is especially indicated in the following situations:

- No histologic diagnosis.
- Rapid development of neurologic dysfunction
- Progression occurs during radiation therapy.
- Recurrence develops after completion of radiation therapy.
- Spinal instability is present.
- Retropulsion of bony fragment

Chemotherapy may be indicated in chemo-sensitive disease, particularly in children. Chemotherapy can be used in combination with radiotherapy for the treatment of spinal cord compression, or alone in adults who are not surgical or radiation candidates, but who have chemo-sensitive tumors, such as lymphoma, small cell carcinoma, myeloma, and germ cell tumors.

In general, the key to a successful outcome in this neurologic emergency is early diagnosis, although a patient's overall prognosis is more dependent on the natural history of the malignancy. The preservation of neurologic function is of obvious importance in this group of patients.

## BONE METASTASES

Bone metastases may develop in up to 50% of patients with malignancy, and 5% to 10% of patients with bone metastases develop pathologic long-bone fractures. The most frequent primary tumors metastasizing to bone are:

- Breast cancer
- Prostate cancer
- Lung cancer
- Multiple myeloma (almost invariably involves bone)
- Kidney cancer
- Malignancies of gastrointestinal origin

Marrow-containing bone, such as the vertebral bodies, pelvis, ribs, and femurs, are the most common sites of bone involvement.

Pain is the most common manifestation of bone metastases and is found in up to 75% of patients. Asymptomatic bone disease may be found during staging procedures or at another unsuspected site during an evaluation for bone pain.

Radionuclide bone scans are sensitive in the detection of bone metastases but are relatively nonspecific. Patients with purely lytic bone disease, however, as in multiple myeloma, may have normal bone scans. Plain radiographs, although considerably less sensitive, are quite specific. Radiographic abnormalities have been described as purely lytic (myeloma, kidney, or thyroid), predomi-

nantly blastic (prostate), or mixed lytic and blastic (breast and lung). CT and MRI scans may be useful for specific indications, particularly in better defining disease of the spine and pelvis.

Biopsy confirmation of a bone metastasis may be required if the abnormality represents the first sign of tumor recurrence or in the presence of a single or otherwise unusual bone abnormality. Multiple bone lesions, in the setting of widely disseminated disease, do not require histologic verification.

The treatment of bone metastases is considered palliative. Treatment goals include relief of pain and preservation of function.

Surgery is usually required for the adequate repair of a pathologic fracture and is often recommended for those patients with radiographic evidence of an impending fracture. The indications for prophylactic surgical intervention, particularly involving a weight-bearing bone (e.g., the femur), include a lytic bone lesion with a diameter of greater than 2 to 3 cm or with more than 50% cortical destruction.

Radiation therapy will relieve pain in up to 90% of patients and may prevent progression of bone destruction or even allow for healing. Its value is limited, however, in patients with widespread bone involvement.

Hormonal therapy in patients with breast and prostate cancer, chemotherapy in patients with breast and prostate cancer, and chemotherapy in patients with hematologic neoplasms and other chemotherapy-sensitive diseases are often effective in achieving temporary control. Recent studies have demonstrated the efficacy of intravenous bisphosphonates in reducing skeletal complications in patients with both multiple myeloma and metastatic breast cancer to bone.

In widespread disease with multiple sites of painful bone involvement, hemibody radiation or the systemic administration of radioisotopes has been used.

## MALIGNANT EFFUSIONS

### Pleural Effusions

Malignant pleural effusions may develop in one of two ways:

- Direct deposition of tumor metastases on the pleural surface, with a resultant exudation of pleural fluid
- Tumor involvement of mediastinal lymph nodes, producing lymphatic obstruction and pleural fluid accumulation

The second mechanism has been described in some patients with lymphoma and lung cancer.

The most common diagnoses in patients with malignant pleural effusions include:

- Breast cancer
- Lung cancer
- Lymphoma

- Ovarian cancer
- Adenocarcinoma of unknown primary site

Although the effusion may be asymptomatic in up to 25% of patients, the clinical presentation includes dyspnea, cough, and chest pain.

Patients may have a preexisting malignancy or may present with a malignant effusion as the first manifestation of disease. An accurate diagnostic confirmation and differentiation from a benign pleural effusion are of obvious prognostic and therapeutic importance.

A thoracentesis with pleural fluid cytology is often the easiest diagnostic maneuver. Biochemical analysis of the pleural fluid may be suggestive but is nonspecific. A closed pleural biopsy may add to the diagnostic yield. Thoracoscopy has recently emerged as an excellent diagnostic tool for pleural effusions. If neoplastic, appropriate treatment is often possible at the time of thoracoscopy as well. It is important to recognize the diagnostic difficulty posed by patients with mesothelioma. Cytology and needle biopsy are often nondiagnostic or confusing in such patients, and thoracoscopy, or even thoracotomy, are usually needed.

Treatment strategies include:

- Thoracentesis
- Pleural sclerosis
- Pleurectomy
- Pleuroperitoneal shunts
- Radiation therapy
- Systemic chemotherapy/hormones

Patients with malignant pleural effusions are usually incurable, and their management strategy should be palliative. Thoracentesis alone is of only temporary benefit unless effective systemic treatment is available, such as in lymphoma or breast cancer. Patients with non-small cell lung cancer will usually require chest tube drainage and pleural sclerosis if permanent control of the effusion is to be expected. The intralpleural instillation of agents such as doxycycline, talc, quinacrine, bleomycin, and various other chemotherapeutic agents has been associated with a successful outcome in 70% to 85% of patients. Those patients with continued fluid reaccumulation despite pleural sclerosis may require pleurectomy or the use of a pleuroperitoneal shunt. Radiation therapy is unfortunately of limited value, except when administered to the mediastinum in patients with extensive mediastinal lymphoma.

### Malignant Pericardial Effusions

Cardiac involvement by malignancy is often an asymptomatic autopsy finding and has been reported in 10% to 15% of patients with malignancy. It is clinically important only if it results in cardiac dysfunction, the most common manifestation being pericardial tamponade. This complication is not usually the first manifestation of malignancy and has been reported most frequently in patients with the following diseases:

- Lung cancer
- Breast cancer
- Leukemia/lymphoma
- Melanoma
- Sarcoma

The etiology may reflect either direct extension from mediastinal tumor (as in lymphoma and lung cancer) or hematogenous dissemination. Despite the dramatic presentation of patients with pericardial tamponade, several of the responsible malignancies are potentially curable, even when involving the heart. As such, an aggressive approach to diagnosis and management is imperative. It is also important that malignant pericarditis be distinguished from both the acute and chronic pericarditis occurring after radiation therapy and from the cardiomyopathy that can result from anthracycline use.

The presence of clinical signs or symptoms suggestive of pericarditis or pericardial tamponade mandates urgent evaluation. Diagnostic options include echocardiography, pericardiocentesis, and pericardial biopsy. Echocardiography is usually diagnostic and can be followed rapidly by a diagnostic/therapeutic pericardiocentesis. Cytologic examination may be positive in 80% of patients with neoplastic involvement. In those patients with lymphoma, however, especially after radiation therapy, pericardial biopsy may be needed for diagnosis.

Treatment strategies include:

- Closed drainage/intrapericardial sclerosis
- Pleuropericardial window/subxiphoid pericardiotomy
- Pericardiectomy
- Radiation therapy
- Systemic chemotherapy

Multiple treatment options have been described. Closed pericardial drainage alone or drainage with intrapericardial sclerosis using doxycycline, talc, or any of several chemotherapeutic agents has proved remarkably effective and often represents the procedure of first choice. If unsuccessful, or if the diagnosis is uncertain, a surgical approach using either a pleuropericardial window or a subxiphoid pericardiotomy has been recommended. Patients with radiosensitive tumors can often be effectively treated using mediastinal radiation therapy. Systemic chemotherapy is appropriate in those patients with sensitive diseases.

## MALIGNANT ASCITES

The development of ascites in any patient requires a vigorous evaluation for etiology. Ascites is considered malignant if it arises from the metastatic deposition of tumor on peritoneal surfaces with the resultant exudation of fluid. Ascites may develop in a patient with malignancy from a number of other causes, however, including:

- Hepatic failure due to tumor replacement
- Chemotherapy toxicity

- Myocardial or pericardial disease
- Vena, caval, or hepatic venous obstruction
- Infection

The therapeutic approach taken obviously depends on the etiology of the ascites.

In patients with ovarian or gastrointestinal cancer, malignant ascites may be either the presenting manifestation of the disease or an end-stage complication. In other tumors, such as breast cancer or lymphoma, malignant ascites usually reflects the progression of an established malignancy.

The diagnostic evaluation includes paracentesis with cultures and cytologic analysis. Abdominal CT scan or ultrasonography is often needed to define the presence of any hepatic abnormality. Rarely, an open peritoneal biopsy may be required.

Therapeutic options in patients with cytologically positive malignant ascites have been limited and relatively unsuccessful:

- Medical management
- Paracentesis
- Intracavitary radiocolloids
- Intraperitoneal chemotherapy
- Systemic chemotherapy
- Peritoneovenous shunts

Unlike patients with malignant pleural or pericardial effusions, palliation is difficult. Medical management, including diuresis and salt restriction, has provided only marginal benefit. Repeated paracentesis is an unsatisfactory solution; it is inconvenient for patients and results in significant protein loss and the risk of infection. The intracavitary administration of radioactive colloids has been attempted in the past with mixed results. Intracavitary sclerosing agents, such as those used for pleural effusions, make little theoretical sense and generally are not beneficial.

Some interest has arisen in the use of intraperitoneal chemotherapy, particularly in neoplasms such as ovarian cancer. Drug penetration is limited, however, and in the presence of bulky, intraperitoneal tumor, this intervention has not been very successful. In patients with breast cancer, ovarian cancer, or lymphoma, systemic chemotherapy may be effective and is indicated.

For those patients with refractory ascites, unresponsive to other measures, peritoneovenous shunting has been moderately effective. Generally, such patients have limited life expectancy and achieve significant palliative benefit from this procedure. Although shunt occlusion is frequent, the development of carcinomatosis or of a coagulopathy has not been common.

## TUMOR LYSIS SYNDROME

Acute tumor lysis syndrome occurs as a result of the release of intracellular contents into the blood stream.

Findings include:

- Hyperphosphatemia
- Hypocalcemia (due to precipitation of calcium phosphate)
- Hyperuricemia
- Hyperkalemia
- Acute renal failure

LDH level is used as a marker for the degree of tumor lysis.

### Etiology

The tumors most frequently associated with the tumor lysis syndrome are the poorly differentiated lymphomas, such as Burkitt's lymphoma, and the leukemias, particularly acute lymphoblastic leukemia and less often acute myeloid leukemia.

Post-treatment tumor lysis syndrome has also been described in patients with multiple myeloma, breast cancer, medulloblastoma, sarcomas, ovarian cancer, squamous cell carcinoma of the vulva, and small cell lung cancer.

Most affected patients receive combination chemotherapy, but steroids alone may be sufficient in patients with lymphoma and lymphoblastic leukemia.

### Pathogenesis

#### Prior to Initiation of Therapy
Spontaneous acute renal failure prior to therapy is may occur and is usually due to *acute uric acid nephropathy*. These patients have increased uric acid production and hyperuricosuria due to the high rate of tumor cell turnover.

#### After Initiation of Therapy
The use of allopurinol before the onset of antitumor therapy has reduced, but not eliminated, the incidence of acute uric acid nephropathy. Acute renal failure following therapy is now more frequently associated with severe *hyperphosphatemia*. Calcium phosphate deposition in the renal parenchyma and vessels may contribute to the decline in renal function in this setting. In rare cases, acute renal failure is induced by xanthinuria because high-dose allopurinol prevents the metabolism of xanthine to uric acid.

An important distinction between spontaneous tumor lysis and that occurring after therapy is the lack of hyperphosphatemia in the spontaneous form. It has been postulated that rapidly growing neoplasms with high cell turnover rates can lead to high uric acid levels through rapid nucleoprotein turnover but that the tumor is able to reutilize released phosphorus for resynthesis of new tumor cells. In contrast, the acute increase in uric acid levels associated with chemotherapy is due to cell destruction; in this setting, no new cancer cells are available to reutilize the large amounts of released phosphorus.

## Management

Effective management of the tumor lysis syndrome is a combination of prophylaxis, prevention, and appropriate dialytic treatment.

## Prophylaxis

Prophylaxis should start at least 2 days before receiving chemotherapy or radiation for a malignancy with rapid cell turnover. Drugs of choice include:

- Allopurinol, orally 600 to 900 mg/day. For those unable to receive oral medications, intravenous allopurinol could be used.
- Fluids. Intravenous hydration should be given to maintain a high urine output (greater than 2.5 L/day).
- Alkalinization of urine. The role of urinary alkalinization with acetazolamide and sodium bicarbonate is less clear. Alkalinization converts uric acid to the more soluble urate salt, thereby diminishing the tendency to uric acid precipitation. Experimental studies, however, suggest that hydration with saline alone is as effective as alkalinization in minimizing uric acid precipitation. Furthermore, alkalinization has the potential disadvantage of promoting calcium phosphate deposition in patients with marked hyperphosphatemia and is therefore not recommended.

## Treatment

### Acute Uric Acid Nephropathy Prior to Chemotherapy

Therapy after the onset of acute renal failure consists of:

- Allopurinol (if it has not already been given)
- Fluids and a loop diuretic in an attempt to wash out the obstructing uric acid crystals
- Sodium bicarbonate should not be given at this time because it is difficult to raise the urine pH in this setting
- Hemodialysis to remove the excess circulating uric acid should be used in those patients in whom a diuresis cannot be induced

The prognosis for complete recovery is excellent if treatment is initiated rapidly. Studies have shown that oliguria due to acute uric acid nephropathy responds rapidly to hemodialysis with the initiation of a diuresis as the plasma uric acid level falls to 10 mg/dL.

### Acute Renal Failure Following Chemotherapy

Marked hyperphosphatemia is usually the precipitating factor in this setting. The rapid recovery of renal function in the oligouric patient requires normalization of phosphorus (and uric acid) levels. The phosphate burden in these patients can vary from 2 to 7 grams per day; as a result, it is frequently necessary to perform hemodialysis at 12- to 24-hour intervals. Continuous arteriovenous hemo-

dialysis (CAVHD) with a high dialysate flow rate and continuous venovenous hemofiltration may also be effective. Phosphorus clearance using CAVHD can reach 40 mL/min at a dialysate flow rate of 4 L/hr. This can lead to the removal of up to 10 grams of phosphorus per day without the rebound hyperphosphatemia often seen after intermittent hemodialysis.

# HYPERCALCEMIA OF MALIGNANCY

Hypercalcemia is the most common life-threatening metabolic disorder in patients with cancer.

## Pathophysiology

The pathophysiologic characteristics of hypercalcemia in the setting of cancer are:

- PTH-related protein (PTHrp): most common
- Vit D3
- Cytokines: TGF$\alpha$, $\beta$, TNF, IL6
- Ostelytic bone lesions

### Treatment

The treatment of hypercalcemia of malignancy follows the same guidelines as hypercalcemia of other causes. Adequate intravenous hydration is mandatory to avert declining renal function and the reabsorption of calcium. Bisphosphonates play an important role in the treatment of hypercalcemia of malignancy.

# REVIEW EXERCISES

**1.** A 55-year-old woman smoker is seen in the emergency room complaining of several days of increasing facial fullness, orthopnea, and swelling in her neck and hands. Physical examination is notable for obvious facial swelling, with conjunctival edema, jugular venous distention, and symmetrical swelling of both upper extremities. Fullness is present in both supraclavicular fosse, but there is no clear lymph node enlargement and the lungs are clear. The patient is tachycardic, but no gallop, murmur, or rub is present. No hepatomegaly, ascites, or pedal edema is present. Chest radiography reveals a right hilar mass.

The patient is admitted to the hospital at midnight, and you order which of the following?
a) An emergency upper extremity venogram
b) An emergency CT scan of the chest
c) An emergency echocardiogram
d) Diuretics and elevation of the head of the bed until the morning

**2.** The next morning, the patient feels better, although she remains quite edematous and cannot lie flat. You order the following test to determine the etiology of the patient's superior vena cava syndrome:

a) CT scan of the chest
b) Thyroid scan
c) Serologic test for syphilis
d) Upper extremity venogram
e) All of the above

**3.** You are called by the radiologist that afternoon with the results of the chest CT scan. This study reveals a large right hilar and mediastinal mass, with evidence of compression of the superior vena cava. Your response is which of the following?

a) Expeditiously proceed to bronchoscope or mediastinoscopy to establish the tissue diagnosis
b) Recognize the risk of invasive diagnostic procedures in patients with superior vena cava syndrome and order sputum cytology
c) Identify this as an incurable malignancy and refer the patient for urgent radiation therapy
d) Identify this as an incurable malignancy and refer the patient for hospice care

**4.** The patient proves to have squamous cell carcinoma of the lung and receives a course of mediastinal radiation therapy. The patient does quite well, noting rapid improvement in both the symptoms and signs of her superior vena cava obstruction. A staging workup subsequently demonstrates evidence of asymptomatic bone metastases in rib, femur, and multiple vertebral bodies. Because the patient is feeling well, she declines any discussion of chemotherapy and is followed in your office. Four months later, the patient calls you with the complaint of a 2-week history of increasing midback pain. The patient is fully ambulatory, but the pain is causing difficulty sleeping. The patient specifically denies any weakness in the lower extremities, radicular pain, or incontinence. You would do which of the following?

a) Suggest a course of acetaminophen with codeine
b) Order an elective bone scan
c) Refer the patient for radiation therapy to the spine
d) Order an MRI of the entire spine

**5.** Your patient has heard about MRI scans and does not want one. Angry that you suggested it, the patient cancels her appointment and begins to take her husband's analgesics. Three days later, you call the patient and are told by her husband that she has fallen several times and is now having difficulty walking. You insist that the patient come to the hospital and obtain an emergent MRI scan, which she then does. The MRI reveals extensive midthoracic vertebral body replacement by tumor, with evidence of spinal cord compression. By the time the patient gets to the hospital, she is unable to walk and has had a single episode of urinary incontinence. You begin high-dose corticosteroids, hospitalize the patient, and recommend which of the following?

a) Immediate neurosurgical intervention
b) Intravenous morphine and hospice referral
c) Immediate radiation therapy

**6.** The patient is treated with radiation therapy and, somewhat to your surprise, makes a significant recovery. The patient regains almost full leg strength and can ambulate with minimal assistance. Physical therapy has been started, but during treatment new discomfort is noted in the patient's right hip. You order plain films that reveal a large lytic lesion of the right hip with cortical involvement but no fracture. In consideration of the patient's deteriorating medical condition, limited ambulatory ability, and life expectancy, you recommend which of the following?

a) Pain medication with continued physical therapy and partial weight bearing
b) Pain medication, physical therapy with partial weight bearing, and radiation therapy to the affected hip
c) Surgical stabilization of the right hip with pain medication and subsequent physical therapy

**7.** Your patient elects to not have surgery but undergoes the radiation and physical therapy with some success. The patient has limited ambulation but is managing at home with a walker. Over the next 6 weeks, the patient gradually improves but then returns to see you in the office, concerned about increasing exertional dyspnea. On examination the patient is afebrile, has a resting tachycardia, but has no facial swelling and no jugular venous distention. No pleural or pericardial rub is present, although diminished breath sounds are noted at the right base. Hepatomegaly ascites and pedal edema are not identified. Hemoglobin is 11.2 g/dL, and chest radiography reveals a new, large, right pleural effusion. The most likely diagnosis is which of the following?

a) Malignant pleural effusion
b) Radiation-induced pleuritis
c) Congestive heart failure
d) Radiation-induced pericardial constriction
e) Pulmonary embolus with infarction

**8.** In the office, you perform a 1-L thoracentesis for slightly bloody fluid, which on analysis proves exudative. Cultures are negative, and cytologies are not diagnostic. The patient feels immediately better after the thoracentesis but is back in the office 3 days later with increasing dyspnea and recurrence of this effusion. Your next step is which of the following?

a) Repeat the thoracentesis with cytology.
b) Repeat the thoracentesis with cytology and perform a closed pleural biopsy.

c) Refer the patient for thoracoscopy.

d) Refer the patient for chest tube drainage and pleural sclerosis.

**9.** In patients with spinal cord compression, which of the following is the best predictor of posttreatment neurologic function?

a) Level of cord compression

b) Degree of cord compression on MRI scans

c) Duration of neurologic symptoms prior to treatment

d) Pretreatment neurologic function

**10.** Tumor lysis syndrome is associated with all the following, *except:*

a) Hypercalcemia

b) Hyperkalemia

c) Hyperphosphatemia

d) Hyperuricemia

## ANSWERS

### 1. d.

The clinical diagnosis of superior vena cava syndrome is clear. Although the presentation is dramatic, it is not life threatening, and the initial management is symptomatic. Emergency diagnostic procedures are rarely indicated.

### 2. a.

Malignancy is the most common cause of superior vena cava syndrome and is suggested by this patient's chest radiograph. Further anatomic definition of the process with a CT scan is in order.

### 3. a.

Invasive diagnostic procedures do not pose any increased risk in patients with superior vena cava syndrome. Although the etiology is likely to be malignant, several of the potential malignant diagnoses are curable with appropriate treatment, and this treatment may include chemotherapy. Aggressive and expeditious attempts to establish a histologic diagnosis are indicated so that the most effective treatment can be initiated in an organized fashion.

### 4. d.

Spinal metastases have already been demonstrated in this patient. The new development of pain suggests the possibility of spinal cord compression and mandates the performance of a whole-spine MRI.

### 5. a or c.

Both surgery and radiation may be utilized in this situation. Surgery is particularly indicated in patients in whom the neurologic weakness develops more acutely (within hours), when histologic diagnosis is not established, there is a failure of radiation, or compression occurs secondary to retropulsion of a bone fragment.

### 6. b or c.

Specific treatment of painful bone disease is almost always indicated. Decisions about the best specific treatment (i.e., radiation therapy or surgery) must consider all facets of the patient's medical condition and disease extent.

### 7. a.

Although all these answers are in the differential diagnosis, the absence of a pleural or pericardial rub makes a malignant pleural effusion most likely.

### 8. d.

In a patient this sick, it may be most prudent to forego further aggressive attempts to confirm the likely diagnosis of a malignant pleural effusion and to proceed directly to appropriate management.

### 9. d.

Pretreatment neurologic function is the best predictor of posttreatment function, hence the importance of early diagnosis and management.

### 10. a.

Tumor lysis syndrome is associated with decreased serum calcium.

## SUGGESTED READINGS

Adelstein DJ. Managing three common oncologic emergencies. *Cleve Clin J Med* 1991;58:457–458.

Adelstein DJ, Hines JD, Carter SG, et al. Thromboembolic events in patients with malignant superior vena cava syndrome and the role of anticoagulation. *Cancer* 1988;62:2258–2262.

Aelony Y, King R, Boutin C. Thoracoscopic talc poudrage pleurodesis for chronic recurrent pleural effusions. *Ann Intern Med* 1991;115: 778–782.

Ahmann FR. A reassessment of the clinical implications of the superior vena cava syndrome. *J Clin Oncol* 1984;2:961–969.

Alcan KE, Zabetakis PM, Marino ND, et al. Management of acute cardiac tamponade by subxiphoid pericardiotomy. *JAMA* 1982;247: 1143–1148.

Berenson JR, Lipton A. Use of bisphosphonates in patients with metastatic bone disease. *Oncology* 1988;12:1573–1579.

Byrne TN. Spinal cord compression from epidural metastases. *N Engl J Med* 1992;327:614–619.

Coleman RE. Skeletal complications of malignancy. *Cancer* 1997;80 [Suppl]:1588–1594.

Daw HA, Markman M. Epidural spinal cord compression in cancer patients: diagnosis and management. *Clev Clin J Med* 2000;67: 497–504.

Gilbert RW, Kim JH, Posner JB. Epidural spinal cord compression from metastatic tumor: diagnosis and treatment. *Ann Neurol* 1978; 3:40–51.

Glover DJ, Glick JH. Managing oncologic emergencies involving structural dysfunction. *CA Cancer J Clin* 1985;35:238–251.

Gough IR, Balderson GA. Malignant ascites. A comparison of peritoneovenous shunting and nonoperative management. *Cancer* 1993;71:2377–2382.

Hausheer FH, Yarbro JW. Diagnosis and treatment of malignant pleural effusion. *Semin Oncol* 1985;12:54–75.

Helms SR, Carlson MD. Cardiovascular emergencies. *Semin Oncol* 1989;16:463–470.

Hillner BE, Ingle JN, Berenson JR, et al. American Society of Clinical Oncology guideline on the role of bisphosphonates in breast cancer. *J Clin Oncol* 2000;18:1378–1391.

Lacy JH, Wieman TJ, Shively EH. Management of malignant ascites. *Surg Gynecol Obstet* 1984;159:397–412.

Loblaw DA, Laperriere NJ. Emergency treatment of malignant extradural spinal cord compression: an evidence-based guideline. *J Clin Oncol* 1998;16:1613–1624.

Maranzano, Latini P, Checcaglini F, et al. Radiation therapy in metastatic spinal cord compression. *Cancer* 1991; 67:1311–1317.

Markman M. Common complications and emergencies associated with cancer and its therapy. *Clev Clin J Med* 1994;61:105–114.

Nielson OS, Munro AJ, Tannock IF. Bone metastases: pathophysiology and management policy. *J Clin Oncol* 1991;9:509–524.

Okamoto H, Shinkai T, Tamakido M, et al. Cardiac tamponade caused by primary lung cancer and the management of pericardial effusion. *Cancer* 1993;71:93–98.

Posner MR, Cohen GI, Skarin AT. Pericardial disease in patients with cancer: the differentiation of malignant from idiopathic and radiation-induced pericarditis. *Am J Med* 1981;71:407–413.

Press OW, Livingston R. Management of malignant pericardial effusion and tamponade. *JAMA* 1987;257:1088–1092.

Rodichok LD, Harper GR, Ruckdeschel JC, et al. Early diagnosis of spinal epidural metastases. *Am J Med* 1981;70:1181–1188.

Ruckdeschel JC, Moores D, Lee JY, et al. Intrapleural therapy for malignant pleural effusions: a randomized comparison of bleomycinand tetracycline. *Chest* 1991;100:1528–1535.

Sahn MA. Malignant pleural effusions. *Clin Chest Med* 1985;6: 113–125.

Schiff D, O'Neill BP, Wang CH, et al. Neuroimaging and treatment implications of patients with multiple epidural spinal metastases. *Cancer* 1998;83:1593–1601.

Schraufnagel DE, Hill R, Leech JA, et al. Superior vena caval obstruction—is it a medical emergency? *Am J Med* 1981;70:1169–1174.

Spiess JL, Adelstein DJ, Hines JD. Multiple myeloma presenting with spinal cord compression. *Oncology* 1988;45:88–92.

Tong D, Gillick L, Hendrickson FR. The palliation of symptomatic osseous metastasis. Final results of the study by the Radiation Therapy Oncology Group. *Cancer* 1982;50:893–899.

Tsang TSM, Seward JB, Barnes ME, et al. Outcomes of primary and secondary treatment of pericardial effusion in patients with malignancy. *Mayo Clin Proc* 2000;75:248–253.

Weissman DE. Glucocorticoid treatment for brain metastases and epidural spinal cord compression: a review. *J Clin Oncol* 1988;6: 543–551.

Willson JKV, Masaryk TJ. Neurologic emergencies in the cancer patient. *Semin Oncol* 1989;16:490–503.

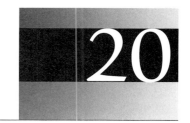

# Gynecologic, Prostate, and Testicular Cancers

*David Peereboom    Maurie Markman*

## GYNECOLOGIC CANCERS

### Cancer of the Cervix

It is interesting that at one time carcinoma of the cervix was the most common cause of cancer death in women. The mortality from this malignancy has decreased more than 50% over the past 30 years, largely due to the widespread use of the Papanicolaou (Pap) smear in routine gynecologic medicine, internal medicine, and family practice.

Several etiologic factors are associated with carcinoma of the cervix, including early initial sexual activity, multiple sexual partners, and prior venereal infections. Experimental and epidemiologic data have provided strong evidence that infection with the human papillomavirus, particularly subtypes 16 and 18, is important in the pathogenesis of this malignancy. More recently, it has been shown that individuals with acquired immunodeficiency syndrome (AIDS) have a high risk for the development of carcinoma of the cervix.

The development of cervix cancer proceeds along a well-defined pathway, from dysplasia to carcinoma in situ (cytologic features of neoplasia, but without an invasion through the basement membrane) to invasive carcinoma. The Pap smear is 90% to 95% accurate in detecting early intraepithelial neoplastic changes. False-negative smear results can be observed in the presence of inflammation, necrosis, or hemorrhage, so all areas observed to be abnormal on visual inspection must be examined via biopsy, regardless of the Pap smear findings.

Standard treatment of carcinoma in situ of the cervix is surgery (total abdominal hysterectomy). Young women wanting to have children may be treated with cervical conization and extremely careful follow-up. More locally advanced cases of carcinoma of the cervix are treated with surgery, radiation therapy, or a combination of the two modalities. Chemotherapy is used mainly in patients with far advanced and metastatic disease. Although responses are observed and may modestly influence survival, they are generally of short duration (less than 4 to 6 months). Of far greater impact are results reported from several randomized trials, which have demonstrated that the use of cisplatin-based chemotherapy in combination with external beam radiation therapy significantly improves overall survival in women with locally advanced cervix cancer.

The importance of finding cancerous changes as soon as possible in the natural history of this disease is highlighted by the fact that the long-term survival for individuals who are diagnosed as having carcinoma in situ is more than 98% to 99%. The survival rate for invasive carcinoma is much less. For patients with advanced cervix cancer, the chances for long-term, disease-free survival are limited.

## Endometrial Cancer

Uterine cancer is the most common gynecologic cancer, causing approximately 9% of all malignancies in women. The incidence of the disease is approximately three times higher than that of cervix cancer. Suggested risk factors include:

- Age
- Late menopause
- Obesity
- Diabetes
- Hypertension

Unopposed exogenous estrogen use has been shown to increase the incidence of endometrial cancer. In contrast, the risk of the disease appears to be decreased by the administration of progesterone. Thus, the use of combination estrogen and progesterone may decrease the risk of endometrial cancer in women receiving this regimen.

The Pap smear identifies approximately 15% to 20% of women with endometrial carcinoma. In most patients, the diagnosis is made through a more extensive evaluation of evacuated tissue after a fractional dilatation and curettage, or direct biopsy. The most common symptom of endometrial cancer is abnormal bleeding in postmenopausal woman.

Endometrial cancer is generally diagnosed at an early stage, a point at which surgery with or without radiation therapy is curative. Hormonal therapy (most commonly employing a progestational agent) or chemotherapy is utilized in the setting of recurrent or metastatic disease.

Concern has been raised regarding the risk of endometrial cancer in individuals receiving tamoxifen, either as a treatment for breast cancer or as a preventive strategy for this malignancy. Women taking tamoxifen who experience any abnormal vaginal bleeding should undergo a careful gynecologic evaluation. Currently, no evidence suggests that a more rigorous screening program is required in this clinical setting. In addition, prophylactic hysterectomy is not recommended for women receiving tamoxifen.

## Ovarian Cancer

Although ovarian cancer is less common than either cancer of the cervix or uterus, it causes more deaths each year in the United States than both of the other gynecologic malignancies combined. Because currently no effective screening test for detecting early stage disease exists, fewer than 10% to 20% of patients are diagnosed with localized disease. Intensive research efforts have been undertaken at a number of centers to find a reliable screening test for ovarian cancer. These have focused on vaginal ultrasonography, circulating tumor antigens (e.g., CA-125), and most recently, proteomics. Whereas screening may be used in patients who have an increased risk for the development of ovarian cancer (i.e., strong family history), such a strategy should not be considered standard clinical practice in most clinical settings.

Although many etiologic factors have been proposed for the development of ovarian cancer (including disordered endocrine function), none has been strongly associated with the disease. It has been noted that approximately 5% of all women with ovarian cancer have a strong family history of the malignancy, suggesting the importance of genetic factors. In the rare circumstance in which a woman has two first-degree relatives with ovarian cancer, she has as much as a 50% chance of developing the malignancy during her lifetime. Two genetic abnormalities, *BRCA-1* and *BRCA-2*, have been demonstrated to be responsible for the large majority of cases of hereditary ovarian cancer. Recently published data suggest the prophylactic removal of the ovaries in women with these specific genetic findings may reduce the subsequent lifetime risk for the development of this malignancy.

Ovarian cancer tends to remain largely confined to the peritoneal cavity for most of its natural history. The disease can be quite widespread throughout the abdomen at the time of diagnosis, however.

In the unusual situation in which ovarian cancer is found to be confined to one ovary (stage 1), surgery without adjuvant chemotherapy can be a reasonable treatment option. Long-term survival in stage 1 ovarian cancer is more than 80% to 90%.

Several well-designed, randomized, controlled trials have revealed that the combination of a platinum agent (carboplatin or cisplatin) plus a taxane (paclitaxel or docetaxel) results in superior objective response rates, progression-free status, and overall survival, compared with nonplatinum, nontaxane regimens previously employed in the management of advanced ovarian cancer. Approximately 70% to 80% of patients experience objective and subjective evidence of a response to chemotherapy, and 50% are found to have no clinical evidence of disease at the completion of therapy. Unfortunately, the disease ultimately recurs in most of these individuals.

In women with persistent or recurrent ovarian cancer after initial chemotherapy, second-line chemotherapy regimens can be used. In view of the extended survival (often in excess of 5 years) for many patients, even with documented progression following primary therapy, it is appropriate to consider ovarian cancer a "chronic disease process," where *cure* is not the ultimate anticipated outcome, but where *prolonged survival of good or excellent quality* is a highly realistic goal of disease management.

## PROSTATE CANCER

Prostate cancer is the most common cancer in American men, comprising 30% of all cases of cancer in American men. The lifetime risk is 1 in 6. Patients aged 40 to 59 have a 1 in 55 chance of being diagnosed with prostate cancer, whereas men aged 60 to 79 have a 1 in 7 chance.

Subclinical prostate cancer is even more common than clinical disease, with 15% to 45% of autopsies in men without any known history of cancer during their life demonstrating the malignancy. This observation raises the important question of the clinical relevance of finding asymptomatic prostate cancer on screening tests in older men. Overall, prostate cancer is a slowly growing malignancy. Thus, simply finding microscopic cancer in an elderly individual should not necessarily be an indication to treat.

Most patients with newly diagnosed prostate cancer present with organ-confined disease as a result of positive screening test. The routes of spread once cancer has gone beyond the prostate are first to the pelvic lymph nodes and then to the bone and bone marrow. Other sites of involvement include the lung and liver.

The following are risk factors for prostate cancer:

- Age greater than 50 years old
- African American race
- Family history
- Twofold risk with one first-degree relative diagnosed with prostate cancer
- Ninefold risk with two first-degree relatives diagnosed with prostate cancer

Among the factors not proven to confer an increased risk are dietary fat and history of vasectomy.

Screening for prostate cancer involves the same goals as screening for any other disease: the detection of early disease in a patient who would suffer from or die of the disease and in whom treatment of early disease prevents mortality and morbidity. For high-risk patients, such as African Americans and patients with a family history (first-degree relatives) of prostate cancer, screening should start at age 40. For other patients, screening is recommended to start at age 50. Those patients who should not be screened include men with a life expectancy of less than 10 years.

The recommended screening technique requires both of the following:

- Serum PSA
- Digital rectal exam (DRE)

It is important to draw the PSA *before* performing a DRE. False elevations of PSAs can occur in the following circumstances:

- Benign prostatic hypertrophy
- Infection, specifically prostatitis
- Any inflammation or irritation of the prostate cancer (e.g., immediately following a digital rectal exam or a needle biopsy of the prostate)

The following represent indications for performing a prostate biopsy. For patients in screening, the following findings are indications for a prostate biopsy:

- Abnormal DRE. Abnormal DRE includes induration of the prostate, either unilaterally or bilaterally, or the finding of a nodule. An abnormal DRE regardless of the PSA requires a biopsy.
- Elevated PSA velocity. The PSA velocity is the rate of rise of the PSA. Any increase in PSA of $>0.75$ ng/mL per year has a $>90\%$ specificity for the detection of prostate cancer, and such patients should be biopsied.
- Elevated free-to-total PSA ratio. The free-to-total PSA can help to distinguish benign prostatic hypertrophy (BPH) from cancer. Men with BPH have a higher fraction of free or unbound PSA. Those with prostate cancer have more PSA bound to α-1 antichymotrypsin. A free-to-total PSA $<0.15$ warrants a prostate biopsy.

Currently, no role is apparent for a spiral computed tomography (CT) scan, positron emission tomography (PET) scan, or a prostate specific membrane antigen (PSMA) radioimmunoscintigraphy scan.

### *Summary on Screening*

African Americans and those with a positive family history should begin screening at age 40; other men should begin screening at age 50. The standard screening modality includes both a DRE and the measurement of a serum PSA; it should be performed in men with an abnormal DRE, elevations in PSA or PSA velocity, or a low free-to-total PSA.

The most common presenting symptom of prostate cancer is the absence of any symptoms, as most men are detected after screening. Patients with symptoms often present with obstructive voiding symptoms (nocturnal frequency, a slow urinary stream, hesitancy, dribbling, and frequent urinary tract infections). Additional symptoms include:

- Hematospermia or decreased ejaculatory volume due to seminal vesicle involvement
- Impotence due to neurovascular bundle invasion
- Pedal edema or lymphedema due to lymph node metastases
- Bone pain due to bone metastases
- Constitutional symptoms including malaise, anorexia, and weight loss

The physical examination for patients with prostate cancer includes abnormalities on the DRE, such as induration, nodules, and extension of disease to the seminal vesicles superiorly or to the pelvic sidewall laterally. It is important to remember that the DRE is commonly normal. Bony tenderness may occur in the vertebral column or the pelvic bones.

Treatment modalities for localized prostate cancer include:

- Radical prostatectomy
- Radiation therapy
- Brachytherapy (interstitial implantation of radioactive seeds)
- Radiation plus hormone therapy for patients with locally advanced disease (i.e., those with prostate cancer beyond the prostate but not having spread to lymph nodes or bone)

For patients with systemic prostate cancer, the mainstay of therapy is hormonal manipulation to block either the production or the action of testosterone. Methods of hormone therapy include:

- Orchiectomy
- LHRH agonists (goserelin, leuprolide)
- Nonsteroidal anti-androgens (bicalutamide, nilutamide, flutamide)

Hormone therapy has a number of side effects that can significantly impact on a patient's quality of life. These include:

- Hot flashes
- Gynecomastia
- Impotence
- Anemia
- Osteoporosis

Osteoporosis in particular is a side effect of long-term hormone therapy for which screening is appropriate, especially for those men who have additional risk factors for osteoporosis. Chemotherapy has an emerging role in the treatment of prostate cancer. Patients for whom chemotherapy is appropriate are men with a good performance status who have progressive disease despite the use of hormonal therapy. Large randomized trials have established docetaxel as the main chemotherapy agent for this patient population.

# TESTICULAR CANCER

Testicular cancer refers to any germ cell tumor that originates in the testicles. The more general term, *germ cell tumor*, can refer to the testicular primary but can also refer to an extragonadal germ cell tumor, such as a mediastinal germ cell tumor. Testis cancers are the most common solid tumor among men aged 15 through 35. Two age peaks occur: 20 to 40 years and over 60 years old. The classification of testicular cancer includes seminoma and nonseminoma (NSGCT). The latter includes embryonal, choriocarcinoma, teratoma, and mixed tumors.

Testicular cancer differs from almost all other cancers in several respects. First, testicular cancer is a cancer for which serum tumor markers ($\alpha$-fetoprotein, $\beta$-HCG, and LDH) are uniquely helpful. For example, an elevated $\alpha$-fetoprotein defines a testicular cancer as a nonseminoma—that is, this marker predicts histologic subtype. In addition, the rate of decline of markers during treatment has prognostic predictive value. Second, testicular cancer is routinely curable even when metastatic. Third, patients with residual or growing masses, usually teratomas, can be cured with surgical resection.

The risk factors for testicular cancer include:

- Cryptorchidism; confers a 20- to 40-fold risk
- Disgenetic gonads; for example, Klinefelter's syndrome (47-XXY) is associated with mediastinal germ cell tumors
- Prior contralateral testis cancer; confers a 500-fold risk of second testis cancer. These tumors occur most often at a median of 3 to 5 years following the primary case

For testicular cancer, no specific screening algorithm has been recommended by large public health groups. Conversely, men aged 15 and older should perform a testicular self-examination on a yearly basis. This recommendation, however, has not been tested in formal clinical trials.

Testicular cancer usually presents with a painless testicular enlargement or mass. A patient who presents with this symptom should undergo a testicular ultrasound to help differentiate a solid mass from a hydrocele or possibly a hernia. The diagnostic test of choice is an ipsilateral inguinal orchiectomy for any solid lesion. A transcrotal biopsy is contraindicated due to violation of tissue planes that may allow additional lymphatic routes of metastatic spread.

Patients may also present with signs or symptoms of metastatic disease. The most common sites of spread include the retroperitoneal lymph nodes, lungs, and mediastinum. Such lesions can present with an abdominal mass, shortness of breath or even hemoptysis. Less common sites of spread include bone, liver, and brain. For a patient with an undifferentiated cancer, the finding of an isochromosome 12P in the tumor tissue is diagnostic of a germ cell tumor.

Prognosis in testicular cancer depends on:

- Histology; seminoma tends to have a slightly better prognosis
- Primary site; mediastinal primary tumors carry a worse prognosis
- Nonpulmonary visceral metastases
- Degree of elevation of tumor markers

For early stage testicular cancer (involvement of the testicle alone), the treatment of choice for seminoma includes a radical orchiectomy plus radiation therapy to the pelvic and retroperitoneal lymph nodes. The radiotherapy eliminates any occult metastatic disease that may have spread to these lymph nodes. For nonseminoma, the treatment of choice includes radical orchiectomy plus a retroperitoneal lymph node dissection, assuming that the tumor markers normalize after the radical orchiectomy. If these patients still have elevated tumor markers, they should receive chemotherapy. Patients who undergo retroperitoneal lymph node dissection and are found to have cancer in those lymph nodes have a survival benefit with the administration of adjuvant chemotherapy. For advanced-stage testicular cancer (overt disease in the pelvic or retroperitoneal lymph nodes or distant metastases), chemotherapy is the initial treatment of choice.

Although chemotherapy confers a high cure rate for testicular cancer, patients live long enough to experience late toxicities. These toxicities are dose- and drug-related and include:

- Pulmonary fibrosis; most often related to bleomycin
- Acute leukemia; most often related to etoposide
- Oligospermia or azospermia
- Raynaud's phenomenon

Fatal toxicities occur in 1% to 5% of patients.

## REVIEW EXERCISES

### QUESTIONS

**1.** A 68-year-old woman is seen in your office for the first time. Which statement is correct concerning the risk of developing cervix cancer in this patient and the role of screening in this population?
**a)** The risk of developing cervix cancer is low and screening is not necessary.
**b)** The risk of developing cervix cancer is high, and the patient should be screened yearly at least until age 80.
**c)** The risk of developing cervix cancer is related to the patient's prior screening history.
**d)** The risk of developing cervix cancer is high, but screening is of no value in the elderly.
**e)** None of the above.

**2.** Which of the following statements concerning cancer of the cervix is incorrect?
**a)** Having a large number of sexual partners protects against the development of cervix cancer.
**b)** Carcinoma in situ is essentially 100% curable.
**c)** Cervix cancer has been associated with AIDS.
**d)** The treatment of metastatic cervix cancer is designed principally to palliate symptoms rather than to result in long-term disease-free control.
**e)** None of the above.

**3.** A 54-year-old female patient is started on estrogens because of significant postmenopausal symptoms. Due to the association between estrogens and endometrial cancer, this patient should

**a)** Undergo a hysterectomy
**b)** Undergo an endometrial biopsy at least every 3 to 4 months while on estrogen therapy
**c)** Never be given progesterone
**d)** Undergo a hysterectomy and bilateral oophorectomy
**e)** None of the above

**4.** A 42-year-old patient asks about screening for ovarian cancer. She has no symptoms suggestive of the disease, and the results of her physical examination are normal. You should
**a)** Ask about her family history of ovarian and breast cancers.
**b)** Strongly recommend yearly screening until at least age 70.
**c)** Recommend a CA-125 blood test and vaginal ultrasonography to be performed within the next 3 to 5 days.
**d)** Inform the patient that screening has proved to be of no value in this disease.
**e)** None of the above.

**5.** A 53-year-old patient is found to have advanced ovarian cancer. She asks for your recommendation regarding treatment. Which one of the following would be an inappropriate statement concerning possible treatment options?
**a)** Cisplatin or carboplatin plus Taxol is the standard chemotherapy treatment strategy in this clinical setting.
**b)** Assuming the patient can tolerate intensive therapy, very high dose chemotherapy with bone marrow transplantation has been proved to result in the best overall outcome in this disease.
**c)** Surgical tumor removal before starting chemotherapy is attempted in most patients with advanced ovarian cancer.
**d)** Approximately 80% of patients with advanced ovarian cancer achieve at least temporary improvement of symptoms after chemotherapy.
**e)** None of the above.

**6.** A 19-year-old patient has an advanced germ cell tumor of the ovary, which has spread to the omentum. All gross disease is removed at the time of surgery. Which one of the following statements concerning this tumor is correct?
**a)** Using cisplatin-based chemotherapy, this individual's chances of survival are between 10% and 20%.
**b)** The administration of chemotherapy will almost certainly result in sterility.
**c)** Compared with epithelial ovarian cancers, germ cell tumors of the ovary have a superior survival.
**d)** Dysgerminomas have the worst prognosis among the germ cell tumors of the ovary.
**e)** None of the above.

**7.** Which of the following is true regarding prostate cancer screening?
a) High-risk men should begin annual screening at age 50.
b) Proper screening includes a digital rectal exam followed by PSA measurement.
c) Spiral CT scan or PSMA radioimmunoscintigraphy scanning are alternative options for screening.
d) Men with a life expectancy less than 10 years should not be screened.

**8.** All of the following men should be referred for prostate biopsy *except*
a) A 47-year-old man with a PSA of 2.1 who feels well and has a firm area on the right lobe of the prostate.
b) An 84-year-old man with a PSA 6.8, free-to-total PSA = 0.25, nocturia for 15 years, and a diffusely enlarged prostate but no new symptoms.
c) A 65-year-old man with a PSA of 5.5, malaise, low-grade fever, dysuria with an enlarged and tender prostate.
d) A 61-year-old man with yearly PSAs of 2.2, 2.6, 2.9, 3.9 who feels well and has a normal prostate examination.
e) b
f) c
g) b and c

**9.** A 63-year-old man presents with a screening PSA of 6.7, no symptoms, and a nodule on the right lobe of the prostate. Transrectal ultrasound and biopsy confirms adenocarcinoma. Treatment options include all of the following, *except*
a) Radical prostatectomy
b) Orchiectomy
c) Radiation therapy, plus 2 years of hormone therapy
d) Radiation therapy (external beam or interstitial implantation of radioactive seeds)

**10.** A 67-year-old man, 4 years status postprostatectomy presents with low back pain and tenderness. His PSA is 85 and a bone scan is positive in multiple areas. The most appropriate treatment is
a) Orchiectomy
b) Radiation therapy to the prostate bed followed by orchiectomy
c) Chemotherapy with docetaxel
d) Bicalutamide (Casodex) followed by goserelin (Zolodex) subcutaneously every 3 months
e) a or d

**11.** Which of the following are side effects of hormone therapy for advanced prostate cancer?
a) Anemia
b) Osteoporosis
c) Impotence
d) All of the above
e) a and c

**12.** A 28-year-old baseball star presents with a painless left testicular mass. Physical exam is otherwise normal. α-Fetoprotein is greater than 400. The most appropriate next step is
a) Testicular ultrasound
b) Ultrasound-guided transcrotal testicular biopsy
c) Inguinal orchiectomy
d) A trial of antibiotics
e) Whole body PET scan

**13.** A 21-year-old man with stage III nonseminomatous germ cell tumor requires chemotherapy. Which of the following might you *not* expect as a late toxicity?
a) Pulmonary fibrosis
b) Biliary sclerosis
c) Azospermia
d) Acute leukemia
e) Raynaud's phenomenon

**14.** A 22-year-old man with testicular cancer comes back to your office 5 months after a radical inguinal orchiectomy and chemotherapy for nonseminomatous germ cell tumor. The patient feels well and has no complaints. His markers have normalized after treatment and remain normal. His markers (α-fetoprotein, β-HCG, and LDH) normalized with treatment and remain normal. A mass is palpated in the left mid-abdomen. This mass is most likely
a) A mature teratoma, best treated with surgical resection
b) Recurrent testicular cancer, best treated with high-dose chemotherapy and autologous stem cell rescue
c) Seminoma, best treated with radiation therapy
d) Chemotherapy-induced chloroma (solid tumor manifestation of acute leukemia), best treated with radiation and chemotherapy

## ANSWERS

**1. c.**
Women who have undergone appropriate Pap smear testing throughout their lives do not require continued testing beyond the age of 70. If testing has not been performed regularly, however, a significant risk of cervix cancer remains even beyond age 70. Such individuals should continue to undergo Pap smear testing for cervix cancer.

**2. a.**
One of the major risk factors for developing cervix cancer is a large number of sexual partners. This fact provides strong supportive evidence for the sexual transmission of an infectious agent that has an important role in the development of this malignancy.

**3. e.**
A specific recommendation for the follow-up of women receiving estrogen replacement as a result of

postmenopausal symptoms is not possible based on currently available data. No convincing evidence suggests, however, that surgery or routine endometrial biopsy is required in women receiving treatment with this agent.

**4. a.**

Currently, no evidence suggests that screening for ovarian cancer reduces mortality from this malignancy. For women with a strong family history of ovarian and breast cancer, however, it certainly can be argued that screening at least has the potential for detecting the disease at an earlier point in time when therapy may be more effective. A woman undergoing such screening must be informed of the limited data supporting this therapeutic strategy.

**5. b.**

The standard treatment for advanced ovarian cancer is surgical debulking, followed by a cisplatin or carboplatin, plus paclitaxel chemotherapy regimen. No evidence suggests that high-dose therapy does anything except increase the toxicity of treatment.

**6. c.**

The overall prognosis of germ cell tumors of the ovary is excellent, certainly compared with epithelial ovarian cancer.

**7. d.**

High-risk men (African Americans or men with a positive family history of prostate cancer) should begin annual screening at age 40; average-risk men should begin screening at age 50. Proper screening includes PSA measurement *before* performance of a digital rectal exam because the DRE can cause a false positive elevation of the PSA. Spiral CT scanning, PET scanning, or PSMA scanning have no established role in screening for prostate cancer. Men with an estimated life expectancy of <10 years do not benefit from screening, because many such patients have clinically unimportant disease (i.e., prostate cancer that will cause neither morbidity nor mortality in their remaining life span).

**8. g.**

The patient with a PSA of 2.1 (a) has an abnormal DRE. Any man in screening who has an abnormal DRE should be referred for a prostate biopsy. The 84-year-old man (b) most likely has benign prostatic hypertrophy, given the free-to-total PSA ratio of 0.25. Those men with a free-to-total PSA of <0.15 have a significantly higher risk of prostate cancer. This patient probably should not have been screened. The 65-year-old man with malaise, fever and dysuria, and a tender prostate gland (c) likely has prostatitis and should return to the office in 2 months for a repeat PSA once the infection has resolved. Therefore, this patient should also not be referred for a prostate biopsy. The 61-year-old man with the rising PSA

and a normal prostate exam (d) has a PSA velocity that exceeds 0.75 ng/mL per year during the last year of screening (PSA rising by 1.0 ng/mL), which puts this patient at high risk for prostate cancer despite the fact that his PSA remains in a normal range.

**9. b.**

Radical prostatectomy (a) and radiation therapy (d) are standard treatments for patients with localized disease. Radiation therapy with a defined duration (e.g., 2 years) or hormone therapy (c) is standard therapy for a patient with locally advanced disease (i.e., cancer that has spread outside the capsule of the prostate into the seminal vesicles). Orchiectomy (b) is an excellent option for systemic prostate cancer (i.e., cancer that has spread to lymph nodes or to bone). The alternative option for androgen ablation is LHRH agonists (e.g., leuprolide or goserelin). The patient in question likely still has organ-confined or locally advanced disease for which orchiectomy is not an appropriate initial therapy.

**10. e.**

Orchiectomy (a) or bicalutamide followed by goserelin (d) represent appropriate initial hormone therapy for patients with systemic disease from metastatic prostate cancer. Bicalutamide is given before goserelin for approximately 10 days to prevent the stimulation of prostate cancer growth that accompanies the transient surge in testosterone production that occurs shortly after the initiation of LHRH agonists (goserelin or leuprolide). The great majority of men have rapid systematic relief, with a radiographic response as well. Radiation to the prostate bed (b) has no role for a patient with metastatic cancer, and therefore, would be performed prior to orchiectomy. Chemotherapy (c) is appropriate for the patient whose disease progresses on hormone therapy.

**11. d.**

Anemia, osteoporosis, and impotence are important side effects of hormone therapy for prostate cancer. The anemia is usually mild and does not require therapy. Osteoporosis is a significant side effect, however, which can lead to compression fractures or fractures of long bones. Men on hormone therapy must be monitored for this complication, and appropriate therapy should be instituted early because these men frequently have multiple risk factors for osteoporosis. Impotence occurs essentially uniformly in men treated with either orchiectomy or LHRH agonists. Few of these men respond to therapy with phosphodiesterase type-5 inhibitors (e.g., sildenafil).

**12. a.**

Testicular ultrasound (a) is the initial diagnostic test of choice for any patient who presents with a testicular mass. Although one might argue that an α-fetoprotein with a level 400 in a young man with a testicular mass is essentially diagnostic of testicular cancer, an ultrasound is still an important first step followed by radical inguinal orchiectomy (c). A transcrotal testicular biopsy (b) is contraindicated due to the violation of tissue planes, which allows alternate lymphatic avenues of metastasis. A trial of antibiotics (d) is not warranted in a patient who has a painless left testicular mass and no testicular tenderness to suggest epididymitis or some other infectious etiology. A whole body PET scan (e) is not a staging procedure at the initial diagnosis of testicular cancer. CT scanning of the chest, abdomen, and pelvis is the standard staging work-up, but would not be pursued before a diagnosis has been confirmed.

### 13. b.

Curative chemotherapy for testicular cancer as well as for other malignancies can cause important late toxicities. Biliary sclerosis, however, is not a known late toxicity. Pulmonary fibrosis (a) occurs in a small fraction and a small percentage of patients treated with bleomycin, most of whom are asymptomatic. Approximately 1% of patients, however, has significant symptoms. Another subgroup of patients develops pulmonary nodules that can be mistaken for lung metastases. Oligospermia (c) commonly exists before the diagnosis of testicular cancer but certainly has a much higher prevalence after the administration of chemotherapy. Acute leukemia (d) is a well-known late sequela of several different types of chemotherapy. Patients with testicular carcinoma receive etoposide, which is one of the agents known to cause this complication. Raynaud's phenomenon (e) occurs in a small subset of patients as well.

### 14. a.

Mature teratoma (a) is a well-known phenomenon that can occur after the successful treatment of nonseminomas, particularly those that contain a component of teratoma. Such a mass is generally curable with surgical resection. Left untreated, these masses can degenerate into malignant teratomas that are not curable. Recurrent testicular cancer (b) can certainly occur but is an unusual phenomenon and, in the setting of tumor markers that remain normal, would be highly unlikely. Seminoma (c) would similarly be extremely unusual after chemotherapy for a nonseminoma. Chemotherapy-induced acute leukemia (d) is a well-described complication of chemotherapy but occurs with a latency of 2 to 9 years. In addition, a patient with acute leukemia and tumor bulk consisting of a chloroma would not generally be asymptomatic.

## SUGGESTED READINGS

### Gynecologic Cancers

Cannistra SA, Niloff JM. Cancer of the uterine cervix. *N Engl J Med* 1996;334:1030–1038.

Koss LG. The Papanicolaou test for cervical cancer detection: a triumph and a tragedy. *JAMA* 1989;261:737–743.

Markman M. Optimizing primary chemotherapy in ovarian cancer. *Hematol Oncol Clin North Am* 2003;17:957–968.

Morris M, Eifel PJ, Lu J, et al. Pelvic radiation with concurrent chemotherapy compared with pelvic and para-aortic radiation for high-risk cervical cancer. *N Engl J Med* 1999;340:1137–1143.

Rubin SC, Sutton GP, eds. *Ovarian Cancer*, 2nd ed. Philadelphia: Lippincott Williams & Wilkins, 2001.

Sirovich BE, Welch HG. Cervical cancer screening among women without a cervix. *JAMA* 2004;291:2990–2993.

### Prostate Cancer

Barry MJ. Clinical practice. Prostate-specific-antigen testing for early diagnosis of prostate cancer. *N Engl J Med* 2001;344(18):1373–1377.

Bolla M, Gonzalez D, Warde P, et al. Improved survival in patients with locally advanced prostate cancer treated with radiotherapy and goserelin. *N Engl J Med* 1997;337(5):295–300.

D'Amico AV, Chen MH, Roehl KA, Catalona WJ. Preoperative PSA velocity and the risk of death from prostate cancer after radical prostatectomy. *N Engl J Med* 2004;351(2):125–135.

Eisenberger M, Partin A. Progress toward identifying aggressive prostate cancer. *N Engl J Med* 2004;351:180–181.

Harris R, Lohr KN. Screening for prostate cancer: an update of the evidence for the U.S. Preventive Services Task Force. *Ann Intern Med* 2002;137(11):917–929.

Messing EM, Manola J, Sarosdy M, et al. Immediate hormonal therapy compared with observation after radical prostatectomy and pelvic lymphadenectomy in men with node-positive prostate cancer. *N Engl J Med* 1999;341(24):1781–1788.

Nelson WG, De Marzo AM, Isaacs WB. Prostate cancer. *N Engl J Med* 2003;349(4):366–381.

Oesterling JE. Age-specific reference ranges for serum PSA. *N Engl J Med* 1996;335(5):345–346.

Vaughn DJ. Hormonal therapy for advanced prostate cancer. *Ann Intern Med* 2000;132(7):584–585.

### Testicular Cancer

Bokemeyer C, Berger CC, Kuczyk MA, Schmoll HJ. Evaluation of long-term toxicity after chemotherapy for testicular cancer. *J Clin Oncol* 1996;14:2923.

Bosl GJ, Motzer RJ. Testicular germ-cell cancer. *N Engl J Med* 1997;337(4):242–253.

IGCCC. International Germ Cell Consensus classification: a prognostic factor-based staging system for metastatic germ cell cancers. *J Clin Oncol* 1997;15:594.

Motzer RJ, et al. National Comprehensive Cancer Network Practice Guidelines in Oncology: Testicular Cancer, Version 1.2002. National Comprehensive Cancer Network, Rockledge, PA, 2001.

Williams SD, Stablein DM, Einhorn LH, et al. Immediate adjuvant chemotherapy versus observation with treatment at relapse in pathological stage II testicular cancer. *N Engl J Med* 1987;317:1433–1438.

Vaughn DJ, Gignac GA, Meadows AT. Long-term medical care of testicular cancer survivors. *Ann Intern Med* 2002;136(6):463–470.

# Leukemia

## 21

*Matt Kalaycio*

The leukemias are hematopoietic malignancies that result in bone marrow failure or immune system dysfunction. Often thought of as either acute or chronic, and myeloid or lymphocytic, the leukemias are in fact a heterogeneous group of malignancies that differ in their molecular pathophysiology, if not always in their histology. These differences are being exploited in modern treatment protocols to improve survival and cure rates. This chapter strives to describe the various leukemias, explains their unique characteristics, and discusses their diagnosis and management.

## ETIOLOGY

The etiology of the vast majority of leukemias is unknown. Clearly, environmental exposures to chemicals such as benzene and ionizing radiation increase the risk of acute leukemia and chronic myelogenous leukemia (CML). No environmental agent, however, has been demonstrated to increase the risk of chronic lymphocytic leukemia (CLL).

In some cases, the etiology of leukemia is known. Several hematologic disorders may transform into acute leukemia. The most common disorder to transform is myelodysplastic syndrome (MDS), but patients with myeloproliferative disorders and aplastic anemia are also at risk. MDS is discussed in greater detail later, but approximately one-third of MDS transforms into acute myelogenous leukemia (AML).

Cancer patients who survive after treatment with chemotherapy are at risk for the subsequent development of high-risk MDS. The risk is particularly high for patients treated with long courses, or high doses, of alkylating agents such as melphalan, busulfan, and cyclophosphamide. The treatment of Hodgkin's disease often uses such agents, and MDS/AML is the most common secondary malignancy associated with the treatment of Hodgkin's disease. Autologous stem cell transplantation for breast cancer or lymphoma may also be complicated by MDS/AML in as many as 10% to 15% of survivors. In contrast, the AML that results from exposure to epipodophyllotoxins, such as etoposide, generally develops in the absence of MDS and has different characteristics, as discussed in the section Secondary Leukemia and the Myelodysplastic Syndromes.

Congenital syndromes such as Down and Klinefelter's syndromes often increase the risk of subsequent acute leukemias. A genetic predisposition to some leukemias also may exist, particularly childhood acute lymphoblastic leukemia (ALL).

## CHRONIC LYMPHOCYTIC LEUKEMIA

Chronic lymphocytic leukemia (CLL) is the most common adult leukemia in Western society. This leukemia increases in incidence with increasing age, and no other etiologic factor has been implicated. As noted previously, patients are often asymptomatic at diagnosis and require no therapy. Often, patients present with lymphadenopathy. An excisional biopsy of the involved lymph nodes demonstrates histologic changes identical to diffuse, small cell lymphocytic lymphoma. There is no meaningful difference in the pathophysiology, complications, and management of CLL and small cell lymphocytic lymphoma, and they are usually considered as a single entity.

Important prognostic information can be determined at diagnosis. Several staging systems have been devised that predict survival based on the extent of disease at diagnosis (Table 21.1). Those patients with low-risk disease often require no therapy and die of unrelated causes. Those patients with high-risk disease have shorter than expected survival, but treatment is not known to alter this fact. Other prognostic factors have been suggested, such as lymphocyte doubling time and $\beta_2$-microglobulin levels, but none has been prospectively validated and none significantly alters treatment recommendations.

CLL may be complicated in several important ways:

- Infection. As noted previously, patients with CLL are predisposed to a variety of infections.
- Autoimmune phenomena. These usually manifest as cytopenias (immune thrombocytopenic purpura).
- Richter's transformation. Transformation into diffuse, large B-cell lymphoma.

Infections are managed as they occur, but prevention with vaccinations and possibly intravenous immunoglobulins is often appropriate. Autoimmune cytopenias, such as immune thrombocytopenic purpura and autoimmune hemolytic anemia, are treated with corticosteroids, as they would be in benign presentations. Richter's transformation carries a poor prognosis, but is treated as any other large cell lymphoma.

**TABLE 21.1**

**STAGING SYSTEMS FOR CHRONIC LYMPHOCYTIC LEUKEMIA**

| Clinical Features | Rai | Modified Rai | Binet | Survival (yr) |
|---|---|---|---|---|
| Lymphocytosis only | 0 | Low risk | | >10 |
| Enlargement of <3 areas[a] | | | A | >10 |
| Enlarged lymph nodes | I | | | 8 |
| Enlarged liver, spleen, or both | II | | | 6 |
| Enlarged lymph nodes + spleen + liver | | Intermediate risk | | 7 |
| Enlargement of 3 areas[a] | | | B | 5 |
| Hgb <11 | III | | | 2.5 |
| Plts <100K | IV | | | 2.5 |
| Hgb <11 and plts <100K | | High risk | | 1.5 |
| Hgb <10, plts <100K, or both | | | C | 2.5 |

Hgb, hemoglobin; Plts, platelets.
[a] The three areas include cervical, axillary, and inguinal lymph nodes, spleen, and liver.

The treatment for CLL is usually successful in inducing at least partial remissions. The elimination of all detectable disease, however, occurs less often, and relapse is inevitable. Traditionally, single-agent alkylating agents, such as chlorambucil, have been used with good effect and minimal side effects. More recently, purine analogs, such as fludarabine, have been shown to increase the remission rate, but at the expense of increased side effects. Survival rates do not seem improved, however, and fludarabine is usually reserved for younger patients.

The prognosis for relapsed patients is relatively poor, with a median survival of less than 2 years. The treatment for relapsed disease may consist of alkylating agents, purine analogs, or monoclonal antibodies, such as alemtuzumab (CamPath), alone or in combination. The role of allogeneic hematopoietic stem cell transplantation is undefined.

## HAIRY CELL LEUKEMIA

Hairy cell leukemia is an uncommon, chronic, B-cell malignancy with unique features. In the United States, 400 to 600 cases are diagnosed each year; the median age of patients is 50 years, with a 4:1 male predominance. Symptoms attributable to pancytopenia or splenomegaly are often present. The leukocyte differential and peripheral smear demonstrate a relative or absolute lymphocytosis with characteristic hairy cells. The bone marrow biopsy is usually hypercellular, with a diffuse infiltrate of hairy cells and increased reticulin, collagen, and fibrosis. Although immunoglobulin levels are normal, antibody-dependent cellular cytotoxicity and cellular immunity are impaired. These immune defects, in association with neutropenia and a characteristic monocytopenia, often lead to unusual infections (e.g., mycobacterial and fungal infections).

Splenectomy improves pancytopenia in two-thirds of patients. Although this procedure temporarily removes the site of platelet and white cell sequestration, it does not prevent continued malignant lymphocyte proliferation, marrow infiltration, or eventual relapse. Patients treated with interferon obtain a partial remission, but relapse within 1 to 2 years after the discontinuation of therapy. Nucleoside analogs have demonstrated promising results. A single cycle of 2-chlorodeoxyadenosine induces prolonged complete and partial remissions in 80% and 20% of patients, respectively.

## CHRONIC MYELOGENOUS LEUKEMIA

Extensive knowledge of the molecular pathophysiologic basis for CML has led to exciting treatment advances. CML is characterized by the Philadelphia chromosome, t(9;22). The translocation of the *ABL* oncogene from chromosome 9 to juxtapose the *BCR* gene on chromosome 22 results in a unique, chimeric fusion gene, *BCR/ABL*, which results in a chimeric protein with autonomous tyrosine kinase activity. This activity directly results in the activation of several intracellular processes that stimulate cellular proliferation and inhibit apoptosis. The malignant clone expands to the exclusion of normal clones and eventually leads to the clinical manifestations of the disease.

Patients may be asymptomatic at presentation, but often present with fever, sweats, weight loss, and bone pain. Physical examination often reveals splenomegaly. Masses composed of hematopoietic tissue—chloromas—may be detected anywhere and signify more advanced disease.

The peripheral blood smear reveals a left-shifted neutrophilic leukocytosis with basophilia and perhaps a few circulating blasts. Red cells and platelets may be either increased or decreased. The diagnosis is confirmed by the demonstration of *BCR/ABL* by cytogenetic analysis or molecular techniques. Patients who present with the clinical features of CML but lack detectable *BCR/ABL* often have another myeloproliferative disorder, such as myelofibrosis or chronic myelomonocytic leukemia. These patients have a poorer prognosis.

CML inevitably transforms to AML, or *blast crisis*, in the absence of therapy designed to eliminate the leukemic clone. The transformation is often heralded by an accelerated phase of disease, characterized by worsening symptoms, progressive splenomegaly, chloromas, and clonal evolution (additional cytogenetic abnormalities in addition to the Philadelphia chromosome). The median survival of patients with CML is 5 to 6 years.

The treatment for CML was strictly palliative in the not-too-distant past. Hydroxyurea effectively controls symptoms and blood counts, but does not suppress the Philadelphia chromosome and, therefore, does not prolong survival or delay blast crisis. Interferon-α also controls symptoms and blood counts. Importantly, however, interferon can suppress the Philadelphia chromosome and thereby improve survival and delay blast crisis. Some patients with low-risk disease have a complete elimination of their Philadelphia chromosome, which may translate into prolonged disease-free survival and potential cure. Interferon, however, does not suppress the Philadelphia chromosome enough in the majority of patients and has significant side effects. Therefore, most patients are not cured by interferon.

Imatinib was developed as a specific inhibitor of the *bcr/abl* tyrosine kinase. In patients refractory to, or intolerant of, interferon, imatinib results in a 100% hematologic remission and at least a 50% cytogenetic remission. In accelerated phase disease and blast crisis, imatinib also results in high complete hematologic remission rates, although the cytogenetic remission rate is lower and relapse is common with more advanced disease. These dramatic results generally occur in the absence of significant side effects. Indeed, for newly diagnosed patients in the chronic phase, imatinib improved remission rates and slowed the rate of progression to accelerated or blast phase when compared to the combination of interferon and cytarabine in a recently published prospective, randomized clinical trial.

Although imatinib represents a major advance in the treatment of CML, the only treatment known to cure CML is allogeneic stem cell transplantation. Patients with chronic-phase CML transplanted within 1 year of diagnosis have a 50% to 70% chance of cure, whether their donor is a human leukocyte antigen (HLA)–matched sibling or matched unrelated donor. Results are poorer for more advanced disease, but cure is still possible even for blast crisis. Transplantation is associated with high treatment-related morbidity and mortality, however, which limits its application to relatively younger patients.

Relapse is unusual after allogeneic transplantation. In contrast, relapse is quite frequent after autologous, syngeneic (identical twin), and T-cell–depleted transplants despite similar pretransplant chemoradiotherapeutic treatment regimens. These observations suggest something unique to the T cells of allogeneic donors that cause antileukemic effects. Supporting evidence for this graft-versus-leukemia effect comes from the observation that relapse is more likely in the absence of graft-versus-host disease (mediated by donor T cells). Direct proof, however, comes from patients with CML who relapsed after an allogeneic transplant and then were reinduced into cytogenetic remission by infusion of donor T cells alone.

The observation of graft-versus-leukemia suggests that CML might be cured in the absence of high-dose chemoradiotherapy if donor T cells successfully engraft in the recipient. T-cell engraftment is indeed possible using immunosuppressive treatments, which are often administered in the outpatient setting with little early morbidity. Separating graft-versus-leukemia from graft-versus-host disease, however, has proven more difficult, and the ultimate role of these nonmyeloablative "mini" transplants is uncertain.

## ACUTE LEUKEMIAS

Gone are the days when clinicians could think of the acute leukemias as either myeloid (AML) or lymphoid (ALL). The French-American-British (FAB) classification system, which subclassified AML and ALL into histologic subtypes, has lost usefulness in the face of newer prognostic categories. Furthermore, the histologic subtypes are subject to poor interobserver agreement and, with the exception of acute promyelocytic leukemia, do not clearly influence treatment decisions. Newer information derived from the study of molecular pathogenesis, cytogenetic and immunophenotypic analysis, and the results of clinical trials has delineated many distinct acute leukemias, each with a specific phenotype and clinical manifestation.

### Acute Promyelocytic Leukemia

The translocation of the promyelocytic leukemia (PML) oncogene on chromosome 15 to the retinoic acid receptor-α (RARα) gene on chromosome 17 results in a novel chimeric fusion protein that binds DNA and interferes with hematopoietic cell differentiation. Normally, RARα binds to DNA where it regulates cellular proliferation with other regulatory proteins. The PML/RARα nuclear-binding protein irreversibly binds corepressor proteins that effectively inhibit the cellular processes necessary for differentiation. Under the inhibition of PML/RARα, the affected leukemic cell's maturation is arrested in the blast or promyelocyte stage. Thus, apoptosis is inhibited and the leukemic blasts accumulate, which ultimately leads to the clinical manifestations of acute promyelocytic leukemia (APL). All-*trans* retinoic acid (ATRA) binds to PML/RARα, induces the unbinding of the corepressors, and allows for subsequent differentiation and apoptosis of the leukemic clone.

The recognition of the molecular pathogenesis of APL is important in that it represents a paradigm for the leukemic transformation of hematopoietic stem cells. Other leukemias caused by translocations have similar pathogeneses. Future treatments for these leukemias will probably involve the inhibition or reversal of these leukemogenic pathways.

APL is characterized by a distinct blast morphology, immunophenotype, and karyotype. The blasts often display numerous Auer rods and show at least some evidence of early differentiation, such as cytoplasmic granules. The blasts also express a distinct pattern of cell surface proteins: CD34-, CD33+, HLA-DR-, and CD13+. Most other myeloid leukemias express HLA-DR and may or may not express CD34. Finally, the pathognomonic feature of APL is the presence of t(15;17) by cytogenetic analysis.

APL is also characterized by an unusual coagulopathy. The coagulopathy has traditionally been considered a form of disseminated intravascular coagulation. The APL coagulopathy, however, manifests with normal levels of antithrombin III, and bleeding is the major complication. One study suggests that the coagulopathy stems from an overexpression of annexin II on the APL blast surface. Annexin II results in the overproduction of plasmin, which may explain the hemorrhagic diathesis. The coagulopathy is treated with intensive transfusion support, including platelets, cryoprecipitate, and fresh frozen plasma. Before ATRA, as many as 30% of patients with APL died from hemorrhage. ATRA reduces the hemorrhagic complications by differentiating the blasts into neutrophils, rather than killing them as chemotherapy does.

The treatment of APL is also different from that applied to other leukemias. APL is uniquely sensitive to the differentiating effects of ATRA. ATRA alone results in an 80% to 90% complete remission rate. In combination with standard chemotherapy, particularly anthracyclines such as daunorubicin and idarubicin, 60% to 80% of patients in remission are cured. Patients who are older than age 60 or present with a white blood count (WBC) greater than 10,000/μL have a worse prognosis, but cure is still possible. For patients who relapse, arsenic trioxide induces a second complete remission in approximately 85% of patients, who are then eligible for potentially curative treatment with an autologous or allogeneic hematopoietic stem cell transplant. The role of arsenic trioxide in less advanced APL is currently under study.

## Core-Binding Factor Leukemia

These leukemias are characterized by translocations that disrupt the function of core-binding factor (CBF), a nuclear binding protein that regulates hematopoiesis in a fashion similar to that of RARα. CBF is composed of two subunits, each of which can be affected by chromosomal translocations that result in leukemogenesis.

One leukemogenic translocation is t(8;21), which juxtaposes the AML1 oncogene to the ETO oncogene, creating a chimeric and leukemogenic CBFα subunit. The resulting leukemia is characterized morphologically by the relatively common observance of Auer rods. Unlike APL, however, this leukemia expresses CD34, CD33, and HLA-DR. Lymphoid antigens, particularly CD19, also may be expressed, with no impact on prognosis. The coexpression of CD56, when present, does connote a worse prognosis, as it does when expressed on other leukemias. Clinically, this leukemia is often associated with granulocytic sarcomas (chloromas).

Another well-characterized translocation is inv(16). This abnormality inverts the CBFβ subunit on the q arm of chromosome 16 to the *MYH11* gene on the p arm. The resulting chimeric CBFβ/MYH11 protein can also be formed by t(16;16) and is leukemogenic in a fashion similar to t(8;21). This leukemia, however, has a unique morphology: The blasts are myelomonocytic, displaying nuclear clefts and cytoplasmic vacuolization. Importantly, dysplastic eosinophils are also evident in marrow aspirates. Thus, this particular leukemia has been referred to as *acute myelomonocytic leukemia with eosinophilia*.

Both t(8;21) and inv(16) result in leukemias that are exquisitely sensitive to cytarabine. Both are almost always induced into remission using standard chemotherapy. Additional cycles of high-dose cytarabine are needed to maintain remission, however. With appropriate treatment, the CBF leukemias are curable in 60% to 70% of cases.

## Secondary Leukemia and the Myelodysplastic Syndromes

The MDSs are malignancies of hematopoietic stem cells that generally occur in the elderly patient population. They usually present as asymptomatic cytopenias and often as macrocytic anemias. They are characterized by inexorable progressively worsening bone marrow failure, but they do not necessarily result in transformation to acute leukemia or death. Treatment is supportive, with blood transfusions and antibiotics for neutropenic infections. Younger patients, however, should be offered potentially curative allogeneic hematopoietic stem cell transplant.

One study has characterized the prognosis of patients with MDS (Table 21.2). The International Prognostic Scoring System uses cytopenias, age, blast percentage, and cytogenetics to classify patients into prognostic groups. Lower-risk disease carries a more favorable prognosis and probably has a different pathophysiology. Emerging evidence suggests that low-risk MDS is characterized by immune dysregulation that, at least in part, explains the cytopenias. Immunosuppressive therapies may reverse the inhibition of normal hematopoiesis and restore blood counts in a minority of cases.

Higher-risk MDS tends to transform into acute leukemia. The secondary leukemias are those that are preceded by hematologic disorders such as MDS or by exposure to stem cell toxins, such as benzene, ionizing radiation, and cytotoxic chemotherapy. Historically, the difference between MDS and AML was made by arbitrary cutoffs for blast percentage. High-risk MDS and secondary leukemia share

## TABLE 21.2
### INTERNATIONAL PROGNOSTIC SCORING SYSTEM FOR MYELODYSPLASTIC SYNDROMES

| Marrow Blast Percentage | Score |
|---|---|
| <5 | 0 |
| 5–10 | 0.5 |
| 11–20 | 1.5 |
| 21–30 | 2.0 |

**Cytogenetic Features (Karyotype)**

| | |
|---|---|
| Good prognosis | 0 |
| Intermediate prognosis | 0.5 |
| Poor prognosis | 1.0 |

**Cytopenias (Hemoglobin <10, Absolute Neutrophil Count <1,500, Platelets <100K)**

| | |
|---|---|
| None or 1 | 0 |
| 2 or 3 | 0.5 |

| Overall Score (Blast + Cytogenetic + Cytopenia Scores) | Median Survival (yr) |
|---|---|
| Low = 0 | 5.7 |
| Low intermediate = 0.5 or 1.0 | 3.5 |
| High intermediate = 1.5 or 2.0 | 1.2 |
| High = >2.5 | 0.4 |

Good prognosis: normal, -Y only, 5q- only, 20q- only; intermediate prognosis: +8, single miscellaneous abnormality, double abnormalities; poor prognosis: complex abnormalities, abnormal chromosome 7.

enough characteristics, however, to be considered the same disease regardless of blast percentage.

Secondary leukemia is characterized by cytogenetic abnormalities that often involve chromosomes 5 and 7. These leukemias are difficult to induce into remission, and survival is short. In fact, secondary leukemias are uniformly fatal in the absence of allogeneic stem cell transplant. These leukemias are also difficult to cure with transplant and are associated with a high relapse rate.

An exception to the rule of poor prognosis in secondary leukemias is the 5q-syndrome. This syndrome tends to occur in female subjects. The syndrome usually presents as a mild anemia, but may also be associated with thrombocytosis. Unlike the other leukemias associated with abnormalities of chromosome 5, the 5q-syndrome carries with it a favorable long-term prognosis, with little likelihood of transformation into acute leukemia.

Another unique secondary leukemia is characterized by abnormalities of chromosome 11q23. Prior exposure to epipodophyllotoxins, such as etoposide used in the treatment of childhood ALL, is associated with an increased risk of leukemias that harbor 11q23 abnormalities, such as t(9;11). Unlike the secondary leukemias induced by alkylating agents (i.e., melphalan), these leukemias are not preceded by a myelodysplastic phase. They are more easily

induced into remission, but similar to the other secondary leukemias, survival is short and transplant is necessary for cure.

## Acute Myelogenous Leukemia in the Older Adult

The incidence of AML increases dramatically with increasing age. Most patients with AML, in fact, are older than age 60. In many respects, AML in the older adult is no different from secondary AML. Both are characterized by dysplastic morphology and harbor similar chromosomal derangements. Both are also characterized by a poor prognosis. The poor prognosis stems from both a more drug-resistant leukemic clone and the inability of older patients to withstand the rigors of induction chemotherapy. To this end, clinical trials have explored the role of adjuvant therapies designed to reduce the morbidity of chemotherapy in this patient population.

A series of clinical trials studied the potential role of hematopoietic growth factors in reducing the period of neutropenia after chemotherapy. When considered as a whole, these studies clearly demonstrate the ability of hematopoietic growth factors to reduce the duration of neutropenia without increasing the risk of relapse. No clear survival benefit was demonstrated, however. Although the hematopoietic growth factors are not considered standard therapy, they are often used to reduce the risk of infection in patients at high risk.

All older patients with AML either fail initial chemotherapy or have a relapse. No effective therapy has been found for these patients. An anti-CD33 monoclonal antibody was linked to calicheamicin, a chemotherapeutic agent too toxic to give as a single agent. The resulting molecule, ozogamicin gemtuzumab, effectively targets $CD33^+$ cells, such as leukemic blasts. For older patients with relapsed AML, approximately 30% achieve a second remission using ozogamicin gemtuzumab.

## Precursor B-Cell Acute Lymphoblastic Leukemia

Precursor B-cell ALL is the most common subtype of ALL and is the subtype generally associated with childhood ALL. Whereas ALL in children is curable in as many as 80% of cases, the same is not true in adult populations. The major contributing factor to poor outcome in adult populations is that adult ALL is associated with adverse clonal cytogenetic abnormalities such as t(9;22) and t(4;11).

ALL typically presents as an acute illness with bone marrow failure, constitutional symptoms, and variable degrees of lymphadenopathy and splenomegaly. The diagnosis is suspected by a histologic review of blood and marrow specimens, but ALL cannot be distinguished reliably from AML on the basis of morphology alone. The best way to discriminate the lineage of acute leukemia is with flow cytometry of the leukemic blasts to determine their immunophenotype. Whereas AML blasts typically express CD33, CD13, and HLA-DR, pre–B-cell ALL blasts typically express CD10, CD19, and tDt.

The treatment of ALL is typically based on the combination of vincristine and prednisone. An anthracycline, such as daunorubicin, is usually included with or without other agents such as L-asparaginase and cyclophosphamide. Remissions are achieved in approximately 80% of patients with any one of a number of induction regimens. Despite intensive postremission treatment, most patients have relapses. The risk of relapse increases with increasing WBC at diagnosis, increasing age, and the presence of adverse, clonal cytogenetics such as t(9;22) and t(4;11). At relapse, adult patients require allogeneic stem cell transplant for cure.

ALL tends to involve sanctuary sites, such as the central nervous system (CNS), more often than does AML. Although the risk of CNS involvement is less in adults compared with children, prophylactic CNS treatment with intrathecal doses of chemotherapy, and sometimes whole brain radiotherapy, is recommended in most modern treatment regimens.

### Precursor T-Cell Acute Lymphoblastic Leukemia

T-cell ALL needs to be considered as a separate entity from pre–B-cell ALL due to its distinct clinical presentation, natural history, and response to treatment. Morphologically, T-cell ALL is indistinguishable from lymphoblastic lymphoma (LBL). There are subtle histologic differences between T-cell and pre–B-cell ALL. Both T-cell ALL and LBL can be distinguished from pre–B-cell ALL by immunophenotype, however. As might be expected, pre–B-cell ALL expresses B-cell antigens such as CD19 and CD 20, but both T-cell ALL and LBL express T-cell antigens such as CD2, CD3, CD4, CD5, CD7, and CD8. T-cell ALL and LBL express similar antigens.

In fact, the only difference between T-cell ALL and LBL is the degree of marrow infiltration. They both are characterized by mediastinal masses and tend to occur in young men. Both are treated identically, with similar results. Most investigators consider them as the same illness.

T-cell ALL, and therefore LBL, has a better prognosis than does pre–B-cell ALL. Relapse only occurs in 30% to 40% of patients with T-cell ALL. Modern treatment regimens that maximize survival in T-cell ALL include cyclophosphamide and higher doses of cytarabine, in addition to intensive CNS prophylaxis.

### Mature B-Cell Lymphoblastic Leukemia

Mature B-cell lymphoblastic leukemia is characterized by an extremely aggressive, rapidly proliferating population of blasts that are identified by a translocations of the *c-myc* oncogene, as occurs in t(8;14) and t(8;22) among others.

The blasts have a distinct morphology that, in the FAB classification system, was labeled L3, or Burkitt's leukemia. The immunophenotype is also distinctive in that surface immunoglobulin is detected, but the cytogenetic abnormality is diagnostic. This leukemia tends to invade the CNS early and requires prophylactic CNS treatment.

Untreated, or treated improperly, B-cell ALL is rapidly fatal, with a short survival time. With appropriate, intensive, short-course chemotherapy, however, cure is the rule rather than the exception.

## MANAGEMENT OF ACUTE LEUKEMIA

Despite the distinctive nature of the individual acute leukemias, some management principles are shared by all of them. Bone marrow failure is universal in the acute leukemias, as a consequence of the leukemia as well as its treatment. The management of the resulting pancytopenia is critical to the success of any treatment program.

### Neutropenic Fever

The incidence of infection increases with more profound and prolonged neutropenia, particularly as the absolute neutrophil count falls below $500/\mu L$. At this degree of neutropenia, the risk of rapidly fatal septicemia is quite high. In contrast to other situations, a fever in the setting of severe neutropenia must be treated empirically to reduce the risk of infectious mortality.

The onset of fever in the neutropenic host should prompt a clinical evaluation looking for a source of infection and the collection of blood and other bodily fluids for culture. Once the cultures are obtained, antibiotics that cover Gram-negative organisms are started empirically, including *Pseudomonas aeruginosa*. The Gram-negative organisms are not the most common infections in this setting, but they are the most virulent. This fact has prompted the study of prophylactic antibiotics for neutropenic patients. The most commonly used agents are the fluoroquinolones, which have been shown to reduce the incidence of Gram-negative infections, but have not been clearly demonstrated to reduce infectious mortality or improve survival.

Gram-positive infections are the most common organisms identified in modern series. These infections are typically less aggressive, however, and empiric therapy is not mandatory. A Gram-positive infection becomes even more likely in the setting of prophylactic antibiotics or an indwelling central venous catheter. Vancomycin is often added to other empiric antibiotics in these situations.

The initial empiric antibiotic regimen of choice depends in large part on the susceptibility patterns of bacteria in the patient's hospital. Whatever regimen is chosen, however, should be broad-spectrum enough to cover a wide variety of organisms, including *P. aeruginosa*. Common regimens include a broad-spectrum penicillin, such as piperacillin in combination with an aminoglycoside. In some situations, monotherapy using agents such as imipenem is appropriate. Cephalosporins should probably be avoided because their long-term use tends to increase the incidence of infections with vancomycin-resistant strains of enterococcus.

If the fever resolves, the antibiotics should be continued until the neutropenia resolves. The aminoglycosides, however, may require replacement after approximately 2 weeks of therapy to avoid ototoxicity. If a specific organism is identified, antibiotics can be changed accordingly. Persistent or recurrent fever in the setting of appropriate broad-spectrum antibiotics suggests fungal infection.

Fungal infections, particularly with *Aspergillus* species, contribute greatly to the infectious morbidity and mortality of patients with prolonged neutropenia. These organisms are notoriously difficult to isolate in culture, but early treatment improves outcome. Therefore, presumed fungal infections must be treated empirically. Fever persisting for more than 4 days in the setting of neutropenia and appropriate antibacterials should be treated with empiric antifungal agents. Traditionally, amphotericin B has been the treatment of choice in this situation, but some studies have suggested that fluconazole or itraconazole can be safely substituted.

Another situation in which fungal infection should be considered is a fever that develops as the neutropenia is resolving. Hepatosplenic candidiasis often presents in this fashion, in association with elevations of alkaline phosphatase. Computed tomography (CT) of the liver and spleen is recommended to demonstrate the typical hypodense parenchymal lesions. Although biopsy of the lesions is recommended for confirmation, the constellation of symptoms and signs in the right setting calls for empiric antifungal therapy.

Other infections are also possible but are either less likely, or less likely to be fatal. *Herpes simplex* infections often complicate the therapy of acute leukemia, and seropositive patients should be treated with prophylactic acyclovir. *Cytomegalovirus* infections are less common, but should be suspected if no other source of infection is identified. *Pneumocystis carinii* complicates the treatment of ALL enough to warrant prophylactic treatment with trimethoprim-sulfamethoxazole.

## Transfusion Support

Although a decision to transfuse should be individualized, certain guidelines pertaining to transfusion support should be followed to avoid complications.

The risks of serious spontaneous bleeding increase rapidly as the platelet count falls below 10,000. Platelet transfusions for platelet counts of less than 10,000 to 20,000 are therefore warranted. These compromised patients are at risk for transfusion-associated graft-versus-host disease resulting from the transfer of lymphocytes in blood products; these patients, especially bone marrow transplantation candidates, should receive irradiated blood products.

Patients may acquire cytomegalovirus through blood transfusions; therefore, previously unexposed patients, especially bone marrow transplantation candidates, should receive cytomegalovirus-seronegative or (preferably) leukocyte-reduced blood products.

Leukocyte reduction is generally performed by filtration. Filtered blood products are associated with less risk of febrile transfusion reactions and may reduce the incidence of alloimmunization. Some authorities suggest that all blood products should be filtered, but this is particularly important in immunocompromised individuals because leukocyte reduction decreases the rate of viral transfer.

Refractory thrombocytopenia caused by alloimmunization may occur in approximately 20% of patients with acute leukemia. No increased incidence exists with cumulative platelet transfusion exposure. Single-donor or HLA-matched platelets may have an increased survival time and may, therefore, be of benefit in this situation.

Red blood cell transfusions also should be filtered and irradiated for the same reasons pertaining to platelet transfusions.

The benefit of granulocyte transfusion is uncertain. The only potential indication for granulocyte transfusion is the patient with a documented infection that is susceptible, but not responding, to appropriate antibiotics.

## REVIEW EXERCISES

### QUESTIONS

**1.** A 35-year-old woman presents to the emergency room with 24 hours of fever and chills. In addition, she complains of increasing fatigue, dyspnea on exertion, and spontaneous bruising.

On physical examination, she appears ill; her vitals are temperature 39.5°C, blood pressure 80/40 mm Hg, pulse 140 bpm, respiration rate 22 breaths/min, petechiae on soft palate, no lymphadenopathy, clear lungs, tachycardia, I/VI systolic ejection murmur, no abdominal mass or hepatosplenomegaly, and scattered petechiae, especially on lower extremities.

Her laboratory values are: hemoglobin, 8.7; platelets, 14,000; WBC, 3,000 with 2% neutrophils, 45% lymphocytes, and 53% blasts; international normalized ratio, 1.1; partial thromboplastin time, 23; fibrinogen, 345.

Her peripheral blood smear shows normochromic, normocytic anemia; thrombocytopenia; rare neutrophils, many blasts.

All of the following are true, *except*

a) Immediate hospitalization is indicated.
b) Antibiotics should be withheld until a source of infection is identified.
c) No evidence is present of a significant coagulopathy.
d) Platelet transfusion is indicated.

**2.** Which of the following is needed to make the diagnosis and predict prognosis?
a) Histologic examination of the blasts
b) Immunophenotype of the blasts
c) Cytogenetic analysis
d) All of the above

**3.** A 25-year-old man presents to the emergency room complaining of dyspnea on exertion for several days. Recently, he has noted frequent nasal congestion and occasional epistaxis. He denies fevers, night sweats, and weight loss and has noted a rash on his legs. He denies any hospitalizations or history of transfusions.

On physical examination, you find a well-developed man in no acute distress; temperature 36.8°C, blood pressure 126/74 mm Hg, respiration rate 20 breaths/min; his oral mucosa has a few petechial hemorrhages, the skin of the pretibial area is covered with petechial hemorrhages, no palpable lymphadenopathy or splenomegaly is present; he is otherwise normal.

His laboratory values are: hemoglobin, 8.3; platelets, 32,000; WBC, 1,100 with 1% neutrophils, 73% lymphocytes, 13% monocytes, and 13% blasts; prothrombin time, 20; international normalized ratio, 2.1; partial thromboplastin time, 40; fibrinogen, 90.

His peripheral smear shows pancytopenia, circulating blasts with Auer rods, and occasional schistocytes. A bone marrow aspirate and biopsy indicate hypercellular with 85% blasts and immature granulocytes.

All of the following statements are true, *except*
a) He probably has acute promyelocytic leukemia.
b) Platelet transfusion is indicated.
c) Fresh frozen plasma is indicated.
d) Antibiotics are indicated.

**4.** A 29-year-old woman presents to your office for a Papanicolaou smear. She is asymptomatic and has a normal physical examination except for a moderately enlarged spleen.

Her laboratory values are: hemoglobin, 11.9; platelets, 671,000; WBC, 227,000 with 55% neutrophils, 7% metamyelocytes, 19% myelocytes, 2% promyelocytes, 2% blasts, 1% eosinophils, 7% basophils, and 3% lymphocytes. A bone marrow chromosome analysis shows 46,XX, t(9;22).

All of the following are true statements, *except*
a) Immediate hospitalization is indicated.
b) Hydroxyurea is indicated.
c) She and her siblings should be tissue typed to consider bone marrow transplantation.
d) Leukophoresis is not indicated.

**5.** A 35-year-old man with AML has been severely neutropenic for 10 days and has been febrile with temperatures greater than 38.5°C for the past 5 days. He has been on piperacillin, gentamicin, and vancomycin for

8 days. No localizing signs of infection are present on examination, and all cultures are negative to date. The most appropriate course of action would be to
a) Continue current antibiotics
b) Change antibiotics to imipenem
c) Add amphotericin B
d) Draw fungal cultures and continue current antibiotics

**6.** A 75-year-old man with a 5-year history of untreated, chronic lymphocytic leukemia presents with fatigue and a peculiar craving for ice. Examination reveals generalized, but small peripheral lymphadenopathy and a barely palpable spleen tip. His laboratory values are: WBC 34,000, Hgb 5.2, and platelets 133,000, reticulocytes 2%, direct Coombs' test negative; LDH and bilirubin normal. The peripheral blood smear demonstrates normocytic red cells and no polychromasia. The most likely cause of anemia in this patient is
a) Pure red cell aplasia
b) Autoimmune hemolytic anemia
c) Bone marrow infiltration with leukemia
d) Gastrointestinal bleeding

**7.** Given this patient's anemia, lymphadenopathy, splenomegaly, and high WBC count, treatment with chemotherapy is indicated.
a) True
b) False

## ANSWERS

**1. b.**
This patient has life-threatening sepsis and must be admitted for fluid resuscitation, a quick evaluation including blood cultures, and the administration of empiric, broad-spectrum intravenous antibiotics. She is anemic, thrombocytopenic, has spontaneous bruising, and is at risk for life-threatening hemorrhage; therefore, she needs transfusion with red blood cells and platelets. Her coagulation tests are normal; therefore, there is no evidence of a coagulopathy.

**2. d.**
All these tests are needed. The morphology of the blasts may be diagnostic in itself. Histochemical staining may also be indicated to improve diagnostic precision. Immunophenotyping is the most important test to determine cell lineage (AML vs. ALL) and may help with prognosis. Cytogenetics is the most important predictor of outcome next to age.

**3. d.**
This patient probably has APL, given the obvious Auer rods and evidence of a significant coagulopathy. Both plasma and platelets are needed to reduce the incidence of fatal hemorrhage. In the absence of fever or other signs of infection, antibiotics are not recommended for

neutropenia. Prophylactic antibiotics are controversial, but have not been shown to improve survival.

## 4. a.

This patient's signs, symptoms, complete blood count, and bone marrow are characteristic of CML. The t(9;22) is the Philadelphia chromosome, which secures the diagnosis. The high WBC requires neither leukophoresis nor hospitalization. Unlike a high blast count, a high neutrophil count does not increase the risk of leukostasis and hyperviscosity syndrome. Hydroxyurea is indicated to reduce the WBC over a period of days to weeks. Hydroxyurea alone, however, will not prevent the progression of CML to blast crisis. The only known curative therapy is bone marrow transplant. Thus, both the patient and her siblings should be tissue typed to determine if marrow transplant is a therapeutic option.

## 5. c.

As the duration of neutropenia increases, the risk of fungal infection increases. This is particularly true in the setting of broad-spectrum antibacterials. This patient is at high-risk for fungal infection. The current antibiotics are failing, thus continuing them with no other changes is inappropriate. A change to imipenem might cover additional bacterial pathogens, but does not address the risk of fungal infection. Fungal infections are difficult to isolate. Clinical studies have clearly demonstrated the importance of *empiric* antifungal therapy. Thus, amphotericin B is the correct choice.

## 6. d

Chronic lymphocytic leukemia is a fairly common lymphoproliferative disorder in the older patient population. Although CLL may be the direct cause of anemia in some patients, it is important to remember that these patients are also at risk for other problems as well. This particular patient has pica, a very specific symptom of iron-deficiency anemia. Even though the red cells are not microcytic, iron-deficiency anemia is still possible, especially if the onset is relatively rapid. Pure red cell aplasia is another possibility, but less likely given the indolent nature of the patient's leukemia and the presence of pica. Similarly, infiltration of the marrow with leukemia in an untreated patient would not likely be enough to induce this degree of anemia given the nonbulky lymph nodes, modest splenomegaly, and modest leukocytosis. The absence of microspherocytes, reticulocytosis, and a

negative Coombs' test make autoimmune hemolytic the least likely cause of anemia in this patient, but AIHA is a common cause of anemia in patients with CLL.

## 7. b

If anemia is due to leukemic infiltration of the bone marrow, with a resulting displacement of other hematopoietic elements, then chemotherapy is indeed indicated. In this case, however, alternative explanations are more likely, and treatment should be directed to the anemia, not the leukemia. Other indications to start therapy are progressive symptoms and rapidly enlarging lymph nodes or splenomegaly.

## SUGGESTED READINGS

Bloomfield CD, Herzig GP, Caligiuri MA, eds. Acute leukemia. *Semin Oncol* 1997;24:1–151.

Cassileth PA, Harrington DP, Appelbaum FR, et al. Chemotherapy compared with autologous or allogeneic bone marrow transplantation in the management of acute myeloid leukemia in first remission. *N Engl J Med* 1998;339:1649–1656.

Copelan EA, McGuire EA. The biology and treatment of acute lymphoblastic leukemia in adults. *Blood* 1995;85:1151–1168.

Druker BJ, Talpaz M, Resta D, et al. Efficacy and safety of a specific inhibitor of the *bcr-abl* tyrosine kinase in chronic myeloid leukemia. *N Engl J Med* 2001;344:1031–1037.

Greenberg P, Cox C, LeBeau MM, et al. International prognostic scoring system for evaluating prognosis in myelodysplastic syndromes. *Blood* 1997;89:2079–2088.

Grimwade D, Walker H, Oliver F, et al. The importance of diagnostic cytogenetics on outcome in AML: analysis of 1,612 patients entered into the MRC 10 trial. *Blood* 1998;92:2322–2333.

The Italian Cooperative Study Group on Chronic Myeloid Leukemia. Long-term follow-up of the Italian Trial of Interferon-α versus conventional chemotherapy in chronic myeloid leukemia 1998; 92:1541–1548.

Koeffler HP, ed. Myelodysplastic syndromes. *Hematol Oncol Clin North Am* 1992;6:485–728.

Mayer RJ, Davis RB, Schiffer CA, et al. Intensive post-remission chemotherapy in adults with acute myeloid leukemia. *N Engl J Med* 1994;331:896–903.

O'Brien SG, Guilhot F, Larson RA, et al. Imatinib compared with interferon and low-dose cytarabine for newly diagnosed chronic-phase chronic myeloid leukemia. *N Engl J Med* 2003;348:994–1004.

Rai KR, Petersen BL, Appelbaum FR, et al. Fludarabine compared with chlorambucil as primary therapy for chronic lymphocytic leukemia. *N Engl J Med* 2000;343:1750–1757.

Rozman C, Montserrat E. Chronic lymphocytic leukemia. *N Engl J Med* 1995;333:1052–1057.

Saven A, Piro L. Newer purine analogues for the treatment of hairy-cell leukemia. *N Engl J Med* 1994;330:691–697.

Sawyers CL. Chronic myeloid leukemia. *N Engl J Med* 1999;340: 1330–1340.

Warrell RP, deThe H, Wang Z, et al. Acute promyelocytic leukemia. *N Engl J Med* 1993;329:177–189.

# Disorders of Platelets and Coagulation

**Steven R. Deitcher**

The human hemostatic system consists of multiple independent yet integrally related cellular and protein components. These components function to maintain blood fluidity under normal conditions and to promote localized, temporary thrombus formation at sites of vascular injury. A normal hemostatic system is the human physiologic defense against exsanguination. An abnormal hemostatic system can result in pathologic bleeding, vascular thrombosis, or both. The hemostatic system comprises six major components: platelets, vascular endothelium, procoagulant plasma protein "factors," natural anticoagulant proteins, fibrinolytic proteins, and antifibrinolytic proteins. Each of these six hemostatic components must be present in a fully functional form and in an adequate quantity to prevent excessive blood loss after vascular trauma and at the same time prevent pathologic thrombosis. The hemostatic system is highly regulated and maintains a delicate balance between a prohemorrhagic state and a prothrombotic state. Any significant acquired or congenital imbalance in the hemostatic "scales" can lead to a pathologic outcome.

Alterations in the quantitative and qualitative status of any hemostatic cellular or protein element can have significant biologic effects. Platelet deficiency (*thrombocytopenia*), platelet adhesion defects, and platelet aggregation disorders are associated with an inability to form an adequate primary hemostatic platelet plug; these conditions can lead to significant mucocutaneous bleeding and posttraumatic, life-threatening hemorrhage. In contrast, a marked increase in platelet count (*thrombocytosis*) and accentuated platelet aggregation (*sticky platelet syndrome*) are associated with thromboembolic events. A deficiency of a procoagulant factor integral to the intrinsic (factors XI, IX, and VIII), extrinsic (factor VII), or common (factors X, V, II, and fibrinogen) pathways of coagulation typically is associated with a variable degree of bleeding tendency. Elevated levels of procoagulant factors, such as factor VIII, fibrinogen, factor XI, and factor VII, on the other hand, are recognized risk factors for vascular disease and thrombosis. A deficiency of natural anticoagulant proteins, such as protein C, protein S, antithrombin III, or heparin cofactor II, is associated with venous thromboembolic disease; to date, a natural anticoagulant protein excess state associated with bleeding has not been described. A defi-

ciency of a fibrinolytic cascade component, such as tissue-type plasminogen activator or plasminogen, and excess plasma levels of the fibrinolytic inhibitor, plasminogen activator inhibitor-1, have been linked to hypercoagulability and thrombosis. A deficiency of fibrinolytic inhibitors, such as α-2 antiplasmin and plasminogen activator inhibitor-1, may precipitate a hyperfibrinolytic bleeding state. A deficiency of endothelial cell–derived von Willebrand's factor (vWF) is associated with altered primary and secondary hemostasis resulting from deficient platelet anchoring at sites of vascular injury and the shortened factor VIII survival characteristic of von Willebrand's disease (vWD). The deficient endothelial cell production of thrombomodulin or release of tissue-type plasminogen activator may be associated with a thrombotic tendency. The balance between these opposing groups of proteins, not the level of any individual factor, seems to be most critical to hemostatic regulation.

## NORMAL HEMOSTASIS

Normal hemostasis can be divided into two major processes of equal importance: *primary hemostasis* and *secondary hemostasis*. Primary hemostasis comprises the reactions needed to form a platelet plug at a site of vascular damage. Secondary hemostasis comprises the reactions needed to generate the cross-linked fibrin required to stabilize the platelet plug and to form a durable thrombus. An understanding of normal hemostasis is required to appreciate fully the disorders of hemostasis and to understand the mechanism of antithrombotic and hemostatic therapeutics. Primary hemostasis consists of three major events:

- Platelet adhesion. After vascular injury, platelets rapidly attach to exposed subendothelial collagen and vWF by means of the platelet surface glycoprotein Ib-IX.
- Platelet activation. After adhering to a site of injury, platelets are stimulated by various agonists [collagen, thrombin, epinephrine, adenosine diphosphate (ADP), and thromboxane $A_2$] to release their granule contents, which further promotes platelet activation and aggregation.

■ Platelet aggregation. Additional platelets are recruited to the site of vascular damage, where they are linked by fibrinogen through the platelet surface glycoprotein IIb-IIIa complex to form a platelet plug.

Secondary hemostasis consists of a series of reactions (*coagulation cascade*) triggered at the same time as platelet plug formation. Factors XI, IX, and VIII form the intrinsic pathway, and factor VII and tissue factor form the extrinsic pathway. Factors X, V, and II (prothrombin) and fibrinogen form the common pathway. Factor VIIIa functions as a cofactor during the activation of factor X to Xa. Factor Va functions as a cofactor during the activation of prothrombin to thrombin. Both the *tenase* and *prothrombinase* complexes require a phospholipid-rich surface, such as a platelet, to facilitate efficient reactions. Once formed, thrombin converts fibrinogen to fibrin, activates additional factor VIII and V, activates factor XIII (fibrin cross-linking factor), and participates as a platelet agonist. The pivotal role of thrombin highlights the potency of antithrombotics, such as heparin and lepirudin, which inactivate thrombin.

Natural anticoagulants function to confine thrombus formation to the sites of vascular injury and limit thrombus size. The two major natural anticoagulants are antithrombin (formerly antithrombin III) and the activated form of protein C. The activity of antithrombin is greatly enhanced by endothelial heparan and pharmacologic heparins. The activity of activated protein C is enhanced by its cofactor, protein S.

Physiologic fibrinolysis is initiated by endothelial cell–derived tissue-type plasminogen activator, which converts plasminogen to plasmin. Plasmin degrades fibrinogen and fibrin, limits the size of a thrombus, and helps clear a thrombus once the inciting vascular injury has been repaired. The fibrinolytic system itself is regulated and localized by antiplasmin and endothelial-derived plasminogen activator inhibitor-1.

## COAGULATION TESTS

The following assays constitute a core panel of tests that are essential to the efficient assessment of a patient's coagulation and platelet status. These tests are readily available at most hospitals on an around-the-clock basis. These in vitro tests are only a reflection of actual in vivo coagulation processes, however. All tests must be interpreted carefully and in light of a particular patient's clinical presentation.

### Activated Partial Thromboplastin Time

The activated partial thromboplastin time (aPTT) is a clot endpoint test that assesses the integrity of the intrinsic and common pathways of coagulation. Individual procoagulant-factor deficiencies and the multiple-factor deficiency state caused by vitamin K deficiency and liver disease result in an aPTT prolongation that can be corrected by mixing patient plasma with an equal volume of normal pooled plasma before performing the test. Alloantibody (in severe congenital hemophilia A patients) factor VIII inhibitors and autoantibody factor inhibitors (in acquired hemophilia) can prolong the aPTT by causing factor deficiency or by interfering with normal factor function. Acquired inhibitors of other coagulation factors are uncommon. Pharmacologic anticoagulants such as heparin and direct antithrombins (hirudin analogues) prolong the aPTT by inhibiting the function of activated factors. Lupus anticoagulants (LAs), a type of antiphospholipid antibody, can prolong the aPTT by interfering with the phospholipid-dependent steps of in vitro coagulation. Unlike factor deficiencies and factor inhibitors, which are associated with bleeding, LAs are associated with a thrombotic tendency.

### Prothrombin Time

The prothrombin time (PT) is a clot endpoint test that assesses the extrinsic and common pathways of coagulation. The PT is widely used to monitor warfarin-based systemic anticoagulation and is primarily a factor VII activity assay. Up to 25% of patients with an underlying LA, however, have a prolonged baseline PT. In vitamin K deficiency, both the aPTT and PT are usually elevated.

### Platelet Count

The platelet count is an integral component of the complete blood cell count and is used to screen for both states of platelet deficiency and platelet excess.

### Peripheral Blood Smear

The peripheral blood smear is required to confirm the results of a machine-derived platelet count, to assess for platelet (clumping) agglutination, and to evaluate for evidence of microangiopathic hemolysis (schistocytes and helmet cells). Microangiopathic hemolysis (red blood cell fragments) should prompt clinicians to assess for disseminated intravascular coagulation (DIC), vasculitis, and thrombotic thrombocytopenic purpura (TTP).

### Bleeding Time

The bleeding time (BT) solely reflects the coagulation elements involved in primary hemostasis (platelet plug formation). The BT prolongs in a linear fashion as the platelet count falls from 100,000/μL to 20,000/μL. The BT is not a "global" test of coagulation and does not predict surgery- or procedure-related bleeding. The value of the BT is operator-dependent and should be performed only by a trained technologist. A new whole blood in vitro assay performed on the platelet function analyzer (PFA)-100 may be preferred to the BT for vWD and platelet function defect screening.

## Thrombin Time (TT)

The thrombin time (TT) is a clot endpoint test that measures the time it takes to convert fibrinogen into fibrin. The TT is prolonged in the setting of fibrinogen deficiency (*hypofibrinogenemia*), fibrinogen dysfunction (*dysfibrinogenemia*), elevated levels of fibrin(ogen) degradation products, and anticoagulation therapy with heparins and direct antithrombins.

## Fibrinogen Level

Most fibrinogen assays measure functional fibrinogen levels using a modification of the TT. Hypofibrinogenemia can result in a prolongation of the aPTT, PT, and TT.

## D-Dimer Level

The D-dimer is a subtype of fibrin(ogen) degradation product. It is also known as a *cross-linked fibrin degradation product* (FDP) and reflects the plasmin-mediated degradation of fibrin that has been covalently cross-linked by factor XIII. Elevated levels of D-dimer reflect the concomitant activation of the coagulation cascades and fibrinolytic pathways. A normal D-dimer essentially rules out the presence of DIC, Gram-negative bacteremia, and acute venous thrombosis (Table 22.1).

The following should be noted:

■ The BT is normal in patients with hemophilia and in those receiving anticoagulants.

■ Factor XII deficiency (intrinsic pathway) results in an elevated aPTT but is not associated with bleeding. Some evidence actually supports the fact that factor XII deficiency results in hypercoagulability.

■ Low-molecular-weight heparins (LMWHs) usually are administered in fixed low doses (*thromboprophylaxis*) or in weight-based doses (*therapeutic anticoagulation*) without the need for laboratory therapeutic monitoring. Special circumstances, such as when managing pregnant, obese, or pediatric patients or those who have renal insufficiency, may warrant monitoring using an antifactor Xa activity assay. A therapeutic antifactor Xa activity level, however, may not reflect the true degree of anticoagulation or correlate with clinical outcomes. LMWH may cause a modest aPTT prolongation but the aPTT should not be used to monitor therapy with this class of anticoagulant.

■ DIC can result not only in an elevated PT and/or aPTT but also in a "short" PT and/or aPTT. The lower-than-normal values can result from the presence of prematurely activated coagulation factors in the plasma of DIC patients, which can rapidly form fibrin in clot endpoint assays.

■ Unlike DIC, patients with TTP usually have normal PT, aPTT, and fibrinogen values.

■ LAs can result in prolonged clot endpoint assays by binding the added phospholipids required for several coagulation reactions. The elevated clotting times do not reflect a bleeding tendency unless concomitant hypoprothrombinemia exists. Up to 25% of persons who have an LA have an elevated baseline PT. Some patients with LAs may have an international normalized ratio of 2.0 or more, even in the absence of oral anticoagulant therapy. LAs are acquired antibodies associated with arterial and venous thrombotic events.

## TABLE 22.1

### COMPARISON OF COAGULATION TEST RESULTS IN SELECTED DISORDERS

| Comparison of Selected Disorders | aPTT | PT | Platelets | BT[a] | TT | Fibrinogen | D-Dimer |
|---|---|---|---|---|---|---|---|
| Immune-mediated thrombocytopenia | ↔ | ↔ | ↓ | ↔ | ↔ | ↔ | ↔ |
| Thrombotic thrombocytopenic purpura | ↔ | ↔ | ↓ | ↑ | ↔ | ↔ | ↔ |
| Disseminated intravascular coagulation | ↑↔ | ↑↔ | ↓ | ↑ | ↑↔ | ↓ | ↑ |
| Aspirin, ticlopidine, or clopidogrel therapy | ↔ | ↔ | ↔ | ↑ | ↔ | ↔ | ↔ |
| Heparin therapy | ↑ | ↔ | ↔ | ↔ | ↑ | ↔ | ↔ |
| Warfarin therapy | ↔ | ↑ | ↔ | ↔ | ↔ | ↔ | ↔ |
| Vitamin K deficiency | ↑ | ↑ | ↔ | ↔ | ↔ | ↔ | ↔ |
| Low-molecular-weight heparin therapy | sl↑ | ↔ | ↔ | ↔ | sl↑ | ↔ | ↔ |
| von Willebrand's disease | ↑ | ↔ | ↔ | ↑ | ↔ | ↔ | ↔ |
| Hemophilia A (factor VIII deficiency) | ↑ | ↔ | ↔ | ↔ | ↔ | ↔ | ↔ |
| Lupus anticoagulant | ↑↔ | ↑↔ | ↔ | ↔ | ↔ | ↔ | ↔ |

↑, increased; ↓, decreased; ↔, normal; aPTT, activated partial thromboplastin time; BT, bleeding time; PT, prothrombin time; sl, slight; TT, thrombin time.
[a]Note that the BT is normal in patients with hemophilia and those receiving anticoagulants.

# SPECIFIC DISORDERS

The following disorders of hemostasis represent relatively common disorders or disorders of extreme importance that should be of particular interest to physicians practicing internal medicine.

## Von Willebrand's Disease

In 1924, Dr. Eric von Willebrand evaluated a family for what appeared to be a previously undescribed bleeding disorder. His observations identified important features that differentiated this new disorder from classic hemophilia. Bleeding was primarily mucocutaneous rather than the hemarthroses or deep muscle hematomas seen in hemophilia. Inheritance was autosomal dominant (involved both sexes) rather than X-linked. Finally, patients of this kindred had prolonged BTs, rather than the normal BTs seen in hemophilia. When he found that their platelet counts were normal, he hypothesized that a qualitative disorder of platelet function existed. Studies performed over the next several years in patients with vWD demonstrated the following:

- Normal platelets did not correct the BT.
- Platelets from patients with vWD were effective when given as platelet transfusions.
- Plasma from normal persons corrected the abnormal BT seen in vWD.

Thus, the abnormality in platelet function was not due to a defect in the platelet itself, but rather to a deficiency of a plasma factor called *vWF*. Endothelial cells and megakaryocytes synthesize and store vWF. This factor plays two major roles in normal hemostasis: (i) vWF is the intercellular bridge that links platelets to injured vascular endothelium through platelet glycoprotein Ib-IX and fibrillar collagen; and (ii) vWF protects bound factor VIII from inactivation, prolongs its intravascular half-life, and may shuttle and concentrate factor VIII at sites of vascular injury. The vWF deficiency or dysfunction (vWD) is the most common inherited bleeding disorder, with an estimated prevalence of between 1 in 1,000 to 1 in 100.

### Clinical Presentation

Mucocutaneous bleeding in the form of epistaxis, menorrhagia, gingival bleeding, and easy bruising is the most common symptom in vWD. Whereas some patients have recurrent spontaneous hemorrhage, most patients with vWD do not have frequent bleeding episodes except after trauma and surgery. Gingival bleeding after dental extraction occurs in approximately 50% of patients. Spontaneous hemarthroses are unusual and occur almost exclusively in patients with severe disease (a complete lack of functional vWF). Unlike hemophilia, affected members of the same family may have variable manifestations of this bleeding disorder, ranging from easy bruising to life-threatening hemorrhages.

### Diagnosis

The vWD most commonly is transmitted in an autosomal dominant fashion; rarely, however, it is inherited as an autosomal recessive trait. The laboratory evaluation of a person suspected of having vWD can be frustrating. Test results may vary in the same patient at different times. If an initial battery of tests is normal but clinical suspicion remains high, testing should be repeated. A relationship exists between vWF levels and the ABO blood groups. Type O patients have the lowest levels, followed by types A, B, and AB. Stress and exercise transiently increase vWF levels, and the hormonal changes that accompany pregnancy may normalize vWF levels even in severely deficient patients. The BT is usually prolonged. The aPTT is often prolonged yet may be normal in patients with mild disease. Depending on the subtype and severity of disease, accelerated factor VIII clearance results in decreased levels of factor VIII coagulant activity, which in turn results in an aPTT prolongation. vWF activity, measured as ristocetin cofactor activity, and vWF antigen are sensitive and specific tests for the detection of vWD. Crossed immunoelectrophoresis determines the multimeric structure present and allows the differentiation of the various types of vWD:

- Type 1 vWD is the most common form of vWD, accounting for approximately 80% of patients. It is inherited as an autosomal dominant trait and represents a partial, quantitative deficiency of vWF. Bleeding is most often posttraumatic, and menorrhagia is a common complaint. Levels of vWF and factor VIII are usually reduced in parallel, and all sizes of vWF multimers are present in reduced amounts.
- Type 2 vWD represents a series of *qualitative* disorders of vWF. Patients with type 2 vWD have normal or only slightly reduced levels of vWF and factor VIII.
- Type 2A vWD involves a variant of vWF that has a decreased platelet-dependent function that is associated with the absence of high-molecular-weight vWF multimers.
- Type 2B vWD comprises vWF variants with increased affinity for platelet glycoprotein Ib-IX, which may result in variable degrees of platelet agglutination and thrombocytopenia.
- Type 2M vWD represents vWF variants with decreased platelet-dependent function that is not caused by the absence of high-molecular-weight vWF multimers.
- Type 2N vWD has vWF variants with markedly decreased affinity for factor VIII caused by a mutation in the factor VIII binding domain. These patients have normal multimeric distributions, normal levels of vWF, and normal ristocetin cofactor activities, but extremely low factor VIII levels. Accordingly, the only abnormality relates to the decrease in factor VIII, and it is possible that some male patients who have previously been diagnosed as mild hemophiliacs actually have this form of vWD. This disorder is often called *autosomal hemophilia*.

- Type 3 vWD represents a profound deficiency of vWF. Patients have severe bleeding. This form of vWD is inherited in an autosomal recessive manner.
- Acquired vWD occurs as a result of the development of inhibitors to vWF and has been described in association with various malignancies: non-Hodgkin's lymphomas, Waldenström's macroglobulinemia, and multiple myeloma. These inhibitors have been associated with intestinal angiodysplasia and have developed in patients with type III vWD who have received multiple transfusions. Acquired vWD also has been described in myeloproliferative disorders.

### Treatment

Treatment options depend on the extent of the bleeding problem and the severity and type of vWD. Antifibrinolytic therapy with ε-aminocaproic acid or tranexamic acid may be sufficient to treat menorrhagia and in patients scheduled to undergo minor oral surgical procedures. Desmopressin acetate (DDAVP) administered by intravenous, subcutaneous, or intranasal routes raises vWF levels in plasma by promoting its release from endothelial cell storage bodies. Not all patients respond adequately to DDAVP, and the response diminishes over time as storage pools are depleted (tachyphylaxis). DDAVP is most effective in patients with type 1 disease, but also has been effective in those with type 2 disease. Ideally, an empiric trial of DDAVP to assess response should be performed before an anticipated operative procedure. Traditionally, its use has not been recommended in type 2B disease because an increase in this particular multimeric structure of vWF may induce excessive thrombocytopenia.

Patients with type 3 disease, patients who have not responded appropriately to DDAVP, and patients who require treatment for more than a few days should receive vWF-containing plasma products. Cryoprecipitate has been the historical mainstay of therapy, but it has the shortcoming of not being treated to reduce viral transmission. Several plasma-derived factor VIII concentrates contain all multimeric forms of vWF and are heat- or solvent detergent–treated to prevent viral disease transmission. A recombinant vWF concentrate is in development.

### Qualitative Platelet Disorders

The presence of vWF acts as the intercellular bridge between the platelet and subendothelium. In its absence or in the presence of an abnormal protein, as in vWD, a platelet adhesion defect is noted. In Bernard-Soulier syndrome, platelet glycoprotein Ib, which functions as a receptor for vWF, is deficient; accordingly, a defect in platelet adhesion results. The paraprotein that accumulates in patients with monoclonal gammopathies, such as multiple myeloma and Waldenström's macroglobulinemia, may bind to platelet membrane glycoprotein receptors and similarly interfere significantly with adhesion.

The sufficient platelet production of ADP and its subsequent release are necessary for normal aggregation. Storage pool disease can result from a decrease in the number of platelet-dense granules, which are ADP storage granules. Other patients have normal granule number and content but have impaired granule "release." Platelet glycoprotein IIb-IIIa is absent in Glanzmann's thromboasthenia. Because glycoprotein IIb-IIIa interacts with fibrinogen to promote platelet aggregation, its deficiency results in a bleeding disorder.

Secondary disorders causing acquired platelet dysfunction include the following:

- Drugs (extremely common and important to recognize)
- Uremia
- Liver disease
- Myeloproliferative and myelodysplastic disorder
- Paraproteinemias (plasma cell malignancies)
- Autoimmune disorders
- Cardiopulmonary bypass

Drugs are the most common cause of acquired platelet dysfunction, with aspirin being the most common offender. Common drugs that interfere with platelet membrane function include the tricyclics, chlorpromazine (Thorazine), cocaine, lidocaine, propranolol, cephalosporins, penicillins, and alcohol. Common drugs that interfere with platelet prostaglandin synthesis include aspirin, nonsteroidal anti-inflammatory drugs (NSAIDs), furosemide, verapamil, hydralazine, methylprednisolone, and cyclosporin A. Aspirin irreversibly impairs platelet function for the life of the platelet, whereas NSAIDs reversibly impair platelet function. Drugs that inhibit platelet phosphodiesterase activity include caffeine, dipyridamole, aminophylline, and theophylline. Drugs that irreversibly block the platelet ADP receptor include ticlopidine and clopidogrel. As may be expected, platelet glycoprotein IIb-IIIa inhibitors, such as abciximab, tirofiban, and eptifibatide, have a dramatic effect on platelet aggregation.

Platelet dysfunction during cardiopulmonary bypass surgery is often severe and multifactorial in nature. Drugs known to interfere with platelet function compound the defects produced by cardiopulmonary bypass–induced platelet activation and storage granule content depletion.

Patients with acute and chronic liver disease often have platelet dysfunction that may occur because of elevated levels of FDPs that compromise platelet function by weakly blocking platelet glycoprotein IIb-IIIa. Abnormalities in aggregation also have been noted.

Platelet dysfunction in uremia is common and may result from altered prostaglandin metabolism and abnormalities in the interaction between vWF and platelet receptors. Effective dialysis, DDAVP, conjugated estrogens, and cryoprecipitate are modes of therapy that, in some instances, have corrected the bleeding tendency associated with uremia. Platelet transfusion, however, is necessary in instances of life-threatening hemorrhage.

## Diagnosis

The BT is the screening test used to assess for platelet function abnormalities. This test is not sensitive, however, and it does not correlate with the risk of bleeding, particularly in operative settings. An abnormal BT is investigated further with platelet aggregometry using agonists such as ADP, epinephrine, collagen, ristocetin, and arachidonic acid. In some cases, the patterns of platelet aggregation seen in response to these agonists are indicative of a specific underlying disease. More commonly, however, the specific mechanism of platelet dysfunction often remains a mystery. Electron microscopy and flow cytometry often are used to assess platelets in more detail.

## Treatment

Life-threatening hemorrhage secondary to platelet dysfunction should be treated with platelet transfusion. Other specific therapy, such as plasmapheresis in the paraprotein-related disorders and dialysis in uremia, should be considered. If a drug is being used that is associated with platelet dysfunction, its use should be discontinued.

# Hemophilia A

The nature and inheritance of hemophilia were recognized as early as biblical times, when rabbis allowed infant boys to be excused from circumcision if two or more of their brothers had suffered fatal bleeding from the procedure. Hemophilia A results from a deficiency or defect of the intrinsic coagulation pathway protein factor VIII. Research suggests that the primary site of factor VIII synthesis is the vascular endothelium. Plasma factor VIII is complexed to and stabilized by vWF. Hemophilia A is an X-linked recessive disorder, making it a disease of males, all of whose sons will be normal and daughters will be obligatory carriers of the trait. Women who are hemophilia A carriers are not usually symptomatic but have a 50% likelihood of having an affected son. In the general population, hemophilia A affects 1 in every 10,000 live male births. This diseases has a relatively high spontaneous mutation rate, and as many as one-fourth to one-third of hemophiliacs may not have a family history of the disorder. The diagnosis of the carrier state may be made by analyzing familial restriction fragment length polymorphisms, ratios of plasma factor VIII activity to vWF activity, or the ratio of antigenic factor VIII to factor VIII functional activity. Women can have "true" hemophilia A only in the setting of Turner's syndrome (XO), extreme lyonization, and if the father is a hemophiliac and mother is a carrier.

## Clinical Presentation

Hemophiliacs with a factor VIII activity level of less than 1% (0.01 U/mL) are classified as *severe*, those with a level between 1% and 5% as *moderate*, and those with levels greater than 5% as *mild*. The severity of disease remains uniform among a kindred. Beginning at an early age,

patients with severe hemophilia experience spontaneous bouts of hemorrhage in the absence of any provocation. Coinheritance of a hypercoagulable state may delay the onset of bleeds in severe hemophiliacs. Patients with moderate or mild disease usually bleed only as a result of trauma and surgery. Hemarthroses and muscle hematomas are the most common bleeding manifestations of hemophilia A. As a result of repeated episodes of hemarthrosis, patients develop a chronic arthropathy, with notable cartilage destruction and synovial lining hyperplasia. The resultant joint destruction results in chronic pain, deformity, disability, and a joint even more susceptible to bleeding. The joints most frequently involved are the knees, elbows, ankles, and shoulders. Small intramuscular hematomas are common and may resolve spontaneously. Large intramuscular bleeds involving the psoas muscles or thigh muscles can result in pseudocyst formation and a compression of vital structures. Because platelet function is normal, bleeding from minor cuts or abrasions is unusual. Intracranial hemorrhage accounts for approximately 20% to 30% of deaths in hemophiliacs.

## Diagnosis

Patients with severe hemophilia A have an elevated aPTT. The PT and BT are normal. A definitive diagnosis rests on the specific assay for factor VIII activity.

## Treatment

The therapy of hemorrhagic episodes revolves around a replacement of factor VIII. Joint bleeds also benefit from rest, immobilization, compression, and elevation. A suitable factor VIII activity target for the control of mild hemorrhage is 30%. Most hemarthroses require replacement to achieve levels of approximately 50%. For life-threatening hemorrhage or in preparation for surgery, levels of 80% to 100% should be achieved. Although cryoprecipitate and fresh frozen plasma (FFP) still may be used as a replacement source of factor VIII, virally inactivated, high-purity plasma-derived and recombinant factor VIII concentrates are the preferred therapeutic agents. Intravenous, subcutaneous, and intranasal DDAVP can effect a rapid release of endogenously synthesized factor VIII from endothelial cell storage sites in patients with mild hemophilia. Because of tachyphylaxis, DDAVP is primarily useful for non--life-threatening bleeds in these patients. Prophylactic factor VIII concentrate therapy is no longer reserved for patients undergoing invasive surgical challenges; now it is provided to hemophiliac children to prevent devastating joint disease.

The major adverse effect of plasma-derived factor VIII concentrates has been the transmission of viral antigens. Hemophiliacs who received repeated treatments during the late 1970s and early 1980s were infected with human immunodeficiency virus (HIV), hepatitis B, and hepatitis C. A significant number of these persons went on to develop acquired immunodeficiency syndrome (AIDS) or chronic liver disease, and to suffer premature death. Current viral inactivation methods, combined with a safer general blood supply, have practically eliminated the risk of HIV and hepatitis C virus transmission. Because nonlipid-enveloped viruses such as hepatitis A and parvovirus B19 have been detected in these products, recombinant factor VIII concentrates have gained great popularity. Despite the persistent fear of viral illness, bleeding remains the most significant source of morbidity and mortality in hemophilia. The other major adverse effect of factor VIII replacement treatment is the formation of alloantibodies against what is perceived by the immune system as a foreign protein. Advances in gene transfer technology will likely facilitate a means of at least converting some severe hemophiliacs into less symptomatic, phenotypic, moderate hemophiliacs.

### Factor VIII Inhibitors in Hemophilia A

The development of a neutralizing alloantibody (inhibitor) to factor VIII remains one of the most devastating complications of severe hemophilia A. Inhibitors develop in at least 21% of hemophilia A patients after as few as 9 to 30 exposures to factor VIII replacement therapy; this occurs predominantly in pediatric age patients. Transient, low-titer inhibitors are most likely of minimal clinical consequence. High-titer (greater than 5 Bethesda units) and high-responding (brisk amnestic response after factor VIII re-exposure) inhibitors place patients at risk for significant morbidity and increased mortality related to bleeding. The treatment of bleeds in hemophiliacs with significant inhibitors is usually accomplished using vitamin K–dependent factor concentrates, such as factor VIII inhibitor bypassing agent, porcine-derived factor VIII concentrate, and recombinant activated factor VII (rFVIIa) concentrate. The financial and social costs associated with increased hospital and outpatient care, increased factor VIII concentrate consumption, school absenteeism, and lost productivity contribute to the overall horror of inhibitor development. The development of less immunogenic factor VIII molecules for the treatment of hemophilia A is targeted at promoting less inhibitor formation.

The induction of immune tolerance (IT) as a successful therapeutic modality for the suppression and eradication of inhibitors in hemophilia A patients has been widely used since it was introduced in 1977. Whereas the last 24 years have seen the use of several permutations of the original IT regimens, daily high-dose factor VIII concentrate infusions remain the centerpiece for most IT. Adjunctive immune modulation therapy has been used sparingly and has consisted of oral corticosteroids, cyclophosphamide, or high-dose intravenous γ-globulin (IVIG). IT regimens used to date have demonstrated similar overall efficacy with regard to IT induction (62% to 81%), but they differ significantly with respect to the time and effort required to achieve successful inhibitor eradication (1.3 to 19.6 months). The longer a patient remains on an IT protocol, the greater the cost of therapy. The longer a patient has an inhibitor, the greater the risk of uncontrollable bleeding. The optimal timing, factor dosing, and duration of IT treatment remain unresolved.

## Hemophilia B and C

Hemophilia B, a coagulation factor IX deficiency, is also an X-linked recessive disorder that is diagnosed by specific factor activity assays and treated using factor concentrates. Patients with hemophilia B rarely develop inhibitors. Both plasma-derived and recombinant monoclonal-antibody purified factor IX concentrates are available in the United States. Hemophilia B is much less common than hemophilia A (1 in 30,000 live male births). Because of its favorable gene size, factor IX is much more likely to be effectively treated by gene transfer technology in the near future.

Hemophilia C is the uncommonly used name for inherited factor XI deficiency. Unlike hemophilia A and B, factor XI deficiency is inherited in an autosomal recessive fashion. Patients with homozygous factor XI deficiency are likely to have factor levels of less than 20% and to be at risk for bleeding. FFP is the major product used for factor XI replacement therapy. Factor XI deficiency seems to be most common in persons of Ashkenazi Jewish descent.

## Acquired Hemophilia

Acquired hemophilia A is a serious immune-mediated hemorrhagic diathesis caused by the development of neutralizing and clearing antifactor VIII antibodies in persons without a pre-existent congenital factor VIII deficiency. Acquired hemophilia A is an uncommon disorder, with an annual incidence of 0.2 to 1.0 cases per million population. Persons older than age 50 years most often are affected; these patients typically present with an unexplained prolongation of the aPTT, accompanied by large ecchymotic lesions, melena, hematuria, deep hematomas, hemarthroses, compartment syndrome, and retroperitoneal or intracranial hemorrhage. Approximately 50% of patients who develop autoimmune antifactor VIII antibodies have an underlying medical condition, such as an autoimmune disease (e.g., rheumatoid arthritis, systemic lupus erythematosus), inflammatory bowel disease, malignancy, or pregnancy. Medications such as sulfonamides, phenytoin, and penicillins also have been implicated. The remaining 50% have idiopathic acquired hemophilia A. Mortality associated with major bleeding episodes approximates 22%. The cornerstone of therapy is the acute control of bleeding using large doses of human factor VIII concentrate to saturate and overcome the inhibitor, factor VIII–bypassing agents, porcine factor VIII concentrate, or recombinant activated factor VII concentrate, combined with immunosuppression to eradicate the inhibitor itself. Inhibitors to other coagulation factors including vWF, factor V, and factor IX have been described but are relatively rare.

## Autoimmune Thrombocytopenic Purpura

Acute immune thrombocytopenic purpura (ITP) is primarily a self-limited disease of children. Acute ITP often follows a viral illness, is associated with profound thrombocytopenia, and uncommonly requires specific therapeutic intervention. Adults can develop acute ITP but more commonly develop chronic ITP. Women are affected by ITP more frequently than men. ITP develops most commonly in persons between the ages of 20 and 40 years.

### Pathophysiology and Diagnosis

Most adults with chronic ITP have platelet-associated immunoglobulin G (IgG) antibodies detectable in their serum. These antibodies may be directed against specific membrane glycoproteins, such as glycoprotein IIIa, IIb, or Ib. These antibodies, therefore, are able to induce a qualitative platelet disorder in addition to inducing accelerated platelet clearance and thrombocytopenia. Platelet-associated IgG is not specific for chronic ITP because it may be detected in settings such as in the presence of solid tumors and lymphoproliferative disorders as well as in normal persons. Antiplatelet antibody testing is not generally recommended. The diagnosis of ITP requires the exclusion of other disorders associated with immune thrombocytopenia, such as connective tissue diseases, lymphoproliferative disorders, and HIV infection. Immune thrombocytopenia is common in HIV-infected patients and results from an immune complex–mediated phenomenon. The consumption of drugs that may be associated with immune thrombocytopenia (quinidine, cimetidine, trimethoprim-sulfamethoxazole) also should be excluded. A peripheral blood smear review is required to rule out artifactual thrombocytopenia resulting from ethylenediaminetetra-acetic acid (EDTA)–induced platelet clumping and processes such as TTP and DIC. A bone marrow examination allows the confirmation of the presence of megakaryocytes, thus confirming that a patient's thrombocytopenia is due to peripheral destruction and not underproduction.

### Treatment

Corticosteroids are the initial treatment of choice in adults with chronic ITP. Treatment is usually reserved for patients with active bleeding or extremely low platelet counts that place them at risk for spontaneous hemorrhage. A response to steroids (prednisone, 1 to 2 mg/kg daily) is generally seen within 7 to 14 days. If a response is seen, treatment should be continued for 2 to 4 additional weeks, and then a slow taper of the steroid begun. In patients refractory to corticosteroids, or whose daily maintenance dose of prednisone is greater than 10 mg, alternative or adjunctive treatments should be considered. Approximately 50% to 60% of patients who respond well, but incompletely, to steroids respond to splenectomy. Pneumococcal and *Haemophilus influenzae* vaccines should be administered 2 to 3 weeks before splenectomy if possible. Splenic irradiation may be considered in patients who are not medically fit for an operation or who refuse the procedure. In patients who do not respond to splenectomy, or who relapse subsequent to an initial response, alternative treatment is indicated.

In the setting of ITP and active bleeding in need of a rapid platelet response, high-dose IVIG may promptly induce an increase in circulating platelet count and improve the response to platelet transfusion. The exact mechanism of action of IVIG in ITP is unknown, but its effectiveness most likely results from a blockade of Fc receptors on reticuloendothelial cells. A second possible mechanism of action would be downregulation of antiplatelet antibody production. Rho(+) immune globulin (anti-D antibodies) infusion also appears to have activity in ITP, without the need for protracted IVIG infusions. Danazol, an attenuated androgen, has been associated with therapeutic responses in ITP. Danazol may be particularly useful in elderly patients who are not good candidates for splenectomy. Protracted danazol therapy of several months' duration is often necessary before a therapeutic response is seen. Danazol also should be considered in patients who relapse after undergoing splenectomy. Immunosuppressive agents (e.g., vincristine, azathioprine, cyclophosphamide, cyclosporin A) have been shown to be effective in selected patients refractory to standard treatments. Their use in association with corticosteroids generally allows the dose of the latter to be significantly reduced. They have the disadvantage, however, of significantly greater toxicities, including myelosuppression and neurotoxicity. Antibody therapy targeted against CD20-bearing B cells also has been successfully used.

If the patient is not bleeding, platelet transfusions are not indicated; however, if serious bleeding problems result, platelet transfusions should not be withheld, and platelet count increases after these transfusions may be seen. As noted, prior therapy with IVIG may increase the therapeutic benefit of platelet transfusions.

In the setting of immune thrombocytopenia in a patient with HIV infection, the use of antiretroviral agents often has produced significant amelioration of the thrombocytopenia. As noted, the underlying pathophysiology of immune thrombocytopenia in HIV infection may be related to immune complex deposition with antibody and viral antigen. If the amount of viral antigen can be reduced, the immune complex deposition also may be reduced and fewer platelets affected.

Many patients with ITP will have unsatisfactory responses to all the therapeutic modalities mentioned previously. These patients may, however, maintain a good quality of life with moderate thrombocytopenia in the range of 30,000/μL to 60,000/μL; if such is the case, no specific therapy is required. Periodically, they may undergo surgical procedures or suffer trauma. During these periods, a reinstitution of high-dose steroid therapy, high-dose IVIG, Rho(+) immune globulin, and platelet transfusions generally provides significant benefit.

## Heparin-Induced Thrombocytopenia

Heparin-induced thrombocytopenia (HIT), also known as the *white clot syndrome*, is a relatively common but under-recognized and potentially devastating immunoglobulin-mediated complication of heparin administration. HIT with thrombosis (HITT) constitutes the major life- and limb-threatening complication of the far more common clinical syndrome known as HIT. The prompt consideration of these paradoxic, thrombotic, adverse drug reactions in patients who develop thrombocytopenia, with or without new or propagating venous and arterial limb thromboses during heparin therapy, is the cornerstone to appropriate HITT diagnosis and limb salvage. An immediate discontinuation of all forms and routes of heparin exposure remains the essential component of HITT treatment.

Typically, HIT develops between 5 and 14 days after the commencement of heparin therapy and produces a variable but often profound thrombocytopenia. A platelet count fall that begins before day 5 of heparin exposure is not likely to represent HIT, except in patients with a recent (within 3 months) heparin exposure. These patients may experience an abrupt onset of thrombocytopenia on re-exposure to heparin as a result of acute platelet activation secondary to circulating HIT IgG. HIT has been noted to develop in up to 3% to 5% of patients exposed to unfractionated (standard porcine- and bovine-derived) heparin. Of these, 36% to 50% of patients with HIT develop life- or limb-threatening thromboses as a result of HITT. The fact that the thrombocytopenia seen in HIT usually resolves within 3 to 7 days of heparin withdrawal is a useful aid to making the diagnosis of HIT. The thrombotic tendency associated with HIT can last for at least 30 days, and HITT can develop well after the discontinuation of heparin and platelet count recovery. HIT and HITT appear to occur infrequently as a result of primary LMWH therapy, but at present, LMWH should not be used for the anticoagulant therapy of patients who have developed HIT or HITT because of a near 100% likelihood of HIT IgG cross-reactivity and anecdotal evidence of clinical syndrome perpetuation.

Immune-mediated HIT must be differentiated from the far more common and benign nonimmune heparin-associated thrombocytopenia. This phenomenon is observed most commonly after large doses of heparin, has an incidence of up to 10%, and is not detected by the usual HIT diagnostic assays. Nonimmune heparin-associated thrombocytopenia is associated with mild thrombocytopenia (rarely less than 100,000 platelets/$\mu$L), which develops within the initial 1 to 2 days of heparin exposure. The platelet count fall may be related to a direct activating effect on platelets by heparin. The platelet count typically normalizes despite continued heparin exposure. Unlike HIT, no significant adverse clinical events, such as thrombosis, are associated with this entity, and heparin administration may be continued.

The pathogenesis of HIT and HITT involves the formation of multimolecular complexes between heparin and platelet factor 4 (PF4), a normal platelet $\alpha$-granule moiety that is released by platelets when they are activated by agonists, including heparin. In some patients, IgG-class antibodies are generated against the heparin:PF4 complexes. The immune complexes comprising heparin, PF4, and anti-heparin:PF4 antibodies interact with platelet Fc-$\gamma$II receptors, thus leading to potent platelet activation, platelet aggregation, procoagulant platelet microparticle formation, and a marked increase in thrombin generation. HIT-associated IgG also has been demonstrated to activate the endothelium in vitro by interacting with heparin:PF4 complexes formed on the endothelial cell surface. Theoretically, this endothelial cell activation may lead to increased tissue factor synthesis, which may contribute further to excess thrombin generation and thrombosis formation. HITT most likely constitutes a more severe and protracted form of HIT, with evidence of macrovascular thrombosis or thrombus-induced end-organ dysfunction.

Thrombosis is the major complication of HIT. Venous thrombosis is more common than arterial thrombosis in HIT patients, especially in patients who receive heparin for postoperative deep venous thrombosis prophylaxis. Extremity deep venous thrombosis is the most frequently encountered venous thrombotic complication in HIT patients, followed infrequently by pulmonary embolism and cerebral sinus thrombosis. Most HIT-associated arterial thromboses involve the extremities, but stroke, myocardial infarction, and renal artery thrombosis related to heparin infusion have been described. HITT after coronary artery bypass grafting may present as bypass graft occlusion, left atrial thrombus formation, valvular thrombosis, or pulmonary embolism. It is reasonable to assume that patients with pre-existing vascular lesions, intravascular catheters, sepsis, and postoperative venous stasis are particularly susceptible to the thrombotic complications of HIT.

Heparin-induced skin lesions have been observed in approximately 10% to 20% of patients who generate HIT IgG in response to subcutaneous heparin injections. The skin lesions develop at heparin injection sites and can range from painful, red plaques to overt skin necrosis. Thrombocytopenia may not develop in most patients with heparin-induced skin lesions, but those who develop skin lesions and thrombocytopenia appear to be at high risk for arterial thrombosis. Other clinical presentations of HIT include heparin "resistance" and adrenal vein thrombosis that leads to hemorrhagic infarction, primarily in patients in the intensive care unit (ICU). The thrombocytopenia that develops in this syndrome is not normally associated with hemorrhagic events, and platelet transfusion may exacerbate the HIT-induced prothrombotic tendency. The identification of any platelet-rich "white clot" during surgical thrombectomy should alert surgeons to the possible existence of HITT.

It is not uncommon for postoperative and critically ill patients to develop thrombocytopenia as a result of events unrelated to HIT. The differential diagnosis of thrombocytopenia that develops in the ICU can be extensive and complex. Thrombocytopenia in this setting can result from hemodilution, nonimmune heparin-associated thrombocytopenia, bacteremia, DIC, and nonheparin medications. HIT always must be considered strongly because a failure to discontinue all heparin promptly and to initiate an effective alternative antithrombotic agent can result in significant morbidity and mortality. HIT may not be the most common cause of thrombocytopenia in ICU patients, but it certainly may be the most limb and life threatening.

Both HIT and HITT usually are associated with a platelet count below the lower limits of normal, which is approximately $150,000/\mu L$ in most laboratories. The diagnosis should be strongly considered in any patient in whom the platelet count falls below 50% of the baseline value after the fifth day of heparin treatment. A 30% fall in baseline platelet count combined with any form of thrombosis in a patient receiving heparin should be considered HITT until proved otherwise. HIT and HITT should be considered clinical diagnoses, and HIT diagnostic assays should be reserved for HIT confirmation and possibly for anticoagulant cross-reactivity testing. Because of the inherent delay in receiving the results of HIT diagnostic assays and the limited availability of such testing at most facilities, HIT management should begin at the earliest clinical recognition of the syndrome.

Both functional and antigenic assays are available to detect HIT IgG. Functional assays detect the ability of a patient whose serum contains HIT IgG to activate normal donor platelets in the presence of heparin. Activation endpoints, such as carbon-14–serotonin release, platelet aggregation, and platelet adenosine triphosphate release (lumi-aggregometry), are used in various assay systems. Antigenic assays based on the ability of patient HIT IgG to bind solid-phase heparin:PF4 complexes (enzyme-linked immunosorbent assay methodology) have been developed and are commercially available for use in the United States. False-negative results in patients who form platelet-activating antibodies that recognize an antigen other than heparin:PF4 complexes and positive HIT IgG detection in patients without any clinical manifestation of HIT illustrate the limitations of the antigenic assay diagnostic method. A quantification of platelet microparticle formation by flow cytometric analysis also has been used to diagnose HIT. Because the ability to make a definitive objective diagnosis of HIT and HITT eludes us, clinical diagnosis remains the "gold standard."

The most essential element in the treatment of HIT and HITT remains the discontinuation of all heparin, including heparin line flushes, subcutaneous heparin, and heparin-coated indwelling catheters. Despite heparin discontinuation and platelet count recovery, patients with isolated, serologically confirmed HIT have an approximately 50% risk of developing a confirmed thrombotic event during the 30-day period after heparin stoppage. The persistent prothrombotic tendency associated with HIT, the presence

of thrombus in HITT, and a patient's original indication for heparin therapy all warrant the use of an alternative anticoagulant agent after heparin cessation. Anticoagulants that have been used with varying degrees of success for the management of patients with HIT and HITT include argatroban (synthetic direct thrombin inhibitor), ancrod (defibrinogenating Malayan pit viper venom), danaparoid sodium (anticoagulant glycosaminoglycan mixture with antifactor Xa activity), recombinant hirudin (medicinal leech-derived direct-antithrombin), low-molecular-weight dextran, and LMWH.

Interest in LMWH as a treatment for HIT stems from the observation that LMWH is less likely than unfractionated heparins to elicit HIT IgG formation and less likely to cause clinical HIT and HITT. Because of a high likelihood for in vitro and in vivo cross-reactivity (80% to 100%) of the HIT IgG for LMWH, this class of anticoagulant may be harmful in patients who already have formed HIT IgG. Danaparoid sodium, composed mainly of heparan sulfate, dermatan sulfate, and chondroitin sulfate, may cross-react with 10% to 20% of HIT sera, but in vivo cross-reactivity is not commonly observed.

Recombinant hirudin (lepirudin) has been approved by the U.S. Food and Drug Administration (FDA) for the treatment of HIT. Lepirudin does not cross-react with heparin, has a short half-life, is able to inactivate clot-bound thrombin, and can be monitored using the ubiquitous aPTT assay. The major drawbacks to lepirudin are the lack of an antidote, the development of clearance-inhibiting antibodies in approximately 40% of treated patients, and the extreme care needed when treating patients with even mild renal insufficiency. Marked bolus and infusion rate reductions are necessary in patients with a creatinine clearance of less than 60 mL/minute (serum creatinine of more than 1.6). Lepirudin is to be avoided completely in the settings of hemodialysis or acute renal failure.

Argatroban is a synthetic lysine analog direct thrombin inhibitor that also has been approved by the FDA for use in patients with HIT. Argatroban does not cross-react with heparin, has a shorter half-life than lepirudin, and can be monitored by aPTT. Argatroban does not induce antibody formation and is safe for use in the setting of renal insufficiency. Argatroban should be avoided in the setting of significant liver dysfunction.

Warfarin anticoagulation may be desired for long-term therapy, but it never should be used as the sole alternative anticoagulant in patients with HIT and HITT. Warfarin has the disadvantages of requiring 5 days or longer to achieve full therapeutic effect and has been associated with venous limb gangrene when used alone. Warfarin treatment is the major factor contributing to the limb amputation caused by a progression of otherwise unremarkable deep venous thromboses to phlegmasia cerulea dolens in HIT patients. The combination of HIT-associated hypercoagulability and warfarin-induced protein C deficiency most likely produces a profound procoagulant state, which causes venous limb gangrene. The existence of this syndrome justifies the absolute need for systemic anticoagulation with an agent like lepirudin or argatroban during the initiation of warfarin anticoagulation in patients with HIT and HITT.

Adjuncts to alternative anticoagulant therapy in the management of HIT and HITT include antiplatelet agents (e.g., aspirin and ticlopidine), high-dose IVIG, and prostacyclin analog (iloprost) infusion. The benefit of these agents is primarily anecdotal in nature. Interest and clinical experience in using parenteral and oral platelet glycoprotein IIb-IIIa inhibitors to reverse or prevent the harmful platelet aggregation found in HIT are mounting. Surgical thromboembolectomy and pharmacologic thrombolysis should be reserved for selected patients. Thromboembolectomy may provide limited benefit in patients with limb artery occlusion because of the diffuse nature of the thrombotic process, which extends into the small vasculature. The administration of thrombolytic agents to patients with HIT and thrombosis offers the benefit of promoting anticoagulation secondary to fibrinogen depletion and FDP accumulation while at the same time lysing the thrombotic obstruction.

Considering the complexity of HIT diagnosis and treatment, HIT prevention must be emphasized. Patients receiving heparin should have platelet count monitoring at baseline and probably every third day between day 5 and day 21 of heparin exposure. Early oral warfarin anticoagulation initiation in patients receiving heparin therapy for an acute thrombosis or atrial fibrillation should allow the duration of heparin exposure to be kept to a minimum and, it is hoped, under 5 days. Appropriate medical record documentation and patient education should help avert heparin re-exposure in patients with a history of HIT or HITT. Re-exposure to heparin in patients with past HIT or HITT should be delayed at least 3 months, kept to a minimum duration to provide succinct anamnesis, and avoided when possible. LMWH may be preferable to unfractionated heparin for both the treatment and prevention of thromboembolic disease because of the greatly reduced likelihood of instigating HIT and HITT.

## Thrombotic Thrombocytopenic Purpura

Thrombotic thrombocytopenic purpura is a multisystem disorder characterized by disseminated microvascular thrombotic phenomenon. TTP and the other thrombotic microangiopathy, hemolytic-uremic syndrome (HUS), are believed to be variants of the TTP-HUS syndrome. The syndrome is characterized by thrombocytopenia, microangiopathic hemolytic anemia, fever, renal dysfunction, and neurologic symptoms. *TTP* usually refers to the disorder that develops in adults in which neurologic symptoms predominate, whereas *HUS* refers to the pediatric disorder in which renal failure predominates. Neurologic signs and symptoms can range from headache to frank coma. Because the anemia in TTP is associated with mechanical

red blood cell damage caused by microthrombi, schistocytes are identified easily on the peripheral smear, and serum lactate dehydrogenase is elevated. An elevated indirect bilirubin, aspartate aminotransferase, or serum glutamic-oxaloacetic transaminase, and reticulocyte count usually accompanies the hemolytic anemia. Thrombocytopenia is universally present and often severe. An elevated serum amylase and lipase level reflects TTP-associated pancreatitis. TTP is most commonly wrongly identified as vasculitis, catastrophic antiphospholipid antibody syndrome, HELLP (*h*emolysis, *e*levated *l*iver enzymes, and *l*ow *p*latelet count), sepsis, ITP, and DIC. TTP, unlike DIC, does not result in abnormal coagulation times and fibrinogen levels. TTP has been associated with HIV infection and the use of drugs such as cyclosporine, mitomycin C, ticlopidine, and clopidogrel.

The cause of TTP has been hotly debated for years. Many believe that a vascular toxin accumulates; others believe a vital inhibitor of platelet aggregation is lacking. Most recently, it was demonstrated that the sera from TTP patients is able to induce apoptosis in cultured human endothelial cells from most organs, except the lungs and liver. This finding supports the notion of a toxic substance and is interesting because TTP rarely affects the lungs and liver. It also was shown that deficiency of an inhibitor of vWF-cleaving protease results in the formation of unusually large vWF multimers and the development of chronic relapsing TTP. Thus, both schools of thought seem to have merit.

### Treatment

Because TTP is a medical emergency, treatment should be initiated as soon as possible, even if one is not completely certain about the diagnosis. Therapy should be undertaken despite the severity of symptoms and the overall status of the patient. It should be continued until a remission occurs or the patient dies. Failure to recognize the diagnosis and provide prompt, effective treatment has been associated with a mortality rate approaching 90%. Even with the best treatment, mortality may be as high as 20% to 30%.

The treatment of choice in patients with TTP is plasma exchange, which combines plasmapheresis with donor plasma infusion. If the equipment necessary for plasmapheresis is unavailable, therapy consisting of plasma infusion alone may be instituted until arrangements can be made for plasmapheresis. In some hands, the use of vincristine has led to an increased response rate. Anecdotal reports of therapeutic benefit from high doses of γ-globulin, corticosteroids, antiplatelet agents, splenectomy, and the infusion of cryosupernatant (plasma minus the vWF-containing cryoprecipitate) have been published. The goal of therapy is the normalization of the neurologic signs and symptoms and of the platelet count, serum lactate dehydrogenase, and peripheral blood smear. If evidence of a therapeutic response from plasma exchange alone is not seen in 3 to 5 days, adjunctive therapies should be considered. Platelet transfusions should be avoided because they may aggravate the underlying pathologic process.

As more and more patients survive, a distinct entity known as *chronic relapsing TTP* has been described. Hematologic abnormalities predominate in these relapsing situations. Patients who relapse are treated similarly to patients with de novo TTP. Splenectomy and periodic prophylactic plasma exchanges may be helpful in this setting.

## Disseminated Intravascular Coagulation

Disseminated intravascular coagulation is a potentially lethal, complex, consumptive coagulopathy associated with a variety of medical and surgical disease states. DIC itself is not a disease but, like fever, is a manifestation of a multitude of underlying disorders. Unlike normal localized coagulation in response to focal vascular injury, DIC represents an exaggerated, poorly controlled systemic response to illness. Whatever the inciting event, procoagulant mechanisms are activated, intravascular fibrin is produced, small-vessel thrombosis occurs, and ischemic organ damage results. A compensatory fibrinolysis develops, and combined with the exhaustion of coagulation factors and thrombocytopenia, a hemorrhagic diathesis may occur.

### Clinical Presentation

Conditions associated with the development of acute DIC include obstetric accidents, such as abruptio placenta and retained dead fetus; bacterial sepsis; massive tissue injury secondary to trauma or burns; and acute leukemia. On the surface, acute DIC primarily appears to be a hemorrhagic disorder. Patients may have bleeding from all vascular access sites and sites of mucosal trauma. One must remember that DIC-associated bleeding results from factor deficiencies and thrombocytopenia caused by diffuse, organ-based, microvascular thromboses.

A more indolent, chronic DIC is associated with solid tumors, connective tissue disorders, and abdominal aortic aneurysms. Because the rate of factor consumption is balanced by a compensatory increased rate of production, chronic DIC is also known as *compensated DIC*. The usual DIC screening tests may be normal in this setting, but the fibrinogen level often is depressed slightly. Hemorrhage may occur when the hemostatic system is stressed by trauma, surgery, or intercurrent infection. In chronic DIC, thrombotic complications may predominate.

### Diagnosis

The PT and aPTT usually are prolonged in patients with DIC. The fibrinogen level is either low or is found to be decreasing on serial measurements. FDPs are present. The most accurate FDP is the D-dimer, which is released only when thrombin is activated to produce fibrin from fibrinogen; secondarily, this fibrin is degraded by plasmin. Monoclonal antibodies to this fused region have been developed that do not cross-react with fibrinogen or other FDPs. Antithrombin, along with other natural anticoagulants, is also consumed in DIC, and thus its levels are diminished. The TT is prolonged by the presence of FDPs and depressed fibrinogen levels. Platelets are consumed during intravascular coagulation, and thrombocytopenia, often severe, results. Red blood cells that encounter strands of fibrin laid across the vessel lumen are sheared, and microangiopathic hemolysis results.

### Treatment

The cornerstone of therapy for DIC is the identification and amelioration of the precipitating cause. If the inciting event is rapidly reversible, supportive therapy may suffice. If bleeding occurs while this goal is pursued, transfusion therapy with cryoprecipitate as a source of fibrinogen, FFP as a source of clotting factors, and platelets to correct the resulting thrombocytopenia may be effective. If the pathologic process that produced this coagulopathy is not readily reversible, or serious refractory bleeding occurs, anticoagulation with heparin or LMWH may be cautiously considered. Anticoagulation in this situation interrupts the consumption of coagulation factors and fibrinogen and may cease clinical bleeding. The goal of therapy is to allow the fibrinogen to increase to a level above 100 to 150 mg/dL. Central nervous system bleeding and severe thrombocytopenia contraindicate the use of heparin. Continued replacement with cryoprecipitate and FFP is indicated. The infusion of antithrombin concentrates in patients with severe DIC seems theoretically sound and prudent. Unfortunately, infusions are often begun too late to accomplish much more than an improvement in laboratory parameters without impacting patient outcome. Activated protein C concentrate has been shown to be effective as an adjunctive treatment in persons with severe sepsis, which is often accompanied by DIC.

In patients who have thrombotic events associated with chronic DIC, particularly in association with a malignancy, anticoagulation with warfarin is often unsuccessful in preventing further thrombotic events. In this situation, the use of heparin or LMWH should be considered.

## HYPERCOAGULABLE STATES

The term *hypercoagulable state* and its synonym *thrombophilia* refer to any inherited or acquired abnormality of the hemostatic system that places a person at increased risk for venous or arterial thrombosis. These abnormalities include elevated levels of selected procoagulant factors (fibrinogen, factor VIII, factor XI, and prothrombin), deficiencies of natural anticoagulant proteins (antithrombins, protein C, and protein S), thrombocythemia, "sticky" platelets, fibrinolytic system derangements, and endothelial cell dysfunction. Any approach to the hypercoagulable patient should include a comprehensive clinical evaluation and a carefully conceived laboratory evaluation. The "best" approach must be individualized to meet the specific needs of an individual patient.

The clinical evaluation is necessary not only to guide acute thrombosis management and screen patients for an idiopathic thrombosis-associated malignancy but also to help determine which patients will benefit most from special coagulation laboratory testing. The clinical evaluation should include an assessment for thrombosis risk factors, such as recent trauma, recent surgical procedures, prior history of thrombosis, family history of thrombosis, pregnancy, exogenous estrogen use (including oral contraceptive pill use), and a history of recurrent fetal loss. A knowledge of a patient's age at the time of a first thrombosis; the location of thrombosis; and whether thromboses involve the arterial vascular tree, venous system, or both, are also important components in the clinical evaluation. Patients who are traditionally considered for hypercoagulable state screening tests include those with a family history of thrombosis, a history of recurrent idiopathic thrombosis, thrombosis at an early age (before the age of 45 years), thrombosis after minimal provocation, thrombosis in an unusual site, and thrombosis in association with a history of early fetal loss. It is of paramount importance that testing include tests of proven value and that the tests are performed only on patients for whom the results will provide a distinct benefit.

Testing rarely impacts acute thrombosis management, but acute thrombosis and its management certainly impact the results and validity of coagulation tests. For this reason, testing typically should be postponed until a course of anticoagulation has been completed and the patient is no longer in a state of acute illness, in which acute-phase protein release is common. Test results should be compared carefully to locally derived normal ranges that reflect the patient population being tested because gender and age may impact the normal range of several plasma protein levels. Testing usually begins with an assessment of the PT, aPTT, clottable fibrinogen, and TT. These widely available tests help to detect LAs and dysfibrinogenemias, which can be associated with a thrombotic tendency. Specialized tests that address hereditary hypercoagulable states in general, and in the setting of idiopathic venous thromboembolism in particular, include activated protein C resistance (factor V Leiden), prothrombin G20210A, antithrombin activity, protein C activity, protein S activity, and plasma homocysteine levels. The first two tests mentioned evaluate more recently described genetic defects that predispose an affected person to primarily venous thrombosis. Because of the low prevalence of these two disorders in Asian and African American populations, it may be most appropriate to limit testing to White patients. A quantification of free (active) and total protein S antigen levels may be required to validate activity assay results. Testing for acquired hypercoagulable states includes tests for anticardiolipin antibodies (ACAs), LAs, and vitamin deficiency–induced hyperhomocysteinemia.

Both inherited and vitamin deficiency–associated hyperhomocysteinemic states are amenable to treatment with folic acid or vitamin $B_{12}$ and vitamin $B_6$. Antiphospholipid antibody (ACA and LA) are of particular importance in the setting of recurrent fetal loss and arterial thrombosis. Because activated protein C resistance, prothrombin G20210A, and hyperhomocysteinemia are the most common abnormalities in selected groups with thrombosis, it is prudent to evaluate each as part of a workup.

In summary, hypercoagulable state testing should be reserved for patients who have had an objectively documented thrombosis and who, after careful clinical history evaluation, are considered most likely to have an underlying coagulation defect. Hypercoagulable state testing might be best reserved for those situations in which the results will significantly impact the choice of antithrombotic therapy, intensity of therapy, duration of therapy, monitoring of therapy, use of estrogen-containing drugs, family planning, and family screening. The entire clinical and family situation must be taken into consideration to ensure that testing is being performed in a setting in which the results will be used specifically to make prophylactic or therapeutic recommendations.

## ANTIPHOSPHOLIPID ANTIBODIES

Among antiphospholipid antibodies, LAs are immunoglobulins that have the ability to prolong phospholipid-dependent coagulation tests. ACAs are immunoglobulins that bind phospholipid-binding proteins such as prothrombin, protein C, and $\beta_2$-glycoprotein-I. LAs and ACAs are distinct types of antiphospholipid antibodies, with only the minority of antibodies capable of functioning as both. Present in 5% to 15% of patients with systemic lupus erythematosus, these antiphospholipid antibodies also can be seen in a variety of clinical conditions, including malignancies, drug reactions, HIV infection, and otherwise healthy individuals.

The prolonged aPTT or PT seen in patients with LAs are an in vitro phenomenon and do not reflect an underlying bleeding tendency. In fact, LAs are strongly associated with an increased risk for recurrent arterial and venous thromboembolic events. Bleeding associated with an LA usually reflects concomitant hypoprothrombinemia or immune thrombocytopenia. The diagnosis of an LA is made by demonstrating the prolongation of a phospholipid-dependent, clot endpoint test such as the aPTT, PT, kaolin clotting time, tissue thromboplastin inhibition test, and dilute Russel viper venom time. The prolongation must not be secondary to a factor deficiency and must be able to be significantly corrected by the addition of saturating quantities of exogenous phospholipids (phospholipid or platelet neutralization). ACAs are detected by enzyme-linked immunosorbent assay. Test results can vary with time. A persistently elevated

ACA titer and consistently detected LA are most clinically significant.

An asymptomatic antiphospholipid antibody patient does not require therapy. The presence of an antiphospholipid antibody in a patient with idiopathic venous thrombosis, however, is associated with one of the highest risks of recurrent thrombosis after warfarin anticoagulation discontinuation. For this reason, it is recommended that such patients receive long-term warfarin therapy.

## REVIEW EXERCISES

### Questions

**1.** A 48-year-old woman has had a stormy course after cholecystectomy. Before surgery, she had poor oral intake, and after surgery she has been receiving broad-spectrum antibiotics. On postoperative day 5, surgical wound site bleeding and prolongation of the PT and aPTT were noted. She has been receiving subcutaneous heparin 5,000 U every 12 hours for deep venous thrombosis prophylaxis. You are consulted to rule out DIC. The test results are PT, 16 seconds (control, 12 seconds); aPTT, 56 seconds (normal range, 28 to 32 seconds); fibrinogen, 326 mg/dL at 0800h (8:00 a.m.) and 354 mg/dL at 2000h (8:00 p.m.) (normal, 200 to 450 mg/dL); TT, 10 seconds (normal, less than 15 seconds); and platelets, $296,000 \times 10^6$/L.

Which of the following is the most likely diagnosis?
a) Intravascular coagulation
b) Heparin effect
c) Vitamin K deficiency
d) Acquired hemophilia A
e) Antithrombin III deficiency

**2.** A 22-year-old man with recent coryzal symptoms becomes lethargic and confused. During his emergency room evaluation, he has a witnessed seizure. He is postictal, pale, icteric, and febrile and has petechiae. His laboratory results include hemoglobin, 6.0 g/dL; platelets, $6,000 \times 10^6$/L; and lactate dehydrogenase, 3,000 IU/L. Coagulation studies, including aPTT, PT, fibrinogen, and D-dimer, are normal.

The initial therapy should consist of which of the following?
a) Low-dose heparin
b) Plasma exchange
c) Platelet transfusion
d) Splenectomy
e) Plasmapheresis and replacement with salt-free albumin

**3.** A 21-year-old woman presents to your emergency room with a dense hemiparesis. Platelet count is $3,000 \times 10^6$/L. Her medical identification necklace says "I have ITP."

Initial management should include which of the following?

a) Platelet transfusion
b) Intravenous corticosteroids
c) IVIG
d) Neurosurgical consultation
e) All of the above

**4.** A 56-year-old man has an uneventful mitral valve replacement. Heparin was given during the surgery and continued postoperatively. On the eighth postoperative day, the patient develops a painful, cold, pulseless leg. His aPTT is noted to be subtherapeutic at 42 seconds, and his platelet count dropped from $110,000 \times 10^6$/L on postoperative day 1 to $55,000 \times 10^6$/L.

The most important step in the initial management is which of the following?
a) To obtain a vascular surgery consultation
b) To increase the dose of heparin to achieve a therapeutic aPTT
c) Platelet transfusions to achieve a platelet count greater than $100,000 \times 10^6$/L
d) To discontinue all heparin immediately
e) To order a heparin-induced platelet aggregation test and begin warfarin so that heparin can be stopped if the test returns positive

**5.** A 70-year-old woman with a history of multiple myeloma develops a pathologic fracture of her femur. PT, aPTT, and platelet count are normal before open reduction and internal fixation of her femur. A life-threatening hemorrhage occurs intraoperatively. An intraoperative coagulation testing reveals a prolonged BT. PT, aPTT, and platelet count remain normal.

Which of the following diagnoses is most likely in this setting?
a) DIC
b) Vitamin K deficiency
c) LA
d) Platelet dysfunction secondary to dysproteinemia
e) Acquired hemophilia A

**6.** What is the most appropriate initial therapy for the patient in the preceding question?
a) Plasmapheresis or exchange
b) FFP infusion
c) Platelet transfusion
d) Factor VIII and vWF concentrate infusion
e) Aspirin

**7.** Which of the following bleeding disorders can be present despite normal screening coagulation studies (PT, aPTT, BT)?
a) Mild vWD
b) Mild hemophilia A
c) Factor XIII deficiency
d) $\alpha_2$-Antiplasmin deficiency
e) All of the above

**8.** A 22-year-old woman has slammed her arm with a car door. A compartment syndrome develops, and in preparation for surgery, a prolonged aPTT is found. She has been evaluated for menorrhagia and easy bruising in the past without a specific diagnosis being made. Other family members of both genders have had similar bleeding problems.

Which is the most likely diagnosis?
a) Mild hemophilia A
b) ITP
c) LA
d) vWD type 1
e) Deficiency of $\alpha_2$-macroglobulin

**9.** A 72-year-old woman develops a massive hematoma after leg trauma. Surgical fasciotomies to treat a compartment syndrome result in profound bleeding. Personal and family histories of bleeding are noncontributory. Laboratory testing reveals a prolonged aPTT that does not correct when mixed with normal plasma and incubated at 37°C for 2 hours. PT, BT, fibrinogen, and platelet count are normal. What test is most likely to confirm the diagnosis?
a) Reptilase time
b) Factor VIII activity assay
c) Peripheral blood smear examination
d) Factor XII activity assay
e) Dilute Russell's viper venom time

**10.** A 68-year-old man undergoes a left total hip arthroplasty because of degenerative joint disease. Despite postoperative prophylactic anticoagulation with LMWH, he develops a left popliteal vein deep venous thrombosis on postoperative day 4. You plan to start intravenous heparin and warfarin to achieve an international normalized ratio between 2 and 3. You recall that heparin and warfarin can adversely influence hypercoagulability testing.

What tests do you order before starting heparin?
a) Factor V Leiden polymerase chain reaction, prothrombin G20210A polymerase chain reaction, and a plasma homocysteine level
b) Protein C, protein S, antithrombin III activity levels
c) LA testing and ACA testing
d) All of the above
e) None of the above

## Answers

**1. c.**
The combination of poor oral intake and broad-spectrum antibiotics that alter gut flora is sufficient to induce vitamin K deficiency. Because factors from the intrinsic pathway (factor IX), extrinsic pathway (factor VII), and common pathway (factors II and X) are affected, a prolongation in both PT and aPTT can be seen. The normal platelet count, TT, and stable fibrinogen over time do not support a diagnosis of DIC. The normal TT rules out a heparin effect. Acquired hemophilia A (factor VIII anti-

body) would not give a prolonged PT. Antithrombin III deficiency results in hypercoagulability and not bleeding.

**2. b.**
This patient has TTP, which requires emergent therapy. The best initial therapy is plasma exchange, which is a combination of plasmapheresis and plasma infusion and is better than plasmapheresis alone. The normal coagulation tests speak against DIC, so low-dose heparin is not a consideration. Platelet transfusions may only exacerbate the situation. Splenectomy may be useful in patients refractory to plasma exchange.

**3. e.**
In the setting of intracranial hemorrhage, everything possible should be used to treat this patient's ITP. Steroids may take a while to become effective. The combination of IVIG to "block" the antibody-mediated clearance of platelets and platelet infusion is advised. Emergent splenectomy also should be considered in this situation.

**4. d.**
If HIT is suspected, all heparin must be stopped immediately. Giving more heparin, infusing platelets, and beginning warfarin are all associated with adverse outcomes in HIT. Vascular surgery consultation and HIT testing may be helpful but should not change the decision to stop all heparin.

**5. d.**
The combination of multiple myeloma, bleeding, and an isolated prolonged BT suggests the possible existence of either a paraprotein-induced qualitative platelet disorder or a vWF inhibitor. The other choices are not supported by the clinical situation or laboratory data.

**6. a.**
The patient is likely to stop bleeding only when the paraprotein level has been markedly reduced by plasmapheresis. Transfused platelets are likely to become impaired rapidly because of the circulating paraprotein. Aspirin will exacerbate the situation.

**7. e.**
Mild factor deficiencies can be difficult to diagnose without performing serial evaluations and obtaining a careful family history. Disorders of fibrin cross-linking (factor XIII deficiency) and fibrinolytic dysregulation ($\alpha_2$-antiplasmin deficiency) are not reflected in the PT, aPTT, or BT.

**8. d.**
The patient's gender, bleeding history, family history, and prolonged aPTT are suggestive of an autosomal dominant disorder. The most common inherited hemorrhagic diathesis, type 1 vWD, fits this case nicely.

**9. b.**
This patient has what sounds like an acquired bleeding disorder caused by an inhibitor. An LA diagnosed by a

prolonged dilute Russell's viper venom time would give the same mixed study results but is not associated with bleeding. Acquired hemophilia most commonly involves factor VIII.

**10. e.**

This patient has had a situational thrombosis. The results of testing are unlikely to impact the duration, intensity, or type of anticoagulation in this setting.

## SUGGESTED READINGS

Brandt JT, Triplett DA, Alving B, et al. Criteria for the diagnosis of lupus anticoagulants: an update. *Thromb Haemost* 1995;74:1185.

Deitcher SR, Caiola E, Jaffer A. Demystifying two common genetic predispositions to venous thrombosis. *Cleve Clin J Med* 2000;67:825.

De Moerloose P, Bounameaux H, Mannucci PM. Screening tests for thrombophilic patients: which tests, for which patient, by whom, when, and why? *Semin Thromb Hemost* 1998;24:321.

Furie B, Limentani SA, Rosenfield CG. A practical guide to the evaluation and treatment of hemophilia. *Blood* 1994;84:3.

George JN, Woolf SH, Raskob GE, et al. Idiopathic thrombocytopenic purpura: a practice guideline developed by explicit methods for the American Society of Hematology. *Blood* 1996;88:3.

Kaufman DW, Kelly JP, Johannes CB, et al. Acute thrombocytopenic purpura in relation to the use of drugs. *Blood* 1993;82:2714.

Rock GA, Shumak KH, Buskard NA, et al. Comparison of plasma exchange with plasma infusion in the treatment of thrombotic thrombocytopenic purpura. *N Engl J Med* 1991; 325:393.

Shaffer LG, Phillips MD. Successful treatment of acquired hemophilia with oral immunosuppressive therapy. *Ann Intern Med* 1997; 127:206.

Warkentin TE, Kelton JG. A 14-year study of heparin-induced thrombocytopenia. *Am J Med* 1996;101:502.

# Anemia  **23**

### *Robert J. Pelley*  *Alan E. Lichtin*

The red blood cell (RBC) mass is maintained in humans as the result of a continuous production of differentiated erythrocytes, generated by erythroid progenitors and stimulated by the hormone erythropoietin. Iron and nutrients, such as vitamin $B_{12}$ and folate, are necessary for RBC production, and energy sources are required to maintain the RBC membrane for RBCs to survive an average of 120 days.

*Anemia* is defined as a reduction in the RBC mass as measured by either the hematocrit or the hemoglobin concentration. *Acquired anemia* is not a disease per se, but rather a sign or symptom of an underlying disease. Because the severity of the anemia does not correlate with the seriousness of the underlying disorder, each patient with anemia deserves a careful evaluation to determine the cause of the anemia.

## CLINICAL FEATURES

Many of the clinical manifestations associated with an anemia are determined by the etiology of the underlying disease that is producing the anemia. If severe enough, all anemias result in symptoms of tissue hypoxia (i.e., the consequence of a low oxygen-carrying capacity of the blood). Therefore, several signs and symptoms are common to all anemias. Weakness, headache, feeling "cold," and exertional dyspnea are common nonspecific symptoms that may be mild if the anemia develops slowly. The presence of physical signs, such

as pallor and tachycardia, can be severe but depends on the patient's previous cardiovascular status. Stress to the cardiovascular system may occur with mild anemia in patients with pre-existing cardiovascular disease; however, even a healthy person begins to have cardiovascular stress at hemoglobin levels of less than 10 g/dL, as a result of the increased cardiac output required to compensate for the reduced oxygen-carrying capacity of the blood.

## EVALUATION

RBCs are made and destroyed constantly. Anemia results when this equilibrium cannot be maintained because of acute or chronic blood loss, failure to produce RBCs, or a shortening of the RBC life span. When anemia is detected, its analysis consists of obtaining old data, gathering an excellent history—especially a drug history—and using physical diagnostic and laboratory methods to classify the anemia and identify its underlying cause. The first step is always to exclude acute blood loss by history and physical examination, including stool guaiac for occult blood loss. Further analyses include a complete blood cell count (CBC) with red cell indices, including a calculation of the mean corpuscular volume (MCV), a review of the peripheral blood smear (PBS), and a corrected reticulocyte count. Results from these initial tests help to determine whether more invasive or expensive testing is required, such as bone marrow aspiration and biopsy or immunoassays.

An important initial step in assessing anemia involves an examination of the PBS, the most cost-effective of hematologic tests. It is useful to correlate the PBS with the RBC indices generated by an automated CBC. The RBC indices should never substitute for an examination of the PBS, however, because the statistical averaging that occurs with an automated CBC loses valuable information about small populations of RBCs. An examination of the PBS reveals more information about specific RBC morphology, dimorphic populations, inclusion bodies, and accompanying white blood cell (WBC) morphology, all of which are not available from an automated CBC.

The corrected reticulocyte count is a useful second test because it serves to divide anemias into two major categories: *hyperproliferative anemias* resulting from the loss or destruction of RBCs, with an associated increased bone marrow activity; and *hypoproliferative anemias*, resulting from decreased bone marrow production. When the underlying cause of an anemia is not readily apparent, the reticulocyte count can be invaluable in interpreting the blood smear and in making an initial assessment as to the etiology of the anemia.

Morphologically, hyperproliferative anemias frequently are macrocytic, with high MCVs resulting from the large size of reticulocytes; however, some anemias caused by chronic hemolysis may result in normocytic morphology or MCVs, which may be in the normal range as a result of averaging between macrocytic reticulocytes and smaller spherocytes. The PBS helps to identify hemolytic anemias rapidly. The presence of spherocytes or schistocytes (fragmented RBCs) may indicate such acquired disorders as immune hemolysis, disseminated intravascular coagulation, or other forms of microangiopathic hemolysis. Inclusion bodies or sickle shapes may indicate hereditary disorders, such as enzymopathies or sickle cell disease. In hypoproliferative anemias, the smear and MCV can be even more informative when RBC size can serve to organize the differential diagnosis. Furthermore, WBC morphology is more likely to be altered in hypoproliferative anemias, in which multiple cell types within the bone marrow may be affected by the same disease process.

## DIFFERENTIAL DIAGNOSES

### Shortened RBC Survival

The causes of shortened RBC survival include:

- Increased reticulocyte count
- Compensated acute blood loss occurring before depletion of iron stores
- Hemolytic anemias
- Immune and autoimmune disorders
- Drugs

- Membrane defects
- Hereditary spherocytosis
- Hereditary elliptocytosis
- Acquired paroxysmal nocturnal hemoglobinuria
- Congenital enzymopathies
- Pyruvate kinase deficiency
- Glucose-6-phosphate dehydrogenase (G6PD) deficiency
- Hemoglobinopathies (sickle cell disorders)
- Mechanical hemolysis
- Heart valves
- Disseminated intravascular coagulation
- Thrombotic thrombocytopenic purpura
- Infections (malaria)
- Decreased reticulocyte count

### Macrocytic Anemias (MCV >100 fl)

Contributing causes to macrocytic anemia include:

- Pernicious anemia (vitamin $B_{12}$ deficiency)
- Folate deficiency
- Alcoholism
- Malabsorption
- Liver disease

### Normochromic, Normocytic (MCV >80 fl, MCV <100 fl)

- Aplastic anemia
- Myelophthisic disorders
- Leukemias
- Lymphomas
- Myeloma
- Myelofibrosis
- Granulomatous diseases
- Lipid storage diseases
- Anemia of chronic disease (anemia of abnormal iron reutilization)
- Anemia of chronic renal failure
- Anemia of endocrine diseases
- Anemia of hepatic failure

### Hypochromic Microcytic (MCV <80 fl)

- Iron deficiency
- Sideroblastic anemia
- Lead intoxication
- Thalassemias
- Anemia of chronic disease (advanced)

## HYPERPROLIFERATIVE ANEMIAS

Hyperproliferative anemias are divided between processes that remove blood cells (i.e., bleeding) and those that destroy blood cells (i.e., hemolysis). The following sections discuss the two most common disorders resulting in RBC destruction: immune hemolysis and unstable hemoglobins.

## Immune Hemolytic Disorders

Immune hemolytic processes can be crudely divided into *autoimmune* processes, in which the patient produces antibodies against RBC surface antigens, and *drug-induced* processes, in which the RBC is frequently an "innocent bystander" in an otherwise typical immune-mediated drug reaction.

All these disorders are characterized by an indirect hyperbilirubinemia, reticulocytosis, marrow erythroid hyperplasia, hemoglobinemia, and perhaps hemoglobinuria. The PBS may have spherocytes, and the haptoglobin protein level may be nearly undetectable because it is removed from the circulation after binding free heme. The Coombs' test will be "directly" positive if antibodies are detected on the patient's circulating RBCs, and it will be "indirectly" positive if antibodies capable of reacting to RBCs are detected only in the serum.

## Immunoglobulin M–Induced Hemolysis

Immunoglobulin M (IgM) antibodies produce "cold hemagglutinin" disease because these antibodies usually only bind or lyse RBCs at lower temperatures. The IgMs frequently are directed against the I antigen or related RBC antigens and result in complement fixation and lysis at temperatures usually below body temperature. The most common cause of cold agglutinins are cross-reactive IgMs resulting from infections (*Mycoplasma pneumoniae*, mononucleosis, cytomegalovirus). They are rarely clinically important. Lymphoproliferative diseases and connective tissue diseases also can produce cold agglutinins, some of which can generate difficult persistent hemolysis.

## Immunoglobulin G–Induced Hemolysis

The immunoglobulin G (IgG) antibodies also can produce a hemolysis of RBCs; however, because they do so at body temperature, the hemolysis is usually clinically more serious. Also, because IgGs bind at warmer temperatures, they are referred to as *warm antibodies*. Although complement may be fixed by the IgGs, the antibody valency is generally inadequate to cause intravascular hemolysis. The RBCs are converted slowly into spherocytes and eventually removed extravascularly in the spleen.

IgG or warm antibody disease is much more likely to produce a clinically apparent anemia, which may be chronic and require treatment. Corticosteroids are the treatment of choice; frequently, these agents already may be in use to treat the connective tissue disease or lymphoma that may be the cause of the warm antibody. Splenectomy is effective treatment in about half of patients for whom corticosteroids fail.

When cold (IgM) hemolysis requires therapy, steroids may help, and plasmapheresis can effectively reduce the intravascular titer of the antibody.

In either situation, a transfusion of RBCs is rarely indicated and always complicated by the difficulty of typing and crossing the patient with compatible blood.

## DRUG-INDUCED IMMUNE HEMOLYSIS

Drugs can contribute to RBC hemolysis in four classic ways. All are diagnosed by taking a careful history.

- Hapten type. In patients receiving high doses of penicillins, hapten type occurs when the drug or its metabolites bind to the RBC and induce an immune response. The antibodies react to a RBC antigen–drug complex and therefore bind only to drug-coated RBCs.
- Quinidine type. The quinidine type IgM antibody reaction is directed most frequently to the drug quinidine when the drug binds to plasma proteins. The antibody then cross-reacts with RBC antigens, resulting in acute hemolysis.
- α-Methyldopa type (Aldomet). The α-methyldopa type reaction is similar to idiopathic warm antibody disease. By an unknown mechanism, one-fourth of patients receiving Aldomet (a drug rarely used now for hypertension) develop IgG autoantibodies directed against the Rh antigens, with 1% suffering some hemolysis. The drug itself is not involved in the antibody–RBC antigen reaction.
- Nonspecific reactions. In rare instances, drugs such as cephalosporines can coat the RBC membrane, resulting in the nonspecific binding of plasma proteins, which may make the Coombs' test positive. Hemolysis is rare.

The removal of the inciting drug is the appropriate treatment and frequently results in rapid improvement. Rarely, corticosteroids are necessary.

## UNSTABLE ERYTHRON (HEREDITARY DISORDERS CAUSING HEMOLYSIS)

The RBC is the most thoroughly studied entity in the human body because of its accessibility and quantity. The result has been a tremendous understanding, at the genetic and biochemical levels, of hereditary disorders affecting hemoglobin (hemoglobinopathies), RBC enzymes (enzymopathies), and the RBC cytoskeleton and structural proteins (spectrin disorders resulting in hereditary spherocytosis).

## Hemoglobinopathies and Sickle Cell Anemia

A point mutation of the β-globin chain at residue 6 substitutes a valine for glutamic acid, thereby altering the net charge and local conformation of the hemoglobin molecule (Hb S). The alteration in charge results in an instability of Hb S when in the deoxygenated state, resulting in insoluble aggregates. These aggregates precipitate into polymers of long rod-like fibers if the concentration of Hb S is sufficiently high. The propagation of these polymers distorts the normally pliant cell membrane into bizarre forms that resemble sickles. These sickle-shaped RBCs are the hallmark of a series of unstable hemoglobins that share a constellation of clinical problems, including hemolytic anemia, small vessel infarction, painful crises, and a predisposition to infections.

Hb S mutations follow recessive inheritance patterns, with the carrier state (sickle trait) being silent; however, patients heterozygous for Hb S, who also have an additional mutant hemoglobin, such as Hb C, D, or O, or thalassemia, manifest a clinically evident sickle syndrome. Diagnosis of Hb S or other hemoglobin mutants is made by electrophoresis of purified Hb. Additionally, reducing agents that deprive cells of $O_2$ promote Hb polymerization and sickling, even in the cells of patients who are Hb AS heterozygotes, thus serving as a screening test (*sickle prep using sodium metabisulfite*).

The therapy of sickle cell anemia and crisis include hydration and analgesia, with early treatment of infections and judicious transfusions.

## Enzymopathies

More than six enzymes involved in glycolysis and adenosine triphosphate production have been identified as hereditary defects capable of inducing hemolytic states. The most common is glucose-6-phosphate dehydrogenase (G6PD) deficiency, which has more than 150 mutant forms. The mutations serve to decrease the half-life of the G6PD protein, which is essential for maintaining the reduced state of the RBC cytoplasm. With time, activity is lost, thus allowing the oxidation and precipitation of aging hemoglobin, with subsequent development of inclusion bodies (Heinz bodies) and hemolysis. Deficiency of G6PD is sex linked and usually manifests in a male subject with episodic hemolysis following oxidative stresses associated with infections or drug ingestions. Because it is the "aged" RBCs that hemolyze, analysis for G6PD levels soon after the hemolytic episode may be misleading and should be delayed to allow the reaccumulation of older cells.

## Cytoskeletal Defects

The cytoskeleton is a complex array of proteins that hold the RBC membrane at the edge of the cell. Its lattice-like state allows the red cell to be pliant enough to navigate the tiny slits in the splenic sinusoids. If a problem is present within the lattice, such as an abnormal structure of spectrin, ankyrin, or band 4.1, a clinical phenotype results in abnormally shaped RBCs. These include hereditary spherocytosis, hereditary elliptocytosis, or hereditary pyropoikilocytosis. These individuals have anemia, elevated indirect hyperbilirubinemia, reticulocytosis, and erythroid hyperplasia of the bone marrow and usually have mild spleen enlargement. After viral infections, anemia worsens and jaundice deepens, sometimes to the point of requiring

transfusion. Bilirubin gallstones occur at a young age. Splenectomy ameliorates the anemia. Moderate to severely affected individuals often have both a cholecystectomy and splenectomy by age 20 to 30 years.

## HYPOPROLIFERATIVE ANEMIAS

Hypoproliferative anemias include those diseases that interfere with RBC production or maturation and lead to an inappropriately low reticulocyte count. Historically, these anemias have been classified by RBC morphology and size. This classification frequently groups physiologically unrelated processes together, but this classification survives because it is an efficient means for clinically diagnosing these anemias.

### Macrocytic Anemias

The two most important disorders in which the MCVs are elevated are vitamin $B_{12}$ deficiency and folate deficiency. Macrocytosis also may be seen in myelodysplasia, alcoholism, liver disease, and persons receiving chemotherapy or phenytoin. The PBS again is valuable in identifying megaloblastic processes ($B_{12}$ and folate deficiency) from processes that produce macrocytosis alone. Usually, not only are hypersegmented neutrophils present, but the RBCs are pleomorphic, containing fragments and other signs of dyserythropoiesis.

#### *Vitamin $B_{12}$ and Folate Deficiency*
Both vitamin $B_{12}$ and folate are involved in DNA synthesis. A deficiency in either leads to dyssynchrony in nuclear and cytoplasmic maturation, producing the RBC macrocytosis and neutrophil hypersegmentation, which are the hallmarks of these disorders. In addition, vitamin $B_{12}$ plays an important role in myelin production, and $B_{12}$ deficiency leads to serious neurologic disorders. Because $B_{12}$ and folate metabolism are closely connected, the administration of folate to $B_{12}$-deficient subjects bypasses and corrects the hematologic abnormalities of vitamin $B_{12}$ deficiency without correcting the neurologic abnormalities. Indeed, the neurologic abnormalities can worsen irrevocably. It is therefore essential to diagnose $B_{12}$ deficiency correctly, and treat with vitamin $B_{12}$ first, before administering any folate.

#### $B_{12}$ Deficiency
Vitamin $B_{12}$ is found in animal products, such as meat, chicken, and fish. On ingestion, $B_{12}$ is bound by an intrinsic factor secreted by gastric parietal cells, and the $B_{12}$-intrinsic factor complex passes into the distal ileum, where it is actively absorbed. $B_{12}$ then is transported by transcobalamins into the liver for storage and then into the erythron. Absolute dietary deficiency can occur in strict ovo-lacto vegetarians. Most deficiencies result from malabsorption. Parietal cell dysfunction occurs either through

the autoimmune process of pernicious anemia or by surgical removal of the stomach. Ileal disease such as Crohn's disease or radiation enteritis, pancreatic insufficiency, blind loop syndromes, and ileal resections likewise result in failure to absorb the $B_{12}$-intrinsic factor complex. Historically, the Schilling's test allowed for the discrimination between a gastric disorder and an ileal disorder, but it is rarely used now. Anti-intrinsic factor and anti-parietal cell antibodies can be measured, but false negatives for pernicious anemia are frequent.

The clinical manifestations of $B_{12}$ deficiency include symptoms attributable to anemia but also include disproportionate fatigue and subtle neurologic symptoms. Some $B_{12}$-deficient persons manifest only mild anemia or macrocytosis, perhaps as a result of folate ingestion. Some of these patients may develop neuropsychiatric symptoms, neuropathies, or difficulties with unconscious proprioception. $B_{12}$ deficiency can lead to "megaloblastic madness," in which patients even may become demented or disoriented.

The therapy for vitamin $B_{12}$ deficiency is simply parenteral administration by monthly intramuscular injections of 100 to 1,000 μg of $B_{12}$, usually after initial repletion of body stores with an injection of 1 mg. This dose is sufficient to reverse the megaloblastosis within days. An improvement in erythropoiesis results in a lowering of serum iron as it is used rapidly and a lowering in serum lactate dehydrogenase, which is elevated as a result of ineffective erythropoiesis and intramedullary hemolysis.

### Folate Deficiency

Many persons are at risk for relative or absolute folic acid deficiency. Those who have diets poor in fresh vegetables, have jejunal malabsorption, or take antagonistic drugs may develop low folic acid levels. Pregnant women are especially susceptible. Folic acid, like $B_{12}$, is also necessary for DNA synthesis and is important in one carbon transfer; but, unlike vitamin $B_{12}$, folate is poorly stored by the body and must be replenished continuously. Unlike liver stores of vitamin $B_{12}$, which may be sufficient for 2 to 5 years, folate stores are minimal, and florid deficiency can develop in 3 months or less.

The anemia of folate deficiency resembles the megaloblastosis of $B_{12}$ deficiency. Diagnosis may be difficult because a small hospital meal, blood transfusion, or intravenous multivitamins may be sufficient to elevate serum levels, thus making any subsequent testing ambiguous. Because RBC folate levels are the last compartment to be replenished and normalized, measuring RBC folate can be diagnostic in situations in which treatment was initiated before diagnosis. Such testing, however, is not universally available.

The most important aspect of folate deficiency is that folate is not involved in myelin production and cannot correct the neurologic deficit of $B_{12}$ deficiency. Therefore, it is critical not to mistake vitamin $B_{12}$ deficiency for folate deficiency.

## NORMOCHROMIC NORMOCYTIC HYPOPROLIFERATIVE ANEMIAS AND ANEMIA OF CHRONIC DISEASE

The anemia of chronic disease can generate RBCs that are microcytic but more frequently may be normocytic. It is defined as an anemia associated with an underlying disorder when no other etiology for the anemia can be identified. Not surprisingly, it is the most common category for anemias within institutions or hospitals. This disorder is characterized by low serum iron, low total iron-binding capacity (transferrin), and a low percent of iron saturation. Often, however, a normal or high ferritin level is found, which, in the presence of a low total iron-binding capacity level, is diagnostic of anemia of chronic disease. It has been labeled by some as the *anemia of abnormal iron reutilization*. Consistent with this, the bone marrow appears normocellular or slightly hypocellular, with poor hemoglobinization but with significant iron within the marrow spaces. Patients with this anemia often have underlying neoplasms, inflammatory disorders, connective tissue diseases (lupus or rheumatoid arthritis), or infectious processes, such as osteomyelitis or tuberculosis. Increasing evidence suggests that cytokines and inhibitory growth factors released during such disease processes may directly inhibit erythropoiesis or make RBC progenitors relatively resistant to normal or mildly elevated erythropoietin levels. Efforts at treating these anemias with exogenous recombinant erythropoietin have met with only modest success. The only effective therapy for this anemia remains the treatment of the underlying disorder.

Other forms of normochromic normocytic anemias tend to be uncommon and usually are associated with clinically obvious conditions, such as hypothyroidism and renal failure, or manifestations of pancytopenia. The anemia of renal failure deserves special mention because it represents an isolated deficiency of erythropoietin. Injections of recombinant erythropoietin correct this anemia as long as iron is given to support erythropoiesis.

## HYPOCHROMIC MICROCYTIC HYPOPROLIFERATIVE ANEMIAS

The microcytic anemias all can be characterized as anemias in which hemoglobin production is somehow deficient. This anemia may be the result of a hereditary inability to produce globin protein chains (thalassemia), to produce heme (sideroblastic anemias), or to supply the iron necessary for heme production (iron deficiency). Of these, iron deficiency is the most common form of impaired heme synthesis on a worldwide basis.

### Iron Deficiency

Worldwide, dietary insufficiency and parasite infestations are leading causes for iron deficiency anemia. In the

United States, the diagnosis of iron deficiency in an adult requires a careful and diligent search for a pathologic source of blood loss. Iron deficiency anemia should be entertained in any anemic patient with microcytosis. Iron deficiency also can accompany other anemias, and if it presents with a macrocytic anemia, a dimorphic condition might exist with normocytic indices. The red cell distribution width (RDW) is an index that measures the variation in RBC size. As the red cell distribution width increases, the variation in RBC size increases, making it likely that severe anisocytosis or a dimorphic population of RBCs is present. In that situation, examination of the PBS is essential. In iron deficiency, the red cell distribution width is high, reflecting the hypochromia, microcytosis, poikilocytes, and fragments that often are present.

People at risk of iron deficiency include infants with low dietary intake, pregnant women, adolescents, and elderly persons. Symptoms of iron deficiency include those common to other anemias, including weakness, lassitude, palpitations, and dyspnea on exertion; however, iron deficiency also produces some unique symptoms in rapidly proliferating tissue. Glossitis, stomatitis, gastric atrophy with abdominal pain, menorrhagia, and fingernail changes all are associated. Pica, or a craving to eat abnormal substances such as starch, ice, or dirt, occurs for unexplained reasons.

Generally, the serum ferritin is the best test for screening for iron deficiency. If the ferritin is below 30 ng/mL in a male patient or 10 ng/mL in a female patient, iron deficiency is present. Because ferritin is also an acute-phase reactant, it may be falsely elevated. Even so, a value of less than 50 μg/mL in the face of inflammation is a strong indicator of iron deficiency. Iron deficiency can be quantified further by measuring the total iron-binding capacity and total iron level, with a calculated percent of transferrin saturation. Finally, the absence of iron within the bone marrow is another way to confirm iron deficiency.

Therapy is straightforward. Iron salts such as ferrous sulfate, gluconate, or fumarate can replete stores in 2 to 6 months. The initial step in treating iron deficiency anemia, however, is to identify the underlying disease and source of blood loss, and then to correct it.

## Thalassemias

The thalassemias are hereditary diseases in which an inadequate or unbalanced production of globin protein chains occurs. α-Thalassemia represents a deficiency in α-chain production and β-thalassemia a reduction in β-chains. The pathologic mechanisms responsible for the decreased protein production generally are the result of hereditary mutations, which either totally delete the genes or result in minimal or no globin RNA production. Afflicted persons have a lifelong microcytic hypochromic anemia that is dependent on the severity of the deficiency. Because there are four copies of the α-globin gene and two copies of the β-globin gene, variations in the production and the clinical spectrum

of disease are vast. For instance, the total lack of α-globin is incompatible with life and results in death in utero during the second trimester. Lack of only one α-globin gene, on the other hand, can be clinically silent and difficult to diagnose. Between these two poles are patients with 50% or less β- or α-globin production who have mild anemias that morphologically resemble iron deficiency, but who obviously do not respond to iron therapy. Over the century, clinicians have classified patients as having either thalassemia major, intermedia, or minor. These terms have no pathologic basis and describe only the severity of the patient's anemia— major means a patient needs transfusions regularly to survive and minor means the individual rarely, if ever, needs a transfusion.

In severe thalassemia, the clinical symptoms present in early childhood and are the result of dyserythropoiesis and bone marrow hypertrophy, rather than anemia. Patients develop bony deformities from marrow hyperplasia and organomegaly from extramedullary hematopoiesis. Oddly, the clinical manifestations of thalassemia relate more to the degree of imbalance between α-globin and β-globin production, which leads to the precipitation of abnormal hemoglobins in the developing RBC and lysis within the marrow. Patients with severe disease rarely survive beyond the age of 30 years. Less severe thalassemias present with fewer manifestations of hyperplastic bones and bone marrow and with more of the classic symptoms and problems of chronic anemia.

The PBS in thalassemia is usually remarkable for hypochromic microcytic cells. Patients with severe disease have manifestations of precipitating hemoglobin in their RBCs, including inclusion bodies and cell fragments resulting from dyserythropoiesis, as well as bizarre forms. Patients with only anemia or thalassemia trait conditions have increased numbers of RBCs (>5 million/μL) and target cells but not fragmented cells from severe intracellular hemoglobin precipitation.

The treatment of thalassemia involves the transfusion of RBCs in severely affected children to reduce their own endogenous bone marrow activity and thus avoid bony hypertrophy and extramedullary hematopoiesis. In adults with anemia, transfusion is again beneficial but can lead to severe iron overload, with consequent heart failure. Finally, patients with thalassemia minor or trait rarely require transfusion but require diagnosis to avoid unnecessary investigations for incorrectly diagnosed iron deficiency.

## REVIEW EXERCISES

### QUESTIONS

**1.** A 31-year-old woman presents with complaints of fatigue, dyspnea on exertion, and tinnitus. The symptoms started a month ago. She had previously been in "perfect health." She has had three normal pregnancies. Her physical examination is remarkable for pallor. The hemoglobin concentration is 7.5 g/dL, the WBC is 6,200, and her platelet count is 550,000/μL. After her last pregnancy 2 years ago, her hemoglobin was normal.

Which of the following tests is the most appropriate first test in the initial evaluation of this patient's anemia?

a) Serum folate and vitamin $B_{12}$ level
b) Review of the PBS
c) Serum ferritin determination
d) Haptoglobin level
e) Coombs' direct and indirect tests

**2.** A 24-year-old Lebanese exchange student comes to the college infirmary with a 3-day history of upper respiratory infection symptoms, cough, purulent sputum, and a low-grade fever. His chest examination is clear, and he is given available trimethoprim-sulfamethoxazole (Bactrim) samples for clinical bronchitis. The following day, he returns with shortness of breath, severe abdominal pain, a high spiking fever, and dark urine. A CBC reveals a hemoglobin of 7 g/dL and a WBC of 12,500. PBS has fragmented RBCs, and distinct "bite cells" are present. The chest radiograph is normal. The patient is admitted to the hospital.

Which of the following statements is true?

a) The Coombs' direct test will be positive.
b) The haptoglobin will be undetectable.
c) A sickle prep screen would be positive.
d) All of the above.

**3.** A 48-year-old man presents with fatigue, weakness, diffuse nonlocalizing abdominal complaints, loss of libido, "funny sensations" in his arms and legs, and depression. He has attempted to medicate himself with "megadoses" of B-complex vitamins as well as vitamin E and β-carotene. He denies any recent alcohol consumption and has had no diarrhea or steatorrhea. He has never had surgery. Physical examination is remarkable for a chronically ill–appearing middle-aged man. The only objective abnormalities include decreased sensation in the legs and decreased proprioception. Initial workup includes a CBC with a hemoglobin of 13 g/dL, MCV of 120, and WBC of 4,500. Platelets were 220,000. The PBS confirms macrocytosis and rare hypersegmented polys. Reticulocyte count is 0.5%. You measure serum $B_{12}$ and folate levels because of the macrocytosis. Folate is greater than 14 (normal >2.0) and $B_{12}$ is 20 (normal >100). Which of the following statements is false?

a) Administration of folate can correct the anemia of $B_{12}$ deficiency.
b) With severe vitamin $B_{12}$ deficiency, pancytopenia can result.
c) Folate administration cannot correct the myelin production defects and neurologic deficits.
d) An oral vitamin $B_{12}$ preparation (Geritol) would have been likely to prevent the patient's neurologic deficits.

**4–6.** Match the following patients with laboratory results (serum iron, total iron-binding capacity, transferrin serum saturation, ferritin, respectively). (Normal values: serum iron, 60 to 160; total iron-binding capacity, 250 to 460; transferrin serum saturation, 24% to 45%; ferritin, 20 to 300.)

a) 220, 260, 85%, 2,560
b) 200, 390, 51%, 840
c) 40, 210, 19%, 400
d) 20, 500, 4%, 12

**4.** A 65-year-old woman on nonsteroidal anti-inflammatory drugs for osteoarthritis with irregular, guaiac-positive stools

**5.** A 48-year-old man with polyarthritis, recent onset diabetes, hyperpigmentation, and cirrhosis

**6.** A 59-year-old woman with long-standing rheumatoid arthritis and anemia

**7.** For a patient with a chronic autoimmune hemolytic anemia (warm IgG antibody) associated with a connective tissue disease, all of the following are appropriate therapy, *except*

a) Daily oral prednisone
b) Plasmapheresis
c) Treatment of the underlying autoimmune disorder
d) Splenectomy

**8.** Which of the following is the most important factor in inducing hemoglobin precipitation?

a) pH
b) $O_2$ partial pressure
c) Hb S concentration
d) Osmolality

**9.** The least likely factor to produce vitamin $B_{12}$ deficiency is

a) Pregnancy
b) Crohn's disease
c) Total gastrectomy for peptic ulcer disease
d) Strict vegetarian diet

**10.** Which laboratory test is most likely to be elevated in iron deficiency anemia?

a) Homocysteine
b) Total iron binding capacity
c) Platelet count
d) Ferritin
e) All of the above

**11.** Chronic transfusion for the treatment of thalassemia major is associated with which of the following?

a) Cirrhosis
b) Cardiomyopathy
c) Hemosiderosis
d) All of the above

## ANSWERS

### 1. b.

A review of the PBS is the single most valuable first step in evaluating an acute anemia. The morphology of the RBCs, the presence of polychromasia (reticulocytes), and platelet morphology can help to focus the differential diagnosis and evaluation immediately. The differential diagnosis for this patient's acute or subacute anemia is broad and includes both gastrointestinal blood loss and diverse causes of hemolysis. The iron studies, folate and $B_{12}$ levels, haptoglobin and Coombs' test are premature and should be ordered according to results of the PBS review and reticulocyte count.

### 2. b.

This patient has clinical G6PD deficiency with acute hemolysis, as manifested by the acute drop in hemoglobin, dark urine, and fragmentation on the PBS. People of Mediterranean descent are more susceptible to rapid severe hemolysis, in contrast to people of African descent. The "bite cells" on the smear are pathognomonic for this condition, which was triggered by the oxidative stress of the sulfa drugs. The precipitating hemoglobin results in RBC stromal damage and acute hemolysis. The haptoglobin level will be low if not undetectable because of its binding to free hemoglobin and removal by the liver. The Coombs' tests, both direct and indirect, are negative because antibodies are not involved in this physical form of hemolysis. Although many antibiotics might produce immune hemolysis, the time course of acute onset within 24 hours goes against any immune process. The sickle preparation will be negative because the precipitation of hemoglobin results in inclusion bodies but not in polymerization with deformity of the RBC architecture. Sickle cells will not be seen unless this patient also has a hemoglobinopathy.

If the G6PD enzyme levels were measured, they would be near normal in the remaining young cells that survived and were not hemolyzed. As these cells age, the enzyme decays and the enzyme levels drop, thus making these cells vulnerable to stress hemolysis. After acute hemolysis, however, the surviving cells usually have normal levels of enzyme.

### 3. d.

This patient most likely has pernicious anemia, an autoimmune disease directed against the intrinsic factor producing parietal cells of the gastric antrum. Almost all vitamin $B_{12}$ deficiency is the result of malabsorption, either because of a lack of intrinsic factor (pernicious anemia) or because of a defective small bowel. Dietary deficiency is very rare and occurs almost exclusively in strict ovo-lacto vegetarians who consume no animal products (vegan). Oral vitamin $B_{12}$ administration cannot overcome the deficit in malabsorption. Schilling's test, which measures the absorption of oral vitamin $B_{12}$, in the presence of exogenous intrinsic factor, can distinguish the etiology of the malabsorption.

Folate administration circumvents the $B_{12}$ defect, in the production of thymidine and DNA synthesis. Therefore, anemia may be ameliorated, and only macrocytosis may exist. Folate does not correct the defect in myelin production, however, so neurologic deficits may exist without hematologic abnormalities.

### 4. d.

### 5. a.

### 6. c.

Serum ferritin and iron levels are frequently used to diagnose iron deficiency states; however, ferritin is an acute-phase reactant and may be elevated to a degree seen in iron overload states in response to inflammation and liver disease. A low serum iron in the presence of an elevated transferrin level and low ferritin are diagnostic of some element of iron deficiency. The ferritin may be falsely elevated in the case of acute inflammation, but rarely will it be greater than 50 µg/L in the face of iron deficiency. On the other hand, the iron level may be low, but if the transferrin level is not elevated, and the ferritin is elevated or in the high normal range, the condition of anemia of chronic disease is most likely present. Rheumatoid arthritis is the best described disease producing this situation. Finally, although in the iron overload condition of hereditary hemochromatosis the ferritin may be extremely high, the transferrin saturation is a much more sensitive and accurate test.

### 7. b.

Plasmaphoresis has not been shown to reliably treat autoimmune hemolytic anemia.

### 8. c.

While all may effect sickling, the Hb S concentration has the greatest effect on precipitation.

### 9. a.

It takes a long time to deplete the body of $B_{12}$ stores.

### 10. b.

Ferritin is low in Fe deficiency. Homocysteine levels are unaffected. Platelet counts may be elevated, but TIBC is almost always increased.

### 11. d.

Self-explanatory.

## SUGGESTED READINGS

Buetler, E. Discrepancies between genotype and phenotype in hematology: an important frontier. *Blood* 2001;98:2597–2602

Beutler E. The common anemias. *JAMA* 1988;259:2433–2437.

Finch CA, Heubers H. Perspectives in iron metabolism. *N Engl J Med* 1982;306:1520–1528.

Freedman ML. Iron deficiency in the elderly. *Hosp Pract* 1986; March: 115–137.

Hebert PC, Fergusson DA. Red blood cell transfusions in critically ill patients. *JAMA* 2002;288:1525–1526

Henry DH, Thatcher N. Patient selection and predicting response to recombinant human erythropoietin in anemic cancer patients. *Semin Hematol* 1996;33[Suppl 1]:2–6.

Jongen-Lavrencic A, Peeters HRM, Vreugdenhil G, et al. Interaction of inflammatory cytokines and erythropoietin in iron metabolism and erythropoiesis in anaemia of chronic disease. *Clin Rheumatol* 1995;14:519–525.

Lindenbaum J, Hilton EB, Savage EG, et al. Neuropsychiatric disorders caused by cobalamin deficiency in the absence of anemia or macrocytosis. *N Engl J Med* 1988;318:1720–1728.

May C, Rivella S, Chadburn A, Sadelain M. Successful treatment of murine β-thalassemia intermedia by transfer of the human β-*globin* gene. *Blood* 2002;99:1902–1908.

Means RT Jr, Krantz SB. Progress in understanding the pathogenesis of the anemia of chronic disease. *Blood* 1992;80:1639–1646.

Mills JL. Fortification of foods with folic acid—how much is enough? *N Eng J Med* 2000;342:1442–1445.

Pietrangelo A. Hereditary hemochromatosis—a new look at an old disease. *N Engl J Med* 2004;350:2383–2397.

Rosenfeld S, Follmann D, Nunez O, Young NS. Antithymocyte globulin and cyclosporine for severe aplastic anemia. *JAMA* 2003;289:1130–1135.

Roy CN, Enns CA. Iron homeostasis: new tales from the crypt. *Blood* 2000;96:4020–4026.

Serjeant GR. *Sickle Cell Disease*. New York: Oxford Medical Publishing, 1985.

Smits LJM, Essed GGM. Short interpregnancy intervals and unfavourable pregnancy outcome: role of folate depletion. *The Lancet* 2001;358:2074–2077.

Vincent JL, Baron J-F, Reinhart K, Gattinoni L, Thijs L, Webb A, Meier-Hellmann A, Nollet G, Peres-Bota D. Anemia and blood transfusion in critically ill patients. *JAMA* 2002;288:1499–1507.

Wald NJ, Law MR, Morris JK, Wald DS. Quantifying the effect of folic acid. *The Lancet* 2001;358:2069–2073.

Wallerstein RO. Laboratory evaluation of anemia. *West J Med* 1987;146:443–451.

Weatherall DJ, Clegg JB. *The Thalassemia Syndromes*, 3rd ed. Oxford: Blackwell Scientific, 1981.

Welch HG, Meechan KR, Goodnough LT. Prudent strategies for elective red blood cell transfusion. *Ann Intern Med* 1992;116: 393–402.

# Breast Cancer

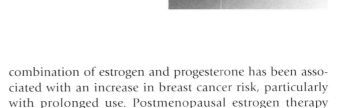

## *Halle C. F. Moore*

Breast cancer is the most common cancer in American women, excluding basal cell and squamous cell cancers of the skin. The annual incidence of invasive breast cancer in the United States currently exceeds 200,000 and the death rate, while improving, remains over 40,000 per year in this country. Despite a rising breast cancer incidence, a reduction in breast cancer mortality has been achieved over the past decades, presumably due to earlier detection and improved therapies. The median age at the time of breast cancer diagnosis is 63 years. Long-term survival following a diagnosis of breast cancer is common, and 5-year survival currently exceeds 85% overall. Breast cancer survivors in the United States number in the millions.

## RISK FACTORS AND SCREENING

The most common risk factor for breast cancer is female gender, with only approximately 1% of breast cancers occurring in men. For a woman, the estimated lifetime risk of being diagnosed with breast cancer is approximately a 1 in 7. Hormonal factors appear to play an important role in the development of breast cancer. Factors associated with prolonged cyclic estrogen exposure, including early menarche, late menopause, nulliparity, and delayed parity, have been associated with an elevated risk of breast cancer. Postmenopausal hormone replacement therapy with a combination of estrogen and progesterone has been associated with an increase in breast cancer risk, particularly with prolonged use. Postmenopausal estrogen therapy alone (without progesterone) has not been clearly implicated in increasing breast cancer risk.

Other risk factors for breast cancer include exposure to therapeutic doses of ionizing radiation and certain findings identified on breast biopsy including lobular carcinoma in situ (LCIS) and atypical hyperplasia. Breast cancer risk increases with increasing age, and approximately two-thirds of breast cancers are diagnosed in women over the age of 55. For the most part, dietary links to breast cancer have not been clearly established, although increased alcohol intake has been associated with increased breast cancer risk. Family history is also an important risk factor, particularly when the affected individual is young, has a first-degree or second-degree relative with breast cancer, or has bilateral breast cancer.

Familial breast cancer syndromes account for approximately 5% to 10% of breast cancer cases. Pathologic mutations in *BRCA-1* and *BRCA-2* are present in approximately 0.33% of the general population, but the frequency of mutations is higher in Ashkenazi Jewish populations. Individuals with *BRCA-1* or *BRCA-2* mutations may have a greater than 80% risk of developing breast cancer by age 70, particularly in families in which the penetrance of the gene is high. *BRCA-1* is located on chromosome 17q21 and also is associated with a significantly increased risk of ovarian cancer, as well as other cancers, including prostate and colon cancers. *BRCA-2* is located on chromosome 13 and has been associated with only a modestly increased risk of ovarian cancer, but with an increased risk of a greater variety of cancer types including prostate, pancreatic, and stomach cancers and melanoma. Both mutations are inherited in an autosomal dominant pattern, although the penetrance of the mutations varies from family to family. No firm data demonstrate the effectiveness of aggressive screening for breast and ovarian cancer in women with known mutations in *BRCA-1* or *BRCA-2*; however, screening often begins from age 25 and may include clinical breast examination, screening mammography, pelvic examination, and ultrasonography every 6 to 12 months. Magnetic resonance imaging (MRI) is potentially useful in the screening of populations at particularly high risk for breast cancer but is costly. Prophylactic mastectomy and prophylactic oophorectomy procedures are frequently discussed with these patients but do not eliminate the risk for developing cancer, and their impact on survival is unclear.

Other familial syndromes that account for a smaller proportion of inherited breast cancer include the Li-Fraumeni syndrome resulting from an inherited *p53* mutation, Cowden's disease, Muir-Torre syndrome, Peutz-Jeghers syndrome, and heterozygosity for the ataxia-telangiectasia gene. These syndromes are characterized by a variety of clinical manifestations including other cancer sites. Whereas the increased breast cancer risk in these patients should be recognized, other manifestations of these syndromes may dominate management of these individuals.

The most important strategy for reducing breast cancer mortality in the general population is thought to be screening. Early detection before the development of symptomatic disease improves the potential for cure of breast cancer. The American Cancer Society recommends that for most women monthly breast self-examination begin at age 20, with clinical breast examination every 3 years until age 39. Women age 40 and older should receive annual clinical breast examination, annual mammography, and should continue monthly breast self-examination. Some controversy exists as to the precise benefit of screening in the 40-year to 49-year age group; however, annual mammography in conjunction with clinical breast examination appears to reduce breast cancer mortality by 25% to 30% in women between the ages of 50 and 69. An upper age cutoff for mammography has not been set, but the screening of elderly women should be individualized, with consideration of comorbid illnesses. Mammography should never substitute for breast examination and a normal mammogram does not rule out the possibility of cancer.

## DIAGNOSIS AND LOCAL THERAPY

Once a suspicious lesion has been detected either mammographically or on breast examination, further evaluation is warranted. Diagnostic imaging, such as ultrasound, may be useful in differentiating solid from cystic lesions. MRI also is being used increasingly in the preoperative evaluation of breast cancer. The mainstay of breast cancer diagnosis, however, is biopsy, which may consist of fine-needle aspiration (FNA), core biopsy, or excisional biopsy. FNA is a relatively simple technique, which can be performed in the office and may confirm a suspicion of cancer. FNA may fail to differentiate between invasive and noninvasive cancer, and a negative FNA result does not rule out the possibility of cancer. An advantage of core needle biopsy over FNA is the ability to obtain enough tissue to evaluate histologic architecture and thus obtain important information about the pathology of the lesion. Excisional biopsy involves removal of the entire lesion of concern and may, at times, serve as the definitive procedure.

The most common histologic types of invasive breast cancer are infiltrating ductal carcinoma and infiltrating lobular carcinoma. The prognosis of both types of breast cancer is similar. Other less common histologies include medullary, tubular, metaplastic, squamous, adenoid cystic, and apocrine carcinomas. Rarely, other types of cancer such as lymphoma and sarcoma can present in the breast and are approached in accordance with their histology.

Noninvasive breast cancer, or ductal carcinoma in situ, is an early form of breast cancer that, theoretically, should not have the ability to metastasize. It is characterized by a malignant epithelial proliferation that is contained within the ductal-lobular system of the breast. Simple mastectomy or local excision, followed in most cases by radiation therapy, is curative. LCIS is not a true cancer, but rather a histologic finding that is associated with an increased risk of breast cancer in either the affected or the contralateral breast. Excision of the LCIS does not appear to alter subsequent cancer risk.

Standard surgical treatment for invasive breast cancer includes either modified radical mastectomy (removal of the breast and an axillary lymph node dissection) or excision of the tumor (lumpectomy or partial mastectomy) with axillary dissection. Ideally, surgical margins on the excised specimen should be free of both invasive and noninvasive cancer. Radiation therapy is recommended for patients at high risk for local recurrence, and indications include breast-conserving surgery, large primary tumors (>5 cm), and extensive lymph node involvement (four or more). The role of the axillary dissection is in evolution and, while once regarded as crucial for local control, is now viewed primarily as a staging procedure. In an effort to limit the morbidity of a full axillary dissection, the sentinel lymph node procedure has been developed. This involves the injection of a radioactive tracer, a blue dye, or both into the affected area of the breast or subdermally to elicit the drainage pattern of the mammary lymphatics. Presumably, the first lymph nodes to pick up the dye or radioactive tracer would also have the highest likelihood of involvement with cancer and, if found to be normal, predict a high likelihood that no further cancer would be identified in the remaining axilla. The finding of tumor in a sentinel lymph node frequently prompts a full axillary lymph node dissection.

## STAGING AND PROGNOSIS

Breast cancer staging uses the TNM (*Tumor, Node, Metastasis*) system as outlined in Table 24.1. In general, stage I, II, and many stage III cancers are operable and considered to be *early breast cancer*. The term *locally advanced breast cancer* most often refers to stage IIIB or IIIC disease

---

**TABLE 24.1**

### AMERICAN JOINT COMMITTEE ON CANCER STAGING FOR BREAST CANCER: TNM SYSTEM

**T (primary tumor size)**
Tis = Carcinoma in situ
T1 = Up to 2 cm in greatest diameter
T2 = Greater than 2 but no greater than 5 cm
T3 = More than 5 cm
T4 = Tumor extends into skin or chest wall or inflammatory changes
**N (regional lymph nodes)**
N0 = No regional lymph node involvement
   (Includes lymph nodes with IHC positive staining as long as no cluster >0.2mm)
N1 = Ipsilateral axillary metastasis involving 1 to 3 lymph nodes and/or internal mammary lymph node involvement detected by sentinel lymph node evaluation, but not clinically apparent.
N2 = Involvement of 4 to 9 ipsilateral axillary lymph nodes or no axillary involvement but clinically apparent internal mammary lymph nodes
N3 = Involvement of 10 or more ipsilateral axillary lymph nodes, or involvement of any ipsilateral axillary lymph nodes plus clinically apparent internal mammary lymph node involvement, or any ipsilateral supraclavicular or infraclavicular lymph node involvement.
**M (distant metastases)**
M0 = No detectable distant metastases
M1 = Any distant metastasis

**Breast Cancer Stage Grouping**

|  | T (Tumor) | N (Nodes) | M (Metastasis) |
|---|---|---|---|
| Stage 0 | Tis | N0 | M0 |
| Stage 1 | T1 | N0 | M0 |
| Stage IIA | T0–1 | N1 | M0 |
|  | T2 | N0 | M0 |
| Stage IIB | T2 | N1 | M0 |
|  | T3 | N0 | M0 |
| Stage IIIA | T0–2 | N2 | M0 |
|  | T3 | N1–2 | M0 |
| Stage IIIB | T4 | N0-2 | M0 |
| Stage IIIC | Any T | N3 | M0 |
| Stage IV | Any T | Any N | M1 |

Adapted with permission from Singletary SE, et al. Revision of the American Joint Committee on cancer staging system for breast cancer. *J Clin Oncol* 2002;20:3628–3636.

---

(which may or may not be operable), and metastatic breast cancer is stage IV. The staging evaluation to assess for the presence of distant disease typically includes chest radiography, routine blood work, and an optional bone scan. Additional studies such as abdominal computed tomographic (CT) scans can be performed in patients perceived to be at relatively high risk for metastatic disease, including those with localizing symptoms or blood test abnormalities. A positron emission tomography (PET) scan is also approved for use in breast cancer staging, but false positive findings can be misleading; whether PET scan can substitute for conventional staging studies is unclear.

Breast cancer mortality increases with the higher stage of disease. Adverse prognostic factors for early stage breast cancer include a greater number of axillary lymph nodes involved, larger tumor size, higher histologic grade of the tumor, negative hormone receptor (estrogen receptor and progesterone receptor) studies, and the presence of *HER2/neu* amplification. Younger patient age also appears to adversely affect prognosis.

## ADJUVANT SYSTEMIC THERAPY

The goal of adjuvant systemic therapy for operable breast cancer is to increase the possibility of cure through the eradication of micrometastases. In general, adjuvant chemotherapy is considered for cancers measuring at least 1 cm or when axillary lymph node involvement is identified. Factors that influence the decision to proceed with chemotherapy include patient age and comorbid conditions, the histologic grade of the tumor, the presence or absence of estrogen receptors and progesterone receptors, as well as the anticipated absolute benefit from chemotherapy, which is dependent on the recurrence risk. In relative terms, traditional chemotherapy regimens can reduce the annual risk of recurrence by approximately 20% in women over age 50 and by approximately 35% in women under age 50. The inclusion of newer agents in modern regimens will likely be associated with greater benefit to adjuvant chemotherapy.

Combination chemotherapy regimens commonly used in the adjuvant treatment of breast cancer are outlined in Table 24.2. The duration of adjuvant chemotherapy is typically 3 to 6 months. Common toxicities of adjuvant

---

**TABLE 24.2**

### ADJUVANT CHEMOTHERAPY REGIMENS

CMF (cyclophosphamide, methotrexate, and 5-fluorouracil)
CAF [cyclophosphamide, Adriamycin (doxorubicin), and 5-fluorouracil]
CEF (cyclophosphamide, epirubicin, and 5-fluorouracil)
AC (doxorubicin and cyclophosphamide)
AC > T (doxorubicin and cyclophosphamide followed by paclitaxel)
TAC (docetaxel, doxorubicin and cyclophosphamide)

chemotherapy for breast cancer include varying degrees of nausea, vomiting, fatigue, myelosuppression, and alopecia. Long-term toxicities include the induction of premature menopause after cyclophosphamide-containing regimens, cardiac toxicity after doxorubicin-containing chemotherapy, and neuropathy following use of the taxanes (paclitaxel or docetaxel). In addition, some chemotherapy drugs have been associated with an increase in the risk of acute leukemia, particularly when used in higher than standard doses.

Like adjuvant chemotherapy, adjuvant hormonal therapy is also used to improve the chance of cure following local therapy for breast cancer and is indicated for individuals whose cancers express estrogen, progesterone, or both receptors. Historically, tamoxifen has been the most widely used hormonal treatment; a 5-year course of tamoxifen can reduce the annual risk of recurrence by nearly 50% in patients with estrogen receptor–positive tumors and is effective regardless of menopausal status. Premenopausal women also benefit from ovarian ablation as adjuvant therapy; however, the value of oophorectomy added to tamoxifen remains a matter of investigation. For postmenopausal women, the selective aromatase inhibitors, which prevent the peripheral conversion of adrenally produced androgens into estrogens are also very effective in the adjuvant setting. Several large randomized clinical trials have demonstrated a benefit to using aromatase inhibitors either as an alternative to or in sequence with tamoxifen in postmenopausal hormone receptor-positive breast cancer. Ongoing studies are evaluating the safety and efficacy of aromatase inhibitors in combination with ovarian ablation in premenopausal hormone receptor-positive breast cancer.

Tamoxifen should also be considered for use in women with ductal carcinoma in situ who have undergone breast conservation because this treatment reduces the risk of local recurrence as well as contralateral new primary breast cancers. The aromatase inhibitors are under investigation for the treatment of postmenopausal DCIS. The common adverse effects of tamoxifen include vasomotor symptomatology and vaginal discharge. The long-term side effects of tamoxifen include increased risks of endometrial cancer, thromboembolic events, and cataracts. Tamoxifen has favorable effects on lipid profiles and on bone mineral density in postmenopausal women. Aromatase inhibitors are also associated with vasomotor symptoms but do not appear to have the same risk of uterine cancer or thromboembolism. Aromatase inhibitors can result in bone density loss and are associated with an increased incidence of musculoskeletal symptoms. For women with invasive breast cancer, the risks of hormonal therapy are generally more than offset by the survival advantage gained by preventing breast cancer recurrence. Their use in noninvasive breast cancer and in the setting of prevention need to be considered more cautiously, given the lack of survival advantage in the latter situations.

## FOLLOW-UP AND SURVEILLANCE FOR INDIVIDUALS WITH BREAST CANCER

Whereas screening for early stage (potentially curable) disease may have an important impact on survival, intensive surveillance to detect metastatic disease has not been shown to significantly affect outcome. The American Society of Clinical Oncology guidelines recommend that careful history and physical examination be performed every 3 to 6 months for 3 years after diagnosis, then every 6 to 12 months for the next 2 years, and annually thereafter. Patients should also continue annual mammography, annual pelvic examination, and monthly breast self-examination. The routine use of tumor marker studies, other blood work, chest radiography, bone scans, or CT scans is not encouraged.

Because long-term survival after a diagnosis of breast cancer is common, it is important that patients continue to receive preventive medicine recommendations and undergo screening for treatable conditions. Examples include screening for colon cancer, cervical cancer, and osteoporosis, as well as preventive strategies for heart disease. Issues relating to menopause may be of particular concern for breast cancer survivors in whom hormone replacement therapy is generally contraindicated.

## METASTATIC BREAST CANCER

Once breast cancer metastasizes to organs outside of the breast and local lymph nodes, cure is unlikely, however, average survival with metastatic breast cancer has improved significantly over the past several decades. Breast cancer tends to be responsive to a variety of therapies including chemotherapy, hormonal therapy, and biologic therapies. Treatment is directed at palliating symptoms and prolonging life. Because prolonged treatment is often required, a selection of agents with favorable toxicity profiles is desirable.

For patients who have estrogen and or progesterone receptor–positive metastatic disease, hormonal therapy is generally preferred over chemotherapy. Factors that predict a higher likelihood of response to hormonal therapy include a long disease-free interval before the development of metastatic disease and disease that is limited to bone, soft tissues, and pleura. In postmenopausal women, the selective aromatase inhibitors appear to be superior to tamoxifen as first-line therapy. Premenopausal women may benefit from the removal of the ovaries or suppression of ovarian function with GNRH agonists. Aromatase inhibitors can be considered in combination with ovarian ablation in premenopausal women. Tamoxifen may be given alone or in combination with ovarian ablation. Hormonal therapy should be continued as long as no evidence of disease progression is present. Patients whose disease has previously responded to a hormonal manipulation have a reasonable chance of responding to subsequent hormonal maneuvers. Commonly used hormonal therapies for metastatic breast cancer are listed in Table 24.3.

Individuals whose cancers are hormone receptor–negative, who have rapidly progressive or organ-threatening disease, and those whose disease is no longer responding to hormonal therapy are candidates for chemotherapy. Chemotherapy drugs for metastatic disease may be given as single agents or in combination. Although the response rates are often higher with combinations of drugs, this may not translate into a survival advantage and may expose patients to unnecessary toxicity. Patients with rapidly progressive visceral disease are most likely to benefit from combination therapy, whereas those with slower paced disease may be successfully treated with single agents given sequentially. A variety of chemotherapy drugs have activity in metastatic breast cancer, and many of these are outlined in Table 24.4.

The current trend toward attempting to specifically target therapies to the cancer is exemplified by the development of trastuzumab (Herceptin) for individuals with metastatic breast cancer overexpressing the *HER2/neu* protein. This monoclonal antibody therapy, although having a favorable toxicity profile, has activity as a single agent in patients with *HER2/neu* overexpressing metastatic breast cancer. When used in combination with standard chemotherapy, a survival advantage is observed over using chemotherapy alone in *HER2/neu* overexpressing metastatic breast cancer. Other monoclonal antibody treatments, as well as other classes of biologic therapies such as angiogenesis inhibitors and inhibitors of the epidermal growth factor receptor (EGFR),

## TABLE 24.4
### CHEMOTHERAPY AGENTS ACTIVE IN METASTATIC BREAST CANCER

Capecitabine
Cyclophosphamide
Docetaxel
Doxorubicin
Epirubicin
5-Fluorouracil
Gemcitabine
Methotrexate
Vinorelbine
Paclitaxel

are currently under investigation for the treatment of metastatic breast cancer.

Symptom control is also an important aspect of managing metastatic breast cancer. Radiation therapy can be useful in palliating painful bony lesions or brain metastases and may be used to prevent an impending fracture or to treat spinal cord compression. Bisphosphonates, such as pamidronate and zolendronate, are useful in preventing skeletal complications from lytic bone metastases.

## BREAST CANCER PREVENTION

Until relatively recently, little knowledge pertained to the means of preventing the development of breast cancer. Currently, options include prophylactic surgery (bilateral mastectomies) and use of the selective estrogen receptor modulator tamoxifen.

Although no large randomized controlled trials have evaluated the effectiveness of prophylactic bilateral mastectomies for the prevention of breast cancer, a retrospective series from the Mayo Clinic suggested at least a 90% reduction in the risk of breast cancer using bilateral prophylactic mastectomy. For most women, however, breast cancer risk does not warrant this permanent and disfiguring option.

The effectiveness of tamoxifen for the prevention of breast cancer was demonstrated in a randomized controlled trial conducted by the National Surgical Adjuvant Breast and Bowel Project. It had previously been observed that women receiving adjuvant tamoxifen for early stage breast cancer had fewer contralateral new primary breast cancers than those who did not receive tamoxifen, suggesting the drug's potential role as a preventive agent for women at high risk for breast cancer. The selection criteria used in the study, National Surgical Adjuvant Breast and Bowel Project P1, are outlined in Table 24.5. In this study, women randomized to receive 5 years of tamoxifen experienced a 49% reduction in the risk of developing invasive breast cancer at a median follow-up time of 54.6 months. Tamoxifen preferentially prevented hormone receptor–positive breast cancer, with

## TABLE 24.3
### HORMONAL TREATMENT FOR METASTATIC BREAST CANCER

**Antiestrogens**

Tamoxifen
Toremifene
Fulvestrant (ER downregulator)
**Ovarian Ablation[a]**

Surgical oophorectomy
Gonadotropin-releasing hormone analogs
**Selective Aromatase Inhibitors[b]**

Anastrozole
Letrozole
Exemestane
**Progestational Agents**

Megestrol acetate
**Androgens**

Halotestin

[a] Active in premenopausal women.
[b] Active in postmenopausal women.

**TABLE 24.5**

**BREAST CANCER RISK CRITERIA FOR NATIONAL SURGICAL ADJUVANT BREAST AND BOWEL PROJECT P1**

Female age 60 or older
OR
Female age 35–59 with lobular carcinoma in situ on prior biopsy
OR
5-Year calculated breast cancer risk of at least 1.66%[a]

[a] Breast cancer risk is calculated using the Gail model, which takes into account the following variables: age, race, number of first-degree relatives with breast cancer, nulliparity or age at first live birth, number of prior breast biopsies, history of atypical hyperplasia on biopsy, and age at menarche.

no reduction in the development of hormone receptor–negative breast cancer. In addition, no difference in survival has been observed between patients who received and did not receive tamoxifen in the setting of prevention.

Raloxifene, like tamoxifen, is a selective estrogen receptor modulator and is currently used in the treatment of postmenopausal women with osteoporosis. In the Multiple Outcomes of Raloxifene trial, a placebo-controlled trial of raloxifene for osteoporosis treatment in postmenopausal women, patients receiving raloxifene were observed to have fewer breast cancers and a trend toward fewer endometrial cancers than those not receiving the drug. It is anticipated, therefore, that this drug may also be useful in breast cancer prevention. Currently, a second prevention trial, the National Surgical Adjuvant Breast and Bowel Project P2, is comparing the safety and effectiveness of raloxifene versus tamoxifen in the prevention of breast cancer. Aromatase inhibitors are also under investigation for the prevention of breast cancer in postmenopausal women at risk.

## REVIEW EXERCISES

### QUESTIONS

**1–4.** Choose the appropriate breast cancer screening/prevention strategy (in addition to regular breast self-examination) for each asymptomatic woman below:

**1.** A 55-year-old woman with no family history of breast cancer or personal history of breast disease

**2.** A 42-year-old woman with LCIS

**3.** A 30-year-old smoker whose great aunt had breast cancer at age 65

**4.** A 28-year-old woman whose sister had bilateral breast cancer in her 30s and mother had ovarian cancer in her 50s

a) Clinical breast examination every 3 years
b) Annual mammography and clinical breast examination
c) Clinical breast examination and mammography every 6 to 12 months
d) Annual mammography, clinical breast examination, and consideration of tamoxifen, 20 mg, daily for 5 years

**5–8.** Choose the most appropriate management for each patient with metastatic breast cancer:

**5.** A 40-year-old premenopausal woman treated with chemotherapy alone for early stage hormone receptor–positive breast cancer 3 years ago develops diffuse bone pain and is found to have multiple lytic bone metastases.

**6.** A 45-year-old woman with hormone receptor–negative breast cancer involving lungs, who has been responding to chemotherapy, develops headache and slurred speech. She is found to have multiple brain metastases.

**7.** A 60-year-old woman with *HER2/neu* overexpressing hormone receptor–negative breast cancer is found to have liver metastases 9 months after the completion of adjuvant doxorubicin-containing chemotherapy.

**8.** A 65-year-old woman has just undergone pleurodesis for a malignant pleural effusion occurring 2 years after completing adjuvant tamoxifen for early stage breast cancer.
a) Refer to radiation therapy.
b) Begin a selective aromatase inhibitor.
c) Initiate trastuzumab in combination with taxane chemotherapy.
d) Recommend bilateral oophorectomy, tamoxifen and monthly zoledronate.
e) Proceed with high-dose chemotherapy and stem cell transplant.

**9.** Which of the following factors in metastatic breast cancer predicts for response to hormonal therapy?
a) Progression of bone disease 3 years after an initial response to prior hormonal therapy
b) Young age
c) Hepatic involvement of breast cancer
d) Persistence of menses following adjuvant breast cancer therapy

**10.** Which of the following most clearly improves the cure rate for a 75-year-old woman who has undergone excision of a 2-cm estrogen receptor–positive left breast cancer?
a) Left axillary dissection or sentinel lymph node procedure
b) Bilateral mastectomies
c) Tamoxifen, 20 mg/day for 5 years

**d)** CMF [cyclophosphamide, methotrexate and 5- fluorouracil] chemotherapy for 6 months

**11.** Adjuvant chemotherapy for early stage breast cancer results in which of the following?
**a)** Prevention of or delay in progression to metastatic disease
**b)** Rapid reduction in cancer-related symptoms
**c)** Decrease in the risk of new primary breast cancers
**d)** All of the above

**12–17.** For each of the following treatments used in patients with early breast cancer, match the associated potential long-term toxicity:

**12.** Tamoxifen

**13.** Anastrozole

**14.** Doxorubicin

**15.** Cyclophosphamide

**16.** Paclitaxel

**17.** Chest-wall radiation therapy
**a)** Congestive heart failure
**b)** Premature menopause
**c)** Uterine cancer
**d)** Neuropathy
**e)** Lymphedema
**f)** Osteoporosis

## ANSWERS

**1. b.**
In women aged 50 to 69 years, annual mammography, in combination with clinical breast examination, appears to reduce breast cancer mortality.

**2. d.**
An individual with LCIS is at increased risk for breast cancer. Individuals over the age of 35 with LCIS were eligible for NSABP-1, a clinical trial that demonstrated a reduction in breast cancer risk using tamoxifen for 5 years. Participants with LCIS appeared to derive particular benefit from tamoxifen, and women under the age of 50 were less likely to experience severe toxicity from tamoxifen. The risks and benefits of chemoprevention with tamoxifen should be discussed with this patient. Screening should include annual mammograms and clinical breast examinations.

**3. a.**
This individual's breast cancer risk is not high enough to warrant intensive screening, and age-appropriate recommendations include breast self-examination and clinical breast examination every 3 years. A baseline mammogram could be considered at age 35; annual mammograms should begin at age 40.

**4. c.**
This individual's family history is suggestive of a hereditary breast cancer syndrome, and intensive surveillance is appropriate. The value of tamoxifen for chemoprevention in this population is unclear. If this patient were to test positive for *BRCA-1* or *BRCA-2*, counseling on the options of prophylactic mastectomies and/or oophorectomy (after completion of childbearing) is appropriate.

**5. d.**
Appropriate first-line hormonal therapy for a premenopausal woman with osseous metastatic breast cancer includes ovarian ablation, tamoxifen, or the combination. An aromatase inhibitor in combination with ovarian ablation would also be reasonable, but is not listed as an option. The addition of a bisphosphonate decreases the risk of fracture and other complications of lytic bone metastases.

**6. a.**
Systemic chemotherapy is unlikely to be effective for the treatment of central nervous system metastases. Whole brain radiation is appropriate in this situation.

**7. c.**
In *HER2/neu* overexpressing metastatic breast cancer, a survival advantage is observed when trastuzumab is combined with paclitaxel or docetaxel chemotherapy.

**8. b.**
Hormonal therapy is appropriate for this patient having presumably hormone receptor–positive metastatic breast cancer limited to the pleura, and a selective aromatase inhibitor is the best option for this postmenopausal woman.

**9. a.**
Response to hormonal therapy for metastatic disease is more likely with estrogen receptor/progesterone receptor–positive disease; long disease-free intervals; older age; disease that is limited to bone, soft tissues, and pleura; as well as disease that has previously responded to hormonal therapy.

**10. c.**
Whereas an axillary node dissection or sentinel lymph node procedure is appropriate for the staging of breast cancer, a survival advantage to such procedures has not been established. Similarly, neither mastectomy nor bilateral mastectomy has demonstrated a survival benefit over breast-conserving surgery. The benefit of chemotherapy in women older than the age of 70 with low-risk disease is unclear; however, a clear benefit in both survival and recurrence-free survival persists with tamoxifen regardless of patient age.

**11. a.**

The purpose of adjuvant chemotherapy is to reduce the risk of recurrence after surgical removal of the cancer. By definition, patients receiving adjuvant chemotherapy do not have symptomatic or detectable disease. Whereas adjuvant tamoxifen has been demonstrated to reduce the risk of contralateral new primary breast cancers, the same effect has not been established with chemotherapy.

**12. c.**

Tamoxifen has estrogen-like effects on the endometrium and, like estrogen, increases the risk of uterine cancer.

**13. f.**

Because of profound lowering of estrogen levels, the aromatase inhibitors can result in bone density loss increasing the risk of osteoporosis and fracture.

**14. a**

Doxorubicin is associated with cardiotoxicity. The effect is related to total (life-time) dose of doxorubicin.

**15. b**

Alkylating agents, including cyclophosphamide, can cause ovarian failure. The risk is increased with higher patient age and higher cumulative drug dose.

**16. d.**

Paclitaxel is associated with a peripheral neuropathy that preferentially affects the long nerves. This effect is usually reversible, but may persist in some patients.

**17. e.**

Local-regional radiation therapy is associated with an increased risk of lymphedema in the affected arm. The risk is increased with axillary radiation and with prior axillary dissection.

## SUGGESTED READINGS

Baum M, Budzar AU, Cuzick J, et al. Anastrozole alone or in combination with tamoxifen versus tamoxifen alone for the treatment off postmenopausal women with early breast cancer. *Lancet* 2002;359:2131–2139.

Chlebowski RT, Hendrix SL, Langer RD, et al. Influence of estrogen plus progestin on breast cancer and mammography in healthy postmenopausal women: the Women's Health Initiative Randomized Trial. *JAMA* 2003:289;3243–3253.

Claus EB, Risch N, Thompson WD. Autosomal dominant inheritance of early-onset breast cancer: implications for risk prediction. *Cancer* 1994;73:643–651.

Collaborative Group on Hormonal Factors in Breast Cancer. Breast cancer and hormone replacement therapy: collaborative reanalysis of data from 51 epidemiological studies of 52,705 women with breast cancer and 108,411 women without breast cancer. *Lancet* 1997;350:1047–1059.

Coombes RC, Hall E, Gibson LJ, et al. A randomized trial of exemestane after two to three years of tamoxifen therapy in postmenopausal women with primary breast cancer. *N Engl J Med* 2004:350;1081–1092.

Cox CE, Haddad F, Bass S, et al. Lymphatic mapping in the treatment of breast cancer. *Oncology* 1998;17:1283–1292.

Early Breast Cancer Trialists' Collaborative Group. Polychemotherapy for early breast cancer: an overview of the randomized trials. *Lancet* 1998;352:930–942.

Early Breast Cancer Trialists' Collaborative Group. Tamoxifen for early breast cancer: an overview of the randomized trials. *Lancet* 1998;351:1451–1467.

Fisher B, Costantino JP, Wickerham DL, et al. Tamoxifen for the prevention of breast cancer: report of the National Surgical Adjuvant Breast and Bowel Project P-1 Study. *J Natl Cancer Inst* 1998;90:1371–1388.

Fisher B, Dignam J, Wolmark N, et al. Tamoxifen in treatment of intraductal breast cancer: National Surgical Adjuvant Breast and Bowel Project B-24 randomized controlled trial. *Lancet* 1999;353:1993–2000.

Goss PE, Ingle JN, Martino S, et al. A randomized trial of letrozole in postmenopausal women after five years of tamoxifen therapy for early-stage breast cancer. *N Engl J Med* 2003:349;1793–1802.

Grodstein F, Stampfer MJ, Colditz FA, et al. Postmenopausal hormone therapy and mortality. *N Engl J Med* 1997;336:1769–1775.

Hartmann LC, Schaid DJ, Woods JE, et al. Efficacy of bilateral prophylactic mastectomy in women with a family history of breast cancer. *N Engl J Med* 1999;340:77–84.

Hortobagyi GN, Theriault RL, Lipton A, et al. Long-term prevention of skeletal complications of metastatic breast cancer with pamidronate. *J Clin Oncol* 1998;16:2038–2044.

Hoskins KF, Stopfer JE, Calzone KA. Assessment and counseling for women with a family history of breast cancer: a guide for clinicians. *JAMA* 1995;273:577–585.

Liede A, Karlan BY, Narod SA. Cancer risks for male carriers of germline mutations in BRCA1 or BRCA2: a review of the literature. *J Clin Oncol* 2004:22;735–742.

MacMahon B, Cole P, Brown J. Etiology of human breast cancer. *J Natl Cancer Inst* 1973;50:21–42.

Morrow M, Schnitt SJ, Harris JR. In situ carcinomas. In: Harris JR, Lippman ME, Morrow M, et al., eds. *Diseases of the Breast.* Philadelphia: Lippincott–Raven, 1996:355–368.

Norton L, Slamon D, Leyland-Jones B, et al. Overall survival (OS) advantage to simultaneous chemotherapy (CRx) plus the humanized anti-HER2 monoclonal antibody Herceptin (H) in HER2-overexpression (HER2+) metastatic breast cancer (MBC). *Proc Am Soc Clin Oncol* 1999;18:127a(abst).

Recommended Breast Cancer Surveillance Guidelines. *J Clin Oncol* 1997;15:2149–2156.

Ries LAG, Eisner MP, Kosary CL, et al., eds. *SEER Cancer Statistics Review, 1973–1997.* National Cancer Institute, NIH Publication No. 00-2789. Bethesda, MD: 2000.

Rosen PP. Invasive mammary carcinoma. In: Harris JR, Lippman ME, Morrow M, et al., eds. *Diseases of the Breast.* Philadelphia: Lippincott–Raven, 1996:393–444.

Singletary SE, Allred C, Ashley P, et al. Revision of the American Joint Committee on cancer staging system for breast cancer. *J Clin Oncol* 2002;20:3628–3636.

Smith-Warner SA, Spiegelman D, Yaun S, et al. Alcohol and breast cancer in women: a pooled analysis of cohort studies. *JAMA* 1998;279:535–540.

WHI Investigators. Risks and benefits of estrogen plus progestin in healthy postmenopausal women: principal results from the Women's Health Initiative Randomized Controlled Trial. *JAMA* 2002;288;321–333.

# Lymphoma

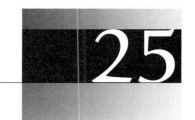

*Brad L. Pohlman*

## HODGKIN LYMPHOMA

Hodgkin lymphoma (or Hodgkin's disease) is a malignant neoplasm involving primarily lymphoid tissue. It has a characteristic histologic appearance, including Reed-Sternberg cells or their variants. Accumulating data suggest that the origin of Reed-Sternberg cells is a precursor B cell. The etiology of Hodgkin lymphoma is not known. Epidemiologic, serologic, and genetic studies have implicated Epstein-Barr virus in some cases. The American Cancer Society estimates that 7,000 new cases and 1,320 deaths will occur in the United States during 2004.

### Clinical Presentation

The most common initial complaint is painless enlargement of cervical, supraclavicular, axillary, or, less often, inguinal lymph nodes. Most patients are asymptomatic, but up to one third of patients have systemic B symptoms (e.g., fevers, night sweats, weight loss). Some patients complain of cough, chest pain, dyspnea, or diminished exercise tolerance attributable to mediastinal or, less commonly, pericardial or pulmonary involvement. Infrequently, patients experience generalized or, less commonly, localized pruritus, which may be associated with a skin rash. Patients with a history of mononucleosis, autoimmune disease, or immunodeficiency, including human immunodeficiency virus (HIV) infection, have an increased incidence of Hodgkin lymphoma. The siblings of young adults with Hodgkin lymphoma have an increased incidence.

An enlargement of supradiaphragmatic lymph nodes is present in most patients. Lymphadenopathy exclusively below the diaphragm occurs in only 5% to 10% of patients. Lymph nodes are usually firm, rubbery, mobile, and nontender. The spleen may be palpable. Laboratory abnormalities are not specific. A moderate to marked leukemoid reaction, monocytosis, eosinophilia, and thrombocytosis are common. Anemia resulting from impaired iron use, lymphopenia, and thrombocytopenia usually occur in patients with more advanced disease. An elevation of the erythrocyte sedimentation rate is present in approximately one-half of patients. Chest radiography commonly demonstrates mediastinal or hilar adenopathy.

## Diagnosis and Staging

The diagnosis of Hodgkin lymphoma requires a biopsy of an involved lymph node or an extralymphatic site. If a superficial lymph node is not accessible, a percutaneous True-cut needle biopsy occasionally may be adequate. A fine-needle aspiration may be adequate to identify other malignancies, such as metastatic carcinoma, but this technique usually cannot distinguish Hodgkin lymphoma from non-Hodgkin lymphoma (NHL) or most benign etiologies. The histologic criteria for diagnosis include a disrupted nodal architecture, Reed-Sternberg cells or variants, and a nonmalignant reactive background. Two major types of Hodgkin lymphoma are recognized: classical (which includes the nodular sclerosis, mixed cellularity, lymphocyte-rich, and lymphocyte-depleted subtypes) and nodular lymphocyte-predominant.

All sites of disease must be identified to stage, plan, and monitor therapy. The staging process should include a detailed history, with particular attention to B symptoms, pruritus, HIV risk factors, and performance status; a complete physical examination, including the size of lymph nodes, liver, and spleen; laboratory evaluation, including a complete blood cell count and differential, Westergren erythrocyte sedimentation rate, liver tests, creatinine and calcium levels, and HIV screening (if risk factors are present); and radiologic studies, including chest radiography and computed tomography (CT) of the chest, abdomen, and pelvis. Patients with suspected advanced-stage disease should have bilateral iliac crest bone marrow biopsies. Positron emission tomography (PET) scan is also useful in some patients. Bipedal lymphangiography or staging laparotomy are no longer utilized. The Ann Arbor staging system is shown in Table 25.1.

## Treatment

The initial treatment of Hodgkin lymphoma depends primarily on the stage, but also may be influenced by the histologic subtype, other prognostic features, and physician or patient preference. Historically, patients with early stage (I and II) disease were treated with extensive radiation therapy. Currently, most of these patients are treated with chemotherapy followed by more limited radiation

## TABLE 25.1
### ANN ARBOR STAGING SYSTEM

| Stage | Definition |
|---|---|
| I | One lymph node region |
| II | Two or more lymph node regions on the same side of the diaphragm |
| III | Lymph node regions on both sides of the diaphragm |
| IV | Extranodal sites |
| A | No B symptom |
| B | Any B symptom (i.e., fever, night sweats, or weight loss) |

therapy. Patients with advanced-stage (III, IV, or bulky II) disease are treated with chemotherapy followed occasionally by radiation therapy (primarily to sites of initially bulky disease). Patients who relapse after radiation therapy alone should receive combination chemotherapy. Patients who relapse after chemotherapy may occasionally be cured with another regimen; however, high-dose chemotherapy with autologous bone marrow or stem cell transplantation offers the best chance for long-term, disease-free survival.

## Prognosis

The prognosis for patients with newly diagnosed Hodgkin lymphoma is predicted by the stage and bulk of disease. Patients with Hodgkin lymphoma that has relapsed after initial radiation therapy have the same prognosis as patients with newly diagnosed advanced-stage disease. Patients with Hodgkin lymphoma that has relapsed following chemotherapy have a worse prognosis (Table 25.2).

Among patients with newly diagnosed advanced-stage disease, a prognostic score identified seven independent poor prognostic features: albumin level of less than 4 g/dL, hemoglobin level of less than 10.5 g/dL, male sex, stage IV disease, age 45 years or older, white blood cell count of 15,000/mm$^3$ or higher, and lymphocyte count below 600/mm$^3$ or less than 8%. The number of poor prognostic features predicts both freedom from progression and overall survival (Table 25.3).

## TABLE 25.2
### PROGNOSIS FOR PATIENTS WITH HODGKIN LYMPHOMA

| Clinical Situation | Overall Survival (%) |
|---|---|
| Stage I–II | 80–95 |
| Stage III–IV | 50–85 |
| Bulky stage I–II | 50–85 |
| Relapse after radiation therapy | 50–85 |
| Relapse after chemotherapy | 20–50 |

## TABLE 25.3
### PROGNOSTIC FEATURES IN HODGKIN LYMPHOMA

| Poor Prognostic Features | Freedom from Progression (%) | Overall Survival (%) |
|---|---|---|
| 0 | 84 | 89 |
| 1 | 77 | 90 |
| 2 | 67 | 81 |
| 3 | 60 | 78 |
| 4 | 51 | 61 |
| 5 | 42 | 56 |

Adapted from Hasenclever D, Diehl V. A prognostic score for advanced Hodgkin's disease. International Prognostic Factors Project on Advanced Hodgkin's Disease. *N Engl J Med* 1998;339(21):1506–1514.

## Complications

In addition to relapse, patients who have been treated for Hodgkin lymphoma are susceptible to a variety of disease-related and treatment-related complications. Because of disease-associated cell-mediated immunodeficiency, prior splenectomy, chemotherapy-induced neutropenia, or steroid administration, these patients are at risk for developing serious bacterial and fungal infections, *Varicella zoster, Pneumocystis carinii* pneumonia, and other opportunistic infections. Up to 50% of patients who receive mantle irradiation develop clinical or subclinical hypothyroidism, which may not be apparent for several years. In addition, up to one-half of these patients develop benign, or rarely malignant, thyroid neoplasms 20 years or longer after treatment. Cardiopulmonary complications from chemotherapy, especially doxorubicin and bleomycin, and mantle irradiation may occur during or months to years after treatment. These complications are more likely to occur in patients who have received both chemotherapy and radiation therapy. Pulmonary complications include acute pneumonitis and chronic restrictive fibrosis. Cardiac complications include acute pericarditis, chronic constrictive pericarditis, acute myocarditis, myocardial dysfunction, valvular heart disease, and accelerated coronary artery disease. Some chemotherapy regimens may cause temporary or permanent azoospermia in males and amenorrhea, sterility, or premature menopause in females. The incidence is higher in women over the age of 25 years and in those who receive chemotherapy and pelvic irradiation. The risk of second malignancies after the treatment of Hodgkin lymphoma is significantly higher than expected for age-matched controls. Of patients who receive extensive radiation therapy, 10% to 20% may subsequently develop solid tumors. The risk continues to increase with time. These tumors, which usually occur within the radiation field, include soft tissue sarcoma; melanoma; and cancer of the head, neck, lung, breast, gastrointestinal tract, and urogenital tract. NHL develops in approximately 5% of patients.

Myelodysplastic syndrome and acute nonlymphocytic leukemia occur mainly as a complication of chemotherapy, particularly following the use of alkylating agents, in 3% to 10% of patients 2 to 10 years after treatment. The short-term and long-term psychosocial sequelae of the diagnosis and treatment of Hodgkin lymphoma often are not discussed. These patients face problems with body image, self-esteem, marriage, interpersonal relationships, sexuality, insurability, employment, and socioeconomic advancement.

## NON-HODGKIN LYMPHOMA

Non-Hodgkin lymphoma is a heterogeneous group of malignant neoplasms arising from the immune system. Although these disorders are discussed together, they actually constitute an array of clinicopathologic entities with widely variable features, behavior, treatment, and prognosis. The American Cancer Society estimates that 54,370 new cases and 196,410 deaths will occur in the United States in 2004. The incidence increases with age, and the median age is 65 years.

Patients with inherited and acquired immunodeficiencies have a significantly increased risk of developing NHL. With few exceptions, the etiology of NHL is unknown. Epidemiologic studies have implicated irradiation, chemotherapy, and some environmental exposures (e.g., pesticides and dark hair dyes). Table 25.4 presents infectious agents that have been strongly implicated in the pathogenesis of certain subtypes of NHL.

### Clinical Presentation

Because NHL may involve any lymphatic or extralymphatic tissue, virtually any presenting symptom is possible. Most patients complain of painless enlargement of one or more superficial lymph nodes. This abnormality may have been present for weeks or months and may have been stable or progressing. Mediastinal lymphadenopathy may cause chest pain, cough, dyspnea, or superior vena cava syndrome. Retroperitoneal or mesenteric lymphadenopathy or splenomegaly may cause abdominal pain or fullness, early satiety, or back pain. Although extranodal involvement is often a manifestation of more extensive nodal disease, some extranodal sites may be the only site involved: *Gastrointestinal tract lymphoma* may lead to abdominal pain or fullness, early satiety, symptoms of complete or partial bowel obstruction, hemorrhage, or perforation; *central nervous system lymphoma* may cause headaches, change in mental status, seizures, focal neurologic deficits; and *cutaneous lymphoma* may result in localized or extensive lesions. Symptoms may be due to involvement of less common sites, such as bone, testis, spinal cord, orbit, and sinus. Patients may complain of symptoms of anemia or thrombocytopenia. Approximately 20% of patients have B symptoms (i.e., fever, night sweats, or weight loss).

The most common physical finding is single or multiple, firm, enlarged, nontender cervical, supraclavicular, axillary, inguinal, or epitrochlear lymph nodes. Splenomegaly is common. Occasionally, a mass may be palpable in the abdomen or pelvis. Waldeyer's ring may be involved. Extranodal involvement (e.g., skin, central nervous system, testis, bone, or orbit) may lead to abnormal findings.

The complete blood count is often normal; however, patients may have mild to moderate anemia (due to gastrointestinal involvement and hemorrhage, impaired iron utilization, or bone marrow involvement), thrombocytopenia (resulting from bone marrow involvement, hypersplenism, or immune thrombocytopenic purpura), or, less commonly, leukopenia. Serum lactate dehydrogenase (LDH) may be mildly or markedly elevated. A monoclonal gammopathy may be present. Imaging studies may show lymphadenopathy, splenomegaly, or parenchymal lesions in any organ.

### Diagnosis and Evaluation

The diagnosis of NHL requires a tissue biopsy. The World Health Organization classification recognizes more than two dozen different types of NHL. The specific types are defined by histology, immunophenotype, and, occasionally, genotype. For non-oncologists, the subtypes of NHL can be divided into two broad categories: *indolent* (i.e., low grade) and *aggressive* (i.e., intermediate and high grade). Examples of each are listed here:

- Indolent lymphomas
  - ☐ Follicular lymphoma
  - ☐ Small lymphocytic lymphoma
  - ☐ Extranodal marginal zone B-cell lymphoma of mucosa-associated lymphoid tissue (MALT)
- Aggressive lymphomas
  - ☐ Diffuse large B-cell lymphoma
  - ☐ Peripheral T-cell lymphoma
  - ☐ Lymphoblastic lymphoma
  - ☐ Burkitt lymphoma

**TABLE 25.4**

**INFECTIOUS AGENTS STRONGLY IMPLICATED IN THE PATHOGENESIS OF CERTAIN SUBTYPES OF NON-HODGKIN LYMPHOMA**

| Infectious Agent | Non-Hodgkin Lymphoma Subtype |
| --- | --- |
| Epstein-Barr virus | Posttransplant lymphoproliferations |
| Epstein-Barr virus | Burkitt lymphoma |
| Human T-cell lymphotrophic virus 1 | T-cell leukemia/lymphoma |
| Human herpesvirus 8 | Primary effusion lymphoma |
| *Helicobacter pylori* | Gastric MALT lymphoma |

The indolent lymphomas account for approximately 50% of cases. Advanced-stage (III or IV) disease accounts for 80%. With few exceptions, these patients are incurable with conventional therapy. Paradoxically, they have a relatively long median survival of 5 to 10 years.

The aggressive lymphomas account for the remaining 50% of cases. Approximately 50% of patients have localized or early stage (I or II) disease. Patients with these subtypes are potentially curable with appropriate therapy. Fewer than 50% are actually cured, however. The median survival is only 1 to 4 years.

The complete evaluation of these patients provides prognostic information and dictates management. The evaluation should include a detailed history, including age, performance status, and HIV risk factors; a complete physical examination, including lymph node regions, liver, and spleen; laboratory evaluation, including a complete blood cell count, differential, liver tests, creatinine, calcium, and LDH levels, and HIV screening (if risk factors are present); radiologic studies, including chest radiography and CT of the chest, abdomen, and pelvis, and occasionally other imaging studies [e.g., magnetic resonance imaging (MRI) or PET scan] that may define other sites of disease; and bone marrow aspirate and iliac crest biopsy(ies). The stage is defined by the Ann Arbor system for Hodgkin lymphoma.

## Treatment

The management of patients with NHL depends on the specific pathologic subtype. Most indolent lymphomas are considered incurable, and treatment is by definition palliative. Some patients may not require any treatment initially, and expectant monitoring of symptoms, physical findings, and radiographic abnormalities may be all that is required. When the patient develops deleterious signs or symptoms (e.g., bulky lymphadenopathy, pain, fever, night sweats, weight loss, anemia, or thrombocytopenia), or progressive disease with impending problems, treatment should be initiated. Patients with localized disease may receive chemotherapy, radiation therapy, or both. Patients with advanced-stage disease usually receive chemotherapy.

Rituximab is a monoclonal antibody that binds specifically to CD20 on benign and malignant B lymphocytes and leads to apoptosis and the activation of immune responses (e.g., complement-dependent cytotoxicity and antibody-dependent cellular cytotoxicity). Approximately 50% of patients with relapsed indolent NHL respond to this agent. Rituximab is often combined with chemotherapy. Two recently approved radiolabeled monoclonal antibodies (yttrium[90] ibritumomab tiuxetan and iodine 131 tositumomab) lead to high response rates and durable remissions even in chemotherapy-refractory and rituximab-refractory patients.

Gastric MALT lymphoma is a unique and uncommon variant of extranodal marginal zone B-cell lymphoma of mucosa-associated lymphoid tissue (MALT), which in-

### TABLE 25.5

**INTERNATIONAL PROGNOSTIC INDEX FOR NON-HODGKIN LYMPHOMA**

| Poor Prognostic Features | Complete Response (%) | 5-Yr Survival (%) |
|---|---|---|
| 0 or 1 | 87 | 73 |
| 2 | 67 | 51 |
| 3 | 55 | 43 |
| 4 or 5 | 44 | 26 |

Adapted from Anonymous. A predictive model for aggressive non-Hodgkin's lymphoma. The International Non-Hodgkin's Lymphoma Prognostic Factors Project. *N Engl J Med* 1993;329(14):987–994.

volves the stomach. Approximately 90% of cases are caused by *Helicobacter pylori*. Infection with this bacterium leads to chronic inflammation in the gastric mucosa, persistent lymphocyte stimulation, and development of an *H. pylori*–dependent (and subsequently independent) monoclonal B-cell proliferation. Remarkably, 50% to 70% of patients with localized gastric MALT lymphoma respond to anti–*H. pylori* therapy.

In general, patients with newly diagnosed, aggressive, localized lymphoma should receive chemotherapy followed by involved field radiation therapy. Patients with newly diagnosed, advanced-stage, aggressive lymphoma should receive chemotherapy. Three large randomized studies show that the addition of rituximab to standard chemotherapy improves survival. For patients who relapse after initial therapy, many salvage chemotherapeutic regimens are available. Patients who respond to salvage chemotherapy should receive high-dose therapy with autologous blood stem cell transplantation.

## Prognosis

The prognosis of patients with newly diagnosed, aggressive NHL is predicted by the International Prognostic Index. This model recognizes five clinical features that independently predict a worse prognosis: age older than 60 years, LDH above normal level, performance status 2 to 4, stage III or IV, and more than one extranodal site of disease (Table 25.5).

## REVIEW EXERCISES

### QUESTIONS

**1.** A 20-year-old woman presents with night sweats, 15-lb weight loss, and painless left neck lumps. Physical examination is remarkable only for multiple, nontender, rubbery, mobile, 1- to 2-cm left cervical lymph nodes. Laboratory studies reveal normocytic, normochromic anemia. CT of the neck confirms the presence of left

cervical and supraclavicular lymphadenopathy. Which procedure has the highest diagnostic yield?
a) Fine-needle aspiration of an enlarged lymph node
b) Core needle biopsy of an enlarged lymph node
c) Excisional biopsy of an enlarged lymph node

**2.** Biopsy reveals classical Hodgkin lymphoma. CT of the chest, abdomen, and pelvis demonstrates thoracic lymphadenopathy and splenic lesions. What is the correct stage?
a) Stage IIA
b) Stage IIB
c) Stage IIIA
d) Stage IIIB

**3.** Which feature predicts a good prognosis?
a) Age 20 years
b) Female sex
c) Both age 20 years and female sex

**4.** A 78-year-old man complains of dyspepsia and 10-lb weight loss during the past several months. Eight years earlier, he had a gastrointestinal bleed, which was attributed to ibuprofen-induced gastritis. His current medications include a cyclooxygenase-2 inhibitor and aspirin. Physical examination is unremarkable. Laboratory studies are normal. Esophagogastroduodenoscopy shows erythema and ulcerations "consistent with medication-induced gastropathy." Biopsies unexpectedly reveal extranodal marginal zone B-cell lymphoma of MALT. Complete staging evaluation demonstrates no other evidence of lymphoma. Which of the following statements is correct?
a) *H. pylori* is probably involved in the development of this patient's lymphoma.
b) *H. pylori* eradication may help his gastritis but not his lymphoma.
c) *H. pylori* is the only infectious agent implicated in lymphomagenesis.

**5.** A 70-year-old woman complains of fatigue and progressive abdominal discomfort during the past 2 months and a "bulk" in her left abdomen during the past week. Her performance status is 1. Physical examination reveals a couple of 1-cm right axillary lymph nodes and a huge left lower quadrant mass. Laboratory studies include a white blood cell of 15.4 with a normal differential, hemoglobin of 10.0, platelets of 370, and LDH of 897 (normal 100 to 220). CT of the chest, abdomen, and pelvis show a few slightly enlarged right axillary lymph nodes and massive retroperitoneal and mesenteric lymphadenopathy. CT-guided core needle biopsy demonstrates diffuse large B-cell lymphoma. Bone marrow biopsy shows no evidence of lymphoma.

This patient's lymphoma is potentially curable with standard therapy.
a) True
b) False

**6.** Which of this patient's presenting features predict a good prognosis?
a) Age 70 years
b) Stage III
c) Elevated LDH
d) Good performance status

## ANSWERS

**1. c.**
The diagnosis of lymphoma requires a histologic examination of a lymph node or involved tissue. The cytologic specimen provided by a fine-needle aspiration is usually inadequate to make a diagnosis of lymphoma, let alone determine the specific subtype. An excisional lymph node biopsy provides the most tissue for the pathologist to evaluate the lymph node and perform any indicated ancillary diagnostic studies.

**2. d.**
Involvement of lymphoid tissue above and below the diaphragm indicates at least stage III. Both lymph nodes and spleen are considered lymphoid tissue. The presence of night sweats and weight loss (i.e., B symptoms) adds the additional letter B.

**3. c.**
The International Prognostic Factors Project identified seven independent poor prognostic features among patients with newly diagnosed, advanced-stage Hodgkin lymphoma: hypoalbuminemia, anemia, male sex, stage IV, age of 45 years or older, leukocytosis, and lymphopenia.

**4. a.**
*H. pylori* is demonstrable in 90% or more of patients with gastric MALT lymphoma. The majority of patients with localized gastric MALT lymphoma respond to the eradication of these bacteria. Other infectious agents (e.g., Epstein-Barr virus) have been implicated in the pathogenesis of several other types of lymphoma.

**5. a.**
Patients with aggressive NHL (e.g., diffuse large B-cell lymphoma) are potentially curable with appropriate therapy. Only a minority of patients are actually cured, however.

**6. d.**
The International NHL Prognostic Factors Project identified five independent poor-risk features among patients with newly diagnosed, advanced-stage, aggressive NHL: age greater than 60 years, performance status 2 to 4, stage III or IV, elevated LDH, and two or more extranodal sites of involvement.

## SUGGESTED READINGS

Canellos GP, Anderson JR, Proper KJ, et al. Chemotherapy of advanced Hodgkin's disease with MOPP, ABVD, or MOPP alternating with ABVD. *N Engl J Med* 1992;327:1478–1484.

Coiffier B, Lepage E, Briere J, et al. CHOP chemotherapy plus rituximab compared with CHOP alone in elderly patients with diffuse large-B-cell lymphoma. *N Engl J Med* 2002;347:235–242.

Diehl V, Franklin J, Pfreundschuh M, et al. Standard and increased-dose BEACOPP chemotherapy compared with COPP-ABVD for advanced Hodgkin's disease. *N Engl J Med* 2003;348:2386–2395.

DeVita VT, Hellman S, Rosenberg SA, ed. *Cancer: Principles and Practice of Oncology.* Philadelphia: Lippincott Williams & Wilkins, 2001: 2215–2387.

Fisher RI, Gaynor ER, Dahlberg S, et al. Comparison of a standard regimen (CHOP) with three intensive chemotherapy regimens for advanced non-Hodgkin's lymphoma. *N Engl J Med* 1993;328: 1002–1006.

Hasenclever D, Diehl V. A prognostic score for advanced Hodgkin's disease. *N Engl J Med* 1998;339:1506–1514.

Jaffe ES, Harris NL, Stein H, et al, eds. *World Health Organization Classification of Tumors: Pathology and Genetics of Tumors of Haematopoietic and Lymphoid Tissues.* Lyon, France: IARC Press, 2001.

Kaminski M, Zelenetz A, Press O, et al. Pivotal study of iodine 131 tositumomab for chemotherapy-refractory low-grade or transformed low-grade B-cell non-Hodgkin's lymphomas. *J Clin Oncol* 2001;19:3918–3928.

McLaughlin P, Grillo-Lopez AJ, Link BK, et al. Rituximab chimeric anti-CD20 monoclonal antibody therapy for relapsed indolent lymphoma: half of patients respond to a four-dose treatment program. *J Clin Oncol* 1998;16:2825–2833.

Miller TP, Dahlberg S, Cassady JR, et al. Chemotherapy alone compared with chemotherapy plus radiotherapy for localized intermediate- and high-grade non-Hodgkin's lymphoma. *N Engl J Med* 1998; 339:21–26.

Philip T, Guglielmi C, Hagenbeek A, et al. Autologous bone marrow transplantation as compared with salvage chemotherapy in relapses of chemotherapy-sensitive non-Hodgkin's lymphoma. *N Engl J Med* 1995;333:1540–1545.

Shipp JA, for The International Non-Hodgkin's Lymphoma Prognostic Factors Project. A predictive model for aggressive non-Hodgkin's lymphoma. *N Engl J Med* 1993;329:987–994.

Witzig TE, Flinn IW, Gordon LI, et al. Treatment with ibritumomab tiuxetan radioimmunotherapy in patients with rituximab-refractory follicular non-Hodgkin's lymphoma. *J Clin Oncol* 2002;20:3262–3269.

# BOARD SIMULATION: Hematology and Medical Oncology

# 26

*Alan E. Lichtin      Brian J. Bolwell      Mohamad A. Hussein
Steven W. Andresen*

This board simulation chapter is divided into three sections. First is a review of plasma cell disorders, which are not discussed elsewhere in this text. This is followed by board simulation questions spanning the fields of hematology and medical oncology and questions from Dr. Steve Andresen's Board Simulation review from the 2004 Board Review course.

## PLASMA CELL DISORDERS

Plasma cell disorders are a group of neoplastic or potentially neoplastic diseases of plasma cells. The clinical manifestations of these disorders result from the uncontrolled and progressive proliferation of plasma cells, the effect of their replacement of normal bone marrow, and the overproduction of certain proteins. Plasma cell disorders are characterized by the secretion of monoclonal proteins (M protein, or paraprotein). M protein can be present when the total protein concentration and quantitative immunoglobulin values are within normal limits. The presence of M protein suggests monoclonal gammopathy of undetermined significance (MGUS), multiple myeloma (MM), primary amyloidosis, Waldenström's macroglobulinemia (WM), or other lymphoproliferative diseases.

## Monoclonal Gammopathy of Undetermined Significance

MGUS is a diagnosis of exclusion. It is characterized by the following clinical features:

- Serum paraprotein concentration less than 3 g/dL
- Fewer than 5% plasma cells in the bone marrow
- Absence of lytic bone lesions and renal insufficiency
- No other evidence of MM
- Stability over time

A review from the Mayo Clinic described 851 patients presenting with M protein in the serum (1). Nearly two-thirds (66%) of these patients had MGUS as a clinical diagnosis; for the remaining patients, the diagnoses included MM (12%), amyloidosis (9%), and non-Hodgkin lymphoma (NHL) (6%). Immunoglobulin G (IgG) was the most common paraprotein, followed by IgM and IgA. MGUS is common; 1% of people older than 50 years and 3% of those older than 70 in the United States have an abnormal paraprotein concentration.

The Mayo Clinic also has analyzed the long-term outcome of 241 MGUS patients (2). Median age at presentation was 64 years. Median M protein concentration was 1.7 g/dL. The outcome for these patients was as follows: no change, 24%; progression to MM, amyloidosis, 22%; and death from unrelated cause, 51%.

Median time to progression was 8 years: The longer patients lived, the more likely was the risk of progression. At 10 years, 17% of the patients had experienced disease progression; at 20 years this figure was 33%.

MGUS has no specific therapy. The monitoring of patients' protein values should occur every 3 to 12 months.

## Multiple Myeloma

The neoplastic proliferation of a single clone of plasma cells characterizes MM. These abnormal cells grow in bone marrow and frequently directly invade adjacent skeletal tissue, resulting in bone destruction. The median age at presentation is 61 years. MM represents 1% of all malignancies. Cytogenetic abnormalities of the bone marrow can be found in 18% to 36% of patients with MM. Interleukin (IL)-6 is a major myeloma cell growth factor in vivo and in vitro.

### Clinical Manifestations
The clinical manifestations of MM can be divided into the following broad categories:

- Plasma cell growth in bone marrow
- Hematologic changes
- Bone destruction
- Neurologic abnormalities
- Immune deficiency
- M protein itself
- Hyperviscosity
- Amyloidosis
- Clotting disorder
- Renal failure

### Skeletal Disease and Plasma Cell Growth in Bone Marrow
The most common presenting symptom of MM is bone pain. This most commonly involves the spine. The pain is often "rheumatic." The characteristic bone changes are lytic lesions (rounded, punched-out areas of bones) found most commonly in vertebral bodies, the skull, ribs, pelvis, humerus, and femur. Occasionally, diffuse osteoporosis is seen on radiography. Bone scans may or may not accurately reflect the destruction seen on plain radiographic films.

MM cells in the bone marrow are influenced by both autocrine and paracrine regulatory cytokines. MM cells secrete a number of cytokines that act on bone marrow stromal cells, which, in turn, secrete factors that contribute to the growth and proliferation of the MM cells. The anchoring of myeloma cells to bone marrow stroma is mediated by the CXCR4 binding of stromal-cell derived factor-1, followed by the upregulation of very late antigen-4. This process initiates a fierce cycle of events that includes bone resorption and the stimulation of myeloma cell growth. Following the adherence of myeloma cells, stromal cells secrete a number of cytokines, including interleukin-1$\beta$ (IL-1$\beta$), IL-6, and tumor necrosis factor (TNF-$\beta$). These cytokines promote the secretion of TNF-related activation-induced cytokines (TRANCE), also known as osteoprotegerin ligand, a member of the TNF family that stimulates the differentiation and proliferation of osteoclasts.

### Skeletal Changes
Research on the mechanisms by which MM cells induce osteolysis has focused on the osteoclast's role in shifting the normal balance between bone formation and bone resorption in favor of resorption. Bone resorption is blocked by bisphosphonates, but the inability of these compounds to repair lytic lesions indicates that a functional defect of osteoblasts is also important in the lytic process. The Wnt signaling pathway has been identified as an important pathway for the growth and differentiation of osteoblasts. Disabling mutations in the gene for the Wnt co-receptor low-density lipoprotein receptor–related protein 5 (LRP5) cause the osteoporosis–pseudoglioma syndrome. In the syndrome of hereditary high bone density, mutations in the LRP5 gene prevent binding of dickkopf1 (DKK1), a soluble inhibitor of Wnt, to LRP5. In a recent study by Tian et al., different patterns of a large number of gene expressions were studied in control subjects and MM patients with and without bony lesions. They noted that DKK1, and its corresponding protein (DKK1), was one of the four genes overexpressed in patients with lytic lesions. As indicated earlier, because of the role of DKK1 as a secreted factor in skeletal pathophysiology, the gene and its product were studied in detail. Immunohistochemical analysis of bone marrow–biopsy specimens showed that only myeloma cells contained detectable DKK1. Elevated DKK1 levels in bone marrow plasma and peripheral blood from patients with MM correlated with the gene-expression patterns of DKK1 and were associated with the presence of focal bone lesions. Recombinant human DKK1 or bone marrow serum containing an elevated level of DKK1 inhibited the differentiation of osteoblast precursor cells in vitro. The production of DKK1, an inhibitor of osteoblast differentiation, by myeloma cells is associated with the presence of lytic bone lesions in patients with MM. Agents modulating this molecule will be of great benefit in managing this devastating complication of the MM. (This discussion may be more detailed than necessary for internal medicine boards,

but it demonstrates how actively this field of interest is progressing.)

A solitary plasmacytoma is found in 2% of patients. Solitary plasmacytoma usually presents in a vertebral body. Conventional treatment consists of radiation therapy; most patients, however, ultimately progress to MM. Disease-free survival at 10 years is only 15% to 25%.

Most neurologic abnormalities associated with MM result from the direct extension by a tumor of skeletal origin. Spinal cord compression is present in 10% of patients, and many have nerve root compression. Peripheral neuropathy is not common in MM; it is usually caused by amyloidosis or hyperviscosity.

Anemia ultimately develops in most patients. This is generally secondary to poor red blood cell (RBC) production. Rouleaux is often present, resulting from the increased amount of globulin in the plasma. Total leukocyte count often is normal, but mild neutropenia occurs in up to 50% of patients. Thrombocytopenia often develops at some point during the disease, either from the myeloma itself or from repeated courses of chemotherapy. When plasma cells predominate among the circulating white blood cells (WBCs), the condition is known as *plasma cell leukemia*. This typically represents a terminal stage of the disease and is associated with a short survival. Primary plasma cell leukemia, unlike MM, is associated with lymphadenopathy, splenomegaly, and fewer lytic bone lesions. In plasma cell leukemia, 60% of patients present with the disease as a primary manifestation; for the remaining 40%, plasma cell leukemia represents a transformation of MM.

### Immunologic Abnormalities

Patients with MM often suffer repeated bouts of infection. The spectrum of infections is similar to that seen in patients with reduced levels of normal immunoglobulins. Encapsulated organisms, such as *Streptococcus pneumoniae* and *Haemophilus influenzae*, are frequent pathogens. After disease progression and therapy, *Staphylococcus aureus* is a common pathogen. More recent reports suggest that Gram-negative organisms now account for up to 50% of septic events later in MM. In addition to decreased levels of immunoglobulin, patients may have abnormalities of B cells and T cells, along with a loss of surface immunoglobulin-positive B cells. CD4 T-lymphocyte levels also are often reduced.

### Effect of Abnormal Paraprotein

The hyperviscosity syndrome results from the presence of serum proteins with a high intrinsic viscosity. This is most commonly seen in WM, but it may occur in MM with IgG or IgA paraprotein. The high viscosity interferes with efficient circulation to the brain, eyes, kidneys, and extremities. Headaches are common. Dizziness, vertigo, and symptoms as severe as stupor and coma can result secondary to intracerebral vascular occlusions. Seizures may develop. Peripheral neuropathy may result secondary to occlusive

changes in small vessels. Occasionally, cardiac failure occurs. High levels of M protein can interfere with coagulation factors and lead to abnormal platelet aggregation and abnormal platelet function. Bruising and purpura are common. Bleeding from the mucous membranes of the mouth, nose, and intestinal tract may also be seen.

### Renal Failure

Proteinuria is present in 90% of patients with MM, and abnormal light chains (Bence-Jones protein) are found in 80%. At diagnosis, the creatinine level is elevated in 50%. Proximal tubules are increasingly damaged by the large protein load. Additionally, large obstructing casts form along tubules. The combination of interstitial fibrosis and hyaline casts surrounded by epithelial cells or multinucleate giant cells constitutes the picture of "myeloma kidney." Besides Bence-Jones proteinuria, other factors that are important causes of renal dysfunction include hypercalcemia and hypercalciuria secondary to bone destruction and immobilization, and hyperuricemia resulting from increased cellular turnover. Nephrotoxic drugs, such as nonsteroidal anti-inflammatory drugs (NSAIDs), may precipitate renal failure. Finally, dehydration may exacerbate renal dysfunction.

### Diagnosis

The criteria for the diagnosis of MM are as follows:

I.
    ☐ A. Plasma cells more than 10% of marrow cells
    ☐ B. Plasmacytoma

II.
    ☐ A. Serum M protein
    ☐ B. Urine M protein
    ☐ C. Osteolytic bone lesions

IA or IB + IIA, IIB, or IIC = MM

### Treatment and Prognosis

Radiation therapy is the treatment of choice for painful bone lesions. It is also indicated for lesions that impair the function of vital structures. For the overall treatment of MM, chemotherapy is the treatment of choice. Most chemotherapeutic protocols employ alkylating agents. It is currently controversial whether multiple alkylating agents are superior to the standard regimen of melphalan (Alkeran) and prednisone. A 60% response rate occurs using most chemotherapeutic schedules. Newer schedules using a continuous infusion of vincristine, doxorubicin (Adriamycin), and dexamethasone may lead to improved response rates. Generally, chemotherapy is continued for approximately 12 months and stops when paraprotein levels are stable. Newer therapy with either autologous or allogeneic bone marrow transplantation (BMT) is promising in younger patients. The best results are seen in those treated earlier in the course of disease.

MM is not curable using standard therapy, and its prognosis is generally poor. Survival is 6 months without therapy. The median survival with therapy is 2 to 3 years. $\beta_2$-Microglobulin levels less than 4 mg/mL correlate with a good prognosis; levels greater than 6 mg/mL portend a poor prognosis. Prognosis is best with IgM disease and worst with IgD myeloma. An elevated lactate dehydrogenase (LDH) level is associated with a poor prognosis.

## Waldenström's Macroglobulinemia

The term *macroglobulinemia* is used to describe a variety of clinical conditions associated with an abnormal M protein of IgM type. The primary disorder is WM, in which a clonal proliferation of abnormal lymphocytes, with or without plasma cells, leads to the production of IgM paraprotein. Occasionally, an abnormal IgM paraprotein can be associated with NHL. Low levels of IgM may be seen in MGUS.

The median age at presentation for WM is 65 years. Symptoms are often related to hyperviscosity and include headaches, weakness, and bleeding. Hepatomegaly or splenomegaly is found in 40% of patients and lymphadenopathy in 30% of patients; 17% have neurologic dysfunction. Renal disorders are not common in WM. Patients are often anemic at presentation. Usually, the WBC count is normal, although occasionally a leukemic phase of macroglobulinemia is seen. Thrombocytopenia is found in approximately 50% of patients. The bone marrow biopsy shows increased numbers of lymphoplasmacytoid cells. These cells more closely resemble lymphocytes, rather than plasma or myeloma cells. Less frequently, patients have a marrow that is more characteristic of myeloma.

No treatment is usually necessary in the early stage of the disease. When symptoms develop, treatment consists of chemotherapy, similar to that used in MM. Plasmapheresis is recommended for symptoms associated with hyperviscosity. Newer drugs, such as fludarabine (Fludara) and pentostatin (Nipent), have been shown to have high response rates in small clinical trials. The median survival of WM is only 4 to 5 years. Death is secondary to progression of the neoplastic process, infections, or cardiac failure.

## REVIEW EXERCISES

The following review exercises discuss a wide array of issues in hematology and medical oncology that are relevant to clinical practice and potentially testable on the internal medicine board examination.

### QUESTIONS

**1.** Which of the following is true of patients with MGUS?
a) Marrow plasma cells greater than 20%
b) Lytic bone lesions
c) Majority progress to MM
d) Reciprocal decreased normal serum immunoglobulin levels
e) Serum paraprotein less than 3 g/dL

**2.** What condition is characterized by levels of Na 130, $K^+$ 4.0, and CL 105?
a) Multiple myeloma
b) Acute myelogenous leukemia (AML)
c) Large cell lymphoma
d) Breast cancer

**3.** Which of the following is true of multiple myeloma?
a) Although renal failure develops in most patients, it is present at diagnosis in only 10%.
b) In contrast to the situation with NHL, an elevated LDH is not an adverse prognostic sign.
c) Most patients with a solitary plasmacytoma at presentation are cured using radiation therapy.
d) Newer chemotherapeutic regimens such as vincristine, doxorubicin (Adriamycin), and dexamethasone cure approximately 30% of patients.
e) The most common presenting symptom of MM is bone pain.

**4–7.** A 28-year-old internal medicine resident on vacation walks into the emergency department (ED) complaining of dyspnea, low-grade fever, and fatigue. The symptoms have been progressive for more than 4 weeks. Physical examination reveals no lymphadenopathy. Lungs demonstrate scattered rhonchi. Hemoglobin (Hgb) is 11.0 g/dL, WBC count is 14,000/mm$^3$ with 85% neutrophils, and platelet count is 420,000/mm$^3$. LDH is 390 U/L. $\beta$-Human chorionic gonadotropin and $\alpha$-fetoprotein levels are normal. A chest radiograph reveals a large mediastinal mass.

**4.** What is the most likely diagnosis?
a) Germ cell tumor
b) Lymphoma
c) Thymoma
d) Lung cancer
e) Sarcoidosis

**5.** What is your next step?
a) Needle biopsy of mediastinum
b) Following the patient closely and repeating chest radiography in 2 weeks
c) Bronchoscopy
d) Mediastinoscopy
e) Thoracotomy

**6.** If the patient's mediastinal mass showed compression of the trachea, the correct procedure would be
a) Bronchoscopy first
b) Mediastinoscopy
c) Thoracotomy

**d)** Prebiopsy radiation therapy
**e)** Immediate combination chemotherapy

**7.** The patient relapses after attaining a complete remission. The appropriate management is
**a)** Repeating a course of the original chemotherapy protocol
**b)** Combination chemotherapy with different drugs
**c)** High-dose chemotherapy with autologous progenitor cell rescue (transplant) after a second remission is obtained

**8.** A 42-year-old woman with follicular small cleaved-cell lymphoma has had waxing and waning cervical and axillary lymphadenopathy since the condition was diagnosed 3 years ago. She presents with fever and a 1-week history of a rapidly enlarging right anterior cervical mass. The patient has a 6-cm mass involving the right anterior cervical chain and bilateral 12-cm axillary and inguinal enlarged lymph nodes. Except for an Hgb level of 10.0 g/dL and a modestly elevated LDH, the results of laboratory studies are normal. Which of the following would you recommend next?
**a)** Combination chemotherapy
**b)** Computed tomography (CT) of the abdomen
**c)** Irradiation of the cervical mass
**d)** Biopsy of the cervical mass
**e)** CT of the neck

**9.** The following are toxicities of cisplatin, *except*
**a)** Renal failure
**b)** Decreased hearing
**c)** Pulmonary fibrosis
**d)** Myelosuppression
**e)** Peripheral neuropathy

**10.** It is 1985, and your last patient in clinic for the day is a 30-year-old man with stage IV Hodgkin's disease (HD) who is receiving combination chemotherapy with mechlorethamine (nitrogen mustard), vincristine (Oncovin), procarbazine, and prednisone (MOPP). His wife, who has never smiled in your presence, called this morning and demanded that the patient be seen because he was "falling apart." You walk into the room and are greeted with a dazed look from the patient and a look of pure hatred from the spouse. You greet them as warmly as possible and ask what the matter is. The patient replies, "I don't know." The spouse says, "You have screwed him all up. Three months ago he was a vital 30-year-old man, on track to be a full partner in his law firm. Now, he is mentally out of it, he has no hair, he complains of numbness of his hands and feet, and he is always nauseated and has lost weight. He can't even have a glass of wine because it causes heavy sweating and headache. You did this to him. I want to know why, and what you propose to do about it." Reluctantly, you admit that the drugs that you chose to

treat his HD probably did cause these symptoms. In fact, one drug can explain all of them. Which drug is it?
**a)** Nitrogen mustard
**b)** Vincristine
**c)** Procarbazine
**d)** Prednisone
**e)** No one drug listed can cause all of the toxicities mentioned

**11.** All of the following are true of fludarabine, *except*
**a)** It is one of the most active drugs used to treat chronic lymphocytic leukemia (CLL).
**b)** It is extremely active in low-grade lymphomas.
**c)** The acute dose-limiting toxic effect of fludarabine is myelosuppression.
**d)** It causes B-cell immunodeficiency.
**e)** It can cause an irreversible neurotoxicity characterized by cortical blindness and coma.

**12.** A 57-year-old woman with AML recently received consolidation therapy consisting of high-dose cytarabine (ara-C; Cytosar-U) (2 g/m$^2$ every 12 hours on Monday, Wednesday, and Friday). Her husband has noticed that she has an ataxic gait. She has no other significant problems and is fully alert.
   Which of the following is true about this clinical situation?
**a)** The toxicity is likely a complication of antibiotic therapy.
**b)** You used the correct dose of ara-C, and the ataxia is a well-described toxicity.
**c)** The patient's symptoms are probably metabolic in nature, secondary to the well-described nephrotoxicity of ara-C.
**d)** The patient's neurologic toxicity is probably a result of central nervous system involvement by leukemia.

**13.** The combination of 5-fluorouracil, adriamycin, and mitomycin C (FAM) was once used for gastric cancer. The reason it has fallen out of favor is reflected by the following case:
   A 50-year-old woman with gastric cancer had been in complete remission for 2 months after combination chemotherapy with 5-fluorouracil (5-FU), doxorubicin (Adriamycin), and mitomycin. She now has early signs of renal failure. Hgb is 8.5 g/dL, platelet count is 25,000/mm$^3$, and WBC count is 9,000/mm$^3$ with a normal differential. Fibrinogen, prothrombin time, and partial thromboplastin time are normal. Peripheral blood smear shows RBC fragments.
   The most likely diagnosis is
**a)** Disseminated intravascular coagulation
**b)** Bone marrow hypoplasia secondary to chemotherapy
**c)** Marrow involvement by cancer
**d)** Hemolytic uremic syndrome
**e)** Hepatic metastases with hypersplenism

**14.** IL-2–based therapy has been shown to result in durable complete remission in
a) Breast cancer
b) Renal cell carcinoma
c) Testicular cancer
d) Colon cancer
e) Non–small cell lung cancer

**15.** The dose-limiting toxicity of cyclophosphamide is
a) Renal
b) Pulmonary
c) Hematologic
d) Cardiac
e) Neurologic

**16.** A woman with metastatic breast cancer presents with fever and shortness of breath. Four weeks ago, she was discharged from another hospital after undergoing autologous BMT. The preparative regimen was high-dose cyclophosphamide, cisplatin (Platinol), and carmustine (BCNU; BiCNU). Before BMT, the patient had known metastatic disease of the lung and liver. She has had an increasing nonproductive cough and substernal discomfort. Physical examination and vital signs are normal. Hgb is 11.8 g/dL, WBC count is 5,800/mm³ with 50% neutrophils and 45% lymphocytes, and platelet count is 98,000/mm³. Levels of hepatic enzymes and serum creatinine are normal. A chest radiograph is unremarkable. Pulse oximetry was 90% on room air. The patient's diffusing capacity for carbon monoxide is 40% of predicted.

Which of the following represents the appropriate next step?
a) Begin a broad-spectrum antibiotic.
b) Give reassurance that it is probably a viral syndrome.
c) Begin administering prednisone.
d) Perform CT of the liver to document progression of hepatic metastases.
e) Obtain an echocardiogram to rule out pericarditis.

**17.** A 50-year-old woman with metastatic breast cancer is seen in the ED with new-onset hematemesis. She has had breast cancer for 18 months. She was progressing with hormonal therapy and was switched to cyclophosphamide, methotrexate, and 5-FU 3 weeks ago. She has metastatic disease to her bone and lungs, with a malignant right pleural effusion; she is taking aspirin for bone pain. On physical examination, temperature is 38.5°C, pulse 120 beats/min, and blood pressure 80/50 mm Hg with orthostatic changes. She has a petechial rash. Right lung examination reveals dullness throughout one half of the examined field. Cardiac examination demonstrates normal first and second heart sounds with a I/VI systolic ejection murmur. Abdominal examination is unremarkable. Hgb is 7.5 g/dL, WBC count is 0.2/mm³, and platelet count is 8,000/mm³. Serum creatinine is

5.2 mg/dL, and blood urea nitrogen is 65 mg/dL. Alkaline phosphatase is minimally elevated; aspartate transaminase (AST; serum glutamic-oxaloacetic transaminase) is normal.

The most likely diagnosis is
a) Hemolytic uremic syndrome
b) Hepatorenal syndrome with hepatic dysfunction secondary to hepatic metastases
c) Bone marrow infiltration by metastatic breast cancer
d) Methotrexate toxicity
e) Cyclophosphamide toxicity

**18.** The combination of 5-FU and leukovorin has been conclusively shown to reduce tumor recurrence in which stage of colon cancer?
a) Stage I
b) Stage II
c) Stage III
d) Stage IV
e) None of the above; nothing has been shown to reduce tumor recurrences in colon cancer

**19.** A 65-year-old man with Dukes stage C colon cancer is being treated with adjuvant 5-FU and levamisole. He is normally an upbeat and optimistic person, but today comes into your office in a wheelchair. His speech is slurred. His son tells you that his father is not doing well. The son reports that the patient has experienced frequent diarrhea with nausea, sensitivity to sunlight, hair loss, and recent problems with gait and slurred speech. The patient appears somewhat somnolent. A complete blood cell count shows mild anemia, leukopenia, and cytopenia. A comprehensive metabolic panel reveals that serum glutamic-oxaloacetic transaminase is elevated to twice the normal upper limit. You confidently tell patient and son that everything will get better in the next 2 weeks and that the next course of chemotherapy simply needs to be delayed.

Which of the following is true?
a) Your arrogance is getting the better of you; this patient is ill, and not all of his symptoms can be explained by drug toxicity.
b) Although 5-FU can certainly cause diarrhea, the remainder of the patient's symptoms (liver toxicity, myelotoxicity, cerebellar toxicity, and alopecia) are not caused by 5-FU.
c) Although 5-FU can cause diarrhea and myelosuppression, the remaining toxicities are not from 5-FU.
d) 5-FU can cause all of the previously mentioned toxicities except cerebellar dysfunction.
e) You are right because all of the previously mentioned toxicities can be caused by 5-FU and likely will improve if chemotherapy is delayed and the doses later reduced.

20. Which of the following is *not* true of interferon-α?
a) Although flu-like symptoms are the most common initial side effect, hepatic toxicity is the most common chronic toxicity.
b) Approximately 30% of patients with Kaposi's sarcoma have an objective response to interferon-α.
c) Most patients experience side effects of interferon-α.
d) Interferon induces cytogenetic remission in chronic myelogenous leukemia (CML), as evidenced by a decrease in the percentage of Philadelphia chromosome–positive cells in the bone marrow.
e) Nausea and anorexia are common initial toxicities.

21. You are stat paged to the ED to see a 25-year-old man with CML who underwent allogeneic BMT 3 months ago from a matched sibling donor. He has known graft-versus-host disease of the skin and liver. His current medications include trimethoprim-sulfamethoxazole, fluconazole (Diflucan), acyclovir (Zovirax), cyclosporine, prednisone, and amoxicillin. As the patient is obtunded, his father, who is with him, gives you a medical history, saying, "My son lives in Los Angeles. He underwent BMT at UCLA. He is visiting us. Today, we were at a baseball game when he stated that he did not feel well and became progressively confused. I called his physician in Los Angeles, and he said that I should bring him here and ask for you."

You state that more information is needed and obtain some blood tests and radiographs. Fortunately, the patient does not have a neutropenic fever and has a normal chest radiograph. Hgb is 8.1 g/dL, WBC count is 2,400/mm$^3$ with 90% neutrophils, and platelet count is 17,000/mm$^3$. Peripheral blood smear shows microangiopathic RBC changes and low platelets. Additionally, creatinine is 2.3 mg/dL; blood urea nitrogen is 40 mg/dL; and the value for AST is two times, bilirubin is three times, and LDH is five times higher than normal.

You should tell the father that
a) Despite the patient's being afebrile and having no physical symptoms, he likely has a central nervous system infection due to profound myelosuppression, and this is likely the cause for his change in mental status.
b) The patient has hepatic failure, which explains his confusion.
c) The patient is experiencing a side effect of prednisone.
d) The patient is experiencing a side effect of cyclosporine.
e) The patient is experiencing a side effect of acyclovir.

22. Paclitaxel (Taxol) is known to cause all the following, *except*
a) A significant incidence of anaphylactic reactions
b) Neurotoxicity

c) Pulmonary toxicity
d) Hematologic toxicity
e) Nausea and vomiting

23. In addition to cardiac toxicity, all the following are common toxicities of doxorubicin, *except*
a) Sterility
b) Radiation recall
c) Extravasation leading to local tissue necrosis
d) Mucositis
e) Neutropenia

24. A 25-year-old woman presents with a clinical history of bruising. Her platelet count is 5,000/mm$^3$, with normal Hgb and WBC counts. Peripheral smear is unremarkable, except for a paucity of platelets.

The most likely diagnosis is
a) Immune thrombocytopenic purpura
b) Glanzmann's thrombasthenia
c) Congenital thrombocytopenia
d) Acute leukemia
e) Posttransfusion purpura

25. The most frequent cause of death in polycythemia vera is
a) Evolution to acute leukemia
b) Vascular thrombosis
c) Bleeding
d) Marrow fibrosis leading to leukopenia leading to infections
e) Cardiac failure

26. You are seeing a 29-year-old woman for pancytopenia; she presented to another hospital 4 weeks ago with jaundice. AST and alanine transaminase values were greater than 2,000 U/L, and bilirubin peaked at 12 U/L. All hepatic serology findings were negative. As her hepatic enzymes improved, she abruptly became pancytopenic and was transferred to your institution. At the time of consultation, Hgb is 6 g/dL, WBC count is 0.2/mm$^3$ with 90% lymphocytes, and platelet count is 25,000/mm$^3$. She had received five units of packed RBCs at the local hospital. Physical examination was remarkable only for scattered ecchymoses and petechiae. A bone marrow aspirate was dry; a bone marrow biopsy showed a profoundly hypocellular marrow (cellularity less than 5%), with the majority of cells being plasma cells and lymphocytes.

The correct diagnosis is
a) Multiple myeloma
b) Aplastic anemia
c) Acute myelogenous leukemia
d) Acute lymphoblastic leukemia
e) Myelofibrosis

27. The most common cause of aplastic anemia is
a) Benzene
b) Hepatitis

c) Chloramphenicol (Chloromycetin)
d) Radiation
e) Idiopathic or unknown

**28.** The therapy of choice for the patient in Question 26 is
a) Allogeneic BMT from an HLA-matched sibling donor
b) Antithymocyte globulin
c) Prednisone
d) Androgens
e) Granulocyte colony-stimulating factor (G-CSF)

**29.** A physician asks you to evaluate his mother, who has been diagnosed with a diffuse large cell lymphoma (DLCL). The physician elected to receive opinions concerning her treatment from physicians at five different cancer centers. All five opinions stated that the patient should receive combination chemotherapy with cyclophosphamide, hydroxydaunomycin (doxorubicin), vincristine (Oncovin), prednisone (CHOP) and rituximab (Rituxan). The patient has received five cycles of CHOP-Rituxan but now presents with prolonged and severe leukopenia. Significant hematologic toxicity developed from the chemotherapy after the third cycle, and the patient was given recombinant G-CSF filgrastim (Neupogen). The physician managing the treatment told her to continue filgrastim daily, which the patient has done for 40 consecutive days. Her last dose of chemotherapy was 4 weeks ago, but her WBC count is still only 1,400/mm$^3$; as a result she has not received the next course of chemotherapy.

The most likely cause of this clinical situation is
a) The patient is old and is experiencing the expected hematologic toxicity from chemotherapy.
b) The patient was treated with chemotherapy while taking G-CSF.
c) The patient probably has marrow involvement by lymphoma.
d) Acute leukemia is developing secondary to chemotherapy.
e) Rituxan induces acute leukemia.

**30.** The most common skin manifestation of patients with mast cell disorders is
a) Porphyria cutanea tarda
b) Erythema of the palms and soles
c) Urticaria pigmentosum
d) Urticaria
e) Café-au-lait spots

**31.** Patients with sickle cell disease may benefit from treatment with hydroxyurea (Hydrea). Studies have shown that hydroxyurea can decrease the incidence of vaso-occlusive crises requiring hospital admission. Problems may exist with the use of this drug, however, including.

a) Leukopenia
b) Thrombocytopenia
c) Induction of AML
d) Dryness and redness of the skin of the extremities
e) All of the above

**32.** A 22-year-old college student has a brief viral syndrome. Two weeks later, she comes to the ED with seizures, temperature of 38°C, petechiae, and jaundice. Platelet count is 4,000/mm$^3$, Hgb 6 is g/dL, and reticulocyte count is 20%; peripheral smear reveals microangiopathic hemolytic anemia and severe thrombocytopenia. Prothrombin time–international normalized ratio is 1.0, partial thromboplastin time is 30 seconds, and fibrinogen is 640.

You should immediately institute
a) Aspirin
b) Hydrocortisone
c) Vincristine
d) Splenectomy
e) Plasma exchange

**33.** A 72-year-old man is seen in the ED with symptoms of right-sided hemiparesis of brief duration. On examination, he is plethoric and has no adenopathy, but his spleen is felt 4 cm below the left costal margin. WBC count is 16,400/mm$^3$ with 80% polymorphonuclear leukocytes, 10% lymphocytes, 5% monocytes, and 5% basophils. Hgb is 20.7 g/dL, hematocrit is 61.0%, and platelets are 199,000/mm$^3$.

You should first institute
a) Plasmapheresis
b) Aspirin
c) Heparin
d) Phlebotomy
e) Hydroxyurea

**34.** A 40-year-old woman presents for preoperative evaluation and is completely asymptomatic. She is found to have a WBC count of 150,000/mm$^3$ with 70% neutrophils, 5% lymphocytes, 5% monocytes, 5% eosinophils, 5% basophils, 3% metamyelocytes, 3% myelocytes, 1% promyelocytes, and 3% blasts. Platelet count is 1,000,000/mm$^3$ and Hgb is 15.0 g/dL. On examination, she has no adenopathy, and her spleen is not palpable. She was to have an elective bunionectomy. This patient has CML.

The initial treatment of choice is
a) Tissue-typing her siblings and, if one is compatible, proceeding to allogeneic BMT
b) Giving interferon-α and monitoring her bone marrow chromosome status every 6 months
c) Giving STI-571 (Gleevec)
d) Giving hydroxyurea followed by interferon-α plus ara-C to maintain the WBC count below normal
e) Giving busulfan

**35.** A perfectly healthy 26-year-old woman visits her new obstetrician for the first time, contemplating becoming pregnant now that she is newly married. Her physical examination is completely normal. WBC count is 9,000/mm$^3$ with a normal differential, Hgb is 13.4 g/dL, and platelet count is 1,200,000/mm$^3$. Further testing shows that on platelet aggregation analysis, her platelets do not aggregate at all to epinephrine. She is completely asymptomatic. She has no headaches, pain or burning in her palms or soles, or hematuria. She is taking no medicines. A workup for causes of secondary thrombocytosis is negative, including an antinuclear antibody test. CT of the chest, abdomen, and pelvis fails to reveal any underlying malignancy. The diagnosis of essential thrombocythemia is established after bone marrow testing shows megakaryocytic hyperplasia and the absence of any chromosomal abnormality. She wishes to become pregnant.

The treatment of choice is

a) Aspirin starting before and continuing through the pregnancy
b) Heparin given subcutaneously starting before and continuing through pregnancy
c) No specific intervention
d) Hydroxyurea therapy first to bring the platelet count down before conception and then stopping therapy once she is found to be pregnant
e) Anagrelide (Agrylin) therapy to normalize the platelet count until she becomes pregnant, then continuing anagrelide through the pregnancy

**36.** A 40-year-old man presents with pneumonia. WBC count is 2,600/mm$^3$, Hgb is 12.7 g/dL, and platelet count is 80,000/mm$^3$ with a normal differential. Hepatosplenomegaly is noted. The pneumonia is treated with an antibiotic, and he does well. Bone marrow aspirate and biopsy show macrophages with eccentrically placed nuclei and cytoplasm with characteristic striations or crinkles. A diagnosis of Gaucher's disease is entertained. An increase in plasma cells also is present, and the patient is found to have a monoclonal spike of 1.5 g/dL. The percentage of plasma cells is 10%, and they are monoclonal by immunohistochemistry.

The definitive test to prove this patient's disorder is

a) Assay of phosphofructokinase activity
b) Assay of glucocerebrosidase activity
c) MRI evaluation of the bone marrow
d) Histologic evaluation of the spleen
e) Assay of α-galactosidase activity

**37.** A 24-year-old man who received a kidney transplant 3 years ago is taking cyclosporine and prednisone for immunosuppression and is doing well. Over a period of several weeks, fever and night sweats develop, and he is found to have an enlarged lymph node. Biopsy of the lymph node is performed, and a post-transplantation lymphoproliferative disorder (B-cell type diffuse large cell lymphoma) is found.

The treatment of choice is

a) CHOP chemotherapy
b) Cyclophosphamide, vincristine, and prednisone therapy
c) Interferon-α
d) Reducing immunosuppression, such as reducing or stopping the cyclosporine
e) Harvesting peripheral stem cells for autologous stem cell transplantation

**38.** A 54-year-old man comes to your office. He feels well, but lately low-grade fevers and some pain in the left side of the abdomen have developed. On examination, minimal adenopathy is present; however, his spleen is felt 12 cm below the left costal margin and is slightly uncomfortable on palpation. WBC count is 1,600/mm$^3$ with 20% neutrophils, 60% lymphocytes (many with a reniform nucleus and enlarged with small projections from the cytoplasm), and the remainder being monocytes and a small number of eosinophils and basophils. Platelet count is 62,000/mm$^3$ and Hgb is 10.0 g/dL. The diagnosis is slowly progressive pancytopenia. Flow cytometry of the peripheral blood demonstrates a portion of B lymphocytes that express monotypic λ-light chains. These B cells also appear to express CD22, CD11, and CD25.

The treatment of choice is

a) Splenectomy
b) Interferon-α
c) Pentostatin
d) Infusion of cladribine (2-chlorodeoxyadenosine; Leustatin) for 7 days
e) CHOP chemotherapy

**39.** A 40-year-old man has a 3-year history of mild but worsening pancytopenia. It is known that his complete blood cell count values were normal before 3 years ago, and they have slowly declined. A bone marrow biopsy shows mild to moderately hypercellular marrow with moderate erythroid hyperplasia; mild dyserythropoiesis and a moderate increase in megakaryocytes are present. His physical examination is completely normal except for slight pallor. WBC count is 2,260/mm$^3$, Hgb is 11.0 g/dL, and platelet count is 110,000/mm$^3$ with a normal differential. Bilirubin is 5.3 mg/dL, with an unconjugated bilirubin of 4.1 mg/dL and a conjugated bilirubin of 1.2 mg/dL; LDH is 2,000 U/L (normal, 100 to 220 U/L) and AST is 97 U/L (normal, 7 to 40 U/L). Ham's and sugar water testing are both positive. The patient has no evidence of a clotting disorder.

You should recommend which of the following?

a) Because the greatest risk to patients with paroxysmal nocturnal hemoglobinuria is thrombosis, the patient should receive prophylactic anticoagulation with warfarin sodium (Coumadin).

b) Because there is no thrombosis at present, the patient should be merely followed and begin anticoagulation if thrombosis occurs.

c) Because the median survival after diagnosis is greater than 10 years, there is no rush to begin anticoagulation in patients.

d) For patients who survive longer than 10 years, some may experience spontaneous clinical recovery; therefore patients require no prophylactic anticoagulation.

e) The patient should be given aspirin.

**40.** A 72-year-old man with CLL, being followed without chemotherapy, has a slowly rising WBC count over 6 years. Hgb and platelet counts have always been normal. At this routine visit, he shows significant pallor but is afebrile. WBC count is 82,000/mm³ with 3% neutrophils and 97% abnormal lymphocytes consistent with CLL cells. Reticulocyte count is 0.2%; platelets are 150,000/mm³. The previous Hgb was 14.2 g/dL, and reticulocyte count 1.7%.

The patient probably has

a) Parvovirus B19 infection

b) CLL infiltration of the bone marrow to the point at which he is unable to have proper erythropoiesis

c) An antierythropoietin antibody

d) Pure red cell aplasia

e) Hypogammaglobulinemia causing pneumococcal sepsis

**41.** A 47-year-old woman comes to your office with a history of fevers, perirectal abscesses, and paronychial infections over the past year. WBC count is 3,900/mm³ with 1% neutrophils and 98% lymphocytes. Comprehensive metabolic profile is completely normal. LDH is normal. On peripheral blood smear, many of the lymphocytes have pinkish cytoplasmic granules.

The patient has

a) Felty's syndrome

b) Large granular lymphocytosis with neutropenia

c) AML

d) Systemic lupus erythematosus

e) Severe combined immunodeficiency syndrome

**42.** A 37-year-old patient with a history of Hodgkin's disease (HD) at age 20 years presents in the ED desperately ill. Part of his evaluation at age 20 included a staging laparotomy. He was given mantle radiation therapy for pathologic stage IIA nodular sclerosing HD. After radiation therapy, he was doing well until 4 hours before coming to the ED, when he began to have pharyngitis and fever, eventually became confused and weak, fainted, and was rushed to the ED. On physical examination, he shows pallor, rigors, and blotchy purplish lesions over his legs; he has neck stiffness. Blood pressure is 60/40 mm Hg, and he is unresponsive. WBC count is 24,000/mm³ with 90% polymorphonuclear

leukocytes and many band forms among them; Hgb is 10 g/dL, and platelet count is 19,000/mm³. A spinal tap shows cloudy fluid. He is rushed to the intensive care unit, where he dies within 12 hours, despite maximal antibiotic and pressor support. This clinical scenario is best explained by which of the following?

a) The patient died of meningococcemia and meningococcal meningitis. At autopsy, one would expect to find Waterhouse-Friderichsen syndrome.

b) The patient's staging laparotomy at age 20 included a splenectomy. This has predisposed the patient to the development of meningococcal disease.

c) Meningococci are bacteria that need to be cleared by opsonin activity, and the splenectomy has decreased the ability of this patient to clear such encapsulated bacteria.

d) Bacteria such as *Escherichia coli* and *Streptococcus pneumoniae* must also be cleared by opsonin activity, and patients after splenectomy can have fulminant sepsis with these organisms.

e) All of the above.

**43.** A 70-year-old woman presents with an Hgb of 9.5 g/dL and has felt weaker over the past 2 years. Platelet count is 450,000/mm³, and WBC count is 4,200/ mm³ with a normal differential except for 3% basophils. On peripheral blood smear analysis, the polymorphonuclear leukocytes appear to be hypogranular, and rarely a Pelger-Huët anomaly is noted. On bone marrow analysis, dysplastic RBC precursors are seen, and the percentage of blasts is increased so that the diagnosis of myelodysplasia is made (refractory anemia). No ringed sideroblasts are observed. Over the next 5 years, she becomes progressively more anemic and requires transfusions despite erythropoietin therapy. During this time, her platelet count remains greater than 250,000/mm³. She eventually dies of progressive neutropenia and infection.

The chromosome anomaly reflected in her initial bone marrow is most likely

a) Monosomy 7

b) t(8;21)

c) Trisomy 8

d) 5q–

e) 20q–

**44.** A 30-year-old man who had received four cycles of etoposide, cis-platinum and, bleomycin for widely metastatic nonseminomatous germ cell testis cancer 5 years previously has been noted to have a slowly rising β-human chorionic gonadotropin (β-HCG) level. Thorough restaging, including brain, chest, abdomen, and pelvis scans are negative. Complete blood count and metabolic studies are normal.

At this point, you should

a) Perform bone marrow test.

b) Inquire about Szechuan food intake.
c) Inquire about marijuana use.
d) Inquire about ephedra intake.
e) Perform abdominal surgery.

**45.** In cancer trials, Phase I studies are performed on patients who have progressed despite standard care. Often, groups of three patients are treated on escalating doses of a new experimental drug. The goal of Phase I studies is to find
a) The efficacy of the new drug
b) The maximally tolerated dose (MTD) of the drug
c) The potential for cure using the drug
d) Whether the drug works for a certain type of cancer
e) Whether a placebo effect occurs

**46.** A 20-year-old man presents with a 2 cm left cervical lymph node. A CAT scan of the abdomen and pelvis and bone marrow aspirate and biopsy are normal. He is asymptomatic. Biopsy of the node shows Reed-Sternberg cells.
   Which of the following statements is correct?
a) He has clinical stage IIA Hodgkin's disease.
b) Chemotherapy will be the initial treatment approach.
c) Radiation treatment to the mediastinal mass is reasonable post-chemotherapy.
d) Sperm banking should be performed prior to initiating therapy.
e) All of the above.

**47.** Six months after completing radiation therapy, he develops abdominal pain. A CAT scan of his abdomen and pelvis demonstrates bulky lymphadenopathy.
   Which of the following statements is correct?
a) No curative therapy is available.
b) Abdominal radiation will likely cure this relapse.
c) Salvage standard chemotherapy will likely cure this relapse.
d) Salvage chemotherapy followed by an autologous stem cell transplant offers the greatest potential treatment benefit.
e) An allogeneic transplant is preferable to an autologous transplant in this setting.

**48.** Two years out, he becomes pancytopenic. His marrow shows 8% blasts.
   Which statement is correct?
a) He has treatment-related myelodysplasia.
b) Cytogenetic abnormalities are unlikely.
c) Palliative measures are the treatment of choice.
d) The risk–benefit ratio for allogeneic transplant makes this approach untenable.
e) Induction chemotherapy for acute leukemia often produces durable remissions.

**49.** He tolerates his preparatory regimen without difficulty and engrafts nicely. However, on day +50, he develops a diffuse maculopapular rash, bloody diarrhea that approaches 2L in a 24-hour period, and a bilirubin of 5. His CMV titer is negative.
   Which of the following statements is correct?
a) He has acute graft-versus-host disease.
b) Donor B-cells are the principle mediators.
c) Steroids should be added to his cyclosporine A.
d) Maintaining adequate nutrition usually is not a problem.
e) Answers a and c are correct.

**50.** A 29-year-old woman is found to have a platelet count of 2 million. The hemoglobin and white blood count are normal. She is healthy, asymptomatic, and has a normal exam.
   Which of the following statements is correct?
a) She likely has essential thrombocytosis (ET) and needs no further studies.
b) She likely has ET and requires immediate therapy.
c) Thrombocytosis may occur with iron deficiency, inflammatory disorders, and malignancies.
d) In ET, interferon is the treatment of choice.
e) All of the above.

**51.** A 50-year-old man presents with progressive weakness, weight loss, and pancytopenia. On physical examination, he has massive splenomegaly. The peripheral smear shows teardrop red cells, and bone marrow evaluation shows fibrosis.
   Which of the following statements is correct?
a) He has myelofibrosis.
b) He should be HLA-typed.
c) Supportive measures are generally the treatment of choice.
d) He may develop acute leukemia.
e) All of the above.

**52.** A 30-year-old woman presents to your office with an erythematous, indurated left breast. She has been previously seen by her family physician and started on an antibiotic. She is no better. You refer her to a surgeon, and a core biopsy done that day demonstrates findings consistent with a breast cancer.
   Which of the following statements is correct?
a) She has inflammatory breast cancer.
b) She requires emergent surgery.
c) Breast conservation is a reasonable option.
d) Routine staging studies are not indicated.
e) All of the above.

**53.** She responds nicely to therapy. At one office visit, however, she brings her 25-year-old sister, who has noticed a "lump" in her left breast and notes that she is 8 weeks pregnant.
   Which of the following statements is incorrect?
a) This is likely a clogged milk duct, and she should be re-evaluated after delivery.

b) Mammography with abdominal shielding can be safely performed.

c) Core biopsy for diagnosis and receptor studies can be safely performed.

d) Modified radical mastectomy or breast conservation can be safely performed in any trimester.

e) Chemotherapy should be avoided during the first trimester and radiation therapy avoided until completion of the pregnancy.

**54.** A 60-year-old male with rheumatoid arthritis presents with severe abdominal pain. His abdomen is distended and ecchymotic areas are noted on his flank. A CT demonstrates a large retroperitoneal hematoma. He has no bleeding history.

Initial coagulation studies include a normal CBC, PT 12, PTT 80 seconds (repeated and remains elevated), and normal BT.

What coagulation study should be ordered next?

a) Mixing study

b) Fibrinogen

c) dRVVT or phospholipid neutralization procedure

d) Platelet aggregation studies

e) All of the above

**55.** The PTT remains prolonged with the mix. The Factor VIII:C activity is 0 and an inhibitor titer is pending. The best treatment approach in this setting is

a) Large doses of Factor VIII concentrate

b) Porcine Factor VIII

c) Treatment will depend on the titer of the inhibitor

d) Recombinant Factor VIIa.

e) Partially or fully activated Factor IX concentrates

**56.** An 18-year-old presents to your emergency room with a left hemiparesis. Her smear shows sickled red cells. Which of the following statements is correct?

a) She likely has a stroke secondary to intracerebral sickling.

b) Transfusion or exchange transfusion will help.

c) Stroke in this setting tends to recur.

d) Chemotherapy may help.

e) All of the above.

**57.** A 60-year-old woman has been found to have mild pancytopenia. She is an Ashkenazi Jew. The only abnormality on physical exam is mild splenomegaly. Her glucoscerebrosidase level is low. Which statement is correct?

a) She has Gaucher's disease.

b) Enzyme replacement therapy is helpful, available commercially, and inexpensive.

c) In selected patients, bone marrow transplantation can be considered.

d) All patients require therapy.

e) Answers a and c.

**58.** A 75-year-old man with long-standing asymptomatic chronic lymphocytic leukemia presents with a hemoglobin of 6 and jaundice. Some red cells are spherocytes. Which statement is correct?

a) The direct Coombs' test will be positive.

b) He has pure red cell aplasia.

c) Erythropoietin is the treatment of choice.

d) His anemia is likely secondary to progressive marrow infiltration.

e) Answers a and c are correct.

**59.** A 57 year-old woman presents with anemia, an IgG κ-paraprotein and diffuse osteolytic lesions. Her marrow shows 60% plasma cells. Which statement is incorrect?

a) She has myeloma and treatment options, while plentiful, remain palliative.

b) Bone marrow transplantation, both in autologous and allogeneic forms, are treatment options.

c) General immunity remains intact.

d) Bisphosphonates and growth factors are often included in supportive therapy.

e) Thalidomide and other antiangiogenic agents have activity.

**60.** A 64-year-old man has multiorgan system dysfunction, failure to thrive, proteinuria, and a very large tongue. Which of the following statements is correct?

a) Tissue is needed for congo red staining.

b) The heart is the most common organ involved.

c) No specific therapy is available.

d) Renal involvement carries the worst prognosis.

e) Answers a and c are correct.

**61.** A 50-year-old woman presents with a 2cm left axillary lymph node, a biopsy of which demonstrates a poorly differentiated carcinoma. Mammogram, ultrasound, MRI, CT scan of the abdomen and pelvis, and a bone scan are all negative or normal. Which of the following statements is correct?

a) Metastatic carcinoma of unknown primary site is uncommon.

b) Extensive diagnostic studies generally reveal the primary site.

c) Chemotherapy is always indicated.

d) This patient should be treated as a stage II breast cancer.

e) Answers a and c are correct.

## ANSWERS

**1. e.**

Twenty percent or more of plasma cells in the marrow, lytic bone lesions, and reciprocal decreases in normal immunoglobulin levels are all characteristic of MM. In the majority of patients, MGUS does not evolve into MM. Serum paraprotein levels are less than 3 g/dL in MGUS.

**2. a.**

The presence of a circulating paraprotein (M protein) is often associated with a decreased anion gap. At serum pH, these proteins act as cations, binding chloride and reducing the sodium–chloride difference.

**3. e.**

The most common presenting symptom of MM is in fact bone pain, most commonly in the spine.

**4. b.**

**5. d.**

**6. d.**

**7. c.**

The chest radiograph shows a large mediastinal mass. In a patient of this age, lymphoma is far and away the most likely diagnosis. HD, diffuse large cell lymphoma, and lymphoblastic lymphoma are the most probable types. A needle biopsy rarely yields a definitive diagnosis of a lymphoma, largely because the underlying cellular architecture is important for an accurate pathologic diagnosis. Thus, an appropriate open or excisional biopsy should be performed. If the chest CT reveals tracheal compression, prebiopsy irradiation therapy should be administered to relieve the compression. The danger of proceeding with a biopsy in the face of external tracheal compression is the risk of tracheal collapse at extubation.

In the case presented, the diagnosis is DLCL, which is curable with primary therapy in approximately 40% of patients. A relapse would be incurable, however, using conventional therapy. The only curative modality is high-dose chemotherapy using autologous progenitor cell rescue.

**8. d.**

This patient has stable adenopathy with the exception of an asymmetric enlarging nodal area. It is likely that this represents the transformation to a more aggressive histology. Biopsy confirmation is essential for additional management. The most likely result of the biopsy is a DLCL.

**9. c.**

It is well known that cisplatin can cause myelosuppression, including severe thrombocytopenia and renal failure. A main dose-limiting toxicity is neurologic dysfunction, however, and it can include peripheral neuropathies or decreased hearing.

**10. c.**

Procarbazine (Matulane) is an oral drug used in the treatment of HD and is part of several chemotherapeutic regimens for NHL. Hematologic toxicity is common, as well as nausea and vomiting. Procarbazine can cause

direct and indirect neurologic effects and is known to induce altered levels of consciousness, including depression, psychosis, and peripheral neuropathy, usually reversible with discontinuation of the drug. Additionally, procarbazine inhibits the cytochrome P450 system. Drugs metabolized by hepatic microsomal enzymes have prolonged half-lives in patients who are receiving procarbazine; the sedative effects of barbiturates and narcotics are therefore potentiated. Some patients report headaches, sweating, and facial flushing when they consume alcohol while taking procarbazine. Procarbazine is also associated with hypersensitivity pneumonitis and is highly teratogenic. Corticosteroids have a number of known side effects, including gastrointestinal irritation, muscle weakness, fluid retention, glucose intolerance, and altered mental status. They do not cause myelosuppression. The main toxicity of vincristine is neurologic, which is dose-related; this usually is a peripheral neuropathy associated with sensory loss, pain, and weakness. Additionally, autonomic neuropathy may occur, resulting in paralytic ileus. Vincristine can also cause local tissue irritation if extravasation occurs; it is not myelosuppressive. Nitrogen mustard is also a local vesicant. Its main toxicities are gastrointestinal (nausea and vomiting), hematologic, and reproductive (sterility).

**11. d.**

Myelosuppression is common with fludarabine, and nausea, vomiting, and hepatocellular toxicity are also acute toxicities. The most serious side effect, however, is an irreversible neurotoxicity characterized by blindness, encephalopathy, and coma. Pathologic findings include a diffuse necrotizing leukoencephalopathy, especially in the occipital lobes. Fludarabine does cause T-cell immunodeficiency, but infections with *Pneumocystis carinii* are rare. It is extremely active in CLL and is also active in other low-grade lymphoid malignancies.

**12. b.**

Myelosuppression is the most common acute toxicity of ara-C. However, high-dose ara-C can cause unique side effects, including diarrhea, conjunctivitis, and possibly pneumonitis. Cerebellar toxicity is well described as a complication of high-dose ara-C. If ataxia begins to develop, ara-C should be discontinued. The neurologic toxicity is usually reversible. Ara-C is not known to cause nephrotoxicity. The dose used in this case is a well-described "high dose" for the treatment of acute leukemia.

**13. d.**

Mitomycin is known to be associated with hemolytic uremic syndrome, which may present weeks or months after the administration of mitomycin. The clinical picture is consistent with hemolytic uremic syndrome. This is not disseminated intravascular coagulopathy because the prothrombin time, partial thromboplastin time, and fibrinogen are normal. Bone marrow hypoplasia is not likely because the WBC count is normal. Bone marrow involvement with metastases would likely result in teardrop cells, not fragments. Hypersplenism rarely results from hepatic metastases and does not cause RBC fragments or renal failure.

**14. b.**
IL-2 in conjunction with lymphokine-activated killer cells has been shown to lead to complete responses in 10% of patients with renal cell carcinoma. It is unclear whether lymphokine-activated killer cells contribute to this response. IL-2 has no demonstrable activity in the other malignancies mentioned. Many toxicities are associated with IL-2. Patients receiving high-dose IL-2 may get a capillary leak syndrome with severe peripheral edema, adult respiratory distress syndrome, and hypotension. Severe rashes are common.

**15. d.**
Cyclophosphamide has no known neurologic or renal toxicity. The latter point is often missed on board examinations. Pulmonary toxicity is possible but rare. Hematologic toxicity is common. The dose-limiting toxicity, especially in the BMT setting, however, is cardiac, with cardiomyopathy and cardionecrosis occurring with doses greater than 200 mg/kg.

**16. c.**
The patient does not have any evidence of metastatic disease at present. Symptoms include substernal discomfort and cough. She has a severe reduction in diffusing capacity for carbon monoxide. All of this is consistent with lung toxicity secondary to BCNU-containing, high-dose chemotherapy regimens. This lung toxicity is commonly seen in women with breast cancer treated with high-dose BCNU. Untreated pulmonary deterioration may be fatal. Prompt initiation of corticosteroids usually restores normal pulmonary function. The initiation of radiation therapy may precipitate this pulmonary toxicity.

**17. d.**
Methotrexate has many toxicities: It is the most commonly mentioned chemotherapy drug on board examinations. Although aspirin is known to elevate methotrexate drug levels, the key to this question is that the patient has a pleural effusion. Methotrexate equilibrates into third-space fluids within hours after intravenous therapy. The clearance of methotrexate from third-space fluids is slow, however, and a retention of methotrexate in third-space fluids results in a prolonged terminal plasma half-life. This may result in serious methotrexate toxicity, which in this case includes serious hematologic and renal toxicity. The patient is critically ill and needs prompt initiation of intravenous antibiotics, fluids,

RBCs, and other intensive supportive care measures. Leucovorin calcium (Wellcovorin) should be initiated and methotrexate levels followed.

**18. c.**
Several studies have confirmed that the combination of 5-FU and leucovorin reduces tumor recurrences and overall death rate for patients with lymph node–positive (stage III) colon carcinoma. The therapy of metastatic disease remains far from optimal, as 5-FU results in an approximately 20% response rate and little, if any, improvement in overall survival. The addition of leucovorin to 5-FU has been shown to improve response rates in metastatic colon cancer, although studies are mixed on whether overall survival is improved.

**19. e.**
The most common toxicities of 5-FU are gastrointestinal and myelosuppressive. The gastrointestinal toxicity is more common when continuous infusions of 5-FU are given, producing stomatitis, nausea, vomiting, and diarrhea. Myelosuppression is more common when bolus 5-FU is given. Hyperpigmentation of the skin is frequently observed. Alopecia and conjunctivitis may occur as well. Cerebellar toxicity is a well-known complication of 5- FU, with symptoms including somnolence, ataxia, slurred speech, and nystagmus.

**20. a.**
Interferon-α has a variety of toxicities. Most patients experience a temporary flu-like illness within the first 2 to 3 weeks of initiation of therapy. Chronic fatigue is the most common chronic toxicity, however. Many other organs may be affected by interferon-α, but most toxicities resolve with discontinuation of therapy.

**21. d.**
The peripheral smear and peripheral blood counts are consistent with thrombotic thrombocytopenic purpura. Cyclosporine commonly causes renal toxicity and occasionally also causes thrombocytopenic purpura, which manifests with thrombocytopenia, anemia, elevated LDH, altered mental status, and RBC fragments on the peripheral blood smear. Neurologic toxicity is an extremely uncommon side effect of acyclovir and is not associated with RBC fragments.

**22. c.**
Paclitaxel is used in the treatment of breast and ovarian cancers. It is known to cause the previously mentioned toxicities, except pulmonary toxicity.

**23. a.**
Although many chemotherapeutic drugs are known to cause sterility, it is unusual for doxorubicin to do so. *Radiation recall* is a phenomenon whereby a local injury may occur after the initiation of radiation therapy in a

patient who has been previously exposed to doxorubicin. This is most commonly seen in radiation therapy above the diaphragm and may result in severe mucositis. Doxorubicin extravasation is a serious problem that can lead to severe local necrosis and damage to underlying nerves, tendons, and muscles. Use of a free-flowing intravenous line and avoidance of veins in the antecubital fossa are essential. If extravasation occurs, the drug should be stopped and an attempt made to aspirate blood from the intravenous line. An application of ice and steroid cream has been reported to reduce the severity of the reaction.

### 24. a.

The only abnormality given is a low platelet count. In the absence of a congenital history, immune thrombocytopenic purpura is the most likely diagnosis. Glanzmann's thrombasthenia is a rare platelet disorder involving an abnormality of platelet membrane IIb/IIIa that causes defective fibrinogen binding to the platelet surface. The platelet count is normal in this disorder, however. The patient has a normal Hgb and WBC count and an unremarkable peripheral smear, which help rule out acute leukemia. No clinical history of transfusions rules out post-transfusion purpura, a rare clinical syndrome in which acute thrombocytopenia develops 7 to 14 days after an RBC transfusion.

### 25. b.

All patients with polycythemia vera have abnormal platelet function. As a result, the most common manifestations of this myeloproliferative disorder are clotting and bleeding. Thrombosis is the cause of death in approximately 40% of patients with polycythemia vera. In addition to deep vein thrombosis of the lower extremities, pulmonary emboli, and cerebrovascular or coronary occlusions, the development of thromboses at unusual anatomic sites is common for patients, including splenic, hepatic, and mesenteric vessels. In one series, 10% of patients presenting with Budd-Chiari syndrome had coexisting polycythemia vera; therefore, polycythemia vera should be excluded in any patient in whom Budd-Chiari syndrome develops. Bleeding is also common in this disease, but does not cause mortality as often as it does thrombotic events. Evolution to leukemia is a well-known complication, although the frequency of leukemic evolution is increased if patients have been treated with alkylating agents or radioactive phosphorous. If patients are treated with phlebotomy alone, the incidence of progression to acute leukemia is approximately 15%. Myelofibrosis with resultant pancytopenia occurs in approximately 10% to 15% of patients and usually develops more than 10 years after the initial diagnosis. Polycythemia vera does not have direct cardiac toxicity, although coronary artery disease may be exacerbated by the thrombotic tendency. A diagnosis of polycythemia vera is made on the following clinical and laboratory criteria:

- Elevated RBC mass with a normal arterial oxygen saturation
- Splenomegaly
- Thrombocytosis
- Bone marrow hypercellularity
- Low serum erythropoietin levels
- Abnormal marrow proliferative capacity as shown by formation of erythroid colonies in the absence of exogenous erythropoietin

Therapy should attempt to maintain the hematocrit in the range of 42% to 45%. Treatment generally consists of phlebotomy with or without hydroxyurea.

### 26. b.

The patient has an aplastic anemia. Hepatitis is the most common infection preceding aplastic anemia, with 4% to 6% of aplastic anemia patients having an antecedent infection. Serologic testing may be negative.

### 27. e.

The vast majority of patients presenting with aplastic anemia have no known etiologic factor. Benzene is known to cause acute leukemia and myelodysplasia, but it also may be associated with aplastic anemia. The actual incidence of aplastic anemia associated with chloramphenicol is exceptionally low. Chloramphenicol does cause reversible, dose-related bone marrow depression. The actual incidence of chloramphenicol-associated aplastic anemia is 1 in 100,000 courses.

### 28. a.

The therapy of choice is allogeneic BMT, which cures approximately 70% of patients with an HLA-matched sibling donor. Antithymocyte globulin is an immunologic therapy that leads to improvement in peripheral blood counts in approximately 50% of patients, although relapses are frequent. Steroids have not been shown to be beneficial in this illness. Hematopoietic growth factors may temporarily improve neutrophil counts, although improvement is transient.

This case represents an actual patient treated several years ago. The problem encountered was HLA typing. The patient's low WBC count, coupled with having received RBC transfusions, made tissue typing problematic. Ultimately, DNA was extracted from hair follicles to perform HLA typing. The patient underwent allogeneic BMT and is alive and well 10 years later.

### 29. b.

Filgrastim stimulates granulocyte cells. It also stimulates the production and release of immature progenitor cells. Clinically, G-CSF has been useful in autologous and allogeneic BMT to stimulate stem cells and enhance neutrophil recovery. It also has been shown to reduce the incidence and severity of febrile neutropenia in selected patients receiving conventional doses of chemotherapy. Given its ability to stimulate the granulocyte series at all levels of maturation, however, receiving filgrastim concomitantly with chemotherapy often causes profound and long-lasting neutropenia. As a result, patients receiving chemotherapy should not receive any hematopoietic growth factors for at least 48 hours. Rituxan also can contribute to neutropenia, especially when used in patients with indolent non-Hodgkin lymphoma, who have received extensive previous therapy.

### 30. c.
Patients with mast cell disorders can have various dermatologic manifestations. Many have a history of urticaria after taking certain drugs. The most common dermatologic manifestation of patients with a histologically confirmed mast cell disorder is urticaria pigmentosum, however. Porphyria cutanea tarda is a separate illness characterized by bullous lesions in sun-exposed areas, particularly the dorsa of the hands; it is due to a partial deficiency of uroporphyrinogen decarboxylase activity. Erythema of the palms and soles is often seen in essential thrombocythemia, a myeloproliferative disorder. Café-au-lait spots are often seen in neurofibromatosis.

### 31. e.
Indeed, hydroxyurea may increase the Hgb F concentration of cells, leading to less intraerythrocyte sickling and a more benign clinical course. All the mentioned complications, however, may be seen as part of therapy in patients with sickle cell disease, and the drug must be used very judiciously.

### 32. e.
This patient has thrombotic thrombocytopenic purpura. The treatment of choice is immediate plasma exchange therapy. Other drugs are given to these patients, but their exact use is unknown. These include aspirin and corticosteroids, but by far, the most efficacious treatment is plasma exchange. Trials have shown that plasma infusion may be equally efficacious; however, thrombotic thrombocytopenic purpura is a heterogenous disease, and the current approach is plasma exchange.

### 33. d.
This patient most likely has polycythemia vera. It would be best to try to find some history about smoking or to determine whether this might be a secondary polycythemia; however, splenomegaly and a high WBC count can certainly be part of the presentation of polycythemia vera. When a patient with polycythemia vera presents with a neurologic event, the best first treatment is phlebotomy. The goal is to lower the hematocrit to less than

45% and keep it there; however, in the acute neurologic setting, the goal is to phlebotomize to the point of relieving the neurologic event. This may or may not occur, and the patient may have permanent sequelae from a stroke-like syndrome.

### 34. c.
This is a controversial area for hematologists today. Interferon-α, with or without ara-C, given to a patient in this age group leads to the disappearance of the Philadelphia chromosome 20% of the time. Some patients who achieve this status may remain free of Philadelphia-positive CML for many years. Most randomized controlled trials comparing interferon with hydroxyurea show a survival advantage with interferon. Alternatively, other controlled clinical trials show no benefit of interferon compared with hydroxyurea. In summary, a survival benefit probably accrues to interferon-based therapy compared with hydroxyurea alone. Busulfan (Myleran) is inferior to hydroxyurea in the maintenance of patients with CML.

If the patient had an HLA-compatible sibling and underwent allogeneic BMT, the risk of early death or complications such as graft-versus-host disease would obtain from the procedure. If the patient survives longer than 5.6 years, allogeneic BMT offers greater benefit than any other therapy, as has been shown in a recent meta-analysis. The American Society of Hematology practice guideline discusses this dilemma in great detail, spelling out all the risks and benefits of each procedure. Autologous stem cell transplantation for this disorder is considered experimental, although advocates for it exist. If an HLA-compatible sibling exists, allogeneic BMT gives most patients probably the best chance of eradicating the Philadelphia chromosome. The risks of this course are early demise and immunologic complications. The new drug STI- 571 (Gleevec) specifically inhibits the protein responsible for the proliferation of the granulocytic series in CML. It is probably the best initial treatment for patients with CML. Some patients treated with ST1-571 have remained Philadelphia chromosome negative for more than 5 years.

### 35. c.
This woman does have essential thrombocythemia diagnosed at a young age. Controversy arises on the management of this disease in completely asymptomatic individuals. Most hematologists would probably adopt a watch-and-wait approach, warning the patient to contact the physician if headaches or erythromelalgia (painful burning of the palms or soles) develop. Again, this is controversial, and other hematologists, seeing this as a potentially life-threatening process, would institute therapy to lower the platelet count. Patients being treated for this disorder should be cautioned not to become

pregnant while taking drugs such as hydroxyurea or ana-grelide. Most women who become pregnant show a decline in their platelet count because plasma volume increases or because gestation may lead to a mild decrease in the platelet count; thus, some of these patients go through pregnancy with a decreased platelet count and are better off. Once formed, however, the fetus can cause compression of pelvic veins, sometimes with an increased risk of thrombophlebitis or deep vein thrombosis. If the patient has headaches, migraine-type headaches, or erythromelalgia, the platelet count should be lowered before the patient becomes pregnant because the placenta can be the source of thrombotic events if the woman is symptomatic. Most young individuals have such pliant vasculature that a platelet count of $1,200,000/mm^3$ can be tolerated without the development of thromboses or, paradoxically, bleeding. The best approach for this individual is to allow her to become pregnant if she wishes to do so, and strongly counsel her to report any symptom that would prompt early intervention. It is wise to involve a high-risk obstetrician in the care of such a patient. Both hydroxyurea and anagrelide (probably to a lesser extent) are teratogens and should be avoided in women of childbearing potential.

### 36. b.

This case demonstrates several problematic features of the diagnosis of Gaucher's disease. First, had this patient been seen before the episode of pneumonia and found to have cytopenia and hepatosplenomegaly, a careful history may have detected issues of bone pain and the person's Ashkenazi Jewish background. With this information, a wise clinician might have ordered a glucocerebrosidase enzyme level and, if finding it low, could have avoided bone marrow aspiration and biopsy. The assay for glucocerebroside activity alone is enough to make the diagnosis now. Because the patient presented with an acute medical problem (pneumonia), however, there was greater urgency in establishing why the patient was cytopenic.

Some patients with Gaucher's disease have a chronic inflammatory aspect to their disorder, and a monoclonal plasma cell dyscrasia develops. Indeed, some cases of myeloma arise in the setting of Gaucher's disease. This is a more worrisome feature and may indicate a worse prognosis than Gaucher's disease alone. This certainly would be reason to treat a patient with enzyme therapy.

α-Galactosidase deficiency is seen in Fabry's disease, a lipid storage disorder. Splenectomy may normalize the counts in a patient with Gaucher's disease, but may be contraindicated early in the course of the disease because the spleen is a site of globoside accumulation. Enzyme replacement therapy has made a dramatic impact in the lives of patients with Gaucher's disease. Indeed, with enzyme replacement, enlarged livers and spleens may shrink, and bone improvements may occur. Initially, the agent was called alglucerase (Ceredase), but with modification of the sugar moieties, it is now called imiglucerase (Cerezyme). Controversy among physicians treating this disorder concerns whether high-dose therapy every 2 weeks is more efficacious than or equally as efficacious as lower dose therapy three times per week. This continues to be an area of contention.

### 37. d.

Some individuals with post-transplantation lymphoproliferative disorder have complete shrinkage and resolution of the lymphoma by reduction of the immunosuppression. The problem is that patients may begin to experience transplanted organ rejection. In renal transplant patients, it is possible to carefully monitor the creatinine level and judiciously reapply immunosuppression if rejection is seen. This must be done in conjunction with a treating nephrologist so that a uniform approach to each individual patient is applied. If continued growth of post-transplantation lymphoproliferative disorder occurs after a reduction of immunosuppression, then chemotherapy is usually the next approach, although some favor interferon-α if progression of disease is noted after reduction of immunosuppression. Rituxan (anti-CD20) may have a role in these patients.

### 38. d.

This patient has hairy cell leukemia. This disorder is rare, but many excellent treatments are available for it, some even curative with the most minimal of interventions. Historically, splenectomy was used to normalize the counts, but the bone marrow process would continue. Interferon-α causes a complete resolution of hairy cells in a fairly high proportion of patients, but the treatment may take many months and is difficult to administer with daily injections. Pentostatin can cause remission with very few courses. The treatment of choice is now cladribine, which may induce a complete cure in up to 50% of patients after a 7-day infusion. Sometimes, a second infusion is needed 3 months after the initial treatment.

### 39. a.

Thrombosis, especially of the hepatic veins, is a serious complication of paroxysmal nocturnal hemoglobinuria, and natural history studies demonstrate that patients with paroxysmal nocturnal hemoglobinuria should receive prophylactic anticoagulation with warfarin. This needs to be tailored somewhat on an individual basis because some patients with paroxysmal nocturnal hemoglobinuria have severe thrombocytopenia, and a greater risk of hemorrhage occurs if warfarin is given. This man represents a borderline case; still, it is probably better for him to take warfarin to maintain an international normalized ratio at a safe enough level (around 2.0) so that thrombocytopenia does not yield too great a risk of hemorrhage.

**40. d.**

Anemia can develop "out of the blue" (rapidly progressive anemia) in patients with CLL for two primary reasons. One is the development of an acquired autoimmune hemolytic anemia, which is usually Coombs' positive and associated with an elevated reticulocyte count. The other is the development of a pure red cell aplasia associated with reticulocytopenia, which this case demonstrates.

Usually, when people have a parvovirus B19 infection, they have had some antecedent febrile illness. Patients with CLL can be hypogammaglobulinemic, making them prone to bacterial infection, such as pneumococcal sepsis, but this patient was not febrile. There is no known association of anything like an antierythropoietin antibody with this clinical scenario.

**41. b.**

This disorder, variably called *large granular lymphocytosis* or *T-cell gamma lymphocytosis*, is a lymphoproliferative disorder of T cells (CD3$^+$ and CD2$^+$), which may exhibit deletion of CD5 and partial deletion of CD7. The CD4-to-CD8 ratio is usually reversed. T-cell receptor gene rearrangement studies often find rearrangements of the T-cell receptor gene. The chronicity of this disorder speaks against it being an acute leukemia. The peripheral blood smear often demonstrates that the majority of these lymphocytes have granules in the cytoplasm. Some patients with this type of disorder may be natural killer cell–positive with CD56 positivity. Typically, bacterial infections develop, and treatment is usually supportive using antibiotics. G-CSF may raise the neutrophil percentage. Some individuals may respond to alkylating agent–based chemotherapy, but this can be risky because it can cause further immunocompromise. A 1% to 2% neutrophil level is often enough to keep these patients active with good functional status (except for periodic infections).

**42. e.**

Patients who have had a splenectomy as part of a staging laparotomy or therapy for a hematologic disorder, such as hereditary spherocytosis or elliptocytosis, are prone to the development of fulminant pneumococcal sepsis or fulminant sepsis with other encapsulated organisms. This scenario occurs in approximately 1% of patients who have had a splenectomy. A patient's condition can deteriorate rapidly, and all such patients need to be warned of this so that they seek immediate medical attention when they feel ill.

**43. d.**

One of the best prognostic chromosome anomalies in myelodysplasia is the 5q– anomaly. This disorder has

actually been called the *5q–syndrome*. Typically, it is seen in older women, and the platelet count is usually elevated at presentation and remains normal for a long time into the course of the myelodysplasia. The 20q– anomaly also carries a good prognosis, but patients usually become thrombocytopenic as time goes on. Monosomy 7 and trisomy 8 have a poor prognosis. The translocation of chromosome 8 to chromosome 21 is an anomaly that is more often associated with AML.

**44. c.**

Marijuana use can raise a man's β-HCG level. The other two listed ingestions are not known to do this. Before resorting to any invasive test, further history or urine drug screening should occur.

**45. b.**

The Phase I studies of a new anticancer drug are really toxicity studies. They are not really done with therapeutic intent. Once a drug's MTD dose has been defined, and if any response or stabilization is noted, researchers establish a Phase II trial to determine if any efficacy is found in a certain tumor type. Placebo-controlled trials are done after Phase I and II trials are completed.

**46. e.**

The Sternberg-Reed cell is likely of B-cell origin and is necessary to make a definitive diagnosis of Hodgkin's disease. In the past, early stage Hodgkin's disease was most frequently treated by relatively large radiation fields. Today, most of these patients are treated by chemotherapy, followed by more limited radiation. Patients with Hodgkin's disease tend to relapse in areas of bulk disease and frequently, particularly with chest disease, post-chemotherapy consolidative radiation therapy to the mediastinum is recommended. Although newer combination chemotherapy programs, for example, ABVD, cause far less sterility in young males, sperm banking should be considered prior to therapy.

**47. d.**

A relapse of Hodgkin's disease within a year following diagnosis portends a poor prognosis. Whereas alternative combination chemotherapy programs often demonstrate significant responses and have a small curative potential, high-dose chemotherapy with hematopoietic transplantation offers the best potential for cure. In this setting, an autologous transplant has less morbidity and mortality than allogeneic transplantation and a substantial improvement in overall survival, as compared to standard chemotherapy programs. Salvage chemotherapy programs are usually administered prior to transplant and act essentially as debulking agents.

**48. a.**

Myelodysplasia or acute nonlymphocytic leukemia occurs in 3% to 10% of patients 2 to 10 years after chemotherapy for Hodgkin's disease. Cytogenetic abnormalities are common, and those related to chromosome 5 and/or 7 portend a poor prognosis. Secondary myelodysplastic syndromes or secondary leukemias, particularly those with these types of cytogenetic abnormalities are best treated with allogeneic transplant, should the patient be a candidate and a match present. In patients not considered candidates for transplant, supportive care, including transfusions and, potentially, growth factors is the standard of therapy for myelodysplasia; induction chemotherapy is utilized for leukemia. Of patients who receive radiation therapy, 10% to 20% may subsequently develop solid tumors. Sarcomas, melanomas, and cancers of the head and neck, lung, breast, and gastrointestinal tract are most frequent. Non-Hodgkin's lymphoma develops in approximately 5% of patients.

### 49. e.

In hematologic malignancies, the myeloablative doses of chemotherapy and/or radiotherapy are potentially augmented by a powerful immune reaction generated by donor cells against residual tumor, best exemplified in acute leukemia as a graft-versus-leukemia (GVL) effect. The relatively high risk of morbidity and mortality in this setting is related to the transplantation of an allogeneic immune system, which causes graft-versus-host disease (GVHD), and the attendant infectious complications related to immunosuppression. Nonmyeloablative transplants (mini) involve less intense preparatory regimens and, accordingly, have less potential toxicity; these are utilized primarily for the graft-versus-tumor effect.

Graft-versus-host disease (GVHD) results from immunocompetent donor T cells interacting with recipient tissues that possess antigens absent from the donor. Major sites of graft-versus-host disease involvement include the skin, liver, and gastrointestinal tract, although any tissue may be involved. GVHD occurs in a stepwise process—recipient tissues are recognized as foreign by the donor immune system, and this is followed by the activation and expansion of effector populations. This leads ultimately to T-cell–mediated cytotoxic damage. GVHD prophylaxis involves either prophylactic immunosuppression or T-cell depletion prior to stem cell infusion, or both. The most common immunosuppressive program involves the use of cyclosporin A or FK506 and methotrexate. Steroids are the mainstay of therapy for the treatment of acute GVHD. Mycophenolate, monoclonal antibodies that target T-cell antigens, and photopheresis are additional techniques that may be helpful. Chronic GVHD occurs 3 months to 2 years post-transplant and characteristically involves the skin, with lichenoid or sclerodermatous skin involvement, and hepatic biliary obstruction.

### 50. c.

Essential thrombocytosis is a clonal disorder manifested by thrombocytosis; it is one of a group of chronic myeloproliferative disorders that include chronic granulocytic leukemia, polycythemia vera, and myelofibrosis with myeloid metaplasia. The diagnosis of essential thrombocytosis is made with increasing frequency, particularly in younger individuals; however, ET is one of the more unusual myeloproliferative disorders. Physical findings are usually limited to splenomegaly, which may be present in 40% of patients. Bleeding or thrombotic episodes are the major causes of morbidity and mortality. Although unpredictable, an increased risk of thrombosis is seen in patients who are older and have had a previous history of thrombosis. Thrombotic complications include erythromelalgia and digital microvascular ischemia, cerebral vascular ischemia, recurrent abortions, and hepatic and portal vein thrombosis. One study suggests that in patients over age 60, or in those who have had a previous episode of thrombosis, control of the platelet count to levels below 600,000/$\mu$L reduces the incidence of thrombotic episodes.

An increased risk of bleeding is seen in patients with extreme thrombocytosis (platelet count greater than 2,000,000/$\mu$L) or when aspirin and NSAIDs are utilized. The most common sites of bleeding are mucosal and gastrointestinal.

In patients with active or recurrent bleeding or thrombosis, platelet cytoreduction therapy results in clinical improvement. Young, asymptomatic patients may not need treatment, but rather expectant observation. When therapy is indicated, options include hydroxyurea, anagrelide, interferon, and plateletpheresis. Indications for prompt platelet reduction therapy include cerebral ischemia or microvascular digital symptoms. Aspirin therapy is controversial in the myeloproliferative disorders but may be helpful, particularly if digital or cerebral vascular ischemia has occurred; however, it may be associated with an increased risk of bleeding. Although the other myeloproliferative disorders have been demonstrated to transform to acute leukemia, this association is less clear in essential thrombocytosis.

The pathogenesis of reactive thrombocytosis is not well defined. It may be associated with inflammatory disorders, however, following episodes of bone marrow suppression, in the post-splenectomy state, and in malignant disorders. Reactive thrombocytosis is not thought to lead to an excess incidence of thrombosis or hemorrhage and, when this does occur, it likely is related to the underlying problem.

Uncommonly, chronic granulocytic leukemia may present solely with a thrombocytosis, and for this reason, the presence of the fusion gene product bcr-abl should be excluded.

**51. e.**

Myelofibrosis is a clonal marrow disorder. The marrow fibrosis is reactive and likely results from cytokines released by abnormal megakaryocytes. The disorder is characterized by anemia, leukocytosis, thrombocytosis, and progressive splenomegaly. Clinical manifestations are produced by a progressive marrow failure, most often characterized by progressive anemia, and increasing symptoms related to splenomegaly. The splenomegaly, and often hepatomegaly, results from extramedullary hematopoiesis. Other sites of extramedullary hematopoietic "tumors" may include the adrenals, lymph nodes, kidneys, lung, and bone, particularly the skull and spinal cord. Foci on serosal surfaces may cause pleural or pericardial effusions or ascites. Portal hypertension may result from the large increase in splenic portal flow.

Chronic myelogenous leukemia could present in a similar fashion, and the presence of the bcr-abl fusion gene should be excluded.

Other disorders associated with marrow fibrosis include metastatic carcinoma, infections (particularly mycobacterial), connective tissue disorders, non-Hodgkin lymphoma, multiple myeloma, chronic lymphocytic leukemia, and malignant histiocytic disorders. In the secondary disorders, treatment of the primary disorder may result in improvement in the fibrosis. No specific therapy is available for myelofibrosis, although some patients may be candidates for allogeneic marrow transplantation.

Many patients will be asymptomatic and not require specific therapy for some time. Otherwise, the therapy includes transfusion for symptomatic anemia. The use of erythropoietin has not been generally successful. Hydroxyurea or other chemotherapeutic agents have been utilized to treat splenomegaly, thrombocytosis associated with the disorder, or symptomatic hematopoietic implants. Radiation therapy can be utilized to control spleen size, and for focal areas of extramedullary hematopoietic tumors. Splenectomy may be useful in selected patients. Interferon may be helpful in treating splenic enlargement and thrombocytosis in selected patients. Major causes of death include infection, hemorrhage, and transformation to acute leukemia.

**52. a.**

Inflammatory breast cancer is a distinct clinical entity. On examination, a diffuse, brawny, erythematous edema of the skin is present, generally without an underlying mass. Dermal lymphatic invasion by malignant cells is the pathologic correlation. Primary surgical therapy results in problems with margins and an excess rate of local recurrence. With preoperative chemotherapy, most patients can proceed to surgery and local radiation postoperatively. In the absence of systemic therapy, patients with inflammatory breast cancer generally do not survive 5 years. With current multimodality programs, however, approximately 50% of patients are alive at 5 years, and approximately 35% are disease free at 10 years.

**53. a.**

Breast cancer may complicate 1 in 1,000 pregnancies. Delays in diagnosis are not uncommon due to difficulties in examining the breast and a low index of suspicion in the young, pregnant patient. Mammography may not be as helpful because of an increased density of the breast associated with pregnancy. The survival of women treated during pregnancy for breast cancer is similar to that seen in the nonpregnant woman.

Mammography can be performed safely throughout pregnancy. Other diagnostic radiologic studies should be avoided, however. Radiation therapy is contraindicated at all times during pregnancy because of the possibility of scatter. Chemotherapy should be avoided during the first trimester because it may lead to an increased risk of abortion, compromised fetal viability, and major organ malformations. Breast conservation can be considered if the cancer develops during the third trimester and subsequent radiation therapy can proceed on schedule or with minimal delay. This is less important if adjuvant chemotherapy is planned subsequent to surgery. If the administration of radiation would be delayed because of the timing of the cancer in pregnancy, consideration should be given to mastectomy.

Immediate reconstruction is generally not feasible, given the increase in anesthesia time, and the difficulty of obtaining symmetry in the pregnant female. A TRAM procedure is contraindicated because of the effect on abdominal musculature. Chemotherapy after the first trimester does not appear to increase the risk of major fetal malformations; however, it may lead to growth retardation and low birth weight. Depending on the situation, adjuvant chemotherapy in the third trimester may be delayed slightly, with the thought of potentially delivering the baby early. Adjuvant tamoxifen has not been demonstrated to be safe during pregnancy.

**54. a.**

Mixing study will distinguish between a factor deficiency and a factor inhibitor as the cause of prolonged PTT.

**55. c.**

Acquired coagulation inhibitors are circulating immunoglobulins, generally of the IgG class. They neutralize the activity of coagulation proteins or accelerate clearances from plasma. They occur as alloantibodies when they arise subsequent to blood product exposure, for example, in patients with hereditary factor deficiencies. They occur as autoantibodies in patients without an antecedent coagulation abnormality. They are rare but may be associated with significant morbidity and mortality.

Mixing studies confirm the presence or absence of an inhibitor, and the Russell viper venom time and phospholipid neutralization procedure are the best tests to exclude the common clinical entity of the lupus anticoagulant. Specific factor assays identify the specific protein.

Inhibitors to factor VIII are most common and may be associated with often severe bleeding manifestations. In contradistinction to patients with congenital factor VIII deficiency (hemophilia A), in which intra-articular hemorrhage is the most common manifestation, intramuscular, gastrointestinal, or retroperitoneal bleeding are most commonly seen.

Fifty percent of patients have no concomitant illness. In the remainder, associated disorders include connective tissue disease, inflammatory bowel disease, malignancy, and medication side effects, such as from penicillin, sulfa, and phenytoin, and inhibitors that arise in the peripartum period.

Inhibitor titers are measured in Bethesda units; patients with inhibitors of less than 5 Bethesda units have low titer inhibitors. All others are high titer.

The treatment options for patients with low-titer inhibitors involve the use of high doses of human factor VIII concentrates or DDVAP in an attempt to overwhelm the inhibitor. Options for patients with high-titer inhibitors include porcine factor VIII concentrate, partially activated or fully activated IX complex concentrates, and recombinant factor VIIa concentrates. These latter approaches bypass the need for factor VIII.

Exchange plasmapheresis may also be helpful in temporarily decreasing antibody titers. Intravenous immune globulin may also be helpful in suppressing factor VIII inhibitors, perhaps related to the presence of anti-idiotypic antibodies in the preparation.

Although most acquired inhibitors spontaneously remit, immunosuppression using steroids, azathioprine, cyclophosphamide, and newer agents, such as cyclosporine A or rituximab, may be helpful in producing a remission or hastening its evolution.

## 56. e.

Sickle cell disease results from a single amino acid substitution in the glutamic acid DNA codon. Molecules of deoxyhemoglobin-S aggregate and become a firm gel. The distorted appearance of the sickled cell is the result of this molecular aggregation. The sickling and unsickling that results from deoxygenation and reoxygenation in the lungs eventually leads to membrane abnormalities, and the cells become irreversibly sickled, which leads to the disease manifestations of both chronic hemolysis and vaso-occlusion. Microvascular vaso-occlusion leads to ischemic bone and abdominal pain. The acute chest syndrome and cerebral infarction occurs similarly. Heart, liver, and eye may also be involved with occlusive events.

Therapy in acute stroke involves decreasing sickling by increasing hemoglobin A levels and decreasing hemoglobin S levels. This is best accomplished by exchange transfusion. Stroke tends to be a recurrent event, and therefore, prophylaxis generally is reasonable using exchange transfusion. The use of chemotherapeutic agents, such as hydroxyurea, increases hemoglobin F levels and may decrease sickling events. The overall utility of this approach is uncertain at this time.

Allogeneic hematopoietic stem cell transplantation and gene therapy offer hope for future curative therapy.

## 57. e.

Gaucher's disease is the most common lipid storage disease, occurring in about 1 in 1,000 Ashkenazi Jews. A deficiency of glucocerebrosidase results in the accumulation of glucocerebroside in cells of the reticuloendothelial system. Splenomegaly commonly occurs and may result in cytopenias. Three forms occur: The most common, type I, is not associated with neurologic symptoms. In types II and III, however, the central nervous system is involved. The diagnosis is based on the demonstration of deficient levels of glucocerebrosidase, which is a $\beta$-glycosidase.

Patients with type I disease generally have a good prognosis. Those severely affected, or those with type III disease, may die as a result of liver disease or bleeding. In type II disease, death is usually due to neurologic sequela. Most patients do not require therapy; however, infusion enzyme replacement is available. Bone marrow transplantation has been utilized in this disorder, and specific gene therapy is under study.

Gaucher's cells are found mainly in the marrow, spleen, and liver.

## 58. a.

Chronic lymphocytic leukemia (CLL) is the most common type of adult leukemia, with 7,000 new cases each year. At diagnosis, 80% to 90% of patients are asymptomatic, and the major decision in managing patients with CLL is when to institute treatment. Staging systems have been devised to help with this decision and generally reflect tumor burden, relying on number of nodal areas involved, the presence of splenomegaly, and cytopenias.

Autoimmune disease may occur, as in the patient noted, with immune hemolysis. Immune thrombocytopenia may also occur. Pure red cell aplasia presumed secondary to autoantibodies also may be a manifestation of the disease. Patients with CLL often have hypogammaglobulinemia, an impaired antibody response to microbes, and increased infection rates. Intravenous gammaglobulin may be helpful in this setting. With progressive duration of disease, this problem worsens. Patients with CLL have an increased risk of second malignancies, which may be epithelial or hematopoietic.

The use of alkalating agents in therapy may enhance the incidence of epithelial neoplasms.

Extramedullary disease may occur in the lung, gastrointestinal tract, and central nervous system.

Generally agreed upon indications for therapy include significant cytopenia, symptomatic lymphadenopathy or hepatosplenomegaly, constitutional symptoms, or extreme lymphocytosis. Autoimmune phenomenon generally respond to steroids and usually suggest the need to treat the underlying disorder.

A plethora of therapeutic agents are available for the treatment of CLL, and what to use when remains an important issue. Treatment options include single alkylating agents such as chlorambucil, purine analogs such as fludarabine or 2-chloro-deoxyadenosine, monoclonal antibodies such as CamPath-1H and rituximab, and combinations of these agents.

Stem cell transplantation, both autologous and allogeneic, has been utilized in this disorder, and nonmyeloablative programs with less treatment-related toxicity may make this approach more viable in the older population of patients with CLL.

Until recently, the goal of therapy has always been one of palliation, however, with the newer treatment modalities available, the goal of attaining a complete remission may become feasible.

### 59. c.

Multiple myeloma is a malignancy of plasma cells that usually produce a monoclonal immunoglobulin. The disease may be indolent or highly aggressive; symptoms may be caused either by tumor mass, which may result in pain, or deposition of protein in organ systems, such as the heart or kidney. $\beta_2$-microglobulin, C-reactive protein, plasma cell labeling index, and abnormalities of chromosome-13 correlate best with tumor burden and prognosis. Chemotherapy with melphalan and prednisone or other combinations results in palliative benefit and a small incidence of complete response. High-dose programs using hematopoietic stem cell transplantation have increased the complete response rate to approximately 50%. The melphalan/prednisone combinations interfere with the harvesting of stem cells, and many authorities believe these agents should be avoided if a patient is a transplant candidate.

Allogeneic bone marrow transplantation can be considered, particularly in younger individuals, with the thought of potentially exploiting a graft-versus-tumor effect.

Nonmyeloablative programs may diminish treatment-related morbidity and mortality. Thalidomide and high-dose glucocorticoid therapy have efficacy in patients who have relapsed subsequent to primary therapy. Radiation to areas of bone pain affords significant palliation. The bisphosphonates are extremely helpful in treating myeloma bone disease. Deficiencies in both cellular and humoral immunity lead to the potential infectious sequela seen in this disorder. Erythropoietin can be a helpful adjunct in the treatment of anemia in myeloma.

Essential monoclonal gammopathy is the presence of a monoclonal immunoglobulin in the serum or of a light chain in the urine, in the absence of a demonstrable malignancy of lymphocytes or plasma cells. Its incidence increases with age, and it is seen in approximately 10% of patients 80 years of age or older. Some of these monoclonal proteins interact with plasma or cell membrane proteins, resulting in problems such as immune hemolytic anemia, acquired von Willebrand's disease, and neuropathies. If these proteins result in symptoms, plasmapheresis and/or immunosuppressive chemotherapy may be indicated. Follow-up is recommended because approximately 1% of cases per year will transform to overt lymphoma or myeloma. All patients considered, 25% remain stable, 50% die of an unrelated cause, and the remaining 25% develop myeloma, lymphoma, amyloidosis, or macroglobulinemia.

### 60. a.

AL amyloid is the most common form of systemic amyloidosis in this country. Estimated incidence is about 1 case per 100,000 people. Most patients present with weakness and weight loss; purpura is commonly seen, particularly in the face. The prognosis depends on the pattern of tissue deposition. Any organ may be involved; however, the kidney is the most common site of AL deposition. Heart, gastrointestinal tract, liver, and peripheral nerves may also be involved. Patients with cardiac involvement have the worst prognosis. Good prognostic indicators are a small number of clonal plasma cells in the marrow and normal renal function. The most common renal manifestation is proteinuria. Cardiac involvement produces diastolic dysfunction, arrhythmias, and congestive heart failure. A sensorimotor neuropathy with deposition in peripheral nerves is the most common neurologic sequela. An autonomic neuropathy may produce severe symptoms. Involvement of the gastrointestinal tract may produce macroglossia and interfere with gastrointestinal motility.

Massive hepatomegaly may occur; however, liver function abnormalities are unusual. Diffuse interstitial or alveolar pulmonary involvement may produce a reticular nodular pattern on radiograph; however, this often is asymptomatic. Articular deposition of AL may produce a clinical syndrome much like seronegative rheumatoid arthritis. Subendothelial deposition in capillaries may produce fragility and cutaneous hemorrhage. Factor X may be bound by AL fibrils and produce clinical bleeding.

Amyloidosis is demonstrated by staining tissue with congo red, which produces a characteristic apple green fluorescence under polarized light. Subcutaneous fat aspiration or a rectal biopsy are reasonable approaches. The biopsy of an organ with impaired function produces the diagnosis and demonstrates that the dysfunction is secondary to the disorder. The amyloid subtype should be diagnosed by immunohistochemistry.

## 61. d.

An unknown primary tumor is a metastatic malignancy whose primary site remains unknown after a good history and physical examination, chest radiograph, and CT scan of the abdomen and pelvis. One must pay particular attention to exclude those cancers that are curable when metastatic, such as germ cell tumor or lymphomas, and tumors that have a good response to therapy, such as breast cancer, prostate cancer, small cell carcinoma of the lung, and ovarian cancer. Exhaustive evaluations are expensive and often unrevealing. Accordingly, evaluations should be tailored to the individual patient's situation. Women with adenocarcinoma in axillary nodes and no evidence of disease elsewhere should be treated as having potentially curable stage II carcinoma of the breast. Women with abdominal carcinomatosis with no evidence of a primary site should be treated as having ovarian carcinoma. Men with unknown primary site adenocarcinomas involving predominantly the bone should be considered to have prostate cancer until proven otherwise.

Patients with squamous cell carcinomas involving cervical nodes usually have a head and neck or possibly lung primary. If a primary tumor cannot be found, they should be treated as having a primary head and neck cancer.

Patients with poorly differentiated carcinomas involving lymph nodes in the mediastinum and/or retroperitoneum may represent a population of patients with extragonadal germ cell tumors. This should be considered in particular with young patients with rapidly growing tumors. Multiple pulmonary nodules may be part of the presentation.

The history and physical examination and interaction between the clinician and the pathologist are the most important facets of this evaluation.

## REFERENCES

### Plasma Cell Dyscrasias

1. Barlogie B, et al. Treatment of multiple myeloma. *Blood* 2004; 103(1):20–32.
2. Berenson JR, Lichtenstein A, Porter L, et al. Efficacy of pamidronate in reducing skeletal events in patients with advanced multiple myeloma. Myeloma Aredia Study Group. *N Engl J Med* 1996;334: 488–493.
3. Boyden LM, Mao J, Belsky J, et al. High bone density due to a mutation in LDL-receptor-related protein 5. *N Engl J Med* 2002; 346:1513–1521.
4. Cadigan KM, Nusse R. Wnt signaling: a common theme in animal development. *Genes Dev* 1997;11:3286–3305.
5. Drach J, Kaufmann H, Urbauer E, et al. The biology of multiple myeloma. *J Cancer Res Clin Oncol* 2000;126:441–447.
6. Gong Y, Slee RB, Fukai N, et al. LDL receptor-related protein 5 (LRP5) affects bone accrual and eye development. *Cell* 2001;107: 513–523.
7. Kyle RA, Lust JA. Monoclonal gammopathies of undetermined significance. *Semin Hematol* 1989;26:176–200.
8. Kyle RA. Benign monoclonal gammopathy—after 20 to 35 years of follow-up. *Mayo Clin Proc* 1993;68:26–36.
9. Lacey DL, Timms E, Tan HL, et al. Osteoprotegerin ligand is a cytokine that regulates osteoclast differentiation and activation. *Cell* 1998;93:165–176.
10. Rajkumar SV. Thalidomide in multiple myeloma. *Oncology* 2000; 14:11–16.
11. Tricot G. New insights into role of microenvironment in multiple myeloma. *Lancet* 2000;355:248–250.
12. Sanz-Rodriguez F, Hidalgo A, Teixido J. Chemokine stromal cell-derived factor-1alpha modulates VLA-4 integrin-mediated multiple myeloma cell adhesion to CS-1/fibronectin and VCAM-1. *Blood* 2001;97:346–351.
13. Roodman GD. Biology of osteoclast activation in cancer. *J Clin Oncol* 2001;19:3562–3571.
14. Tian E, Zhan F, Walker R, et al. The role of the Wnt-signaling antagonist DKK1 in the development of osteolytic lesions in multiple myeloma. *N Engl J Med* 2003;349:2483–2494.

## SUGGESTED READINGS

Attal M, Harousseau JL, Stoppa AM, et al. A prospective, randomized trial of autologous bone marrow transplantation and chemotherapy in multiple myeloma. *N Engl J Med* 1996;335: 91–97.

Drucker BJ, Talpaz M, Resta D, et al. Efficacy and safety of a specific inhibitor of the bcr-abl tyrosine kinase in chronic myeloid leukemia. *N Engl J Med* 2001;344:1031–1037.

Dunbar CE, Nienhuis AW. Multiple myeloma: new approaches to therapy. *JAMA* 1993;269:2412–2416.

George JN, Woolf SH, Raskob GE, et al. Idiopathic thrombocytopenic purpura: a practice guideline developed by explicit methods for the American Society of Hematology. *Blood* 1996; 88:3–40.

Gregory WM, Richards MA, Malpas JS. Combination chemotherapy versus melphalan and prednisolone in the treatment of multiple myeloma: an overview of published trials. *J Clin Oncol* 1992; 10:334–342.

Greipp P. Advances in the diagnosis and management of myeloma. *Semin Hematol* 1992;29[Suppl 2]:24–44.

Heaney ML, Golde DW. Myelodysplasia. *N Engl J Med* 1999;340: 1649–1660.

Hillmen P, Lewis SM, Bessler M, et al. Natural history of paroxysmal nocturnal hemoglobinuria. *N Engl J Med* 1995;333:1253–1258.

Loeffler J, Leopold K, Recht A, et al. Emergency prebiopsy radiation for mediastinal masses: impact on subsequent pathologic diagnosis and outcome. *J Clin Oncol* 1986;4:716–721.

Loughran TP. Clonal disorders of large granular lymphocytes. *Blood* 1993;82:1–14.

Philip T, Guglielmi C, Hagenbeek A. Autologous bone marrow transplantation as compared with salvage chemotherapy in relapses of chemotherapy-sensitive non-Hodgkin's lymphoma. *N Engl J Med* 1995;333:1540–1544.

Sawyers CL. Chronic myeloid leukemia. *N Engl J Med* 1999;340: 1330–1340.

Silver RT, Woolf SH, Hehlmann R, et al. An evidence-based analysis of the effect of busulfan, hydroxyurea, interferon, and allogeneic bone marrow transplantation in treating the chronic phase of chronic myeloid leukemia: developed for the American Society of Hematology. *Blood* 1999;94:1517–1536.

Steinberg MH. Management of sickle cell disease. *N Engl J Med* 1999; 340:1021–1030.

# BOARD SIMULATION: Cellular Morphology

## 27

*Andrew J. Fishleder*

This chapter reviews the abnormal red blood cell (RBC) and white blood cell (WBC) morphology encountered in common hematologic disorders. Case histories are provided to test your knowledge of cellular morphology with clinical correlation. The answers to the questions posed in each case are listed at the end of the chapter. A discussion concerning the morphology of the correct answer and the differential possibilities listed in the questions below is provided in the associated text. Details regarding individual clinical conditions and their therapies are covered elsewhere in this book.

## CASE 1

1. A 20-year-old man presents with weakness and fatigue. A complete blood cell count reveals a hemoglobin level of 9.0 g/dL. The peripheral smear (see Fig. 27.1) is most consistent with
   a) Thalassemia minor
   b) Immune hemolytic anemia
   c) Cold agglutinin disease
   d) Postsplenectomy
   e) Unstable hemoglobin with oxidative hemolysis

## CASE 2

2. A 35-year-old woman presents to the emergency department with confusion. Her hemoglobin level is 7.0 g/dL, platelet count is 20,000/mm³, and the prothrombin time and partial thromboplastin time are normal. In conjunction with the peripheral blood smear (see Fig. 27.5), the most likely diagnosis is
   a) Immune thrombocytopenic purpura
   b) Disseminated intravascular coagulopathy
   c) Thrombotic thrombocytopenic purpura
   d) Aortic valve disease
   e) Acute promyelocytic leukemia (FAB M3)

## CASE 3

3. A 25-year-old man is found to have a hemoglobin of 10.0 g/dL at routine physical examination. The peripheral smear (see Fig. 27.7) is most consistent with
   a) Hemoglobin C trait
   b) Sickle cell trait
   c) Renal failure
   d) Iron deficiency
   e) Myelofibrosis

## CASE 4

4. A 55-year-old man presents with a skin rash, pancytopenia, and mild splenomegaly. The peripheral smear (see Fig. 27.12) is most consistent with
   a) Aplastic anemia
   b) Drug reaction
   c) Sézary's syndrome
   d) Myelodysplasia
   e) Hairy cell leukemia

## CASE 5

5. A 40-year-old woman presents with fatigue, mild splenomegaly, lymphadenopathy, and a WBC count of 20,000/mm³. The peripheral smear (see Fig. 27.17) is most consistent with
   a) Acute lymphoblastic leukemia
   b) Chronic lymphocytic leukemia (CLL)
   c) Infectious mononucleosis
   d) Adult T-cell leukemia/lymphoma
   e) Plasma cell leukemia

## CASE 6

6. A 45-year-old man presents with mild splenomegaly and a WBC count of 30,000/mm³. The peripheral smear (see Fig. 27.19) is most consistent with
   a) Bacterial infection
   b) CLL
   c) Chronic myelogenous leukemia
   d) Essential thrombocythemia
   e) Acute myelogenous leukemia

## CASE 7

**7.** A 60-year-old man has a hemoglobin level of 9.0 g/dL, a mean corpuscular volume of 110 fl, and pancytopenia. Bone marrow was obtained for evaluation. The cell demonstrated by Prussian blue (iron) stain (see Fig. 27.22) can be seen in all of the following, except
   **a)** Myelodysplasia
   **b)** Alcohol abuse
   **c)** Megaloblastic anemia
   **d)** Hemochromatosis
   **e)** Postchemotherapy

## RED BLOOD CELL MORPHOLOGY

Figure 27.1 is remarkable for the presence of small, round RBCs with dense hemoglobin and no central pallor. These cells are called *spherocytes*. The larger blue-gray RBCs noted in the blood smear are reticulocytes, indicating a bone marrow response to the anemia. Spherocytes are seen most commonly in immune hemolysis and hereditary spherocytosis, but also can be seen in other conditions (Table 27.1). It is important to remember that immune hemolysis is associated with spherocytes but not with RBC fragments.

The variably sized clumps of RBCs (Fig. 27.2) indicate the presence of a cold agglutinin in this patient. Spherocytes may be seen in cold agglutinin disease when an immune hemolytic component is present. Cold agglutinins can alter peripheral blood indices, thus causing a spurious decrease in RBC count and an increase in mean corpuscular volume, mean corpuscular hemoglobin, and mean corpuscular hemoglobin concentration. RBC morphology and indices revert to normal after warming of the blood sample.

Dense, purple inclusions within RBCs are called *Howell-Jolly bodies* (Fig. 27.3). These DNA inclusions are seen after

### TABLE 27.1
### CONDITIONS ASSOCIATED WITH SPHEROCYTES

Immune hemolysis
Hereditary spherocytosis
Postsplenectomy
Post-transfusion
Severe burns
Oxidative hemolysis
Fragmentation hemolysis

splenectomy and in conditions that compromise splenic function.

Figure 27.4 demonstrates the "bite cells" characteristic of oxidative hemolysis. These RBCs typically have one or more concave indentations in the RBC membrane, secondary to removal of denatured hemoglobin by the reticuloendothelial system. Bite cells can be seen in patients with oxidative hemolysis caused by unstable hemoglobins; RBC enzyme defects, such as glucose-6-phosphate dehydrogenase deficiency; or drugs with oxidative capacity, such as sulfonamides.

Numerous RBC fragments and only rare platelets are apparent in Figure 27.5. RBC fragments can be seen in a variety of hematologic disorders (Table 27.2). The concomitant presence of thrombocytopenia and RBC fragments suggests thrombotic thrombocytopenic purpura, disseminated intravascular coagulopathy, or hemolytic-uremic syndrome, although megaloblastic anemia and autoimmune vasculitis cannot be excluded. In the latter condition, thrombocytopenia may be autoimmune-related, whereas RBC fragments result from intravascular trauma in damaged blood vessels. Conversely, traumatic hemolysis secondary to heart valve disease demonstrates RBC fragments without thrombocytopenia. In contrast, immune thrombocytopenic purpura is

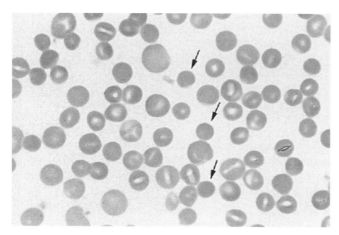

**Figure 27.1** Peripheral blood smear: spherocytes (*arrows*). (See Color Fig. 27.1.)

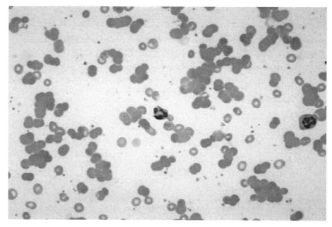

**Figure 27.2** Peripheral blood smear: aggregates of red blood cells in cold agglutinin disease. (See Color Fig. 27.2.)

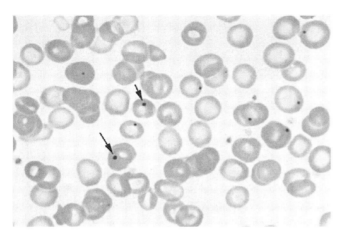

**Figure 27.3** Peripheral blood smear: Howell-Jolly bodies (*arrows*) within red blood cells. (See Color Fig. 27.3.)

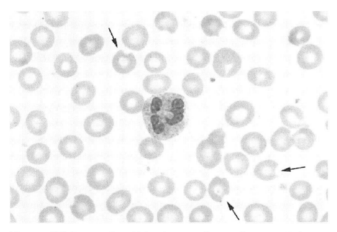

**Figure 27.4** Peripheral blood smear: bite cells (*arrows*) characteristic of oxidative hemolysis. (See Color Fig. 27.4.)

| TABLE 27.2 |
| --- |
| **CONDITIONS ASSOCIATED WITH RED BLOOD CELL FRAGMENTS** |

Diffuse intravascular coagulation
Thrombotic thrombocytopenic purpura
Hemolytic-uremic syndrome
Heart valve disease
Vasculitis
Megaloblastic anemia
Severe burns

associated with decreased platelets but no evidence of RBC fragments.

As demonstrated in Figure 27.6, patients with megaloblastic anemia may also have decreased platelets and RBC fragments, although hypersegmented polymorphonuclear leukocytes and oval macrocytes typically also are seen. The decrease in platelets is secondary to an inadequate production by megaloblastic bone marrow, whereas the RBC fragments result from defective erythropoiesis.

Abnormal RBCs called *target cells* have a central core of dense hemoglobin surrounded by a zone of otherwise normal RBC pallor (Fig. 27.7). Target cells are a nonspecific finding seen in a variety of disorders (Table 27.3). In particular, hemoglobin C disease, hemoglobin C trait, hemoglobin SC disease, and sickle cell anemia are all associated with target cells. It should be noted that patients with sickle cell trait have normal blood smear morphology. In addition, although iron deficiency anemia may be associated with target cells, RBCs in iron deficiency are typically pale, small, and varied in size and shape. Target cells are not seen as a result of renal failure.

Figure 27.8 demonstrates the target cells, as well as misshapen RBCs, consistent with sickle cells. Sickle cells are

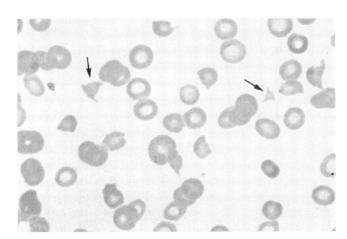

**Figure 27.5** Peripheral blood smear: Red blood cell fragments (*arrows*). (See Color Fig. 27.5.)

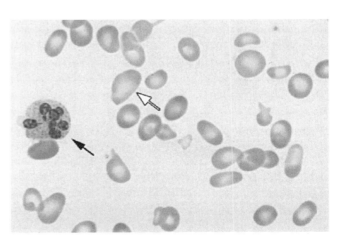

**Figure 27.6** Peripheral blood smear: hypersegmented neutrophil (*dark arrow*) and oval macrocyte (*open white arrow*). (See Color Fig. 27.6.)

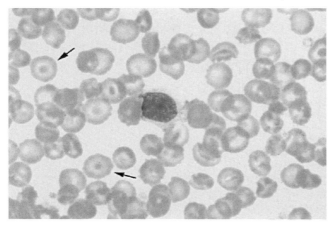

**Figure 27.7** Peripheral blood smear: target red blood cells (*arrows*). (See Color Fig. 27.7.)

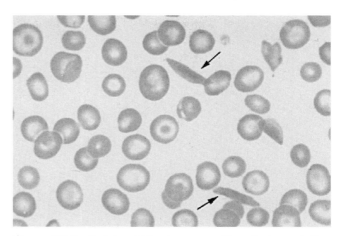

**Figure 27.8** Peripheral blood smear: sickle cells (*arrows*). (See Color Fig. 27.8.)

variable in shape, but diagnostic forms are typically elliptical with pointed ends. They may be seen in sickle cell anemia, sickle beta-thalassemia, and hemoglobin SC disease, but are not seen in sickle cell trait.

Teardrop RBCs (Fig. 27.9) are most commonly associated with conditions causing bone marrow fibrosis, including myeloproliferative disorders, myelodysplasia, and metastatic carcinoma. They are also commonly seen in patients receiving cyclosporine (Sandimmune).

The presence of many pale RBCs indicates poor hemoglobinization (Fig. 27.10). The associated variation in RBC size (as measured by an increased red cell distribution width) and shape is consistent with iron deficiency anemia. RBC hypochromasia and microcytosis are also seen in thalassemia minor, although the red cell distribution width is typically normal, indicating a more uniform RBC size distribution (Fig. 27.11).

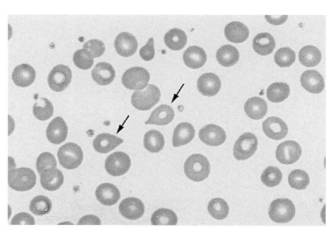

**Figure 27.9** Peripheral blood smear: teardrop red blood cells (*arrows*). (See Color Fig. 27.9.)

## WHITE BLOOD CELL MORPHOLOGY

The lymphoid cell shown in Figure 27.12 is consistent with that seen in hairy cell leukemia. Classic hairy cells have a ragged cytoplasmic border, light blue-gray cytoplasm, and

**TABLE 27.3**

**CONDITIONS ASSOCIATED WITH TARGET CELLS**

Liver disease
Postsplenectomy
Thalassemia
Iron deficiency
Hemoglobinopathies

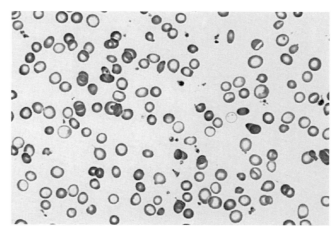

**Figure 27.10** Peripheral blood smear: numerous red blood cells demonstrating increased central pallor and moderate variation in size indicative of iron deficiency anemia. (See Color Fig. 27.10.)

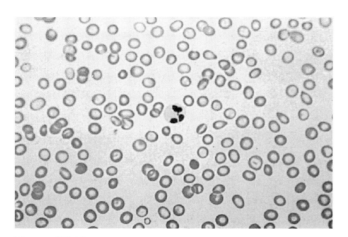

**Figure 27.11** Peripheral blood smear: a uniform population of pale red blood cells seen in thalassemia minor. (See Color Fig. 27.11.)

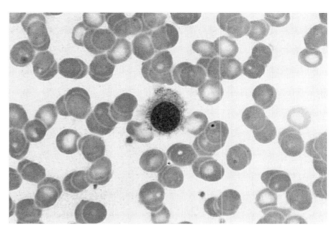

**Figure 27.12** Peripheral blood smear: single lymphoid cell demonstrating irregular cytoplasmic border seen in hairy cell leukemia.

immature nuclear chromatin. Tartrate-resistant acid phosphatase activity can be demonstrated cytochemically, and flow cytometry demonstrates a characteristic immunophenotype of CD22$^+$, CD11C$^+$, and CD25$^+$. Clinically, patients with hairy cell leukemia typically present with pancytopenia and splenomegaly.

Pancytopenia with a markedly hypocellular bone marrow (less than 10%) is typical of aplastic anemia (Fig. 27.13A). In contrast, the cellularity of normal bone marrow typically ranges between 30% and 70%, depending on the patient's age (Fig. 27.13B).

Sézary's cells are abnormal T cells that typically demonstrate a high nucleus-to-cytoplasm (N/C) ratio with fine nuclear convolutions (Fig. 27.14). Immunophenotypically, these cells are positive for CD2$^+$, CD3$^+$, and CD4$^+$ but are negative for the pan T-cell marker CD7.

A high WBC count with increased numbers of small mature lymphocytes is consistent with CLL (Fig. 27.15). Smudge cells may be prominent in the blood smear, and associated immune hemolysis or immune thrombocytopenia may be noted. Flow cytometry characteristically reveals an immunophenotype of CD19$^+$, CD23$^+$, and CD5$^+$ in B-cell CLL.

The reactive lymphocytes seen in infectious mononucleosis and other viral infections typically have a low N/C ratio with a moderate amount of cytoplasm (Fig. 27.16). The cell nuclei are mature, with smudged chromatin, although occasional immature nucleolated cells may be seen. Characteristically, reactive lymphocytes demonstrate scalloped cytoplasmic borders and often have dark-blue cytoplasm. Natural killer cells and CD8$^+$ T-suppressor cells with faintly granular cytoplasm may be seen in

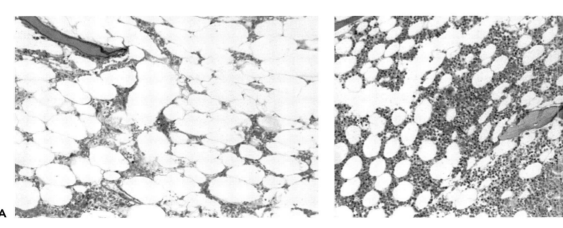

**Figure 27.13** **(A)** Hypocellular bone marrow biopsy sample from a patient with aplastic anemia. **(B)** Normocellular bone marrow biopsy sample from healthy control.

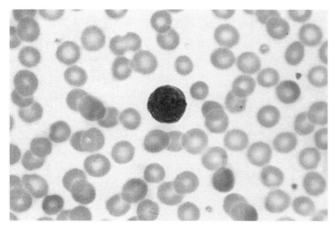

**Figure 27.14** Peripheral blood smear: hyperchromatic lymphoid cell consistent with Sézary's cell.

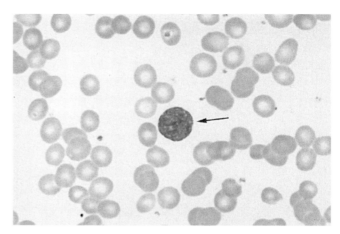

**Figure 27.17** Peripheral blood smear: small blast seen in acute lymphoblastic leukemia (*arrow*).

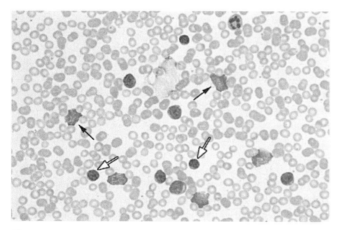

**Figure 27.15** Peripheral blood smear: mature lymphocytes (*open white arrows*) and smudge cells (*dark arrows*).

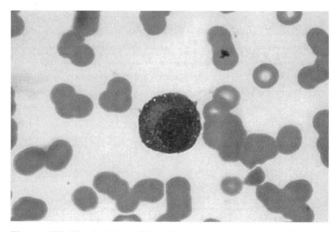

**Figure 27.18** Peripheral blood smear: single plasma cell.

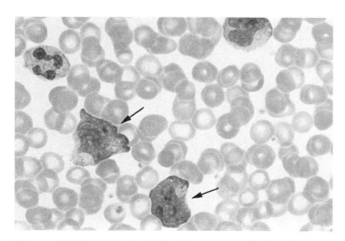

**Figure 27.16** Peripheral blood smear: reactive lymphocytes seen in infectious mononucleosis (*arrows*).

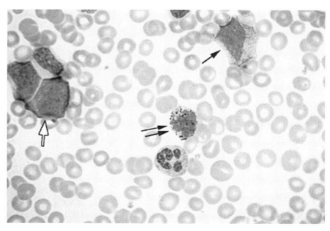

**Figure 27.19** Peripheral blood smear: granulocytic leftward shift with myelocytes (*dark arrow*) and blast (*open white arrow*), as well as a basophil (*double dark arrow*).

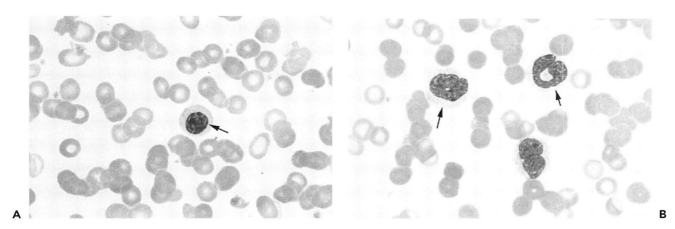

**Figure 27.20** Peripheral blood smear: single hyposegmented (*arrow*) **(A)** and hypogranular (*arrows*) **(B)** neutrophils.

increased number. These reactive cells are seen in infections with Epstein-Barr virus and cytomegalovirus, as well as in drug reactions. Serologic confirmation of the diagnosis is necessary.

The lymphoblasts seen in acute lymphoblastic leukemia FAB L1 have a high N/C ratio and fine nuclear chromatin (Fig. 27.17). L1 blasts are most commonly seen in childhood acute lymphoblastic leukemia.

In plasma cell leukemia, circulating plasma cells are typically immature and comprise more than 20% of circulating WBCs (or an absolute count greater than 2,000/mm³) (Fig. 27.18). These cells have a low N/C ratio, an eccentric nucleus, and a pale perinuclear Golgi zone. Mature plasma cells may normally be found circulating in association with reactive processes.

Figure 27.19 demonstrates a peripheral blood smear that is most consistent with chronic myelogenous leukemia. Patients with chronic myelogenous leukemia typically have an elevated WBC count with a prominent granulocytic leftward shift, including circulating metamyelocytes, myelocytes, promyelocytes, and scattered blasts. Basophilia and sometimes eosinophilia typically are seen, and these help to distinguish chronic myelogenous leukemia from left-shifted reactive processes, such as bacterial infections.

Patients with myelodysplasia commonly have pancytopenia that may be accompanied by dysplastic granulocytes. These abnormal WBCs may have nuclear hyposegmentation (Fig. 27.20A) or cytoplasmic hypogranularity (Fig. 27.20B).

Figure 27.21 shows a peripheral blood smear from a patient with acute myelogenous leukemia. Patients typically display circulating blasts with low N/C ratios and variable cytoplasmic granulation. The presence of Auer's rods is diagnostic of a myelogenous origin.

A bone marrow preparation with Prussian blue stain for iron shows a classic ringed sideroblast (Fig. 27.22). The

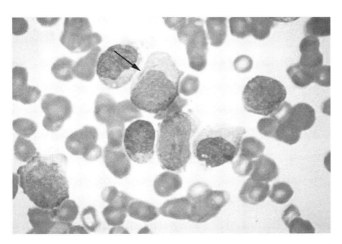

**Figure 27.21** Peripheral blood smear: blast with Auer's rod (*arrow*).

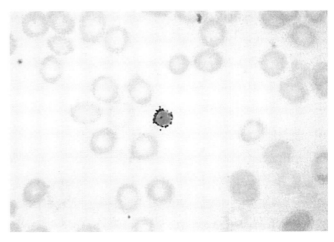

**Figure 27.22** Bone marrow biopsy sample stained with Prussian blue demonstrating a ringed sideroblast.

blue granules surrounding the red nucleus represent iron accumulation within RBC mitochondria. Ringed sideroblasts are characteristically seen in myelodysplasia, although they may also be seen in conditions such as megaloblastic anemia and after chemotherapy.

## ANSWERS

1. b.

2. c.

3. a.

4. e.

5. b.

6. c.

7. d.

## REVIEW EXERCISES

### QUESTIONS

**1.** Spherocytes are seen in each of the following, *except*
a) Immune hemolysis
b) Traumatic hemolysis
c) Postsplenectomy
d) Thalassemia minor
e) Severe burns

**2.** RBC fragments are *not* typically seen in which of the following?
a) Disseminated intravascular coagulopathy
b) Prosthetic heart valve dysfunction
c) Immune hemolysis
d) Severe megaloblastic anemia
e) Vasculitis

**3.** RBCs are seen in each of the following, *except*
a) Metastatic carcinoma involving the bone marrow
b) Aplastic anemia
c) Myelofibrosis
d) Renal transplant recipient on cyclosporine
e) Myelodysplasia

**4.** Pancytopenia is characteristically seen in each of the following disorders, *except*
a) Aplastic anemia
b) $CD22^+$, $CD11C^+$, $CD25^+$ lymphoproliferative disorder

c) $CD19^+$, $CD23^+$, $CD5^+$ lymphoproliferative disorder
d) Myelodysplasia
e) Postchemotherapy

**5.** The peripheral blood in chronic myelogenous leukemia typically demonstrates each of the following, *except*
a) Elevated WBC count
b) Myeloid leftward shift
c) Basophilia
d) Prominent lymphocytosis
e) Scattered circulating blasts

### ANSWERS

**1. d.**
Thalassemia minor is characterized by a relatively uniform population of microcytic RBCs. Target cells may be seen, but spherocytes are not. All the other conditions listed may demonstrate spherocytes in the peripheral blood.

**2. c.**
Immune hemolysis is characterized by the presence of circulating spherocytes. RBC fragments are not seen in immune hemolysis.

**3. b.**
Teardrop RBCs are usually associated with bone marrow fibrosis, although they also may be seen in patients being treated with cyclosporine. These RBCs are not typically seen in aplastic anemia.

**4. c.**
B-cell CLL is characterized by a lymphocytosis with an immunophenotype of $CD19^+$, $CD23^+$, and $CD25^+$. In contrast, hairy cell leukemia typically is associated with pancytopenia, and the atypical lymphoid cells are $CD22^+$, $CD11C^+$, and $CD25^+$.

**5. d.**
Chronic myelogenous leukemia is associated with an increased WBC count composed of left-shifted granulocytic elements, not lymphocytes. CLL is associated with a prominent lymphocytosis.

## SUGGESTED READINGS

Kapff CT, Jandl JJ. *Blood, Atlas and Source Book of Hematology,* 2nd ed. Boston: Little, Brown, 1991.
Miale J. *Laboratory Medicine, Hematology.* St. Louis: Mosby, 1982.

# Palliative Medicine

**28**

*Susan LeGrand*

Palliative medicine (PM) is a growing specialty that focuses on ensuring the best quality of life for individuals living with advanced, ultimately terminal illness. It is recognized as a subspecialty in the United Kingdom and Canada, and it is awaiting recognition in the United States. More hospitals are starting palliative care programs, in response to articles published in the medical literature that document the cost benefits accrued from decreasing ICU days and resource utilization. As our population ages, more people will need these services. Despite this trend, the education curricula for PM remain limited at best. Teaching in medical schools and residency programs is minimal, and supervision by faculty without the appropriate skills fails to reinforce what may have been learned in lectures or rotations. Nonetheless, primary PM skills are fundamental to good internal medicine and subspecialty care.

Palliative medicine services will be available more readily as increasing numbers of trainees complete fellowships and start consultation services. Tertiary care in major centers, with the research and education responsibility necessary for any specialty, will also continue to grow.

This chapter defines PM, differentiates it from hospice care, and discusses the Medicare hospice benefit. The chapter then focuses on several key skills and addresses several controversies associated with primary palliative medical care, namely (i) effective use of opioids, (ii) care of the dying, and (iii) hydration at end-of-life. This is not a comprehensive review of these topics, and appropriate references for further review are included.

## PALLIATIVE CARE DEFINED

The World Health Organization (WHO) defines palliative care as care that "improves the quality of life for patients and families who face life-threatening illness, by providing pain and symptom relief, spiritual and psychosocial support from diagnosis to the end-of-life and bereavement." Palliative medicine is the physician specialty that participates with other team members including nursing, social workers, pastoral care, and others to provide palliative care as defined by WHO as:

- Providing relief from pain and distressing symptoms
- Affirming life and regards dying as a normal process
- Intending neither to hasten or postpone death

- Integrating psychologic and spiritual aspects of care
- Offering a support system to help patients live as actively as possible until death
- Using a team approach to address the needs of patients and their families, including bereavement counseling, if indicated
- Enhancing quality of life and also may positively influence the course of illness
- Being applicable early in the course of illness, in conjunction with other therapies that are intended to prolong life, such as chemotherapy or radiation therapy, and includes those investigations needed to better understand and manage distressing clinical complications

## PALLIATIVE MEDICINE SKILL SET

Excellent PM requires skills in seven different areas:

- Communication. It is fundamental that palliative care workers possess the ability to sensitively communicate prognosis, discuss the goals of care when cure is not possible, and explore an individual's hopes and values as end-of-life approaches. Good communication is necessary for good medical care in general, and yet evidence abounds that it is lacking. All other skills depend on good communications.
- Decision making. To do everything possible for every patient may require no thought. Knowing what can be done and then deciding based on an individual's goals, values, and disease status what should be done is much more complex.
- Symptom management. Knowledge of the different treatments (nonpharmacologic, pharmacologic, and interventional techniques) available to improve symptoms is fundamental. A 1,000-patient database found that, on average, PM patients have 11 symptoms with a range of 1 to 27. Symptoms include both physical and psychologic problems.
- Prevention and management of complications. This can be as simple as an air mattress to relieve pain and prevent decubitus ulcers in a cachetic patient to asking an orthopedic surgeon to prophylactically pin a high-risk lytic lesion in the arm of a cancer patient.
- Psychosocial issues. The management of social and practical concerns that affect patients and families is

critical. A comprehensive assessment of family structure, dynamics, coping styles, cultural and religious influences, financial status, social support systems, and other issues is invaluable in determining not only appropriate discharge plans but also in facilitating better communication, decision making, and symptom control.

- Care of the imminently dying. Despite the common misconception that caring for the dying is all that PM does, care of the dying is a specific skill set that is clearly appropriate for every physician caring for acutely or chronically ill people.
- Bereavement. After the death of an individual in palliative care, the bereaved include not only the family members but the program staff, volunteers and, if in a facility, their staff. The needs of these individuals are managed by bereavement support services in a team fashion.

Both hospice and PM identify their unit of care as patient and family (as defined by the patient). An advanced disease does not occur only to an individual, but affects all those involved with that person. The emotional coping of the caregivers likewise impacts the health and symptoms of the patient. The effective exploration of goals of care, symptoms, coping strategies, decision making, and other issues cannot occur without an active understanding of the social and emotional circumstances of all involved. This fundamental need also leads to another key feature of both programs: an interdisciplinary team approach. The necessity of nursing, social work, and pastoral care involvement in identifying these issues cannot be overstated.

## PALLIATIVE MEDICINE VERSUS HOSPICE

Palliative medicine grew from the hospice movement and, as such, shares many key features. One simple fundamental difference exists between the two disciplines, and that is life expectancy. In the United States, access to insurance payment for hospice care requires:

- A terminal diagnosis
- An anticipated life expectancy of less than 6 months
- Patient and family acceptance of a goal of care that is focused on comfort rather than life prolongation

None of this is required for PM. It may comfortably coexist with active "curative" therapy, and if or when those treatments are of little value, PM can become the predominant approach and facilitate the transition to hospice when appropriate.

## HOSPICE CARE

One of the most misunderstood issues surrounding hospice is the question of life expectancy. Good hospice care requires time for relationships to develop between the patient and her family and the team members, with a minimum of 90 days preferred. Currently, more than 30% of hospice patients die less than 2 weeks after referral. This is crisis intervention, not hospice care. In the late 1990s, concern arose about abuse of hospice services with patients surviving for years on the Medicare benefit. Since that time, the Office of the Inspector General (OIG) has tried to reassure physicians that they are not at risk of investigation with good-faith estimates. The OIG acknowledges the difficulty of prognostication, particularly with noncancer diagnoses. The hospice benefit was designed on a cancer model, in which the disease trajectory follows a consistent downhill course once active treatment of the malignancy stops. Noncancer diagnoses characterized by periodic exacerbation with improvement, even though the overall course is progressive decline, are much more difficult to predict. Guidelines recommended by the National Hospice and Palliative Care Organization have been shown to be incapable of predicting 6-month life expectancy and yet are commonly used by hospice agencies for documentation.

The question a referring physician should ask is not when the patient will die, but would they be surprised if death occurred within 6 months. If that would not be a surprise, and a primary focus on comfort would be an appropriate goal of care, then that person could be referred to hospice care. The physician is certifying to a probability that death will occur within that time frame, not offering a guarantee. There is no penalty for patients who survive longer, nor is there a limit on the number of days an individual can be on the Medicare benefit. Prolonged time in hospice is an opportunity to reassess the original referral. Recertification every 2 to 3 months is required. If patients improve (or goals change), and hospice is truly no longer appropriate, a physician may revoke hospice and then readmit the patient when or if decline occurs.

Most private insurers have benefits similar to Medicare. Some policies have a more limited approach, with either a set number of visits or a specific dollar amount available. To create a useful service, these policies require more discussion with the company by social workers or discharge planners, often utilizing home care benefits that may be less restricted. Currently, no "palliative medicine benefits" are outside standard insurance payments (although this issue is under consideration by some companies). Physicians bill as they would any other patient, using the time spent rather than E/M documentation for the prolonged counseling that may be required. Hospitalizations are coded using the primary diagnosis and any complications that occur, as would be done on any other admission.

Hospice, like an HMO, is a capitated benefit. Hospice is paid a set amount per inpatient per day per patient to provide for all care related to the admitting diagnosis. For example, a patient with congestive heart failure admitted to hospice with a diagnosis of lung cancer will not have his heart medications paid for, but any medications, testing, or other services needed for the lung cancer will be covered. A patient admitted for heart failure would be provided with cardiac medications. Any care ordered for the admitting diagnosis is paid for by the hospice—laboratory studies, radiology studies, durable medical equipment, hospitalization—from a current daily benefit of approximately $115 (exact amount varies by region). Longer stays in hospice help agencies recoup the initial costs involved in establishing care. Most hospices have formularies of preferred medications to limit costs also.

Another confusing issue is that patients "give up" when they go on hospice care. Significant variability exists on what services hospices will provide. Each physician must learn the policies of the agencies they utilize. Some consider transfusion appropriate symptom management if it improves dyspnea or fatigue, whereas others consider it life-prolonging therapy and not part of hospice care. Ultimately, the decision to use a particular medication, hospitalization, or intervention is between the patient and his family and his physician. The patient may always revoke hospice and return to his standard insurance if, after discussion, he wishes to receive something that hospice does not provide. Therefore, a patient does not "give up" anything.

## Hospice Benefit versus Home Care

In the short term, to qualify for benefits, hospice patients can actually be healthier than home care patients. To qualify for home care services, a patient must:

- Be homebound. Visits to the physician are allowed, but the ability to travel independently beyond the home setting renders a patient ineligible for hospice care.
- Have a skilled nursing need, such as complicated dressing, physical therapy, short-term teaching for diabetic education, new tube feedings, and the like.
- Have a documented medical need for any equipment requested, such as minimum oxygen saturation values for home oxygen support.
- Meet the first two criteria to be approved for home care aide services.

Because hospice is a capitated system, none of that is required. Hospice patients may have a bed, standard wheelchair, or oxygen if they think it is helpful. They may continue to travel or work if they wish. Home care aides can be available to assist basic care needs, regardless of what other services are required. The involvement of the team may provide enough care to allow a person to remain in their home alone, or for a family to continue to care for their loved-one, even when no skilled needs exist. Twenty-four-hour, seven-day-a-week availability by phone with a potential for a home visit after hours also provides a sense of security that can prevent emergency room visits and hospitalizations.

## EFFECTIVE USE OF OPIOIDS

The decision of whether to use opioids for a particular person is beyond the scope of this chapter. The goal for this section is the correct use of opioids once initiated; therefore, fundamental principles will be outlined. Physicians are encouraged to review the repeatedly validated WHO guidelines for pain management. Successful pain control in 80% to 90% of patients has been documented when these guidelines are utilized.

### Definitions

- Three troublesome definitions continue to interfere with the appropriate management of pain, particularly in advanced disease:
  - Addiction. Also called *psychologic dependence*, addiction is a relatively rare occurrence in those without prior tendency to addictive behaviors. Certainly, in advanced malignancy and at end-of-life, this concern is irrelevant. Prior or current drug dependency does not prohibit the use of opioids in these settings, but does require careful follow-up, preferably by a specialist in the field.
  - Dependence. Physical dependence necessitates a taper to prevent a withdrawal syndrome if or when a medication is no longer indicated. This is an aspect of the pharmacology of a particular medication and is not unique to opioids (the same rationale applies to selective serotonin reuptake inhibitors, benzodiazepines, barbiturates, etc.).
  - Tolerance. The need for an increasing dosage of medication for the same level of effect. Tolerance to the pain-relieving effects of opioids has been shown to be clinically irrelevant in malignancy, although it may be more problematic in chronic nonmalignant pain. In malignancy, a need for increased medication is generally secondary to increased pain. Tolerance rapidly develops to most side effects of opioids, with the notable exception of constipation.

### Principles for Use of Opioid Medications

#### Pain Assessment

In prescribing opioid medications, a careful pain assessment is needed, including:

- Location, radiation, and description of pain (i.e., sharp, burning, etc.)
- Severity assessment, using any one of a variety of pain scales
- Time course of the pain (constant vs. intermittent) and any precipitating factors
- Assessing and documenting each site and type of pain separately

■ Documentation of any past or present medication use, including degree and duration of response and side effects

### Selecting Appropriate Medication

Choose a medication appropriate to the severity of the pain (see Fig. 28.1 and Table 28.1, using the following general guidelines:

■ Moderate or severe cancer-related pain (>4 on a scale of 0–10) should be managed with a Step 2 or 3 medication. Step 2 medications have a dose ceiling secondary to the combination product (acetaminophen or ASA) or toxicity (tramadol). Step 3 medications do not have a dose ceiling and may be increased as needed until adequate pain control is obtained.
■ It is not necessary to start at Step 1 and progress to Step 3 although this may be appropriate in nonmalignant pain. In cancer-related pain, the choice of medication is determined by the severity of the pain. For example, a cancer patient whose baseline pain is 8 should receive morphine even if opioid naïve.

### Contraindicated Medications

Certain medications are *not* recommended for chronic pain management. These include:

## WHO's Pain Relief Ladder

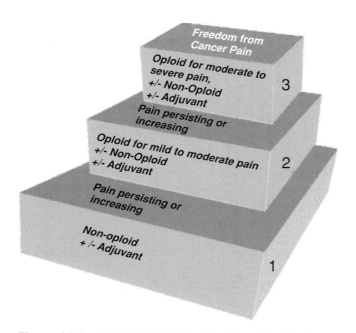

**Figure 28.1**   WHO's Pain Relief Ladder. Reproduced with permission from the World Health Organization: http://www.who.int/cancer/palliative/painladder/en/.

| TABLE 28.1 | | |
|---|---|---|
| **MEDICATIONS ON THE WHO PAIN RELIEF LADDER** | | |
| **Step 1** | **Step 2** | **Step 3** |
| Aspirin | Codeine | Morphine |
| Acetaminophen | Tramadol | Hydromorphone |
| NSAID | Hydrocodone/ASA | Oxycodone |
| | Hydrocodone/APAP | Fentanyl |
| | Oxycodone/ASA | Levorphanol |
| | Oxycodone/APAP | Methadone |
| ± Adjuvant | ± Adjuvant | ± Adjuvant |

■ Meperidine. Meperidine has a toxic metabolite that causes seizures and delirium. Some hospitals have removed it completely from their formulary to prevent usage. It has no advantage over other less toxic opioids.
■ Agonist/antagonist agents. Agonist/antagonist agents have ceiling effects and an increased incidence of psychotomimetic effects. Although they may be used in opioid naïve individuals, their use in someone on chronic opioids can provoke withdrawal.
■ Codeine. Codeine is more constipating and has an increased incidence of psychotomimetic effects. It is a pro-drug that requires metabolism to the active agent, however, 10% of the population lacks the enzyme needed for conversion.
■ Propoxyphene. Propoxyphene has been demonstrated to have no advantage over placebo in controlled trials. It is considered one of the most misused medications in the elderly.

### Continuous Pain Relief

Constant pain requires constant medication. This can be accomplished by sustained release products or the scheduled dosing of immediate release products. A recent study of opioid errors (unpublished data) found this to be one of the more common problems with opioid prescribing. Despite constant pain, a person is given PRN pain medications. If treating an opioid naïve person as an outpatient, the initiation of PRN dosing for 24 to 48 hours to determine the need is reasonable, when promptly converted to sustained release once dose has been determined.

The initial opioid chosen (+/− an adjuvant) should be titrated until a therapeutic effect is obtained or an intolerable side effect develops. Further guidelines include:

■ No indication is present for more than one sustained release opioid
■ Immediate release medications should be the same opioid when possible (exception: fentanyl)

Dosing should be based on the pharmacology of the medication and the patient report of efficacy and duration of effect:

- Immediate release opioid medications (excluding methadone), alone or in combination, have an effective half-life of 3 to 4 hours. Therefore, every 4-hour dosing is preferred. Tramadol is dosed every 6 hours. Half lives may be prolonged in the elderly, but PRN dosing should still be at the shorter interval. If the medication lasts longer, it will not be requested. If it does not, it will be available.
- The oral sustained release products are *never* dosed PRN. The most commonly prescribed medications (generic SR morphine, MS Contin, Oramorph, and Oxycontin) can usually be dosed every 12 hours. An occasional individual will experience end-of-dose failure with a consistent report of increased pain prior to each scheduled dose. This may be managed by an increase in dose or a change to an 8-hour schedule. Compliance is much better on twice daily dosing. Similar problems can occur with transdermal fentanyl, with reports of worsening pain control on the third day. Patches may need to be changed at 48 to 60 hours. Changing patches more often than 48 hours is not recommended.

Patients on sustained release medications or continuous parenteral infusions must also have immediate release medications or bolus doses available for breakthrough pain.

The use of adjuvant analgesic agents, such as nonsteroidal anti-inflammatory drugs (NSAIDs), anticonvulsants, and tricyclic antidepressants, should be tailored to the specific characteristics of the pain. For example, adding an NSAID for musculoskeletal pain, an anticonvulsant or tricyclic for neuropathic pain, or a muscle relaxant/antispasmodic agent for cramps may be appropriate.

A frequent reassessment of the efficacy of the medication chosen, side effects, and need for breakthrough dosing is important because adjustments in management are frequently required. Patients should keep diaries of their usage of medication. Physicians must assess the baseline pain control, which includes the number of breakthrough doses required. The efficacy of the breakthrough dose should be assessed separately. If frequent breakthrough dosing is required, then an increase in scheduled medication may be appropriate. If breakthrough dosing is never needed, then a decrease in dose might be tolerated. When adjusting medications, phone call follow-up in several days, with clinic visit in 1 to 2 weeks, is needed.

It is important to anticipate and manage common side effects, particularly nausea, sedation, and constipation. Tolerance will develop to all these, except constipation. Patient education on the possibility of these side effects and the fact that they will resolve if given time can prevent premature discontinuation. Any patient started on opioid medications *must* also be placed on an aggressive bowel regimen, usually including a stool softener and a stimulant. Failure to start bowel regimens was another common error in a recent trial.

### Choice of Opioid Medication

Despite small studies (often with pharmaceutical funding) that suggest the superiority of one opioid or another for pain control or minimalizing side effects, in reality only minimal differences exist between opioids (except methadone). There are, however, significant differences in cost. In the absence of clinically relevant efficacy or toxicity differences, then cost should be a major factor in choosing medications. Most individuals can be successfully managed with a less expensive opioid (i.e., generic morphine). If unacceptable side effects develop, then conversion to more expensive products such as SR Oxycodone or transdermal fentanyl would be appropriate. A patient report of an "allergic reaction" to morphine is more often a side effect, such as nausea or pruritis. Rechallenge is usually appropriate because tolerance will develop. If the prior reaction was delirium or confusion, then alternate medications should be used. Physicians prescribing opioids should know the relative costs of the products because an inability to afford the medication is a known cause of poor pain control.

## CARE OF THE DYING

The sensitive, ethically appropriate care of the dying is not limited to prescribing a morphine drip. Specific symptoms commonly associated with dying need to be assessed and managed individually. The physician also has a responsibility to the family whose subsequent bereavement will be affected by how the dying process occurs and the education they receive in preparation for the death. The National Consensus Project developed clinical practice guidelines for quality palliative care and has recommended the following steps in care of the imminently dying:

- Recognize the transition to the actively dying phase when possible; communicate and document this appropriately to patient, family, and staff.
- Address end-of-life concerns, hopes, fears, and expectations openly and honestly in a socially, culturally, and age-appropriate manner.
- Assess and document with appropriate frequency the symptoms at end-of life. Treatment is based on patient and family preferences.
- Revise the care plan to reflect the unique needs of the patient and family at this phase. Needs for higher intensity and acuity of care are met and documented.
- Document and meet wishes for care setting at death, if possible. Any inability to meet this preference is reviewed and documented.

- Educate family regarding the signs and symptoms of approaching death in a developmentally and culturally appropriate manner.
- Offer hospice care, if not already in place.

The signs and symptoms of imminent death are similar regardless of the specific underlying cause. In the last 48 hours of life, three problems predominate: *pain, respiratory symptoms* including dyspnea and secretions, and *restlessness* or what is commonly called terminal delirium. The ethical principle of double effect allows the use of medication up to and including sedation to manage a symptom. When symptoms are assessed and managed appropriately, potentially life-threatening levels of medication are not needed. It is important to address the goals of care for each person because for some, the maintenance of consciousness is paramount even if associated with more physical suffering.

## General Recommendations

Once it is clear that the dying process has actively begun, certain general recommendations apply:

- All medications except those needed for symptom management should be stopped. The only exception is anticonvulsant medications if seizure were a significant risk. An alternative anticonvulsant, such as lorazepam, may be needed once swallowing problems occur.
- Medications for anticipated symptoms (even if not yet present) should be ordered on an as-needed (PRN) basis. If they are used frequently, then scheduled administration and/or continuous infusion may be needed.
- As swallowing becomes impaired, alternative routes of administration will be required. In hospital settings, a conversion to subcutaneous routes is preferable. In the home setting, rectal or sublingual administrations are acceptable alternatives. Hospice agencies often can advise on which products can be effectively used by these routes.
- Any laboratory or radiologic orders should be discontinued.
- Routine vital sign checks may be stopped.

## Pain Management

Individuals with pre-existing pain concerns may develop pain crises as death approaches, thus necessitating a rapid increase in medication to re-establish adequate control. Those who have never had pain are unlikely to suddenly develop it in the last hours of life if basic needs, such as bowel and bladder management, are addressed. Therefore, the common practice of starting a morphine infusion in those without pain (or dyspnea) symptoms as management of dying is incorrect. Morphine in the absence of a specific symptom may produce toxicity without benefit.

Providing a PRN order for low-dose morphine, however, provides nursing options if pain were to occur.

## Respiratory Symptoms

Dyspnea in the last hours of life can be a difficult symptom to manage without sedation. Opioids are the medication of choice and will improve the sensation to a degree without sedation. Combination therapy with chlorpromazine in uncontrolled trials has been helpful also. Oxygen support is controversial, but clearly contributes little other than a normalization of oxygen saturation, when possible. The maintenance of a normal $O_2$ saturation frequently does not resolve dyspnea because mechanical issues such as muscle weakness rather than hypoxemia are the more important etiologic factors. If needed, the timing of sedation is the patient's choice. Opioids should not be used for sedation, as noted in the Pain Management section. Suggested medications are discussed in the section on restlessness.

Secretions, commonly called the *death rattle*, are a symptom of more concern to families than patients. Often the individual is no longer conscious and therefore not distressed, but the sound can be quite troubling for those sitting vigil. Therefore, treatment is reasonable. Positioning on either side can eliminate some sounds, but anticholinergic medications such as hyoscyamine, glycopyrrolate, or scopalamine also have been shown to help. These medications can be given via sublingual (hyoscyamine, glycopyrrollate), subcutaneous (glycopyrrolate), or transdermal (scopalamine) routes.

## Terminal Delirium

This is the most common intractable symptom requiring sedation at end-of-life. Although maintaining consciousness is reasonable, when an individual is confused without reversible cause, or if searching for a cause is not within the goals of care, then control of the symptom becomes primary. Easily treated causes such as fecal impaction and urinary retention should be excluded. Unfortunately, in the last days of life, control may only be accomplished with sedation. It is quite distressing for families to see a loved one thrashing, moaning, or crying out, so treating the symptom is critical.

Differentiating pain and delirium can be difficult when patient report is not available. Moaning is not always pain. Physicians must use their best guess based on the physical appearance, pre-existing pain complaints, and family and nursing impressions. Medications used for sedation include the benzodiazepines, phenothiazines (particularly chlorpromazine), and barbiturates. Doses are titrated until comfort is achieved, and then maintained either scheduled or PRN depending on need. Because opioid medications can cause delirium, particularly if renal function is declining, increasing these medications for delirium may exacerbate the problem.

# HYDRATION AT END-OF-LIFE

Hydration in the last days of life is a controversial subject even within the field of PM. The debate centers on the burden–benefit ratio. In 1997, a systematic review found inadequate data from which to draw firm conclusions on the balance of burden and benefit. Consensus confirms that the discontinuation of parenteral fluids in the dying is a legal and ethical choice. Parenteral fluid support is a medical intervention like any other, which may be stopped if not appropriate to the patient and/or family goals of care. In considering the administration of fluids in the last days of life, what is the goal? Do fluids help achieve that goal? Goals might include comfort, prevention or treatment of symptoms, and prolongation of life.

## Comfort

Do fluids contribute to comfort at end of life? An alternative question is, does dehydration cause discomfort? A prospective evaluation of the intake in advanced cancer patients found that 60% drank less than 500 cc/day in the days prior to death. The only symptom experienced was dry mouth, and this was effectively managed with local measures. No difference in comfort level was observed related to fluid consumption. Another study found that although 70% of dying cancer patients experienced thirst, it was satisfied with mouth care and small amounts of oral fluid. Therefore, fluids do not necessarily contribute to comfort. Dehydration may also stimulate endogenous opioids.

Fluids can cause discomfort in several ways:

- The need for IV access, which may require repetitive sticks
- The development of edema because hypoalbuminemia is common
- An increased frequency of urination, which may require painful movement or catheterization
- An accumulation of pulmonary secretions

If one looks at a goal of comfort only, then fluids probably cause more distress.

## Prevention and Management of Symptoms

Those who advocate the use of fluids do so to achieve this goal. If renal insufficiency develops, some medications (particularly certain opioid metabolites) may accumulate and lead to neurotoxicity. Hydration can prevent or reverse this and potentially avoid an agitated delirium. In the setting of an unexplained deterioration in mental status, a time-limited trial of 1 to 1.5 L of fluid over 24 hours is reasonable. If mental status improves, then maintenance can continue. If no change occurs, then fluids can be stopped.

## Prolongation of Life

A question to ask is whether one is prolonging life or the dying process. There is little question that allowing dehydration to occur may shorten life if the expectancy is several weeks or more. In someone with hours or a few days to live, it is unlikely to change the time course. Fluids may however, prolong the dying process and the suffering.

Arguments against and for hydration at the end of life are listed here:

- Arguments against Hydration
  □ The only symptom, dehydration, can be managed effectively with local measures
  □ Increased discomfort occurs from the intravenous access
  □ Prolongs the dying process
  □ Increases secretions and/or edema
- Arguments for Hydration
  □ Can be administered via hypodermoclysis (subcutaneous) or proctoclysis (retention enema), thus avoiding the discomfort of intravenous administration
  □ May improve delirium

The decision to use fluids in the dying must be individualized. This is a very emotional topic, complicated by recent communications from Pope John Paul II (2004) suggesting that fluids and artificial nutritional support must be provided to all and should never be stopped regardless of the circumstances. Although these statements are in direct contradiction to legal and medical opinions (American Medical Association, American Nurses Association, American Academy of Neurology), they may be relevant to devout Catholic families. Ultimately, the family must be able to live with whatever they choose. Physicians can counsel on the medical reality (i.e., dehydration not painful) that families often do not understand. The pros and cons should be sensitively discussed without bias, based on the physician's personal belief system. If fluid support is continued, it should be at relatively low rates (1 to 1.5 L/day) to avoid excessive edema. The need can be readdressed at a later time, particularly if fluid accumulation in the lungs should occur.

# CONCLUSION

The care of those with advanced disease requires the same attention to detail needed throughout the life span. Sensitive communication that includes patient and families, honest discussion of the goals of care, and management of the disease symptoms are critical. The growth of PM as a field will increase the number of physicians skilled in this aspect of care, but primary care specialists must learn to manage the majority of patients in this phase of life, seeking consultation for difficult cases. Dying is a normal part of life, not a physician failure. A patient dying unprepared, however, with uncontrolled symptoms, in a hospital when she wanted to be home, *is* a physician failure.

## SUGGESTED READINGS

Abrahm J. Pain management for dying patients. How to assess needs and provide pharmacologic relief. *Postgrad Med* 2001;110(2): 99–100.

Adam J. ABC of palliative care. The last 48 hours. *BMJ* 1997;315(7122): 1600–1603.

American Board of Internal Medicine Committee on Evaluation of Clinical Competence. *Caring for the Dying: Identification and Promotion of Physician Competency*. Philadelphia: American Board of Internal Medicine, 1998.

American College of Physicians-American Society of Internal Medicine End-of-Life Care Consensus Panel. Ethics manual. Fourth edition. *Ann Intern Med* 1998;128(7):576–594.

American Geriatric Society Panel on Persistent Pain in Older Persons. The management of persistent pain in older persons. *J Am Geriatr Soc* 2002;50(6 Suppl):S205–224.

American Geriatrics Society Ethics Committee. The care of dying patients: a position statement from the American Geriatrics Society. *J Am Geriatr Soc* 1994;43(5):577–578. (http://www.americangeriatrics.org/products/positionpapers/careofd.shtml.)

American Geriatrics Society Panel on Chronic Pain in Older Persons. The management of chronic pain in older persons. *J Am Geriatr Soc* 1998;46(5):635–651.

American Medical Association Council on Ethical and Judicial Affairs, 2003. Elements of Quality Care for Patients in the Last Phase of Life. (www.ama-assn.org/ama/pub/category/7567.html.)

American Medical Directors Association (2000). White paper on hospice in long-term care. Columbia, MD:http://www.amda/com/library/whitepapers/hospiceinltc/index.htmhttp://www.amda.com/.

American Nurses Association *Foregoing Nutrition and Hydration*. Washington, D.C.: American Nurses Association, 1991. (http://www.ana.org.)

American Pain Society Quality of Care Committee. Quality improvement guidelines for the treatment of acute pain and cancer pain. *JAMA* 1995;274(23):1874–1880.

American Pain Society Task Force on Pain, Symptoms and End of Life Care (n.d.). Treatment of pain at the end of life: a position statement from the American Pain Society. www.ampainsoc.org/advocacy/treatment.htm.

American Society of Clinical Oncology End of Life Task Force. Cancer care during the last phase of life. *J Clin Oncol* 1998;16:1986–1996.

Asch DA, Faber-Langendoen K, et al. The sequence of withdrawing life-sustaining treatment from patients. *Am J Med* 1999;107(2): 153–156.

Back AL, Arnold RM, et al. Teaching communication skills to medical oncology fellows. *J Clin Oncol* 2003;21(12):2433–2436.

Baer WM, Hanson LC. Families' perception of the added value of hospice in the nursing home. *J Am Geriatr Soc* 2000;48(8):879–882.

Baluss ME. Palliative care: ethics and the law. In: Berger AM, Porenoy RK, Weissman DE, eds. *Principles and Practice of Palliative Care and Supportive Oncology*. Philadelphia: Lippincott Williams & Wilkins 2002;902–914.

Barry LC, Kasl SV, et al. Psychiatric disorders among bereaved persons: the role of perceived circumstances of death and preparedness for death. *Am J Geriatr Psychiatry* 2002;10(4):447–457.

Bascom PB, Tolle SW. Care of the family when the patient is dying. *West J Med* 1995;163(3):292–296.

Beel A, McClement SE, et al. Palliative sedation therapy: a review of definitions and usage. *Int J Palliat Nurs* 2002;8(4):190–199.

Benedetti C, Brock C, et al. NCCN practice guidelines for cancer pain. *Oncology* 2000;14(11A):135–150.

Bennett MI. Death rattle: an audit of hyoscine (scopolamine) use and review of management. *J Pain Symptom Manage* 1996;12:229–233.

Billings JA. Comfort measures for the terminally ill. Is dehydration painful? *J Am Geriatr Soc* 1985;33(11):808–810.

Billings JA. What is palliative care? *J Palliat Med* 1998;1(1):73–78.

Block SD. Perspectives on care at the close of life. Psychological considerations, growth, and transcendence at the end of life: the art of the possible. *JAMA* 2001;285(22):2898–2905.

Boyle DM, Abernathy G, et al. End-of-life confusion in patients with cancer. *Oncol Nurs Forum* 1998;25:1335–1343.

Bozzetti F, Amadori D, et al. Guidelines on artificial nutrition versus hydration in terminal cancer patients. European Association for Palliative Care. *Nutrition* 1996;12(3):163–167.

Braun TC, Hagen NA, et al. Development of a clinical practice guideline for palliative sedation. *J Palliat Med* 2003;6(3):345–350.

Breitbart W, Cohen K. Delirium in the terminally ill. In: Chochinov HM, Breitbart W, eds. *Handbook of Psychiatry in Palliative Medicine*. New York: Oxford University Press: 2000;75–90.

Brett AS, Jersild P. "Inappropriate" treatment near the end of life: conflict between religious convictions and clinical judgment. *Arch Intern Med* 2003;163(14):1645–1649.

Brody H, Campbell ML, et al. Withdrawing intensive life-sustaining treatment-recommendations for compassionate clinical management. *N Engl J Med* 1997;336(9):652–657.

Bruera E, Belzile M, et al. Volume of hydration in terminal cancer patients. *Support Care Cancer* 1996;4(2):147–150.

Buckman R. *How to Break Bad News: A Guide for Health Care Professionals*. Baltimore, MD: John Hopkins University Press, 1992.

Cain JM. Practical aspects of hospice care at home. *Best Pract Res Clin Obstet Gynaecol* 2001;15(2):305–311.

Campbell M. *Forgoing Life-Sustaining Therapy: How to Care for the Patient Who is Near Death*. Aliso Veigo, CA: American Association of Critical Care Nurses, 1998.

Cherny NI, Portenoy RK. Sedation in the management of refractory symptoms: guidelines for evaluation and treatment. *J Palliat Care* 1994;10(2):31–38.

Cleeland CS, Gonin R, et al. Pain and treatment of pain in minority patients with cancer. *Ann Intern Med* 1997;127:813–816.

Cleeland CS, Gonin R, et al. Pain and its treatment in outpatients with metastatic cancer. *N Engl J Med* 1994;330(9):592–596.

Clever SL, Tulsky JA. Dreaded conversations: moving beyond discomfort in patient-physician communication. *J Gen Intern Med* 2002; 17(11):884–885.

Cohen SR, Leis A. What determines the quality of life of terminally ill cancer patients from their own perspective? *J Palliat Care* 2002; 18(1):48–58.

Cohen SR, Mount BM. Quality of life in terminal illness: defining and measuring subjective well-being in the dying. *J Palliative Care* 1992;8(3):40–45.

Conill C, Verger E, et al. Symptom prevalence in the last week of life. *J Pain Symptom Manage* 1997;14(6):328–331.

Costantini M, Higginson IJ, et al. Effect of a palliative home care team on hospital admissions among patients with advanced cancer. *Palliat Med* 2003;17(4):315–321.

Council on Ethical and Judicial Affairs AMA. Decisions near the end of life. *JAMA* 1992;267:2229–2233.

Council on Ethical and Judicial Affairs AMA. Medical futility in end-of-life care. *JAMA* 1999;281(10):937–941.

Council on Scientific Affairs AMA. Good care of the dying patient. *JAMA* 1996;275(6):474–478.

Covinsky KE, Goldman L, et al. The impact of serious illness on patients' families. SUPPORT Investigators. Study to Understand Prognoses and Preferences for Outcomes and Risks of Treatment. *JAMA* 1994;272(23):1839–1844.

Cowan JD, Palmer TW. Practical guide to palliative sedation. *Curr Oncol Rep* 2002;4(3):242–249.

Dixon S, Fortner J, et al. Barriers, challenges, and opportunities related to the provision of hospice care in assisted-living communities. *Am J Hosp Palliat Care* 2002;19(3):187–192.

Du Pen SL, Du Pen AR, et al. Implementing guidelines for cancer pain management: results of a randomized controlled clinical trial. *J Clin Oncol* 1999;17(1):361–370.

Early BP, Smith ED, et al. The needs and supportive networks of the dying: an assessment instrument and mapping procedure for hospice patients. *Am J Hosp Palliat Care* 2000;17(2):87–96.

Edmonds P, Karlsen S, et al. A comparison of the palliative care needs of patients dying from chronic respiratory diseases and lung cancer. *Palliat Med* 2001;15(4):287–295.

Ellershaw J, Smith C, et al. Care of the dying: setting standards for symptom control in the last 48 hours of life. *J Pain Symptom Manage* 2001;21(1):12–17.

Ellershaw J, Ward C. Care of the dying patient: the last hours or days of life. *BMJ* 2003;326(7379):30–34.

Ellershaw JE, Sutcliffe JM, et al. Dehydration and the dying patient. *J Pain Symptom Manage* 1995;10(3):192–197.

Emanuel LL, von Gunten CF, et al. Education for Physicians on End-of-Life Care (EPEC) Curriculum. Chicago: American Medical Association, 1999. (http://www.ama-assn.org/ama/pub/category/2910.html.)

Fainsinger R, Bruera E. The management of dehydration in terminally ill patients. *J Palliat Care* 1994;10(3):55–59.

Fainsinger RL, Bruera E. When to treat dehydration in a terminally ill patient? *Support Care Cancer* 1997;5(3):205–211.

Fainsinger R, Miller MJ, et al. Symptom control during the last week of life on a palliative care unit. *J Palliat Care* 1991;7(1):5–11.

Fallowfield L. Communication with the patient and family in palliative medicine. In: Doyle D, Hanks G, Cherny N, Calman K, eds. *Oxford Textbook of Palliative Medicine*. Oxford: University Press: 2004;101–107.

Field MJ, Cassel CK, eds. *Approaching Death: Improving Care at the End of Life*. Washington, D.C.: Institute of Medicine, National Academy Press, 1997.

Flowers B. Palliative care for patients with end-stage heart failure. *Nurs Times* 2003;99(11):30–32.

Foley KM, Carver AC. Palliative care in neurology. *Neurol Clin* 2001;19(4):789–799.

Freeborne N, Lynn J, et al. Insights about dying from the SUPPORT project. The Study to Understand Prognoses and Preferences for Outcomes and Risks of Treatments. *J Am Geriatr Soc* 2000;48(5 Suppl):S199–205.

Friedman BT, Harwood MK, et al. Barriers and enablers to hospice referrals: an expert overview. *J Palliat Med* 2002;5(1):73–84.

Furst CJ, Doyle D. The terminal phase. In: Doyle D, Hanks G, Cherny N, Calman K, eds. *Oxford Textbook of Palliative Medicine*. Oxford: Oxford University Press: 2004;1117–1133.

Gage B, Miller SC, et al. Synthesis and analysis of Medicare's Hospice benefit, executive summary and recommendations, 2000. Washington, DC: U.S. Department of Health and Human Services. (aspe.hhs.gov/daltcp/reports/samhbes.htm.)

Goetschius SK. Caring for families: the other patient in palliative care. In: Matzo ML, Sherman DW, eds. *Palliative Care Nursing: Quality Care to the End of Life*. New York: Springer Publishing Company: 2001;245–274.

Goodlin SJ, Winzelberg GS, et al. Death in the hospital. *Arch Intern Med* 1998;158(14):1570–1572.

Greenstreet W. The concept of total pain: a focused patient care study. *Br J Nurs* 2001;10(19):1248–1255.

Grossman SA, Benedetti C, et al. National Comprehensive Cancer Network practice guidelines for cancer pain. *Oncology* 1999;13:33–44.

Hallenbeck J. Terminal sedation: ethical implications in different situations. *J Palliat Med* 2000;3(3):313–320.

Hanson LC, Henderson M. Care of the dying in long-term care settings. *Clin Geriatr Med* 2000;16(2):225–237.

Harris JT, Suresh Kumar K, et al. Intravenous morphine for rapid control of severe cancer pain. *Palliat Med* 2003;17(3):248–256.

Hastings Center. *Guidelines on the Termination of Life-Sustaining Treatment and the Care of the Dying*. Bloomington, IN: Hastings Center, 1987.

Higginson IJ, Sen-Gupta G, et al. *Changing Gear–Guidelines for Managing the Last Days of Life in Adults. The Research Evidence*. London: Working Party on Guidelines in Palliative Care, The National Council for Hospice and Palliative Care Services, 1997.

Hospice and Palliative Nurses Association. *Hospice and Palliative Care Clinical Practice Protocol: Terminal Restlessness*. Pittsburgh, PA.: Hospice and Palliative Nurses Association, 1997.

Jaycox A, Carr DB, et al. *Management of Cancer Pain: Clinical Practice Guideline, No 9*. Rockford, MD: Agency for Health Care Policy and Research Publication No. 94-0592, U.S. Department of Health and Human Service, 1994.

Jaycox A, Carr DB, et al. New clinical-practice guidelines for the management of pain in patients with cancer. *N Engl J Med* 1994;330(9):651–655.

Jansen LA, Sulmasy DP. Proportionality, terminal suffering and the restorative goals of medicine. *Theor Med Bioeth* 2002a;23(4-5):321–337.

Jansen LA, Sulmasy DP. Sedation, alimentation, hydration, and equivocation: careful conversation about care at the end of life. *Ann Intern Med* 2002b;136(11):845–849.

Jennings B, Ryndes T, et al. Access to hospice care: expanding boundaries, overcoming barriers. *Hasting Cent Rep* [Suppl] 2003;33(2).

Kane RL, Klein SJ, et al. The role of hospice in reducing the impact of bereavement. *J Chronic Dis* 1986;39(9):735–742.

Kayser-Jones J, Schell E, et al. Factors that influence end-of-life care in nursing homes: the physical environment, inadequate staffing, and lack of supervision. *Gerontologist* 2003;43(Spec No 2):76–84.

Keay TJ, Schonwetter RS. The case for hospice care in long-term care environments. *Clin Geriatr Med* 2000;16(2):211–223.

Koenig BA. Cultural diversity in decision-making about care at the end-of-life. Approaching Death: Improving Care at the End of Life: 1997;363-382.

Krakauer EL. Responding to intractable terminal suffering. *Ann Intern Med* 2000;133(7):560; discussion 561–562.

Krakauer EL, Penson RT, et al. Sedation for intractable distress of a dying patient: acute palliative care and the principle of double effect. *Oncologist* 2000;4(1):53–62.

Larson DG, Tobin DR. End-of-life conversations: evolving practice and theory. *JAMA* 2000;284(12):1573–1578.

Lawlor PG. Delirium and dehydration: some fluid for thought? *Support Care Cancer* 2002;10(6):445–454.

Leland JY. Death and dying: management of patients with end-stage disease. *Clin Geriatr Med* 2000;16(4):875–894.

Lichter I, Hunt E. The last 48 hours of life. *J Palliat Care* 1990;6(4):7–15.

Lo B, Quill T, et al. Discussing palliative care with patients. ACP-ASIM End-of-Life Care Consensus Panel. American College of Physicians-American Society of Internal Medicine. *Ann Intern Med* 1999;130(9):744–749.

McCann RM, Hall WJ, et al. Comfort care for terminally ill patients. The appropriate use of nutrition and hydration. *JAMA* 1994;272(16):1263–1266.

Milch RA. The dying patient: pain management at the hospice level. *Curr Rev Pain* 2000;4(3):215–218.

Miller SC, Gozalo P, et al. Hospice enrollment and hospitalization of dying nursing home patients. *Am J Med* 2001;111(1):38–44.

Miller SC, Kinzbrunner B, et al. How does the timing of hospice referral influence hospice care in the last days of life? *J Am Geriatr Soc* 2003;51(6):798–806.

Miller SC, Mor V, et al. Hospice enrollment and pain assessment and management in nursing homes. *J Pain Symptom Manage* 2003;26(3):791–799.

Miller SC, Mor V, et al. Does receipt of hospice care in nursing homes improve the management of pain at the end of life? *J Am Geriatr Soc* 2002;50(3):507–515.

Miller SC, Mor V, et al. The role of hospice care in the nursing home setting. *J Palliat Med* 2002;5(2):271–277.

Munley A, Powers CS, et al. Humanizing nursing home environments: the relevance of hospice principles. *Int J Aging Human Dev* 1982;15(4):263–284.

National Consensus Project for Quality Palliative Care, 2004. Clinical Practice Guidelines for Quality Palliative Care. (www.nationalconsensusproject.org.)

National Hospice and Palliative Care Organization. (http://www.nhpco.org/files/public/facts_and_figures_0703.pdf.)

Norton SA, Talerico KA. Facilitating end-of-life decision-making: strategies for communicating and assessing. *J Gerontol Nurs* 2000;26(9):6–13.

Novak B, Kolcaba K, et al. Measuring comfort in caregivers and patients during late end-of-life care. *Am J Hosp Palliat Care* 2001;18(3):170–180.

O'Neill J, Fallon M. ABC of palliative care. Principles of palliative care and pain control. *BMJ* 1997;315(7111):801–804.

Pantilat SZ. End-of-life care for the hospitalized patient. *Med Clin N Am* 2002;86(4):749–770.

Patrick DL, Curtis JR, et al. Measuring and improving the quality of dying and death. *Ann Intern Med* 2003;139(5 Pt2):410–415.

Pickett M, Yancey D. Symptoms of the dying. In: McCorkle R, Grant R, Frank-Stromborg M, Baird S, eds. *Cancer Nursing: A Comprehensive Textbook.* Philadelphia, PA: W.B. Saunders Company, 1998;1157–1182.

Portenoy RK. Cancer pain management. *Semin Oncology* 1993; 20(2 Suppl 1):19–35.

Portenoy RK. Pharmacologic management of cancer pain. *Semin Oncology* 1995;22(2 Suppl 3):112–120.

Portenoy RK. The physical examination in cancer pain assessment. *Semin Oncology Nurs* 1997a;13(1):25–29.

Portenoy RK. Treatment of temporal variations in chronic cancer pain. *Semin Oncology* 1997b;24(5 Suppl 16):S16–17–12.

Portenoy RK, Hagen NA. Breakthrough pain: definition, prevalence and characteristics, *Pain* 1990;41(3):273–281.

Portenoy RK, Lesage P. Management of cancer pain. *Lancet* 1999; 353(9165):1695–1700.

Post LF, Dubler NN. Palliative care: a bioethical definition, principles, and clinical guidelines. *Bioethics Forum* 1997;13(3):17–24.

Rabow MW, Hauser JM, et al. Supporting family caregivers at the end of life: "they don't know what they don't know." *JAMA* 2004; 291:483–492.

Reynolds K, Henderson M, et al. Needs of the dying in nursing homes. *J Palliat Med* 2002;5(6):895–901.

Rousseau P. Management of symptoms in the actively dying patient. In: Berger AM, Portenoy RK, Weissman DE, eds. *Principles & Practice of Palliative Care & Supportive Oncology.* Philadelphia: Lippincott Williams & Wilkins, 2002;789–798.

Sarhill N, Walsh D, et al. Evaluation and treatment of cancer-related fluid deficits: volume depletion and dehydration. *Support Care Cancer* 2001;9(6):408–419.

Silveira MJ, DiPiero A, et al. Patients' knowledge of options at the end of life: ignorance in the face of death. *JAMA* 2000;284(19): 2483–2488.

Smith TJ, Coyne P, et al. A high-volume specialist palliative care unit and team may reduce in-hospital end-of-life care costs. *J Palliat Med* 2003;6:699–705.

Steiner N, Bruera E. Methods of hydration in palliative care patients. *J Palliat Care* 1998;14(2):6–13.

Steinhauser KE, Christakis NA, et al. Factors considered important at the end of life by patients, family, physicians, and other care providers. *JAMA* 2000;284(19):2476–2482.

Sullivan AM, Lakoma MD, et al. The status of medical education in end-of-life care. *J Gen Intern Med* 2003;18:685–695.

Sulmasy DP. A biopsychological-spiritual model for the care of patients at the end of life. *Gerontologist* 2002;42 Spec No 3: 24–33.

Sulmasy DP, Ury WA, et al. Responding to intractable terminal suffering. *Ann Intern Med* 2000;133(7):560–562; disc. 561–562.

Sykes N, Thorns A. Sedative use in the last week of life and the implications for end-of-life decision making. *Arch Intern Med* 2003; 163:341–344.

Teno JM, Fisher ES, et al. Medical care inconsistent with patients' treatment goals: association with 1-year Medicare resource use and survival. *J Am Geriatr Soc* 2002;50(3):496–500.

Teno JM, Weitzen S, et al. Persistent pain in nursing home residents. *JAMA* 2001;285(16):2081.

Teno JM (2003). Facts on Dying: Policy relevant data on care at the end of life. Center for Gerontology and Healthcare Research at Brown Medical School. (http://www.chcr.brown.edu/dying/future.htm.)

The AM, Hak T, et al. Collusion in doctor-patient communication about imminent death: an ethnographic study. *BMJ* 2000;321(7273): 1376–1381.

Thielemann P. Educational needs of home caregivers of terminally ill patients: literature review. *Am J Hosp Palliat Care* 2000;17(4): 253–257.

Thorns A. Sedation, the doctrine of double effect and the end of life. *Intern J Palliat Nurs* 2002;8(7):341–343.

Thorns A, Sykes N. Opioid use in last week of life and implications for end-of-life decision-making. *Lancet* 2000;356(9227):398–399.

Tierney RM, Horton SM, et al. Relationships between symptom relief, quality of life, and satisfaction with hospice care. *Palliat Med* 1998;12(5):333–344.

Tolle SW, Rosenfeld AG, et al. Oregon's low in-hospital death rates: what determines where people die and satisfaction with decisions on place of death? *Ann Intern Med* 1999;130(8):681–685.

Tolle SW, Tilden VP, et al. Family reports of barriers to optimal care of the dying. *Nurs Res* 2000;49(6):310–317.

Truog RD, Berde CB, et al. Barbiturates in the care of the terminally ill. *N Engl J Med* 1992;27(23):1678–1682.

Truog RD, Cist AF, et al. Recommendations for end-of-life care in the intensive care unit: The Ethics Committee of the Society of Critical Care Medicine. *Crit Care Med* 2001;29(12):2332–2348.

Ventafridda V, Ripamonti C, et al. Symptom prevalence and control during cancer patients' last days of life. *J Palliat Care* 1990;6(3): 7–11.

Vig EK, Davenport NA, et al. Good deaths, bad deaths, and preferences for the end of life: a qualitative study of geriatric outpatients. *J Am Geriatr Soc* 2002;50(9):1541–1548.

Viola RA, Wells GA, et al. The effects of fluid status and fluid therapy on the dying: a systematic review. *J Palliat Care* 1997;13(4):41–52.

Von Gunten CF. Discussing hospice care. *J Clin Oncol* 2002a;20(5): 1419–1424.

Von Gunten CF, Ferris FD, et al. The patient-physician relationship. Ensuring competency in end-of-life care: communication and relational skills. *JAMA* 2000;284(23):3051–3057.

Vullo-Navich K, Smith S, et al. Comfort and incidence of abnormal serum sodium, BUN, creatinine and osmolality in dehydration of terminal illness. *Am J HospPalliat Care* 1998;15(2):77–84.

Wein S. Sedation in the imminently dying patient. *Oncology* 2000; 14:585–592.

World Health Organization. *Cancer Pain Relief.* Geneva: World Health Organization, 1996.

World Health Organization. *Symptom Relief in Terminal Illness.* Geneva: World Health Organization, 1998.

World Health Organization. *Palliative Care.* Geneva: World Health Organization, 2002. (www.who.int/hiv/topics/palliative/ Palliative-Care/en/.)

Yan E, Bruera E. Parenteral hydration of terminally ill cancer patients. *J Palliat Care* 1991;7(3):40–43.

Yedidia MJ, MacGregor B. Confronting the prospect of dying. Reports of terminally ill patients. *J Pain Symptom Manage* 2001;22(4): 807–819.

# Rheumatology

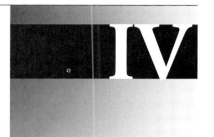

# Acute Monoarticular Arthritis

## 29

*Brian F. Mandell*

Acute monoarticular arthritis represents a medical urgency because of the possibility of joint infection, which can result in total loss of joint function. Additionally, septic arthritis may be the initial manifestation of systemic bacterial infection. Bacterial septic arthritis, in most series, is associated with a >10% mortality. The appropriate diagnosis of specific crystal-induced arthritis will direct long-term management decisions. The treatment of crystal-induced arthritis and hyperuricemia should be individualized, taking into consideration medical comorbidities as well as the anticipated frequency and potential adverse effects of treating acute flares of crystal disease in the future.

## ETIOLOGY

In an unpublished series of 64 hospitalized and emergency department patients with acute monoarticular or oligoarticular arthritis, 17% had documented bacterial infection (Fig. 29.1). The majority of patients had uric acid or calcium pyrophosphate crystal-induced arthritis. It is impossible to distinguish between crystal-induced and septic arthritis on clinical grounds alone. Hence, the possibility of bacterial infectious arthritis dictates the diagnostic approach to the patient with acute monoarticular or oligoarticular arthritis.

## DIAGNOSIS

### History

A thorough history should be obtained, with a focus on several specific issues. Quite frequently, patients describe a history of trauma before their presentation with acute joint swelling and pain. A careful discussion regarding the mechanism and severity of injury, as well as the timing in relationship to the presentation with acute arthritis, is mandatory. Often, it can be determined that the history of trauma bears no relationship to the acute arthritis. Joint trauma alone rarely elicits a striking inflammatory articular response. The general history surrounding the onset of the arthritis should be explored. The presence of an acute migratory arthralgia prodrome is consistent with infection, including rheumatic fever, disseminated gonorrhea, bac-

teremia, and viral infections. Prolonged systemic features before the onset of arthritis also are consistent with a chronic infection, such as bacterial endocarditis or viral hepatitis. Patients should be questioned about prior episodes of arthritis in the same or different joints. Patients with *Borrelia burgdorferi* infection (Lyme disease), crystal disease, psoriasis, enteropathic arthritis, spondylitis, and, occasionally, other syndromes may have a history of prior episodes of self-limited monoarticular or oligoarticular arthritis. Careful questioning should focus on exposure to intravenous drugs or to sexual contact with partners with such exposure, use of medications, or potential exposure to viral hepatitis or human immunodeficiency virus (HIV) infection. Patients living in an area endemic for Lyme disease should be questioned regarding time spent outdoors during the spring, summer, or early autumn months, and a history of any annular rashes.

### Physical Examination

A careful physical examination should be undertaken. An entire musculoskeletal screening evaluation should be performed. Although the patient may only complain of single joint pain, physical examination may reveal multiple inflamed joints, coexistent tenosynovitis, or enthesitis. Mucosal surfaces should be carefully examined for the presence of ulcers or inflammation. The conjunctivitis of Reiter's syndrome (urethritis, arthritis, and conjunctivitis) is typically mild and asymptomatic. Extremities should be examined for purpura or digital infarcts. Psoriatic lesions should be sought in typical but often unrecognized areas (gluteal crease, scalp, behind ears, and umbilicus).

A careful physical examination should focus on distinguishing between bursitis and other soft tissue periarticular pain syndromes and true inflammatory arthritis (Fig. 29.2). Septic bursitis in these areas can be associated with a surrounding erythema or edema and can mimic true joint involvement or cellulitis.

Certain syndromes have a predilection for involving the tendon sheath, as well as the joint structures. Acute tenosynovitis, particularly when accompanying acute arthritis, should prompt a consideration of the diagnosis of infection with *Neisseria gonorrhoeae* or *Haemophilus influenzae*, crystal disease, mycobacterial infection (particularly atypical mycobacteria, such as *Mycobacterium marinum*), and specific

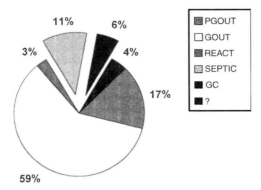

**Figure 29.1** Etiology of acute arthritis. GC, gonococcal arthritis; PGOUT, pseudogout; REACT, reactive arthritis; SEPTIC, septic arthritis. Graduate Hospital, Philadelphia: 64 hospitalized patients. (Mandell BF, unpublished.)

fungal infections, such as sporotrichosis. The sausaging of digits (dactylitis) suggests the diagnosis of psoriasis, sarcoidosis, spondylitis, and reactive arthritis; but if in a single digit, soft tissue infection must also be considered.

Constitutional symptoms are not sensitive or specific enough to establish the diagnosis of septic arthritis or distinguish infectious from crystal-induced arthritis. A study of 43 patients with documented bacterial arthritis predominantly due to *Staphylococcus aureus* revealed the following constitutional markers and their frequency:

- Leukocytosis, 42%
- Temperature >38°C, 41%
- Erythrocyte sedimentation rate (ESR) <30 mm/hr, 24%
- Rigors, 21%

Conversely, a study of documented crystal-induced arthritis found the following:

- Temperature >38°C in 29% of patients with gout (one patient had a maximum temperature of 39.4°C)

- Temperature >38°C in 38% of patients with documented pseudogout
- Temperature >38°C in 50% of patients with polyarticular crystal arthritis

Thus, fever and leukocytosis are neither sensitive nor specific findings in septic arthritis.

## Imaging and Laboratory Studies

Initial laboratory and radiographic studies have limited diagnostic value in the setting of acute monoarticular arthritis, and should be kept to a minimum. The laboratory study of choice is synovial fluid analysis. The distinction between crystal-induced and bacterial arthritis cannot be made reliably with studies from peripheral blood. Radiographs are of initial value if significant trauma or osteomyelitis is suspected, but they play no role in the initial distinction of acute crystal-induced versus bacterial arthritis: The presence of chondrocalcinosis does not exclude the possibility of infection as the etiology of the acute arthritis.

A measurement of serum urate values also is of no diagnostic value in determining the etiology of acute arthritis. The diagnostic test of choice in patients with acute monoarticular arthritis is synovial fluid analysis with cell count, polarized microscopy, and culture. Invariably, patients with infectious or crystal-induced arthritis have synovial fluid leukocytosis with a striking neutrophil predominance (Fig. 29.3). The absolute cell count or neutrophil differential count does not distinguish between septic and crystalline arthritis, however.

The accurate initial diagnosis of monoarticular arthritis rests entirely on the arthrocentesis and a few synovial fluid studies. (A single drop of synovial fluid—as little as that contained in the hub of the needle in an initially presumed "dry tap"—may be sufficient to allow the diagnosis.) The following procedure can be used:

1. Place a single drop of synovial fluid on a glass slide and cover with a coverslip.

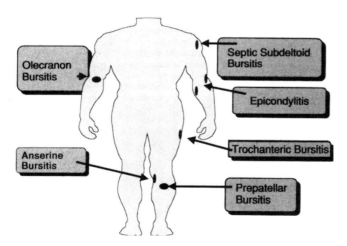

**Figure 29.2** Acute soft tissue problems.

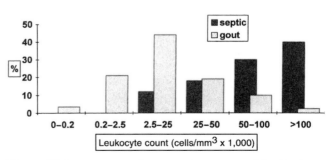

**Figure 29.3** Diagnosis of septic arthritis: synovial fluid leukocytosis. (Reproduced with permission from Krey PR, Bailen DA. Synovial fluid leukocytosis: a study of extremes. *Am J Med* 1979; 67:436–442.)

2. Perform a wet-preparation microscopic analysis using the 40× objective. Estimate the cell count, with one cell per high-power field equaling ~500 cells/mm³.
3. Perform polarized microscopy on the same wet preparation to check for crystals.
4. Remove the coverslip, gently heat-fix the fluid, then perform a Gram's stain.

The Gram's stain permits a differential cell count of polymorphonuclear neutrophils versus mononuclear cells, as well as staining of bacteria. If the fluid is inflammatory, with >7,500 cells/mm³, more than 80% neutrophils, and no crystals evident, the fluid should be sent for culture and the patient treated for potential septic arthritis, unless an obvious alternative diagnosis is apparent. Only rarely will a bacterial infection occur with lower cell counts. Infected joints frequently have synovial fluid white cell counts of <50,000/mm³. Common conditions, such as uncomplicated osteoarthritis, do not cause inflammatory fluids to this degree. If the fluid is not inflammatory by these criteria, and no crystals are observed, cultures still should be undertaken if the patient is febrile or other concerns exist for the possibility of infection, including potential periarticular osteomyelitis. If the fluid is bloody, an evaluation for possible intra-articular injury or synovial tumor should be considered. Intracellular fat droplets suggest the possibility of an intra-articular fracture. Thrombocytopenia, unlike coagulation factor deficiencies, usually is not associated with spontaneous joint hemorrhage. Synovial fluid should be examined promptly, if possible, for the presence of crystals.

If prompt analysis is not possible, the fluid should be maintained in a sterile tube in the absence of anticoagulants, pending polarized microscopic evaluation. Alternatively, the fluid can be placed on a glass slide, the coverslip sealed in place with nail polish, and the fluid examined the next day. It should be noted that crystals (especially calcium pyrophosphate) may not be identified on examination as a result of observer inexperience, a limited number of crystals in the fluid, or other undetermined reasons. Hence, if no crystals are initially seen in an inflammatory fluid without etiology, repeat joint aspirations and evaluation of the fluid by polarized microscopy is mandatory. Alizarin stain may help confirm the presence of calcium-containing crystals, although this test is not available uniformly. In immunocompromised patients, it may be of value to save some of the fluid for special studies, including fungal and mycobacterial culture or polymerase chain reaction (PCR) analysis for *Ureaplasma* organisms (in patients with hypogammaglobulinemia). Routinely obtaining cultures for tuberculosis or fungal infection at the time of initial presentation is not warranted. Some reports demonstrate positive cultures from tissue obtained by synovial biopsy when the fluid culture was negative; however, this procedure is not routinely employed. PCR may occasionally be of value when looking for specific infections.

# SPECIFIC ACUTE MONOARTICULAR ARTHRITIS CONDITIONS

## Gouty Arthritis

Acute urate crystal arthritis is the most common cause of monoarticular arthritis in most reported series (Fig. 29.1).

### Etiology

A review of the natural history of gouty arthritis in older literature reveals that 90% of first attacks are monoarticular, and 60% occur in the first metatarsophalangeal joints (podagra). Approximately 60% of patients may have a recurrence within 1 year; however, 7% may never have another recurrence. Subcutaneous uric acid tophi or radiographic findings of joint damage are rare at the outset of the disease, despite the fact that the synovial tissues are undoubtedly already saturated with uric acid. It is crucial to recognize that attacks of acute gout can be elicited by abrupt changes in serum urate levels, whether up or down. Attacks frequently occur with a normal or even low serum urate value. Figure 29.4 summarizes serum urate level data at times of an acute gouty attack, demonstrating that patients may have a low, normal, or high serum urate level at the time of an attack.

### Pathogenesis

The pathogenesis of an acute gouty attack is reasonably well understood. The cartilage matrix and synovium are saturated with uric acid, a process usually occurring over years of exposure to elevated levels of urate, above the saturation point (approximately 7 mg/dL) in physiologic fluids. In some patients, this supersaturation becomes extreme and results in subcutaneous deposits (tophi) or synovial deposits, setting in motion a local granulomatous inflammatory response that invades adjacent bone, causing erosive changes and reactive bone proliferation in these areas. Factors favoring the nucleation of the uric acid crystals into tophi are not well described. Radiographs in long-standing gouty arthritis may demonstrate the presence of erosions, often at sites away from the joint margins, and reactive bone (overhanging edge) in the absence of significant joint space narrowing. This should be distinguished from the joint space narrowing seen in rheumatoid arthritis, which may occur before the onset of significant erosions.

As urate leaches out of the supersaturated synovium and cartilage into the synovial fluid because of a decrease in the serum urate level or microtrauma to the joint, it may crystallize into phlogistic structures. The ability of crystals to induce an inflammatory response can be modified by coating them with lipoproteins, immunoglobulins, or other proteins present within the synovial fluid. The crystals are phagocytized by synovial lining cells, neutrophils, or mononuclear cells within the synovial fluid. After phagocytosis, these cells produce several chemokines that can elicit and amplify the inflammatory response.

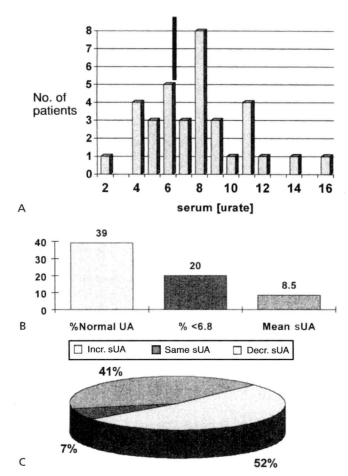

A

B

C

**Figure 29.4** **(A)** Serum urate at the time of acute polyarticular gout. **(B)** Serum urate at the time of acute articular gout in 59 men with documented gout. **(C)** Serum urate at the time of an attack compared with an intercritical period. sUA, serum uric acid; UA, uric acid. (Reproduced with permission: **(A)** from Hadler NM, Franck WA, Bress NM, et al. Acute polyarticular gout. *Am J Med* 1974;56:715–716; **B** and **C** from Schlesinger N, Baker DG, Beutler AM, et al. Serum uric acid during bouts of acute gouty arthritis. *Arthritis Rheum* 1996;39S:348.)

Inflammatory mediators include leukotriene B₄, a crystal-induced protein chemotactic factor (not well defined), inter-leukin-8, interleukin-1, and probably other granule contents and chemokines. Colchicine can suppress the release and synthesis of many of these mediators. Urate crystals activate in neutrophils at least one tyrosine kinase that is sensitive to inhibition by colchicine. Crystals also upregulate the expression of cyclooxygenase-2 in mononuclear cells. Complement and Hageman factor, although activated by urate crystals, do not seem to be necessary for the development of the acute inflammatory response in animals. Complement may be involved, however, in modulating the expression of acute crystal-induced inflammation. The experimental injection of urate crystals under the skin or into the joints of humans is sufficient to elicit the acute inflammatory response (Fig. 29.5). Urate crystals can be found in the fluid obtained from the asymptomatic joints

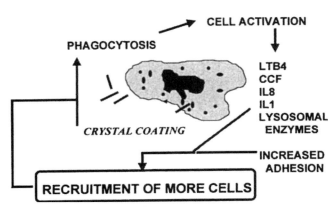

**Figure 29.5** Crystal-induced arthritis. CCF, crystal-induced chemotactic factor; IL1, interleukin-1; IL8, interleukin-8; LTB4, leukotriene B4.

of patients with a history of gout, despite the absence of significant inflammation. Why the inflammatory response is blunted in this setting is a matter of conjecture, but intriguing in vitro studies suggest that mononuclear cells exposed to crystals mature into macrophages that exhibit a phenotype that is less responsive to crystal induced activation. Additionally, as noted above, the crystals themselves are modulated during the course of the attack by acquiring a coating of different proteins.

### Syndromes of Gouty Arthritis

Several distinct phases occur in the clinical expression of gout. Acute arthritis is usually monoarticular, but it may be oligoarticular or even polyarticular. The initial attack is rarely polyarticular. If untreated, the frequency and severity of attacks tends to increase over time. The attacks tend to last longer and involve additional joints. Initially, there is a predominance of lower extremity joint involvement; however, over time, upper extremity joints may become involved (Fig. 29.6). Case reports describe spine involvement,

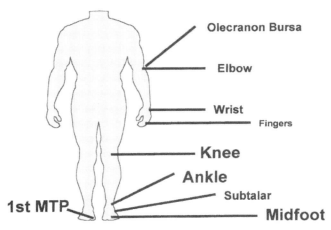

**Figure 29.6** Gout: common sites of involvement. MTP, metatarsophalangeal.

enthesitis, bursitis, and recurrence in prosthetic joints. Flares may involve osteoarthritic Heberden's nodes of the distal finger joints, causing inflammatory finger nodules. This has been best described in postmenopausal, elderly women using thiazide diuretics.

Between attacks (intercritical periods), patients with gout may be totally asymptomatic. Nonetheless, if synovial fluid is obtained at these times, urate crystals still may be found floating in the slightly inflammatory synovial fluid, generally not within cells. Chronic treatment with colchicine lowers the white cell counts in these fluids. Chronic hypouricemic therapy decreases the likelihood of detecting crystals, likely due to the reduced urate burden within the joint. Saturnine gout occurs in the setting of interstitial renal disease, historically in patients who have significant lead exposure resulting from ingestion of illicitly distilled liquor.

Attacks of acute gouty arthritis can be precipitated by changes, either up or down, in serum urate levels. Documentation of hyperuricemia is *not* equivalent to the diagnosis of acute gouty arthritis in an individual patient. Many patients have hyperuricemia without ever having an attack of gouty arthritis. Additionally, hyperuricemia per se is not necessarily associated with any organ damage, including the development of progressive renal disease. A strong statistical (population-based) association exists, however, between elevated levels of serum urate and the development of urate nephrolithiasis and gouty arthritis, coronary artery disease, hypertension, and metabolic syndrome X. In one experimental rat model, mild acute hyperuricemia was shown to elicit the development of hypertension.

Not all crystal-induced arthritis is due to uric acid. Calcium pyrophosphate crystals can cause attacks that totally mimic gout (pseudogout), but they can also cause several other syndromes. Radiographic finding of calcium deposition within menisci and other intra-articular cartilage has been termed *chondrocalcinosis* and may be asymptomatic or associated with inflammatory arthritis. Attacks may be infrequent, or a pseudorheumatoid syndrome may develop with a chronic symmetric polyarthritis due to low-grade, crystal-induced inflammation. Some metabolic diseases have been associated with atypical distribution and early onset of osteoarthritis, perhaps owing to the presence of calcium pyrophosphate crystals. The best known of these is hemochromatosis, which causes low-grade inflammation in the wrists and second and third metacarpophalangeal joints with a radiographic pattern consistent with osteoarthritis. Several systemic diseases have been associated with the occurrence of calcium pyrophosphate deposition, including:

- Hyperparathyroidism
- Hypothyroidism
- Hypophosphatasia
- Hypomagnesemia

- Gout
- Amyloidosis
- Prior joint trauma
- Prior joint surgery
- Hemochromatosis

Both gout and pseudogout attacks are common in the postoperative setting.

Hemochromatosis is emphasized because the gene for hemochromatosis may be present in as much as 10% of the population. Manifestations include a mildly inflammatory osteoarthritis-like arthropathy with predominant metacarpophalangeal involvement, with or without chondrocalcinosis. Prominent metacarpophalangeal involvement is not typical of classic osteoarthritis. The arthropathy may precede the recognition of visceral organ iron overload. Unlike the favorable liver and heart response to early initiation of chelation treatment, phlebotomy may not induce a remission of hemochromatosis-related joint symptoms. Nonetheless, a recognition of hemochromatosis due to the presence of the unique joint syndrome may preserve organ function by prompting early therapy. Skin pigmentation is due to the deposition of melanin, not iron. Cardiomyopathy, hepatic cirrhosis, and endocrine disturbances, including diabetes mellitus and hypogonadism, are also manifestations of hemochromatosis.

Other crystal-induced arthropathies include (rare) oxalate-induced arthritis in patients on dialysis for treatment of chronic renal insufficiency, and arthritis induced by hydroxyapatite crystals. Hydroxyapatite crystals have been associated with a chronic disease known as *Milwaukee shoulder*. This disease tends to affect elderly women, producing severe chronic rotator cuff disease and shoulder effusions composed of an enormous amount of synovial fluid containing few cells and multiple aggregates of apatite crystals. The clinical manifestations include asymptomatic large effusions or severe pain and chronic disability due to shoulder dysfunction. The knees also may be involved similarly.

### Treatment

Conservative indications for the treatment of hyperuricemia include prophylactic therapy to prevent the tumor lysis syndrome and treatment of recalcitrant gouty arthritis in patients in whom there is significant concern over the use of drugs for acute therapy. Patients who have documented soft tissue tophi or joint erosions owing to uric acid deposits should also be treated with hypouricemic agents. Some clinicians suggest that patients who have had more than one attack of gouty arthritis should be treated with hypouricemic agents because it is implicit in the pathophysiology of an attack that the joint structures are already saturated with uric acid. The concern over this therapy is the potential side effects of hypouricemic therapy. Allopurinol, an inhibitor of xanthine oxidase (the key synthetic enzyme in the uric acid pathway), is generally well tolerated; however, the medication has been associated with life-threatening hypersensitivity reactions and the Stevens-Johnson syndrome. Uricosuric agents, such as probenecid, are well tolerated but are harder to use effectively. For maximal efficacy, patients must ingest significant amounts of fluid and use the medication several times daily. Before initiating any therapy to lower the serum urate level, clinicians should be absolutely certain of the diagnosis of gout, which means synovial fluid analysis should have documented the presence of uric acid crystals. Strong consideration should be given to initial simultaneous prophylactic anti-inflammatory therapy using medications such as colchicine or nonsteroidal anti-inflammatory drugs (NSAIDs) because drug-induced hypouricemia may precipitate an attack of gout. The frequency at which this occurs is not defined. Hypouricemic therapy should not be introduced in the setting of an acute attack, nor should it be discontinued while an attack is under way, due to the belief that abrupt changes in serum urate levels may further prolong the attack or induce another attack.

Abnormally low levels of serum urate can be found in select clinical situations including:

- Syndrome of inappropriate antidiuretic hormone secretion
- High-dose salicylate therapy
- Renal tubular diseases (e.g., Wilson's disease, Fanconi's syndrome)
- Starvation
- Alcohol withdrawal

Hypouricemia also has been described in several other disorders and circumstances:

- Xanthine oxidase deficiency syndromes
- Severe liver disease
- Overhydration
- Total parenteral nutrition
- Following use of iodinated contrast agents

Agents or conditions that induce hyperuricemia include:

- Low-dose aspirin
- Diuretics
- Cyclosporine
- Organic acidosis
- Acute ethanol exposure
- Pyrazinamide
- Ethambutol

Hyperuricemia develops in the overwhelming majority of patients because of insufficient renal excretion rather than overproduction. Disorders associated with the hyperproduction of uric acid (more than 1 g urate excreted daily while on a normal diet) include hereditary enzymopathies, such as hypoxanthine-guanine phosphoribosyl transferase deficiency, and proliferative disorders, such as psoriasis or Paget's disease of bone. Most commonly, the specific etiology for the inefficient excretion of uric acid is not demonstrable. Polycystic kidney disease, Bartter's syndrome,

Down syndrome, starvation, and lead nephropathy have been associated with a reduced excretion of uric acid. Most likely, the reduced excretion is due to the inefficient function of either a voltage-sensitive or anion exchange transporter in the proximal tubule. These transporters have been identified, and it is possible that functional polymorphisms of one or both genes can explain the inefficient uric acid excretion with resultant hyperuricemia. The necessity of obtaining a 24-hour urine collection in all gouty patients to quantify uric acid excretion is arguable, unless the use of a uricosuric agent is being considered. Because the occurrence of stones can be precipitated, uricosurics should be avoided in the minority of patients who "overproduce" and thus excrete large amounts of uric acid. If 24-hour uric acid collections are performed, they should be done at least twice prior to making clinical decisions based on the result because of possible physiologic variability in uric acid excretion. Xanthine oxidase inhibition can effectively lower the serum urate level in overproducers as well as underproducers. Therapy should be initiated with *low* doses of allopurinol and slowly increased over weeks to achieve the target level of urate (approximately 6 mg/dL). Approximately 50% of patients may require more than 300 mg daily to reach this target. If this target level of serum urate is not attained, it is unlikely that tophi will be resorbed. Other xanthine oxidase inhibitors and uricase are in clinical development.

Acute crystal arthritis has many treatment options. Probably any NSAID at high dose is capable of treating an acute attack. Aspirin is generally avoided because of its striking effects on urate excretion and the significant side effects associated with high-dose therapy. Concerns over the use of nonselective NSAIDs include renal and platelet dysfunction and gastric toxicity. Additionally, NSAIDs are general antipyretics. Parenteral use of NSAIDs is no safer than oral use, and (in my opinion) parenteral ketorolac has a poor risk-benefit ratio because it is one of the most gastrotoxic NSAIDs. COX-2 selective NSAIDs are likely as effective as the nonselective NSAIDs when used in high doses, are slightly GI safer, and do not affect platelet function. The selective COX-2 inhibitors do, however, share with older NSAIDs the side effects of fluid retention and renal toxicity. Corticosteroid therapy, either oral or parenteral, is quite effective, but should be provided in moderate (not low) doses. Parenteral adrenocorticotropic hormone, although it elicits variable cortisol secretion and has more fluid retentive properties than prednisone, has been suggested by some authors as a viable therapeutic option. It has been proposed that adrenocorticotropic hormone (ACTH) may also have anti-inflammatory effects via its interaction with peripheral (nonadrenal) receptors. Concerns about corticosteroid use include:

- Masking signs of infection
- Exacerbation of diabetes
- Decreased wound healing in the postoperative setting (theoretical)
- Diagnostic confusion resulting from the leukocytosis induced by the corticosteroids

Intra-articular corticosteroids are effective; however, in virtually all patients, joint infection should be ruled out by synovial fluid culture before intra-articular administration. Colchicine is an effective prophylactic drug and also can be used to treat crystal-induced arthridites, such as gout or pseudogout. The older oral administration regimen of one tablet (0.6 mg) every hour until relief or gastrotoxicity develops (usually diarrhea) is generally unacceptable to patients because the diarrhea usually occurs at the same time or slightly before clinical relief is obtained. Intravenous colchicine (1–2 mg initial dose) is an effective therapy for many patients with acute attacks of crystal disease, but it *can be extremely toxic* if inappropriate doses are used, and thus many authors have decried its use. Colchicine should not be used as acute therapy in patients with hepatic or renal disease without a significant decrease in the dosage (if it is used at all).

In patients who suffer frequent attacks, multiple regimens are potentially of value for prophylaxis. Colchicine, 0.6 to 1.8 mg daily, can be used; diarrhea may limit the dosing. In patients with renal insufficiency, colchicine use can result in a reversible neuromuscular toxicity; this should be regularly monitored by history, examination, and occasional creatine phosphokinase measurement. The dosage must be decreased in this setting. Daily NSAIDs are not ideal as chronic prophylactic therapy because of their side-effect profile. In general, dietary manipulations are not likely to provide an enormous change in the serum uric acid level; the one exception to this is cautioning patients about intermittent binge ethanol use. In one epidemiologic study, beer and hard liquor ingestion was associated with a greater risk of hyperuricemia and gout (wine was not). Acute ethanol ingestion causes fluctuations in serum uric acid levels and has been associated with acute gouty attacks.

## GOUTY ARTHRITIS IN TRANSPLANTATION PATIENTS

Special note should be made of the occurrence of severe gouty arthritis in patients receiving transplanted organs. Cyclosporine is seemingly the risk factor, rather than the transplant itself, at least in part because this drug induces hyperuricemia. The course of gout in transplantation patients is more rapidly progressive than in patients not taking cyclosporine. Tophi develop much earlier than expected, and early involvement of the joints of the upper extremity and even the axial skeleton frequently occurs. Multiple potential toxicities exist in the treatment of transplantation patients, including drug interactions between NSAIDs and cyclosporine and between allopurinol and azathioprine. These drug interactions must be closely monitored. The increasing use of mycophenolic acid as a maintenance antirejection therapy simplifies the management of transplant-associated gout.

## SEPTIC ARTHRITIS

Bacterial infection is an uncommon (~15%) cause of acute arthritis. Nonetheless, associated morbidity and potential mortality mandate its prompt exclusion as the cause of acute arthritis. The distribution of affected joints is shown in Figure 29.7. Fibrocartilage joints, such as the sternoclavicular, sacroiliac, and acromioclavicular joints, are involved with infections in specific settings. These joints are prone to infection after persistent bacteremia, particularly with Gram-negative organisms. Patients with a history of intravenous drug use or intravenous catheters (e.g., total parenteral nutrition, hemodialysis, apheresis) are at particular risk.

### Etiology

In most series, staphylococci and streptococci are the most common organisms causing septic arthritis. Disseminated gonococcemia is also a frequent cause of septic arthritis in some populations. The diagnosis of septic arthritis cannot be made with certainty without the culture of synovial fluid. Fever, leukocytosis, rigors, and an elevated erythrocyte sedimentation rate (ESR) are neither specific nor sensitive for the diagnosis of septic arthritis. A positive Gram's stain may be seen in only a slight majority of cases of nongonococcal septic arthritis; thus, a negative Gram's stain does not exclude the possibility of infection.

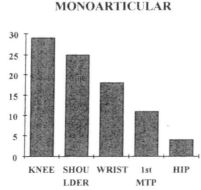

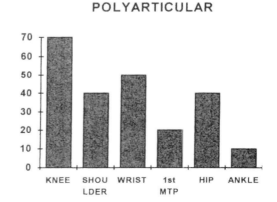

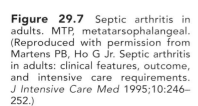

**Figure 29.7** Septic arthritis in adults. MTP, metatarsophalangeal. (Reproduced with permission from Martens PB, Ho G Jr. Septic arthritis in adults: clinical features, outcome, and intensive care requirements. *J Intensive Care Med* 1995;10:246–252.)

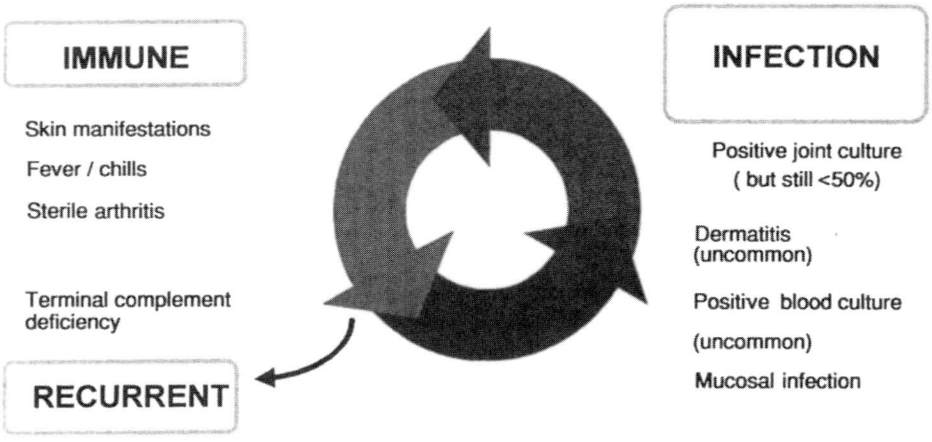

**Figure 29.8** Spectrum of disseminated gonococcal infection.

Disseminated gonococcal infection produces skin lesions and tenosynovitis more commonly than purulent arthritis. The arthritis often follows a syndrome of migratory myalgia and arthralgia. The synovial fluid Gram's stain is usually negative in disseminated gonococcal arthritis, and culture is usually negative as well. Why synovial fluid culture results are negative may relate in part to the difficulty in growing the organism, as well as to the pathophysiology by which arthritis can be induced by immune complexes containing gonococcal antigens without live organisms (Fig. 29.8).

## Specific Conditions Related to Septic Arthritis

### Lyme Disease

Lyme disease results from a tick-transmitted infection by the spirochete *B. burgdorferi*. Frequently, there is a history of an initial characteristic rash, erythema chronicum migrans. Erythema chronicum migrans appears as single or multiple target-like lesions with central clearing. Studies suggest that the overwhelming majority of patients with Lyme disease have a rash at the onset of their illness. This rash may be associated with a flu-like syndrome and symptoms of aseptic meningitis. Fluctuating neurologic syndromes, including facial palsy, may develop shortly thereafter. Cardiac conduction disease, which can fluctuate but may include complete heart block, also occurs. The joint involvement is a monoarticular or oligoarticular, remittent or intermittent, large-joint arthritis. It does not cause a symmetric polyarthritis of small joints, as in rheumatoid arthritis. It is associated with inflammatory joint fluid. The provisional diagnosis of Lyme disease must include the following factors:

- Opportunity for exposure to a suitable tick vector
- Clinical pattern of symptoms consistent with described disease manifestations
- Positive enzyme-linked immunosorbent assay (ELISA) supported by a positive Western blot test result (multiple borrelia-associated bands)

Seronegative Lyme disease is extremely uncommon, and this diagnosis should be entertained only with a great deal of caution. Fibromyalgia, although described in persons who have had Lyme disease, is not a symptom complex suggestive of active infection and does not warrant long-term antibiotic therapy. Circulating antibodies persist for years, and their presence does not warrant chronic or repeated antibiotic administration.

## CULTURE-NEGATIVE AND CRYSTAL-NEGATIVE ACUTE ARTHRITIS

If monoarticular arthritis is not initially found to be due to crystals, and if bacterial culture results are negative in the absence of prior antibiotic use, the differential diagnosis should then include:

- Gonococcal infection
- Lyme disease (if potential exposure was possible; the absence of a concurrent rash does not exclude this diagnosis)
- Mycobacterial infection
- Fungal infection
- Reactive arthritis

Undiagnosed systemic diseases, such as psoriasis or inflammatory bowel disease, also can cause acute or chronic monoarticular arthritis. Periarticular osteomyelitis should also be considered.

## Reactive Arthritis

Reactive arthritis is generally a diagnosis of exclusion at the time of first presentation with monoarticular arthritis. The arthritis is presumably reactive to infection elsewhere in the body. The joint fluids are sterile, although some investigators have suggested that specific bacterial antigens, which localize to the synovium and are not successfully cleared, cause the synovitis. Organisms associated with reactive arthritis include *Chlamydia, Salmonella,*

*Clostridium difficile,* and *Yersinia.* Patients with reactive arthritis may have other features of Reiter's syndrome, including mild conjunctivitis or uveitis, allergic or infectious urethritis, balanitis, psoriasiform skin lesions, or oral ulcerations. The pattern of joint involvement is often large-joint (knee) with a lower-extremity predominance; joint fluid may be extremely inflammatory. Sausage digits, enthesitis, and asymmetric sacroiliac involvement may also occur.

## Viral Arthritis

Viral infections also have been associated with acute arthritis. Viral arthritis often is associated with a pseudorheumatoid distribution of involved joints. Some forms of viral arthritis (varicella-zoster virus, cytomegalovirus, herpes simplex virus type 1, HIV), however, have been associated with monoarticular or oligoarticular arthritis. Rubella-associated arthritis affects female more frequently than male subjects and occurs in 50% to 60% of patients following natural infection and perhaps in 50% of patients following immunization. Approximately one-third of patients having joint symptoms retain these symptoms for approximately 1 year. Parvovirus (fifth disease in children) has been associated with arthritis and arthralgia in adults, usually in a polyarticular pattern and usually without the typical skin eruption that is seen in children. Transient rheumatoid factor may occur in these patients. Parvovirus infection also has been associated with aplastic crises in patients with chronic hemolysis or HIV infection. Hepatitis B and C viruses have been associated with joint symptoms, with or without cryoglobulinemia, which can totally mimic acute rheumatoid arthritis. In one report, an increased frequency of distal finger joint involvement occurred with hepatitis B. The arthritis can be associated with the prodromal phase or in the setting of chronic active hepatitis. It also can be associated with a polyarteritis nodosa syndrome. Hepatitis C–induced arthritis frequently occurs in association with cryoglobulinemia and a high-titer rheumatoid factor; it may be present in patients who have only a minimal elevation in transaminases. HIV infection has been associated with an acute, extremely painful oligoarthritis associated with minimally inflammatory or noninflammatory synovial fluid. Marked hyperesthesia of the joint capsule may be present.

### Diagnosis

The diagnosis of gonococcal infection is frequently made by culture from alternative sites, predominantly the urogenital tract. It must be noted, however, that the absence of pelvic symptoms (or physical findings) in no way excludes the possibility of disseminated gonococcemia (Fig. 29.9).

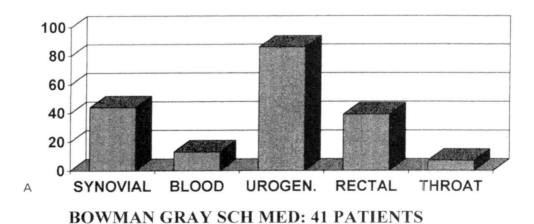

**Figure 29.9** **(A,B)** Positive culture results in patients with gonococcal arthritis. ESR, erythrocyte sedimentation rate; MIG, migratory; UROGEN, urogenital. (Reproduced with permission from Wise CM, Morris CR, Wasilauskas BL, et al. Gonococcal arthritis in an era of increasing penicillin resistance: presentations and outcomes in 41 recent cases, 1985–1991. *Arch Intern Med* 1994;154: 2690–2695.)

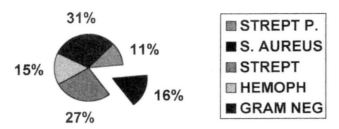

**Figure 29.10** Polyarticular infections in patients without rheumatoid arthritis: nongonococcal causative organisms. Polyarticular disease was present in 6% of all infected patients from a selected series. GRAM NEG, Gram-negative; HEMOPH, *Haemophilus*; STREPT P., *Streptococcus pneumoniae*; STREPT, *Streptococcus*.

The appropriate evaluation of a patient with potential disseminated gonococcemia should include:

- Blood and joint fluid cultures
- Cervical cultures (vaginal cultures in postmenopausal women)
- Rectal and pharyngeal cultures

The absence of rectal or pharyngeal symptoms does not obviate obtaining samples from these areas for culture. Patients with disseminated gonococcemia may have multiple joints involved. Other bacterial causes of nongonococcal polyarticular infections in patients without underlying rheumatoid arthritis are shown in Figure 29.10. The gold standard for diagnosing septic arthritis is the microbiologic identification of an organism in the synovial fluid or tissue.

### Treatment

The treatment of suspected septic arthritis should not be delayed until culture results are available. If the diagnosis of infection is considered, the joints should be treated as a closed-space infection, using parenteral systemic antibiotics and adequate local drainage. The percutaneous drainage of a joint is adequate if it can be performed efficiently. Hip joints are difficult to aspirate, and open drainage is usually used. Until a diagnosis is certain, the percutaneous drainage of an affected joint should be performed daily or as often as necessary to attempt to maintain an effusion-free joint. Successful antibiotic therapy is usually accompanied by a decrease in cell counts; the synovial white blood cell count generally decreases by 50% each day. Initially, the joint should be splinted for pain control and joint protection; however, as the inflammation resolves over subsequent days, passive and then active physical therapy should be introduced as quickly as possible to preserve joint function. If disseminated gonococcemia is suspected, NSAIDs or other anti-inflammatory drugs should be withheld until the diagnosis is confirmed because a favorable response to antibiotics may be necessary to support the diagnosis of gonorrhea when cultures are negative; a response to NSAID therapy may cause diagnostic confusion. There is no role for intra-articular antibiotics. At present, no data suggest that any alternative drainage approach (e.g., lavage, arthroscopy, or arthrotomy) is routinely superior to adequate percutaneous drainage in adults. In patients with underlying joint damage (RA), delayed diagnosis, or immunosuppression, however, I frequently employ arthroscopic drainage in the hopes of removing damaged tissue nidus for recalcitrant infection. Until a diagnosis is confirmed by culture, each aspirated joint fluid sample should be evaluated for the presence of crystals using polarized microscopy because crystals may have been missed on the initial evaluation. Recommended antibiotic regimens vary according to local bacterial resistance profiles and patient demographics. A general empiric antibiotic regimen for treating septic arthritis could involve:

- Young healthy patients: treat for gonococcal and staphylococcal infection
- Patients with underlying joint disease, prolonged hospitalization, prior antibiotic use, urinary tract infections, or prostate disease: treat for methicillin-resistant *Staphylococcus aureus* and Gram-negative bacteria
- Patients with a history of intravenous drug abuse: consider HIV issues, treat for *Pseudomonas* and methicillin-resistant *S. aureus*

If Lyme disease is suspected or confirmed and disease stage identified, treatment options include:

- Presence of erythema chronicum migrans: on clinical grounds, treat for 21 to 28 days (do not wait for antibody testing) using doxycycline, 100 twice daily, amoxicillin, 500 three times daily, or erythromycin, 250 to 500 four times daily
- Stage 2: neurologic/cardiac disease: treat for 14 to 28 days with intravenous penicillin, 20 million U daily, intravenous ceftriaxone (Rocephin), 1 g every 12 hours, or doxycycline, 100 mg twice daily.

Thirty days of therapy in 38 patients with arthritis caused by Lyme disease produced the following results:

- Doxycycline, 100 twice daily: response in 18 of 20
- Amoxicillin/probenecid, 500 four times daily: response in 16 of 18

Note that although the majority of patients responded to this regimen in less than 1 month, response may take 3 months.

## REVIEW EXERCISES

### QUESTIONS

**1.** A 56-year-old white man presents to the emergency department with a 2-day history of increasing right wrist pain and associated swelling. He denies a history of prior episodes of arthritis or any antecedent trauma. His only medication is a diuretic for the treatment of hypertension. He was recently hospitalized for a transurethral prostate resection for benign prostatic hypertrophy. His older brother has been diagnosed with gout.

The most useful diagnostic tests for this patient include

a) Radiography of the wrist
b) Serum uric acid level
c) Complete blood cell count with differential and ESR
d) b and c
e) None is particularly useful

2. A 56-year-old man is found to have a serum uric acid level of 9.4 mg/dL. Clear-cut indications for treatment with allopurinol include

a) A 24-hour urinary urate excretion >1,000 mg
b) A creatinine value of 2.6 mg/dL
c) A history of two episodes of documented gouty arthritis in the past 2 years
d) A requirement for chronic hydrochlorothiazide
e) None of the above

3. All of the following conditions may be associated with hypouricemia, *except*

a) Syndrome of inappropriate antidiuretic hormone secretion
b) High-dose salicylate therapy
c) Wilson's disease
d) Lactic acidosis
e) Early alcohol withdrawal

4. Preoperative medical consultation was requested for a 56-year-old white, insulin-dependent, diabetic man with peripheral vascular disease and osteomyelitis and septic arthritis of the fourth toe. Pain, redness, and swelling were noted for 6 weeks and were only minimally responsive to an oral antibiotic. Drainage of pus reportedly had increased over the previous week. ESR was 54 mm/hr, and the white blood cell count was 10,500/mm$^3$. Bone scan was positive in three phases, and radiographs showed periarticular proximal interphalangeal bone erosion with patchy sclerosis and demineralization of the phalanx.

As the medical consultant, you recommend

a) Preoperative angiogram, an approach for glucose management, and consideration for spinal anesthesia
b) Percutaneous (needle) bone cultures with the patient off antibiotics, plus the above preoperative evaluation
c) Culture of a sinus tract for sensitivities and 3 days of preoperative intravenous antibiotics, plus the above preoperative evaluation
d) Full re-examination of pus, including microscopy, before the above preoperative evaluation

5. A 26-year-old African American woman presents with a chief complaint of foot pain. Examination reveals ankle joint arthritis. She is afebrile and otherwise symptom-free.

She has a documented history of sickle cell anemia. Synovial fluid reveals a white blood cell count of 18,000/mm$^3$ with 86% neutrophils. No crystals are seen. She is treated with a broad-spectrum antibiotic but experiences only minimal improvement after 3 days. Synovial cultures after 72 hours are negative.

The presumptive diagnosis is

a) Gout
b) Salmonella arthritis
c) Avascular necrosis
d) Gonococcal arthritis
e) Reactive arthritis

## ANSWERS

**1. e.**
The major differential diagnosis is between acute crystal disease and infection. The only reliable way to distinguish these is by synovial fluid analysis and culture.

**2. e.**
Asymptomatic hyperuricemia in general need not be treated. No firm evidence exists that treating hyperuricemia in this range prevents renal disease or other end-organ dysfunction in the absence of any symptoms, laboratory dysfunction, or related problems (e.g., nephrolithiasis).

**3. d.**
Organic acidosis produces mild hyperuricemia, not hypouricemia. The causes of hypouricemia include syndrome of inappropriate antidiuretic hormone secretion, renal tubular disorders, very high-dose aspirin therapy, hydration, and the administration of radiocontrast agents.

**4. d.**
As the medical consultant, it is worthwhile to review the primary data whenever possible. In this case, examination of the "pus" revealed that the infection was actually a draining uric acid tophus.

**5. d.**
Seventy-two hours is not always sufficient time to observe a dramatic response to antibiotics. Whereas salmonella or other routine bacterial infections would have been expected to have been recognized in bacterial culture, gonococcus often is not isolated from joint fluid. Gout is more common in sickle cell patients, but the diagnosis of gout should not be made in this setting in the absence of visualized crystals. Avascular necrosis does *not* elicit an inflammatory synovial fluid response.

## SUGGESTED READINGS

Cucurull E, Espinoza LR. Gonococcal arthritis. *Rheum Dis Clin North Am* 1998;24:305–321.
Donatto KC. Orthopedic management of septic arthritis. *Rheum Dis Clin North Am* 1998;24:275–286.

George TM, Mandell BF. Gout in the transplant patient. *J Clin Rheumatol* 1996;1:328–334.

George TM, Mandell BF. Individualizing the treatment of gout. *Cleve Clin J Med* 1996;63:150–155.

Ho G, DeNuccio M. Gout and pseudogout in the hospitalized patient. *Arch Intern Med* 1993;153:2787–2790.

Johnson RJ, Kivlign SD, Kim YG, et al. Reappraisal of the pathogenesis and consequences of hyperuricemia in hypertension, cardiovascular disease, and renal disease. *Am J Kidney Dis* 1999;33:225–234.

Lin KC, Lin HY, Chai P. The interaction between uric acid level and other risk factors on the development of gout among asympto-matic hyperuricemic men in a prospective study. *J Rheumatol* 2000;27:1501–1505.

Lipkowitz MS, Leal-Pinto E, Rappaport JZ, et al. Functional reconstitution, membrane targeting, genomic structure, and chromosomal localization of a human urate transporter. *J Clin Invest* 2001;107:1103–1115.

Lossos IS, Yossepowitch O, Kandel L, et al. Septic arthritis of the glenohumeral joint. *Medicine (Baltimore)* 1998;77:177–187.

Pioro MH, Mandell BF. Septic arthritis. *Rheum Dis Clin North Am* 1997;23:239–258.

Schlapbach P. Bacterial arthritis: are fevers, rigors, leukocytosis, and blood cultures of diagnostic value? *Clin Rheumatol* 1990;9:69–72.

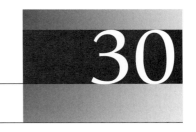

# Osteoarthritis and Polyarticular Arthritis

## 30

*David E. Blumenthal*

The differential diagnosis of musculoskeletal pain is broad. Pain can result from pathology in the articular cartilage, synovium, ligaments, tendons, fibrocartilage, bursae, skeletal muscle, periosteum, bone, peripheral nerves, and nerve roots. This chapter reviews chronic diseases of the articular cartilage and synovium.

## OSTEOARTHRITIS

Osteoarthritis (OA) is also known as degenerative arthritis or degenerative joint disease (DJD). Some physicians prefer the term osteoarthrosis because inflammation is not a prominent feature of the disease. OA usually begins to appear in mid-life and is almost universal in the elderly. The radiographic prevalence of OA in the DIP joint rises rapidly between age 40 and 60 years, and reaches a prevalence of about 60% of men and 75% of women by age 75 years.

OA can be further classified into primary osteoarthritis, which occurs frequently with normal aging, and secondary osteoarthritis, where another medical condition has caused or accelerated the loss of articular cartilage.

### Primary Osteoarthritis

Primary OA occurs in a characteristic distribution. Note that some joints are infrequently affected by primary OA.

| Common site of OA | Uncommon site of OA |
|---|---|
| Distal interphalangeal (DIP) joint | Metacarpal phalangeal (MCP) joint |
| Proximal interphalangeal (PIP) joint | Wrist |
| 1st carpometacarpal (CMC) joint | Elbow |
| Acromioclavicular (AC) joint | Shoulder (glenohumeral) joint |
| Cervical spine | Ankle |
| Lumbar spine | |
| Hip | |
| Knee | |
| First metatarsal phalangeal (MTP) joint | |

OA is a disease of articular (hyaline) cartilage. With aging, the water content of the cartilage increases and the content of glycosaminoglycans decreases. The concentrations and activities of matrix metalloproteinases are increased, with a subsequent degradation of collagen and proteogylcans. The cartilage becomes thin, fissured, frayed, and less able to cushion the joint and provide a smooth gliding surface during joint movement. The adjacent bone is exposed to greater forces and reinforces itself by producing osteophytes at the margins of the joint and subchondral sclerosis. Synovial fluid may migrate under pressure through pits in the articular cartilage and result in subchondral cysts. OA is not a simple consequence of "wear and tear" or weight bearing. The ankle is exposed to at least as much weight as the knee, yet it rarely shows signs of OA. Obesity is a risk factor for OA of the knee, and a lesser risk for OA of the hip, but is not a risk factor for OA in other joints.

Patients with OA experience "mechanical" symptoms: The affected joint becomes more painful with use and improves with rest. There may be some stiffness on arising in the morning, but it usually lasts 30 minutes or less. There are no systemic symptoms, and local signs of inflammation are absent. *Gelling*, or a stiffening of the joints during periods of rest, is mild. This history contrasts with that of inflammatory arthritis, as discussed later.

The physical examination reveals bony osteophytes on the margins of the joint. The joint is cool, and the overlying synovium is not usually thickened or inflamed. Crepitus, a sensation of friction within the joint, may be felt with joint motion. The range of motion of the joint is diminished, and angulation deformities may be apparent, especially at the DIPs and PIPs of the fingers, the 1st MTP, and the knees. A synovial cyst (ganglion) may be seen in the vicinity of the joint, particularly in the fingers.

Radiographs show an asymmetric loss of joint space, subchondral sclerosis, marginal osteophytes, and subchondral cysts.

## Secondary Osteoarthritis

Secondary OA is suspected when a joint that is not commonly involved by primary OA shows evidence of OA on physical examination and radiographs. In secondary OA, a primary disorder causes the loss of articular cartilage and the appearance of OA in a joint where it would not ordinarily be expected to occur. Evidence of OA in an unexpected location should prompt a search for the underlying cause. The causes of secondary osteoarthritis include:

- Dysplasia, congenial or acquired
- Trauma
- Osteonecrosis
- Infection
- Chronic inflammation
- Hemarthroses, especially hemophilia
- Metabolic disorders
  - □ Acromegaly
  - □ Hemochromatosis
  - □ Ochronosis
  - □ Calcium pyrophosphate dihydrate deposition disease (CPPD arthropathy)
- Joint hypermobility
- Mucopolysaccharidoses
- Neuropathy [e.g., neuropathic (Charcot) joint]

## Treatment of OA

Pain can be relieved using analgesics. Acetaminophen should be the first analgesic offered to most patients. Some patients report superior pain relief with nonsteroidal anti-inflammatory agents (NSAIDs), which can be considered if acetaminophen is ineffective. Nonselective NSAIDs are more likely to cause adverse effects in the elderly, and should be used with caution. COX-2–selective NSAIDs are less likely to cause gastric bleeding, but are otherwise not preferable to nonselective NSAIDs. The nutrient glucosamine may provide pain relief and the possible preservation of articular cartilage. Weight reduction will help OA of the knee and hip. Quadriceps muscle strengthening is beneficial in OA of the knee. An assistive device such as a cane or walker will transfer some of the body weight from the affected lower extremity. Refractory OA of the knee can be treated with viscosupplementation, the intra-articular injection of synthetic hyaluronic acid. If conservative measures fail, an orthopedic surgeon can offer the patient arthrodesis (fusion) or arthroplasty (replacement). Arthrodesis is most useful for the ankle, wrist, spine, and 1st MTP. Arthroplasty is most useful for the hip, knee, and shoulder.

# POLYARTICULAR INFLAMMATORY ARTHRITIS

The hallmark of inflammatory arthritis is inflammation of the synovium. In contrast to the patient with a mechanical joint problem such as OA, the patient with inflammatory arthritis will have "inflammatory symptoms." In addition to joint pain, the patient will complain of morning stiffness that lasts more than 1 hour. The joints feel better with use, and the worst periods are during the night and on arising in the morning. Gelling is prominent. An examination of the joint will reveal warmth, tenderness, joint swelling (a mixture of synovial thickening and joint effusion), loss of function, and occasionally erythema. The presence of inflammatory cytokines and other mediators can lead to systemic symptoms, such as fatigue, malaise, weight loss, and fever. The differential diagnosis of polyarticular arthritis is broad, as listed below. The connective tissue diseases, vasculitides, Lyme disease, and the varieties of crystal-induced arthritis are reviewed in other chapters.

## Differential Diagnosis of Polyarticular Inflammatory Arthritis

The differential diagnoses of polyarticular inflammatory arthritis include:

- Rheumatoid arthritis
- Spondyloarthropathies
- Connective tissue diseases
- Vasculitis
- Polyarticular gout
- Polyarticular CPPD (pseudogout)
- Polymyalgia rheumatica
- Viral arthritis
- Lyme disease
- Sarcoidosis
- Adult-onset Still's disease
- Rheumatic fever
- Serum sickness
- Subacute bacterial endocarditis
- Cryoglobulinemia

# RHEUMATOID ARTHRITIS

Rheumatoid Arthritis (RA) is the most prevalent chronic inflammatory arthritis, affecting about 1% of the population worldwide. Women are affected two to four times as frequently as men. HLA-DR4 is a risk factor.

## Pathophysiology

In RA, an unknown stimulus causes hyperplasia of the resident macrophages and fibroblasts of the synovium and angiogenesis (ingrowth of new blood vessels). The macrophages and fibroblasts secrete inflammatory mediators, including tumor necrosis factor (TNF), interleukin-1 (IL-1), interleukin-6 (IL-6), interleukin-8 (IL-8), prostaglandins, leukotrienes, and nitric oxide. These inflammatory mediators attract B and T lymphocytes into the synovium and neutrophils into the synovial fluid. The synovium becomes an enlarged mass of inflammatory cells and fibroblasts, called *pannus*, that has the potential to damage nearby bone, ligaments, tendons, and articular cartilage. The neutrophils elaborate metalloproteinases, which assist in the degradation of nearby tissues. With time, the articular cartilage thins, ligaments slip, tendons weaken, and the characteristic deformities and disabilities of RA appear.

RA is not merely an articular disease. The inflammation can be accompanied by a variety of extra-articular manifestations, including:

- Rheumatoid nodules
- Interstitial lung disease
- Pleuropericarditis
- Sjögren's syndrome
- Scleritis/episcleritis/corneal melt
- Digital infarcts
- Vasculitis
- Felty's syndrome
- Lower extremity ulcers
- Amyloidosis

## Diagnosis

Rheumatoid arthritis is usually a symmetric, polyarticular arthritis, although it may sometimes be asymmetric and oligoarticular early in the course of the disease. Symptoms are those of inflammatory arthritis. The synovium is warm and thickened, and joint effusions are common. With time, characteristic deformities appear, such as swan-neck and boutonniere deformities of the fingers, volar subluxation of the carpus, loss of full extension of the elbows and full abduction of the shoulders, valgus angulation at the knees and ankles, and pes planus.

Laboratory testing shows the features of a chronic inflammatory disease. The erythrocyte sedimentation rate (ESR) and C-reactive protein are high, serum albumin is low, and an anemia of chronic disease often is present. The serum rheumatoid factor (RF), an IgM antibody that recognizes immunoglobulin G (IgG) as its antigen, will be present in 75% to 85% of patients,. Patients with the serum RF often are called *seropositive*, whereas those who lack RF are called *seronegative*. Seropositive patients generally have a more aggressive arthritis and are at greater risk for the extra-articular manifestations of the disease. A positive RF can be seen in a variety of chronic inflammatory and infectious diseases, and in otherwise healthy elderly patients. RF should not be used as a screening test in low-risk populations and should be interpreted with caution if the history and physical examination are atypical for RA. Antibodies to cyclic citrullinated peptide (anti-CCP) are highly specific for RA (96%–98%) with a sensitivity of about 50%.

Radiographs initially show periarticular osteopenia and soft tissue swelling. As the disease progresses, a symmetric loss of joint space and periarticular erosions appear. The erosions are caused by the synovial pannus invading the periarticular bone.

## Treatment

Medications used in RA attempt to decrease the synovial inflammation, and thereby relieve pain, improve joint function, and preserve articular and periarticular tissues. Salicylates and NSAIDs can provide some relief of inflammation and pain, but are seldom sufficient. Selective COX-2 inhibitors may offer less risk of NSAID gastropathy, but they do not appear to be more efficacious than traditional NSAIDs for RA. Corticosteroids, such as prednisone and methylprednisolone, are potent inhibitors of inflammation, but their chronic use can lead to a variety of unacceptable adverse effects, including weight gain, arterial hypertension, glucose intolerance, ocular cataracts, opportunistic infection, and osteoporosis. Intra-articular corticosteroids can provide effective treatment of an injected joint, with fewer systemic effects. Disease modifying antirheumatic drugs (DMARDs) are used to control the synovial inflammation so that corticosteroid use can be avoided or minimized. The traditional DMARDs are listed below. Of these, methotrexate is probably the most efficacious. Potential adverse effects include mucositis, nausea, diarrhea, bone marrow suppression, hepatocellular injury, cirrhosis, pneumonitis, and opportunistic infection. Methotrexate should not be used in patients with hepatic, renal, or bone marrow disease, and it should be used with caution in patients with lung disease. Sulfasalazine is often effective, but sulfa allergy and frequent gastrointestinal intolerance limit its usefulness. Hydroxychloroquine is well tolerated and commonly prescribed in combination with other DMARDs, but as a single agent, it will seldom provide adequate control of the synovitis. Clinical studies have demonstrated efficacy for minocycline, cyclosporine, leflunomide, etanercept, infliximab, adalimumab, and anakinra. Leflunomide is an inhibitor of dihydro-orotate dehydrogenase, an important enzyme in the de novo synthesis of pyrimidines. The efficacy of leflunomide is similar to methotrexate; possible adverse effects include reversible alopecia, rash, diarrhea, and increased hepatic transaminases. Etanercept, infliximab, and adalimumab are blockers of TNF. Etanercept is a polypeptide comprised of two soluble TNF receptors fused to the Fc portion of IgG. It binds to TNF, thus preventing it from interacting with TNF receptors on the surface of immune cells. The adverse effects of etanercept may include irritation at the site of injection and increased susceptibility to infection. Infliximab and adalimumab are monoclonal antibodies that bind TNF as their antigen. Infliximab is given by intravenous infusion three times during the first 6 weeks, then every 2 months thereafter. Adalimumab is given by subcutaneous injection every 14 days. Anakinra is a recombinant IL-1 receptor antagonist, which blocks the biologic effect of IL-1. It is given daily by subcutaneous injection. Single-agent therapy is often insufficient, and many patients are treated using combinations of antirheumatic drugs. The combinations of methotrexate + sulfasalazine + hydroxychloroquine, and methotrexate + cyclosporine have each been shown to be superior to single DMARD therapy in comparative trials. Infliximab is generally used in combination with methotrexate to decrease the likelihood that the patient will develop antibodies against the drug. Other combinations frequently encountered in clinical use include methotrexate + leflunomide, and etanercept + either methotrexate or leflunomide. Parenteral gold, oral gold, and penicillamine are seldom used now because so many superior options are available.

Patients receiving therapy with the anti-TNF therapies are at increased risk for the reactivation of latent mycobacterial infections.

Traditional DMARDs used to treat RA include:

- Methotrexate (MTX)
- Sulfasalazine (SSZ)
- Hydroxychloroquine (HQ)
- Azathioprine (AZA)
- Oral Gold (auranofin)
- IM Gold
- Penicillamine

Newer anti-inflammatory therapies used to treat RA include:

- Minocycline
- Cyclosporine (CSA)
- Leflunomide (LF)
- Etanercept
- Infliximab
- Adalimumab
- Combination Therapy
  - ☐ MTX + SSZ + HQ
  - ☐ MTX + CSA
  - ☐ MTX + LF
  - ☐ MTX or LF + etanercept or adalimumab
  - ☐ MTX + infliximab

The extra-articular manifestations of RA are often treated with the same immunosuppressive agents used for the synovitis. Vasculitis and vision-threatening eye disease may require treatment with cyclophosphamide. Mechanical pain caused by joint damage is treated with analgesics. Arthrodesis or arthroplasty may be effective in relieving pain in a damaged joint. Surgical synovectomy may provide temporary relief of the synovitis in the surgically treated joint, but it provides no benefit for the other inflamed joints or the systemic features of the disease, and therefore is of limited value.

# THE SPONDYLOARTHROPATHIES

The spondyloarthropathies include ankylosing spondylitis, psoriatic arthritis, Reiter's syndrome, and enteropathic arthritis. This group of diseases share several common features:

- Risk of sacroiliitis and spondylitis
- Peripheral arthritis often asymmetric
- Enthesopathy: inflammation of tendon insertions
- Risk of inflammatory eye disease
- Association with HLA-B27

## Ankylosing Spondylitis (AS)

Ankylosing spondylitis is most commonly seen in young males (M:F 3:1). The typical patient experiences the onset of inflammatory pain in the low back or buttocks in the late teens or twenties. Onset of symptoms always occurs prior to age 40. Inflammation usually begins in the sacroiliac joints and ascends the spine. With time, slender calcifications called *bridging syndesmophytes* extend from one vertebral body to the next, resulting in a fusion of the spine. Peripheral arthritis is seen in about 25% of patients, usually in the hips or shoulders. Patients with AS are at risk to develop inflammation of the aortic root, with resulting aortic insufficiency, iritis/uveitis, and apical pulmonary fibrosis.

### Diagnosis

History reveals buttock, back, neck, or peripheral joint pain that has the typical features of an inflammatory process: most severe symptoms in the morning, more than 1 hour morning stiffness, improvement with increasing activity and worsening with rest, "gelling" with inactivity. Family history often reveals other affected family members, particularly in male first-degree relatives. Physical examination may reveal a loss of lumbar or cervical lordosis, loss of range of motion in the spine including an abnormal Schober's test, diminished chest expansion, peripheral arthritis, and evidence of extra-articular manifestations of the disease.

HLA-B27 is a risk factor for developing ankylosing spondylitis, with positive tests in 80% to 98% of Caucasian patients. Testing for HLA-B27 is seldom clinically useful, however. HLA-B27 is present in 6% to 8% of the population in the United States, and only 1% to 2% of those who carry the HLA-B27 antigen develop ankylosing spondylitis. Thus, testing for HLA-B27 in low-risk populations has a low positive predictive value. The test is even less useful in African Americans, in whom only about 50% of patients with AS carry HLA-B27. Other blood tests often show elevated acute phase reactants and anemia of chronic disease.

Plain radiographs show bilateral sacroiliitis, loss of lumbar and cervical lordosis, squaring of vertebral bodies, and bridging syndesmophytes that eventually result in a fusion of the entire spine. In the early stages of the disease, a radionuclide bone scan may show evidence of sacroiliitis or spondylitis before any abnormalities can be appreciated on plain radiographs.

### Treatment

NSAIDs are often used to control the stiffness and pain. Sulfasalazine and methotrexate can be used to control peripheral joint synovitis, but they are less effective for the spondylitis. Blockers of TNF, as used in RA, can be quite effective in refractory cases. None of the available therapies has been proven to prevent the inevitable fusion of the spine. Patients are advised to perform extension exercises and maintain proper posture so that fusion can occur in a functional position.

## Psoriatic Arthritis

Psoriatic arthritis can present with a variety of clinical patterns: (i) symmetric, polyarticular, resembling seronegative RA; (ii) isolated DIP arthritis; (iii) asymmetric, oligoarticular; (iv) arthritis mutilans, where the PIPs and DIPs are so severely damaged that the fingers become a "main en lorgnette" or opera-glass hand with collapsible digits; and (v) any of the above, with sacroiliitis or spondylitis. The cutaneous psoriasis need not be severe and is often subtle. An occasional patient may have the typical features of psoriatic arthritis prior to the appearance of the cutaneous disease, which can lead to difficulties with diagnosis.

### Diagnosis

Psoriatic arthritis is usually diagnosed on clinical grounds when a patient with evidence of cutaneous psoriasis develops the symptoms and signs of an inflammatory arthritis. Psoriatic arthritis has a number of features that distinguish it from RA. Evidence of the cutaneous disease usually is present: well-demarcated erythematous plaques with superficial scale that bleed on gentle scraping, nail pitting, and onycholysis. The DIPs are commonly involved in psoriatic arthritis, rarely in RA. Enthesopathy occurs in psoriatic arthritis, and the combination of enthesopathy and synovitis leads to dactylitis, also called a "sausage digit." Such diffuse swelling of a digit is characteristic of the spondyloarthropathies, and is not seen in RA. Sacroiliitis and spondylitis are not seen in RA, but occur in 20% to 40% of patients with psoriatic arthritis. Psoriatic patients lack serum RF, and the extra-articular manifestations of psoriatic arthritis resemble those of other spondyloarthropathies; psoriatic patients do not develop rheumatoid nodules, vasculitis, or Felty's syndrome. Radiographs in psoriatic arthritis are more likely to show DIP involvement, periostitis, growth of bone at tendon insertions (enthesophytes), and a pencil-in-cup deformity in an interphalangeal joint (the more proximal phalanx is whittled to a point and the more distal phalanx is flared at its base).

### Treatment

Milder cases of psoriatic arthritis can be controlled using NSAIDs. More widespread or destructive arthritis is usually treated using DMARDs, as in RA. Methotrexate, leflunomide, sulfasalazine, etanercept, infliximab, adalimumab, and cyclosporine are all options for more severe disease.

## Reiter's Syndrome

Reiter's syndrome occurs when an at-risk individual encounters an antigen, leading to "reactive arthritis" and autoimmune attack on other body tissues. HLA-B27 is present in approximately 80% of affected individuals and appears to be the leading risk factor for the disease. Post-venereal Reiter's occurs after exposure to *Chlamydia trachomatis*. Post-dysenteric Reiter's occurs after exposure to Salmonella, Shigella, Campylobacter, Yersinia, or occasionally *Clostridium difficile*. The classic triad consists of arthritis, sterile urethritis, and conjuctivitis, with an onset of symptoms about 2 to 4 weeks after exposure to the microorganism. Affected individuals may develop sacroiliitis and spondylitis; unlike ankylosing spondylitis, the sacroiliitis may be unilateral, and some areas of the spine may be spared. The bridging osteophytes may be more bulky than the delicate syndesmophytes seen in ankylosing spondylitis. The peripheral arthritis is often asymmetric and oligoarticular, with a lower extremity predominance. Of Reiter's patients, 15% to 30% will develop chronic arthritis. Enthesopathy and dactylitis are common, usually presenting as sausage digits, achilles tendon inflammation, and plantar fasciitis ("lover's heel"). Keratoderma blenorrhagicum is a characteristic skin rash, mainly on the palms and soles, that is indistinguishable from pustular psoriasis both in its appearance and its histopathology. Onycholysis similar to that of psoriasis may be seen, but nail pitting is absent in Reiter's syndrome. Circinate balanitis is an ulcerative lesion of the glans penis. Approximately 20% of Reiter's patients will eventually experience anterior uveitis.

Treatment of Reiter's syndrome is usually with NSAIDs. The disease usually subsides within 6 months, but in 15% to 30% of cases, it may become chronic. The post-dysenteric form of the disease is more likely to become chronic. Sulfasalazine and methotrexate can be used for chronic arthritis, and a trial of minocycline or doxycycline may be beneficial for post-venereal forms of the disease. Blockers of TNF may be considered for refractory disease.

## Enteropathic Arthritis

Arthritis can occur in association with either ulcerative colitis or Crohn's disease. In patients with inflammatory bowel disease, 10% to 20% will develop a nonerosive oligoarticular arthritis of the large joints. Knee involvement is most common, followed by ankles, elbows, shoulders, and wrists. Sacroiliitis and spondylitis occur in about 15% of patients with inflammatory bowel disease. The peripheral joint arthritis often flares in concert with flares of the bowel disease. Activity of the sacroiliitis and spondylitis is usually independent of the bowel disease. The peripheral arthritis is often successfully treated by the same medications used for the bowel disease, which may include corticosteroids, sulfasalzine, methotrexate, azathioprine, or infliximab.

Arthritis may also be seen in association with other bowel disorders, including intestinal bypass, gluten-sensitive enteropathy, Whipple's disease, and collagenous colitis.

## POLYMYALGIA RHEUMATICA

Polymyalgia rheumatica (PMR) is a nonerosive arthritis that affects primarily the elderly. The typical patient is a Caucasian woman with a mean age of 70 years. The ratio of women to men is about 2:1. The disease is very rarely seen prior to age 50, and is uncommon in African Americans and Asians.

PMR is characterized by stiffness, primarily in the shoulders, upper back, neck, hips, proximal thighs, and low back. Symptoms are usually most severe during the night and on arising in the morning, and the gelling phenomenon is prominent. Fever, weight loss, fatigue, and malaise are common. Some patients will have simultaneous giant cell arteritis and report the headaches, jaw claudication, and scalp tenderness typical of that disease. Arthritis of peripheral joints can occur, but if synovitis of the hands and wrists is a major feature of the illness, then a diagnosis of rheumatoid arthritis may be more appropriate.

The diagnosis is usually made clinically. Laboratory evaluation often shows anemia of chronic disease and an acute phase response, but the ESR can be normal in 20% to 25% of patients. One should keep in mind that the ESR increases with age, and that an ESR as high as 40 mm/hr may be normal for a 70-year-old woman.

Occasionally, patients obtain satisfactory relief of symptoms using NSAIDs, but most will require corticosteroids. Prednisone dosed at 10 to 20 mg daily usually provides prompt relief of symptoms. The prednisone dose is then tapered to the lowest effective dose. Disease activity often subsides between 6 months and 5 years after onset, but exacerbations requiring an intensification of therapy are common. Because the typical patient usually has multiple risk factors for osteoporosis prior to instituting corticosteroid therapy, attention should be paid to detecting, treating, and preventing osteoporosis. Patients who cannot taper the prednisone to a dose that is acceptable for long-term use should be considered for steroid-sparing immunosuppressive therapy. The ideal steroid-sparing strategy for PMR has not yet been defined, but a trial of methotrexate may be considered, although trial-based data for its successful use is warranting.

The practitioner should take care to differentiate PMR from RA because the former diagnosis carries a risk of giant cell arteritis, and the latter diagnosis carries the risk of joint damage if DMARDs are not prescribed. Fibromyalgia is also common in the elderly and has a clinical presentation that can seem quite similar to PMR. Distinguishing between these two conditions is vital because of the risks of chronic corticosteroid therapy in the elderly.

## VIRAL ARTHRITIS

True synovitis can be caused by a variety of viruses, including Parvovirus B19, acute hepatitis B, chronic hepatitis C, rubella, mumps, and the enteroviruses. With the exception of chronic hepatitis C, viral arthritis is usually self-limited, with resolution of symptoms within 3 months. A positive test for RF commonly is seen in chronic hepatitis C, especially if cryoglobulins are present, which can lead to a mistaken diagnosis of RA.

The diagnosis of viral arthritis is possible if the patient's presentation and exposure history suggest a recent viral illness. Serology can be used to confirm the presence of IgM antibodies or recent seroconversion.

Treatment is supportive. NSAIDs are usually sufficient for relief of symptoms. The arthritis of chronic hepatitis C may respond to treatment of the underlying viral infection with interferon-α or ribavirin.

## SARCOID ARTHRITIS

Arthritis is seen in 15% of sarcoidosis patients. It usually occurs in the first 6 months of the illness and is usually self-limited and nonerosive. Sarcoidosis may present with a triad of acute arthritis, bilateral hilar adenopathy, and erythema nodosum, which is called Lofgren's syndrome.

The acute arthritis can be oligoarticular or polyarticular, but is rarely monarticular. The ankles are almost always involved, followed in frequency by the knees, wrists, and elbows. Treatment with NSAIDs is usually sufficient, and the arthritis usually resolves within 3 to 4 months.

Chronic arthritis is uncommon. When seen, it usually is in patients with skin, lung, or bone involvement who have been ill for at least 6 months. The patient often needs immunosuppressive treatment for involvement of other organ systems. Corticosteroids are the first line of therapy, with methotrexate, cyclosporine, and other cytotoxic medications used as steroid-sparing agents. Blockers of TNF can be considered for refractory disease.

## ADULT-ONSET STILL'S DISEASE

The systemic-onset type of juvenile rheumatoid arthritis called Still's disease also can occur in adults. Some patients will give a prior history of Still's disease in childhood. The illness is a systemic, inflammatory, multisystem disease characterized by fever, weight loss, skin rash, pleuropericarditis, hepatosplenomegaly, and lymphadenopathy. The body temperature returns to normal between the once or twice daily fever spikes. The rash is often salmon-pink in color and may be evanescent, most notable at times of fever. Polyarticular inflammatory arthritis is common, but the arthritis may not be a prominent feature of the disease.

Laboratory evaluation generally reveals an exuberant acute phase response, with high sedimentation rate, C-reactive protein and platelet count, low albumin, and anemia of chronic disease. The WBC count often is greater than 15,000, and increased levels of hepatic enzymes are found in the serum. Serum ferritin may be strikingly elevated. Antinuclear antibodies (ANA) and RF are negative.

NSAIDs may be effective in some patients, but many require corticosteroids. Methotrexate is an effective steroid-sparing agent.

## RHEUMATIC FEVER

Rheumatic fever is a late complication of Group A streptococcal pharyngitis. It usually is not seen after Group A strep infection of other anatomic sites, such as the skin, genital tract, or lung. Certain M serotypes confer a greater likelihood of developing rheumatic fever. Symptoms typically occur 1 to 5 weeks after pharyngeal infection, at a time when throat cultures are negative.

The modified Jones criteria are used to diagnose rheumatic fever in children. A diagnosis of rheumatic fever is considered likely if two major criteria, or one major and two minor, are met, plus evidence of an antecedent streptococcal infection.

The modified Jones criteria include:

- Major Criteria
  - ☐ Carditis
  - ☐ Polyarthritis
  - ☐ Chorea
  - ☐ Erythema marginatum
  - ☐ Subcutaneous nodules
- Minor criteria
  - ☐ Arthralgia
  - ☐ Fever
  - ☐ Increased ESR
  - ☐ Increased CRP
  - ☐ Prolonged PR interval

The arthritis is more commonly seen in large joints, is migratory, and not additive. Typically, a joint will be inflamed for less than 1 week, improve, and the arthritis will appear in another joint. Pain and tenderness are often out of proportion to the observed physical findings. The arthritis improves rapidly after treatment with aspirin or NSAIDs.

The carditis is typically a pancarditis, and may present as heart block, a new murmur or evidence of valvular insufficiency, cardiomegaly, congestive heart failure, or pericarditis.

The subcutaneous nodules are similar in appearance and location to rheumatoid nodules, but often are smaller and resolve in 1 to 2 weeks.

Erythema marginatum is a pink to light red rash with a sharp outer border that typically appears on the trunk or proximal extremities and spreads centrifugally with central clearing. The face is usually spared.

A patient can develop sudden, purposeless, involuntary movements, known as *Sydenham's chorea*. These abnormal movements cease when the patient falls asleep. Chorea is often associated with generalized weakness and emotional lability.

Antecedent streptococcal infection is sometimes established by finding prior record of a positive throat culture before the onset of rheumatic fever symptoms. Often, however, the patient has no recollection of a prior pharyngitis, and throat cultures obtained at the time that rheumatic fever is manifest are usually negative. Serologic studies, including antibodies to streptolysin O, hyaluronidase, and DNAase B, can be helpful, especially if more than one of these tests are positive.

The diagnosis in adults can be difficult because chorea and erythema marginatum are rare, and carditis and subcutaneous nodules are less common than in childhood rheumatic fever.

Aspirin or NSAIDs are usually sufficient treatment for acute rheumatic fever. Glucocorticoids may be used for severe carditis. Penicillin or erythromycin is used to eradicate any lingering streptococcal infection.

Patients who have recovered from rheumatic fever may have a recurrence if streptococcal pharyngitis recurs. Repeated bouts of rheumatic carditis can cause additive injury to the heart valves. All patients who have recovered from rheumatic fever should be given antibiotic prophylaxis with either IM benzathine penicillin G, oral penicillin VK, or oral erythromycin. Recommendations vary on the duration of prophylaxis. For most patients, it should be continued until at least age 21 and for at least 5 years after the last attack of acute rheumatic fever. Some physicians recommend lifelong prophylaxis.

## REVIEW EXERCISES

### QUESTIONS

**1.** A 32-year-old sailor reports pain in the joints and dysuria. The right 4th toe is diffusely swollen, and the right ankle and left knee are warm, with pain on range of motion. The left eye is red. Urinalysis shows 25 to

30 WBC/hpf and 1 to 2 RBC/hpf. Urine culture and urethral swab for gonococcal infection are both negative. What is the diagnosis?

**a)** Acute gout

**b)** Adult-onset Still's disease

**c)** Reiter's syndrome

**d)** Polymyalgia rheumatica

**e)** Acute rheumatic fever

**2.** A 67-year-old man complains of gradually worsening knee pain for 5 years. He now can walk only 50 meters before stopping because of knee pain. Morning stiffness is 20 minutes. The right knee is cool with moderate crepitus, a small effusion, and range of motion from 5 degrees to 90 degrees. On weight bearing, he has a moderate varus deformity. What is your plan?

**a)** NSAIDs and a knee brace

**b)** Trial of prednisone 20 mg/d for one week

**c)** Check ESR and serum RF

**d)** Arthrocentesis to rule out gout

**e)** Order radiographs and refer to orthopedics

**3.** A 35-year-old woman is admitted for dyspnea. Upon examination, she has decreased breath sounds at the left lung base, and synovial thickening in her MCPs, PIPs, wrists, and ankles. The olecranon bursa is diffusely swollen with embedded nodules. Her laboratory results are Hgb 11.2, plt 545K, ESR 102, CRP 7.4, ANA + 1:160, and RF 168 (normal 0–20). A chest radiograph shows left pleural effusion. A thoracentesis reveals exudate, pH 7.38, and glucose 24 mg/dL. What is the most likely diagnosis?

**a)** Systemic lupus erythematosus

**b)** Bacterial endocarditis with empyema

**c)** Adult-onset Still's disease

**d)** Lyme carditis

**e)** Rheumatoid arthritis

## ANSWERS

### 1. c.

The diffusely swollen toe likely represents a sausage digit, suggesting that the illness is likely to be a spondyloarthropathy. The triad of arthritis, conjunctivitis, and sterile urethritis is diagnostic of Reiter's syndrome. The treating physicians wisely did appropriate cultures to rule out disseminated gonococcal infection, which can also cause arthritis, urethritis, and conjunctivitis.

### 2. e.

The history and examination suggest a gradual deterioration of the knee without the symptoms and signs of an inflammatory process. The typical history and physical examination is sufficient to make a diagnosis of osteoarthritis. Because the patient can only walk 50 meters at a time and has a marked loss of range of motion of the knee, one can conclude that the OA is rather advanced and the quality of life significantly diminished. Surgery is probably inevitable, and there is little to be gained by instituting conservative therapy in the hope of postponing surgery. If this 67-year-old man does not have a contraindication to surgery, it would be reasonable to consider total knee arthroplasty at this point . NSAID use can be hazardous in the elderly, and should be used cautiously only when acetaminophen has failed.

### 3. e.

The joint examination suggests a polyarticular inflammatory arthritis. The swollen olecranon bursa with embedded nodules is typical of RA. Gout can cause olecranon bursitis with embedded tophi, but polyarticular tophaceous gout would be uncommon in a 35-year-old woman. Evidence suggests an acute phase response, further suggesting the presence of a systemic inflammatory disease. Patients with seropositive RA are at risk for extra-articular manifestations of the disease, including rheumatoid nodules and pleuropericarditis. A positive ANA is not unusual in rheumatoid arthritis, and does not by itself suggest the presence of lupus. The exudative pleural effusion with a low glucose is typical of rheumatoid arthritis. Although bacterial endocarditis can present as a systemic inflammatory illness with arthritis and a positive RF, the normal pH of the pleural fluid suggests that the low glucose is not caused by an empyema.

## SUGGESTED READINGS

Abril A, Cohen MD. Rheumatologic manifestations of sarcoidosis. *Curr Opin Rheumatol* 2004;16:51–55.

Dieppe P, Brandt KD. What is important in treating osteoarthritis? Whom should we treat and how should we treat them? *Rheum Dis Clin North Am* 2003;29:687–716.

Fautrel B, Zing E, Golmard JL, et al. Proposal for a new set of classification criteria for adult-onset Still disease. *Medicine* 2002;81: 194–200.

Flores D, Marquez J, Garza M, et al. Reactive arthritis: newer developments. *Rheum Dis Clin North Am* 2003;29:37–59.

Goldbach-Mansky R, Lipsky P. New concepts in the treatment of rheumatoid arthritis. *Ann Rev Med* 2003;54:97–216.

Kiratiseavee S, Brent LH. Spondyloarthropathies: using presentation to make the diagnosis. *Cleve Clin J Med* 2004;71:184–185,189, 192–194.

Weyand CM, Goronzy JJ. Giant-cell arteritis and polymyalgia rheumatica. *Ann Intern Med* 2003;139:505–515.

Williamson L, Bowness P, Mowat A, et al. Lesson of the week: difficulties in diagnosing acute rheumatic fever-arthritis may be short lived and carditis silent. *BMJ* 2000;320:362–365.

# Systemic Autoimmune Diseases

31

*Karen E. Rendt*

The healthy immune system performs the monumental task of protecting an individual from a barrage of infectious organisms, both external and internal, on an ongoing basis. The cellular elements of the immune system are able to identify and eliminate foreign antigens with impressive specificity and efficiency, and generally do this without harming the host tissue. This requires the immune system to be able to distinguish self from nonself. Sometimes, however, self becomes the antigenic target, and autoimmune disease results. In some forms of autoimmunity, only one organ is targeted, such as the skin in pemphigus vulgaris or the thyroid in Hashimoto's thyroiditis. This chapter focuses on illnesses in which multiple organ systems are targeted, specifically systemic lupus erythematosus (SLE), antiphospholipid antibody syndrome (APAS), progressive systemic sclerosis (scleroderma), Sjögren's syndrome, and the idiopathic inflammatory myopathies.

The diagnosis of these systemic autoimmune illnesses is based primarily on history and clinical examination findings. Laboratory work, including specialized serologic tests such as antinuclear antibodies (ANA), rheumatoid factor (RF), and complement, is rarely diagnostic; rather, in most instances, serologies add support to a working diagnosis and provide information about disease activity. Because many of the systemic autoimmune diseases are uncommon to rare, a physician in general medical practice may encounter only a few patients with any given illness over the course of years. Variable patterns of presentation further challenge the likelihood of early diagnosis. Prompt referral to a rheumatologist when an autoimmune disease is suspected is desirable, not only in terms of facilitating the diagnosis and appropriate treatment of the patient, but also in terms of being cost effective by avoiding unnecessary and expensive data gathering.

## SYSTEMIC LUPUS ERYTHEMATOSUS

Systemic lupus erythematosus (SLE) is the prototypical autoimmune disease characterized by the development of a variety of autoantibodies in the setting of protean clinical manifestations that potentially affect multiple organ systems. The disease is quite variable from patient to patient however, and may even vary in the same patient over time. Both sexes are affected, though the female to male ratio is

approximately 8 to 1 during the reproductive years (between age 15 and 40), and the ratio normalizes somewhat to 2 to 1 in the older and younger age groups.

The pathogenesis of SLE has not been established. Although the hallmark of SLE is the presence of ANA, the role of these antibodies in the pathogenesis of lupus is not clear. Unlike myasthenia gravis, in which antiacetylcholine receptor antibodies are clearly responsible for the interference in neuromuscular function and resultant weakness, the autoantibodies of SLE (anti-SSA, -SSB, -Sm, and -RNP) do not for the most part appear to cause direct tissue injury or dysfunction. Antibodies to dsDNA, on the other hand, have been implicated in immune complex formation as a mechanism for chronic glomerulonephritis. A number of factors are likely to play a role in the development of lupus. These include:

- Genetic predisposition
- Hormonal influences
- Environmental triggers
- Infectious agents
- Drugs

A role for genetics in SLE is suggested by data taken from twins studies, in which a higher degree of concordance for lupus is observed among monozygotic twins when compared with dizygotic twins. Furthermore, first-degree relatives of patients with SLE are at a higher risk of developing SLE themselves. A first-degree relative of a patient with SLE is also at higher risk for developing other autoimmune diseases such as rheumatoid arthritis, Sjögren's syndrome, and Hashimoto's thyroiditis. The HLA markers DR2 and DR3 are over-represented in the SLE population compared with normal controls, although the risk conferred by carrying these haplotypes is not large. Congenital complement deficiency is also a risk factor for the development of SLE. This is particularly true in those persons born with a deletion of one or more of the four alleles of the gene for the fourth component of complement (C4). Persons who have deletions in other early components of the complement cascade are also at very high risk for developing SLE. Conversely, complement deficiency is quite rare, and the majority of patients with SLE develop the disease for other reasons. Finally, specially bred strains of mice, such as NZB/NZW $F_1$ mice (offspring of New Zealand Black crossed with New Zealand white mice) develop ANA, αDNA antibodies, and glomerulonephritis resulting in premature death, thus demonstrating that the genetic manipulation of a strain of mouse creates a model of human lupus.

The role of sex hormones has long been implicated based on the observation that SLE is more common in women compared with men, and the imbalance between the sexes is greatest during the reproductive years. This suggests that estrogen may play some role in the genesis of autoimmunity. In the NZB/NZW F$_1$ murine model of SLE, female infant mice can be protected from developing glomerulonephritis by the administration of androgens, and likewise the administration of estrogens to male infant mice leads to the premature development of glomerulonephritis.

A role for infectious agents has been suggested, and one candidate agent is Epstein-Barr virus. Recent epidemiologic data linked this infection to childhood-onset SLE. Unanswered is the question as to cause and effect, in that patients who develop lupus as children might be more prone to the development of EBV infection because of their altered immunity.

Environmental triggers are believed to play a role, based on the observation that ultraviolet light can trigger an exacerbation of cutaneous lupus and even systemic flares in some susceptible individuals. L-canavaline, an amino acid found in alfalfa sprouts, can trigger flares in a primate model of SLE. Diets low in saturated fats have a protective effect in murine models of lupus.

Finally, certain medications are associated with the development of drug-induced lupus syndromes. Among these are procainamide, hydralazine, isoniazid, methyldopa, chlorpromazine, quinidine, and a number of other agents. The features associated with drug-induced lupus generally remit, however, once the offending agent is removed.

The syndrome that we recognize as SLE is, in fact, a spectrum of illnesses resulting from the influence of some triggering exposure(s) in genetically susceptible individuals.

## Manifestations of SLE

Systemic lupus erythematosus can affect virtually any organ system in the body, and the presentation can vary considerably from patient to patient. This can make identification and accurate diagnosis of the patient with SLE a challenge. The American College of Rheumatology has established 11 features of SLE to assist in the identification of patients. A patient is said to have a high likelihood of having SLE if that person exhibits four of the 11 features, which include:

- Malar rash
- Discoid rash
- Photosensitivity
- Oral ulcers
- Serositis

- Arthritis
- Renal involvement
- Neurologic involvement
- Hematologic abnormalities
- Positive ANA
- Evidence of immunologic dysfunction as revealed by false positive VDRL, positive anti-double-stranded DNA antibody, positive anti-Sm (Smith) antibody, or presence of an antiphospholipid antibody

The cutaneous manifestations of lupus can be divided into lupus-specific rashes and non-lupus–specific rashes. The lupus specific rashes include acute cutaneous lupus (malar rash), subacute cutaneous lupus erythematosus (SCLE), and discoid lupus (DLE). Acute lupus erythematosus presents as a very photosensitive malar rash, with erythema over the malar eminences, bridging the nose and sparing the nasolabial folds. Other sun-exposed areas of the face, such as the forehead and chin, may be involved. The lesions are frequently raised due to cutaneous edema. It typically occurs in the setting of a systemic flare of disease. It typically heals without scarring. About 50% of patients with lupus experience a malar rash as part of their syndrome. The rash must be distinguished from other causes of facial erythema, such as rosacea, dermatomyositis, contact dermatitis, seborrheic dermatitis, polymorphous light eruption, cutaneous sarcoid, and other illnesses. Discoid lesions are generally circular, erythematous plaques, with hyperkeratotic scaling, follicular plugging, and an area of central epidermal atrophy. These lesions tend to affect the scalp, face, arms, and upper trunk and tend to be more chronic. Discoid lupus usually exists by itself in the absence of other systemic features, though 10% of patients with discoid lupus will eventually develop SLE. The discoid lesions tend to heal with scarring. Subacute cutaneous lupus is another photosensitive rash, which might appear as a papulosquamous eruption, psoriasiform eruption, or as an annular or polycyclic rash, with a predilection for the face, upper trunk, and arms. It generally heals without scarring. Many, but not all, patients with subacute cutaneous lupus harbor antibodies to SSA (Ro) and tend not to have antibodies to double-stranded DNA, Smith, and RNP.

Many other dermatologic conditions, which are not specific for lupus, may be seen in the patient with lupus. These include livedo reticularis, bullous skin disease, panniculitis, oral ulcers, alopecia, urticaria, purpura, Raynaud's phenomenon, and digital ulcerations.

The musculoskeletal features of lupus include arthralgias, which affect the majority of patients. A subset of these will experience true arthritis, with joint swelling, synovitis detected by the examining healthcare worker, and even deformities in the small joints of the hands. The hand deformities of long-standing lupus may have the appearance of those seen in rheumatoid arthritis, with MCP subluxation and swan neck deformities of the fingers. Unlike rheumatoid arthritis, these deformities are generally reducible, not fixed. Bony erosions on hand radiograph are unusual in lupus. Avascular necrosis (AVN), particularly of the humeral head, femoral head, tibial plateau, and ankle, occurs in 5% to 10% of patients. Corticosteroid therapy accounts for most of the cases; others may be due to antiphospholipid antibodies, fat emboli, and vasculitis. Pain localized to a single joint with a fairly acute onset, especially in the absence of other signs of articular disease or lupus activity, should raise the concern for AVN. Although a unilateral presentation is typical, AVN is frequently detectable in the contralateral joint by plain radiography or magnetic resonance imaging (MRI). Early detection is crucial to a favorable outcome; a delay in diagnosis increases the likelihood of the patient needing a total joint replacement.

Inflammatory muscle disease occurs in 5% to 10% of patients, heralded by proximal muscle weakness and an elevated creatine phosphokinase (CPK). Electromyogram (EMG) results vary from being normal to revealing the typical changes of myositis, including spontaneous fibrillations, short-amplitude, polyphasic, short-duration potentials. In the patient with an established diagnosis of lupus, a muscle biopsy is generally unnecessary. A careful review of the patient's medication list is prudent, however, to avoid overlooking a drug-induced myopathy (especially from corticosteroids, antimalarials, or hyperlipidemic agents) because treatment of lupus-related myositis will necessitate an introduction or increase in steroid dose, or addition of a second agent in some cases.

About 30% to 40% of patients with lupus also develop secondary fibromyalgia during the course of their illness. Features of fibromyalgia syndrome, including arthralgias, myalgias, and morning stiffness, must be differentiated from symptoms related to lupus. A careful examination of joints (absence of synovial thickening or joint effusions in fibromyalgia) and muscle strength (generally effort-related in fibromyalgia, as opposed to proximal weakness in the patient with lupus myositis or steroid myopathy) will help to distinguish lupus symptoms from fibromyalgia symptoms. "Pain all over," pain in widespread structures such as skin, and a nonrestorative sleep pattern is consistent with fibromyalgia. Labwork [erythrocyte sedimentation rate (ESR), hemoglobin, complement levels] may help to distinguish symptoms of active lupus from symptoms of active fibromyalgia.

The identification of renal involvement from lupus is especially important because renal disease is a major predictor of morbidity and mortality. Lupus nephritis is the most feared complication of renal disease. The World Health Organization (WHO) has established six classifications of lupus nephritis based on the histopathology of renal biopsy sections as follows:

- WHO IA: normal by all microscopic techniques
- WHO IB: normal by light microscopy with immune complex deposition demonstrated by electron microscopy or immunofluorescence

- WHO II: mesangial disease
- WHO IIIA: focal segmental GN
- WHO IIIB: focal proliferative GN
- WHO IV: diffuse proliferative GN
- WHO V: membranous GN
- WHO VI: advanced sclerosing nephropathy

Most patients who develop end-stage renal disease requiring dialysis have WHO class III or IV histology, and it is important to identify these patients early and consider the aggressive management of their disease to prevent end-stage renal disease. For many years, the standard therapy, dating back to studies done at the National Institutes of Health (NIH) in the early 1980s, consisted of corticosteroids (1 mg/kg prednisone or equivalent) with a monthly bolus of intravenous cyclophosphamide ($\sim$750 mg/m$^2$). This combination of therapy had proved more efficacious for prolonging renal and patient survival than either drug given alone. Concerns over the short-term and long-term toxicities of this regimen, however, have since prompted trials of other agents, such as mycophenylate mofetil and azathioprine, either as maintenance therapy after induction of remission by cyclophosphamide and steroids, or as induction agents themselves, in place of cyclophosphamide.

Most patients with WHO Class II (mesangial) disease do not require specific treatment of their renal lesion. The optimal strategy for treatment of WHO Class V (membranous) disease has not been established. In the patient with WHO Class VI, advanced glomerulosclerosis, the risks of immunosuppressive treatment generally outweigh the benefits.

The prevalence of renal disease should not be underestimated. Most patients with lupus are found to have renal involvement when systematic renal biopsies are done, as in a study protocol. Some patients will even demonstrate different histologic types of lupus nephritis in different portions of their renal biopsy. Furthermore, a more benign histologic type can evolve to a more aggressive type over time. All these factors can make the accurate classification and selection of treatment for the patient challenging. Most patients, regardless of histology, will have some degree of proteinuria as well, and the proteinuria may only improve partially with treatment of the underlying nephritis. The implications of long-term proteinuria after treated nephritis still are not known.

Because the treatment of lupus nephritis is associated with significant side effects, it is desirable to limit the use of these regimens to patients who are likely to benefit from treatment. Knowing the WHO classification is not enough; if the disease process is relatively recent in onset, a better outcome will be realized than if the same lesion is discovered and treated at a later stage, when more scarring or atrophy has occurred. Recognizing that reversibility is an important factor, the biopsy specimens can be graded according to their "activity" and "chronicity" features. Activity features include those abnormalities that would be expected to be reversible with immunosuppressive therapy, such as glomerular tuft proliferation, interstitial infiltration, leukocyte infiltrates throughout the glomerulus, cellular crescent formation, karyorrhexis and fibrinoid necrosis, and hyaline thrombi. Other features, such as fibrous crescents, interstitial fibrosis, tubular atrophy, and glomerulosclerosis, are included among the chronicity features that would not be expected to be reversible with treatment and, therefore, portend a poor outcome.

In assessing the patient with possible lupus nephritis, it should be noted that standard office urinalysis is superior to assessment of the blood urea nitrogen (BUN) levels, creatinine levels, or the 240-hour protein collection to detect the presence of underlying renal disease. An active sediment is defined by the presence of red cell casts, or hematuria or pyuria in the absence of infection. The finding of an active sediment should prompt aggressive investigation into the nature of the patient's renal status, including consideration of kidney biopsy. Consultation with a rheumatologist and nephrologist is helpful in this area. Renal function may decline precipitously, so time is of the essence.

Other renal manifestations of lupus include interstitial nephritis and renal vein thrombosis. Interstitial nephritis may be associated with tubular dysfunction [concentration defects, the syndrome of inappropriate ADH secretion or dilutional hyponatremia (SIADH)] and acute renal failure. Renal vein thrombosis may occur in the setting of nephrotic syndrome or APAS.

The cardiac manifestations of lupus include pericardial, myocardial, and valvular disease. Pericardial disease is the most common cardiac manifestation, and can range from asymptomatic pericardial rubs, thickening observed in echocardiograms, or acute chest pain syndromes. Small pericardial effusions are frequent and usually asymptomatic. Larger pericardial effusions may occur and occasionally lead to tamponade. Pericardial fluid analysis may look very similar to that found in bacterial pericarditis, with leukocytosis, predominantly neutrophilic, and decreased glucose levels.

Libman-Sacks endocarditis is a verrucous nonbacterial endocarditis, in which vegetations of variable size form, usually on the ventricular undersurface of the posterior leaflet of the mitral valve. Sometimes they extend to the ventricular mural endocardium. Though the mitral valve is most often affected, the Libman-Sacks lesion can occur on any valve. Histologically, proliferating endothelial cells and myocytes are seen, with scattered mononuclear cells and variable degrees of necrosis. Neutrophils are conspicuously absent; their presence raises the question of infectious endocarditis. Libman-Sacks lesions are typically too small to be detected in transthoracic echocardiography. Rare complications of valvular disease include embolic phenomena and valvular stenosis or insufficiency.

Myocarditis may occur with lupus, but the incidence as indicated in necropsy is much higher than premorbid clinical complaints would have suggested. Coronary artery disease is frequently seen in lupus and is a leading cause of premature death. This generally is not due to coronary vasculitis but instead to an accelerated atherosclerosis, possibly a result of treatment with corticosteroids, or related to hypertension, hyperlipidemia, or chronically elevated levels of homocystine, which are higher in lupus patients as a group compared with normals.

The pulmonary manifestations of lupus include alveolar hemorrhage syndrome, which may be heralded by rapidly progressive respiratory insufficiency, associated with a falling hemoglobin, diffuse alveolar infiltrates on chest radiograph, and increased $D_LCO$ on pulmonary function tests. Hemoptysis may be present in only half of affected patients. This catastrophic event may occur in the face of ongoing immunosuppression. Acute lupus pneumonitis is another form of acute respiratory distress, presenting with alveolar infiltrates on chest radiograph and frequently fever. Pulmonary hypertension and pulmonary embolism may occur in lupus, especially in association with APAS. *Shrinking lung syndrome* is a poorly defined and rare syndrome characterized by diaphragmatic muscle weakness without a true intrinsic pathology of the lungs.

The hematologic manifestations of lupus include leukopenia (<4,000 white cells per $cm^3$), lymphopenia (<1,500 lymphocytes per $cm^3$), thrombocytopenia (<100,000 platelets per $cm^3$), and anemia. Although, classically, the anemia is described as being a Coombs' positive hemolytic anemia, it is actually more common for the patient with lupus to have anemia of chronic disease. Chronic use of nonsteroidal therapy might also lead to iron deficiency anemia through occult gastrointestinal blood loss. Finally, many patients with lupus are functionally hyposplenic, and consideration of a prophylactic Pneumovax inoculation is appropriate in this patient group.

The neurologic and psychiatric manifestations of lupus are protean (Table 31.1).

## TABLE 31.1
### CENTRAL NEUROLOGIC AND PSYCHIATRIC MANIFESTATIONS OF SLE

Stroke
Seizures
Transverse myelitis
Headache
Psychosis
Aseptic meningitis
Organic brain syndrome
Demyelinating disease
Others

**Peripheral neurologic and psychiatric manifestations of SLE**
Mononeuritis multiplex
Acute inflammatory demyelinating polyneuropathy
Plexopathy
Others

These neurologic and psychiatric manifestations of SLE include severe catastrophic events such as transverse myelitis, seizures, and stroke, as well as less morbid events such as cranial neuropathy or peripheral neuropathy. Depression is frequently found in lupus patients. A more subtle cognitive abnormality or organic brain syndrome may be seen. Psychosis may occur, sometimes exacerbated by high-dose corticosteroids. Cerebral infarcts and transverse myelitis generally result not from vasculitis, but from bland vasculopathy or thrombosis. Less commonly, emboli, hemorrhage, or true small-vessel vasculitis can cause ischemic injury. The putative role of ANA is as yet unclear because the histopathologic findings of neuropsychiatric SLE are generally unimpressive. For each of these entities, one must carefully consider non-lupus etiologies and rule them out appropriately. For example, changes in cognitive functioning may be a result of neuropsychiatric lupus, but may also occur in the setting of infection [central nervous system (CNS) or systemic], electrolyte disturbances, uremia, medication side effects [especially from nonsteroidal anti-inflammatory drugs (NSAIDs), steroids], or primary psychiatric diseases.

Imaging techniques such as computed tomography (CT) scanning and MRI can help to exclude space-occupying lesions and infarcts, and MRI is superior in assessing acute ischemic injury, such as recent stroke or transverse myelitis. Single photon emission CT (SPECT) imaging measures the energy utilization of tissue, but is limited by lack of specificity. In particular, SPECT scanning may not distinguish lesions of active disease from those of prior injury.

The utility of ANA testing, such as antiribosomal P protein antibodies, remains unclear. Although associated with both depression and psychosis in lupus, the assay is usually a "send-out" test, and becomes available long after a working diagnosis is made and a treatment regimen is initiated. Antiphospholipid antibodies, especially anticardiolipin antibodies and an assay for lupus anticoagulant, should be sought in the patient with stroke syndromes, transverse myelitis, or multi-infarct dementia.

Serologic abnormalities are the hallmark of systemic lupus, the most prevalent abnormality being a positive ANA test. The ANA is found to be positive in 97% to 100% of patients with lupus. That subgroup once described as being "ANA negative" is shrinking in prevalence as assays improve and there is an improved understanding of the APAS, which historically may have accounted for some of the so-called ANA negative lupus patients. Although ANA is a very sensitive test for detecting patients with lupus, it is lacking in specificity because ANA is found in many other disease states. Positive ANAs are seen in other autoimmune diseases, such as rheumatoid arthritis, Sjögren's syndrome, polymyositis and dermatomyositis, scleroderma, Grave's disease, Hashimoto's thyroiditis, primary biliary cirrhosis, and chronic active hepatitis. Patients with hematologic malignancies may demonstrate a positive ANA. Some patients with certain neurologic disorders, such as myasthenia gravis

and multiple sclerosis, exhibit positive ANAs. Relatives of patients with autoimmune disease will not uncommonly demonstrate a positive ANA. Patients exposed to certain drugs, such as procainamide, may develop an asymptomatic positive ANA (or evolve to symptomatic drug-induced lupus). Furthermore, otherwise healthy individuals with no apparent risk factors for developing a positive ANA may have a positive ANA with a prevalence of roughly 5% to 7%. The prevalence increases with age.

Anti-double-stranded DNA antibodies are relatively specific for lupus, especially if they are found in high titer. Anti-single-stranded DNA antibodies are found in normal controls as well as lupus patients and have no diagnostic utility. Of the extractable nuclear antigens, the presence of antibodies to Smith antigen (Sm) have the greatest specificity for lupus, but the sensitivity of only 30% to 40% hampers their clinical utility when trying to make a diagnosis. The autoantibodies to SSA, SSB, and RNP are seen in a number of autoimmune diseases and are not specific for lupus. Furthermore, antibodies to Smith, RNP, SSA, and SSB do not change reliably with disease activity, and longitudinal monitoring is not indicated. The presence of anti-SSA is associated with some SLE clinical subtypes, including patients with subacute cutaneous lupus erythematosus and patients with complement deficiency. Women who have antibodies to SSA are at increased risk for having a child affected by the congenital or neonatal lupus syndrome, characterized by transient neutropenia, transient skin rash, and complete heart block, which is permanent and requires the insertion of a pacemaker. Antiribosomal P-protein is associated with the neuropsychiatric manifestations of lupus as well as liver and renal involvement, but the test is done in only a few reference centers and is not very practical on a clinical basis because of relatively low sensitivity and lengthy turn-around time. Other laboratory studies that may be useful in assessing the patient with lupus include complement levels, particularly C3 and C4. In some, but not all, patients with lupus, the C3 and C4 levels will fall at the time of a flare and return to normal during disease quiescence. Hence, complement levels can help to follow disease activity. Likewise, the rise in anti-DNA levels may portend an impending flare, and as the flare resolves, the anti-DNA levels fall again toward their baseline range. Not all lupus patients, however, demonstrate anti-double-stranded DNA antibodies. The ANA, in contrast, does not change significantly between periods of disease activity and quiescence, and generally, repeated measures of the ANA are not indicated in the follow-up of the patient. Acute phase reactants such as ESR and C-reactive protein (CRP) are of use in those patients in whom elevations have been previously correlated with illness or flare. In some individuals, the ESR and CRP do not rise impressively with flare, and in some individuals discordance exists between ESR and CRP during flare. Therefore, these tests have greatest utility in the management of an individual patient in whom prior flare characteristics (lab profile, etc.) are known.

## Treatment of Lupus

The treatment of lupus includes nonpharmacologic as well as pharmacologic therapy. Patient education is paramount, and patients should be advised to avoid exposure to ultraviolet light. Broad-brimmed hats and sun block are encouraged. Fatigue is a common problem in patients with lupus, and it is helpful to advise patients to pace themselves in their activities and to take naps if necessary. At the same time, because many patients develop secondary fibromyalgia, an aerobic exercise program is also generally recommended. Pneumococcal vaccine should be administered.

In terms of pharmacologic therapy, simple analgesic and low-dose nonsteroidals can be helpful in patients with arthralgias and mild arthritis. Occasionally, patients with lupus will manifest aseptic meningitis upon exposure to ibuprofen, but due to the availability of over-the-counter ibuprofen, many patients have already demonstrated tolerability to this medication prior to seeing a physician. Hydroxychloroquine (Plaquenil) is a useful agent for the management of the constitutional symptoms, fatigue, dermatologic manifestations, and articular manifestations of the disease. Although it is not indicated as first-line therapy for major organ involvement, data suggest that hydroxychloroquine may help to prevent major organ flares in patients who continue to take the drug on a long-term basis. Prednisone is reserved for more serious organ or life-threatening complications such as severe hematologic dyscrasias, renal involvement, neurological involvement, and some cases of refractory serositis. Because of the numerous side effects of long-term steroid use, the minimal effective dose should be used to control the disease process. Methotrexate is a useful adjunct to treatment of arthritis and myositis.

Cyclophosphamide is generally reserved for major organ-threatening or life-threatening flares particularly affecting the CNS or kidneys. The side effects of cyclophosphamide include marrow suppression, hemorrhagic cystitis, stomatitis, hair loss, nausea, vomiting, and an increased risk of eventually developing lymphoma, leukemia, and bladder cancer. For all these reasons, the use of cyclophosphamide should be confined to serious manifestations of lupus.

Azathioprine and mycophenylate mofetil are generally associated with fewer and less severe side effects than cyclophosphamide, and as such may be preferable for maintaining control of lupus nephritis and other major organ manifestations.

## Systemic Lupus versus Drug-induced Lupus

Drug-induced lupus is a syndrome of lupus-like illness associated with the ingestion of a particular medication. The syndrome has been well described with procainamide use, and numerous other drugs including hydralazine, α-methyldopa, isoniazid, quinidine, chlorpropamide, minocycline, and others. Clinical manifestations include fever, malaise, arthralgias, pleurisy, pericarditis, rashes, and cytopenias. It is unusual to see hypocomplementemia, renal disease, CNS disease, or a false positive venereal disease research laboratory (VDRL) in drug-induced lupus. Serologically, positive ANA is seen in both disorders, as is a positive anti-single-stranded DNA antibody. Antibodies to histone H2b are well described in procainamide-induced lupus; however, antibodies to histone also occur in the majority of systemic lupus patients as well and therefore do not have a discriminatory value. Anti-double-stranded DNA antibodies are generally not found in drug-induced lupus, however they are only found in about half of patients with systemic lupus, with a slightly higher prevalence among patients tested during flare, and a somewhat lower prevalence of patients tested during periods of no disease flare. The treatment of drug-induced lupus requires a recognition of the syndrome and the discontinuation of the offending drug. Most symptoms will resolve on their own with removal of the drug. For particularly symptomatic patients, a limited course of low-dose prednisone or nonsteroidal therapy may be appropriate.

## ANTIPHOSPHOLIPID ANTIBODY SYNDROME

Antiphospholipid antibody syndrome is a syndrome characterized by recurrent arterial and/or venous thromboses, recurrent fetal loss, and thrombocytopenia in association with sustained elevated titers of antiphospholipid antibodies. The term *antiphospholipid antibodies* actually encompasses a family of antibodies that have in common their in vitro binding to phospholipid or protein-phospholipid complexes. Phospholipids include such molecules as phosphatidylinositol, phosphatidylserine, phosphatidylglycerol, phosphatidylcholine, cardiolipin, and other entities. Some antiphospholipid antibodies were functionally characterized as *lupus anticoagulants*, a doubly troublesome term because the antibodies are not confined to the lupus patient population and are, in fact, associated with a hypercoagulable state. Historically, however, they were identified because of their ability to induce a prolongation of phospholipid-dependent coagulation assays, including the activated partial thromboplastin time (aPTT), kaolin clot time, dilute Russell Viper Venom time (dRVVT), and other tests of coagulation that are phospholipid dependent. Later refinement of antibody detection techniques led to enzyme-linked immunoabsorbent assays (ELISAs) for specific antibodies to cardiolipin and β-2-glycoprotein-I. β-2-Glycoprotein-I ($\beta_2$GP-I) is a naturally occurring circulating anticoagulant that has affinity for anionic phospholipids; some investigators feel that antibodies to $\beta_2$GP-I are the most pathogenic for APAS. No single assay has 100% sensitivity for APAS, however, and specificity varies as well. Furthermore, evidence is emerging that other members of the coagulation cascade (protein C, protein S, prothrombin, etc.) may be antigenic targets in some patients with APAS.

Therefore, the question arises: How extensive should laboratory evaluation be in assessing the patient with suspected APAS? A recent session of the International Symposium on Antiphospholipid Antibodies recommended that initial testing consist of a lupus anticoagulant assay (usually the aPTT) plus an anticardiolipin ELISA. If these tests are negative or equivocal, then further testing with other coagulation tests (i.e., DRVVT, aro), $\beta_2$GP-I ELISA, or assays for other phospholipids can be pursued. When checking the anticardiolipin antibody assay, results are reported in terms of immunoglobulin M (IgM), IgG, and sometimes IgA units. Clinically, the manifestations of primary or secondary APAS correlate best with moderate to high levels of IgG anticardiolipin antibodies. The significance of IgM or IgA anticardiolipin antibodies is less clear.

The antiphospholipid antibody syndrome is divided into primary and secondary forms, the latter occurring in patients with systemic lupus. Clinically, the frequencies of thrombotic events, thrombocytopenia, and fetal loss are similar between the two groups, but neutropenia, low C4 levels, and Coombs'-positive hemolytic anemia are more frequently seen in secondary APAS. Other less common manifestations of APAS include seizures, transverse myelitis, pulmonary hypertension, and aortic insufficiency. Livedo reticularis, a blotchy violaceous discoloration of the legs, is not uncommonly seen in this disorder, but may also be seen in patients with cholesterol emboli syndrome and polyarteritis nodosa.

Antiphospholipid antibodies can also be found in a number of different patient populations, including patients with HIV infection (50% to 75%), patients with other autoimmune diseases (rheumatoid arthritis, Sjögren's syndrome, inflammatory myopathy), patients with chronic infectious (syphilis, leishmaniasis, leptospirosis, others), patients taking medications known to induce a drug-induced lupus illness, and even in healthy controls. Patients with drug-induced antiphospholipid antibodies generally do not have clinical manifestations of APAS.

Because this syndrome has only been recognized for 20 years, much is yet to be learned regarding "best treatments" for specific clinical scenarios. A lack of ample trial data precludes an evidence-based approach for many situations; however, based on recommendations presented at the latest International Congress of Antiphospholipid Antibody Syndrome, September 2002, the following comments are offered. Asymptomatic patients who are detected to have antiphospholipid antibody on incidental laboratory evaluation (e.g., preoperative testing reveals an elevated aPTT that fails to correct with mixing and normalizes with the addition of excess phospholipid, thus identifying a lupus anticoagulant) should be placed on daily low-dose (81 mg) aspirin indefinitely, unless contraindications (e.g., allergy) exist, in which case the patient should simply be observed. In the immediate perioperative period, prophylactic heparin can be used instead of aspirin. The recommendation of chronic low-dose aspirin is offered as well to the asymptomatic pregnant woman who is known to be anticardiolipin antibody positive. If that patient also has an obstetric history suggestive of APAS (prior miscarriage, especially if more than one and especially if occurring at a time other than the first trimester), then treatment may also include low-dose subcutaneous heparin along with low-dose aspirin for the duration of the pregnancy. In persons who have had a clinical event such as a deep vein thrombosis (DVT) or an arterial thrombosis, full anticoagulation should be employed. The duration and intensity of anticoagulation, however, is unresolved. It is recognized that the risk of recurrent thrombosis after completing a course of therapeutic anticoagulation is higher than in the general population, prompting experts to recommend a longer duration of treatment than in the general population. No consensus arises, however, on the duration of this treatment because data is lacking to address the relative benefit versus risk of long-term anticoagulation. It is also uncertain as yet whether repeated determinations of antiphospholipid antibody should be used to guide the duration of anticoagulant therapy. Finally, the target international normalized ratio (INR) is also subject to debate. Retrospective studies suggest a high INR offers extra benefit, whereas a recent prospective trial did not confirm this.

Catastrophic APAS is manifested by widespread thromboses developing rapidly in multiple organ systems, and it is associated with a high mortality rate. The onset is typically abrupt, generally becoming manifest in less than 1 week. No standardized protocols for treatment exist, but aggressive management with steroids, full anticoagulation, and plasmapheresis has been employed.

## SCLERODERMA (PROGRESSIVE SYSTEMIC SCLEROSIS)

Scleroderma is a rare disorder, striking 2 to 10 persons per million per year. The female to male ratio is less striking than that of lupus, at only 3:1. The onset of disease is generally between ages 30 and 50 and is typically heralded by Raynaud's phenomenon, with the later development of sclerodactyly and skin thickening and fibrosis over the hands, arms, legs, face, and trunk. As the skin thickening progresses, range of motion is lost in the underlying joints, with secondary muscle atrophy and weakness. Late complications of the musculoskeletal disease include joint contractures, muscle atrophy, and skin ulceration over the contracted joints. Internal organ involvement is common, including pulmonary complications of interstitial lung disease, cardiac arrhythmias due to microscopic areas of ischemia, rapidly progressive renal failure, and gastrointestinal complications of gastric dysmotility, esophageal dysmotility, and gut hypomotility.

Limited scleroderma or CREST syndrome (*c*alcinosis cutis, *R*aynaud's phenomenon, *e*sophageal dysmotility, *scl*erodactyly, *t*elangiectasia), is characterized by more restricted cutaneous disease, with skin thickening progressing no more proximally than the elbows and knees, but still occurring on the face. Renal involvement and pulmonary fibrosis are much less common in CREST syndrome when compared to diffuse scleroderma, but pulmonary hypertension is more likely. The characteristic autoantibody association is with anticentromere antibody, present in 95% of patients with CREST. In diffuse scleroderma, antibodies to topoisomerase I (anti-Scl-70) are found in about 70% of patients.

The pathogenesis of scleroderma is unclear. It is known that fibroblasts taken from the skin of scleroderma patients continue to produce excessive amounts of Type I collagen, the major collagen component of skin, even after several passages in tissue culture. T cells in patients with scleroderma release cytokines such as transforming growth factor-$\alpha$ (TGF$\alpha$) and interleukin-2 (IL-2) that stimulate fibroblast activity. A role for vascular abnormalities is suggested by the observations that (i) the earliest fibrosis of the skin is seen in perivascular areas, and (ii) Raynaud's phenomenon, a vasospastic event, is present at the outset in 95% of patients with scleroderma. Later in the disease, obliteration of the vessel lumen and a net loss of the capillary bed in the affected tissue occurs. Sclerosing illnesses associated with the ingestion of particular substances (toxic oil syndrome from contaminated rapeseed oil ingestion in Spain; eosinophilia-myalgia syndrome from adulterated tryptophan supplements) prompt consideration of an ingested toxin to explain scleroderma, but such an agent has not been identified to date.

Although the cutaneous disease is certainly disabling, the threat to long-term survival in scleroderma and CREST is the course of major organ involvement. For many years, renal disease was the major determinant of survival, with the majority of early (<2 years) deaths attributable to scleroderma renal crisis. Scleroderma renal crisis is a form of rapidly progressive renal insufficiency that affects about 10% of patients with diffuse scleroderma. It tends to occur within the first 4 years of illness, and patients who have rapidly progressive cutaneous disease appear to be at higher risk. The complication is heralded by the sudden onset of severe hypertension, although it should be noted that in 10% of patients with scleroderma renal crisis, the blood pressure can remain in the normal range. A microangiopathic hemolytic anemia and thrombocytopenia in the setting of rising BUN and creatinine levels is the classic clinical picture. The urinalysis is typically bland, although non-nephrotic proteinuria and hematuria may occur. The use of systemic corticosteroids has been suggested to be a risk factor for the development of scleroderma renal crisis; hence, some rheumatologists recommend minimizing or avoiding corticosteroid therapy if possible. Scleroderma renal crisis was the major cause of mortality in scleroderma until the early 1980s, when angiotensin-converting enzyme (ACE) inhibitors became available. The prompt initiation of ACE inhibitors at the diagnosis of renal crisis is associated with a dramatically enhanced renal and patient survival (patient survival <15% at 1 year without ACE inhibitors, 76% at 1 year with ACE inhibitors). Scleroderma renal crisis rarely recurs. Even with appropriate therapy, however, some patients, particularly those who are >55 years or present with congestive heart failure (CHF), may still have a poor outcome (permanent dialysis or death).

Cardiac disease in scleroderma arises from microscopic areas of reversible ischemia that eventually lead to a pathologic finding of contraction-band necrosis. This lesion can predispose to aberrant or delayed conduction, re-entrant arrhythmias, and CHF.

Pulmonary disease has emerged as the major cause of mortality since scleroderma renal crisis has become more manageable. Interstitial inflammation may start early in the disease and lead to alveolitis and, eventually, interstitial fibrosis with impairment in oxygen transfer and restrictive lung physiology. Pulmonary function testing (PFT) with $D_LCO$, high-resolution CT scanning, and bronchoalveolar lavage (BAL) help to establish the diagnosis. Retrospective analyses available to date suggest that the treatment of patients with alveolitis using cyclophosphamide results in a normalization of BAL results and a slower progression of lung disease compared with patients with untreated alveolitis.

Nearly the entire gastrointestinal tract is at risk for involvement from scleroderma. Xerostomia is common because as many patients have secondary Sjögren's syndrome; thrush may result. Esophageal dysmotility is a prominent feature of diffuse scleroderma and CREST, and it results in reflux esophagitis, esophageal stricture, Barrett's esophagus, or esophageal cancer. Gastric dysmotility can result in early satiety. Small bowel involvement, from atrophy of smooth muscle fibers, leads to hypomotility, bacterial overgrowth, dilatation, and pseudo-obstruction. Malabsorption and failure to thrive may result from the bacterial overgrowth. Large-mouth diverticula are found at the small or large bowel. Pneumatosis cystoides intestinalis is an unusual complication of scleroderma characterized by multiple air-filled blebs infiltrating the wall of the colon. These are asymptomatic unless rupture occurs, which usually leads to peritonitis.

## Treatment for Scleroderma

At present, the treatment of scleroderma is directed toward individual disease manifestations because an effective treatment for the fibroproliferative process has not been established. Raynaud's phenomenon is managed using calcium channel blockers, occasionally $\alpha$-1-blockers, topical nitrates, or in severe refractory cases, digital sympathectomy. ACE inhibitors, as mentioned, are organ- and life-saving in the treatment of scleroderma renal crisis. Cyclophosphamide suggestively has been shown in retrospective studies to be of use in treating alveolitis caused by scleroderma, with improvement in pulmonary function testing and clinical symptomatology (shortness of breath). The endothelin-1 antagonist bosentan is approved for the treatment of pulmonary hypertension and has proven efficacious in patients with scleroderma and CREST having this complication. The esophageal manifestations respond to typical agents for reflux and acid control, such as omeprazole and lansoprazole. Propulsid has been removed from the market, but is available on a "compassionate basis" for selected patients, and other prokinetic agents such as metoclopramide or erythromycin may be helpful. For secondary Sjögren's syndrome, a trial of pilocarpine 5 mg four times a day or cevimeline 30 mg three times a day taken with food can be effective. A scheduled rotation of antibiotics (taken for the first 10 days of each month using each of two antibiotics in alternating months) helps to control bacterial overgrowth and resultant symptoms of diarrhea, bloating, and malabsorption. The use of corticosteroids carries with it the concern of precipitating scleroderma renal crisis, but may be indicated for complications such as inflammatory myopathy and alveolitis.

# SJÖGREN'S SYNDROME

Sjögren's syndrome is a chronic autoimmune exocrinopathy characterized by the infiltration of exocrine glands (especially salivary and lacrimal glands) by lymphocytes, leading to acinar disruption, scarring, and eventual failure of glandular function. The clinical symptoms that result include the "sicca complex" of dry mouth (xerostomia) and dry eyes (xerophthalmia), often with salivary gland (parotid and/or submandibular gland) enlargement. In addition, patients can develop dryness of the throat (xerotrachea), dry skin, vaginal dryness, and other symptoms from exocrine gland inflammation. Sjögren's syndrome is also characterized by disregulated B-cell function, with autoantibody production, hypergammaglobulinemia, and an increased risk of developing a malignant transformation in the form of non-Hodgkin B-cell lymphoma.

Sjögren's syndrome is classified as being primary if it is not associated with any other autoimmune disease. Secondary Sjögren's syndrome is frequent, and often unappreciated, in patients with lupus, rheumatoid arthritis, scleroderma, and inflammatory myopathy. Primary Sjögren's syndrome may occur at any age, but the peak age of onset is between 30 and 50 years, with a female predominance (F:M = 9:1).

The extraglandular involvement of primary Sjögren's syndrome reflects the systemic nature of this autoimmune disease. Pulmonary involvement includes interstitial lung disease, alveolitis, xerotrachea, and pseudolymphoma. The gastrointestinal associations include primary biliary cirrhosis, subclinical pancreatitis, and atrophic gastritis. Vitamin deficiencies and malabsorption result from the gastric and pancreatic disease. Renal effects include interstitial nephritis with hyposthenuria distal, renal tubular atrophy (RTA),

and nephrogenic diabetes insipidus. Patients frequently have arthralgias and sometimes a nonerosive arthritis. One-third experience Raynaud's phenomenon. Autoimmune thyroid disease is present in one-third of patients.

Small- and medium-size vessel vasculitis, with manifestations of palpable purpura, ulcerations, gangrene, mononeuritis multiplex, and mesenteric arteritis, may be seen. Nervous system involvement can manifest in many ways, including aseptic meningitis, ataxia, transverse myelopathy, optic neuropathy, and stroke syndromes. Patients who experience optic neuropathy or other discrete neurologic events over time might be diagnosed with multiple sclerosis if the other features of Sjögren's are not recognized. Further confusion arises because the spinal fluid in a patient with neurologic manifestations of Sjögren's syndrome, as in SLE, can indeed exhibit evidence of local immunoglobulin synthesis, including oligoclonal bands on agarose-gel electrophoresis. MRI scanning in these patients reveals discrete white-matter lesions best seen on $T_2$-weighted images.

Patients with primary Sjögren's syndrome are also at a forty-fourfold increased risk for the development of non-Hodgkin lymphoma, particularly those with lymphadenopathy, splenomegaly, and parotid gland swelling.

The differential diagnosis of salivary gland enlargement is broad, with sicca symptoms occurring in some entities. Infectious causes of salivary gland enlargement include viruses (mumps, EBV, CMV, Coxsackie A, HIV, Hepatitis C, and influenza), mycobacteria (tuberculosis), fungi (histoplasmosis, actinomycosis), and bacteria (staph, strep). Acute viral and bacterial parotitis is usually painful. Infiltrative disorders, such as sarcoidosis and amyloidosis, may cause painless, gradual parotid swelling. Endocrine disorders, such as diabetes and types II, IV, and V hyperlipidemia, can cause chronic painless salivary gland enlargement with dry mouth. Malnutrition states such as alcoholism, anorexia, bulimia, and pancreatitis can lead to salivary gland enlargement, which can develop abruptly with refeeding. Although Sjögren's syndrome may cause bilateral or unilateral salivary gland enlargement, unilateral enlargement should also raise the suspicion of a neoplasm such as lymphoma or primary salivary adenocarcinoma. Laboratories will help to differentiate the above disorders. In primary Sjögren's syndrome, the ANA is positive in more than 90% of affected patients. The presence of antibodies to SSA or Ro occurs in about 80% of patients, with antibodies to SSB or La occurring slightly less frequently at 60% to 70%. Serum protein electrophoresis often shows a diffuse hypergammaglobulinemia, but suppression of IgM levels has been described with the onset of lymphoma. Acute phase reactants are variably elevated, and RF is present in roughly 60%. Schirmer's testing is an assessment of tear production, easily performed in the office, in which strips of filter paper are inserted into the unanesthetized eye between the lower lid and the eyeball. After 5 minutes, a minimum of 5 mm of wetting should have occurred. The patient may also undergo ophthalmologic examination using topical staining of the cornea by rose bengal stain, which allows the appreciation of corneal erosions or abrasions, frequent sequelae of chronic dry eyes. The assessment of salivary gland inflammation is performed via minor salivary gland biopsy from the inner aspect of the lower lip. Infiltration of the glands by focal aggregates of lymphocytes are supportive in establishing a diagnosis of Sjögren's syndrome. A biopsy of the major salivary glands is generally not performed unless a neoplasm is suspected. Parotid gland biopsy carries the risk of facial nerve injury.

The treatment of Sjögren's syndrome is largely symptomatic. For sicca symptomatology, education of the patient and supportive measures are usually sufficient. Patients should be encouraged to use eye drops on a regular basis (three times a day or more) because they frequently underestimate the degree of drying of the cornea. Oral moisturizers such as artificial saliva are not very palatable, and as a result, patients often suffer from the lack of saliva and its antibacterial properties, leading to rampant dental caries and loss of teeth. Close follow-up with a dental specialist is important. Sialogogues such as pilocarpine and cevimeline are used to stimulate salivary flow. Patients must be informed that it may take 6 weeks or more for the secretagogue action to become appreciable. Contraindications to use of pilocarpine include narrow angle glaucoma. Hydroxychloroquine (Plaquenil) may be useful in some patients with constitutional and musculoskeletal complaints. For patients who have organ-threatening dysfunction, such as mononeuritis multiplex, CNS disease, or vasculitis, the use of steroids and/or cytotoxics are necessary. The patient with pancreatic insufficiency may benefit from pancreatic enzyme replacement. Whereas many patients carry beverages and hard candy to relieve dry mouth, they should be advised to use sugarless products that do not promote tooth decay.

## IDIOPATHIC INFLAMMATORY MYOPATHIES

The idiopathic inflammatory myopathies include seven disorders:

- Polymyositis (PM)
- Dermatomyositis (DM)
- Inclusion body myositis
- Idiopathic inflammatory myopathy associated with malignancy
- Childhood PM/DM
- Amyopathic dermatomyositis
- Overlap syndromes with other collagen vascular diseases

Of these seven, polymyositis and dermatomyositis are the most commonly encountered entities in a general medicine practice, although they are uncommon illnesses with an annual incidence of 2 to 10 new cases per million per-

sons. Mean age of onset is 45 years, and women are affected twice as often as men; however, the genders are equally affected in the pediatric population. These disorders share several clinical features, including gradually progressive proximal muscle weakness that is usually painless. Occasionally, patients will present with aching in the muscles associated with their proximal muscle weakness, but these patients are the exception to the rule. Patients complain of a subacute onset (3 to 6 months) of weakness involving the proximal muscle groups. Stair climbing and arising from a squat or seated position become difficult due to hip girdle weakness. Keeping the arms raised, to shave or shampoo, becomes difficult. Patients may feel as if their limbs are becoming heavier. Hoarseness and nasal regurgitation reflect pharyngeal muscle involvement. In addition to the complaint of weakness, the patient with dermatomyositis has cutaneous clues to the diagnosis. Periorbital edema and heliotrope rash over the eyelids is typical of dermatomyositis. Gottron's papules, which are flat-topped whitish to violaceous nonpruritic lesions overlying the MCP and PIP joints, are pathognomonic for this illness. The rash must be distinguished from the erythematous rash that may occur in SLE, which also has a predilection for the dorsum of the hands, but appears on the dorsum of the phalanges and tends to spare the MCP and PIP areas. Vasculitic rashes may appear, particularly on the elbows. More common in children with dermatomyositis than in adults is dystrophic calcification in the soft tissues of the extremities or trunk, a condition known as *calcinosis cutis*. Calcinosis cutis can lead to the breakdown of the overlying skin and secondary infection. Periarticular involvement leads to joint contractures. The *shawl sign* is an erythematous flat rash that occurs in the V of the anterior chest and neck and drapes across the shoulder girdle posteriorly, like a shawl. Nail-fold capillary abnormalities are also frequently seen in dermatomyositis, with capillary loop bushy dilatation and tortuosity. These can be seen with the unaided eye or with the use of the ophthalmoscope and a drop of immersion oil placed on the cuticle area.

The differential diagnosis of idiopathic inflammatory myopathy includes other conditions that might cause a patient to present to his physician complaining of "weakness." Such conditions include nonmyopathic processes such as arthritis, CHF, anemia, uremia, and neurologic problems. These are usually easily discerned through careful physical examination and basic laboratory testing. In the patient with true muscular weakness on manual resistive testing, however, one must consider a number of other causes of myopathy (Table 31.2).

The laboratory hallmark of polymyositis and dermatomyositis is a striking elevation of CPK, usually over 1,000 or even over 10,000 mg/dL. CPK-MB elevation is also seen, released by regenerating skeletal muscle fibers. Laboratories do not distinguish between CPK-MB of myocardial origin versus regenerating skeletal muscle. Cardiac troponin-I, however, does reasonably differentiate between injury of

## TABLE 31.2

### DIFFERENTIAL DIAGNOSIS OF INFLAMMATORY MYOPATHY

Drugs/Toxins (see Table 31.3)

Infection
    Bacterial, mycobacterial, fungal, viral, parasitic, treponemal

Metabolic myopathy
    Glycogen storage diseases
    Carnitine deficiency
    Carnitine palmitoyltransferase deficiency

Endocrinopathy
    Hypothyroidism
    Hyperthyroidism
    Hyperparathyroidism
    Cushing syndrome
    Vitamin D deficiency

Polymyalgia rheumatica

Sarcoidosis

Fibromyalgia

Neuromuscular disorders
    Amyotrophic lateral sclerosis, muscular dystrophy, myasthenia gravis

myocardial origin from that of skeletal origin. Less sensitive and specific markers for inflammatory myopathy include aldolase, aspartate aminotransferase (AST), serum glutamic-oxaloacetic transaminase (SGOT), alanine transaminase (ALT), serum glutamate pyruvate transaminase (SGPT), and ESR. Aldolase is an enzyme found in the glycolytic pathway, downstream of phosphofructokinase. It is found in muscle

## TABLE 31.3

### DRUGS/TOXINS ASSOCIATED WITH MYOPATHY

Amiodarone
Chloroquine
Cimetidine
Clofibrate
Colchicine
Corticosteroids
Danazol
Ethanol
Gemfibrozil
HMG-CoA reductase inhibitors
Hydralazine
Ipecac
Ketoconazole
Nicotinic acid
Penicillamine
Procainamide
Rifampin
Vincristine
Zidovudine

fast-twitch fibers, but also in liver, kidney, brain, intestines, and fetal tissue. AST and ALT can be elevated into the several hundred range. It is helpful to keep this in mind because many multichannel chemistry batteries, such as the comprehensive metabolic panel (CMP), or chemistry screens, such as the SMA-20, do not include CPK as a routine test. In a patient who has elevations of "liver function" tests (AST and ALT) without an obvious hepatic source, consider checking a CPK and assessing muscle strength.

Laboratory studies more specific for inflammatory myopathy are the so-called myositis specific autoantibodies (MSAs). These include the members of the antisynthetase family, anti-Jo-1, anti-PL-7, anti-PL-12, and anti-OJ. Anti-Jo-1 antibodies are found in 20% of patients with polymyositis. The other autoantibodies are seen less frequently. These antibodies are each directed against a different amino acid transfer RNA synthetase. Amino acid transfer RNA synthetases are cystoplasmic enzymes that serve as shuttles for specific amino acids in the assembly of proteins. Anti-Jo-1, for example, is directed against histidyl transfer RNA synthetase. The antisynthetase syndrome is characterized by inflammatory myopathy occurring with fever, inflammatory arthritis, interstitial lung disease, Raynaud's phenomenon, and a roughened, fissured rash on the palmar aspect of the fingers/hands (mechanic's hands).

In addition to laboratory testing, the work-up of the patient with a suspected inflammatory myopathy generally includes neuroelectrodiagnostic studies and muscle biopsy. Electromyography reveals characteristic abnormalities including: (i) insertional irritability, (ii) bizarre polyphasic potentials, (iii) absence of full interference pattern on muscle recruitment, and (iv) normal nerve conduction studies. One side of the body is examined by EMG and, based on the results of the test, a muscle from the contralateral side may be biopsied. On histology, the muscle tissue reveals variable degrees of mononuclear cell infiltrate. The histologic features can be patchy, hence an open muscle biopsy is preferable to needle biopsy. In polymyositis, the lymphocytic infiltrates are present throughout the fascicles, whereas in dermatomyositis, they tend to be perifascicular and associated with perifascicular muscle atrophy. A variable degree of myophagocytosis is present, as is centralization of nuclei. Some fibers appear atrophic, and the regeneration of fibers occurs. Special histochemical stains rule out metabolic myopathies, and electron microscopy helps to identify inclusion body myositis and other less common entities.

The treatment of the idiopathic inflammatory myopathies starts with corticosteroids, generally prednisone, at a dose of 1 mg/kg per day taken orally in the morning. Treatment at this dose level is continued until a substantial fall in the CPK occurs. The patient's clinical response in terms of constitutional symptoms and weakness is usually fairly rapid. Once a laboratory response is achieved, a very gradual tapering schedule can begin, although it should be noted that by 6 months of therapy, the dose of prednisone is still roughly half the original starting dose. This emphasizes the rather slow pace of the taper that is employed in managing this illness. A rapid taper frequently results in a recurrence of the disease state. Second-line agents, such as methotrexate or azathioprine, can be added when patients require higher doses of steroids than are acceptable. Intravenous immunoglobulin (IVIg) has also been used with success in cases of refractory dermatomyositis. Hydroxychloroquine can be useful for the cutaneous manifestations of dermatomyositis.

It is not uncommon to be faced with the problem of recurrence of proximal muscle weakness after several months of moderate-dose to high-dose prednisone therapy. The question arises whether this represents a flare in the patient's underlying disease due to steroid tapering or whether the patient has developed an iatrogenic complication, that of steroid myopathy. Steroid myopathy mimics PM/DM clinically because the proximal muscles are more affected than the distal muscles. Typically, this is a painless weakness similar to the original inflammatory myopathy. Lower extremities such as hip flexors, quadriceps, and hamstrings tend to be affected to a greater degree than the proximal muscle groups in the upper extremities. Unlike a flare of PM/DM, however, CPK and other enzyme levels are normal in steroid myopathy. A muscle biopsy generally reveals noninflammatory findings. Primarily, steroid myopathy affects Type II fibers, those that are fast twitch or glycolytic in energy utilization, unlike PM/DM, which affects both Type I and Type II muscle fibers. Type II atrophy may also be seen in post inflammatory states and disuse atrophy, however, so the finding remains nonspecific. MRI with short inversion time inversion recovery (STIR) imaging is potentially useful in differentiating muscle edema (caused by active inflammation) from lipomatosis (caused by steroid therapy). If the clinical judgment is that the patient is experiencing a steroid myopathy, then the steroid taper should continue or be accelerated slightly. If, on the other hand, the clinical judgment is that the patient's new onset of weakness represents a flare of polymyositis or dermatomyositis, then treatment must be intensified, and a second-line agent must be considered.

An association between inflammatory myopathy and internal malignancy has been recognized for over a century. The stronger association appears to be with dermatomyositis, but a slight risk is also noted by some authors in patients with polymyositis. The type of malignancy generally reflects the expected malignancies for that patient's age and sex, though non-Hodgkin lymphoma is over-represented in both sexes, and ovarian cancer is over-represented in women. No consensus exists on the extent of the "malignancy work-up" at time of myositis diagnosis. Certainly, the patient should have a thorough history, physical examination, and baseline laboratory assessment, with age-appropriate cancer screening (mammography, for example) and follow-up on any abnormalities. Consider CT scanning of the chest, abdomen, and pelvis, because of the increased risk of non-Hodgkin lymphoma and ovarian

cancer. In patients with a concurrent malignancy, a recurrence of malignancy is often associated with recurrent myositis.

## REVIEW EXERCISES

### QUESTIONS

**1.** A 28-year-old woman presents with a 3-month history of fatigue, patchy hair loss, Raynaud's phenomenon, and joint stiffness, pain, and swelling in the small joints of the hands, the wrists, elbows, and knees. Your examination reveals normal vital signs, several shallow oral ulcers, frontal hair loss, and synovitis at the PIPs, MCPs, and wrist joints.

The most important test to obtain at this point is
a) Anti-double-stranded DNA antibodies
b) Anti-single-stranded DNA antibodies
c) Anti-Smith antibody
d) Microscopic examination of the urinalysis
e) Rheumatoid factor

**2.** A 48-year-old man has been followed for gradually progressive skin thickening, which began in the hands, and spread centrally to now extend to the upper arms, trunk, and face. He has been maintained on calcium channel blockers for Raynaud's phenomenon, although his borderline-low blood pressure has not allowed optimal dosing of the medicine for the vasospasm. He presents for a routine visit with increasing fatigue, some exertional shortness of breath, and a blood pressure of 160/100.

Your first action is
a) Arrange for pulmonary function testing to be done
b) Increase the calcium channel blocker
c) Order CBC with peripheral smear, serum creatinine, and institute treatment with an ACE-inhibitor
d) Order CBC with peripheral smear, serum creatinine, and institute treatment with D-penicillamine

**3.** Match the medication with the appropriate side-effect association (use each answer once):

| Medication | Side Effect |
|---|---|
| 1. Procainamide | a) Avascular necrosis of the femoral head |
| 2. Penicillamine | b) Acute narrow-angle glaucoma |
| 3. Pilocarpine | c) Acute onset pleurisy, fever, and joint pain |
| 4. Prednisone | d) Myasthenia gravis |

**4.** Match the physical exam finding with the appropriate diagnosis; use each answer once.
**1.** Rash over dorsum of the phalanges between the MCPs and PIPs
**2.** Rash over the dorsum of the MCPs and PIPs

3. Tendon friction rubs over the dorsum of the hands
4. Glossitis
a) Diffuse scleroderma
b) SLE
c) Sjögren's syndrome
d) Dermatomyositis

5. All of the following statements are true *except*
a) Patients with Sjögren's syndrome are at increased risk for development of Hodgkin's lymphoma.
b) Patients with dermatomyositis are at an increased risk for development of non-Hodgkin's lymphoma.
c) Patients with Sjögren's syndrome are at increased risk for development of non-Hodgkin's lymphoma.
d) Patients with lupus who have completed standard treatment for diffuse proliferative glomerulonephritis are at increased risk for development of bladder cancer.

6. Measures of lupus disease activity include all but
a) Anti-double-stranded DNA antibody levels
b) ANA levels
c) C3 (third component of complement)
d) C4 (fourth component of complement)

## CASE PRESENTATION

A 39-year-old woman presents to your office with concerns that she may have SLE because her younger sister has been recently diagnosed with that condition by another physician. Your patient describes fatigue, hair loss in the comb but no patchy "bald spots," a weight gain of 20 pounds in the past 6 months, and achy joints and muscles. She feels weak, and reports shortness of breath with minimal exertion (one flight of stairs). Her past medical history reveals Hashimoto's thyroiditis diagnosed 6 years ago, and she has been on thyroxine since then, although she has not had follow-up for that condition in over a year. She also has hypercholesterolemia and takes pravachol. Her social history reveals cigarette smoking, one pack per day, which she explains helps her to defray the stress of her job (she works full-time in a family owned restaurant as the business manager, shopper and part-time cook). The family history is notable for her father having committed suicide after a long struggle with depression. Her mother has thyroid disease and rheumatoid arthritis; her sister has recently diagnosed SLE, and her twin teenage sons are healthy, but have recently been on a brief detention from school after being caught drinking alcohol on the school premises. On review of systems, she denies Raynaud's phenomenon, hematuria, or pleurisy, but reports occasional painful mouth ulcers, dry mouth and dry eyes, trouble sleeping, and irregular and heavy menses.

Your examination reveals a BP of 135/85, pulse regular at 90, afebrile. Weight is 100 kg. Skin shows mild

eczema on the hands, with dry skin. The oral mucosa and hair density on the scalp both appear unremarkable. Eyes are moist, and Schirmer's testing documents 14 mm wetting OU. No enlargement of the thyroid, cervical lymph nodes, or major salivary glands is present. Chest and abdominal examinations are normal. The musculoskeletal exam reveals full strength in the distal muscle groups, but break-away testing proximally, with the patient complaining of soreness in the muscles on manual resistive testing. Tenderness is noted on palpation of the PIP, MCP, and wrist joints, without distinct synovitis, although the hands are somewhat chubby. The articular range of motion is normal throughout, with the patient remarking that the shoulders, neck, and hips feel achy during these maneuvers. The patient has tenderness to soft tissue palpation at 12 tender points.

7. Which of the following statements is true?
a) Stress may be playing a very significant role in this patient's presenting complaints.
b) A positive ANA will help establish a diagnosis of SLE in this patient.
c) Antibodies to SSA (Ro) and SSB (La) are likely to be present.
d) A normal CPK would rule out statin-related myopathy.

8. The least useful test on this visit would be
a) TSH
b) CPK
c) CBC
d) ANA

9. A treatment plan at the end of the first visit (before laboratory data available) would reasonably include which of the following?
a) Addition of prednisone, 5 to 10 mg/d
b) Discontinuation of pravachol
c) Decrease the thyroxine dose
d) Addition of hydroxychloroquine, 200 mg twice a day

## ANSWERS AND EXPLANATIONS

**1. d.**
The finding of an abnormal NA, suggesting glomerulonephritis, will dramatically alter therapy.

**2. c.**
This is scleroderma renal crisis, a true medical emergency.

**3. c, d, b, a.**

**4. b, d, a, c.**

**5. a.**
No explanation necessary.

**6. b.**
The ANA does not reliably fluctuate with disease activity.

## 7. a.

This patient presents, as many do, with many nonspecific complaints and with few objective findings. Even the manual resistive testing results are subjective to a degree because they depend on patient effort, which is determined in part by patient pain. The physician must consider a differential diagnosis that includes anemia (from heavy menses), hypothyroidism, statin-induced myopathy (which may occur with a normal CPK), and fibromyalgia (as suggested by the poor sleep, tender points, and stressful family/social situation). Other etiologies to consider include depression, smoking-related pulmonary disease, idiopathic inflammatory myopathies, and other disorders, the work-up for which will be guided by the first battery of test results.

## 8. d.

Although the patient is naturally concerned about SLE, she does not display any objective findings that would suggest this illness, and an ANA will not be helpful at this time because she might well have a positive ANA related to her Hashimoto's thyroiditis, and as a family member of someone with SLE. Likewise, with the lack of objective findings, SSA and SSB autoantibodies are unlikely to be positive.

## 9. b.

On the initial visit, counseling for stress reduction, smoking cessation, and weight loss would be in order. A pravachol "drug-holiday" would determine whether the myalgias and weakness were related to a statin side-effect. There is no immediate indication for corticosteroids nor hydroxychloroquine.

## SUGGESTED READINGS

### Systemic Lupus Erythematosus

Balow JE and Austin HA. Maintenance therapy for lupus nephritis—something old, something new. *N Engl J Med* 2004;350:1044–1046.

Cameron JS. Lupus nephritis. *J Am Soc Nephrol* 1999;10:413–424.

Chan TM, et al. Efficacy of mycophenolate mofetil in patients with diffuse proliferative lupus nephritis. *N Engl J Med* 2000;343:1156–1162.

Contreras G, et al. Sequential therapies for proliferative lupus nephritis. *N Engl J Med* 2004;350:971–980.

Dooley MA, Falk RJ. Immunosuppressive therapy of lupus nephritis. *Lupus* 1998;7:630–634.

Elkon K, Weissbach H, Brot N. Central nervous system function in systemic lupus erythematosus. *Neurochem Res* 1990;15:401–406.

James JA, Kaufman KM, Farris AD, et al. An increased prevalence of Epstein-Barr virus infection in young patients suggests a possible etiology for systemic lupus erythematosus. *J Clin Invest* 1997;100:3019–3026.

Korbet SM, Lewis EJ, Schwartz M, et al. Factors predictive of outcome in severe lupus nephritis. *Am J Kidney Dis* 2000;35:904–914.

Laman SD, Provost TT. Cutaneous manifestations of lupus erythematosus. *Rheum Dis Clin North Am* 1994;20:95–107.

Mandell BF. Cardiovascular involvement in systemic lupus erythematosus. *Semin Arthritis Rheum* 1987;17:126–141.

Santos-Ocampo AS, Mandell BF, Fessler BJ. Alveolar hemorrhage in systemic lupus erythematosus. *Chest* 2000;118:1083–1090.

Sibbitt WL, Jung RE, Brooks WM. Neuropsychiatric systemic lupus erythematosus. *Comp Ther* 1999;25(4):198–208.

Wallace DJ, Hahn BH, eds., *Dubois' Lupus Erythematosus*, 4th edition. Philadelphia: Lea & Febiger, 1993.

### Antiphospholipid Antibody Syndrome

Alarcon-Segovia D, et al. Prophylaxis of the antiphospholipid syndrome: a consensus report. *Lupus* 2003;12:499–503.

Bartholonew JR, Kottke-Marchange K. Monitoring anticoagulation therapy in patients with the lupus anticoagulant. *J Clin Rheumatol* 1998;4:307–311.

Esplin MS. Management of antiphospholipid syndrome during pregnancy. *Clin Obstet Gynecol* 2001;44:20–28.

Pierangeli SS, Gharavi AE, Harris N. Testing for antiphospholipid antibodies: problems and solutions. *Clin Obstet Gynecol* 2001;44:48–57.

Shoenfeld Y. Systemic antiphospholipid syndrome. *Lupus* 2003;12:497–498.

Valesini G, Pittoni V. Treatment of thrombosis associated with immunological risk factors. *Ann Med* 2000;32:41–45.

Vianna JL, Khamashta MA, Ordi-Ros J, et al. Comparison of the primary and secondary antiphospholipid syndrome: a European multicenter study of 114 patients. *Am J Med* 1994;96:3–9.

### Scleroderma

Cohen S, Laufer I, Snape WJ, et al. The gastrointestinal manifestations of scleroderma: pathogenesis and management. *Gastroenterology* 1980;79:155–166.

Helfrich DJ, Banner B, Steen VD, et al. Normotensive renal failure in systemic sclerosis. *Arthritis Rheum* 1989;32:1128–1134.

Rubin LJ, et al. Bosentan therapy for pulmonary arterial hypertension. *N Engl J Med* 2002;346:896–903.

Silver RM, Miller KS, Kinsella MB, et al. Evaluation and management of scleroderma lung disease using bronchoalveolar lavage. *Am J Med* 1990;88:470–476.

Steen VD, Costantino JP, Shapiro AP, et al. Outcome of renal crisis in systemic sclerosis: relation to availability of angiotensin converting enzyme (ACE) inhibitors. *Ann Intern Med* 1990;113:352–357.

White B, Moore WC, Wigley FM, et al. Cyclophosphamide is associated with pulmonary function and survival benefit in patients with scleroderma and alveolitis. *Ann Intern Med* 2000;132: 947–954.

### Sjögren's Syndrome

Alexander EL, Malinow K, Lejewski JE, et al. Primary Sjögren's syndrome with central nervous system disease mimicking multiple sclerosis. *Ann Intern Med* 1986;104:323–330.

Alexander EL, Beall SS, Gordon B, et al. Magnetic resonance imaging of cerebral lesions in patients with the Sjögren syndrome. *Ann Intern Med* 1988;108:815–823.

Davidson BKS, Kelly CA, Griffiths ID. Ten-year follow up of pulmonary function in patients with primary Sjögren's syndrome. *Ann Rheum Dis* 2000;59:709–712.

Kassan SS, Thomas TL, Moutsopoulos HM, et al. Increased risk of lymphoma in sicca syndrome. *Ann Intern Med* 1978;89:888–892.

Johnson R, Haga H, Gordon TP. Current concepts on diagnosis, autoantibodies and therapy in Sjögren's syndrome. *Scand J Rheumatol* 2000;29:341–348.

### Idiopathic Inflammatory Myopathy

Bohan A, Peter JB, Bowman RL, et al. A computer-assisted analysis of 153 patients with polymyositis and dermatomyositis. *Medicine* 1977;56:255–286.

Bunch TW. Polymyositis: a case history approach to the differential diagnosis and treatment. *Mayo Clin Proc* 1990;65:1480–1497.

Callen JP. Dermatomyositis. *Lancet* 2000;355:53–57.

Cherin P, Herson S, Wechsler B, et al. Efficacy of intravenous gamma-globulin therapy in chronic refractory polymyositis and dermatomyositis: an open study with 20 adult patients. *Am J Med* 1991;91:162–168.

Dalakas MC. Molecular immunology and genetics of inflammatory muscle diseases. *Arch Neurol* 1998;55:1509–1512.

Dalakas MC. Therapeutic approaches in patients with inflammatory myopathies. *Semin Neurol* 2003;23:199–206.

Hill CL, Zhang Y, Sigurgeirsson B, et al. Frequency of specific cancer types in dermatomyositis and polymyositis: a population-based study. *Lancet* 2001;357:96–100.

Kiely PDW, Bruckner FE, Nisbet JA, et al. Serum Skeletal troponin I in inflammatory muscle disease: relation to creatine kinase, CKMB and cardiac troponin I. *Ann Rheum Dis* 2000;59:750–751.

Rendt K. Inflammatory myopathies: narrowing the differential diagnosis. *Cleve Clin J Med* 2001;68:505–519.

# Systemic Vasculitis

## Leonard H. Calabrese    Gary S. Hoffman

The term *vasculitis* refers to a heterogeneous group of disorders sharing, to varying degrees, the pathologic features of a vascular inflammation that may be so severe that it progresses to vessel and tissue necrosis. Although vasculitis may stem from a variety of pathogenetic mechanisms, the primary vasculitides generally encompass syndromes that are suspected or proven to be immune mediated. This chapter reviews our current understanding of pathogenesis, classification, and the clinical spectrum of these disorders and provides a diagnostic and therapeutic approach to each disorder.

## ETIOLOGY AND PATHOGENESIS

Under normal circumstances, leukocytes only enter and pass through the walls of the smallest vessels (capillaries and postcapillary venules). They negotiate this passage between junctions of endothelial cells. In transmigrating into tissue to eliminate debris, foreign antigens, or apoptotic cells, the small vessels are not injured. In vasculitis, however, the leukocytes and their products leave the vascular lumen and damage the vessel wall itself (vasculitis). Whether necrosis is present or not, this constitutes the first step in vasculitis.

Since 1990, considerable progress has been made in understanding vascular inflammation. Before the mid-1980s, most theories of pathogenesis focused on the role of immune complexes (ICs). With the refinement of laboratory techniques, however, it has become apparent that IC deposition in tissues and vessels only explains the initiation of injury in a subset of patients with these diseases. Other mechanisms of vascular inflammation have been elucidated, and evidence supports at least five mechanisms in different types of vasculitis:

- IC deposition [serum sickness, hypersensitivity vasculitis (HV), Henoch-Schönlein purpura (HSP), vasculitis complicating viral and certain bacterial infections, cryoglobulinemia, or systemic lupus erythematosus (SLE)]
- Antibody targeting specific vascular structures (antibasement membrane disease, Goodpasture's syndrome)
- Antibody-associated diseases that target nonvascular structures: antineutrophil cytoplasmic antibodies (ANCA) not associated with IC deposition [including Wegener's granulomatosis (WG), microscopic polyangiitis (MPA), Churg-Strauss syndrome or disease (CSD)]
- Cell-mediated (primarily mononuclear cells) tissue injury [giant cell arteritis (GCA), Takayasu's arteritis (TA)]
- Combined mechanisms (WG, MPA, CSD)

Supporting evidence for circulating ICs in certain vasculitic conditions includes the following:

- Animal models of IC disease
- Identification of IC in tissues
- Identification of IC in the sera of patients with necrotizing vasculitis
- Identification of discrete antigens responsible for certain IC disorders

In humans, the identification of ICs in sera and tissues is supportive of their importance in certain diseases. In particular, the diseases within the HV group have the most strongly supported IC pathogenesis. True HV frequently follows exposure to a discrete antigen by 7 to 10 days and is often accompanied by evidence of IC activation and immunoglobulin or IC deposition in involved tissues.

### Antibody-Associated Disease

The discovery of ANCA in 1982 has been an important contribution. The presence of ANCA in an appropriate clinical setting has important implications for diagnosis and may enhance our understanding of pathogenesis in certain forms of vasculitis. ANCA were first identified with the use of indirect immunofluorescent (IIF) techniques in a small number of patients with crescentic glomerulonephritis (GN) and vasculitis. This was followed by the observations of a Dutch group that noted ANCA were frequently present in patients with WG and had an approximate correlation with disease activity. Since then, many investigators have confirmed and extended these findings, as well as documented the presence of ANCA in patients with a form of crescentic GN, MPA, and CSD, in which few or no ICs are present.

ANCA are divided on the basis of their immunofluorescent pattern and antigenic specificity:

- Diffuse cytoplasmic pattern (C-ANCA)
- Perinuclear pattern (P-ANCA)

The antigen almost always responsible (at least 80%) for the typical C-ANCA pattern is proteinase-3 (PR-3), a 29-kDa serine protease. The antigen most often associated with the P-ANCA pattern is the enzyme myeloperoxidase (MPO). For the latter example, however, the association is less robust. The P-pattern may also represent antibodies binding to lactoferrin, elastase, lysozyme, azurocidin, cathepsin G, and other enzyme antigens. MPO and PR-3 are located in the $\alpha$ or azurophilic granules of granulocytes and the cytosolic granules of monocytes. P-ANCA reactivity by immunofluorescence alone is nonspecific and, in the majority of patients, is owing to antinuclear antibodies (ANA) or cytoplasmic antigens other than MPO.

The classical ANCA-associated diseases share certain characteristics: vasculitis, with some neutrophilic component to the initial inflammatory infiltrate and crescentic GN, with scant or no IC deposition. Although only 50% to 90% of all cases are positive for ANCA, the following disorders have become known as ANCA-associated vasculitides:

- WG
- MPA
- CSD
- Idiopathic rapidly progressive crescentic GN

Although the sensitivity of ANCA in these diseases may vary, the best association has been with WG, in which antibodies have been noted in approximately 90% of patients with severe active multisystem disease, including GN. Antibodies to MPO are more likely to be found in patients with isolated renal disease (i.e., idiopathic rapidly progressive GN). The specificity of these assays depends on their technical performance attributes (whether done by immunofluorescence only or solid-phase assay). Most experts agree that the ANCA test is incomplete if it is only performed by IIF. If IIF is positive, an antigen-specific assay should be performed to determine if the reaction is to PR-3, MPO, or neither. A large number of conditions, including infections [e.g., endocarditis, sepsis, human immunodeficiency virus (HIV), malaria, tuberculosis], malignancies, and nonvasculitic, immune dysfunctional diseases (e.g., rheumatoid arthritis, systemic lupus, sclero-

derma, primary sclerosing cholangitis, ulcerative colitis, Kawasaki's disease, etc.) may be associated with antibody production to leukocyte antigens other than PR-3 or MPO and, rarely, even to PR-3 or MPO. Thus, IIF alone may be falsely positive and clinically misleading. In laboratories that perform IIF and antigen-specific assays, an IIF and PR-3 or MPO dual-positive is associated with a specificity of >95% for WG or MPA, respectively.

Given the moderately high sensitivity (~70%) and high specificity (>95%) under certain circumstances, antibodies against PR-3 or MPO can replace the need for biopsy proof of WG or MPA. These circumstances include a very high pretest probability for the presence of disease (on a clinical basis) and a confirmation against competing, mimicking diagnoses, especially infection. Although some investigators have suggested that these tests may be useful to monitor disease activity, most believe that the relationships between ANCA titers and clinically important events is too crude to allow ANCA to play a primary role in treatment decision making.

At present, it is uncertain whether ANCA are directly pathogenic, although evidence from sophisticated animal models and in vitro experiments suggest that this is likely. Evidence that is primarily in vitro suggests that this may be the case. Under certain circumstances, ANCA are capable of binding to activated neutrophils and enhancing the release of their toxic products. MPO and PR-3 released from neutrophils may bind to endothelial cells and cause injury by a direct action of the enzymes or by binding antibody that is already bound to neutrophils. Whether endothelial cells manufacture and express PR-3 remains a matter of controversy.

## Cellular-Mediated Vascular Injury

Neither GCA nor TA exhibits significant evidence of circulating ICs or specific antibodies. Their pathology is more suggestive of a cell-mediated injury. Both diseases involve macrophage and lymphocyte infiltration of the vessel wall. Mononuclear cells access the elastic (aorta and its primary branches) and medium-sized muscular arteries (temporal, coronary, distal extremity, etc.) via the vasa vasorum of the adventitia. The vasa vasorum usually remain unaffected. As the infiltrate migrates toward the primary lumen, the cytokine-mediated and enzyme-mediated destruction of muscle cells and elastic fibers ensues. If the vessel is slow to respond in regard to myointimal proliferation and the formation of fibrotic scar, aneurysm formation may follow. In general, if the aortic root is affected, then aneurysm formation is common. If aortic branch vessel disease occurs, the result is most often vascular stenosis.

## Immunoproliferative Disorders

Several vascular inflammatory disorders demonstrate strong evidence of being lymphoproliferative disorders; in particular, these include syndromes of benign lymphocytic angiitis and lymphomatoid granulomatosis/polymorphic reticulosis. These conditions are angiocentric and predominantly T-cell infiltrates, with little propensity for vessel necrosis. Frequently, they are the forerunners of frank T-cell lymphomas within the vascular wall (i.e., angiocentric lymphoma). Recent studies using gene rearrangement have demonstrated the clonal nature of many of these cases, even in the presence of morphologically benign disease.

Finally, it should be appreciated that most vasculitic syndromes represent admixtures of these proposed mechanisms. Among the best examples is WG, in which ANCA may play a role, but mounting evidence for macrophage and T-cell (especially Th1 type) injury is the focus of new therapies. In other settings, endothelium may be injured initially by antibody or ICs, leading to endothelial activation, secretion of cytokines, or increased display of adhesion molecules; this later becomes the focus for cell-mediated pathologic damage. In Kawasaki's disease, strong evidence suggests endothelial activation and cytokine release. A clearer understanding of the pathologic mechanisms involved in these syndromes will facilitate more specific therapies, including biologic response modifiers.

## CLASSIFICATION

The inciting causes of most forms of vasculitis remain unknown, and the features of pathogenesis are often incompletely understood. Consequently, the clinician has had to combine a knowledge of the typical clinical characteristics and pathologic features of each disease to derive a working diagnosis on which to base treatment. Many classifications have been put forth in an effort to facilitate this process. Most schemes continue to be works in progress. Although they have been useful to ensure the homogeneity of patients for clinical studies, these classification schemes cannot substitute for a thorough knowledge of each illness. The following classification represents an admixture of several classification schemes, taking into account some features of vessel size and clinical features:

- Polyarteritis nodosa (PAN): classic (exclusively medium vessel disease)
- Immune complexes scant or absent group (small to medium vessels), ANCA-associated
- MPA
- WG
- CSD
- IC-mediated diseases
- True HV
- HSP
- Cryoglobulinemia
- Hypocomplementemic vasculitis

- Vasculitis associated with malignancy
- Vasculitis associated with a primary immune dysfunctional systemic disease
- Large vessel, mononuclear cell inflammatory disease
- GCA
- TA
- Overlap disorders
- Miscellaneous conditions
- Primary angiitis of the central nervous system (CNS)
- Behçet's disease
- Others

Recently, several newer classification schemes were proposed by the American College of Rheumatology and an international cooperative group, but neither group has significantly advanced an understanding of the relationships among these disorders.

## CLINICAL PRESENTATION AND DIAGNOSIS

As a group, the vasculitides remain formidable challenges to physicians from a diagnostic and therapeutic perspective. Diagnostically, the signs and symptoms of vasculitis are generally nonspecific because they represent vascular ischemia, regardless of the cause. Certain vasculitic syndromes present greater diagnostic challenges than others because of the nature and distribution of their target-organ involvement. For example, when the skin is involved, such as in the HV group, it is apparent that vasculitis is the underlying process, but a greater challenge is to determine the precise etiology and thus the prognosis and treatment. In the absence of the typical signs of vasculitis, such as a characteristic rash or signs of peripheral ischemia, systemic vasculitis may mimic a wide variety of nonvasculitic diseases. Warning signs or symptoms of systemic vasculitis include the following:

- Fever of unknown origin (FUO) with constitutional symptoms
- Unexplained multisystem disease
- Unexplained inflammatory arthritis
- Unexplained myalgias
- Suspicious rash
- Mononeuritis multiplex
- Unexplained end-organ ischemia
- GN

When a careful work-up for other causes is unrevealing, these findings should alert clinicians to the possibility of systemic vasculitis. Certain of these signs or symptoms have a greater degree of sensitivity or specificity, depending on the clinical situation. For example, mononeuritis multiplex in the absence of diabetes or trauma is highly specific and should always be considered indicative of vasculitis until proved otherwise. Other signs, such as unexplained myalgias or arthritis, are relatively nonspecific and may be mimicked by a wide variety of conditions.

## SPECIFIC SYSTEMIC VASCULITIS CONDITIONS

### Polyarteritis Nodosa

First described more than 100 years ago by Kussmaul and Maier, PAN is an uncommon disease affecting small-sized and medium-sized muscular arteries. In classic PAN, capillaries and venules are spared. The general characteristics of PAN include:

- More common in men than women (~2:1)
- Most common between 40 and 60 years of age, although can occur at any age

#### Pathophysiology

PAN has been reported in association with hepatitis B and has thus been considered to be IC in origin. Most authorities would reserve the term *PAN* for only those patients who do not have a known association with an infection, malignancy, or other primary illness. Thus, these PAN-like conditions would be referred to as *endocarditis-associated vasculitis*, *hepatitis B–associated vasculitis*, etc. Only approximately 5% to 10% of patients with purely medium-sized vessel vasculitis have evidence of hepatitis B, whereas the remaining patients represent a syndrome of idiopathic disease that in time will be subclassified when the etiology is better understood. Diseases that have been associated with a PAN-like syndrome include:

- Hairy cell leukemia
- Endocarditis
- Connective tissue disease (rheumatoid arthritis, SLE, scleroderma, Sjögren's syndrome, etc.)
- Drug abuse
- HIV infection

In the presence of these other systemic diseases, a diagnosis of primary idiopathic PAN cannot be made.

#### Clinical Presentation and Pathologic Features

The clinical and pathologic features of PAN reflect medium-sized vessel disease and include the following:

- Common features
  □ Cardiac, gastrointestinal (GI), CNS, and peripheral nervous system disease
  □ Hypertension
- Fever and constitutional symptoms
  □ Livedo reticularis
- Uncommon features
  □ Eosinophilia, allergy, and lung disease
- Absent features
  □ GN

  □ Pulmonary hemorrhage
  □ Palpable purpura

#### Diagnosis

##### Angiography and Biopsy

The presence of the cardinal signs and symptoms of vasculitis may be the first clue to its presence. The diagnosis must be based on characteristic angiographic findings or biopsy (tissue evidence of vasculitis).

Significant debate arises over which is the first test to choose in the process of diagnosing this condition; however, several generalizations can be made:

- Studies or biopsies of clinically normal organs are usually unrewarding. If a biopsy is to be performed, features of disease should be present at that site, whether there be clinical, laboratory, or imaging abnormalities.
- Consider a biopsy of nodular or tender skin lesions, tender muscles, or peripheral nerve in the setting of neuropathy.
- Consider mesenteric and renal angiography if appropriate signs or symptoms are present (e.g., pain, blood in stools, abnormal hepatic or pancreatic enzymes, new onset hypertension). Approximately 70% to 80% of patients with PAN will have abnormal angiograms, with 75% of these patients demonstrating classic multiple microaneurysms.

##### Laboratory Studies

No specific laboratory tests are available for PAN. The most sensitive laboratory findings are elevations in levels of acute-phase reactants, including erythrocyte sedimentation rate (ESR). Elevated white blood cell count and anemia are also frequently present. Circulating ICs and hypocomplementemia are helpful when present, but these are absent in the majority of patients. ANCA (both PR-3 and MPO) are generally absent. The following generalizations regarding laboratory tests for PAN can be made:

- They are mostly useful for ruling out other diagnoses (e.g., infection, malignancy, coagulopathy).
- Acute-phase reactants and a complete blood cell count, if normal, have a high negative predictive value.
- ICs, complement, and autoantibodies are of limited use.

#### Prognosis

Prognostic factors in PAN include the following:

- Poor prognostic markers [5-factor score (FFS)]
  1. GI involvement
  2, 3. Renal involvement (proteinuria, azotemia)
  4. Cardiomyopathy
  5. CNS involvement

In addition, patients older than 50 years had worse outcomes.

In one large series of 278 patients with PAN, MPA, or CSD, mortality at 7.3 years (mean) was 31%. Patient

**TABLE 32.1**

**OUTCOME IN PATIENTS WITH POLYARTERITIS NODOSA**

| Intervention | 5-Yr Survival (%) |
|---|---|
| None | <15 |
| Corticosteroids | 55–70 |
| Corticosteroids and cyclophosphamide | >80 |

mortality could be stratified based on FFS risk, however. The greater the number of critical organs involved, the worse the prognosis. This may serve as a guide for treatment.

If PAN is untreated, the 5-year survival rate is 10% to 15% (Table 32.1). With the use of corticosteroids, the 5-year survival rate can improve to 50%. In recent years, combination therapy with CP and high doses of corticosteroid has been reported to increase the 5-year survival rate to 80% or more. The advantage of adding CP to corticosteroids becomes more obvious with increasing disease severity.

PAN-like disease associated with hepatitis B appears to have a more serious prognosis. A recent study from France suggested that therapy with interferon-$\alpha$ may provide a higher rate of recovery for this subset of patients.

### Treatment

The treatment of PAN generally adheres to the principles of therapy for systemic vasculitis outlined in the final section of this chapter. Glucocorticoids alone may be indicated for people with limited or non–life-threatening disease. The presence of an underlying viral infection such as HBV, HCV or HIV (present in less than 5% of patients) requires special considerations on the need for combined therapy of both the inflammatory and infectious process.

## Immune Complex Scant or Absent (Pauci-immune) Vasculitis of Small- and Medium-Sized Vessels

A family of vasculitic diseases that are often considered together include Wegener's granulomatosis (WG), Churg-Strauss disease (CSD), and microscopic polyangiitis (MPA). These conditions are characterized by the following:

- Shared renal lesion of pauci-immune, crescentic, necrotizing GN
- Propensity for renal and pulmonary involvement (pulmonary-renal syndrome)
- Varying frequency of ANCA
- High rate of relapse (especially when renal involvement is present)

The diseases may be clinically distinct or difficult to distinguish.

## Microscopic Polyangiitis

The European literature is replete with descriptions of MPA. MPA generally refers to a vasculitis that involves small vessels (i.e., capillaries, venules, arterioles, and small arteries), with little or no IC deposition. MPA has a predilection for the lungs, which pathologically display capillaritis without granuloma formation (distinguishing it from WG). It is frequently associated with ANCA (anti-MPO). Differentiation from WG may be difficult at times when the pathology is not classically abnormal. At times, MPA may resemble PAN because larger vessels may also be involved in MPA. When diffuse pulmonary hemorrhage occurs, MPA has a very poor prognosis, comparable to that of WG.

Characteristics include the following:

- Nongranulomatous vasculitis involving small and sometimes medium vessels
- Renal involvement common (rapidly progressive GN)
- Pulmonary involvement common (alveolar hemorrhage)
- ANCA positive in 50% to 80%
- Angiographic abnormalities uncommon (although most cases not studied by angiography)

The treatment of MPA should generally follow the principles of therapy outlined at the end of the chapter.

## Wegener's Granulomatosis

Wegener's granulomatosis affects 1 in 20,000 to 30,000 Americans. It is characterized by upper and lower respiratory disease and GN, plus the pathologic features of necrotizing, granulomatous inflammation with and without vasculitis. Many other organ systems also may be involved. This disorder, if untreated, in its fully expressed form is uniformly fatal. Combined treatment with corticosteroids and CP, however, can achieve long-term remissions in the vast majority of patients.

The clinical manifestations of WG include:

- Prominent constitutional symptoms
- Upper and/or lower respiratory tract symptoms such as rhinitis, epistaxis, sinusitis, otitis media, hearing loss, cough, hemoptysis, tracheitis, subglottic stenosis, and shortness of breath
- Pulmonary and renal disease can vary from being minor and asymptomatic to severe
- Renal disease occurs in a minority at presentation but is present in the majority over time
- Other target organs: eyes, ears, skin, CNS or peripheral nervous system, and joints

### Diagnosis

In the past, the diagnosis of WG depended on the appropriate clinical picture and a compatible biopsy. Sampling error and the patchy nature of the underlying pathology have made the interpretation of biopsy material problematic. Characteristic pathologic findings include:

- Granuloma formation
- Necrotizing vasculitis
- Tissue necrosis, especially in a "geographic pattern"

Because these features may also be in seen in the setting of infection, all biopsies should be evaluated with that in mind (cultures and special stains for infectious agents).

Nasal biopsy often shows only nonspecific inflammation or necrosis, but in approximately 50% of cases, necrotizing vasculitis, granulomatous inflammation, or both, can be identified. Renal biopsy generally demonstrates a segmental, necrotizing, crescentic GN of the pauci-immune variety (indistinguishable from that found in MPA and idiopathic rapidly progressive GN). Percutaneous renal biopsy occasionally shows vasculitis outside the glomerulus. Open lung biopsy is more invasive but gives a higher yield of ~90% characteristic features. Use of antibody detection to PR-3 (i.e., C-ANCA) can replace the need for tissue confirmation in limited circumstances when the pretest probability of disease is high (Table 32.2). Meticulous attention must be given to ruling out underlying infection. As previously noted, the diagnosis of WG has been greatly enhanced by the development of ANCA testing.

### Treatment

The treatment of WG relies on the principles of therapy outlined at the end of this chapter. In general, patients with life-threatening disease are treated with a combination of high-dose prednisone and CP until remission is achieved; they are then "stepped down" to an antimetabolite, such as methotrexate or azathiprine, for the duration of therapy. Methotrexate therapy may be substituted for CP as primary therapy in patients who do not have immediately life-threatening disease and who have a serum creatinine level of less than or equal to 2.0 mg/dL. Of final note, trimetho-

prim-sulfamethoxazole has been demonstrated to be efficacious in decreasing the rate of upper respiratory flares and may be incorporated into the regime, especially in those with disease limited to the upper airways. It is generally agreed, however, that this therapy should not be applied as primary therapy to any patient with a significant risk of morbidity (i.e., with features beyond mild upper airway disease).

### Prognosis

Untreated, patients with typical WG survive a mean of 5 months. Survival is greatly improved with combination therapy (CP and prednisone). Treatment-related morbidity develops in 50% of patients.

## Churg-Strauss Disease (Syndrome)

Churg-Strauss disease is also known as *allergic angiitis* and *granulomatosis*. CSD was first described in 1951, in a group of patients with necrotizing vasculitis, a history of adult-onset asthma, and striking eosinophilia. CSD is clinically more rare than PAN or WG. In one study from the United Kingdom, the annual incidence was estimated to be 3.1 per 1.0 million population. CSD has a predilection for small vessels and medium-sized muscular arteries. The upper airways (sinusitis, allergic rhinitis) and lungs are nearly always involved. Other common sites of disease include the skin, GI tract, heart, peripheral nervous system, and kidneys. CSD should be suspect in any person with recent-onset asthma who develops palpable purpura or cutaneous infarction, peripheral neuropathy, GI ischemia, cardiomyopathy, or nephritis. The laboratory hallmark of CSD is peripheral eosinophilia, which is generally greater than 1,500 cells/mm$^3$. Finally, recent epidemiologic studies have provided data incriminating the use of leukotriene inhibitors in triggering some cases of CSD. These studies are problematic, however, given that their use in an asthmatic population often leads to decreased glucocorticoid use, thus perhaps unmasking latent CSD. Despite these criticisms, occasional patients have been reported who have relapsed upon rechallenge with these agents, thus leading most clinicians to avoid their use if at all possible in patients with CSD.

In summary, CSD is marked by the following features:

- Allergic rhinitis/sinusitis, ~70%
- Asthma (or history of asthma), 100%
- Pulmonary infiltrates, ~70%
- Cardiomyopathy, ~50%
- Peripheral neuropathy, ~65%
- CNS involvement, ~25%, seizures, coma, infarction, confusion, and hydrocephalus
- Myalgias or arthralgias, ~50%
- GN, ~40%

Vasculitis may be preceded by asthma and/or allergic rhinitis for many years.

### TABLE 32.2

**HIGH PRETEST PROBABILITY OF WEGENER'S GRANULOMATOSIS**

| C-ANCA | P-ANCA |
|---|---|
| >95% PR-3 | 85% ANA |
| 5% other | 10% MPO |
| Cytoplasmic/ethanol | 5% Non-MPO |
| Cytoplasmic/formalin | Cathepsin G |
| Lactoferrin | — |
| Others | |
| Ethanol (P) | |
| Formalin (C) | |

ANA, antinuclear antibodies; C-ANCA, diffuse cytoplasmic pattern antineutrophil cytoplasmic antibody; MPO, myeloperoxidase; P-ANCA, perinuclear antineutrophil cytoplasmic antibodies.

*Pathology*

CSD is a small- to medium-sized vessel disease that may progress to fibrinoid necrosis, infiltration with eosinophils, and granuloma formation.

*Treatment*

The initial treatment for CSD is generally a high-dose corticosteroid following the principles of therapy outlined at the end of the chapter. Cytotoxic drugs, such as CP, are reserved for patients with critical organ system involvement (see Prognosis section under Polyarteritis Nodosa) or those with disease refractory to corticosteroids. In a recent series of 64 patients with CSD, at a mean period of 7.3 years follow-up, 69% had survived.

## "Hypersensitivity" Vasculitis Group

The concept that hypersensitivity mechanisms could result in vasculitis was first proposed by Zeek and colleagues in 1948. HV may follow exposure to drugs or serum or be related to recent infection. In many cases, however, no evidence exists for such factors playing a role. The most frequent feature of HV is involvement of the skin (palpable purpura and maculopapular lesions). Skin biopsies usually reveal small-vessel (capillaries and venules) inflammation, with leukocytoclasis (nuclear fragmentation).

*Pathogenesis*

The etiology of this group of disorders is diverse, but strong evidence suggests that most cases have IC deposits in vessels. ICs also can be often detected in the serum.

*Diagnosis*

Various disorders may present with palpable purpuric or macular skin lesions and have occult evidence of other diagnoses or develop the features of other illnesses over time. Examples include WG, MPA, SLE, and other systemic immune disorders. As a consequence, such findings should serve as the clinical starting point for the differential diagnosis:

- Idiopathic HV (functionally at bottom of list, after all else ruled out)
- Drug-induced HV
- Infection-associated vasculitis
- HSP
- Cryoglobulinemia
- Connective tissue–associated vasculitis
- Malignancy-associated vasculitis
- Urticarial hypersensitivity
- Cutaneous manifestations of systemic vasculitis (i.e., MPA, WG, CSD)
- Livedo vasculitis
- Erythema elevatum diutinum
- Other forms of systemic necrotizing vasculitis

*Treatment*

True HV, caused by an exposure to exogenous antigen, is the most common syndrome within the HV group. Diverse antigens have been incriminated:

- Drugs
- Infectious agents
- Chemicals
- Immunizations
- Insect bites
- Foreign proteins

The clinical course of patients with HV is variable and usually self-limiting. In some cases, HV can be recurrent or chronic. Cutaneous disease may be associated with constitutional symptoms (fever, malaise, weight loss) or visceral inflammation. When precipitating events are identified, a pattern of illness usually develops 7 to 10 days after exposure and resolves within a 4- to 6-week period.

The treatment of true HV should focus primarily on removal of the inciting antigen. If the antigen is a drug, it should be discontinued, and if an infection is incriminated, it should be treated. Many patients require no treatment, whereas patients with more severe disease may require antihistamines, colchicine, corticosteroids, or, for severe cases, the addition of cytotoxic drugs.

## Henoch-Schönlein Purpura

Henoch-Schönlein purpura is a syndrome characterized by palpable purpura and varying degrees of polyarthralgias, arthritis, myalgias, GI ischemia, and GN. Constitutional symptoms such as fever, malaise, and anorexia may be present. HSP is most common in children, although adults may be affected as well. The median age of onset is 4 years. Tissue injury is mediated by immunoglobulin A–containing (less often immunoglobulin G) ICs, which can be identified within the tissues, especially the kidney. Biopsies of the skin reveal (as with HV) leukocytoclastic vasculitis. In ~60% of cases, a preceding infection has been implicated as a disease trigger. Suspected agents include streptococci, mycoplasmic pneumonia, *Yersinia*, *Legionella*, *Helicobacter pylori*, Epstein-Barr virus, hepatitis B, varicella, adenovirus, cytomegalovirus, and parvovirus B19. As with HV, allergens and drugs have been implicated as well.

The treatment of HSP depends on its severity. Mild disease requires essentially no therapy, whereas life-threatening visceral disease may require corticosteroids and possibly even cytotoxic drugs. In controlled trials, the use of these agents has not been demonstrated to prevent or improve the course of nephritis in HSP patients. A recent study suggested that intravenous γ-globulin may be effective in stabilizing (but not improving) renal function in HSP and immunoglobulin A nephropathy (Rostoker et al., 1994).

## Cryoglobulinemia

Much progress has been made in the understanding of cryoglobulinemia in the past 3 years. Cryoglobulins are characterized on the basis of their content:

- Type I: monoclonal (containing a single immunoglobulin)—most often seen in the presence of lymphoproliferative diseases such as B-cell malignancies
- Type II: mixed (containing a monoclonal and polyclonal immunoglobulin) or monoclonal—often considered to be of unknown or "essential" origin
- Type III: mixed or polyclonal

Recently, an association was established between hepatitis C virus (HCV) infection and type II mixed cryoglobulinemia. This association was based on the following:

- Serologic evidence of exposure to HCV in 90% of cases previously thought to be "essential"
- Evidence of active HCV infection
- Concentration of HCV RNA and antibodies to HCV within the cryoglobulin
- HCV deposition in blood vessels or kidneys

Previously, most cases of type II were believed to be idiopathic. There have been rare reports of HBV associated with cryoglobulinemia, but these represent only a minority of cases. Many studies have now confirmed that HCV RNA is found in the serum and cryoprecipitate in the majority of patients with type II cryoglobulinemia. Estimates range from 30% to 98%, depending on the techniques used. With the use of molecular techniques (polymerase chain reaction), HCV has been identified and found to be present up to 1,000-fold in the cryoprecipitate. It is controversial whether an HCV antibody can be identified in the cryoprecipitate.

The signs and symptoms in patients with HCV-associated cryoglobulinemia include the following (Table 32.3):

- Palpable purpura
- Arthralgia
- Weakness
- Peripheral neuropathy
- GN (most frequently membranoproliferative)
- Hepatomegaly and/or splenomegaly
- Skin ulcers

The association of HCV and cryoglobulinemia has provided the rationale for more specific treatment using interferon-α, which is approved to treat chronic active hepatitis secondary to HCV infection. Preliminary reports suggest that the majority of patients with cryoglobulinemia and HCV may favorably respond to a treatment course lasting 3 months or longer. Some patients have sustained long-term remissions (up to 40 months) after discontinuing interferon. A recent controlled trial has demonstrated clinical improvement in the majority of patients; however, all patients experienced relapse after discontinuation of interferon.

Traditional therapies for type II cryoglobulinemia were directed at decreasing the formation or deposition of cryoglobulins and relied on immunosuppression and apheresis. After a time, a moderate risk exists for the development of lymphoproliferative disease with this condition, and thus alkylating agents (e.g., CP) should be avoided wherever possible. Although the overall prognosis for patients with type II cryoglobulinemia is good, the prognosis depends on the severity of visceral involvement, especially in regard to the kidneys. No controlled trials have been undertaken of any agents used in the treatment of cryoglobulinemia. Most investigators agree that apheresis is useful in controlling many of the acute manifestations, but cryoglobulin levels are quick to rebound after discontinuation of treatment. Other therapies reported to have been palliative include anti-inflammatory drugs, antihistamines, and intravenous immunoglobulin IVIg. The following points should be considered when selecting therapy:

- Controlled studies of steroids, cytotoxic agents, or apheresis have not been conducted.
- Morbidity and mortality are related to the severity of organ involvement.
- A high rate of lymphoproliferative transformation occurs.
- Antiviral (interferon-α plus ribavirin) therapy has been associated with clinical improvement and may be appropriate for some patients.
- In the presence of active HCV infection, the use of prolonged immunosupression may have adverse effects on the underlying infectious process.
- HCV-infected patients with symptomatic cryoglobulinemia should be co-managed by a skilled hepatologist and a therapist knowledgable in the use of immunsupressive drugs.

## TABLE 32.3
### MIXED CRYOGLOBULINEMIA: CLINICAL PROFILE

| Manifestation | Frequency (%) |
| --- | --- |
| Palpable purpura | 80–100 |
| Arthralgia | 50–90 |
| Weakness/fatigue | 70–100 |
| Glomerulonephritis | 20–75 |
| Polyneuropathy | 20–70 |
| Liver involvement[a] | 60–90 |
| Cryoglobulins in chronic hepatitis | 40–70 |

[a] Lymphoproliferative disease (B-cell non-Hodgkin lymphoma).

## Giant Cell Arteritis Group

Temporal arteritis or GCA of the elderly increases in frequency with age. GCA is seldom seen before 50 years of age. It is relatively uncommon in African Americans. Classic symptoms include:

- Severe unusual headache and/or scalp tenderness
- Transient visual disturbances (amaurosis fugax)
- Blindness
- Jaw claudication
- Polymyalgia rheumatica in 50% of patients
- Large vessel–related ischemia (arm claudication) or aortic aneurysms (thoracic much greater than abdominal)
- Fever, malaise, or weight loss

This picture is even more characteristic when it occurs in a patient with polymyalgia rheumatica. The relationship between these two conditions is complex; pure examples of each are well recognized, and the coexistence of these conditions occurs in more than 50% of cases. Increasing evidence indicates that GCA is a more severe form of polymyalgia rheumatica (i.e., they are part of a continuum of vascular inflammatory disease).

Temporal arteritis is a granulomatous inflammation of the arterial wall with destruction of the internal elastic lamina and giant cell formation. Diagnosis depends on a temporal artery biopsy. If clinical suspicion is high and vision is threatened, this condition should be treated as a medical emergency, using high doses of corticosteroids. Negative biopsy results do occur because lesions tend to be patchy in nature. The ESR is usually markedly elevated, although 10% to 20% of cases may have a normal ESR. Serum IL6 levels, a reflection of macrophage activation, appear to be more sensitive than the ESR and C-reactive protein but at present are not commercially available for routine use.

The treatment of temporal arteritis consists of high doses of prednisone, 40 to 60 mg/day for ~4 weeks, then tapering to the lowest dose that maintains freedom from symptoms and suppression of the ESR. Many patients require treatment for many years. In patients resistant or highly dependent on glucocorticoids, there are few desirable options for the clinician. Several recent controlled trials of steroid-sparing agents, such as methotrexate, have yielded mixed results.

## Takayasu's Arteritis

Takayasu's arteritis (TA) is a form of large-vessel vasculitis that occurs mostly in young women. Prevalence is ~2.6 cases per 1 million population. Although it has been first and most often described in Asia, it has also been reported to occur in young individuals of many other races, including African Americans and Whites. Men may be affected as well, and they make up 10% to 20% of most series. Other than this demographic peculiarity, little distinguishes TA as a nosologic entity from generalized GCA of the elderly with large-vessel involvement. The latter may occur in 15% to >90% of GCA cases. This range is broad because of the different means of identifying large vessel disease in different series (clinical vs. postmortem).

Some characteristics of TA include:

- Large-vessel granulomatous arteritis, primarily affecting the aorta and its branches. A predilection exists for aortic arch vessels, especially the subclavian arteries.
- Clinical features generally reflect extremity or end-organ (enteric, cardiac, CNS) ischemia resulting from a stenosis of involved arteries. The aortic arch is more prone to aneurysm formation than stenosis.
- Systemic or constitutional and musculoskeletal symptoms and headache each occur in ~50% of cases.

Among 60 patients (median age, 25 years) described by Kerr (1995), a variable presentation occurred, ranging from asymptomatic to catastrophic. In addition:

- Stenosis was present in 98% and aneurysms in 27%.
- ESR was not a reliable guide for disease activity.
- Surgical specimens showed active disease in 44% of patients who were believed to be clinically inactive.
- Bypass surgery was palliative but often followed by partial restenosis in ~30% of cases.
- Angioplasty for stenotic lesions was followed by partial or complete restenosis in ~45% of cases.
- Glucocorticoids with or without cytotoxics failed to control the disease in 25% of patients.

The most common presentation is claudication of the upper extremities. An involvement of the aorta occurs in ~65% of cases and may lead to aneurysm formation (especially root, with aortic regurgitation) or stenosis (especially abdominal aorta). Lightheadedness and, rarely, strokes may be due to multivessel disease of carotids and vertebral arteries. GI ischemia may result from stenoses and occlusion of the celiac or mesenteric arteries. Hypertension may affect 32% to 93% of cases and is usually due to renal artery stenosis or occlusion. In some parts of Asia, TA is the most common cause of childhood hypertension. Coronary artery involvement is less common but, when present, is usually due to proximal vessel stenoses.

The histopathologic features of TA are identical to those of GCA of the elderly. Laboratory studies are not particularly helpful, and, although the ESR is usually elevated, it may be normal in the presence of active disease.

### Treatment of Giant Cell Arteritis

The treatment for GCA and TA is corticosteroids. Cytotoxic drugs, including methotrexate, may be useful in refractory cases. Surgical intervention is often required in TA and has been reported to be successful.

It is critical to recognize that the treatment of TA does not merely consist of the use of immunosuppressive agents. Hypertension must be recognized and controlled if serious morbidity is to be avoided in the forms of hypertensive heart disease, stroke, or renal failure. The continuity of flow from the aortic root to extremity vessels must be anatomically defined. A stenotic lesion may be responsible for a misleading low-extremity cuff blood pressure compared to the central aortic arch pressure. Occasionally, all extremity pressures are misleading because of bilateral subclavian (or innominate), iliac, and femoral stenoses. A stenotic abdominal aorta may also cause leg pressures to be misleading. Severe extremity claudication, severe aortic regurgitation, or coronary artery disease may require surgical therapy. The complexity of these cases requires a team approach that includes generalists, rheumatologists, and vascular specialists in imaging and surgery if the patient is to have the best possible outcome.

## Polyangiitis Overlap Syndrome

The term *polyangiitis overlap syndrome* is intended to recognize the imprecise nature of current classification systems that are based on descriptive anatomy, symptoms, and histopathology without benefit of more precise information about etiology and pathogenesis. "Overlap" also recognizes that patients exist who may have features of multiple entities that have been named and reviewed, such as a concurrence of HV and GCA, WG and PAN, or TA and cutaneous vasculitis.

## PRINCIPLES OF THERAPY FOR SYTEMIC VASCULITIS

The therapy of systemic vasculitis involves more than just focusing on the vascular inflammatory process. Regardless of the type of vasculitis being treated, the physician must consider the following:

- Treatment of events caused by disease itself (e.g., hypertension, organ ischemia, tissue necrosis)
- Patient-associated variables (e.g., corticosteroid-aggravated diabetes, heart failure, or mental status changes)
- Disease activity, which may change during the course of treatment and require adjustment in therapies
- Treatment toxicity, which may require new medications, changes in the initial plan, or choices of interventions
- *Pneumocystis carinii* pneumonia prophylaxis, which should be part of any program of immunosuppressive therapy that is likely to produce significant lymphopenia
- Osteoporosis prophylaxis or treatment, which should be part of all protocols
- Cancer, which may complicate the use of certain therapies
- Bladder complications, which may follow extended use of cyclophosphamide

Treatment of systemic vasculitis occurs in three phases:

- Acute phase: initial control of disease
- Subacute phase: tapering of immunosuppression to limit treatment- and disease-associated comorbidities
- Consolidation phase: minimization of long-term toxicity and ultimate discontinuation of therapy

Successful outcomes are highly dependent on a meticulous monitoring for complications of therapy as well as careful assessments for following disease activity.

The therapy of systemic vasculitis varies depending on severity, prognosis, and rate of disease progression. Certain types of vasculitis may be self-limiting and merely require careful monitoring (HSP, some cases of HV). Treatment should always be individualized. General guidelines for the treatment of the more severe vasculitides (including PAN, WG, CSD, MPA, and all forms refractory to steroids alone) include the initial use of one or more of the following agents:

- Corticosteroid (prednisone) or equivalent, 1 mg/kg in the acute phase with a tapering of dose (part of all protocols)
- Cyclophosphamide, 2 mg/kg orally (daily CP remains the most effective proven therapy for severe disease. Higher doses can be used in the first 3 to 4 days of treatment in disparate circumstances).
- Cyclophosphamide P, 0.5 to 1.0 g/m$^2$ intravenously every 3 to 4 weeks.

## Step-Down Therapy

A recent advance in the efforts to reduce treatment-related morbidity and mortality is the employment of the so-called "step down" approach. This strategy takes advantage of the potency of the alkyator class of drugs and their ability to induce remissions in patients with life-threatening forms of disease by limiting the time to which patients are exposed to them. In general, when cyclophosphamide therapy is initiated, it is continued only for as long as necessary to achieve a remission from all signs of active disease. This generally takes about 3 months but may be shorter or much longer depending on the individual case. This is then followed by switching to a less toxic agent, such as methotrexate, azathioprine, or mycophenolate, for the duration of therapy. A series of studies have demonstrated the safety and efficacy of this approach, and most now consider this to be the standard of care.

For patients with non–life-threatening presentations, methotrexate may be substituted for cyclophosphamide as primary therapy. The dose is generally 15 mg to start, with titration up to 25 mg/week depending on intervening toxicity (avoid if serum creatinine >2 mg/dL).

Cyclophosphamide toxicity may cause or contribute to the following:

- Infections, especially because of profound immunosuppression that occurs with the combination of cyclophosphamide + corticosteroids [One should try to avoid severe leukopenia (total white blood cells <3,500/mm$^3$, absolute neutrophil count <1,500/mm$^3$) but expect lymphopenia.]
- Drug-induced cystitis, which can rarely be hemorrhagic
- Gonadal dysfunction, sterility

- Bladder cancer
- After extended use, lymphoproliferative and myeloproliferative diseases
- Miscellaneous: nausea, vomiting, rash, hepatitis, and hypersensitivity reactions
- Biologic therapies such as inhibitors of TNF, monoclonal antibodies and others should be considered experimental at the present time

## REVIEW EXERCISES

### QUESTIONS

**1.** Symptoms and signs that may lead to a diagnosis of underlying systemic necrotizing vasculitis include
a) Mononeuritis multiplex
b) FUO
c) Unexplained end-organ ischemia
d) Red blood cell casts in the urine
e) All of the above

**2.** A 50-year-old man was admitted with a 3-month history of fever, weight loss, abdominal pain, and hypertension. A detailed FUO workup was unrevealing. Pertinent physical findings included a blood pressure of 220/120 mm Hg, livedo reticularis on the legs, footdrop on the left, and absent pinprick sensation in the lower legs. Laboratory study results included an ESR of 100 mm/h, a creatinine level 2.2 mg/dL, microscopic hematuria, and an aspartate transaminase level of twice normal.

PAN is suspected. After consideration of the diagnostic yield and the risks, the logical next step would be
a) Skin biopsy
b) Percutaneous renal biopsy to demonstrate vasculitis of extraglomerular vessels
c) Abdominal angiography
d) Sural nerve biopsy

**3.** The differential diagnosis for the rash shown in Figure 32.1 includes
a) Drug-associated vasculitis
b) Vasculitis with malignancy
c) HSP
d) Subacute bacterial endocarditis
e) a and b
f) All of the above

**4.** The following may be said about the ANCA test:
a) C-ANCA representing antibodies to PR-3 are highly correlated with a diagnosis of WG.
b) P-ANCA by immunofluorescence is less sensitive and specific for a diagnosis of WG or MPA.
c) A rise in ANCA titers alone should clearly justify an escalation of immunosuppressive therapy.

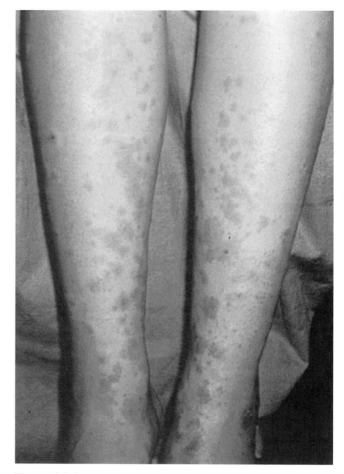

**Figure 32.1** Rash. (See Color Fig. 32.1.)

d) a and b
e) a, b, and c

**5.** Which of the following statements about cryoglobulinemia is correct?
a) The most common clinical finding is a vasculitic rash.
b) If the cryoglobulin is composed only of a monoclonal immunoglobulin, it is generally associated with an underlying malignancy.
c) The most common associated condition is an underlying infection with HBV.
d) a and b
e) a, b, and c

In questions 6–9, indicate whether each of the following statements about biopsies and vasculitis is true (T) or false (F).

**6.** A skin biopsy that reveals small vessel, leukocytoclastic vasculitis is a reliable measure of the qualitative features of vessel disease in other organs (i.e., is predictive of only small vessel disease elsewhere).

T _____  F _____

**7.** Open biopsies of abnormal visceral organs in patients with systemic vasculitis are supportive or compatible with the diagnosis of vasculitis in approximately two-thirds of cases.

T _____    F _____

**8.** A lung biopsy that reveals necrotizing granulomatous inflammation and vasculitis supports the diagnosis of *only* WG or, if eosinophils are present, Churg-Strauss syndrome.

T _____    F _____

**9.** Visceral angiography provides diagnostic information that is as revealing as a biopsy of involved organs.

T _____    F _____

**10.** Vasculitis associated with hepatitis B or C or HIV may have a phenotypic appearance similar to
a) PAN and MPA
b) CSD
c) WG
d) GCA

## ANSWERS

**1. e.**
The diagnosis of vasculitis begins with clinical suspicion. There are relatively few findings of high diagnostic specificity for systemic necrotizing vasculitis, but suspicion should mount in the presence of presumptive signs or "red flags" for vasculitis. These include FUO with constitutional symptoms; unexplained multisystem organ disease; unexplained inflammatory arthritis; unexplained myalgias; a suspicious rash, in particular palpable purpura; peripheral neuropathies, especially mononeuritis multiplex; unexplained end-organ ischemia, including cardiac, CNS, and GI; and GN. Although none of these findings is specific for systemic vasculitis, the presence of any one or more should lead to increasing suspicion of the disease.

**2. d.**
This patient presents a clinical picture highly suspicious for systemic necrotizing vasculitis, in particular PAN. Each diagnostic test outlined in the question should be considered in terms of sensitivity, specificity, and risk. A skin biopsy is sensitive but nonspecific because vasculitis of the skin can be caused by so many different conditions. On occasion, a nodular subcutaneous lesion may have characteristic features. Palpable purpura is less specific, and leukocytoclastic vasculitis may occur in many conditions. Percutaneous renal biopsy in this setting is insensitive for demonstrating vasculitis of the extraglomerular vessels. Abdominal angiography has increased sensitivity, but in the presence of severe hypertension and azotemia, it carries unacceptable risks.

Lastly, sural nerve biopsy, although somewhat morbid and invasive, has an increasing diagnostic yield (>60%), particularly in the presence of objective neurologic signs and symptoms.

**3. f.**
The rash shown in Figure 32.1 is palpable purpura. It is highly specific for small-vessel cutaneous vasculitis but is unrevealing of an underlying nosologic diagnosis. Drug-associated vasculitis is an extremely common cause of small-vessel vasculitis. Vasculitis associated with malignancies is most frequently found in the setting of an underlying lymphoproliferative disease. A small-vessel vasculitis such as this would be characteristic. HSP is characterized not only by such a rash but also by the presence of abdominal pain and GN. It is most frequently seen in children but may also be seen in adults. Subacute bacterial endocarditis has a variety of extracardiac complications, the majority of which are mediated by ICs. A small-vessel vasculitis would not be unusual in subacute bacterial endocarditis, although it is rare for this to be the dominant and presenting finding of the disorder. Many other conditions can be seen with this type of rash, including a variety of connective tissue diseases (e.g., rheumatoid arthritis and systemic lupus), other types of infections, cryoglobulinemia secondary to HCV infection, and a variety of miscellaneous systemic diseases.

**4. d.**
ANCA testing has been a step forward in the diagnostic process for certain forms of systemic vasculitis. The test is generally performed by immunofluorescence but increasingly is also performed by antigen-specific assays. In the majority of cases, an immunofluorescent pattern of C-ANCA is associated with antibodies to the lysosomal enzyme PR-3. It is highly correlated with the diagnosis of WG, being more than 80% sensitive and more than 95% specific in the presence of active untreated and widespread disease. P-ANCA by immunofluorescence, however, is not only less sensitive for the diagnosis of WG (present in only a small percentage of cases) but also relatively nonspecific. The P-ANCA pattern can be mimicked by a variety of antibodies, including ANA. The antibodies of interest in the diagnosis of systemic vasculitis responsible for the P-ANCA pattern of immunofluorescence are those directed against MPO, another lysosomal enzyme. ANCA test results by immunofluorescence should always be confirmed by an antigen-specific assay. Finally, although the major use of ANCA is in the diagnosis of related conditions, some correlation exists with disease activity. ANCA titers are not in and of themselves justification for the modification of therapy. A clinical evaluation of end-organ damage is still the "gold standard" for determining modifications of therapy.

### 5. d.

Cryoglobulinemia and cryoglobulinemic vasculitis result from immunoglobulins and other proteins that precipitate from serum at temperatures lower than 37°C. Cryoglobulins are characterized on the basis of their content as type I (monoclonal), type II (mixed or monoclonal), or type III (polyclonal). The finding that the vast majority of cases of mixed cryoglobulinemia are associated with underlying HCV infection has been a major breakthrough in the understanding of this complex disease.

Patients with cryoglobulinemia from any underlying cause may have a variety of end-organ manifestations. A small-vessel vasculitis, most often manifesting as palpable purpura, is the most frequent finding. Arthralgia and arthritis are also common. With considerable frequency, patients also have GN, peripheral neuropathy, and a variety of other complications.

### 6. f.

The presence of leukocytoclastic vasculitis of capillaries and post-capillary venules does not preclude the involvement of larger vessels (arteries and veins) in other sites. Examples can be seen in WG, MPA, Behçet's disease, viral-associated vasculitides, lupus vasculitis, and other diseases.

### 7. T.

Skip lesions—the lack of uniform involvement of vessels and organs—are responsible for not finding vasculitis in 100% of all biopsies in patients with unequivocal vasculitis.

### 8. F.

These findings may also occur in granulomatous infections such as those due to tuberculosis, atypical mycobacteria, or fungal diseases.

### 9. F.

Angiography is not as specific as histopathology. Vessels may become stenotic or aneurysmal due to processes other than vasculitis [e.g., Ehlers-Danlos syndrome (type IV), infection, fibromuscular dysplasia, atherosclerosis, etc.].

### 10. a.

The same size vessels may be affected in PAN, MPA, and viral vasculitides, especially those due to hepatitis and HIV. Thus, the disease phenotypes of PAN and MPA should have as part of their assessment viral diagnostic studies.

## SUGGESTED READINGS

Gross WL. Churg-Strauss syndrome: update on recent developments. *Curr Opin Rheumatol* 2002;14:11–14.

Hoffman GS, Specks U. Antineutrophil cytoplasmic antibodies. *Arthritis Rheum* 1998;41:1521–1537.

Hoffman GS, Weyend CM, eds. *Inflammatory Diseases of the Blood Vessels.* New York: Marcel Dekker, 2002.

Jennette CJ, Falk R. Small vessel vasculitis. *N Engl J Med* 1997;337:1512.

Langford C. Management of systemic vasculitis. *Best Pract Res Clin Rheumatol* 2001;15:281–297.

Proceedings of the 10th International Vasculitis and ANCA workshop. *Cleve Clin J Med* 2002;(Suppl 2)69:II, 1–191.

Vassilopoulos D, Calabrese LH: Hepatitis C virus infection and vasculitis: implications of antiviral and immunosuppressive therapies. *Arthritis Rheum* 2002;46(3):585–597.

# Selected Musculoskeletal Syndromes

# 33

## *Brian F. Mandell*

Musculoskeletal pain is one of the most frequently listed chief complaints of patients seeing family practice physicians and general internists. Although some of these complaints relate to osteoarthritis or inflammatory joint disease, the majority are due to soft-tissue musculoskeletal syndromes. Many of these pain syndromes are self-limited or reversible with short-term therapy. A clinical recognition of specific syndromes limits the need for expensive diagnostic testing. In particular, recognizing specific syndromes obviates the need for laboratory evaluation or musculoskeletal imaging. Although the pathophysiology of many of these syndromes is poorly understood, accumulated experience permits the clinical diagnosis of discrete syndromes and allows for empiric, therapeutic interventions.

Despite the common occurrence of these syndromes, controlled clinical outcome studies are rarely reported in the medical literature.

# HIP GIRDLE SYNDROMES

Pain in the hip region in elderly patients is frequently attributed to hip osteoarthritis. In the elderly, as well as in young patients, however, a focused examination of the painful area may delineate one of several nonarticular pain syndromes. True hip joint discomfort is classically present in the inguinal crease or felt deep in this area. Occasionally, true hip joint pain is felt primarily in the deep gluteal area or radiating down the thigh as far as the knee. Hip joint pain may be elicited by passive range of motion of the hip joint, but is not usually reproduced by palpation. Examination should include:

- Passive internal rotation
- Passive external rotation
- Passive abduction
- Passive flexion
- Passive posterior extension

This last motion, undertaken with the patient lying on his or her abdomen, is frequently neglected. It is uncommon for isolated hip (joint) disease to manifest only as lateral hip pain reproducible with pressure over the trochanteric area.

## Lateral Hip Pain

The syndrome of lateral hip pain, reproduced with deep pressure to this area, has generally been termed *trochanteric* or *pseudotrochanteric bursitis*. A differential diagnosis of this lateral hip pain syndrome exists, but most commonly it is attributed to trochanteric bursitis.

Examination of the area is best undertaken with the patient lying on the contralateral side with the upper leg flexed toward the chest and adducted across the body, with the medial aspect of the upper knee resting on the table. This pulls the soft tissue overlying the trochanteric area fairly taut, permitting easier examination. The superficial trochanteric bursa directly overlies the trochanteric prominence, and this area should be gently palpated. The deep trochanteric bursa area is proximal and slightly posterior and sits in a deep groove. It can be easily palpated in this position. A reproduction of the patient's pain with firm pressure in these areas warrants a clinical diagnosis of trochanteric bursitis. Eliciting tenderness that does not mimic the patient's pain syndrome is not diagnostic.

This syndrome is exceedingly common and often does not respond to nonsteroidal anti-inflammatory drug (NSAID) therapy. It may respond dramatically to local infiltration with lidocaine and a deposit steroid. Injection should be made deep within this tissue, but not into the periosteum because this provokes extreme discomfort in the patient (As with all steroid injections, the patient should be forewarned about the possibility of infection, as well as atrophy or skin discoloration.) The syndrome of trochanteric bursitis is often precipitated by mechanical factors, including primary hip or knee disease, pes planus or other foot disorders, and altered gait because of low back pain or new shoes. Mimics of this syndrome with radiation of pain into the same anatomic area include:

- High lumbar radiculopathy
- Hip abductor muscle strain
- Entrapment neuropathy
- Stress fractures of the femoral neck or pelvis

If the pain is attributable to trochanteric bursitis, the local infiltration of several milliliters of lidocaine or bupivacaine (Marcaine) will provide at least transient, and usually complete, relief of the discomfort. Patients will report that they are able to lie comfortably on this side, which they were not able to do prior to the injection. The inclusion of corticosteroids in the injection provides lasting relief in approximately 70% of patients, perhaps for as long as several months. If a gait disturbance or hip disease is present, the pain will likely return. For isolated trochanteric bursitis, pain relief may be indefinite after a single injection (or occasionally several injections). Failure of two (or at most, three) injections to relieve the pain should prompt an aggressive search for other etiologies of the pain, including a generalized myofascial pain syndrome such as fibromyalgia.

The coexistence of trochanteric pain with degenerative disease of the spine or the hip must be noted, although the exact relationship between these conditions is not clear. If pain radiates down the leg from the trochanteric bursa and can be elicited by firm pressure along the fibrous tissue surrounding the muscle bundles (fascia lata), then physical therapy directed at stretching this fibrous muscle area should also be provided. Gluteal tendonitis frequently coexists with trochanteric bursitis. The anatomic bursa is rarely actually distended with fluid (by imaging), but septic trochanteric bursitis has been reported.

The lasting value of physical therapy modalities, including ultrasonography, transcutaneous electrical nerve stimulation unit application, iontophoresis, or deep heat, has not been clearly established.

## Gluteal Pain

Gluteal pain can be caused by strain in the gluteal muscles or a bursitis involving the bursa overlying the ischial prominence and under the gluteal muscles.

Ischial bursitis is best diagnosed with the patient standing and forward flexed at the hips; the area of tenderness can be easily palpated by pressure along the ischial prominence. Gluteal bursitis can be elicited by deep palpation along the gluteal muscles with the muscles pulled taut while the patient is in a lateral position.

Piriform syndrome is a controversial entity, presumably caused by spasms of the piriformis muscle. Patients complain of moderate, severe, or even disabling lateral buttock pain. Deep palpation of the piriformis muscle in the lateral upper quadrant of the buttock area or, more specifically, by rectal wall examination, is considered to be diagnostic. Pain may radiate posteriorly to the upper portion of the thigh. Patients may walk with an antalgic gait. Pain may be elicited with forced internal rotation of the hip against resistance. Treatment, which also is controversial, may include physical therapy or local injection.

## Meralgia Paresthetica

Entrapment of the lateral femoral cutaneous nerve causes the syndrome of meralgia paresthetica. Entrapment usually occurs overlying the superior iliac spine under the inguinal ligament. The clinical syndrome is usually marked by an area of intense dysesthesia, often with numbness on careful pinprick examination in a patch of skin in the anterior thigh. It can be associated with rapid weight gain, as can be seen in pregnancy, or with use of a tight, constraining belt. Treatment is supportive. No additional evaluation is necessary. It is not associated with systemic disease. It should be remembered, however, that herpes zoster may be heralded by an area of dysesthesia without visible skin lesions.

## KNEE PAIN

Similar to the situation in the hip, pain surrounding the knee frequently is attributed to osteoarthritis of the knee, especially in the elderly. Pain in the knee area can be referred from the hip joint, the lumbar spine, and (rarely) from the foot in patients with significant pes planus and tightened calf muscles.

Examination of the knee should include evaluation for:

- Crepitus
- Synovial thickening or fluid
- Reproduction of pain with pressure and movement of the patella
- Mechanical stability
- Popliteal fullness
- Specific bursitis or tendonitis

An extremely common cause of regional knee pain, especially in patients with osteoarthritis of the medial compartment of the knee or with pes planus, is pain in the area of the pes anserine bursa. Patients with this syndrome frequently complain of pain localized to the medial aspect of the leg slightly below the joint line. Pain is frequently exacerbated by the act of rising from a low chair, walking up steps, and occasionally in bed at night as the two knee areas touch together. Patients may describe the need to sleep with a pillow between their legs at night to avoid the painful pressure of their knees touching together. Pain can be elicited by gentle palpation approximately 1 cm below the joint line on the medial aspect of the leg. It is most important to be certain that the pain that is elicited with firm, but not extreme, palpation is the exact pain that the patient experiences; tenderness to palpation alone is not sufficient to make this diagnosis.

This syndrome frequently does not respond to NSAID therapy, but strikingly responds to local injection. The pain can be debilitating, but it is often dramatically and immediately relieved by a local infiltration of lidocaine. Corticosteroid is frequently included in the injection mixture.

Prepatellar bursitis is a frequent cause of swelling in the knee area. The area of swelling may appear as a fluctuant mass immediately anterior to the patella. This is frequently a result of trauma and is an occupational hazard of patients who work in a kneeling position. The aspiration of the traumatically induced serosanguinous fluid may relieve the discomfort; however, this bursa can be inflamed owing to infection (most frequently *Staphylococcus aureus*) or gout. Infection frequently is associated with surrounding cellulitis and may mimic joint inflammation. The bursa does not communicate with the joint; care should be taken to distinguish this entity from actual arthritis. An attempt at true knee joint aspiration should not be undertaken unnecessarily, especially through an overlying cellulitis. Recurrent bursitis may be relieved by intrabursal steroid injection once infection has been excluded.

## ELBOW AREA

The olecranon bursa separates the skin from the olecranon process. Frequently, after minor trauma (such as friction or resting of the elbow on a hard surface), the bursa may be distended with sterile, noninflammatory, often serosanguinous fluid. In this case, it may respond to drainage and the injection of a local corticosteroid preparation (once infection has been excluded). The bursa may be involved with urate-crystal–induced inflammation or occasionally with infection, similar to the pre-patella bursitis of the knee. Cell counts in septic bursitis are generally much lower than in septic arthritis. Frequently, a surrounding cellulitis is present, with pitting edema of the soft tissue. *S. aureus* is the most common infecting agent.

Specific pain syndromes in the area of the lateral or medial epicondyles of the elbow—tennis and golfer's elbow, respectively—are extremely common. Both of these pain syndromes are believed to be caused, in part, by frequent and vigorous use of the forearm muscles. Lateral epicondylitis may be reproduced by palpation to the specific area surrounding the lateral epicondyle, but more specifically, pain can be elicited by resisted, active extension of the middle finger. Pain will radiate specifically to the area of the lateral epicondyle and often to the forearm. Epicondylitis may respond to rest, use of a forearm band, and NSAID therapy. Infiltration of the area with a mixture of lidocaine and a low dose of deposit corticosteroid preparation may be of value in providing more rapid relief, but long-term outcome in most series is identical to treatment with physical therapy alone. Surgical intervention is rarely required. Care must be taken when injecting the medial epicondyle area to avoid the median nerve. Ultrasound high-energy therapy has been shown in some studies to be of benefit. Carpal tunnel syndrome can cause radiation of discomfort up the forearm toward the elbow region.

## THE HAND

Carpal tunnel syndrome, caused by the compression of the median nerve as it travels through the carpal canal, is common. Frequent associations include:

- Diabetes mellitus
- Trauma
- Pregnancy
- Hypothyroidism
- Repetitive palm trauma
- Synovitis of the wrist (most commonly from rheumatoid arthritis)

Association is also recognized with primary and dialysis-related (not secondary) amyloidosis. The development of carpal tunnel syndrome as an overuse syndrome is debatable. The clinical recognition of the syndrome is by:

- Reproduction of dysesthesias in the appropriate distribution by pressure over the carpal canal (distal to the wrist crease at the base of the palm)
- Elicitation of the symptoms with percussion in the same area by finger or reflex hammer (Tinel's sign)
- Phalen's maneuver

Early in the course of the syndrome, neurologic deficits are not present; however, two-point discrimination and detailed sensory testing over the area of the thumb, index, and middle finger may demonstrate sensory loss. Dysesthesias are occasionally described to occur in all five digits or as extending proximally up the arm. The diagnosis can be confirmed after it has been present for a significant period of time, using nerve conduction testing. In a recent Swedish study, however, 20% of *asymptomatic* volunteers had abnormal conduction of their median nerve compatible with carpal tunnel syndrome.

Initial treatment should include splinting the wrist in a slightly hyperextended, near-neutral position. A local injection of corticosteroid into the carpal canal may provide relief but should be performed only by someone with experience and knowledge of the anatomy. Surgical treatment is usually (but not always) curative if nerve

damage has not occurred, but large outcome studies are not available.

*De Quervain's tenosynovitis*, a common cause of pain on the radial aspect of the hand, is frequently described by the patient as thumb or wrist pain. This can occur as a sporadic pain syndrome but is frequently induced by repetitive resisted motion of the thumb. The condition may occur with increased frequency in women caring for a newborn infant. Typical clinical presentation consists of pain overlying the radial styloid radiating into the thumb and occasionally up the forearm. Visible swelling and erythema may be present over the tendon sheath of the extensor pollicis brevis. Pain can be elicited by resisted abduction of the thumb or by having the patient place the thumb inside a closed fist with gentle movement of the fist by the examiner in an ulnar direction. Pain is elicited over the radial styloid. This syndrome should be distinguished from osteoarthritis of the metacarpophalangeal joint at the base of the thumb. The initial treatment of the tendonitis can be conservative, with use of a custom-made resting thumb splint and NSAID therapy. Some authors have proposed primary infiltration of the tendon sheath with a corticosteroid-lidocaine mixture. Care should be taken with the injection to avoid the snuffbox area and the radial artery.

*Trigger finger* can occur owing to the presence of noninflammatory fibrous nodules in the flexor tendon sheath of the palmar tendons. Patients describe the finger(s) as being stuck in a flexed position, with the need to be forcibly extended, eliciting a resultant sharp, painful pop. Frequently, patients may awaken with their finger or thumb "stuck" in a flexed position. Treatment can include passive splinting of the involved finger in an extended position, with or without local infiltration of corticosteroid into the flexor sheath nodule. This should result in the shrinkage of the nodule and less triggering. Progressive fibrosis of the flexor tendons, with contracture and nodularity of the palmar fascia, results in *Dupuytren's contractures*. Most trigger fingers do not evolve into this syndrome. Nonsurgical treatment is usually effective, and surgical intervention is rarely required. Acute severe palmar fasciitis has been rarely associated with carcinoma of the ovary and lung.

## SHOULDER AREA

Acute shoulder pain in the absence of trauma is most frequently caused by rotator cuff disease (periarthritis) rather than true shoulder joint disease. Glenohumeral synovitis occurs in the setting of rheumatoid arthritis and polymyalgia rheumatica (mild synovitis and bursitis). Periarthritis can occur in young, active people and in anyone after overuse of the musculature of the shoulder girdle. Pain from periarthritis is frequently described as worsened by specific motions, particularly with extension of the arm. Sharp pain with abduction or full arm motion is termed *impingement* and is often caused by pressure on an inflamed tendon sheath on a bone, osteophyte, or ligamentous structure in the area of the shoulder girdle. Passive joint motion on examination is not as painful as active or resisted motion. Attempts should be made at delineating the specific involved tendon using resistive stressing of the individual tendons of the rotator cuff. The most common form of rotator cuff tendonitis involves the supraspinatus tendon. This can be evaluated by having the patient elevate his arm with the thumb pointed toward the ground; the examiner applies downward pressure, and the patient resists this motion. Pain is usually referred to the deltoid and upper arm region.

Generally, pain with passive motion of the glenohumeral joint within the normal range of motion does not elicit pain in the absence of glenohumeral synovitis. An examination of the shoulder should also routinely include palpation of the acromioclavicular and sternoclavicular joints. Acromioclavicular osteoarthritis can cause pain when the patient reaches across his body in the anterior plane or reaches far behind his back, as when putting on a jacket. Cervical radiculitis also can refer to the shoulder area. Posterior pain can be due to a periscapular trigger point or scapulocostal syndrome. Pain from this latter syndrome, reproduced by pressure in a trigger point underneath the medial aspect of the scapula on the chest wall, may radiate down the arm and across the chest. Pain can also be referred to the shoulder area from within the thorax or a subdiaphragmatic, hepatic, or splenic process; in this case pain is not generally reproduced by active or passive shoulder motion.

The treatment of shoulder periarthritis and rotator cuff tendonitis can be accomplished with a course of NSAID therapy or the injection of corticosteroid and anesthetic into the subacromial space. Injection into the space from the lateral approach through the subacromial bursal area is the safest approach. Physical therapy, with emphasis on range of motion, should be emphasized to avoid the development of adhesive capsulitis (more common in patients with diabetes).

## LUMBAR CANAL STENOSIS

Lumbar canal stenosis (spinal stenosis) occurs in the setting of degenerative joint and disc disease. It is characterized by the subacute or occasionally acute onset of bilateral leg and back discomfort. The leg discomfort may occur in a pattern of pseudoclaudication of calves or thighs and can mimic vascular ischemia. Because this syndrome occurs in an elderly population, it frequently coexists with the physical findings of peripheral vascular disease. Deep tendon reflexes may be preserved; specific nerve root symptoms are usually not elicited.

Diagnosis is generally made by magnetic resonance imaging (MRI) of the lumbar canal. In the absence of cauda equina syndrome, marked neurologic deficits are not generally appreciated. The pain can be quite limiting to the patient's activity and is frequently associated with lumbar pain.

Conservative treatment is successful in many patients, with the focus on extension-oriented physical therapy. Surgical intervention is a reasonable option for patients who fail conservative therapy. Some patients may find the use of subcutaneous calcitonin helpful for the relief of pain, although this should be viewed as experimental therapy.

## FIBROMYALGIA

Fibromyalgia is a generalized pain syndrome. It occurs in patients of all ages and seemingly occurs at an increased frequency in patients with underlying systemic disease such as rheumatoid arthritis, systemic lupus erythematosus, multiple sclerosis, and inflammatory bowel disease.

Neurologic complaints of dysesthesia are common; however, objective neurologic abnormalities on physical and electrical examination are absent. No inflammatory markers are present through laboratory testing. Synovitis is notably absent in primary fibromyalgia. Quite frequently, an associated subjective sleep disturbance is reported, with a complaint of not feeling refreshed in the morning. Patients frequently describe multiple awakenings during the night. Mild dryness of eyes or mouth is a frequent complaint. The presence of multiple discrete myofascial tender points on examination is characteristic; the presence of these tender points is required to make an unequivocal diagnosis. Pressure should be applied to a degree that the fingernail of the examiner is noted to barely blanch with the pressure. Neutral points also should be evaluated. The number of involved tender points and the intensity of tenderness may vary dramatically between different examinations. The tender points are frequently in areas of common myofascial pain syndromes previously described (trochanteric, gluteal, pes anserine); the distinguishing characteristic of the fibromyalgia syndrome is the generalized nature of this pain sensitivity. In the absence of discrete tender points, the diagnosis should be made with trepidation because these features often overlap those of patients having chronic fatigue syndrome. These tender points may not be elicited on any given examination day, however, and in some patients tender points are not prominent.

Clinical recognition of this pain syndrome should dramatically limit the need for laboratory testing. Serologic testing has no role in a patient who has no features of specific autoimmune disease (e.g., systemic lupus erythematosus or rheumatoid arthritis). Care should be taken when making this diagnosis, however, to exclude by detailed history and physical examination the presence of an underlying disorder such as hypothyroidism or primary depression. Many patients with fibromyalgia have features of depression with somatization; however, not all patients are clinically depressed.

Treatment is directed at the maintenance of normal activities; reversal of the abnormal sleep cycle with the use of low doses of soporific tricyclic antidepressants, if not contraindicated; and sparse, judicious use of medications such as cyclobenzaprine (Flexeril), acetaminophen, and NSAIDs. Chronic use of NSAIDs should be discouraged. Narcotics, corticosteroids, and most other chronic pain medications should be avoided. Regular aerobic exercise is believed to be of value in maintaining patient function. The distinction between fibromyalgia and chronic fatigue syndrome can be difficult, if not impossible; the conditions are frequently treated in a similar manner.

# REVIEW EXERCISES

## QUESTIONS

**1.** A 56-year-old overweight woman with radiographic osteoarthritis of the right knee presents with a chief complaint of increasing, limiting knee pain, most notable when rising from a chair or toilet, walking up stairs, and in bed at night. Examination reveals valgus deformity with walking, minimal cool-knee effusions, and tenderness to palpation (which mimics the pain) at the medial aspect of the joint, approximately 2 inches distal to the joint line. You suggest
**a)** Full-dose NSAID trial (patient has been using over-the-counter preparations)
**b)** Quadriceps-focused strengthening regimen
**c)** Intra-articular steroid injection
**d)** Steroid injection of anserine bursa
**e)** a and b

**2.** A 32-year-old previously healthy secretary complains of recent (3 months) onset of progressive pain in her right arm involving the second and third fingers, forearm, and upper arm. It awakens her from sleep and worsens while driving. It is at times associated with painful tingling. Physical examination reveals normal neck motion, negative Spurling's and Adson's test results, and normal shoulder examination results. Test results of pulses, deep tendon reflexes, pinprick, strength, and elbow are normal. A likely diagnostic test is
**a)** Nerve conduction of the distal median nerve
**b)** MRI of the cervical spine
**c)** Upper extremity angiography
**d)** Chemical sympathetic block

**3.** A 64-year-old former construction worker presents with increasing exertional bilateral calf pain and leg tingling. Leg symptoms have been present for 1 year but have worsened after his recent myocardial infarction during cardiac rehabilitation. He could only walk 0.4 mile on the treadmill because of leg pain. He

switched to an exercise cycle, on which he could ride for 3 miles. Physical examination demonstrated decreased left distal pulses and a left iliac bruit, with normal foot temperature, color, deep tendon reflexes, pinprick, and strength. The study with high yield for diagnosis is
**a)** Angiography
**b)** Abdominal ultrasonography
**c)** Spinal MRI
**d)** Electromyography

**4.** A 28-year-old woman presents 2 months postpartum complaining of 4 months of left-thigh burning pain. She was told of carpal tunnel syndrome during her pregnancy and has been wearing wrist splints but is now concerned regarding the possibility of multiple sclerosis. Physical examination reveals bilateral wrist Tinel's sign with a positive Phalen's maneuver. The results of hip examination are normal, with negative straight-leg raise. Deep tendon reflexes are preserved. No motor weakness is detected. There is an area approximately the size of a hand with marked dysesthesias to light touch on the anterior lateral left thigh. In addition to clinical diagnosis, a positive test result would include
**a)** Electromyography of the sacral plexus
**b)** Tinel's sign over the lateral inguinal ligament
**c)** Pelvic computed tomography scan
**d)** Cerebrospinal fluid oligoclonal bands

**5.** A 42-year-old woman, with a diagnosis of rheumatoid arthritis for 2 years (fairly well controlled on hydroxychloroquine, nabumetone, and 2.5 mg prednisone daily), 8 months after the birth of a healthy boy, presents for a routine visit complaining of increasing "pain all over." She describes an increase in morning stiffness of her back, neck, and hands; trouble sleeping; and difficulties with painful flares after exposure to any drafts or physical exertion. The erythrocyte sedimentation rate (ESR) is 22 mm/hour, and the rheumatoid factor (RF) is present in high titer. Joint examination shows multiple tender, nonswollen joints; normal grip strength; bilateral trochanteric bursitis, gluteal tenderness, and costochondritis; and anserine bursitis. The course of action should be to
**a)** Increase prednisone for 10 days, then taper.
**b)** Add methotrexate.
**c)** Add a tricyclic plus physical therapy.
**d)** b and c.

## ANSWERS

**1. d.**
The pes anserine bursitis should be treated. Patients with osteoarthritis of the knee have many causes of pain. Anserine bursitis is one of the more common nonarticular ones. It is particularly common in overweight

patients with valgus deformity. Pain is reproduced by local pressure. It often does not respond to NSAIDs but does respond to local injection. Osteoarthritis is not usually a cause of nocturnal pain in bed; however, patients with anserine bursitis get relief by relieving the pressure of their legs touching by sleeping with a pillow between their knees.

### 2. a.

The patient has carpal tunnel syndrome. Nerve conduction of the median nerve would likely provide the diagnosis. Local provocative testing with Tinel's sign, Phalen's maneuver, or direct compression might also provide suggestive information. Prolonged keyboard typing may be a risk factor. Other tests are not warranted based on the history and examination, which do not suggest radiculopathy, thoracic outlet, or reflex sympathetic dystrophy or Raynaud's syndrome. Causes include wrist synovitis, hypothyroidism, diabetes mellitus, pregnancy, trauma, primary amyloidosis, acromegaly, and possibly polymyalgia rheumatica.

### 3. c.

Although MRI of the spine has limited specificity for diagnosing disc disease and back pain, it is excellent for diagnosing spinal stenosis. This patient has peripheral vascular disease, but the positional aspects of claudication symptoms argue for the presence of neurogenic, not vascular, claudication. Spinal stenosis frequently coexists with peripheral vascular disease, and neurologic examination is often normal for age. Osteoarthritis of the spine is common. Physical therapy is often effective; surgery may be curative.

### 4. b.

The patient has meralgia paresthetica caused by entrapment of the lateral femoral cutaneous nerve, which often occurs as it exits through the lateral inguinal ligament. It can be diagnosed clinically and usually requires no workup or treatment. It may accompany weight gain, the wearing of constricting garments, or overtight seat belts. Often self-limiting, it may respond to local steroid injection. A differential diagnosis might include pre-zoster neuralgia.

### 5. c.

The patient has fibromyalgia. The diagnosis is most likely secondary fibromyalgia, perhaps precipitated by the stress of a newborn child in the house. The symptoms will not respond to intensified therapy for the rheumatoid arthritis. A detailed examination will likely reveal additional myofascial trigger points. Education is another key element of the therapy.

## SUGGESTED READINGS

Anderson BC, Manthey R, Brouns MC. Treatment of Du Quervain's tenosynovitis with corticosteroids: a prospective study of the response to local injection. *Arthritis Rheum* 1991;34:793–798.

Goldenberg DL. Fibromyalgia and chronic fatigue syndrome: are they the same? *J Musculoskel Med* 1990;7:19–28.

Kang I, Han SW. Anserine bursitis in patients with osteoarthritis of the knee. *South Med J* 2000;93:207–209.

Mandell BF. Avascular necrosis of the femoral head presenting as trochanteric bursitis. *Ann Rheum Dis* 1990;49:730–732.

Pace JB, Nagle D. Piriform syndrome. *West J Med* 1976;124:435–439.

Shbeeb MI, O'Duffy JD, Michet CJ Jr, et al. Evaluation of glucocorticosteroid injection for the treatment of trochanteric bursitis. *J Rheumatol* 1996;23:2104–2106.

Smith DL, McAfee JH, Lucas LM, et al. Treatment of nonseptic olecranon bursitis: a controlled, blinded prospective trial. *Arch Intern Med* 1989;149:2527–2530.

Swezey RL. Pseudo-radiculopathy in subacute trochanteric bursitis of the subgluteus maximus bursa. *Arch Phys Med Rehabil* 1976; 57:387–390.

Traycoff RB. "Pseudotrochanteric bursitis": the differential diagnosis of lateral hip pain. *J Rheumatol* 1991;18:1810–1812.

# BOARD SIMULATION: Rheumatic and Immunologic Diseases

**34**

*Raymond J. Scheetz, Jr.*

The following questions have one best answer.

## CASE 1

A 65-year-old white man presents to his physician with complaints of gradually worsening weakness in his arms and legs over the preceding 4 months. He also complains of weakness in his hands and forearms that causes him to have difficulty in grasping and holding some objects. He has fallen down unexpectedly on three occasions. He has no family history of muscle disease. His examination reveals anterior thigh and forearm muscle atrophy, with proximal and distal muscle weakness worse on the left side; the results of his neurologic examination are normal (Fig. 34.1). His creatine phosphokinase (CPK) level is 620 U (normal is less than 220 U), and his aspartate aminotransferase level is 80 U (normal is less than 40 U). An electromyogram shows myopathic motor unit potentials in the right upper and lower extremities. A muscle biopsy reveals fibrosis, a mild mononuclear cell infiltrate, some variation in fiber size, and rimmed vacuoles in several myofibers.

### Questions

1. The most likely diagnosis is
a) Adult-onset muscular dystrophy
b) Drug-induced myopathy
c) Inclusion body myositis
d) Occult malignancy with paraneoplastic myopathy
e) Adult acid maltase deficiency

2. The best initial therapy in this case is
a) An intensive physical therapy program
b) Prednisone, 40 mg every morning
c) Prednisone, 60 mg every morning and methotrexate, 15 mg every week
d) Prednisone, 60 mg and azathioprine, 100 mg every morning
e) Levothyroxine (Synthroid), 0.15 mg every morning

3. Examination of muscle tissue by electron microscopy (Fig. 34.2) would be likely to reveal:

a) Psammoma bodies
b) Calciphylaxis
c) Microtubular filaments in the vacuolar inclusions
d) Sarcolemmal membrane interruptions
e) Negri bodies

## CASE 2

A 28-year-old African-American woman has pain and swelling in her metacarpophalangeal (MCP) and proximal interphalangeal (PIP) joints of 1 month duration, intermittent rash on her face and forearms, and three episodes of pleuritic chest pain associated with fever to 38.4° C, each episode lasting 3 to 4 days. On examination, she has synovitis in the MCPs and PIPs, an erythematous confluent rash on the forearms, and 1+ edema in each leg (Fig. 34.3). Blood pressure is 160/100 mm Hg.

### Questions

4. The most likely diagnosis would be
a) Rheumatoid arthritis
b) Reiter's syndrome
c) Polyarteritis nodosa
d) Systemic lupus erythematosus
e) Behçet's syndrome

Initial laboratory studies yield the following results: white blood cell (WBC) count 3,800/mm³; hematocrit, 28%; Westergren erythrocyte sedimentation rate (ESR), 62 mm/hour; urinalysis 2+ protein, 3+ blood; C4 complement 6 IU/mL (normal = 16−64 ); creatinine, 1.4 mg/dL; antinuclear antibody (ANA), 1:640, homogeneous pattern; antineutrophil cytoplasmic antibody negative. Microscopic examination of a fresh, early morning urine specimen discloses 25 to 35 red blood cells (RBCs) per high-power field (hpf), 3 to 5 WBCs/hpf, and 3 to 5 RBC casts/hpf. A chest radiograph reveals small bilateral pleural effusions. Anti-DNA is 150 (normal is less than 50).

5. Your next diagnostic maneuver should be
a) Electromyography
b) Echocardiogram

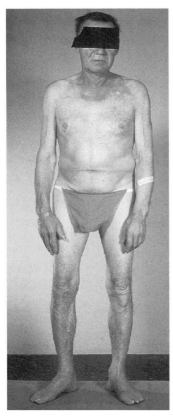

**Figure 34.1** Appearance of patient in Case 1. (See Color Fig. 34.1.)

c) Computed tomography (CT) of sinuses
d) Renal biopsy
e) Capillaroscopy

**6.** Renal biopsy shows a crescentic necrotizing proliferative glomerulonephritis (Fig. 34.4). The best treatment for this patient would be
a) Prednisone, 1 mg/kg daily, oral cyclophosphamide, 2 mg/kg daily, and apheresis
b) Azathioprine, 1 mg/kg daily

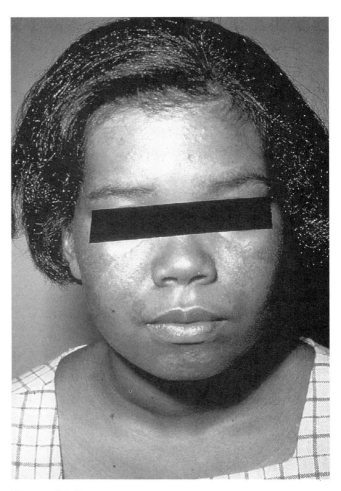

**Figure 34.3** Confluent facial rash of patient in Case 2. (See Color Fig. 34.3.)

c) Prednisone, 1 mg/kg daily, and monthly intermittent intravenous cyclophosphamide, 0.70 g/m$^2$
d) Oral prednisone, 40 mg daily
e) Oral prednisone, 40 mg daily, and oral methotrexate, 10 mg/week

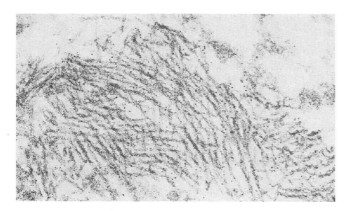

**Figure 34.2** Electron microscopic findings of patient in Case 1.

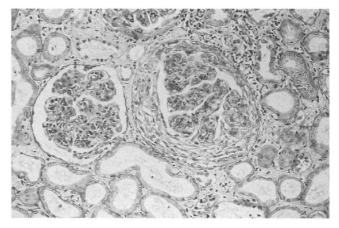

**Figure 34.4** Renal biopsy of patient in Question 6. (See Color Fig. 34.4.)

The patient receives 6 months of prednisone and intravenous cyclophosphamide, then two more intravenous treatments of cyclophosphamide over the next 6 months. At the end of 1 year of treatment, her urine shows no protein, no blood, and no RBC casts. She is maintained on hydroxychloroquine sulfate, and prednisone is tapered and discontinued. One year later she develops severe headaches, periodic confusion, and has a grand mal seizure. Spinal fluid studies show 80 mg/dL protein, 10 WBCs (all lymphocytes), and negative cultures. Magnetic resonance imaging (MRI) of the brain reveals multiple unidentified bright objects in a periventricular distribution.

**7.** The best initial treatment would be
**a)** Intravenous methotrexate, 2.5 mg/week, and phenytoin
**b)** Azathioprine, 3 mg/kg per day
**c)** Intravenous methylprednisolone, 1 g for 3 days, then 1 mg/kg per day orally, and phenytoin
**d)** Prednisone, 0.5 mg/kg per day, and phenytoin
**e)** Cyclophosphamide, 3 mg/kg per day orally, and phenytoin

## CASE 3

A 64-year old man complains of pain and swelling of 5 days duration in his right knee. Examination shows tenderness, swelling, warmth, and mild erythema of the right knee, all other joints being normal.

**8.** The most appropriate initial action should be
**a)** Aspiration and synovial fluid analysis and culture
**b)** Radiography of the right knee
**c)** Immediate injection of methylprednisolone into the right knee
**d)** Measurement of serum uric acid
**e)** Testing of complete blood count, sedimentation rate, and C-reactive protein

**9.** Synovial fluid studies reveal weakly positive rhomboidal birefringent crystals (Fig. 34.5), and right knee

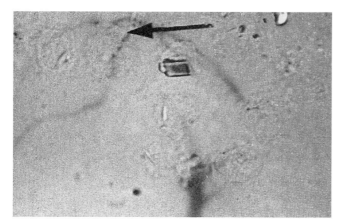

**Figure 34.5** Crystals (*arrow*) found in knee of patient in Question 9. (See Color Fig. 34.5.)

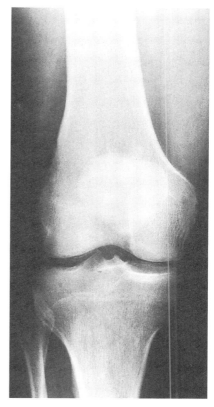

**Figure 34.6** Knee radiograph of patient in Question 9.

radiographs reveal chondrocalcinosis (Fig. 34.6). Appropriate treatment could include all the following, *except*
**a)** Injection with methylprednisolone
**b)** Use of a nonsteroidal anti-inflammatory drug (NSAID)
**c)** Ice, rest, and elevation
**d)** Institution of allopurinol
**e)** Further aspiration if joint effusion persists

**10.** Concommitant illnesses in individuals with calcium pyrophosphate crystal deposition disease may be associated with all the following, *except*
**a)** Brown urine on alkalinization
**b)** Kayser-Fleischer rings
**c)** Elevated serum calcium and low serum phosphorous
**d)** Elevated serum ferritin
**e)** Markedly low serum C4 and C3 complements

## CASE 4

A 34-year-old woman presents with a 1-year history of Raynaud's phenomenon (Fig. 34.7). On examination, she is noted to have sclerodactyly and facial telangiectasia. Further questioning reveals that she has symptoms of acid reflux when supine at night.

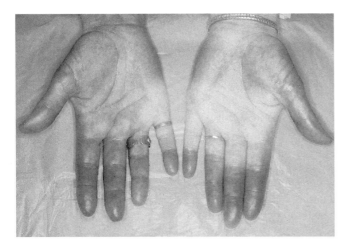

**Figure 34.7**    Hands of patient in Case 4. (See Color Fig. 34.7.)

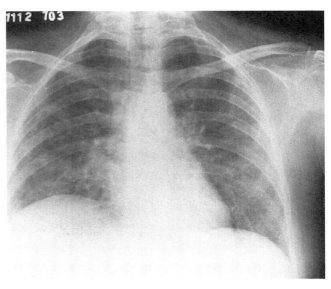

**Figure 34.8**    Chest radiograph of patient in Question 13.

**11.** The most likely diagnosis is
**a)** Polymyositis
**b)** Rheumatoid arthritis
**c)** Buerger's disease
**d)** Systemic lupus erythematosus
**e)** CREST syndrome

**12.** The most likely laboratory abnormality to be found in this patient is
**a)** Antineutrophil cytoplasmic antibody
**b)** Rheumatoid factor
**c)** Anticentromere antibody
**d)** Anti-SCL 70 antibody
**e)** Elevated uric acid

## CASE 5

A 52-year-old man with progressive systemic sclerosis (scleroderma) gradually develops significant shortness of breath. Pulmonary function tests are normal, except for a decrease in diffusion capacity. Chest radiograph reveals early changes consistent with pulmonary fibrosis (Fig. 34.8), and a high resolution CT scan of the chest shows patchy areas of ground-glass infiltrate in the bases.

**13.** The best means of additional evaluation is
**a)** Ventilation/perfusion lung scan
**b)** Pulmonary angiogram
**c)** Blood-gas determinations
**d)** Bronchoalveolar lavage
**e)** Serial chest radiographs

**14.** Bronchoalveolar lavage reveals a WBC count of 432/mm³ with 56% polymorphonuclear cells and 31% lymphocytes. The best treatment for his pulmonary condition is
**a)** Oral azathioprine, 1 mg/kg per day
**b)** Intravenous methotrexate, 50 mg/week

**c)** Oral methotrexate, 25 mg/week
**d)** Oral cyclophosphamide, 2 mg/kg per day
**e)** Prednisone, 4 mg/kg per day

## CASE 6

A 65-year-old woman presents with pain and swelling of 18 months duration in both knees. She notes crepitus in her knee joints, and the right knee has collapsed on two occasions. Her primary care physician has given her naproxen, then sulindac, with minimal improvement. On examination, she has bony hypertrophy at the knee joints with bilateral genu valgus deformities, decreased flexion to 100 degrees bilaterally, and small, bland knee effusions (Fig. 34.9). She also has thumb carpometacarpal joint enlargement and squaring, as well as Heberden's and Bouchard's nodes.

**15.** The most likely diagnosis is
**a)** Rheumatoid arthritis
**b)** Gout
**c)** Osteoarthritis
**d)** Pseudogout
**e)** Paget's disease

**16.** Appropriate initial therapy could include all of the following, *except*
**a)** Tylenol, 650 mg four times daily
**b)** Quadriceps muscle strengthening
**c)** Use of elastic knee braces when ambulatory
**d)** Prednisone, 10 mg every morning
**e)** Modification of physical activities

**17.** On failure to improve, second-line therapy for osteoarthritis of the knees could include all the following, *except*

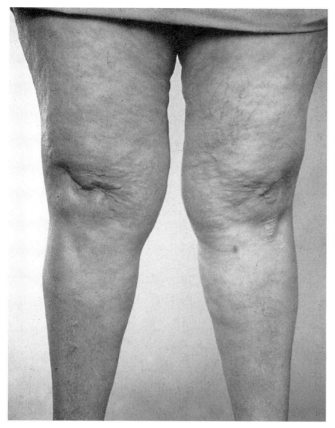

**Figure 34.9**  Appearance of knees of patient in Case 6. (See Color Fig. 34.9.)

a) Injection of knee joints with corticosteroids
b) Joint lavage
c) Injection of knee joints with sodium hyaluronate
d) Oral methotrexate, 7.5 mg weekly
e) Total knee replacement

## CASE 7

A 62-year-old woman has had rheumatoid arthritis involving multiple joints for 17 years. She has been taking hydroxychloroquine, 200 mg daily; prednisone, 5 mg daily; and methotrexate 7.5 mg once a week. She presents with a right foot drop of 4 days duration, as well as ulcerative skin lesions of 1 week's duration over the distal legs and feet (Fig. 34.10).

**18.** The most appropriate test would be
a) Serum ceruloplasmin level
b) Antineutrophil cytoplasmic antibody
c) Gastrocnemius muscle and sural nerve biopsy
d) Serum rheumatoid factor (RF)
e) Serum creatine phosphokinase

**19.** A sural nerve and gastrocnemius muscle biopsy demonstrate evidence of necrotizing vasculitis

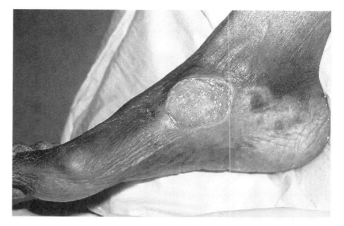

**Figure 34.10**  Foot ulceration of patient in Case 7. (See Color Fig. 34.10.)

(Fig. 34.11). The most appropriate therapy would be
a) Increase methotrexate to 10 mg/week orally.
b) Increase prednisone to 10 mg/day orally.
c) Discontinue methotrexate; start cyclophosphamide, 2 mg/kg per day orally; and increase prednisone to 1 mg/kg per day.
d) Discontinue methotrexate; start azathioprine, 0.5 mg/kg per day orally and increase prednisone to 20 mg/day.
e) Continue same treatment and add leflunomide, 10 mg/day.

Questions 20 through 30 may have multiple correct answers.

## CASE 8

A 58-year-old diabetic man develops pain and swelling in his MCP joints and knees. The sedimentation rate is 27 mm/hour, the serum ferritin is 862 mg/dL, and his RF is

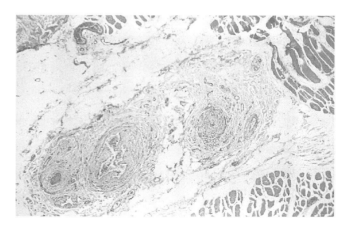

**Figure 34.11**  Sural nerve biopsy in patient in Question 19. (See Color Fig. 34.11.)

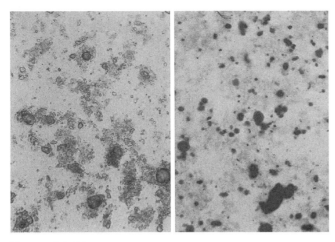

**Figure 34.12** Joint fluid stained with alizarin red S in Case 9 (See Color Fig. 34.12.)

negative. A synovial biopsy of his left knee stained for iron is positive.

**20.** Appropriate actions by the physician would include:
**a)** Family counseling
**b)** Use of colchicine
**c)** Use of methotrexate
**d)** Institution of phlebotomies
**e)** Use of an NSAID
**f)** Institution of radiation therapy

## CASE 9

An 84-year-old woman is seen for severe right shoulder pain. She has a large effusion, and a radiograph shows erosive changes in the humeral head, which is displaced from the glenoid. Aspirated joint fluid stained with alizarin red S shows the findings seen (Fig. 34.12)

**21.** Which of the following statements is (are) true in this case?
**a)** These clumps of crystals contain apatite (basic calcium crystals).
**b)** Knees are never involved in this process.
**c)** Both shoulders are affected in 50% of patients.
**d)** Treatment may include NSAIDs, aspiration and /or injection, and surgery.
**e)** Colchicine and allopurinol are effective treatments.

## CASE 10

A 42-year-old woman presents with bilateral ankle and knee pain and swelling of 2 months duration. She denies diarrhea and rectal bleeding. A synovial biopsy from her right knee shows noncaseating granulomata.

**22.** In a patient with such a biopsy result you might expect which of the following?
**a)** Abnormal delayed hypersensitivity skin tests
**b)** A negative PPD skin test
**c)** A history of uveitis
**d)** A primary Ghon complex and bilateral apical pleural thickening on chest radiograph
**e)** Hyperpigmented maculopapular skin lesions
**f)** Sterile leukocyturia

## CASE 11

A 23-year-old woman complains of pain and swelling of the right elbow. A biopsy is eventually performed; the pathology reveals red blood cells, hemosiderin deposits, giant cells, and foam cells.

**23.** Based on these finding, you might expect
**a)** Synovial fluid to contain an excessive number of RBCs
**b)** A fairly good response to radiation therapy
**c)** A fairly good response to synovectomy
**d)** An excellent response to colchicine
**e)** A good response to isoniazid and rifampin
**f)** Cultures to reveal a definitive diagnosis

## CASE 12

An 18-year-old man presents with a swollen ankle (Fig. 34.13). He has no other joint complaints.

**24.** Appropriate evaluation might include
**a)** Delayed hypersensitivity skin tests
**b)** Chest radiograph
**c)** Muscle biopsy
**d)** Proctosigmoidoscopy
**e)** Synovial fluid aspiration and study

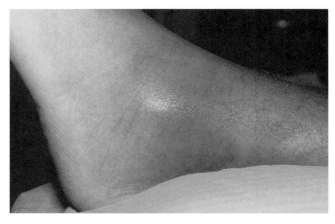

**Figure 34.13** Ankle of patient in Case 12. (See Color Fig. 34.13.)

## CASE 13

A 45-year-old carpenter reports malaise, weakness, weight loss, and generalized aching for 3 months. His temperature is 37.8°C, and blood pressure is 160/95 mm Hg. His knees are tender but not swollen. He has a right wrist drop, weakness of the right knee extensors, and absence of the right knee tendon reflex. Laboratory results are hematocrit, 35%; WBC count, 12,000/mm$^3$; Westergren ESR, 54 mm/h; aspartate aminotransferase, 45 mg/dL; CPK normal; RF, negative; ANA, negative; urine protein, 600 mg/24 hours; and urine RBCs, 25/hpf.

**25.** The most likely diagnosis is:
a) Rheumatoid arthritis
b) Systemic lupus erythematosus
c) Polymyositis
d) Progressive systemic sclerosis
e) Polyarteritis nodosa

## CASE 14

A 25-year-old woman had pain on moving her left elbow for 1 day, then pain in her right third MCP joint, followed by pain in her right knee. Examination discloses an uncomfortable young woman with a temperature of 37.2°C. Her right wrist is swollen and tender, and flexion and rotation of the left hip cause pain. Erythematous lesions with a central blister are noted on the dorsum of the left hand and on the left thigh. Aspirated fluid from her right wrist is cloudy and contains 37,000 leukocytes/mm$^3$, 80% of which are neutrophils.

**26.** Which of the following would be most likely to establish the diagnosis?
a) A lupus erythematosus cell test
b) A latex fixation test for rheumatoid factor
c) Determination of the antistreptolysin-0 titer
d) A culture of cervical secretions
e) A smear and culture of synovial fluid

## CASE 15

A 20-year-old nurse complains of stiff, swollen fingers of 1-week duration. Examination discloses tenderness and slight swelling of the proximal interphalangeal joints of the second, third, and fourth digits bilaterally. The laboratory results are hematocrit, 39%; leukocyte count, 7,000/mm$^3$; Westergren ESR, 25 mm/h; and rheumatoid latex titer, 1:40.

**27.** The differential diagnosis should include
a) Rheumatoid arthritis
b) Systemic lupus erythematosus

c) Acute viral hepatitis B
d) Postrubella vaccination reaction

## CASE 16

A young Arab from Jordan presents with severe headache and visual disturbances. He has bilateral papilledema, oral mucosal ulcers, and a single 4-cm scrotal ulcer. Bilateral anterior uveitis is noted and is thought to have been present for several months. Oral and scrotal ulcers have been recurring over the past year.

**28.** Additional manifestations of this illness that might occur in the future include all of the following, *except*
a) Thrombophlebitis
b) Arthritis
c) Widespread secondary amyloidosis
d) Skin lesions resembling erythema nodosum over the pretibial area
e) A syndrome resembling multiple sclerosis

**29.** Which of these statements is true concerning hepatitis B infection?
a) Acute polyarthritis usually follows the appearance of jaundice.
b) Urticaria may accompany acute polyarthritis.
c) Serum complement levels are usually elevated in patients with acute polyarthritis.
d) Necrotizing vasculitis occurs in patients with persistent hepatitis B antigenemia.
e) Glomerulophritis may be associated with hepatitis B infections.

**30.** The laboratory reports that a patient in the hospital has a serum urate level of 1.6 mg/dL. This patient might have:
a) Had a cholecystogram showing stones.
b) Had an upper GI study showing a duodenal diverticulum.
c) Had a chest radiograph showing a right upper lobe mass.
d) Been taking colchicine.
e) Been taking allopurinol.

**31.** The anemia of giant cell arteritis responds to treatment with:
a) Prednisone
b) Vitamin B$_{12}$
c) Oral iron
d) Parenteral iron
f) Salicylates

**32.** The differential diagnosis of sore throat, fever, and polyarthritis should include all the following, *except*
a) Gonococcal arthritis
b) Rheumatoid arthritis
c) Dermatomyositis

**d)** Systemic lupus
**e)** Psoriatic arthritis

**33.** Shoulder-hand syndrome may be associated with all the following, *except*
**a)** Myocardial infarction
**b)** Cervical disc disease
**c)** Laennec's cirrhosis
**d)** Cerebral vascular accident
**e)** Anticonvulsant drugs

**34.** The management of Charcot's arthropathy of the knee in a diabetic could include all the following, *except*
**a)** Immobilization
**b)** Total knee joint replacement
**c)** Restriction of weight bearing
**d)** Mechanical supports
**e)** Arthrodesis

**35.** Treatment with methotrexate has been associated with
**a)** Stomatitis
**b)** Pancytopenia
**c)** Liver dysfunction
**d)** Deposition of mercury in synovial lining cells.

**36.** Joint fluid is found to have a WBC of 20,000/mm³, 90% of which are neutrophils, 10% monocytes, no crystals, decreased complement, and a glucose of 45 mg/dL. The most likely diagnosis is
**a)** Gout
**b)** Osteoarthritis
**c)** Rheumatoid arthritis
**d)** Pseudogout

**37.** Joint fluid is found to have WBC of 12,000/mm³, 72% neutrophils, and 28% mononuclears, free and intracellular strongly negative birefringent crystals, and normal complement. The most likely diagnosis is
**a)** Gout
**b)** Osteoarthritis
**c)** Rheumatoid arthritis
**d)** Pseudogout

**38.** Joint fluid is found to have WBC of 850/ mm³, 25% of which are neutrophils, 75% mononuclears, no crystals, normal complement, and cartilage fibrils are noted. The most likely diagnosis is
**a)** Gout
**b)** Osteoarthritis
**c)** Rheumatoid arthritis
**d)** Pseudogout

**39.** Joint fluid is found to have WBC of 5,000/ mm³, 45% neutrophils, 55% mononuclears, free and intracellular weakly positive rhomboidal birefringent crystals, and normal complement. The most likely diagnosis is

**a)** Gout
**b)** Osteoarthritis
**c)** Rheumatoid arthritis
**d)** Pseudogout

## CASE 17

**40.** A 28-year-old man has rash, edema of his feet, and arthritis of his knees and ankles for 6 weeks. He has had some recent upper abdominal pain, and his stools have been dark for 3 or 4 days. His rash is confined to the legs and consists of purpuric lesions varying from bright red to dark purple. Platelets are normal on peripheral blood smear. The most useful initial diagnostic test would be
**a)** A urinalysis
**b)** A latex test for RF
**c)** Skin biopsy with immunofluorescent studies
**d)** A synovial biopsy
**e)** A sedimentation rate

**41.** The basic pathologic lesion accounting for the skin and probably the GI manifestations in this same patient is
**a)** Nerve fiber degeneration
**b)** A defect in platelet function
**c)** Degeneration of collagen fibers in the wall of blood vessels
**d)** A consumptive coagulopathy
**e)** A small vessel vasculitis

**42.** The most useful diagnostic test for determining the prognosis of the disorder in this same patient is
**a)** A platelet count
**b)** Urinalysis
**c)** Electrocardiogram
**d)** Skin biopsy
**e)** Gastroscopy

**43.** Finally, this same disorder in children differs from its counterpart in adults in that:
**a)** It is usually a mild or subclinical disorder in children.
**b)** Intussusception is common in children with the disorder but rare or absent in the adult.
**c)** The kidneys are rarely involved in the adult.
**d)** The skin is rarely involved in children.

## ANSWERS AND EXPLANATIONS

**1. c.**
This diagnosis should be suspected because of the rimmed vacuoles on biopsy, proximal and distal muscle weakness, and a relatively small increase in muscle enzymes.

**2. b.**
Inclusion body myositis is relatively resistant to treatment attempts, so lower doses of prednisone are generally tried.

If fairly conservative treatment fails, aggressive treatment may simply lead to therapeutic complications.

**3. c.**
These are typical electron microscopic findings in inclusion body myositis.

**4. d.**
Rash is not common in rheumatoid arthritis or Behçet's syndrome, and pleurisy rarely occurs in Reiter's syndrome or polyarteritis nodosa.

**5. d.**
Renal biopsy should be considered to make a firm diagnosis of lupus nephritis to determine appropriate therapy, although it is not always necessary if hypertension, an active urine sediment, and low complements are present.

**6. c.**
Prednisone at 1 mg/kg per day and monthly intermittent intravenous cyclophosphamide at 0.70 g/m$^2$ have been determined to be the best combination of safety and effectiveness for treatment of lupus nephritis.

**7. c.**
The findings described are typical of systemic lupus erythematosus (SLE) cerebritis. The best treatment is 1 g intravenous methylprednisolone (Solu-Medrol) for 3 days followed by 1 mg/kg per day prednisone and phenytoin for seizures.

**8. a.**
Aspiration and synovial fluid analysis and culture is the most appropriate initial action. The immediate injection of methylprednisolone into the right knee would not be appropriate when the diagnosis is not clear. Radiography of the knee, and testing complete blood cell count, sedimentation rate, C-reactive protein, and uric acid may all yield helpful information, but should be done after synovial fluid analysis.

**9. d.**
Allopurinol plays no role in the treatment of calcium pyrophosphate crystal deposition disease. All other measures listed are appropriate.

**10. e.**
Low complements, characteristic of immune complex disease, are not seen in pseudogout. Brown urine on alkalinization (ochronosis), Kayser-Fleischer rings (Wilson's disease), elevated calcium and low phosphorous (hyperparathyroidism), and elevated ferritin (hemochromatosis) are occasionally associated with pseudogout.

**11. e.**
CREST causes Raynaud's phenomenon, esophageal symptoms, sclerodactyly, and telangiectasia. Sclerodactyly and telangiectasia are not seen in Buerger's disease.

**12. c.**
Anticentromere antibody is characteristic of CREST syndrome.

**13. d.**
Bronchoalveolar lavage indicates whether alveolitis is present in progressive systemic sclerosis (scleroderma).

**14. d.**
Oral cyclophosphamide, 2 mg/kg per day, has been shown to be useful in the treatment of alveolitis associated with progressive systemic sclerosis (scleroderma).

**15. c.**
The clinical findings are typical of osteoarthritis.

**16. d**
Prednisone is not used to treat osteoarthritis. All other measures listed are appropriate.

**17. d.**
Methotrexate is not used to treat osteoarthritis. All other measures listed are appropriate.

**18. c.**
Gastrocnemius muscle and sural nerve biopsy would be useful to confirm the diagnosis of vasculitis.

**19. c.**
Cyclophosphamide, 2 mg/kg per day orally with prednisone at 1 mg/kg per day would be the most appropriate treatment of rheumatoid necrotizing vasculitis.

**20. a, d, and e.**
The patient has a positive synovial iron stain, in addition to diabetes, an elevated ferritin, and MCP involvement, characteristic of hemochromatosis. Family counseling is appropriate because hemochromatosis is a hereditary disease. Phlebotomy can be used to decrease the iron load, and NSAIDs can improve joint symptoms.

Colchicine is unlikely to improve joint symptoms; methotrexate could aggravate hepatic disease, and radiation therapy has no role in treatment of hemochromatosis.

**21. a, c, and d.**
The slide depicts Milwaukee shoulder joint fluid findings. The crystals found in Milwaukee shoulder are primarily hydroxyapatite, and bilateral shoulder involvement often is present.

Treatment using NSAIDs, aspiration and/or injection, and surgery are all appropriate treatments.

Answers b and e are incorrect because the knees are often involved in Milwaukee shoulder syndrome, and colchicine and allopurinol do not have the same efficacy as in gout.

**22. b, c, and e.**
The synovial biopsy shows findings typical of sarcoidosis: the negative PPD, uveitis, and hyperpigmented maculopapular skin lesions are all characteristic of sarcoidosis. Answers a, b, and f are incorrect because delayed

hypersensitivity skin tests are normal in 80% of patients with sarcoidosis; Ghon complex and apical pleural thickening are characteristic of tuberculosis, not sarcoidosis, and a sterile leukocyturia is also characteristic of tuberculosis.

### 23. a, b, and c.

The biopsy shows pigmented villonodular synovitis (PVS) with giant cells, RBCs and hemosiderin-laden macrophages. Synovial fluid in PVS is often hemorrhagic, and radiation and/or synovectomy may be helpful in treating. Answers d, e, and f are incorrect because neither colchicine nor antituberculous treatment is effective, and no infectious cause for PVS has been discovered.

### 24. a, b, d, and e.

The slide shows ankle synovitis. Chest radiography can be reveal sarcoidosis. Inflammatory bowel disease may cause lower extremity synovitis, often involving the ankles. Synovial analysis can determine whether inflammatory fluid or another type of synovial fluid is present.

Myositis would be an unlikely cause of ankle swelling.

### 25. e.

Arthralgia, myalgia, fever, hypertension, wrist drop, peripheral neuropathy, anemia, leukocytosis, ESR, proteinuria, and hematuria are very suggestive of polyarteritis nodosa.

Answers a, b, c, and d are incorrect because proteinuria and hematuria would be unusual in rheumatoid arthritis; leukocytosis would be unusual in SLE, polyneuropathy and proteinuria would be unusual in polymyositis; and fever and polyneuropathy would be unusual in progressive systemic sclerosis.

### 26. d.

The case description is typical of gonococcal arthritis-dermatitis syndrome.

### 27. a, b, c, and d.

The clinical description is that of acute synovitis.

### 28. e.

The case described is typical of Behçet's syndrome, which does not cause symptoms typical of multiple sclerosis.

### 29. b, d, and e.

Utricaria often accompanies acute polyarthritis prior to onset of jaundice. A significant percentage of patients with necrotizing vasculitis will have persistent hepatitis B antigenemia. Immune complex glomerulonephritis may accompany hepatitis B infection.

Answers a and c are incorrect because the polyarthritis precedes jaundice, and complement levels will usually be depressed in this immune complex disease.

### 30. a, c, and e.

Uric acid levels can be influenced by oral cholesystographic agents, which may have a urate lowering effect in some patients; lung tumors, which may secrete substances causing inappropriate ADH syndrome, thus

leading to hypouricemia; and allopurinol use, which lowers urate levels.

Answers b and d are incorrect because neither bowel contrast agents nor colchicine affect the uric acid level.

### 31. a.

Prednisone helps resolve the inflammation associated with giant cell arteritis causing the anemia. All others are incorrect because they have no affect on anemia-related inflammation.

### 32. e.

Psoriatic arthritis does not cause sore throat and would rarely cause fever. All the other four could cause such symptoms. Disseminated gonococcal syndrome could cause polyarthritis, fever, and gonococcal pharyngitis. Rheumatoid arthritis is often polyarticular, and it may cause fever and cricoarytenoid inflammation. Dermatomyositis may cause polyarthritis and fever and is often preceded by polyarthritis, fever, and aphthous pharyngitis. Lupus may cause mouth ulcers, fever, and arthritis.

### 33. c.

Cirrhosis is not associated with shoulder-hand syndrome but all the others have been associated by unknown mechanisms, perhaps by neurovascular reflexes.

### 34. b.

Total joint replacement is not done ordinarily in a Charcot joint because insensitivity to pain would lead to early prosthetic failure from overuse of the joint.

Answers a, c, d, and e are acceptable treatment for Charcot's joints.

### 35. a, b, and c.

All these and a number of other side effects can be observed with methotrexate therapy, but the deposition of mercury is not characteristic of methotrexate therapy.

### 36. c.

Rheumatoid arthritis. The elevated white count with increased polys, low complement, and low glucose are very typical of rheumatoid synovial fluid.

Gout is incorrect because no crystals are seen. The white count is too high for osteoarthritis and pseudogout is not likely because no crystals are seen.

### 37. a.

These characteristics are typical of urate. Osteoarthritis is not correct because the white count is too high and crystals are present; rheumatoid arthritis is incorrect because crystals are present and complement is normal; and pseudogout is incorrect because the crystals described are not characteristic of CPPD, but the opposite.

### 38. b.

Osteoarthritis is characterized by the very low white count and especially by the cartilage fibrils that were noted, all other three being less likely.

**39. d.**

These crystals are characteristic of pseudogout. They are weakly positively birefringent and have a more rhomboidal shape, instead of the long needle-like shape of urate crystals.

**40. c.**

The case described is fairly typical of Henoch-Schonlein purpura, and so a skin biopsy is quite helpful. A urinalysis might help but is nonspecific. The purpuric rash is a bit atypical for rheumatoid arthritis unless the person also has leukocytoclastic vasculitis. A synovial biopsy is not necessary for diagnosis and would probably be nonspecific and the ESR is very nonspecific.

**41. e.**

Leukocytoclastic vasculitis is a small-vessel vasculitis and very typical of that seen in Henoch-Schonlein purpura. Answers a, b, c, and d are not operative in HSP.

**42. b.**

Hematuria, suggestive of renal involvement, is the most important prognosticator here. None of the others is very helpful in determining prognosis.

**43. b.**

In children, intussusception is a very characteristic occurrence in HSP and all the others are false statements.

## SUGGESTED READINGS

Banker BQ, Engel AG. The plymyositis and dermatomyositis syndromes. In: Engel AG. Banker BQ, eds. *Myology*, vol. 2. New York: McGraw-Hill, 1986:1385–1422.

Ben-Dov I, Berry E. Acute rheumatic fever in adults over the age of 45 years: an analysis of 23 patients together with a review of the literature. *Semi Arthritis Rheum* 1980;10:100–110.

Bluestone R. Rheumatological complications of some endocrinopathies. *Clin Rheum Dis* 1975;1:95–107.

Brogadir SP, Schimmer BM, Myers AR. Spectrum of the gonococcal arthritis-dermatitis syndrome. *Semin Arthritis Rheu* 1979;8:177–183.

Calabrese LH, Mitsumoto H, Chou SM. Inclusion body myositis presenting as treatment–resistance polymyositis. *Arthritis Rheu* 1987;30:397–403.

Cream JJ, Gun JM, Peachey RDG. Schönlein-Henoch purpura in the adult. *QJM* 1970;39:461–484.

Dubois EL, Wallace DJ. Clinical and laboratory manifestations of SLE. In: Wallace DJ, Dubois EL, eds. *Lupus Erythematosus*. Philadelphia: Lea & Febiger, 1987:317–449.

Edwards CQ, Griffen LM, Goldgar D, et al. Prevalence of hemochromatosis among 11, 065 presumably healthy blood donors. *N Engl J Med* 1988;318: 1355–1362.

Espinoza LR, Spilberg I, Osterland CK. Joint manifestations of sickle cell disease. *Medicine* 1974;53:295–305.

Fam AG, Pritzker KPH, Stein JL, et al. Apatite-associated arthropathy: a clinic study of 14 cases and of 2 patients with calcific bursitis. Jl. *Rheumatol* 1979;6:461–471.

Fauci AS, Haynes BF, Katz P. The spectrum of vasculitis: clinical, pathologic, immunologic, and therapeutic considerations. *Ann Intern Med* 1978;89:660–676.

Gilbert MS. Musculosketetal manifestations of hemophilia. *Mt Sinai J Med* 1977;44:339–358.

Halverson PB, Carrera GF, McCarty DJ. Milwaukee shoulder syndrome. Fifteen additional cases and a description of contributing factors. *Arch Intern Med* 1990;150:677–682.

Hunder GG, Allen GL. Giant cell arteritis: a review. *Bull Rheum Dis* 1978–1979;29:980–986.

Hurd ER. Extra-articular manifestations of rheumatoid arthritis. *Semin Rheum Dis* 1979; 8:151–176.

Masi AT. Classification of systemic sclerosis (scleroderma). In: Black CM, Myers AR, eds. *Systemic Sclerosis (Scleroderma)*. New York; Gower Medical, 1985:7–15.

McCarty DJ. Calcium pyrophosphate dehydrate crystal deposition disease, 1975. *Arthritis Rheum* 1976;19:275–285.

McEwen C, DiTate D, Lingg C, et al. Ankylosing spondylitis and spondylitis accompanying ulcerative colitis, regional enteritis psoriasis, and Reiter's disease: a comparative study. *Arthritis Rheum* 1971;14:291–318.

Michet CJ Jr., McKenna CH, Lutura HS, et al; Relapsing polychondritis. *Ann Intern Med* 1896;104:74–78.

Myers BW, Masi AT. Pigmented villonodular synovitis and tenosynovitis: a clinical epidemiologic study of 166 cases and literature review. *Medicine* 1980;59:223–238.

Neustadt DH. Intra-articular and steroid therapy. In: Moskowitz RW, Howell DS, Goldberg VM, Mankin HF, eds. *Osteoarthritis, Diagnosis and Management*, 2nd ed. Philadelphia: WB Saunders, 1992: 493–510.

Salerni R, Rodman GP, Leon DF, et al. Pulmonary hypertension in the CREST syndrome variant of progressive sclerosis (scleroderma). *Ann Intern Med* 1977;86:394–399.

Smith PH, Beun RT, Sharp J. Natural history of rheumatoid cervical luxations. *Ann Rheum Dis* 1972;31:431–439.

Strongwater SL. Overview and clinical manifestation of inflammatory myositis: polymyositis and dermatomyositis. *Mt Sinai Med* 1988; 55:435–446.

Spilberg I, Siltzbach LE, McEwen C. The arthritis of sarcoidosis. *Arthritis Rheum* 1969;12:126–137.

Yu TF. Diversity of clinical features in gouty arthritis. *Semin Arthritis Rheum* 1984;13:360–368.

# Pulmonary and Critical Care Medicine

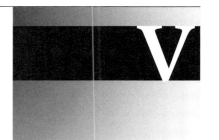

# Venous Thromboembolic Diseases

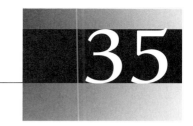

*Steven R. Deitcher*

Venous thromboembolic disease is the third most common cardiovascular disease after atherosclerotic heart disease and stroke. It has been estimated that between 500,000 and 2 million venous thromboembolic events (VTEs), including calf vein thrombosis, proximal deep venous thrombosis (DVT), and pulmonary embolism (PE), occur annually in the United States alone. It is estimated that up to 50% of DVTs are asymptomatic or go undetected. Antemortem diagnosis may actually be made in fewer than one third of patients with suspected PE. In autopsy-based studies, PE has been identified as the proximate cause or contributor to death in 15% to 30% of all patients. In general, VTEs are a major cause of sudden death and in-hospital morbidity and mortality. The extremely high incidence of DVT and PE likely reflects inadequate attention to VTE prophylaxis in high-risk surgical settings and the medically ill patient, in particular.

The spectrum of clinical outcomes secondary to venous thrombosis depends on the extent, location, and setting of the index event. The major clinical consequences of extremity DVT include the post-thrombotic syndrome (chronic swelling, stasis dermatitis, stasis ulceration, and venous claudication all secondary to venous insufficiency) and PE. The major clinical consequences of PE include chronic dyspnea, pulmonary hypertension, pulmonary infarction, and death. DVT restricted to the calf veins uncommonly results in a clinically important PE and is rarely associated with a fatal outcome. In contrast, inadequately treated DVT involving the popliteal or more proximal leg veins is associated with a 20% to 50% risk of clinically relevant recurrence and is strongly associated with both symptomatic and fatal PE. In untreated patients, death from PE occurs most frequently within 24 to 48 hours of initial presentation. All-cause mortality rates in treated patients with PE as high as 11% at 2 weeks and 17% at 3 months have been reported. Even small PE in patients with emphysema, cardiac disease, or lung involvement with malignancy may result in death. Any VTE in a patient with a contraindication to anticoagulation presents a therapeutic challenge and greater likelihood of adverse outcome. In part, for these reasons, calf DVT, proximal DVT, and PE have been considered distinct manifestations of thromboembolic diseases.

This chapter focuses on the diagnostic and therapeutic challenges of the full spectrum of venous thromboembolic disease routinely encountered by the general internist. The information is presented in a case-based format and key points likely to be addressed by a comprehensive examination are highlighted. The *hot tips* will, it is hoped, serve as a useful tool for review.

## SUPERFICIAL VENOUS THROMBOSIS DIAGNOSIS AND TREATMENT

### Case 1

A 56-year-old woman presents complaining of a painful, red, linear lesion involving her leg. Examination reveals a tender, palpable cord involving the medial aspect of the left thigh. Compression ultrasound demonstrates a left greater saphenous vein thrombosis within 5 cm of the saphenofemoral junction. Ultrasonographic evidence of DVT is absent. She denies a history of past DVT and superficial venous thrombosis (SVT). She has not received any recent intravenous therapy and is unaware of any significant varicose veins. She has no symptoms of PE. Her only current medication is a calcium channel blocker prescribed for mild hypertension. Her family history is notable for DVT in a maternal aunt.

### Questions
1. What is the most appropriate treatment for this woman's superficial thrombosis?
   a) Nonsteroidal anti-inflammatory drugs (NSAIDs) and warm compresses
   b) Intravenous heparin followed by oral anticoagulation (warfarin) for 6 to 12 weeks
   c) Low-molecular-weight heparin (LMWH) followed by oral anticoagulation for 3 to 6 months
   d) Placement of an inferior vena cava (IVC) filter
   e) Serial ultrasound to monitor for entry into the femoral vein

2. In addition to your preferred method of treatment, which of the following would you perform?
   a) Testing for inherited and acquired hypercoagulable states
   b) Whole-body computerized tomography (CT) in search of an occult malignancy
   c) An antinuclear antibody (ANA) test in search of an autoimmune disorder

d) All of the above

e) None of the above

## Hot Tips

■ Remember that the *superficial femoral vein* is a *deep* vein, whereas the *greater saphenous vein* is a *superficial* vein.

## Discussion

Thrombosis involving the superficial veins of the lower or upper extremities is often viewed as a common but insignificant form of venous thrombosis and thus neglected by clinicians. SVT may be at the mild end of the venous thromboembolic disease spectrum with regard to morbidity secondary to limb compromise and PE, but it may be a strong indicator of underlying hypercoagulability or malignancy. The diagnosis of SVT is often made on the basis of an area of tenderness, cord, and erythema overlying a superficial vein. SVT is not uncommon in the upper extremities after an indwelling catheter (intravenous) and in the lower extremities at sites of varicose veins. The progression of SVT into the deep venous system has been reported to occur in 7% to 44% of cases. The most common location for the progression from SVT to DVT to occur is at the junction between the greater saphenous vein (a superficial leg vein) and the common femoral vein (a proximal deep leg vein). In patients with SVT, PE in general and symptomatic PE in particular have been found in 33% and 10% of cases, respectively. The proximity of an SVT to the junction between the involved superficial vein and its connection to the deep venous system does not seem to impact the likelihood of PE. Several reports have described an association between SVT and concomitant DVT.

Typically, NSAIDs and warm compresses are adequate treatment for SVT symptom control. When the deep system is involved, or symptomatic PE is diagnosed, standard anticoagulant therapy is indicated. Because of the reported high rate of progression from SVT to DVT (3.6% by day 12), many physicians treat SVT with anticoagulants for a variable length of time. Short-term (8–12 days) prophylactic-intensity LMWH, treatment-intensity LMWH, and tenoxicam (an NSAID) have been shown to reduce DVT rates compared to placebo. Anticoagulants, such as heparin and LMWH, may help relieve symptoms related to vessel inflammation but are probably best reserved for individuals with recurrent SVT or documented DVT. Serial ultrasound to detect meaningful SVT progression seems prudent in selected cases, such as those with SVT already present at the saphenofemoral junction. Inherited risk factors for thrombosis are found more commonly in persons with SVT than in controls, but testing has not been shown to warrant an alteration in treatment, impact the rate of progression, or support the need for serial ultrasound. Despite the fact that SVT has been associated with adenocarcinoma, searching for occult cancer with CT scans is not recommended. An age- and gender-appropriate cancer screening, though, does seem reasonable.

## Answers and Explanations

**1. a and e.**

SVT can be diagnosed on the basis of history and physical examination, but compression ultrasound is useful to confirm the diagnosis and look for concomitant DVT.

Anticoagulation is not generally recommended for SVT unless it is recurrent or associated with DVT and PE. Whether NSAIDs or a brief course of anticoagulation should be prescribed to all SVT patients will require further trials.

**2. b.**

Recurrent and migratory thrombophlebitis including SVT may be a sign of occult malignancy and warrants an age- and gender-appropriate patient cancer screening.

## CALF DEEP VENOUS THROMBOSIS DIAGNOSIS AND TREATMENT

### Case 2

A 33-year-old man with Crohn's disease presents with right calf pain and swelling 2 days after being discharged from the hospital for an inflammatory bowel disease flare associated with documented gastrointestinal blood loss. He has a history of central venous access device–associated venous thrombosis during past hospitalizations and past courses of total parenteral nutrition. Compression ultrasonography of both legs reveals right posterior tibial and soleal vein acute thrombosis. The popliteal, superficial femoral, common femoral, and distal external iliac veins demonstrate no findings suggestive of thrombosis.

### Questions

3. Compression ultrasonography is an appropriate initial means of imaging for calf DVT.

a) True

b) False

4. What is the most appropriate treatment for this man's isolated calf DVT?

a) NSAIDs and warm compresses

b) Intravenous heparin followed by oral anticoagulation (warfarin) for 6 to 12 weeks

c) LMWH followed by oral anticoagulation for 3 to 6 months

d) Serial ultrasound (twice weekly for 2 to 3 weeks) to monitor for proximal extension

e) Placement of an IVC filter

## Discussion

### Hot Tips

- Calf DVT is not necessarily benign in nature and requires anticoagulant therapy or serial ultrasound surveillance to detect proximal thrombus extension.
- Risk factors for any DVT include advanced age, immobilization, prior VTE, major abdominal and orthopedic surgery, pregnancy, cancer, obesity, varicose veins, myocardial infarction, congestive heart failure, respiratory tract infections, inflammatory diseases, estrogen containing medications, and hypercoagulable states.
- Pain, swelling, redness, and increased warmth limited to the calf do not rule out a more proximal DVT.

It is perceived by many that calf DVT is uncommon and of limited clinical significance. This misunderstanding and underappreciation of the morbidity and mortality associated with calf DVT has resulted in a lack of clear consensus on the optimal management strategy for this thrombotic disease. Contemporary clinical studies have revealed that isolated calf DVT may account for as few as 6.2% of all symptomatic acute DVT and as many as 43% of all acute VTEs. Studies also have demonstrated that, although calf DVT and proximal DVT may be considered separate diseases at their outset, 15% to 25% of calf DVT propagate and convert into a proximal DVT. Symptomatic and asymptomatic calf DVT appears to propagate with an equal frequency. Such "proximal conversion" renders what was initially a calf DVT just as dangerous as any proximal DVT. Proximal conversion has been shown to occur within the initial 2 weeks after diagnosis in the majority of cases and warrants treatment accordingly.

Although 6 months of anticoagulation has been shown to be superior to 6 weeks' duration of therapy in patients with proximal DVT, the shorter course of therapy has *not* been shown to be significantly inferior in patients with initial distal thrombosis. Situational calf DVT (DVT with a clear precipitant, such as an inflammatory bowel disease flare and prolonged bed rest) can be safely treated for only 6 weeks, assuming the precipitating illness or event has resolved. IVC filter placement is not recommended for calf DVT in most circumstances.

### Answers and Explanations

#### 3. a.
Compression ultrasound is an acceptable initial imaging technique for calf DVT diagnosis. Idiopathic calf DVT, like idiopathic proximal DVT, may be the initial presentation of occult malignancy, and appropriate history, physical examination, and screening tests should be performed to detect cancer at its earliest stage.

Despite past reports of inadequate ultrasound sensitivity and specificity for calf DVT, newer imaging hardware and software have made calf DVT diagnosis very feasible by experienced vascular ultrasound technologists.

#### 4. d.
Although the primary goals of proximal DVT treatment include the prevention of DVT recurrence and PE, it is believed that the most essential goal of calf DVT treatment should be to prevent early proximal conversion. Current treatment approaches for isolated calf DVT range from identical intensity and duration of anticoagulant therapy, as is used for proximal DVT, to a complete lack of any pharmacologic therapy at all. Acceptable management, which falls between these extremes, includes serial duplex ultrasound surveillance, with therapy begun only in the event of proximal conversion, and abbreviated courses of standard anticoagulation. Surveillance consists of noninvasive imaging twice weekly for typically no more than 3 weeks (this includes the usual period for proximal conversion). The limitations of serial surveillance, however, include cost, compliance, and convenience. Serial surveillance seems especially prudent in situations such as recent gastrointestinal bleeding, in which the risk of anticoagulation would likely exceed the benefit.

## VENOUS THROMBOSIS DIAGNOSIS

### Case 3

A 54-year-old woman with a history of varicose veins presents complaining of progressive left leg pain and swelling of 3 days' duration, as well as vague right lateral pleuritic chest pain without significant shortness of breath. She has no known history of past VTEs. Her family history is noncontributory. She has taken hormone replacement therapy for the past 5 years without a recent dose increase. A chest radiograph performed in the emergency department reveals clear lung fields and a lack of obvious rib fracture. Your pretest clinical suspicion for DVT is high and for PE is intermediate. A rapid D-dimer assay is notable for an elevated concentration of D-dimer.

#### Questions
**5.** What is the most appropriate initial means of evaluating this woman for an acute lower extremity DVT?
a) Iodine$^{125}$–radiolabeled fibrinogen leg scanning
b) Ascending contrast venography
c) Compression ultrasound
d) Magnetic resonance imaging
e) No further testing needed because the positive D-dimer test is diagnostic of acute DVT

**6.** What is the most appropriate initial means of evaluating this woman for acute PE?
a) Radionucleotide ventilation/perfusion (V/Q) lung scanning

b) Helical (spiral) CT
c) Pulmonary angiography
d) Transesophageal echocardiography
e) No further testing is needed because the positive D-dimer test is diagnostic of acute PE

### *Discussion*

### Hot Tips

- DVT can present with limb pain, swelling, redness, warmth, or a palpable cord, or it can be *asymptomatic*. One should not rule-in or rule-out DVT based on clinical grounds alone.
- Compression ultrasonography performed by a skilled operator is very sensitive and specific (>95%), especially for acute symptomatic DVT and proximal DVT.

Failure to accurately and promptly diagnose DVT and PE can result in excess morbidity and mortality due to post-thrombotic syndrome, pulmonary hypertension, and recurrent VTEs. Conversely, unnecessary anticoagulation therapy provides risk in the absence of any tangible benefit. Therefore, the proper and timely diagnosis or exclusion of DVT and PE is imperative to ensure optimal patient clinical outcome.

Because the signs and symptoms of PE, including chest pain (70% of patients), shortness of breath (25%), cough (40%), tachypnea (70%), tachycardia (33%), syncope (5%), and signs of DVT (10%), are nonspecific, the purely clinical diagnosis is challenging and discouraged. In fact, a high clinical suspicion alone accurately predicts for PE in only 68% of cases. An individualized approach to PE diagnosis based on patients' clinical presentation, comorbidities, chest radiograph, and the availability of imaging and interpretive expertise seems prudent. Pulmonary angiography is the historical gold standard for PE diagnosis, to which all other imaging modalities have been compared. PE is diagnosed by the identification of an intraluminal filling defect or arterial cutoff demonstrated in two imaging planes (perpendicular views). Interinterpreter variability can be high, and the sensitivity for peripheral, subsegmental PE has been questioned. The advantages of pulmonary angiography include the ability to perform adjunctive procedures, such as suction thrombectomy, local catheter-directed thrombolysis, and IVC filter placement, at the same time as the diagnostic procedure. The procedure, however, is invasive and associated with death, major complications, and minor complications in 0.5%, 1.0%, and 5.0% of cases, respectively. Pulmonary angiography is most often used as a second-line diagnostic modality, especially in patients with an indeterminate scan.

The perfusion scan is the most frequently ordered diagnostic test in those with clinically suspected PE. The perfusion study (Q scan) is performed using an intravenous injection of macroaggregated particles of technetium[99m]-labeled human serum albumin. Any obstruction to arterial flow is viewed as an area of nonperfusion or underperfusion, termed a *perfusion defect*. The performance of ventilation scintigraphy (V scan) in individuals with abnormal Q scans helps improve test specificity. A V scan involves the inhalation of a radioactive gas or aerosolized technetium[99m] that provides an image of all ventilated portions of the lung. Based on the presence and extent of matched (absence of both perfusion and ventilation) and unmatched (absence of perfusion with preserved ventilation) defects, the scan can be interpreted using published criteria as either normal, low probability, indeterminate probability, or high probability for PE. The high negative predictive value of a normal or near normal scan alone essentially excludes (<5% probability) PE. The high positive predictive value (approximately 90%) of a high-probability scan alone has led most physicians to consider such a scan as diagnostic of PE. A nondiagnostic (indeterminate) scan, one that is interpreted as low or intermediate probability, neither confirms nor refutes the diagnosis of PE and is best interpreted in the context of clinical suspicion and additional testing. For example, in patients in whom a low clinical suspicion for PE exists and who have a low probability scan, PE is unlikely. Other combinations of clinical probability and scan result usually warrant the performance of additional testing before a suitable diagnosis can be achieved. Patients with suspected PE, in whom treatment is withheld on the basis of a low pretest clinical probability and a nondiagnostic scan, have been shown to have a very low (1.7%) 3-month thromboembolic risk *as long as* lower extremity compression ultrasound does not reveal proximal DVT.

The high prevalence of nondiagnostic studies and the failure of many physicians to establish a clinical probability for the likelihood of PE before obtaining and interpreting the scan are significant limitations to its use as a diagnostic tool. In the Prospective Investigation of Pulmonary Embolism Diagnosis study, 73% of scans were nondiagnostic. This number may be as high as 90% in patients with underlying chronic obstructive pulmonary disease or other underlying pulmonary processes that can result in an abnormal chest radiograph. The scan is an appropriate "first test" to evaluate a patient with suspected PE. The procedure is noninvasive and associated with a limited exposure to radiation. In addition, it is widely available, and most radiologists have extensive experience with its use. If the baseline chest radiograph is abnormal, if there is a history of significant underlying pulmonary disease, or if there a history of prior PE, however, the scan may not provide the necessary information to diagnose or exclude acute PE.

Some investigators have suggested that spiral CT replace scanning as the initial test of choice for PE diagnosis. Others advocate that it should be used as the confirmatory test of choice in place of a pulmonary angiogram. Still others believe additional comparative data are needed before widespread spiral CT use is warranted. With spiral CT, PE is diagnosed by identifying a filling defect in the pulmonary arteries. When compared with scintigraphy or pulmonary angiography, the sensitivity and specificity of spiral CT have ranged from 53% to 100% and 78% to 100%, respectively. Spiral CT is best used to identify thrombus within the main pulmonary arteries, lobar pulmonary arteries, and first-order segmental branches of the pulmonary artery. A normal spiral CT does not rule out PE and, like scanning, should be combined with an assessment of clinical probability and other diagnostic tests to arrive at a diagnosis.

Whether subsegmental PE is clinically significant and necessary to definitively detect has been debated and is a central issue to consider when choosing a PE diagnostic modality. Data from the Prospective Investigation of Pulmonary Embolism Diagnosis suggest that only 6% of PEs are subsegmental. The effects of a subsegmental PE may be negligible in patients with normal cardiopulmonary function. A subsegmental PE could be disastrous in a patient with decreased cardiopulmonary reserve or severe underlying lung disease, however. The danger of fatal recurrent PE in patients with an initial subsegmental event also is always present. Two recent meta-analyses that evaluated the use of spiral CT in the diagnosis of PE suggested that there was currently insufficient evidence to rely on a negative spiral CT scan to justify withholding anticoagulation or to support the insignificance of undetected subsegmental PE. In patients unable to cooperate with breath holding, breathing artifacts can change the orientation and the diameter of vessels. The presence of hilar lymphadenopathy or other mediastinal soft tissue mass may mimic the appearance of PE. Any shunt, whether due to a patent foramen ovale or intrapulmonary circulation from pleuroparenchymal disease, or a left-to-right cardiac shunt with prominent bronchopulmonary circulation, may make the CT scan more difficult to accurately interpret. One benefit of spiral CT is that up to 67% of scans can lead to or support an alternative diagnosis to explain a patient's presenting symptoms. Therefore, spiral CT may be the optimal initial test in patients with an abnormal baseline chest radiography.

Increased plasma concentrations of D-dimer reflect thrombus formation and concomitant fibrinolytic cascade activation. Because of its derivation from lysed thrombus and not from circulating fibrinogen, D-dimers have been extensively studied as a VTE diagnostic tool. Monoclonal antibody–based D-dimer assay methodologies differ with regard to ease of use, turn-around time, cost, sensitivity for PE, and specificity for PE. Traditional quantitative enzyme-linked immunosorbent assays (ELISAs) and rapid enzyme-linked immunosorbent assay–derived assays have the best sensitivity and negative predictive value for DVT and PE. Many disparate conditions can lead to an elevation in D-dimer. These conditions include VTE, myocardial infarction, pneumonia, sepsis, disseminated intravascular coagu-

lation, liver disease, malignancy, surgery, hemorrhage, and trauma. Thus, D-dimer testing may be specific for cross-linked fibrin degradation products, but cross-linked fibrin degradation products are not specific for PE. To put it simply, a positive D-dimer assay is of limited diagnostic use, whereas a negative test (D-dimer level of <500 ng/mL) essentially excludes venous thromboembolism.

Some centers use D-dimer testing as a stand-alone VTE screening test that, if not elevated, obviates the need for any radiographic imaging test. Other centers reserve D-dimer testing for patients with nondiagnostic initial imaging studies before pursuing more invasive testing. The specificity of D-dimer testing is particularly low in the very elderly suspected of having PE (9% in patients older than 80 years). In cancer patients, who are at high risk for VTEs because of the hypercoagulability of malignancy, D-dimer testing may lack sensitivity, specificity, and adequate negative predictive value for PE exclusion. Therefore, D-dimer testing is best reserved for otherwise healthy outpatients suspected of acute VTE.

### Answers and Explanations

#### 5. c.
For suspected DVT involving the arms or legs, compression ultrasound is the preferred initial imaging test. A diagnosis of DVT is based on the inability to completely compress a venous segment. Acute DVTs result in dilated, and often thickened, veins filled with uniformly echogenic material. Loss of flow phasicity, direct thrombus visualization, and aberrations on color flow imaging are less validated means of diagnosing DVT. Ultrasonography is noninvasive, rapid, and readily available at most hospitals. It is highly sensitive and specific for DVT when performed in symptomatic patients by experienced ultrasonographers. Screening compression ultrasound in asymptomatic patients is less accurate. Another limitation of ultrasound is the inability to diagnose pelvic vein thrombosis. Venography remains the "gold standard" test but is invasive and requires intravenous contrast. Magnetic resonance imaging (MRI) is an effective but costly means of diagnosing DVT. The role of nuclear medicine imaging for DVT remains to be defined.

#### 6. a or b.
PE can present with pleuritic chest pain, dyspnea, palpitations, syncope, dysrhythmias, hemoptysis, pleural effusion, or can be *asymptomatic* (silent PE). One should not rule-in or rule-out PE based on clinical grounds alone.

Radionucleotide Q lung scanning is sensitive but not specific for PE and is indeterminate in up to 73% of cases. Combining a Q scan with a radionucleotide V scan improves specificity. The combination of scanning with an assessment of pretest clinical suspicion improves specificity even more.

A normal or near normal scan alone essentially rules out PE. A low-probability scan combined with a low pretest clinical suspicion is unlikely to represent PE. A high-probability scan alone is accepted by most clinicians as diagnostic of PE. Most patients with an indeterminate scan (result other than normal/near normal or high-probability) will require further diagnostic evaluation regardless of the degree of clinical suspicion.

Helical (spiral) CT can diagnose PE involving the main, lobar, and segmental branches of the pulmonary arteries. A normal helical CT does not rule out subsegmental PE. Because helical CT is able to detect other thoracic pathology (alternative diagnosis in 40%) in addition to PE, it may be preferred in patients with abnormal baseline chest radiographs.

The D-dimer test is highly sensitive, but it is not specific for thrombosis. A negative test essentially rules out thrombosis; a positive test essentially means nothing.

## DEEP VENOUS THROMBOSIS TREATMENT

### Case 4

The patient from the last case is found to have an acute left common femoral, superficial femoral, and popliteal vein DVT on compression ultrasound examination. Her scan is interpreted as normal. She is able to ambulate without significant difficulty. She has a normal neurologic examination and no evidence of blood in her stool. Her pedal pulses are normal. Serum creatinine, liver function tests, hematocrit, and platelet count are all within normal limits. She is an active woman and would like to avoid hospitalization if possible. Like any patient, she wants the "best" treatment.

### Questions

**7.** Which of the following treatment strategies would *not* be acceptable?
a) Admission for at least 5 days of heparin and conversion to oral warfarin
b) Admission for 1 to 2 days of heparin followed by outpatient LMWH and conversion to oral warfarin
c) Admission for at least 5 days of LMWH and conversion to oral warfarin
d) Outpatient LMWH and conversion to oral warfarin
e) Inpatient or outpatient commencement of warfarin alone

### Discussion

### Hot Tips

- Initial treatment of DVT with LMWH is as safe and effective as treatment with heparin, but facilitates a shorter length of hospital stay.

Before selecting an approach to DVT management, one must clearly appreciate the goals of therapy. The goals of DVT management include (i) prevention of embolization, (ii) prevention of thrombus extension, (iii) prevention of early and late recurrence, (iv) restoration of venous patency, and (v) prevention of the post-thrombotic syndrome. Supportive care alone (i.e., doing nothing) accomplishes none of these goals. The placement of an IVC filter effectively prevents all PE in the short run but probably at the expense of a greater long-term DVT recurrence rate. Intravenous activated, partial thromboplastin time–adjusted, unfractionated heparin and weight-based LMWH effectively prevent embolization, extension, and recurrence. LMWH appears to be slightly but significantly better than standard heparin at restoring venous patency. Catheter-directed thrombolytic therapy is the most effective means of completely restoring patency but is associated with excessive bleeding and significant cost. Thrombolysis is best reserved for iliofemoral DVT in the young and those with extensive thrombosis resulting in venous limb gangrene (phlegmasia cerulea dolens).

Several prospective, randomized, controlled trials have demonstrated the efficacy and safety equivalency of unfractionated heparin and LMWH for the treatment of DVT. The major advantage of subcutaneous LMWH is its ability to be self-administered at home without the need for therapeutic monitoring. This translates into a significant reduction in mean hospital length of stay (6.5 days vs. 1.1 days). Patients may be started on LMWH in the hospital and then discharged in an accelerated fashion to continue their conversion to oral warfarin or treated exclusively in the outpatient setting. LMWHs are associated with less osteopenia, less heparin-induced thrombocytopenia, and less nonspecific protein binding than unfractionated heparin. Meta-analyses have demonstrated a survival advantage in those patients with acute DVT who have been treated initially with LMWH versus those treated initially with heparin. This overall survival advantage seems to be derived primarily from a survival advantage imparted on cancer patients with DVT.

The anticoagulant effects of LMWHs are not completely reversed by protamine sulfate.

Fondaparinux (synthetic heparin pentasaccharide) has been shown to be equivalent to heparin for the treatment of acute PE and equivalent to the LMWH enoxaparin for the treatment of acute DVT. Ximelagatran (oral direct thrombin inhibitor) also has been shown to be equivalent to enoxaparin in the setting of acute DVT. Ximelagatran has the potential to provide both acute and chronic phase anticoagulation without the need for therapeutic monitoring. Periodic liver function testing during ximelagatran treatment seems prudent.

Regardless of one's choice of heparin or location of initial therapy, a few key treatment issues must be noted:

- Treatment with heparin or LMWH should be begun as soon as possible. A delay in achieving a therapeutic intensity of initial parenteral therapy may negatively impact a patient's long-term VTE recurrence rate.
- Weight-based initial dosing of heparin (80 U/kg bolus followed by 18 U/kg per hour), with subsequent dose adjustments based on a standardized nomogram, allows a therapeutic activated partial thromboplastin time to be reached quickly. Weight-based LMWH dosing is the standard of care.
- Heparin and LMWH therapy must overlap oral warfarin therapy for a minimum of 4 days, and ideally until a stable target range (2.0 to 3.0) international normalized ratio (INR) has been achieved.

The INR, not the prothrombin time or prothrombin time ratio, should be used to monitor warfarin therapy. Monitoring at least every 4 weeks is recommended. More frequent monitoring helps maintain the INR within the target range for a greater amount of time.

Warfarin therapy *alone* is contraindicated in the setting of acute thrombosis because of the inherent delay in achieving therapeutic anticoagulation and the theoretical transient exacerbation of hypercoagulability caused by a rapid reduction in protein C functional activity. This warfarin-induced paradoxical hypercoagulability may explain warfarin-induced skin necrosis and warfarin-induced limb gangrene in patients with heparin-induced thrombocytopenia.

Warfarin therapy can be started as soon as a therapeutic level of heparin or LMWH has been reached (usually within 24 to 48 hours of therapy initiation). Bolus dosing of warfarin does not help to more quickly achieve a target INR. Initial dosing with 2.5 to 7.5 mg/day (based on patient weight and nutritional status) seems prudent.

Because of its teratogenic effects, warfarin therapy is contraindicated in pregnancy.

Patients at increased risk for bleeding probably should be treated initially in an inpatient setting. Such patients include those with active bleeding (including occult stool blood), a history of recent surgery, past gastrointestinal tract or neuraxial bleeding, recent trauma or stroke, concomitant regular NSAID use, thrombocytopenia, and renal insufficiency. Severe renal dysfunction (creatinine clearance of <30 mL/min) results in a 25% or greater reduction in LMWH clearance and thus results in drug accumulation.

LMWH therapy may not be suitable for the morbidly obese. Most reported clinical trials have enrolled patients weighing less than or equal to 120 kg. Monitored heparin therapy may be the safest choice for the morbidly obese with acute DVT.

Therapeutic monitoring of LMWH therapy using the antifactor Xa activity assay is not indicated in most patients. An exact therapeutic range has not been carefully determined. Adjusting the dose of LMWH based on such testing may not be superior to simple weight-based dosing.

The optimal duration of anticoagulation has been widely studied and debated. For idiopathic DVT, 3 months of therapy is better than 4 weeks, and 6 months is better than 6 weeks. In short, the risk of VTE recurrence is very low as long as therapeutic anticoagulation is continued. Only the 3% to 4% annual risk of major hemorrhage secondary to warfarin prevents physicians from prescribing long-term anticoagulation with abandon. Anticoagulation for 3 to 6 months is generally prescribed for individuals with a first DVT. Recurrent DVT after the completion of a course of anticoagulation usually warrants long-term therapy. Patients with persistent risk factors for thrombosis, such as an antiphospholipid antibody, hyperhomocysteinemia, incurable malignancy, or a deficiency of a natural anticoagulant (protein C, protein S, and antithrombin), usually benefit from long-term therapy.

The recently published PREVENT (Prevention of Recurrent Venous Thromboembolism) trial compared low-intensity oral warfarin with placebo for the secondary prevention of venous thrombosis, following a standard course of therapy for an index idiopathic DVT with or without PE. Warfarin with a target INR between 1.5 and 2.0 monitored every 8 weeks resulted in a 64% reduction in thrombosis recurrence rate without a significant difference in major bleeding rate. PREVENT also showed that factor V Leiden heterozygotes have the same risk of thrombosis recurrence as patients with two normal factor V alleles. Thus, in the absence of a persistent and potent prothrombotic state like cancer, antithrombin deficiency, homozygous factor V Leiden, and lupus anticoagulant, long-term, low-dose warfarin may provide the optimal blend of efficacy and safety.

### Answers and Explanations

**7. e**

Never begin warfarin without first achieving a therapeutic intensity of anticoagulation using another agent.

A 4-day minimum heparin/LMWH and warfarin overlap is warranted, and the heparin or LMWH should be continued until a stable INR of between 2.0 and 3.0 has been achieved. High-risk patients are best treated in the hospital with a drug that can be readily monitored, adjusted, and reversed.

A "bolus" of warfarin does not help to achieve a stable INR between 2.0 and 3.0 any faster than starting with lower doses, and it may actually promote transient hypercoagulability.

Therapeutic-intensity warfarin should be continued for at least 3 to 6 months (and longer in select patients).

## WARFARIN FAILURE

### Case 5

The same patient presents 3 months into her course of oral warfarin anticoagulation with right leg swelling and pain, as well as pleuritic chest pain, fever, and dyspnea on exertion. Compression ultrasound reveals a new acute right common femoral vein DVT.

Scanning reveals multiple new segmental "mismatches" highly suggestive of PE. A review of her anticoagulation clinic records reveals a stable INR between 2.3 and 3.2 (target, 2.5; range, 2.0 to 3.0) on each of her weekly tests. She denies recent trauma, travel, surgery, or new illness. Initial clinical assessment reveals that she is hemodynamically stable and not in pulmonary distress.

### Question

**8.** How would you treat this patient's recurrent thromboses?

a) Admission for intravenous heparin or LMWH and increase the warfarin dose to achieve an INR between 3.0 and 4.0

b) Admission for intravenous heparin or LMWH and discharge the patient on treatment-dose LMWH

c) Increase the warfarin dose to achieve an INR between 3.0 and 4.0 without any heparin or LMWH

d) Continue the current warfarin and insert an IVC filter

### Discussion

### Hot Tips

- Warfarin failure should alert the clinician to a possible underlying lupus anticoagulant or malignancy.
- Widely fluctuating INR values may represent patient noncompliance, dietary indiscretion, or drug–drug interactions.
- LMWH therapy is an acceptable alternative to warfarin in the setting of recurrent VTE despite documented INR values within the desired target range.

Warfarin "failure" implies that a patient has developed a recurrent VTE despite being treated with warfarin and maintaining a target INR between 2.0 and 3.0. The following causes for warfarin failure should be considered:

- Widely fluctuating or difficult-to-control INRs, resulting in an excessive amount of time spent with an INR below 2.0. Dietary indiscretion and the addition of new medications should be sought.
- Presence of a lupus anticoagulant that interferes with the accurate quantification of the INR.
- A persistent and potent thrombotic predisposition, such as adenocarcinoma, may render an INR of 2.0 to 3.0 inadequate. In general, the intensity of antithrombotic therapy must match and offset the intensity of any prothrombotic tendency.

### Answer and Explanation

**8. b.**
If a patient develops a recurrent VTE in the face of a below-target (below 2.0) INR, this is not warfarin failure.

In this setting, reinstitution of heparin or LMWH until the INR can be properly targeted and regulated is acceptable. If a lupus anticoagulant is detected, an alternative means of anticoagulation monitoring is indicated. If a persistent and potent prothrombotic state exists, one can either aim for a higher target INR or switch to an alternative anticoagulant. Aiming for an INR in the range of 3.0 to 4.0 is empiric, most likely associated with greater bleeding, and still associated with wide INR fluctuations. Switching to weight-based, treatment-dose LMWH seems justified. IVC filter placement will solely prevent further PE in the short run and will serve as a nidus for subsequent thrombosis in the long run. Fondaparinux and ximelagatran may also be acceptable alternatives in the near future.

## PULMONARY EMBOLISM

### Case 6

A 29-year-old physician presents complaining of acute onset chest pain and dyspnea. The symptoms developed while he was brushing his teeth before leaving his home to take the American Board of Internal Medicine–certifying examination. He felt like he might "pass out." He denies leg symptoms, history of cancer, family history of thrombosis, recent surgery, and past similar symptoms. An evaluation at a local emergency department reveals a respiratory rate of 28, a regular pulse of 110, and a blood pressure of 100/50. An electrocardiogram does not reveal evidence of cardiac ischemia. A lung scan is "highly probable" for PE. Compression ultrasound reveals a left popliteal acute DVT.

### Questions

**9.** Which of the following treatment strategies would be most acceptable?

a) Inpatient heparin and conversion to oral warfarin

b) Outpatient LMWH and conversion to oral warfarin

c) Placement of an IVC filter and no anticoagulation

d) Placement of an IVC filter plus inpatient heparin and conversion to oral warfarin

e) Thrombolysis with recombinant tissue plasminogen activator followed by anticoagulation as in choice (a) above

**10.** He develops melena on day 2 of heparin and is found to have gastritis on endoscopy. In addition to stopping heparin and starting $H_2$ blockade, the best treatment strategy includes which of the following?

a) IVC filter placement and no further anticoagulation

b) IVC filter placement now and restarting of heparin in the hospital once the gastritis has resolved

c) IVC filter placement now and outpatient LMWH with warfarin once the gastritis has resolved

d) Nothing

## Discussion

### Hot Tips

- Approximately 40% of patients with acute DVT have perfusion lung scan abnormalities suggestive of PE even in the absence of cardiopulmonary symptoms.
- LMWHs are not currently approved by the U.S. Food and Drug Administration for outpatient PE treatment.
- LMWHs have been shown to be equivalent to unfractionated heparin with regard to safety and efficacy for PE treatment in the inpatient setting.
- Lysis clears PE faster than anticoagulation alone but may not result in less long-term morbidity or mortality.
- IVC filters protect against PE in the short run and may actually increase the risk of recurrent DVT in the long run.
- IVC filters are not required in all PE patients and are intended to protect against fatal PE in patients who cannot receive anticoagulants or who develop PE despite anticoagulation.
- IVC filters, unlike anticoagulation, do not prevent thrombus extension or thrombus recurrence.

Thrombolysis has been shown to decrease pulmonary artery pressures and clear PE more rapidly than standard anticoagulant therapy. Survival does not appear to be significantly affected, however. Thrombolysis is probably best reserved for the acute treatment of PE patients with significant hemodynamic or respiratory compromise. Conflicting data exist on whether patients with evidence of right ventricular dysfunction, in particular, benefit from thrombolysis. The obvious major risk of thrombolytic therapy is bleeding.

### Answers and Explanations

#### 9. a.

In general, acute PE should be treated in the same fashion as acute DVT. It is actually advisable to start anticoagulation at the time of suspected PE even before diagnostic testing has been performed. LMWH has been shown to be safe and effective in patients with acute PE treated in-hospital. Outpatient treatment of PE seems reasonable but has not been formally studied to date. The placement of an IVC filter at the time of PE diagnosis is usually reserved for those with an absolute contraindication to anticoagulation. Many physicians, however, place filters in patients with underlying cardiac or pulmonary disease who are perceived as being at risk for death should they develop a second PE.

#### 10. b.

It is important to note that active bleeding may be a treatable and transient contraindication to anticoagulation. An IVC filter should not be viewed as an equivalent

substitute to anticoagulation in the setting of acute VTE, and it is certainly not an "insurance policy" against subsequent PE. In patients with filters placed because of bleeding, appropriate anticoagulation should begin as soon as the bleeding source has been properly and completely treated. Because of the significant risk of rebleeding, such a patient should have his anticoagulation begun in the hospital.

## VENOUS THROMBOEMBOLIC DISEASE ADJUNCTIVE CARE

### Case 7

A 67-year-old man presents with acute-onset leg pain and swelling. He lacks PE symptoms. He takes no medications. His parents are deceased, he was an only child, and he has no children. His mother died of a "blood clot" at the age of 66 years. His father died of prostate cancer at the age of 77 years. Besides occasional epigastric "aches," he feels well. He quit smoking 10 years ago and does not drink. Compression ultrasound reveals an acute proximal DVT. History and physical examination are otherwise normal. He weighs 80 kg, has a serum creatinine level of 0.9, a platelet count of 280,000/mm$^3$, and a normal digital rectal examination. He is treated as an outpatient with enoxaparin, 80 mg subcutaneously every 12 hours, and oral warfarin with a target INR of 2 to 3.

### Question

**11.** Which of the following statements is true?
a) Prescription of compression stockings will reduce his risk of developing post-thrombotic syndrome by approximately 50%.
b) Because of an approximate 10% risk of being diagnosed with cancer within 1 year of DVT diagnosis, full-body CT scanning is indicated.
c) A comprehensive hypercoagulable state work-up will impact his acute DVT management.
d) All of the above.
e) None of the above.

### Discussion

### Hot Tips

- A comprehensive clinical evaluation including history, physical examination, chest radiograph, screening labs, and other testing as indicated by age, gender, or previous test findings is indicated to detect most cancers.
- Post-thrombotic syndrome develops in up to 50% to 80% of DVT patients, typically within the first 2 years

of diagnosis. Severe post-thrombotic syndrome is associated with recurrent ulcers, disability, and great expense.

■ Know why you are ordering hypercoagulation testing before doing so.

The post-thrombotic syndrome develops in up to 50% to 80% of all patients with DVT. This syndrome was once thought to be a late complication of DVT, but it is now known that the majority of cases develop within 2 years of the index acute DVT. Treatment typically focuses on the control of pronounced dependent edema and the tedious healing of venous stasis ulcers. It may take months and thousands of dollars to heal one ulcer, only to have recurrent ulceration within 1 year in approximately one-fourth of cases. Prevention is a must. Many have hoped that the early restoration of venous patency through thrombolytic therapy would translate into less post-thrombotic syndrome. Clinical trial evidence to this effect is still absent.

The likelihood of being diagnosed with a cancer within 1 year of an idiopathic DVT ranges between 2.5% and 22.6%. Most of these cancers are diagnosed during the index hospitalization for DVT and likely represent the underlying cause for the DVT itself. Thus, not only does cancer promote hypercoagulability and clinical thrombosis, but idiopathic clinical thrombosis is a harbinger of cancer. A complete medical history, physical examination including digital rectal examination, chest radiograph, and basic laboratory testing are sufficient to uncover the majority of these thrombosis-associated cancers. Abnormal findings warrant further laboratory and imaging studies. Head-to-toe CT scanning is excessive and expensive. With the mounting popularity of outpatient strategies for VTE management, physicians must be sure to not overlook the importance of performing a thorough clinical assessment as a means of diagnosing cancer in its early stages.

With regard to hypercoagulable state testing, physicians often focus too much on their ability to find an abnormality and focus too little on how the results of such testing will impact management and help the patient. Testing just to "see what one will find" is not acceptable. The results of testing rarely, if ever, impact acute VTE management. Testing may be best delayed until the patient has completed a course of anticoagulant therapy and has returned to a baseline state of health. A good rule is to obtain testing only if the results will impact at least one of the following:

■ Type of anticoagulant therapy
■ Intensity of anticoagulant therapy
■ Duration of anticoagulant therapy
■ Patient prognosis
■ Family screening
■ Family planning
■ Concomitant medication use

False-positive results in the acute setting may actually adversely affect patient management.

### Answer and Explanation

**11. a.**

The only modality shown to significantly reduce the incidence of all degrees of post-thrombotic syndrome is compression garment therapy. The prescription of fitted, below-knee, 30- to 40-mm Hg graduated compression stockings within weeks of an acute DVT has become an integral part of overall DVT management.

## VENOUS THROMBOEMBOLIC DISEASE PREVENTION

### Case 8

While on call, you admit or consult on five patients:

1. A 38-year-old woman scheduled to undergo a total hip replacement
2. A 90-year-old vital man admitted for nursing home placement because of "advancing Alzheimer's"
3. A 50-year-old man admitted because of congestive heart failure and suspected lobar pneumonia
4. A 37-year-old woman receiving treatment with oral warfarin because of an acute DVT 1 month ago, admitted now with cellulitis
5. A 62-year-old man with newly diagnosed pancreatic cancer admitted for chemotherapy and radiation therapy

### Question

**12.** In which of these patients would you advise pharmacologic DVT prophylaxis?
a) 1, 3, and 5
b) 2, 3, and 5
c) 1, 2, and 5
d) All of them
e) None of them

### Discussion

### Hot Tips

■ The mastery of preventing DVT and PE in surgical patients and the medically ill is as important as the mastery of evolving treatment regimens.
■ LMWHs are at least as effective and safe as unfractionated heparin and clearly superior in the setting of orthopedic surgery.
■ Acutely ill medical patients are at significant risk for venous thrombosis (14.9% total; 5% proximal DVT) within 14 days of admission (5.5% with prophylaxis).

- Major risk factors are age, cancer, history of thrombosis, major surgery, congestive heart failure, sepsis or major infections, myocardial infarction, bed rest of more than 72 hours, inflammatory bowel disease, advanced age, and so forth.

- If physicians focused more on VTE prophylaxis, we would spend much less time emphasizing the methods for VTE diagnosis and treatment. It has been shown in a study of general surgery residents that the key to proper prophylaxis is the recognition of risk factors for thrombosis. An appreciation of risk factors and the results of recent trials are essential to the internist. Medically ill patients (predominantly those immobilized with severe cardiopulmonary disease) have a 14.9% risk of developing DVT within 14 days of admission in the absence of active prophylaxis. The DVT rate is reduced to 5.5% by the addition of a once-daily dose of LMWH (enoxaparin, 40 mg) without a significant increase in bleeding risk. Other studies have demonstrated the equivalency between LMWH and heparin, 5,000 U administered three times a day.

### Answer

**12. a.**

Joint replacement surgery, congestive heart failure, and active cancer place patients are at very high risk of VTE. Patients who are not acutely ill and immobilized should be encouraged to ambulate frequently. Patients already receiving therapeutic-intensity anticoagulation derive no added benefit from the addition of prophylactic-intensity therapy. In patients who cannot receive pharmacologic prophylaxis, thromboembolism deterrence stockings and/or pneumatic antiembolism stockings should be used.

## Pre-Test and Post-Test Questions

**13.** Superficial thrombophlebitis requires the same treatment as DVT.
a. True
b. False

**14.** Calf DVT can propagate into the proximal veins and cause PE.
a. True
b. False

**15.** A patient with acute leg pain, swelling, redness, and an increased concentration of D-dimer can be diagnosed with DVT based solely on clinical grounds.
a. True
b. False

**16.** Patients with DVT and *any* abnormality upon hypercoagulable state testing require life-long anticoagulation.
a. True
b. False

**17.** Post-thrombotic syndrome following DVT is common and is associated with disability and significant health care cost.
a. True
b. False

### Answers

**13. b.**

**14. a.**

**15. b.**

**16. b.**

**17. a.**

## SUGGESTED READINGS

Brandjes DPM, Buller HR, Heijboer H, et al. Randomised trial of effect of compression stockings in patients with symptomatic proximal-vein thrombosis. *Lancet* 1997;349:759–762.

Chengelis DL, Bendick PJ, Glover JL, et al. Progression of superficial venous thrombosis to deep vein thrombosis. *J Vasc Surg* 1996; 24:745–749.

Comerota AJ, Aldridge SC. Thrombolytic therapy for deep venous thrombosis: a clinical review. *Can J Surg* 1993;36:359–364.

Cornuz J, Pearson SD, Creager MA, et al. Importance of findings on the initial evaluation for cancer in patients with symptomatic idiopathic deep venous thrombosis. *Ann Intern Med* 1996;125: 785–793.

Decousus H, Leizorovicz A, Parent F, et al. A clinical trial of vena caval filters in the prevention of pulmonary embolism in patients with proximal deep-vein thrombosis. *N Engl J Med* 1998;338: 409–415.

Deitcher SR, Caiola E, Jaffer A. Demystifying two common genetic predispositions to venous thrombosis. *Cleve Clin J Med* 2000; 67:825–836.

Deitcher SR, Gomes MPV. Hypercoagulable state testing and malignancy screening following venous thromboembolic events. *Vasc Med* 2003;8:33–46.

Deitcher SR, Olin JW, Bartholomew J. How to use low-molecular weight heparin for outpatient management of deep vein thrombosis. *Cleve Clin J Med* 1999;66:329–331.

Garg K, Sieler H, Welsh CH, et al. Clinical validity of helical CT being interpreted as negative for pulmonary embolism: implications for patient treatment. *AJR Am J Roentgenol* 1999;172:1627–1631.

Ginsberg JS, Wells PS, Kearon C, et al. Sensitivity and specificity of a rapid whole-blood assay for D-dimer in the diagnosis of pulmonary embolism. *Ann Intern Med* 1998;129:1006–1011.

Gould MK, Dembitzer AD, Doyle RL, et al. Low-molecular-weight heparins compared with unfractionated heparin for treatment of acute deep vein thrombosis. A meta-analysis of randomized, controlled trials. *Ann Intern Med* 1999;130:800–809.

Hull RD, Raskob GE, Pineo GF, et al. Subcutaneous low molecular weight heparin compared with continuous intravenous heparin in the treatment of proximal deep vein thrombosis. *N Engl J Med* 1992;326:975–988.

Kimmerly WS, Sellers KD, Deitcher SR. Graduate surgical trainee attitudes toward postoperative thromboprophylaxis. *South Med J* 1999;92:790–794.

Levine M, Gent M, Hirsh J, et al. A comparison of low molecular weight heparin administered primarily at home with unfractionated heparin administered in the hospital for proximal deep vein thrombosis. *N Engl J Med* 1996;334:677–681.

Meignan M, Rosso J, Gauthier H, et al. Systematic lung scans reveal a high frequency of silent pulmonary embolism in patients with proximal deep venous thrombosis. *Arch Intern Med* 2000;160: 159–164.

Moll S, Ortel TL. Monitoring warfarin therapy in patients with lupus anticoagulants. *Ann Intern Med* 1997;127:177–185.

PIOPED Investigators, The. Value of the ventilation/perfusion scan in acute pulmonary embolism. Results of the Prospective Investigation of Pulmonary Embolism Diagnosis (PIOPED). *JAMA* 1990;263:2753–2759.

Prandoni P, Lensing AW, Buller HR, et al. Deep-vein thrombosis and the incidence of subsequent symptomatic cancer. *N Engl J Med* 1992;327:1128–1133.

Raschke RA, Reilly BM, Guidry JR, et al. The weight-based heparin dosing nomogram compared with a "standard care" nomogram: a randomized controlled trial. *Ann Intern Med* 1993;119:874–881.

Ridker PM, Goldhaber SZ, Danielson E, et al. Long-term, low-intensity warfarin for the prevention of recurrent venous thromboembolism: a randomized, double-blind, placebo-controlled trial. *N Engl J Med* 2003;348:1425–1434.

Samama MM, Cohen AT, Darmon JY, et al. A comparison of enoxaparin with placebo for the prevention of venous thromboembolism in acutely ill medical patients. Prophylaxis in Medical Patients with Enoxaparin Study Group. *N Engl J Med* 1999;341:793–800.

Schulman S, Rhedin A-S, Lindmaker P, et al. A comparison of six weeks with six months of oral anticoagulant therapy after a first episode of venous thromboembolism. *N Engl J Med* 1995;332:1661–1665.

Schulman S, Granqvist S, Holmstrom M, et al., and the Duration of Anticoagulation Trial Study Group. The duration of oral anticoagulant therapy after a second episode of venous thromboembolism. *N Engl J Med* 1997;336:393–398.

Simonneau G, Sors H, Charbonnier B, et al. A comparison of low-molecular-weight heparin with unfractionated heparin for acute pulmonary embolism. *N Engl J Med* 1997;337:663–669.

# Lung Cancer

# 36

*Alejandro C. Arroliga*     *Atul C. Mehta*

As the leading cause of cancer death in the United States, lung cancer continues to be a major health hazard: During the decade of 1990 to 2000, lung cancer mortality decreased in men by 1.7% but unfortunately, the mortality increased in women by 1%. In the United States, in 2004, 25% of all cancer deaths in women and 32% of all cancer deaths in men were caused by lung cancer. Although the death rate was expected to have peaked in the 1990s, it will remain very high over the next two to three decades.

Lung cancer continues to be the most common fatal malignancy in both genders. The American Cancer Society estimates that 173,770 new cases of bronchogenic carcinoma were diagnosed in 2004, and it is estimated that 160,440 persons died of the disease. The World Health Organization (WHO) estimates that 2 million cases of bronchogenic carcinoma will occur annually, worldwide.

## ETIOLOGY OF LUNG CANCER

Approximately 90% of all lung cancers are linked to smoking. Cigarette smoking is by far the most important risk factor for bronchogenic carcinoma. The relationship between smoking and bronchogenic carcinoma has been appreciated since the 1950s. In general, smokers have 10 to 25 times the incidence of lung cancer compared with nonsmokers. Fewer than 20% of cigarette smokers develop lung cancer, however, and it may be that other factors play a role in the disease. When smokers quit, they experience a progressive

decline in lung cancer risk that is noticeable 5 years after they stop smoking; after 15 years of abstinence, the risk of developing lung cancer is near that of a life-long nonsmoker. (Cigar smokers also are at higher risk of developing aerodigestive tract cancers, including bronchogenic carcinoma. The relative risk of lung cancer is 2.14 in cigar smokers versus nonsmokers.)

Many factors are clearly related to a high risk of developing bronchogenic carcinoma:

- Number of cigarettes smoked
- Duration in years of smoking
- Early age at initiation of smoking
- Depth of inhalation
- Tar and nicotine content in the cigarettes smoked

Women who smoke up to 9 cigarettes per day have 4 times the risk for death from lung cancer as nonsmokers; those who smoke one to two packs per day have more than 20 times the risk. Smoking among women decreased from 33% in the 1970s to 25% in the 1990s, whereas smoking among men declined from 43% to 28% in the same time period. Unfortunately, no decrease in smoking has been observed among those 18 to 24 years of age, suggesting that increased advertising and sales promotion by the tobacco industry is successfully reaching this age group. The prevalence of smoking among adolescents has remained unchanged (or even increased slightly) in the past few years. For example, in 1991, 28% of high school seniors had smoked within the previous 3 days. By 1993, the proportion had increased to 30%. Smoking among college students has increased dramatically during the last decade. Of adults aged 18 to 24 years, 45% had used tobacco in the past year and 33% are current users of tobacco. It has been estimated that every day, 3,000 more young people become regular smokers. A person who has not started smoking as a teenager is unlikely to ever become a smoker. Therefore, it is important that our efforts should be directed at preventing young people from starting to smoke.

Second-hand smoking also increases the risk of bronchogenic carcinoma. The effect of passive smoking and lung cancer risk, under conditions of domestic exposure, increases a nonsmoker's low risk by about 30%. The significance of this lies not in the magnitude of the risk for any passive smoker exposed individually, which is quite small, but in the number of excess cancer deaths owing to the frequency of such environmental exposure in the general population. It is estimated that second-hand smoking from spouses of heavy smokers may explain 3,000 to 5,000 lung cancer deaths in the United States every year.

The carcinogenic substances in cigarette smoke are only partially understood. More than 40 carcinogens have been identified in cigarette smoke, including:

- Polycyclic aromatic hydrocarbons
- Nickel
- Vinyl chloride
- Aldehydes
- Catechols
- Peroxides
- Nitrosamines

Evidence suggests that the formation of benzo-(a)-pyrene causes strong and selective adduct formation at guanine positions in codons 157, 248, and 273 of the p53 gene. This, in turn, appears to shape the p53 mutational spectrum in lung cancer, providing a direct etiologic link between a chemical carcinogen present in cigarette smoke and human cancer.

The use of filter-tipped, low-tar, and low-nicotine cigarettes does not reduce the risk of lung cancer because smokers increase the number of cigarettes smoked and the depth of inhalation with these cigarettes, thus resulting in an increased nicotine and carcinogen intake. It has been suggested as well that the use of mentholated cigarettes actually increases the relative risk of lung cancer over non-mentholated cigarettes by 1.45 in men; in effect, this suggests that mentholation increases the lung cancer–causing effect of cigarette smoking in men.

Other well-documented lung carcinogens include:

- Asbestos
- Ionizing radiation
- Chromium
- Nickel
- Mustard gas
- Vinyl chloride
- Arsenic

- Isopropyl oil
- Hydrocarbons
- Chloroethyl ether

Many of these materials have a carcinogenic effect that is additive or synergistic with cigarette smoke. For example, asbestos exposure in nonsmokers increases the incidence of bronchogenic cancer by three- to fivefold, but in smokers, this risk may be increased seventy- to ninetyfold.

Radon gas, the decay product of uranium in the earth, has been recognized as a carcinogen for many years. The interaction with cigarette smoking is synergistic. It is estimated that indoor and outdoor radon exposure, in conjunction with past or current cigarette smoking, may explain up to 20,000 lung cancer deaths in the United States, or roughly 5% to 10% of new lung cancer cases. The life-time risk of a nonsmoker is 1 in 357; if all radon was removed from all homes, this risk would decrease to 1 in 492. A life-long nonsmoker in a home with a high level of radon may have a life-time lung cancer risk of about 1 in 100; for a pack-a-day smoker, the risk increases to 1 in 14. With the removal of all radon from homes, the pack-a-day smoker's risk would decrease to about 1 in 20.

Less well-established risk factors include:

- Air pollution
- Idiopathic pulmonary fibrosis and pneumoconiosis
- Lung scar
- Genetic determinants (such as elevated pulmonary cytochrome P450 enzymes)
- Vitamin A deficiency
- Vitamin E deficiency

## PATHOPHYSIOLOGY OF LUNG CANCER

The four histopathologic categories of bronchogenic carcinoma are:

- Non–small cell lung cancers
- Adenocarcinoma (30%–35%)
- Squamous cell carcinoma (30%–32%)
- Large cell carcinoma (10%)
- Small cell carcinoma (20%–25%)

All four major cell types of lung cancer have been associated with cigarette smoking.

The increased incidence of adenocarcinoma may be attributed in part to a more frequent appearance in women, changes in environmental exposures, and modifications in the histologic classification. Adenocarcinomas form acinar or glandular structures. Bronchoalveolar cell carcinoma, an uncommon subtype of adenocarcinoma (3% of all invasive lung malignancies), has unique histologic and clinical presentations. Bronchoalveolar cell carcinoma might present as an isolated nodule, but occurs in multicentric forms. The carcinoma arises from terminal bronchoalveolar regions and grows along alveolar walls, rather than invading the lung structure directly.

Squamous cell carcinomas are composed of flattened or polygonal, stratified, epithelial cells that form intercellular bridges and elaborate keratin. The tumor tends to be bulky, usually an intrabronchial granular or polypoid mass that obstructs the lumen. Squamous cell carcinoma is the cell type more prone to cavitation, although in recent years, a higher incidence of cavitated adenocarcinoma has been reported.

Large cell carcinomas are composed of pleomorphic cells with variably enlarged nuclei and prominent nucleoli with abundant cytoplasm. They do not show squamous or glandular differentiation by light microscopy. The diagnosis of large cell carcinoma might be overestimated because tumors without clear differentiation often are classified as large cell tumors. Most of these tumors, similar to adenocarcinoma, are peripheral lesions unrelated to bronchi except for continuous growth. The metastatic pattern of large cell carcinoma is similar to adenocarcinoma, with cerebral metastases in half of the cases.

Squamous cell carcinoma, adenocarcinoma, and large cell carcinoma belong to the clinical category of non–small cell lung cancer. They are separated from the small cell lung cancer group because the therapy is different. Small cell lung cancer was felt to originate from the neuroectoderm, but actually may develop from a common pulmonary stem cell, with secondary differentiation into a cell type with neural characteristics. From the histologic point of view, small cell carcinoma is a very cellular tumor with scanty cytoplasm and little stroma. Small cell carcinoma expresses many neurohormones that may act locally or may have systemic effects. Approximately 80% of small cell tumors are central in location and are found mainly in a submucosal area. The small cell tumors are characterized by a rapid clinical growth, and they may spread quickly into mediastinal lymph nodes without involving the respiratory tract. Metastatic dissemination on clinical presentation is common in these tumors.

## CLINICAL PRESENTATION OF LUNG CANCER

In general, the clinical presentation of bronchogenic carcinoma depends on the cell type. Adenocarcinoma and large cell carcinoma tend to spread systemically relatively early in their course. Squamous cell carcinoma frequently invades locally prior to systemic spread. Small cell lung cancer has a very aggressive behavior, with mediastinal and extrathoracic spread at the time of presentation. In the cases of mixed tumors, the behavior depends on the predominant cell type.

Approximately 15% of all patients are asymptomatic at the time of diagnosis; the tumor is found incidentally as a chest radiograph abnormality. As many as 40% of patients present with cough, whereas 70% to 80% develop cough during the course of the disease. A change in the character of the cough in a smoker is a significant clinical manifestation and should trigger the search for a neoplasm. Streaky hemoptysis is present in 60% of patients, and wheezing, dyspnea, stridor, obstructive pneumonitis, and vague chest pain are occasionally symptoms at the time of presentation. Bronchorrhea is an uncommon initial presentation of bronchoalveolar cell carcinoma; when it is present (20% of patients), it indicates extensive lung involvement.

Other signs and symptoms resulting from local tumor spread include:

- Hoarseness owing to involvement of the left recurrent laryngeal nerve, resulting in vocal cord paralysis
- Superior vena cava syndrome secondary to compression or invasion of the superior vena cava
- Pleural effusion owing to direct malignant invasion of the pleural space
- Mediastinal lymphatic obstruction or a parapneumonic effusion
- Esophageal obstruction
- Pericardial involvement
- Myocardial involvement
- Vertebral invasion

In cases of superior sulcus tumors (Pancoast's tumors), the direct invasion of the apex of the lung causes C7/T2 neuropathy and Horner's syndrome.

Extrathoracic manifestation of bronchogenic carcinoma may be attributable to direct tumor infiltration (metastasis) or to the nonmetastatic complications known as *paraneoplastic syndromes*. Metastatic disease commonly involves:

- Thoracic lymph nodes
- Central nervous system (CNS)
- Liver
- Bone
- Adrenal glands
- Various areas of the lung

Bone and CNS involvement usually are symptomatic. Small cell carcinoma predominantly involves bone marrow (up to 50% of the cases) with or without peripheral hematologic abnormalities.

Paraneoplastic syndromes occur in 10% to 15% of patients with bronchogenic carcinoma. Paraneoplastic syndromes are manifestations of malignancies not caused by the direct invasion of the tumor, infection, or side effects of the therapy of the primary tumor. The paraneoplastic syndromes most commonly present in bronchogenic carcinoma include:

- Hypercalcemia of malignancy
- Syndrome of inappropriate antidiuresis
- Ectopic Cushing's syndrome
- Paraneoplastic neurologic syndromes

The hypercalcemia of malignancy is predominantly associated with squamous cell carcinoma, although it may be caused by adenocarcinoma and large cell carcinoma. Present in 15% to 20% of patients with advanced bronchogenic carcinoma, hypercalcemia is caused by the tumor's secretion of a protein called parathyroid hormone–related peptide in 85% of the cases. The peptide, which has characteristics and functions similar to that of parathyroid hormone, increases osteoclast activity, with resulting increased resorption of bone. The management of hypercalcemia of malignancy in patients with bronchogenic carcinoma includes hydration, inhibition of bone resorption by the administration of bisphosphonates, and treatment of the malignancy. Other treatment options include the use of calcitonin and plicamycin.

Inappropriate antidiuresis is caused by the ectopic secretion of arginine vasopressin. Atrial natriuretic factor and inappropriate thirst play an important role in the pathogenesis of this syndrome. The management of patients with inappropriate antidiuresis includes the treatment of the small cell carcinoma, water restriction, and administration of demeclocycline and fludrocortisone. In severe symptomatic hyponatremia, the use of hypertonic saline and furosemide administration may be needed. The rapid correction of the hyponatremia, however, may lead to central nervous system complications such as central pontine myelinolysis.

Ectopic Cushing's syndrome is caused by the secretion of propiomelanocortin, a precursor of adrenocorticotropic hormone. The treatment of the ectopic Cushing's syndrome includes the management of the tumor, as well as administration of adrenal enzyme inhibitors such as ketoconazole, metyrapone, and aminoglutethimide. The administration of the somatostatin analog octreotide has shown some efficacy. Bilateral adrenalectomy may be considered in selected cases of refractory disease.

Paraneoplastic neurologic syndromes, present in 1% to 3% of patients with small cell lung cancer, are more commonly associated with small cell lung cancer. The most common of these fascinating disorders is the Eaton-Lambert syndrome. Other paraneoplastic neurologic disorders include subacute cerebellar degeneration, subacute sensory neuronopathy, and limbic encephalitis, polyneuropathy, and cancer-associated retinopathy.

# DIAGNOSIS OF LUNG CANCER

## Screening

Mass screening of high-risk patients with serial chest radiographs and sputum cytology has showed a favorable impact on survival in patients with localized tumors. No significant improvement in overall survival for lung cancer has been noted when all the patients entered into the studies were analyzed, however. Consequently, no consensus exists that high-risk patients should undergo yearly chest radiography or sputum cytology. Nevertheless, for the individual high-risk patient concerned about cancer, it may be

reasonable to screen periodically, especially if the patient has multiple risk factors (such as a smoker who has been exposed to asbestos and radon). In the presence of significant chronic obstructive airway disease, a yearly chest radiograph may be helpful.

More recently, low-dose spiral computed tomography (CT) has been found helpful in the early diagnosis of bronchogenic carcinoma. Low-dose spiral CT is a promising technique that allows the complete imaging of the chest in one breath-hold. Currently, however, no guideline supports the routine screening of patients with low-dose spiral CT, and this technique cannot be recommended for routine practice until further study clearly demonstrates greater benefit than potential harm.

## Diagnostic Studies

### Radiography

Most asymptomatic lung cancers are detected on plain chest radiographs. Lesions smaller than 5 to 6 mm in diameter are rarely noticed in the chest radiograph. In general, the radiographic appearance of a lesion will not distinguish between a benign or malignant process. The radiographic characteristic suggestive of a malignancy includes lobulation and margins that are shaggy and ill-defined. Adenocarcinoma usually presents as a peripheral lung mass and represents 40% of all peripheral lung tumors. At least 50% of the lesions are less than 4 cm in diameter.

Bronchoalveolar cell carcinoma presents as a solitary nodule, numerous small unilateral or bilateral nodules, or a lobar or segmental unilateral or bilateral consolidation with or without air bronchograms.

The majority of squamous cell carcinomas (65%) are centrally located and may cause:

- Partial or complete obstruction of the airways with radiographic changes of atelectasis
- Postobstructive pneumonia
- Lung abscess
- Bronchiectasis
- Mucoid impaction

When squamous cell carcinoma presents in a peripheral location, the tumor usually cavitates and may resemble a lung abscess.

Large cell carcinoma is more frequently peripheral (72%) and tends to be sharply defined. The majority of lesions are more than 4 cm in diameter on presentation.

Small cell lung cancer is a predominantly central lesion and presents as a hilar mass. The lesions almost never cavitate. Although the primary lesion does not tend to obstruct, the metastatic adenopathy can cause external compression of airways, with a consequent atelectasis or postobstructive pneumonia. Small cell lung cancer occasionally occurs peripherally.

Approximately 30% of all bronchogenic carcinomas present as a solitary nodule. Solitary pulmonary nodules are characterized by a single lesion up to 3 cm in diameter, surrounded by lung parenchyma. In the United States, the number of nodules resulting from bronchogenic carcinoma is approximately 55,000 to 111,000 per year.

Approximately 40% to 50% of solitary nodules are malignant. These malignancies are primarily bronchogenic carcinoma, but a small number (10%) are solitary metastatic deposits, and approximately 2% to 3% are carcinoid tumors. Most of the malignant solitary nodules are large cell carcinoma and adenocarcinoma. Small cell carcinoma and squamous cell carcinoma rarely present as a solitary nodule. Benign nodules are almost always infectious granulomas. Other less common etiologies include hamartomas, other benign tumors, and noninfectious granulomas.

Establishing the etiology of solitary pulmonary nodules is a major clinical challenge. The goal in the management of a patient with a solitary pulmonary nodule is to identify malignant nodules that need surgery while avoiding thoracotomy in those with benign nodules. Absence of growth in the size of the solitary pulmonary nodule for more than 24 months is considered a reliable sign of benignity. The presence of characteristic patterns of calcification—such as homogenous, popcorn, laminated, and central calcification—is considered evidence of benignity. If the solitary nodule is noncalcified and the pattern of growth in the preceding 2 years cannot be determined, the probability of cancer based on the clinical features (predictive variables) must be assessed. Important clinical features suggestive of malignancy include:

- Size of the nodule (>3 cm)
- Age of the patient (patients under age 35 usually have benign nodules)
- Smoking history
- History of previous malignancy
- Radiologic characteristics of the edge of the nodule
- Presence or absence of occult calcification determined by CT

The imaging techniques more commonly used in the evaluation of a solitary nodule include chest radiography and CT. Obtaining previous chest radiographs is probably the most important diagnostic maneuver in the evaluation of a patient with a solitary nodule. As noted, a lesion that has remained stable in size for more than 2 years is more likely to be benign. Benign nodules, usually of infectious etiology, tend to grow fast (i.e., faster than malignancies), with a doubling time of less than 21 days. CT allows better visualization of the nodule than does chest radiography, provides better definition of the margins, and better helps detect calcifications and the presence of multiple lesions.

In addition to chest radiography and CT, other imaging techniques that have been used in the evaluation of patients with solitary nodules include magnetic resonance imaging (MRI) and positron emission tomography (PET). MRI has no role in the routine evaluation of the patient with a solitary pulmonary nodule. The PET scan uses the uptake of 2[F-18]-fluoro-2-deoxy-D-glucose to measure the uptake of glucose metabolism in the malignant tissue. A sensitivity of 96% and specificity of 93% has been reported in patients with indeterminate nodules, but PET scanning has significant limitations and probably is inadequate to evaluate small nodules of 1 cm or less. CT and PET scans may be useful to rule out malignancy in those patients with a lung nodule who are at low to moderate risk for malignancy. If a patient is at high risk for lung cancer, however, the false negative rate may remains unacceptable. In these cases, tissue diagnosis is indicated.

If the noncalcified nodule is still of undetermined etiology after all the above studies, and the probability of cancer is high, then a biopsy via transthoracic needle aspiration or thoracotomy is a reasonable diagnostic choice, depending on the wishes of the patient. If the probability of cancer is high, immediate thoracotomy has the highest expected utility. In patients with low probability of cancer, however, a "wait and watch" strategy is favored.

### Tissue Diagnosis

Currently available methods for the tissue diagnosis of suspected lung cancer include:

- Sputum cytology
- Fiberoptic bronchoscopy
- Transthoracic needle aspiration
- Thoracotomy

Other techniques, potentially useful in selected cases, include thoracentesis (pleural biopsy), pleuroscopy, and mediastinoscopy.

Sputum cytology is occasionally helpful in the diagnosis of central squamous and small cell carcinomas. The results are variable and the interpretation may be technically difficult. A negative sputum cytology result does not rule out the presence of bronchogenic carcinomas in the appropriate setting.

### Bronchoscopy

Flexible fiberoptic bronchoscopy (FFB) is helpful in the diagnosis of central airway lesions. In this setting, FFB is diagnostic in 90% of the cases. In cases of peripheral lesions (tumor visible on chest radiography but not on FFB), FFB has a diagnostic yield of 40% to 80% using transbronchial biopsy, brushings and washings, and biplanar fluoroscopy. This result is significantly lower than the yield in central lesions. The size of the lesion is the best determinant of diagnostic yield in peripheral lesions:

- Lesions less than 2 cm in diameter: 28% to 30% yield
- Lesions greater than 2 cm in diameter: 64% yield
- Lesions greater than 4 cm in diameter: 80% yield

The complications of FFB, which are infrequent (5%), include hemorrhage, pneumothorax, laryngospasm, and transient hypoxemia.

### Transthoracic Needle Aspiration Biopsy

Transthoracic needle aspiration biopsy has been used to diagnose lung masses and mediastinal lesions. Needle aspiration complements bronchoscopy in establishing the diagnosis of lung abnormalities. The diagnostic yield of percutaneous transthoracic needle aspiration is greater than 90% for peripheral lesions, but the frequency of complications is increased, reportedly 25% to 30%. Up to 15% of patients require treatment with a chest tube to re-expand the lung. Some of the features associated with lower diagnostic rates are smaller lesion size and central location.

It is important to emphasize that a negative result, unless it indicates a specific benign diagnosis, such as hamartoma, cannot be used to rule out carcinoma. If no contraindication exists (pulmonary and cardiac status, no evidence of metastatic disease), one should proceed to thoracotomy.

## Staging

After tissue diagnosis, staging is important to assess the extent of local and distant disease. Accurate staging is crucial in the selection of therapy and for prognostic purposes—the ultimate prognosis of patients with lung cancer depend largely on the stage of disease at the time of the diagnosis. The TNM system is used to stage non–small cell bronchogenic carcinoma. The TNM classification has been revised recently to provide greater specificity for identifying patient groups, and now more accurately reflects survival among homogenous groups:

- Resectable tumors
  - Stage IA (T1N0M0)
  - Stage IB (T2N0M0)
  - Stage IIA (T1N1M0)
  - Stage IIB (T2N1M0)
  - Stage IIB (T3N0M0)
  - Selected Stage IIIa (T3N1M0) or (T1–3N2M0)
- Unresectable tumors
  - Stage IIIB (any T, N3, M0)
  - Stage IV (any T, any N, M1)

Small cell lung cancer generally is not included in the TNM classification because the majority of these tumors are in advanced stage at the time of the diagnosis. Small cell lung cancer has two stages:

- Limited disease (implies that the tumor is confined within a radiation port)
- Extensive disease (implies disseminated disease beyond a radiation port)

Clinical staging starts with a careful clinical history and complete physical examination. The history and examination are highly cost-effective staging tools. An examination of the hilar and mediastinal areas is a key step in the staging process; CT scan of the chest is useful in this situation because it offers significant advantages compared with standard chest radiography. If the lymph node has a transverse diameter on CT scan of <1 cm, the likelihood of finding metastatic tissue is in the range of 3% to 16%. Nodes that have a diameter of 1 to 2 cm, however, have metastatic disease in 70% of cases and those of >2 cm have a greater chance of being malignant. When a lymph node is enlarged on CT, histologic examination is needed before assuming tumor involvement. Transbronchial needle aspiration, transthoracic needle aspiration, and mediastinoscopy are some of the techniques that have been used to sample mediastinal lymph nodes. Mediastinoscopy remains the standard for the purpose of mediastinal staging in non–small cell carcinoma patients. CT and MRI of the chest are of value in detecting chest wall or pleural involvement in patients with lung cancer. MRI has been found to be helpful, especially for patients who have superior sulcus tumors, for delineating vascular and neural invasion, and for patients with tumor invasion of the pericardium and heart. PET imaging has high sensitivity and specificity for assessing the presence of tumor within mediastinal lymph nodes.

## COMPLICATIONS OF LUNG CANCER

The majority of lung cancers metastasize to the liver, CNS, bone, adrenal glands, and supraclavicular lymph nodes. The detection of extrapulmonary metastases begins with a thorough history and physical examination. Suspicious symptoms include weight loss, anorexia, neurologic symptoms, and localized bone pain. Laboratory data, including liver function tests, alkaline phosphatase, and calcium, are necessary and will indicate the need for further workup.

Frequently used imaging techniques include CT scan of the chest, which includes liver and adrenal glands and bone and liver–spleen scans. A CT scan of the CNS is probably only justified in patients with adenocarcinoma. Patients with other types of non–small cell lung cancer do not need a routine CT scan of the head unless there is clinical suspicion of CNS involvement.

In small cell lung cancer, extrathoracic staging is particularly important. In these patients, routine scans of bone, liver–spleen, and the head are necessary to detect tumor spread. Bone marrow aspiration and biopsy often are used to detect tumor at this site. In patients with obvious metastases, however, examination of the bone marrow is not necessary.

## TREATMENT OF LUNG CANCER

### Non–Small Cell Lung Cancer

The three major treatment modalities for a patient with non–small cell lung cancer are surgical resection, radiation therapy, and chemotherapy.

Surgical resection is the treatment of choice because it offers the best prospect of long-term survival. Unfortunately, only one-third of patients have resectable disease at the time of diagnosis. The overall 5-year survival rates for all stages of surgically resected lung cancer is in the range of 40%:

- Stage IA and IB: 5-year survival of 67% and 57 respectively
- Stage IIA and IIB: 5-year survival of 55% and 39% respectively
- Stage IIIa: 5-year survival of 26%

Unfortunately, the majority of patients with non–small cell lung cancer present with locally advanced (stage IIIB) or metastatic (stage IV) disease that is not curable through surgery. All patients with non–small cell lung cancer should be evaluated for potential resection as initial therapy. Surgical procedures include pneumonectomy, lobectomy, segmentectomy, wedge resection, and sleeve bronchoplasty. Lobectomy is the surgical procedure of choice for patients with stage I and some stage II lung cancers. An evaluation of pulmonary reserve must be done using pulmonary function tests in patients undergoing resection for lung surgery. A preoperative forced expiratory volume in 1 second ($FEV_1$) value of greater than 2 L or greater than 80% of predicted indicates a good lung reserve, and the patient may tolerate up to a pneumonectomy. Patients who have an $FEV_1$ value less than 80% of predicted need a quantitative perfusion scan to predict postoperative lung function. A postoperative predicted $FEV_1$ of less than 40% of normal predicted, postoperative predicted DLCO of less than 40%, and presence of significant dyspnea suggests the potential for high morbidity and mortality in patients undergoing lung resection.

Non–small cell lung cancers are relatively unresponsive to chemotherapy. Conversely, radiation therapy is effective in decreasing the size of local tumors in patients with non–small cell and small cell lung cancer. Radiation therapy is useful as a palliative measure, especially in patients who have obstruction of airways, compression of vital chest structures by the tumors, pain, or hemoptysis. Radiation therapy may be curative in fewer than 15% of patients with stage I non–small cell lung cancer.

### Small Cell Lung Cancer

The treatment of small cell carcinoma remains nonsurgical in the vast majority of patients because of the high frequency of the metastases at the time of diagnosis. In most cases, small cell lung cancer is sensitive to both chemotherapy and radiation therapy. The agents most commonly used for patients with small cell lung cancer include:

- Cisplatin and carboplatin
- Etoposide
- Vinorelbine
- Paclitaxel
- Docetaxel
- Gemcitabine
- Irinotecan

The majority of patients with limited disease have a complete response to chemotherapy. Only 15% to 20% of these patients with limited disease survive 3 years, however. Thoracic radiation is used in combination with chemotherapy to control local recurrence in patients with limited disease. Elective cranial irradiation has been used in complete responders to chemotherapy to treat occult brain metastasis.

In the uncommon patient with small cell lung cancer who presents with an isolated lung nodule, surgical resection is considered the treatment of choice, followed by adjuvant chemotherapy, with a cure rate of up to 50%.

Patients with extensive disease are treated with chemotherapy. The survival rate is 5% at 3 years.

## PREVENTION OF LUNG CANCER

The most effective way to prevent lung cancer is to prevent smoking. Every physician has the duty to advise every patient about quitting the smoking habit. Several agents are helpful in smoking cessation. The use of bupropion either alone or in combination with nicotine replacement is associated with a high abstinence rate and with a 20% continuous abstinence rate at 1 year versus 6% in patients given placebo. Other modalities, such as psychotherapy and consultation programs, may be of help as well.

Other modalities of prevention, such as chemotherapy prevention for lung cancer using β-carotene and vitamin A, have not shown significant benefit in reducing the incidence of bronchogenic carcinoma.

### SUGGESTED READINGS

Deslauriers J, Gregoire J. Surgical therapy of early non-small cell lung cancer. *Chest* 2000;104S–109S.

Evans TL, Donahue DM, Mathisen DJ, et al. Building a better therapy for stage IIIA non-small cell lung cancer. *Clin Chest Med* 2002;23: 191–207.

Gerber RB, Mazzone P, Arroliga AC. Paraneoplastic syndromes associated with bronchogenic carcinoma. *Clin Chest Med* 2002;23: 257–264.

Gould MK, Maclean CC, Kushcner WG, et al. Accuracy of positron emission tomography for diagnosis of pulmonary nodules and mass lesions. A metaanalysis. *JAMA* 2001;285:914–924.

Hoffman PC, Mauer AM, Vokes EE. Lung cancer. *Lancet* 2000;355: 479–485.

Hurt RD, Ebbert JO. Preventing lung cancer by stopping smoking. *Clin Chest Med* 2002;23:27–36.

Jain P, Kathawalla SA, Arroliga AC. Managing pulmonary nodules. *Cleve Clin J Med* 1998;65:315–326.

Jeenal A, Tiwari RC, Murray T, et al. Cancer statistics, 2004. *CA Cancer J Clin* 2004;54:8–29.

Johnson BE. Management of small cell lung cancer. *Clin Chest Med* 2002;23:225–239.

Jorenby DE, Leischow SJ, Nides MA, et al. A controlled trial of sustained release bupropion, a nicotine patch, or both for smoking cessation. *N Engl J Med* 1999;340:685–691.

Mazzone P, Jain P, Arroliga AC, Matthay RA. Bronchoscopy and needle biopsy techniques for diagnosis and staging of lung cancer. *Clin Chest Med* 2002;23:137–158.

Mountain CF. Revisions in the international system for staging lung cancer. *Chest* 1997;111:1710–1717.

Mountain CF, Dresler CM. Regional lymph node classification for lung cancer staging. *Chest* 1997;111:1718–1723.

Patz EF Jr, Swensen SJ, Herndon JE 2nd. Estimate of lung cancer mortality from low-dose spiral computed tomography screening trials: implications for current mass screening recommendations. *J Clin Oncol* 2004;22:2202–2226.

Rigotti NA, Lee JE, Wechsler H. US college students' use of tobacco products: results of a national survey. *JAMA* 2000;284:699–705.

Smith-Bilello K, Murin S, Matthay RA. Epidemiology, etiology, and prevention of lung cancer. *Clin Chest Med* 2002;23:1–25.

Tanoue LT, Ponn RB. Therapy for stage I and stage II non-small cell lung cancer. *Clin Chest Med* 2002;23:173–190.

Travis WD. Pathology of lung cancer. *Clin Chest Med* 2002;23:65–81.

# Obstructive Lung Disease: Asthma and Chronic Obstructive Pulmonary Disease

**37**

*Mani S. Kavuru     Loutfi S. Aboussouan*

Bronchial asthma and chronic obstructive pulmonary disease (COPD) represent major causes of morbidity in the United States. Asthma affects 3% to 5% of the U.S. population. An estimated 24 million Americans are afflicted with COPD. Although asthma is not a leading cause of death, it is responsible for approximately 1% of all visits to physicians and results in approximately 500,000 hospital admissions per year. COPD was the fourth leading cause of death in the United States, with approximately 119,000 deaths in 2000. Therefore, both of these disorders are quite common and pose a significant burden on healthcare resources, and represent a great measure of human suffering. It is essential for the general internist, as well as the pulmonary subspecialist, to be very familiar with the nuances of management. History, physical examination, and simple ancillary studies (e.g., chest radiograph and spirogram) are usually adequate to establish a diagnosis of asthma or COPD and initiate proper management.

Chronic airflow obstruction is a feature of asthma, chronic bronchitis, emphysema, cystic fibrosis, and other bronchiectatic syndromes. The discussion here is limited to the typical adult patient with asthma and COPD. It is most essential to distinguish patients with bronchial asthma from the usual adult smoker with COPD because the prognosis and emphasis on certain types of management are quite different (e.g., asthma is characterized by exquisite steroid responsiveness).

## ASTHMA

Asthma is a chronic, episodic disease of the airways; it has protean manifestations and is best viewed as a syndrome. Important features of this syndrome include:

- Episodic symptoms
- Airflow obstruction with a reversible component
- Bronchial hyper-responsiveness to a variety of nonspecific and specific stimuli
- Airway inflammation
- A tendency toward atopic and allergic inheritable disease

All these features need not be present. Although some features overlap between asthma and COPD, it is important to understand the distinctions between these conditions:

- Asthma typically occurs in younger individuals who are nonsmokers.
- The asthmatic's baseline level of functioning, exercise tolerance, and spirometric parameters are usually better preserved between episodes than are those of individuals with COPD.
- The presence of extrinsic triggers, seasonal variability, family history, allergic rhinitis, and positive skin test results or atopy may be helpful in solidifying an initial diagnosis of asthma.

- Physiologically, asthmatics have a normal diffusing capacity, whereas patients with emphysema have a diffusing capacity reduced in proportion to the severity of airflow obstruction.

## Etiology

### Epidemiology

Data from the Centers for Disease Control (CDC) indicate that 15 million American adults suffer from asthma. The annual rate of asthma mortality, which increased between 1980–1995, has plateaued or decreased more recently. The evolving consensus from a number of retrospective studies is that several risk factors contribute to poor outcomes and fatal asthma:

- Patients with prior serious asthma, requiring emergency room visits or mechanical ventilation, are at the greatest risk.
- Factors that interfere with compliance and access to medical care are important. In the United States, the mortality rate from asthma for African Americans is three times that for whites.
- Inadequate objective assessment of asthma severity by pulmonary function testing or peak flow measurements appears to be frequently noted in patients who die from asthma.
- Inadequate treatment with either inhaled or systemic corticosteroid is also a frequently described finding.

Therefore, underdiagnosis or underestimation of asthma severity is an important contributing factor in asthma-related fatality. Despite these recent trends, asthma remains a relatively infrequent cause of death.

In the early 1990s, a number of studies suggested a potential role of β-agonist aerosols in the increasing asthma mortality rate. The hypothesis was that excessive or regularly scheduled use of β-adrenergic bronchodilators can actually worsen asthma, perhaps contributing to morbidity and mortality. More recent studies have indicated that the regular administration of β-agonist aerosols does not directly cause worse asthma control. Recent studies indicate that polymorphisms for the β-adrenergic receptor gene exist in a subset of patients (perhaps 15%). It is likely that certain variants (i.e., Arg/Arg homozygotes at position 16) do not will tolerate chronic β-agonist administration. If patients require an increasing number of puffs of β-agonist aerosols, this is usually a marker for the need for more effective anti-inflammatory therapy. β-Agonist aerosols remain a critical part of the regimen for acute emergency room management of bronchial asthma. For chronic maintenance therapy, it is best to use β-agonist aerosols on an as-needed basis.

## Pathogenesis

In recent years, the central role of airway inflammation in the pathogenesis of asthma has been established. The mech-anism by which airway inflammation is related to bronchial reactivity remains unclear. A classic model is that of an allergic asthmatic challenged with an inhaled antigen to which the patient is sensitive. This challenge may result in a biphasic decline in respiratory function. The early asthmatic response may occur within minutes and resolve within 2 hours. The early asthmatic response is thought to be related to the release of preformed mediators (perhaps from mast cells) and is abolished by pretreatment with β-agonists (but not with corticosteroids). A late asthmatic response usually occurs within 6 to 8 hours and may last for 24 hours or longer. The late asthmatic response is classically associated with airway hyper-reactivity and airway inflammatory cell influx; it can be inhibited by pretreatment with corticosteroids (but not β-agonists). Cromoglycates may block both responses.

The current paradigm is that asthma is not simply bronchospasm but involves a complex cascade of inflammatory events that involves cellular, epithelial, neurogenic, and various biochemical mediators. In addition to the mast cells and eosinophils, the T lymphocyte (TH2) has been added as an important regulator of inflammation. The TH2 lymphocytes appear to mediate allergic inflammation in atopic asthmatics by a cytokine profile that involves interleukin-4 (which directs B lymphocytes to synthesize immunoglobulin E) and interleukin-5 (which is essential for the maturation of eosinophils), along with interleukin-13. Current thinking suggests that asthma is characterized by a TH2 rather than a TH1 response. Other effector cells implicated in asthmatic inflammation include mast cells, eosinophils, epithelial cells, and macrophages. Immunoglobulin E may be an important trigger for activating effector cells. The products of arachidonic acid metabolism also have been implicated in airway inflammation and have been the target of pharmacologic antagonism. Prostaglandins (PGs) are generated by the cyclo-oxygenation of arachidonic acid, and leukotrienes are generated by the lipoxygenation of arachidonic acid. The proinflammatory agents include all the leukotrienes and PGD2, PGF2α, and thromboxane. PGE2 and $PGI_2$ (prostacyclin) are believed to be protective and produce bronchodilation.

Most recently, research has focused on airway remodeling, which represents irreversible or permanent changes that may occur over time in asthmatic airways. It is tempting to speculate that long-standing asthma, especially if airway inflammation is not treated or inadequately treated, leads to basement membrane collagen deposition and subepithelial fibrosis. Currently, this remains speculative, and the relationship between airway inflammation and remodeling is unknown, as is how often remodeling occurs and how effectively anti-inflammatory therapy can avoid remodeling.

## Clinical Presentation

The history and physical examination are important for several reasons:

- They confirm a diagnosis and exclude mimics, such as upper airway obstruction (UAO) and congestive heart failure.
- They assess the severity of airflow obstruction and the need for admission to a hospital.
- They identify factors that might place a patient at particular risk for poor outcome.
- They identify comorbid diseases that may complicate the management, such as sinusitis, gastroesophageal reflux, and avoidable external triggers.

The cardinal symptoms of asthma include episodic dyspnea, chest tightness, wheezing, and cough. Some patients may present with atypical symptoms, such as cough alone (cough-equivalent asthma) or only dyspnea on exertion. It is essential to specifically inquire about nocturnal symptoms because this is often ignored.

The most objective indicator of asthma severity is the measurement of airflow obstruction by spirometry or peak expiratory flow. Both the $FEV_1$ and peak expiratory flow yield comparable results. The National Asthma Education Prevention Program, in its Expert Panel Report II (updated on the web, 2002), set forward the grading of asthma severity based on the frequency of symptoms, peak flows, and need for inhaled β-agonists into four categories: mild-intermittent, mild-persistent, moderate-persistent, and severe-persistent.

Hyperinflation, the most common finding on a chest radiograph, has no diagnostic or therapeutic value. A chest radiograph should not be obtained unless complications of pneumonia, pneumothorax, or an endobronchial lesion are suspected. The correlation of severity between acute asthma and arterial blood gases is poor. Mild to moderate asthma is typically associated with respiratory alkalosis and mild hypoxemia on the basis of ventilation–perfusion mismatching. Severe hypoxemia is quite uncommon. Normocapnia and hypercapnia imply severe airflow obstruction, with an $FEV_1$ of usually less than 25% of predicted. Recent data suggest that hypercapnia in the setting of acute asthma does not necessarily mandate intubation or suggest a poor prognosis.

Numerous parameters from the physical examination and airflow measurement, either separately or as a composite score, have been evaluated to assess the severity of acute asthma and the need for hospital admission. It is true that physical findings such as pulsus paradoxus (inspiratory decline in systolic blood pressure of more than 12 mm Hg), accessory muscle use including sternocleidomastoid muscle retraction, a respiratory rate of >30 breaths/minute, and a heart rate of >130 beats/minute are generally associated with more severe airflow obstruction. None of these signs alone or in combination, however, is specific or sensitive.

Spirometry in an asthmatic typically shows obstructive airway disease with reduced expiratory flows that improve upon the administration of bronchodilator therapy (i.e., reduced $FEV_1$/forced vital capacity ratio). Typically, an improvement in either $FEV_1$ or forced vital capacity occurs with the acute administration of an inhaled bronchodilator (12% and 200 mL). The absence of a bronchodilator response, however, by no means excludes asthma. The shape of the flow–volume loop may provide insight into the nature and location of airway obstruction. With disorders that cause UAO, classically, a plateau occurs in either limb of the flow–volume loop during periods of maximal flow. Specifically, the loop shows a flattening of the inspiratory limb with variable extrathoracic UAO, likely caused by a lesion involving the glottic or subglottic area. Flattening of the expiratory limb is seen with variable intrathoracic UAO, such as a mid- or distal tracheal lesion. A fixed UAO produces a box-like flattening of both inspiratory and expiratory limbs. In patients with atypical chest symptoms of unclear etiology (cough or dyspnea alone), a variety of challenge tests may help to identify the presence of airway hyper-reactivity. By far the most commonly used agents are methacholine or histamine, which give comparable results. Exercise, cold air, and isocapnic hyperventilation—other approaches that require complex equipment—have a lower sensitivity. In a patient with known asthma, there is no indication for a challenge procedure. The methacholine challenge test is very sensitive, but it is nonspecific and can occur in a variety of other conditions, including COPD.

## Treatment

The National Asthma Education Prevention Program Expert Panel Report II provides an excellent algorithmic framework for the management of bronchial asthma. The general goals of asthma therapy include:

- Maintain normal activity levels, including exercise
- Maintain near normal pulmonary function tests
- Prevent chronic and troublesome symptoms or recurrent exacerbations of asthma
- Avoid adverse effects from asthma medications

Overall, asthma treatment has four key components:

- Measure lung function both initially and during periodic evaluation, including home peak expiratory flow monitoring
- Educate patients
- Avoid asthma triggers by controlling the environment
- Treat the condition pharmacologically

The pharmacologic treatment for asthma can be classified as *symptomatic therapy* ("relievers") using bronchodilators (β-agonists, theophylline) and *anti-inflammatory therapy* ("controllers") using corticosteroids, cromolyn, nedocromil, antileukotrienes, and anti-immunoglobulin E (IgE).

The therapy is further classified as acute versus chronic maintenance therapy. The National Asthma Education Prevention Program outlines detailed guidelines for stepwise management using these agents. For the mildest asthma (mild-intermittent), the guidelines recommend as-needed use of one to two puffs of a β-agonist aerosol. Cromolyn may alternatively be used before exposure to a variety of triggers, such as exercise or allergen.

For all asthmatics with persistent asthma (symptoms more than one to two times per week), the mainstay of maintenance therapy is inhaled corticosteroids. These agents should be used in adequate doses to fully control the symptoms. Numerous studies have shown that inhaled steroid therapy provides an effective symptomatic control of chronic asthma, as well as the reversal of a number of parameters of airway inflammation.

With the current paradigm of asthma as a chronic inflammatory disorder of the airways, inhaled corticosteroids have assumed the role of first-line therapy for all patients with persistent asthma (mild, moderate, severe). Over the past 5 to 10 years, the trend in the use of inhaled steroids has been to use higher and higher doses, especially in the more severe asthmatics. This is predicated on the hypothesis that a dose–response effect exists for these agents. Although quite a number of studies support this hypothesis, debate continues. It is well documented that higher doses of inhaled corticosteroids facilitate a reduction in systemic corticosteroids in severe asthma. Another trend has been the use of inhaled corticosteroids at an earlier stage of asthma. Some data suggest that this might improve the long-term $FEV_1$ by preventing subepithelial fibrosis. Several studies suggest that less frequent dosing, such as once or twice a day, may be equally effective. The less frequent dosing has clear-cut benefits in terms of compliance. Some studies have shown a cost advantage to asthma care through the use of inhaled corticosteroids. A recent case-controlled study indicates that the use of inhaled steroid maintenance therapy (i.e., one canister per month) is associated with lower asthma mortality.

Currently, five specific inhaled corticosteroids are approved in the United States for the maintenance therapy of asthma. The two newest agents include fluticasone (Flovent) and budesonide (Pulmicort Turbuhaler). The National Institutes of Health Expert Panel Report II provides a table of comparative-dose inhaled steroids needed to achieve similar clinical effect. In general, the more potent agents, such as fluticasone, have the advantage of dosing with far fewer puffs per day to accomplish the same clinical benefit. This has a significant advantage in terms of compliance.

A recent development in chronic asthma maintenance therapy is a concept of combination therapy to produce either additive or synergistic effects. A variety of studies show that groups of mild to moderate asthmatics who remain symptomatic on low to intermediate doses of inhaled corticosteroids clearly benefit from the addition of a long-acting inhaled bronchodilator, in addition to the dose of inhaled steroid (rather than doubling the dose of the inhaled steroid). A natural extension of this concept of combination or concurrent therapy has been the development of a new inhaled product that combines both flutica-

sone and salmeterol into a single device. This has recently become available as a Diskus device (Advair), with the medication packaged as a nonchlorofluorocarbon dry powder preparation. This product is available in three different steroid dose strengths, Advair 100/50 (green), 250/50 (yellow), and 500/50 (red). Several recent pivotal studies indicate that the combination product is superior to the individual components in patients with mild and moderately severe chronic asthma. The study by Kavuru et al. is a randomized controlled trial of Advair 100/50; administered as a dry powder inhaler, one puff twice a day markedly improved a variety of outcomes, including $FEV_1$ and the probability to have an asthma exacerbation over 12 weeks, compared with each of the individual components separately or placebo.

A number of studies have examined the usefulness of inhaled steroids plus other agents, including theophylline and leukotriene antagonists. These studies have strongly indicated that the benefits of combination therapy using these other agents are not as dramatic as with the addition of the long-acting inhaled bronchodilator. The exact molecular mechanism whereby the combination of inhaled steroids and long-acting β-agonists synergistically improve asthma control is not fully known. Preliminary data indicate that the β-agonists facilitate the steroid effect, whereas the steroids upregulate the β-agonist receptors. Preliminary data also indicate that the long-acting bronchodilators do not have a masking effect of the underlying airway inflammation.

Recent data suggest that inhaled steroids probably do not cure asthma in the sense that symptoms promptly return if these agents are stopped. These agents clearly reduce airway hyper-reactivity (unlike oral corticosteroids). In general, with the use of low-dose inhaled corticosteroid therapy (less than 1,000 μg/day), systemic complications appear to be negligible. The oral pharyngeal complications of inhaled steroid therapy, such as candidiasis, dysphonia, and hoarseness, are usually mild. The use of a spacer device (or a powder preparation) and routine rinsing of the mouth help to minimize these side effects. Data suggest that systemic effects may occur with the use of higher dosages (more than 1,200 μg/day) of inhaled corticosteroids. Definitely, certain biochemical parameters of the hypothalamic-pituitary-adrenal axis (24-hour urinary free cortisol, morning serum cortisol, and adrenocorticotropic hormone stimulation test) and bone metabolism (serum osteocalcin and urinary hydroxyproline) may be affected. The clinical importance, however, of these effects in terms of bone growth, likelihood for osteoporosis, or fractures is not known.

Data over the past 10 years suggest that the cysteinyl leukotrienes are involved in the pathogenesis of asthma. Three agents that antagonize the leukotriene pathway have been approved for use as maintenance therapy for mild persistent asthma. Zileuton is a synthesis inhibitor that blocks the 5-lipoxygenase enzyme. Zafirlukast and montelukast are selective, competitive receptor antagonists at the LTD4 and LTE4 level. Early clinical trials suggest that these agents have beneficial effects in mild to moderate asthma compared with placebo. The exact place for antileukotrienes in the chronic maintenance therapy for asthma remains to be established. The Expert Panel Report II indicates a possible role for these agents, as an alternative to inhaled corticosteroids, in the initial therapy of mild persistent asthma. Also, the Expert Panel Report II indicates a possible role for these agents as adjunctive therapy (in addition to inhaled steroids) for added asthma control at any level of severity for persistent asthma. These agents have effects on early and late asthma response. Therefore, they act as a bronchodilator within 1 to 3 hours after administration and as an anti-inflammatory agent having a response over 2 to 4 weeks. The magnitude of increase in $FEV_1$ at 4 weeks is approximately 14% above that of the placebo. Several published studies directly comparing currently available inhaled corticosteroids with the antileukotrienes indicate that the inhaled steroids have more potent effects, especially in patients with moderate–severe disease. The antileukotrienes facilitate a reduction in the need for inhaled β-agonists and inhaled corticosteroids, thereby minimizing certain side effects. Also, these oral agents may improve compliance, when compared with the metered-dose inhalers. Antileukotrienes may be particularly beneficial as the drug of choice in a small subset of patients with aspirin-sensitive asthma.

Omalizumab (Xolair), the first selective anti-IgE agent, is a unique humanized monoclonal anti-IgE antibody that binds with high affinity to the receptor-binding site on IgE. Omalizumab binds the free IgE in the serum and reduces the serum level of IgE by over 95% after a single dose. The rationale for the use of anti-IgE in allergic asthmatic inflammation is that free soluble IgE would not be available to bind to the surface of effector cells and will avoid cross-linking by an allergen and the subsequent downstream release of preformed inflammatory mediators. Omalizumab was approved by the U.S. Food and Drug Administration (FDA) in 2003 for use in patients with chronic moderate-to-severe persistent asthma who are symptomatic despite moderate or high doses of inhaled corticosteroids. Corticosteroids are atopic, and whose IgE levels are in the range of 30 to 700 IU/mL. Several randomized placebo-controlled trials indicate that omalizumab lowers the acute exacerbation rate when added to conventional therapy for chronic asthma. This drug is administered subcutaneously once every 2 or 4 weeks. The dose is determined uniquely by the patient's ideal body weight as well as the serum IgE level. This drug is quite expensive (as most monoclonal antibodies are), and the exact place in long-term asthma management remains to be established. For patients who require frequent inpatient care for asthma, however, this agent appears to be a rational alternative.

A minority of patients continue to have troublesome asthma symptoms, with frequent exacerbations requiring hospital stays despite maximal conventional therapy. The literature suggests that this is a small subset, perhaps less than 10% to 15% of all asthmatics. The reversible factors that contribute to the subset of steroid-dependent asthma include:

- Patient noncompliance
- Poor self-management strategies by the patient
- Inadequate control of allergen burden at home
- Suboptimal inhaler technique
- Suboptimal pharmacotherapy prescription by the physician

Exciting research has begun into the concept of pharmacogenetics, or the presence of variant genotypes or polymorphisms that modify disease phenotype or response to different classes of drugs. The most widely studied is the β-adrenergic receptor gene, in which >15 known variants exist, several of which are associated with poor response to an agonist. Ongoing research explores the relative steroid resistance in a subset of these difficult-to-control asthmatics. Several factors—including steroid metabolism, steroid receptor alternate splice variants, and a variety of intracellular factors—are being studied. It appears that steroid metabolism and steroid receptor polymorphisms are likely to be an explanation in a small minority of patients only. Several polymorphisms also occur in the enzymes involved in leukotriene metabolism. The clinical significance of this burgeoning area of pharmacogenetics to the practicing clinician remains to be established.

The placebo arm of a number of studies has clearly shown that a compulsive traditional management plan, with frequent follow-up (perhaps in an asthma center), can reduce the need for oral steroids by 40% to 50% in steroid-dependent asthma. The literature is replete with numerous studies demonstrating the efficacy of alternative anti-inflammatory therapies that provide a steroid-sparing effect in these individuals. Gold salts, methotrexate, cyclosporine, colchicine, troleandomycin, chloroquine, intravenous γ-globulin, and dapsone are some of the agents that have been investigated. Overall, no alternative anti-inflammatory agent has been proved to be superior to inhaled corticosteroids in the treatment of asthma, and the use of these therapies should be restricted to clinical trials only.

## CHRONIC OBSTRUCTIVE PULMONARY DISEASE

The Global Initiative for Chronic Obstructive Lung Disease (GOLD) report defines COPD as "a disease state characterized by airflow limitation that is not fully reversible. The airflow limitation is usually both progressive and associated with an abnormal inflammatory response of the lungs to noxious particles or gases."

Although most adult patients with COPD exhibit features of both chronic bronchitis and emphysema, neither is included in the current definition of COPD, which highlights instead the importance of airflow limitation on

**TABLE 37.1**

## CLASSIFICATION OF COPD SEVERITY (FROM THE GOLD REPORT)

| Stage | Characteristics |
|---|---|
| 0: At risk for COPD | Normal spirometry<br>Chronic symptoms (cough, sputum production) |
| I: Mild COPD | $FEV_1/FVC$ <70%<br>$FEV_1$ ≥80% predicted<br>With or without chronic symptoms (cough, sputum production) |
| II: Moderate COPD | $FEV_1/FVC$ <70%<br>50% ≤$FEV_1$ <80% predicted<br>With or without chronic symptoms (cough, sputum production) |
| III: Severe COPD | $FEV_1/FVC$ <70%<br>30% ≤$FEV_1$ ≤50% predicted<br>With or without chronic symptoms (cough, sputum production) |
| IV: Very severe COPD | $FEV_1/FVC$ <70%<br>$FEV_1$ <30% predicted or $FEV_1$ ≤50% predicted plus chronic respiratory failure |

morbidity and mortality. COPD severity is also classified based on the degree of airway obstruction (Table 37.1). Nevertheless, both chronic bronchitis and emphysema remain useful diagnoses from epidemiologic and clinical standpoints. Chronic bronchitis is clinically defined (based on the Ciba Guest Symposium report of 1959) as chronic cough with sputum production, occurring on most days for at least 3 months of the year for at least 2 successive years. Emphysema is anatomically defined as an abnormal permanent enlargement of the air spaces distal to the terminal bronchiole, accompanied by destruction of their walls, and without obvious fibrosis.

Several different anatomic types of emphysema occur, the most common being the typical smoking-related centriacinar emphysema. This centriacinar emphysema (synonyms are *centrilobular* or *proximal acinar*) involves the dilatation of the air space between the terminal bronchiole and the first- and second-generation respiratory bronchiole. The other major type of emphysema, panacinar or panlobular emphysema, is usually seen in association with the inherited $\alpha_1$-antitrypsin deficiency.

## Etiology

### Epidemiology, Risk Factors, and Natural History

Overall, smoking is the single most important risk factor for COPD. About 15% to 20% of COPD occurs in never-smokers, however, and only about 20% of ever-smokers develop COPD. Although host factors may explain these findings, current concepts also emphasize the total burden of inhaled particles as an exposure risk factor (Table 37.2). In

the general nonsmoking population, the $FEV_1$ percentage predicted follows a unimodal distribution. Among cigarette smokers, the distribution is shifted leftward, to lower $FEV_1$ values. A longitudinal study from East Boston, with a 10-year follow-up, suggested that asymptomatic nonsmoking males showed a prolonged period of either slow growth or plateau phase between ages 23 and 35. Age-related decline in lung function began after this period and occurred at a rate of 20 to 30 mL/year. Although most heavy smokers have a slightly reduced $FEV_1$, only 10% to 15% have a significant chronic obstructive airflow limitation (i.e., $FEV_1$ of less than 65%). In nonsusceptible smokers, the decline in $FEV_1$ is similar to that of nonsmokers. In the small subset of susceptible smokers, an accelerated decline in $FEV_1$ occurs of approximately 70 to 150 mL/year.

The Intermittent Positive-Pressure Breathing Trial Group followed a cohort of 985 patients with established COPD who had a postbronchodilator $FEV_1$ of approximately 40% for a 3-year period. They noted an average mortality of 23% over the 3-year period and found the postbronchodilator $FEV_1$ and the patient's age as the most accurate predictors of death. A slightly increased risk is also present with an elevated resting heart rate, untreated hypoxemia, and hypercapnia. A recent study identifies a composite index combining body-mass index, airflow obstruction, dyspnea, and exercise capacity (the BODE index) as better than the $FEV_1$ in predicting the risk of death in COPD. Respiratory tract infections do not influence the overall course of the disease. Early evidence suggests that increased baseline airway hyper-responsiveness may imply a better prognosis. This remains controversial and is contrary to the so-called Dutch hypothesis, which holds that in patients with increased bronchodilator responsiveness, an accelerated $FEV_1$ decline occurs with time. For example, in data from the Lung Health Study, methacholine responsiveness was found to be an important predictor of the progression of airway obstruction in continuing smokers with early COPD.

## Pathogenesis

Overwhelming evidence suggests that cigarette smoking is causally related to emphysema. The exact component in

**TABLE 37.2**

## RISK FACTORS FOR COPD (FROM THE GOLD REPORT)

| Host factors | Genes (e.g., $\alpha_1$-antitrypsin deficiency)<br>Airway hyper-responsiveness<br>Lung growth |
|---|---|
| Exposures | Tobacco smoke (both active and passive)<br>Occupational exposure to dust and chemicals<br>Indoor and outdoor air pollution<br>Infections<br>Socioeconomic status |

smoke that is responsible for this process is unknown. The lung destruction in emphysema is generally explained by the protease–antiprotease hypothesis: It is believed that in a normal nonsmoking individual, a fine balance exists between the elastolytic proteinases and the endogenous agents that inhibit their activity. Specifically, proteinases involved in COPD include those produced by neutrophils (elastase, cathepsin G, and proteinase-3) and macrophages (cathepsins B, L, and S) and various matrix metalloproteinases (MMP). Alternatively, major antiproteinases providing a screen against the deleterious effects of proteinases include $\alpha_1$-antitrypsin, secretory leukoproteinase inhibitor, and tissue inhibitors of MMPs. It appears that cigarette smoke affects both arms of this balance, thus producing severe lung destruction by a so-called two-hit concept. Components in smoke oxidize $\alpha_1$-antitrypsin as well as directly stimulate neutrophils to produce elastases. Most adult smokers with severe emphysema have serum $\alpha_1$-antitrypsin levels within normal limits. This leads to the notion that additional, poorly understood endogenous antiproteases exist, and/or that the protease–antiprotease hypothesis is only one mechanism for the establishment of COPD.

For example, as is apparent from the new definition of COPD, inflammation is now considered a key component of the pathogenesis of emphysema. Important differentiating characteristics from the inflammation found in asthma are outlined in Table 37.3.

A third mechanism in the pathogenesis of COPD is oxidative stress, which can promote cellular dysfunction, damage the extracellular matrix, and unfavorably affect both arms of the proteinase–antiproteinase balance.

The $\alpha_1$-antitrypsin–deficient form of emphysema occurs in a minority (2% to 3%) of adult patients and should be suspected in those who present with the following features:

- Early-onset emphysema (younger than 50 years)
- Emphysema with minimal smoking history
- Predominantly basilar bullous emphysema
- Family history of emphysema, liver disease, or panniculitis
- Emphysema occurring with liver disease

The diagnosis of $\alpha_1$-antitrypsin deficiency is made by measuring the serum $\alpha_1$-antitrypsin level followed by Pi typing for confirmation. The threshold level for emphysema (less than 80 mg/dL or 11 $\mu$M) usually is seen only in patients with the Pi*ZZ phenotype (homozygotes). In addition to cigarette smoking and $\alpha_1$-antitrypsin deficiency, there are a number of rare causes for COPD:

- Hypocomplementemic urticarial vasculitis syndrome
- Intravenous methylphenidate (Ritalin) abuse
- Ehlers-Danlos or Marfan's syndrome
- Salla disease
- $\alpha_1$-Antichymotrypsin deficiency
- Human immunodeficiency virus (HIV) infection
- Systemic necrotizing vasculitis
- Variant of the gene for tumor necrosis factor (TNF$\alpha$)

## Clinical Presentation

The cardinal symptoms of COPD include dyspnea and cough, with or without sputum production and wheezing. Symptoms are usually chronic (i.e., of at least 3 to 5 years' duration) and slowly progressive. Patients may give a history of a variable course with occasional acute exacerbations interspersed with periods of stable or slowly progressive illness. The variability in the symptoms is not nearly as dramatic as in young patients with typical asthma, however, in whom the periods between acute exacerbations are quite symptom-free.

Physical examination is tailored to establish whether a patient has an acute exacerbation of her illness and whether a concomitant illness is contributing to symptoms. Although some patients exhibit the classic body habitus of either a "pink puffer" (type A) or a "blue bloater" (type B), most adult patients with COPD exhibit features of both. The lung examination is most remarkable for a decrease in the intensity of breath sounds, prolonged expiratory phase, and occasional scattered wheezes on forced expiration. Rales usually are not present. Heart sounds usually are distant and difficult to appreciate. The presence of right ventricular strain or failure can be ascertained by a loud pulmonic

**TABLE 37.3**

**COMPARISON OF INFLAMMATION IN ASTHMA AND COPD (FROM THE GOLD REPORT)**

| Characteristic | COPD | Asthma |
|---|---|---|
| Cells | Neutrophils<br>Large number of macrophages<br>Increase in CD8+ T lymphocytes | Eosinophils<br>Small increase in macrophages<br>Increase in CD4+ Th2 lymphocytes<br>Activation of mast cells |
| Mediators | LTB4, IL-8, TNF$\alpha$ | LTD4, IL-4, IL-5 |

component of the second heart sound, a right ventricular heave, elevated neck veins, a pulsatile liver, and edema in the lower extremities. Clubbing of the fingers is not usually present in smoking-related COPD, and its presence should strongly suggest a complicating illness such as lung cancer, pulmonary fibrosis, chronic infection, or liver disease.

Although the chest roentgenogram may offer clues supporting a diagnosis of obstructive airway disease, its primary importance is in excluding important concomitant diseases, such as pulmonary nodules, congestive heart failure, or pulmonary fibrosis. Computed tomography (CT) scan of the chest shows certain typical features but is not necessary for the diagnosis.

Pulmonary function testing is essential to establish a diagnosis of COPD and its severity (Table 37.1). The typical spirometric abnormalities in COPD consist of a reduction in the $FEV_1$ and in the ratio of the $FEV_1$ to the forced vital capacity. The single-breath diffusing capacity for carbon monoxide is usually reduced in emphysema and has a good correlation with the extent of anatomic destruction in emphysema.

Many patients with COPD have a significant response to the acute administration of inhaled bronchodilators (an increase in $FEV_1$ of 12% and 200 mL). Clearly, the presence of bronchodilator response itself is not adequate to distinguish asthma from COPD. Also, a methacholine provocation test result may be positive in more than 60% of patients with COPD, so this also does not distinguish COPD from asthma. There is no indication for this challenge test in patients with known COPD.

## Treatment

The management of stable COPD is considered separately from treatment during acute exacerbations. The critical interventions that have been shown to prolong survival and affect the natural history of the underlying disease are oxygen therapy for the chronically hypoxemic patient and perhaps smoking cessation. All other management strategies have less compelling data to suggest long-term measurable benefit, either in terms of survival or other criteria, such as rate of decline in $FEV_1$. Proposed guidelines from the GOLD report, tailoring the treatment of COPD to stage of disease, are shown in Table 37.4.

The commonly used therapy for stable COPD includes prevention (smoking cessation, annual flu vaccination, and vaccination for pneumococcus every 6 years), supplemental oxygen if indicated, inhaled bronchodilators, and, in a small subset, theophylline preparations and inhaled or systemic corticosteroids. In a meta-analysis of exercise performance studies, the overall effect favored pulmonary rehabilitation, with specific benefits including an 11% to 33% increase in maximal work rate, a 9% increase in maximal oxygen consumption, a 38% to 85% increase in exercise endurance time, and increases in 6-minute walk distance by 38 to 96 meters. Pulmonary rehabilitation did not improve $FEV_1$ or survival, however.

The current database showing survival advantage for supplemental oxygen therapy in chronically hypoxemic patients is largely based on two landmark studies: the Nocturnal Oxygen Therapy Trial and the British Medical Research Council trial. Both studies included patients with severe but stable COPD and resting hypoxemia. The combined results from these studies suggest that continuous oxygen therapy for 24 hours or 12 hours confers a definite survival benefit. Other significant findings included improvement in quality of life and neuropsychiatric function, exercise tolerance, reduction in secondary polycythemia, and reduced pulmonary artery pressure in selected groups of patients. Although the exact mechanism for the survival benefit is unknown, it is probably through improved pulmonary vascular resistance. Patients with a resting room air alveolar oxygen tension of less than 55 mm Hg or an $SpO_2$ by pulse oximetry of less than 88% should be given supplemental oxygen. These criteria should be checked during a period of clinical stability rather than during an acute exacerbation. In patients with alveolar oxygen tension between 55 mm Hg and 59 mm Hg, the additional clinical features of chronic hypoxemia and end-organ damage should be present.

The pharmacotherapy for COPD is mostly used to accomplish symptom control rather than to affect the natural history of the disease (i.e., unlike inhaled steroids in asthma). A stepwise therapy is usually followed, using one or a combination of inhaled bronchodilators, based on disease severity (Table 37.4). The three bronchodilators primarily used and currently available are anticholinergic

## TABLE 37.4

### COPD THERAPY BY STAGE (FROM THE GOLD REPORT)

| 0: At Risk | I: Mild | II: Moderate | III: Severe | IV: Very Severe |
|---|---|---|---|---|
| Avoidance of risk factors; vaccination | Add short-acting bronchodilator when needed | Add regular treatment with one or more long-acting bronchodilator, add rehabilitation | Add inhaled glucocorticosteroids if repeated exacerbations | Add long-term O2, consider surgical options |

agents, $\beta_2$-selective adrenergic agents (both short- and long-acting), and theophylline preparations.

A variety of studies document the efficacy of each of these agents in the management of stable COPD, either alone or in combination. All three classes of bronchodilators have been shown to produce improvement in symptoms and exercise capacity in COPD, usually without a significant chronic increase in $FEV_1$. Most symptomatic patients are usually treated with short-acting inhaled $\beta$-agonists (usually albuterol). As in asthma, recent data indicate that the regularly scheduled administration of $\beta$-agonists is not superior to as-needed or on-demand use. It appears that patients with COPD have a significantly increased cholinergic bronchomotor tone.

The human lung has three subtypes of muscarinic cholinergic receptors (M1, M2, and M3). The M2 subtype is postganglionic and is the only type that protects against bronchoconstriction. Both atropine and ipratropium are nonselective and inhibit all three subtypes. A multicenter study suggested that ipratropium showed a bronchodilator effect superior to that of metaproterenol in patients with severe COPD. Over the past 10 years, ipratropium has achieved the status of first-line maintenance therapy for COPD. Results of the Lung Health Study I (prospective evaluation of smoking cessation $\pm$ ipratropium over 5 years) were disappointing in that the benefits of ipratropium were modest, occurred during year 1 only, and improvement in lung function was lost within weeks of stopping therapy. It has the advantage of being safe and free of side effects, however. It is inconvenient to administer (available only as a metered-dose inhaler and requiring two to six puffs four times a day) and is not as potent because it is nonselective (inhibits M2 receptor as well as M1 and M3). A recently approved anticholinergic agent, tiotropium bromide (Spiriva), is long acting and may be more potent (has some M1 and M3 selectivity). Several recent studies indicate its superiority over ipratropium. Also, a recent randomized trial suggests that theophylline improves respiratory function and dyspnea in patients with severe COPD.

Numerous studies have examined the role of oral corticosteroid therapy in patients with stable COPD. A recent meta-analysis by Callahan et al. surveyed 33 original studies of oral corticosteroid use in the literature and selected 15 studies that met some preselected criteria of study quality. Callahan et al. concluded that stable COPD patients receiving steroids have a 20% or greater improvement in baseline $FEV_1$, approximately 10% more often than similar patients receiving placebo alone. Unfortunately, no satisfactory clinical predictors for response are apparent. In general, steroid use in these patients should be considered as an empirical trial, patient response should be objectively assessed, and benefits should be weighed against the well-known side effects of corticosteroid use. Current guidelines do not recommend the long-term use of corticosteroids in stable COPD due to the risk of skeletal muscle myopathy and other side effects.

Four randomized, large studies have examined the effect of inhaled steroids versus placebo on the annual rate of decline in $FEV_1$, with a minimum follow-up of 3 years (Copenhagen City lung study, European Respiratory Society Study on Chronic Obstructive Pulmonary Disease trial, Inhaled Steroids in Obstructive Lung Disease study, and Lung Health Study II). These studies did not show a beneficial effect for inhaled steroids on lung function decline. Current evidence and guidelines, however, recommend the use of inhaled corticosteroids to reduce the exacerbation rate and improve the health status in individuals with Stage III or IV COPD (FEV 1 <50%) who have repeated exacerbations (e.g., three exacerbations in the preceding 3 years). Additionally, in at least three randomized trials, the combination of an inhaled corticosteroid with an inhaled long-acting $\beta_2$-agonist improved lung function and dyspnea compared to the individual components. Mucokinetic agents, such as organic iodides, have not been shown to have objective benefit in COPD. $\alpha_1$-Antitrypsin augmentation therapy is used in nonsmoking younger patients with severe $\alpha_1$-antitrypsin deficiency and associated emphysema. The efficacy of this therapy is unproved, although observational studies show that augmentation therapy decreases the rate of decline of $FEV_1$, reduces infections, improves survival, and reduces markers of lung inflammation. Human-pooled plasma-derived $\alpha_1$-antitrypsin is administered by intravenous infusion weekly, biweekly, or monthly. The recommended weekly dose is 60 mg/kg, and the monthly dose is 250 mg/kg.

The two most common causes of COPD exacerbations are infections of the tracheobronchial tree and air pollution, although as many as one-third of exacerbations have no identified cause. Acute exacerbations of COPD are often managed in a hospital setting, using aggressive aerosolized and intravenous pharmacotherapy with the agents discussed above. Repeated inhaled $\beta$-agonists (either nebulized or by metered-dose inhaler) are preferred over anticholinergics because the onset of action is more rapid. Systemic corticosteroids are usually given during acute exacerbations of COPD (either in the outpatient setting or in the hospital), and good evidence suggests that they accelerate the recovery and restoration of lung function. The efficacy of antibiotic therapy in exacerbations of COPD is a topic of several studies and some controversy. In general, patients with a change in sputum, fever, and new infiltrate are optimal candidates for antibiotics, with the choice of agent directed at local patterns of sensitivity to *Streptococcus pneumoniae*, *Haemophilus influenzae*, and *Moraxella catarrhalis*. *Pseudomonas aeruginosa* may also play a role in severe COPD. There is probably no need for a routine sputum culture. The vast majority of patients with COPD exacerbation can be successfully managed using this therapy alone.

Perhaps 5% to 10% of COPD patients either fail this therapy or initially present with acute respiratory failure requiring intensive care, and perhaps 20% to 60% require ventilatory support, either noninvasively or following intubation and invasive mechanical ventilation. Several randomized controlled trials have shown that, in selected patients, noninvasive positive pressure ventilation was successful in 80% to 85%, and reduced mortality and hospitalization. Extensive literature documents the intensive care unit (ICU) management of COPD patients; this topic is beyond the scope of this discussion. Previously, the prognosis for patients with acute respiratory failure secondary to COPD exacerbation alone, without complicating illness, was believed to be quite favorable. Recent studies suggest that exacerbation of COPD with admission to an ICU is associated with a hospital mortality rate of 24%. For patients 65 years and older, the 1-year mortality rate is 30% to 59%. In patients with COPD exacerbation and hypercapnia ($PaCO_2$ of $\geq 50$ mm Hg), 1- and 2-year mortality rates are 43% and 49%, respectively. An episode of acute respiratory failure caused by an exacerbation of COPD appears not to significantly alter the overall prognosis of the disease, which is largely dictated by the $FEV_1$ and age.

## Surgery for Emphysema

A variety of surgical techniques have been applied to a small subset of patients with advanced or end-stage COPD. Surgical resection of lung tissue in emphysema is "counterintuitive" and is based on the premise that advanced emphysema is characterized by very large, baggy lungs (with hyperinflation and reduced elastic recoil), along with respiratory muscles that are at a mechanical disadvantage because of hyperinflation. A variety of surgeries have been performed, including localized resection or bullectomy for focal giant bullae and lung volume reduction surgery (LVRS) (or bilateral pneumectomy or pneumoplasty). A variety of approaches have been used to perform LVRS, including a thoracoscopic approach using laser resection, median sternotomy using bilateral LVRS, or unilateral LVRS. This procedure has sometimes been used as a bridge during the consideration of lung transplantation. Presently, all these techniques should be considered experimental, and they should be considered for a small subset of patients who have very advanced emphysema, who remain symptomatic despite maximum medical therapy and oxygen, and whose nonpulmonary medical status is very good. Lung transplantation is an extremely limited surgical option, largely because of the scarcity of donors. This has partly contributed to consideration of alternative surgical procedures such as LVRS.

The physiologic mechanism for the benefit of LVRS in emphysema is probably mediated by increasing the elastic recoil of the lungs and reducing the resting and expiratory lung volumes. This restores the normal outward circumferential force on the airways, thus reducing resistance to expiratory airflow. In addition, improvements probably occur in the configuration of the diaphragm and intercostal muscles and in a greater contribution by the abdom-

inal musculature to total volume. Currently, the selection criteria for LVRS are controversial but the following features have been proposed to be associated with improved outcome in a systematic review with expert opinion:

- Smoking-related emphysema
- Heterogeneous emphysema on computed tomography (i.e., surgically accessible "target" areas)
- Bilateral LVRS
- Good general fitness/condition
- Thoracic hyperinflation

Additionally, in the randomized National Emphysema Treatment Trial Research Group (NETT) study, survival was improved with LVRS, compared to medical therapy in patients with both predominantly upper-lobe emphysema and low baseline exercise capacity. Other favorable features include age <75 years, $FEV_1$ between 20% and 40% of predicted, evidence of hyperinflation (RV >150%, TLC >100% of predicted), $PaO_2$ >45 mm Hg, $PaCO_2$ <60 mm Hg, postrehabilitation 6-min walk >140 m. Selected unfavorable resection criteria include pulmonary hypertension (PA systolic >45 mm Hg, PA mean >35 mm Hg), $FEV_1$ <20% of predicted, lung diffusion capacity (DLCO) level of <20% of predicted, homogeneous emphysema, non–upper lobe predominant emphysema, and high achieved wattage on postrehabilitation cycle ergometry.

Several surgical series using LVRS have indicated short-term improvement of $FEV_1$ between 50% and 82% at 6 months, along with reduced dyspnea and improved exercise tolerance and quality of life. The procedure does carry significant complications, however, including a 90-day surgical mortality of 5.2% in non–high-risk patients, as compared to 1.5% in medically treated patients, and a mean hospital stay of 7 to 10 days, often due to prolonged air leak (in approximately 40% to 50% of the patients). The few studies with long-term outcomes suggest that, over time, lung volumes return to near preoperative baseline and dyspnea worsens, although the loss of 6-min walk distance appears to be slower than other functional measures.

Lung transplantation remains an alternative for a few patients with advanced disease who meet the selection criteria noted below. Single-lung transplantation has emerged as a transplant procedure of choice for patients with COPD. The American Thoracic Society and European Respiratory Society recommend the following COPD-specific guidelines for the selection of lung transplantation candidates:

1. $FEV_1$ of <25% of predicted (without reversibility), and/or
2. Resting, room air $PaCO_2$ of >55 mm Hg, and/or
3. Elevated $PaCO_2$ with progressive deterioration requiring long-term oxygen therapy, and/or
4. Elevated pulmonary artery pressure with progressive deterioration

# REVIEW EXERCISES

## QUESTIONS

1. Which of the following is the most important variable to correct in patients with severe COPD (either acute or chronic)?
a) $Pa_{CO_2}$
b) pH
c) Hypoxemia
d) Pulmonary hypertension
e) Cardiac output

2. Which one of the following has been shown to increase survival in patients with severe COPD?
a) ICU care and mechanical ventilation
b) Systemic steroids during acute exacerbations
c) Long-term oxygen therapy
d) Smoking cessation
e) Chronic therapy with bronchodilators

3. All the following regarding asthma therapy are correct, *except*
a) Case control studies indicate that regular use of inhaled steroids reduces asthma mortality.
b) Chronic maintenance anti-inflammatory is indicated in all patients with persistent asthma.
c) A variety of novel therapies are under development for asthma.
d) Head-to-head studies have proved that inhaled steroids are the best therapy for all patients with asthma.

4. Antileukotrienes may have particular benefit in which subset of asthmatics?
a) Aspirin-sensitive asthma
b) Allergic bronchopulmonary aspergillosis
c) Prednisone-dependent asthma
d) Allergic asthma
e) Occupational asthma

5. Which one of the following statements does not belong with the other choices?
a) Bilateral vocal cord paralysis
b) Postextubation stridor
c) Factitious (or functional) asthma
d) Variable extrathoracic upper airway obstruction
e) Flattening of the expiratory limb of flow–volume loop

## ANSWERS

### 1. c.
The overriding concern should be to improve tissue oxygen delivery. Although supplemental oxygen may contribute to hypercapnia (mostly by affecting ventilation–perfusion mismatching rather than the suppression of hypoxic drive), correcting hypoxemia ($Pa_{O_2}$

60 mm Hg, $Sa_{O_2}$ of 90%) is critical. The mechanism whereby chronic oxygen improves survival is probably by reducing pulmonary hypertension. The best way to reduce pulmonary artery pressures is to correct hypoxemia.

### 2. c.
All the answer choices are reasonable therapies for COPD, but only ambulatory home oxygen for more than 12 hours/day has been unequivocally shown to improve survival (in appropriate candidates who have baseline hypoxemia). In the Nocturnal Oxygen Therapy Trial, survival in the continuous oxygen group was 75% versus 54% in the control group at 36 months (oxygen 12 hours/day).

### 3. d.
All agents approved for asthma (cromoglycate, inhaled steroids, antileukotrienes) have shown objective benefit compared with placebo. Limited head-to-head studies do exist, but those available indicate that the magnitude of improvement is higher for inhaled steroids, especially for patients with severe asthma. These agents have the potential for systemic side effects. Therefore, for any given patient, therapy should be individualized.

### 4. a.
The leukotriene pathway is particularly important in patients with aspirin-induced asthma. Studies show the effectiveness of leukotriene antagonists.

### 5. e.
With variable extrathoracic UAO (i.e., bilateral vocal cord paralysis, postextubation stridor, functional vocal cord adduction), the flow–volume loop would show flattening of the inspiratory limb.

## SUGGESTED READINGS

### Asthma

Broide DH. Molecular and cellular mechanisms of allergic disease. *J Allergy Clin Immunol* 2001;108:S65–S71.

Elias JA, Lee CG, Zheng T, et al. New insights into the pathogenesis of asthma. *J Clin Invest* 2003;111:291–297.

Guidelines for the Diagnosis and Management of Asthma–Update on Selected Topics 2002. U.S. Department of Health and Human Services, National Institutes of Health; 2002. NIH Publication No. 02-5075. (http://www.nhlbi.nih.gov/guidelines/asthma/index.htm.)

Kavuru M, Melamed J, Gross G, et al. Salmeterol and fluticasone propionate combined in a new powder inhalation device for the treatment of asthma: A randomized, double-blind, placebo-controlled trial. *J Allergy Clin Immunol* 2000;105;1108–1116.

Mannino DM, Homa DM, Akinbami LJ, et al. Surveillance for asthma–United States, 1980–1999. In: *MMWR Surveill Summ*, March 29, 2002.

Palmer LJ, Silverman ES, Weiss ST, et al. Pharmacogenetics of asthma. *Am J Respir Crit Care Med* 2002;165;861–866.

Reiss TF, Chervinsky P, Dockhorn RJ, et al. Montelukast, a once daily leukotriene receptor antagonist in the treatment of chronic asthma; a multicenter randomized double-blind trial. *Arch Intern Med* 1998;158:1213–1220.

Soler M, Matz J, Townley R, et al. The anti-IgE antibody omalizumab reduces exacerbations and steroid requirement in allergic asthmatics. *Eur Respir J* 2001;18(2):254–261.

Szefler S, Weiss S, Tonascia J, et al. Long-term effects of budesonide or nedocromil in children with asthma. The CAMP Research Group. *N Engl J Med* 2000;343:1054–1063.

Weiss ST. Eat dirt–The hygiene hypothesis and allergic diseases. *N Engl J Med.* 2002;347;930–931.

### Chronic Obstructive Pulmonary Disease

Anthonisen NR, Connett JE, Kiley JP, et al. Effects of smoking intervention and the use of an inhaled anticholinergic bronchodilator on the rate of decline of $FEV_1$: the Lung Health Study. *JAMA* 1994;272:1497–1505.

ATS statement: standards for the diagnosis and care of patients with chronic obstructive pulmonary disease. *Am J Respir Crit Care Med* 1995;152[Suppl]:78–121. Update 2004 available at http://www.thoracic.org/COPD. Accessed May 30, 2004.

Callahan CM, Dittus RS, Katz BP. Oral corticosteroid therapy for patients with stable chronic obstructive pulmonary disease. A meta-analysis. *Ann Intern Med* 1991;114:216–223.

Casaburi R, Briggs DD Jr, Donohue JF, et al. The spirometric efficacy of once-daily dosing with tiotropium in stable COPD: a 13-week multicenter trial. *Chest* 2000;118:1294.

Celli BR, Cote CG, Marin JM, et al. The body-mass index, airflow obstruction, dyspnea, and exercise capacity index in chronic obstructive pulmonary disease. *N Engl J Med* 2004;350:1005–1012.

Connors AF, Dawson NV, Thomas C, et al. Outcomes following acute exacerbation of severe chronic obstructive pulmonary disease. *Am J Respir Crit Care Med* 1996;154:959–967.

Fein AM, Braman SS, Casaburi R, et al. Lung volume reduction surgery: official statement of the American Thoracic Society. *Am J Respir Crit Care Med* 1996;154:1151.

Fishman A, Martinez F, Naunheim K, et al. A randomized trial comparing lung-volume-reduction surgery with medical therapy for severe emphysema. *N Engl J Med* 2003;348:2059–2073.

Geddes D, Davies M, Koyama H, et al. Effect of lung-volume-reduction surgery in patients with severe emphysema. *N Engl J Med* 2000;343:239.

Global Initiative for Chronic Obstructive Lungs Disease (GOLD). Available at www.goldcopd.com. Accessed May 30, 2004.

Hill NS. Noninvasive ventilation: does it work, for whom, and how? *Am Rev Respir Dis* 1993;147:1050–1055.

International guidelines for the selection of lung transplant candidates. *Am J Respir Crit Care Med* 1998;158:335.

Kotlke TE, Battista RN, DeFriese GH, et al. Attributes of successful smoking cessation interventions in medical practice: a meta analysis of 39 controlled trials. *JAMA* 1988;259:2882–2889.

Lacasse Y, Wong E, Guyatt GH, et al. Meta-analysis of respiratory rehabilitation in chronic obstructive pulmonary disease. *Lancet* 1996;348:1115–1119.

Lung Health Study Research Group. Effect of inhaled triamcinolone on the decline in pulmonary function in chronic obstructive pulmonary disease. *N Engl J Med* 2000;343:1902.

Mannino DM, Gagnon RC, Petty TL, et al. Obstructive lung disease and low lung function in adults in the United States: data from the National Health and Nutrition Examination Survey, 1988–1994. *Arch Intern Med* 2000;160:1683–1689.

Mannino DM, Homa DM, Akinbami LJ, et al. Chronic obstructive lung disease surveillance–United States, 1971–2000. *MMWR Surveill Summ* 2002;51(6):1–16.

Niewoehner DE, Erbland ML, Deupree RH, et al. Effect of systemic glucocorticoids on exacerbations of chronic obstructive pulmonary disease. Department of Veterans Affairs Cooperative Study Group. *N Engl J Med* 1999;340:1941–1947.

Ries AL, Kaplan RM, Limberg TM, et al. Effects of pulmonary rehabilitation on physiologic and psychological outcomes in patients with chronic obstructive pulmonary disease. *Ann Intern Med* 1995;122:823–832.

Rutten-van Molken M, van Doorslaer E, Jansen M, et al. Costs and effects of inhaled corticosteroids and bronchodilators in asthma and COPD. *Am J Respir Crit Care Med* 1995;151:975–982.

Saint S, Bent S, Vittinghoff E, et al. Antibiotics in chronic obstructive pulmonary disease exacerbations: a meta-analysis. *JAMA* 1995; 273:957–960.

Sciurba FC, Rogers RM, Keenan RJ, et al. Improvement in pulmonary function and elastic recoil after lung-reduction surgery for diffuse emphysema. *N Engl J Med* 1996;334:1095.

Stoller JK, Aboussouan LS. Intravenous augmentation therapy for AAT deficiency: Current understanding. *Thorax* 2004;59:708–712.

Tarpy SP, Celli BR. Long-term oxygen therapy. *N Engl J Med* 1995; 333:710–714.

Thompson WH, Nielson CP, Carvalho P, et al. Controlled trial of oral prednisone in outpatients with acute COPD exacerbation. *Am J Respir Crit Care Med* 1996;154:407–412.

Weinmann GG, Hyatt R. Evaluation and research in lung volume reduction surgery. *Am J Respir Crit Care Med* 1996;154:1913–1918.

# Interstitial Lung Disease                    38

## Jeffrey T. Chapman

The term *interstitial lung disease* (ILD) refers to a heterogeneous group of disorders that present in a similar manner, rather than a specific diagnosis. These disorders generally are progressive, inflammatory, or scarring processes that affect the interstitium to a greater extent than the airways or air spaces. In general, these diseases are considered together because of their common clinical, radiographic, and physiologic picture. Because these diseases usually are considered together as part of a differential diagnosis, the term ILD is a clinically useful starting point. One must keep in mind, however, that within this category there exist many diverse diseases with unique clinical characteristics, causes, treatments, and prognoses.

Figure 38.1 illustrates the distinction made between the pulmonary parenchymal interstitium as opposed to the conducting airways and airspaces (alveoli).

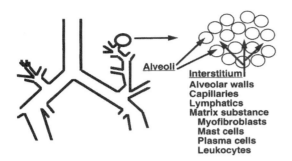

**Figure 38.1** The conducting airways and the gas exchange components (alveoli and interstitium) of the lung.

## ETIOLOGY OF INTERSTITIAL LUNG DISEASE

The ILDs are quite numerous and varied and may be difficult to organize into a usable conceptual framework. When evaluating a patient with ILD of uncertain etiology, it is helpful to consider diseases in the following categories; examples are given of specific types within each category:

- Occupational ILD
  - □ Asbestosis
  - □ Silicosis
  - □ Coal workers' pneumoconiosis
- Iatrogenic ILD
  - □ Anti-inflammatory agents (e.g., methotrexate, gold)
  - □ Chemotherapeutic agents (e.g., bleomycin, bis-chloroethylnitrosourea)
  - □ Nitrofurantoin and other drugs
  - □ Radiation therapy
  - □ Connective tissue disease–associated ILD
  - □ Rheumatoid arthritis
  - □ Scleroderma
  - □ Polymyositis/dermatomyositis
  - □ Sjögren's syndrome
  - □ Systemic lupus erythematosus (SLE)
- Granulomatous ILD
  - □ Sarcoidosis
  - □ Pigeon fancier's lung
  - □ Farmer's lung
  - □ Humidifier lung
  - □ Environmental fungi
- Smoking-related ILD
- Respiratory bronchiolitis–associated ILD
  - □ Desquamative interstitial pneumonia
- Idiopathic interstitial pneumonias
  - □ Idiopathic pulmonary fibrosis (IPF)
  - □ Nonspecific interstitial pneumonia
  - □ Cryptogenic organizing pneumonia
- Other, unclassifiable entities
  - □ Lymphangioleiomyomatosis
  - □ Eosinophilic granuloma (histiocytosis X)

- □ Chronic eosinophilic pneumonitis
- □ Pulmonary alveolar lipoproteinosis
- □ Various vasculitides
- □ Inflammatory bowel disease
- □ Hepatic cirrhosis

Although the final two categories, idiopathic and unclassified entities, include a fairly large number of diseases, this way of approaching ILDs helps to guide the proper history and physical examination. If you consider each of these categories, you will ask the right questions and be alert to the relevant signs.

## DIAGNOSIS OF ILD

### History

Given the wide variety of diseases and exposures that can be associated with ILD, the history is critically important in the evaluation of a patient with ILD. The history should include questions regarding symptoms such as cough and dyspnea or symptoms of connective tissue disease. The description of the onset of these symptoms, their duration, and the general cadence of the illness may also help narrow the diagnostic possibilities. Clearly, these patients should be asked about significant occupational exposure such as asbestos, silica, or carcinogens. One must also investigate environmental exposures, looking for possible antigenic sources, which could lead to chronic hypersensitivity pneumonitis. This includes questions related to mold or mildew in the home environment, pets (especially birds), and hobbies. In addition, it is important to take a careful medication history, looking for agents that may be associated with drug-induced lung disease. A focused review of systems is necessary to rule out ILD associated with systemic disorders.

### Physical Examination

The physical examination in patients with ILD is fairly nonspecific. One tends to find crackles on examination of the chest. Clubbing and signs of *cor pulmonale* are late signs in ILD. One must also look for signs of connective tissue disease, including skin rash, joint changes, hair loss, or muscle weakness.

### Radiography

The chest radiograph in ILD is also generally nonspecific. Diffuse reticular or reticulonodular opacities may be seen in association with reduced lung volumes. These findings may be subtle at first and progress gradually. It is not uncommon for the radiologist to read "chronic" changes only. This is sometimes taken to mean that these chronic changes are not significant. Despite the fact that the chest radiograph changes shown in many of the ILDs are chronic and slowly progressive, however, these diseases may be quite serious and merit further evaluation. Significant clinical deterioration can occur in the setting of unchanging or minimally changing "chronic" abnormalities. Another common pitfall in the analysis of chest radiographs in patients with ILD is the assumption that the decreased lung volumes resulted because "the patient didn't take a deep breath." In general, routine chest films are taken after deep inspiration. Occasionally, miscommunication between the technician and the patient may result in a film being taken anywhere in the respiratory cycle. If the radiography reports on a particular patient consistently comment on poor inspiration, however, one must consider the possibility that a restrictive lung disease is present, leading to small lung volumes despite appropriate inspiratory effort.

Although chest radiography in the ILDs generally is nonspecific, particular patterns or associated findings seen on the radiograph may be helpful in narrowing the diagnostic possibilities. For example, asbestos-related lung disease may be associated with pleural plaques or pleural effusions in addition to the reticulonodular infiltrates and reduced lung volumes. In general, the reticulonodular infiltrates in asbestosis are seen in a lower zone distribution.

The distribution of chest radiograph abnormalities may suggest certain diagnoses. Diseases that tend to involve predominantly the upper lung zones include silicosis, chronic hypersensitivity pneumonitis, sarcoidosis, eosinophilic granuloma (also known as histiocytosis X), and ankylosing spondylitis. Diseases that tend to have a lower zone distribution include IPF, asbestosis, and the ILDs associated with various connective tissue diseases. Chronic eosinophilic pneumonia is a disease that classically has a peripheral distribution. The chest radiograph in chronic eosinophilic pneumonia is said to appear as the "radiographic negative of congestive heart failure." When reticular or reticulonodular infiltrates demonstrate straight borders and are present within the ports of prior radiation therapy, radiation pneumonitis is the likely diagnosis.

The character of the infiltrates also may suggest certain disease entities. Cystic changes may be seen in lymphangioleiomyomatosis, in eosinophilic granuloma, and in the later stages of lung diseases of various etiologies, so-called end-stage honeycombing. The presence of Kerley B lines should suggest the possibility of lymphangitic carcinoma or chronic interstitial edema. Nodular infiltrates are seen in sarcoidosis, silicosis, coal workers' pneumoconiosis, bronchiolitis obliterans, miliary distributions of various infections, and carcinoma.

Other aspects of the chest radiograph also may help to suggest certain diagnoses. Although most of the ILDs are associated with decreased lung volumes, several may result in the remarkable combination of diffuse reticular infiltrates along with normal or increased lung volumes. These include lymphangioleiomyomatosis, eosinophilic granuloma, chronic hypersensitivity pneumonitis, and

sarcoidosis. In this setting, one must also consider the possibility that two disease processes are present, namely any ILD along with significant smoking-related emphysema. The presence of a pneumothorax should raise the possibility of eosinophilic granuloma or lymphangioleiomyomatosis or tuberous sclerosis–related lung disease. The presence of a pleural effusion should raise the possibility of rheumatoid arthritis, asbestosis, carcinoma, or lymphangioleiomyomatosis. Likewise, pleural plaques are an indication of asbestos exposure and raise the possibility of asbestosis. Hilar adenopathy may be seen in sarcoidosis, silicosis, and carcinoma.

One must keep in mind that a small fraction of patients with ILD indeed have a normal chest radiograph. This has particularly been reported in chronic hypersensitivity pneumonitis. The use of high-resolution computed tomography (CT) scanning has been increasing in the evaluation of patients with ILD. High-resolution CT can be quite helpful regarding the documentation of the extent of disease and in guiding subsequent open lung biopsy. Occasionally, certain high-resolution CT findings can suggest a specific diagnosis, as in eosinophilic granuloma, lymphangioleiomyomatosis, or pulmonary alveolar lipoproteinosis. Although exact correlations between high-resolution CT scan appearance and both pathologic findings and response to therapy are lacking, patients with more so-called ground glass opacities generally tend to respond better to therapy than do those with extensive honeycomb lung.

## Pulmonary Function Testing

The physiologic evaluation of the patient with ILD should include full pulmonary function testing and arterial blood gases. Occasionally, physiologic findings may yield clues to the diagnosis. In addition, this testing allows an estimate of the current disease severity and provides a baseline for future decision making.

In general, the ILDs result in a restrictive pulmonary physiology characterized by a reduced forced expiratory volume in 1 second ($FEV_1$) and forced vital capacity (FVC). The ratio of $FEV_1$ to FVC remains normal or may be, in fact, supranormal. The lung volumes are reduced, and the diffusing capacity is reduced. The diffusing capacity may improve somewhat when corrected for lung volume but tends not to return to the normal range. The pressure–volume curve, in which transpulmonary pressure is plotted against lung volume, is a test that can be performed in most pulmonary function laboratories (Fig. 38.2). It is not commonly performed as a matter of routine procedure, however, because it requires the placement of an esophageal balloon with which to measure intrathoracic pressures. The pressure–volume curve demonstrates the increased elastic recoil that is seen with these restrictive lung diseases. At any particular lung volume, the transpulmonary pressure is markedly increased, reflecting the "stiffness" of these patients' lungs. This is

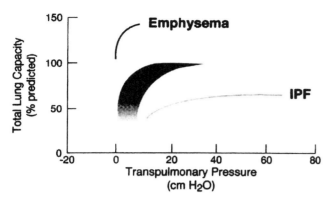

**Figure 38.2** Pressure-volume curve of pulmonary compliance. IPF, idiopathic pulmonary fibrosis.

exactly the opposite of what occurs in emphysema, in which the destruction of pulmonary parenchyma leads to a loss of elastic recoil. Thus, in emphysema, the lung volumes are generally elevated, and at any particular lung volume, the transpulmonary pressure is much smaller than expected.

This concept of opposing effects on elastic recoil forces raises the subject of a common pitfall in the diagnosis of ILD. In a patient who is a heavy smoker and has increased interstitial markings on chest radiography, one must keep in mind the possibility that two disease entities, emphysema and ILD, are present. Because of the opposing physiologic effects of the ILD and the emphysema, the severity of the overall disease may be underestimated based solely on spirometry and lung volumes. This is because the elastic properties of the lung (its stiffness) greatly influence both the dynamic flow rates and the measured lung volumes. Thus, a patient who is severely disabled from a combination of emphysema and IPF may have preserved spirometry and lung volumes. In such a patient, however, the diffusing capacity is usually quite low, and this should be a clue to this possibility.

### Laboratory and Other Studies

Baseline complete blood cell count and metabolic profiles are useful to establish a baseline and predict the side effects to possible therapies. Directed laboratory studies such as rheumatoid factor (RF), antinuclear antibodies (ANA), erythrocyte sedimentation rate (ERS), and HLA-B27 are useful to exclude secondary causes of ILD, when guided by the patient's symptoms.

### Bronchoscopy

Bronchoscopy is most useful in its ability to help rule out infection, granuloma, and malignancy. Occasionally, the bronchoalveolar lavage (BAL) cytology may be diagnostic, as in pulmonary alveolar lipoproteinosis, lymphangitic carcinoma, and eosinophilic granuloma. Past research has

shown that CD4 to CD8 T-cell ratios can suggest certain diagnoses such as sarcoidosis (elevated CD4) and hypersensitivity pneumonitis (elevated CD8). In IPF, elevated lavage neutrophils or eosinophils suggest a lack of response to steroids. The transbronchial biopsy specimens obtained through bronchoscopy are usually too small to make definitive diagnoses of most of the ILDs. One may, however, be able to obtain a diagnosis in patients with lymphangitic carcinoma or granulomatous diseases such as sarcoidosis or hypersensitivity pneumonitis.

### Surgical Lung Biopsy

In many patients, a diagnosis can be made after clinical and radiologic evaluation; however, some patients require a surgical lung biopsy to obtain large tissue samples and secure a pathologic diagnosis. The thoracoscopic approach is generally quite well tolerated, even in fairly significantly impaired patients. The specific location for the lung biopsy should be discussed ahead of time with the surgeon. It is best to biopsy two or three locations in the lung and avoid areas of the lung that appear to exhibit end-stage honeycombing on CT scan because this is a nonspecific pathologic finding. It is better to perform a biopsy on those areas that seem to be involved with ground glass opacities or even those areas that appear normal on the high-resolution CT scan because these areas may give the most diagnostic information to the pathologist.

## SPECIFIC INTERSTITIAL LUNG DISEASE ENTITIES

### Idiopathic Pulmonary Fibrosis

IPF is a specific disease entity that is characterized by progressive fibrosis of the lung parenchyma. The incidence of IPF is approximately 5 to 25 per 100,000, and its onset is usually between the ages of 40 and 70 years. Patients typically present with insidious, progressive dyspnea on exertion and cough. Physical examination reveals bilateral "Velcro" rales and, in advanced disease, clubbing of the digits. The chest radiograph typically shows reduced lung volumes and reticulonodular infiltrates, predominantly in a peripheral and basilar distribution. Pulmonary function testing demonstrates restrictive pulmonary physiology with decreased diffusing capacity for carbon monoxide. The histopathologic finding is termed *usual interstitial pneumonitis* (UIP).

No treatment has been proven to prolong survival in IPF, and a minority of patients demonstrate a physiologic or subjective improvement with treatment. It is unclear to what extent treatment may help to slow the progressive scarring, but it is usually with this intention that treatment is initiated. The most commonly used initial treatment is corticosteroids, begun at high doses (e.g., prednisone at

0.5 mg/kg daily). Unfortunately, few patients demonstrate an objective or subjective response to treatment with prednisone, and many patients develop significant symptoms. Cytotoxic agents, such as cyclophosphamide or azathioprine, are generally considered second-line choices and are used when patients may be suspected to benefit from prolonged immunosuppression. Antifibrotic agents, such as colchicine or D-penicillamine, have been tried but represent minimal benefit if any. Although treatment has not been proven to prolong survival, it has been observed that those patients who respond to therapy (with physiologic improvement) tend to live longer than nonresponders. Regardless of treatment, IPF is a progressive disease with an approximate survival of 2 to 5 years postdiagnosis.

Experimental therapies are emerging for IPF, but none has been proven as yet to attenuate the progressive decline in lung function or improve survival.

## Sarcoidosis

Sarcoidosis is a multisystem granulomatous disorder of unknown etiology. It commonly presents as an asymptomatic chest radiograph finding. Serum angiotensin-converting enzyme levels may be elevated, but this test lacks sufficient sensitivity and specificity to be used as a diagnostic test. Angiotensin-converting enzyme levels may be helpful in certain cases, particularly in following response to treatment. Transbronchial biopsy is diagnostic in 85% to 90% of patients with parenchymal abnormalities (80% if only hilar adenopathy is present). Chronic beryllium disease can mimic sarcoidosis clinically and pathologically and is excluded by history or lymphocyte proliferation tests when necessary. Given the side effects of corticosteroids, the treatment of asymptomatic patients is usually unwarranted. The treatment of sarcoidosis with corticosteroids is indicated for patients with progressive pulmonary function test abnormalities, hypercalcemia, or significant extrathoracic involvement (e.g., eye, central nervous system, or cardiac). Treatment also may be considered in patients with significant symptoms that are clearly attributable to the disease. When necessary, steroid-sparing agents are used (methotrexate, chloroquine, or pentoxifylline).

The radiographic stages of sarcoidosis are:

- Stage 0—normal chest radiograph
- Stage 1—hilar lymphadenopathy
- Stage 2—hilar lymphadenopathy and parenchymal infiltrate
- Stage 3—parenchymal infiltrates without adenopathy

Common sites of sarcoidosis involvement include:

- Hilar lymph nodes
- Pulmonary parenchyma
- Skin (erythema nodosum, lupus pernio)
- Ocular system
- Cardiac system (arrhythmias, dilated cardiomyopathy)
- Central nervous system (facial nerve palsy, cranial mass, seizures)
- Hepatic granulomas often present, usually not end-stage liver disease
- Bone
- Parotid or lacrimal glands
- Kidney (renal impairment associated with hypercalcemia)

## Asbestosis

*Asbestos-related lung disease* is a term used to encompass all the pulmonary complications of asbestos exposure, including pleural processes and rounded atelectasis, in addition to interstitial disease. This is in contrast to the term *asbestosis*, which should be reserved for patients with true pulmonary parenchymal fibrosis (which may or may not occur along with other asbestos-related changes). The diagnostic criteria for asbestosis are:

- Dyspnea
- Persistent crackles on examination
- Restrictive lung disease on pulmonary function testing
- Characteristic chest radiographic abnormalities
- Sufficient asbestos exposure

No effective therapy exists for progressive asbestosis. Steroids are not recommended, and if the patient is too old for lung transplantation, as is typical given the 30-year lead-time, symptom relief through the use of oxygen is the only therapy.

Asbestos exposure alone increases the risk of lung cancer only minimally (1.5 to 3.0 times). Asbestos exposure *and* cigarette smoking, however, act synergistically to greatly increase the risk of cancer.

Asbestos exposure also may result in benign asbestos pleural effusions (BAPE) or an entity known as *rounded atelectasis*. BAPE may be asymptomatic or may be associated with acute chest pain, fever, and dyspnea. Generally, a shorter lag time exists between the initial asbestos exposure and the development of BAPE (<15 years) than is seen with other manifestations of asbestos exposure. The effusions are characteristically exudative and are often bloody. In a patient with a history of asbestos exposure and a bloody pleural effusion, the major differential diagnostic concern is that of malignant pleural effusion, particularly associated with mesothelioma, another asbestos-related disease. The clinical course of BAPE is that of spontaneous resolution, often with recurrences, and treatment is drainage to reduce for symptoms. Rounded atelectasis typically presents as a pleural-based parenchymal mass that may be mistaken for carcinoma. The characteristic CT features, however, such as evidence of local volume loss, pleural thickening, and the "comet tail" appearance of bronchi and vessels curving into the lesion may be used to help distinguish rounded atelectasis from carcinoma.

## Silicosis

Silicosis is a lung disease attributed to the inhalation of silicon dioxide or silica. The diagnosis is usually based on a characteristic chest radiograph, in patients with a history of exposure. Those in the following occupations are most frequently affected:

- Mining
- Tunneling
- Quarrying
- Foundry work
- Sandblasting
- Ceramic work
- Stonework

Silicosis may be divided into three distinguishable entities: acute silicosis, accelerated silicosis, and chronic silicosis. These are differentiated by presentation and have important prognostic consequences.

Acute silicosis occurs in subjects with high-level fine dust exposure over days to months. The chest radiograph shows air space disease, which may progress to adult respiratory distress syndrome. The histopathology resembles pulmonary alveolar proteinosis.

Accelerated silicosis occurs after 5 to 15 years of dust exposure. The chest radiograph shows upper zone reticulonodular infiltrates. Pulmonary function impairment may be present and may progress to respiratory failure. The histopathology shows nodules with interstitial fibrosis.

Chronic silicosis results after chronic, lower level exposure occurring over decades. Pulmonary function abnormalities may or may not be present and may not progress. Pathology shows silicotic nodules in upper lobes and hila.

Complicated silicosis, sometimes referred to as *progressive massive fibrosis*, may occur with the consolidation of silicotic nodules into upper lobe masses, which progress despite the cessation of exposure. Mycobacterial superinfection may occur in all three types of silicosis, may be difficult to treat, and may occur with either tuberculosis or atypical mycobacteria. Underlying rheumatoid arthritis may increase the risk of developing silicosis in exposed individuals; scleroderma is associated with silica exposure. It is unclear whether silicosis is a risk factor for lung cancer.

## Iatrogenic Interstitial Lung Disease

Myriad offending agents exist for iatrogenic ILD, some well established, some only in case reports. Drug-induced ILD may be acute, subacute, or chronic. Multiple histologic patterns that have been attributed to drug exposure include the following:

- Lymphoplasmacytic pneumonitis
- Eosinophilic infiltration
- Granulomatous inflammation
- Pulmonary alveolar proteinosis-like lesion
- Bronchiolocentric or vascular inflammation

The diagnosis is based on suspicion and is often difficult to prove. The following sections describe some of the more common drugs that may induce ILD.

### Methotrexate

Lung injury may develop at any time while on methotrexate therapy. The histopathology is that of interstitial pneumonitis. Granulomas, an uncommon finding in drug-induced lung disease, may be present. Occasionally, peripheral eosinophilia and hilar lymphadenopathy may occur. The ILD is usually reversible upon discontinuation of the drug, with or without corticosteroids. Interestingly, the ILD does not always recur if methotrexate is reinstituted.

### Bleomycin

Bleomycin lung injury is probably the most common chemotherapy-related pulmonary toxicity. Risk factors for the development of lung injury include age older than 70 years, more than 450 U total dose, prior thoracic radiation therapy, and subsequent exposure to high fractional inspired oxygen. The chest radiograph usually shows mixed interstitial and alveolar infiltrates. Parenchymal nodules on the chest radiograph may falsely suggest metastatic disease. Once fibrosis is established, there is no treatment.

### Radiation Pneumonitis

Radiation pneumonitis may be divided into acute and chronic varieties. Acute radiation pneumonitis occurs 1 to 6 months after radiation therapy. Presenting symptoms are cough, dyspnea, fever, and chest pain. Treatment usually employs corticosteroids, if the symptoms or impairment is significant. Interestingly, the radiographic abnormalities can occur outside the radiation port. Chronic radiation pneumonitis is characterized by progressive parenchymal fibrosis in areas of prior radiation. No correlation exists with the presence or severity of prior acute injury. Symptoms depend on the extent of lung involved and may include cough and dyspnea. Treatment with corticosteroids is often attempted when symptoms are significant, although corticosteroids are of uncertain benefit.

### Nitrofurantoin

Two types of nitrofurantoin pulmonary toxicity exist: acute and chronic. The acute syndrome occurs hours to days after initiation of the medication. It is characterized by fever, dyspnea, cough, and leukocytosis, with or without eosinophilia. Chest radiography shows mixed interstitial and alveolar markings with or without pleural effusion. Treatment consists of discontinuing the drug. Chronic toxicity is unrelated to the acute syndrome. The symptoms and chest radiograph may mimic IPF. Treatment also consists of discontinuing the drug. Corticosteroids may be useful.

### Amiodarone

Amiodarone toxicity most commonly presents with insidious cough and dyspnea. Occasionally, the presentation may be more acute, suggesting bacterial pneumonia. Histologic features include foamy alveolar macrophages and lamellar cellular inclusions. Toxicity usually occurs with doses of more than 400 mg every day for more than 1 month, although cases have been reported in patients taking only 200 mg every day. The findings on chest radiography are variable, with mixed interstitial and alveolar infiltrates that may be focal or diffuse. Chest CT scan may show infiltrates that have a higher attenuation than soft tissue, a finding that relates to the iodine content of the compound. Treatment consists of discontinuing the drug, with or without the addition of corticosteroids.

# CONNECTIVE TISSUE DISEASE–ASSOCIATED INTERSTITIAL LUNG DISEASE

ILD may be a manifestation of various connective tissue diseases. Some of the more common entities and their characteristic presentations are discussed in the following sections.

## Interstitial Lung Disease Associated with Rheumatoid Arthritis

Although rheumatoid arthritis is more common in women, the associated ILD is more common in men with rheumatoid arthritis. Joint involvement may limit the patient's activity; therefore, more severe lung disease may be present by the time the symptoms of lung disease become apparent. Most commonly, the ILD develops in patients with established rheumatoid arthritis, but lung disease may occasionally predate joint symptoms. The severity of the lung disease is not correlated with severity of joint symptoms. A surgical biopsy may reveal any of several pathologic findings, with UIP being the most common. Bronchiolitis also may be seen. Treatment is with steroids and steroid-sparing agents.

## Interstitial Lung Disease Associated with Lupus

Patients with SLE may develop an associated acute lupus pneumonitis or a chronic, progressive ILD. The acute pneumonitis is characterized by acute dyspnea, cough, and fever. In up to one-half of patients, the acute pneumonitis may be the presenting manifestation of lupus. Acute lupus pneumonitis may be recurrent. The chronic ILD is much less common. It is characterized by slowly progressive dyspnea and cough and diffuse reticulonodular infiltrates on chest radiography. The histopathologic finding is UIP.

## Interstitial Lung Disease Associated with Scleroderma

Patients with scleroderma may develop ILD, pulmonary hypertension, or both. The incidence of ILD appears to be fairly high, based on autopsy studies, and all patients should be screened. A poor correlation exists between the severity of the pulmonary and cutaneous manifestations.

## Interstitial Lung Disease Associated with Polymyositis and Dermatomyositis

No correlation exists between the severity of the ILD and the muscle disease. A surgical lung biopsy may reveal any of several histopathologies, including bronchiolitis obliterans with organizing pneumonia, UIP, and diffuse alveolar damage. The presence of Jo-1 antibody may identify a subset of polymyositis and dermatomyositis patients with ILD.

## Interstitial Lung Disease Associated with Sjögren's Syndrome

The pathology of ILD related to Sjögren's syndrome often involves lymphocytes (lymphocytic interstitial pneumonitis, pseudolymphoma, or lymphoma). Other pathologic findings include UIP, bronchiolitis obliterans with organizing pneumonia, and constrictive bronchiolitis. Airway disease due to proximal airway drying resulting in chronic cough and mucous plugs is also common.

# TREATMENT OF INTERSTITIAL LUNG DISEASE

The treatment of patients with ILD depends on the specific disease entity, as described previously. Many of these diseases, particularly the most common entities such as IPF and connective tissue disease–associated ILD, are characterized by progressive inflammation and fibrosis. For this reason, anti-inflammatory agents are commonly used. The most frequently used agent is prednisone or another corticosteroid preparation. In general, fairly high doses (e.g., 0.5 to 1.0 mg/kg per day) are used. In certain instances, such as in patients with contraindications to the use of steroids or when disease progression occurs despite the use of prednisone, cytotoxic agents often are used. Such agents would include cyclophosphamide or azathioprine. Some of the ILDs are not thought to respond to anti-inflammatories and have unique treatments. Examples of these include lymphangioleiomyomatosis, which usually is treated with hormonal manipulation (such as medroxyprogesterone), or pulmonary alveolar lipoproteinosis, which is treated with whole lung lavage.

Other general treatment measures usually include supplemental oxygen therapy, physical and occupational therapy, and the removal of the patient from any etiologic exposure that can be identified. Lung transplantation is an option for patients who have end-stage ILD without significant comorbidities.

## PROGNOSIS OF INTERSTITIAL LUNG DISEASE

As with therapy, the prognosis of ILD depends greatly on the specific disease entity. Many of these diseases are characterized by a slowly progressive loss of lung function over months to years. The pace of the decline may be slowed by treatment, but for many diseases, progression occurs despite treatment. For example, although some patients with IPF may seem to respond to therapy with subjective or objective improvements, the disease is almost uniformly fatal, with death occurring after a mean interval of 3 to 5 years after diagnosis. Likewise, ILD associated with connective tissue disease tends to have a poor prognosis. The clinical course of patients with chronic hypersensitivity pneumonitis is more variable. In general, the disease is more responsive to steroids acutely, and the disease may stabilize, especially if the patient is removed from the exposure.

The ILDs are a broad category of lung diseases. They tend to share common clinical, radiographic, and physiologic features, but have many unique characteristics. Arriving at a specific diagnosis may be challenging and requires careful evaluation and open lung biopsy. Treatment often entails anti-inflammatory therapy using corticosteroids or cytotoxic agents.

## REVIEW EXERCISES

### QUESTIONS

**1.** Which of the following chest radiographic findings is inconsistent with the diagnosis of asbestosis?
a) Presence of pleural plaques
b) Presence of pleural effusion
c) Reticulonodular infiltrates
d) Upper-lobe predominance
e) Reduced lung volumes

**2.** Which one of the following statements regarding IPF is incorrect?
a) IPF most commonly affects patients in the sixth and seventh decades of life.
b) There is a familial variety of IPF.
c) The histology of IPF is indistinguishable from that seen in rheumatoid arthritis.
d) Clubbing is a late finding in IPF.
e) Corticosteroids are the only proven effective therapy for IPF.

**3.** Which one of the following statements is incorrect?
a) Obtaining an occupational history is imperative before diagnosing a patient with sarcoidosis.

b) An elevated serum angiotensin-converting enzyme level is not diagnostic.
c) Sarcoidosis can involve any organ system.
d) The presence of sarcoid granulomas in the pulmonary parenchyma is an indication for treatment.
e) The most common presentation is an asymptomatic chest radiograph abnormality.

**4.** Which one of the following statements is incorrect?
a) BAPE is one of the earliest manifestations of asbestos exposure.
b) Pleural thickening in a patient with asbestos exposure indicates asbestosis.
c) Pleural plaques almost never result in symptoms or physiologic impairment.
d) Mesothelioma may develop in patients with brief, low-level exposure to asbestos.
e) Rounded atelectasis is a benign manifestation of asbestos exposure that can be mistaken for a malignancy.

**5.** Which one of the following statements is incorrect?
a) Three patterns of silicosis exist: acute, accelerated, and chronic (classic).
b) Silicosis shows a predominantly lower zone distribution on the chest radiograph.
c) Progressive massive fibrosis is a complication of silicosis.
d) An increased incidence of tuberculosis occurs in patients with silicosis.
e) An increased incidence of rheumatoid arthritis and scleroderma occurs in patients with silicosis.

**6.** Which one of the following statements is incorrect?
a) Methotrexate pulmonary toxicity may not recur on reinitiation of the drug.
b) Using supplemental oxygen after administration can prevent bleomycin pulmonary toxicity.
c) Radiation pneumonitis may mimic infectious pneumonia (cough, fever, chest pain, dyspnea).
d) Nitrofurantoin pulmonary toxicity may mimic IPF.
e) Pneumonitis caused by amiodarone may appear denser than surrounding soft tissue on a CT scan.

**7.** Which one of the following statements is incorrect?
a) ILD is more common in men with rheumatoid arthritis than in women with rheumatoid arthritis.
b) Fifty percent of patients presenting with acute lupus pneumonitis have had no history of lupus.
c) A good correlation exists between the severity of the cutaneous and pulmonary manifestations of scleroderma.
d) Jo-1 antibody is associated with the presence of ILD in patients with polymyositis.
e) ILD associated with Sjögren's syndrome often involves lymphocytic infiltration.

## ANSWERS

### 1. d.

Asbestosis is characterized by the presence of reticulonodular infiltrates in a lower zone distribution. As the disease progresses, volume loss often occurs in the lower lobes. The presence of pleural disease, although not sufficient to make the diagnosis of true asbestosis, may be seen in patients with asbestos exposure and is therefore not inconsistent with the diagnosis of asbestosis.

### 2. e.

Answers a through d are all correct. This question is meant to emphasize the fact that although corticosteroid treatment may result in subjective or objective improvements, it has not been proven to improve survival.

### 3. d.

Making a histologic diagnosis of sarcoidosis is not considered sufficient reason to treat with steroids. Commonly accepted indications for treatment include significant symptoms or progressive loss of lung function. The involvement of critical extrapulmonary organs also may prompt treatment.

### 4. b.

This question is meant to emphasize the fact that the term *asbestosis* should be reserved for patients with evidence of pulmonary parenchymal scarring. Pleural disease does not merit the diagnosis of asbestosis.

### 5. b.

The distribution of abnormalities on the chest radiograph may be helpful in narrowing the differential diagnosis. Silicosis is associated with radiographic changes in the upper lobes.

### 6. b.

The administration of supplemental oxygen is a risk factor for the development of bleomycin pulmonary toxicity.

### 7. c.

As with many of the connective tissue disease–associated ILDs, no real correlation exists between the severity of the ILD and the extrapulmonary manifestations.

# Pleural Diseases

*Atul C. Mehta    Raed A. Dweik*

A pleural effusion is among the most frequently encountered problems in chest medicine. One estimate places the annual incidence of pleural effusion in the United States at approximately 1 million persons.

An accumulation of pleural fluid is not a specific disease, but rather a reflection of underlying pathology. Pleural effusion may result from many different pulmonary or systemic diseases. The task facing the contemporary clinician is little different from that outlined by Osler in 1892: In the diagnosis of pleuritic effusion, the first question is, Does a fluid exudate exist? The second question is, What is its nature?

## DIAGNOSIS OF PLEURAL EFFUSION

Clinical symptoms (dyspnea or pleuritic pain) or signs (diminished breath sounds and dullness to percussion) may suggest the presence of a pleural effusion. Chest radiographic techniques are important in confirming the presence of pleural effusion and in detecting associated abnormalities that may provide important information regarding etiology (Fig. 39.1).

## Imaging Studies

### Conventional Chest Radiography

The standard posteroanterior and lateral chest radiographs remain the most important techniques for the initial diagnosis of pleural effusion (Fig. 39.1). The distribution of free pleural fluid around the normal lung is influenced primarily by gravity and lung elastic recoil and, to a lesser extent, by *capillary attraction* between the pleural surfaces, which creates the meniscus-shaped upper border. Fluid first gravitates to the inferior portion of the hemithorax and lies between the hemidiaphragm and the inferior surface of the lung. Small fluid collections are best appreciated by an inspection of the posterior costophrenic angle on the lateral radiograph. Larger fluid collections completely obscure the hemidiaphragm on both projections

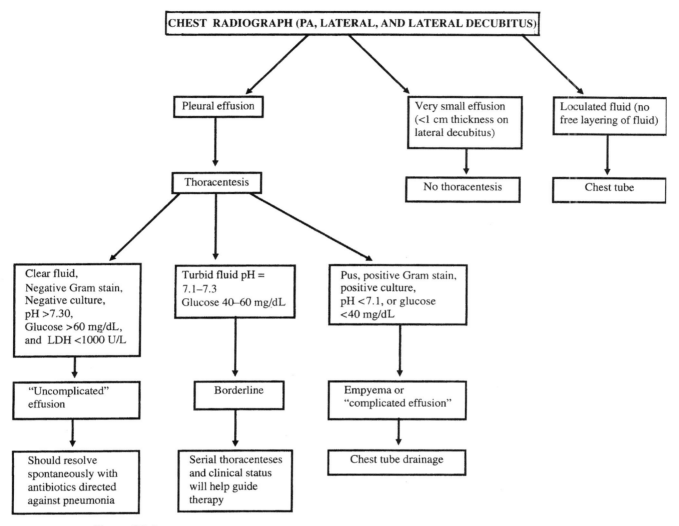

**Figure 39.1** Approach to parapneumonic effusion. LDH, lactate dehydrogenase; PA, posteroanterior.

and assume a typical appearance. Most fluid collects around the lateral, anterior, and posterior thoracic wall; less fluid collects along the mediastinal surface of the lung because there is relatively less elastic recoil in this region (the lung is fixed at the hilum and pulmonary ligament).

Occasionally, relatively large pleural effusions may remain confined to the infrapulmonary location (*subpulmonic effusion*). Such effusions may give the radiographic appearance of elevation of the hemidiaphragm. When a subpulmonic effusion occurs on the left side, its presence is suggested by the separation of the *pseudohemidiaphragm* from the gastric bubble. A lateral decubitus roentgenogram is extremely valuable in the detection of subpulmonic effusions.

Lateral decubitus films are also useful in distinguishing *free* pleural fluid from the *loculated* pleural effusion (fluid confined by fibrous pleural adhesions). Pleural effusions might be overlooked on supine or semierect roentgenograms (e.g., portable radiograph obtained in the intensive care unit) because the only abnormality may be a vague increase in radiographic density over the hemithorax.

The lateral decubitus roentgenogram can detect effusions as small as 15 mL. The standard posteroanterior and lateral roentgenogram can detect roughly 250 mL. The "moderate" pleural effusion (1,000 mL) extends upward approximately one-third or one-half of the hemithorax, typically obscuring the hemidiaphragm.

## Other Radiographic Techniques
### Ultrasound
Thoracic ultrasound is a rapid and safe technique for defining and localizing pleural fluid. A major advantage over conventional roentgenograms is the ability of ultrasound to differentiate the solid components (e.g., tumor or fibrous peel) from the liquid components of a pleural process. Ultrasound is also valuable in detecting subpulmonic or subphrenic pathology and differentiating these abnormalities (i.e., by evaluating the relationship of

radiographic densities to the diaphragm). A major use of ultrasound is to guide thoracentesis needles into small or loculated pleural effusions, thereby increasing the yield and safety of thoracentesis. Portable ultrasound units can be brought to the bedside of extremely ill patients.

### Computed Tomography

Computed tomographic (CT) examination of the thorax is a major advance in the evaluation of pleural disease. The cross-sectional tomographic image allows the evaluation of complex situations in which the anatomy cannot be fully assessed by plain films or ultrasound. For instance, CT scans are helpful in distinguishing empyema from lung abscess, in detecting pleural masses (e.g., mesothelioma, plaques), and in outlining loculated fluid collections.

## Laboratory Studies

### Transudate versus Exudate

Although the history, physical examination, and radiographic studies may provide important clues to the etiology of a pleural effusion, almost all cases should be evaluated through a diagnostic thoracentesis. After obtaining fluid, the first diagnostic step is to classify the effusion as a transudate or an exudate by using the protein and lactate dehydrogenase (LDH) values of serum and pleural fluid (Table 39.1). As described by Light et al., this method is 99% accurate (1). Previous methods, which used cut-off values for pleural fluid total protein (3.0 g/100 mL) or specific gravity (1.016), are considerably less accurate (60% to 90%).

In more recent years, newer criteria have been explored in diagnosing exudative effusions. As outlined in Table 39.2, the more recent criteria use cholesterol levels in the pleural fluid and have a lower threshold for LDH. Although the newer criteria offer no diagnostic improvement over Light's criteria, they offer the distinct advantage that phlebotomy is not required (2). These criteria rely on cholesterol levels and on the absolute values of LDH and protein in the pleural fluid rather than on their ratios to the serum values. Furthermore, cholesterol levels in the pleural fluid may be helpful in diuretic-treated congestive heart failure (CHF), a transudate that can be inaccurately classified as an exudate by the traditional Light's criteria due to high protein levels (3 to 4 g/dL).

**TABLE 39.1**

**TRANSUDATE AND EXUDATE CLASSIFICATION**

| | Fluid/ Serum Protein | | Fluid/ Serum LDH | | Fluid LDH |
|---|---|---|---|---|---|
| Transudate | <0.5 | and | <0.6 | and | <200 |
| Exudate | ≥0.5 | or | ≥0.6 | or | ≥200 |

LDH, lactate dehydrogenase.

**TABLE 39.2**

**NEWER CRITERIA FOR CLASSIFICATION OF EXUDATES AND TRANSUDATES**

| | LDH | Cholesterol | Protein |
|---|---|---|---|
| Transudate | <45%* | <45 mg/dL | <2.9 g/dL |
| Exudate | >45%* | >45 mg/dL | >2.9 g/dL |

* Of serum upper limit of normal.

### Transudates

Transudates are formed secondary to elevations in hydrostatic pressure or reductions in colloid osmotic pressure within the systemic or pulmonary circulation. Causes of transudates include:

- Congestive heart failure (CHF)
- Nephrotic syndrome
- Cirrhosis with ascites
- Peritoneal dialysis
- Atelectasis (early)
- Urinothorax

Pleuropulmonary disease rarely exists with transudates, which is why the finding is so important. Further analysis of the pleural fluid, or a pleural biopsy, is unlikely to provide positive information and probably can be avoided. A study by Peterman and Speicher (3) supports this approach: 83 transudates were evaluated, with 725 further tests. Only nine of these follow-up test results were positive, and seven gave false-positive results.

Nonetheless, it is important to maintain some wariness before dismissing a transudative effusion. The clinician must remain alert to the few instances in which a transudate may be associated with underlying lung disease. Early atelectasis may be associated with a transudate. Also, it is well documented, but often unappreciated, that some patients with malignant pleural effusions have transudative fluids (4). Most of these patients have concomitant CHF, nephrotic syndrome, or the early stage of mediastinal lymph node involvement with malignancy.

### Exudate

Exudative effusions signal the presence of disease involving the lungs or pleura. The following are important or common causes of exudates:

- Malignancy
- Bacterial and fungal infection
- Collagen vascular disease
- Parapneumonic effusion (pleural reaction to pneumonia)
- Pulmonary embolus
- Chylothorax (thoracic duct disruption)
- Uremia
- Asbestos exposure

- Thoracic lymphatic obstruction (e.g., lymphoma, radiation)
- Pancreatitis
- Empyema
- Tuberculosis (TB)
- Viral infections
- Yellow-nail syndrome
- Postcardiotomy syndrome
- Subdiaphragmatic abscess
- Esophageal rupture
- Atelectasis (chronic)
- Idiopathic causes

Exudative effusions should not be ignored, and attempts to establish the diagnosis should be undertaken. Additional studies of pleural fluid, such as cell count and differential, cytology, Gram's stain, cultures, and glucose, amylase, pH, antinuclear antibodies (ANA), and complement levels, may help to establish the etiology. Pleural biopsy sometimes may help to establish the cause of an exudative effusion. Biopsy specimens should be examined histologically (tumor, granuloma) and sent for culture (TB, fungal).

### Specific Tests of Pleural Fluid
#### Glucose
The pleural fluid glucose level of transudates and most exudates is similar to that of serum. There are few causes of a very low pleural fluid glucose (<25 mg/100 mL). Such a finding is seen with rheumatoid disease, TB, empyema, and tumors with extensive pleural involvement. The latter two conditions are usually obvious by the clinical setting or other pleural fluid findings; therefore, a low glucose level may be an important first clue to TB or rheumatoid disease. It has been reported that an intravenous glucose infusion raises the pleural fluid glucose level in TB but not in rheumatoid disease.

#### Amylase
A high pleural fluid amylase usually indicates pancreatitis or esophageal rupture. Isoenzymes can be used to distinguish pancreatic amylase from salivary gland amylase; however, the clinical setting usually separates these two entities. Also, the fluid pH is low with esophageal rupture and normal in pancreatitis. Approximately 10% of malignant effusions may have elevations of amylase.

#### pH
The pH of the small amount of pleural fluid present in normal persons is approximately 7.64. A low pleural fluid pH (i.e., <7.30) may be seen with infected parapneumonic effusions, frank empyema, malignancy, collagen vascular disease, TB, esophageal rupture, and urinothorax (the only cause of a low pH transudative effusion). Effusions from other causes almost always have a pH greater than 7.30. It is essential that pleural fluid for pH analysis be aspirated anaerobically and transported on ice. A falsely high pH

results if the fluid is exposed to room air, and a falsely low pH results if the fluid is not kept on ice. The pH is stable for 1 to 2 hours at 0°C. The major use of pleural fluid pH is in the management of parapneumonic effusions, as popularized by R. W. Light (see Parapneumonic Effusions, later in this chapter); however, the pH may provide no independent information in this regard beyond that which can be learned by measuring pleural fluid glucose (5).

## Diagnostic Aspects of Certain Exudative Effusions

### Collagen Vascular Disease
Systemic lupus erythematosus (SLE) and rheumatoid disease are important causes of pleural effusion. Up to 75% of SLE patients have pleural involvement during the course of their disease. Frequently, the effusion is the only radiographic abnormality in these patients. Lupus effusions are characteristically small to moderate in size but are associated with significant pleuritic pain (pleurisy). Pleuritis may be an important first manifestation of SLE; in approximately 6% of patients, pleural effusion is an isolated first sign, and in an additional 30% of patients, only minor antecedent symptoms are present.

The pleural fluid ANA titer may be helpful in separating SLE effusions from effusions caused by other etiologies, even in patients with known SLE. A pleural fluid ANA ratio greater than 1:160 or a pleural fluid to serum ANA ratio greater than 1.0 indicates lupus pleuritis (6). Although these criteria appear to be highly specific, they are not highly sensitive (some patients with SLE pleuritis will not fulfill them). The presence of LE cells in pleural effusions is highly specific for SLE or drug-induced lupus, and this finding has been reported to precede the appearance of LE cells or ANA in serum by several months in some patients; however, the finding of LE cells may not have a high sensitivity. The presence of a speckled staining pattern usually suggests an alternate diagnosis.

Pleural effusions occur in approximately 5% of patients with rheumatoid arthritis. Unlike SLE, the effusions are often asymptomatic, may be quite large, and often persist for many months without change. Interestingly, rheumatoid effusions are more common in men, despite the fact that rheumatoid disease is more common in women. Usually, effusions occur in patients with high serum rheumatoid factor (RF) titers and rheumatoid nodules. Pleural fluid RF titers are not helpful because they may be elevated in pneumonia, TB, malignancy, and SLE. "Silent empyema" is a risk, especially in steroid-treated patients. SLE and rheumatoid effusions may have low complement levels and high levels of immune complexes, but these findings are not completely specific (tumors, empyema).

### Tuberculosis
The most common form of TB effusion is a "hypersensitivity" reaction that occurs in the postprimary phase of the

initial infection. Other evidence of infection is usually lacking. Although these exudates usually resolve spontaneously, approximately 30% of patients develop active disease within 5 years. The diagnosis is difficult and usually requires a pleural biopsy, in which the pleura is examined histologically for granulomas and acid-fast bacilli, and cultured for TB. Pleural-fluid analyses (acid-fast bacilli and culture) are positive in only 20% to 25% of cases; pleural biopsies increase the yield to 55% to 80%.

### Chylothorax

A disruption of the thoracic duct (e.g., by trauma, surgery, tumor) leads to a chylothorax. The "milky" appearance is characteristic, but occasionally a chronic TB or rheumatoid effusion has this appearance (*pseudochylothorax*). A true chylothorax has a high fat content (>400 mg/100 mL), mostly triglycerides. The chylothorax, in contrast, has low fat and high cholesterol levels. A pleural fluid triglyceride level above 110 mg/dL indicates a probable chylothorax, whereas a level below 50 mg/dL essentially rules out chylothorax. In borderline situations (pleural fluid triglyceride level between 50 and 100 mg/dL), lipoprotein electrophoreses of the pleural fluid is helpful; the finding of chylomicrons in the fluid establishes the diagnosis of chylothorax.

### Urinothorax

Urinothorax is a relatively rare disorder in which urine collects in the pleural space because of ipsilateral urinary tract obstruction. The diagnostic triad is transudate, low pH (<7.30), and a pleural fluid to serum creatinine ratio greater than 1.0.

### Malignancy

Pleural fluid cytology is positive in 60% to 90% of patients with effusion secondary to involvement of the pleura by tumor, except for mesothelioma, in which its sensitivity is only 32%. Remember that bronchogenic cancer may cause effusion owing to atelectasis, pneumonia, or lymphatic obstruction, without involving the pleura. Carcinoembryonic antigen may help to differentiate malignant from benign effusions in some cases, but the sensitivity and specificity of this test is not high enough to make it useful in routine evaluation. Mesothelioma appears to be the only cause of an extremely high hyaluronic acid level, although this finding may not be sensitive. In one study, immunocytometry proved helpful in the diagnosis of lymphoma in an idiopathic pleural effusion in which conventional cytologic and histopathologic techniques were nondiagnostic (7).

### Asbestosis

The entity of *benign asbestos effusion* is well recognized, and its natural history is better defined. These effusions are often bloody but are otherwise nonspecific exudates. The peak incidence is approximately 10 to 15 years after the onset of asbestos exposure (somewhat earlier than the other pleural complications of asbestos). Approximately one-third of patients are asymptomatic; the remaining cases may have pleuritic discomfort, mild fever, or dyspnea. The effusions persist for a mean of 4 months and then resolve spontaneously in most patients. A variable amount of pleural fibrosis often results. Approximately one-third of patients may have recurrent effusion or persistent pleural pain. Few cases of mesothelioma have occurred in these patients, and usually only after an interval of several years. Thus, benign asbestos pleurisy does not seem to be an indicator for an increased risk of mesothelioma. The diagnosis of benign asbestos pleurisy is by history of asbestos exposure and exclusion of other causes.

### Amyloidosis

Amyloidosis can be accompanied by pleural effusion in up to 30% of patients. These effusions are usually transudative and probably most often are caused by CHF; however, one report suggests that amyloid deposition can be found on pleural biopsy specimens in a high percentage of these patients, suggesting that pleural biopsy may be a reasonably sensitive technique in the diagnosis of systemic amyloidosis (8). Furthermore, some patients with pleural amyloidosis have otherwise unexplained exudative effusions, raising the possibility that amyloid deposits may play a causative role in pleural fluid formation.

### Acquired Immunodeficiency Syndrome

Pleural effusion in hospitalized acquired immunodeficiency syndrome (AIDS) patients is not uncommon (27%). Bacterial infection (30%), *Pneumocystis carinii* (15%), and TB (8%) are the most common causes. Kaposi's sarcoma and hypoalbuminemia are the most common noninfectious causes.

### Pleural Effusions after Coronary Bypass Grafting

Approximately 175,000 patients undergo coronary artery bypass grafting (CABG) each year in the United States. Approximately 50% of these patients develop small pleural effusions in the immediate postoperative period. Most post-CABG effusions are left-sided and resolve spontaneously without specific therapy; however, approximately 1% of patients have large pleural effusions (occupying >25% of the hemithorax). These large effusions are usually left-sided or, if bilateral, the left side effusion is much larger than the right. In one large study, the following causes were found to contribute to large post-CABG effusions:

- 24% (7/29) CHF
- 7%  (2/29) Constrictive pericarditis
- 3%  (1/29) Pulmonary embolism
- 66% (19/29) No discernible cause
- 42% (8/19) Bloody
- 58% (11/19) Nonbloody

## TABLE 39.3

**DEFINITIVE DIAGNOSES BASED ON PLEURAL FLUID ANALYSIS**

| Diagnosis | Criteria |
|---|---|
| Urinothorax | pH <7, *transudate*, pl/s creat. >1.0 |
| Empyema | Pus, positive Gram's stain or culture |
| Malignancy | Positive cytology |
| Chylothorax | Triglycerides >110 mg/dL, chylomicrons |
| TB, fungal | Positive stains, cultures |
| Hemothorax | Hct. >50% of blood |
| Peritoneal dialysis | Prot. <1g/dL, gluc. 300–400 mg/dL |
| Esophageal rupture | pH <7, high amylase (salivary) |
| Lupus pleuritis | LE cells, pl/s ANA >1.0 |

The bloody pleural effusions post-CABG probably were related to bleeding within the pleural space. These bloody effusions achieved a maximum size within 1 month after CABG, were frequently eosinophilic, had high levels of LDH, and usually resolved after one or two thoracenteses. Nonbloody pleural effusions, on the other hand, reached their maximum size more than 1 month after surgery, were mostly lymphocytic, had lower levels of LDH, and were difficult to manage because of recurrence despite multiple thoracentesis, chest tube drainage, and pleurodesis.

Table 39.3 lists some clinical situations in which the pleural fluid analysis can provide a definitive diagnosis of the underlying etiology, whereas Table 39.4 gives examples of the more common scenario, in which the pleural fluid analysis can provide clues to the etiology rather than a definitive diagnosis.

## TABLE 39.4

**CLUES FROM PLEURAL FLUID ANALYSIS**

| Criteria | Possible Diagnoses |
|---|---|
| Lymphocytosis (>50%) | TB, malignancy |
| Eosinophilia (>10%) | Air, blood, (BAPE), drug-induced |
| | Churg-Strauss, parasitic/fungal, malignancy |
| Glucose <60 (or <50% of serum) | TB, esophageal rupture, malignancy |
| Glucose <30 | Empyema, rheumatoid arthritis |
| High amylase (pl/s >1.0, or higher than UL in serum) | Pancreatitis, pseudocyst, pancreatic cancer (10–30× serum level, pancreatic) |
| | Esophageal rupture (5× serum level, salivary), malignancy, ruptured ectopic pregnancy |

pl, Pleural, s, serum, BAPE, benign asbestos pleural effusion.

## TREATMENT OF PLEURAL EFFUSIONS

### Therapeutic Thoracentesis

When a pleural effusion is large enough to cause symptoms (usually dyspnea) and specific therapy of the underlying etiology is ineffective or too slow, a "therapeutic" thoracentesis is indicated. If fluid reaccumulates and symptoms recur, thoracentesis can be repeated two or three times; however, the repetitive removal of large amounts of fluid over a short period is discouraged because of potential complications from protein loss and fluid shifts. More definitive therapy, such as the instillation of a pleural sclerosing agent, usually is indicated when a symptomatic pleural effusion rapidly recurs after a few attempts at drainage using thoracentesis.

In general, no more than 1,000 to 1,500 mL of fluid should be removed at one time. Removal of more fluid risks the development of edema in the underlying lung (*reexpansion pulmonary edema*) or rapid fluid shift from the intravascular space into the pleural space (*post-thoracentesis shock*). Both phenomena appear to be related, in part, to creating excessive negative pleural pressures during thoracentesis. If desired, pleural fluid pressures can be measured directly on a periodic basis during thoracentesis by using an Abrams needle connected to a three-way valve and a manometer. Fluid can be safely withdrawn until a pressure of approximately −20 cm water is reached (measured in the eighth or ninth posterior intercostal space). This technique has allowed up to 4 L of effusion to be withdrawn safely at one time. Because removal of 1.0 to 1.5 L is usually enough to provide at least temporary relief of dyspnea, measuring pleural fluid pressures during thoracentesis is generally unnecessary.

Dyspnea secondary to pleural fluid accumulation probably is related more to intrathoracic volume changes than to chemoreceptor input. Even in instances in which thoracentesis provides relief of dyspnea, a temporary decrease in arterial oxygenation often occurs. The magnitude and duration of hypoxia bear a rough correlation to the amount of fluid removed. Hypoxia may last 12 hours or longer. Thus, if a large amount of fluid is removed, or the patient has a low baseline arterial oxygenation level, supplemental nasal oxygen probably should be given for several hours after a thoracentesis.

### *Transudates*

Pleural effusions secondary to heart failure, ascites, or nephrotic syndrome usually can be managed with appropriate medical therapy, such as diuretics and sodium restriction. Acutely, therapeutic thoracentesis allows time for medical management. Rarely, recurrent symptomatic pleural effusions complicate cirrhosis or nephrosis despite optimal medical therapy; doxycycline sclerosis of the pleural cavity (see Pleural Sclerosis, later in this chapter) usually is successful.

*Exudates*

Parapneumonic Effusions

The management of parapneumonic effusions represents a particular challenge to the clinician. These exudative effusions often accompany bacterial pneumonias, but they usually resolve spontaneously with appropriate antimicrobial therapy of the pneumonia. A minority, probably a subset of those that become infected, progresses to empyema (frank pus in the pleural space) and subsequent loculation and fibrosis of the pleura. Treatment at this late stage may require several tube thoracostomies or even surgical decortication. These complications usually can be prevented by early and complete drainage of the pleural space with a single chest tube; however, the indiscriminate universal application of tube thoracostomy constitutes unnecessary therapy for most patients with parapneumonic effusions. Thus, the task is to intervene with tube thoracostomy selectively, but early enough to be definitive.

All parapneumonic effusions should be evaluated immediately by thoracentesis. An exception may be extremely small parapneumonic effusions (fluid layer seen on lateral decubitus chest film <1 cm thick), which rarely cause complications. The following findings are all indications for complete drainage of the pleural space:

- Presence of *frank pus* (admittedly a loosely defined term)
- Bacteria on Gram's stain
- Evidence of loculation (by chest roentgenography)

Thoracentesis may be adequate for complete pleural space drainage in some instances, but usually tube thoracostomy is required. Conversely, effusions that are sterile and not turbid in appearance do not require aggressive intervention; however, many parapneumonic effusions are "borderline," occupying a position between these extremes.

The use of fluid pH level analysis has been advocated as a means of evaluating these borderline effusions. The literature, however, does not support the use of a single "cut-off" pH value as a predictor. Furthermore, misinterpretation is possible if fluid specimens for pH analysis are not kept anaerobic and on ice. Nevertheless, a low pH (<7.0 to 7.2) usually indicates a fluid with high potential for loculation, whereas a high pH (>7.3) suggests an extremely low risk for complications. In cases that are doubtful, a serial evaluation of the pleural fluid may help to guide therapy. All parameters (e.g., appearance, Gram's stain, white blood cell count, glucose, protein, LDH, pH) should be evaluated on each thoracentesis. In this setting, a declining pH would argue for tube drainage. Pleural loculation can occur rapidly (i.e., within <24 hours) with certain infections; serial evaluation should not be allowed to delay necessary therapy. At times, two or three thoracenteses should be used in the first day. Finally, it is better to err on the side of early tube drainage rather than risk incomplete drainage of an infected parapneumonic effusion. Table 39.5 gives a suggested approach to the classification and management of parapneumonic effusions.

### TABLE 39.5

**SUGGESTED APPROACH TO CLASSIFICATION AND MANAGEMENT OF PARAPNEUMONIC PLEURAL EFFUSION**

| | pH | Glucose | Gram's Stain/ Culture | Management |
|---|---|---|---|---|
| Simple | >7.2 | >40 mg/dL | Negative | Antibiotics |
| Borderline | 7–7.2 | >40 mg/dL | Negative | Serial thoracentesis |
| Complicated | <7 | <40 mg/dL | Negative | Tube thoracostomy |
| Empyema | <7 | <40 mg/dL | Positive | Tube thoracostomy |

## Malignant Effusions

A variety of malignancies can lead to pleural effusion, usually secondary to direct extension or metastases of the tumor to the pleura. Breast and lung cancers are the most frequent, but many others, including pancreas, colon, esophageal, and ovarian cancers, also can involve the pleura. Lymphomas, in contrast, frequently cause pleural effusion without a direct involvement of the pleura, probably through central obstruction of lymphatics.

The first step in controlling malignant effusions is radiation therapy or systemic chemotherapy, if appropriate for the tumor. With lymphomas, the use of mediastinal radiation (1,400 to 2,600 rad) is usually effective, even when the chest roentgenogram shows no evidence of central lymph node involvement. Radiation therapy directed to the pleura usually is not appropriate therapy for malignant effusions because of unavoidable exposure of the lung parenchyma. Chemotherapy for carcinomas is usually not effective in controlling malignant effusions, except with some breast, ovarian, or small cell lung cancers.

Needle aspiration is an important early step to assess whether symptoms are relieved by fluid removal and to determine the rate of fluid reaccumulation. Most malignant effusions recur rapidly within 3 or 4 days. Prolonged drainage by tube thoracostomy may be tried but fails in at least 50% of cases.

### *Pleural Sclerosis*

In patients with uncontrolled and symptomatic malignant effusions, pleural symphysis achieved through the instillation of a "sclerosing" agent is indicated. Pleural sclerosis should be attempted only if the lung expands fully after fluid removal. Agents that can be instilled into the pleural cavity to achieve pleural sclerosis include doxycycline, talc slurry, bleomycin, and quinacrine.

We believe these agents work by producing a chemical serositis that heals through fibrosis, rather than through a direct antitumor effect. This is probably true even for most of the antineoplastic agents that have been used. Regardless of what agent is used, proper technique is essential for success. The pleural cavity should be drained completely of fluid to avoid dilution of the sclerosing substance. More important, the visceral and parietal pleura must be approximated closely, obliterating the pleural space, so that fibrotic healing achieves pleural symphysis and thus prevents the recurrence of the effusion.

The ideal sclerosing agent would be readily available at low cost, have a low morbidity and toxicity, and be highly effective. Doxycycline appears to be the agent of first choice. With proper technique, doxycycline sclerosis is 80% to 90% effective:

1. Evacuate the pleural cavity by tube thoracostomy at low suction (approximately 15 to 20 cm of water).
2. Order a chest radiograph to verify the position of the tube, clearance of pleural fluid, and re-expansion of the lung.
3. Premedicate the patient with a narcotic analgesic 30 to 60 minutes before sclerosis.
4. Instill 15 to 20 mg/kg of doxycycline in 80 mL of saline, combined with 20 mL of 1% lidocaine, into the chest tube.
5. Flush the tube with 20 mL of saline.
6. Clamp the tube (no suction).
7. Place the patient in a prone, supine, right decubitus, left decubitus, and sitting position for 4 to 5 minutes each (20 to 25 minutes). Repeat each position for 30 minutes each (2.5 hours).
8. Unclamp the tube and connect to low suction.
9. Continue until drainage is less than 100 to 150 mL/day (this may take 3 to 5 days).
10. Remove the tube.

Side effects are mild. Approximately one-third of patients have a low-grade febrile response. Chest pain is unpredictable; sometimes it is absent and at other times it is rather severe; however, the pain is self-limited, lasting 30 to 45 minutes. Generally, pain can be prevented by premedication with parenteral narcotics and the concurrent administration of intracavitary lidocaine. Some have advocated giving the intracavitary lidocaine 30 minutes before instilling doxycycline, but this is probably unnecessary. The effectiveness of doxycycline sclerosis is not diminished by peripheral neutropenia because a white-cell inflammatory response is not necessary for its action.

Treatment failures usually are related to an inability to approximate the pleural surfaces during doxycycline administration, which may be owing to *atelectasis* (central bronchial obstruction because of tumor) or to a "trapped lung" encased by either a fibrotic visceral pleura or massive tumor involvement. The last circumstance may be suggested when a malignant effusion has an extremely low pH and glucose.

If doxycycline is contraindicated because of allergy or other reasons, bleomycin appears to be a good choice. Although experience with this agent is limited, instillation

is well tolerated and often effective. Systemic side effects have not been reported.

Talc is quite effective in producing pleural symphysis. Traditionally, this agent has been introduced as a dry powder abrasive (*talc poudrage*) at open thoracotomy or insufflated through a chest tube. Because even the latter approach usually is done with the patient under general anesthesia, use of talc has been limited; however, a bedside technique using the instillation of a talc saline suspension has been advocated. In this method, 10 g of talc United States Pharmacopeia (USP) powder (previously gas sterilized and aerated) is suspended in 250 mL of sterile saline solution. This step can be accomplished using a bulb syringe and sterile plastic cup. The suspension is administered with tube thoracostomy in a manner analogous to doxycycline sclerosis. Because instillation of talc may be painful, narcotic premedication should be given. Talc pleurodesis has rarely been associated with acute pneumonitis and adult respiratory distress syndrome.

### Surgical Therapy

Parietal pleurectomy and, if necessary for a trapped lung, decortication of the visceral pleura are both definitive procedures that give a 100% response rate; however, mortality is high (up to 5% to 10%) and morbidity may be great (air leaks after decortication). Thus, these procedures should be applied selectively. Surgery generally should be limited to cases in which sclerosis has failed or lung expansion is prevented by a thickened pleura. Important considerations before resorting to surgery include:

- Good condition of the underlying lung
- Low tumor burden outside the chest
- Expected long-term survival
- General medical condition good enough for major surgery

When a malignant cause for pleural effusion is discovered at thoracotomy, it is usually appropriate to attempt pleural abrasion, talc poudrage, or pleurectomy at that time.

## Chylothorax

The accumulation of chyle in the pleural space is usually secondary to disruption of the thoracic duct by trauma (surgical or nonsurgical) or by malignancy. A congenital form also exists. Most "idiopathic" adult cases are thought to be caused by unrecognized mild trauma. Chylothorax is differentiated from pseudochylothorax by its high triglyceride and low cholesterol content.

Chylothorax may cause dyspnea; other local complications are rare. Chyle is bacteriostatic, and infections rarely occur. Furthermore, chyle does not seem to be highly fibrogenic. The major problem is the nutritive and immunologic cost of the continuous loss of thoracic duct contents. Chyle is high in protein, electrolytes, fat, fat-soluble vitamins, and lymphocytes. Cell-mediated immunity assessed by skin tests and graft survival decreases at 3 to 6 weeks of continuous drainage. Furthermore, the theoretic problem of a permanent loss of T lymphocytes in adults who have little thymic activity is present. Before modern nutritional and surgical therapy, chylothorax had a 50% mortality.

The flow within the thoracic duct is highly dependent on diet, especially fat intake. Normal lymph flow is approximately 2.5 L daily (1.38 mL/kg per hour); in starvation, it may decrease to 300 to 500 mL. Dietary manipulation that decreases lymph flow rate is important for the healing of thoracic duct lesions and forms the rationale for conservative therapy. Of note, medium chain triglycerides (MCT) are absorbed through the portal venous system, whereas long chain triglycerides are carried by lymph. Thus, lymph flow is greatly reduced if dietary fat is limited to MCT.

### Conservative Therapy

Initially, two or three thoracenteses are done to assess the reaccumulation rate. If leakage continues, tube thoracostomy drainage should be instituted. Concurrently, oral intake should be limited to an MCT diet (e.g., MCT oil). If necessary, lymph flow is reduced further by using venous hyperalimentation and avoiding oral intake. Of course, this is much less convenient and carries a risk of infection and other complications. Chyle itself should not be reinfused intravenously because of the possibility of venous thrombosis or fatal anaphylaxis.

Pleural sclerosis is usually avoided because it may complicate subsequent surgical therapy if this proves necessary. If a patient is not a surgical candidate, pleural sclerosis may be attempted when dietary manipulation fails.

### Surgical Therapy

Surgical therapy consists of ligation of the thoracic duct. Two general approaches are available. The duct can be ligated most easily through a right thoracotomy at the level of T8 to T10, where it usually exists as a single trunk. Alternatively, closure may be attempted directly at the leakage site. Both locating the site (despite the use of dyes to stain the lymph) and sealing the leak may be technically difficult, however. Furthermore, the duct has to be ligated both above and below the leak because of rich anastomotic communications. With either choice, ligation of the thoracic duct has few adverse consequences because lymph reaches the venous system by alternate channels.

### Choice of Therapy

The major difficulty is deciding how long to try conservative therapy before resorting to surgery. There is no easy answer; each case must be individualized. A few generalizations may help. Congenital chylothorax in neonates usually responds well to conservative management. With

chylothorax owing to malignancies, radiation or systemic chemotherapy may halt chyle leakage in up to two-thirds of lymphomas and in one-half of carcinomas; furthermore, unless relatively long-term survival is expected, therapy should remain conservative. Traumatic chylothorax eventually ceases spontaneously in approximately 50% of cases; however, it is difficult to predict this outcome. In trauma and other causes of chylothorax, the rate of chyle loss should help to guide therapy. If chyle loss is low (i.e., <0.25 mL/kg per hour), a longer trial of conservative therapy will be feasible. If chyle loss is dramatic (>2 mL/kg per hour), conservative therapy will likely be less effective and should be abandoned earlier. As a general rule, it is reasonable to try 1 to 4 weeks of conservative therapy before resorting to surgery.

## Effusions of Indeterminate Etiology

The etiology of some pleural effusions remains obscure even after thoracentesis and two or three closed pleural biopsies have been done on separate occasions. A careful general clinical examination, including appropriate laboratory tests (purified protein derivative, ANA, and rheumatoid factor) or radiographs (CT of the thorax), may provide important clues; however, the cause often remains perplexing. At this point, the clinician is faced with a choice of observing the patient or proceeding with thoracoscopy or thoracotomy. A case for taking the conservative approach derives from the fact that many of these effusions (roughly half) resolve spontaneously and no disease is apparent on long-term follow-up, but that leaves the other half, who have carcinoma, mesothelioma, lymphoma, or other serious diseases.

If the patient looks well and has no fever, pain, or weight loss, careful observation may be warranted. If indications of underlying disease are present, an aggressive diagnostic approach is warranted. Some information in the literature supports the general soundness of this approach. It should be noted, finally, that even a negative exploratory thoracotomy does not rule out occult malignancy as a cause for pleural effusion.

## Other Effusions

Moderate- or large-sized hemothorax should be evaluated promptly and completely. Blood in the pleural space may lead to fibrin deposition, thus causing adhesions and a limitation of lung expansion. Furthermore, as a practical point, tube thoracostomy helps evaluate the rate or recurrence of bleeding. Small hemothoraces usually resolve spontaneously without residua.

The treatment of pleural effusions associated with collagen vascular diseases is directed against the underlying disease. Lupus effusions usually are not large enough to cause symptoms; rather, pain from the pleuritis heralds the process. Appropriate analgesics or anti-inflammatory medications are given. Rheumatoid effusions may present with dyspnea and require therapeutic thoracentesis. Clinically "silent" empyemas may occur in rheumatoid patients on corticosteroids and require tube thoracostomy drainage. Effusions owing to pulmonary thromboembolism or pancreatitis require no specific therapy for the effusion itself.

### Asbestosis

Asbestos exposure may lead to benign, often serosanguineous, exudative effusions. The diagnosis is difficult to make and usually must be presumptive based on history and by ruling out other causes. These effusions resolve spontaneously, but often leave behind a thickened pleura. It is not known whether aggressive drainage of the effusion prevents this sequela.

### Tuberculous Effusions

Tuberculous effusions may occur early in the course of the infection, often as part of an otherwise occult process. Such tuberculous pleurisy is usually self-limited, clearing without treatment. Up to one-half of untreated patients, however, subsequently develop active disease elsewhere within 5 years. Thus, antituberculous therapy with an appropriate drug regimen is indicated. Often therapy must be presumptive, pending the results of pleural fluid and biopsy cultures. If the effusion is large and symptomatic, the concurrent use of systemic corticosteroids may have a salutary effect. TB also may involve the pleura by direct spread from active disease of lung, lymph nodes, or bone. Frank tuberculous empyema requires chest tube drainage.

### Pneumothorax

*Pneumothorax*, or an accumulation of air in the pleural space, is seen in association with certain lung diseases (see following list), or it may occur without underlying lung disease (primary pneumothorax). Common causes of secondary pneumothorax include the following:

- Malignancy
- Infection (e.g., TB, cystic fibrosis, *P. carinii* pneumonia)
- Chronic obstructive pulmonary disease and asthma
- Trauma
- Congenital disorders
- Iatrogenic
- Transthoracic needle aspiration
- Subclavian vein puncture
- Thoracentesis
- Transbronchial biopsy
- Pleural biopsy
- Mechanical ventilation
- Aerosolized pentamidine
- Other
- Endometriosis (catamenial pneumothorax)
- Lymphangioleiomyomatosis

Primary spontaneous pneumothorax can occur in otherwise healthy patients with no underlying lung disease. The

incidence of primary spontaneous pneumothorax is 9 cases per 100,000 persons per year with a 6:1 male-to-female ratio. The incidence is higher in smokers. Compared with nonsmokers, the relative risk of pneumothorax in men is seven times higher in light smokers (1 to 12 cigarettes per day), 21 times higher in moderate smokers (13 to 22 cigarettes per day), and 102 times higher in heavy smokers (>22 cigarettes per day). Table 39.6 lists helpful classifications and definitions for pneumothorax based on an American College of Physicians consensus statement.

### Treatment

Simple observation may be all that is needed in patients who have no evidence of tension pneumothorax, are not symptomatic (no dyspnea, no hypoxemia), and in whom the pneumothorax occupies less than 15% of the hemithorax. The site of the leak usually closes, and the air in the pleural space is gradually absorbed. Supplemental oxygen can enhance the rate of pleural air absorption.

### TABLE 39.6
### PNEUMOTHORAX CLASSIFICATIONS AND DEFINITIONS

Spontaneous: no antecedent traumatic or iatrogenic cause
Primary spontaneous: no clinically apparent underlying lung abnormalities
Secondary spontaneous: clinically apparent underlying lung disease
Size: determined by distance from the lung apex to the ipsilateral thoracic cupola at the parietal surface as determined by an upright standard radiograph
☐ Small pneumothorax: <3 cm apex-to-cupola distance
☐ Large pneumothorax: >3 cm apex-to-cupola distance
Patient age groups (yr)
☐ Young, 18–40
☐ Older, >40
Clinical stability
☐ Stable patient: all of the following present—respiratory rate, <24 breaths/min; heart rate, >60 or <120 beats/min; normal blood pressure; room air oxygen saturation, >90%; and patient can speak in whole sentences between breaths
☐ Unstable patient: any patient not fulfilling the definition of stable
Drainage tube sizes
☐ Small, 14 F
☐ Moderate, 16–22 F
☐ Large, 24–36 F
Simple aspiration: insertion of a needle or cannula with removal of pleural air followed by immediate removal of the needle or cannula
Sclerosis (pleurodesis) procedure
☐ Chemical pleurodesis: intrapleural instillation of a sclerosing agent through a chest tube or percutaneous catheter
☐ Open or surgical pleurodesis: performed with a thoracoscope or through a limited or full thoracotomy

Adapted with permission from Colice GL, Curtis A, Deslauriers J, et al. for the American College of Chest Physicians Parapneumonic Effusions Panel. Medical and surgical treatment of parapneumonic effusions: an evidence-based guideline. *Chest* 2000;118:1158–1171.

| **TABLE 39.7** |
|---|
| **MANAGEMENT OF SPONTANEOUS PNEUMOTHORAX** |

Primary spontaneous pneumothorax
- ☐ Stable patients with small pneumothoraces
- ☐ Observe in the emergency department for 3–6 h
- ☐ Discharge home if a repeat radiography excludes progression
- ☐ Follow-up radiograph within 12 h to 2 d to document resolution

Stable patients with large pneumothoraces
Hospitalize in most instances with insertion of a small-bore catheter (14 F) or a 16–22 F chest tube
Catheters or tubes may be attached either to a Heimlich valve or to a water seal device
If the lung fails to re-expand quickly, suction should be applied to a water-seal device
- ☐ Unstable patients with large pneumothoraces
- ☐ Hospitalize with insertion of a chest catheter to re-expand the lung
- ☐ Most patients should be treated with a 16–22 F standard chest tube
- ☐ A 24–28 F standard chest tube may be used if the patient requires positive-pressure ventilation

Secondary spontaneous pneumothorax
- ☐ All should be hospitalized
- ☐ Patients may be observed or treated with a chest tube, depending on the extent of their symptoms and the course of their pneumothorax

Adapted with permission from Colice GL, Curtis A, Deslauriers J, et al. for the American College of Chest Physicians Parapneumonic Effusions Panel. Medical and surgical treatment of parapneumonic effusions: an evidence-based guideline. *Chest* 2000;118:1158–1171.

Although simple aspiration may be sufficient in some patients (especially those with primary pneumothorax), tube thoracostomy is the treatment of choice for most patients with secondary, large, or symptomatic pneumothoraces (Table 39.7). Small-caliber tubes (9 F) can be used for iatrogenic pneumothorax following procedures and for primary spontaneous pneumothorax. Most patients with secondary (other than iatrogenic) or large pneumothoraces require a standard size (28 F) tube thoracostomy for effective treatment.

Patients with recurrent pneumothorax may benefit from pleurodesis. The pneumothorax recurrence rate decreases significantly after pleurodesis compared with the rate for management with chest tube alone (13% versus 36%, respectively). Video-assisted thoracoscopy should be considered in patients who do not respond to these therapies or who have occupations in which the development of pneumothorax may be dangerous (e.g., airplane pilots or deep-sea divers). Because of the association of pneumothorax with smoking, all patients with pneumothorax should be strongly advised to stop smoking.

### Tension Pneumothorax

In tension pneumothorax, the pressure of air in the pleural space exceeds ambient pressure throughout the respiratory cycle. Tension pneumothorax may result in acute respiratory failure, hemodynamic compromise, and cardiopulmonary arrest. If tension pneumothorax is suspected, a large-bore needle should be inserted immediately in the affected side to allow immediate relief of the tension until tube thoracostomy can be performed.

## REVIEW EXERCISES

### QUESTIONS

**1.** A 30-year-old man presents with acute, excruciating, right-flank and lower chest pain, nausea, and vomiting. His past medical history is notable for one episode of hematuria 1 year ago. He has a family history of a twin sister with sarcoid. On examination, the patient is in distress with pain, right flank tenderness, and upper-quadrant guarding. Right dullness and pleural rub is present. His chest radiograph shows a moderate right effusion. A kidney and upper bladder film is not obtainable. An analysis of the pleural fluid reveals an amber fluid, with a pH of 6.9; LDH, 40 IU/dL; protein, 0.5 g/dL; and hemoglobin, +1.

After administration of adequate analgesia, which would be the most appropriate action?
a) Ultrasound of gallbladder and pancreas
b) Ventilation–perfusion scan
c) Closed pleural biopsy
d) Urology consult
e) Upper endoscopy

**2.** A 70-year-old man with a history of insulin-dependent diabetes mellitus, alcohol abuse, severe gastroesophageal reflux disease, emphysema, and benign prostatic hyperplasia requiring an indwelling catheter and frequent courses of intravenous antibiotics presents with high-grade fever, congestion, cough productive of thick, yellow, blood-tinged sputum, and right pleuritic chest pain.

On examination, you are presented with an ill-looking man with right upper lung consolidation and right base dullness. His chest radiograph shows right upper lobe alveolar infiltrate with cavity and moderate right effusion. Laboratory findings show leukocytosis with left shift. His arterial blood gas analysis shows pH, 7.32; $P_{CO_2}$, 52; arterial oxygenation, 80 on 3 L forced inspiratory oxygen.

His pleural fluid is thick, yellow, and purulent; laboratory findings are pH, 7.82; glucose, 30 mg/dL; LDH, 1,050 IU/dL.

What would be the most appropriate immediate action?
a) Urine culture and sensitivity; replace Foley
b) Continuous broad-spectrum positive/negative intravenous antibiotics
c) Thoracic surgery consult for open thoracostomy

d) Tube thoracostomy

e) Stop antacid, order esophagogastroduodenoscopy

**3.** A 60-year-old white man presents with bilateral, vague, nonpleuritic chest pain and mild shortness of breath; no fever, cough, or night sweats. On history taking, 15 months ago, this patient had right effusion that resolved spontaneously; 5 years ago, he had occasional bilateral wrist pain, treated with aspirin. An annual purified protein derivative test was negative 3 months ago. On examination, you find bibasilar dullness and a hard nodule on the nose. His chest radiograph shows bilateral moderate pleural effusion.

The pleural fluid analysis reveals a white blood cell count of 2,000/mm³; polymorphonuclear leukocytes, 90%; pH, 7.05; LDH, 1,000 IU/dL; protein, 4 g/dL; glucose, 5 mg/dL.

Based on the most likely diagnosis, what would be the most appropriate action?

a) Isoniazid, 300 mg; rifampin, 600 mg; ethambutol, 900 mg daily

b) Prednisone, 40 mg daily

c) Bilateral chest tube placement

d) Intravenous ceftazidime and gentamicin

e) Close observation for spontaneous resolution of fluid

**4.** A 30-year-old woman presents with slowly progressing shortness of breath of 6 months duration. Her past medical history includes pneumothoraces, one on either side, 4 weeks apart 1 year ago.

On examination, she has increased dullness in the left base, right basilar crackles, and small ascites. Her chest radiograph shows hyperinflated lungs, vague interstitial changes, and left effusion. A pleural tap reveals milky white fluid, with triglycerides, 200 mg/dL.

The most likely diagnosis is which of the following?

a) Lymphoma

b) Catamenial pneumothorax

c) Gorham's syndrome

d) Lymphangioleiomyomatosis

e) Histiocytosis X

**5.** A 63-year-old man in a wheelchair presents with crippling rheumatoid arthritis. His annual chest radiograph revealed moderate bilateral effusion. No chest pain, cough, or shortness of breath is present

You review his old radiographs and observe bilateral subpulmonic effusions for 5 years. His purified protein derivative test is negative. His pleural fluid is milky white and shiny; the analysis reveals a white blood cell count of 2,000/mm³, 90% L; glucose, 16 mg/dL; LDH, 1,200 IU/dL; triglycerides, 30 mg/dL; cholesterol, 150 mg/dL; large amount of cholesterol crystals.

What would be the most appropriate action?

a) Start MCT diet

b) Lymphangiography

c) Serology for *Wuchereria bancrofti* infestation

d) Bilateral pleuroperitoneal pump

e) Conservative treatment

**6.** A 70-year-old man with a history of CHF, on optimal medication, underwent thoracentesis in the emergency department for large right effusion using a 16-gauge spinal needle (3.5 L of serosanguinous fluid was removed uneventfully). Minutes after the procedure, the patient developed progressive shortness of breath and needed 100% fractional inspired oxygen.

On examination, you observe tachypnea, right-lung wheeze and basilar rales; his blood pressure is 100/70 mm Hg; pulse, 100 beats per minute.

What would be the most appropriate statement regarding the event?

a) Place large-bore chest tube for tension pneumothorax

b) Transfuse 2 U of pack cells for hemothorax

c) Lasix, 60 mg intravenously

d) Intrapleural pressure monitoring could have avoided the event

e) Check creatine phosphokinase and ventilation–perfusion lung scan

**7.** What is the most important mechanism for the relief of dyspnea after thoracentesis?

a) Arterial oxygen pressure

b) Placebo effect

c) Intrathoracic volume

d) Forced expiratory volume, forced vital capacity

e) Static lung compliance

**8–13.** Match each of the following pleural effusions with the appropriate diagnosis:

| Pleural/ Serum Protein Ratio | Pleural/ Serum LDH Ratio | pH | Glucose (mg/dL) | Triglycerides (mg/dL) |
|---|---|---|---|---|
| 8. 0.1 | 0.4 | 6.9 | 10 | 0 |
| 9. 0.6 | 0.7 | 7.4 | 100 | 10 |
| 10. 0.7 | 1.2 | 7.3 | 93 | 335 |
| 11. 0.4 | 0.4 | 7.4 | 88 | 30 |
| 12. 0.7 | 5.1 | 7.2 | 25 | 50 |
| 13. 0.8 | 2.2 | 7.0 | 50 | 15 |

a) Urinothorax

b) Pulmonary embolism

c) Chylothorax

d) CHF

e) Rheumatoid effusion

f) Empyema

**14–18.** Match the following pleural effusions with the appropriate management strategy in a patient with pneumonia:

| | Glucose (mg/dL) | pH | LDH (U/L) | Gram's Stain | Culture |
|---|---|---|---|---|---|
| 14. | 70 | 7.30 | 250 | Negative | Negative |
| 15. | 55 | 7.15 | 1,000 | Negative | Negative |
| 16. | 35 | 6.90 | 1,000 | Negative | Negative |
| 17. | 30 | 7.00 | 1,000 | Positive | Pending |
| 18. | 30 | 7.00 | 1,000 | Negative | Positive |

a) Simple parapneumonic effusion; treat with appropriate antibiotics
b) Borderline parapneumonic effusion; needs serial thoracentesis in addition to antibiotics
c) Complicated parapneumonic effusion; needs tube thoracostomy in addition to antibiotics
d) Empyema; needs tube thoracostomy in addition to antibiotics

19. A 35-year-old man who smoked one pack per day for 20 years was diagnosed with AIDS 4 years ago. He is allergic to sulfa and receives aerosolized pentamidine for *P. carinii* pneumonia prophylaxis. He was doing well until a few days before admission, when he started developing progressive shortness of breath. His respiratory status deteriorated quickly, requiring intubation and mechanical ventilation. The next day, the respiratory therapist called because the patient had developed high airway pressures. This was also associated with a drop in the patient's blood pressure and arterial oxygen saturation. When you examine the patient, you notice decreased air entry on the left side with a deviation of the trachea to the right.
     What should you do next?
a) Order chest radiography.
b) Add 10 cm $H_2O$ of positive end-expiratory pressure.
c) Insert a chest tube in the right lung.
d) Insert a large-bore needle in the second intercostal space on the left.
e) Place the patient on his side with the left side down.

## ANSWERS

**1. d.**
Urinothorax based on transudate with acidic pH.

**2. d.**
Proteus empyema, urea-splitting property leads to ammonia production and an increased pH.

**3. b.**
This is rheumatoid effusion.

**4. d.**
The chylothorax with interstitial changes in a young woman would suggest lymphangioleiomyomatosis.

**5. e.**
This is a pseudochylothorax.

**6. d.**
The patient develops pulmonary edema following drainage of a large volume of a chronic pleural effusion.

**7. c.**

**8. a.**
The only transudate with acidic pH.

**9. b.**
An exudate with a normal pH.

**10. c.**
High triglyceride ($>110$ mg/dL) diagnostic of chylothorax.

**11. d.**
A transudate characteristic of CHF.

**12. e.**
An exudate with low pH and extremely low glucose typical of rheumatoid arthritis.

**13. f.**
Similar to 12, but pH is much lower as is seen in empyema.

**14. a.**

**15. b.**

**16. c.**

**17. d.**

**18. d.**

**19. d.**
The patient has signs of tension pneumothorax on the left.

## REFERENCES

1. Light RW, MacGregor MI, Luchsinger PC, et al. Pleural effusions: the diagnostic separation of transudates and exudates. *Ann Intern Med* 1972;77:507–513.
2. Costa M, Quiroga T, Cruz E. Measurement of pleural fluid cholesterol and lactate dehydrogenase. *Chest* 1995;108:1260–1263.
3. Peterman TA, Speicher CE. Evaluating pleural effusions: a two-stage laboratory approach. *JAMA* 1984;252:1051–1053.
4. Sahn SA. Malignant pleural effusions. *Clin Chest Med* 1985;6: 113–125.
5. Potts DE, Taryle DA, Sahn SA. The glucose-pH relationship in parapneumonic effusions. *Arch Intern Med* 1978;138:1378–1380.
6. Good JT, King TE, Antony VB, et al. Lupus pleuritis: clinical features and pleural fluid characteristics with special reference to pleural fluid antinuclear antibodies. *Chest* 1983;84:714–718.
7. Kavuru MS, Tubbs R, Miller ML, et al. Immunocytometry in the diagnosis of lymphoma in an idiopathic pleural effusion. *Am Rev Respir Dis* 1992;145:209–211.
8. Kavuru MS, Adamo JP, Ahmad M, et al. Amyloidosis and pleural disease. *Chest* 1990;98:20–23.

## SUGGESTED READINGS

### General

Chretien J, Bignon J, Hirsch A, eds. The pleura in health and disease. In: *Lung Biology in Health and Disease.* New York: Marcel Dekker, 1985.

Light RW, ed. Pleural diseases. *Clin Chest Med* 1985;6:1.

Sahn SA. The pleura. *Am Rev Respir Dis* 1988;138:184–234.

### Thoracentesis

Brandstetter RD, Cohen RP. Hypoxemia after thoracentesis: a predictable and treatable condition. *JAMA* 1979;242:1060–1061.

Brown NE, Zamel N, Aberman A. Changes in pulmonary mechanics and gas exchange following thoracentesis. *Chest* 1978;74:540–542.

Estenne M, Yernault J-C, Troyer A. Mechanism of relief of dyspnea after thoracentesis in patients with large pleural effusions. *Am J Med* 1983;74:813–819.

Sprung CL, Loewenherz JW, Baier H, et al. Evidence for increased permeability in reexpansion pulmonary edema. *Am J Med* 1981;71:497–500.

### Diagnostic Aspects

Adelman M, Albelda SM, Gottlieb J, et al. Diagnostic utility of pleural fluid eosinophilia. *Am J Med* 1984;77:915–920.

Good JT, Taryle DA, Maulitz RM, et al. The diagnostic value of pleural fluid pH. *Chest* 1980;78:55–59.

Hammersten JF, Honska WL, Limes BJ. Pleural fluid amylase in pancreatitis and other diseases. *Am Rev Tuberc* 1959;79:606.

Heffner JE. Evaluating diagnostic tests in the pleural space. Differentiating transudates from exudates as a model. *Clin Chest Med* 1998;19:277–293.

Hunder GG, McDuffie FC, Huston KA, et al. Pleural fluid complement, complement conversion, and immune complexes in immunologic and non-immunologic diseases. *J Lab Clin Med* 1977;90:971–980.

Jay SJ. Diagnostic procedures for pleural disease. *Clin Chest Med* 1985;6:33–48.

Klockars M, Pettersson T, Riska H, et al. Pleural fluid lysozyme in human disease. *Arch Intern Med* 1979;139:73–79.

Light RW, MacGregor MI, Ball WC, et al. Diagnostic significance of pleural fluid pH and $P_{CO_2}$. *Chest* 1973;64:591–596.

Pettersson T, Riska H. Diagnostic value of total and differential leukocyte counts in pleural effusions. *Acta Med Scand* 1981;210:129–135.

### Pleural Biopsy

Boutin C, Astoul P. Diagnostic thoracoscopy. *Clin Chest Med* 1998;19:295–309.

Mezies R, Charbonneau M. Thoracoscopy for the diagnosis of pleural disease. *Ann Intern Med* 1991;114:271–276.

Poe RH, Israel RH, Utell MJ, et al. Sensitivity, specificity, and predictive values of closed pleural biopsy. *Arch Intern Med* 1984;144:325–328.

### Radiographic Evaluation

McLoud TC. CT and MR in pleural disease. *Clin Chest Med* 1998;19:261–276.

Pugatch RD, Spirn PW. Radiology of the pleura. *Clin Chest Med* 1985;6:17–32.

Ravin CE. Thoracentesis of loculated pleural effusions using grey scale ultrasonic guidance. *Chest* 1977;61:666–668.

### Parapneumonic Effusions and Empyema

Colice GL, Curtis A, Deslauriers J, et al. for the American College of Chest Physicians Parapneumonic Effusions Panel. Medical and surgical treatment of parapneumonic effusions: an evidence-based guideline. *Chest* 2000;118:1158–1171.

Lew DP, Despont J-P, Perrin LH, et al. Demonstration of a local exhaustion of complement components and of an enzymatic degradation of immunoglobulins in pleural empyema: a possible factor favoring the persistence of local bacterial infections. *Clin Exp Immunol* 1980;42:506–514.

Light RW. Management of parapneumonic effusions. *Arch Intern Med* 1981;141:1339–1341.

Light RW, Rodriguez RM. Management of parapneumonic effusions. *Clin Chest Med* 1998;19:373–382.

Light RW, Girard WM, Jenkinson SG, et al. Parapneumonic effusions. *Am J Med* 1980;69:507–512.

Potts DE, Levin DC, Sahn SA. Pleural fluid pH in parapneumonic effusions. *Chest* 1976;70:328–331.

Varkey B, Rose HD, Kutty K, et al. Empyema thoracis during a ten-year period. *Arch Intern Med* 1981;141:1771–1776.

Wiedemann HP, Reynolds HY. Humoral immune defenses in bacterial infection of the pleural spaces. In: Chretien J, Bignon J, Hirsch A, eds. *The Pleura in Health and Disease.* New York: Marcel Dekker, 1985:347–368.

### Malignant Effusions

Austin EH, Flye MW. The treatment of recurrent malignant pleural effusion. *Ann Thorac Surg* 1970;28:190–203.

Bitran JD, Brown C, Desser RK, et al. Intracavitary bleomycin for the control of malignant effusions. *J Surg Oncol* 1981;16:273–277.

Bouchama A, Chastre J, Gaudichet A, et al. Acute pneumonitis with bilateral pleural effusion after talc pleurodesis. *Chest* 1984;86:795–797.

Canto A, Ferrer G, Romagosa V, et al. Lung cancer and pleural effusion: clinical significance and study of pleural metastatic locations. *Chest* 1985;87:649–652.

Ceyhar BB, Demiralp E, Celirel T. Analysis of pleural effusions using flow cytometry. *Respiration* 1996;63:17–24.

Decker DA, Dines DA, Payne WAS, et al. Significance of a cytologically negative pleural effusion in bronchogenic carcinoma. *Chest* 1978;74:640–642.

Dewald GW, Hicks GA, Dines DE, et al. Cytogenetic diagnosis of malignant pleural effusions: culture methods to supplement direct preparations in diagnosis. *Mayo Clin Proc* 1982;57:488–494.

Gupta N, Opfell RW, Padova J, et al. Intrapleural bleomycin versus tetracycline for control of malignant pleural effusion: a randomized study. *Proc Am Assn Cancer Res Am Soc Clin Oncol* 1980; 23:C189.

Heffner JE, Standerfer RJ, Torstveit J, et al. Clinical efficacy of doxycycline for pleurodesis. *Chest* 1994;105:1743–1747.

Leff A, Hopewell PC, Costello J. Pleural effusion from malignancy. *Ann Intern Med* 1978;88:532–537.

Livingston RB, McCracken JD, Trauth CJ, et al. Isolated pleural effusion in small cell lung carcinoma: favorable prognosis. *Chest* 1982;81:208–211.

Nystrom JS, Dyce B, Wada J, et al. Carcinoembryonic antigen titers on effusion fluid: a diagnostic tool? *Arch Intern Med* 1977;137:875–879.

Ostrowski MJ, Halsall GM. Intracavitary bleomycin in the management of malignant effusions: a multicenter study. *Cancer Treat Rep* 1982;66:1903–1907.

Prakash UBS, Reiman HM. Comparison of needle biopsy with cytologic analysis for the evaluation of pleural effusion: analysis of 414 cases. *Mayo Clin Proc* 1985;60:158–164.

Renshaw AA, Dean BR, Antman KH, et al. The role of cytologic evaluation of pleural fluid in the diagnosis of malignant mesothelioma. *Chest* 1997;111:106–109.

Rerger HW, Maher G. Decreased glucose concentration in malignant pleural effusions. *Am Rev Respir Dis* 1971;103:427–429.

Rinaldo JE, Owens GR, Rogers RM. Adult respiratory distress syndrome following intrapleural instillation of talc. *J Thorac Cardiovasc Surg* 1983;85:523–526.

Rittgers RA, Loewenstein MS, Feinerman AE, et al. Carcinoembryonic antigen levels in benign and malignant pleural effusions. *Ann Intern Med* 1978;88:631–634.

Sahn SA. Malignancy metastatic to the pleura. *Clin Chest Med* 1998;19:351–361.

Whitcomb ME, Schwarz MI. Pleural effusion complicating intensive mediastinal radiation therapy. *Am Rev Respir Dis* 1971;103:100–106.

### Collagen-Vascular Diseases

Halla JT, Schrohenloher RE, Volanakis JE. Immune complexes and other laboratory features of pleural effusions: a comparison of rheumatoid arthritis, systemic lupus erythematosus, and other diseases. *Ann Intern Med* 1980;92:748–752.

Hunder GG, McDuffie FC, Hepper NG. Pleural fluid complement in systemic lupus erythematosus and rheumatoid arthritis. *Ann Intern Med* 1972;76:357–363.

Khare V, Baetlige B, Larg S, et al. ANA in pleural fluid. *Chest* 1994;106:866–871.

Pettersson T, Klockars M, Hellstrom P-E. Chemical and immunological features of pleural effusions: comparison between rheumatoid arthritis and other diseases. *Thorax* 1982;37:354–361.

Sahn SA. Immunologic diseases of the pleura. *Clin Chest Med* 1985;6:83–102.

Sahn SA, Kaplan RL, Maulitz RM, et al. Rheumatoid pleurisy: observations on the development of low pleural fluid pH and glucose level. *Arch Intern Med* 1980;140:1237–1238.

### Asbestos

Epler GR, McLoud TC, Gaensler EA. Prevalence and incidence of benign asbestosis pleural effusion in a working population. *JAMA* 1982;247:617–622.

Nishimura SL, Broaddus VC. Asbestos-induced pleural disease. *Clin Chest Med* 1998;19:311–329.

Robinson BWS, Musk AW. Benign asbestos pleural effusion: diagnosis and course. *Thorax* 1981;36:896–900.

### Esophageal Rupture

Bellman MH, Rajaratnam HN. Perforation of the esophagus with amylase-rich pleural effusion. *Br J Dis Chest* 1974;68:18–22.

Dye RA, Laforet EG. Esophageal rupture: diagnosis of pleural fluid pH. *Chest* 1974;66:454–456.

Sherr HP, Light RW, Merson MH, et al. Origin of the pleural fluid amylase in esophageal rupture. *Ann Intern Med* 1972;76:985–986.

### Urinothorax

Miller KS, Wooten S, Sahn S. Urinothorax: a cause of low pH transudative pleural effusions. *Am J Med* 1988;85:448–449.

Stark DD, Shaves JG, Baron RL. Biochemical features of urinothorax. *Arch Intern Med* 1982;142:1509–1511.

### Chylothorax

Sassoon CS, Light RW. Chylothorax and pseudochylothorax. *Clin Chest Med* 1985;6:163–171.

Teba L, Dedhia HV, Bowen R, et al. Chylothorax review. *Crit Car Med* 1985;13:49–52.

### Miscellaneous

Fine NL, Smith LRE, Sheedy PF. Frequency of pleural effusions in mycoplasma and viral pneumonias. *N Engl J Med* 1970;283:790–793.

George RB, Penn RL, Kinasewitz GT. Mycobacterial, fungal, actinomycotic, and nocardial infections of the pleura. *Clin Chest Med* 1985;6:63–75.

Hansen RM, Caya JG, Clowry LJ Jr, et al. Benign mesothelial proliferation with effusion: clinicopathologic entity that may mimic malignancy. *Am J Med* 1984;77:887–892.

Hiller E, Rosenow EC III, Olsen AM. Pulmonary manifestations of the yellow nail syndrome. *Chest* 1972;61:452–458.

Hughson WG, Friedman PJ, Feigin DS, et al. Postpartum pleural effusion: a common radiologic finding. *Ann Intern Med* 1982;97:856–858.

Weil PH, Margolis IB. Systematic approach to traumatic hemothorax. *Am J Surg* 1981;142:692–694.

Weiss JM, Spodick DH. Association of left pleural effusion with pericardial disease. *N Engl J Med* 1983;308:696–697.

### Postcardiac Injury

Stelzner TJ, King TE, Antony VB, et al. The pleuropulmonary manifestations of the postcardiac injury syndrome. *Chest* 1983;84:383–387.

### Pleural Effusions Post–Coronary Artery Bypass Grafting

Light RW, Rogers JT, Cheng D, et al. Large pleural effusions occurring after coronary artery bypass grafting. *Ann Intern Med* 1999;130:891–896.

### Pulmonary Embolism

Brown SE, Light RW. Pleural effusion associated with pulmonary embolization. *Clin Chest Med* 1985;6:77–81.

Bynum LJ, Wilson JE III. Characteristics of pleural effusions associated with pulmonary embolism. *Arch Intern Med* 1976;136:159–162.

### Indeterminate Effusions

Ansari T, Idell S. Management of undiagnosed persistent pleural effusions. *Clin Chest Med* 1998;19:407–417.

Black LF. Pleural effusions [Editorial]. *Mayo Clin Proc* 1981;56:210–212.

Canto A, Rivas J, Saumench J, et al. Points to consider when choosing a biopsy method in cases of pleurisy of unknown origin. *Chest* 1983;84:176–179.

Gunnels JJ. Perplexing pleural effusion. *Chest* 1978;74:390–393.

Ryan CJ, Rodgers RF, Unni KK, et al. The outcome of patients with pleural effusion of indeterminate cause at thoracotomy. *Mayo Clin Proc* 1981;56:145–149.

### Acquired Immunodeficiency Syndrome

Beck JM. Pleural disease in patients with acquired immune deficiency syndrome. *Clin Chest Med* 1998;19:341–349.

Joseph J, Strange C, Sahn SA. Pleural effusions in hospitalized patients with AIDS. *Ann Intern Med* 1993;118:856–859.

### Pneumothorax

Baumann MH, Strange C, Heffner JE, et al. for the ACCP Pneumothorax Consensus Group. Management of spontaneous pneumothorax: an American College of Chest Physicians Delphi Consensus Statement. *Chest* 2001;119:590–602.

Bense L, Eklund G, Wiman LG. Smoking and increased risk of contracting spontaneous pneumothorax. *Chest* 1987;92:1009–1012.

Jantz MA, Pierson DJ. Pneumothorax and barotrauma. *Clin Chest Med* 1994;15:75–91.

Light RW. Management of spontaneous pneumothorax. *Am Rev Respir Dis* 1993;148:245–248.

Light RW, O'Hara VS, Moritz TE, et al. Intrapleural tetracycline for the prevention of recurrent spontaneous pneumothorax. *JAMA* 1990;264:2224–2230.

## 40

# BOARD SIMULATION:
## Critical Care Medicine

*Alejandro C. Arroliga*

This simulation and discussion introduces some concepts regarding the pathophysiology and management of a patient with the acute respiratory distress syndrome (ARDS), hypotension, and shock.

## CASE 1: DAY 1

A 40-year-old man was admitted 1 day previously with a diagnosis of right lower lobe pneumonia. Now he is agitated, tachypneic, tachycardic, febrile, and hypotensive (80/60 mm Hg). He has crackles in both lungs and is oliguric (20 mL/hour).

### Question

**1.** All of the following statements regarding ARDS are true, *except*
**a)** Survival is about 60% to 70%.
**b)** If patients survive, lung function improves to normal or near normal.
**c)** ARDS is associated with low lung compliance.
**d)** Most patients die of severe hypoxemia.

### Discussion

Acute respiratory distress syndrome (ARDS) is often progressive and is characterized by the presence of bilateral lung infiltrates and hypoxemia in the absence of left ventricular failure. Patients with ARDS have stiff lungs (low total respiratory compliance), which are difficult to inflate, thus increasing the work of breathing. These patients have been classified into two groups: those with acute lung injury, in which the patient has moderate to severe hypoxemia [arterial oxygen pressure ($Pao_2$): inspired oxygen fraction ($Fio_2$) of $<300$ and $>201$] and ARDS ($Pao_2$: $Fio_2$ $<200$). The incidence of ARDS has been estimated to be 65 per 100,000 per year; more recent estimates, however, suggest that the incidence is in the range of 13.5 per 100,000 per year.

The etiology of ARDS is diverse and includes *direct* and *indirect* causes. The most common direct causes are aspiration and infections (pneumonia). The most common indirect causes are sepsis and trauma. Independent of the cause, the alveolar-capillary membrane is injured and suffers alteration to its permeability, resulting in flooding of the alveoli (edema) and the alteration of the surfactant quality and quantity. The end result is alveolar collapse. In pathologic specimens, diffuse alveolar damage is present, with abundant inflammatory cells (neutrophils and macrophages), erythrocytes, hyaline membranes, and proteinacious edema fluid. These process cause disruption of the alveolar epithelium. If the stimuli continue, fibroproliferative changes occur, causing progressive lung damage. In patients who survive, the hypoxemia slowly resolves and lung compliance improves.

The severity of the alteration to normal physiology is associated with the prognosis of the patients with ARDS. For example, an elevated alveolar dead-space, probably caused by the injury to the pulmonary capillaries, and with obstruction due to thrombosis and inflammation, is associated with increased risk of dying.

### Answer and Explanation

**1. d.**
Some series reported survival rates in the range of 60%, and only a minority (fewer than 10% in the acute setting) of the patients die of hypoxemia. Interestingly, patients who survived tended to recover normal or near-normal lung function, although patients with severe ARDS sometimes were left with some degree of restrictive defect. The pulmonary function abnormalities, however, correlate with a reduction in health-related quality of life. It is important to note that persistent functional disability may be present in a significant percentage of patients who survive ARDS. Up to 50% of the patients were not working 1 year after being discharged from the intensive care unit (ICU), despite improvement in lung function. Most of these patients have significant functional limitation due to muscle wasting and muscle weakness.

## CASE 1: LATER THAT DAY

The patient from Case 1 was intubated because of severe hypoxemia [arterial blood gas (ABG) pH, 7.30; $PaCO_2$, 24 mm Hg; $PaO_2$, 42 mm Hg]. The patient was started on assisted controlled ventilation, with a tidal volume of 600 mL, $FiO_2$ of 1.0. Repeated arterial blood gas (ABG) analysis after intubation showed pH, 7.32; $PaCO_2$, 22 mm Hg; $PaO_2$, 50 mm Hg.

### Question

2. The next step includes the following measures, *except*
a) Sedation
b) Optimization of cardiac output
c) Optimization of hemoglobin
d) Addition of positive end-expiratory pressure (PEEP)
e) Addition of extracorporeal membrane oxygenation (ECMO) and nitric oxide (NO) to improve survival

### Discussion

In ARDS, adequate sedation, nutrition, skin care, attention to details like optimal fluid and electrolyte management, and adequate prophylaxis for venous thromboembolism and upper gastrointestinal bleeding are essential.

Mechanical ventilation is important in patients with ARDS. The objectives of mechanical ventilation are to reverse hypoxemia, relieve acute respiratory acidosis, and reduce the work of breathing, ventilatory muscle fatigue, and oxygen consumption. The ARDS Network studied 861 patients with ARDS and acute lung injury who were assigned to two groups. Patients were ventilated with volume-cycle, assist-controlled ventilation. One group received conventional mechanical ventilation (12 cc per Kg of predicted body weight), and the study group received low-tidal volume ventilation (6cc per Kg of predicted body weight). The patients assigned to the low-tidal volume had a reduction in mortality of 22%, from 39.8% to 31%. Based on this evidence, it is suggested that patients with ARDS be ventilated using low-tidal volume, 6 cc per Kg of predicted body weight.

A common way to improve oxygenation in patients with ARDS is through the use of positive end-inspiratory pressure (PEEP). PEEP improves oxygenation in 3 out of 4 patients with acute lung injury or ARDS. PEEP helps in the recruitment of atelectatic areas of the lung; however, it may overdistend normally aerated areas of the lung. Recently, the ARDS Clinical Trials Network reported a study of 549 patients who were randomized to receive a low level of PEEP (mean of $8 \pm 3$ cm of water) or a higher level of PEEP ($13 \pm 3$ cm of water). All the patients received a tidal volume of 6 mL/kg of predicted body weight. The clinical outcomes, including mortality, were similar between both groups. The amount of PEEP used should be enough to avoid end-expiratory collapse but not so high that it decreases the venous return and the cardiac output.

The optimal level of hemoglobin in patients with ARDS is not known. The use of a liberal strategy for packed red blood cells transfusion (to keep hemoglobin between 10 g/dL and 12 g/dL), however, has not been found to be associated with a better outcome in intubated patients receiving mechanical ventilation when compared with a restrictive red blood cells transfusion strategy that keeps hemoglobin in the range of 7 g/dL to 9 g/dL.

### Answer and Explanation

**2. e.**
The management of patients with ARDS is supportive. ECMO and NO have not been shown to improve survival in randomized trials. The administration of nitric oxide has been associated with some improvement in the gas exchange (improved oxygenation) but no improvement in the survival or in the duration of ventilatory support.

## CASE 1: DAY THREE

In the intensive care unit (ICU), this same patient developed bilateral pneumothoraces on day 3 of his hospital stay. At 4 p.m., the patient became hypotensive and tachycardic, and his hypoxia worsened.

### Question

3. You are at the bedside and will do all the following, *except*
a) Check peak and plateau pressures
b) Give 500 mL of normal saline and increase $FiO_2$ to 1.0
c) Check the chest tubes and obtain a chest radiograph
d) Obtain an electrocardiogram (ECG) and auscultate the patient's chest
e) Obtain blood cultures

### Discussion

The causes of hypotension in patients in the ICU are varied. Some of the most frequent causes include hypovolemia, tension pneumothorax, acute myocardial events (arrhythmia and ischemia), sepsis, and cardiac tamponade. Pneumothorax and other air leaks are present in 10% in patients receiving mechanical ventilation for ARDS. In the presence of a pneumothorax, the compliance of the respiratory system will decrease and the peak and plateau pressures will increase. Obviously, checking that chest tubes are permeable and obtaining a chest radiograph are essential to rule out pneumothorax.

PEEP, either external (given by the ventilator) or auto-PEEP (present more frequently in patients with severe obstructive airway diseases), is an important cause of hypotension because PEEP can decrease the venous return, with a subsequent drop in the cardiac output.

The syndrome of shock is present when the circulatory system is unable to maintain adequate cellular perfusion. If shock is not reversed, irreversible cellular damage will occur. The management of hypotension and shock in the ICU is of great importance. The majority of patients will need the administration of fluids and/or pressors. The goal is to keep a mean systemic blood pressure of 65 mm Hg; however, other parameters, such as urinary output, skin perfusion, mental status, and heart rate, are very important. Crystalloids and colloids are the two groups of fluid given to patients in shock. There is no difference in outcome between the use of colloids or crystalloids, although several meta-analyses have suggested that crystalloid resuscitation is associated with a lower mortality in trauma patients and that the administration of albumin does not reduce mortality in patients with hypovolemia, burns, or hypoalbuminemia and may increase mortality. Recently, in a study of 6,997 patients randomized to receive either albumin (4%) or normal saline for intravascular fluid resuscitation, no difference occurred in mortality rate, days in the ICU and in the hospital, days on mechanical ventilation, or in the number of days of renal-replacement therapy.

The two vasopressors most frequently used in patients with shock—most commonly septic shock—are dopamine and norepinephrine. In patients who are not responsive to aggressive fluid administration (boluses of 12 cc/Kg of isotonic saline solution), dopamine and norepinephrine are effective.

## Answer and Explanation

3. e.
Although nosocomial infections are frequent in patients admitted to the ICU, obtaining blood cultures in a patient in shock is important but not essential.

## CASE 1: DAY 4

The patient from Case 3 is still hypotensive, his white blood cell count (WBC) is 15,000/mm³, and his hemoglobin is 10 g/dL.

## Question

4. What would you do next?
a) Duplex of extremities and echo
b) Adrenocorticotrophic hormone (ACTH) stimulation test
c) Give another 500 mL of normal saline and start dopamine
d) Tranfuse 2 U of packed red blood cells (PRBCs)
e) Both a and c

## Discussion

The most important part of the management of venous thromboembolism is prevention. Unfortunately, in some studies, data suggest that up to 20% of patients do not receive prophylaxis. In our ICU, the modalities most frequently used for prevention are low-dose heparin and pneumatic calf compression. Low-molecular weight heparin has been used as well.

The management of hypotension and shock is important. Shock requires aggressive therapy, with adequate volume infusion in the case of hypovolemic and distributive shock, and of vasopressors and inotropes in the case of cardiogenic shock. We prefer the rapid infusion of crystalloids to replenish the intravascular volume and packed red blood cells in the presence of hemorrhage. No clinical advantage accrues to the use of colloids in patients to increase intravascular volume.

## Answer and Explanation

4. e.
Deep venous thromboembolism (DVT) occurs in 18% to 30% of patients admitted to the ICU. It is important to make the diagnosis, and ultrasound of the upper and lower extremities is probably the most important initial step in making a diagnosis of DVT. An evaluation with a ventilation–perfusion scan or with a spiral computed tomography (CT) is helpful in making a diagnosis of pulmonary embolism, although in 2004, pulmonary angiography was still the gold standard for making a diagnosis of pulmonary embolism.

Echocardiography is important in the management of the hypotensive patient in the ICU. Echocardiography can guide the clinician about the status of the right ventricle, which is dilated and overloaded in the case of pulmonary embolism with pulmonary hypertension, or underfilled in the case of hypovolemia. The diagnosis of cardiac tamponade or ventricular segmental abnormalities in the case of ischemia is important as well.

## CASE 1: DAY 7

The patient has been stable for 3 days. He is being treated with erythromycin and sedated with lorazepam. He became agitated and was given haloperidol. Suddenly, he became hypotensive, and his pulse is not palpable. The ECG tracing is shown (ventricular tachycardia) in Figure 40.1.

The patient is still hypotensive; his WBC is 15,000/mm³; hemoglobin, 10 g/dL.

## Question

5. You will do all of the following, *except*
a) Cardioversion-defibrillation
b) Administer magnesium intravenously

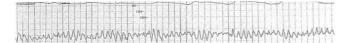

**Figure 40.1** The electrocardiographic trace in this patient is consistent with a type of ventricular tachycardia called *torsades de pointes*. This type of ventricular tachycardia is characterized by QRS complexes of changing amplitude that appear to twist around an isoelectric line and occur at a rate of 200 to 250 beats per minute. The tachycardia may terminate spontaneously, or it can go to ventricular standstill or a new episode of torsades. Frequently, in the critically ill patient, ventricular fibrillation may supervene. Although several predisposing factors have been cited, the most common predisposing factors in critically ill patients include brady-cardia, electrolyte abnormalities, and use of drugs such as cis-apride, phenothiazines, and butyrophenones (haloperidol). The most important aspect of management in this patient is to avoid the arrhythmias by aggressive correction of electrolyte abnormalities, including hypokalemia, hypocalcemia, and hypomagnesemia. It is important to pay attention to drug interactions. In the hemo-dynamically unstable patient, electric cardioversion is essential.

c) Increase the dose of haloperidol and erythromycin
d) Correct hypocalcemia, hypokalemia, and alkalosis

## Discussion

This question highlights an important topic of critical care medicine: drug interactions. An important effect of drug interaction in the critically ill patient is hypotension caused by partial adrenal insufficiency. This drug interaction occurs in patients receiving drugs that can increase the activity of the P450 system (e.g., phenytoin, phenobarbital). When the P450 system is activated, the metabolism of steroids increases, creating a state of partial adrenal insufficiency. This drug interaction should be suspected in patients receiving medication that can increase the metabolism of the P450 system and who present with persistent hypotension in the absence of other etiologies.

## Answer and Explanation

**5. c.**
Erythromycin and haloperidol, drugs commonly used in the ICU, are known to increase the QT interval. Patients with underlying ischemic heart disease and with electrolyte and acid–base abnormalities are more likely to develop this complication. Phenothiazines and cisapride can prolong the QT interval as well.

## CASE 1: DAY 9

The patient, in his ninth day in the ICU, becomes hypotensive and oliguric. His excreted fraction of sodium (FeNa) is greater than 1, but he is "positive" by 10 L. A pulmonary artery catheter was inserted until a wedge pressure was obtained at 35 cm and was read as 20 mm Hg (Fig. 40.2). Based on the tracing and reading, the senior medical resident on call gave 160 mg of furosemide, and the patient became more hypotensive.

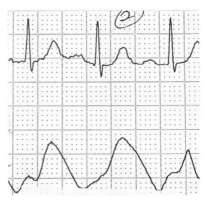

**Figure 40.2** A frequent problem in the reading or interpretation of the data generated with catheterization of the right side of the heart is proper identification of the waveform in the different chambers of the heart. In this case, the physician failed to recognize that the catheter never went to the pulmonary artery and stayed in the right ventricle. Passage from the right ventricle into the pulmonary artery is evidenced by an increase in the diastolic pressure (the diastolic pressure of the pulmonary artery is higher than the diastolic pressure of the right ventricle). The pulmonary artery waveform has a systolic pressure wave and a diastolic trough. The pulmonary artery waveform also has a dicrotic notch caused by the closure of the pulmonary valve; this can be identified on the terminal part of the systolic pressure wave.

## Question

**6.** What is your next step?
a) Check hemodynamic readings.
b) Add dobutamine and norepinephrine (Levophed).
c) Give 320 mg of furosemide and afterload reducer.
d) Increase PEEP to decrease the preload.

## Discussion

The possibility of catheterizing the right ventricle at the bedside and obtaining pressures on the right side of the heart revolutionized critical care medicine. The pulmonary artery catheter provides information useful for the management of respiratory and circulatory failure and for the assessment of intravascular volume. Unfortunately, available studies show that a significant proportion of clinicians working in the ICU cannot correctly interpret the data obtained with the catheter or cannot recognize errors in the tracing and in the measurements taken with the catheter.

## Answer and Explanation

**6. a.**
In this case, the clinician failed to recognize that reaching a wedge at 35 cm in an average-sized patient is unlikely. The right ventricle should be reached at 30 to 40 cm from the subclavian or internal jugular veins. The pulmonary artery can be reached if the catheter is inserted an additional 10 to 15 cm. The other important information that was not recognized in this case was the fact that the waveform changes when the catheter moves from the

right ventricle to the pulmonary artery. The diastolic pressure is higher in the pulmonary artery, and a dicrotic notch due to pulmonary valve closure should be noted in the pulmonary artery waveform.

The usefulness of the pulmonary artery catheter has been controversial. Several observational and retrospective studies suggest that the use of the catheter may be associated with an increase rate of morbidity and mortality. The increased morbidity and mortality found in these observational studies may be directly associated with the catheter use (mechanical complications) or may be due to errors in the interpretation of the data generated by the catheter. Finally, it is possible that the use of the pulmonary artery catheter is a mark of aggressive physician management in the ICU, and this aggressive management is associated with a higher rate of complications and mortality. A randomized study by the ARDS Network is ongoing to assess the efficacy of the pulmonary artery catheter versus central venous catheter management in reducing the morbidity and mortality in patients with ARDS and acute lung injury.

All clinicians must be aware of the complications that can occur with use of a pulmonary artery catheter. Examples of these complications include line infections, complications of insertion (pneumothorax and hematomas), cardiac arrhythmias, cardiac perforation, venous thromboembolism, rupture of the pulmonary artery, infarction of lung parenchyma, and knotting of the catheter. It is imperative that all physicians involved in the care of the critically ill must be adequately educated in the insertion, interpretation of the data, and use of the pulmonary artery catheter.

## SUGGESTED READINGS

Artigas A, Bernard GR, Carlet J, et al. The American-European consensus conference on ARDS Part 2. *Am J Respir Crit Care Med* 1998; 157:1332–1347.

Bernard GR, Artigas A, Brigham KL, et al. The American-European consensus conference on ARDS: Definitions, mechanisms, relevant outcomes, and clinical trial coordination. *Am J Respir Crit Care Med* 1994;149:818–824.

Choi PTL, Yip G, Quinonez LG, et al. Crystalloids vs. colloids in fluid resuscitation: a systematic review. *Crit Care Med* 1999;27:200–210.

Coulter TD, Wiedemann HP. Complications of hemodynamic monitoring. *Clin Chest Med* 1999;20:249–267.

Connors AF Jr, Speroff T, Dawson NV, et al. The effectiveness of right heart catheterization in the initial care of critically ill patients. *JAMA* 1996;276:889–897.

Hebert PC, Blajchman MA, Cook DJ, et al. Do blood transfusion improve outcomes related to mechanical ventilation? *Chest* 2001; 119:1850–1857.

Herridge MS, Cheung AM, Tansey CM, et al. One-year outcomes in survivors of the acute respiratory distress syndrome. *N Engl J Med* 2003;348:683–693.

Legere BM, Dweik RA, Arroliga AC. Venous thromboembolism in the intensive care unit. *Clin Chest Med* 1999;20:367–384.

Nuckton TJ, Alonso JA, Kallet RH, et al. Pulmonary dead-space fraction as a risk factor for death in the acute respiratory distress syndrome. *N Engl J Med* 2002;346:1281–1286.

Orme J Jr, Romney JS, Hopkins RO, et al. Pulmonary function and health-related quality of life in survivors of acute respiratory distress syndrome. *Am J Respir Crit Care Med* 2002;167:690–694.

Romac DR, Albertson TE. Drug interactions in the intensive care unit. *Clin Chest Med* 1999;20:385–399.

Sandur S, Stoller JK. Pulmonary complications of mechanical ventilation. *Clin Chest Med* 1999;20:223–247.

Task Force of the American College of Critical Care Medicine, Society of Critical Care Medicine. Practice parameters for hemodynamic support of sepsis in adult patients in sepsis. *Crit Care Med* 1999; 27:639–660.

Taylor RW, Zimmerman JL, Dellinger RP, et al. Low-dose inhaled nitric oxide in patients with acute lung injury. A randomized controlled trial. *JAMA* 2004;291:1603–1609.

The SAFE Study Investigators. A comparison of albumin and saline for fluid resuscitation in the intensive care unit. *N Engl J Med* 2004; 350:2247–2256.

The National Heart, Lung and Blood Institute ARDS Clinical Trials Network. Higher versus lower positive end-expiratory pressures in patients with the acute respiratory distress syndrome. *N Engl J Med* 2004;351:327–336.

Tobin MJ. Advances in mechanical ventilation. *N Engl J Med* 2001; 344:1986–1996.

Ware LB, Matthay MA. The acute respiratory distress syndrome. *N Engl J Med* 2000;342:1334–1349.

Wiedemann HP, Matthay MA, Matthay RA. Cardiovascular and pulmonary monitoring in the intensive care unit (I, II). *Chest* 1984; 85:537–545, 656–668.

## 41

# BOARD SIMULATION:
## Pulmonary Medicine

*James K. Stoller*

The typical questions posed in board certification examinations include those addressing the following:

- Common features of uncommon diseases
- Uncommon features of common diseases
- Disease associations, especially those that require integrated knowledge of diagnosis, treatment, and complications of therapy
- Knowledge of established therapies, even if relatively uncommon
- Integration of knowledge (e.g., associating classic disease symptoms with pathologic and radiographic manifestations, associating pathologic findings with treatments of choice or complications of therapy)

As a general rule, the questions posed in board examinations are meant to discriminate between the majority of examinees who will pass the examination and a minority (approximately 15% to 20% over past years) who will not succeed. The questions are psychometrically validated to achieve this level of discrimination and to serve the goal of a predetermined pass criterion (e.g., 70% correct responses).

## CASES 1–5

Five cases are presented for your consideration. Each of the following patients has some degree of respiratory distress. Match the patient profiles to the correct patterns of the flow–volume loop shown in Figure 41.1

- *Patient Profile 1.* The patient is a 55-year-old man with history of multiple trauma, adult respiratory distress syndrome, and prolonged intubation.
- *Patient Profile 2.* The patient is a 65-year-old man with long-standing rheumatoid arthritis and cricoarytenoid involvement.
- *Patient Profile 3.* The patient is a 40-year-old woman with painful ears, saddle-nose deformity, and arthralgias.
- *Patient Profile 4.* The patient is a 45-year-old woman with "factitious asthma" presenting as stridor.
- *Patient Profile 5.* The patient is a 30-year-old man with relapsing polychondritis and expiratory wheezing.

## Questions

1. What is the flow–volume loop pattern for patient 1?
2. What is the flow–volume loop pattern for patient 2?
3. What is the flow–volume loop pattern for patient 3?
4. What is the flow–volume loop pattern for patient 4?
5. What is the flow–volume loop pattern for patient 5?

## Discussion

Recognizing the patterns of an abnormal flow–volume loop can be helpful in determining the presence and position of upper airway obstruction. In understanding the flow–volume loop, it is important to recognize that *positive flow* (i.e., above the horizontal line) denotes expiration, and *negative flow* (below the horizontal; Fig. 41.1, pattern 1) denotes the inspiratory limb.

The flow–volume loop is a different way of graphically presenting the information gathered in a spirogram or volume–time tracing. Specifically, in determining the flow rate (i.e., in liters per second), the slope of the volume–time tracing is taken. The first derivative of volume with respect to time represents flow. The flow rate or slope of the volume–time tracing then is plotted against the volume (which is on the *vertical axis* of the volume–time tracing) but is transposed to become the *horizontal axis* of a flow–volume loop. Thus, the expiratory limb of the flow–volume loop is an algebraic transformation of the volume–time tracing; however, the inspiratory limb of the flow–volume loop is not depicted on a volume–time tracing (which is confined to expiration). To obtain the inspiratory component, the patient must inspire from residual volume to total lung capacity. In addition to the normal flow–volume loop (Fig. 41.1, pattern 1), three characteristic deviations from the normal flow–volume loop suggest various forms of upper airway obstruction (Fig. 41.1, patterns 2, 3, and 4).

*Pattern 2* represents dynamic intrathoracic upper airway obstruction, *pattern 3* represents dynamic extrathoracic upper airway obstruction, and *pattern 4* represents fixed upper airway obstruction. The descriptor *dynamic* denotes that the airway lesion is floppy or malacic, and so the degree of airway blockage will be affected by the transmural pressure gradient (across the airway wall). To understand

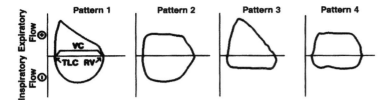

**Figure 41.1**   Patterns of the flow–volume loop. RV, respiratory volume; TLC, total lung capacity; VC, vital capacity.

these three variant patterns of the flow–volume loop, one must consider the pressure gradient across the airway walls during inspiration and expiration (Figs. 41.2 and 41.3). During inspiration, intrapleural pressure is negative; thus, atmospheric gas flows into the lung across a gradient from higher to lower pressures. The situation reverses during exhalation. During exhalation, as intrapleural pressure becomes more positive relative to atmospheric pressure, gas leaves the lung and moves to the outside atmosphere, which is now lower in pressure. With this in mind, it stands to reason that any fixed obstruction to airflow in the upper airway will produce a decrease in flows during both inspiration and expiration, causing flow to decrease in both limbs of the flow–volume tracing (Fig. 41.1, pattern 4). Thus, as in the patient profile, flow is decreased during both expiration and inspiration, giving rise to the characteristic flattening of both the inspiratory and expiratory limbs. In contrast to the situation with fixed airway obstruction, dynamic airflow can occur in the upper airway. To understand more clearly how dynamic airflow obstruction affects the shape of the flow–volume loop, it is important to recognize that dynamic airflow obstruction can occur in the extrathoracic upper airway (e.g., caudal to the thoracic inlet). As shown in Figure 41.1, pattern 3, dynamic extrathoracic upper airway obstruction is characterized by a flattening of the inspi-

ratory limb of the flow–volume loop, with preservation of a normal expiratory limb. Examples of such conditions might include tracheomalacia of the extrathoracic upper airway or vocal cord paralysis. In contrast, dynamic intrathoracic obstruction produces a flattening of only the expiratory limb of the flow–volume loop (Fig. 41.1, pattern 2). Examples of conditions that cause dynamic intrathoracic upper airway obstruction include tracheomalacia of the intrathoracic airway or tumors that straddle the main carina. Figures 41.2 and 41.3 graphically review the pathophysiology of dynamic upper airway obstruction.

## Answers and Explanations

### 1. Pattern 4.
In patient profile 1, the patient is a 55-year-old man with a history of multiple trauma, adult respiratory distress syndrome, and prolonged intubation. This is the first of the cases calling on the reader to recognize an upper airway lesion and to match this with the appropriate pattern of the flow–volume loop. In this first case, the patient has fixed laryngotracheal obstruction resulting from prolonged intubation, complicating adult respiratory distress syndrome (ARDS). Overall, the frequency of clinically significant upper airway obstruction following prolonged

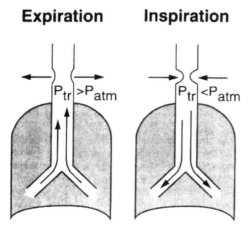

**Figure 41.2**   Effect of expiration and inspiration on dynamic or nonfixed extrathoracic airway obstruction. **(Left)** During forced expiration, intratracheal pressure ($P_{tr}$) exceeds the pressure around the airway ($P_{atm}$) or atmospheric pressure, lessening the obstruction. **(Right)** During forced inspiration, when pressure around that airway is greater, the obstruction worsens. (Reproduced with permission from Kryger MH, Bode F, Antic R, et al. Diagnosis of obstruction of the upper and central airways. *Am J Med* 1976; 61:85–93.)

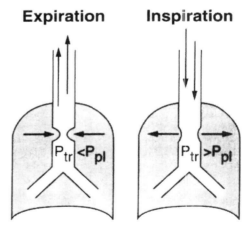

**Figure 41.3**   Effects of expiration and inspiration on dynamic or nonfixed intrathoracic airway obstruction. **(Left)** During forced expiration, pressure exerted around the airway ($P_{pl}$, or pleural pressure) may exceed intratracheal pressure ($P_{tr}$), worsening the obstruction. **(Right)** During forced inspiration, intratracheal pressure is greater, relieving the obstruction. (Reproduced with permission from Kryger MH, Bode F, Antic R, et al. Diagnosis of obstruction of the upper and central airways. *Am J Med* 1976;61:85–93.)

intubation is 5% to 15%, although controversy still exists regarding whether the risk of laryngeal injury increases as the duration of intubation lengthens.

Upper airway obstruction after prolonged intubation may result from several different lesions, including vocal cord stricture (especially at the posterior glottic chink) and tracheal stenosis, either at the site of the tracheostomy stoma or at the site of the cuff on the endotracheal tube. Because upper airway obstruction complicating prolonged intubation usually consists of granulation tissue, the airway obstruction is usually characterized by fixed upper airway obstruction, as demonstrated by pattern 4 in Figure 41.1. This pattern shows a flattening of both the expiratory and inspiratory limbs of the flow–volume loop. In contrast, a fixed lesion is constant and shows airflow limitation both on inspiration and expiration. In this terminology, *extrathoracic* denotes a position along the airway cephalad of the thoracic inlet and *intrathoracic* denotes an airway lesion caudal to the thoracic inlet as far down as the main carina.

### 2. Pattern 4.

Patient profile 2 presents a 65-year-old man with long-standing rheumatoid arthritis and cricoarytenoid involvement. The best answer is Figure 41.1, pattern 4, denoting fixed extrathoracic upper airway obstruction. This case demonstrates the consequences of arthritis or ankylosis of the cricoarytenoids, which can cause upper airway obstruction in patients with rheumatoid arthritis. In a series by Lawry and colleagues (1), the prevalence of inspiratory difficulty was 29% among 45 patients with rheumatoid arthritis.

### 3. Patterns 2, 3, or 4.

Patient profile 3 is of a 41-year-old woman with painful ears, saddle-nose deformity, and arthralgias. This profile describes the scenario of upper airway involvement in relapsing polychondritis, clinical features of which include recurrent inflammation primarily affecting the nose, respiratory tract, ears, and joints. Notably, 25% of patients with relapsing polychondritis present with respiratory tract complaints, and 50% of patients have respiratory tract symptoms sometime during the course of their illness. Laryngotracheal involvement is responsible for 10% of deaths by pneumonia or by upper airway compromise in patients with relapsing polychondritis. The spectrum of upper airway lesions may include acute inflammation, fibrosis, or dissolution of cartilage and malacia. As a result, the flow–volume loop abnormalities may include fixed upper airway obstruction as well as dynamic intrathoracic or extrathoracic obstruction.

As such, the correct answer in this case may be patterns 2, 3, or 4 in Figure 41.1, all of which are possible. In the absence of more defining symptoms, such as inspiratory stridor (which would suggest dynamic extrathoracic upper airway obstruction) or expiratory wheezing (which might favor dynamic intrathoracic

upper airway obstruction), any of the abnormal patterns is an acceptable answer.

### 4. Pattern 3.

Patient profile 4 presents a 45-year-old woman with "factitious asthma" presenting as stridor. The correct pattern is 3 in Figure 41.1, characterized by a flattening of the inspiratory limb only. The cause of factitious asthma is vocal cord dysfunction. A spectrum of functional vocal cord problems has been observed, including paradoxic inspiratory closure and paradoxic expiratory closure. As noted, paradoxic inspiratory closure would be more likely to present as stridor and to be characterized by a flattening of the inspiratory limb of the flow–volume loop.

### 5. Pattern 2.

Finally, patient profile 5 presents a 30-year-old man with relapsing polychondritis and expiratory wheezing. The correct flow–volume loop abnormality is Figure 41.1, pattern 2. In this case, unlike patient profile 2, the presence of expiratory wheezing should suggest the presence of intrathoracic upper airway obstruction.

## CASES 6–10

Five more cases are presented for your consideration. Each patient has been evaluated for pulmonary function. Match the appropriate patient to the best pulmonary function test profile in Table 41.1. Note that each pulmonary function test profile may be used once, more than once, or not at all.

- *Patient Profile 6.* The patient is a 25-year-old man with von Recklinghausen's disease.
- *Patient Profile 7.* The patient is a 62-year-old man 2 days post–coronary artery bypass grafting (CABG).
- *Patient Profile 8.* The patient is a 35-year-old obese man with nocturnal cough.
- *Patient Profile 9.* The patient, a 45-year-old woman, has a cirrhotic child.
- *Patient Profile 10.* The patient, a 60-year-old man, smokes one or two packs of cigarettes per day.

### Questions

**6.** What are the results of the pulmonary function test for patient 6?

**7.** What are the results of the pulmonary function test for patient 7?

**8.** What are the results of the pulmonary function test for patient 8?

**9.** What are the results of the pulmonary function test for patient 9?

**10.** What are the results of the pulmonary function test for patient 10?

## TABLE 41.1
### PULMONARY FUNCTION TEST RESULTS

| FEV$_1$ (% Predicted)[a] | FEV (% Predicted) | Forced Vital Capacity (Sit to Supine) | Total Lung Capacity (%) | Diffusing Capacity of the Lung for Carbon Monoxide (% Predicted) |
|---|---|---|---|---|
| 1.60 | 78 | 19 | 73 | 83 |
| 2.50 | 52 | 11 | 65 | 60 |
| 3.84 | 91 | 8 | 90 | 90 |
| 4.52 | 81 | 12 | 105 | 70 |
| 5.45 | 55 | 27 | 70 | 55 |

[a] FEV$_1$, forced expiratory volume in 1 second.

## Discussion

## Answers and Explanations

### 6. Test Profile 2.

Patient profile 6 presents a 25-year-old with von Recklinghausen's disease. The most appropriate pulmonary function test profile is number 2, demonstrating pulmonary restriction characterized by a total lung capacity of 65% of predicted, a proportionate decline in the diffusing capacity (60% of predicted), and proportionate decreases in forced expiratory volume in 1 second (FEV$_1$) and forced vital capacity (FVC), such that the FEV$_1$/FVC is preserved. Also, the change in FVC going from sitting to a supine position is normal (i.e., <20%). This pulmonary function profile is characteristic of extrathoracic pulmonary restriction, such as might be seen by the kyphoscoliosis that accompanies von Recklinghausen's disease in up to 20% of patients.

Notably, in approximately 5% of affected persons, the kyphoscoliosis is clinically significant. The sine qua non of restrictive lung disease is decreased total lung capacity. In this case, the proportionate decrease in the diffusing capacity suggests extrathoracic disease, rather than a parenchymal restrictive lung disease, for example, interstitial lung disease.

### 7. Test Profile 5.

Patient profile 7 presents a 62-year-old man 2 days after undergoing CABG surgery. The most appropriate pulmonary function test result profile is number 5. As in previous cases, this is a pattern depicting extrathoracic pulmonary restriction with decreased total lung capacity. Unlike the former case, the decrease in the FVC on moving from the sitting to supine posture exceeds the normal upper boundary of 20%. In this case, the cause is bilateral diaphragmatic paralysis, causing an accentuated decline in the FVC on lying down, as the diaphragm is pushed into the chest by the abdominal contents. This case demonstrates the phenomenon of "frostbitten" phrenic nerves, which may complicate CABG surgery [as a result of bathing the phrenic(s) in cold cardioplegia solution or ischemia] in up to 5% of cases.

Unilateral diaphragmatic paralysis is more common than bilateral diaphragmatic paralysis, and unilateral paralysis is usually not apparent clinically. When both phrenic nerves are affected, however, the patient exhibits marked orthopnea accompanied by the decline in FVC, as noted already.

### 8. Test Profile 1.

Patient profile 8 presents a 35-year-old obese man with nocturnal cough. Pulmonary function profile 1 is the best choice and indicates a pattern of airflow obstruction (i.e., a disproportionate decrease in FEV$_1$ compared with FVC). In this case, the patient's obesity likely accounts for the mild restrictive lung disease (total lung capacity 73% of predicted, below the 80% predicted that is the lower limit of normal). In fact, this case presents combined restrictive and obstructive lung disease, the differential diagnosis of which includes asthma with obesity as well as eosinophilic granuloma of lung (histiocytosis X), sarcoidosis, lymphangioleiomyomatosis, and congestive heart failure. In this case, the patient's nocturnal cough is a manifestation of asthma.

In fact, nocturnal symptoms accompany asthma in up to one-third of patients and frequently dominate the clinical presentation. Management strategies may include the use of inhaled corticosteroids and or long-acting inhaled β-agonists (e.g., salmeterol).

### 9. Test Profile 3 or 4.

Patient profile 9 is that of a 45-year-old woman with a cirrhotic child. The case is meant to prompt consideration of severe (e.g., PI*ZZ homozygous) α$_1$-antitrypsin deficiency. In this regard, the best pulmonary function profile is number 4, demonstrating a pattern of airflow obstruction with a suggestion of alveolar-capillary unit loss, demonstrated by the mild decrease in the diffusing capacity. Overall, this pattern suggests lung parenchymal loss consistent with emphysema, rather than asthma alone.

$\alpha_1$-Antitrypsin deficiency is an autosomal codominant condition. The major pulmonary manifestation is emphysema, but persons who have the Z allele also may develop cirrhosis and hepatoma, related to the inadequate secretion of Z protein from the hepatocyte.

This case also invites consideration of the causes of a decreased diffusing capacity for carbon monoxide. The diffusing capacity is a measurement of gas transfer across the alveolar-capillary units, which may be decreased when a loss occurs of pulmonary vasculature (e.g., pulmonary vascular disease or lung resection) or loss of lung parenchyma (as may be seen in emphysema or interstitial lung disease). Because the uptake of carbon monoxide by erythrocytes requires adequate red blood cells with hemoglobin avid for carbon monoxide, the diffusing capacity also will be decreased in the face of anemia or prior carbon monoxide poisoning (which creates a back pressure that decreases further uptake of carbon monoxide by red blood cells).

Pulmonary features that should lead to the consideration of severe $\alpha_1$-antitrypsin deficiency include emphysema at an early age (e.g., under the age of 45 years), emphysema in the absence of antecedent smoking, emphysema with a positive family history of lung or liver disease, and radiographic changes showing basilar hyperlucency (in contrast to the more apical distribution of emphysema changes in "garden variety" emphysema unrelated to $\alpha_1$-antitrypsin deficiency).

### 10. Test Profile 3 or 4

Patient profile 10 presents a 60-year-old man who smokes one to two packs of cigarettes per day. Pulmonary function profile 3 is considered the best choice, although profile 4 (characteristic of emphysema) would be acceptable. Pulmonary function profile 3 represents normal lung function, emphasizing that, although cigarette smoking can cause an accelerated decline in $FEV_1$, most cigarette smokers escape accelerated airflow obstruction. In fact, "susceptible" smokers with accelerated airflow decline are said to make up approximately 10% to 15% of all smokers. Even in susceptible smokers, the cessation of cigarette smoking slows the rate of decline of lung function to that of non-smokers, although the recovery of lost lung function after smoking cessation is uncommon.

## CASES 11–15

Five additional cases are presented for your consideration. Match the five patient profiles with the appropriate room air arterial blood gas pattern in Table 41.2. As before, each arterial blood gas pattern in Table 41.2 may be used once, more than once, or not at all.

### TABLE 41.2

### ROOM AIR ARTERIAL BLOOD GASES

| | Partial Pressure of Oxygen in Arterial Blood (mm Hg) | Arterial Pressure of Carbon Dioxide (mm Hg) | pH |
|---|---|---|---|
| 1. | 50 | 65 | 7.30 |
| 2. | 60 | 60 | 7.20 |
| 3. | 50 | 65 | 7.37 |
| 4. | 85 | 28 | 7.51 |
| 5. | 65 | 35 | 7.42 |

- *Patient Profile 11.* The patient is a 70-year-old man with fasciculations and upper motor neuron disease.
- *Patient Profile 12.* The patient is a 50-year-old man with dyspnea and panniculitis.
- *Patient Profile 13.* The patient is a 48-year-old man who is a heavy smoker and experiences acute confusion.
- *Patient Profile 14.* The patient is a 45-year-old woman who has sustained neck trauma.
- *Patient Profile 15.* The patient is a 25-year-old man, seen 3 weeks after a skiing accident and tibial fracture.

### Questions

**11.** What is the appropriate room air arterial blood gas pattern for patient 11?

**12.** What is the appropriate room air arterial blood gas pattern for patient 12?

**13.** What is the appropriate room air arterial blood gas pattern for patient 13?

**14.** What is the appropriate room air arterial blood gas pattern for patient 14?

**15.** What is the appropriate room air arterial blood gas pattern for patient 15?

### Discussion

In interpreting room air arterial blood gases, a calculation of the alveolar–arterial oxygen gradient is helpful. Table 41.3 depicts this calculation. Normal values of the alveolar–arterial oxygen gradient are age dependent, as depicted in Figure 41.4. A useful mnemonic for the mean age-specific alveolar–arterial oxygen gradient is (age/4 + 4), with the upper limit value of the age-specific alveolar–arterial oxygen gradient roughly calculated by the equation (age/4 + 4) + 10 mm Hg. A calculation of the alveolar–arterial oxygen gradient is useful in approaching the differential diagnosis of hypoxemia. Six causes of hypoxemia should be remembered: anatomic shunt, ventilation–perfusion (V/Q) mismatch, diffusion impairment, hypoventilation, inhaling a decreased inspired oxygen fraction, and diffusion–perfusion impairment (e.g., as seen in the hepatopulmonary

## TABLE 41.3

### ALVEOLAR–ARTERIAL OXYGEN GRADIENT (AaDO$_2$)

**Calculate the Alveolar Oxygen Tension (Pao$_2$)**

PaO$_2$ = (P$_B$−47)FIO$_2$−[(PaCO$_2$)/(resp quotient)]
P$_B$ = barometric pressure (e.g., 760 mm Hg)
PaCO$_2$ = arterial CO$_2$ tension
Resp quotient = Respiratory quotient (moles CO$_2$ produced per mole of O$_2$ consumed, usually 0.8)
Subtract PaO$_2$ (arterial oxygen tension)
AaDO$_2$ = P$_{A}$O$_2$−PaO$_2$

FIO$_2$, fraction of inspired oxygen.

syndrome). Of these six causes, diffusion–perfusion impairment is uncommon and is confined to patients with hypoxemia caused by the hepatopulmonary syndrome. Hypoxemia relating to inhaling decreased inspired oxygen fractions occurs only when the patient is exposed to high altitude or when a hypoxic gas mixture is breathed at sea level. Among the other four causes of hypoxemia (anatomic shunt, V/Q, diffusion impairment, and hypoventilation), the age-specific alveolar–arterial oxygen gradient is increased

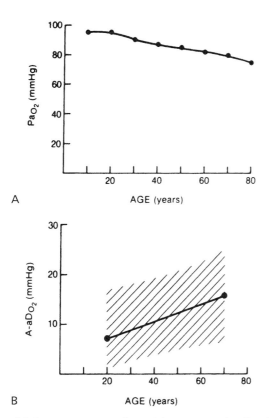

**Figure 41.4** **(A)** Variations of arterial oxygen tension (Pao$_2$) with age. **(B)** Variations of alveolar–arterial oxygen gradient (A – aDO$_2$) with age; mean values for A – aDO$_2$ = 2.5 + 0.21 × age; bold line indicates mean values; shaded area + 2 SD. (Reproduced with permission from Tisi G. *Pulmonary Physiology in Clinical Medicine.* Baltimore: Williams & Wilkins, 1980:78.)

for all causes except hypoventilation, in which the alveolar–arterial oxygen gradient is normal.

## Answers and Explanations

### 11. Pattern 3 or 5.

Patient profile 11 presents a 70-year-old man with fasciculations and upper motor neuron disease. The clinical scenario is intended to elicit the diagnosis of amyotrophic lateral sclerosis (ALS), a degenerative disease of the motor neurons that is slowly progressive and is associated with extrathoracic pulmonary restriction as well as blood gases reflecting hypoventilation or the effect of ventilation–perfusion ratio (V/Q) mismatch. In this instance, the most appropriate blood gas pattern would be profile 3 or 5.

Profile 3 represents a pattern of pure hypoventilation, which may be seen in neuromuscular diseases such as ALS. Alternately, patient profile 5 represents hypoxemia with hypocapnia (i.e., chronic respiratory alkalosis). In arterial blood gas profile 5, the alveolar–arterial oxygen gradient is widened, consistent with mismatch or anatomic shunt.

Using a rule-of-thumb equation (Table 41.3) for calculating the room air alveolar–arterial oxygen gradient: 149 – [partial pressure of oxygen in arterial blood (PaO$_2$) + arterial pressure of carbon dioxide (PaCO$_2$) (1.25)], the alveolar–arterial oxygen gradient in blood gas profile 3 is 149 – [50 + 65 (1.25)], or 18 mm Hg, which is normal for a 70-year-old man. Therefore, for a 70-year-old patient, arterial blood gas profile 3 indicates hypoventilation, which might accompany neuromuscular disease such as amyotrophic lateral sclerosis. In contrast, the value of the room air alveolar–arterial oxygen gradient for blood gas profile 5 is 40 mm Hg, which is elevated even for a 70-year-old man. Such a profile might be seen in neuromuscular disease, in which atelectasis is causing mismatch, thus resulting in hypoxemia without hypoventilation.

### 12. Pattern 5.

Patient profile 12 presents a 50-year-old man with dyspnea and panniculitis. The case is meant to suggest α$_1$- antitrypsin deficiency characterized by panniculitis and emphysema. Arterial blood gas profile 5 is considered the best answer, indicating hypoxemia with chronic respiratory alkalosis on the basis of long-standing mismatch.

### 13. Pattern 1.

Profile 13 presents a 48-year-old heavy smoker with acute confusion. The history of heavy smoking is meant to suggest severe chronic obstructive lung disease. Such a patient might demonstrate chronic hypoxemia with chronic hypercapnia and compensated respiratory acidosis. The presence of acute confusion, however, suggests an acute worsening of respiratory acidosis, as best demonstrated by the arterial blood gas profile 1.

### 14. Pattern 2.

Patient profile 14 presents a 45-year-old woman who has had neck trauma. Spinal cord injury above the level of C3, resulting in acute hypoventilation, should be considered. The expected arterial blood gas profile is that of hypoventilation with acute respiratory acidosis, best represented by arterial blood gas profile 2. In this case, a pH of 7.20 indicates acute respiratory acidosis and the room air alveolar– arterial oxygen gradient is 14 mm Hg, again demonstrating hypoventilation.

### 15. Profile 4.

Patient profile 15 presents a 25-year-old man 3 weeks after a skiing accident and tibial fracture. The clinical setting should suggest the possibility of an acute pulmonary embolism. An acute respiratory alkalosis with a widened alveolar–arterial oxygen gradient would be expected and is best demonstrated by arterial blood gas profile 4. In this case, the alveolar–arterial oxygen gradient is 29 mm Hg, which is above normal for a 25-year-old man. This case serves as a reminder that patients with acute pulmonary emboli may not demonstrate hypoxemia, but that the alveolar–arterial oxygen gradient is usually (but not uniformly) elevated.

## CASES 16–20: RECOGNIZING DISEASE ASSOCIATIONS

Questions on the board examinations are less likely to address straightforward associations, such as common complications of commonly used medications and common medical manifestations of common illnesses. In the spirit of simulating the types of questions posed by the board examination, the following sections of the Pulmonary Board Simulation are meant to resemble more board-like problems.

In the following exercise, the reader is asked to match the lung diseases in the left column with the associated condition or conditions on the right. More than one condition in the right column can be associated with each lung disease on the left, and associating one of the conditions in the right column with the lung disease on the left does not preclude the associated condition from being matched with other lung diseases on the left.

| Lung Disease | Associated Condition |
| --- | --- |
| 16. PI*ZZ $\alpha_1$-antitrypsin deficiency | Hepatoma |
| 17. Intrapulmonary vascular dilatations | Hepatic cirrhosis |
| 18. Pulmonary arteriovenous malformation | Lymphangioleiomyomatosis |
| 19. Pulmonary hypertension | Hereditary hemorrhagic telangiectasis |
| 20. Chylous pleural effusion | |

## Questions

**16.** Which associated condition or conditions are associated with PI*ZZ $\alpha_1$-antitrypsin deficiency?

**17.** With which associated condition on the right is there an association with intrapulmonary vascular dilatations?

**18.** With which associated condition(s) are pulmonary arteriovenous malformations matched?

**19.** With which associated condition is pulmonary hypertension best matched?

**20.** With which associated condition(s) is a chylous pleural effusion related?

## Answers and Explanations

### 16. Hepatoma and hepatic cirrhosis.

Since the early description of $\alpha_1$-antitrypsin deficiency, hepatic complications were recognized as a feature of PI*ZZ homozygous $\alpha_1$-antitrypsin deficiency in approximately 12% of affected persons. The spectrum of liver diseases includes cirrhosis, hepatoma, and neonatal jaundice. Indeed, the complications of $\alpha_1$-antitrypsin deficiency pose a challenge to the internist assessing the patient with idiopathic cirrhosis, although liver complications are far more common in children with $\alpha_1$-antitrypsin deficiency. In this context, homozygous PI*ZZ $\alpha_1$-antitrypsin deficiency sometimes causes neonatal jaundice progressing to liver failure and, as such, $\alpha_1$-antitrypsin deficiency is the second most common indication for liver transplantation in children. Unlike the mechanism of lung destruction in $\alpha_1$-antitrypsin deficiency (which is due to unopposed elastolytic activity in the lung interstitium), liver disease seems to result from the intrahepatocyte accumulation of unsecreted Z-type $\alpha_1$-antitrypsin. The Z mutation is caused by a single amino acid substitution at position 342 of the 394 amino acid glycoprotein, which is $\alpha_1$-antitrypsin. The substitution of a lysine for a glutamic acid residue at position 342 causes abnormal folding as the protein is secreted from the endoplasmic reticulum for glycosylation and packaging at the Golgi apparatus. Abnormal folding allows polymerization within the hepatocyte (a process called *loop-sheet polymerization*), which impairs the normal secretion of the protein from the liver into the bloodstream. As such, liver disease in Z-type $\alpha_1$-antitrypsin deficiency is more akin to a hepatic inclusion disease (e.g., Gaucher's disease) than it is due to unopposed proteolytic breakdown of the liver parenchyma.

Increasing evidence suggests that PI*ZZ-type persons who develop liver disease have abnormal processing of the unsecreted protein. Current understanding suggests that persons at risk for liver disease are less able to clear the unsecreted protein than PI*ZZ individuals not destined to develop liver disease, although the pathogenetic mechanism by which the accumulation of intrahepatocyte protein leads to cirrhosis or hepatoma remains unknown.

Although more than 100 alleles for the $\alpha_1$-antitrypsin protein have been identified, the PI*ZZ homozygous state accounts for 95% of all clinically recognized severe $\alpha_1$-antitrypsin deficiency. Other rare phenotypes that also can give rise to liver disease include PI*M malton and PI* Siyama.

Those aspects of $\alpha_1$-antitrypsin deficiency that lend themselves to being tested in the context of a board examination include (i) emphysema with early age of onset or emphysema without concomitant cigarette smoking; (ii) emphysema presenting with basilar hyperlucency on the chest radiograph (versus the more expected clinical changes of emphysema seen with the more common type of $\alpha_1$-antitrypsin–replete cigarette smoking–related emphysema); (iii) the occurrence of liver disease as noted previously, characterized by the presence of inclusion bodies within the hepatocyte; such inclusion bodies stain positively with periodic acid–Schiff and are resistant to digestion by diastase; and (iv) the autosomal codominant inheritance pattern of $\alpha_1$-antitrypsin deficiency.

### 17. Hepatic cirrhosis.

This question asks the examinee to recognize the hepatopulmonary syndrome as a complication of chronic liver disease, usually cirrhosis, of various causes. The hepatopulmonary syndrome is a disease characterized by a widened alveolar–arterial oxygen gradient, often with associated dyspnea or platypnea (breathlessness that develops on upright posture). The physiologic and pathologic hallmark of the hepatopulmonary syndrome is the development of intrapulmonary vascular dilatations, which are sometimes apparent on plain chest radiographs as a "spongy" interstitial pattern of the lung bases.

Prevalence estimates suggest that the hepatopulmonary syndrome occurs in up to 40% of patients with chronic liver disease, but it is often subclinical in that it has a relatively small impact on gas exchange or symptoms. Conversely, the hepatopulmonary syndrome can be quite debilitating and can outstrip the symptomatic impact of liver disease on these patients. In such instances, liver transplantation is considered for the treatment of the underlying hepatopulmonary syndrome, rather than the end-stage liver disease alone. Various series suggest that the associated hypoxemia and its symptomatic consequences can completely reverse following liver transplantation, although predicting this response remains difficult.

The diagnosis of the hepatopulmonary syndrome requires clinical suspicion as well as the demonstration of right-to-left intrapulmonary shunt, which is often evaluated using contrast-enhanced echocardiography,

using either agitated saline or (less commonly) indocyanine. The visualization of "bubbles" of agitated saline within the left heart chambers is an abnormal finding and demonstrates right-to-left shunt. The timing of the appearance of bubbles in the left heart chambers indicates whether the shunt is *intracardiac* (when bubbles appear within 3 beats of injection) or *intrapulmonary* (bubbles appear for 4 to 6 beats after injection as a result of the need for bubbles to traverse the pulmonary circulation before appearing in the left heart chambers). This so-called *bubble echocardiogram* is highly sensitive for the presence of the hepatopulmonary syndrome, but it lacks specificity in that many patients lacking clinically significant manifestations of the hepatopulmonary syndrome show evidence of a positive "bubble study."

### 18. Hepatic cirrhosis and hereditary hemorrhagic telangiectasia.

Question 18 asks the reader to recognize that hereditary hemorrhagic telangiectasia (otherwise known as Osler-Weber-Rendu syndrome) is accompanied by various arteriovenous malformations, including pulmonary arteriovenous malformations in 5% to 15% of affected persons.

In addition, hepatic cirrhosis is considered correct because intrapulmonary vascular dilatations, a hallmark feature of hepatopulmonary syndrome, are a type of arteriovenous malformation in the lung.

First recognized by Rendu in 1896, *hereditary hemorrhagic telangiectasia* is an autosomal-dominant disease, with variable penetrance, characterized by the development of vascular abnormalities in various organs. The most common manifestation is epistaxis due to nasal telangiectasia, usually with onset by the age of 21 years. Telangiectasias characterized by small lesions, usually on the lips, tongue, or fingers, are of later onset. The subject of this question is the development of pulmonary arteriovenous malformations, which occur in 5% to 15% of persons with hereditary hemorrhagic telangiectasia. These arteriovenous malformations are often multiple and are located in the lower lobes of the lung. Chest radiographic features include smooth, nodular densities, sometimes with "vascular feeder" vessels entering the pulmonary "nodule." Hypoxemia may result from the concomitant right-to-left shunt, as can platypnea. Several points emphasize the importance of recognizing pulmonary arteriovenous malformations. First, clinical suspicion of a vascular abnormality is important to avoid attempted biopsy, which could be accompanied by serious bleeding. Second, clinical recognition is important because pulmonary arteriovenous malformations allow venous blood to enter the systemic arterial circulation without normal filtration by the lung vasculature. As such, patients with pulmonary arteriovenous malformations complicating the Osler-Weber-Rendu syndrome are at risk for brain abscess. This risk has led to the clinical recommendation that pulmonary arteriovenous malformations should be ablated, either surgically or by embolization. Such embolization therapy can reverse hypoxemia, and it also lessens the risk of brain abscess.

The diagnostic criteria for the hereditary hemorrhagic telangiectasia syndrome include the presence of at least two of the following diagnostic criteria:

- Recurrent epistaxis
- Telangiectasias outside the nose
- Autosomal dominant inheritance
- Visceral involvement either of lung, gastrointestinal tract, or brain

Specifically, the brain and gastrointestinal tract also can be the site of vascular abnormalities that predispose to bleeding or vessel rupture, with associated neurologic consequences.

### 19. Hepatic cirrhosis.

This question asks the reader to recognize the association between hepatic cirrhosis and pulmonary hypertension, another pulmonary manifestation of chronic liver disease. Unlike the hepatopulmonary syndrome, in which pulmonary vascular resistance is actually decreased (because arteriovenous channels open), pulmonary hypertension complicating hepatic cirrhosis has been called the *hepatopulmonary syndrome.* Less common than the hepatopulmonary syndrome, portopulmonary hypertension occurs in 3% to 5% of patients with chronic liver disease. The pathophysiology is poorly understood, but the presence of portal hypertension is required, and portopulmonary hypertension has been described in cases of portal hypertension in the absence of substantial parenchymal liver damage (e.g., hepatic vein thrombosis).

The question also invites the reader's understanding of the etiologies of pulmonary hypertension, which can be considered according to an anatomic schema. Starting with the left ventricle, left-sided congestive heart failure or ventricular hypertrophy with a noncompliant left ventricle can cause pulmonary hypertension. Diseases affecting the mitral valve, including mitral stenosis, mitral regurgitation, and left atrial myxoma, also may contribute to pulmonary hypertension. Diseases of the pulmonary veins, such as pulmonary vein thrombosis (e.g., pulmonary veno-occlusive disease), and diseases encasing the pulmonary veins (e.g., fibrosing mediastinitis, neoplasm) can cause pulmonary hypertension. Diseases of the pulmonary capillaries, such as pulmonary hemangiomatosis, also are a consideration. Diseases causing a constriction of the pulmonary arteries, such as hypoxic states with secondary pulmonary vasoconstriction, can cause pulmonary hypertension.

Pulmonary thromboembolic disease is an important consideration, as are diseases causing primary vasospasm of the pulmonary arteries. Examples include collagen–vascular diseases, such as scleroderma and systemic lupus erythematosus, human immunodeficiency virus infection, and diet pills (including the European drug called aminorex and dexfenfluramine, which has been withdrawn), as well as true "primary" pulmonary hypertension, which denotes pulmonary arterial pressure elevation in the absence of an alternative explanation. Diseases causing increased flow through the pulmonary artery, such as atrial or ventricular septal defects, can cause pulmonary hypertension and should be considered in the differential diagnosis.

### 20. Lymphangioleiomyomatosis.

Chylous pleural effusion, as commonly seen in lymphangioleiomyomatosis and other conditions (see following discussion), is characterized by the presence of chyle within the pleural fluid. The source of chyle is the thoracic duct, so a chylous pleural effusion reflects a disruption of the thoracic duct or interruption of normal lymph flow.

A defining characteristic of chylothorax is the presence of chyle, most frequently demonstrated by the presence of triglyceride level exceeding 110 mg/dL within the pleural fluid. Conversely, a triglyceride level below 50 mg/dL is thought to exclude chylothorax, and triglyceride values between these values (50 to 110 mg/dL) are equivocal and require validation by demonstrating other elements of chyle, for example, chylomicrons. Chylomicrons can be demonstrated through lipoprotein electrophoresis.

A common, but not universal, feature of chylothorax is the milky appearance of the fluids, although dietary avoidance of complex fats can cause chylothoraces to lack this suggestive feature.

The causes of chylothorax characteristically involve a disruption or interruption of normal lymph flow. Neoplasm represents the most common cause, most frequently lymphoma. Surgical or other trauma represents another common etiology, including the possibility of disruption of the thorax duct by the placement of a central venous catheter into the right neck. Congenital and idiopathic causes constitute a third broad group, as do miscellaneous causes. Among the miscellaneous causes, pulmonary lymphangioleiomyomatosis figures prominently, along with tuberculosis, sarcoidosis, Behçet's syndrome with superior vena cava obstruction, and Gorham's syndrome, a rare disease of children and young adults characterized by the intraosseous development of vascular or lymphatic channels contributing to bone lysis.

Among the known etiologies of chylous pleural effusion, only lymphangioleiomyomatosis appears among the choices given. Hence, this is the preferred answer.

Lymphangioleiomyomatosis is an uncommon condition occurring almost exclusively in women and characterized by a proliferation of smooth muscle in the lung interstitium. Common presenting symptoms include dyspnea and pneumothorax, but chylous pleural effusion, chyloptysis (the expectoration of chylous material), and chylous ascites have been described. The presumed mechanism is lymphatic obstruction by the known smooth muscle proliferation. One other testable feature of lymphangioleiomyomatosis is the fairly characteristic appearance of the high-resolution chest computed tomography (CT), showing a reticulonodular interstitial infiltrate characterized by diffuse cystic changes. Although characteristic of lymphangioleiomyomatosis, cysts also may occur in eosinophilic granuloma of lung, a distinction that may require lung biopsy. Finally, patients with lymphangioleiomyomatosis may demonstrate associated renal angiomyolipomas, which are hamartomatous tumors of the kidneys, also seen in association with tuberous sclerosis.

## CASE 21

A 45-year-old man with known insulin-dependent diabetes mellitus has developed infection causing diabetic ketoacidosis. With this episode, his electrolytes are as follows: sodium, 145 mEq/L; chloride, 90 mEq/L; potassium, 5.1 mEq/L; and bicarbonate, 16 mEq/L. His anion gap (delta) is 29. Arterial blood gases are drawn on room air because he is tachypneic. The arterial blood gasses show $PaO_2$, 70 mm Hg; $PaCO_2$, 40 mm Hg; and pH, 7.28. In addition to his anion gap metabolic acidosis, you are called on to assess whether his respiratory response is appropriate for the clinical condition.

### Question

21. Specifically, is this a simple metabolic acidosis? Is he compensating appropriately for the metabolic acidosis?
a) Yes
b) No

### Discussion

The assessment of whether the respiratory response to a metabolic acidosis is appropriate can be aided by using the "Winter's equation." The Winter's equation predicts the $PCO_2$ for observed serum bicarbonate with the following relationship:

$$PCO_2 = [1.5 \, (HCO_3^-) + 8] \pm 2$$

The Winter's equation was derived from studying a population of patients with metabolic acidosis of various types and performing a regression equation of the observed $PCO_2$ against the measured serum bicarbonate values. None of these patients had intrinsic pulmonary disease, neuromuscular disease, or other insults that would cause respiratory depression or stimulate respiratory drive (e.g., aspirin overdose, liver disease).

## Answer and Explanation

### 21. b.

No, the patient has a complex acid–base disorder with an anion gap metabolic acidosis, a respiratory acidosis, and a concomitant antecedent metabolic alkalosis.

Specifically, in the current case, the patient's serum bicarbonate is 16 mEq/L, suggesting that an inappropriate respiratory response would be a $PCO_2$ of [1.5 (16) + 8] ± 2, or 30 to 34 mm Hg.

The patient's observed $PCO_2$ is 40 mm Hg, higher than expected, and indicates a respiratory acidosis in addition to the metabolic acidosis. Further assessment of the case indicates the presence of metabolic alkalosis as well. Using the concept of the "delta delta" (as discussed in Chapter 53), we can determine what the patient's serum bicarbonate was before he experienced this metabolic acidosis. Specifically, to have an elevated anion gap of 29 [which exceeds the upper limits of normal (12) by 17], the patient would have had a serum bicarbonate 17 mEq/L higher than the currently observed value of 16 mEq/L, or 33 mEq/L. In other words, to get to the current serum bicarbonate of 16 mEq/ L, 17 mEq/L of bicarbonate was eliminated by the patient's current acid load. The serum bicarbonate value of 33 mEq/L at that time suggests a slight metabolic alkalosis before the current illness. The Winter's equation used to determine an appropriately compensated $PCO_2$ response to a metabolic acidosis is clinically important because it allows the clinician to assess whether the patient may be experiencing respiratory failure. In the current case, although the $PCO_2$ is 40 mm Hg and is within the normal range, the presence of a respiratory acidosis on top of a metabolic acidosis raises some concern about the possibility of ventilatory failure and would cause the clinician to observe the patient closely over the short term with regard to worsening hypercapnia.

## CASE 22

You are asked to evaluate a plain chest radiograph showing an upper lobe infiltrate.

### Question

22. Which of the following diseases is *least likely* to present with an upper lobe infiltrate?
a) Rheumatoid arthritis
b) Asbestosis
c) Histoplasmosis
d) Tuberculosis
e) Ankylosing spondylitis

### Discussion

This question tests the reader's awareness of classic radiographic patterns. Indeed, the distribution of infiltrates on the plain chest radiograph is often helpful in focusing the differential diagnosis because diseases may have classic radiographic "signatures." At the same time, clinical variability requires that the astute clinician recognizes the possibility of exceptions to every clinical "rule."

## Answer and Explanation

### 22. b.

As prompted by this question, several diseases are characterized by upper lobe distribution and others by a lower lobe distribution. Examples of "upper lobe diseases" include tuberculosis (especially reactivation), histoplasmosis (which can mimic tuberculosis), and the upper lobe, usually bilateral fibrocavitary changes that may accompany ankylosing spondylitis and rheumatoid arthritis. Other upper lobe processes include Pancoast tumors, which by definition involve the stellate ganglion and may present with a Horner's syndrome and evidence of a brachial plexopathy, and melioidosis due to *Burkholderia pseudomallei*, a Gram-negative bacterium often contracted from soil exposure in Asia.

Classic lower lobe processes include idiopathic pulmonary fibrosis (characterized by increased interstitial markings, which are more pronounced at the bases than at the apices of the lung and which abut the pleuropulmonary interface, often accompanied by honeycomb changes), asbestosis (which may be accompanied by calcified pleural plaques indicating asbestos exposure), pulmonary histiocytosis X (also known as pulmonary Langerhans cell histiocytosis and eosinophilic granuloma of lung, and in which the costophrenic angles are often spared), and emphysema due to severe deficiency of $\alpha_1$-antitrypsin (in which the emphysematous changes almost invariably involve the lung bases, often more so than the apices, thus distinguishing $\alpha_1$-antitrypsin deficiency from the usual causes of emphysema, such as centriacinar smoking-related emphysema, in which the apices are often preferentially affected).

Finally, the radiographic signatures of lung diseases can vary by whether the infiltrates are more central or peripheral. Examples of diseases characterized by central infiltrates include congestive heart failure and pulmonary alveolar proteinosis. In contrast, chronic eosinophilic pneumonia, an illness classically affecting middle-aged women and characterized by pulmonary eosinophilia and bronchospasm, has been described as having a "photo-negative appearance," meaning that the periphery of the lung may show more dense infiltrates than the central areas of the lung. Another classically peripheral process is the "Hampton's hump" that may accompany pulmonary embolism, and which represents an area of pulmonary infarction in an area whose blood supply has been compromised by the embolism.

## REFERENCE

1. Lawry GV, Finerman, ML, Hanafee WN, et al. Laryngeal involvement in rheumatoid arthritis. A clinical, laryngoscopic, and computerized tomographic study. *Arthritis Rheum* 1984;27:873–882.

## SUGGESTED READINGS

Aboussouan LS, Stoller JK. Diagnosis and management of upper airway obstruction. *Clin Chest Med* 1994;15:35–53.

Albert MS, Dell RB, Winters RW. Quantitative displacement of acid-base equilibrium in metabolic acidosis. *Ann Intern Med* 1967; 66:312–322.

Alpha-1 Antitrypsin Deficiency Task Force. American Thoracic Society/European Respiratory Society Statement: Standards for the diagnosis and management of individuals with alpha-1 antitrypsin deficiency. *Am J Respir Crit Care Med* 2003;168:818–900.

Kryger MH, Bode F, Antic R, et al. Diagnosis of obstruction of the upper and central airways. *Am J Med* 1976;61:85–93.

Light RW. Chylothorax and pseudochylothorax. In: *Pleural Diseases*, 3rd ed. Baltimore: Williams & Wilkins, 1995:284–295.

McFarlane MJ, Imperiale TF. Use of the alveolar-arterial oxygen gradient in the diagnosis of pulmonary embolism. *Am J Med* 1994; 96:57–62.

Miller RD, Hyatt RE. Obstructing lesions of the larynx and trachea: clinical and physiologic characteristics. *Mayo Clin Proc* 1969; 44:145–161.

Narins RD, Emmett M. Simple and mixed acid-based disorders: the practical approach. *Medicine* 1980;59:161–187.

Stein PD, Goldhaber SZ, Henry JW. Alveolar-arterial oxygen gradient in the assessment of acute pulmonary embolism. *Chest* 1995; 107:139–143.

Stoller JK. Clinical features of alpha-1 antitrypsin deficiency. *Chest* 1997;111:1235–1285.

Stoller JK. Spirometry: a key diagnostic test in pulmonary medicine. *Cleve Clin J Med* 1992;59:75–78.

# Endocrinology

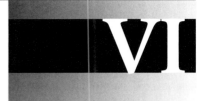

# Thyroid Disorders

## Charles Faiman

## 42

Thyroid hormone secretion is regulated by the hypothalamo–pituitary–thyroid axis (Figure 42.1), which has the following characteristics:

- Approximately 25% of the circulating triiodothyronine ($T_3$) is derived from direct secretion by the thyroid gland; the remainder comes from peripheral conversion.
- Reverse $T_3$, which is biologically inert, is produced instead of active $T_3$ in the sick euthyroid state and in the fetus.
- Circulating thyroid hormones are mainly bound to proteins:
  - Thyroxine-binding globulin (TBG) binds both thyroxine ($T_4$) and $T_3$.
  - Prealbumin (TBPA, also called *transthyretin*) binds only $T_4$.
  - Albumin binds both $T_4$ and $T_3$.
  - 99.97% of $T_4$ and 99.7% of $T_3$ are bound.
- The free hormone is active.

## THYROID FUNCTION TESTS

Thyroid function tests include:

- Thyroid-stimulating hormone (TSH) (sensitive/ultra-sensitive), the best single indicator of thyroid function
- Total $T_4$
- $T_4$ uptake ($T_4U$) or $T_3$ resin uptake ($T_3RU$) (estimates of binding)
- Free thyroxine index (FTI), adjusted for serum protein binding
- Free $T_4$ ($FT_4$)
- Total $T_3$
- Free $T_3$

Factors that alter binding or binding capacity result in alterations in total $T_4$ and total $T_3$:

- Changes in TBG influence both $T_4$ and $T_3$ values
- Changes in TBPA influence $T_4$ values only

The following conditions are associated with TBG excess:

- Pregnancy
- Drug use (estrogen, tamoxifen, raloxifene, heroin, methadone, perphenazine)
- Acute hepatitis

- Chronic active hepatitis
- Acute intermittent porphyria
- Hereditary conditions

The following conditions are associated with TBG deficiency:

- Excess androgens
- Acromegaly
- Hypoproteinemia
- Nephrotic syndrome
- Chronic liver disease
- Glucocorticoids (large doses)
- Hereditary conditions

The measurement of the binding proteins by a $T_4U$ test or $T_3RU$ test and calculation of the FTI help to correct for the effect of changes in the binding proteins on thyroid hormone levels. Newer assays of $FT_4$ are at least equal to the FTI and, in some cases, better. $FT_4$ by equilibrium dialysis remains the gold standard, but it is too expensive for routine clinical use.

Important points for the clinician to remember:

- A high $T_4U$ test (or low $T_3RU$ test) indicates that thyroid hormone–binding sites are present in excess, which can be caused by:
  - Excessive binding protein (see previous discussion)
  - Diminished occupancy (hypothyroidism)
- A low $T_4U$ (or high $T_3RU$ test) indicates that thyroid hormone–binding sites are deficient because of:
  - Diminished binding protein (see previous discussion)
  - Excessive occupancy (hyperthyroidism)

Drugs or conditions (e.g., sick euthyroidism) that interfere with thyroid hormone protein–binding are listed in Tables 42.1 through 42.3.

Thyroid function tests are readily interpretable in ambulatory patients, but are often not helpful or may be confusing in the hospitalized sick patient.

### Tests for Hypothyroidism

Thyroid function tests for diagnosing hypothyroidism include:

- TSH (0.4–4.5 μU/mL, normal); the upper limit of normal remains controversial, with values as low as 2.5 to 3.5 having been advocated but not generally accepted:

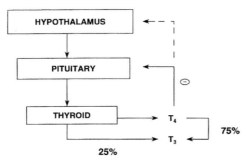

**Figure 42.1** Hypothalamo-pituitary-thyroid axis. $T_3$, triiodothyronine; $T_4$, thyroxine.

□ >10–20 μU/mL, diagnostic (caveats: newborn or recovery phase of sick euthyroidism)

□ 4.5–10.0 μU/mL, borderline or subclinical hypothyroidism (may be normal for geriatric population), assess for goiter; order $T_4$, FTI, or $FT_4$; order thyroid microsomal antibodies (TMA); decide on replacement therapy versus observation

□ Beware that normal (or low) values can be seen with pituitary (secondary) or hypothalamic (tertiary) hypothyroidism

■ FTI or $FT_4$
  □ May also be used as primary test
  □ Less discriminating
■ $T_3$ is of no value
■ Radioactive iodine uptake (RAIU) is not indicated and may mislead
■ Consider TMA as a cause of hypothyroidism/goiter

## Tests for Hyperthyroidism

Thyroid function tests for diagnosing hyperthyroidism include:

■ TSH
  □ Normal, 0.4–4.5 μU/mL
  □ Suppressed, <0.02–0.1 μU/mL (depends on assay sensitivity)

---

### TABLE 42.2
### EUTHYROID HYPOTHYROXINEMIA

Decreased thyroxine-binding globulin production
Severe systemic illness
Glucocorticoids
Androgens
Familial X-linked (many variants)
Excessive thyroxine-binding globulin loss
Protein-losing enteropathy
Nephrosis
Jejunoileal bypass
Inhibition of protein binding
Systemic illness (free fatty acids and tissue factor)
Dilantin (in vitro, possibly not in vivo)
Salicylates
Furosemide
Fenclofenac

---

□ 0.1–0.4 μU/mL, consider:
  □ Early autonomy
  □ Slight overreplacement
  □ Drug side effects (e.g., steroids, dopamine)
  □ Pregnancy (first trimester)
■ FTI or $FT_4$: helpful particularly if TSH is low
■ $T_3$ or $FT_3$ (if TSH suppressed and FTI or $FT_4$ normal)
  □ Think of early hyperthyroidism or thyroid extract treatment

## Tests for Euthyroid Sick Syndrome

Thyroid function tests for diagnosing euthyroid sick syndrome include:

■ $T_4$, normal (N), or ↑
■ $T_4U$, ↓ or N
■ $T_3RU$, ↑ or N
■ FTI or $FT_4$, N, or ↓
■ $T_3$, ↓
■ Reverse $T_3$, ↑
■ TSH, N, or ↓ (↑ in recovery phase)

---

### TABLE 42.1
### FACTORS INHIBITING $T_4$ TO $T_3$ CONVERSION

Systemic illness (acute or chronic)
Caloric deprivation (fasting, anorexia nervosa, or protein-calorie malnutrition)
Surgery
Newborn
Aging
Drugs [glucocorticoids, propranolol (high doses), amiodarone, propylthiouracil]
Contrast media (ipodate, iopanoic acid)

$T_3$, triiodothyronine; $T_4$, thyroxine.

---

### TABLE 42.3
### EUTHYROID HYPERTHYROXINEMIA

Binding protein abnormalities [excess binding to thyroxine-binding globulin, thyroxine-binding prealbumin, or albumin (rare to $T_4$ antibodies)]
Transient hyperthyroxinemia of acute medical or psychiatric illness
Decreased peripheral conversion of $T_4$ to $T_3$, especially by propranolol or amiodarone
Amphetamine ingestion
Tissue resistance to thyroid hormone

$T_3$, triiodothyronine; $T_4$, thyroxine.

In the euthyroid sick syndrome, response to thyrotropin-releasing hormone is normal or blunted. TRH testing is of little or no value with the advent of sensitive TSH assays, except as a test for pituitary function (TSH and prolactin reserve).

No more vexing problem arises in the interpretation of thyroid function tests than the euthyroid sick syndrome. The information in this chapter is a guide, but it does not represent an absolute interpretation because overlap in test results is common, and confounding factors are frequent. Therefore, clinical acumen is critical. Because isolated TSH deficiency is uncommon (isolated secondary hypothyroidism), it is important to look for other signs of hypopituitarism; however, gonadotropins also may be suppressed during the acute stress and starvation state. The new tests of $FT_4$ have problems similar to those of FTI in this syndrome. The changes in thyroid function tests reflect the severity of illness.

Mortality is inversely proportional to total $T_4$ in euthyroid medical intensive care unit patients. $T_4$ treatment of patients with severe nonthyroidal illness and low $T_4$ does not help, however, and could possibly harm.

## Other Thyroid Tests

Other diagnostic thyroid tests include:

- TMA, also called *thyroid peroxidase* (TPO) antibodies
- Thyroglobulin (Tg) antibodies
- Thyroid receptor antibodies, stimulating [thyroid-stimulating immunoglobulins (TSI)] and receptor binding
- Tg
- Serum or urinary iodide
- RAIU
- Thyroid scan (RAI or pertechnetate)
- Thyroid ultrasound
- Fine-needle biopsy

The measurement of serum Tg, the protein that is iodinated to make $T_4$ and $T_3$, can reveal either increased or decreased thyroid activity: Elevated Tg levels reflect increased secretory activity by or damage to the thyroid, and low Tg levels indicate a paucity of thyroid tissue or suppressed activity.

The test is useful in the diagnosis of thyrotoxicosis factitia. The highest Tg levels are seen in metastatic differentiated nonmedullary thyroid carcinoma; therefore, the test also is useful in monitoring patients with thyroid cancer (see Thyroid Nodules and Cancer, later in this chapter). Beware of artifacts caused by the presence of antithyroglobulin antibodies.

The measurement of serum thyroid antibodies provides additional information on antimicrosomal (peroxidase) and antithyroglobulin, and TSH receptor–stimulating antibodies. Antimicrosomal (peroxidase) antibodies and antithyroglobulin antibodies are occasionally useful in the management of hypothyroidism and in screening for the polyglandular autoimmune syndrome. TSH receptor–stimulating antibodies, the cause of thyrotoxicosis in Graves' disease, may help to predict remission of this disease following treatment with antithyroid drugs.

Thyroid scanning and RAIU are less helpful because patients with hypothyroidism can have low, "normal," or high RAIU, and patients with hyperthyroidism can have low, "normal," or high RAIU. The RAIU is clinically useful only in the differential diagnosis of hyperthyroidism, in the calculation of radioiodine dosage, and in concert with a scan, in the management of thyroid carcinoma. Note that RAIU gives you a number; a scan gives you a picture.

# SCREENING FOR THYROID DYSFUNCTION

## Neonatal Screening

Neonatal screening programs, usually based on heel-prick blood TSH assays, are mandatory in most states in the United States and in most developed countries. The prevention of cretinism (1:4,000 live births) is far more cost effective using TSH assays than were the original phenylketonuria screening programs.

The following problems may be encountered:

- Location, institution, and maintenance of therapy in neonates with abnormal test results
- Need for new strategies to help differentiate the physiologic neonatal TSH surge from pathologic primary hypothyroidism (not a problem when studies are done on or after 3 days of life)
- Rare cases of hypothalamic-pituitary hypothyroidism missed unless a simultaneous $T_4$ assay is performed

## Adult Screening

Who should be screened? Keep in mind that to screen for a disease assumes that detecting the disease is beneficial to the patient and that screening itself is not harmful to those without the disease. Even in hypothyroidism, in which therapy is easy, the costs of screening a large population are not trivial. Therefore, screening should be performed only in populations with a reasonably high prevalence of thyroid dysfunction, such as women over the age of 40 years and patients admitted to specialized geriatric units. There is little reason to screen the general population, either in the ambulatory setting or on hospitalization. The issue of the treatment of subclinical thyroid disease is controversial. Data are accumulating, however, to indicate that subclinical thyroid disease is common (5% to 10% in population surveys) and is worth delineating from a cost-effectiveness point of view (1,2). Because undiagnosed hypothyroidism in pregnancy may adversely affect fetal neurologic development, screening for thyroid deficiency during pregnancy also may be warranted (3).

**TABLE 42.4**

**SUMMARY OF RECOMMENDED TESTS FOR THYROID DYSFUNCTION**

| Condition | Type | Recommended Tests | Additional Tests |
|---|---|---|---|
| Hypothyroidism | Primary | TSH | Thyroid microsomal antibody |
| | Pituitary/hypothalamic | $T_4$-FTI or free $T_4$ | Pituitary function (e.g., cortisol) |
| Hyperthyroidism | Various | TSH | $T_4$-FTI, free $T_4$, $T_3$ |
| | | Radioactive iodine uptake scan | |
| | | TSH receptor antibodies | |
| Sick euthyroid | | TSH, free $T_4$, $T_3$ | Pituitary function |
| Thyroid cancer | Papillary/follicular | Thyroglobulin, TSH | $T_4$-FTI, free $T_4$, $T_3$ |
| Screening | Neonatal | TSH | $T_4$ |
| | Adult | TSH | |

FTI, free thyroxine index; $T_3$, triiodothyronine; $T_4$, thyroxine; TSH, thyroid-stimulating hormone.

How should screening be done? High-sensitivity TSH screening is probably the most effective way to screen ambulatory populations, because it has superior test characteristics, because primary hypothyroidism is the most common form of abnormal thyroid function (far more common than secondary hypothyroidism), and because primary hyperthyroidism is far more common than secondary hyperthyroidism.

In outpatients, the sensitivity and specificity of $FT_4$ and FTI is approximately 90% in the diagnosis of hyperthyroidism, whereas the sensitivity and specificity of the high-sensitivity TSH assay is approximately 99%. The operating characteristics of these tests are far worse in hospitalized patients, in whom the specificity of the TSH assay is particularly low (Table 42.4).

## HYPOTHYROIDISM

Hypothyroidism is the clinical disorder that results from insufficient thyroid hormone action.

### Etiology

Hypothyroidism is a common disease, more prevalent in women (1% to 2% prevalence) than in men (0.1% prevalence). In one large study from England, 25% to 30% of patients were iatrogenic. Hypothyroidism is particularly common in elderly persons. Congenital hypothyroidism occurs in 1 of every 4,000 newborns. The causes of hypothyroidism can be subdivided into three groupings (common causes are italicized):

- Primary (thyroid cause)
  - Agenesis
  - Destruction of gland
  - Surgical removal

  - *Irradiation* (therapeutic radioactive iodine for thyrotoxicosis or external irradiation therapy for nonthyroid malignant disease of the neck)
  - Autoimmune disease (Hashimoto's disease)
  - *Idiopathic atrophy* (possibly after autoimmune disease)
  - Replacement by cancer or other infiltrative process
  - Inhibition of synthesis and release of thyroid hormone
  - Iodine deficiency
  - Excess iodide in susceptible individuals
  - Antithyroid drugs
  - Lithium
  - Inherited enzyme defects
- Transient causes
  - After surgery or therapeutic radioactive iodine
  - Postpartum
  - In the course of thyroiditis
- Secondary to pituitary or hypothalamic disease
  - Resistance to thyroid hormones

### Clinical Presentation

The clinical presentation of hypothyroidism depends on the pathogenesis: sudden onset (e.g., after thyroidectomy) versus gradual decline (e.g., owing to idiopathic atrophy). In the former, the clinical onset relates to the serum half-life of $T_4$ (1 week) and occurs in a matter of weeks. In the latter, decreases in thyroid hormone levels may take place over years. In addition, the clinical picture depends on the age of the patient. Because thyroid hormone is essential for brain development, a neonatal onset has different manifestations from an adult onset.

Symptoms of hypothyroidism include:

- Constitutional symptoms (weakness, fatigue, lethargy, and sleepiness)
- Mental slowness
- Cold intolerance

- Muscle aches
- Paresthesias (especially carpal tunnel syndrome)
- Diminished sweating
- Hoarseness
- Weight gain
- Constipation
- Hair loss
- Menstrual dysfunction (usually heavy, frequent menses, rarely amenorrhea, and galactorrhea)

The signs of hypothyroidism include:

- Dry, coarse, cold skin
- Edema of eyelids
- Puffy hands and swelling of feet (myxedema)
- Coarse hair and hair loss
- Thick tongue
- Slow speech
- Hoarse voice
- Slow movements
- Pseudomyotonia (delayed relaxation phase of deep tendon reflexes)
- Sallow, pale complexion

Note that many of these features are common in normal aging.

Myxedema coma represents the end stage of hypothyroidism or the combination of severe hypothyroidism, plus one or more complicating factors. The pathophysiology involves:

- Respiratory failure
- Decreased cardiac output
- Anemia
- Hypothermia
- Hypoglycemia
- Hyponatremia
- Thyroid hormone deficiency

Respiratory dysfunction plays an important role in the development of most cases of myxedema coma. Hypothyroidism affects the respiratory system at all levels, from the respiratory center to peripheral oxygen delivery. Respiratory center depression manifests by impaired responses to hypercapnia and hypoxia and results in hypoventilation and a diminished ability to respond to acute hypoxemia-producing insults.

## Diagnosis

In the diagnosis of hypothyroidism, laboratory study manifestations include:

- Increased serum creatine phosphokinase and cholesterol
- Decreased serum sodium
- Electrocardiogram (low voltage, bradycardia)

Primary hypothyroidism caused by Hashimoto's thyroiditis is associated with other autoimmune diseases, for example, autoimmune adrenal insufficiency and the polyglandular autoimmune syndrome.

Two vital questions to answer in making the diagnosis of hypothyroidism are: Is the patient hypothyroid? If the patient is hypothyroid, is the cause primary or secondary? The answer to the latter question has important implications for therapy, as outlined in the preceding section.

## Treatment

The treatment of hypothyroidism is two-pronged: to administer thyroid hormone and to treat the underlying disease. The causes of secondary and tertiary hypothyroidism (i.e., hypothyroidism attributable to pituitary or hypothalamic insufficiency) often require therapy directed at both the causes and the effects of thyroid hormone deficiency. The causes of primary hypothyroidism (i.e., diseases directly affecting the thyroid gland) do not, as a general rule, require treatment directed at the cause. Rather, the key in treatment is therapy directed toward amelioration of the effects of thyroid hormone deficiency.

The treatment of hypothyroidism is simple: Administer thyroid hormone. Levothyroxine ($LT_4$) is the preparation of choice. Its advantages include that the patient given $T_4$ develops a substantial peripheral pool of $T_4$, which turns over more slowly than does $T_3$ and provides a buffer against lapses in the ingestion of medication. In addition, the pool of $T_4$ acts as a continuous source of $T_3$, thereby maintaining a stable $T_3$ serum concentration.

When first diagnosed, hypothyroidism is usually of long duration and seldom requires rapid reversal. Therefore, the restoration of a normal metabolic state may be undertaken gradually. The untreated hypothyroid patient is extremely sensitive to small doses of thyroid hormone. In the hypothyroid patient with long-standing hypothyroidism, high-dose $T_4$ may precipitate a myocardial infarction or congestive heart failure.

*In secondary hypothyroidism, it is important to treat adrenal insufficiency, if present, before thyroid replacement.*

Conversely, no untoward risk is present in initiating therapy with full replacement doses of $LT_4$ (estimated at 1.6 μg/kg body weight) in most younger adult patients with hypothyroidism. In the pediatric age group, requirements are considerably higher. Monitoring therapy is best accomplished by means of the high-sensitivity TSH assay, with the aim of restoration to the normal range. Because of the inherent lag of TSH in the system, no dose adjustments based on the TSH value should be made for a minimum 6-week interval. On clinical grounds, however, small dose adjustments working toward total replacement can be made safely at 2-week intervals in elderly patients and in those with a precarious cardiac status.

In hypothalamic-pituitary hypothyroidism, TSH determinations are of no value. Monitoring is best accomplished by using an FTI or $FT_4$ assay. If hyperthyroxinemia develops, the $T_3$ radioimmunoassay should be used to determine whether overtreatment has occurred (values should be <130 to 140 ng/dL; normal, 80 to 170 ng/dL). Overtreatment may result in accelerated osteopenia.

The following additional considerations should be noted in patients on LT$_4$ therapy:

- Use the same brand-name drug (avoid generics).
- Monitor compliance and dosage requirements at 6- to 12-month intervals.
- Beware of the concomitant use of preparations that may interfere with absorption [soybean, infant formula; soy milk in adults (4), cholestyramine, sucralfate (polyaluminum hydroxide), antacids (aluminum hydroxide), or iron] or with metabolism [anticonvulsants (phenytoin or carbamazepine) or rifampin]. The effects of anticonvulsants are complex; TSH values remain the best guide (except in hypothalamic-pituitary hypothyroidism).

One study suggests that replacement therapy with combined LT$_4$ plus LT$_3$ may be preferable to treatment with LT$_4$ alone (5); however, three more recent studies provide strong evidence against this notion (6–8). Accordingly, this approach is not recommended.

In the past, hypothyroidism has been considered a contraindication for surgery; however, the intraoperative and perioperative risks tend to be minor and can be managed preemptively (9).

# HYPERTHYROIDISM

Hyperthyroidism is a common clinical condition (10).

## Etiology

As with most thyroid disorders, hyperthyroidism is much more common in women than men. A cross-sectional study of autoimmune thyroid disease in an English community revealed a prevalence of established hyperthyroidism of 2% in women and an annual incidence of 3 in 1,000 women. The causes of hyperthyroidism can be subdivided into three groupings:

- Primary thyroid overproduction [RAIU elevated or high normal, unless iodide pool is expanded, such as recent radiocontrast, Jod-Basedow (iodide-induced hyperthyroidism)]:
  □ Graves' disease
  □ Toxic multinodular goiter (Plummer's disease)
  □ Toxic adenoma (uninodular Plummer's disease)
  □ Thyroid carcinoma (metastatic)
  □ Human chorionic gonadotropin–mediated
  □ Trophoblastic disease
  □ Hyperemesis gravidarum
- TSH receptor abnormality (enhanced human chorionic gonadotropin recognition)
  □ Fetal/neonatal

- TSH-mediated
  □ Pituitary adenoma
  □ Pituitary thyroid hormone resistance
  □ Iodide excess
  □ Intrinsic TSH receptor abnormality
  □ Thyroid damage (RAIU low)
  □ Subacute (painful, de Quervain's) thyroiditis
  □ Painless and postpartum thyroiditis
  □ Amiodarone (clinical significance is uncertain)
  □ Nonthyroidal disease (RAIU low)
  □ Exogenous hormone use (excessive dose; factitious use)
  □ Accidental exposure (laced hamburgers)
  □ Struma ovarii (extremely rare)

## Clinical Presentation

Symptoms of hyperthyroidism include:

- Nervousness
- Fatigue
- Weakness
- Palpitations
- Heat intolerance
- Increased sweating
- Dyspnea
- Hyperdefecation
- Insomnia
- Poor concentration
- Infrequent, scanty menses

Signs of hyperthyroidism include:

- Weight loss
- Proximal myopathy
- Tachycardia, arrhythmias
- Warm, moist skin
- Tremor
- Eye conditions (stare, lid lag, and lid retraction)
- Emotional lability
- Hyperactive deep tendon reflexes
- Radiologic evidence of thymic enlargement in Graves' disease (11)

*Thyroid storm*, which represents the extreme form of hyperthyroidism, presents with:

- Exaggerated typical signs
- Exaggerated typical symptoms
- Fever
- Changes in neurologic function (delirium)

## Diagnosis

A biochemical diagnosis of suppressed TSH and elevated circulating T$_4$ or T$_3$ requires an RAIU test (a thyroid scan also may prove useful) to confirm the diagnosis and aid in the treatment plan. Contraindications to the use of RAIU in testing or therapy include:

- Pregnancy
- Lactation
- Iodide (nonradioactive) overload
- Intercurrent illness or therapy (which precludes waiting for the test to be done)

A positive thyroid receptor antibody test can be helpful in such situations.

## GRAVES' DISEASE

In 1835, Robert Graves published a report of three patients with cardiac palpitations and goiter. One of the three patients also had exophthalmos. This condition is now recognized as the most common cause of noniatrogenic hyperthyroidism in the United States. Three major manifestations of the disease appear:

- Hyperthyroidism with diffuse goiter
- Ophthalmopathy (eye disease)
- Dermopathy (pretibial myxedema)

Several lines of evidence support the role of hereditary factors in the development of Graves' disease in the children and siblings of patients with Graves' disease. The presence of certain human leukocyte antigens is associated with an increased incidence of Graves' disease; in particular, the HLA-DR3 antigen in white persons may confer a fourfold risk for the development of the disease. An increased incidence of other autoimmune disorders (e.g., Hashimoto's thyroiditis, pernicious anemia, myasthenia gravis, and Addison's disease) also occurs in patients with Graves' disease and their family members. The disease occurs most frequently between the ages of 20 and 40 years, and it has a marked female sex preponderance (approximately 3–8:1). Therapy may consist of iodine-131 ($^{131}$I), antithyroid drugs or, rarely, surgery (see following discussion). Symptomatic treatment with β-blockers also is useful.

### Hyperthyroidism with Diffuse Goiter

The thyrotoxicosis and goiter of Graves' disease result from stimulation of the gland by autoantibodies (immunoglobulins of the IgG class). These autoantibodies are polyclonal and collectively are referred to as TSIs. The antigen to which these are directed is the TSH receptor, or a region adjacent to it, on the plasma membrane. The binding of these immunoglobulins to the TSH receptor mimics the action of TSH, stimulating adenyl cyclase and thereby initiating a chain of reactions that leads to thyroid growth, increased vascularity, and hypersecretion of hormone.

### Ophthalmopathy

The ophthalmopathy (eye disease) of Graves' disease is probably present to some degree in most patients, although only approximately one third to one half of patients have obvious symptoms or signs of eye disease. Symptoms include:

- Pain
- Lacrimation
- Photophobia
- Blurred vision
- Double vision

Signs of opthalmopathy include:

- Periorbital edema
- Lid edema
- Lid lag
- Chemosis
- Ophthalmoplegia
- Proptosis
- Corneal ulcerations
- Optic neuropathy

### Dermopathy

Infiltrative dermopathy (skin disease) occurs in only approximately 1% of patients with Graves' disease. The pretibial myxedema (most common site) is a consequence of the accumulation of acid mucopolysaccharides and lymphocytes, and the presentation is quite variable. The etiology is not known.

## AUTOIMMUNE THYROID DISEASE

Autoimmune thyroid disease can be viewed as a spectrum of diseases in individuals and in their family members (Fig. 42.2). The clinical presentation of the disorder, according to this view, depends on the morphologic state of the gland and the mixture of circulating antibodies at any particular point in time. The antibodies include:

- Microsomal (TMA, TPO)
- Tg
- Thyroid-damaging

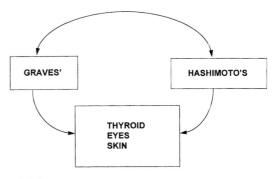

**Figure 42.2**  Spectrum of autoimmune thyroid disease.

- Receptor-binding [stimulating (TSI), blocking, binding]
- Growth-promoting (may be independent from stimulating)

Thus, Graves' disease may "burn out" to become hypothyroidism; receptor-blocking antibodies may result in transient hypothyroidism, giving way to Graves' hyperthyroidism when TSI prevails, and different family members may have different presentations.

## TOXIC MULTINODULAR GOITER (PLUMMER'S DISEASE)

Toxic multinodular goiter is a disorder in which hyperthyroidism arises in a multinodular goiter, usually of longstanding duration. The development of this type of goiter probably starts with the appearance of local areas of autonomous thyroid hyperplasia within individual follicles, followed by their continued replication and growth. The process is accompanied by areas of involution, so functional and anatomic heterogeneity (nodules) appears. If the autonomous regions grow and function sufficiently, hyperthyroidism ensues. Because this process is a slow one, the typical age of appearance of hyperthyroidism tends to be older than in Graves' disease, usually past the age of 50 years. Therapy may consist of $^{131}$I (high, multiple doses may be required) or occasionally surgery; antithyroid drugs may be used, but therapy must be permanent.

## TOXIC ADENOMA

Toxic adenoma, considered to be a true benign tumor of the thyroid gland, is a far less common cause of thyrotoxicosis than Graves' disease or toxic multinodular goiter. Adenomatous tissue develops in the thyroid, which secretes thyroid hormone autonomously, without stimulation by TSH or other thyroid stimulators. This condition tends to occur in patients in their 30s and 40s, somewhat younger than those with toxic multinodular goiter. A single palpable nodule is found on physical examination; a radioactive iodine scan reveals uptake of the isotope only in the adenoma, resulting in a "hot" nodule. (The excess circulating thyroid hormone suppresses TSH secretion and the nonautonomous areas of the thyroid gland; therefore, neither take up iodine or produce thyroid hormone.) Therapy usually consists of $^{131}$I or surgery.

## IODIDE-INDUCED THYROTOXICOSIS (JOD-BASEDOW PHENOMENON)

Jod-Basedow phenomenon refers to iodide-induced hyperthyroidism. (*Jod* is German for iodine and *von Basedow* was one of the early describers of thyrotoxicosis.) This condition occurs most commonly in patients with underlying thyroid disease, who reside in areas of iodide deficiency, and who subsequently receive a load of exogenous iodide (e.g., iodide-containing contrast dye). The pathogenesis, although unclear, is thought to be due to an overproduction of thyroid hormone by autonomously functioning thyroid tissue when presented with excess substrate (iodide). This is the only form of thyrotoxicosis in which ongoing overproduction of thyroid hormone by the thyroid gland occurs, associated with a low RAIU. This occurs because the radioactive isotopic iodide is diluted by large quantities of circulating stable iodide; therefore, only a small quantity of the radioisotope is taken up by the gland. Therapy consists of removing the source of iodide. Occasionally, surgery is necessary (especially in amiodarone-induced hyperthyroidism).

## SUBACUTE THYROIDITIS (DE QUERVAIN'S, GRANULOMATOUS THYROIDITIS)

Subacute thyroiditis is a painful inflammatory process involving the thyroid gland. It results in an elevation of the serum concentration of thyroid hormone into the thyrotoxic range. A history of viral illness often precedes onset, and a number of different viruses have been shown to be associated. The inflammation in the thyroid gland results in the destruction of the follicular epithelium, with the subsequent discharge of large amounts of preformed thyroid hormone into the circulation. Histologically, infiltration of the interstitial areas by histiocytes and lymphocytes occurs; these often appear to congregate into *giant cells*. The characteristic feature of subacute thyroiditis is a painful, tender, mildly enlarged thyroid gland. Systemic manifestations, such as fever, fatigue, and malaise, are also common. Half of patients experience symptoms of hyperthyroidism. Laboratory abnormalities include an extremely high erythrocyte sedimentation rate (ESR) and an extremely low RAIU (the damaged follicles are unable to concentrate iodine). Moreover, the suppressed TSH resulting from the release of excessive amounts of preformed thyroid hormone (the thyroid gland usually has a month's supply of thyroid hormone stored) leads to inactivity even of the undisrupted thyroid follicles. The course of subacute thyroiditis is self-limited, with complete recovery being the general rule. Therapy is primarily supportive and directed toward relief of symptoms (aspirin and β-blockers). Occasionally, glucocorticoids are necessary, but relapses may occur when the glucocorticoids are stopped.

## PAINLESS THYROIDITIS

Painless thyroiditis is another inflammatory condition of the thyroid in which preformed thyroid hormone is discharged from damaged follicles into the circulation. The association in most patients with high titers of antimicrosomal antibodies suggests an autoimmune pathogenesis. Painless thyroiditis occurs most commonly in postpartum women. The course is quite similar to that of subacute thyroiditis, except for the absence of pain and thyroidal tenderness. The RAIU is similarly low, although the ESR usually is normal. Therapy is primarily supportive.

## TREATMENT OF THYROTOXICOSIS

### Radioactive Iodine

The administration of $^{131}$I results in thyroid damage through two different mechanisms: acute radiation thyroiditis and chronic gradual thyroid atrophy. Acute cell death leads to an inflammatory response, with infiltration by granulocytes and mononuclear cells. The eventual result is a progressive atrophy associated with an obliterative endarteritis and interstitial fibrosis that occurs over a period of years. The usual dose of $^{131}$I for the treatment of Graves' disease results in the delivery of 7,000 to 10,000 rad to the thyroid bed. The treatment for toxic multinodular goiter or toxic adenoma generally requires higher doses of $^{131}$I. Therapy with $^{131}$I is safe, with the only major side effect being the frequent development of hypothyroidism in patients with Graves' disease. Posttreatment hypothyroidism has been thought to be quite uncommon with toxic multinodular goiter or toxic adenoma.

In the latter two conditions, after destruction of autonomously functioning tissue, follicles that were previously suppressed (and thus did not take up the radioiodine) resume normal function. One study suggests, however, that eventual hypothyroidism may be seen in as many as 30% of $^{131}$I-treated solitary toxic adenoma patients (12). Fears that $^{131}$I therapy is a risk factor for thyroid or other neoplasms have proved unfounded. The gonadal radiation exposure following a standard dose of $^{131}$I is less than 3 rad (approximately the same as for an intravenous pyelogram or a barium enema) and thus does not pose a risk for an increased incidence of genetic defects in the offspring of treated patients. Because iodine crosses the placenta and is also excreted in breast milk, $^{131}$I therapy is absolutely contraindicated in pregnant women or breastfeeding mothers because destruction of the fetal or neonatal thyroid gland may be the consequence. One disadvantage of this form of therapy is that amelioration of the thyrotoxicosis may take up to 3 months or longer. Therefore, for patients who are quite symptomatic, treatment both before and after radioiodine therapy may be necessary using other agents (e.g., antithyroid drugs or β-blockers).

Radioiodine therapy for Graves' hyperthyroidism has been reported to increase the development or worsen already present ophthalmopathy, when compared with therapy using antithyroid drugs. This worsening of ophthalmopathy is often transient and may be prevented through the use of prednisone (13). Cigarette smoking, a known

risk factor for the development of Graves' ophthalmopathy, appears not only to aggravate the eye risk due to radioiodine therapy but also to have a negative impact on the treatment of the eye disease through prednisone or orbital radiotherapy (14). $^{131}$I therapy is not effective in treating conditions in which thyrotoxicosis is not a consequence of overproduction of thyroid hormone by the thyroid gland (e.g., subacute thyroiditis).

### Antithyroid Drugs (Propylthiouracil or Methimazole)

The mechanism of action of antithyroid drugs is the inhibition of thyroid hormone biosynthesis through the blocking of iodine oxidation, organification, and iodotyrosine coupling, all reactions that are catalyzed by TPO. An additional mechanism of action, unique to propylthiouracil, is the inhibition of peripheral conversion of $T_4$ to $T_3$. This particular effect is useful in patients who are extremely thyrotoxic. In addition to their antithyroid effects, both drugs have immunosuppressive activity and thus may ameliorate the underlying pathogenetic process in Graves' disease. Because these drugs inhibit thyroid autoantibody production, their use in Graves' disease for a 12-month period is associated with long-term remission in approximately 30% to 40% of cases.

These drugs do not alter the underlying pathogenetic process in toxic multinodular goiter or toxic adenoma; therefore, life-long term therapy is required for these conditions. Some improvement in symptoms is usually apparent after 1 to 2 weeks of therapy and is substantial after 4 to 6 weeks of treatment. This fairly rapid onset of action makes antithyroid drug therapy particularly useful for toxic patients before definitive treatment with $^{131}$I or surgery.

Adverse drug reactions occur in as many as 5% to 10% of patients treated with antithyroid medication. The most common side effect is a rash, occurring in 3% to 5% of patients. The most serious side effect, *agranulocytosis* (the complete absence of circulating granulocytes), is seen in 0.5% of patients. It occurs abruptly and, although it is reversible with cessation of the drug, may result in serious illness or even death, especially in older patients. Patients must be cautioned to discontinue the drug and report for a white blood count immediately on the advent of a severe sore throat or fever. Monitoring white blood counts in anticipation is of no value and is not recommended.

### Surgery

The surgical removal of abnormally functioning thyroid tissue is usually definitive, although there may be 10% of patients with Graves' disease in whom thyrotoxicosis recurs after subtotal thyroidectomy. The prevalence of postoperative hypothyroidism (up to 40%) and other surgical complications (vocal cord paralysis owing to recurrent laryngeal nerve damage or permanent hypoparathyroidism) makes surgery less than ideal as a form of therapy and rarely the first choice, although in expert hands surgical complications are minimal.

## β-Blocking Agents

Many of the symptoms and signs of thyrotoxicosis are similar to those of excessive β-adrenergic stimulation. These manifestations are ameliorated when pharmacologic agents that block the β-receptor are used (e.g., propranolol). These agents, therefore, are extremely useful in treating some of the symptoms of thyrotoxicosis until definitive therapy of the underlying cause is effective or a transient pathogenetic process resolves (e.g., subacute thyroiditis). Caution must be exercised in patients with a history of asthma or in the presence of cardiac failure.

## SUBCLINICAL THYROID DISEASE

This controversial topic was studied in detail by a panel of 13 experts in endocrinology, epidemiology, and preventive services. The consensus guidelines (15) and clinical applications (16) were published in 2004. The major conclusions are quoted verbatim:

"Data supporting associations of subclinical thyroid disease with symptoms or adverse clinical outcomes or benefits of treatment are few. The consequences of subclinical thyroid disease (serum TSH 0.15–0.45 μU/mL or 4.5–10.0 μU/mL) are minimal, and we recommend against routine treatment of patients with TSH levels in these ranges. There is insufficient evidence to support population-based screening. Aggressive case finding is appropriate in pregnant women, women older than 60 years, and others at risk for thyroid dysfunction."

## THYROIDITIS

### Acute Suppurative Thyroiditis

Bacterial infection of the thyroid is rare. It presents with pain, fever, and other signs of infection.

### Subacute Thyroiditis

Subacute thyroiditis is a cause of thyrotoxicosis (see preceding discussion).

### Hashimoto's Thyroiditis

Hashimoto's (lymphocytic) thyroiditis, an autoimmune disorder, is a common cause of *goiter* (enlarged thyroid) and hypothyroidism. It is more frequent in women and may run in families. It is associated with autoimmune disorders involving other endocrine glands, such as Addison's disease (adrenal insufficiency) and insulin-dependent diabetes

mellitus, and involving other systems, such as rheumatoid arthritis. The pathogenesis involves cell-mediated immunity. In addition, thyroid autoantibodies against Tg and the microsome TPO enzyme are found, although their significance in vivo is not clear.

In Hashimoto's, the titer of antimicrosomal antibodies is usually greater than 1:400. Pathologically, diffuse lymphocytic infiltration by germinal centers, fibrosis, and obliteration of the thyroid follicles are observed. Abnormalities in thyroid hormone biosynthesis include an organification defect demonstrable by the perchlorate discharge of radioiodine. Abnormal iodoproteins may be released. As long as intact follicles remain, iodine trapping is preserved.

This disorder frequently produces a goiter, and some patients develop hypothyroidism. Some patients with Graves' disease may have histologic features of Hashimoto's thyroiditis, giving rise to the basically meaningless term *Hashitoxicosis* (see Autoimmune Thyroid Disease, earlier in this chapter).

### Painless Thyroiditis

Painless thyroiditis most commonly occurs postpartum. It may have a typical three-phase course—hyperthyroidism, hypothyroidism, and then a return to the euthyroid state—or it can present with hypothyroidism or hyperthyroidism alone. Women with antimicrosomal antibodies are more likely to develop this disease: Some clinicians advocate measuring TMA in pregnancy, especially in the presence of goiter, and monitoring thyroid status routinely in the puerperium. At present, however, no compelling evidence supports such a practice.

## DRUGS AND THYROID DYSFUNCTION

### Lithium

Lithium causes primary hypothyroidism. Also, lithium therapy has been associated with hyperthyroidism and hypercalcemia, and it can cause nephrogenic diabetes insipidus.

### Amiodarone

Amiodarone causes both hypothyroidism and hyperthyroidism. The former is more common in persons with antimicrosomal antibodies. The latter probably has more than one cause: iodine-induced thyrotoxicosis and drug-induced thyroid damage.

The therapy of the hypothyroidism should include cautious thyroid hormone replacement; patients on amiodarone have significant heart disease. Hyperthyroidism therapy may be difficult because antithyroid drugs are often ineffective. The combination of high-dose propylthiouracil and potassium perchlorate (not routinely available) has been effective in some patients. Surgery sometimes is necessary.

# THYROID NODULES AND CANCER

## Thyroid Nodules

Thyroid nodules occur commonly and may be single or multiple. Most are benign. The major issue for the clinician is to determine which nodules are likely to be malignant and require surgical removal. Most thyroid nodules are "cold" on thyroid scans, thus scanning is not very helpful.

Those clinical features raising the likelihood of malignancy include:

- Male sex
- Family history (especially of multiple endocrine neoplasia type II, which includes medullary thyroid carcinoma)
- History of radiation treatment to the head and neck, especially in childhood or adolescence
- Hoarseness or vocal cord paralysis
- A single nodule or a dominant nodule in a multinodular gland
- Lymphadenopathy

  Diagnostic techniques include:

- Fine-needle biopsy
  □ Most cost effective
  □ Various techniques
  □ Need experienced cytologist
- Ultrasound: beware the incidental nodule(s)
- RAIU scan is of limited value
- Chest radiography
- Tg

The best diagnostic approach involves fine-needle aspiration biopsy, which has excellent sensitivity and specificity. There are some limitations, especially in the diagnosis of follicular neoplasms, because cytologic differentiation between adenoma and carcinoma cannot be done with any certainty. Such lesions should be removed.

The therapy of nontoxic nodular thyroid disease is controversial (17). $LT_4$ suppressive therapy has been used with variable results. Nodules that continue to enlarge despite $LT_4$ therapy, even with negative cytology, merit surgical removal. Compressive symptoms and signs similarly demand surgical attention. The use of radioiodine therapy for symptomatic nontoxic multinodular goiter in Europe has gained little attention in the United States or Canada.

## Thyroid Cancer

The major types of thyroid cancer are:

- Primary
  □ Papillary
  □ Follicular
  □ Anaplastic
  □ Medullary (sporadic, familial, multiple endocrine neoplasia type II)
  □ Hürthle cell
- Mixed
- Secondary
  □ Lymphoma

*Papillary* and *follicular cancers*, which tend to be relatively slow growing, account for the vast majority of cases (18). Papillary cancer tends to metastasize to lymph nodes, whereas follicular cancer tends to have earlier hematogenous spread, primarily to lung and bone.

*Anaplastic cancer*, which presents with a rapidly growing mass, has a dismal prognosis.

*Medullary cancer* is a tumor of C cells and is associated with calcitonin production. It can be sporadic, familial, or occur as part of multiple endocrine neoplasia type II. Family members should be screened.

*Thyroid lymphoma* appears to be increasing in frequency. It may occur in a gland involved with Hashimoto's thyroiditis.

The treatment of the common cancers (papillary or follicular) usually includes surgery (near total thyroidectomy is recommended, although some centers recommend more conservative surgery), ablative $^{131}I$ therapy, and $LT_4$ suppression of TSH (19). Serial serum Tg determinations are of value in monitoring disease eradication or recurrence.

The periodic withdrawal of suppressive $LT_4$ therapy permits endogenous TSH to rise and to stimulate any residual thyroid tissue, as demonstrated by whole body scans or serum Tg determinations. Further therapy with $^{131}I$ can be administered, within limits, as required. Regrettably, $LT_4$ withdrawal can be associated with unwanted and sometimes serious morbidity. Recombinant human TSH is available for use to identify patients with residual tumor tissue; this agent avoids the need to render patients hypothyroid. To date, the results obtained in identifying residual tumor tissue are less sensitive compared with those following withdrawal of thyroid hormone.

# REVIEW EXERCISES

## QUESTIONS

**1.** A patient being screened for intermittent diarrhea has a $T_4$ (total) value of 19.6 μg/dL (normal, 5.0–10.5). No other features of hyperthyroidism are present; no goiter is present. A $T_4U$ test is elevated at 2.01 (normal, 0.8–1.20), whereas the $T_3RU$ test is subnormal at 15% (normal, 25%–35%). The FTI is calculated to be 9.8 (normal, 5.0–10.5). What single test would be most helpful in delineating the patient's thyroid status?
**a)** TSH
**b)** Thyroid receptor antibodies
**c)** Serum $T_3$
**d)** Serum $FT_4$ equilibrium dialysis
**e)** None of the above

**2.** The serum TSH test result is 3.0 μU/mL (normal, 0.4–5.5). No drugs or hepatic disease explain the findings. What is the best working diagnosis?
a) Antibodies against circulating $T_3$
b) Hereditary increase in TBG production (X- linked)
c) Hereditary increase in TBPA production
d) All of the above
e) None of the above

**3.** A patient with primary hypothyroidism has been stable (normal TSH) on replacement $LT_4$ (dose, 1.6 μg/kg of body weight) for several years. On annual follow-up, the following laboratory tests are obtained: $T_4$, 14.1 μg/dL (normal, 5.0–10.5); TSH, 23.4 μU/mL (normal, 0.4–5.5). She saw a gastroenterologist 6 months previously for nonsteroidal anti-inflammatory drug–related gastritis and takes an iron preparation and occasional antacids. Which is the most likely diagnosis?
a) Malabsorption of $LT_4$ owing to concomitant use of antacids and iron
b) Progressive loss of endogenous thyroid function
c) Development of thyroid hormone resistance
d) Poor compliance this past year with attempt to "catch up" with excessive $LT_4$ intake recently
e) None of the above

**4.** The development of Graves' hyperthyroidism following the presence of Hashimoto's hypothyroidism is best explained by which of the following?
a) The finding of histopathologic changes of Hashimoto's thyroiditis in Graves' thyroid glands
b) Graves' hyperthyroidism as a natural phase of Hashimoto's disease
c) That the two disorders are part of the spectrum of autoimmune thyroid disease, the clinical manifestations of which are dependent on the mixture of circulating polyclonal antibodies and the morphologic state of the gland at a particular point in time
d) All of the above
e) None of the above

**5.** You are asked to see a 75-year-old white man who was admitted to the psychiatric ward with a diagnosis of delirium. The history obtained from the wife revealed that he was well until 6 months before admission. He has had a 30-lb weight loss with a poor appetite since that time. No history is present of any medication, recent investigations involving radiocontrast media, goiter, or neck discomfort. No family history of thyroid disease is present. On physical examination, he is afebrile; he looks cachectic but is not pigmented; no features of infiltrative eye changes are present; the thyroid gland is prolapsed, but may be just palpable on swallowing. The pulse rate is irregular at 120 beats per minute. The electrocardiogram shows atrial fibrillation. The serum $T_4$ is 19.7 μg/dL (normal, 5.0–10.5) with a serum TSH less than 0.02 μU/ mL (normal, 0.4–5.5).

The next step in diagnosis is to order
a) Serum $T_3$
b) 24-Hour RAIU
d) 24-Hour RAIU and scan
d) Thyroid-stimulating antibodies
e) Thyroid microsomal (TPO) antibodies

**6.** Management of the patient in the preceding question should include all of the following, *except*
a) β-Blockers
b) Digoxin
c) Coumadin
d) Propylthiouracil
e) Stress doses of glucocorticoids

## ANSWERS

**1. a.**
The aim of the question is to help gain understanding of the role of free (nonprotein bound) thyroid hormone in regulating TSH secretion. The hypothalamo-pituitary unit "reads" the free hormone level, not the total hormone level, which is subject to changes owing to alterations in protein binding (TBG, TBPA, albumin, or conditions that may interfere with binding).

In practice, FTI can be calculated from total $T_4$ and an estimate of protein binding ($T_4U$ or $T_3RU$; $T_4U$ measures binding directly, whereas $T_3RU$ provides an index of unbound hormone). Automated $FT_4$ assays are replacing these more indirect indices; the gold standard, $FT_4$ by equilibrium dialysis, is available in some reference laboratories but is rarely needed. Thus, serum TSH in this patient should provide the best indicator of thyroid function status and is independent from thyroid hormone protein–binding abnormalities.

**2. b.**
The aim of the question is to explore thyroid hormone binding in more detail. The major normal thyroid hormone–binding proteins are TBG and TBPA. Certain drugs and conditions can alter these levels or binding capacity. Antibodies against $T_4$ and $T_3$ rarely occur in patients who have Hashimoto's thyroiditis (haptenic autoantigen). Hereditary increases in TBG (binds both $T_4$ and $T_3$) or TBPA (binds $T_4$ only) occur uncommonly. The increases in thyroid hormone–binding capacity in this patient are reflected by both the $T_4U$ (high) and the $T_3RU$ (low) tests. Antibodies against $T_3$ would be expected to lower the $T_3RU$ test results, but not affect the $T_4U$ test; increased TBPA levels would result in increased $T_4U$ values, but not affect $T_3RU$ values (because $T_3$ does not bind to the TBPA ligand).

**3. d.**
The aim of this question is to help understand the time lag in the hypothalamo-pituitary-thyroid axis. Although TSH secretion may be acutely altered by stress, illness,

or drugs, the major regulation is based on the integrated thyroid hormone exposure over the preceding 2 to 5 weeks. Although iron preparations and aluminum-containing compounds can interfere with $T_4$ absorption, the elevated serum $T_4$ level argues against this notion. Similarly, a progressive loss of thyroid function would be expected to lead to low or low-normal $T_4$ values. Although acquired thyroid hormone resistance may occur hypothetically, no clinical descriptions of such disorders exist. The correct answer is not a rare occurrence: Patients often wish to please their healthcare provider, even if it means not being perfectly honest on occasion.

### 4. c.

The aim of this question is to gain understanding of the concept that the correct answer helps to explain this, as well as a number of other clinical conditions (see Autoimmune Thyroid Disease, earlier in this chapter).

### 5. c.

The aim of the question is to reinforce the clinical presentation of elderly patients with thyrotoxicosis and their management. Although weight loss despite a generous appetite is characteristic in the younger adult, anorexia is not an uncommon finding in the elderly. Cachexia in an "apathetic" patient should be considered. (Concomitant Addison's disease in a patient with known thyroid autoimmunity is a "distractor" in the current case presentation; the lack of pigmentation was intended to get the reader back on focus.) A cardiac dysrhythmia (usually atrial fibrillation) or congestive heart failure may be the major feature(s). The most common cause of hyperthyroidism in this age group is toxic multinodular goiter (sometimes iodide induced), but the absence of a goiter may be seen in up to 25% of elderly patients (5% in young adults).

Serum $T_3$ may be of academic interest (and occasionally a higher $T_4$:$T_3$ ratio may help to discriminate thyroiditis or toxic multinodular goiter from Graves' hyperthyroidism), but it is generally reserved for cases in which total $T_4$ and $FT_4$ values are normal. Thyroid-stimulating antibodies are of minor value in ruling out Graves' disease (usually a positive family history is obtained), but this diagnosis can be inferred from an elevated RAIU and diffuse scan. TMAs are a less expensive but less specific surrogate for Graves' disease. The RAIU is necessary to discriminate thyroid hyperfunction [autonomous nodule(s), receptor antibody, TSH, or human chorionic gonadotropin driven] from subacute or silent thyroiditis, iatrogenic, or factitious causes. (Recent exposure to radiocontrast media or iodine-containing drugs or pregnancy may preclude its use, however.) A scan is of particular value when the clinician is unsure of the size and nature of the thyroid gland.

### 6. e.

β-Blockers and propylthiouracil are helpful as primary therapy for hyperthyroidism in the elderly.

Propylthiouracil is initiated only after the diagnosis is confirmed by an RAIU (and scan, if necessary). RAI therapy may cause a transient worsening (radiation thyroiditis) of the hyperthyroidism and is often postponed in elderly patients until euthyroidism is attained (and antithyroid medication transiently withdrawn for 2 to 3 days before $^{131}$I treatment). Digoxin is helpful to control the heart rate in atrial fibrillation. Coumadin is indicated in preventing embolic consequences of atrial fibrillation. The only drug not indicated without more data (the patient was not in "thyroid storm") is the glucocorticoid.

## REFERENCES

1. Canaris GJ, Manowitz NR, Mayor G, et al. The Colorado thyroid disease prevalence study. *Arch Intern Med* 2000;160:526–534.
2. Danese MD, Powe NR, Sawin CT, et al. Screening for mild thyroid failure at the periodic health examination: a decision and cost-effectiveness analysis. *JAMA* 1996;276:285–292.
3. Haddow JE, Palomaki GE, Allan WC, et al. Maternal thyroid deficiency during pregnancy and subsequent neuropsychological development of the child. *N Engl J Med* 1999;341:549–555.
4. Bell DSH, Ovalle F. Use of soy protein supplement and resultant need for increased dose of levothyroxine. *Endocr Pract* 2001;7:193–194.
5. Bunevicius R, Kazanavicius G, Zalinkevicius R, et al. Effects of thyroxine as compared with thyroxine plus triiodothyronine in patients with hypothyroidism. *N Engl J Med* 1999;340:424–429.
6. Walsh JP, Shiels L, Lim EM, et al. Combined thyroxine/liothyronine treatment does not improve well-being, quality of life, or cognitive function compared to thyroxine alone: a randomized controlled trial in patients with primary hypothyroidism. *J Clin Endocrinol Metab* 2003;88:4543–4550.
7. Sawka AM, Gerstein HC, Marriott MJ, et al. Does a combination regimen of thyroxine ($T_4$) and 3,5,3′–triiodothyronine improve depressive symptoms better than $T_4$ alone in patients with hypothyroidism? Results of a double-blind, randomized, controlled trial. *J Clin Endocrinol Metab* 203;88:4551–4555.
8. Clyde PW, Harari AE, Getka EJ, et al. Combined levothyroxine plus liothyronine compared with levothyroxine alone in primary hypothyroidism; a randomized controlled trial. *JAMA* 2003;290:2952–2958.
9. Ladenson PW, Levin AA, Ridgway EC, et al. Complications of surgery in hypothyroid patients. *Am J Med* 1984;77:261–266.
10. Cooper DS. Hyperthyroidism. *Lancet* 2003;362:459–468.
11. Bergman TA, Mariash CN, Oppenheimer JH. Anterior mediastinal mass in a patient with Graves' disease. *J Clin Endocrinol Metab* 1982;55:587–588.
12. Goldstein R, Hart IR. Follow-up of solitary autonomous thyroid nodules treated with $^{131}$I. *N Engl J Med* 1983;309:1473–1476.
13. Bartalena L, Marcocci C, Bogazzi F, et al. Relation between therapy for hyperthyroidism and the course of Graves' ophthalmopathy. *N Engl J Med* 1998;338:73–78.
14. Bartalena L, Marcocci C, Tanda ML, et al. Effect of cigarette smoking on treatment outcome of Graves' eye disease in patients receiving radioiodine ablation. *Ann Intern Med* 1998;129:632–635.
15. Surks MI, Ortiz E, Daniels GH, et al. Subclinical thyroid disease: scientific review and guidelines for diagnosis and management. *JAMA* 2004;291:228–238.
16. Col NF, Surks MI, Daniels GH. Subclinical thyroid disease: clinical applications. *JAMA* 2004;291:239–243.
17. Hermus AR, Huysmans DA. Treatment of benign nodular thyroid disease. *N Engl J Med* 1998;338:1438–1447.
18. Schlumberger JM. Papillary and follicular thyroid carcinoma. *N Engl J Med* 1998;338:297–306.
19. Wartofsky L, Sherman SI, Gopal J, et al. The use of radioactive iodine in patients with papillary and follicular thyroid cancer. *J Clin Endocrinol Metab* 1998;83:4195–4203.

## SUGGESTED READING

Barbot N, Calmettes C, Schuffenecker I, et al. Pentagastrin stimulation test and early diagnosis of medullary thyroid carcinoma using an immunoradiometric assay of calcitonin: comparison with genetic screening in hereditary medullary thyroid carcinoma. *J Clin Endocrinol Metab* 1994;78:114–120.

Borst GC. Euthyroid hyperthyroxinemia. *Ann Intern Med* 1983;98: 366–378.

Borst GC, Eil C, Burman KD. Euthyroid hyperthyroxinemia. *Ann Intern Med* 1983;98:366–378.

Brent GA, Hershman JM. Thyroxine therapy in patients with severe nonthyroidal illnesses and low serum thyroxine concentration. *J Clin Endocrinol Metab* 1986;63:1–8.

Burrow GN, Fisher DA, Larsen PR. Mechanisms of disease: maternal and fetal thyroid function. *N Engl J Med* 1994;331:1072–1078.

Campbell NRC, Hasinoff BB, Stalts H, et al. Ferrous sulfate reduces thyroxine efficacy in patients with hypothyroidism. *Ann Intern Med* 1992;117:1010–1013.

Cavalieri RR, Gerard SK. Unusual types of thyrotoxicosis. *Adv Intern Med* 1991;36:271–286.

Char DH. The ophthalmopathy of Graves' disease. *Med Clin North Am* 1991;75:97–119.

Cooper DS. Antithyroid drugs. *N Engl J Med* 1984;311:1353–1362.

Cooper DS. Subclinical hypothyroidism. *Adv Endocrinol Metab* 1991; 2:77–88.

Dayan CM. Interpretation of thyroid function tests. *Lancet* 2001;357: 619–624.

De los Santos ET, Starich GH, Mazzaferri EL. Sensitivity, specificity, and cost-effectiveness of the sensitive thyrotropin assay in the diagnosis of thyroid disease in ambulatory patients. *Arch Intern Med* 1989;149:526–532.

DeGroot LJ. Long-term impact of initial and surgical therapy on papillary and follicular thyroid cancer. *Am J Med* 1994;97:499–500.

Docter R, Krenning EP, de Jong M, et al. The sick euthyroid syndrome: changes in thyroid hormone serum parameters and hormone metabolism. *Clin Endocrinol* 1993;39:499–518.

Dolan JG. Hyperthyroidism and hypothyroidism. In: Panzer RJ, Black ER, Griner PF, eds. *Diagnostic Strategies for Common Medical Problems.* Philadelphia: American College of Physicians, 1991: 375–384.

Doria R, Jekel JF, Cooper DL. Thyroid lymphoma: the case for combined modality therapy. *Cancer* 1994;73:200–206.

Farrar JJ, Toth AD. Iodine-131 treatment of hyperthyroidism: current issues. *Clin Endocrinol* 1991;35:207–212.

Fisher DA. Screening for congenital hypothyroidism. *Trends Endocrinol Metab* 1991;2:129–133.

Gharib H, Goellner JR. Fine-needle aspiration biopsy of the thyroid: an appraisal. *Ann Intern Med* 1993;118:282–289.

Hamburger JI. The various presentations of thyroiditis: diagnostic considerations. *Ann Intern Med* 1986;104:219–224.

Helfand M, Crapo LM. Monitoring therapy in patients taking levothyroxine. *Ann Intern Med* 1990;113:450–454.

Helfand M, Crapo LM. Screening for thyroid disease. *Ann Intern Med* 1990;112:840–849. (See letters to the editor: *Ann Intern Med* 1990; 113:896–897.)

Klein I, Levey GS. Unusual manifestations of hypothyroidism. *Arch Intern Med* 1984;144:123–128.

Klein I, Ojamaa K. Thyroid hormone and the cardiovascular system. *N Engl J Med* 2001;344:501–509.

Ladenson PW, Braverman LE, Mazzaferri EL, et al. Comparison of administration of recombinant human thyrotropin with withdrawal of thyroid hormone for radioactive iodine scanning in patients with thyroid carcinoma. *N Engl J Med* 1997;337: 888–896.

Lazarus JH, Othman S. Thyroid disease in relation to pregnancy. *Clin Endocrinol* 1991;34:91–98.

Ledger GA, Khosla S, Lindor NM, et al. Genetic testing in the diagnosis and management of multiple endocrine neoplasia type II. *Ann Intern Med* 1995;122:118–124.

Liel Y, Sperber AD, Shang S. Nonspecific intestinal adsorption of levothyroxine by aluminum hydroxide. *Am J Med* 1994;97: 363–365.

Lips CJM, Landsvater RM, Hoppener JWM, et al. Clinical screening as compared with DNA analysis in families with multiple endocrine neoplasia type 2A. *N Engl J Med* 1994; 331:828–835.

Mandel SJ, Larsen PR, Seeley EW, et al. Increased need for thyroxine during pregnancy in women with primary hypothyroidism. *N Engl J Med* 1990;323:91–95.

Mandel SJ, Brent GA, Larsen PR. Levothyroxine therapy in patients with thyroid disease. *Ann Intern Med* 1993;119:492–502.

March DE, Desai AG, Park CH, et al. Struma ovarii: hyperthyroidism in a postmenopausal woman. *J Nucl Med* 1988;29:263–265.

Mazzaferri EL. Long-term impact of initial surgical and medical therapy on papillary and follicular thyroid cancer. *Am J Med* 1994;97: 418–428.

Mazzaferri EL. Management of a solitary thyroid nodule. *N Engl J Med* 1993;328:553–559.

McDougall IR. Graves' disease: current concepts. *Med Clin North Am* 1991;75:79–95.

Mendel CM. The free hormone hypothesis; a physiologically based mathematical model. *Endocrinol Rev* 1989;10:232–274.

Mulligan DC, McHenry CR, Kinney W, et al. Amiodarone-induced thyrotoxicosis: clinical presentation and expanded indications for thyroidectomy. *Surgery* 1993;114:1114–1119.

Ozata M, Suzuki S, Miyamoto T, et al. Serum thyroglobulin in the follow-up of patients with treated differentiated thyroid cancer. *J Clin Endocrinol Metab* 1994;79:98–105.

Pineda JD, Lee T, Ain K, et al. Iodine-131 therapy for thyroid cancer patients with elevated thyroglobulin and negative diagnostic scan. *J Clin Endocrinol Metab* 1995;80:1488–1492.

Refetoff S, Lever EG. The value of serum thyroglobulin measurement in clinical practice. *JAMA* 1983;250:2352–2357.

Rosenbaum D, Davies TF. The clinical use of thyroid autoantibodies. *Endocrinologist* 1992;2:55–62.

Ross DS. Subclinical thyrotoxicosis. *Adv Endocrinol Metab* 1991;2: 89–105.

Schectman JM, Pawlson LG. The cost-effectiveness of three thyroid function testing strategies for suspicion of hypothyroidism in a primary care-setting. *J Gen Intern Med* 1990;5:9–15.

Sherman SI, Tielens ET, Ladenson PW. Sucralfate causes malabsorption of L-thyroxine. *Am J Med* 1994;96:531–535.

Slag MF, Morley JE, Elson MK, et al. Hypothyroxinemia in critically ill patients as a predictor of high mortality. *JAMA* 1981;245:43–45.

Stagnaro-Green A. Postpartum thyroiditis: prevalence, etiology, and clinical importance. *Thyroid Today* 1993;16:1–11.

Surks MI, Sievert R. Drugs and thyroid function. *N Engl J Med* 1995;333:1688–1694.

Surks MI, Smith PJ. Multiple effects of 5,5'-diphenylhydantoin on the thyroid hormone system. *Endocrinol Rev* 1984;5:514–524.

Surks MI, Chopra IJ, Mariash CN, et al. American Thyroid Association guidelines for use of laboratory tests in thyroid disorders. *JAMA* 1990;263:1529–1532.

Tachman ML, Guthrie GP Jr. Hypothyroidism: diversity of presentation. *Endocr Rev* 1984;5:456–465.

Van Middlesworth L. Effects of radiation on the thyroid gland. *Adv Intern Med* 1989;34:265–284.

Weetman AP, McGregor AM. Autoimmune thyroid disease: further developments in our understanding. *Endocrinol Rev* 1994;15: 788–830.

Wiener JD. A systematic approach to the diagnosis of Plummer's disease (autonomous goitre), with a review of 224 cases. *Neth J Med* 1975;18:218–233.

Weiss RE, Refetoff S. Thyroid hormone resistance. *Annu Rev Med* 1992; 43:363–375.

Woeber KA. Thyrotoxicosis and the heart. *N Engl J Med* 1992;327: 94–98.

Wong TK, Hershman JM. Changes in thyroid function in nonthyroidal illness. *Trends Endocrinol Metab* 1992;3:8–11.

Yassa R, Saunders A, Nastase C, et al. Lithium-induced thyroid disorders: a prevalence study. *J Clin Psychiatry* 1988;49:14–16.

# Androgenic and Reproductive Disorders

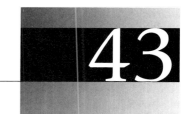

*Adi E. Mehta*

## FEMALE REPRODUCTIVE DISORDERS

Androgen excess is one of the most common endocrine disorders in women, affecting 2% to 8% of all women, and it is the most common cause of anovulatory infertility. The clinical manifestations can vary significantly, from dermatologic manifestations, such as hirsutism or acne, to menstrual irregularities, amenorrhea, and, rarely, virilization. Prognostically, whereas the short-term manifestations are a cosmetic nuisance and can cause great psychologic and emotional distress because of relatively reduced fecundity, the long-term morbidity and mortality are marked and expensive, causing diabetes, dyslipidemia, and cardiovascular disease.

### Androgenic Disorders

#### Anatomy and Physiology of Androgenic Sources
The ovaries and adrenal glands are the source of androgens in women. Androgens may be secreted, in small amounts, as biologically active androgens or may serve as precursor compounds for conversion to active androgens in the periphery. Both ovaries and adrenals produce the hormones in response to their tropic hormones [luteinizing hormone (LH) and adrenocorticotropic hormone (ACTH), respectively], but the androgens cannot act as powerful negative-feedback control hormones for the pituitary. Thus, their secretion is not self-controlled.

The major products of adrenal secretion are dehydroepiandrosterone sulfate (DHEAS), dehydroepiandrosterone, and androstenedione; the major ovarian secretory product is androstenedione. Approximately half the circulating levels of testosterone in women are secreted from both glandular sources, whereas the rest is made by peripheral conversion of 17-ketosteroids in the liver, skin, and adipose tissue.

#### Transport in Serum
The bulk of active androgen (and estradiol, E2) is tightly bound in the circulation to sex hormone–binding globulin (SHBG) of hepatic origin. Lesser binding to albumin also occurs. Thus, only small amounts of free (unbound) sex

steroids are present. SHBG production by the liver is influenced by the androgen-to-estrogen balance, as well as by thyroid hormone. Estrogen and thyroid hormone stimulate SHBG production. Androgen is inhibitory.

#### Biologic Activity of Androgens
The major biologically active androgen in most target tissues is dihydrotestosterone, which is formed by the conversion of testosterone under the influence of 5-α reductase, which is present in the skin and external genitalia. The effect of androgen on target tissues is thought to be mediated by the ratio of free testosterone to free E2 in the circulation. Thus, simple measurements of total testosterone or E2 may be misleading.

The SHBG multiplier effect can be summarized as follows:

- Hepatic SHBG production is influenced by the androgen-to-estrogen status.
- Binding kinetics for testosterone and E2 to this protein are different. (As SHBG concentration falls under an androgenic influence, a greater increment in unbound testosterone occurs, compared with unbound E2.)
- Androgen excess begets androgen excess.

#### Clinical Presentation of Androgenic Disorders
The clinical presentation of androgenic disorders in women is relatively classic and restrictive in focus. The most common presentation is with a complaint of hirsutism, possibly with acne, and irregular and infrequent menses. Obesity is not an uncommon associated finding in such individuals.

#### Specific Androgenic Disorders
##### Polycystic Ovary Syndrome
The 1990 National Institutes of Health consensus criteria define polycystic ovary syndrome (PCOS) as the invariable presence of chronic oligoovulation or anovulation associated with hyperandrogenism (i.e., signs of androgen excess, such as acne, alopecia, or hirsutism, even without clearly elevated serum androgen levels) in the absence of other known causes of androgen excess, such as congenital

adrenal hyperplasia, tumor, or hyperprolactinemia. Although there may be associated abnormal ovarian morphology, abnormal gonadotropins, or abnormal insulin regulation, these do not have to be invariably present to make the diagnosis.

*Pathophysiology.* The pathophysiology of PCOS is unclear, but numerous theories exist. Most point to the establishment of a vicious cycle of events, possibly initiated by the presence of two phenomena normally occurring in puberty that, in the predisposed person, sets this cycle in motion: an early increase in LH and androgen levels, and insulin resistance. Three proposed theories encompass both phenomena:

- The *LH theory* hypothesizes a primary neuroendocrine defect that causes an exaggerated LH pulse frequency in amplitude.
- The *insulin theory* hypothesizes that PCOS is initiated by the familial presence of decreased peripheral insulin sensitivity and resultant hyperinsulinemia, which is further aggravated by the physiologic insulin resistance induced by puberty. Such hyperinsulinemia inhibits the production of insulin-like growth factor 1 (IGF-1) binding protein and SHBG in the liver. This results in an increased concentration of free IGF-1. In the ovary, both insulin and IGF-1, working in synergy with LH, stimulate thecal androgen production, possibly by stimulating an existing defect in insulin receptor autophosphorylation: Instead of the usual tyrosine phosphorylation, a unique change occurs in the phosphorylation of the insulin receptor by serine, causing it to have an increased basal activity but decreased insulin responsivity. Thus, both the increased insulin levels and the higher androgen levels lower SHBG, thus further increasing free androgens.
- The *ovarian theory* hypothesizes that a genetic defect exists in the ovary, leading to increased steroidogenic activity, characterized by a dysregulation of the ovarian P450 C17 enzyme, which increases androgen production, especially in the presence of serine phosphorylation.

Predispositions to the development of PCOS include the following:

- A family history of non–insulin-dependent diabetes mellitus
- Maternal gestational diabetes mellitus
- Borderline adrenal hyperplasia accentuated by the pubertal adrenarche
- Occult hypothyroidism
- Childhood obesity

In the PCOS-predisposed person, LH and androgen levels are higher, whereas in the healthy person, ovulating cycles decrease LH and attenuate the insulin resistance of puberty; in PCOS-predisposed persons, this does not occur. Thus, PCOS is sometimes termed *hyperpuberty*.

Clinical PCOS frequently presents as hirsutism (70% to 75%), oligomenorrhea (50%), and resulting infertility. Obesity and insulin resistance leading to diabetes may be present (30% to 40%). Biochemically, an elevation of LH values is frequent (up to 75%), and some schools emphasize an elevated LH-to-follicle-stimulating hormone (FSH) ratio (more than 2:1 or 3:1). Androgens, especially ovarian androgens, are elevated, and adrenal androgens (DHEA) may have up to a twofold increase.

*Metabolic Consequences.* The following summarizes the metabolic consequences of PCOS:

- Insulin resistance is present in a large percentage of women with PCOS.
- Insulin resistance can be present in nonobese women with PCOS as well as in obese women with PCOS, although a percentage of lean women with PCOS are not insulin resistant.
- The insulin resistance manifests more peripherally in muscle than in the liver.
- Insulin potentiates LH-stimulated androgen production from the theca and stroma of the ovary.
- The ovary is not resistant to insulin in the face of the peripheral muscle and adipose tissue insulin resistance.
- Acanthosis nigricans, a marker of insulin resistance, can be seen but may fade with the reduction of circulating androgens.
- An increased waist-to-hip ratio is commonly associated with the elevated androgens.

The proposed theoretic basis of PCOS appears in Figure 43.1.

The late consequences of acne, hirsutism, PCOS, and relative subfecundity include the following:

- Infertility
- Hyperlipidemia

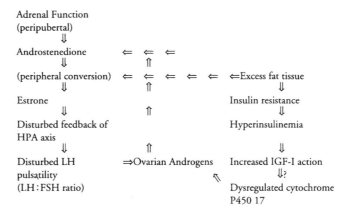

**Figure 43.1** The proposed theoretic basis of polycystic ovary syndrome. FSH, follicle-stimulating hormone; HPA, hypothalamic-pituitary-adrenal; IGF-I, insulin-like growth factor–I; LH, luteinizing hormone.

- Hypertension
- Late development of non–insulin-dependent diabetes mellitus
- Increased risk of endometrial and breast cancer
- Cardiovascular disease

These later associations with hyperlipidemia, hypertension, and non–insulin-dependent diabetes mellitus form the metabolic syndrome as defined in the NCEP-ATP III Guidelines, which predispose to premature cardiac disease.

## Hirsutism

Hirsutism—excess terminal (sexual) hair in a woman—is characterized by two types of hair: (i) vellus (small diameter, soft texture, and nonmedullated); and (ii) terminal (large diameter, coarse, medullated), usually found in sex hormone–sensitive skin. This hair is androgen dependent for growth.

***Etiology of Hirsutism.*** The causes of hirsutism and virilization include:

- Genetic, racial, atavistic causes (e.g., Mediterranean women)
- Iatrogenic causes
- Drug side effects
  - Hormones ("the pill," anabolic steroids)
  - Diphenylhydantoin
  - Hexachlorobenzene
  - Diazoxide
  - Cyclosporine
  - Minoxidil (nonsteroid drugs cause hypertrichosis)
- Adrenal conditions
  - Congenital adrenal hyperplasia (adult-onset variant)
  - Benign and malignant tumors
  - Cushing's syndrome
  - Prolactin or growth hormone excess
- Ovarian conditions
  - Idiopathic hirsutism
  - PCOS (Stein-Leventhal)
  - Stromal hyperthecosis (likely a more severe variant of PCOS)
  - Virilizing neoplasms
  - Ovarian steroidogenic block
  - Hermaphroditism
  - Human chorionic gonadotropin (hCG)
  - Peripheral androgen overproduction
  - Obesity
- Other

***Diagnosis of Hirsutism and Virilization.*** In diagnosing hirsutism and virilization, the clinician must attempt to answer several important questions:

*Is hirsutism present? Is it because of androgen excess?*
*Hypertrichosis*, which is nonsexual excessive hair growth (i.e., due to ethnic causes, in malnutrition, owing to nonsteroid drugs), is not associated with virilism. Hirsutism is defined as excessive sexual hair growth (pubic, axillary, abdominal, chest, and facial). This hair is coarse and pigmented.

*What is the degree of virilism?*
Acne and hirsutism are the earliest (and frequently the only) signs of excessive circulating androgen(s).

Anovulation and oligomenorrhea–amenorrhea manifest relatively early in ovarian conditions, but tend to appear later in adrenal disorders. Frontal balding, clitoromegaly, low-pitched voice, and increased muscularity indicate marked androgenic stimulation.

*What are the points of importance for differential diagnoses?*

- Onset
  - Peripubertal: usually benign
  - Prepubertal or late postpubertal: more ominous
- Progression
  - Slow or static: benign
  - Progressive: malignant
- Family history: positive points to benign
- Libido enhancement of recent onset: inauspicious
- Medication use
- Menstrual regularity: uncommon in face of excess androgen

*What is the source of androgen?*

- Rule out exogenous sources
- Rule out neoplasia; sudden onset and rapid progression suggests neoplasm, abdominal or pelvic masses
- High androgen levels (i.e., 17-ketosteroids, DHEAS, testosterone)
- Cushing's disease: rare among obese, hirsute women (adult-onset congenital adrenal hyperplasia may be common); produces excess androgen

Other functional syndromes may have an ovarian or adrenal origin (at present, these cannot be distinguished by dynamic stimulation or suppression tests; indeed, having ruled out organic disease, the definition of the precise source has little practical significance).

***Laboratory Tests.*** Laboratory tests used to diagnosis hirsutism or virilization include:

- Serum DHEAS or urinary (24-hour) 17-ketosteroids (useful to rule out adrenal neoplasms)
- Serum testosterone
  - Into the normal male range (>8 nmol/L) in ovarian (or adrenal) neoplasms
  - Mild to moderately elevated in most cases of PCOS
  - Normal or borderline high (slightly >2 nmol/L) in idiopathic hirsutism
- 17-OH-progesterone (may pick up an occasional adult congenital adrenal hyperplasia case)
- Index of free testosterone or testosterone-to-SHBG ratios where available (often elevated, even when total testosterone levels are normal)

- Other steroids (e.g., androstenedione or metabolites) are of little additional help
  - 5-Androstanediol glucuronide of questionable additional benefit
  - Serum prolactin (elevations may be associated with PCOS)
- Thyroid function tests (hirsutism may be seen in primary hypothyroidism)
- Anatomic studies generally are not indicated

**Treatment of Hirsutism.** The treatment regimen for hirsutism includes:

- Treat organic disease
- Weight loss by diet and exercise in obese women to reduce androgens and insulin
- Medical therapy
  - Glucocorticoids
  - Estrogen/progestin (birth control pill)
  - Antiandrogens
  - Cyproterone acetate and estrogen (birth control pill)
  - Spironolactone
  - Flutamide
  - Finasteride
  - Cimetidine
  - Gonadotropic [gonadotropin-releasing hormone (GnRH)] analogs
  - Ketoconazole
  - Local application of steroids
  - Progesterone
  - Cyproterone
  - Spironolactone
- Local treatment
  - Shaving
  - Chemical depilatories
  - Wax depilation
  - Bleaching
  - Electrolysis
  - Laser removal of hair
- Ovulation induction (if the major complaint is infertility)

The most commonly used insulin sensitizers are metformin and troglitazone. By increasing insulin sensitivity and lowering insulin levels, insulin sensitizers have been shown to reduce androgens and restore menstrual cyclicity or reestablish responsivity to inducers of ovulation. Although earlier therapy for hirsutism—whether of PCOS origin or idiopathic in women not interested in fertility—was an oral contraceptive pill (OCP) containing an antiandrogen, increasing reports now indicate that insulin sensitizer therapy with or without an OCP may be of greater benefit both for the present and for the future in terms of preventing the progression of disease to features of the metabolic syndrome.

Reassurance and support is essential to good outcomes because treatment requires patience and perseverance; most treatments require 8 to 14 months to achieve a clinical effect.

### Amenorrhea

Amenorrhea is the absolute lack of menses for more than 3 months in a woman with previously regular cycles (secondary amenorrhea) or no menses by the age of 16 years (primary amenorrhea).

**Diagnosis.** It is important to ascertain whether amenorrhea is primary or secondary, and whether it is anatomic, owing to hormonal or functional hormone dysregulation, or because of other endocrine or systemic illnesses. The classification breakdown for amenorrhea includes:

- Anatomic
- Primary
  - Congenital uterine absence
  - Cryptomenorrhea
- Secondary
  - Asherman's syndrome
  - Iatrogenic
  - Hysterectomy/oophorectomy
- Chromosomal
  - XO/XO mosaic (Turner's syndrome)
  - XY androgen insensitivity
- Hormonal/functional (could be primary but more frequently secondary)
  - Pregnancy
  - Prolactin excess
  - Androgen excess
  - Weight loss
  - Excessive exercise
  - Anorexia nervosa
  - Excessive weight gain
  - Emotional stress
  - Hypopituitarism
  - Ovarian failure
- Other illnesses (usually secondary amenorrhea, occasionally primary)
- Other endocrine diseases
  - Hyperthyroidism/hypothyroidism
  - Adrenal disease
  - Diabetes mellitus
  - Chronic systemic illnesses
  - Crohn's disease
  - Ulcerative colitis
  - Rheumatoid arthritis

**Laboratory Studies.** After ruling out pregnancy as a cause for the amenorrhea, an evaluation of gonadotropin, estrogen, androgens, prolactin, and thyrotropin levels, general chemistry, and a complete blood cell count usually are required. In primary amenorrhea or amenorrhea occurring after only a few irregular cycles in young persons, a karyotype also is indicated.

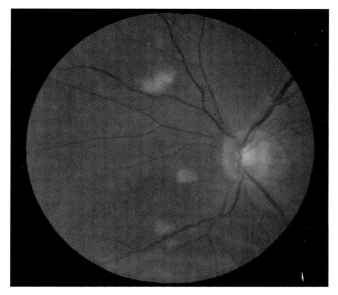

**Figure 5.1** Cotton-wool spots. (This figure appears in black and white on page 57.)

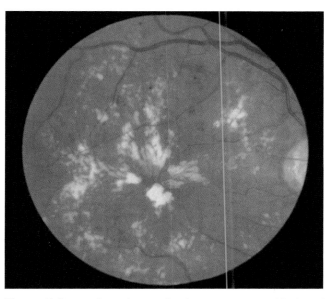

**Figure 5.2** Hard exudates. (This figure appears in black and white on page 57.)

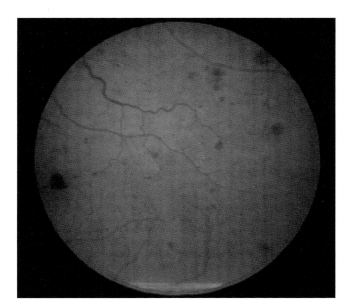

**Figure 5.3** Intraretinal hemorrhages. (This figure appears in black and white on page 57.)

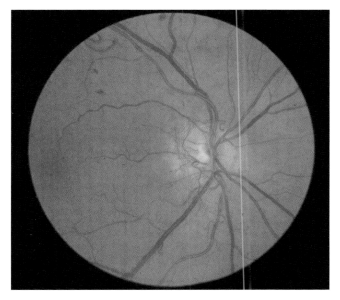

**Figure 5.4** Neovascularization of the disc. (This figure appears in black and white on page 57.)

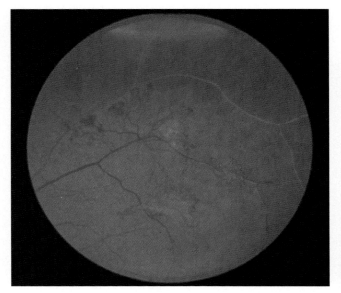

**Figure 5.5** Neovascularization elsewhere is seen along the superotemporal arcade of the left eye, as well as a sclerotic vessel (white vessel in top portion of figure). (This figure appears in black and white on page 58.)

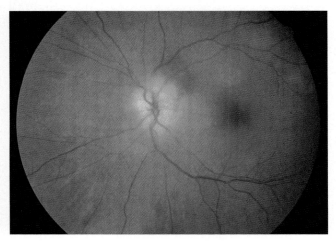

**Figure 5.6** Pallid optic nerve edema in giant cell arteritis. (This figure appears in black and white on page 58.)

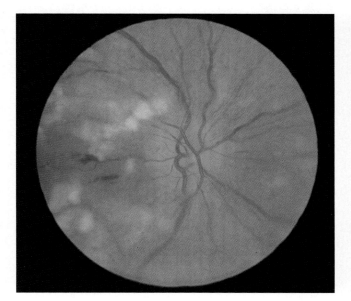

**Figure 5.7** The edematous optic nerve is surrounded by cotton-wool spots and intraretinal hemorrhages in malignant hypertension. (This figure appears in black and white on page 59.)

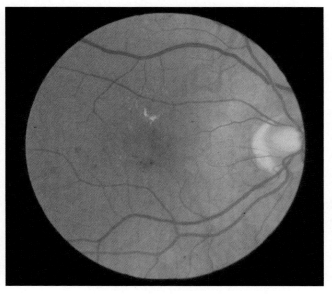

**Figure 5.8** Background diabetic retinopathy consisting of dot hemorrhages and hard exudates. (This figure appears in black and white on page 59.)

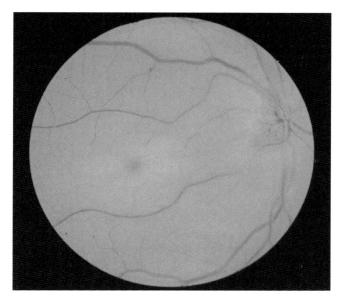

**Figure 5.10** The retina is edematous, and there is a cherry-red spot in the macula of a patient with central retinal artery occlusion. (This figure appears in black and white on page 61.)

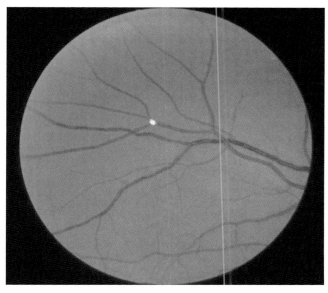

**Figure 5.11** Hollenhorst's plaque. (This figure appears in black and white on page 61.)

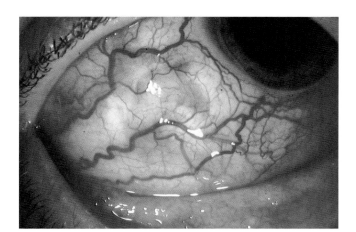

**Figure 5.13** Avascularity of the sclera leads to scleromalacia in a patient with rheumatoid arthritis. (This figure appears in black and white on page 62.)

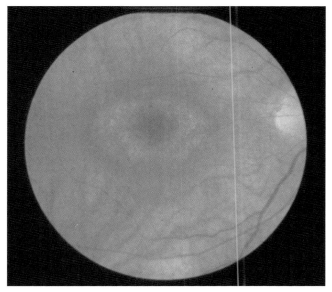

**Figure 5.14** Bull's-eye of hydroxychloroquine pigmentary maculopathy. (This figure appears in black and white on page 62.)

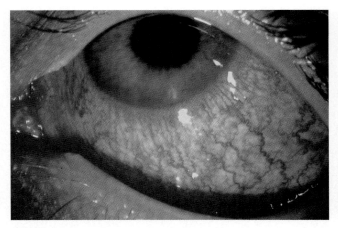

**Figure 5.15** Marked conjunctival injection and ciliary flush in acute iritis. (This figure appears in black and white on page 62.)

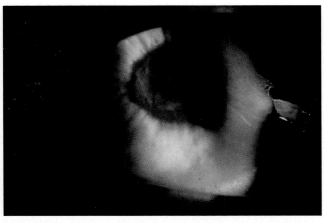

**Figure 5.16** The anterior lens capsule is covered by a fibrinous exudate in a patient with HLA-B27–associated acute iritis. (This figure appears in black and white on page 63.)

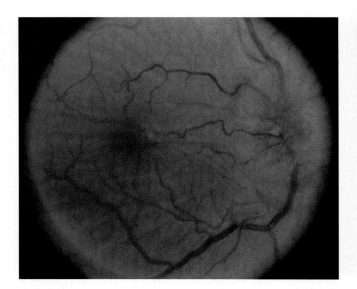

**Figure 5.17** Fundus photograph shows a swollen optic nerve and choroidal folds secondary to compression by enlarged muscles in a patient with thyroid optic neuropathy. (This figure appears in black and white on page 63.)

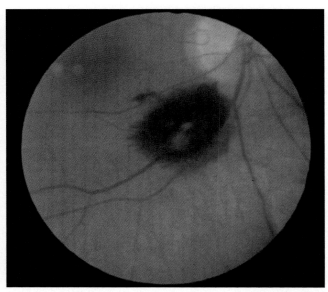

**Figure 5.18** Leukemic retinopathy characterized by intraretinal and preretinal hemorrhages. (This figure appears in black and white on page 63.)

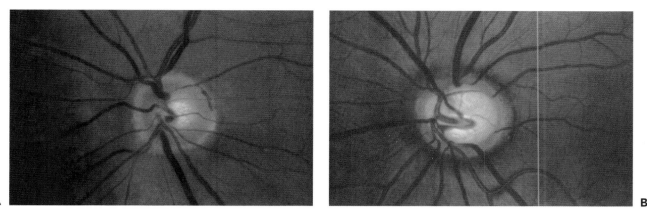

**Figure 5.20** **(A)** Normal optic nerve. **(B)** Glaucomatous optic nerve. (This figure appears in black and white on page 64.)

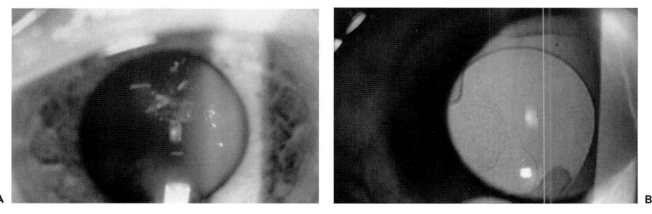

**Figure 5.21** **(A)** Cataract. **(B)** Intraocular lens implant. (This figure appears in black and white on page 66.)

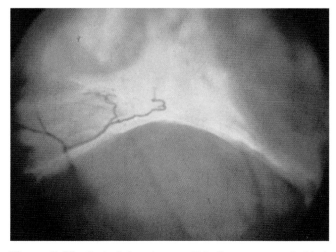

**Figure 5.22** Retinal detachment. (This figure appears in black and white on page 66.)

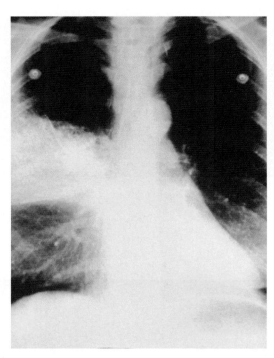

**Figure 18.3** Chest x-ray of patient in Case 6. (This figure appears in black and white on page 233.)

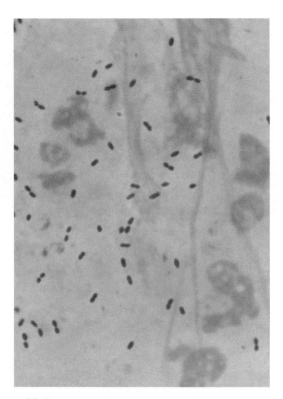

**Figure 18.4** Sputum Gram's stain of patient in Case 6. (This figure appears in black and white on page 233.)

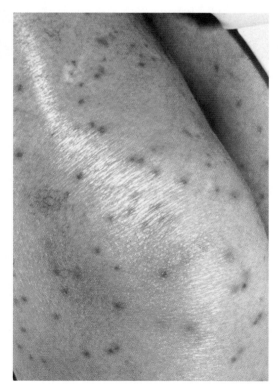

**Figure 18.5** Erythematous, nonblanching, nonpruritic, macronodular rash of patient in Case 6. (This figure appears in black and white on page 234.)

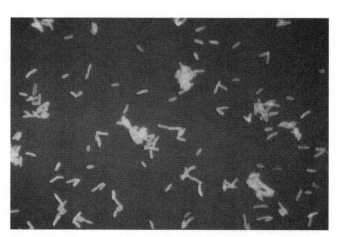

**Figure 18.9** Finding for Case 9. (This figure appears in black and white on page 238.)

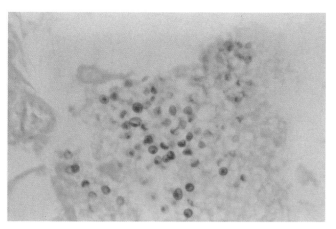

**Figure 18.10** Finding for Case 9. (This figure appears in black and white on page 239.)

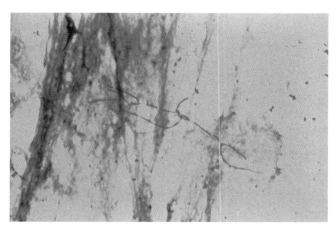

**Figure 18.11** Finding for Case 9. (This figure appears in black and white on page 239.)

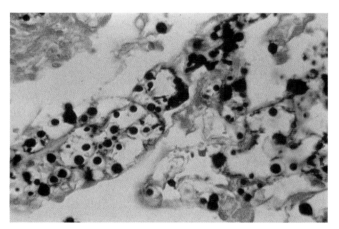

**Figure 18.12** Finding for Case 9. (This figure appears in black and white on page 239.)

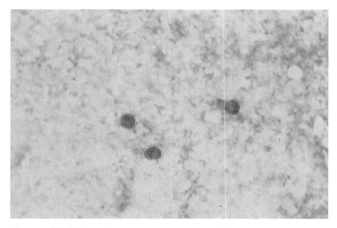

**Figure 18.13** Pathogen in Case 10. (This figure appears in black and white on page 241.)

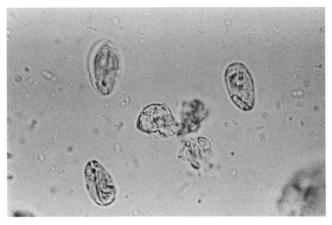

**Figure 18.14** Pathogen in Case 10. (This figure appears in black and white on page 241.)

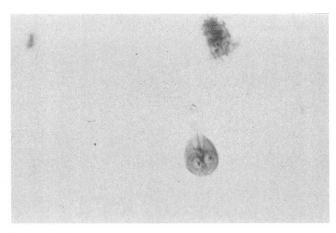

**Figure 18.15** Pathogen in Case 10. (This figure appears in black and white on page 241.)

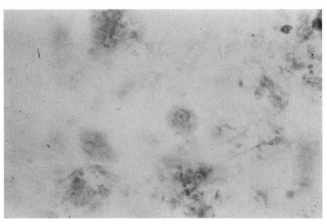

**Figure 18.16** *Entamoeba histolytica* trophozoite. (This figure appears in black and white on page 242.)

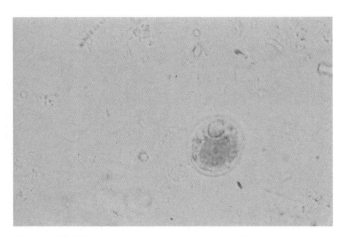

**Figure 18.17** *Entamoeba histolytica* cyst. (This figure appears in black and white on page 242.)

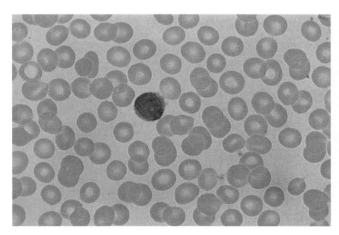

**Figure 18.18** Smear for patient 1. (This figure appears in black and white on page 244.)

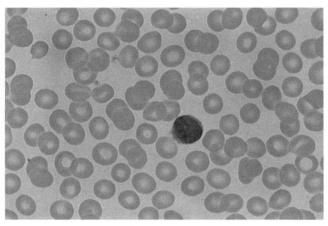

**Figure 18.19** Smear for patient 2. (This figure appears in black and white on page 245.)

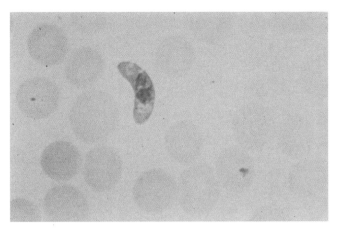

**Figure 18.20** Smear for patient 3. (This figure appears in black and white on page 245.)

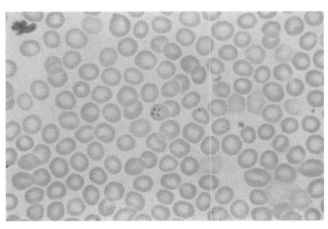

**Figure 18.21** Smear for patient 4. (This figure appears in black and white on page 245.)

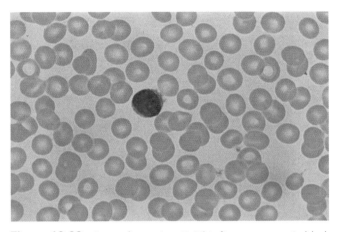

**Figure 18.22** Smear for patient 5. (This figure appears in black and white on page 245.)

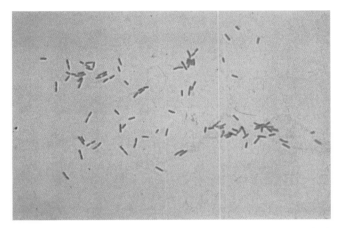

**Figure 18.23** Pathogen in Case 12. (This figure appears in black and white on page 250.)

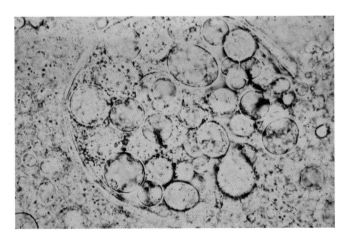

**Figure 18.24** Pathogen in Case 12. (This figure appears in black and white on page 250.)

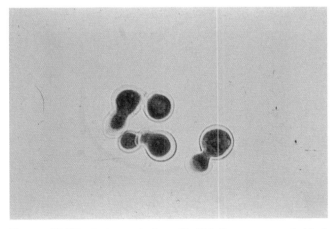

**Figure 18.25** Pathogen in Case 12. (This figure appears in black and white on page 250.)

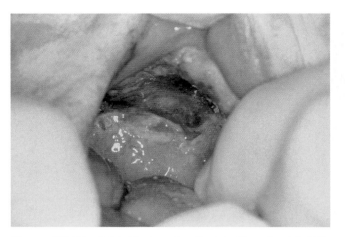

**Figure 18.26** Palatal lesion of patient in Question 54. (This figure appears in black and white on page 252.)

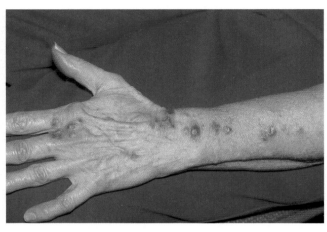

**Figure 18.27** Left arm lesions of patients in Questions 56 and 57. (This figure appears in black and white on page 252.)

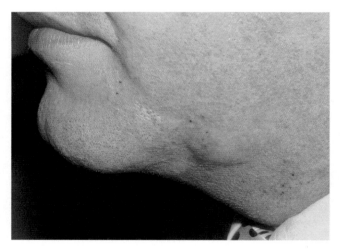

**Figure 18.28** Left mandibular lesion of patient in Question 58. (This figure appears in black and white on page 252.)

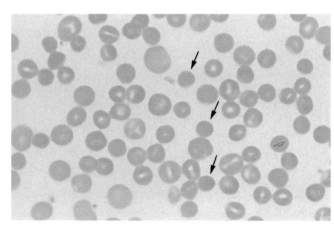

**Figure 27.1** Peripheral blood smear: spherocytes (*arrows*). (This figure appears in black and white on page 342.)

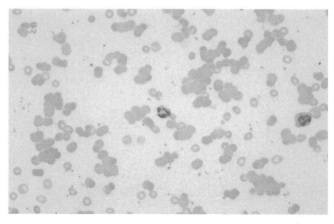

**Figure 27.2** Peripheral blood smear: aggregates of red blood cells in cold agglutinin disease. (This figure appears in black and white on page 342.)

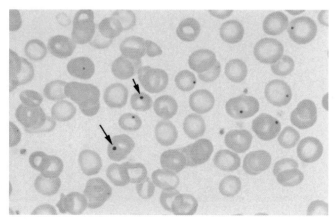

**Figure 27.3** Peripheral blood smear: Howell-Jolly bodies (*arrows*) within red blood cells. (This figure appears in black and white on page 343.)

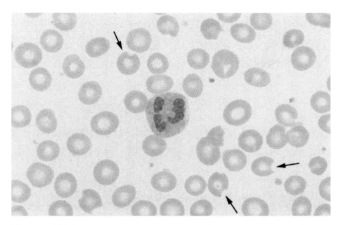

**Figure 27.4**  Peripheral blood smear: bite cells (*arrows*) characteristic of oxidative hemolysis. (This figure appears in black and white on page 343.)

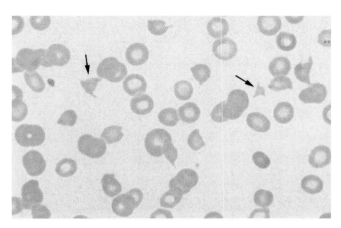

**Figure 27.5**  Peripheral blood smear: red blood cell fragments (*arrows*). (This figure appears in black and white on page 343.)

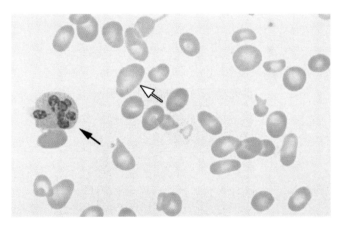

**Figure 27.6**  Peripheral blood smear: hypersegmented neutrophil (*dark arrow*) and oval macrocyte (*open white arrow*). (This figure appears in black and white on page 343.)

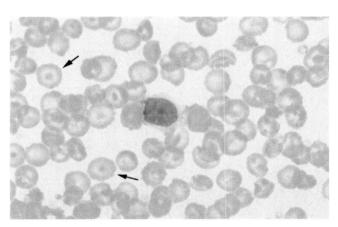

**Figure 27.7**  Peripheral blood smear: target red blood cells (*arrows*). (This figure appears in black and white on page 344.)

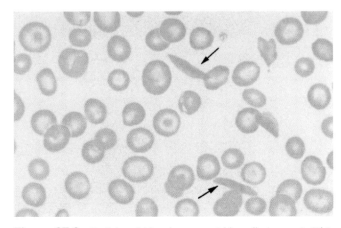

**Figure 27.8**  Peripheral blood smear: sickle cells (*arrows*). (This figure appears in black and white on page 344.)

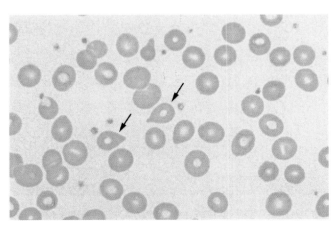

**Figure 27.9**  Peripheral blood smear: teardrop red blood cells (*arrows*). (This figure appears in black and white on page 344.)

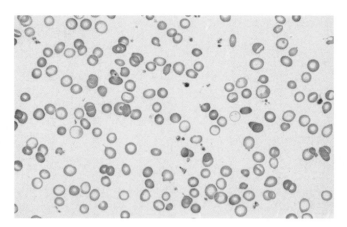

**Figure 27.10** Peripheral blood smear: numerous red blood cells demonstrating increased central pallor and moderate variation in size indicative of iron deficiency anemia. (This figure appears in black and white on page 344.)

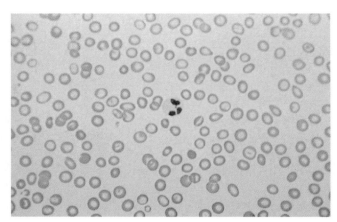

**Figure 27.11** Peripheral blood smear: a uniform population of pale red blood cells seen in thalassemia minor. (This figure appears in black and white on page 345.)

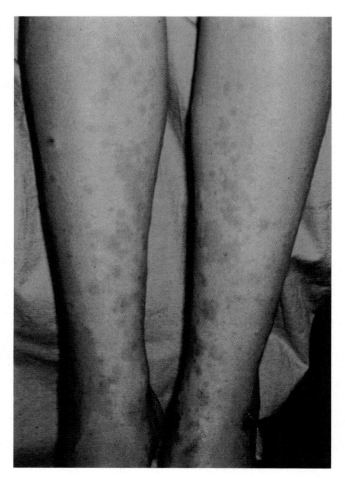

**Figure 32.1** Rash. (This figure appears in black and white on page 404.)

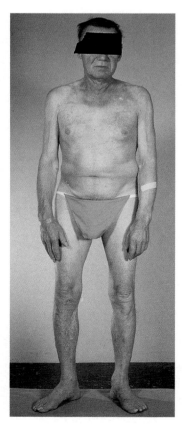

**Figure 34.1** Appearance of patient in Case 1. (This figure appears in black and white on page 414.)

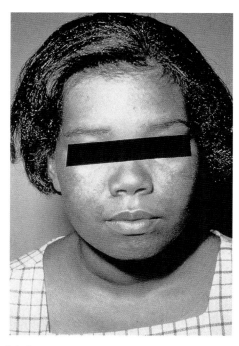

**Figure 34.3** Confluent facial rash of patient in Case 2. (This figure appears in black and white on page 414.)

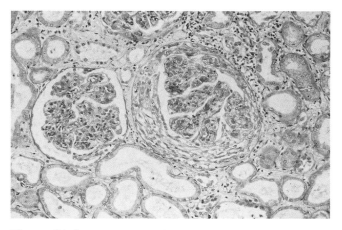

**Figure 34.4** Renal biopsy of patient in Question 7. (This figure appears in black and white on page 414.)

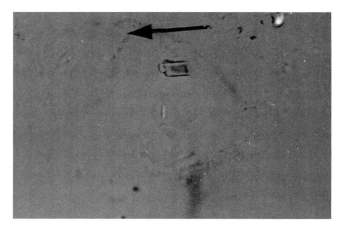

**Figure 34.5** Crystals (*arrow*) found in knee of patient in Question 11. (This figure appears in black and white on page 415.)

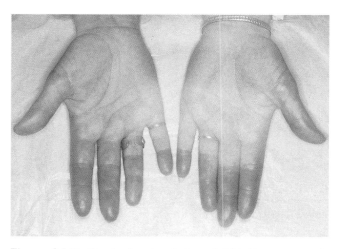

**Figure 34.7** Hands of patient in Case 4. (This figure appears in black and white on page 416.)

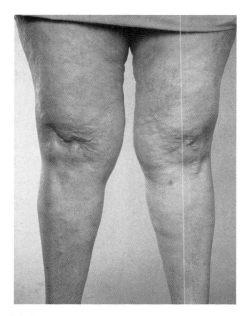

**Figure 34.9** Appearance of knees of patient in Case 5. (This figure appears in black and white on page 417.)

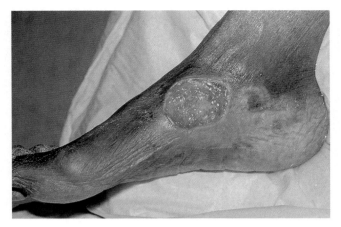

**Figure 34.10** Foot ulceration of patient in Case 6. (This figure appears in black and white on page 417.)

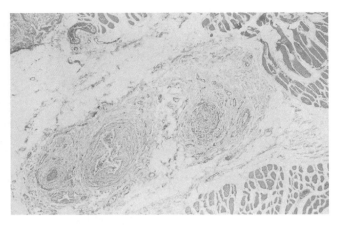

**Figure 34.11** Sural nerve biopsy in patient in Question 21. (This figure appears in black and white on page 417.)

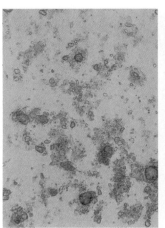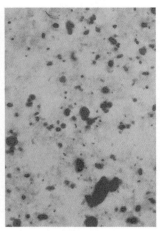

**Figure 34.12** Joint fluid stained with Alizarin Red S in Case 8. (This figure appears in black and white on page 418.)

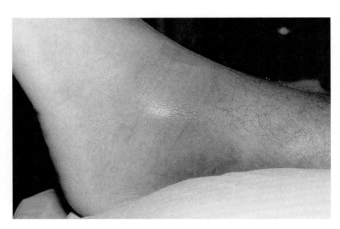

**Figure 34.13** Ankle of patient in Case 11. (This figure appears in black and white on page 418.)

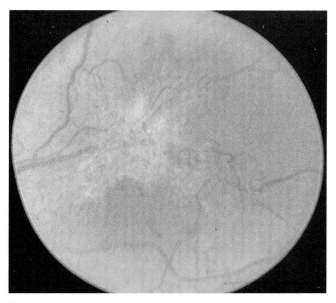

**Figure 48.1** Diabetic retinopathy. (This figure appears in black and white on page 566.)

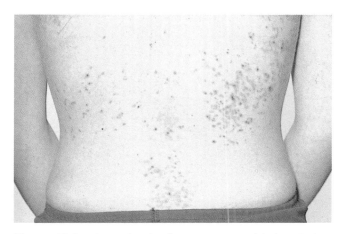

**Figure 48.2** Skin rash. (This figure appears in black and white on page 566.)

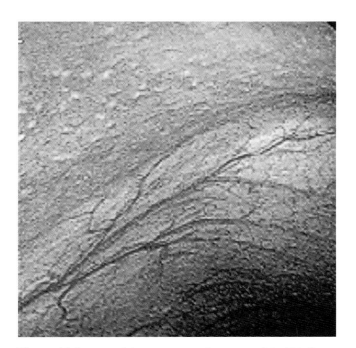

**Figure 60.1** Line of demarcation in ulcerative colitis. (This figure appears in black and white on page 727.)

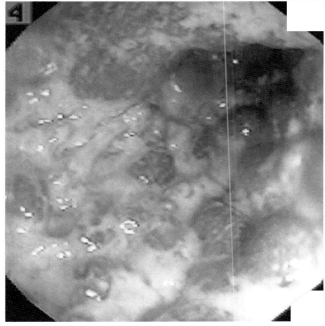

**Figure 60.2** Severe Crohn's disease. (This figure appears in black and white on page 729.)

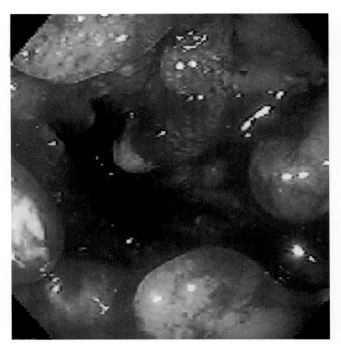

**Figure 62.1** Endoscopic photograph for the patient described in Question 14. (This figure appears in black and white on page 748.)

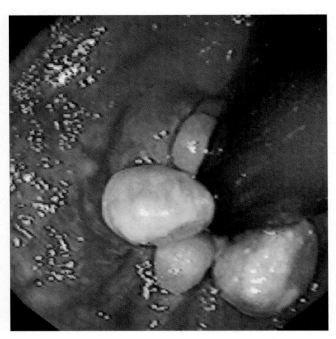

**Figure 62.2** Retroflexed view in the rectum of the patient described in Question 15. (This figure appears in black and white on page 748.)

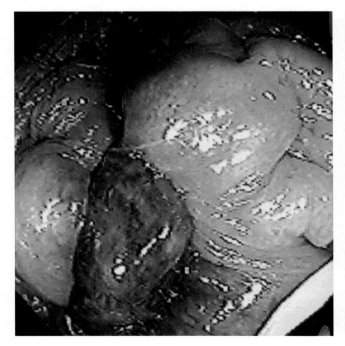

**Figure 62.3** Endoscopic photograph for the patient described in Question 16. (This figure appears in black and white on page 748.)

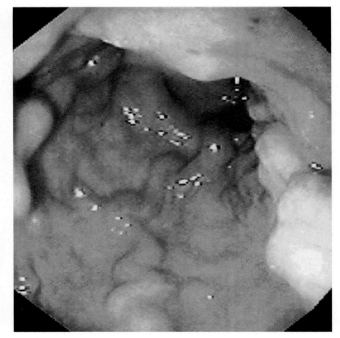

**Figure 62.4** Photograph from screening flexible sigmoidoscopy performed on the patient described in Question 17. (This figure appears in black and white on page 749.)

*Treatment.* The treatment of amenorrhea is groomed to the individual patient's requirements and may include simple gonadal steroid replacement; correcting the underlying etiologic disorder, if possible; psychiatric or psychosocial support; and the reestablishment of puberty using exogenous medications or hormones or the newer reproductive technologies. It is important to remember that the presence of the Y chromosome in a phenotypic female subject requires the operative removal of the gonads because they are considered precancerous.

## Premature Ovarian Failure

Growing evidence in the literature indicates that premature ovarian failure (POF) is multifactorial and encompasses a spectrum of clinical presentations, including:

- Permanent hypergonadotropic amenorrhea
- The apparent presence of a prematurely early perimenopausal state
- A condition waxing and waning from normogonadotropic menstrual cycles
- Hypergonadotropic amenorrhea

*Etiology.* The mean age at menopause in North America, 52 years, appears to be unrelated to the age of menarche or to parity, ethnic extraction, nutrition, or environmental factors. Menopause, owing to ovarian failure and the virtual absence of primordial follicles in the ovary, is characterized by low E2 levels, amenorrhea, and sustained elevation of gonadotropin levels. The final cessation of menses may be preceded by 2 to 10 years of progressively irregular cycles with prolonged intermenstrual intervals. During this time, gonadotropins, particularly FSH, may be variably elevated, but E2 levels are usually normal, ovulation is sporadic, and hot flashes are common.

Studies indicate a correlation between the size of the residual follicular stock and the preservation of more normal menstrual function at this stage. Although the primary cause of cessation of menstrual function is no doubt because of the disappearance of ovarian follicles, the nature of pituitary–ovarian interrelationships and a change in the ovarian milieu may help to explain the apparent gonadotropin resistance and relative infertility at this stage.

Because fewer than 2% of women reach menopause before the age of 40 years, this is the currently accepted cutoff for the definition of premature menopause. The etiology of POF is outlined in Table 43.1.

The classification of POF based on the presence or absence of follicles on an ovarian biopsy (at a particular time point) may be overly simplistic because the factors that govern the number of endowed ova, the rate of follicular atresia, the changes in ovarian steroid and peptide hormone production, and the intraovarian milieu as a function of age remain poorly understood.

## TABLE 43.1

### ETIOLOGIC CLASSIFICATION OF PREMATURE OVARIAN FAILURE

Chromosomal
- ☐ X-linked: Turner's syndrome and variants
- ☐ Familial long arm X deletion
- ☐ Triple X syndrome
- ☐ Autosomal
- ☐ Trisomy 13
- ☐ Trisomy 18

Enzymatic defects
- ☐ 17 hydroxylase deficiency
- ☐ Galactosemia

Gonadotropin apparatus defects
- ☐ Abnormal gonadotropin molecules
- ☐ Abnormal gonadotropin receptors

Infection
- ☐ Tuberculosis
- ☐ Mumps
- ☐ Others

Iatrogenic
Surgery
Chemotherapy
Irradiation
Vascular
Torsion/hemorrhage
Immunologic
Deficiency
Ataxia-telangiectasia
DiGeorge's syndrome
Autoimmune diseases
Oophoritis
Idiopathic
- ☐ With follicles
- ☐ Resistant ovary syndrome
- ☐ Afollicular

*Autoimmune Oophoritis.* Circulating antibodies against some ovarian component (including gonadotropin receptors) define the condition of autoimmune oophoritis in patients presenting with primary or secondary hypoestrogenic, hypergonadotropic amenorrhea, and the biopsy-proven presence of ovarian follicles. This occurs in 15% to 40% of such patients. Follicular lymphocytic infiltration, often transient, also may be found in ovarian biopsy specimens, particularly during the early evolution of the condition.

Variables, such as the type of antigen used, assay technique, and the time of testing in relationship to disease onset, appear to be of critical importance in the detection of this disorder. This concept should not seem surprising in light of identical issues that apply to the prototypic autoimmune glandular disease, Hashimoto's thyroiditis. In this condition, the antibody mix is heterogenous (organ damaging, antienzyme, growth promoting, receptor agonist, receptor blocking), the antibody mix is not fixed in proportion with time (the response varies with the antibody mix and the state of the thyroid gland at a particular time, and so transient or permanent hypofunction of the thyroid gland may occur), and the antibodies may disappear after organ death.

The coexistence of autoimmune POF in patients with Addison's disease may be as frequent as 25% and may relate to the presence of antibodies directed against the common steroidogenic enzymes shared by the two organs. The association of POF with hypothyroidism is less frequent but more so than in the general population. As with type I diabetes mellitus and Hashimoto's thyroiditis, there is an HLA-DR3 locus association with autoimmune oophoritis.

***Idiopathic Premature Ovarian Failure and the Resistant Ovary Syndrome.*** A significant proportion of women with POF, in whom circulating autoantibodies are either not detected or not looked for, and for whom no other cause has been identified, are defined as having idiopathic POF. If ovarian follicles are present, the term *resistant ovary syndrome* has been used to define the condition. The presence or absence of follicles in patients presenting with POF is pivotal, not only for establishing a diagnosis but also in delineating therapeutic options.

***Diagnosis.*** The patient history and physical examination may help to establish the diagnosis of POF. Documentation requires the presence of hypoestrogenemic hypergonadotropism, especially on more than on one occasion. A karyotype is mandatory in primary amenorrhea and can be helpful in secondary amenorrhea as well. Searching for antibodies may be helpful; a positive finding opens up a number of therapeutic options. Testing is generally not available, however, and the procedures have not been standardized.

Establishing the presence or absence of primordial follicles in the ovary is crucial. The gold standard has been a full-thickness biopsy of the ovary to look for primordial follicles. The results are qualitative, however, and presume appropriate representation in the specimen obtained, the major disadvantage of such biopsies. Moreover, the ensuing potential risk of adhesions and mechanical infertility is added to the already existing infertile state. Thus, attempts have been made to use the noninvasive transvaginal ultrasound to document the presence of follicles. The data are still preliminary as to the usefulness and accuracy of such an evaluation.

***Treatment.*** In the 1990s, the impetus to find methods to treat POF was obtunded or lost through the availability of successful egg donation, in vitro fertilization, and embryo-transfer programs. In persons who desire biologic offspring, the whole question of our ability to differentiate

better the heterogenous group of POF patients is crucial if successful (and presumably less costly) treatment programs are to evolve.

Those patients with no primordial follicles, if clearly defined, is really untreatable except by donor in vitro fertilization techniques. Those patients with immunologic abnormalities and discernible primordial follicles might benefit from such therapies as high-dose glucocorticoids or plasmapheresis.

Other patients might benefit from megadoses of exogenous gonadotropins or short-term downregulation by estrogen.

Estrogens also may act by ameliorating the autoimmune process. Such regimens have been variably reported to yield successful pregnancies. A more recent approach has been the downregulation by GnRH agonists, followed by attempts at ovulation induction using exogenous gonadotropins.

Overall, the success of therapeutic intervention has been remarkably small, and most schools of thought are that such attempts are futile. The easy, safe, and highly successful egg donation and in vitro fertilization programs have, therefore, mainly replaced all such endeavors.

# MALE ENDOCRINE DISORDERS

## Male Hypogonadism

Male hypogonadism is defined as the failure to produce testosterone or sperm.

### Etiology

Hypogonadism is usually classified as primary or secondary, according to its cause:

- Primary
  - Genetic disease
  - Klinefelter's syndrome
  - Androgen-resistance syndrome
  - Steroidogenic enzyme defects
  - Congenital anorchia
  - Infection
  - Iatrogenic causes
  - Drug side effects
  - Chemotherapy
  - Radiation
  - Vasectomy
  - Toxin exposure
    - Mercury
    - Cadmium
- Secondary
  - Endocrine disorders
  - Pubertal delay
  - Hypopituitarism
  - Hypothalamic
  - Kallmann's syndrome

☐ Hyperprolactinemia
☐ Adrenal gland dysfunction
☐ Thyroid gland dysfunction
☐ Systemic illness
☐ Malnutrition
☐ Weight loss
☐ Anorexia nervosa
☐ Cancer
☐ Drug abuse

### Specific Hypogonadism Conditions

#### Klinefelter's Syndrome

Klinefelter's syndrome is a chromosomal disorder characterized by the presence of one or two extra X chromosomes, XXY or XXXY. Klinefelter's syndrome occurs in about 1 in 500 male births. The characteristics of the disorder include:

- Variable androgen deficiency is present
- On average, patients are taller, with disproportionate lower segment growth
- Small testes
- Azoospermia
- Gynecomastia
- Hypergonadotropic hypogonadism

**Uncommon Testicular Disorders.** Table 43.2 presents uncommon testicular disorders.

### TABLE 43.2
### UNCOMMON TESTICULAR DISORDERS

| Testicular Disorder | Association/Cause |
| --- | --- |
| Hypogonadotropic hypogonadism | Craniofacial anomalies |
| Congenital deafness | |
| Intellectual impairment | |
| Cerebellar ataxia | |
| Laurence-Moon-Biedl syndrome | |
| Prader-Willi syndrome | |
| Hemochromatosis | |
| Anorexia nervosa | |
| Excessive exercise | |
| Primary hypogonadism | Myotonic dystrophy |
| Noonan's syndrome | |
| Reifenstein's syndrome | |
| Androgen receptor defects | |
| Absent vasa deferentia | Cystic fibrosis |
| Zero motility (cilial defects) | Kartagener's syndrome |
| Varicocele | Renal carcinoma |
| Renal malformations | |
| Testicular infarction/orchitis | Polyarteritis nodosa |
| Hemophilia | |
| Sickle cell anemia | |
| Brucellosis | |
| Gonorrhea | |

**Clinical Presentation.** Peripubertally, hypogonadism presents as an absence of secondary sex characteristics, including:

- Small testes
- Penis indicating a lack of development
- Eunuchoid proportions (arm span >5 cm longer than height)

Postpubertally, the cardinal features are:

- Decreased libido
- Impotence
- Loss of secondary sexual hair
- Wrinkled skin
- Testicular atrophy
- Little change in penile size

**Diagnosis.** In laboratory investigation, a check for gonadotropins, prolactin, and testosterone is needed. If the patient is found to be hypogonadotropic with or without hyperprolactinemia, a standard evaluation should be done to rule out hypothalamic or pituitary abnormality. If the patient is hypergonadotropic, karyotyping should be done.

**Treatment.** The treatment of male hypogonadism usually is geared to replacement. In hypogonadotropic persons, fertility may be stimulated by the use of gonadotropins.

#### Erectile Dysfunction

Erectile dysfunction (ED), formerly termed *impotence*, is the consistent inability to achieve or maintain an erection sufficient for satisfactory sexual activity.

In the United States, ED is estimated to affect as many as 30 million men. The incidence of ED increases with age, but it is not a necessary consequence of aging. It may be significantly underdiagnosed because of a reluctance on the part of patients to discuss the problem with their equally reluctant caregivers.

Simplistically, ED can be organic or psychogenic, although most cases have a combination of the two. Some of the causes of ED include:

- Inflammation
- Mechanical injury
- Psychologic disorders
- Occlusive-vascular disorders
- Traumatic or operative injury
- Endurance-related disorders
- Neurologic disorders
- Chemical exposures
- Endocrine disorders

Up to 35% (in one study) of patients with impotence have an endocrine cause, usually an easy diagnosis to make and relatively easy and gratifying to treat. Common endocrine causes include hypogonadotropic hypogonadism (Kallmann's syndrome), hypergonadotropic hypogonadism

(Klinefelter's syndrome), hyperprolactinemia, and diabetes mellitus.

In hyperprolactinemia, the impotence is thought to develop through two mechanisms:

- A direct feedback of prolactin on the GnRH neurons in the hypothalamus by the ultra-short-loop feedback (the major operative mechanism) whereby GnRH pulsatility, and thus LH pulsatility, is dampened, slowed, and thereby made significantly dysfunctional. Consequently, no stimulation of the testes occurs, and hypogonadotropic hypogonadism ensues.
- A direct effect on the "libidigenous" center by prolactin, and a resultant decreased sexual interest and drive. Thus, testosterone supplementation alone is not always or totally effective in restoring libido and potency, and normoprolactinemia usually is required for the full effect of testosterone to be manifested.

Diabetes mellitus is probably the most common cause of impotence. Whereas the patient's age is a factor (i.e., older men are more likely to develop impotence than younger men), the duration of diabetes is also an important variable in the tendency to develop impotence. The longer the duration of diabetes, the higher the incidence of impotence. Etiologically, the impotence of diabetes is caused by the combination of vasculopathy and neuropathy, the relative contribution of each being variable in any one patient. Psychogenic factors may play a significant role early in the disorder: The expectation and fear of failing after one failure commonly worsen the problem initially, and the decreased sensation of orgasm and ejaculation because of neuropathy and retrograde ejaculation takes its toll. Actual hormonal deficiency secondary to diabetes is rare.

***Physiology of Erection and Pathophysiology of Erectile Dysfunction.*** Penile erection occurs because of a series of events that cause a relaxation of the smooth muscle in the corpus cavernosa. Noradrenergic, noncholinergic neurons acting on the endothelial cells generate nitric oxide, which activates guanylate cyclase and fosters the change of guanosine triphosphate to cyclic guanosine monophosphate (cGMP). cGMP causes relaxation and penile erection; however, cGMP is rapidly metabolized by phosphodiesterase-5 to GMP, and thus relaxation and erection are not maintained. Any agent causing an increase in nitric oxide, and therefore activation to cGMP, or alternatively slowing the breakdown of cGMP by inhibiting phosphodiesterase-5, causes and maintains penile erection.

***Diagnosis.*** The clinical aspects to be considered in the evaluation of impotence include an evaluation of hormonal function, both by history (libido, hair growth, gynecomastia, previous fertility, and history of alcohol or drug abuse) and by physical examination (hair distribution, body habitus, testes size, prostate size, visual fundi and fields, evidence of other endocrinopathy, and evidence of other illnesses). In the investigation of impotence, in addition to an evaluation of testosterone, gonadotropin, and prolactin levels, it is important to evaluate vascular integrity using Doppler flow studies and neurogenic integrity by the snap gauge test or the more cumbersome nocturnal penile tumescence evaluation. There is no place for an oral glucose tolerance test in the evaluation of impotence. A growing body of evidence shows that the presence of ED is a powerful indicator for the presence of various cardiovascular risk factors and, in fact, may reveal clinically significant but still silent cardiovascular disease in as many as 60% of ED patients. Thus, asking the question may reveal more than just an easily treated, personally embarrassing, awkward situation.

***Treatment.*** The goal of treatment is to find the underlying cause, if possible. Otherwise, testosterone replacement, if needed, can be quite helpful. If no clear cause is found, attempts to induce erection remain the mainstay. Herbal remedies, such as ginseng, have been tried with low and variable success rates, rarely exceeding 20% to 30%. In the same vein, yohimbine, an α-adrenergic receptor blocker, has had variable and low rates of success (33% in one study). Venous arterial microsurgery is rarely indicated or successful. Penile prostheses have been used with good success, and numerous rigid, semirigid, or inflatable prostheses are available and in use. External mechanical devices, such as vacuum-constrictive pumps, can be used but tend to detract from the spontaneity of the sexual act. The standby therapies with the greatest patient acceptance rates have been transurethral prostaglandin application [alprostadil (MUSE)] and the intracavernosal injection of papaverine or prostaglandin E2. The former was associated with a painful urethritis that limited its use, and the latter suffers from the disadvantage of injections and the lack of spontaneity.

Most recently, the advent of sildenafil citrate (Viagra) has revolutionized the whole picture of ED. Sildenafil is an inhibitor of phosphodiesterase-5 and therefore allows cGMP to persist and maintain erection. The ease of administration (orally) and the high chance of success (60% to 85% in various reports), irrespective of the cause of the ED, have fostered a lot of discussion and "coming out of the closet" of patients with ED. The shorter the duration of ED, the greater the chance of success. Furthermore, because by itself it will not cause erection, but is dependent on physical intimacy to induce erection, the spontaneity is better established. Side effects are minimal, consisting of occasional headaches and a temporary blue visual haze at the highest dosage because of blockage of the phosphodiesterase in the retina. Reports of myocardial infarctions occurring while a patient is taking sildenafil are thought to be more likely due to the untoward and unusual resumption of sexual intimacy rather than a direct effect of the drug on the diseased myocardium. Because of the intimate relationship of nitrous oxide to the process of generating cGMP, and the ubiquity of that biochemical mechanism, however, patients taking nitrates may not use PDE-5 inhibitors. These agents also behave like nitrate donors and therefore predispose to severe hypotension if used concurrently. (Using a nitrate spray on the shaft of the penis can cause erection, but it also induces a headache in the partner because of transvaginal absorption of nitrate during intercourse.) In summary, the use of sildenafil has tended to decrease the ancillary testing of ED. Although this may be of economic benefit, it must be stressed that a good history and physical, a marginal hormonal evaluation if indicated, and good hygiene, in terms of the treatment of underlying causes, cannot be replaced by the generalized and thoughtless use of sildenafil.

### Gynecomastia

Gynecomastia is defined as palpable glandular tissue below the areola in males.

Gynecomastia is caused either by increased estrogen or decreased androgens. Estrogens stimulate breast tissue; androgens inhibit breast tissue. Thus, the ratio of estrogen to androgen determines the degree of stimulation. More important, in the absence of androgens, it requires extremely small concentrations, even below those measurable by conventional assays, to stimulate mammary growth. Estrogen, in men, is derived from the peripheral conversion of precursors like androstenedione and testosterone. LH and hCG stimulate E2 secretion by the testes.

***Diagnosis.*** The evaluation of gynecomastia usually demands a methodologic search to establish the following:

- Presence
- Associations
- Speed of development
- Progression
- Systemic illnesses
- Associated drugs
- Genital abnormalities

***Physical Examination.*** The physical examination must rule out a malignancy with a good detailed examination, including a detailed testicular examination and a mammogram if the index of suspicion is high.

***Laboratory Studies.*** Laboratory evaluation may be unnecessary in asymptomatic, nontender gynecomastia. If the physical evaluation reveals pain, rapid growth, or a large size, laboratory evaluation should include testosterone, LH, hCG, DHEAS, or urinary 17-ketosteroids levels, as well as E2, prolactin, thyroid, and liver functions.

***Differential Diagnosis.*** The differential diagnosis of gynecomastia includes:

- Physiologic
  - Newborn
  - Pubertal
  - Aging
- Pathologic
  - Increased estrogens
  - Tumors
    - Adrenal
    - Testes (Leydig cell tumors)
    - Choriocarcinoma
  - Ectopic gonadotropin
  - Ectopic placental-like hormone
  - Cirrhosis
  - Hyperthyroidism
  - Decreased androgen effect
  - Hypogonadism
  - Klinefelter's syndrome
  - Mumps
  - Cytotoxic chemotherapy
  - Irradiation
  - Androgen insensitivity
  - Refeeding
  - Chronic renal failure/dialysis
- Pharmacologic
  - Estrogens
  - Aromatizable androgens
  - hCG
  - Antiandrogens
  - Psychotropics-phenothiazines
  - Methyldopa
  - Reserpine
  - Spironolactone
  - Cimetidine
  - Ketoconazole
  - Cyproterone
  - Flutamide
  - Estrogen-like agents
    - Digitalis
    - Marijuana
  - Others
  - Central nervous system acting
- Miscellaneous
  - Idiopathic
  - Pseudogynecomastia (mimics appearance of normal breast)
  - Lipomastia (adipose-related)
  - Neoplasm

Among newborns, 60% to 90% have gynecomastia, likely secondary to placental estrogen exposure; this feature regresses over weeks. Among pubertal boys, 50% to 70% have unilateral or bilateral gynecomastia, thought to be secondary to the preponderance of estrogen production over testosterone and the earlier achievement of normal adult values of estrogen; this condition regresses in most cases.

Among elderly men, 4% may have gynecomastia at autopsy, likely secondary to a decrease in testosterone with aging, whereas E2 is still maintained, possibly by increased peripheral conversion.

Tumors, whether producing de novo estrogen or its precursors (adrenal or Leydig cell testicular tumors) or producing hormones such as hCG, which stimulate the testes to produce estrogen, cause gynecomastia.

Gynecomastia in cirrhosis is thought to occur because of two mechanisms: an increased peripheral conversion owing to decreased clearance of androstenedione, and an alcohol-mediated suppression of testosterone production by the suppression of the hypothalamic-pituitary-adrenal system.

Hyperthyroidism induces SHBGs, thereby increasing the level of total testosterone and E2. Free testosterone remains normal, but free E2 is increased because of the increased androstenedione available for peripheral conversion.

Gynecomastia associated with hypogonadism is secondary to the increased E2 to testosterone ratio.

Refeeding seems to induce a "second puberty," and the mechanism of gynecomastia is the same as that seen in pubertal gynecomastia. This is also thought to be one of the factors that cause gynecomastia in chronic renal failure or dialysis.

**Treatment.** The treatment of gynecomastia is usually to address the underlying cause, if any (which generally helps to resolve the problem), and to reassure the patient if the cause is likely physiologic or residual. If no obvious etiology is found, follow-up and observation are all that is indicated. It must be remembered that the resolution of the problem still may leave a mass of fibrous tissue. The treatment regimen may include the following:

- Androgen (testosterone), danazol, or antiestrogens, although medical treatments are not frequently used
- Prevention by radiation before estrogen treatment has been advocated by a few
- Surgery and a reduction mammoplasty remain the most appropriate treatment of significant, psychologically damaging gynecomastia, although the words of Nuhall are appropriate and bear keeping in mind: "In the absence of pain, rapid change in size, eccentric, or hard breast mass or testicular mass, no further evaluation of gynecomastia in men is necessary"

# REVIEW EXERCISES

## QUESTIONS

Match the hormone profile, taken in the morning, to the disease in these women with acne and hirsutism:

**1.** ACTH 22, cortisol 35, DHEAS 5.6, testosterone 75, thyroid-stimulating hormone (TSH) 0.5, $T_4$ 6.4

**2.** ACTH 22, cortisol 19, DHEAS 3.6, testosterone 72, TSH 3.4, $T_4$ 6.4

**3.** ACTH <1, cortisol 5, DHEAS 0.9, testosterone 12, TSH 0.6, $T_4$ 6.4

**4.** ACTH 38, cortisol 14, DHEAS 5.6, testosterone 78, TSH 0.9, $T_4$ 7.3

**5.** ACTH <5, cortisol 42, DHEAS 9.8, testosterone 112, TSH 0.5, $T_4$ 7.8

**6.** ACTH 16, cortisol 21, DHEAS 2.5, testosterone 66, TSH 9.8, $T_4$ 6.2
a) Primary hypothyroidism
b) Exogenous steroids
c) Polycystic ovary disease
d) Adrenal carcinoma
e) Congenital adrenal hyperplasia
f) Cushing's disease

Match the disease scenario with the hormone profile:

**7.** A 21-year-old woman with primary amenorrhea and no sense of smell

**8.** A 19-year-old woman with short stature, primary amenorrhea, and webbed neck

**9.** A 24-year-old woman with treated schizophrenia, presenting with amenorrhea

**10.** A 23-year-old with postpill amenorrhea

**11.** A 26-year-old with headaches, visual blurring, and amenorrhea
a) LH <2, FSH <2, prolactin 683
b) LH <2, FSH <2, prolactin 68
c) LH <2.0, FSH <2.0, prolactin 6
d) LH 2.3, FSH 3.1, prolactin 18
e) LH 23, FSH 47, prolactin 8

Match the hormonal profile to the case presented:

**12.** A 26-year-old, tall, young man with gynecomastia, microphallus, and small, soft testes (<3 cc)

**13.** A 24-year-old, tall, young man with widely spread teeth, goiter, skin tags, microphallus, and small, normal-sized testes (6 to 7 cc)

**14.** A 19-year-old, tall, young man with bilateral inguinal hernia and an empty scrotum

**15.** A 25-year-old, tall, young man with a history of pubertal mumps orchitis, a normal-sized penis, and normal testes (8 to 10 cc)

**16.** A 22-year-old, tall, young man with microphallus, small testes (4 to 5 cc), and no sense of smell
a) LH <2, FSH <2, testosterone 25, prolactin 7, growth hormone 11
b) LH <2, FSH 2.3, testosterone 48, prolactin 38, growth hormone 18

c) LH 3.8, FSH 23, testosterone 389, prolactin 7, growth hormone 0.9

d) LH 13.6, FSH 13.8, testosterone 176, prolactin 9, growth hormone 0.6

e) LH 76, FSH 95, testosterone 92, prolactin 12, growth hormone 1.6

**17.** Impotence is commonly seen in which of the following?

a) Diabetes mellitus

b) Congenital adrenal hyperplasia

c) Schizophrenia that is well controlled

d) Androgen insensitivity syndrome

e) a and c only

f) b and d only

g) All of the above

**18.** Gynecomastia is commonly seen in which of the following?

a) An XY individual with bilateral inguinal scars and a total lack of secondary sexual hair

b) An XY individual with well-treated and controlled salt-losing congenital adrenal hyperplasia

c) An XY individual with spider nevi, asterixis, and ascites

d) An XY individual who is the "timid" member of a homosexual couple

e) a and c only

f) b and d only

g) All of the above

**19.** A 27-year-old Italian woman presents for evaluation of hirsutism and a 2-year history of irregular heavy menses. Menarche was at age 13, and her periods were always irregular, except when she was on birth control pills (ages 18 to 24 years). Thelarche and adrenarche were normal. She noted the onset of significant acne at the age of 17 years, for which she was treated with antibiotics and isotretinoin (Accutane). Accutane had to be discontinued because of severe hypertriglyceridemia. At about the same time, she noted the development of hirsutism, which has slowly progressed. She had been trying to become pregnant for the past 3 years.

On examination, her weight is 170 pounds; height, 5 ft, 3 in. She has hyperpigmentation of the neck and axillary folds; a small goiter; and hirsutism on the chin, upper lip, and side of her face, as well as periareolar and periumbilical coarse, dark terminal hair. Her blood pressure is 120/82 mm Hg. Waist to hip ratio is 0.95 and no striae. Liver edge is palpable 1 cm below the costal margin.

The differential diagnosis in this case would include

a) Genetic hirsutism

b) Adult-onset congenital adrenal hyperplasia

c) Polycystic ovarian disease

d) Cushing's syndrome

e) a, b, and c

f) a and c

g) All of the above

**20.** In this same case, the appropriate laboratory tests include the following

a) Serum DHEAS, testosterone, free testosterone

b) Serum TSH, prolactin

c) Serum 17 hydroprogesterone

d) Gonadotropins and $E_2$

e) a, b, and c only

f) All of the above laboratory tests

**21.** A 26-year-old woman presents for evaluation of amenorrhea of 6 months' duration. She had a normal menarche at age 12 and normal puberty. Her menses had become progressively lighter over the past 2 or 3 years and occurred 4 to 9 weeks apart before amenorrhea. She has been under a significant amount of stress in the past 2 years, completing her medical degree, competing on the university gymnastic team, and experiencing the breakup of a long-term relationship. She has never taken birth control pills and has never been pregnant. She denies galactorrhea; she has had a 15-pound weight loss; and has no hirsutism, acne, or headache. She was diagnosed with Hashimoto's hypothyroidism at age 16, for which she is on L-thyroxine with a normal serum TSH over the years.

Laboratory examination showed an FSH of 4 IU/L, an LH of 2 IU/L, and a prolactin of 12 mg/mL, with a serum TSH of 10.8 μU/mL, testosterone 42 ng/dL, and DHEAS 3.3 ng/mL. The remaining biochemistry was normal.

Which of the following would *not* be in the differential diagnosis?

a) Functional amenorrhea secondary to stress, weight loss, and exercise

b) Hypothyroidism

c) PCOS

d) POF

**22.** A 26-year-old man presents with primary infertility. He has been married for 4 years and has been trying to father a child for 3 years. He has no difficulty with sexual function. Past and family history is unremarkable, and he is on no medications and does not smoke, drink, or take any street drugs. He is 6 ft, 2 in tall (the tallest in his family), weighs 264 pounds, has an arm span of 80 in, and has a pubis-to-heel length of 39 in. He has bilateral gynecomastia; a 2.5-in penis partially embedded in the mons; bilateral small, soft testes; and sparse, but present, secondary sexual hair growth. His testosterone value is 210 ng/dL (normal >220 ng/dL), and he is azoospermic.

Your diagnosis is

a) Klinefelter's syndrome

b) Congenital hypoorchia

c) Postsubclinical mumps orchitis

**d)** Kallmann's syndrome
**e)** Pubertal hyperprolactinemia

**23.** In this same case, does our young man with primary infertility, no sexual dysfunction, and azoospermia with small testes but nearly low-normal testosterone need treatment with testosterone?
**a)** Yes
**b)** No

**24.** A 52-year-old man presents with a complaint of impotence. He reports progressively increasing difficulty, first with maintaining and later with achieving an erection. He is an attorney, married for 24 years, has four children, the youngest age 16, and has no verbalized stress. He was found to have hypertension about 6 years before and suffered a myocardial infarction 4 years earlier. He has been controlled on β-blockers and a thiazide diuretic, has no angina and no arrhythmias, and has well-controlled blood pressure. He has no other symptoms of note. He has a family history of diabetes, hyperlipidemia, hypertension, and heart disease. He does not smoke and only drinks socially.

Examination shows weight, 180 pounds; height, 5 ft, 9 in. Blood pressure is 135/84 mm Hg and pulse is 68 bpm and regular, with an occasional extra systole. Liver is palpable 1 cm below the costal margin, with a span of 17 cm. No bruits are present. Bilateral lipomastia is noted. Genital examination reveals a normal penis and testicles that measure 4.5 to 3.1 cm bilaterally. A small varicocele is present on the right side. The prostate is mildly enlarged with an intact median groove. Fundi and fields are normal.

The required laboratory evaluation would include which of the following?
**a)** Gonadotropins, testosterone, and thyroid function tests
**b)** Testosterone, prolactin, TSH
**c)** Liver, kidney, electrolyte, glucose panel
**d)** Oral glucose tolerance test
**e)** a and c only
**f)** b and c only
**g)** b, c, and d

**25.** Which further evaluations are needed?
**a)** A snap gauge
**b)** Nocturnal penile tumescence study
**c)** Magnetic resonance imaging of the head
**d)** a and c only
**e)** All of the above
**f)** None of the above

**26.** Which is the treatment option in this case?
**a)** T shots
**b)** Bromocriptine
**c)** Intravenous injection of papaverine
**d)** Discontinuation of propranolol (Inderal) and thiazides

**e)** Penile prosthesis placement
**f)** Reassurance and support with no treatment

## ANSWERS

**1. f.**
Cushing's disease matches the laboratory values of ACTH 22, cortisol 35, DHEAS 5.6, testosterone 75, thyroid-stimulating hormone (TSH) 0.5, $T_4$ 6.4

**2. c.**
Polycystic ovary disease matches the laboratory values of ACTH 22, cortisol 19, DHEAS 3.6, testosterone 72, TSH 3.4, $T_4$ 6.4

**3. b.**
Exogenous steroid use matches the laboratory values of ACTH <1, cortisol 5, DHEAS 0.9, testosterone 12, TSH 0.6, $T_4$ 6.4

**4. e.**
Congenital adrenal hyperplasia matches the laboratory values of ACTH 38, cortisol 14, DHEAS 5.6, testosterone 78, TSH 0.9, $T_4$ 7.3

**5. d.**
Adrenal carcinoma matches the laboratory values of ACTH <5, cortisol 42, DHEAS 9.8, testosterone 112, TSH 0.5, $T_4$ 7.8

**6. a.**
Primary hypothyroidism matches the laboratory values of ACTH 16, cortisol 21, DHEAS 2.5, testosterone 66, TSH 9.8, $T_4$ 6.2

**7. c.**

**8. e.**

**9. b.**

**10. d.**

**11. a.**

**12. e.**

**13. b.**

**14. d.**

**15. c.**

**16. a.**

**17. e.**

**18. e.**

**19. e.**
No clinical evidence given for Cushing's disease.

**20. e.**
Gonadotropins and $E_2$ are no clinical help.

**21. d.**
Gonadotropins indicate that this is impossible.

**22.** a.

**23.** a.

Yes. The patient needs treatment to stop continued stimulation of the testes, which synthesize $E_2$ and contribute to gynecomastia.

**24.** f.

**25.** a.

A snap gauge gives almost the same information as nocturnal penile tumescence evaluation.

**26.** d.

If possible, these should be changed to other medications to determine whether they are contributing to the problem.

## SUGGESTED READINGS

### Female

Barbieri RL. Hyperandrogenic disorders. *Clin Obstet Gynecol* 1990;33: 640–659.

Barnes R, Rosenfeld RL. The polycystic ovary syndrome: pathogenesis and treatment. *Ann Intern Med* 1989;110:386–399.

Biffignandi P, Massucchetti D, Molinatti GM. Female hirsutism: pathophysiological considerations and therapeutic implications. *Endocr Rev* 1984;5:498–513.

Brodie BL, Wentz AC. Late onset congenital adrenal hyperplasia: a gynecologist's perspective. *Fertil Steril* 1987;48:175–188.

Lobo RA. Hirsutism in polycystic ovary syndrome: current concepts. *Clin Obstet Gynecol* 1991;36:817–826.

McKenna TJ. Pathogenesis and treatment of polycystic ovary syndrome. *N Engl J Med* 1988;318:558–562.

Rittmaster RS, Loriaux DL. Hirsutism. *Ann Intern Med* 1987;106: 96–107.

Yen SSC. The polycystic ovary syndrome. *Clin Endocrinol (Oxf)* 1980;12: 177–207.

### Menstrual Disorders

Dalkin AC, Marshall JC. Medical therapy of hyperprolactinemia. *Endocrinol Metab Clin North Am* 1989;18:259–276.

Reindollar RH, Novak M, Tho SP, et al. Adult-onset amenorrhea: a study of 262 patients. *Am J Obstet Gynecol* 1986;155:531–543.

### Premature Ovarian Failure

Mehta AE, Matwijiw L, Lyons EA, et al. Noninvasive diagnosis of resistant ovary syndrome by ultrasonography. *Fertil Steril* 1992;57: 56–61.

### Male

Braunstein GD. Gynecomastia. *N Engl J Med* 1993;328:490–495.

Glass AR. Gynecomastia. *Endocrinol Metab Clin North Am* 1994;23: 825–827.

Krane RJ, Goldstein L, Saenz De Tejada I. Impotence. *N Engl J Med* 1989;321:1648–1659.

# Diabetes Mellitus: Control and Complications

# 44

## Robert S. Zimmerman     S. Sethu K. Reddy

Diabetes mellitus (DM) affects more than 7 million people in the United States, and as many as 8 million others may not be aware that they have DM. DM is a complex metabolic condition, with major health and social ramifications. In recent years, many advances have been made that have increased the ability to achieve optimal metabolic control of DM, while a wealth of accumulated data show that improved control delays the long-term complications of the disease.

## ETIOLOGY

DM can be broadly classified as follows:

- Type 1: insulin-dependent DM
- Type 2: noninsulin-dependent DM

- Gestational
- Other
  - Pancreatic disease, hormonal disease, drugs
  - Rare genetic forms, insulin-receptor abnormalities
  - Impaired glucose tolerance (IGT)

In North America, most individuals with DM have either type 1 DM or type 2 DM. Both types involve a tremendous interaction between genetic endowment and environment (Table 44.1).

## Type 1 Diabetes Mellitus

A positive correlation appears to exist between the incidence of type 1 DM and the distance away from the

## TABLE 44.1
### FEATURES OF TYPE 1 VERSUS TYPE 2 DIABETES MELLITUS

| Feature | Type 1 | Type 2 |
|---|---|---|
| Prevalence (%) | 0.4 | 6.6 |
| Annual incidence in United States | 15,000 | 500,000 |
| Ketosis prone | ++++ | + |
| Anti–islet cell antibody | +++ | − |
| Anti-GAD antibody | ++++ | − |
| Prevalence of other autoimmune conditions | +++ | − |
| Usual age of onset (yr) | <30 | >40 |
| Prevalence of obesity | + | ++++ |
| Family history | + | ++++ |
| HLA linkage | DR3, DR4 | − |
| DQ β-polymorphism | ++ | − |
| Insulin secretion | Absent | Abnormal |
| Insulin resistance | − | +++ |

The symbols −, +, ++, +++, ++++, indicate relative strength of association with type of diabetes.

equator. Finland has the highest incidence, whereas southern European countries have a lower incidence, and Mediterranean countries an even lower incidence. Whether this is related to different genetic backgrounds or to environmental factors is unknown. No male–female differences are known.

Type 1 DM, predominantly affecting those younger than 30 years, is associated with an absolute insulin deficiency owing to the chronic autoimmune destruction of pancreatic beta cells. These individuals need insulin for survival.

In genetically susceptible individuals, this autoimmune process, which can be detected by the presence of antibodies to various components of β-cells (e.g., insulin, glutamic acid decarboxylase, phosphotyrosine, phosphatase), results in the gradual deterioration of insulin production. During this phase (which may last longer than 10 years), no evidence of hyperglycemia may be apparent; at a later time, a critical event, such as surgery or a viral illness, may result in the acute deterioration of pancreatic function and result in acute severe hyperglycemia.

The presence of a gene(s) within the major histocompatibility complex is essential to the development of type 1 DM. More than 90% of whites with type 1 DM express either HLA-DR3 or HLA-DR4. However, 40% of the nondiabetic population also express one of these alleles. This genetic linkage has been further enhanced by studies showing that 96% of patients with type 1 DM are homozygous for amino acid nonaspartate/nonaspartate at position 57 of the DQ-β-chain. Despite such great progress in the understanding of the genetic susceptibility to type 1 DM, the approximately 60% discordance of type 1 DM in identical twins suggests an important role for

environmental factors. These environmental factors may be nutritional components, such as cow's milk, viral infections, or chemical toxins. Having a first-degree relative with type 1 DM increases one's risk of type 1 DM tenfold. Type 1 DM will not develop in 95% of these individuals, however.

Because type 1 DM is an autoimmune disease, its prevention has focused on immune intervention. Various immunosuppressives and immunomodulators have been tested in multicenter trials. Some early studies from Australia and the United States (using azathioprine [Imuran] with or without prednisone in subjects with recent-onset type 1 DM) were favorable, but further study has been abandoned in favor of safer immunotherapies.

Cyclosporine (Sandimmune) has been evaluated in two large and two small double-blind, placebo-controlled studies, as well as in later open studies. In patients with recent-onset type 1 DM, insulin-free remission rates of 18% to 24% at 12 months were observed, but no remissions were evident at 24 months, despite continued cyclosporine therapy.

Intensive insulin therapy and oral insulin were thought to possibly preserve pancreatic insulin secretion in new-onset type 1 DM patients. The results of the Diabetes Prevention Trial for type 1 DM did not prove to preserve β-cell function. Other potential interventions include induction of tolerance to islet cells by oral antigens (including insulin itself), avoidance of cow's milk in infancy, newer immunomodulatory agents, and free-radical scavengers.

## Type 2 Diabetes Mellitus

Type 2 DM accounts for about 85% of the diabetic population. At present, type 2 DM is believed to be the result of many years of insulin resistance, leading to disordered pancreatic insulin secretion and, in turn, to fasting hyperglycemia. Quite often, weight gain (particularly central obesity), physical inactivity, and a high-fat diet exaggerate the insulin resistance and may accelerate the development of type 2 DM. Individuals with type 2 DM may require insulin therapy for improved control of glucose levels; they are then labeled as "insulin-requiring" type 2 DM. In most Westernized countries, the risk for the development of type 2 DM continues to increase with age, resulting in an approximately 30% prevalence of type 2 DM in the geriatric population. In many aboriginal communities, the incidence of type 2 tends to peak before age 50 years.

Genetic risk for type 2 DM can be illustrated by the differences in the risk for the development of type 2 DM related to the familial prevalence of type 2 DM. If both parents have type 2 DM, offspring have a 50% chance for its developing, whereas the risk declines to 20% if only one parent has type 2 DM. If an identical twin has type 2 DM, the risk is estimated to be more than 90%.

Striking differences occur in the prevalence of type 2 DM among different ethnic groups. For example, Native

Americans of the Pima tribe in the southwestern United States have a greater than 30% prevalence of type 2 DM, whereas Americans of European ancestry have approximately a 5% prevalence. Environment, however, is equally important in the development of type 2 DM. Within an ethnic group, the prevalence of type 2 DM varies, depending on the presence of obesity, physical inactivity, and dietary composition, as well as whether living conditions are urban or rural. Studies of Japanese Americans, aboriginals of North America, Asian immigrants to Europe, Mexican Americans, and natives of the South Pacific have confirmed the importance of these risk factors.

Obesity, particularly central obesity, and elevated insulin-to-glucose ratios have generally been considered to be important risk factors. It should be noted that a family history of type 2 DM also connotes a higher than usual risk for the development of type 2 DM in the obese. Physical activity may also be important. Bjorntorp et al. (1992) showed that physically trained insulin-resistant obese subjects could decrease their plasma insulin values by almost 50% without decreasing body fat. Helmrich et al. (1991) studied lifestyle habits and health factors in 1962, and again in 1976, in a cohort of 5,990 men. DM developed in 202 men during the 14 years. The incidence of DM decreased by 41% in patients doing the highest level of physical activity (greater than 3,500 kcal per week) compared with those doing the lowest level (less than 500 kcal per week). This effect was independent of other risk factors. A high body mass index (BMI) (greater than 26) was the strongest predictor of type 2 DM. Tuomilehto et al. (2001) demonstrated that diet and exercise resulting in 3.5 to 5.5 kg weight loss after 2 years resulted in a 58% decreased incidence of diabetes in patients with impaired glucose tolerance. Metformin 850 mg twice daily resulted in a 31% reduction in the development of diabetes in a second group of patients with impaired glucose tolerance (Diabetes Prevention Program Research Group 2002). Because diabetes prevention is greater with diet and exercise, it is the first line of treatment to prevent diabetes.

Molecular defects in the insulin receptor, glucose transporters, and the insulin gene have been reported in different DM syndromes, but none appears to cause the common form of type 2 DM. Recently, the glucokinase gene, hepatocyte nuclear factors 4-$\alpha$, 1-$\alpha$, and 1-$\beta$, as well as insulin promoter factor 1 and neurogenic differentiation factor 1, have been associated with different types of maturity-onset DM of the young.

### Secondary Diabetes Mellitus and Diabetes due to Pancreatic Destruction

Secondary DM may present in individuals with the following conditions:

- Chronic pancreatitis
- Cystic fibrosis

- Hemochromatosis
- Pancreatectomy

Conditions associated with elevated counterregulatory hormones—pheochromocytoma, acromegaly, and Cushing's syndrome—may also precipitate DM. Drugs may also cause hyperglycemia; these include glucocorticoids, thiazide diuretics, phenytoin (Dilantin), interferon-$\alpha$, pentamidine (Pentam 300 or NebuPent), and diazoxide (Proglycem or Hyperstat I.V.).

## COSTS OF DIABETES MELLITUS: MORBIDITY

The prognosis for an individual with type 2 DM may be affected by:

- Inherent background morbidity pattern of the nondiabetic in his or her population
- Competing risks
- Pattern of risk factors
- Quality and quantity of available healthcare
- Possible differences in etiology of the patient's type 2 DM

More than 10 studies have documented an excess mortality in type 2 DM; several studies have estimated a 5- to 10-year loss in life expectancy in patients older than 40 years. DM is the leading cause of blindness in adults 25 to 74 years old in Europe and North America. Women appear to be predisposed to retinopathy, and Blacks appear to be at more risk than whites. DM also is the leading cause of end-stage renal disease, which also has major implications for a patient's quality of life. DM, which also may have an adverse effect on productivity, leads to a greater use of healthcare resources. The life expectancy of children with type 1 DM is about 75% of that of nondiabetics.

The direct and indirect costs of DM are extremely high. In the United States, it has been estimated that DM care costs more than $100 billion per year, with patients with DM requiring two to three times the cost of healthcare of individuals without DM.

## DIAGNOSIS

### Screening

Individuals with the following characteristics should be screened for DM:

- Increased number of risk factors
- Obesity
- Family history of type 2 DM
- History of gestational DM or giving birth to infant weighing more than 9 lb
- Hypertension
- Cardiovascular disease (CVD)

- Belonging to a high-risk ethnic group
- Increasing age (greater than 45 years)

Screening should be accomplished using a fasting plasma glucose test. The use of the oral glucose tolerance test (OGTT) and testing for levels of insulin and C-peptide cannot be recommended, except for research trials. Because the methods for measuring glycosylated hemoglobin (HgbA$_{1c}$) are not standardized, it is not recommended for diagnosing DM. Screening on a population basis cannot be recommended.

### Oral Glucose Tolerance Test

The OGTT is a useful tool when appropriately used, but it is often overused and rarely leads to a change in management decisions. Patients need to fast for 8 hours (abstaining from caffeine and nicotine) before receiving 75 g of glucose (for adults) or 1.75 g/kg (for children). The total volume is between 250 and 300 mL and should be ingested over 5 minutes. Patients should not be malnourished and should have eaten at least 150 g of carbohydrate per day for at least 3 days before the test. They should be ambulatory and not acutely ill. The formal OGTT in pregnant women requires a 100-g glucose load and is extended to 3 hours. It should be kept in mind that plasma glucose values are about 15% higher than whole-blood glucose values. The discussion below uses plasma glucose values.

### Interpretation of the OGTT

The most recent clinical practice guidelines of the American Diabetes Association uses the following diagnostic criteria. For most individuals with DM, the designation should be either type 1 or type 2.

The classification should be based on an etiologic basis rather than on the type of treatment.

Two fasting plasma glucose levels greater than 126 mg/dL (7 mM) indicate the presence of DM. If the 2-hour postprandial value is greater than 200 mg/dL, the patient is deemed to have DM (Table 44.2). Fasting glucose levels of ≥100 and <126 mg/dL indicate impaired fasting glucose (IFG). During an OGTT, 2-hour postprandial glucose levels between 140 and 200 mg/dL indicate IGT. Of patients with IGT, DM will develop in 1% to 5% per year. However, 50% of patients with IGT will have a normal OGTT if repeated in 6 months.

### Variables Affecting the OGTT

The reproducibility of OGTT results is notoriously poor. Several studies have shown that repeat testing of the same individual may result in blood glucose levels that vary by 18 to 27 mg/dL. There is no doubt that this variability is caused by changes in nutritional status, weight, medications, use of caffeine or nicotine, and the normal physiologic variability of glucose metabolism. Thus, some investigators advocate that at least two OGTTs are needed to properly classify a patient.

In addition, as one ages, the prevalence of glucose intolerance increases dramatically. In the geriatric population, up to 30% may have DM. Aging is associated with the delayed absorption of glucose but, more important, also with delayed glucose-induced insulin secretion and insulin resistance at the level of the liver and skeletal muscle. The major disturbance appears to be insulin-mediated glucose uptake. It is also worth noting that although the total weight may not change as one ages, the weight distribution may be altered to a central-obesity pattern. Such a pattern has been linked to insulin resistance and related disorders.

A careful medical history must always be obtained to assess the risk of DM. It should include the use of the following medications that adversely affect glucose tolerance:

- Diazoxide
- Furosemide (Lasix)
- Thiazides
- Glucocorticoids
- Oral contraceptives
- Adrenaline
- Isoproterenol (Isuprel)
- Nicotinic acid
- Phenytoin (Dilantin)
- Tacrolimus
- Cyclosporin

If necessary, these medications may need to be withdrawn (if possible).

**TABLE 44.2**

**INTERPRETATION OF ORAL GLUCOSE TOLERANCE TEST**

| | Normal | Impaired Glucose Tolerance | DM | DM (pregnancy) |
|---|---|---|---|---|
| Fasting (mg/dL) | <110 | <126 | <126 | <105 |
| 0.5, 1.0, or 1.5 h postprandial (mg/dL) | | | | .190 |
| 2 h postprandial (mg/dL) | <140 | 140–200 | >200 | .165 |
| 3 h postprandial (mg/dL) | | | | .145 |

Other Potential Uses of the OGTT

**Reactive Hypoglycemia.** It has become common practice to perform a 5-hour, prolonged OGTT in patients who have apparent hypoglycemic symptoms postprandially. Several studies have shown significant inconsistencies between symptoms and the presence of hypoglycemia. Other studies have confirmed the inadequacies of the OGTT in the workup of hypoglycemia.

**Pregnancy.** Gestational DM is characterized by a diabetic state first detected during a pregnancy. The prevalence of gestational DM has varied from 0.15% to 12.3%, depending on the study group and the set of diagnostic criteria. In North America, gestational DM has been reported to be associated with a higher frequency of metabolic abnormalities, higher birth weights, and increased morbidity and mortality. In the United States, the relative risk of perinatal mortality of gestational diabetic women compared with that of normal control women was 2.2.

The Fourth International Workshop Conference on Gestational Diabetes Mellitus recommends screening all pregnant women with a 50-g OGTT at 24 to 28 weeks. If the 1-hour postload glucose level is greater than 140 mg/dL, then a 3-hour, 100-g OGTT should be performed. This diagnostic algorithm seems to be the most cost-effective in North America. The formal OGTT during pregnancy uses a 100-g glucose load. Two of the three postprandial glucose levels need to be met or exceeded to make the diagnosis of gestational DM (1 hr $\geq$180, 2 hr $\geq$155, 3 hr $\geq$140).

**Patients with Apparent Complications of Diabetes.** Rarely, patients present with retinopathy, neuropathy, or nephropathy that is suggestive of diabetic complications, but they may have equivocal plasma glucose levels. In such situations, an OGTT can be performed to definitively confirm or refute the diagnosis of DM.

**Epidemiologic Research.** In the study of the natural history of DM, the OGTT is an invaluable tool. It has been used in many population-based studies to determine the prevalence of DM and associated risk factors.

## TREATMENT

### Dietary Management

Dietary management is the cornerstone of DM care and should be used in conjunction with exercise to promote a healthy lifestyle. Hopefully, this leads to the maintenance of a lower or ideal body weight, decreased insulin resistance, and improved control of hyperglycemia, dyslipidemia, and hypertension. Individuals with DM should be referred to a registered dietitian for detailed, practical advice. Physicians can help greatly by inquiring about a patient's lifestyle and imparting good nutritional principles. Having three balanced meals per day, enjoying a variety of foods, and spacing meals 4 to 6 hours apart is helpful. Including high-fiber and low-fat items in food choices, as well as moderating the intake of simple sugars, will further the overall goal of reducing the complications of DM. Dietary instructions often depend on the "state" of the patient. The rigor of the lifestyle changes will depend on the following (Table 44.3):

- Age
- Comorbid conditions (e.g., pregnancy or renal failure)
- Activity levels
- Metabolic targets

A maintenance diet is approximately 25 kcal/kg of ideal body weight. The simplest way to calculate the ideal body weight is to use the BMI formula:

$$BMI \text{ weight (kg)/height (m)}^2$$

## TABLE 44.3
### SUMMARY OF NUTRITIONAL RECOMMENDATIONS

| Nutrient Type | Recommended Intake | Sources |
|---|---|---|
| Carbohydrates | 50%–55% of total daily energy intake | Mainly complex carbohydrates, high in fiber<br>Bread, cereals, fruits<br>Vegetables<br>Milk<br>Cakes, muffins |
| Protein | 60.8 g/kg of ideal body weight | Meat, fish, poultry<br>Legumes, tofu, cheese, milk |
| Fat/cholesterol | Up to 30% of total daily energy intake<br>Less than 10% saturated<br>>10% polyunsaturated<br>>10% monounsaturated | Saturated fat: butter, dairy products, animal fats, margarine<br><br>Cholesterol: animal products, egg yolk, organ meats, milk |

An optimal BMI is less than 25. A BMI greater than 27 is considered obesity. One kilogram of weight loss is 7,500 to 8,000 kcal; thus, reducing energy intake by 500 to 1,000 kcal per day should result in 0.5 to 1 kg of weight loss per week.

Alcohol may be consumed only in moderation, and salt intake should be restricted in patients with hypertension or nephropathy. Artificial sweeteners such as aspartame, cyclamates, and acesulfame potassium may be consumed and are safe in the amounts used in most diets. (Often, patients focus only on the sugar component and do not realize that although they are eating a low-sugar food, they may be ingesting excess fat.) The focus of a diabetic diet has shifted away from pure avoidance of sugars to a more complete, healthy, risk-reduction nutrition plan. The American Diabetic Association's (ADA) dietary recommendation allows a diabetic to ingest up to 10% of daily energy intake from simple carbohydrates.

A fat substitute now available consists of a sucrose core with six to eight fatty acids (sucrose polyester or olestra), making the molecule too large to be absorbed. Concerns with the use of this product are related to gastrointestinal (GI) side effects and a possible decreased absorption of fat-soluble vitamins. At present, the U.S. Food and Drug Administration (FDA) has approved its use in snack foods only. Used judiciously, this may allow many patients with DM to meet their nutritional goals in fat reduction. Some preliminary evidence suggests that orlistat (Xenical), a drug which impairs fat absorption, may assist in weight loss and in improving glycemic levels.

## Exercise: Benefits and Risks

Exercise has many effects—psychosocial, cardiovascular, and metabolic—that may benefit patients with DM. The benefits of exercise include:

- Improving quality of life and sense of well-being
- Enhancing work capacity
- Ameliorating cardiovascular risk factors, such as hypertension and obesity
- Favorably altering the lipid profile
- Reducing serum triglyceride levels
- Raising high-density lipoprotein (HDL)-cholesterol levels (To significantly change the HDL-cholesterol level, moderate-to-heavy exercise, equivalent to running 4 to 8 miles per day, is required.)
- Achieving ideal body weight (Interestingly, improvements in insulin sensitivity may be evident, independent of the weight loss.)

A myth exists that exercise alone will normalize metabolic control. In type 1 DM, exercise has not been shown to significantly improve glycemic control. It is, however, a useful adjunct to nutritional and pharmacologic therapy. Exercise plays an important role in the management of type 2 DM.

In the fasting state, skeletal muscles obtain energy from fat, whereas in the fed state, glycogen is first consumed, followed by anaerobic glycolysis. This process is most important during a short burst of exercise, but as the exercise continues, glucose uptake rises to almost 20 times the basal rate. With prolonged exercise, free fatty acids become the major substrate for muscle energy production. Insulin levels are usually lower during exercise, allowing more glycogenolysis, but the insulin is more effective at stimulating peripheral glucose uptake.

### Acute Effect

In patients with well-controlled DM, exercise may lower glucose levels because patients are well insulinized and hepatic glucose production is suppressed. Patients with poorly controlled disease, however, are underinsulinized; hepatic glucose production in response to stress hormones is unchecked, and skeletal muscle glucose uptake is diminished. This results in an increase in glucose levels and may even lead to ketosis. Prolonged strenuous exercise (exceeding 80% of maximum capacity) may also lead to the elevation of blood sugars.

### Delayed Effect

Muscle glycogen stores are depleted after 40 to 60 minutes of moderately intense exercise. After exercise, glucose flux across muscle increases significantly, which may lead to delayed hypoglycemia.

### Risks of Exercise

Exercise carries potential risks, as does any therapeutic maneuver. The action of hypoglycemic medications, including sulfonylureas and insulin, may be enhanced through exercise, with resultant hypoglycemia. Because patients with DM are more likely to have heart disease, symptomatic and asymptomatic, the risk of arrhythmia or ischemic episodes is also increased. In elderly persons, antigravity exercise may aggravate degenerative joint disease or more likely lead to soft tissue injuries. In patients with active retinopathy, strenuous exercise may precipitate intraocular hemorrhage or retinal detachment.

### Relative Contraindications to Exercise

Before beginning an exercise program, patients and physicians must be aware of some relative contraindications:

- Poor metabolic control
- Significant microvascular or macrovascular disease
- Severe peripheral neuropathy
- Hypoglycemic unawareness
- Cardiac autonomic neuropathy

These problems must be corrected as much as possible before an individualized, safe exercise program can be developed.

### Practical Tips

The type of exercise remains a patient's choice, but an improvement in insulin sensitivity and a reduction in

## TABLE 44.4
### TARGETS OF CONTROL

|  | Goals | Action If: |
|---|---|---|
| Premeal glucose (mg/dL) | 80–120 | <80 or >140 |
| Bed-time glucose (mg/dL) | 100–140 | <100 or >160 |
| HgbA1c (normal range, 4%–6%) | <7% | >8% |
| Blood pressure (mm Hg) | <135/85 |  |
| LDL-cholesterol (mg/dL) | <100 mg/dL |  |

cardiovascular risk are evident after relatively mild training. Although aerobic exercise is preferred, resistance exercise in selected patients is safe and also improves glucose control. Exercise sessions should last for about 20 to 40 minutes, and systolic blood pressure during exercise should be kept to less than 180 to 200 mm Hg. Patients should exercise at least three times weekly.

Planning and foresight are essential. The ability and willingness to self-monitor blood glucose is also crucial. In general, it is better to exercise after meals. Blood glucose should be checked before and after exercise, and a source of carbohydrate should be readily available. Dehydration must be avoided. Depending on the time of exercise, a reduction will be necessary in either the intermediate-acting or short-acting insulin. It is preferable to use the abdomen for insulin injections because absorption of insulin in this area is least affected by exercise.

## Standards for Glucose Control

It is necessary to determine whether a patient's blood glucose control is adequate using dietary and exercise therapy, or whether pharmacologic therapy should be initiated. Because the diagnosis of DM rests on a fasting blood glucose greater than 126 mg/dL, the goal should be a fasting glucose less than 80 to 120 mg/dL. An acceptable HgbA$_{1c}$ target is less than 7% (normal range, 4% to 6%). These

criteria could also be used with regard to the later initiation of insulin therapy. In fact, the ADA currently recommends the goals shown in Table 44.4.

## Oral Agents

### Sulfonylureas

The sulfonylureas are derived from sulfonamides; thus about a 15% chance of allergy to a sulfonylurea exists for patients with a history of allergy to sulfonamides. The sulfonylureas chiefly increase insulin secretion in response to glucose by inhibiting potassium efflux from pancreatic β-cells, which results in a depolarization of the cell membrane. Prolonged therapy leads to increased insulin sensitivity, but the mechanisms for this are poorly understood. It is well known that hyperglycemia exacerbates insulin resistance; conversely, the normalization of glucose levels reduces the degree of insulin resistance. Sulfonylureas are also known to inhibit hepatic glucose production (Table 44.5). The newer extended-release preparations and glimepiride (Amaryl) appear not to raise fasting insulin levels and thus have a lower incidence of hypoglycemia. Potency is a relative variable and is reflected by the actual dose size of the medication.

Approximately one-third of patients with type 2 DM initially do not respond to sulfonylureas (primary failure), and of those who respond, 5% to 10% per year have secondary failure. Many primary failures may be caused by using the drugs in inappropriate patients. The characteristics of responders include:

- Age greater than 40 years
- Duration of DM less than 5 years
- 110% to 160% of ideal body weight
- No previous insulin therapy or good control with less than 40 U per day
- Fasting plasma glucose level less than 180 mg/dL

Older obese patients with a mild elevation of blood glucose are ideal candidates for sulfonylureas. Secondary failure

## TABLE 44.5
### SULFONYLUREAS

| Sulfonylureas (mg/day) | Relative Potency | Duration of Action (h) | Dose Range (mg/day) | Risk of Hypoglycemia |
|---|---|---|---|---|
| Tolbutamide (Orinase) | 1 | 6–10 | 500–3,000 | <1% |
| Chlorpropamide | 6 | 24–72 | 100–500 | 4%–6% |
| Glyburide | 150 | 18–24 | 1.25–20 | 4%–6% |
| Glyburide (extended release) | 300 | 24 | 12 | <4% |
| Glipizide (Glucotrol) | 75 | 12–24 | 2.5–40 | 5% |
| Glipizide (extended release) | 150 | 24 | 5–20 | <4% |
| Glimepiride (Amaryl) | 300 | 24 | 1–8 | <1.7% |

may be related to decreasing pancreatic function but is often caused by noncompliance with lifestyle changes.

Fewer than 2% of patients taking a sulfonylurea will discontinue therapy because of adverse side effects. A 1% of 3% prevalence of GI side effects exists, and a less than 0.1% prevalence of hematologic and dermatologic side effects is possible. Patients should be warned of a possible disulfiram-like reaction if alcohol is ingested. This is observed more frequently with chlorpropamide than with other agents; chlorpropamide may also cause the syndrome of inappropriate antidiuretic hormone secretion (IADHS) with symptomatic hyponatremia.

The risk of severe hypoglycemia is about 0.22 per 1,000 patient-years compared with 100 per 1,000 patient-years for insulin. Prolonged hypoglycemia while using glyburide or chlorpropamide may be caused by these drugs' metabolites, which also have a hypoglycemic effect. Risk factors for sulfonylurea-induced hypoglycemia include:

- Age greater than 60 years
- Poor renal function decreased
- Poor nutrition
- Interaction with drugs such as insulin, alcohol, salicylates, phenylbutazone, sulfonamides, warfarin (Coumadin), allopurinol, and β-blockers

### Meglitinides

The first clinically useful compound of this class of agents, which is derived from benzoic acid, is repaglinide (Prandin). It stimulates the sulfonylurea receptor at a site different from that of the sulfonylurea-binding site and increases glucose-stimulated insulin secretion within 10 minutes. The duration of action is 3 to 4 hours; thus, dosing is three times daily before meals. Doses range from 0.5 to 4 mg. There appears to be little risk of severe hypoglycemia. Repaglinide may be used in combination with metformin (Glucophage). Repaglinide is metabolized by the liver into inactive metabolites and thus can be used in patients with renal failure without any concern regarding prolonged hypoglycemia.

Nateglinide is a D-phenylalanine derivative that also binds to the sulfonylurea receptor at a binding site different from that of the sulfonylurea binding site. It increases glucose-stimulated insulin secretion. It is taken before each meal at a dose of 120 mg. Its peak action is at 1 hour, and elimination half-life is 1.5 hours.

### Biguanides

The only biguanide available is metformin. It does not bind to plasma proteins and is eliminated solely via the renal route. With a half-life of 2 to 4 hours, metformin, 500 to 1,000 mg, is given with meals up to three times daily, to a maximum dosage of 2,000 mg per day. It does not cause hypoglycemia (it does not work by enhancing pancreatic insulin secretion). It may increase insulin sensitivity or affect glucose metabolism directly. Metformin also

can have an anorectic effect, which may be beneficial for obese patients with type 2 DM. It also has been shown to lower plasma triglyceride levels.

Metformin may be used as a first-line medication, or it can be combined with a sulfonylurea or insulin. Its chief side effects are GI (up to 20% of patients), but these can be minimized by starting at a low dose and gradually increasing it as tolerance develops. These side effects include dyspepsia, anorexia, diarrhea, and an unpleasant metallic taste. Lactic acidosis is potentially a major side effect, and thus metformin should be avoided in patients with cirrhosis, alcoholism, heart failure, or renal failure. The FDA recommends that patients with creatinine values greater than 1.5 mg/dL (1.4 mg/dL for women) should not take metformin. It should also be avoided in patients with heart failure treated with digozin or furosemide.

### α-Glucosidase Inhibitors

Acarbose (Precose) and miglitol (Glyset) are pseudotetrasaccharides that inhibit α-glucosidases in the brush border of the small intestine. These enzymes are responsible for the digestion of starch, dextrins, maltose, and sucrose into monosaccharides, which can then be absorbed. Acarbose and miglitol reduce postprandial hyperglycemia and are currently approved for use in patients with type 2 DM. Side effects may include flatulence and diarrhea, but these diminish with continued use of the agents. The α-glucosidase inhibitors can be safely combined with other oral agents. Starting dosage is 25 mg once daily, gradually increased to three times daily; the dosage may be increased to 50 mg three times daily with meals. The expectation is that $HgbA_{1c}$ may be reduced by an absolute level of about 0.75% to 1.0% (normal range, 4% to 6%). In patients with higher levels of $HgbA_{1c}$, however, the effect may be greater.

### Thiazolidenediones

The thiazolidenediones, a family of compounds known as *insulin sensitizers*, increase insulin sensitivity in fat, skeletal muscle, and liver. They have no effect on insulin secretion. They modestly reduce fasting and postprandial glucose levels in obese patients with type 2 DM. These agents are generally well tolerated. They may increase plasma volume in some patients. They should be avoided in those with liver disease and in those with heart failure (class III).

Rosiglitazone (Avandia) may be prescribed at a dose of 4 to 8 mg per day, and pioglitizone (Actos) can be prescribed at a dose of 15 to 45 mg/d. Clinical trials prior to FDA approval showed no increase in hepatotoxicity with rosiglitazone or pioglitizone compared to placebo, but the FDA recommends that liver enzymes be checked initially and periodically, thereafter. These agents may be used as initial monotherapy or as part of combination therapy. Pioglitizone may be more effective at lowering triglycerides than rosiglitazone.

### Therapy Using Several Oral Agents

Certainly, no benefit is derived from prescribing two sulfonylureas at the same time, and a greater chance of side effects is possible. A sulfonylurea or repaglinide, however, can be combined with metformin for improved glucose control. No additive effects occur when a sulfonylurea is added to a meglitinide. A thiazolidinedione can be added to all other classes of hypoglycemic agents. The α-glucosidase inhibitors may be combined with any other oral agent. Another oral agent is normally added if a patient is already taking a maximum dose of the initial oral agent. At this stage in a patient's disease, it would be prudent to advise insulin therapy in the near future. The potential for hypoglycemic episodes increases with the use of multiple medications. Thus, multidrug therapy initially may best be supervised by a specialist.

In a patient already taking a biguanide and sulfonylurea, the addition of a thiozolidinedione may reduce glucose levels by 50 to 75 mg/dL, depending on the severity of baseline hyperglycemia. In patients already on sulfonylureas, these agents could be added but should not replace the sulfonylureas.

## Insulin Therapy

The success of insulin therapy depends on the judicious and appropriate use of the variety of available insulins (Table 44.6).

Insulin lispro (Humalog) and aspart (Novolog) have:

■ A very rapid dissociation into monomers after subcutaneous injection; thus they begin to work within 15 minutes
■ An action for 3 to 4 hours only
■ A half-life apparently unaffected by increases in dose (unlike regular insulin)
■ The possibility of combination with other insulin preparations, such as NPH, Lente, or extended insulin zinc (Ultralente)
■ The same potency, unit for unit, as regular insulin but with different onset and duration

## TABLE 44.6
### COMMONLY USED INSULIN PREPARATIONS

| Type | Onset (h) | Peak (h) | Duration (h) |
| --- | --- | --- | --- |
| Rapid | | | |
| Insulin lispro | 0.25 | 1 | 3–4 |
| Short | | | |
| Regular | 0.5 | 2–4 | 5–7 |
| Intermediate | | | |
| NPH | 1–2 | 6–12 | 14–24 |
| Lente | 1–2 | 6–12 | 18–24 |
| Long | | | |
| Ultralente | 4–6 | 18–24 | 32–36 |

Insulin lispro and aspart have been extensively studied in individuals with type 1 or type 2 DM. It is easily accepted by patients because of the convenience of not having to take insulin injections 30 to 45 minutes before a meal. Nocturnal hypoglycemic events are less common, and postprandial glucose values are significantly lower than with regular insulin. No increase in antibody response to insulin lispro occurs.

Some modifications with respect to the timing of intermediate-acting insulins in combination with insulin lispro may be required. Insulin lispro and aspart are often used in insulin pump therapy.

Glargine insulin has a duration of 24 hours. It cannot be mixed with other insulins, and it is the only clear long-acting insulin. Its main role is as an adjuvant in patients using short-acting insulin before each meal.

Special premixed insulin preparations (e.g., 30% regular/70% NPH and 50% regular/50% NPH) may be useful for patients who have very stable DM or who might have difficulties with mixing insulins manually. Penlike delivery systems have also increased the convenience and rapidity of learning insulin administration.

The noted time frames are quite variable and can fluctuate by 20% to 30% between individuals and even within the same individual. Factors that decrease or delay the action of insulin injections include:

■ Higher dose of insulin
■ Higher glucose levels preinjection
■ Site of absorption (thigh more than arm more than abdomen)
■ Cooler temperature of skin
■ Sedentary (versus exercise)
■ Hepatic and renal degradation
■ High titers of anti-insulin antibodies (rare)

The side effects of insulin include hypoglycemia and lipohypertrophy. Allergic phenomena include both local and systemic skin reactions and lipoatrophy.

Dosage regimens may start simply and increase in complexity, depending on a patient's target goals and motivation. More intensive regimens require more frequent self-monitoring of blood glucose. Blood glucose monitoring and insulin adjustments caveats include:

■ Morning glucose level reflects the evening intermediate insulin dose.
■ Lunch glucose level reflects the morning rapid/short acting insulin dose.
■ Supper/dinner glucose level reflects the morning intermediate insulin dose.
■ Bed-time glucose level reflects the presupper rapid/short acting insulin dose.
■ Most individuals will require two to four injections per day.

Insulin may be combined with sulfonylureas, metformin, thiazolidenediones or α-glucosidase inhibitors.

The most common regimen is the use of bedtime NPH insulin or glargine with daytime oral agents.

### Initiating Insulin Therapy

Most patients begin insulin therapy with approximately 0.3 to 0.5 U/kg per day. Typically, two-thirds of the insulin is given in the morning and one-third in the evening. If both intermediate- and rapid-acting insulins are needed, typically two-thirds is intermediate and one-third is regular. Insulin regimens include:

- Phase I
  □ Morning (AM) intermediate only or
  □ Bedtime (HS) intermediate only or
  □ HS Ultralente or glargine only or
  □ HS intermediate plus oral agent during the day
- Phase II
  □ Intermediate insulin twice daily (before breakfast and supper) or
  □ Intermediate insulin twice daily (before breakfast and hs)
- Phase III
  □ Add regular insulin before breakfast plus supper
- Phase IV
  □ Regular before meals hs intermediate or
  □ Regular before meals plus hs long-acting or
  □ Insulin-pump therapy

## COMPLICATIONS

### General Mechanisms

The chronic hyperglycemia to which individuals with DM are exposed is paramount in the etiology of diabetic complications. Hyperglycemia may play a role via several mechanisms:

- Nonenzymatic glycosylation of protein structures, leading to altered blood vessel function
- Conversion of glucose to sorbitol via intracellular aldose reductase enzyme, leading to an accumulation of sorbitol, which in turn can have several deleterious effects on cellular function
- Adverse effects on coagulability, platelet function, atherogenic potential of lipoproteins
- Increased susceptibility to free oxygen radical–induced damage

### Diabetes Control and Complications Trial

The results of the Diabetes Control and Complications Trial (DCCT) (1993), a historic study designed to test whether chronic hyperglycemia is related to the development of complications in type 1 DM, clearly demonstrated that intensive treatment delays the onset and progression of long-term complications in patients with type 1 DM without complications or with early complications. More than 1,400 individuals, 13 to 39 years of age, with type 1 DM, were entered into the study, and more than 99% of them completed it. One-half of the subjects were enrolled in a standard treatment program (twice daily insulin injections), whereas the remainder were intensively treated. Intensive therapy included:

- More frequent doses of insulin per day or insulin-pump therapy
- Self-adjustment of insulin according to meal content, exercise activity, and glucose levels
- Frequent dietary instructions and monthly clinic visits

The standard treatment group's goals were to remain clinically well and symptom-free, whereas the goal of the intensive-treatment group was the normalization of blood glucose levels. This regimen required a great deal of commitment from both the volunteer subjects and the diabetes healthcare teams.

Intensive therapy resulted in an average HgbA1c of 7.2, whereas standard therapy achieved an average of 9.2%. It reduced clinically meaningful eye changes by 34% to 76%, and the first appearance of any eye changes by 27%. Evidence of kidney complications was reduced by 35% and nerve damage by 60%. Subjects in the intensive treatment group were three times more likely to have severe hypoglycemic reactions. Intensive therapy did not, however, worsen quality of life.

Patients with the following characteristics may not be good candidates for intensive therapy:

- Inability to comply with intensive treatment
- Age younger than 13 years
- Elderly with established severe complications
- Significant heart disease
- Hypoglycemic unawareness
- Repeated severe hypoglycemia (more than two episodes in the previous 2 years) (relative contraindications)
- End-stage complications

### Kumamoto Study

The Kumamoto Study by Okhubo et al. (1995) compared the incidence and progression of microvascular complications in 110 Japanese patients with type 2 DM, treated with intensive insulin therapy, with the incidence and progression of complications in conventionally treated patients with type 2 DM. The intensively treated group had a $HgbA_{1c}$ of 7.1%, whereas the conventionally treated group had a mean $HgbA_{1c}$ of 9.4%. Reductions in the progression of retinopathy and nephropathy, similar to the rates observed in the DCCT, were observed in the intensively treated group. Thus, intensive therapy also appears to be beneficial to patients with type 2 DM.

## Wisconsin Epidemiologic Study of Diabetic Retinopathy

The Wisconsin Epidemiologic Study of Diabetic Retinopathy (WESDR) by Klein et al. (1989), a population-based study with a longitudinal follow-up of 2,990 subjects with DM, revealed a significant relationship between baseline $HgbA_{1c}$ and all aspects of retinopathy, microalbuminuria, and gross proteinuria. In both the type 1 and type 2 DM groups, the WESDR showed a similar relationship between $HgbA_{1c}$ and lower extremity amputation, as well as all-cause mortality.

## United Kingdom Prospective Diabetes Study

The United Kingdom Prospective Diabetes Study (UKPDS, 1998), begun in 1977, recently reported some initial findings with respect to glucose and blood pressure control and their impact on microvascular and macrovascular complications. More than 4,000 newly diagnosed subjects with type 2 DM were enrolled and randomized to either conventional policy (fasting glucose goal of 270 mg/dL) or intensive policy (fasting glucose goal of 108 mg/dL). Therapeutic choices included sulfonylureas, insulin, or metformin. Subjects were also randomized to either tight blood pressure control (150/85 mm Hg) or less tight blood pressure control (less than 180/105 mm Hg) with captopril (Capoten) or atenolol. The clinical implications of the UKPDS include:

- Glucose lowering reduces the risk of retinopathy and nephropathy.
- Glucose lowering did not significantly reduce the risk of coronary heart disease (CHD) in the sulfonylurea and insulin groups.
- All glucose lowering drugs (sulfonylureas, metformin, insulin) have a comparable effect on reducing diabetic complications. In obese patients, metformin may have a greater benefit in reducing diabetic complications. Metformin was the only agent that significantly reduced the risk of CHD in this study.
- Reducing blood pressure with either a β-blocker or an angiotensin converting enzyme (ACE) inhibitor reduces the risk of *both* microvascular and macrovascular complications and overall mortality.

## Smoking

Despite numerous public strategies to educate people about the hazards of smoking and tobacco consumption, many individuals with DM smoke. In the United States, the 1988 Behavioral Risk Factor Surveillance System reported that the prevalence of smoking in the diabetic population was the same as in the general population. It was also noted that young African Americans with DM (18 to 34 years of age) who had not completed high school had higher rates of smoking than controls.

In view of the overall health of individuals with DM, cigarette smoking is an important cause of increased complications from DM and in DM-associated morbidity and mortality. Several prospective cohort studies lend support to this conclusion. Yudkin calculated that smoking cessation would prolong life by 3 years in a man with DM, whereas aspirin and antihypertensive therapy would prolong life by only 1 year.

## Microvascular Complications

### Retinopathy

DM is responsible for 8% of cases of blindness in the United States and is the leading cause of blindness in the 20- to 64-year age range. The most common form of retinopathy is nonproliferative (background) retinopathy consisting of microaneurysms, intraretinal hemorrhages, or exudates. Infarction of the nerve layer of the retina may occur, causing cotton-wool exudates. This ischemia is thought to play a role in the eventual proliferation of new, friable vessels from the retina into the vitreous. This latter phase is termed *proliferative retinopathy* and is associated with vitreous hemorrhages, retinal scarring, and potential retinal detachment. An altered expression of various local growth factors within the retina is thought to mediate the vascular changes in the retina. Macular edema is also more prevalent in those with DM and may occur with or without proliferative retinopathy. Patients should be referred to an ophthalmologist at the time of diagnosis of type 2 DM, whereas referral to an ophthalmologist should be made 5 years after the diagnosis of type 1 DM if the patient is asymptomatic.

The most important risk factors for retinopathy include:

- Duration of DM
- Glycemic control
- Hypertension

Depending on the stage of retinopathy, management includes the following options:

- Appropriately frequent funduscopic examination (more often during pregnancy)
- Improved control of hyperglycemia and hypertension
- Early laser treatment
- Vitrectomy

Aspirin therapy has no adverse ophthalmic effects.

### Nephropathy

Renal failure is a major cause of mortality in patients with DM. In the United States, approximately one in three patients on dialysis has DM. Whereas retinopathy eventually occurs in almost all patients with DM, clinical nephropathy develops in about 40% of patients with type 1 DM and in less than 20% of those with type 2 DM. The most important risk factors for nephropathy include:

- Duration of DM
- Glycemic control
- Hypertension
- Smoking
- Hypercholesterolemia

Recent prospective studies lend support to the hypothesis that smoking accelerates nephropathy in patients with DM. In a clinic-based prospective study by Chase et al. (1991), the odds ratio for the development of significant albuminuria was 2.2 times higher in smokers than nonsmokers. Most other studies also confirm this finding. Recent interest has focused on the polymorphism of various genes linked to hypertension, such as the angiotensin-converting enzyme (ACE) gene. Proteinuria, which is 15 times more frequent in diabetics than nondiabetics, worsens the prognosis and is a prognostic factor with respect to renal failure and macrovascular disease.

In 1996, the National Kidney Foundation recommended that all individuals with DM, 12 to 70 years of age, undergo urine testing for albumin at least annually. Ideally, individuals should be metabolically stable. Heavy exercise, urinary tract infection, acute febrile illness, or heart failure may transiently increase urinary albumin excretion. Nonsteroidal anti-inflammatory drugs and ACE inhibitors should be avoided during screening.

A 24-hour or overnight (8- to 12-hour timed) collection is the most sensitive screening method. Albumin excretion rates greater than 30 mg per 24 hours or greater than 20 mg per minute indicate diabetic nephropathy when confirmed on at least two urine samples. Because timed-collections are often impractical, the recommendation of using the albumin-to-creatinine ratio was made. A urinary albumin-to-creatinine ratio of 30 to 300 mg/g indicates the presence of microalbuminuria. Various national guidelines have recommended testing for microalbuminuria at the time of type 2 DM diagnosis and 5 years after the diagnosis of type 1 DM (Table 44.7).

In most circumstances, the blood pressure should be lower than 140/90 mm Hg, but in the presence of microalbuminuria, it should be 130/85 mm Hg or lower. The first measures should be to improve blood glucose control, to achieve an optimal body weight and smoking cessation, and to follow the proper life-style. Subsequently, ACE inhibitors, calcium channel blockers, and α-blockers may be used. In the presence of microalbuminuria, an ACE inhibitor is generally favored. Trials have shown that captopril can reduce the need for dialysis and delay adverse outcomes in Type 1 diabetics. Similar effects in Type 2 diabetics have recently been shown for several angiotensive receptor blockers.

### Neuropathy

Neuropathy, one of the most common complications of DM, can affect the sensory, motor, and autonomic nervous systems. Painful symptoms or paresthesias develop in some patients. For peripheral painful neuropathy, simple analgesics, tricyclic antidepressants, phenytoin, and carbamazepine (Tegretol) have been used, but newer, potentially helpful agents include topical capsaicin (Zostrix), mexiletine (Mexitil), and gabapentin (Neurontin). Other causes of neuropathy should always be ruled out before DM is assumed to be the cause.

### TABLE 44.7

**NATURAL HISTORY OF DIABETIC NEPHROPATHY**

| Stage | Renal Pathology | Albumin Excretion | GFRa | Management |
|---|---|---|---|---|
| Diagnosis | Normal or renal hypertrophy | None | Increased | Improve glucose control |
| 3–15 years | 1. Basement membrane thickening 2. Increased mesangial matrix 3. Glomerulosclerosis | Microalbuminuria (30–300 mg/24 h) | Normal | 1. As above 2. Monitor and treat hypertension |
| Incipient nephropathy | Advancing glomerulosclerosis | Macroalbuminuria | Normal | 1, 2, and 3. Restrict protein |
| Nephrotic syndrome | Progression | >1.5 g/24 h | Normal or decreased | 1, 2, 3, and 4. Diuretic therapy |
| End-stage renal disease | Loss of tubular function | | Progressively decreasing | 1, 2, 3, 4, and 5. Manage renal failure |

a GFR, glomerular filtration rate.

Hypoglycemic unawareness, a sign of autonomic dysfunction, is often present in individuals with type 1 DM for more than 15 years. At this point, intensive control of DM is dangerous, and appropriately higher targets for blood glucose control should be set.

Symptoms of postural hypotension are associated with a poor prognosis in patients with DM. Traditionally, norepinephrine bitartrate (Levophed), fludrocortisone acetate (Florinef acetate), or proamitine have been used. Patients may also respond to low doses of a β-blocker. For associated nocturnal diarrhea, once infectious causes have been ruled out, clonidine (Catapres) or a bile acid sequestrant may be helpful.

Autonomic dysfunction may affect the GI or genitourinary systems, resulting in constipation, gastroparesis, diabetic diarrhea, erectile dysfunction, or a neurogenic bladder.

It is crucial to always consider causes other than DM in the etiology of any neuropathy.

## Macrovascular Complications

Atherosclerotic vascular disease is a major cause of morbidity and mortality in patients with DM. For patients with type 1 DM, more than one third of mortality is owing to cardiac and cerebrovascular diseases; for patients with type 2 DM, two thirds of mortality is the result of macrovascular disease.

In the classic Whitehall study, a clearly increased mortality from CHD was observed in glucose-intolerant individuals and in diabetics. Age and blood pressure are the strongest risk factors related to subsequent death from CHD. Cigarette smoking, dyslipidemia, and hyperinsulinemia are also important co–risk factors in DM. Other factors associated with the development of macrovascular disease are high fibrinogen levels and the presence of cataracts.

### Clinical Presentation

Both the incidence and the extent of atherosclerosis are greater in individuals with DM. Within any artery, the disease also may be diffuse. Although infarct size may not differ from that of nondiabetics, complications after myocardial infarction (MI) occur more frequently in the diabetic population. In a prospective study, Yudkin et al. (1988) showed that a patient's metabolic control before MI had an impact on early mortality:

- 23% mortality with normal HgbA$_{1c}$
- 33% mortality with HgbA$_{1c}$ of 7.5% to 8.5%
- 63% mortality with HgbA$_{1c}$ greater than 8.5%

A greater late-mortality also occurs after MI. These features are no doubt owing to coexisting changes in the hearts of patients with DM (e.g., cardiomyopathy, autonomic neuropathy, and more diffuse atherosclerotic disease).

Women with DM tend to be at a relatively higher risk than men. The Framingham Study reported that the average adjusted incidence of intermittent claudication was 12.6 per 1,000 for diabetic men and 8.4 per 1,000 for diabetic women, compared with 3.3 per 1,000 and 1.3 per 1,000 for nondiabetic men and women, respectively. One potential reason for the absence of protection against atherosclerotic disease in diabetic women is the markedly different lipid profiles evident in these patients. Quite often, they exhibit elevated triglycerides and lower HDL-cholesterol levels.

### Coronary Artery Bypass Surgery

Although coronary artery bypass grafting (CABG) is efficacious in diabetics with CHD (criteria are the same for diabetic as for nondiabetic patients), many studies have shown that diabetics will have more associated risk factors, poorer left ventricular function, and a poorer long-term prognosis. The Bypass Angioplasty Revascularization Investigation by Jacobs et al. (1998), involving 1,829 patients needing a first revascularization, reported that the 5-year mortality rate with CABG in a subgroup of 353 drug-treated diabetics was 19% compared with 35% for angioplasty. The 5-year mortality rate for the remaining subjects was 9%. Mortality was not due to acute complications of the procedures.

Compelling evidence exists for the role of hyperglycemia in accelerating atherosclerosis, but well documented evidence suggests that individuals with IGT but without DM (as defined by national and international guidelines) have much higher rates of CVD. This implies that individuals with IGT of any degree are at increased risk of CVD. In addition, the duration of type 2 DM does not correlate very highly with the incidence of CVD. This latter observation may reflect the lack of early diagnosis of DM in asymptomatic individuals.

The risk of CVD in a particular patient also depends on his ethnic origin. For example, Japanese with DM have a lower prevalence of atherosclerosis, when compared to diabetics of Scots origin. On the other hand, Japanese who have migrated to Hawaii have a higher incidence of CVD than those still living in Japan, underscoring the tremendous interplay between inherited and environmental factors.

## Pregnancy

Pregnancy complicated by pre-existing DM carries a 10- to 20-fold increased risk of congenital malformations. These include neural tube defects and cardiac defects. Excellent control after conception leads to a dramatic decrease in complications, but a two- to threefold increase in congenital malformations still remains. It is highly advisable that excellent metabolic control be instituted before pregnancy. Metabolic complications affecting the fetus, such as perinatal death, hypoglycemia, hypocalcemia, respiratory distress syndrome, and jaundice, are reduced in prevalence to levels observed in normal pregnancies. Sufficient animal data demonstrate the toxic effects of ketones on central nervous system development, thus ketosis should be actively prevented.

The white classification of diabetic pregnancies has been useful in predicting outcomes. Unfavorable variables include:

- Increasing age
- Increasing duration of DM
- Retinopathy
- Nephropathy
- CHD

Gestational DM occurs in approximately 2% to 3% of pregnancies. In North America, screening for DM is recommended for all pregnant women between the 24th and 28th weeks of gestation, according to guidelines outlined in the discussion of OGTT (see above). By definition, a woman should not have DM postpartum. No increase in congenital malformations occurs, but there does appear to be an increase in macrosomia and neonatal hypoglycemia. Management is usually with diet, exercise, and insulin (if necessary). Oral agents are not used. Some preliminary evidence suggests that insulin resistance may later develop in the infants of diabetic mothers.

## Hypoglycemia

### Diabetes-Associated Hypoglycemia

Hypoglycemia associated with DM is often caused by a mismatch of caloric intake to insulin peaks. Physicians must take a careful history, being particularly attentive to the following:

- Late or missed meals
- Exercise
- Excessive insulin or sulfonylurea
- Hypoglycemic unawareness
- Gastroparesis
- Use of alcohol or sedatives
- Renal or hepatic impairment
- Coincidental hypoadrenalism or hypopituitarism

### Nondiabetes-Associated Hypoglycemia

The symptoms of nondiabetes-associated hypoglycemia may be either adrenergic or neuroglycopenic, with the adrenergic signs occurring earlier, at glucose levels less then 50 mg/dL. Clinically, a distinction must be made between fasting and reactive hypoglycemia. Fasting hypoglycemia implies a pathologic cause, whereas reactive hypoglycemia tends to be a functional, benign phenomenon.

The gold standard test is the 72-hour fast to measure serial glucose and insulin levels. At the time of hypoglycemia or symptoms, the C-peptide level is also determined. This is critical for ruling out exogenous insulin as a cause. Sulfonylureas may increase C-peptide levels, and thus should be screened for in a 24-hour urine test.

The liver is of prime importance in the etiology of hypoglycemia. Thus, GH or cortisol deficiencies, severe malnutrition, excessive alcohol consumption, and liver failure may be associated with reduced hepatic glucose output. Sulfonylureas, quinine, pentamidine, disopyramide (Norpace), or monoamine oxidase inhibitors may

increase insulin levels. Rarely, anti-insulin receptor antibody or anti-insulin antibody may be linked to hypoglycemia. A thorough history and physical examination can rule out many of these causes.

An insulinoma is favored in the presence of fasting symptoms and an insulin-to-glucose ratio greater than 0.3 mU/L/ mg/dL; an elevated C-peptide level is very supportive. An insulinoma should be localized preoperatively or intraoperatively using laparoscopic ultrasound of the pancreas. Fewer than 10% of these tumors are multiple and associated with multiple endocrine neoplasia type I syndrome.

## REVIEW EXERCISES

### QUESTIONS

**1.** A 55-year-old businessman comes to your office complaining of fatigue. He denies any weight change but has nocturia one or two times a night. His 75-year-old mother is a diabetic; his father died of premature heart disease at 60 years of age. He has a history of hypertension treated with hydrochlorothiazide, 50 mg per day. Physical examination reveals that he is 50% above his ideal body weight; his blood pressure is 135/90 mm Hg, but is otherwise unremarkable. Fasting plasma glucose is 120 mg/dL, sodium 143 mEq/L, potassium 3.1 mEq/mL, chloride 100 mEq/L, bicarbonate 26 mEq/L, blood urea nitrogen (BUN) 12 mg/dL, and creatinine 1.1 mg/dL. HgbA$_{1c}$ is 6.0% (normal range, 4% to 6%).

Which of the following is false?
a) With a normal HgbA$_{1c}$, he is unlikely to have DM.
b) An OGTT is not indicated.
c) Risk factors for DM include his family history, obesity, hypertension, and hypokalemia.
d) His hypokalemia should be corrected before retesting his plasma glucose level.
e) He would benefit from weight reduction, increased exercise, and improved dietary habits.

**2.** The above patient returns to your office 6 months later, having missed several return appointments. Despite following your lifestyle prescription, he continues to be fatigued, has experienced a 10-pound weight loss, and presents with polydipsia, polyuria, and blurred vision. He has been monitoring his capillary blood glucose, and it has consistently been greater than 250 mg/dL. You diagnose DM and examine him more closely.

Which of the following features favors type 1 DM?
a) Presence of vitiligo
b) Obesity and age of 55 years
c) Negative for islet cell antibodies
d) Family history of DM
e) C-peptide levels at upper limit of normal

**3.** The dietitian is on holiday, and you must counsel the patient regarding nutrition. Which of the following recommendations would you *not* make?

**a)** Avoid all sweet foods.

**b)** Encourage 50% carbohydrates, less than 30% fat, and 20% protein.

**c)** Do not take vanadium or chromium supplements.

**d)** Increase fiber intake and decrease amount of saturated fat.

**e)** Space caloric intake over the whole day.

**4.** This patient is interested in increasing his physical activity. He wonders how exercise will affect his DM. Which of the following is false?

**a)** Exercise may acutely increase his blood glucose level.

**b)** Exercise may acutely decrease his blood glucose level.

**c)** Exercise may not benefit his glucose control if he has type 2 DM.

**d)** Exercise may not benefit his glucose control if he has type 1 DM.

**e)** Exercise will have to be individualized according to his previous habits and the presence of any diabetic complications.

**5.** The patient's sister, who is visiting from out of town, is also known to have type 2 DM and hypertension. She is treated with glyburide, 10 mg twice daily, and her fasting blood glucose averages 160 mg/dL, with her HgbA$_{1c}$ at 8.8%. She seeks your counsel. Physical examination is unremarkable except for moderate obesity. Fasting glucose is 200 mg/dL, BUN 25 mg/dL, and creatinine 1.9 mg/dL; electrolytes and liver enzymes are normal.

Which of the following would be reasonable recommendations, in addition to improving her dietary habits and exercise regimen?

**a)** Discontinue glyburide.

**b)** Add metformin, 500 mg twice daily after meals.

**c)** Add acarbose, 25 mg three times daily.

**d)** Add vosiglitazone, 4 mg daily.

**6.** On a clinic visit 5 years later, the patient in Question 1 is noted to have microalbuminuria. Your review indicates he has type 2 DM, a blood pressure of 140/90 mm Hg, and a HgbA$_{1c}$ of 9.0%. He is being treated with an ACE inhibitor and a maximum dose of glyburide.

Which of the following options would be your management?

**a)** Intensify the antihypertensive regimen.

**b)** Intensify glucose control only.

**c)** Begin insulin-injection therapy.

**d)** Aim to lower blood pressure and blood glucose.

**7.** Ten years later, the patient is noted to have orthostatic hypotension. No signs or symptoms of heart failure or respiratory distress are present. Sitting blood pressure is 130/75 mm Hg. He is afebrile.

Which of these is *not* compatible with his presentation?

**a)** Insomnia

**b)** Constipation

**c)** Supine blood pressure of 150/95 mm Hg

**d)** Gastroparesis

**e)** Persistent resting sinus tachycardia

## ANSWERS

**1. a.**

A normal HgbA$_{1c}$ does not exclude DM.

**2. a.**

Vitiligo is an autoimmune condition and more likely to occur with type 1 DM.

**3. a.**

Some simple sugars are allowed (up to 15% of total calories), provided the overall dietary intake is appropriate.

**4. c.**

Exercise is very important for controlling type 2 DM.

**5. d.**

Glyburide should not be discontinued but could be reduced. With an elevated creatinine, metformin should not be prescribed. One should start a patient on acarbose (Precose), slowly and gradually increasing dosage. Rosiglitazone could be used, starting at 4 mg daily.

**6. d.**

Both glycemic control and blood pressure control are key factors in the development of diabetic nephropathy.

**7. e.**

All are symptoms and signs of autonomic neuropathy, except insomnia.

## SUGGESTED READINGS

Becker K, ed. *Principles and Practice of Endocrinology and Metabolism*, 2nd ed. Philadelphia: JB Lippincott Co, 1995.

Bjorntorp P. New concepts in the relationship obesity—non-insulin dependent diabetes mellitus. *Eur J Med* 1992;1:37–42.

Brenner BM, Cooper ME, deZeeuw D, et al. Effects of losartan on renal and cardiovascular outcomes in patients with type 2 diabetes and nephropathy. *N Engl J Med* 2001;345:861–869.

Carel JC., Landais P., Bougneres P. Oral insulin does not prevent type 1 diabetes. *NIDDK* 2003;1–3.

Chase HP, Garg SK, Marshall G, et al. Cigarette smoking increases the risk of albuminuria among subjects with type 1 diabetes. *JAMA* 1991;265:614–617.

Diabetes Prevention Trial-Type 1 Diabetes Study Group. Effects of insulin in relatives of patients with type 1 diabetes mellitus. *N Engl J Med* 2002;346:1685–1691.

Gerich JE. Oral hypoglycemic agents. *N Engl J Med* 1989;321: 1231–1245.

Helmrich SP, Ragland DR, Leugn RW, et al. Physical activity and reduced occurrence of NIDDM. *N Engl J Med* 1991;325:147–152.

Jacobs AK, Kelsey SF, Brooks MM, et al. Better outcome for women compared with men undergoing coronary revascularization: a report from the bypass angioplasty revascularization investigation. *Circulation* 1998;98:1279–1285.

Jarrett RJ. Cardiovascular disease and hypertension in diabetes mellitus. *Diabetes Metabolism Rev* 1989;5:547.

Kannel WB, McGee DL. Diabetes and cardiovascular risk factors: The Framingham Study. *Circulation* 1979;59:8–13.

Klein R, Moss SE, Klein BE, et al. Relation of ocular and systemic factors to survival in diabetes. *Arch Intern Med* 1989;149:266–272.

Lewis E., Hunsicker LG., Clarke, WR., et al. Renoprotective effect of the angiotensin-receptor antagonist irbesartan in patients with nephropathy due to type 2 diabetes. *N Engl J Med* 2001;345:851–860.

Metzger BE, Coustan DR. Summary and recommendations of the Fourth International Workshop-Conference on Gestational Diabetes Mellitus. The Organizing Committee. *Diabetes Care* 1998;21(Suppl 2):B161–B167.

Okhubo Y, Kishikawa H, Araki E, et al. Intensive insulin therapy prevents the progression of diabetic microvascular complications in Japanese patients with non-insulin dependent diabetes mellitus: a randomized, prospective 6-year study. *Diabetes Res Clin Pract* 1995;28:103–117.

Oswald T, et al. *The Physician's Guide to Type 2 diabetes: Diagnosis and Treatment.* American Diabetes Association, 1996.

Report of the expert committee on the diagnosis and classification of diabetes mellitus. *Diabetes Care* 1997;20:1183–1197.

Parving HH, Lehnert H, Brochner-Mortensen J, et al. The effect of irbesartan on the development of diabetic nephropathy in patients with type 2 diabetes. *N Engl J Med* 2001;345:870–878.

Tuomilehto J, Lindstrom J, Eriksson JG, et al. Prevention of type 2 diabetes mellitus by changes in lifestyle among subjects with impaired glucose tolerance. *N Engl J Med* 2001;344:1343–1350.

UK Prospective Diabetes Study Group. Intensive blood-glucose control with sulphonylureas or insulin compared with conventional treatment and risk of complications in patients with type 2 diabetes (UKPDS 33). *Lancet* 1998;352:837–853.

UK Prospective Diabetes Study Group. Tight blood pressure control and risk of macrovascular and microvascular complications in type 2 diabetes: UKPDS 38. *BMJ* 1998;317:703–713.

Yudkin JS. How can we best prolong life? Benefits of coronary risk factor reduction in non-diabetic and diabetic subjects. *BMJ* 1993;306:1313–1318.

Yudkin JS, Oswald GA. Determinants of hospital admission and case fatality in diabetic patients with myocardial infarction. *Diabetes Care* 1988;11:351–358.

Zinman B. Physiologic replacement of insulin. *N Engl J Med* 1989;321:363–370.

# Adrenal Disorders

**45**

**S. Sethu K. Reddy**    **Rossana D. Danese**

The adrenal gland consists of the medulla and the cortex. The cortex is further divided into the zona reticularis, the zona fasciculata, and the zona glomerulosa (Fig. 45.1). The medulla produces norepinephrine and epinephrine. The zonae fasciculata and reticularis produce cortisol and androgens [mainly dehydroepiandrosterone (DHEA-S)], whereas zona glomerulosa produces aldosterone. As a result of the absence of 17-hydroxylase in the zonal glomerulosa, cortisol and androgens cannot be produced in that layer.

The zonae reticularis and fasciculata are under the control of adrenocorticotropic hormone (ACTH), released by the pituitary gland in response to hypothalamic corticotropin-releasing hormone (CRH). CRH, in turn, is regulated by cortisol negative feedback, stress, and a circadian rhythm. Besides increasing the synthesis of cortisol, ACTH is trophic for the adrenal gland, so that a lack of ACTH results in atrophy of the zonae fasciculata and reticularis. Although ACTH has some effect on aldosterone production, the zona glomerulosa is predominantly under the control of renin. Understanding the anatomy and physiology of the adrenal gland is crucial to understanding its hypofunction and hyperfunction.

## ADRENAL INSUFFICIENCY

### Etiology

Clinical adrenal insufficiency (AI) results from hypofunction of the adrenal cortex. This may be due to destruction of the adrenal gland itself [Addison's disease (AD) or primary AI] or to a lack of ACTH (secondary AI) or CRH. The most common cause of AD in adults is autoimmune destruction of the adrenal gland (80%). This often is seen in association with other autoimmune diseases, including Hashimoto's thyroiditis, Graves' disease, or type I diabetes mellitus. AI is known as type II autoimmune polyglandular syndrome. (Type I autoimmune polyglandular syndrome, more commonly seen in children, consists of AD, hypoparathyroidism, and mucocutaneous candidiasis.) In addition to the polyglandular syndromes, other clues to the presence of autoimmune AI include:

- Chromosome disorders (Down's, Klinefelter's, and Turner's syndromes)
- Alopecia
- Vitiligo

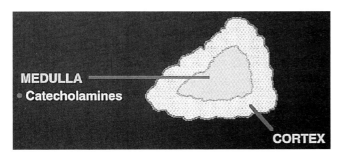

**Figure 45.1** The adrenal gland.

| TABLE 45.1 ADRENAL INSUFFICIENCY (AI): SIGNS AND SYMPTOMS | Primary AI | Secondary AI |
|---|---|---|
| *Cortisol deficiency* Anorexia/nausea/vomiting Weight loss/fatigue Myalgia/arthralgia Hypotension Hyponatremia | Yes | Yes |
| *Androgen deficiency* Loss of axillary and pubic hair (usually women only) | Yes | Yes |
| *Aldosterone deficiency* Hyperkalemia Orthostasis | Yes | No |
| *ACTH excess* Hyperpigmentation | Yes | No |

- Other autoimmune disorders (pernicious anemia, chronic active hepatitis, myasthenia gravis, primary hypogonadism)

In addition to autoimmune disease, other causes of primary AI in adults include:

- Infection
  - □ Viral
  - □ Mycobacterial
  - □ Fungal
- Hemorrhage/infarction
- Anticoagulants/coagulopathy
- Sepsis
- Thrombosis
- Metastatic cancer: breast, lung, gastrointestinal, renal
- Infiltrative disorders: amyloidosis, sarcoidosis, hemochromatosis
- Adrenoleukodystrophy/adrenomyeloneuropathy
  - □ Affecting young men (X-linked)—abnormal accumulation of very-long-chain fatty acids in adrenal cortex, brain, testes, and liver
- AI and central nervous system (CNS) demyelination

Currently, the acquired immunodeficiency syndrome (AIDS) is the most common cause of infectious adrenal destruction, while the antiphospholipid syndrome (lupus anticoagulant) is increasingly being recognized as a cause of adrenal hemorrhage.

Secondary AI is a result of adrenal gland atrophy from ACTH deficiency. This most often results from:

- Pituitary corticotroph atrophy owing to previous exogenous glucocorticoid use
- Hypopituitarism
- Isolated ACTH deficiency (usually postpartum)

## CLINICAL PRESENTATION

The underlying etiology of AI determines its clinical presentation (Table 45.1). Under the regulation of ACTH, cortisol and adrenal androgens are lost in both primary and secondary AI. Aldosterone production, predominantly regulated by renin, remains intact in secondary AI. Therefore, hyperkalemia and profound dehydration with orthostatic hypotension are seen in primary AI only. Likewise, hyperpigmentation of the skin or mucus membranes (secondary to increased ACTH) is seen in primary AI only. Consequently, the absence of hyperkalemia or hyperpigmentation does not exclude AI.

In addition to hyponatremia and hyperkalemia, laboratory abnormalities in AI may include:

- Hypoglycemia (usually chronic)
- Hypercalcemia
- Eosinophilia
- Lymphocytosis

## DIAGNOSIS

The diagnosis of AI is made by demonstrating diminished responsiveness of the hypothalamic-pituitary-adrenal (HPA) axis to stimulation. A morning cortisol value less than 3 μg/dL (assuming normal cortisol-binding globulin) can be sufficient to make the diagnosis; however, the cosyntropin (Cortrosyn) (ACTH) stimulation test is usually required and is the gold standard:

| Time 0 minutes | Baseline cortisol |
|---|---|
| Cosyntropin, 250 mg intramuscularly or intravenously | |
| Time 30 or 60 minutes | Cortisol |

A rise in the cortisol level to 18 μg/dL is a normal response. If an abnormal response is obtained, an ACTH level then determines primary (high ACTH) versus secondary disease (normal or low ACTH).

In secondary AI, however, the ACTH-stimulation test is not always abnormal. Adequate ACTH may be present to prevent adrenal gland atrophy (thereby resulting in a response to the supraphysiologic dose of ACTH used in the ACTH-stimulation test), but the HPA axis may not be able to respond to stress. In patients with suspected secondary AI and a normal ACTH-stimulation test, CRH is available to assess ACTH responsivity. In addition, the insulin tolerance test or the metyrapone test evaluate the integrity of the HPA axis by its response to hypoglycemia or inhibited cortisol synthesis, respectively. Though not widely used yet, some investigators find that a 1 microgram ACTH stimulation test may be more sensitive at detecting mild adrenal insufficiency.

## TREATMENT

The treatment of AI is replacement of the deficient hormones. The following agents may be used in treating AI:

- Hydrocortisone, 30 mg every day
- Prednisone, 7.5 mg every day
- Dexamethasone, 0.75 mg every day

Cortisol, 20 mg in the morning and 10 mg in the evening, or prednisone, 5 to 7.5 mg daily, provides dramatic relief of symptoms. To prevent Cushing's syndrome, however, the smallest dose needed to control the patient's symptoms should be used. For a minor illness, the glucocorticoid dose should be doubled for as short a time as needed. For a major stress, parenteral hydrocortisone, 200 to 400 mg daily, is given initially and then rapidly tapered. Aldosterone replacement is required in primary AI only; it is given as fludrocortisone acetate (Florinef Acetate), 0.05 to 0.2 mg daily. The dose is adjusted according to the patient's blood pressure and potassium level. Adrenal androgens are not replaced.

In undiagnosed patients with suspected adrenal crisis, dexamethasone, 2 to 4 mg intravenously or intramuscularly, should be given along with saline and glucose. Dexamethasone does not interfere with the cortisol assay. The ACTH-stimulation test should then be done as soon as possible.

In the management of secondary AI caused by previous exogenous steroids, glucocorticoids with short half-lives (usually cortisone) should be given as larger doses in the morning and smaller doses in the evening. The evening doses are gradually tapered, as symptoms permit, to allow overnight hypothalamic-pituitary "desuppression" and a rise in ACTH level. This leads to a return of adrenal gland function; when morning cortisol reaches 10 μg/dL, replacement glucocorticoid generally can be discontinued. Stress glucocorticoids, however, should be given until a ACTH-stimulation test is normal. The recovery of the HPA axis from glucocorticoid suppression generally requires 6 to 12 months.

## HYPOALDOSTERONISM

Hypoaldosteronism results from decreased aldosterone production by the zona glomerulosa of the adrenal cortex. This may be due to deficient renin stimulation or defective aldosterone production, despite renin stimulation (Table 45.2). In adults, the most common cause of primary hypoaldosteronism is AD. Renal insufficiency (or type IV renal tubular acidosis) is the most common cause of secondary hypoaldosteronism. Children and young adults may have adrenal cortex enzyme deficiencies causing hypoaldosteronism.

The symptoms and signs of mineralocorticoid deficiency include hyperkalemia and metabolic acidosis. Blood pressure may be low, normal, or high. Serum sodium may be normal or low. If necessary, the diagnosis may be established by aldosterone levels that fail to rise with standing or volume depletion with diuretics.

The treatment of hypoaldosteronism involves mineralocorticoid replacement using fludrocortisone, 0.05 to 0.2 mg daily, with dose adjustments based on blood pressure and potassium levels. Patients with hypertension or congestive heart failure are treated with loop diuretics.

## LATE-ONSET CONGENITAL ADRENAL HYPERPLASIA

Congenital adrenal hyperplasia (CAH), due to deficiency of an enzyme in the cortisol synthesis pathway, occurs in three variant forms:

- Classic CAH
- Simple virilizing CAH
- Late-onset CAH

Late-onset CAH results in a relative cortisol deficiency and increased ACTH levels. Cortisol production is normalized, but at the expense of adrenal hyperplasia and increased androgens. Therefore, late-onset CAH presents with peripubertal (or later) evidence of androgen excess (acne, hirsutism, menstrual irregularities, infertility) and adrenal hyperplasia or nodules. AI is not present.

**TABLE 45.2**
**ETIOLOGY OF HYPOALDOSTERONISM**

| Defective aldosterone secretion | Defective aldosterone stimulation |
|---|---|
| High renin | Low renin |
| Adrenal insufficiency | Renal insufficiency |
| Critically ill patient syndrome | Diabetes mellitus, pyelonephritis, gout |
| Heparin | NSAIDs, β-blockers |
| ACE inhibitors | Autonomic insufficiency |
| | Acquired immunodeficiency syndrome |

The most common (relative) enzyme deficiency is 21-hydroxylase, resulting in an accumulation of 17-hydroxy-progesterone (17-OHP). In this case, screening for late-onset CAH may include:

■ Random early morning follicular phase 17-OHP
■ Stimulated (by cosyntropin) 17-OHP

Late-onset CAH is best treated with low-dose glucocorticoid to lower ACTH and androgens.

## CUSHING'S SYNDROME

### Etiology

Cushing's syndrome is a result of glucocorticoid excess. Endogenously, this may be due to increased ACTH secretion by the pituitary gland (Cushing's disease) or ectopically, or to autonomous cortisol secretion by an adrenal tumor. The most common cause of Cushing's syndrome, however, is the exogenous use of glucocorticoids.

### Clinical Presentation

The clinical features of Cushing's syndrome are listed in Table 45.3. With respect to specificity for Cushing's syndrome, thinning of the skin, purple striae, and bruising are the best clinical signs. Hypokalemia, edema, and hyperpigmentation are more commonly seen in ectopic ACTH secretion, in which ACTH and cortisol levels tend to be much higher.

### Diagnosis

The diagnosis of Cushing's syndrome revolves around the inability to suppress the HPA axis. Two screening tests are employed:

■ 24-Hour urine collection for free cortisol and creatinine (UFC)
■ Overnight dexamethasone suppression test (ODST), in which dexamethasone, 1 mg, is given at 11 p.m. and a serum cortisol is drawn the following morning: Cortisol less than 5 μg/dL is a normal (or negative) response

The 24-hour UFC is more specific but is also more cumbersome. The value may be elevated in depression, acute illness, and alcoholism. The 1-mg ODST is easy to perform but has several false-positive and false-negative responses. The causes of a false-positive test result include increased cortisol-binding globulin (high circulating estrogen), depression, acute illness, and alcoholism. Drugs that increase the metabolism of dexamethasone [rifampin, phenobarbital, and phenytoin (Dilantin)] may also result in a false-positive response. False-negative tests may be seen in Cushing's disease or cyclic intermittent Cushing's syndrome.

## TABLE 45.3

### SIGNS AND SYMPTOMS OF CUSHING'S SYNDROME

| Clinical Feature | Approximate Prevalence (%) |
| --- | --- |
| Obesity | |
| General | 80–95 |
| Truncal | 45–80 |
| Hypertension | 75–90 |
| Menstrual disorders | 75–95 |
| Osteopenia | 75–85 |
| Facial plethora | 70–90 |
| Hirsutism | 70–80 |
| Impotence/decreased libido | 65–95 |
| Neuropsychiatric symptoms | 60–95 |
| Striae | 50–70 |
| Glucose intolerance | 40–90 |
| Weakness | 30–90 |
| Bruising | 30–70 |
| Kidney stones | 15–20 |
| Headache | 10–50 |

### Differential Diagnosis

If an abnormal result is obtained by either the 24-hour UFC or the 1-mg ODST, the pseudo-Cushing's state of alcoholism or endogenous depression should first be sought by a careful history, physical examination, and laboratory evaluation. A repeat UFC during alcohol abstention should be normal. If necessary, the low-dose DST may document true hypercortisolism. Dexamethasone, 0.5 mg orally every 6 hours, is administered for 48 hours, while a 24-hour UFC, including 17-hydroxysteroids (17-OHCS), is collected before and on the second day of dexamethasone. Failure to suppress 24-hour urine 17-OHCS to less than 4 mg or the UFC to less than 25 μg suggests pathologic hypercortisolism, although pseudo-Cushing's states occasionally cannot be suppressed. (Urinary 17-OHCS level is less essential because of the advent of the UFC, but the UFC is not yet as well standardized.) Once true Cushing's syndrome has been documented, an ACTH level separates ACTH-dependent from ACTH-independent disease:

■ ACTH-dependent hypercortisolism
  □ Cushing's disease
  □ Ectopic ACTH
  □ Ectopic CRH
■ ACTH-independent hypercortisolism
  □ Adrenal adenoma
  □ Adrenal carcinoma
  □ Nodular adrenal hyperplasia
  □ Exogenous glucocorticoids

A low ACTH level prompts computed tomography (CT) of the adrenal to look for a tumor or nodules. A normal or elevated ACTH value suggests Cushing's disease or ectopic ACTH production; these can be differentiated using the high-dose (8 mg) ODST. If a morning cortisol level suppresses by 50% in response to 8 mg of dexamethasone the evening before, the diagnosis is presumed to be Cushing's disease. The specificity is not 100%, however; many occult bronchial carcinoid tumors with ACTH secretion can suppress in response to high-dose dexamethasone.

Magnetic resonance imaging (MRI) is not definitive for distinguishing pituitary from nonpituitary tumors, since 50% of Cushing's disease patients have occult pituitary adenomas. Furthermore, up to 10% of patients may have false-positive pituitary scans (pituitary "incidentaloma"). Inferior petrosal sinus sampling (enhanced with CRH) may be necessary; an elevated sinus-to-peripheral ACTH gradient suggests Cushing's disease.

### Treatment

It should be apparent that the diagnostic workup for Cushing's syndrome can have many pitfalls. False-positive screening tests, pseudo-Cushing's states, modest specificity of the high-dose DST, and pituitary imaging can all lead to an erroneous diagnosis. It is important to correctly diagnose Cushing's disease because the most appropriate treatment is transsphenoidal pituitary adenomectomy performed by an experienced neurosurgeon, although radiation therapy, ketoconazole (Nizoral) or bilateral adrenalectomy may be needed in some cases. Resection or chemotherapy of the underlying tumor is the treatment for adrenal neoplasia and ectopic ACTH production.

## HYPERALDOSTERONISM

Excess aldosterone results in hyperaldosteronism with hypertension, hypokalemia, and metabolic alkalosis. This may be associated with Cushing's syndrome, particularly in patients with adrenal carcinoma. Isolated primary hyperaldosteronism, marked by an elevated aldosterone level and suppressed plasma renin activity (PRA), accounts for 1% to 2% of patients with hypertension; the presence of spontaneous hypokalemia or a potassium level of less than 3.0 mEq/L on diuretics should prompt an evaluation.

Once hypokalemia is corrected and interfering drugs discontinued [diuretics, angiotensin-converting enzyme (ACE) inhibitors, and β-blockers], the ratio of aldosterone (ng/dL) to PRA (ng/mL per h) is a simple screening test. A ratio greater than 20 is quite sensitive but not specific. Because the ratio can swing widely with small changes in PRA, some rely on a 24-hour urinary aldosterone levels as an indicator of excess aldosterone secretion. The saline suppression test confirms the diagnosis. (The test involves a determination of aldosterone and PRA before and after the administration of 2 L of normal saline: Normal patients suppress aldosterone to less than 5 ng/dL.) A persistently elevated aldosterone-to-PRA ratio after captopril (Capoten) also may be used to confirm the diagnosis.

The next step is to differentiate adrenal adenoma from hyperplasia. An adenoma can be differentiated by CT findings, increased 18-hydroxycorticosterone levels, or bilateral adrenal vein catheterization. Spironolactone (Aldactone), an aldosterone antagonist, is the treatment of choice for patients with hyperplasia, small adenomas, or contraindications to surgery.

## OTHER MINERALOCORTICOID EXCESS SYNDROMES

The pathogenesis of several mineralocorticoid excess syndromes has recently been elucidated. Dexamethasone-suppressible hyperaldosteronism is an entity that should be suspected in a young patient with elevated aldosterone, suppressed renin, and an appropriate family history. Through the development of a hybrid gene, the enzyme that catalyzes the final steps of aldosterone synthesis becomes regulated by ACTH. Treatment with dexamethasone suppresses ACTH and subsequently excess aldosterone production.

In patients with suppressed PRA and low aldosterone, a mineralocorticoid other than aldosterone is present. In the syndrome of apparent mineralocorticoid excess, seen in young adults, the mineralocorticoid has been identified as cortisol (which normally has little mineralocorticoid effect). Normally, cortisol is inactivated to cortisone in the renal tubular cell by 11β-hydroxysteroid dehydrogenase. A deficiency of this enzyme allows cortisol to bind to the mineralocorticoid receptor, resulting in hypertension, hypokalemia, and suppressed PRA. Natural licorice (glycyrrhizic acid) is now known to inhibit 11β-hydroxysteroid dehydrogenase, thus explaining licorice-induced hypermineralocorticoidism.

Excess sodium itself serves to suppress PRA and causes hypertension in Liddle's syndrome. In this familial syndrome, the constitutive activation of the kidney's epithelial sodium channel results in increased sodium resorption and potassium excretion, independently of any mineralocorticoid. Spironolactone is therefore ineffective; triamterene (Dyrenium) is the treatment of choice.

## PHEOCHROMOCYTOMA

### Clinical Presentation

Pheochromocytoma arises usually in the adrenal medulla. It accounts for approximately 0.1% of hypertensive patients. This tumor should be especially suspected in multiple endocrine neoplasia type II (MEN IIA and MEN IIB), in which disease is frequently bilateral:

- MEN IIA
  - Pheochromocytoma
  - Medullary thyroid carcinoma
  - Hyperparathyroidism

- MEN IIB
  - ☐ Pheochromocytoma
  - ☐ Medullary thyroid carcinoma
  - ☐ Mucosal neuromas
  - ☐ Marfanoid habitus

The neuroectodermal syndromes also have an increased incidence of pheochromocytoma:

- Neurofibromatosis
- Neurofibromas
- Cafe-au-lait spots
- Cerebelloretinal hemangioblastosis
- Renal cell cancer
- Retinal angioma
- CNS hemangioblastoma
- Tuberous sclerosis
- Seizures
- Mental deficiency
- Adenoma sebaceum

The triad of headaches, palpitations, and diaphoresis in the presence of hypertension is classic for pheochromocytoma. Other signs and symptoms include:

- Postural hypotension
- Tachycardia
- Weight loss
- Pallor
- Hyperglycemia
- Anxiety
- Nausea/vomiting
- Constipation
- Tremulousness

Silent pheochromocytomas are more frequently recognized, presenting as adrenal incidentalomas. Cocaine abuse may be mistaken for pheochromocytoma.

## Diagnosis

Screening for pheochromocytoma consists of a 24-hour urine collection for catecholamines and catecholamine metabolites (metanephrines and vanillymandelic acid). Plasma catecholamines may also be useful; plasma norepinephrine greater than 2,000 pg/mL is specific for pheochromocytoma. Borderline or indeterminate results require further testing. The clonidine (Catapres) suppression test is used to confirm the diagnosis in patients with indeterminate urine or plasma studies. (The test involves the measurement of plasma catecholamines before and 3 hours after clonidine, 0.3 mg, is administered orally: A normal response is a plasma norepinephrine level less than 500 pg/mL or a 50% decrease from baseline.) The glucagon stimulation test may also be used; an increase in blood pressure and plasma catecholamines strongly suggests pheochromocytoma. The sensitivity of this test is limited, however, and it is potentially dangerous (hypertensive crisis). Chromogranin

A, a neuropeptide secreted with the catecholamines, is reasonably sensitive for pheochromocytoma but of poor specificity; it is elevated with even minor degrees of renal insufficiency and cosecreted with many hormones.

Once the diagnosis is biochemically established, radiographic localization is indicated. Although CT is the initial choice, MRI may be especially useful because pheochromocytoma can be markedly hyperintense (white) on T2-weighted images. Scanning with iodine-131-labeled metaiodobenzylguanidine (MIBG) is most specific and particularly useful for extraadrenal (10%) and malignant metastatic tumors (10%).

The treatment of a pheochromocytoma is resection after appropriate operative preparation (volume loading and adrenergic receptor blockade). Calcium channel blockers may also be effective.

## INCIDENTALLY DISCOVERED ADRENAL MASS

Incidental adrenal masses are common, detected in approximately 2% of patients having abdominal CT. The differential diagnosis of such masses includes:

- Functioning or nonfunctioning adenoma
- Functioning or nonfunctioning carcinoma
- Pheochromocytoma
- Metastasis from tumors at other sites (especially malignant melanoma, lung, breast, and gastrointestinal cancers)
- Myelolipoma
- Cyst
- Focal enlargement in hyperplastic gland (e.g., Cushing's disease, CAH)
- Pseudoadrenal mass arising from nearby organs

Management of an incidentaloma is controversial; clinical judgment is required. Patients should first be clinically evaluated for evidence of adrenal hormone production (cortisol, androgens, aldosterone, catecholamines). If the tumor appears to be clinically nonfunctional, most endocrinologists still screen biochemically for pheochromocytoma because of the associated morbidity and mortality. Several investigators also recommend dexamethasone suppression testing to exclude preclinical Cushing's syndrome. These patients will not have the classic signs or symptoms of hypercortisolism but will have evidence of HPA axis dysfunction, such as loss of diurnal rhythm. The long-term implications of preclinical Cushing's syndrome are unknown, and the optimal management is therefore controversial; however, at a minimum, these patients must be identified before adrenal surgery because postoperative AI may develop.

Despite an absence of hormone excess, nonfunctional tumors greater than 4 to 6 cm should be resected owing to an increased risk of malignancy; nonfunctional tumors measuring 4 cm and less can be further evaluated radiographically to determine the likelihood of benign disease. The attenuation value, obtained from a noncontrast CT scan, is a measure of a tumor's lipid content. A value less than 10 Hounsfield units (HU) suggests fat density and is specific for adenoma. Masses of indeterminate attenuation value (10 to 20 HU) can be further classified by opposed-phase MRI. Masses inconsistent with adenoma by CT or MRI require repeated follow-up with CT to assess growth, or fine-needle aspiration (FNA) biopsy.

## REVIEW EXERCISES

### QUESTIONS

**1.** A 40-year-old white woman with a history of severe asthma and Hashimoto's thyroiditis reports 2 months of fatigue, anorexia, nausea, weight loss, and myalgia. Her examination is remarkable only for a blood pressure of 98/60 mm Hg and a pulse of 98 beats/min without orthostasis. She shows no hyperpigmentation. Sodium is 130 mEq/L, potassium 4.5 mEq/L, chloride 105 mEq/L, and bicarbonate 24 mEq/L. ACTH-stimulation tests shows cortisol at 5.8 μg/dL at T 0 minute and 13.2 μg/dL at T 60 minutes.

Which of the following is correct?
a) The most likely cause of her AI is AD.
b) The most likely cause of her AI is prior exogenous corticosteroid use.
c) She does not have AI because her ACTH-stimulation tests is normal.
d) She will require treatment with prednisone, 7.5 mg daily, and fludrocortisone, 0.1 mg daily.

**2.** You are treating a 58-year-old man with hypopituitarism following radiation therapy for craniopharyngioma. He is taking hydrocortisone sodium succinate, 15 mg daily, levothyroxine, 0.15 mg daily, and testosterone injections, 200 mg every 2 weeks. He feels weak and tired. His examination is remarkable only for a blood pressure of 95/58 mm Hg. Sodium is 131 mEq/L, potassium 4.8 mEq/L, thyroid-stimulating hormone (TSH) 0.23 μIU/mL, and FTI 9.0 μg/dL.

Which of the following would you do next?
a) Decrease levothyroxine
b) Increase testosterone
c) Add fludrocortisone
d) Increase hydrocortisone
e) Begin desmopressin acetate (DDAVP)

**3.** A 63-year-old woman whom you are treating for hypertension, osteoarthritis, gout, recurrent deep vein thrombosis, and a 10-year history of type 2 diabetes mellitus has a potassium level of 6.2 mEq/L at a follow-up appointment. Serum aldosterone is 1.8 ng/dL.

Which of the following is false?
a) A β-blocker and nonsteroidal anti-inflammatory drugs (NSAIDs) may be contributing to the hyperkalemia.
b) An ACE inhibitor may be contributing to the hyperkalemia.
c) Long-term heparin may be contributing to hypoaldosteronism.
d) Prednisone will likely be required as treatment.

**4.** A 37-year-old woman presents to you for evaluation of weight gain and hirsutism of several years' duration. Her gynecologist has prescribed an oral contraceptive for oligomenorrhea. She has noted easy bruising, but no muscle weakness. On examination, she weighs 240 lb, with central obesity. Blood pressure is 144/92 mm Hg. She has significant facial hair, mild acne, multiple thin whitish striae on her abdomen, and a small buffalo hump. Her proximal muscle strength is normal. A random glucose level is 183 mg/dL, and potassium is 3.9 mEq/L. Her gynecologist sends you the results of an ODST (morning cortisol of 6.2 μg/dL) and a random ACTH level (25 pg/mL).

Which of the following would you do next?
a) Order MRI of the pituitary.
b) Order CT of the adrenals.
c) Obtain a 24-hour UFC.
d) Perform a high-dose (8 mg) dexamethasone suppression test.

**5.** A 50-year-old woman on chronic warfarin therapy for a previous pulmonary embolus was recently started on an acetylsalicylic acid (ASA) containing analgesic for joint pain. She suddenly developed severe abdominal pain and, by the time she was taken to the emergency department, she was partially obtunded, hypotensive, and pale. Hemoglobin was found to be 8 mg/dL.

What would you do next?
a) Check INR
b) Do a one-hour ACTH stimulation test
c) Intravenous saline and dexamethasone
d) Do a blood type and match
e) Abdominal CT

**6.** A 52-year old-woman is referred to you by her urologist for a 3-cm right adrenal mass detected on abdominal CT. Her weight has been stable, and she has generally felt well. She has not noted hirsutism, acne, proximal myopathy, or easy bruising, but she has felt depressed lately. She also has had diaphoresis and occasional headaches, but no palpitations. Her last menstrual period was 6 months earlier. She has a 2-year history of diabetes mellitus that is well controlled by diet. Her last mammogram 8 months earlier was negative, and no breast masses are present. She smokes one pack of cigarettes daily. Blood pressure is 135/85 mm Hg, pulse

95 beats/min, and weight 174 pounds; she has no buffalo hump, supraclavicular fat, or abdominal striae. Proximal muscle strength is normal. Stool is negative for occult blood. Complete blood cell count and chemistry profile are normal.

Which of the following would you do next?
a) Obtain a 24-hour UFC
b) Determine the aldosterone-to-PRA ratio
c) Obtain serum DHEAs and androstenedione levels
d) Obtain a 24-hour urine collection for catecholamines and metanephrines
e) All of the above

**7.** A 68-year-old man presents for evaluation of a 2.5-cm adrenal mass. History and physical examination are negative for malignancy and overproduction of any adrenal hormones. A biochemical evaluation for pheochromocytoma is negative. No data are present regarding CT attenuation value, and MRI opposed-phase imaging is not available.

Which of the following would you recommend?
a) Surgery
b) FNA biopsy of the mass
c) Conventional MRI
d) Follow-up CT in 3 to 6 months

## ANSWERS

### 1. b.

This case illustrates the differences between primary and secondary AI in clinical presentation and treatment. In secondary AI, the renin–aldosterone axis is intact; therefore hyperkalemia and metabolic acidosis are not seen, and fludrocortisone is not required for treatment.

### 2. d.

This case also illustrates secondary AI and inadequate glucocorticoid replacement. Physiologic hydrocortisone replacement is 20 to 30 mg daily. No data suggest the need for desmopressin or increased testosterone. Levothyroxine doses should not be adjusted by the TSH in secondary disease.

### 3. d.

This case illustrates several conditions associated with hypoaldosteronism. Although AI can be associated with hypoaldosteronism, no suggestion of AI is present from the history presented, and it is more likely that medications are the cause. A heparin preservative (chlorbutol) can inhibit aldosterone synthesis, whereas NSAIDs (through the inhibition of prostacyclin, a vasodilator and renin secretagogue) and β-blockers suppress renin release.

### 4. c.

This case illustrates the evaluation of Cushing's syndrome. Generally, the 24-hour UFC is the best screening test; the 1-mg ODST is easier to perform but has more false-positive results, including increased cortisol-binding globulin owing to the estrogen in oral contraceptives. Radiographic imaging is not indicated until the diagnosis is established biochemically.

### 5. c.

This patient likely has adrenal insufficiency from an adrenal hemorrhage, through the potentiation of warfarin by ASA. Intravenous fluids and dexamethasone can be life-saving; then other options can be considered. Dexamethasone does not cross-react with cortisol in the radio immune assay. All the choices are reasonable but answer c should be performed first.

### 6. d.

This case illustrates the work-up of an incidental adrenal mass. Biochemical testing should be influenced by clinical findings. If no evidence of hormone production is apparent through history and physical examination, a biochemical screening for pheochromocytoma should nonetheless be done.

### 7. d.

Surgery is not recommended for incidental adrenal masses unless they are large (greater than 4 to 6 cm). A FNA biopsy can be diagnostic but should be used only when an immediate answer is needed and an experienced radiologist is available. FNA biopsy can diagnose metastatic disease but cannot always distinguish adrenal carcinoma from adenoma. Conventional MRI cannot distinguish metastasis from adenoma; only opposed-phase imaging (chemical-shift imaging) can do this. When CT or MRI cannot provide a definite diagnosis (metastasis versus adenoma), follow-up CT is indicated.

## SUGGESTED READINGS

Bravo EL. Primary aldosteronism: issues in diagnosis and management. *Endocrinol Metab Clin North Am* 1994;23:271–283.
Byny RL. Withdrawal from glucocorticoid therapy. *N Engl J Med* 1975; 1:30–32.
Grinspoon SK, Biller BM. Clinical review 62: laboratory assessment of adrenal insufficiency. *J Clin Endocrinol Metab* 1994;79:923–931.
Gross MD, Shapiro B. Clinical review 50: clinically silent adrenal masses. *J Clin Endocrinol Metab* 1993;77:885–888.
Kong MF, Jeff CW. Eighty-six cases of Addison's disease. *Clin Endocrinol* 1994;41:757–761.
Orth DN. Cushing's syndrome. *N Engl J Med* 1995;332:791–803.

# 46

# Pituitary Disorders and Multiple Endocrine Neoplasia Syndromes

**S. Sethu K. Reddy**     **Amir H. Hamrahian**

The pituitary gland is divided into two lobes, the anterior lobe (developed from Rathke's pouch) and the posterior lobe (developed as a diverticulum growing downward from the base of the hypothalamus).

The pituitary gland weighs from 500 to 1,000 mg and sits in the sella turcica, immediately behind the sphenoid sinus. It has anterior and posterior bony walls and a bony floor. Above it is a layer of dura (diaphragma sella), and then the optic chiasm, hypothalamus, and third ventricle. Laterally, on each side, is the cavernous sinus, inclusive of the internal carotid artery and cranial nerves III, IV, $V_1$, $V_2$, and VI. The optic chiasm may be anterior (15%), above (80%), or behind the sella (5%).

In the 1930s, it was hypothesized that releasing hormones traveled from the hypothalamus to the pituitary via the hypothalamic-pituitary portal system, but it was not until the mid-1960s that these releasing hormones were isolated and identified. The first releasing hormone to be identified was thyrotropin-releasing hormone (TRH). In subsequent years, other releasing hormones were identified (Table 46.1). All pituitary hormones are under positive stimulatory effect from the hypothalamus, except prolactin (PRL), which is under tonic inhibitory effect through dopamine acting as a PRL release-inhibiting factor (PIF).

Magnetic resonance imaging (MRI) is the best method for visualizing hypothalamic-pituitary anatomy because the optic chiasm, vascular structures, and tumor extension to cavernous sinuses can be well visualized using MRI, when compared to other imaging techniques.

## PITUITARY TUMORS

Pituitary tumors may present with either hypofunction or hyperfunction, as well as symptoms directly related to the mass effect of the tumor (Table 46.2). Since the advent of computed tomography (CT), microadenomas have been designated arbitrarily as equal or less than 10 mm in diameter, and macroadenomas as greater than 10 mm in diameter. They are almost always benign. Pituitary adenomas are rarely associated with parathyroid and pancreatic hyperplasia or neoplasia as part of the multiple endocrine

neoplasia type I (MEN I) syndrome. Pituitary carcinomas are very rare, but metastases from other organs may occur.

About 30% of pituitary adenomas are prolactinomas; 15% are growth hormone (GH)–producing, 10% are adrenocorticotropin hormone (ACTH)–producing, 10% are glycoprotein-producing, and less than 1% secrete thyroid-stimulating hormone (TSH). Nonfunctioning pituitary adenomas, or more appropriately named nonsecretory adenomas, represent about 25% of pituitary tumors. On morphologic examination, most of these adenomas reveal granules containing glycoprotein hormones or their subunit.

Impingement on the optic chiasm or its branches by pituitary pathology may result in visual field defects, with the most common being bitemporal hemianopsia. A lateral extension of the pituitary mass to the cavernous sinuses may result in diplopia, ptosis, or altered facial sensation. Among the cranial nerves, third nerve palsy is the most common.

Autopsy studies suggest that up to 20% of normal individuals harbor incidental pituitary microadenomas that are pathologically similar in distribution to those that present clinically. The initial work-up should be limited and include serum prolactin and insulin-like growth factor-1 (IGF-1) level testing. Other screening tests may be performed depending on clinical feature, such as obtaining 24-hour urinary free cortisol in a patient with clinical features suggestive of Cushing's disease. The adenoma must be followed yearly by MRI, increasing the duration between imaging studies, if size remains stable.

## HYPOPITUITARISM

Pituitary adenomas are the most common cause of hypopituitarism, but other causes including parasellar diseases, inflammatory disorders, following pituitary surgery or radiation therapy, and head injury also must be considered. The usual consequence of pituitary hormones deficiency secondary to a mass effect is in the following order: GH, luteinizing hormone (LH), follicle-stimulating hormone (FSH), TSH, ACTH, and prolactin. Prolactin deficiency is uncommon except in those with pituitary infarction.

## TABLE 46.1

### INTERACTION OF HYPOTHALAMIC REGULATORY HORMONES, PITUITARY HORMONES, AND PERIPHERAL HORMONES FROM TARGET GLANDS

| Hypothalamic Hormones | Pituitary Hormones | Target Gland | Feedback Hormone |
|---|---|---|---|
| TRH | TSH | Thyroid | T4,T3 |
| LHRH | LH | Gonad | E2, Test |
| LHRH | FSH | Gonad | Inhibin, E2, Test |
| GHRH, SMS | GH | Multiorgans | IGF-1 |
| PIF | Prolactin | Breast | ? |
| CRH, ADH | ACTH | Adrenal | Cortisol |

ACTH, adrenocorticotropin hormone; ADH, antidiuretic hormone; CRH, corticotropin-releasing hormone; E2, estradiol; FSH, follicle-stimulating hormone; GH, growth hormone; GHRH, growth hormone–releasing hormone; GnRH, gonadotropin-releasing hormone; IGF-1, insulin-like growth factor 1; LH, luteinizing hormone; PIF, prolactin release inhibiting factor; SMS, somatostatin; T3, triiodothyronine; T4, thyroxine; Test, testosterone; TRH, thyrotropin-releasing hormone; TSH, thyroid-stimulating hormone.

Isolated deficiencies of various anterior pituitary hormones have also been described.

Growth hormone deficiency is now recognized as a pathologic state in adults, and more patients with GH deficiency undergo GH replacement. The symptoms of GH deficiency in adults include decreased muscle strength and exercise capacity, decreased bone density, and reduced sense of well being (e.g., diminished libido, social isolation). Patients with GH deficiency have increased body fat, particularly intraabdominally, and decreased lean body mass compared with normal adults. A trial of GH replace-

ment in adults with documented GH deficiency and symptoms, or metabolic abnormalities suggestive of GH deficiency, is indicated. The treatment of GH deficiency has shown to have a favorable effect on lipid profile and to result in decreased carotid intima thickness. The most common side effects of GH therapy include fluid retention, carpal tunnel syndrome, and arthralgia. These side effects are usually dose related and improve with dose reduction.

Gonadotropin deficiency may be secondary to a pituitary disorder, hypothalamic deficiency of luteinizing hormone–releasing hormone (LHRH), or a functional abnormality such as hyperprolactinemia, anorexia nervosa, and severe disease state. In women, gonadotropin deficiency causes infertility and menstrual disorders, including amenorrhea. It is often associated with lack of libido and dyspareunia. In men, hypogonadism is diagnosed less often because decreased libido and impotence may be considered as a function of aging. Hypogonadism is often diagnosed retrospectively when a patient presents with mass effect. Osteopenia is a consequence of long-standing hypogonadism and usually responds to hormone replacement therapy.

The symptoms of secondary adrenal insufficiency are similar to primary adrenal insufficiency, with one important difference. Mineralocorticoid secretion is mainly regulated by the renin and angiotensin system and is preserved in patients with pituitary disorders. For this reason, the symptoms are more chronic in nature and include malaise, loss of energy, anorexia, and hypoglycemia. An acute illness may precipitate vascular collapse and be life threatening if unrecognized. Hyperkalemia is not a feature of secondary adrenal insufficiency.

TSH deficiency is a relatively late finding in patients with pituitary disorders, having symptoms similar to those of primary hypothyroidism including malaise, leg

## TABLE 46.2

### CLINICAL MANIFESTATIONS OF PITUITARY TUMORS

| Mass Effects | Endocrine Effects | |
|---|---|---|
| | Hyperpituitarism | Hypopituitarism |
| Headaches | GH: Acromegaly | GH: Short stature in children, Increased fat |
| Chiasmal syndrome | PRL: Hyperprolactinemia | mass, osteoporosis, decreased strength, |
| Hypothalamic syndrome | ACTH: Cushing's disease | and quality of life |
| Disturbances of thirst, appetite, satiety, | Nelson's syndrome | PRL: failure of postpartum lactation |
| sleep, and temperature regulation | LH/FSH: Mostly present with mass effect | ACTH: hypocortisolism |
| Diabetes insipidus | but may result in gonadal dysfunction | LH or FSH: hypogonadism |
| SIADH | TSH: hyperthyroidism | TSH: hypothyroidism |
| Obstructive hydrocephalus | | |
| Cranial nerves III, IV, $V_1$, $V_2$, and | | |
| VI dysfunction | | |
| Temporal lobe dysfunction | | |
| CSF rhinorrhea | | |

ACTH, adrenocorticotropin hormone; CSF, cerebrospinal fluid; FSH, follicle-stimulating hormone; LH, luteinizing hormone; PRL, prolactin; SIADH, syndrome of inappropriate secretion of antidiuretic hormone; TSH, thyroid-stimulating hormone.

cramps, lack of energy, and cold intolerance. The degree of hypothyroidism depends on the duration of thyrotropin deficiency.

## PROLACTINOMA

The pituitary content of PRL is approximately 100 μg but can increase ten- to twentyfold during pregnancy and lactation. Although breast tissue is the most important target organ for PRL, PRL receptors have been identified in various tissues, including liver, kidney, ovaries, testes, prostate, and seminal vesicles. Dopamine is the major inhibitor of PRL secretion, and any mechanisms that interrupt dopamine transport from the hypothalamus to the pituitary can lead to elevated levels of PRL.

Hyperprolactinemia is the most common pituitary disorder. Observational studies in patients with microprolactinomas indicate that serum prolactin concentration or adenoma size increase in only a minority of patients over time. Past estrogen therapy has been suggested as a cause of prolactinoma formation, but careful case-cohort studies have found no evidence that oral contraceptives induce the development of prolactinomas. The clonal analysis of tumor DNA indicates that prolactinomas are monoclonal in origin.

Hyperprolactinemia impairs pulsatile gonadotropin release (LH and FSH), likely through an alteration in hypothalamic LHRH secretion. Women of reproductive age usually present with oligomenorrhea, amenorrhea, galactorrhea, and infertility. Those with long-standing amenorrhea are less likely to have galactorrhea, secondary to long-standing estrogen deficiency. Men and postmenopausal women usually come to medical attention because of mass effect, such as headaches and visual field defects. Many men with hyperprolactinemia do not report any sexual dysfunction, but once treated effectively for hyperprolactinemia, the majority realize the presence of problems including decreased libido and erectile dysfunction. Men with long-standing hypogonadism may have decreased beard and body hair, with soft but usually normal size testes (if hypogonadism starts before completion of puberty, testes will be small). Patients with microadenomas have a higher frequency of headaches compared with control subjects.

A drug history is a very important part of the initial evaluation of patients with elevated prolactin level because some medications are associated with hyperprolactinemia and their discontinuation (if possible) will avoid any further and often expensive work-up. Other common conditions associated with elevated prolactin levels include pregnancy and hypothyroidism (Table 46.3). A serum prolactin level above 200 μg/L is indicative of a prolactin-producing pituitary tumor, although rare exceptions occur. Conversely, a serum prolactin level below 200 μg/L in the presence of a large pituitary adenoma is suggestive of stalk compression. The PRL level usually correlates with the size of the tumor. Stimulatory tests, including a TRH stimulation test to determine whether an elevated prolactin is the result of a prolactinoma, are nonspecific and cannot be used to diagnose or exclude a tumor.

Bromocriptine mesylate (Parlodel) and cabergoline (Dostinex) are potent inhibitors of PRL secretion and often result in tumor shrinkage. The suppression of prolactin secretion through dopamine agonists depends on the number and affinity of dopamine receptors on the lactotroph adenoma. A substantial decrease in the prolactin level usually occurs, even when serum prolactin levels do not normalize. These medications should be initiated slowly because side effects often occur at the beginning of treatment. The most common side effects include nausea, headache, dizziness, nasal congestion, and constipation. It may take up to 6 months before testosterone levels increase and normal sexual function is restored in men

## TABLE 46.3

### DIFFERENTIAL DIAGNOSIS OF HYPERPROLACTINEMIA

| Physiologic | Pathologic | Pharmacologic |
|---|---|---|
| Pregnancy | Prolactinoma | Antipsychotic medication |
| Postpartum | Acromegaly (GH and prolactin cosecretion) | Tricyclic antidepressant |
| Newborn | | Some SSRIs, including fluoxetine and fluvoxamine |
| Stress | Pituitary stalk lesion or compression secondary to mass effect | |
| Hypoglycemia | | Methyldopa, reserpine, verapamil |
| Sleep | Hypothyroidism | Metoclopramide |
| Intercourse | Renal failure | Estrogen, antiandrogens |
| Nipple stimulation | Liver disease | H2 blockers (especially intravenous preparation) |
| | Chest wall trauma (burn, shingles) | |
| | Spinal nerves or cord lesions | Opiates, cocaine |
| | Ectopic prolactin secretion (very rare) | Protease inhibitors |

GH, growth hormone; SSRI, selective serotonin reuptake inhibitor.

successfully treated for prolactinomas. Prolactin appears to have an independent effect in men on libido because exogenous testosterone works poorly in restoring libido in those who continue to have elevated prolactin levels.

Although patients with microprolactinomas can sometimes be followed without therapy, patients with macroprolactinomas always must be treated. Patients with good response to dopamine agonist therapy may be weaned from them with no increase in prolactin concentration. For this reason, it would be reasonable to try a "drug holiday" after several years of therapy with close follow-up.

Medical therapy during pregnancy often stirs debate about the continuation of bromocriptine. Tumor-related complications are seen in about 15% of pregnancies, and in only 5% of women with microadenomas. A sensible approach would be to stop bromocriptine when pregnancy is confirmed, and then follow the clinical status with visual-field examinations. If any evidence for mass effect presents, bromocriptine may be reinstituted.

Medical therapy with dopamine agonists is the first-line treatment for prolactinoma. Surgery, typically, transsphenoidal resection, is reserved for those who cannot tolerate or do not respond to medical therapy. Even in patients with mass effect, including visual field defects, dopamine agonist are first-line therapy because a rapid improvement in symptoms is observed in a majority of patients. The main advantage of surgery is the avoidance of chronic medical therapy. Radiation therapy may be considered for patients who poorly tolerate dopamine agonists and who are not likely to be cured by surgery (e.g., tumor invasion of cavernous sinuses).

## ACROMEGALY

Acromegaly occurs at a rate of 3 to 4 cases per million per year, with a mean age at diagnosis of 40 years in men and 45 years in women. The GH secreting tumors tend to be more aggressive in younger patients. Classical clinical features include:

- Coarsening of facial features
- Prominent jaw and frontal sinus
- Broadening of hands and feet
- Hyperhidrosis
- Macroglossia
- Signs of hypopituitarism
- Diabetes mellitus (10% to 25%)
- Skin tags (screening for colonic polyps required)
- Hypertension (25% to 30%)
- Cardiomyopathy (50% to 80%)
- Carpal tunnel syndrome
- Sleep apnea (5%)

In more than 98% of cases, acromegaly is caused by GH-secreting pituitary tumors (rarely by ectopic GHRH secretion). These tumors are mainly carcinoids and pancre-

atic islet cell tumors. Patients with acromegaly have 3.5-fold increased mortality rate, with cardiovascular disease being the most common cause of death. Somatotrope adenomas appear to be monoclonal in origin. A stimulatory GTP-binding protein mutation in a $Gsp_l\alpha$ subunit in GH cells, leading to continuous GH secretion, has been shown to cause acromegaly.

Due to the pulsatile nature of GH secretion, random GH levels can overlap in acromegalic patients and controls. Therefore, a random GH level is usually inadequate to establish the diagnosis. IGF-1 has a longer plasma half-life than GH and is an excellent initial screening test for those suspected of acromegaly. An elevated IGF-1 level in a clinical setting suggestive of acromegaly almost always confirm the diagnosis. The IGF-1 level may be falsely low in patients with poorly controlled diabetes, hypothyroidism, and malnutrition and should not be used to exclude the diagnosis. The oral glucose tolerance test remains the gold standard to confirm the diagnosis. Normal individuals suppress their GH level to less than 1 µg/L (using chemiluminescent assays) within 2 hours after ingestion of 75 g oral glucose solution.

In the case of ectopic acromegaly, elevated GHRH can be measured in blood to confirm the diagnosis (usually >200 ng/mL). As an exception, patients with hypothalamic GHRH0-secreting tumors may have normal GHRH levels, probably secondary to the direct release of GHRH to the hypophyseal portal system. In patients with GH-secreting pituitary adenoma, the GHRH level is low or undetectable.

The early detection of cardiovascular disease (CVD) is of particular importance because CVD is the primary cause of mortality in these patients. Patients with acromegaly have an increased risk of colon polyps, with the potential for an increased risk of malignancy. Thus, acromegaly patients should undergo colonoscopy every 3 to 5 years until more data about the frequency of such screening tests are available. It is not clear if more rigorous screening for a variety of cancers, including breast, lung, or prostate cancer, is indicated.

In acromegaly, the primary aims of treatment include relieving symptoms, reducing tumor bulk, normalizing IGF-1 and GH dynamics, and preventing tumor regrowth. The medical treatment of acromegaly has gained significance as the limitations of radiation therapy has become evident. Current medical therapies for acromegaly include dopamine agonist, somatostatin analogs, and GH receptor antagonist. The normalization of IGF-1 is seen in only 10% to 15% of patients treated with dopamine agonists and is more likely with pituitary tumors cosecreting GH and prolactin. Octreotide (a somatostatin analog) and its long-acting preparation (Sandostatin LAR) lower and normalize IGF-1 in 90% and 65% of acromegalic patients, respectively. The long-term observations of patients on somatostatin analogs have shown no evidence for tachyphylaxis. Some degree of tumor shrinkage in up to 50% of patients is expected, although in most cases less than 50% shrinkage occurs in tumor size. The most common side effects are gastrointestinal, including diarrhea, abdominal pain, and nausea. The most serious side effect of somatostatin analogs is cholelithiasis, seen in up to 25% of patients. Its long-term management is similar to those with cholelithiasis in the general population, and routine ultrasonographic screening is not indicated.

The U.S. Food and Drug Administration (FDA) recently has approved the GH antagonist Somavert, which normalizes IGF-1 in more than 95% of patients. Liver function tests and follow-up MRI at intervals that closely monitor tumor size is recommended.

A surgical approach is the treatment of choice in patients presenting with pituitary microadenoma or when the tumor is confined to the sella; in experienced hands, surgery results in a cure in as many as 90% of patients. Even in those not cured by surgery, tumor debulking usually results in improvement of symptoms and lowering of IGF-1 levels. Radiation therapy almost always induces a decrease in tumor size and GH level, but the cure rate after conventional radiotherapy has been disappointing. Radiosurgery (gamma knife) seems to be superior to conventional radiation therapy, but large studies with strict cure criteria, including normalization of IGF-1 and long-term safety profiles, are lacking.

## CUSHING'S DISEASE AND ECTOPIC ACTH SYNDROME

An ACTH-secreting pituitary adenoma is the most common cause of endogenous Cushing's syndrome (60%), with the rest being adrenal (25%) or ectopic (15%) in origin. The following findings are suggestive of hypercortisolism state:

- Central obesity
- Muscle wasting with proximal muscle weakness
- Unexplained osteopenia or osteoporosis
- Spontaneous ecchymosis
- Purplish wide striae (>1cm)
- Hypokalemia
- Serial photographs show change in appearance

Other findings, which are less helpful in discriminating patients with and without Cushing's, are hypertension, abnormal glucose tolerance, menstrual irregularities, and psychiatric disturbances, including depression. Women with Cushing's disease typically have fine facial lanugo hair and may have acne and temporal scalp hair loss secondary to increased adrenal androgen secretion. A 3- to 6-year delay in the diagnosis of patients with Cushing's disease usually occurs, and it may be possible to date the onset of the disease by determining which scars are pigmented due to excess secretion of ACTH and other melanotropins.

A 24-hour urinary free cortisol measurement is the single best test for diagnosing Cushing's syndrome. Because of

the significant overlap between normal individuals and those with Cushing's, random serum cortisol has no role in diagnosis of Cushing's syndrome. A 1 mg overnight dexamethasone suppression test with a morning cortisol level below 1.8 μg/dL virtually rules out the disease but has a false-positive rate of as high as 40%. A combination of low-dose dexamethasone suppression test and CRH stimulation test has been shown to have 100% diagnostic accuracy in an National Institutes of Health (NIH) study. This test may have a significant value in establishing the diagnosis in those with pseudo-Cushing and elevated 24-hour urinary free cortisol. Other tests useful in establishing the diagnosis of Cushing's disease include midnight serum and salivary cortisol (Fig. 46.1).

Once the diagnosis of Cushing's syndrome has been established, the next step is to find out whether it is ACTH dependent (Fig. 46.1). Although undetectable or low ACTH levels are consistent with adrenal etiology, low-normal ACTH levels may be seen in both adrenal Cushing's disease and those with ACTH-secreting pituitary adenoma. The CRH stimulation test is used to differentiate between the two; no significant change in ACTH and cortisol levels following CRH stimulation occurs in adrenal Cushing's disease. Although ACTH level tend to be higher in those with ectopic Cushing's syndrome compared with patients having pituitary disease, considerable overlap occurs. A high-dose (8 mg) dexamethasone suppression test (HDDST) and/or CRH stimulation test are helpful in differentiating between the two. Patients with ectopic Cushing's disease do not suppress their cortisol level during high HDDST, and no significant rise occurs in ACTH

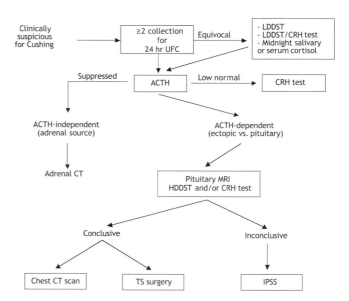

**Figure 46.1**  Cushing's evaluation: work-up algorithm. ACTH, adrenocorticotropin hormone; CRH, corticotropin-releasing hormone; UFC, urinary free cortisol; LDDST, low-dose dexamethasone suppression test; HDDST, high-dose dexamethasone suppression test; TS, transsphenoidal; IPSS, inferior petrosal sinus sampling.

and cortisol following CRH stimulation. The gold standard test to differentiate pituitary Cushing's disease from an ectopic ACTH-producing tumor is inferior petrosal sinus sampling. This test should be only performed by an experienced neuroradiologist, and it is essential to note that it cannot be used to make the diagnosis of Cushing's syndrome because the result in patients with Cushing's disease may be similar to normal individuals.

Ectopic ACTH syndrome is the most frequent and best studied of the ectopic hormone syndromes. Most tumors associated with ectopic ACTH syndrome are carcinomas and have a poor prognosis. These tumors usually present with a rapid-onset syndrome (within 6 months) associated with profound muscle weakness, hyperpigmentation, hypertension, hypokalemia, and edema. Hyperpigmentation is thought to be due to cosecretion of β-melanocyte–stimulating hormone (β-MSH), one of the byproducts of ACTH synthesis. Some benign tumors, such as carcinoids or islet cell tumors, have been shown to cause ectopic ACTH syndrome; these are difficult to differentiate from the pituitary causes of Cushing's syndrome. This difficulty is exaggerated by radiologic investigations of the sella that are often negative or shows a microadenoma, which is seen in up to 20% of normal individuals in autopsy series.

The surgical (transsphenoidal) removal of ACTH-secreting pituitary tumor is the treatment of choice. The availability of an experienced surgeon is crucial, with an 80% to 90% remission rate following surgery. An undetectable postoperative cortisol level without steroid use is considered to be a good marker for long-term cure. A period of temporary adrenal insufficiency occurs, following successful surgery; this insufficiency usually lasts for 6 to 12 months, but may be as long as 2 years in duration. For those not cured by the surgery, other options include a second resection and radiation therapy. Patients whose tumor is unresponsive to these therapies may then be offered medical or surgical adrenalectomy. Ectopic ACTH-producing tumors should be resected if possible.

Medical treatment includes octreotide, which may inhibit ectopic ACTH secretion. Mitotane (Lysodren) is perhaps the most effective adrenolytic agent. Other medications, such as aminoglutethimide (Cytadren), ketoconazole (Nizoral), or metyrapone (Metopirone), are useful as temporizing agents only.

## NONFUNCTIONAL OR GLYCOPROTEIN-SECRETING TUMORS

Nonfunctional or glycoprotein-secreting pituitary tumors are usually clinically silent because they are inefficient in secreting hormones and lack a clinically recognizable syndrome. They usually come to attention because of mass lesion manifestations, including headache and visual field defect. Patients may present with varying degrees of hypopituitarism due to mass effect. Rarely, an FSH adenoma may

cause amenorrhea in a woman, or an LH adenoma may cause precocious puberty in a boy. The diagnosis is confirmed by the measurement of either intact glycoprotein hormones or their α and β subunits.

The transsphenoidal surgical approach is standard, especially if visual function is abnormal. Radiation therapy is used in those with significant residual tumor or evidence of tumor recurrence. Octreotide may be helpful in reducing tumor hypersecretion, but further studies are required to assess whether it has any effect on tumor size. Dopamine agonists, such as bromocriptine and cabergoline, have been used in high doses, but clinical responses (i.e., changes in tumor size or visual symptoms) occur in less than 10% of patients.

In summary, the efficacy of the medical therapy in patients with nonfunctional or glycoprotein-secreting pituitary adenoma is not established, but may be used in an attempt to reduce tumor hypersecretion and size, especially in those who are not a surgical candidate.

## TSH-SECRETING PITUITARY TUMORS

The clinical picture in patients with TSH-secreting pituitary adenoma includes pituitary mass lesion, hyperthyroidism, and goiter. The most important biochemical feature of TSH-secreting pituitary tumors is the elevation of thyroid hormone levels in the presence of normal or elevated TSH level. For this reason, any patient presenting with endogenous hyperthyroidism and an elevated or normal TSH should be further evaluated for the presence of a TSH-secreting pituitary adenoma. Elevated serum prolactin and α subunit favor the diagnosis of a thyrotrope adenoma and cast doubt on a diagnosis of thyroid hormone resistance syndrome. Octreotide is especially useful in reducing hormone hypersecretion, but its effect on tumor size is not well studied. Antithyroid medications may be used to make the patient euthyroid before surgical resection of the tumor is attempted.

## LYMPHOCYTIC HYPOPHYSITIS

Lymphocytic hypophysitis is an autoimmune disease that often presents in women during or after pregnancy. The clinical manifestations are secondary to hypopituitarism, adrenal insufficiency, or may be caused by a pituitary mass effect. The serum prolactin level is elevated in more than half of patients, but it may be decreased. Other autoimmune endocrine disorders, including Hashimoto's thyroiditis and Addison's disease, have been seen with increased frequency in such patients. Although the diagnosis may be suspected on clinical ground in a pregnant or postpartum woman, a surgical biopsy may be needed to confirm the diagnosis. Isolated ACTH deficiency has been described in some of patients, and its presence should alert the physician to the possibility of lymphocytic hypophysitis as an underlying disorder. Some patients recover fully, whereas others may need selective hormone replacement. For this reason, patients must be assessed at regular intervals for the necessity of continued hormone replacement.

## EMPTY SELLA

The diagnosis of empty sella syndrome is increasingly made owing to the prevalence of CT and MRI. Pituitary fossa enlargement is secondary to a communication between the pituitary fossa and the subarachnoid space, which causes remodeling and enlargement of the sella. Although a primary empty sella is the result of a congenital diaphragmatic defect, a secondary empty sella may result from previous surgery, irradiation, or infarction of a preexisting tumor. Most patients have no pituitary dysfunction, but a wide spectrum of pituitary deficiencies have been described, especially in those with secondary empty sella. Coexisting tumors may occur. Management usually comprises reassurance and hormone replacement, if necessary. Surgery is rarely indicated, unless cerebrospinal fluid rhinorrhea is present.

## PITUITARY APOPLEXY

Pituitary apoplexy is an endocrine emergency resulting from a hemorrhagic infarction of the pituitary, usually associated with a preexisting pituitary tumor. A variety of predisposing conditions, including bleeding disorders, diabetes mellitus, pituitary radiation, pneumoencephalography, mechanical ventilation, and trauma have been described. The clinical manifestations of this syndrome are related to the rapid expansion and compression of the pituitary gland and the perisellar structures, leading to hypopituitarism, visual field defects, and cranial nerve palsies. An extravasation of blood or necrotic tissue into the subarachnoid space may cause clouding of consciousness, meningismus, and fever. If pituitary apoplexy is suspected, anterior pituitary insufficiency should be presumed, and the patient must be treated accordingly. Glucocorticoids, in a dose adequate to the degree of stress and presumptive cerebral edema, are the treatment of choice. Any evidence of sudden visual-field defects, oculomotor palsies, hypothalamic compression, or coma should lead to immediate surgical decompression. The recovery of a variety of pituitary hormone deficiencies following surgery have been documented, and all patients should be reevaluated for possible recovery of their pituitary hormone axes.

*Sheehan's syndrome* is the result of an ischemic infarction of the normal pituitary gland, which leads to hypopituitarism secondary to postpartum hemorrhage and hypotension. Patients have a history of failure to lactate postpartum, failure to resume menses, cold intolerance, or fatigue. Some women may have an acute crisis mimicking apoplexy within 30 days postpartum. Subclinical central diabetes insipidus (DI) often is present.

## MULTIPLE ENDOCRINE NEOPLASIA SYNDROMES

The MEN syndromes are rare, but their recognition is crucial because it is important to promptly treat the patient and identify affected family members. The MEN syndromes are all inherited as an autosomal-dominant trait. It is essential that treating physician be alert to their various clinical presentations and use the available molecular DNA testing for diagnostic confirmation.

MEN syndromes include:

- MEN I
- MEN II
- MEN IIA
- MEN IIB
- Familial Medullary Thyroid Cancer (FMTC)

MEN I syndrome, which may involve an anterior pituitary tumor, usually manifests in the fourth or fifth decades. Its prevalence is about 2 per 100,000. The parathyroid glands (80% to 90%), the pancreas (80%), and the pituitary (65%) may be involved. Gastrinoma (Zollinger-Ellison syndrome) is the most common pancreatic tumor (70%), followed by insulinoma. Pancreatic tumors may secrete gastrin, insulin, vasoactive intestinal polypeptide (Werner-Morrison syndrome), serotonin, glucagon, somatostatin, pancreatic polypeptide, or GHRH. Carcinoid tumors are also associated with MEN I and MEN II syndromes. Hyperparathyroidism is the initial manifestation in the majority of patients, and it is clinically and biochemically similar to that of primary hyperparathyroidism in the general population. It is estimated that 1% to 2% of all cases of primary hyperparathyroidism is caused by MEN I syndrome. Pituitary tumors occur in a distribution similar to that of isolated pituitary adenomas.

From the findings of molecular biologic studies, it appears that a mutation at the q13 locus in chromosome 11 results in the loss of a tumor suppressor product. If the q13 locus is lost from both chromosomes 11, it leads to a homozygous deficiency of the suppressor protein. This suppressor protein has been termed *menin*, and it has been isolated. Until the utility of measuring the levels of this protein has been tested, clinical management must include genetic counseling, careful gathering of family history, and screening of first-order relatives. Monitoring calcium, PRL, and glucose levels at 1- to 2-year intervals beginning at age 15 years is recommended.

The clinical spectrum of MEN IIA, in order of frequency, includes medullary thyroid cancer, pheochromocytoma, and hyperparathyroidism. Cutaneous lichen amyloidosis has been described in some families and is considered a component of the syndrome. Early diagnosis through screening of family members at risk is essential because total thyroidectomy can cure or prevent medullary thyroid cancer. MEN IIB syndrome consists of medullary thyroid cancer, pheochromocytoma, and multiple mucosal neuromas. Familial medullary thyroid cancer is a variant of MEN type II A, in which only a strong predisposition for medullary thyroid cancer exists, without the other components of the syndrome. A mutation of the *RET* protooncogene appears to be strongly correlated with the presence of disease in MEN II syndrome. Screening for this gene has largely supplanted calcium injection or pentagastrin (Peptavlon) stimulation of calcitonin levels as a screening test.

## POSTERIOR PITUITARY

The posterior pituitary acts as a repository for antidiuretic hormone (ADH, vasopressin) and oxytocin. ADH secretion is regulated by serum osmolality, as well as plasma volume. Small increments in serum osmolality greater than 290 mOsm/kg lead to the prompt secretion of ADH. A greater than 10% plasma volume decrease, however, will override any osmolar stimulus (e.g., a severely dehydrated individual can thus be hyponatremic). Nausea, vomiting, pain, nicotine, and caffeine can increase ADH secretion. It should be noted that ADH is a potent vasoconstrictor, whereas the clinically safer desmopressin (DDAVP) is an ADH analog with pure antidiuretic action.

To establish the diagnosis of DI, a measurement of 24-hour urine volume and osmolality is taken during ad libitum fluid intake. DI is established if urine volume is more than 50 ml per kg body weight, with a concomitant osmolality of <300 mOsm/kg. At the same time, polyuria due to an osmotic agent such as glucose should be excluded.

Central DI is a polyuric syndrome secondary to inadequate ADH secretion and the inability to concentrate the urine. Patients have a normal response to the administration of vasopressin. Maximum urine output due to complete ADH deficiency is 18 L per day, and urine volume in excess of this indicates excess fluid intake. Central DI has many causes including:

- Familial predisposition
- Trauma or postsurgical insult
- Granulomatous disease
- Tumors
- Craniopharyngioma
- Pituitary tumors
- Metastatic cancer
- Infectious causes
- Vascular causes
- Aneurysms
- Sheehan's syndrome

- Autoimmune disorders
- Idiopathic causes

Conscious patients with DI usually have sufficient thirst to maintain a normal serum sodium in spite of polyuria. In this situation, a standard water deprivation test should be performed, during which time patients are allowed no fluid to drink while their serum levels are closely monitored. When two consecutive voided urine osmolalities differ by less than 10% or when 5% of body weight is lost, 5 U of aqueous vasopressin (or 2 micrograms of DDAVP IV) is given intravenously. Urine osmolality testing is repeated in 30 and 60 minutes.

Desmopressin administration following dehydration elicits the following responses:

- A greater than 50% rise in urine osmolality with minimal urine concentration during the test in spite of dehydration—central DI
- Little or no rise in urine osmolality with minimal urine concentration during the test in spite of dehydration—nephrogenic DI
- Less than 10% increase in urine osmolality without achieving maximal urine concentration (but often above plasma osmolality) during the test—primary polydipsia

Serum ADH levels at the end of the fast and before administration of vasopressin may help to differentiate between partial central and nephrogenic DI because both may have a modest concentration of urine with dehydration and a more than 10% increase in urine osmolality in response to vasopressin. It is noteworthy that patients with psychogenic polydipsia have a diluted medullary concentrating gradient, and a partial nephrogenic DI may develop. Some conditions associated with nephrogenic DI include familial tubulointerstitial renal disease, electrolytes disorder (hypokalemia and hypercalcemia), drug side effects (e.g., lithium, demeclocycline), and pregnancy.

The posterior pituitary is gadolinium-enhanced on MRI and is a good assay of ADH reserve, keeping in mind that up to 20% normal individuals do not have a bright spot. Partial central DI may be treated with chlorpropamide or thiazides, whereas complete central DI must be treated with desmopressin. The drug is available in subcutaneous, oral, and nasal spray. The exact dosing and timing must be individualized.

## REVIEW EXERCISES

### QUESTIONS

**1.** A 25-year-old shoe salesman reports frontal headaches for 6 months. Four months ago, his primary care physician diagnosed hypothyroidism. His free thyroxine ($FT_4$) level is 0.4 ng/dL µg/dL (normal, 0.7–2.0 ng/dL), and his TSH level is 0.41 mIU/mL (normal, 0.4–5.5 mIU/mL). He also reports some loss of energy, leg cramps, and dry skin.

What other history should you obtain?
a) Change in body hair distribution and fat distribution
b) Symptoms of erectile dysfunction
c) Visual-field disturbances
d) Symptoms of polydipsia
e) All of the above

2. An MRI of the sella turcica reveals a 2-cm mass. Visual fields appear normal by confrontation, but under Goldmann perimetry, they show bilateral superior-temporal defects to the color red. Laboratory findings include normal blood urea nitrogen (BUN), creatinine, and electrolyte levels; a testosterone level of 30 ng/dL (normal, 200–1,000 ng/dL); LH, 2 mIU/mL (normal, 1–7 mIU/mL); FSH, 1.5 IU/mL (normal, 2–10 mIU/mL); morning cortisol, 4.5 μg/dL (normal, 5–26.9 μg/dL); and PRL, 400 ng/mL (normal, less than 15 ng/mL).

Which of the following is false?
a) The patient has secondary hypogonadism.
b) The patient is likely to have cortisol deficiency.
c) The patient's GH reserve is probably normal.
d) The patient has a prolactinoma.

3. What is the best course of action for the patient in Question 2, after adequate replacement with hydrocortisone and thyroid hormone?
a) Emergency transsphenoidal removal of pituitary adenoma
b) Initiate dopamine agonist therapy
c) Gamma knife surgery
d) Testosterone, 200 mg intramuscularly every 2 weeks

Match the following case scenarios with the most compatible laboratory findings (each laboratory result is used only once).

4. A 25-year-old chronic schizophrenic woman with galactorrhea

5. A 25-year-old man with impotence, galactorrhea, and visual-field defect

6. An 18-year-old man with delayed puberty, anosmia, and appropriate bone density

7. A 45-year-old man with worsening diabetes control, coarsening features, and skin tags

8. A 40-year-old woman with headaches, normal menses, no visual-field defect, and CT head scan suggesting an empty sella
a) Low testosterone, low LH and FSH, and normal PRL of 15 ng/mL
b) Elevated IGF-1 level
c) Normal TSH and PRL response to TRH, normal LH and FSH response to LH-RH, normal cortisol and GH response to insulin-induced hypoglycemia

d) Normal T$_4$ and TSH, and PRL of 50 ng/mL
e) Low testosterone, low LH and FSH, and PRL of 250 ng/mL

9. Which of the following tests does not have any role in establishing the diagnosis of Cushing's syndrome?
a) Midnight salivary cortisol
b) 24-hour urinary free cortisol
c) Midnight serum cortisol
d) Random serum cortisol
e) Low-dose dexamethasone suppression test

10. A 45-year-old white female with clinical findings suggestive of Cushing's syndrome has been found to have two elevated UFCs of 220 and 300 (normal, 2–70 mg/24 hr); her ACTH level is 55 (normal, 5–50 pg/mL), and her pituitary MRI shows a 3 mm adenoma.

Which of the followings is the *best* next course of action?
a) Repeat 24-hour urinary free cortisol
b) Transsphenoidal surgery
c) Low-dose dexamethasone suppression test
d) High dose dexamethasone suppression and/or CRH test
e) Midnight serum cortisol level

11. Which of the following is *not* seen with increased frequency in patients with newly diagnosed acromegaly?
a) Cholelithiasis
b) Goiter
c) Sleep apnea
d) Galactorrhea
e) Colon polyps

12. A 65-year-old man with a history of macroadenoma develops severe retroorbital headache, nausea, and vomiting with change in mental status. On examination, right third nerve palsy with stiff neck is present; his blood pressure is 170/90 mm Hg. An emergency MRI of the brain shows hemorrhage in the pituitary adenoma, which is enlarged in size.

What is the *best* next course of action?
a) Emergency transsphenoidal surgery
b) Dexamethasone 2 mg intravenously every 6 hours
c) Nitroprusside drip to keep systolic blood pressure between 140 and 160 mm Hg systolic
d) Broad spectrum antibiotic
e) Dopamine agonist

## ANSWERS

1. e.
The low T$_4$, with an inappropriate TSH level in an individual who is clinically hypothyroid, should prompt a search for hypothalamic-pituitary dysfunction. The clinical situation must be considered. A low total T$_4$ and a normal TSH may also be observed in the sick euthyroid syndrome. Elderly euthyroid men are also more likely to have a low TSH as a benign finding.

**2. c.**

In the presence of pituitary tumors, the pituitary gland sequentially loses the ability to secrete GH, LH, FSH, TSH, and ACTH. This patient has secondary hypogonadism, hypothyroidism, and likely hypoadrenalism. It is almost certain that GH secretion is abnormally low. GH deficiency often goes undetected in adults, and thus gonadotropin deficiency is a presenting symptom. Because irregular menses often leads to medical investigation, women often present earlier with small pituitary tumors.

**3. b.**

Medical therapy with a dopamine agonist is the first-line therapy for patients with prolactinomas, even in those with visual field defect, because it is very effective and has a rapid onset of action. Most patients, including those with mass effect, report improvement in their symptoms. Although this patient's hypogonadism is likely secondary to mass effect and not due to elevated prolactin level, the recovery of gonadotropin axis is possible following a decrease in the size of the pituitary adenoma and a normalization of prolactin. For this reason, testosterone therapy may be delayed, but with close evaluation of patient response to therapy. The patient also must be monitored for recovery of his thyrotropin and corticotropin axes in future.

**4. d.**

This patient likely has drug-induced hyperprolactinemia. Major tranquilizers and other medications, such as metoclopramide (Reglan) and high doses of haloperidol, methyldopa, reserpine, estrogens, and opiates are likely to elevate PRL levels.

**5. e.**

Men with prolactinomas often present with a gradual onset of symptoms. Any pituitary tumor may lead to hypogonadism and gynecomastia but subsequently only hyperprolactinemia leads to galactorrhea.

**6. a.**

The presence of anosmia and hypogonadism is suggestive of a developmental midline defect (Kallmann's syndrome). This disorder of hypogonadotropic hypogonadism affects 1 in 10,000 to 60,000 individuals. After suitable priming with LHRH, the pituitary can secrete LH and FSH.

**7. b.**

The measurement of IGF-1 has become a convenient screening test for acromegaly. An elevated IGF-1 level in a clinical setting suggestive of acromegaly almost always confirms the diagnosis. In patients with poorly controlled diabetes and malnutrition, the IGF-1 level may be falsely low and should not be used to exclude the diagnosis. The oral glucose tolerance test remains the gold standard to confirm the diagnosis.

**8. c.**

This patient has an empty sella syndrome, which is often associated with normal pituitary function. Occasionally, isolated or multiple hormonal deficiencies may be present.

**9. d.**

Because of the significant overlap between normal individuals and those with Cushing's syndrome, random serum cortisol has no role in the diagnosis of Cushing's syndrome. All other answers may be used to establish a diagnosis of Cushing's syndrome. Twenty-four-hour urinary free cortisol is the best initial screening test to establish the diagnosis.

**10. d.**

The diagnosis of Cushing's syndrome has been established in this patient with two significantly elevated 24-hour urinary free cortisol tests (>3 times upper normal). A slightly elevated ACTH level excludes adrenal origin, but may be seen in both Cushing's disease and ectopic ACTH-producing tumors. The next step to differentiate between the two is the high-dose dexamethasone suppression and/or CRH stimulation test. If the result is not conclusive, inferior petrosal sinus sampling should be done in an experienced center. The presence of a 3 mm pituitary adenoma is suggestive of a pituitary source for ACTH, but it may be seen in up to 20% of normal individuals as an incidentaloma.

**11. a.**

Cholelithiasis is not part of the clinical picture seen in patients with acromegaly caused by excess GH secretion. Although mostly asymptomatic, cholelithiasis and gallbladder sludge are the most serious side effects of somatostatin analogs, and may occur in up to 25% of patients on chronic therapy.

**12. b.**

High-dose steroid therapy is the initial step in treating patients with pituitary apoplexy. The steroid dose must be adequate for presumptive ACTH deficiency and cerebral edema due to acute mass effect. Patients with altered mental status and neurologic deficits are immediate candidates for surgery, once high-dose steroid has been initiated.

## SUGGESTED READINGS

Bichet DG. Diabetes insipidus and vasopressin. In: Moore WT, Eastman RC, eds. *Diagnostic Endocrinology.* Toronto: BC Decker, 1990:111–124.

Katznelson L, Klibanski A. Prolactin and its disorders. In: *Principles and Practice of Endocrinology and Metabolism,* 2nd ed. Philadelphia: JB Lippincott, 1995.

Melmed S. Acromegaly. *N Engl J Med* 1990;322:966–977.

Molitch ME. Thorner MO, Wilson C. Therapeutic controversy: Management of prolactinomas. *J Clin Endocrinol Metab* 1997;82: 996.

Melmed S, Kleinberg D. Anterior pituitary. In: Larsen RP, Kronenberg HM, Melmed S, Polonsky KS, eds. *Williams Textbook of Endocrinology*, 10th ed. Philadelphia: WB Saunders, 2003:177–279.

Vance ML. Hypopituitarism. *N Engl J Med* 1994;330:1651–1662.

Yanovski JA, Cutler GB, Chrousos GP, et al. Corticotropin-releasing hormone stimulation following low-dose dexamethasone administration. A new test to distinguish Cushing's syndrome from pseudo-Cushing's states. *JAMA* 1993;269:2232–2238.

# Metabolic Bone Disease and Calcium Disorders

# 47

## *Angelo A. Licata*

## HYPERCALCEMIA

The extent of a patient's symptoms from hypercalcemia depends directly on two major factors: the duration of the hypercalcemic process and the rapidity of its development. The more chronic and slowly progressive the rise in serum calcium, the less likely that the patient will be aware of it. If the hypercalcemic process arises rapidly, within weeks to months, symptoms develop that are generally of a neurologic or musculoskeletal nature. The diagnosis of hypercalcemia is separated into two major areas: parathyroid-related and non-parathyroid–related; both are discussed in this chapter.

### Clinical Presentation

The symptoms of hyperparathyroid hypercalcemia have taken on a vastly different presentation over the last two to three decades:

- Asymptomatic (up to 80%)
- Symptomatic (20%)
- Renal stones (colic), mental status changes, gastritis (ulcers), pancreatitis, constipation, malaise-fatigue-weakness-arthralgia, and bone pain or fractures are some of the symptoms noted in patients. Mild symptoms can be so nonspecific in early disease that a firm diagnosis may be missed.

Most patients with hyperparathyroidism are asymptomatic. The detection of abnormalities in serum calcium by routine chemical assays now identifies patients many years before symptoms arise. Historical descriptions of hyperparathyroidism, however, emphasize symptoms such as osteitis fibrosa cystica (bone pain and arthralgia), renal stone disease, gastric ulcers, pancreatitis, decreased mental status, and weakness.

In patients with other causes of hypercalcemia, the unique presentation of hyperparathyroidism may not be the clinical presentation. An abrupt onset of lethargy, confusion, fatigue, and even outright coma is often the presentation of many patients whose calcium level rises abruptly. In these cases, hypercalcemia occurs so rapidly that problems such as renal stone disease may not have time to develop. Manifestations of bowel dysfunction may be present, however, such as pain or constipation, and generalized muscular weakness. Older patients are more likely to be overcome by these symptoms; younger individuals tolerate higher levels of hypercalcemia with fewer symptoms.

### Diagnosis

Textbook descriptions of hypercalcemia list extensive causes of this condition:

- Primary hyperparathyroidism
- Cancer [e.g., tumors secreting parathyroid hormone–related protein (PTH-rp) or ectopic vitamin D, bone metastases]
- Endocrine disorders (e.g., thyrotoxicosis, oversecretion of vasoactive intestinal polypeptide, Addison's disease, pheochromocytoma)
- Granulomatous diseases
- Drugs (e.g., thiazides, lithium, antiestrogens, vitamins A and D)
- Familial hypocalciuric hypercalcemia
- Parenteral nutrition
- Immobilization
- Milk-alkali syndrome
- Acute and chronic renal insufficiency

A workable approach to this diagnosis separates the causes into two major areas:

- Parathyroid
- Nonparathyroid [hypervitaminosis D (endogenous or exogenous); malignancy (metastatic or humoral)]

The nonparathyroid causes of hypercalcemia are related to vitamin D–mediated or malignant processes. Intoxication with exogenous vitamin D is seen because the vitamin is used to treat osteoporosis. Endogenous hypervitaminosis D usually arises from granulomatous diseases, such as sarcoidosis, but granuloma located in any part of the body may cause this form of hypercalcemia.

Malignant diseases also produce hypercalcemia. Some malignant diseases, such as breast cancer, cause skeletal destruction. Others, such as myeloma and epidermal (squamous) tumors, make chemical (humoral) substances that increase bone metabolism and bone destruction. Myelomas release interleukins and cytokines within the bone marrow from plasma cells, stimulating osteoclastic activity and ultimately bone turnover and calcium loss. Originally, squamous or epidermal tumors were shown to produce PTH-rp. This substance increases bone loss and renal tubular reabsorption of calcium and is distinct from true parathyroid hormone (PTH). Many other types of tumors are known to produce this protein, but they may not all cause hypercalcemia.

## Laboratory Study: Parathyroid Hormone Assay

The introduction of the intact-PTH assay, which uses sophisticated chemical techniques, has virtually eliminated those problems noted in the past concerning the differentiation of parathyroid disease from other forms of hypercalcemia (e.g., ectopic) that might be caused by PTH-rp. This new assay clearly differentiates hyperparathyroidism from other disorders. The normal range of PTH is 10 to 65 pg/mL for a serum calcium level of 8.5 to 10.5 mg/dL. Values greater than the normal reference interval, in combination with a high calcium value, are diagnostic of hyperparathyroidism. In the non-PTH–mediated causes of hypercalcemia, no measurable intact PTH should be present.

## Differential Diagnosis

The workup for hypercalcemia can be accomplished simply by using the algorithm shown in Figure 47.1. The level of PTH measured indicates a parathyroid or nonparathyroid problem. Primary hyperparathyroidism is differentiated from other causes by finding a measurable or increased value with an increase of serum calcium. If no measurable hormone is found, vitamin D intoxication or a malignancy is probably present. The serum phosphorus level can sometimes help make the distinction between these processes: When the serum phosphorus level is elevated or high normal, a vitamin D–mediated process is suspected (if renal function is normal). In some cases of metastatic disease to

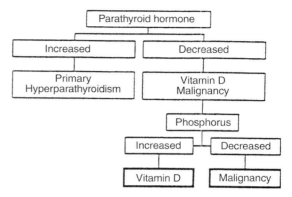

**Figure 47.1**   Diagnostic algorithm for hypercalcemia.

bone, an elevation in serum calcium and phosphorus may be present, due to bone destruction, but this should not be a diagnostic difficulty because the history, physical examination, and radiologic examinations help identify this problem. When the phosphorus level is low, a humoral agent from a cancer is often suspected, the most common being PTH-rp.

For purposes of board examinations, the algorithm in Figure 47.1 can be quite useful to quickly focus one's thinking, although the algorithm may oversimplify the diagnostic process. Various permutations and combinations of secondary diseases can very well cloud the reality of the diagnosis.

## Treatment

The treatment of hypercalcemia is directed toward resolving acute symptoms and instituting the long-term control of the underlying process.

The treatment of acute symptoms begins with saline hydration to increase the excretion of sodium and calcium in the urine. Adequate hydration is mandatory to avert declining renal function and its secondary reabsorption of calcium. Loop diuretics [furosemide (Lasix)] have been considered first-line therapy in the past, but this is not the major approach taken today. Intravenous doses of a bisphosphonate—pamidronate disodium (Aredia) 60 to 90 mg, etidronate disodium (Didronel) 7.5 mg/kg, or zolendric acid (Zometa ) 1 or 2 mg—are used to control the hypercalcemic process; zolendric acid is the most potent, with pamidronate a close second and etidronate the weakest. Pamidronate and etidronate require infusions over several hours, whereas zolendric acid can be given as a bolus over a few minutes. The use of a diuretic agent in hypercalcemia may be risky if the patient has not been sufficiently hydrated. Worsening dehydration in the face of diuretic use can actually promote worsening hypercalcemia, renal shutdown, and even death.

Steroid use in the treatment of hypercalcemia is helpful for specific disorders, such as hypervitaminosis D and myeloma, but it is ineffective in parathyroid disease.

## TABLE 47.1
### LONG-TERM CONTROL OF HYPERCALCEMIA

| Cause | Treatment |
|---|---|
| Parathyroid disease | Surgery |
| | No curative medication |
| Vitamin D related | Steroids |
| Malignancy | Control of symptoms |
| | Chemotherapy for underlying tumor |
| | Steroids |

Injectable calcitonin has been used in the past with some success to control hypercalcemia, but it lacks the prolonged responses seen with the potent bisphosphonate drugs. The dosage range for calcitonin is 7 to 10 U/kg body weight per day. Side effects from the administration of this drug, including nausea and vomiting, limit its usefulness. Nasal spray calcitonin and oral bisphosphonates are not efficacious.

The long-term control of hypercalcemia is directed toward eradicating the underlying disease (Table 47.1). Parathyroid surgery is curative in almost all patients with primary disease. Steroid therapy is curative for problems of vitamin D intoxication and certain tumors. Other forms of chemotherapy for cancer may offer long-term control of the hypercalcemic process. For malignancy-related hypercalcemia, however, the weekly or monthly administration of an intravenous bisphosphonate is useful when the underlying disease cannot be completely eradicated. Oral phosphates (e.g., Neutra-Phos) do not work well over the long term; intestinal side effects limit the possible dose and tolerability. Adequate hydration is obviously mandatory. In some cases, added salt in the diet, with a low dose of a loop diuretic, can keep a patient asymptomatic.

## HYPOCALCEMIA AND OSTEOMALACIA

Osteomalacia is the hallmark of poor skeletal mineralization owing to hypocalcemia, hypophosphatemia, or both. Symptoms range from subtle and obscure complaints to muscle weakness and overt bone pain upon palpation or movement.

### Pathophysiology

Overt fractures and pseudofractures are the sign of insufficient mineralization. Osteomalacia due to hypocalcemia and/or hypophosphatemia arises from the following causes:

- Vitamin D deficiency
- Dietary lack
- Deprivation of sunlight
- Malabsorption
- Increased catabolism

- Decreased formation metabolites of vitamin D
- Phosphate depletion
- Renal tubular disorders
- Neoplasm
- Secondary hyperparathyroidism

Endogenous vitamin D arises from the ultraviolet-light irradiation of epidermal cholesterol. A deprivation of sunlight causes vitamin D deficiency, but dietary sources of vitamin D substitute for endogenous forms. In situations in which a dietary lack of this vitamin occurs, or in which abnormalities in the gastrointestinal tract prevent its absorption, a deficiency may arise. Any gastrointestinal disease that alters absorption can lower serum levels of vitamin D. Likewise, increased catabolism of vitamin D produces a relative deficiency of vitamin D. (This occurs when drugs stimulate liver mitochondrial cytochrome P450 and increase the catabolism of vitamin D.) Likewise, renal failure decreases the serum concentration of bioactive vitamin D (1,25-dihydroxyvitamin D).

Phosphorus depletion, an uncommon cause of osteomalacia, may be an isolated finding or may be combined with hypocalcemia. Vitamin D deficiency causes hypophosphatemia and hypocalcemia. Renal tubular disorders cause a primary phosphorus leak or a widespread abnormality, such as that noted in Fanconi syndrome. In either case, the correction of the phosphorus leak is very difficult. Rare mesenchymal tumors also cause osteomalacia because they block production of active vitamin D. The surgical removal of these tumors reverses the process. When severe, secondary hyperparathyroidism also causes hypophosphatemia.

### Diagnosis

#### Laboratory Studies
The primary findings of osteomalacia include:

- Hypocalcemia
- Hypophosphatemia
- Hyperphosphatasia (defined as increased alkaline phosphatase)

Upon testing, increased total serum alkaline phosphatase is not invariably present in all patients. The degree to which serum alkaline phosphatase is elevated is directly proportional to the underlying changes in bone metabolism. A bone-specific alkaline phosphatase assay is also used, but may not be immediately available routinely. New assays for bone collagen fragments in the urine or serum are supplanting the old insensitive assays, such as hydroxyproline. These tests measure the N- or C-telopeptides of α-1 bone collagen. Other tests analyze the urinary pyridinoline or deoxypyridinoline cross-links of collagen. These are more sensitive than older urine hydroxyproline tests. Secondary findings include decreased urinary calcium and phosphorus; however, urinary phosphorus increases in cases of renal tubular leak and secondary hyperparathyroidism. Other laboratory findings arise from the underlying diseases.

The laboratory data in osteomalacia can be summarized as follows:

- Primary findings
  - ☐ Decreased calcium or phosphorus, or both
  - ☐ Variable increase in alkaline phosphatase
- Secondary findings
  - ☐ Decreased urinary calcium or phosphorus
  - ☐ Increased PTH
  - ☐ Other disease-specific changes

## Differential Diagnosis

Figure 47.2 contains a useful clinical algorithm with which to establish the general categories of hypocalcemia. The presence of hypocalcemia prompts evaluation for albumin first. Decreased levels of serum albumin cause a corresponding decrease in total serum calcium levels. Every gram of albumin binds 0.8 mg of calcium; hence, a given serum calcium level must first be corrected for serum albumin level. (Serum ionized calcium does not respond to changes in serum albumin.) If the serum albumin level is normal, then the presence of hypocalcemia is real. The ambient phosphorus level thereafter serves to differentiate the causes of hypocalcemia quite nicely. With normal phosphatemia or hypophosphatemia, intestinal disease is probable. Suitable workup is therefore undertaken in that respect. In the presence of increased phosphorus, parathyroid disease or renal disease is the main cause. Serum creatinine differentiates these two possibilities. In renal disease, the level is elevated; in parathyroid disease, it is normal.

Hypoparathyroidism is a very rare phenomenon. Primary hypoparathyroidism—clearly the most rare of the disorders—generally arises early in life. It is associated with either an autoimmune phenomenon of other endocrine glands or embryologic atresia of the parathyroid gland. Secondary hypoparathyroidism is more common. Postoperative hypoparathyroidism may occur after neck surgery for parathyroid, thyroid, or malignant diseases. In some patients, it may develop years after neck surgery.

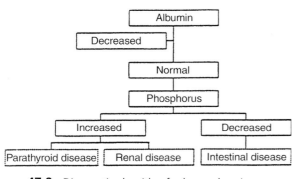

**Figure 47.2** Diagnostic algorithm for hypocalcemia.

Acute hypoparathyroidism is unusual. Infiltrated diseases of the parathyroid gland are rare. Several subtypes of "apparent" hypoparathyroidism are even more rare. In pseudohypoparathyroidism, for example, the appropriate secretion of PTH is present, but this hormone cannot act because of dysfunction in its target-organ receptor. Another form of apparent hypoparathyroidism arises in intestinal dysfunction and magnesium malabsorption and deficiency. A low magnesium level causes the poor synthesis and secretion of PTH, poor activity of the hormone at its receptor sites, and poor production of vitamin D. True hypoparathyroidism would not cause osteomalacia or bone disease, but in pseudohypoparathyroidism, in which there are defective receptors in the kidneys, one may actually see normal receptors in the bone that respond to PTH, thus causing osteitis.

## Treatment

Treatment options for hypocalcemia include:

- Correction of the underlying disease
- Calcium supplementation
- Empiric therapy (i.e., 2 g elemental calcium, tablet or liquid preparations
- Meal timing
- Vitamin D supplements
- Ergocalciferol (Calciferol)
- Calcifediol (Calderol) (not currently available)
- Calcitriol

It is essential to address first the underlying disease process causing vitamin D and phosphorus abnormalities. Calcium supplementation is used if dietary sources are limited. Dairy products are essential because they provide 80% of daily calcium needs. The minimum daily requirement for men and premenopausal women is 1,000 mg of elemental calcium. In its absence, calcium supplements are needed. Most supplements are carbonate salt, which provides more calcium per tablet (40% by weight) than other calcium supplements. The carbonate salt may not be absorbed well in patients with achlorhydria. The citrate salt has a theoretic advantage because it is absorbed more efficiently in all patients, regardless of gastric acidity. No data show how effective citrate salts might be in situations in which intestinal dysfunction occurs.

Another consideration is the use of a liquid calcium supplement. Liquids may be more easily absorbed than tablets. In general, generic brands of calcium should be as readily bioavailable as brand names, but this may not always be the situation. Studies have indicated that the dissolution or breakdown of calcium tablets in 1 or 2 oz of warm (i.e., body temperature) household vinegar is a good sign of the relative bioavailability in the stomach.

Vitamin D supplementation for patients who are vitamin D deficient, or who may need assistance in the absorption of calcium, is the next consideration. The cheaper forms of the vitamin are generally the cholecalciferol or ergocalciferol derivatives, precursors to the 25- and 1,25-hydroxyl derivatives. These vitamins are available in 50,000-U doses per capsule. In profound hypocalcemia from hypoparathyroidism, for example, the number of required daily units may range from 50,000 to 500,000. In simple cases of hypocalcemia and osteomalacia, the dosage may be as small as 50,000 U/week. The most potent vitamin D forms, 25-hydroxyvitamin D (calcifediol) and 1,25-dihydroxyvitamin D (calcitriol), are more expensive, but they are safer to use. If evidence of hypercalcemia exists, the discontinuation of these potent vitamins restores eucalcemia within days. In patients who cannot absorb oral medications, the use of injectable vitamin D is mandatory. Ergocalciferol is generally the vitamin used, although an intravenous form of calcitriol is available and is used primarily for dialysis patients.

# OSTEOPOROSIS

## Pathophysiology in women

Osteoporosis is a multifactorial disease that ultimately leads to insufficiency of skeletal strength and increased susceptibility to fracture from relatively minor or nontraumatic causes. It is histologically manifested by thinning, perforation, and breakage of the trabecular plates within the interior of bone, resulting in a subsequent lack of compression strength. The disease is divided into a primary disorder and secondary disorders.

Primary osteoporosis occurs from high bone turnover secondary to estrogen deficiency at the time of menopause; later in life, several additional factors aggravate the menopausal bone loss and cause insufficient osteoblastic activity. Attendant abnormalities include decreased calcium absorption and vitamin D metabolism and increased PTH levels. This distinction between menopausal and postmenopausal problems is somewhat artificial because a blending of pathologic processes may occur across all ages.

Secondary causes of osteoporosis run the gamut of many diseases. The suggested readings cover these topics in greater depth.

The pathophysiology of osteoporosis can be viewed from four major standpoints:

- Genetic
- Nutritional
- Hormonal
- Lifestyle

### Genetic Impact

Osteoporosis has a genetic component; it occurs in families and affects women and men. Of all risk factors discussed in the literature, the most clinically robust is a family history of osteoporosis. This fact alone often pinpoints individuals who have evidence of bone deficiency (osteopenia) without evidence of clinical fracture. Epidemiologic studies clearly indicate that the daughters of individuals with osteoporosis have osteopenia, even in their early years, whereas the daughters of patients without osteoporosis have normal bone mass for age. Racial differences, too, are clearly notable. Osteoporosis is present more often in white and Asian American women than in African American women when population studies are reviewed. Individual African American women can certainly develop this disease either as a primary or secondary problem.

### Nutritional Impact

The major nutritional factor involved in osteoporosis is calcium insufficiency. The debate still rages whether calcium is a causal or promoting factor. A deficiency of dairy products in the diet leads to insufficiency of calcium because these products are the greatest nutrient source of calcium. Most people require 1,000 mg of elemental calcium daily. Postmenopausal women may require more calcium because of a relative inability to efficiently absorb it; the generally recommended dose is 1,500 mg or more.

The effects of calcium on the skeleton are directly related to an individual's age. A degree of bone loss is attributable to the aging process, the exact details of which are not well understood. This degree of loss is small (approximately 0.1% yearly). It tends to arise after 30 years of age and in the later years of life, usually approximately 10 or more years after menopause. Calcium supplementation is helpful in controlling bone metabolism due to the aging process. Immediately around the time of menopause, however, and for 5 to 10 years afterward, calcium supplementation cannot control the turnover of bone. This period is associated with a high degree of bone loss from osteoclastic activity secondary to estrogen deficiency.

The overuse of other substances, such as alcohol and tobacco, has a negative influence on bone metabolism and must be considered in osteoporosis.

Nephrolithiasis does not develop in most individuals when the calcium content in the diet is increased. The body regulates calcium absorption so that hypercalciuria and stone disease generally do not occur. If a preexisting problem with hypercalciuria is present, however, or a patient or family history of renal stones is noted, the patient should be evaluated for hypercalciuria before and, more important, after supplementation is started. A simple test for hypercalciuria can uncover potential problems before they lead to stone disease.

### Hormonal Impact

Hormonal factors have long been known to be an associated problem in osteoporosis. With loss of estrogen, postmenopausal women have increased production and activity of osteoclasts and secondary increased bone turnover and loss. Estrogen and antiosteoclastic drugs are the most useful treatments for women with osteoporosis at this time because they target osteoclasts, whereas calcium alone is not sufficient. During menopause, bone-loss rates might be 10 to 20 times higher than the rate associated with the aging process.

Pubertal development should also be considered. Estrogen is a major stimulant of bone growth in adolescent girls. Any aberrations in growth at this time will ultimately lead to insufficiency of bone in adult life. Adolescent development directly determines the peak bone mass that each individual will have. The inability to attain this during adolescence leads to a less than maximally calcified adult skeleton.

### Lifestyle Impact

An individual's lifestyle and exercise pattern are also intimately related to overall skeletal strength. Increasing muscle mass and strength concurrently increases skeletal mass. The dilemma facing clinicians is the amount and types of exercise needed to promote a healthy skeleton. In premenopausal women, especially, too much as well as too little exercise is risky. Too much exercise causes amenorrhea and bone weakening. Exercise maximizes peak bone mass during adolescence, helps maintain adult bone mass, and attenuates loss because of the aging process.

## Pathophysiology in men

Many of the causes of primary osteoporosis in women have an analogous cause in men—hypogonadism (testosterone deficiency), poor pubertal development, dietary factors, genetic inheritance, and activity deficiency. The primary form of osteoporosis often arises in men later in life. A large number of men developing this problem before the sixth or seventh decades may have secondary causes (see Table 47.2). Twenty percent of hip fractures occur in men. Surprisingly, the one-year mortality for men with these fractures is almost 50%, compared with about 20% for women.

---

**TABLE 47.2**
**COMMON SECONDARY CAUSES OF OSTEOPOROSIS IN MEN**

Glucocorticoids, alcohol, hypogonadism (45%)
Primary or idiopathic (35%–45%)
Other causes (15%–20%)
  Gastrointestinal
  Hypercalciuria
  Drug side effects (anticonvulsants, glucocorticoids, antigonadotrophins, alcohol, tobacco)
  Hyperparathyroidism
  Neoplasia (monoclonal gammopathy)
  Other endocrine diseases (hypogonadism, hypercortisolism, hyperprolactinemia, acromegaly)
  Metabolic/genetic (Marfan's syndrome, homocystinuria, hypophosphatasia, osteogenesis imperfecta)

## DIAGNOSIS OF OSTEOPOROSIS

The diagnosis of primary osteoporosis in its early asymptomatic stage was a challenge until the introduction of dual-energy x-ray absorptiometry (DEXA) scans for the measurement of bone density. An abnormal (i.e., low) bone density, however, is not sufficient to make this diagnosis. Many nonosteoporotic bone problems cause an abnormal density.

Early osteoporosis produces no symptoms; finding it obviously is a challenge. By the time fractures, back pain, height loss, and kyphosis develop, there is little challenge in diagnosing it because these are the hallmarks of a disease that has gone unchecked for years. Osteopenia noted on radiographs usually indicates a loss of at least 20% to 30% of bone mass, which represents approximately 10 years of silent osteoporosis. In most cases of asymptomatic disease, routine health screening blood test results are normal. The new bone markers mentioned earlier do not diagnose osteoporosis; they only indicate an abnormality in bone metabolism.

Bone densitometry results are the single most important factor in the prediction of fractures in patients who have osteoporosis. Decreased bone density is a necessary but not sufficient reason for fractures. This testing (which costs from $75 to $200) is performed at the initiation either of a diagnostic workup or of therapy, and then repeated 1 or 2 years later to assess the results of therapy. The federal government guidelines provide insurance coverage for testing women over 65 years of age and allow rechecking every 2 years, with limited exceptions. Most insurers follow this protocol. Younger women with significant risks, however, should be checked before this age. The usual considerations for densitometry include the following factors:

- Family history
- Atraumatic fractures
- Steroid use
- Back pain
- Monitoring of therapy
- Decision point for hormone replacement therapy

These measurements focus on the rapid turnover of trabecular bone in the spine or femoral neck, where bone is lost earliest. Bone density measurements at these sites more than 2.5 standard deviations (SD) below peak mass (commonly called the young normal value) identify osteoporosis according to the World Health Organization guidelines. The risk of fracture rises exponentially with a decline in the SD. Values between −1.0 and −2.5 SD below peak bone mass are classified as osteopenic, an intermediate zone that has lower prognostic significance for fracture. Values greater than −1.0 SD are classified as normal. The chance of fracture with density values in this range is even lower than with values classified as osteopenic. Having said this, however, one must never assume that an absolutely safe, fracture-free density exists. These are population data; an individual patient can fracture at any value given the right circumstances.

## Treatment

The therapy for primary osteoporosis in women includes:

- Calcium supplementation with or without vitamin D
- Exercise
- Skeletal pharmacologic agents
- Antiresorptives (e.g., estrogen, calcitonin, and bisphosphonates—alendronate sodium, risedronate sodium)
- Anabolic drugs (parathyroid hormone)

### Antiresorptive Therapy

All therapies used to date are antiresorptive in nature; they work against osteoclasts and reduce bone turnover and loss. Estrogen controls the local production of those bone marrow cytokines that stimulate osteoclastic bone resorption; thus, its use in menopause. Calcitonin, the first antiosteoclastic drug used in practice, affects osteoclast membrane structure. The bisphosphonates have several actions on osteoclast function: They inhibit osteoclast membrane cholesterol synthesis, increase apoptosis, inhibit the proton pump, and prevent adherence to the bone surface.

Calcitonin is a drug long recognized for the treatment of osteoporosis. The injectable form has been supplanted by the nasal spray. Both forms yield modest increases in spinal density, but not as great as those from estrogen or the bisphosphonates. The average increase is 1% to 3%. No significant increase is seen in hip density.

Bisphosphonate drugs hold a major place in the treatment of osteoporosis. These potent antiresorptives affect osteoclastic function, decrease bone turnover, and increase bone mass to varying degrees. Alendronate (Fosamax), the first approved bisphosphonate, increases bone density in the spine (about 6% to 7%) and hip (about 4%) and prevents vertebral and hip fractures. Both the 10 mg daily and the weekly 70 mg tablets produce equivalent effects. A weekly 70 mg liquid dose is now available. Lower doses (35 mg weekly) prevent the development or progression of osteoporosis in much the same fashion as estrogen does. Risedronate (Actonel) is the latest bisphosphonate agent approved for the treatment of osteoporosis. It is available as a daily 5 mg tablet and a weekly 35 mg dose. It also will increase spinal and hip density to about the same extent as alendronate. Its tolerability may be better for patients with gastroesophageal disease. Both drugs reduce fracture risk at the spine and hip from 40% to 60%. The greatest rate of reduction occurs in patients who have had previous fractures.

Estrogen has been recognized as a useful therapy to prevent osteoporosis since the 1950s. In women with an intact uterus, it is combined with a progestin to stop the development of endometrial hyperplasia and reduce the risk of endometrial cancer. The usual daily dose is 0.625 mg of conjugated estrogen or its equivalent. Corresponding doses of progestin are between 2.5 mg and 5.0 mg. These may be given cyclically or daily. Cyclical use produces menses to varying degrees. Daily combined use prevents it. The influence of the progestin on lipid and cardiovascular function is only beginning to be understood. Women with a prior hysterectomy generally do not use progestin, although some believe it has skeletal benefit. Some women complain of premenstrual symptoms from progestin, which limits its use.

Hormone replacement therapy in the treatment of osteoporosis is now under question as a result of the information from The Women's Health Initiative (WHI). This study was a federally sponsored program to evaluate the effect of estrogen plus progestin (E+P) and estrogen (E) alone (hysterectomized patients) on heart disease and invasive breast cancer. Secondary areas of interest were strokes, pulmonary embolism, colorectal cancer, hip fractures, and deaths due to other causes.

The E+P arm was stopped prematurely due to an increased incidence of breast cancer. Concurrently, the prevalence of coronary heart disease, stroke, and thromboembolic events increased. Hip and vertebral fractures declined by about one-third. Colorectal cancer declined 37%. Controversy about the results remains, primarily due to the average age of the patients, the years since menopause, and the possibility that the patients may have had early asymptomatic cardiovascular disease. Data on the E arm is just beginning to appear and may be available within the year. As a result of the study, new FDA labeling for combined drug therapy states that the chronic use of conjugated estrogen and progestin should not be used as primary prevention of cardiovascular disease. Its use should be limited to the short-term treatment of vasomotor symptoms. A risk–benefit analysis for each patient should be discussed to decide on its optimal use.

Estrogen patches are also used to provide replacement therapy. Although they have not been available as long as the oral agents, the patches can prevent osteoporosis. Clinical evidence shows protection from fractures as well. Cessation of estrogen causes bone loss to the degree at which it would have occurred in menopause. Hence, other approaches for long-term therapy are mandatory. Low-dose alendronate and risedronate can prevent osteoporosis. Likewise the selective estrogen receptor modulator drugs (SERM) or "antiestrogen" drugs have become a substitute for estrogen.

SERM agents are modeled on the drugs used in the treatment of breast cancer. These agents are estrogen antagonists in the uterus and breasts, but estrogen agonists in the heart, blood vessels, liver (i.e., with regard to lipid profile), and bone. Raloxifene hydrochloride (Evista) is the first such drug available for clinical use. Ongoing studies show favorable effects on skeletal density, vertebral fracture rate, and lipid profile. Menstruation, breast pain, and uterine hyperplasia do not occur. Recent preliminary data (still to be confirmed by muticentered trials) are a reduction in the incidence of breast cancer and cardiovascular disease in high-risk patients. Its daily dosage (60 mg) reduces vertebral fractures about 40% to 50%. Preliminary postmarketing data suggest an effect on nonvertebral fracture reduction, but the original pivotal study did not support this because the incidence of this type fracture was so low.

## Efficacy of Fracture Reduction

A great deal of data exist about fracture reduction. The efficacy of a therapy is based not only on suitable changes in density but also on reduction in fracture rates. The newly approved therapies reduce vertebral fractures from 20% to 60%, depending on the study. Calcitonin has the lowest rate of fracture reduction, estrogen and raloxifene an intermediary rate, and alendronate and risedronate the highest. Reduction in hip fractures is more tenuous for most drugs, but the bisphosphonates clearly show the advantage. Therapeutic trials of calcitonin do not display the protective effect on hip fractures in the studies performed to date. The WHI study does show that the E+P arm had a significant reduction in hip and vertebral fractures. All studies show that the greatest benefit arises in patients who have had prior fractures.

## Therapy for Osteoporosis in Men

The FDA has approved use of alendronate and teriparatide (PTH 1-34, see below) in men.

These drugs cover primary or idiopathic problems, however, the secondary causes of osteoporosis are the major issues for younger men. Only after these disorders are treated might it be necessary to resort to the FDA-approved drugs. The appropriate intake of calcium and vitamin D is as important for men as it is for women.

### Anabolic Therapy

Teriparatide is the first anabolic class drug approved for the treatment of osteoporosis in men. Its active agent is the 1-34 N-terminal fragment of parathyroid hormone. This type drug directly affects osteoblastic cells, produces thicker and more plate-like trabeculae, and increases bone volume and connectivity among trabeculae. Paradoxically, this arises because the drug is used as a solitary subcutaneous daily injection. Longer daily exposure to the skeleton, as occurs in primary hyperparathyroidism, promotes activity of osteoclasts and subsequent bone loss. The pivotal study showed a 60% to 65% reduction in new vertebral fractures by 18 months of use and about a 50% to 55% reduction in nonvertebral fractures. No significant long-term effects were noted on serum or urine calcium. The study was originally planned to run for 2 to 3 years, but toxicology concerns in rats prompted suspension of

the study at a median 18-month point. In animal studies, rats developed dose dependent osteosarcoma when given daily doses of the drug, from infancy to old age, at three to sixty times the therapeutic dose. It is unlikely that this observation has significant bearing on therapeutic human use. Both men and women can use this drug, if the prescribing physician feels the patient is at risk for fractures, has failed other therapies, or is intolerant of other therapies. The daily 20 microgram injection is delivered from a metered pen device. Other anabolic drugs are presently under study.

## PAGET'S DISEASE OF BONE

Paget's disease of bone is most often an incidental finding during routine radiographs taken for other purposes. It may be present in as many as 3% to 5% of the population older than 50 years. Generally, Paget's disease is monostotic, asymptomatic, and discovered incidentally during the workup of other problems. With spread of the disorder, bone deformity and pain may arise. Most commonly, the pelvic, femoral, cranial, and vertebral bones are affected, although any and all bones may be involved.

In the absence of significant clinical findings, most patients do not seek medical care. Only after pain and skeletal deformity arise do most patients seek assistance. Cranial nerves may become involved when skeletal deformity of the cranial vault occurs. More commonly, cranial nerve VIII is affected, although all cranial nerves may be involved in very severe cases. A higher incidence of fractures is seen because the skeletal structure, although appearing more massive, is actually architecturally weaker. Osteosarcoma is an extraordinarily rare complication.

The biochemical evaluation of the disorder usually shows the presence of increased alkaline phosphatase, with normal calcium and phosphorus levels. With immobilization, hypercalcemia may arise, although this is not an invariable finding.

The treatment of Paget's disease of bone is generally directed toward the control of pain and the underlying pagetic process. Unfortunately, most patients are seen late in the course of the disorder, when anatomic skeletal deformities are beyond treatment with the usual antiresorptive drugs. Calcitonin was the first therapy available to treat this disease. The bisphosphonates are now first-line therapy. Alendronate (40 mg daily) or residronate (30 mg daily) are usually used. They are given for 3 to 6 months or longer if serum alkaline phosphatase or bone markers of skeletal collagen do not return to normal. Intravenous pamidronate or zolendric acid are other options. Any tolerated and effective analgesic may be used to manage pain, although the control of the underlying pagetic process may completely eradicate the pain.

## REVIEW EXERCISES

### QUESTIONS

**1.** A 35-year-old man reports a 10-year history of renal stone disease and diffuse arthralgia. He is otherwise healthy and uses no vitamins, minerals, or drugs. Review of systems is normal, but a tibial radiograph shows a lesion at the midshaft. Serum data include a calcium level of 11.8 mg/dL (normal, 8.5–10.5 mg/dL); phosphorus, 2.9 mg/dL (normal, 2.5–4.5 mg/dL); creatinine, 1.0 mg/dL (normal, 0.5–1.3 mg/dL); intact PTH, 87.0 pg/mL (normal, 10–65 pg/mL); and calcitriol, 52.0 pg/mL (normal, 13–60 pg/mL).

All the following are true, *except*

**a)** Treatment with pamidronate is not necessary.
**b)** Adenomectomy is curative in most cases.
**c)** Recurrence is unlikely.
**d)** The chronicity of the problem argues for the presence of a neoplastic disorder.
**e)** Steroids will not control the problem.

**2.** A 53-year-old woman presents with generalized pain, muscle weakness, and weight loss. She uses estrogen and progestin for menopausal symptoms after surgery for gynecologic cancer, which was also treated with radiation and chemotherapy. She has lost 60 pounds over 3 to 5 years. She has diffuse pain in all bones on examination. Her gait is painful, and her muscles are tender to touch. Baseline laboratory data show a hemoglobin level of 10.3 g/dL; calcium, 5.2 mg/dL; phosphorus, 2.8 mg/dL; albumin, 3.5 g/dL; creatinine, 1.0 mg/dL; alkaline phosphatase, 226 IU/L; immunoreactive PTH, 206 pg/mL (normal, 10–65 pg/mL); calcitriol, 35 pg/mL (normal, 15–52 pg/mL); and urine calcium, 3 mg/day (normal, 100–300 mg/ day).

She is given calcium and vitamin D, and the urine calcium rises to 15 mg daily. She calls and says that she has bruises on her arms and legs.

All the following are false, *except*

**a)** She has celiac disease.
**b)** She requires surgery for the hyperparathyroidism.
**c)** Her serum carotene is likely elevated.
**d)** Increased oral calcium and vitamin D are the only therapy needed.
**e)** Increased uncalcified osteoid should be found.

**3.** A spinal deformity is noted on the radiograph of a 73-year-old woman who was seen for back pain and spinal compression fracture. She was previously healthy, except for a cholecystectomy. She is a heavy tobacco and perhaps alcohol user and was on a golf outing when the incident occurred. She is being treated with calcium and analgesics. On examination, she is emaciated and has severe pain in the lumbar region. Radiograph of the spine shows a fracture at L2.

Laboratory data show a calcium level of 8.6 mg/dL; alkaline phosphatase, 100 IU/L; protein, 6.0 g/dL; hemoglobin, 10 g/dL; and an erythrocyte sedimentation rate of 100 mm/hour.

Which of the following would you do next?

**a)** Continue analgesics
**b)** Start estrogen and extra calcium
**c)** Evaluate the problem further
**d)** Start alendronate
**e)** Start calcitonin and physical therapy

### ANSWERS

**1. d.**
The chronicity of renal stone disease combined with the increased serum calcium, decreased phosphorus, increased PTH, and high-normal calcitriol is typical of hyperparathyroidism. The radiographic finding of a brown tumor or cyst typifies the bone disease (osteitis fibrosa cystica) of hyperparathyroidism. The best treatment is parathyroidectomy. Hyperplasia is an unusual finding.

**2. e.**
The patient has radiation-induced bowel dysfunction—malabsorption and osteomalacia. Bone will have large amounts of uncalcified osteoid. The secondary hyperparathyroidism is not treated by surgery. Celiac disease is less likely given the clinical facts. Carotene will be low from the poor absorption. More oral therapy is less likely to work in this case. Parenteral treatment is needed.

**3. c.**
A diagnosis of osteoporosis was made. When the patient was originally seen, she was quite ill-appearing. Her laboratory test results showed anemia and an increased erythrocyte sedimentation rate. Serum calcium level was low normal, and the alkaline phosphatase high normal. The best response to the question is to evaluate the problem further. None of the answers deals with the critical issue of the abnormal test results. Primary osteoporosis is not associated with any chemical abnormality. An elevated erythrocyte sedimentation rate and anemia are harbingers of other problems. Starting the patient on analgesics to temporize and control some of her discomfort might be reasonable, but clearly more needs to be done. The use of estrogen and calcium or alendronate or physical therapy and calcitonin is a long-term solution if the problem proves to be primary osteoporosis. In this particular case, the patient's disorder was much more ominous than evident by the compression deformity on the radiograph; the compression deformity was the result of an erosive tumor.

## SUGGESTED READINGS

Baker DE. Alendronate and risedronate: what you need to know about their upper gastrointestinal tract toxicity. *Rev Gastroenterol Dis* 2002;2:20–33.

Body JJ. Current and future directions in medical therapy: hypercalcemia. *Cancer* 2000;88:3054–3058.

Boonen S. Haentjensp, et al. Preventing osteoporotic fractures with antiresorptive therapy: implications of microarchitectural changes. *J Intern Med.* 2004;255:1–12.

Bourke E, Delaney B. Assessment of hypocalcemia and hypercalcemia. *Clin Lab Med* 1993;13:157–181.

Brown EM. The pathophysiology of primary hyperparathyroidism. *J Bone Miner Res* 2002;17 Suppl 2:N24–9, Review.

Campion J, Maricic MJ. Osteoporosis in men. *Am Fam Physician* 2003; 67:1521–1526.

Carroll MF, Schade DS. A practical approach to hypercalcemia. *Am Fam Physician* 2003; 67: 1959–1966.

Chesnut CH III, Silverman S, Andriano K, et al. A randomized trial of nasal spray salmon calcitonin in postmenopausal women with established osteoporosis: the prevent recurrence of osteoporotic fractures study. PROOF Study Group. *Am J Med* 2000;109: 267–276.

Clementt D, Spencer CM. Raloxifene: a review of its use in postmenopausal osteoporosis. *Drugs* 2000;60:379–411.

Cohen S, Levy RM, Keller M, et al. Risedronate therapy prevents corticoid induced bone loss: a twelve-month multicenter randomized double blind placebo controlled parallel group study. *Arthritis Rheum* 1999;42:2309–2318.

Delmas PD. Markers of bone turnover for monitoring treatment of osteoporosis with antiresorptive drugs. *Osteoporosis Int* 2000;11: S66–S76.

Doggrell SA. Present and future pharmacotherapy for osteoporosis. *Drugs Today* 2003;39:633–657.

Esbrit P. Hypercalcemia of malignancy—new insights into an old syndrome. *Clin Lab* 2001;47:67–71.

Fogelman I, Blake GM. Different approaches to bone densitometry. *J Nucl Med* 2000;41:2015–2025.

Harris ST, Watts NB, Genant HK, et al. Effects of risedronate treatment on vertebral and nonvertebral fractures in women with postmenopausal osteoporosis. *JAMA* 1999;282:1344–1352 [see bibliography for further references].

Hausemann HJ, Rizzoli R. A comprehensive review of treatments for postmenopausal osteoporosis. *Osteoporos Int* 2003;14:2–12.

Igbal MM. Osteoporosis: epidemiology, diagnosis, and treatment. *South Med J* 2000;93:2–18.

Khan A, Bilezikian J. Primary hyperparathyroidism: pathophysiology and impact on bone. *CMAJ* 2000;163:173–175.

Lang P, Steiger P, Faulker K, et al. Osteoporosis: current techniques and recent developments in quantitative bone densitometry. *Radiol Clin North Am* 1991;29:49–76.

Licata AA. Osteoporosis in men. *Cleve Clin J Med* 2003;70:247–254.

Maricic M, Chen Z. Bone densitometry. *Clin Lab Med* 2000;20: 469–488.

Marx SJ. Hyperparathyroid and hypoparathyroid disorders. *N Engl J Med* 2000;343:1863–1875.

McIlwain HH. Glucocorticoid induced osteoporosis: pathogenesis, diagnosis, and management. *Prev Med* 2003;36:243–249.

Miller PD, Baran DT, Bilezikian JP, et al. Practical clinical application of biochemical markers of bone turnover: consensus of an expert panel. *J Clin Densitometry* 1999;2:323–432.

Neer RM, Arnaud CD, Zanchetta JR, et al. Effect of parathyroid hormone (1-34) on fractures and bone mineral density in postmenopausal women with osteoporosis. *N Engl J Med* 2001;344: 1434–1441.

Orwoll E, Ettinger M, Weiss S, et al. Alendronate for the treatment of osteoporosis in men. *N Engl J Med* 2000;343:604–610.

Reid IR. Bisphosphonates; new indications and methods of administration. *Curr Opin Rheumatol* 2003;15:458–463.

Roe EB, Chiu KM, Arnaud CD. Selective estrogen receptor modulators and postmenopausal health. *Adv Intern Med* 2000; 45: 259–278.

Sharma OP. Hypercalcemia in granulomatous disorders: a clinical review. *Curr Opin Pulm Med* 2000;6:442–447.

Silverman S. Calcitonin. *Clin Endocrinol Metabol N Amer* 2003;32: 273–284.

Siris E. Alendronate in the treatment of osteoporosis: a review of the clinical trials. *J Womens Health Gend Based Med* 2000;9:599–606.

Strewler GJ. The parathyroid hormone-related protein. *Endocrinol Clin North Am* 2000;29:629–645.

Umland EM, Boyce EG. Risedronate: a new oral bisphosphonate. *Clin Ther* 2001; 23:1409–1421.

Watts NB. Treatment of osteoporosis with bisphosphonates. *Rheum Dis Clin N Amer* 2001;27:197–214.

# BOARD SIMULATION: Endocrinology

# 48

## S. Sethu K. Reddy

## QUESTIONS

**1.** A 40-year-old patient with type I diabetes mellitus (DM) has a blood pressure of 150/95 mm Hg, a pulse of 96 beats/minute, a glycosylated hemoglobin (HgbA$_{1c}$) level of 10%, and elevated triglycerides.

Which class of antihypertensive agents should be avoided in this patient?

**a)** Angiotensin-converting enzyme (ACE) inhibitors

**b)** Angiotensin II receptor blockers

**c)** Calcium channel blockers

**d)** $\alpha$-Adrenergic blockers

**e)** $\beta$-Adrenergic blockers

**2.** A 40-year-old patient with type I DM has a blood pressure of 150/95 mm Hg, a pulse of 96 beats/minute, an HgbA$_{1c}$ level of 10%, and elevated triglycerides.

Which class of antihypertensive agents would most consistently help lower triglycerides in this patient?

**a)** ACE inhibitors

**b)** Angiotensin II receptor blockers

c) Calcium channel blockers
d) α-Adrenergic blockers
e) β-Adrenergic blockers

**3.** A 37-year-old white man with type I DM has a blood pressure of 140/90 mm Hg, an HgbA$_{1c}$ level of 8.6%, urinary albumin excretion rate of 45 μg/minute (normal, less than 30 μg/min), and normal electrolyte levels.

Which of the following should be started to treat his blood pressure?
a) Clonidine hydrochloride (Catapres), 0.1 mg at bedtime
b) Captopril (Capoten), 12.5 mg three times daily
c) Propranolol hydrochloride (Inderal), 20 mg three times daily
d) Doxazosin mesylate (Cardura), 1 mg twice daily
e) Diltiazem hydrochloride (Cardizem), 60 mg three times daily

**4.** A 40-year-old white man with a 27-year history of type I DM on a four-times-daily insulin regimen complains of nausea, diarrhea, and postprandial hypoglycemia.

Which of the following laboratory tests may help establish a diagnosis?
a) Gastric emptying study
b) Serum electrolyte levels
c) Cosyntropin (Cortrosyn) stimulation test
d) All of the above
e) None of above

**5.** Figure 48.1 shows what type of diabetic retinopathy?
a) None
b) Background with macular edema
c) Preproliferative with cotton-wool exudates
d) Preproliferative with hard exudates
e) Proliferative diabetic retinopathy

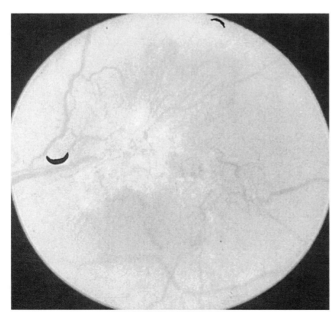

**Figure 48.1** Diabetic retinopathy. (See Color Fig. 48.1.)

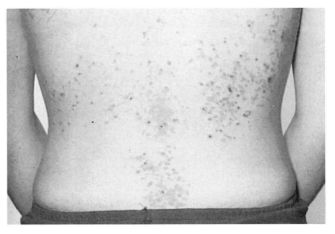

**Figure 48.2** Skin rash. (See Color Fig. 48.2.)

**6.** A 45-year-old white woman with type II DM presents with a skin rash (Fig. 48.2).

Which of the following should be done?
a) Refer to dermatology for a biopsy.
b) Check HgbA$_{1c}$ and treat as appropriate.
c) Start metronidazole hydrochloride, 250 mg three times daily.
d) Start prednisone, 40 mg daily, and taper over 10 days.
e) Admit the patient for intravenous antibiotics.

**7.** Using the values given in the table below, which is the most likely lipid profile associated with the situation in Question 6? (TC, total cholesterol; TG, triglycerides; HDL-C, high-density lipoprotein cholesterol; LDL-C, low-density lipoprotein cholesterol; all values are mg/dL.)

|    | TC | TG | HDL-C | LDL-C |
|----|----|----|-------|-------|
| a) | 200 | 100 | 40 | 140 |
| b) | 3,000 | 10,000 | 13 | 45 |
| c) | 450 | 100 | 40 | 390 |
| d) | 225 | 540 | 25 | 110 |
| e) | 500 | 480 | 35 | 385 |

**8.** Which of the following drugs or drug classes would best treat the associated lipid disorder from Question 7?
a) HMG-CoA reductase inhibitor
b) Niacin
c) Bile acid sequestrant
d) Fibric acid derivative
e) Probucol (Lorelco)

**9.** A patient is referred to you with the following thyroid indices: thyroxine (T$_4$), 15.5 μg/dL (normal, 4–10.8 μg/dL), and thyroid-stimulating hormone (TSH), 5 μIU/mL (normal, 0.4–5.0 μIU/mL).

Which of the following situations is least compatible with this profile?
a) Thyroid hormone resistance
b) Symptoms of hyperthyroidism and a TSH adenoma

**c)** Oral contraceptive use
**d)** Acute hepatitis
**e)** Subacute thyroiditis with symptoms of hyperthyroidism for the past 4 weeks

**10.** A 25-year-old woman presents with classic symptoms of hyperthyroidism, an elevated $T_4$, and a suppressed TSH.

Which of the following best confirms the diagnosis of Graves' disease?
**a)** Increased radioactive iodine uptake (RAIU) by the thyroid
**b)** Stare and lid lag
**c)** Pretibial myxedema
**d)** Positive antimicrosomal (antithyroid peroxidase) antibodies
**e)** Family history of Graves' disease

**11.** A woman with Graves' disease has been treated with propylthiouracil (PTU), 100 mg three times daily, for the past 2 months. Her symptoms have abated, her pulse is 72 beats/minute, and she has gained 5 lb. Her $T_4$ is 11.0 μg/dL (normal, 4.0–10.8 μg/dL) and TSH is still less than 0.03 μIU/mL (normal, 0.4–5.0 μIU/mL).

What do you do now?
**a)** Increase the PTU until TSH returns to normal.
**b)** Reassure her that her weight gain will stop.
**c)** Add propranolol to the regimen.
**d)** Stop the PTU.
**e)** Do not make any changes and reassess in 6 to 8 weeks.

**12.** You are asked to see a patient in the intensive care unit for pneumonia after gastrointestinal surgery. His $T_4$ level is 3.9 μg/dL (normal, 4.0–10.8 μg/dL) and his TSH level is 2.5 μIU/mL (normal, 0.4–5.0 μIU/mL).

Which of the following is false?
**a)** He should be started on levothyroxine to rapidly correct the problem until the pneumonia resolves.
**b)** He should have thyroid function tests in 2 to 3 months.
**c)** His triiodothyronine level will be low.
**d)** His free $T_4$ level will be normal.
**e)** An RAIU test and thyroid scan are of no value.

**13.** A 50-year-old woman with a 5-year history of menopausal symptoms is evaluated for osteoporosis prevention. She has a family history of breast cancer and refuses hormone replacement therapy. She has a 20-year history of hyperprolactinemia treated with bromocriptine mesylate (Parlodel) with good success. Her spinal bone density has declined from 1.12 to 0.92 g/cm² in 5 years.

Options for her care include all the following, *except*
**a)** Daily etidronate disodium (Didronel)
**b)** Alendronate sodium (Fosamax)
**c)** Calcium
**d)** Etidronate disodium cyclically
**e)** Calcitonin (intranasally)

**14.** An 85-year-old man is admitted for hypercalcemia. He is comatose and anuric. Calcium is 15.1 mg/dL, phos-

phorus 2.0 mg/dL, creatinine 6.0 mg/dL, carbon dioxide 18 mEq/L, alkaline phosphatase 184 IU/L, and intact parathyroid hormone (PTH) 110 pg/mL. He has been ill for 6 months and has lost 30 lb. He has a 20-year history of renal stones.

Therapy may include all the following, *except*
**a)** Furosemide (Lasix)
**b)** Prednisone
**c)** Saline hydration
**d)** Intravenous pamidronate disodium (Aredia)

**15.** A 73-year-old woman has severe pain with walking. She has a history of ovarian cancer many years ago, treated with a total abdominal hysterectomy and postoperative radiation. Her weight has gradually declined approximately 30 lb but has remained stable for 5 years. Her legs hurt with movement. A bone scan shows multiple hot spots in the ribs and right femur. Erythrocyte sedimentation rate is 5 mm/hour, alkaline phosphatase is 550 IU/L, creatinine is 0.8 mg/dL, and calcium is 7.5 mg/dL.

Which of the following is most likely to be correct?
**a)** Bone biopsy results: osteomalacia; PTH: low; phosphorus: high
**b)** Bone biopsy results: metastatic cancer; PTH: normal; phosphorus: normal
**c)** Bone biopsy results: osteoporosis; PTH: normal; phosphorus: low
**d)** PTH: high; 25-hydroxyvitamin D: low; urine calcium: low
**e)** Bone biopsy results: osteomalacia; PTH: high; carotene: high

**16.** A 35-year-old woman has had epilepsy since adolescence and has been treated with a variety of anticonvulsants. Recently, she suffered rib and spinal fractures during a seizure. Her menstrual periods are irregular. She has been taking an oral contraceptive. Serum calcium is 8.6 mg/dL, phosphorus is 3.0 mg/dL, and alkaline phosphatase is 110 IU/L. Her bone density is more than 2 standard deviations below norms for her age.

Which is the best option to offer her?
**a)** Cyclical etidronate with repeat bone mineral densitometry (BMD) in 6 months
**b)** Daily alendronate with repeat BMD in 6 months
**c)** Vitamin D and calcium with repeat BMD in 1 to 2 years
**d)** Calcium with repeat BMD in 1 to 2 years
**e)** Intranasal calcitonin with repeat BMD in 1 year

**17.** A 55-year-old man has a 20-year history of hypoparathyroidism after thyroidectomy. He has been eucalcemic with daily administration of calcium lactate and 150,000 U ergocalciferol (Calciferol). Until recently, efforts to self-wean from these drugs caused mild tetany. One year ago, he discontinued his calcium and vitamin D without the development of tetany. His only other medical problem is cigarette smoking. His weight has decreased 5 lb, but he has no other complaints. Calcium is 10.0 mg/dL, and phosphorus 3.1 mg/dL. You order a chest radiograph.

Which of the following additional tests would you *not* order initially?
a) Tuberculin skin test
b) Serum electrolyte levels and osmolality
c) PTH-related peptide level
d) ACE level
e) Colonoscopy

18. Which of the following patients would be likely to require treatment with fludrocortisone acetate (Florinef Acetate)?
a) A 23-year-old woman with Hashimoto's thyroiditis and type I DM who is having recurrent hypoglycemia despite decreasing doses of insulin
b) A 63-year-old man with bitemporal hemianopsia who presents with decreased libido, impotence, cold intolerance, and anorexia/nausea
c) A 34-year-old hyperkalemic, pregnant woman with lupus anticoagulant on long-term heparin but with no evidence of adrenal hemorrhage on computed tomography
d) Two of the above
e) All of the above

19. A 35-year-old man reports muscle weakness. He has hypertension treated with hydrochlorothiazide. His family history is positive for early onset hypertension. Potassium is 2.9 mEq/L and bicarbonate 34 mEq/L. Further evaluation shows suppressed plasma renin activity and low aldosterone level.

Which of the following is least likely?
a) Cushing's syndrome
b) Liddle's syndrome
c) Licorice ingestion
d) Adenoma of the zona glomerulosa
e) Renal artery stenosis

20. A 22-year-old woman has headaches. Magnetic resonance imaging (MRI) suggests a 3-mm pituitary nodule. She has no symptoms of hormone excess or deficiency. Serum prolactin (PRL) is 16 ng/mL (normal, less than 15 ng/mL).

Appropriate management would be
a) Bromocriptine, 1.25 mg orally at bedtime
b) Referral to a radiotherapist
c) Referral to a neurosurgeon
d) Continued observation of PRL levels
e) Repetition of MRI in 1 month

21. A 40-year-old man presents with a history of headaches, impotence, and difficulty with his vision.

Which of the following defects rules out a pituitary tumor as the cause of his symptoms?
a) Homonymous hemianopsia
b) Unilateral visual loss

c) Bitemporal hemianopsia
d) None of the above
e) a and b only

22. Which of the following patients is least likely to manifest elevated PRL levels?
a) A 25-year-old woman with chronic schizophrenia
b) A 45-year-old woman with reflux esophagitis on cisapride (Propulsid)
c) A 50-year-old man with peptic ulcer disease and heartburn taking metoclopramide hydrochloride (Reglan)
d) A 53-year-old woman with shingles along the T5 distribution
e) A 42-year-old woman with cold intolerance and a goiter

23. The wife of a patient whom you are following because of his recent history of hyperparathyroidism and a gastrinoma contacts you. She is concerned about their children, who are 20 and 25 years of age.

What screening would you perform in these adult children?
a) Calcitonin level
b) Calcium level
c) PRL level
d) Glucose level
e) Gastrin level

24. A 30-year-old woman has a 3-month history of polyuria. Serum glucose is 95 mg/dL. After fluid restriction, urine osmolality is 500 mOsm/kg and plasma osmolality is 295 mOsm/kg. After the patient is given a test dose of desmopressin acetate, urine osmolality rises to 750 mOsm/kg.

Which of the following is the likely diagnosis?
a) Psychogenic polydipsia
b) Complete central diabetes insipidus (DI)
c) Nephrogenic DI
d) Partial central DI
e) No DI

25. A 54-year-old nonsmoker presents with hyperpigmentation.

Which of the following scenarios is least compatible with this presentation?
a) History of left adrenalectomy for a benign nodule
b) Recent emigration from Vietnam and a positive purified protein derivative tuberculin test result
c) History of previous Cushing's syndrome treated with bilateral adrenalectomy
d) Chest radiograph showing a new right upper lobe lesion

26. A 30-year-old accountant with a recent diagnosis of prolactinoma complains of impotence as his main problem. He is wondering how such a small tumor can cause this.

Which is the best explanation for his symptoms?

a) PRL has a deleterious effect on the testes and reduces testosterone production.

b) PRL decreases adrenal androgens.

c) PRL inhibits gonadotropin-releasing hormone secretion.

d) By its effect on salt and water excretion, PRL has direct vascular effects on penile blood flow.

e) PRL increases the conversion of testosterone to estradiol.

**27.** A 19-year-old woman with primary amenorrhea associated with short stature and a webbed neck is most likely to have which of the following laboratory profiles? (LH, luteinizing hormone; FSH, follicle- stimulating hormone.)

| | LH (mIU/mL) | FSH (mIU/mL) | PRL (ng/mL) |
|---|---|---|---|
| a) | <2 | <2 | 683 |
| b) | <2 | <2 | 68 |
| c) | <2 | <2 | 6 |
| d) | 2.3 | 3.1 | 18 |
| e) | 23 | 47 | 8 |

**28.** An 18-year-old postpubertal woman presents with primary amenorrhea and galactorrhea.

Which of the following should her initial laboratory evaluation include?

a) Serum PRL level and thyroid function tests

b) β-Human chorionic gonadotropin (β-hCG) level, serum PRL level, and thyroid function tests

c) Serum PRL level and MRI of pituitary

d) Growth hormone level, thyroid function tests, and gonadotropin levels

e) β-Human chorionic gonadotropin (β-hCG) level and mammogram

**29.** A 33-year-old woman reports a 5-month history of secondary amenorrhea and galactorrhea.

Which of the following should her initial laboratory evaluation include?

a) Serum PRL level and thyroid function tests

b) β-Human chorionic gonadotropin (β-hCG) level, serum PRL level, and thyroid function tests

c) Serum PRL level and MRI of pituitary

d) Growth hormone level, thyroid function tests, and gonadotropin levels

e) β-Human chorionic gonadotropin (β-hCG) level and mammogram

**30.** A 46-year-old woman has had type I DM for 3 years. Her self-monitoring blood glucose (SMBG) meter has recently been calibrated. She has no signs or symptoms of hypoglycemia. She is taking neutral protamine Hagedorn (NPH) insulin, 30 μ in the morning and 10 μ before supper. Glucose is 170 mg/dL and HgbA$_{1c}$ is 8.9% (normal, 4–6%). Her SMBG record is very neat and shows the following: breakfast, 95 to 130 mg/dL; lunch, 100 to

136 mg/dL; supper, 100 to 130 mg/dL; and bedtime, 90 to 117 mg/dL.

How would you manage her DM at present?

a) Monitor glucose less often and have patient return in 6 months.

b) Continue present treatment.

c) Disregard her SMBG records; review her diet, lifestyle, and insulin regimen; and aim for improved glucose control.

d) Book an eye clinic appointment and review in 6 months.

e) Have her purchase a new SMBG meter.

**31.** A 39-year-old white woman has a 4-year history of episodic weakness and hunger relieved by food, especially at night and in the morning. The symptoms are increasing in frequency, and she has gained 100 lb. She had a capillary glucose level of 30 mg/dL during one episode. She has a family history of hypothyroidism; she is gravida 2, para 2. On physical examination, she weighs 220 lb and is 5 ft, 4 in. tall; otherwise, the examination is negative.

Which would be the most useful test?

a) Insulin antibody levels

b) Insulin tolerance test

c) Oral glucose tolerance test with glucose, insulin, and C-peptide levels

d) 72-Hour fast with glucose, insulin, C-peptide levels

e) Adrenocorticotropic hormone (ACTH) stimulation test

**32.** A 24-year-old white man with a 6-year history of type I DM is brought to the emergency department in a coma; he is febrile and stuporous. Pulse is 120 beats/minute, blood pressure is 100/50 mm Hg, respiration rate is 20 per minute, and breath is "fruity." Plasma glucose is 527 mg/dL, sodium 130 mEq/L, potassium 3.6 mEq/L, chloride 95 mEq/L, bicarbonate 14 mEq/L, blood urea nitrogen 30 mg/dL, creatinine 1.4 mg/dL, calcium 9.8 mg/dL, and phosphorus 1.0 mg/dL. Arterial blood gas findings are pH 7.18, PO$_2$ 85 mm Hg, and PCO$_2$ 24 mm Hg.

Which of the following is least essential in your management?

a) Potassium chloride replacement

b) Intravenous normal saline at 500 to 1,000 mL/hour

c) Potassium phosphate replacement

d) Chest radiograph

e) Intravenous regular insulin

**33.** A patient is taking 20 U of isophane insulin (NPH) and 10 U of regular insulin in the morning. Average or typical capillary SMBG readings are as follows: breakfast, 150 mg/dL; lunch, 110 mg/dL; supper, 180 mg/ dL; bedtime, 145 mg/dL.

What would be the best initial adjustment?

a) Add some regular insulin at supper.

b) Increase morning NPH insulin.

c) Increase morning NPH and regular insulin.
d) Add some regular insulin at supper and some NPH insulin at bedtime.
e) Add NPH insulin at supper.

**34.** A 36-year-old man with type I DM for 15 years presents with brittle diabetes. He has a history of proliferative retinopathy and was recently diagnosed with hypertension, for which he is taking captopril. $HgbA_{1c}$ is 7% (normal, 4–6%); blood urea nitrogen, 25 mg/dL; creatinine, 1.4 mg/dL; sodium, 135 mEq/L; potassium, 6.0 mEq/L; chloride, 104 mEq/L; and bicarbonate, 28 mEq/L. Electrocardiogram is normal.

Which is your best option?
a) Perform ACTH stimulation test.
b) Begin sodium polystyrene sulfonate (Kayexalate).
c) Admit for electrocardiographic monitoring.
d) Change to a different antihypertensive drug.
e) Order Doppler ultrasonographic study of the renal arteries.

**35.** Which of these scenarios involving XY individuals is least compatible with the presence of gynecomastia?
a) Bilateral inguinal scars and absence of secondary sexual hair
b) Well-controlled salt-losing congenital adrenal hyperplasia
c) Presence of spider nevi, asterixis, and ascites
d) Competitive bodybuilding
e) Hyperaldosteronism treated with spironolactone (Aldactone)

**36.** A 19-year-old woman has primary amenorrhea. Which of the following is false in your evaluation?
a) Obtaining a karyotype is essential.
b) Asherman's syndrome is a possibility.
c) Measurement of PRL and FSH levels would be helpful.
d) A pregnancy test is necessary.
e) The patient may be an XY male.

**37.** A 21-year-old woman has irregular menses, increasing facial hair, and acne.

Which of the following is not indicated in your initial approach?
a) The onset and progression of her symptoms should be determined.
b) An ultrasonogram of the ovaries should be ordered.
c) A high ratio of luteinizing hormone to follicle-stimulating hormone might point to polycystic ovary syndrome.
d) An ACTH stimulation test might yield the diagnosis.
e) The patient should be assured that you will be able to improve her symptoms and signs in the next 6 to 9 months.

**38.** A 36-year-old white woman has a 2-cm thyroid nodule detected on routine physical examination.

Which of the following is the best initial approach to her management?
a) Measurement of TSH level and fine-needle aspiration biopsy
b) Measurement of TSH level, and RAIU test and scan
c) Measurement of TSH and thyroglobulin levels
d) RAIU test and scan
e) Referral to a surgeon for removal

**39.** A 55-year-old white man comes for evaluation of episodic hypertension. His family history reveals a brother who had "neck surgery" and takes cortisone.

Which of the following is the most appropriate screening test panel for this multiple endocrine neoplasia syndrome?
a) Thyroglobulin and catecholamines
b) Testing of patient and brother for *RET* protooncogene mutation
c) Calcitonin, calcium, and catecholamines
d) PRL, calcitonin, calcium, and gastrin
e) Catecholamines, PRL, and insulin

## ANSWERS

**1. e.**
Of all the listed antihypertensive agents, β-blockers are the only agents that may raise serum triglyceride levels. Some of the newer β-blockers with intrinsic sympathomimetic activity may be less likely to affect serum triglyceride levels. If the patient also has hypoglycemic unawareness, β-blockers should be avoided.

**2. d.**
ACE inhibitors, angiotensin II receptor blockers, and calcium channel blockers would be relatively neutral, whereas α-adrenergic blockers have been shown to lower triglyceride levels and raise high-density lipoprotein cholesterol levels. Of course, β-blockers would be the least favored (see Question 1).

**3. b.**
In an individual with type I DM, hypertension, and microalbuminuria, the use of ACE inhibitors is favored because of their additional effect on intraglomerular hypertension. It should be noted, however, that any method of lowering blood pressure will lead to improvement in albumin excretion rates. Of course, improvement in glucose control is also crucial.

**4. d.**
Individuals with type I DM are more likely to experience other autoimmune disorders, including Addison's disease. Chronic DM may also cause autonomic neuropathy, and if the gastrointestinal system is involved, the patient may experience constipation initially and then symptoms of gastroparesis, widely fluctuating blood glucose values, or diarrhea.

**5. e.**

Figure 48.1 shows fronds of new blood vessels. These vessels are more friable and more likely to bleed. It is thought that retinal hypoxia and the resulting local secretion of growth factors results in the neovascularization. Early laser therapy may preserve vision and reduce the degree of subsequent neovascularization.

**6. b.**

This woman has eruptive xanthoma that may be related to severe hypertriglyceridemia secondary to uncontrolled DM. There is no need for antibiotics, hospital admission, or a skin biopsy. Prednisone would not alleviate the rash and may actually worsen the hypertriglyceridemia.

**7. b.**

In an individual with eruptive xanthoma, the serum triglyceride level is usually higher than 1,000 mg/dL. Remember that most laboratories report a calculated low-density lipoprotein cholesterol level, and triglyceride levels greater than 450 to 500 mg/dL invalidate the Friedwald's formula.

**8. d.**

Such dyslipidemias are best treated by a low-fat diet intended to maintain an ideal body weight and by improved glycemic control. If the mixed dyslipidemia (with much higher triglyceride levels) is still present, then a fibric acid derivative such as gemfibrozil (Lopid) is indicated. Other potential choices include niacin or atorvastatin calcium (Lipitor) if the degree of mixed dyslipidemia is more modest.

**9. e.**

If the individual is euthyroid, one must consider thyroid hormone resistance as well as causes of increased thyroid-binding globulin levels, such as oral contraceptive use or acute hepatitis. If the individual is hyperthyroid, it is possible that a TSH adenoma may be the cause because the level of TSH is inappropriate for primary hyperthyroidism. With subacute thyroiditis, if the patient has elevated levels of thyroid hormone, the TSH level should be suppressed below the normal range.

**10. c.**

Increased RAIU only suggests increased thyroid activity, and a stare and lid lag may be observed in cases of hyperthyroidism of any cause. Antimicrosomal antibodies are nonspecific, and a family history of Graves' disease is suggestive but not confirmatory. Pretibial myxedema develops only in patients with Graves' disease. These patients also invariably have proptosis.

**11. e.**

In the management of hyperthyroidism, as one normalizes the thyroid hormone levels, the TSH may remain suppressed, sometimes for more than 6 months.

Therefore, TSH level is not a good indicator for adjustment of therapy during initial treatment. This individual has clearly improved and is becoming euthyroid. One would not increase PTU, add propranolol, or stop PTU. Weight gain is a common problem during the treatment of hyperthyroidism, and the patient should be adequately informed of such a possibility.

**12. a.**

This is a case of sick euthyroid syndrome. Although the low $T_4$ and triiodothyronine levels are signs of a poor prognosis, thyroid replacement has no value. Free $T_4$ levels, especially if checked by an equilibrium dialysis method, will be normal. An RAIU test and scan are never of value in the diagnostic workup of hypothyroidism.

**13. a.**

All the suggested agents are useful in the management of osteoporosis except daily etidronate. Daily etidronate may cause osteomalacia. Calcium alone will help reduce age-related osteoporosis but not menopause-related osteoporosis. In combination with other agents, however, calcium supplementation is helpful.

**14. b.**

This man appears to have severe hyperparathyroidism that is unlikely to respond to glucocorticoids. The current standard therapy for treating severe hypercalcemia is adequate hydration followed by intravenous pamidronate.

**15. d.**

This woman most likely has hypocalcemia related to osteomalacia secondary to vitamin D deficiency. This leads to increased PTH secretion. Malabsorption is the likely cause, and thus carotene levels may be expected to be low.

**16. c.**

This woman has osteomalacia, probably secondary to presumed phenytoin (Dilantin) therapy, and thus would most likely benefit from vitamin D and calcium therapy. Six months is too soon to repeat the BMD.

**17. e.**

Because this man does not require vitamin D and calcium therapy for his chronic hypoparathyroidism, one must be suspicious of another source of vitamin D. Sarcoidosis, tuberculosis, or a malignancy must be considered. All the investigations would be helpful, except colonoscopy.

**18. d.**

Answer a describes a patient with possible Addison's disease. Answer c describes a person with possible isolated hypoaldosteronism. Both may benefit from fludrocortisone therapy. Answer b describes a man with hypopituitarism, and thus mineralocorticoid supplementation is not necessary.

**19. e.**
Renal artery stenosis is associated with increased plasma renin activity. The other causes are associated with decreased plasma renin activity.

**20. d.**
This woman likely has a nonfunctioning pituitary microadenoma. There is no need for therapy at present. The PRL elevation is trivial and should be followed only.

**21. d.**
A pituitary tumor may cause any of the described visual field defects, depending on whether the tumor impinges on the optic nerve, optic chiasm, or optic tract.

**22. b.**
Any of patients described may show elevated PRL levels, except patient b. Cisapride is not known to cause hyperprolactinemia. The use of major tranquilizers or metoclopramide, thoracic shingles, and hypothyroidism all may be associated with elevated PRL levels.

**23. b.**
The patient appears to have multiple endocrine neoplasia 1 syndrome, and thus hypercalcemia is most likely to precede other manifestations of this syndrome.

**24. d.**
This woman appears to partially concentrate her urine with water deprivation and then has a further response to desmopressin. This suggests partial central DI.

**25. a.**
A left adrenalectomy should not result in elevated ACTH levels and hyperpigmentation. Immigrants from Asia are more likely to have tuberculosis and thus are more likely to have bilateral adrenalitis. The scenario in answer c describes Nelson syndrome, in which an individual with an ACTH adenoma is treated with bilateral adrenalectomy, which results in very high levels of ACTH and severe hyperpigmentation. Lung malignancies, in particular small cell carcinoma, are associated with ectopic ACTH syndrome and hyperpigmentation.

**26. c.**
PRL does not have a direct effect on androgen production, and in humans has no effect on salt and water balance. It is thought to inhibit gonadotropin-releasing hormone secretion.

**27. e.**
This scenario describes Turner's syndrome, in which primary ovarian failure is associated with elevated gonadotropins.

**28. b.**
The β-hCG level should always be checked in any amenorrheic patient to rule out pregnancy. Checking the PRL and thyroid hormone levels is reasonable.

**29. b.**
See explanation for Question 28.

**30. c.**
It is important to rely on the HgbA$_{1c}$ value as well as the SMBG record to assess glycemic control. Often, patients report only the better glucose levels. When one observes discordant results, one should look for alternative explanations. In this situation, the HgbA$_{1c}$ is more reliable, and thus the patient's control must be reassessed and therapy intensified.

**31. d.**
This woman appears to have fasting hypoglycemia, and the gold standard test remains a prolonged fast with measurement of glucose, insulin, and C-peptide levels. Many physicians check the C-peptide level basally and again if hypoglycemia (plasma glucose less than 50 mg/dL) develops. One should never rely on capillary blood glucose levels, and it is always important to document the Whipple triad.

**32. c.**
In a patient with diabetic ketoacidosis, infusing fluids, administering insulin, avoiding hypokalemia, and ruling out a possible inciting cause are lifesaving. Although the patient is probably depleted of phosphate, phosphate replacement using intravenous potassium phosphate is not beneficial and has not been shown to improve outcome.

**33. b.**
The highest glucose levels occur at supper, which reflects the morning NPH insulin effect. The first step would be to increase the morning NPH insulin dose and reassess the patient in a few days. Reducing the pre-supper glucose levels may have further salutary effects on later glucose levels.

**34. d.**
In this scenario, a patient with chronic DM presents with hyperkalemia while taking an ACE inhibitor. The potassium level is not critical, and the next step would be to change to another class of antihypertensive agents.

**35. b.**
Hypogonadism, chronic liver disease, and use of anabolic steroids and spironolactone could cause gynecomastia. Salt-losing congenital adrenal hyperplasia is not linked to gynecomastia.

**36. b.**
Asherman's syndrome describes secondary amenorrhea due to uterine scarring.

**37. b.**
The presence or absence of cystic changes in the ovaries is not necessary to make a diagnosis of polycystic ovary syndrome. A rapid onset of symptoms or severe symp-

toms, often associated with extremely high androgen levels, would suggest a possible adrenal or ovarian tumor.

### 38. a.

One should confirm a euthyroid status, and then a fine-needle aspiration biopsy is indicated. If the biopsy results reveal obvious suspicious cells or increased numbers of follicular cells, one would proceed to surgical exploration.

### 39. b.

For possible multiple endocrine neoplasia type 2 syndrome, screening for a mutation in the *RET* protoonco-gene has become the gold standard. If there is linkage in the family, and screening of an asymptomatic family member is positive for the mutation, that individual should have a thyroidectomy because the risk for medullary cancer is extremely high.

## ACKNOWLEDGMENT

Questions were contributed by members of the Department of Endocrinology (Drs. B. J. Hoogwerf, R. Danese, C. Faiman, A. E. Mehta, A. Licata, and S. Reddy), Cleveland Clinic Foundation.

# Nephrology and Hypertension

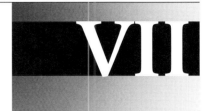

# Acute Renal Failure

**49**

*Joseph V. Nally, Jr.*

Acute renal failure (ARF) is a common problem in the contemporary practice of hospital-based medicine. Prospective studies demonstrated that 2% to 5% of all patients admitted to a general medical-surgical hospital will develop ARF. In selected patients in the intensive care unit (ICU) setting, the incidence may exceed 20%. Marked increases in both morbidity (which prolong hospitalization) and mortality occur in the patient who develops ARF. The high frequency of occurrence and substantial morbidity and mortality of ARF demand a logical approach to prevention and early diagnosis, as well as prompt recognition and management of its complications.

ARF is defined as a rapid decrease in renal function characterized by progressive azotemia (best measured by serum creatinine), which may or may not be accompanied by oliguria. ARF can be diagnosed with certainty when the patient's prior renal function is known and a decrement is documented. It is important to distinguish the three major causes of ARF: prerenal azotemia; postrenal azotemia or obstruction of the urinary tract; and intrinsic renal disease (1). Distinguishing among the three basic categories of ARF is a challenging clinical exercise. The importance of differentiating the major causes of ARF must be stressed because the initial evaluation and management of the ARF patient is tailored to the particular cause. Because the majority of all hospital-acquired ARF is secondary to acute tubular necrosis (ATN), special emphasis will be placed on ATN.

## PRERENAL AZOTEMIA

Prerenal azotemia is caused by a transient renal hypoperfusion that may induce both azotemia and urinary sodium avidity. Prerenal azotemia may be encountered in both the volume-depleted and volume-overloaded patient (Table 49.1). True volume depletion may result from renal or extrarenal losses. In the volume-overloaded patient having edematous states such as cirrhosis, nephrosis, and congestive heart failure, prerenal azotemia may occur because the kidney perceives that the vascular tree is underfilled, thus resulting in renal hypoperfusion. In addition, prerenal azotemia may occur owing to high-grade bilateral renal artery stenosis.

The pathophysiology of prerenal azotemia relates to the reduction in renal blood flow. Renal hypoperfusion stimu-lates both the sympathetic nervous system and renin-angiotensin system to cause renal vasoconstriction and sodium avidity. Furthermore, hypotension is a powerful stimulus to the release of an antidiuretic hormone, which mediates water reabsorption. Hence, urine production is characterized by low volume, decreased concentration of urinary sodium, and increased urinary excretion of creatinine with a high urine osmolality. Microscopy results of the urinary sediment are usually bland. In essence, prerenal azotemia is "a good kidney looking at a bad world."

The therapy for prerenal azotemia is directed at optimizing volume status using isotonic fluids. In patients with edematous disorders who have prerenal azotemia, special efforts are directed at treating the underlying disease states (i.e., heart failure, cirrhosis) and optimizing systemic hemodynamics and renal perfusion.

## POSTRENAL AZOTEMIA

Obstruction of the urinary tract may cause ARF. To be the cause of azotemia, urinary tract obstruction must involve the outflow tract of both normal kidneys, unless preexisting renal dysfunction is present, in which case the obstruction may involve only a single kidney. Patients with acute urinary tract obstruction may present with hematuria, flank or abdominal pain, or signs of uremia. A high index of suspicion for urinary tract obstruction should exist for patients with prior abdominal or pelvic surgery, neoplasia, or radiation therapy. Although oliguria or anuria suggests complete obstruction, partial obstruction may exist in the presence of adequate urinary output. The presence of marked oliguria or anuria is a powerful diagnostic clue that suggests urinary tract obstruction, severe ATN with cortical necrosis, and bilateral vascular occlusion. Lesions that may cause obstruction can be either intrinsic or extrinsic to the genitourinary tract (Table 49.2).

If urinary tract obstruction is a diagnostic consideration, renal ultrasonography is sensitive and specific (90% to 95%) in confirming the diagnosis of hydronephrosis. This test may be operator dependent, so the experience of the radiologist is crucial. False-negative test results may be seen with periureteral metastatic disease or retroperitoneal fibrosis. Abdominal computed tomography (CT) or retrograde pyelography may be helpful in this circumstance. If

**TABLE 49.1**
## PRERENAL ACUTE RENAL FAILURE

A. Cardiac Causes: Primary Decrease in Cardiac Output
  1. Acute disorders: myocardial infarction, trauma, arrhythmias, malignant hypertension, tamponade, acute valvular disease (e.g., endocarditis)
  2. Chronic disorders: valvular diseases, chronic myocardiopathies (ischemic heart disease, hypertensive heart disease)
B. Volume Depletion
  1. Gastrointestinal losses: vomiting, diarrhea, fistulas
  2. Renal: salt-wasting disorders, overdiuresis
C. Redistribution of Extracellular Fluid
  1. Hypoalbuminemic states: nephrotic syndrome, advanced liver disease, malnutrition
  2. Physical causes: peritonitis, burns, crush injury
  3. Peripheral vasodilatation: sepsis, antihypertensive agents
  4. Renal artery stenosis (bilateral)

urinary tract obstruction is a diagnostic consideration, renal ultrasonography should be performed because obstruction represents a potentially reversible cause of ARF.

## INTRINSIC RENAL DISEASE

The major causes of ARF owing to intrinsic renal disease include acute glomerulonephritis, acute interstitial nephritis (AIN), and ATN. Because ATN is by far the most common cause of ARF that develops in the hospital setting, special emphasis is given to that condition.

**TABLE 49.2**
## POSTRENAL ACUTE RENAL FAILURE

A. Ureteral and Pelvic
  1. Intrinsic Obstruction
    Blood clots
    Stones
    Sloughed papillae
    Fungus balls
  2. Extrinsic Obstruction
    Malignancy
    Retroperitoneal fibrosis
    Iatrogenic: inadvertent ligation
B. Bladder
    Stones
    Blood clots
    Prostatic hypertrophy or malignancy
    Bladder carcinoma
    Neuropathic
C. Urethral
    Strictures
    Phimosis

## Acute Glomerulonephritis

The importance of urinalysis in the evaluation of patients with ARF cannot be overemphasized: Physicians must develop skill and expertise in interpreting the microscopic findings of urinalysis. In cases of ARF owing to intrinsic renal disease, such skills are critical. The presence of proteinuria, hematuria, and red blood cell casts are pathognomonic of glomerulonephritis. The differential diagnosis of rapidly progressive glomerulonephritis is beyond the scope of this review (see the section on acute glomerulonephritis in Chapter 50). Evaluation usually includes the performance of a renal biopsy, as well as a detailed serologic evaluation for the presence of systemic vasculitis, collagen vascular disease, and infectious processes. Specific therapies tailored to the disease entity diagnosed after this thorough evaluation may be lifesaving.

## Acute Interstitial Nephritis

The diagnosis of ARF owing to AIN also may be suggested, upon microscopy of the urinalysis sample, by the presence of sterile pyuria, white blood cell casts, and eosinophiluria on Hansel's stain. AIN may be secondary to a variety of drugs, including penicillins, methicillin, cephalosporin, nonsteroidal anti-inflammatory drugs, cimetidine, phenytoin, phenobarbital, allopurinol, interferon-$\alpha$, and diuretics. The clinical syndrome may be quite variable, although it is likely to involve an abnormal urinary sediment (proteinuria and pyuria), eosinophilia/eosinophiluria, and fever. Skin rash is seen in approximately 25% of cases. The specific diagnosis of AIN as a cause of ARF should lead to the discontinuation of possibly offending medications. If the renal insufficiency does not resolve in days to weeks, renal biopsy results may confirm the diagnosis of AIN. In selected cases, a trial of steroid therapy may hasten recovery of renal function, yet prospective trials evaluating the efficacy and safety of steroid therapy are lacking.

## ACUTE TUBULAR NECROSIS

### Incidence and Etiology of ATN

Overall, ARF may affect 2% to 5% of patients in a tertiary care hospital, and the incidence of ARF in the surgical or medical ICU may exceed 20% to 30% in selected high-risk patient populations (Table 49.3).

The vast majority of all hospital-acquired ARF is secondary to ATN. In Madrid, Liano and colleagues observed that the causes of ARF in a multicenter tertiary care hospital setting were ATN 45%, prerenal disease 21%, acute or chronic renal failure 13%, urinary tract infection 10%, glomerulonephritis and vasculitis 4%, AIN 2%, and atheroembolic renal disease 1%. Renal hypoperfusion and renal ischemia are the most common causes of ATN, although nephrotoxic insults from various agents are recognized with increasing frequency. As

## TABLE 49.3
### FREQUENCY OF ARF IN DIFFERENT CLINICAL SETTINGS

| | Percentage Mild ARF (SCr[a] <3 mg/dL) | Percentage Severe ARF (SCr >5 mg/dL) |
|---|---|---|
| Open heart surgery | 5–20 | 2–5 |
| Abdominal aortic aneurysm resection | | |
|     Emergency | 30–50 | 15–25 |
|     Elective | 5–10 | 2–5 |
| Severe trauma | 10–20 | 1–5 |
| Neonatal ICU admission | 17 | 6 |
| Aminoglycoside drug administration | 5–20 | 1–2 |
| Admission to general medical/ surgical unit | 4–10 | 1–2 |

[a] SCr = serum creatinine.

shown in Table 49.3, the incidence of ARF in the ICU and after extensive vascular surgery, such as aortic aneurysm repair or coronary artery bypass grafting, is significant. Because "volume is the primal scream of the kidney," renal ischemia is the leading cause of ARF in this population. Agents (either endogenous or exogenous) that may be toxic to the kidney in any clinical setting are summarized in Tables 49.4 and 49.5.

Table 49.4 lists endogenous nephrotoxic products. Of note, pigment nephropathy may be suspected in the appropriate clinical situation (posttraumatic or atraumatic after intoxications) in which the discrepancies of hematuria by dipstick and the absence of red blood cells on urinary microscopy exist.

The combination of renal hypoperfusion and the nephrotoxic insult of myoglobin or hemoglobin within the proximal tubule may result in ATN. Early recognition of this disorder is crucial because a forced alkaline diuresis is indicated to minimize nephrotoxicity. Similarly, the tumor lysis syndrome may be suspected in the appropriate clinical setting when marked hyperuricemia and hyperuricosuria, as well as crystalluria, are recognized. A forced alkaline diuresis may limit nephrotoxicity and is usually recommended prophylactically before an aggressive chemotherapy regimen.

The list of potential exogenous nephrotoxic agents is exhaustive (see Table 49.5). Simply stated, when a patient develops ATN while receiving medications, each medication should be reviewed for the possibility of nephrotoxicity. Commonly seen nephrotoxins in the hospitalized patient include:

- Radiographic contrast material
- Antibiotics (especially aminoglycosides and amphotericin B)
- Chemotherapeutic agents (especially cis-platinum and ifosfamide)
- Nonsteroidal anti-inflammatory drugs (NSAIDs)
- Angiotensin-converting enzyme (ACE) inhibitor
- Angiotensin receptor blockers (ARBs)

More recently, the potential nephrotoxicity of newer agents, such as acyclovir, protease inhibitors, recombinant interleukin-2, interferon, and selected chemotherapeutic agents, is being appreciated.

In the contemporary practice of hospital-based medicine, the recognition of ARF in two special patient populations deserves special comment.

### Human Immunodeficiency Virus and ATN

Patients with human immunodeficiency virus infection may develop ARF due to the same causes as uninfected patients, but protease inhibitors have been associated with the development of ARF. Ritonavir and indinavir (as well as acyclovir, foscarnet, and sulfadiazine) have been associated with a reversible ARF, thought to occur secondary to crystalluria and intrarenal obstruction. In addition, patients treated with indinavir may present with renal colic; indinavir renal stones have been associated with urinary tract obstruction.

## TABLE 49.4
### ARF RELATED TO ENDOGENOUS NEPHROTOXIC PRODUCTS

**Pigment Nephropathy**
Myoglobin
Hemoglobin[a]
Methemoglobin[a]

**Intrarenal Crystal Deposition**
Uric acid
Calcium
Oxalate

**Tumor-Specific Syndromes**
Tumor lysis syndrome
Plasma cell dyscrasias (e.g., myeloma kidney)

[a] Questionable direct nephrotoxic effect.

## TABLE 49.5
### CAUSES OF EXOGENOUS TOXIC ACUTE RENAL FAILURE

| | |
|---|---|
| *Antibiotics* | Interferon-α or γ-1-B |
| Aminoglycosides | *HIV protease inhibitors* |
| Cephalosporin | Indinavir |
| Sulfonamide, co-trimoxazol | Ritonavir |
| Tetracyclines | *Organic solvents* |
| Amphotericin B | Glycols (ethylene glycol, |
| Polymyxin, colistin | diethylene glycol) |
| Bacitracin | Halogenated hydrocarbons |
| Pentamidine | (CCl4, tetra- and |
| Vancomycin | trichloro-ethylene) |
| Acyclovir | Aromatic hydrocarbons |
| Foscarnet | (toluene) |
| *Anesthetic agents* | Aliphatic-aromatic |
| Methoxyflurane | hydrocarbons (Vaseline, |
| Enflurane | kerosene, turpentine, |
| *Contrast media* | paraphenylene |
| Diatrizoate | diamine) |
| Iothalamate | *Heavy metals* |
| Bunamiodyl | *Poisons* |
| Iopanoic acid | Insecticide (chlordane) |
| *Antiulcer regimens* | Herbicides (paraquat, |
| Cimetidine | diquat) |
| Excess of milk-alkali | Rodenticide (elemental P) |
| *Analgesics* | Mushroom |
| Nonsteroidal anti- | Snake bites[a] |
| inflammatory drugs | Stings[a] |
| (NSAIDs) | Bacterial toxins[a] |
| *Diuretics* | *Chemicals* |
| Mercurials | Aniline |
| Ticrynafen | Hexol |
| Others | Cresol |
| *Chemotherapeutic and* | Chlorates |
| *immunosuppressive agents* | Potassium bromate |
| Cis-platinum | *Recreational drugs[b]* |
| Carboplatin | Heroin |
| Ifosfamide | Amphetamines |
| Methotrexate | *Miscellaneous* |
| Mitomycin | Dextrans |
| 5-azacytidine | EDTA |
| Nitrosourea | Radiation |
| Plicamycin | Silicone |
| Cyclosporine A and | Epsilon-amino caproic |
| tacrolimus (FK506) | acid[a] |
| D-penicillamine | ACE inhibitors |
| Recombinant IL-2 | |

[a] Direct toxicity or indirect systemic effects (shock, intravascular hemolysis, or coagulation).
[b] Slow onset of renal failure, unless associated with rhabdomyolysis.

### Bone Marrow Transplantation and ATN

ARF may be quite common following bone marrow transplantation in some centers. Several nephrologic syndromes may be encountered at various time frames following bone marrow transplantation. In the perioperative period, ATN due to tumor lysis syndrome, bone marrow infusion, sepsis, or antibiotics (especially aminoglycoside and amphotericin B) is likely. At days 10 to 16, ARF is commonly attributed to hepatic venoocclusive disease resulting from endothelial cell injury from radiation or chemotherapy. Clinically, the presentation of this entity mimics hepatorenal syndrome. After 4 to 12 months, ARF may be due to hemolytic uremic syndrome, possibly related to cyclosporine A or radiation therapy. Therapies with plasma exchange have been disappointing.

## Pathophysiology of ATN

Several pathogenic mechanisms have been proposed to account for the abnormalities noted in ARF secondary to ATN. Of note, two significant dichotomies exist regarding the renal physiology and pathology of ATN.

The first dichotomy is a striking reduction in glomerular filtration rate (GFR) in oliguric ARF that is accompanied by a more modest decline in renal plasma flow. This dichotomy of GFR and renal plasma flow reductions suggests a contribution, at least in part, of an intense afferent arteriole vasoconstriction.

The second dichotomy relates to the pathology of ATN. The distribution of the tubular necrosis appears patchy, and the degree of necrosis does not correlate clinically with the level of renal dysfunction. These observations may be reconciled by understanding the pathologic location of early ATN. In general, the renal cortex is well perfused and well oxygenated. The corticomedullary junction is much less well oxygenated, however, and oxygen demand and oxygen supply are nearly equal under basal conditions. Following a hypotensive or hypoxic insult, oxygen demand exceeds supply, and ATN develops in the energy-rich, thick ascending limb of Henle in the corticomedullary junction. This imbalance may account for the patchy nature seen pathologically on a renal cross-sectional biopsy sample.

Ischemic and toxic insults may result in identical clinical syndromes associated with azotemia. The pathophysiologic mechanisms postulated for ARF include:

- Tubular backleak of glomerular filtrate
- Tubular obstruction owing to debris or casts
- Vascular theories invoking afferent arteriolar vasoconstriction (i.e., the renin-angiotensin system)
- Diminished permeability of the glomerular membrane

Disorders of intracellular adenosine triphosphate and calcium metabolism; membrane and phospholipase abnormalities; abnormalities of tubular cell polarity and cytoskeletal function; and the generation of free radical oxygen species and proteases may all be significant in the tubular damage of ATN.

A knowledge of the basic processes involved in the development of ATN is a prerequisite to an understanding of contemporary therapies directed at limiting renal damage and promoting more rapid renal recovery. The sentinel biochemical event in renal ischemia is the depletion of adenosine triphosphate, which is the major energy currency for cellular work. Adenosine triphosphate depletion results in impaired function of the plasma membrane and intracellular adenosine triphosphatases that are vital to normal cell function. As a consequence of these defects, cell swelling and high intracellular levels of calcium result. As the name suggests, ischemic ATN is characterized by renal tubular cell injury. Because obvious necrosis is not a cardinal histopathologic finding in ATN, sublethal injury is important. The sublethal injury to tubular cells leads to aberrations in the cytoskeletal organization of tubular cells, with subsequent loss of cell polarity.

After sublethal injury, the kidney has a remarkable capacity for repairing its normal structure and function. Renal recovery from ATN is a relatively new concept, with great potential for clinical application. Increased mitotic activity and epithelial regeneration are notable features of ATN. Certain aspects of renal recovery duplicate events in renal development. A number of growth factors play a role in recovery. Epidermal growth factor, insulin-like growth factor-1, and hepatocyte growth factor have been shown to limit renal injury and accelerate renal recovery in experimental ischemic ATN.

## Diagnosis of ATN

The diagnostic tools available to the clinician include:

- A thorough history and physical examination to assess volume status, potential nephrotoxic insults, and evidence of systemic disease
- Urine output
- Urinalysis
- Urine electrolytes
- Radiologic and renal ultrasonography evaluation

The schema for evaluating the patient with ARF is outlined in Table 49.6. The urine output may be a clue to the diagnosis of ARF. The presence of marked oliguria or anuria might suggest urinary tract obstruction, renovascular occlusion, or cortical necrosis. In contrast, nonoliguric

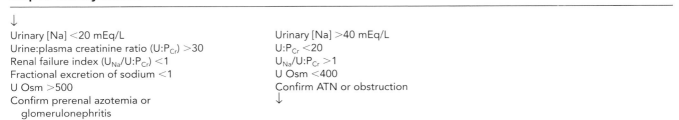

## TABLE 49.6
### DIAGNOSIS OF ACUTE RENAL FAILURE

**Step 1: History and Physical Examination**

↓

| Prerenal | Renal | Postrenal |
|---|---|---|
| Volume depletion; congestive heart failure; severe liver disease or other edematous states | ATN AIN AGN | Palpable bladder or hydronephrotic kidneys; enlarged prostate; abnormal pelvic examination; large residual bladder urine volume; history of renal calculi |

**Step 2: Urine Sediment**

↓

| Eosinophils ↓ | RBC casts ↓ | No abnormalities ↓ | Renal tubular epithelial cells and "muddy-brown" casts ↓ |
|---|---|---|---|
| Suspect AIN | Glomerulonephritis or vasculitis | Suspect prerenal or postrenal azotemia | Suspect ATN |

**Step 3: Urinary Indices**

↓

| | |
|---|---|
| Urinary [Na] <20 mEq/L | Urinary [Na] >40 mEq/L |
| Urine:plasma creatinine ratio (U:P$_{Cr}$) >30 | U:P$_{Cr}$ <20 |
| Renal failure index (U$_{Na}$/U:P$_{Cr}$) <1 | U$_{Na}$/U:P$_{Cr}$ >1 |
| Fractional excretion of sodium <1 | U Osm <400 |
| U Osm >500 | Confirm ATN or obstruction |
| Confirm prerenal azotemia or glomerulonephritis | ↓ |

**Step 4: Therapeutic Challenge**

↓

| Correct prerenal or postrenal factors | Urine volume <500 mL/day | Optional trial of furosemide to convert oliguric to nonoliguric ARF |
|---|---|---|

U Osm = urine osmolarity.

## TABLE 49.7
### ARF URINARY SEDIMENT

| Bland or Scant Findings | Granular Casts | RBCs, RBC Casts | Epithelial and White Blood Cells, WBC Casts | Crystalluria |
|---|---|---|---|---|
| *Vasculitides* | *ATN* | *Glomerulonephritis* | *Eosinophiluria present* | *Uric acid* |
| Preglomerular vasculitis | Pigmented | RPGN | Acute interstitial | Tumor lysis syndrome |
| Hemolytic-uremic syndrome | coarsely granular | Small vessel vasculitis | nephritis likely | |
| | casts common | | | |
| *Scleroderma* | | | | |
| *Renovascular diseases* | | *Interstitial nephritis* | *Eosinophiluria absent* | *Calcium oxalate* |
| Arterial thrombosis or emboli | | Rarely seen | Acute interstitial | Penthrane toxicity |
| | | | nephritis still possible | |
| | | | | Glycol |
| Prerenal azotemia | | *ATN* | *Pyelonephritis* | |
| | | Rarely seen | Severe, with abscesses | |
| Postrenal azotemia | | | | |

ARF is recognized with increased frequency, and the careful monitoring of serum creatinine in at-risk patients is of paramount importance.

An examination of the urinalysis sample is fundamental to the evaluation of the patient with ARF. Simple urinalysis may distinguish the cause of ARF among the various possibilities. Table 49.7 highlights the various urinary abnormalities associated with the clinical diagnoses. For example, proteinuria, hematuria, and red blood cell casts are pathognomonic of glomerulonephritis. The classic sediment for ATN includes pigmented (muddy brown) granular casts and renal tubular epithelial cells, which may be seen in nearly 80% of cases of oliguric ARF.

A determination of urinary chemistries may be helpful in determining the etiology of ARF. Urine sodium ($U_{Na}$), creatinine ($U_{creat}$), and osmolality should be measured, and either the fractional excretion of sodium ($FE_{Na}$) or the renal failure index (RFI) should be calculated, using the following equation:

$$FE_{Na} = \frac{\dfrac{U_{Na}V}{P_{Na}}}{\dfrac{U_{creat}V}{P_{creat}}} \times 100\% \quad \text{or} \quad RFI = \frac{U_{Na} \times P_{creat}}{U_{creat}}$$

where $P_{Na}$ is plasma sodium, $P_{creat}$ is plasma creatinine, and V is urine volume.

Note that a low $FE_{Na}$ (or RFI) may be associated with either prerenal azotemia or acute glomerulonephritis. These entities could be separated clinically by examination of the urinalysis. Conditions associated with prerenal azotemia have a bland urinalysis result, whereas proteinuria, red blood cells, and red blood cell casts are seen in acute glomerulonephritis. Both ATN and obstruction may be associated with an increased $FE_{Na}$ or RFI. Here again, the urinalysis results are key. ATN is associated with a classic sediment containing pigmented coarsely granular casts; in obstruction, however, the urinalysis results often are bland.

The radiologic evaluation in ARF might include renal ultrasonography, plain frontal supine radiography of the abdomen, and retrograde urography. The value of renal ultrasonography in the evaluation of possible urinary tract obstruction was discussed earlier. Such studies as intravenous pyelography or abdominal CT, which use contrast material, should be avoided because of potential nephrotoxicity.

## Stages of ATN

The oliguric phase usually begins less than 24 hours after the inciting incident and may last for 1 to 3 weeks. Urine volume averages 150 to 300 mL/day. The oliguric phase may be prolonged in the elderly. During this phase, the clinician must be alert for the expected complications, with special emphasis on metabolic consequences, gastrointestinal bleeding, and infection.

The diuretic phase is characterized by a progressive increase in urine volume, a harbinger of renal recovery. The serum creatinine may continue to increase for another 24 to 48 hours, however, before it reaches a plateau and decreases. Severe polyuria during this phase is seen less frequently now. Careful management during this phase is crucial because up to 25% of deaths from ARF may occur in this phase, usually related to fluid and electrolyte abnormalities, as well as infection. Finally, the recovery phase ensues. Renal function returns to near baseline, but abnormalities of urinary concentration and dilution may persist for weeks or months.

## Treatment of ATN

During the initial evaluation, it is imperative to search for reversible causes, such as volume depletion, obstruction, and vascular occlusion. During the initial stages, a trial of parenteral hydration using isotonic fluids may correct ARF secondary to prerenal causes. In early established ARF secondary to ATN, a trial of a loop diuretic may be warranted. A recent retrospective observational study suggested that the use of loop diuretics in patients with ARF may be associated with a delayed recovery of renal function and increased mortality (2). Nevertheless, pharmacologic intervention to convert oliguric ATN to nonoliguric ATN is a salutary clinical goal. In general, increases in urinary volume make it easier to address problems of volume overload, hyperkalemia, and metabolic acidosis.

Increases in urine volume also may provide room for supplemental total parenteral nutrition in the critically ill patient. Morbidity, the need for dialysis, and mortality may be less prevalent in the nonoliguric form of ATN. Unfortunately, very few prospective, randomized trials have adequately tested this hypothesis (3). In particular, the data available for "renal dose" dopamine therapy in oliguric ARF are surprisingly scant. In fact, the only such prospective trial reported concerns ARF caused by malaria. If considered, a trial of "renal dose" dopamine should be used after a clinical challenge of parenteral hydration and a loop diuretic agent. If the treatment is unsuccessful, dopamine should be tapered off within 24 hours. More recently, a prospective, randomized trial using atrial natriuretic peptide (ANP) in patients with ATN (oliguric and nonoliguric) has been reported. Overall, no benefit on morbidity and mortality was established using ANP. In a subset of patients with oliguric ATN, however, clinical improvement was seen with ANP infusion. A subsequent trial in this select population did not demonstrate clinical benefit. In sum, ANP is not recommended as therapy for ARF.

Once the clinical diagnosis of ATN is made, conservative medical management is in order (Table 49.8). This includes attempts to minimize further renal parenchymal injury, ensure the provision of adequate nutrition, maintain the metabolic balance, and promote the recovery of renal function. Optimizing the patient's volume status is imperative, particularly in patients with oliguric ARF. Protein restriction and the maintenance of essential amino acids and carbohydrate intake may limit catabolism and help maintain nitrogen balance. Dietary phosphorous and potassium may be restricted. Medications should be adjusted for the level of renal dysfunction.

Dialysis (either hemodialysis or peritoneal dialysis) may be instituted when clinically indicated. The indications for acute dialysis include:

- Volume overload
- Severe hyperkalemia
- Severe, uncorrectable metabolic acidosis
- Pericarditis
- Selected poisonings
- Uremic symptomatology

Intermittent hemodialysis provides a rapid treatment of hyperkalemia and volume overload. Newer dialytic tech-

## TABLE 49.8

### CHECKLIST OF CONSERVATIVE MEASURES IN THE MANAGEMENT OF ARF

Fluid balance
    Careful monitoring of intake/output and weights
    Fluid restriction
Electrolytes and acid–base balance
Prevent and treat hyperkalemia
Avoid hyponatremia
Keep serum bicarbonate >15 mEq/L
Minimize hyperphosphatemia
Treat hypocalcemia only if symptomatic or if intravenous
    bicarbonate is required
Uremia and nutrition
Restrict protein (0.5 g/kg/day) but maintain caloric intake; consider
    forms of nutritional support
Carbohydrate intake at least 100 g/day to minimize ketosis and
    endogenous protein catabolism
Drugs
Review all medications
Stop magnesium-containing medications
Adjust dosage for renal failure; readjust with improvement of GFR

niques using biocompatible membranes and the use of bicarbonate dialysis and controlled ultrafiltration may allow better treatment tolerance in the hemodynamically unstable patient. Prospective, controlled trials in patients with ARF treated with different modalities are not available for comparison to offer definitive therapeutic guidelines, however. A recent trial comparing daily versus every other day intermittent hemodialysis suggested a survival benefit for daily therapy (4).

## Prognosis of ATN

The prognosis of ATN depends on the underlying primary disease that resulted in the ARF, as well as any complications that arise during the bout of ARF (e.g., infection, cardiovascular complications, gastrointestinal bleeding, or central nervous system effects). The mortality rate for patients with ATN is nearly 50%. This pessimistic outlook has changed little in the past four decades, despite the advent of effective dialysis. Mortality rates remain high, despite the effective control of uremia, because we are caring for an older, sicker population with severe concomitant illnesses. Mortality rates of as high as 75% have been reported in several series in the ICU population. Higher mortality rates are seen in elderly patients and in patients with respiratory failure, multiorgan failure with severe forms of oliguric ATN, preexisting chronic diseases, and systemic hypotension. Leading causes of death include bronchopulmonary infections, sepsis, cardiovascular disease, and bleeding disorders. Of patients who survive ATN, nearly half will have a complete recovery of renal function, and a majority of the remainder has an incomplete recovery

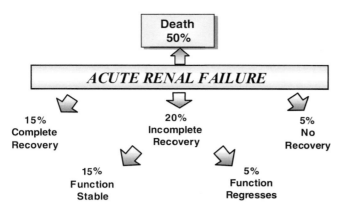

**Figure 49.1**  Prognosis of ATN.

(Fig. 49.1). Only approximately 5% to 10% of all ARF patients require chronic maintenance dialysis. In short, with ARF "you either die or you get better."

## Prevention of ATN

Because the management of ATN is primarily one of conservative care and support, special attention should be focused on the prevention of ARF. Patients at high risk (i.e., patients with preexisting azotemia, the elderly, and volume-depleted individuals) warrant careful clinical consideration of the relative risks and benefits of diagnostic or therapeutic interventions that have a potential for nephrotoxicity. This is especially true for patients at risk undergoing cardiac catheterization or other diagnostic studies that require the use of intravenous contrast material. Two interventions deserve comment.

A study by Solomon and coworkers confirmed that prestudy intravenous hydration with saline was critical in lessening the nephrotoxic effect for patients with preexisting azotemia (4). The addition of either a loop diuretic or mannitol did not improve outcome.

Rudnick et al. published a prospective, randomized trial of nearly 1,200 well-hydrated patients undergoing cardiac catheterization to examine the effects of the newer nonionic contrast material (5). Patients were stratified for the absence or presence of azotemia (serum creatinine greater than or equal to 1.5%) or diabetes mellitus. In patients without azotemia (with or without diabetes mellitus), the incidence of contrast-induced renal dysfunction was low (less than 1%

to 2%) with either the ionic or nonionic contrast material. In contrast, in those with preexisting azotemia, a 50% reduction in contrast-associated renal dysfunction was seen when the nonionic material was used.

These data suggest that in azotemic patients who require cardiac angiography, a protocol of intravenous hydration and the use of a nonionic contrast material appear warranted. Furthermore, seven randomized controlled trials suggest that pretreatment with acetylcysteine may attenuate contrast injury in at-risk patients (6,7).

## REFERENCES

1. Liano F, Pascual J. Epidemiology of acute renal failure: a prospective, multicenter, community-based study. Madrid Acute Renal Failure Study Group. *Kidney Int* 1996;50:811–818.
2. Cosentino F. Drugs for the prevention and treatment of acute renal failure. *Cleve Clin J Med* 1995;62:248–253.
3. Mehta RL, Pascula MT, Soroko S, et al. Diuretics, mortality, and nonrecovery of renal function in acute renal failure. *JAMA* 2002; 288:2547.
4. Solomon R, Werner C, Mann D, et al. Effects of saline, mannitol, and furosemide to prevent acute decreases in renal function induced by radiocontrast agents. *N Engl J Med* 1994;331:1416–1420.
5. Rudnick MR, Goldfarb S, Wexler L, et al. Nephrotoxicity of ionic and nonionic contrast media in 1196 patients: a randomized trial. The Iohexol Cooperative Study. *Kidney Int* 1995;47: 254–261.
6. Birck R, Krzossok S, Markowetz F, et al. Acetylcysteine for prevention of contrast nephropathy: Meta-analysis. *Lancet* 2003;362:598.
7. Tepel M, Van Der Giet M, Schwarzfeld C, et al. Prevention of radiographic-contrast-agent-induced reduction in renal function by acetylcysteine. *N Engl J Med* 2000;343:180.

## SUGGESTED READINGS

Allgren RL, Marbury TC, Rahman SN, et al. Anaritide in acute tubular necrosis. *N Engl J Med* 1997;336:828–871.
Denton MD, Chertow GM, Brady HR. "Renal-dose" dopamine for the treatment of acute renal failure: scientific rationale, experimental studies and clinical trials. *Kidney Int* 1996;50:4–14.
Klahr S, Miller SB. Current concepts: acute oliguria. *N Engl J Med* 1998;338:671–675.
Lake EW, Humes HD. Acute renal failure including cortical necrosis. In: Glassock RJ, Massry SG, eds. *Textbook of Nephrology*, 3rd ed. Baltimore: Williams & Wilkins, 1995:984–1003.
Miller TR, Anderson RJ, Linas SL, et al. Urinary diagnostic indices in acute renal failure. A prospective study. *Ann Intern Med* 1978;89: 45–50.
Schiffl H, Lang SM, Fischer R. Daily hemodialysis and the outcome of acute renal failure. *N Engl J Med* 2002;346:305.
Thadhani R, Pascual M, Bonventre JV. Acute renal failure. *N Engl J Med* 1996;334:1448–1460.
Vijayan A, Miller SB. Acute renal failure: prevention and nondialytic therapy. *Semin Nephrol* 1998;18:523–532.

# Parenchymal Renal Disease

## 50

### Gerald B. Appel

Parenchymal renal diseases affect many millions of persons in the United States and worldwide. In 2000, in the United States, more than 300,000 persons were in end-stage renal disease (ESRD) programs, largely as a result of renal involvement by parenchymal diseases. One form of glomerular damage alone, diabetic glomerulonephropathy, affects millions of people, with a cost of billions of dollars annually. In the United States and worldwide, glomerular disease associated with hepatitis C virus (HCV) and human immunodeficiency virus (HIV) is a major health problem. Fortunately, progress in the diagnosis and treatment of common forms of idiopathic nephrotic syndrome (NS), such as focal glomerulosclerosis and membranous nephropathy (MN), has been striking in the last decade. Table 50.1 shows the incidence of idiopathic NS.

The mechanisms of both glomerular and tubulointerstitial injury are quite varied. In glomerular disease, immune-mediated renal injury is a major initiating pathogenetic mechanism of glomerular damage. In diabetic nephropathy and amyloidosis, other mechanisms of damage to the glomerular capillary wall are clearly at work. In tubulointerstitial disease, the primary insult may be immunologic (e.g., drug-induced acute interstitial nephritis), toxic-metabolic (e.g., analgesics, oxalate, etc.), or vascular (e.g., sickle cell disease and atheroemboli). The end result is damage to the tubules and interstitial space of the kidney, with eventual interstitial scarring and fibrosis.

## NORMAL GLOMERULUS

Each glomerulus, the basic filtering unit of the kidney, consists of a tuft of anastomosing capillaries formed by the branchings of the afferent arteriole. The millions of glomeruli within each kidney comprise approximately 5% of the kidney's weight and provide 2 m$^2$ of filtering surface. Each glomerulus consists of a combination of cellular elements (endothelial cells, mesangial cells, visceral and parietal epithelial cells) and extracellular matrix [the glomerular basement membrane (GBM) and mesangial matrix]. The endothelial cells lining the lumens of the glomerular capillaries have a highly fenestrated cytoplasm attached to the internal aspect of the GBM. These cells possess a variety of histocompatibility antigens, express Fc and C3b receptors that allow the adhesion of macrophages and complement

activation, and produce and secrete numerous vasoactive substances [including antihemolytic factor (factor VIII), thrombin receptors, prostacyclin, and heparin-like growth factors]. They may contribute to the synthesis and maintenance of the GBM.

The mesangium or central stalk region of the glomerulus is composed of both matrix and cells. It is important for mechanical support, transport of molecules out of the capillary loops, and the contractile nature of the glomerular capillaries. The mesangial matrix consists predominantly of type IV collagen, fibronectin, laminin, and proteoglycans. Mesangial cells may proliferate and produce vasoactive substances, including prostaglandins, oxygen radicals, platelet-derived growth factor, and so on.

The GBM is composed of a central dense layer (lamina densa) and more lucent outer and inner layers (lamina rara interna and lamina rara externa). The GBM is chemically composed of type IV collagen and a variety of proteins including entactin, laminin, and fibronectin. The GBM is highly negatively charged and provides both a size- and charge-selective barrier to the passage of circulating macromolecules.

The visceral epithelial cells contain numerous extensions called *foot processes*, which interdigitate with the foot processes of neighboring visceral epithelial cells and are tightly bound to the lamina rara externa of the GBM. The visceral epithelial cells are coated with a highly anionic layer of sialoprotein and are important in the synthesis of many of the components of the GBM. The parietal epithelial cells are simple, flat cells that line the Bowman capsule.

## HISTOPATHOLOGIC TERMS

Understanding renal histopathology requires the knowledge of only a few terms. When dealing with the entire kidney, if all glomeruli are involved, a process is called *diffuse* or *generalized*; if only some glomeruli are involved, the process is called *focal*. When dealing with the individual glomerulus, a process is called *global* if the whole glomerular tuft is involved and *segmental* if only part is involved. The terms *proliferative*, *sclerosing*, and *necrotizing* are often used [e.g., focal and segmental sclerosing glomerulonephritis (GN); diffuse global proliferative lupus nephritis (LN)]. Extracapillary proliferation or crescent formation

**TABLE 50.1**

**INCIDENCE OF IDIOPATHIC NEPHROTIC SYNDROME IN ADULTS**

MCD—5%
FSGS—20%–25%
MN—25%–30%
MPGN—<5%
Other proliferative and sclerosing glomerulonephritides—15%–30%

is caused by the accumulations of macrophages, fibroblasts, proliferating epithelial cells, and fibrin within the Bowman space.

## CLINICAL MANIFESTATIONS OF GLOMERULAR DISEASES

Certain findings common to many glomerular diseases focus the differential diagnosis of unknown parenchymal renal diseases toward a glomerular origin. These include the presence of erythrocyte casts, dysmorphic erythrocytes, or both, in the urinary sediment and the presence of large amounts of albumin in the urine. In normal humans, the urinary excretion of albumin is less than 50 mg daily. Although increases in urinary protein excretion may come from the filtration of abnormal circulating proteins (such as light chains in multiple myeloma) or from the deficient proximal tubular resorption of normally filtered low-molecular-weight proteins (such as $\beta_2$-microglobulin), the most common cause of proteinuria, and specifically albuminuria, is glomerular injury. Protein excretion in proteinuria associated with glomerular disease may range from several hundred milligrams to more than 30 g daily. In some diseases associated with heavy proteinuria, such as minimal-change NS, albumin is the predominant protein found in the urine. In these diseases, the proteinuria is said to be highly "selective." In other glomerular diseases [such as focal segmental glomerulosclerosis (FSGS) and diabetes], the proteinuria, although still largely composed of albumin, contains many higher-weight molecular proteins as well and is said to be "nonselective" proteinuria. When proteinuria exceeds 3 to 3.5 g daily, patients commonly develop hypoalbuminemia, hyperlipidemia, edema, and other manifestations described as NS.

Although a small number of erythrocytes may appear in the urine of normal individuals, urinary excretion of more than 500 to 1,000 erythrocytes/mL defines abnormal hematuria. Although hematuria is common in many glomerular diseases, it is not, of course, specific for glomerular pathology. However, those erythrocytes that pass through gaps in the GBM and must undergo the osmotic changes imposed as they pass down the tubules become deformed. These dysmorphic erythrocytes are highly suggestive of glomerular pathology. Likewise, red blood cell casts, which form when erythrocytes pass the glomerular capillary barrier and become enmeshed in a proteinaceous matrix in the tubules, are highly suggestive of glomerular disease.

## NEPHROTIC SYNDROME

Nephrotic syndrome is defined by more than 3.0 to 3.5 g of protein in the urine daily accompanied by hypoalbuminemia, edema, and hyperlipidemia. In clinical practice, many nephrologists refer to "nephrotic range" proteinuria regardless of whether their patients have the other manifestations of the full NS because the latter are consequences of the proteinuria. Nephrotic proteinuria is always due predominantly to albuminuria.

Hypoalbuminemia is, in part, a consequence of urinary protein loss. It is also due to the catabolism of filtered albumin by the proximal tubule, as well as to redistribution of albumin within the body. The salt and volume retention in NS may occur through two different major mechanisms. In the classic theory, proteinuria leads to hypoalbuminemia, a low plasma oncotic pressure, and intravascular volume depletion. Subsequent underperfusion of the kidney stimulates the priming of sodium-retentive hormonal systems, such as the renin-angiotensin-aldosterone axis, which causes increased renal sodium and volume retention. In the peripheral capillaries, with normal hydrostatic pressures and decreased oncotic pressure, transcapillary fluid leakage and edema occur. In some patients, however, the intravascular volume has been measured and has been found to be increased along with the suppression of the renin-angiotensin-aldosterone axis. In an animal model of unilateral proteinuria created by the unilateral infusion of the aminonucleoside puromycin, evidence suggests a primary renal sodium retention at a distal nephron site, due to altered responsiveness to atrial natriuretic factor. Here, only the proteinuric kidney retains sodium and volume, and at a time when the animal is not yet hypoalbuminemic. Thus, local factors within the kidney may account for the volume retention of NS.

Epidemiologic studies strongly support an increased risk of atherosclerotic complications in conjunction with NS, related in part to the hyperlipidemia of the NS. Most patients have elevated levels of total and low-density lipoprotein cholesterol, and most have low or normal high-density lipoprotein cholesterol levels. Levels of lipoprotein(a) are elevated in patients with NS and revert to normal upon remission of proteinuria. Antihyperlipidemic medications are effective in favorably altering lipoprotein levels in NS. Aggressive therapy, especially with statins, to lower total cholesterol to 200 mg/dL and low-density lipoprotein cholesterol to 100 mg/dL has been recommended.

The initial evaluation of the patient with NS includes laboratory tests to define whether the patient has primary, idiopathic NS, or NS due to a secondary cause (e.g., measurement of fasting blood sugar, antinuclear antibodies, serum complement, etc.). Once secondary causes have been excluded, the treatment of the adult nephrotic patient usually requires a renal biopsy to define the pattern of glomerular involvement. In adults, NS is one of the most common conditions requiring renal biopsy. In virtually every study defining the role of the renal biopsy, those patients with heavy proteinuria are most likely to benefit in terms of a change from the prebiopsy diagnosis and in terms of changes in prognosis and therapy.

## Minimal-Change Disease

Minimal-change disease (MCD), also known as "nil" disease and as part of the older entity of "lipoid nephrosis," is the most common pattern of idiopathic NS in children and comprises approximately 5% of idiopathic NS in adults. Patients typically present with periorbital and peripheral edema. Although the onset of the disease is coincident with upper respiratory tract infections and allergies in some adults, most cases have no precipitating event. Severe proteinuria is typical, and values of less than 3.0 g of protein daily are uncommon. In children, the proteinuria is highly selective, whereas in adults selectivity of the proteinuria is less reliable. Up to 30% of adults with MCD also have hypertension and microscopic hematuria, although active urinary sediment with erythrocyte casts is not found. Many patients have mild to moderate azotemia related to intravascular volume depletion.

In true MCD, histopathology typically reveals no glomerular abnormalities in the light microscopic examination (hence the acronym "nil" disease, "nothing in light microscopy"). The tubules may show lipid droplet accumulation from absorbed lipoproteins (hence the older term *lipoid nephrosis*). Immunofluorescence staining and electron microscopy both show an absence of immune deposits. The GBM is normal, and an effacement or "fusion" of the visceral epithelial foot processes is noted along the entire distribution of every capillary loop.

The course of MCD in both children and adults is often one of relapses and responses to additional treatment. From 90% to 95% of children experience a remission of NS when treated with corticosteroids for 8 weeks. In adults, the response rate is somewhat lower, with 75% to 85% of patients responding to regimens of prednisone given daily (60 mg/day) or on alternate days (120 mg every other day). The time to clinical response may be slower in adults, and they should not be considered to be steroid resistant until no response has been observed after 16 weeks of treatment. Tapering of the steroid dose should begin 1 to several weeks after complete remission and should continue gradually over 1 to 2 months. Both children and adults are likely to have at least one relapse once steroids have been discontinued. Approximately 50% of children and 30% of adults experience relapse by 1 year, and the number increases to almost 80% and 50% by 5 years. Most clinicians treat the first relapse with a regimen similar to the initial treatment

regimen. Those patients who experience a third episode, or who become dependent on steroids (i.e., the prednisone dose cannot be decreased beyond a certain level without recurrence of proteinuria), may be successfully treated with a short course (2 to 4 months) of the alkylating agent cyclophosphamide (1.5 to 2.0 mg/kg per day). Up to 50% of patients who are so treated have a prolonged remission of NS (at least 5 years). The response rate is lower among steroid-dependent patients. Potential side effects include marrow suppression, alopecia, hemorrhagic cystitis, risk of infection, and gonadal toxicity. An alternative to an alkylating agent is low-dose cyclosporine (4 to 6 mg/kg per day), but this carries a potential risk of nephrotoxicity and a higher potential relapse rate.

## Focal Segmental Glomerulosclerosis

Over 20% of adults with idiopathic NS have FSGS. The incidence of FSGS has been dramatically increasing, and it is the most common pattern of idiopathic NS in African Americans. FSGS may be either idiopathic or secondary to a number of differing conditions (e.g., heroin nephropathy, HIV nephropathy, sickle cell nephropathy, reflux nephropathy, remnant kidneys, and the healed phase of focal GN, among others).

Patients with idiopathic FSGS typically present with either asymptomatic proteinuria or edema. Although the NS is present at presentation in two-thirds of adults, protein excretion may vary from less than 1 g/day to levels as high as 20 to 30 g/day. Proteinuria is typically nonselective. Hypertension is found in 30% to 50% and microscopic hematuria in 25% to 75% of these patients. The glomerular filtration rate (GFR) is decreased at presentation in 20% to 30% of patients. Complement levels and the results of other serologic tests are normal in FSGS.

The histologic diagnosis of FSGS depends on identifying within only some of the glomeruli (focal) those areas of glomerulosclerosis restricted to only some part of the glomerular tufts (segmental lesions). By immunofluorescence staining, immunoglobulin M (IgM) and C3 are commonly found in the areas of glomerular sclerosis and are felt to result from the entrapment of immunoglobulin and complement, components rather than from true immune complex deposition. By electron microscopy, fusion or effacement of the foot processes is found to some extent in all the glomeruli, even those unaffected by areas of segmental sclerosis, and no electron-dense immune deposits are present. In biopsy specimens taken early in the course of FSGS, when the GFR is preserved, few glomeruli with segmental sclerosing lesions are present, and almost no global glomerulosclerosis is seen. As renal function declines, repeat biopsy specimens will show many glomeruli with segmental or global sclerosis.

Although variable, the course of unresponsive FSGS is usually one of progressive proteinuria and declining GFR. Patients with asymptomatic proteinuria typically develop

NS over time. Only a minority of patients experience a spontaneous remission of proteinuria. Eventually, most patients develop ESRD in 5 to 20 years from presentation. Some patients with the collapsing variant (or malignant FSGS) have a more rapid course to ESRD in 2 to 3 years. Idiopathic FSGS may recur in the transplanted kidney and is then manifested by the occurrence of severe proteinuria and NS.

The treatment of FSGS in adults is controversial. Few randomized, controlled trials exist on which to base judgments. In general, patients with a sustained remission of their NS are unlikely to progress to ESRD, whereas those with unremitting NS are likely to progress. Risk factors suggesting a higher rate of progression to renal failure include heavier proteinuria, elevated creatinine levels, presence of interstitial scarring on biopsy specimens, African American race, and lack of responsiveness to an initial course of steroids. In older studies, only a small percentage of patients had a remission of proteinuria after treatment with corticosteroids or other immunosuppressives, and the relapse rate after treatment was high. Recent studies using more intensive and especially more prolonged immunosuppressive regimens with steroids or cytotoxics (cyclophosphamide 1 to 2 mg/kg per day) or both have achieved up to a 60% remission rate, with preservation of long-term renal function. A recent randomized, blinded controlled trial of cyclosporine (4 to 6 mg/kg per day for 6 months) in patients with steroid-resistant FSGS showed both a higher remission rate with treatment as well as better preservation of renal function at 4 years after therapy. Even patients whose disease is unresponsive to cytotoxic agents may show response to this therapy. Some patients, however, experience relapse when the therapy is stopped.

At present, many clinicians would not use immunosuppressive therapy for patients with subnephrotic levels of proteinuria and little damage apparent in renal biopsy specimens, treating these patients with angiotensin-converting enzyme (ACE) inhibitors or adrenergic receptor binders (ARBs) to reduce proteinuria and its side effects. For FSGS patients with NS and risk of progressive renal failure, a prolonged course of corticosteroids or other immunosuppressive medication would be used in the hopes of inducing a remission of the NS and preventing eventual ESRD.

### Membranous Nephropathy

Membranous nephropathy is the most common pattern of idiopathic NS in white Americans. It typically presents with the onset of proteinuria leading to periorbital and pedal edema. Hypertension and microhematuria are not infrequent findings, but renal function and GFR are usually normal at presentation. MN is the most common pattern of idiopathic NS to be associated with thrombotic events and especially with renal vein thrombosis. The presence of sudden flank pain, deterioration of renal function, or symptoms of pulmonary emboli in a patient with MN should prompt an investigation for renal vein thrombosis. In certain elderly patients with MN, an underlying carcinoma may be the occult cause of the renal lesion.

The course of MN is variable. In general, renal survival is more than 75% at 10 years. A spontaneous remission rate also occurs, which varies from 20% to 30%. The slow progression and spontaneous remission rate have confounded clinical treatment trials. Both a retrospective study and a controlled clinical trial suggested that short-term corticosteroid therapy led to a reduction in the number of patients progressing to renal insufficiency. Another study found that prolonged therapy with corticosteroids led not only to preservation of renal function but also to remissions of the NS. These studies have been criticized: Two of them lacked a control group, and a third study (a controlled trial) had an extremely rapid rate of progression toward renal insufficiency in the control group, which conferred an advantage on those patients receiving corticosteroids. Other studies have shown no benefit of corticosteroid regimens on the course of MN. A randomized well-performed controlled trial of pulse methylprednisolone followed by oral prednisone for 1 month alternating with 1 month of oral chlorambucil, each repeated for a total duration of 6 months of treatment, has reported a larger number of total remissions and better preservation of renal function. Other recent controlled studies using cytotoxic agents also have shown similar beneficial results. The use of cyclosporine in a double-blind randomized controlled trial of patients with steroid-resistant MN also has yielded higher remission rates than placebo.

At present, most clinicians treat only those subsets of MN patients who, in retrospective studies, have been found to have the highest rate of progression to renal failure (men, older patients, and those with a greater degrees of proteinuria). Whether to use corticosteroids, cytotoxic agents, cyclosporine, or a combination of therapies depends on the clinician's preference.

## ACUTE GLOMERULONEPHRITIS

### Immunoglobulin A Nephropathy

Immunoglobulin A (IgA) nephropathy was originally believed to be an uncommon and benign form of glomerulopathy (Berger's disease). It is now recognized as the most frequent form of idiopathic GN worldwide (comprising 15% to 40% of primary GN in parts of Europe and Asia) and clearly can progress to ESRD. In geographic areas where renal biopsies are commonly performed for milder urinary findings, a higher incidence of IgA nephropathy has been noted. In the United States, some centers report IgA nephropathy to comprise up to 20% of all primary GN. Although men with the disorder outnumber women, and the peak occurrence is in the second to third decade of life,

IgA nephropathy can occur in patients of both genders and all ages.

The diagnosis of IgA nephropathy is established by finding glomerular IgA deposits either as the dominant or codominant immunoglobulin on immunofluorescent microscopy. In addition to IgA, deposits of C3 and immunoglobulin G (IgG) are common. The light microscopic picture may vary from one of minimal change to mesangial proliferation to crescentic GN. The most common picture is mesangial hypercellularity. By electron microscopy, electron-dense deposits are typically found in the mesangial and paramesangial areas. The pathogenesis of IgA nephropathy is unknown. Although the predominant antibody appears to be composed of polymeric IgA1 originating in the secretory-mucosal system, the antigen to which it is directed is unknown. Environmental antigens, such as viral or other pathogens, and diet-related antigens have been proposed but remain unproven as causes. Which factors subsequent to the deposition of immune complexes containing IgA lead to the inflammatory and sclerosing glomerular features of the disease are also unknown.

IgA nephropathy often presents with one of two syndromes: asymptomatic microscopically apparent hematuria or proteinuria, or both (most common in adults), or episodic gross hematuria after upper respiratory tract and other infections or exercise (most common in children). The course of IgA nephropathy is variable. Most patients show no decline in GFR over decades, whereas some develop NS, hypertension, and renal failure. Hypertension is present in 20% to 50% of patients. Increased serum IgA levels do not correlate with the course of the disease.

Factors predictive of a poor outcome in IgA nephropathy may include:

- Older age at onset
- Absence of gross hematuria
- Presence of hypertension
- Persistent and severe proteinuria
- Male sex
- A reduced GFR and elevated serum creatinine level
- Certain histologic features on renal biopsy specimens, including severe proliferation and sclerosis, severe tubulointerstitial damage, and extracapillary glomerular proliferation (i.e., crescent formation)

Renal survival is estimated at 85% to 90% at 10 years and 75% to 80% at 20 years.

The treatment of IgA nephropathy has included efforts to prevent antigenic stimulation or the entry of environmental stimulants, including the use of broad-spectrum antibiotics (e.g., doxycycline), tonsillectomy, and dietary manipulations to eliminate certain dietary antigens (e.g., gluten). With few exceptions, these attempts have not been successful. The benefits of treatment with glucocorticoids and other immunosuppressives are far from clear for most patients with IgA nephropathy. In a recent controlled trial of

6 months of corticosteroid therapy in patients with progressive IgA nephropathy, the treated group had improved renal function over 5 years of follow-up. Other efforts at immunosuppression have included combinations of cyclophosphamide, dipyridamole, and warfarin sodium, which may have given beneficial effects in some patients when chronically administered for years. Immunosuppressive therapy using cytotoxic agents and pulse methylprednisolone (Solumedrol) has also been used for patients with crescentic lesions. At least one recent trial of Ω-fish oils has shown improved renal survival and decreased proteinuria in IgA nephropathy, but two smaller trials showed no beneficial effect of treatment. In all trials, the use of ACE inhibitors has been shown to be beneficial in reducing proteinuria and probably the progression to renal failure. With no clearly proven therapy, many clinicians choose to give only blockers of the renin-angiotensin system (e.g., ACE inhibitors or adrenergic receptor binders) to most patients with IgA nephropathy and reserve therapy for only those patients at highest risk for progression to renal failure.

## Idiopathic Membranoproliferative Glomerulonephritis

Idiopathic membranoproliferative GN (MPGN), or mesangiocapillary GN, is an uncommon glomerular disease that may present in three histologic forms, depending on where the electron-dense deposits are located along the GBM (MPGN types 1, 2, and 3). In series in which biopsies are performed, it comprises only a small percentage of glomerular disease.

By light microscopy, the lesions of types 1, 2, and 3 MPGN look the same and include diffuse mesangial proliferation, infiltration of the glomerular tuft by mononuclear cells, and exaggeration of the lobular pattern of the glomerular tufts with reduplication of the basement membrane, which results in a double contour or "tram track" appearance. By immunofluorescent assay, diffuse granular GBM deposits of C3 and often of IgG, IgA, and IgM are present. Electron microscopy clearly distinguishes the three patterns of MPGN. Type 1 has subendothelial and mesangial deposits. Type 2 has broad, dense, intramembranous deposits along the GBM, Bowman capsule, and tubular basement membranes. Type 3 has subepithelial deposits and intramembranous deposits in addition to subendothelial and mesangial deposits.

The pathogenesis of the idiopathic forms of this type of GN is by definition unknown. By light microscopy, similar patterns of glomerular damage have been seen in association with certain infectious agents (HCV), autoimmune disease (systemic lupus erythematosus, or SLE), and disease of intraglomerular coagulation. Idiopathic MPGN is a rare disease, and many patients with this lesion develop SLE or are found to test positive for HCV with cryoglobulinemia. Type 2 MPGN, also known as *dense deposit disease*, has been called an autoimmune disorder, with an autoantibody (an

IgG, C3 nephritic factor) directed against C3bBb, the alternate pathway C3 convertase. Because degradation of the enzyme is prevented, increased activation and consumption of complement are noted in dense deposit disease.

Although MPGN may present with asymptomatic microhematuria and proteinuria in some patients, most patients present with NS. Other patients may present with an acute nephritic picture with active urinary sediment, renal insufficiency, and hypertension. Most patients have low complement values. Most studies have found similar results for the various patterns of MPGN and have treated them as one disease entity. Attempts to treat MPGN have included the use of corticosteroids and other immunosuppressive medications, and the use of anticoagulants and antiplatelet agents to minimize glomerular damage from coagulation. No therapy has been conclusively proven to be effective in adults with MPGN. In children, long-term corticosteroid therapy has led to more remissions of NS and the preservation of renal function.

## Rapidly Progressive Glomerulonephritis

Rapidly progressive GN (RPGN) comprises a group of glomerulonephritides that have in common a progression to renal failure in a matter of weeks to months and the presence of extensive extracapillary proliferation (i.e., crescent formation) in a large percentage of the glomeruli. RPGN thus includes renal diseases with different etiologies, pathogeneses, and clinical presentations. RPGN has been divided into three patterns, defined by immunologic pathogenesis: type I, characterized by anti-GBM disease; type II, characterized by immune complex deposition (e.g., SLE, poststreptococcal GN, etc.); and type III, characterized by the absence of immune deposits or anti-GBM antibodies (i.e., pauci-immune). Many cases in the latter group fall into the category of antineutrophil cytoplasmic antibody (ANCA)–positive RPGN. In the past, with the exception of those with postinfectious RPGN, prognosis was generally poor for most patients, regardless of pathogenesis. This prognosis has dramatically changed for some patterns of RPGN.

### Anti–Glomerular Basement Membrane Disease

Anti-GBM disease is caused by circulating antibodies that are directed against the noncollagenous domain of type IV collagen and that damage the GBM. This leads to an inflammatory response, to breaks in the GBM, and to the formation of a proliferative and often crescentic GN. If the anti-GBM antibodies cross-react with and cause damage to the basement membrane of pulmonary capillaries, the patient develops pulmonary hemorrhage and hemoptysis. The association of anti-GBM antibody–mediated damage to the kidneys and lungs is called *Goodpasture's syndrome*. The disease most commonly affects young adults, and men are far more commonly affected than women. The presentation is a nephritic picture with hypertension, edema,

hematuria and active urinary sediment, and reduced renal function. Renal function may deteriorate from normal to dialysis-requiring levels in a matter of days to weeks. Patients with pulmonary involvement may have life-threatening hemoptysis. The course of the disease, once it has progressed to renal failure, is usually one of permanent renal dysfunction. If treatment is started early in the course of the disease, patients may regain considerable kidney function.

The pathology of anti-GBM disease shows a proliferative GN, often with severe extracapillary involvement of the Bowman space by crescent formation. By immunofluorescent study, a linear deposition of immunoglobulin is present along the GBM. Electron microscopy does not show any electron-dense deposits.

The treatment of type I RPGN mediated by anti-GBM antibodies includes intensive therapy to reduce the production of anti-GBM antibodies (using immunosuppressive agents such as cyclophosphamide or azathioprine and corticosteroids) combined with plasmapheresis to remove circulating anti-GBM antibodies. Therapy is most effective in patients who have less extensive crescent formation and who have a preserved GFR. Some patients with advanced renal failure, however, even those requiring dialysis, have responded to this form of treatment. Rapid intensive therapy is necessary to prevent irreversible renal damage.

### Immune Complex Rapidly Progressive Glomerulonephritis

Type II RPGN, associated with immune complex–mediated damage to the glomeruli, may occur within a spectrum of diseases from primary glomerulopathies, such as IgA nephropathy and MPGN, to postinfectious GN to SLE. The treatment of IgA nephropathy and MPGN is discussed earlier. Most cases of postinfectious GN resolve with successful treatment of the underlying infection. Here, the potential hazards of immunosuppressive treatment and the limited data available on its benefit should prompt caution in the use of this therapeutic option. The treatment of severe SLE is dealt with in a later section.

### Pauci-immune Rapidly Progressive Glomerulonephritis and Vasculitis-Associated Rapidly Progressive Glomerulonephritis

Patients with pauci-immune type III RPGN include those with and without evidence of systemic vasculitis. Patients often present with progressive renal failure and a nephritic picture with hematuria, oliguria, and hypertension. Many patients have circulating antibodies directed against neutrophil cytoplasmic antigens (ANCA). Patients who test positive for perinuclear ANCA more often have a clinical picture akin to polyarteritis (with arthritis, skin involvement with leukocytoclastic angiitis, and constitutional and systemic signs), whereas those who test positive for C-ANCA are more likely to have granulomatous disease associated with the GN (akin to Wegener's granulomatosis). Considerable overlap occurs between these groups. As in all forms of RPGN, renal function may deteriorate rapidly. An elevated serum creatinine level and the presence of hypertension are risk factors for poor renal outcome. In a study by Falk et al. of the course of ANCA-associated GN and systemic vasculitis, no difference in renal or patient survival was noted between patients with isolated renal disease and those with systemic involvement. With the use of oral cyclophosphamide in addition to corticosteroids, diseases such as Wegener's granulomatosis and polyarteritis nodosa have shown markedly improved survival rates. For example, in the National Institutes of Health (NIH) series of 158 patients with Wegener's granulomatosis, more than 90% experienced marked improvement, and 75% experienced a complete remission. These excellent results includes some patients with crescentic GN, and only 11% of these patients eventually required dialysis. More recently, successful results have been reported with the use of steroids plus cytotoxic agents, even in oliguric patients and those who are already dialysis dependent. It is clear that pauci-immune RPGN has the most favorable response rate of all patterns of RPGN. It responds well to a number of different immunosuppressive regimens, including pulse steroids and cyclophosphamide given orally or intravenously. The therapeutic regimen of choice and the optimal duration of therapy must be determined in controlled trials.

## GLOMERULAR INVOLVEMENT IN SYSTEMIC DISEASES

### Diabetes Mellitus

Diabetic nephropathy is the most common cause of ESRD in the United States, with more than 40% of all new ESRD patients having diabetes. From 25% to 40% of individuals with insulin-dependent (type I) diabetes develop nephropathy. The course is characterized initially by glomerular hyperfiltration with a normal serum creatinine level but with microalbuminuria, then by progressively increasing proteinuria and NS, and a slow decrease in GFR. Recent evidence supports a similar renal course for those with non–insulin-dependent (type II) diabetes. The glomerular histopathologic changes in both are similar, with thickening of the GBM, mesangial sclerosis, nodular intercapillary glomerulosclerosis (Kimmelstiel-Wilson nodules), and microaneurysms of the glomerular capillaries.

Recent studies have documented dramatic improvement in altering the progression of diabetic renal disease through a variety of interventions, including control of hyperglycemia, control of blood pressure, and the use of ACE inhibition and angiotensin II receptor blockers. Poor glycemic control is associated with an increased incidence of nephropathy. The Diabetes Control and Complication Trial documented decreased retinopathy and nephropathy

in the incidence of fixed microalbuminuria and clinical proteinuria among patients with type I diabetes treated with intensive glucose control. In patients with type I diabetes, blood pressure control using a variety of antihypertensives leads to decreased proteinuria and a slowing of the rate of GFR decline. In diabetic persons, the use of ACE inhibitors has been shown to reduce microalbuminuria and clinical proteinuria in both proteinuric and nephrotic patients with type I and type II diabetes. In a trial involving more than 400 individuals with type I diabetes with protein excretion of more than 500 mg daily and a serum creatinine level of less than 2.5 mg/dL, the use of captopril three times a day led to amelioration of the decline in GFR, compared with that in control patients, despite comparable blood pressure control in the latter group. In a smaller study involving patients with type II diabetes who had milder proteinuria, the group receiving ACE inhibitors had better-preserved renal function and less proteinuria at 5 years follow-up. The use of angiotensin II receptor antagonists also decreases proteinuria in nephrotic patients. Two large randomized blinded trials, each enrolling more than 1,500 patients with adult-onset diabetes and proteinuria, have shown less progression to renal failure with use of angiotensin II receptor blockers. Studies treating diabetic animals and humans with agents to prevent the cross-linking of advanced glycosylation end products have also been promising, showing reduction in GBM thickening and proteinuria.

### Systemic Lupus Erythematosus

Renal involvement greatly influences the disease course and choice of treatment of lupus patients. The incidence of clinically detectable renal disease varies from 15% to 75% of patients with SLE. Histologic evidence of renal involvement in SLE is found in the vast majority of biopsy specimens when studied by light microscopy, immunofluorescence, and electron microscopy, even in the absence of clinical renal disease. The World Health Organization (WHO) classification of LN has been used successfully for both clinical and research activities. The WHO classes correlate well with the clinical picture of the patients at biopsy. These classes also help define the clinical course of the patient and provide a guide to therapy.

Patients with WHO class I (normal) biopsy specimens are extremely rare. Such biopsy results are found only in patients without clinical renal findings very early in the course of their disease. Patients with WHO class II (mesangial involvement) biopsy specimens usually have only mild clinical renal disease. These patients are virtually never nephrotic but may have active serologic findings. They have an excellent long-term prognosis and require no treatment directed at their renal lesions. Patients with WHO class III lesions (focal proliferative LN) have more active sediment changes, increased proteinuria, and often active serologic findings. Approximately one-fourth are nephrotic and, in some, the lesions transform or evolve into a class IV pattern. Patients with WHO class IV (diffuse proliferative) LN have the most severe renal involvement, with active sediment, hypertension, heavy proteinuria, frequent NS, and often a reduction of GFR. They have the worst prognosis. Patients with WHO class V (membranous) lesions usually present with NS sometime before fulfilling the American Rheumatism Association criteria for SLE. These patients are typically nephrotic, with inactive serologic findings. Although their short-term prognosis is good, they can progress to renal failure over many years. Membranous LN is the only pattern commonly associated with renal vein thrombosis.

In general, all patients with class IV lesions on biopsy deserve vigorous therapy for their LN. Many patients with class III LN (especially those with active necrotizing lesions and large amounts of subendothelial deposits) also would benefit from such therapy. The optimal therapy for patients with class V lesions is less clear. Standard vigorous treatment of severe LN now includes the use of steroids plus cyclophosphamide, usually given as monthly intravenous boluses. Intravenous pulse methylprednisolone has been shown to be less effective than intravenous cyclophosphamide in preventing long-term renal failure. Plasmapheresis proved unsuccessful in a major clinical controlled trial of more than 80 patients with severe LN.

Currently, a regimen of once-monthly intravenous cyclophosphamide (Cytoxan) therapy has been used for class IV LN. The author and others have found this regimen of monthly intravenous cyclophosphamide therapy with rapid steroid taper to give good short-term results, with a rapid resolution of serologic and clinical abnormalities, decreases in proteinuria and remissions of the NS, and stabilization of serum creatinine level. A recent trial by the NIH has found similar efficacy for this regimen.

Initial trials with cyclosporine in more than 100 SLE patients have shown promising results. Yet, due to poor patient selection, poor study design, or concurrent therapy, conclusions about this form of treatment remain speculative.

## Amyloidosis

Amyloidosis is a generic term for a group of diseases in which the extracellular deposition of one of a number of insoluble fibrillar proteins occurs in a characteristic β-pleated sheet configuration. One of the two most common forms of amyloidosis is primary amyloidosis, now called *light chain–associated (AL) amyloidosis*, due to a plasma-cell dyscrasia that overproduces a monoclonal immunoglobulin light chain. Of AL amyloid patients, 20% have overt myeloma, whereas 10% to 15% of myeloma patients have AL amyloidosis. AL fibrils are derived predominantly from the variable portion of the light chain. Two-thirds to four-fifths of patients with AL amyloid who

have a monoclonal protein have overproduction of a λ-light chain. Renal involvement is one of the most common manifestations of AL amyloid, usually presenting as heavy albuminuria and the NS.

Secondary amyloidosis (synonymous with AA amyloidosis) is associated with high circulating levels and the deposition of the nonimmunoglobulin serum amyloid A protein (a 12-kd high-density lipoprotein apoprotein synthesized by hepatocytes as an acute-phase reactant in disease states). AA amyloidosis occurs in chronic infections and inflammatory states, including rheumatoid arthritis, ankylosing spondylitis, tuberculosis, osteomyelitis, and intravenous drug abuse. Renal amyloidosis presents with proteinuria and NS, and progresses to renal insufficiency and renal failure in the majority of cases.

Amyloid deposits are predominantly found within the glomeruli and often appear as amorphous, eosinophilic extracellular nodules. They also may be found deposited in the tubular basement membranes, the interstitium, and the vessels. They stain positively with Congo red and under polarized light display apple-green birefringence. Under electron microscopy, amyloid appears as nonbranching rigid fibrils 8 to 10 nm in diameter.

No specific effective therapy is available for renal amyloidosis. In patients with AL amyloidosis, both chemotherapy directed at the abnormal clone of B cells (e.g., melphalan and prednisone) and colchicine have been shown to have beneficial results. In a study at the Mayo Clinic, Kyle et al. found that of 100 patients with primary amyloidosis treated with either melphalan and prednisone or colchicine, the chemotherapy treatment was superior. Some patients with primary amyloidosis, however, have responded with complete remissions of their NS using either regimen. In the majority of the cases, the amyloidosis has been progressive, and organ system involvement continues. Survival times of 1 or 2 years are typical for treated patients with AL amyloidosis. Dialysis, using either hemodialysis or peritoneal dialysis, and transplantation have been effective in small numbers of patients with primary amyloidosis and ESRD. Recently, bone marrow transplantation has been used to treat patients with AL amyloidosis.

## Human Immunodeficiency Virus Infection

More than 200,000 cases of acquired immunodeficiency syndrome (AIDS) have occurred in the United States, and more than 40,000 deaths due to this disease. Some cities, such as New York City, have reported more than 10,000 cases of AIDS, and up to 500,000 persons in the New York metropolitan area have been reported to be infected with the virus. Many studies have found populations of intravenous drug abusers to have a 60% to 85% carriage rate for HIV. Infection with this virus has been associated with a number of patterns of renal disease, including acute renal failure and a unique form of glomerulopathy now called *HIV nephropathy*.

## Acute Renal Failure

The course of disease in patients with acute renal failure and AIDS has been described by a number of investigators. Rao et al., at Downstate Medical Center, have reported the disease course in 23 such patients, and Valeri et al. reviewed 88 episodes of acute renal failure in 449 AIDS patients at Bellevue Hospital in New York City. The most common precipitating factors for acute renal failure in both studies included medications [pentamidine isethionate, aminoglycosides, trimethoprim-sulfamethoxazole, nonsteroidal anti-inflammatory drugs (NSAIDs)] and pyrexia and dehydration superimposed on sepsis, hypotension, and respiratory failure. Dialysis support is indicated for the AIDS patient with acute renal failure.

## Human Immunodeficiency Virus Nephropathy

Several histologic patterns of glomerulopathy have been seen in patients with AIDS or HIV infection. These include minimal-change pattern, mesangial hyperplasia, glomerulopathies associated with immune complex deposition or IgA deposition or both, and, most important, HIV nephropathy. HIV nephropathy is a unique pattern of glomerulopathy in HIV-infected patients characterized by heavy proteinuria and a rapid progression to renal failure; it has characteristic ultrasonographic and renal biopsy findings. HIV nephropathy is a better term than AIDS nephropathy because this glomerulopathy may occur in patients with AIDS and AIDS-related complex, as well as in asymptomatic HIV carriers. Although HIV nephropathy has a prevalence of only 3% to 7% in unselected autopsy series, it is by far the most common lesion found in HIV-infected patients undergoing renal biopsy. The classic clinical features of HIV nephropathy include a higher incidence among African Americans, heavy proteinuria (usually with NS), renal insufficiency and a rapid progression to ESRD, and large echogenic kidneys on ultrasonography.

Clinical and histologic data suggest that HIV nephropathy and heroin nephropathy are distinct entities (Table 50.2).

The pathology of HIV nephropathy shows several features distinct from classic FSGS or heroin nephropathy. On light microscopy, diffuse global glomerulosclerosis and collapse is common, with striking visceral epithelial cell hypertrophy showing large cytoplasmic vacuoles and resorption droplets. Severe tubulointerstitial changes also occur, with interstitial inflammation, edema, microcystic dilatation of tubules, and severe tubular degenerative changes. On electron microscopy, tubuloreticular inclusions are prevalent in the glomerular endothelium.

The optimal treatment of HIV nephropathy remains unclear. At present, triple highly active antiretroviral therapy is indicated for all patients. Likewise, ACE inhibitors are helpful as long as the potassium and creatinine levels do not rise markedly. The use of any immunosuppressive therapy remains controversial. Dialysis and support seem appropriate for those patients with HIV nephropathy but without the full-blown AIDS syndrome. Whether dialysis support prolongs useful life once AIDS has developed is open to debate.

## Hepatitis C Virus Infection

The incidence of HCV infection varies in different geographic locations from 0.3% in Canada and northern Europe, to 0.6% in the United States, to 1.2% to 1.5% in Japan and southern Europe, to 3.5% to 7.0% in parts of Africa. In high-risk groups, the incidence is much higher: 60% to 90% of persons with hemophilia, 60% to 70% of intravenous drug abusers, and as many as 15% to 25% of certain dialysis populations.

## Cryoglobulinemia and Hepatitis C Virus

HCV infection has been associated with arthritis, sicca symptoms, corneal ulcerations, porphyria, autoimmune thyroiditis, polyarteritis, as well as mixed cryoglobulinemia associated with immune complex GN. Cryoglobulinemia refers to a pathologic condition caused by the production of circulating immunoglobulins that precipitate on cooling and resolubilize on warming. Cryoglobulinemia is associated with a variety of infections, as well as collagen-vascular disease and lymphoproliferative diseases. Cryoglobulins

### TABLE 50.2

#### HUMAN IMMUNODEFICIENCY VIRUS (HIV) NEPHROPATHY VERSUS HEROIN NEPHROPATHY

|  | HIV Nephropathy | Heroin Nephropathy |
| --- | --- | --- |
| Epidemiology | One-third to one-half intravenous drug abusers | All intravenous drug abusers |
| Pathology | Collapsing FS and GS on light microscopy | Classic focal segmental glomerular sclerosis |
| Progression to end-stage renal disease | Rapid | Moderate |

FS, focal sclerosis; GS, global sclerosis.

have been divided into three major groups based on the nature of the circulating immunoglobulins. In type I cryoglobulinemia, the cryoglobulin is a single monoclonal immunoglobulin, usually without associated antibody activity. This type is found most often in patients with myeloma and Waldenström macroglobulinemia. Both type II and type III cryoglobulinemia are characterized by mixed cryoglobulins, containing a least two immunoglobulins. In type II, a monoclonal IgM immunoglobulin is directed against polyclonal IgG and has rheumatoid factor activity. In type III, the antiglobulin is polyclonal, with both polyclonal IgG and IgM in most cases. To establish a diagnosis of cryoglobulinemia, the offending cryoglobulins must be demonstrated. The cryoglobulin must be solubilized in a warmed blood sample until the test is run. Hypocomplementemia, especially of the early components C1q to C4, is a characteristic and often helpful finding.

In the past, no clear etiology was apparent in 30% of all mixed cryoglobulinemias, and the name "essential mixed cryoglobulinemia" was appropriate. The disease was uncommon but not rare, and it occurred predominantly in adult women. The systemic manifestation of mixed cryoglobulinemia include weakness, malaise, Raynaud's phenomenon, arthralgia and arthritis, hepatosplenomegaly presenting with abnormal liver function test results in two-thirds to three-fourths of patients, peripheral neuropathy, and purpuric-vasculitic skin lesions. In up to one-fourth to one-third of patients, an acute nephritic condition with hematuria, hypertension, proteinuria, and acute renal insufficiency develops. An oliguric, RPGN is present only rarely, and approximately 20% of patients present with NS. In the majority of patients with renal involvement, the disease has a slow, indolent renal course characterized by proteinuria, hypertension, hematuria, and renal insufficiency.

Recent reports have clearly documented HCV as a major cause of cryoglobulin production in many, if not most, patients previously believed to have essential mixed cryoglobulinemia. Antibodies to HCV antigens have been documented in the sera, and HCV RNA and anti-HCV antibodies are enriched in the cryoglobulins of these patients.

### Pathogenesis and Pathology
The pathogenesis and pathology of hepatitic C virus cryoglobulin glomerulonephritis and hepatitic C virus membranoproliferative glomerulonephritis is similar.

In cryoglobulinemia, immunoglobulin complexes deposit in the glomeruli, binding complement and inciting a proliferative response. The serum cryoglobulin clearly has been shown to participate in the formation of the glomerular immune complex. Not all patients with HCV infection and GN have detectable cryoglobulins in the serum and the classic histopathology of cryoglobulinemic MPGN. Mesangial proliferative GN (often with IgA deposits), MN, diffuse proliferative GN, a sclerosing GN, and especially MPGN resembling idiopathic type 1 MPGN all have been reported. Although patients with hepatitis B

virus infection most commonly have the membranous pattern of glomerulopathy, the MPGN pattern is most common with HCV infection. Patients with HCV and MPGN typically present with proteinuria and often NS. At least 30% to 40% of these patients do not have detectable cryoglobulins. Only one-half of these patients have symptoms suggestive of cryoglobulinemia (purpura, arthritis, etc.). Only 20% have signs of liver disease, but as many as two-thirds have mild elevations of transaminase levels. Once again, total hemolytic complement C3, and especially C4, is depressed. The pathology of HCV MPGN is similar to that of idiopathic type 1 MPGN in most cases, although some patients have subepithelial deposits as well (type 3 MPGN pattern) and some have sclerosing features.

### Treatment of Hepatitic C Virus Glomerulonephritis
Recent studies involving patients with HCV-related cryoglobulinemic GN have evaluated the use of interferon-α or combined interferon and ribavirin and have shown improvement of both renal and liver disease. In these studies, patients had decreased proteinuria and improved GFR. The number of patients studied so far is small, however. In one trial by Misiani et al., involving 53 patients with HCV-associated type II cryoglobulinemia, the 27 patients treated with recombinant interferon-α for 6 months showed significant improvement in cutaneous vasculitis, circulating cryoglobulin levels, and renal function. Clinical response correlated closely with the disappearance of HCV from the blood. Other groups have shown patients to have decreasing proteinuria and normalization of liver function test results, but to have no major improvements in GFR. Relapses after the discontinuance of therapy occurred in most patients. Longer treatment, for up to 1 year, using interferon-α or higher-dose therapy is being tried in patients with an initial response to treatment. In some patients with severe progressive renal disease, immunosuppressive therapy clearly has been used successfully. The potential benefits of immunosuppressive therapy must be weighed against the potential hazards of activating viral replication.

## DRUG-INDUCED ACUTE INTERSTITIAL NEPHRITIS

In recent years it has become clear that not all acute interstitial nephritides (AINs) are caused by bacterial invasion of the kidney. Among the common types of AIN is drug-induced AIN. The distinct clinical picture, pathology, and clinical course of this form of acute renal failure has been defined especially from the study of patients receiving β-lactam antibiotics of the penicillin or cephalosporin classes.

The renal histology reveals predominantly edema and interstitial infiltrates of mononuclear cells and eosinophils without marked fibrosis and with only patchy tubular damage. In general, glomerular and vascular changes are not prominent. More than 50 medications have been associated with AIN, and the list of offending drugs grows each year.

## Penicillin

Despite the numerous implicated drugs, the β-lactam antibiotics—the penicillins and cephalosporins—remain among the foremost offenders. It is apparent that all agents of the β-lactam group are capable of producing this lesion. β-Lactam–related AIN occurs in all decades of life. The dosage of the β-lactam antibiotic has usually not been excessive; however, the duration of therapy is often prolonged, with more than three-fourths of patients receiving more than 10 days of therapy and more than one-third receiving more than 20 days of therapy.

The clinical features of penicillin-associated AIN include the hypersensitivity triad of rash (43%), secondary fever (77%), and eosinophilia (80%). Fewer than one-third of patients have the complete triad at diagnosis, however, and one must not wait for this full picture to develop before making a presumptive diagnosis of drug-related AIN. Of the urinary findings, mild proteinuria and pyuria are common but not specific. Nephrotic-range proteinuria and urinary red blood cell casts are rare in this nonglomerular disease and can usually be explained by incidental concomitant glomerular pathology. Hematuria is a cardinal feature of penicillin-associated AIN; it is present in more than 90% of cases and is macroscopic in one-third. The finding of urinary eosinophiluria on Wright's or Hansel's stain of the urinary sediment is often present. Although its significance (sensitivity and specificity) remains unclear at present, a recent study suggests eosinophiluria, in which eosinophils comprise more than 5% of the total urinary leukocytes, to be strongly suggestive of AIN. Eosinophiluria has also been noted in RPGN, cystitis, and prostatitis. The majority of patients have nonoliguric renal failure and never have less than 400 mL of urine volume per day. Recently, gallium scanning has been suggested as a screening test to distinguish drug-induced AIN from renal failure due to acute tubular necrosis.

The histopathology shows patchy tubular damage, interstitial edema, and infiltrates of mononuclear cells and often eosinophils. Of the 40 cases reported using immunofluorescence analysis, only 11 clearly showed the presence of immunoglobulins, complement, or both along the tubular basement membranes or within the interstitium. Electron microscopy has only rarely shown electron-dense deposits along the tubular basement membranes.

Although the pathogenesis of penicillin-associated AIN remains to be defined, good evidence suggests an allergic–immunologic mechanism of renal damage. The small number of patients afflicted despite the extensive use of these drugs; recurrences on rechallenge with another β-lactam drug; the hypersensitivity features of rash, fever, and eosinophilia; and the histopathologic features found in

## TABLE 50.3

### SERUM COMPLEMENT LEVELS IN GLOMERULAR DISEASES

*Diseases with Reduced Complement Levels*
Postinfectious GN (poststreptococcal GN, subacute bacterial endocarditis, visceral abscesses) SLE
Cryoglobulinemia
Idiopathic MPGN

*Diseases Associated with Normal Serum Complement Levels*
Minimal-change NS, focal segmental glomerular sclerosis, MN
  IgA nephropathy, Henoch-Schönlein purpura
Anti-GBM disease
Pauci-immune RPGN, polyarteritis nodosa, Wegener's granulomatosis

---

many cases all support an allergic–immunologic mechanism. The first step may be the binding of drug hapten to kidney structural protein, either tubular or interstitial. Subsequently, a humoral response, with the development of anti–tubular basement membrane antibodies to combined drug hapten and kidney protein, may damage the kidney. In most cases, no evidence suggests such a response (negative immunofluorescent staining results, normal serum complement levels lack of circulating anti–tubular basement membrane or anti–drug antibodies), and a cell-mediated cytotoxic reaction may be the cause of ultimate renal damage. As recently elucidated by Nielson, the pathogenesis may actually be far more complex. Table 50.3 shows the serum complement levels of various glomerular diseases.

The treatment of penicillin-associated AIN includes prompt discontinuation of the drug and avoidance of rechallenge with other β-lactam agents that may lead to a recrudescence of hypersensitivity symptoms and renal failure. Dialysis and good supportive care are crucial because the majority of patients recover good renal function. The use of corticosteroids is controversial. Anecdotal reports of dramatic reversal of renal failure and two partially controlled studies support their use, but rigorous proof of their benefit is lacking, and the hazards of steroid therapy in such a population are well recognized. The use of other immunosuppressive agents remains unproven and has been reported in isolated cases only.

## Other Antimicrobial Agents

Drug-induced AIN has been well documented in several cases of sulfonamide use. Of special concern, the widely used antimicrobial combination of trimethoprim-sulfamethoxazole can produce this form of renal damage. Rifampin use is associated with a unique pattern of acute renal failure. In more than 60 patients who received either intermittent or discontinuous therapy, on rechallenge with rifampin there occurred the sudden onset of fever, flank pain, hematuria, and acute renal failure. Histopathologic findings range from those of classic AIN to a picture indistinguishable from that of ATN. It is clearly wise to avoid the intermittent or discontinuous use of this drug. The quinolone antibiotics have been well documented to produce AIN.

## Diuretics

Diuretics, including the thiazides and chlorthalidone, furosemide, and ticrynafen, have all been well documented to cause AIN. This is a rare occurrence, usually found in patients with prior renal disease (NS, hypertension). Patients present with the classic hypersensitivity features of rash, fever, and eosinophilia. The AIN responds readily to discontinuance of the drug and corticosteroid therapy.

## Nonsteroidal Anti-inflammatory Drugs

The NSAIDs may produce salt and water retention, decreased renal blood flow and GFR, and hyperkalemia associated with hyporenin hypoaldosteronism, perhaps all due to inhibition of prostaglandins. They also can cause an AIN that presents with a number of unique features. The population developing AIN is usually the older age group (fifties to eighties), despite the fact that many young patients receive these drugs. Patients typically have a prolonged exposure to the drugs (months to years) before developing AIN. The hypersensitivity features of rash, fever, and eosinophilia are rare, as are hematuria and eosinophiluria. This is true even when AIN with interstitial eosinophilia is found on renal biopsy. Perhaps the peripheral hypersensitivity features of the disease are modified by the analgesic-antipyretic nature of these drugs. Finally, AIN caused by the NSAIDs has frequently been associated with minimal-change NS. The drug-induced nature of this lesion is clear: "minimal change" is the exclusive pattern of NS reported (despite the fact that it comprises less than 20% of idiopathic NS in this age group); its onset coincides with the onset of ARF from AIN. The NS and AIN remit several weeks after discontinuance of the NSAID, regardless of whether steroid therapy is given. Why AIN caused by NSAIDs should uniquely be associated with minimal-change NS is not known.

## Other Drugs Associated with Acute Interstitial Nephritis

The widely used drug cimetidine has caused an AIN pattern of renal failure, as has the uricosuric antiplatelet agent sulfinpyrazone. Virtually no area of medical therapy is free from medications that can produce AIN. Greater awareness of the clinical picture and course of AIN will surely implicate an increasing number of medications, but may also lead to appropriate interventions for this reversible form of acute renal failure.

## MEDICATION-INDUCED CHRONIC INTERSTITIAL NEPHRITIS

The use of certain medications has been associated with the development of chronic renal insufficiency and chronic interstitial damage. In general, the relationship between the drug use and the renal lesions often has been more difficult to define than that of drug-induced AIN. This is related in part to the slower disease process and its insidious nature and to the complexity of the medication regimens of many of the patients developing such lesions. Several important groups of medications indicted as causing chronic interstitial nephritis include the analgesics phenacetin, acetaminophen, and aspirin; lithium; and the antineoplastic chemotherapeutic agents cisplatin, methyl-cyclohexylchloroethylnitrosourea and bis-chloroethylnitrosourea.

Analgesic agents have been extensively used in over-the-counter preparations in recent decades, and concern about their nephrotoxic potential has generated considerable attention and controversy. The incidence of analgesic nephropathy varies greatly among countries and even within regions of one country. In general, those countries with a higher per capita consumption of phenacetin and other analgesic compounds have had a higher incidence of analgesic nephropathy. Recent studies have documented analgesic nephropathy as the cause of ESRD in more than 16% of ESRD patients in West Germany, 18% of ESRD patients in Belgium, and 13% of all ESRD patients in Australia. In the United States, reports vary from an incidence of more than 10% in the Southeast to a low of only a few percent elsewhere. The exact nature of the offending analgesic or combinations of analgesics remains to be defined. Dubach's well-controlled study involving more than 600 middle-aged Swiss working women clearly documented a higher incidence of renal insufficiency as well as an increased mortality due to urinary tract disease and cardiovascular disease in a phenacetin-consuming population. A recent retrospective case-control study in North Carolina also found significantly more renal disease in consumers of analgesics than in the control population. The risk of renal disease was increased with daily consumption of phenacetin and acetaminophen, but not with the daily use of aspirin. This study confirms the risk of renal damage with phenacetin (which has been removed from most analgesic preparations in the United States), but raises the strong possibility that acetaminophen, the major metabolite of phenacetin, is also nephrotoxic.

The characteristic patient who develops analgesic nephropathy is a middle-aged woman (women outnumber men 4:1), with chronic headaches or arthritic problems, who has consumed large amounts of compounds containing phenacetin, acetaminophen, or aspirin on a daily basis for many years. The ingestion of at least 1 g or more daily of these analgesics for longer than 2 to 3 years is felt to be the minimum dose-time requirement to produce clinical analgesic nephropathy. Systemic symptoms such as malaise, weight loss, emotional and psychiatric disorders, anemia, and peptic ulcer disease may be related in part to the syndrome of analgesic nephropathy and in part to the population that uses these medications excessively. Diagnosis is often difficult because most patients do not consider these over-the-counter preparations to be medications and to have potential side effects. Renal findings relate to chronic interstitial disease and may include nocturia and polyuria, sterile pyuria, urinary tract infections, acidification defects, a predisposition to volume depletion, renal colic and hematuria, and hypertension. Renal insufficiency may be present in asymptomatic patients and is often progressive if analgesic consumption is continued. The finding of papillary necrosis on intravenous pyelography, ultrasonography, or computed axial tomography is helpful in establishing the diagnosis.

Lithium salts, widely used to treat affective disorders, have been associated with a number of renal abnormalities, most prominently a nephrogenic diabetes insipidus–polyuria syndrome. Although reductions in the GFR and chronic interstitial nephritis have been attributed to lithium use, the relationship is not clearly established. In a composite review of studies covering almost 500 patients receiving lithium, only 15% were found to have a reduced creatinine clearance. Likewise, in a review of studies examining ethylenediaminetetraacetic acid clearances in more than 500 patients, the GFR was found to be reduced in only 17%. In those patients with a reduced GFR, the reduction was mild, with most patients having GFRs of 60 to 75 mL/minute. Clearly, even the renal dysfunction of these patients cannot all be attributed to lithium use because psychiatric patient populations not receiving lithium have been noted to have reduced GFRs and chronic changes in renal biopsy specimens when compared with normal subjects. Many studies have also failed to document a positive correlation between duration of lithium treatment and the reduction in GFR. In studies examining longer durations of treatment (6.5 to 10 years), however, a positive correlation has been noted. Only a few prospective studies have investigated the effects of lithium on a reduction in GFR, and although no significant change in GFR has been noted, the duration of follow-up has been short. In some studies, the renal biopsy specimens of lithium-treated patients with normal GFRs have shown focal interstitial fibrotic changes.

Overall, the use of lithium for many years is probably associated with some degree of decline in the GFR and interstitial damage. The damage is usually mild to moderate and appears to occur only after the prolonged use of lithium. The contribution to renal disease from other psychotropic medications or from other factors associated with the affective disorders of these patients remains to be defined.

*Cis*-platinum, an antineoplastic agent widely used to treat a variety of carcinomas and germ cell tumors, may cause both acute renal failure and, less frequently, chronic

renal insufficiency. In those patients suffering chronic renal damage, interstitial fibrosis and chronic inflammatory changes have been noted on renal biopsy. The nitrosourea compounds methyl-cyclohexylchloroethylnitrosourea and bis-chloroethyl-nitrosourea can both produce dose-related nephrotoxicity and chronic interstitial nephritis. Renal biopsy specimens from patients experiencing renal damage after receiving these medications have shown severe tubular atrophy, glomerulosclerosis, and interstitial fibrosis with chronic inflammatory infiltrates. In some patients, the chronic tubulointerstitial damage has led to ESRD.

Cyclosporine and tacrolimus, two potent immunosuppressive agents widely used in transplantation, can cause not only acute renal damage but also chronic tubulointerstitial fibrosis. This is often associated with drug-related microvascular damage to the arterioles of the kidney. These agents can produce a chronic form of tubulointerstitial damage in a band-like pattern within the kidney, called "striped fibrosis." This has been seen in both transplant populations and patients without prior renal disease who are taking this immunosuppressive medicine for autoimmune conditions. It is usually associated with a decreased GFR and renal insufficiency.

## SUGGESTED READINGS

### Glomerular Disease and Nephrotic Syndrome—General

Appel GB. Glomerulonephritis. In: Goldman L, Bennett JC, ed. *Cecil Textbook of Medicine*, 21st ed. Philadelphia: WB Saunders, 2000: 586–594.
Appel GB. Immune complex glomerulonephritis, deposits with interest. *N Engl J Med* 1993;328:505–506.
Maschio G, Alberti D, Janin G, et al. Effect of the angiotensin-converting enzyme inhibitor benazepril on the progression of chronic renal insufficiency. *N Engl J Med* 1996;334:939–945.
Orth SR, Ritz E. The nephrotic syndrome. *N Engl J Med* 1998;338: 1202–1211.
Radharkrishnan J, Appel AS, Valeri A, et al. The nephrotic syndrome, lipids, and risk factors for cardiovascular disease. *Am J Kidney Dis* 1993;22:135–142.

### Minimal-Change and Focal Segmental Glomerulosclerosis

Appel GB. Focal segmental glomerulosclerosis. In: Greenberg A, ed. *Primer on Kidney Disease*. New York: Academic Press, 2001:160–164.
Cattran D, Appel GB, Hebet L, et al., for the North American Nephrotic Syndrome Study Group. A randomized controlled trial of cyclosporine vs. placebo in adults with FSGS. *Kidney Int* 1999; 56:2220–2226.
D'Agati V. Nephrology Forum. The many masks of FSGS. *Kidney Int* 1994;46:1223–1241.
Haas M, Spargo BH, Coventry S. Increasing incidence of FSGS among adult nephropathies: a 20-year renal biopsy study. *Am J Kidney Dis* 1995;26:740–750.
Matalon A, Valeri A, Appel GB. Treatment of focal segmental glomerulosclerosis. *Semin Nephrol* 2000;20:309–317.
Ponticelli C, Passerini P. Treatment of nephrotic syndrome associated with primary glomerulonephritis. *Kidney Int* 1994;46:595–604.
Rydell JJ, Korbet SM, Borok RZ, et al. FSGS in adults: presentation, course, and response to treatment. *Am J Kidney Dis* 1995;25: 534–542.

Savin VJ, Artero M, Sharma R, et al. Circulating factor associated with increased glomerular permeability to albumin in recurrent focal segmental sclerosis. *N Engl J Med* 1996;334:878–882.

## Membranous Nephropathy

Cattran DC, Appel GB, Hebert L, et al. for the North American Nephrotic Syndrome Study Group. Cyclosporine in membranous nephropathy: a randomized trial. *Kidney Int* 2001;59: 1484–1490.

Gedded CC, Cattran D. The treatment of membranous nephropathy. *Semin Nephrol* 2000;20:299–309.

Hogan SL, Muller KE, Jennette JC, et al. A review of therapeutic studies of idiopathic membranous glomerulopathy. *Am J Kidney Dis* 1995;25:862–875.

Lewis E. Idiopathic membranous nephropathy—to treat or not to treat. *N Engl J Med* 1993;329:127–128.

Ponticelli C, Zucchelli P, Passerini P, et al. A 10 year follow-up of a randomized study with methylprednisolone and chlorambucil in idiopathic membranous nephropathy. *Kidney Int* 1995;48:1600–1605.

Ponticelli C, Zucchelli P, Passerini P, et al. Methylprednisolone plus chlorambucil as compared with methylprednisolone alone for the treatment of idiopathic membranous nephropathy. *N Engl J Med* 1992;327:599–603.

Schieppati A, Mosconi L, Perna A, et al. Prognosis of untreated patients with idiopathic membranous nephropathy. *N Engl J Med* 1993;329:85–89.

## Immunoglobulin A Nephropathy

Cattran DC, Greenwood C, Ritchie S. Benefits of angiotensin-converting enzyme inhibitor therapy in patients with severe immunoglobulin A nephropathy: a comparison to patients receiving treatment with other antihypertensive agents and to patients receiving no therapy. *Am J Kidney Dis* 1994;23:247–254.

Donadio J, Bergstrahl EJ, Offord KP, et al., for the Mayo Nephrology Collaborative Group. A controlled trial of fish oils in IgA nephropathy. *N Engl J Med* 1995;331:1194–1199.

Julian B. Treatment of IgA-nephropathy. *Semin Nephrol* 2000;20: 277–286.

Pozzi C, Bolasco PG, Fogazzi GB, et al. Corticosteroids in IgA nephropathy: a randomized controlled trial. *Lancet* 1999;353: 883–887.

## Membranoproliferative Glomerulonephritis

Donadio J, Offord K. Reassessment of treatment results in membranoproliferative glomerulonephritis, with emphasis on life-table analysis. *Am J Kidney Dis* 1989;6:445–451.

Tarshish P, Bernstein J, Tobin J, et al. Treatment of mesangiocapillary glomerulonephritis with alternate-day prednisone: a report of the international study of kidney disease in children. *Pediatr Nephrol* 1992;6:123–130.

## Rapidly Progressive Glomerulonephritis

Bolton K. Treatment of ANCA negative RPGN. *Semin Nephrol* 2001;20: 244–256.

Couser WG. Rapidly progressive glomerulonephritis: classification, pathogenetic mechanisms, and therapy. *Am J Kidney Dis* 1988;6: 449–464.

De'Oliviera J, Gaskin G, Dash A, et al. Relationship between disease activity and ANCA concentration in long-term management of systemic vasculitis. *Am J Kidney Dis* 1995;25:380–389.

Falk R, Hogan S, Carey T, et al. Clinical course of anti-neutrophil cytoplasmic autoantibody-associated glomerulonephritis and systemic vasculitis. *Ann Intern Med* 1990;113:656–663.

Falk R, Jennette C. Anti-neutrophil cytoplasmic autoantibodies with specificity for myeloperoxidase in patients with systemic vasculitis and idiopathic necrotizing and crescentic glomerulonephritis. *N Engl J Med* 1988;25:1651–1657.

Falk R, Nachman P, Hogan S, et al. ANCA glomerulonephritis and vasculitis. *Semin Nephrol* 2000;20:233–244.

Glassock RJ. Intensive plasma exchange in crescentic glomerulonephritis: help or no help? *Am J Kidney Dis* 1992;20:270–275.

Herody M, Bobrie G, Gouarin C, et al. Anti-GBM disease: predictive value of clinical histological and serological data. *Clin Nephrol* 1993;5:249–255.

Hoffman G, Kerr G, Leavitt R, et al. Wegener's granulomatosis: an analysis of 158 patients. *Ann Intern Med* 1992;116:488–498.

Kunis C, Kiss B, Williams G, et al. Intravenous "pulse" cyclophosphamide therapy of crescentic glomerulonephritis. *Clin Nephrol* 1992;1:1–7.

Nachman PH, Hogan SL, Jennette JC, et al. Treatment response and relapse in ANCA-associated microscopic polyangiitis and glomerulonephritis. *J Am Soc Nephrol* 1996;7:23–32.

Pusey CD, Rees AJ, Peters DK, et al. Plasma exchange in focal and necrotizing glomerulonephritis without anti-GBM antibodies. *Kidney Int* 1991;40:757–763.

## Hepatitis C Virus

Appel GB. Immune-complex glomerulonephritis—deposits plus interest. *N Engl J Med* 1993;328:505–506.

D'Amico G, Ferrario F. Cryoglobulinemic glomerulonephritis: a MPGN induced by hepatitis C virus. *Am J Kidney Dis* 1995;25: 361–369.

Jefferson JA, Johnson R. Treatment of hepatitis C associated GN. *Semin Nephrol* 2000;20:286–293.

Johnson RJ, Gretch DR, Yamabe H, et al. Membranoproliferative glomerulonephritis associated with hepatitis C virus infection. *N Engl J Med* 1993;328:465–470.

Johnson RJ, Wilson R, Yambe H, et al. Renal manifestations of HCV infection. *Kidney Int* 1994;46:1255–1263.

Misiani R, Bellavita P, Fenili V, et al. Interferon alpha therapy in cryoglobulinemia associated with HCV. *N Engl J Med* 1994;330: 751–756.

Roth D. Hepatitis C virus: the nephrologist's view. *Am J Kidney Dis* 1995;25:3–16.

## Severe Systemic Lupus Nephritis

Appel GB, D'Agati V. Renal involvement in systemic lupus erythematosus. In: Massary S, Glassock R, eds. *Text of Kidney Disease*. Baltimore: Williams & Wilkins, 1999:787–797.

Austin HA, Balow J. Treatment of lupus nephritis. *Semin Nephrol* 2000; 20:265–277.

Boumpas DT, Austin HA, Vaughn EM, et al. Controlled trial of pulse methylprednisolone versus two regimens of cyclophosphamide in severe lupus nephritis. *Lancet* 1992;340:741–745.

Gourley MF, Austin HA, Scott D, et al. Methylprednisolone and cyclophosphamide, alone or in combination, in patients with lupus nephritis. *Ann Intern Med* 1996;125:549–557.

Lewis EJ, Hunsicker LG, Lau SP, et al., for the Lupus Collaboration Study Group. A controlled trial of plasmapheresis in severe lupus nephritis. *N Engl J Med* 1992;326:1373–1379.

Radhakrishnan J, Valeri A, Kunis C, et al. Use of cyclosporin in systemic lupus. *Contrib Nephrol* 1995;114:59–72.

Zimmerman R, Radhakrishnan J, Valeri A, et al. Advances in the treatment of lupus nephritis. *Ann Rev Med* 2001;52:63–78.

## Human Immunodeficiency Virus Nephropathy

Carbone L, D'Agati V, Cheng J-T, et al. Course and prognosis of human immunodeficiency virus-associated nephropathy. *Am J Med* 1989;87:389–395.

D'Agati V, Appel GB. HIV infection and the kidney. *J Am Soc Nephrol* 1997;8:138–153.

D'Agati V, Suh JI, Carbone L, et al. Pathology of HIV-associated nephropathy: a detailed morphologic and comparative study. *Kidney Int* 1989;35:1358–1370.

Humphreys MH. HIV associated glomerulosclerosis. *Kidney Int* 1995; 48:311–320.

Rao TK, Friedman EA. Outcome of severe acute renal failure in patients with acquired immunodeficiency syndrome. *Am J Kidney Dis* 1995;25:390–398.

## Amyloidosis and Light Chain Deposition Disease

Heilman RL, Velosa JA, Holley K, et al. Long-term follow-up and response to chemotherapy in patients with light chain deposition disease. *Am J Kidney Dis* 1992;20:34–41.

Kyle RA, Gertz MA, Greipp PR, et al. A trial of three regimens for primary amyloidosis: colchicine alone, melphalan and prednisone, and melphalan, prednisone, and colchicine. *N Engl J Med* 1997; 336:1202–1207.

Skinner M, Anderson JJ, Simms R, et al. Treatment of 100 patients with primary amyloidosis: a randomized trial of melphalan, prednisone, and colchicine, versus colchicine alone. *Am J Med* 1996; 100:290–298.

## Diabetes Mellitus

American Diabetes Association Treatment of Hypertension in Diabetes (Consensus Statement). *Diabetes Care* 1996;19[Suppl 1]:S107–S113.

Appel GB. Preventing or slowing the progression of diabetic nephropathy. *Baylor Univ Med Cent Proc* 1999;12:3–6.

Bennett PH, Haffner S, Kasiske BL, et al. Screening and management of microalbuminuria in patients with diabetes. *Am J Kidney Dis* 1995;25:107–112.

Brownlee M. Advanced protein glycosylation in diabetes and aging. *Ann Rev Med* 1995;46:223–234.

Clark CM, Lee DA. Prevention and treatment of the complications of diabetes mellitus. *N Engl J Med* 1995;332:1210–1217.

Diabetes Control and Complication Trial Research Group. The effect of intensive treatment of diabetes on the development and progression of long-term complications in insulin-dependent diabetes mellitus. *N Engl J Med* 1993;329:977–986.

Hansson L, Zanchetti A, Carruther SG, et al. Effect of intensive BP lowering and low-dose aspirin in patients with hypertension: principal results of the Hypertension Optimal Treatment (HOT) randomized trial. *Lancet* 1997;351:1755–1762.

Lewis EJ, Hunsicker L, Bain RP, et al. The effect of angiotensin-converting enzyme inhibition on diabetic nephropathy. *N Engl J Med* 1993;329:1456–1462.

Mogenson CE, Keane WF, Bennett PH, et al. Prevention of diabetic renal disease with special reference to microalbuminuria. *Lancet* 1995;346:1080–1084.

Remuzzi A, Perico N, Amuchastegui CS, et al. Short- and long-term effect of angiotensin II receptor blockade in rats with experimental diabetes. *J Am Soc Nephrol* 1993;4:40–49.

Results of two randomized trials of ARBs in type II DM (RENAAL and IDNT). Paper presented at: American Society HBP; May 2001.

Soulis T, Cooper ME, Vranes D, et al. Effects of aminoguanidine in preventing experimental diabetic nephropathy are related to the duration of treatment. *Kidney Int* 1996;50:627–634.

The Sixth Report of the Joint National Committee on Prevention, Detection, Evaluation, and Treatment of High Blood Pressure. *Arch Intern Med* 1997;157:2413–2446.

Tuomilehto J, Ratenyte D, Birknhager WH, et al., for the Systolic Hypertension in Europe Trial Investigators. Effects of calcium-channel blockade in older patients with diabetes and systolic hypertension. *N Engl J Med* 1999;340:677–684.

## Tubulointerstitial Diseases

Elseviers MM, De Broe ME. Controlled study of analgesic abuse in Belgium. *Kidney Int* 1995;48:1912–1919.

Henrich WL, Agodoa LE, Barrett B, et al. Analgesics and the kidney: summary and recommendations to the Scientific Advisory Board of the National Kidney Foundation. *Am J Kidney Dis* 1996;27: 162–166.

Segasothy M, Samad SA, Zulfigar A, et al. Chronic renal disease and papillary necrosis associated with the long-term use of NSAIDs as the sole or predominant analgesic. *Am J Kidney Dis* 1994;24:17–24.

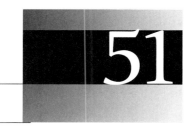

# Hallmarks of Essential and Secondary Hypertension

*Martin J. Schreiber, Jr.    Donald G. Vidt*

A number of pathophysiologic factors have been implicated in the development of hypertension, thus making selective mechanistically based antihypertensive therapy difficult for most patients (1). In a broad sense, increased sympathetic nervous system activity, autonomic imbalance (increased sympathetic tone, abnormally reduced parasympathetic tone), vascular remodeling, arterial stiffness, and endothelial dysfunction contribute to both the development and maintenance of hypertension. Increased sympathetic activity may stem from alterations in baroflex and chemoreflex pathways, both peripherally and centrally. The renin-angiotensin system plays a major role in vascular remodeling (the alterations in structure, mechanical properties, and function of small arteries) and critical target organ damage (myocardial fibrosis, renal injury). In addition, arterial stiffness, a primary contributor to increased vascular resistance especially with advancing age, results from continued collagen deposition, smooth muscle hypertrophy, and changes in the elastin media fibers. Whereas intact vascular endothelium is critical to maintaining vascular tone (relaxation and contraction), we know that multiple insults (decreased nitric oxide synthesis, increased endothelin, estrogen deficiency, high dietary salt intake, diabetes mellitus, tobacco usage, and increased homocysteine) can damage vascular endothelium and are important clinically. These factors or conditions disrupt normal endothelial function and initiate the cascade of cardiovascular events that results in atherosclerosis, thrombosis, and heart failure.

## CLINICAL APPROACHES TO HYPERTENSION

Hypertension prevalence is increasing in the United States, occurring in 20% of the population and in more than two-thirds of individuals over 65 years of age. Recent data support the contention that hypertension control rates remain low. Hypertension prevalence is highest among non-Hispanic Blacks and women, and increases with age and elevated body mass index (BMI) (2).

Over the last 5 years, several landmark clinical trials have assessed the impact of different therapeutic agents on outcome in hypertension. These studies highlight the importance of treatment selection in the individual patient with hypertension (3). The findings from these trials, coupled with the recent recommendations of the Seventh Report of the Joint National Committee on the Prevention, Detection, Evaluation and Treatment of High Blood Pressure (JNC VII) (4,5), underscore the importance of recognizing up-to-date blood pressure (BP) classification, selecting the appropriate agents for the clinical setting, and achieving effective target BP lowering.

The new classification of BP for adults 18 years or older in JNC VII defines a (prehypertension category and combines stages II and III, as delineated in the JNC VI Report (Table 51.1)(6). When considering the number of patients with a BP of 120 to 139/80 to 89 mm Hg, prehypertension represents a major public health problem. Vigorous attempts at lifestyle modifications should be undertaken for individuals categorized as prehypertensive. Patients

with systolic BPs between 120 and 140 mm Hg are not entirely free from a potential cardiovascular event; these prehypertensive individuals have a higher risk for developing hypertension than those with systolic BPs <120 mm Hg. Figure 51.1 depicts the importance of matching the initial drug selection with the stage of hypertension and the presence or absence of compelling indications (heart failure, diabetes mellitus type 1 and 2, proteinuria, renal disease, isolated hypertension, myocardial infarction, etc.). The presence of compelling indications not only emphasizes renewed attention to drug selection, but also denotes a need to achieve a more significant decrease in BP (<130/80 mm Hg) in settings of diabetes, chronic kidney disease (CKD) plus proteinuria, congestive heart failure (CHF), and in minority populations.

Findings from recent clinical trials (Table 51.2) illustrate specific caveats for therapeutic selection in high-risk patients for cardiovascular disease (7), for those with diabetic renal disease (8,9), and in high-risk ethnic groups (i.e., African Americans; 10). For patients with essential hypertension and at high risk for cardiovascular disease, the use of diuretic therapy resulted in outcomes at least equivalent to the use of ACE inhibitors or calcium channel blockers (CCBs) without diuretics in the Antihypertensive and Lipid-Lowering Treatment to Prevent Heart Attack Trial (ALLHAT) study (11). Dihydropyridine calcium blockers should not be used as monotherapy in patients with proteinuric renal disease, whether associated with diabetes mellitus or hypertension. Recent clinical trials with metoprolol and newer vasodilating β-blockers (carvedilol and bucindolol) have shown benefit when added to standard therapy, including ACE inhibitors (12,13). For patients with type 1 diabetes, ACE inhibitor therapy is the cornerstone of treatment. ACE inhibitors and angiotensin II

### TABLE 51.1

**BLOOD PRESSURE (BP)\* CLASSIFICATION AND MANAGEMENT FOR ADULTS AGED 18 YEARS AND OLDER**

| BP Classification | SBP, mm Hg | | DBP, mm Hg | Lifestyle Changes | Initial Drug Therapy Compelling Indications | |
|---|---|---|---|---|---|---|
| | | | | | Without | With |
| Normal | <120 | and | <80 | Encourage | | |
| Pre HYTN | 120–139 | or | 80–89 | Yes | No | Yes[a] |
| Stage 1 HYTN | 140–159 | or | 90–99 | Yes | Yes[b] | Yes[c] |
| Stage 2 HYTN | >160 | or | >100 | Yes | Yes[d] | Yes[e] |

SBP, systolic blood pressure; DBP, diastolic blood pressure; HYTN, hypertension.
\* Treatment determined by highest BP category.
[a] Treat patients with chronic kidney disease or diabetes to BP goal of <130/80 mm Hg.
[b] Thiazide-type diuretic for most; may consider angiotensin-converting enzyme (ACE) inhibitor, angiotensin II receptor blocker (ARB), β-blocker, calcium channel blocker (CCB), or combination.
[c] Other antihypertensive drugs (diuretic, ACE inhibitor, ARB, β-blocker, CCB) as needed.
[d] Two-drug combination for most (usually thiazide-type diuretic and ACE inhibitor or ARB or β-blocker or CCB). Initiation of combined therapy should be used cautiously in those at risk for orthostatic hypotension.
[e] Other antihypertensive drugs (diuretic, ACE inhibitor, ARB, β-blocker, CCB) as needed.
[From JNC VII (4).]

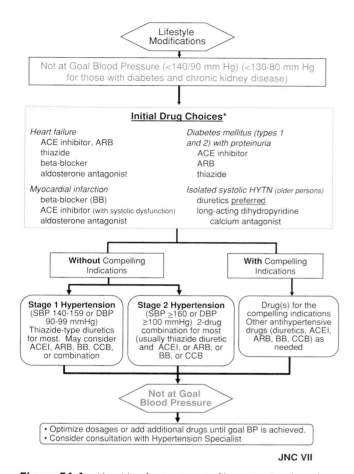

**Figure 51.1** Algorithm for treatment of hypertension (based on randomized controlled trials). (Adapted with permission from Abbott KC, Bakris GL. What have we learned from the current trials? *Med Clin North Am* 2004;88:189–207.) ACE, angiotensin-converting enzyme; ARB, angiotensin II receptor blocker; CCB, calcium channel blocker; HYTN, hypertension.

receptor blockers (ARBs) have demonstrated favorable results in both diabetic and nondiabetic renal disease. The greatest benefit for slowing the progression of type 2 diabetes with renal disease can be seen using ARBs, based on findings from the Reduction of Endpoints in NIDDM with the Angiotensin II Antagonist Losartan (RENAAL) and Irbesartan Diabetic Nephropathy Trial (IDNT) studies (14,15).

Because patients with CKD (serum creatinine greater than or equal to 1.4 mg/dL) are just as likely to die from cardiovascular disease as from ESRD, hypertension should be aggressively controlled (16). The risk for cardiovascular and renal disease events starts at systolic BP levels less than 115 mm Hg (17). ACE inhibitors or ARBs should be used in CKD patients whenever possible, even in settings of abnormal creatinine. An increase in baseline serum creatinine of approximately 35% while on these agents is acceptable, unless clinically resistant hyperkalemia develops. Hypertensive patients with CKD of <30 mL/min per

1.73 m2 will require increasing doses of loop diuretic, in combination with other agents, to optimize volume, a critical determinant of elevated BP. The development of microalbuminuria is associated with abnormal vascular reactivity, salt sensitivity, increased presence of target organ damage, and loss of nocturnal dipping in BP (18). An elevated urine albumin-to-creatinine ratio heralds the need for aggressive BP control.

Effective BP control can be achieved in the majority of patients with hypertension, but more than two (2.7 to 3.8) medications may be needed to reach target BP levels (19). When BP is >20/10 mm Hg above target, consideration should be given to initiating therapy using two drugs. Extensive clinical experience with available antihypertensive agents suggests that any single drug preparation will control only 30% and 65% of patients treated, whereas the addition of a second or third drug to the regimen can improve control rates into the range of 90% to 95%. Patients should return for monthly follow-up until the BP goal is achieved. Serum potassium and creatinine should be monitored at least twice per year (20).

Among older persons, systolic BP (SBP) is a better predictor of events (coronary heart disease, cardiovascular disease, heart failure, stroke, ESRD, and all-cause mortality) than is diastolic BP (DBP). The initial goal of treatment in older patients should be the same as in younger individuals—namely, to achieve a BP below 140/90 mm Hg. The concept of a J curve for mortality with exaggerated BP lowering may be of greatest important in the elderly. Findings from both the Systolic Hypertension in the Elderly Program (SHEP) trial (21) and the Rotterdam Study (22) suggest that an increased cardiovascular risk may exist in the lowest strata of BP and that reducing SBP to below 130 mm Hg or DBP to below 65 mm Hg may not represent optimal strategy in the elderly.

Electrocardiographic and/or echocardiographic evidence of left ventricular hypertrophy (LVH) is associated with increased risk of coronary disease, ventricular arrhythmias, and sudden death (23,24) and requires optimal target BP. Most of the antihypertensive drugs used for initial therapy of hypertension induce regression of LVH

Because the risk of heart disease and stroke increases with age among women, increasing attention has been focused on the nearly 30 million American women over age 50 years. In women 50 to 64 years of age, 47% have high BP—this figures increases to 58% in women 65 to 74 years of age, to 75% for those 75 years and older. African American women have a death rate from hypertension that is approximately 4.5 times higher than the rate for white women, which makes hypertension the probable cause of up to 20% of all deaths in hypertensive African American women. No evidence suggests that women respond differently from men to the risk reduction effect of antihypertensive drugs (25), and the JNC VII guidelines should be applied equally to women.

**TABLE 51.2**

**SUMMARY OF CV AND KIDNEY OUTCOME TRIALS (2001–2004)**

| Study | Population | Special Note(s) | Impact on Clinical Practice |
|-------|-----------|-----------------|----------------------------|
| ALLHAT | North American subjects >55 y | α-Blocker terminated due to excess risk for hospitalized CHF | Hypertensive patients respond as well or better to diuretics compared to other agents ACE inhibitors, CCB |
| RENAAL | Type 2 diabetics, 31–70 y with nephropathy | Controlling BP may require 3 or 4 antihypertensive agents | Greater reduction in proteinuria for losartan vs. placebo |
| IDNT | Type 2 diabetics, hypertensive, proteinuria | | Lower risk of SCr doubling with irbesartan vs. amlodipine or placebo |
| AASK | African Americans, 18–70 y, hypertensive with renal disease | Amlodipine arm terminated due to excess risk of ESRD/death vs. ramipril | Patients with proteinuria should not receive DHP CCB as monotherapy. Lower than usual BP control did not slow progression of renal disease. ACE inhibitors more effective at slowing progression (CCB, β-blocker) |

Y, year(s); CHF, congestive heart failure; ACE, angiotensin-converting enzyme; CCB, calcium channel blocker; SCr, serum creatinine; ESRD, end-stage renal disease; DHP CCB, dihydropyridine calcium channel blocker; BP, blood pressure.
Trial Names: ALLHAT, Antihypertensive and Lipid-Lowering Treatment to Prevent Heart Attack Trial; RENAAL, Reduction of Endpoints in NIDDM with the Angiotensin II Antagonists Losartan; IDNT, Irbesartan Diabetic Nephropathy Trial; AASK, African American Study of Kidney Disease and Hypertension.

## GENETICS OF HYPERTENSION

Hypertension results from a complex interaction of genetic, environmental, and demographic factors. Variations in BP result from the contributions of many different genes (polygenaic) (26). In most patients with essential hypertension, genetic profiling is not currently beneficial in the diagnostic evaluation. Exceptions are the occasional cases of secondary hypertension, for which clinical data and biochemical profiling may point to anatomic or functional aberrations, such as abnormal function of the adrenal hormones or abnormal receptor response. Although the majority of cases of essential hypertension are considered polygenaic and are characterized by a complex mode of inheritance, rare cases of simple Mendelian forms of high BP occur in which a single gene defect may be largely responsible for the hypertensive phenotype. Improved techniques of genetic analysis (i.e., genetic-wide linkage analysis) have aided in the search for genes that contribute to the development of primary hypertension. The genetic causes of hypertension, although uncommon in the general population with elevated BP, may be more frequent in selective hypertensive populations, particularly in those patients with resistant hypertension. Genome scans have identified regions of specific human chromosomes that influence BP. These regions are called blood pressure quantitative trait loci (QTL) (e.g., chromosome 6.2).

From the clinical prospective, a family with a history of hypertension can be a surrogate marker for undefined risk factors shared by the family. Risk factors such as obesity, dyslipidemia, and insulin resistance are predictive of future hypertension. Having a single first-degree relative with hypertension is only a weak predictor of hypertension, whereas a finding of greater than or equal to two relatives with hypertension at an early age (before 55 years), identifies a smaller subset of families who are at much higher risk for the future development of hypertension (27).

Several locations for hypertensive genes previously reported include chromosome arms 1q, 2p, 2q, 8p, 17q, and 18q. Genes encoding angiotensinogen expression seem to be closely related to hypertension, in addition to B2-adrenoreceptor, aldosterone synthetase, and the G protein in the angiogenic II AT1 receptor genes. Several genes have been identified with specific salt interactions, as in glucocorticoid-remedial hypertension and apparent mineralocorticoid excess (28); the α-adducin gene is associated with an increased risk of renal tubular absorption of sodium, and angiotensinogen gene polymorphism (A-G substitution and methionine to threonine amino acid substitution) has been linked to an increase in plasma levels of angiotensinogen (29).

Gene-to-drug interactions may explain the heterogeneity of BP responses to different antihypertensive agents. α-Adducin responds best to thiazide diuretics; those with Met235 thr angiotensinogen respond best to ACE inhibitor; and CCB and specific G-protein genes impart a response to β-blockers and diuretics (30).

A number of syndromes represent genetic mutations of single-gene forms of hypertension. These include glucocorticoid remedial hypertension (chimeric gene formation; autosomal dominant), 11-β hydroxylase (mutation in gene encoding), 17-α-hydroxylase deficiency, Liddle's syndrome (mutation in the sodium channel gene), hypertension exacerbated by pregnancy, syndrome of apparent mineralocorticoid excess, and pseudohypoaldosteronism (31). Human atrial naturetic peptide (hANP) is an attractive gene for linking specific population groups to an associated increased risk for hypertension. Polymorphisms of the angiotensinogen gene have been detected in hypertensive patients and in the children of hypertensive parents.

Advances in molecular biology and newer technologies make likely the possibility of gene expression profiling being applied to hypertensive research, diagnosis, and treatment selection in the future (32).

## SIGNIFICANCE OF SYSTOLIC, DIASTOLIC, AND PULSE PRESSURE

A shift in emphasis from DBP to SBP has occurred over the last decade (33–35). A reanalysis of the Framingham Heart Study using longer follow-up data and more extensive cardiovascular data tracking showed that at all levels of systolic pressure, even within a normal range, the level of the SBP accurately predicted coronary heart disease (CHD)(36). In addition, these data also suggest that the pulse pressure (SBP–DBP) is a major independent predictor of CHD. A wide pulse pressure is a marker for large artery stiffness and for vascular aging (arteriosclerosis). Elevated coronary arterial calcifications scores are associated with arterial stiffness and increased pulse pressure (37). Age is a determinant of pulse pressure importance in hypertension. A growing body of evidence supports pulse pressure readings as an important predictor in patients older than 65 years of age (38,39). Furthermore, pulse pressure may be a strong predictor of cardiovascular risk in the presence of compromised ventricular function with normal or low SBP (40).

Therefore, DBP, SBP, and pulse pressure are important in staging hypertension at different ages. Earlier generations of physicians favored the importance of DBP over SBP, in part because hypertension was apparently a young person's disease. With the aging of the population, hypertension has become a disease of older patients, specifically reflected by isolated systolic hypertension (ISH). As arteries stiffen and pulse wave amplification decreases with aging, a general shift in elevation occurs from DBP to SBP, and eventually in some, to pulse pressure as predictors of cardiovascular risk (41).

Situations occur in which pulse pressure does not represent arterial stiffness (a discrepancy between central and brachial pulse pressure) increased cardiac output, variable heart rate, and vasodilation. Therefore, pulse pressure cannot replace SBP as a single measure of CHD risk. SBP and DBP together are frequently superior to SBP alone in predicting cardiovascular risk. From a practical standpoint, physicians should first measure SBP (i.e., especially in the middle-aged healthy and elderly cohorts), and then adjust risk upward for pulse pressure if there is a discordantly low DBP (i.e., post–myocardial infarction, heart failure, ESRD, etc.). Only in the presence of a discordantly low DBP does pulse pressure embellish SBP in predicting cardiovascular risk.

## EVALUATION

A complete history, physical examination, basic serum chemistries analysis, urinalysis, and electrocardiogram (EKG) are recommended for the initial evaluation of a hypertensive patient. The urinalysis is especially important because of the impact renal disease has on the treatment selection and target goals for BP lowering.

Specific aspects of the patient's history should entail family history, early cerebrovascular hemorrhagic stroke (if younger than 60 years), nonprescription medication use (nonsteroidal anti-inflammatory drugs, diet pills, decongestants, appetite suppressants, herbal therapy), birth control pills, alcohol or street drug use, and sleep history. The physician should always be alert to history or physical examination findings that suggests a secondary cause for the hypertension.

The physical examination should include two or more BP measurements, separated by 2 minutes, with the patient either supine or seated and after standing for at least 2 minutes, in accordance with recommended techniques. BP should be verified in the contralateral arms; if values are different, the higher value should be used. Measurements of height, weight, and waist circumference should be obtained. Special attention should be directed to fundoscopic examination; presence or absence of carotid bruits or distended neck veins; thyroid enlargements; and an examination of the heart, lungs, abdomen, and extremities. Particular attention should be directed to peripheral pulses, the presence of abdominal bruits, and the presence or absence of edema. A neurologic assessment should also be performed.

In most cases, the presence of significant arteriosclerosis or arteriovenous nicking on fundoscopic examination indicates that the BP has been elevated for more than 6 months. Arteriolar changes are the most common manifestation of hypertensive retinopathy. The mean ratio of arteriole-to-venular (AV) diameter in nonhypertensive patients is 0.84. This ratio progressively decreases with increased mean arterial BP. AV nicking can be detected where branch retinal arteries cross over veins. The thickened arteriole wall compresses the thin-walled vein and causes a tapering or "nicked" appearance.

A basic laboratory evaluation should include a urinalysis, complete blood count, blood chemistries (potassium,

sodium, creatinine, fasting glucose, uric acid, total cholesterol and high-density lipoprotein cholesterol, and an
EKG). An elevated uric acid level predicts the development
of hypertension and is frequently present in patients with
hypertension; the degree of elevation also correlates with
the degree of BP elevation. Uric acid also may have a pathogenic role in progressive renal disease.

Ambulatory blood pressure monitoring (ABPM), EKGs,
and the assessment of plasma renin activity are not indicated for the routine evaluation of most hypertensive
patients at the first visit. ABPM may be useful in separating
those patients who require antihypertensive therapy from
those who can be managed by lifestyle modifications.
Higher ambulatory SBP or DBP predicts cardiovascular
events even after adjustment for classic risk factors (42). In
select situations (i.e., white coat hypertension, nocturnal
hypotension with treatment), ABPM may be helpful.

## REFRACTORY HYPERTENSION

Refractory hypertension is defined as the persistence of
out-of-office BP levels greater than 140/90 mm Hg for
most patients, or above 130/80 mm Hg for those with diabetes mellitus and renal insufficiency (abnormal GFR, proteinuria), or above 140 mm Hg for those with ISH.
Refractory hypertension falls into two broad categories:
apparent resistance or true resistance (Table 51.3; 43).

Refractory hypertension is present in approximately
10% of patients in a primary care setting and in more than
30% of patients seen in subspecialty clinics. Suboptimal
therapeutic regimens are the major cause for apparent
refractory hypertension (Fig. 51.2; 44). More intensive therapy, with an emphasis on the targeted control of volume
using diuretic therapy, can achieve goal BP levels in a significant percentage of patients with apparent resistant
hypertension (45).

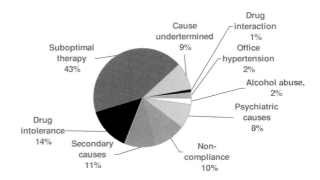

**Figure 51.2** Of 436 patients treated at a hypertension clinic, 92 (21%) had refractory hypertension. In 83 patients, a cause was identified, the most frequent being suboptimal therapy. Blood pressure was brought under control or improved in 58 patients. (Adapted with permission from Yakovlevitch M, Black HR. Resistant hypertension in a tertiary care clinic. *Arch Intern Med* 1991;151:1786.)

An awareness of the association between sleep-
disordered breathing, sleep apnea, and hypertension has
increased over the past few years (46). Both hypoxia and
$CO_2$ retention excite central and peripheral chemorecep-
tors that activate the renin angiotensin system; this can
lead to vasoconstriction and increased BP. Typically, the
onset of sleep is associated with a significant decrease in BP
of 10% to 20% in normotensive individuals. Patients with
disrupted sleep patterns, however, do not experience a nocturnal dip in BP; when these patients are treated with continuous positive airway pressure (cPAP), the nocturnal dip
in BP is restored (Fig. 51.3; 47).

## SECONDARY HYPERTENSION

For those hypertensive patients resistant to treatment using
two or more agents, a number of clinical clues can suggest
the possible presence of secondary hypertension. Table 51.4
divides the causes of secondary hypertension into four
broad categories. Secondary hypertensive disorders can be
effectively treated or cured, thus leading to the partial or
complete normalization of resistant hypertension in most
patients.

### Coarctation of the Aorta

Although coarctation of the aorta may cause left ventricular failure in early life, adults with coarctation are often
asymptomatic (48,49). As a result, the medical history may
be of little help in suggesting the presence of coarctation
unless the diagnosis is suspected in association with other
congenital malformations, such as bicuspid aortic valve,
patent ductus or ventricular septal defect, and mitral valve
abnormalities. The most common location for a coarctation

| TABLE 51.3 | |
|---|---|
| **CAUSES OF REFRACTORY HYPERTENSION** | |
| **Apparent Resistance** | **True Resistance** |
| Cuff-related artifacts | Excess plasma volume |
| Pseudohypertension | Associated conditions* |
| Non-adherence to therapy | Drug-related causes† |
| Prescription errors | Secondary hypertension |

* Obesity, insulin resistance, ethanol excess, sleep apnea.
† Drug–drug interactions and specific drugs that may produce refractory hypertension include: nonsteroidal anti-inflammatory drugs (NSAIDs), sympathomimetic drugs (decongestants, appetite suppressants), corticosteroids, chlorpromazine, over-the-counter dietary substances (e.g., ephedra, ma-huang, bitter orange), tricyclic antidepressants, cocaine, amphetamines, cyclosporine, tacrolimus, erythropoietin, anabolic steroids, monamine oxidase inhibitors, oral contraceptives, licorice, and some chewing tobaccos.

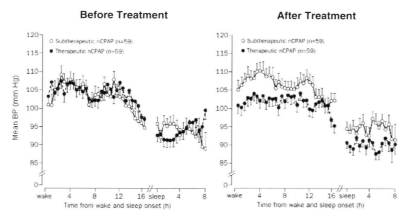

*therapeutic vs. subtherapeutic CPAP (1 cm $H_2O$) over a 1-month period.

**Figure 51.3**   Randomized trial comparing treated and untreated men with sleep apnea. Treatment consisted of therapeutic vs. subtherapeutic CPAP (1 cm H2O) over a 1-month period. Bars denote standard errors for every 30-minute period, synchronized to wake and sleep times. Reproduced with permission from Pepperell JC, Ramdassingh-Dow S, Crosthwaite N, et al. Ambulatory blood pressure after therapeutic and subtherapeutic nasal continuous positive airway pressure for obstructive sleep apnoea: a randomised parallel trial. *Lancet* 2002;359:204.

is distal to the left subclavian artery, but it may occasionally involve the origin of the left subclavian artery and may be missed if BPs are not checked in both upper extremities and at least one lower extremity. Absent or reduced pulses in the legs, together with a BP that is lower in the legs than in the arms, are obviously valuable clues to diagnosis. SBPs are elevated disproportionately to the DBP, resulting in the wide pulse pressure and bounding pulses proximal to the coarctation. A thrill may be observed in the suprasternal notch, together with palpable pulsations or auscultated bruits over the intercostal arteries.

Additional screening studies should include chest radiographs looking for the "three-sign" (i.e., proximal aorta, coarctated segment with poststenotic dilation, and indentation of the aortic knob). For diagnosis and localization, two-dimensional EKG, aortography, and magnetic resonance imaging (MRI) may be helpful. Management should consist of surgical repair or angioplasty.

## Primary Aldosteronism

Primary aldosteronism is the most common cause of hypertension caused by an endocrinopathy. The most common cause of primary aldosteronism is an aldosterone-producing adenoma (70% to 80%). Glucocorticoid remediable hypertension (GRA), adrenal hyperplasia, and adrenal carcinoma are other considerations, however. The best clues to the presence of primary aldosteronism include hypertension with spontaneous hypokalemia (less than 3.5 mEq/L), hypertension with provoked hypokalemia (less than 3.0 mEq/L during diuretic therapy), and hypertension with difficultly in maintaining normokalemia despite potassium supplementation.

Primary aldosteronism should be considered in any patient with both refractory hypertension and hypokalemia with inappropriate kaliuresis (KU greater than 30 mEq/L in 24 hours). One should be especially suspicious of primary aldosteronism if potassium is less than 3.5 mEq/L despite potassium supplementation, ACE inhibitor or ARB therapy, and/or potassium sparing diuretic administration. In addition, patients may develop muscle spasms, periodic paralysis, or metabolic alcholosis. The clinician must remember that not all patients with primary aldosteronism have hypokalemia; 7% to 38% of patients with primary aldosteronism may have normal serum potassium (50). Those individuals with hypertension and renal potassium wasting can be differentiated into high-renin and low-renin states (Table 51.5). Usually, the plasma renin concentration is less

## TABLE 51.4
### CLUES TO SECONDARY HYPERTENSION

Renal
    Renal artery stenosis
    Renal parenchymal
    Obstruction
    Polycystic kidney disease
Endocrine
    Cushing's syndrome
    Adrenogenital syndrome
    Pheochromocytoma
    Adrenal and adrenal-like
    Acromegaly
    Hypercalcemia
    Liddle's syndrome
    Gordon's syndrome

Coarctation of the Aorta

Other
    Preeclampsia
    Acute intermittent porphyria
Thyroid (hyperthyroid, hypothyroid)
Drugs

## TABLE 51.5

### BIOCHEMICAL CLASSIFICATION OF PATIENTS WITH HYPERTENSION, HYPOKALEMIA, AND RENAL POTASSIUM WASTING*

| HIGH Renin States | LOW Renin States[†] |
|---|---|
| Renovascular disease | Conn's syndrome[‡] |
| Malignant hypertension | Bilateral adrenal hyperplasia |
| Renin-secreting tumors | Glucocorticoid remediable hypertension (GRA)[§] |
| | Mineral corticoid excess syndrome |
| | Licorice ingestion |
| | Liddle's syndrome[¶] |

* >20 mEq/d.
[†] <1 ng/mL per hour.
[‡] Aldosterone-secreting adrenal adenoma.
[§] Children, early onset severe hypertension, history of early hemorrhagic stroke, ACTH regulates aldosterone secretion and renin angiotensin system is suppressed. Suppression of ACTH with glucocorticoids decreases aldosterone and cures the hypertension. High 16 hydroxycortisol/18 oxycortisol.
[¶] Hypertension, decreased potassium, alkalosis, decreased aldosterone, sodium channel mutation.

than 1 ng/mL per hour in mineralocorticoid excess, low renin states.

The best screening test for primary aldosteronism is the plasma aldosterone (PA)/plasma renin activity (PRA) ratio (51). Patients with hypokalemia and resistant hypertension should undergo measurement of both PRA and aldosterone concentration. Both specific medications (52) and a variability of PA levels may affect the accuracy of the ratio. All diuretics should be discontinued 1 to 2 weeks prior to laboratory workup of hypokalemia. If the patient has uncontrolled hypertension, calcium channel blocker (CCB), or a non–atenolol β-blocker may be used. Although doxazosin and irbesartan have the least impact on the ratio, atenolol may lead to an increased rate of false-positive aldosterone-to-renin ratios. Spironolactone and ACE inhibitors also adversely affect this ratio. Physicians may be confused by values measured as PRA versus direct renin measurement. The direct renin divided by eight is roughly equivalent to the PRA. An elevated PA/PRA ratio alone does not establish a diagnosis of primary aldosteronism, and the diagnostic suspicion should be confirmed by demonstrating inappropriate aldosterone secretion.

Table 51.6 lists the laboratory workup for patients with hypertension, hypokalemia, and kaliuresis. A high renin value does not rule out primary aldosteronism. The most important test in diagnosing primary aldosteronism is the 24-hour urinary aldosterone excretion rate. Those specific situations that warrant salt-loading (greater than 200 mEq/day) include individuals with hypertension and normal PA, with a PRA less than or equal to 1.0, those with high PA and normal-high PRA, and those with spontaneous hypokalemia who have normal PA and normal PRA.

## TABLE 51.6

### HYPERTENSION; HYPOKALEMIA ($K_S$ <3.5 MEQ/L) WITH KALIURESIS ($K_V$ >30 MEQ/HR)

**Laboratory Workup**

Serum electrolytes
Serum creatinine, urea
Plasma aldosterone, cortisol, PRA
24-Hour urinary Na, K, Cr, aldosterone, and free cortisol
High-salt diet (UNa> 250 mEq/L per 24 hrs)*
    Normal PA with PRA ≤1.0
    High PA with normal/high PRA
    Normal PA and PRA with spontaneous hypokalemia

* Plasma aldosterone 22 ng/dL, plasma renin activity (PRA) 0.7 ng/mL, urinary aldosterone 14 μg/24 hrs (test = PA >22 ng/dL; AER >14 μg/24 hrs).

Individuals warranting salt-loading can be placed on a high-salt diet (1 level teaspoon of salt each day for 5 days). The urinary aldosterone excretion rate should be determined on days 4 and 5, along with creatinine, potassium, and sodium measurements. If the sodium concentration is less than 250 mEq in 24 hrs, mild increases in urinary aldosterone excretion rate may represent inadequate suppression.

Combining urinary aldosterone levels with urinary free cortisol results can distinguish nonaldosterone mineralocorticoid excess from aldosterone mineralocorticoid excess (Table 51.7). Liddle's syndrome is an autosomal dominant disorder resulting in the low-normal urinary excretion of aldosterone, increased kaliuresis secondary to increased collecting tubular sodium reabsorption, and normal urinary free cortisol measurements. The increased sodium reabsorption in collecting tubules results in increased potassium secretion and hypokalemia. Amiloride or triamterene have been used to close the sodium channels and correct the defect clinically. Patients with Liddle's syndrome usually present with hypertension, hypokalemia, and metabolic acidosis at an early age. Liddle's syndrome can be differentiated from congenital renal hyperplasia and 11-β hydroxysteroid dehydrogenate deficiency (OHSD) by comparing urinary aldosterone with urinary free cortisol values in addition to the clinical presentation.

11-β-OHSD results in the excessive activation of mineralocorticoid receptors (MR) by a steroid dependence on adrenocorticotropic hormone (ACTH), rather than by the conventional mineralocorticoid agonist; the steroid appears to be cortisol. The MRs in the distal nephron have equal affinity for both aldosterone and cortisol, but are normally protected from cortisol by the presence of 11-β dehydrogenase, which inactivates cortisol to cortisone. The 11-18 hemiacetal structure of aldosterone protects it from the action of 11-β dehydrogenase, so that aldosterone gains specific access to the receptors. When this mechanism is defective, either

**TABLE 51.7**

**COMBINING URINARY ALDOSTERONE LEVELS WITH URINARY FREE CORTISOL RESULTS CAN DISTINGUISH NONALDOSTERONE MINERALOCORTICOID EXCESS FROM ALDOSTERONE MINERALOCORTICOID EXCESS**

| Urinary aldosterone | Steroid values | Urinary Free Cortisol | | |
|---|---|---|---|---|
| | | Low | Normal | High |
| | Low-normal | Congenital adrenal hyperplasia | Liddle's syndrome | 11 β-OHSD |
| | | | Exogenous mineralocorticoids | Cushing's syndrome |
| | High | | | GR |
| | | | Primary aldosterone | Adrenal cancer |
| | | | GRA | Primary aldosteronism with Cushing's |

OHSD, hydroxysteroid dehydrogenate deficiency; GR, glucocorticoid remedial; GFR, glucocorticoid remedial aldosteronism.

because of congenital 11-β-OHSD or enzyme inhibition (licorice or carbenoxolone), then intrarenal levels of cortisol increase and cortisol causes inappropriate activation of MR. This results in antinatriuresis and kaliuresis associated with hypertension and hypokalemia. Plasma cortisol concentrations in 11-β-OHSD usually are not elevated. The laboratory abnormalities and symptoms are reversed by spironolactone or dexamethasone, but are exacerbated by physiologic doses of cortisone.

Licorice-induced hypermineralocorticoidism has both low PA and low PRA levels. The glycyrrhetinic acid inhibits the enzyme 11-β dehydroxyase steroid dehydrogenase, thus allowing cortisol to act as the major endogenous mineralocorticoid avidly binding to the MR and inducing inappropriate kaliuresis. It is interesting to note that essential hypertension patients are more sensitive to the inhibition of 11-β hydroxysteroid dehydrogenase by licorice than normotensive subjects, and this inhibition causes more clinical symptoms in women than in men (53). Licorice-containing compounds include antipeptic ulcer medication, carbenoxylone sodium, antituberculosis medication, p/aminosalicylic acid, the French alcoholic beverage Boisson de coco, chewing tobacco (54), and some Asian herbal preparations. Diagnosis depends on the elicitation of a thorough history and laboratory evidence of hypokalemia. In general, a regular daily intake of 100 mg of glycyrrhetinic acid produces adverse effects in sensitive individuals, whereas the consumption of 400 mg/day produces adverse effects in most subjects (55).

GRA is an inherited autosomal dominant disorder that mimics primary aldostoneronism. GRA should be suspected in any patient with primary aldosterone–like presentation who presents with positive family history and primary aldosteronism, early age (under 21 years) of onset of hypertension, and severe hypertension with early death of affected members from cerebrovascular accident. GRA is usually associated with bilateral adrenal hyperplasia.

Patients with GRA have ACTH-sensitive aldosterone production occurring in the zona fisciculata rather than in the zona glomerulosa, which is the normal site of production. The isoenzyme in the zona glomerulosa catalyzes the conversion of deoxycorticosterone to corticosterone and of 18-hydroxycorticosterone to aldosterone. The hybrid gene in GRA results from a genetic mutation that allows for a topic expression of aldosterone synthesis activity in the ACTH-regulated zona fisciculata that normally produces cortisol. Usually, the plasma potassium concentration is normal in over one-half of patients with GRA, in contrast to the pattern seen most commonly with primary aldosteronism. Genetic testing using molecular biologic techniques can detect a chimeric gene responsible for GRA. Standard laboratory testing includes dexamethasone suppression testing and increases in 18-hydroxycortisol and 18-oxycortisol levels. The administration of dexamethasone in doses of 2 mg in 24 hrs (0.5 mg every 6 hrs) usually results in remission of hypertension and hyperkalemia within 7 to 10 days. The suppression of ACTH with exogenous glucocorticoid should correct the metabolic defect and control hypertension in GRA. The use of spironolactone and/or amiloride may be supplemental treatment in addition to exogenous glucocorticoid therapy.

The adrenal computed tomography (CT) scan is helpful in differentiating among adrenal adenoma, adrenal hyperplasia, or adrenal carcinoma. Usually, adrenal carcinomas are large (greater than 5 cm) versus a hypodense unilateral macroadenoma (greater than 1 cm) versus abnormalities in both glands (representative of adrenal hyperplasia). Hounsfield units greater than 10 usually indicate adrenal carcinoma, whereas Hounsfield units less than 10 most likely suggest an adrenal adenoma. The difference in density results from a vascular tumor versus a lipid-rich adenoma.

Adrenal vein sampling after the administration of ACTH is most useful when no adrenal abnormality exists on CT scan or MRI, or when an asymmetric abnormality is present in both glands. The sampling of the adrenal vein is technically difficult and may be restricted to experienced centers. It is important to assess both aldosterone and cortisol values at the time of sampling from the right and left adrenal gland and high and low inferior vena cava (adrenal CT with 3-mm cuts). To be certain the samples are from the adrenal veins, cortisol should also be sampled at the same time. Serum cortisol concentrations should be roughly the same in both adrenal veins and approximately tenfold higher than in the peripheral vein. The aldosterone concentrations should be two times higher from the adrenal vein versus periphery.

Medical therapy with eplerenone (selective aldosterone receptor antagonist) or spironolactone can be used in patients with bilateral adrenal adenomas, adenomas unable to be surgically excised (poor surgical risk), in individuals with adrenal hyperplasia, and in those with significant responses to aldosterone receptor antagonists who do not want surgery. Surgical removal of an aldosterone-producing adenoma leads to normotension and the normal restoration of normal potassium homeostasis in most patients. Adrenal adenomas may be removed laparoscopically. Patients may require drug treatment for 3 to 6 months prior to surgery. Selective hypoaldosteronism usually occurs after aldosterone-producing adenoma removal.

## Cushing's Syndrome

Clinical clues to Cushing's syndrome include a history of recent change in facial appearance and considerable weight gain, together with complaints of weakness, muscle wasting, peripheral bruising, impotence, and, in women, amenorrhea and hirsutism (56). Typical physical features include truncal obesity, moon face, plethora, and typical purplish skin stria.

Screening and laboratory studies may indicate glucose intolerance or frank diabetes mellitus, and occasionally neutrophilia with relative lymphocytopenia. Pathologic fractures of a rib are common. A dexamethasone suppression test may be helpful. For diagnosis and localization, a 24-hour urine/free cortisol test, CT, and radioimmunoassay of plasma ACTH may be helpful.

The standard of care for most cases of Cushing's syndrome is surgical resection of a pituitary gland or an ectopic source of adrenocorticotropic hormone, or the removal of a cortisol-producing adrenal cortical tumor. Transsphenoidal pituitary adenomectomy or radiation therapy to the pituitary bed may be considered in selected cases.

## Pheochromocytoma

Of patients with pheochromocytoma, 80% present with headache, 57% with sweating, 48% with paroxysmal hypertension, 39% with persistent hypertension, and 64% have palpitations. Those individuals who warrant a workup for pheochromocytoma include patients with:

- Episodic symptoms of headache, tachycardia, diaphoresis
- A family history of pheochromocytoma or a MEN syndrome
- Unexplained paroxysms of tachy/brady arrhythmias, and/or hypertension during intubation or induction of anesthesia
- Prolonged or unexplained hypotension after surgery
- Adverse cardiovascular responses to the ingestion or inhalation of certain drugs including anesthetic agents, glucagon, ACHT, thyrotropin-releasing hormone, antidopaminergic agents, miloxane, phenothiazine, guanethedine, and tricyclic antibiotics

Figure 51.4 illustrates the approach to using plasma catecholamines and urinary metanephrines in the evaluation of patients suspected of having pheochromocytoma (57). The measurement of fractionated plasma free metanephrines is the best test for familial pheochromocytoma, whereas 24-hour urinary metanephrines and catecholamines provide adequate sensitivity with low false-positive rates for sporadic pheochromocytoma. A number of medications interfere with the biochemical diagnosis of pheochromocytoma. Methylglucamine results in a decrease in metanephrines, whereas asotalol increases metanephrine concentration. ARBs, ACE inhibitors, and bromocryptine decrease catecholamine values, whereas $\alpha$-1 blockers, $\beta$-blockers, and labetalol increase catecholamine values. Methyldopa and monamine oxidase inhibitors decrease vanillylmandelic acid (VMA) values, whereas neldixic acid and anileridine increase VMA values. Phenothiazine, methyldopa, and tricyclic antibiotics have varying effects on these tests. When blood specimens are drawn under standardized conditions, a total plasma catecholamine of greater than or equal to 2,000 pg/mL is diagnostic of pheochromocytoma, whereas a value of less than 500 pg/mL rules out pheochromocytoma.

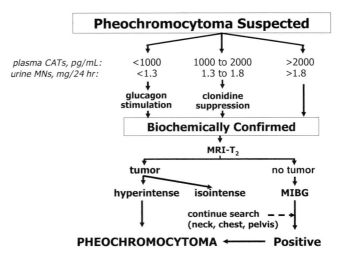

**Figure 51.4** Pheochromocytoma suspected. Reproduced with permission from Bravo EL. Pheochromocytoma. *Cardiol Rev* 2002; 10:44.

For localization, CT scan and MRI are equally sensitive (98% versus 100%), whereas $I^{131}$ metaiodobenzylguanidine iothalamate (MIBG) has excellent specificity (100%) but lower sensitivity (85%). Typically, pheochromocytomas are hyperdense to the liver on T2-weighted images, whereas benign tumors are isodense. If no tumor is detected in a highly suspicious setting, by either CT or MRI, then MIBG scintigraphy should be used.

A provocative test is employed when the clinical findings are highly suggestive of pheochromocytoma, but the blood pressure is normal or slightly increased and plasma catecholamines are between 500 and 1,000 pg/mL. The glucagon test has a high specificity (100%) but low sensitivity (81%). Drugs that inhibit central sympathetic outflow (i.e., clonidine, provocryptine, haloperidol, methyldopa) may decrease plasma catecholamines in normal and hypertensive subjects, but have little effect on the excessive catecholamine secretion by pheochromocytoma. A clonidine suppression test is used for a patient whose plasma catecholamine level is between 1,000 and 2,000 pg/mL, with and without hypertension. A normal clonidine suppression test requires a fall of plasma catecholamines from baseline of at least 50% and below 500 pg/mL.

Pheochromocytomas may develop in about 50% of patients with multiple endocrine neoplasia (MEN) type 2a and type 2b, 25% of patients with Von Hippel–Lindau (VHL) type 2, and 5% with Von Recklinghouse disease (neurofibromatosis). In patients with Von Recklinghouse disease and hypertension, however, a pheochromocytoma has been identified in more than one-third of patients.

Arteriography and/or venous sampling for plasma concentrations are rarely indicated, except in situations in which the biochemical and clinical evidence point strongly to pheochromocytoma and yet the noninvasive techniques persistently fail to localize the tumor sites.

CCBs (nifedipine, verapamil, or diltiazem) are used with or without selective α-1 receptor blockers (ARBs; prazosin, terazosin, doxazasine) in the preoperative management of pheochromocytoma patients. The CCBs relax arterial smooth muscle and decrease peripheral vascular resistance by inhibiting the norepinenephrine-mediated release of intracellular calcium and/or calcium transmembrane influx. These agents do not usually produce the overshoot hypotension seen with nonselective α-adrenergic blockade. Selective ARBs do not enhance norepinenephrine release and usually are not associated with reflex tachycardia. Therefore, CCBs or selective α-1 receptor blockers are effective and safe without the patient experiencing the adverse effects that are associated with the relatively nonspecific, complete, and prolonged α-1 blockade using phenoxybenzamine. Phenoxybenzamine, traditionally used to counteract the sudden release of massive quantities of catecholamines during surgical intervention, is associated with dramatic hypertension during tumor manipulation and is therefore used less today than previously.

Current medications and surgical techniques have significantly decreased the risk of surgical intervention in pheochromocytoma. Laparoscopic surgery can be used successfully in the majority of cases for tumor removal. Patients who undergo laparoscopic versus traditional surgery usually have a shorter postoperative course and earlier resumption of normal activities.

Several prognostic factors have been suggested for characterizing patients with malignant pheochromocytoma. These characteristics include large tumor size, local tumor extension at the time of surgery, and a DNA-ploidy pattern with DNA-diploid being benign and DNA-anuloploidy tetraploidy having a more progressive nature (58).

## Renal Parenchymal Disease

Hypertension is one of the main contributing factors to progressive renal injury. Lowering the BP level to below that recommended for patients with essential hypertension slows the progression of renal injury. Patients with renal parenchymal disease usually present with renal insufficiency, proteinuria, or hematuria (59,60). Renal parenchymal disease is a common secondary cause of hypertension, although not often reversible. The clinical clues of renal parenchymal disease are easily detected with a carefully performed urinalysis and screening tests of renal function (serum creatinine and blood urea nitrogen). Verifying proteinuria using sulfosalicylic acid is important because it detects protein light chains present in dysproteinemic states. Urinary protein should be quantitated with a 24-hour collection to establish the significance of the proteinuria. Additional screening studies may include the determination of 24-hour urine protein levels and renal ultrasonography. For diagnosis and localization, assessment of the iothalamate glomerular filtration rate and renal biopsy may be helpful.

Baseline SBP is a stronger predictor than DBP of renal outcome in patients with type 2 diabetes mellitus and in diabetic nephropathy. Patients with the highest baseline pulse pressure have the highest risk for nephropathy progression and experience the greatest risk reduction when SBP is lowered to <140 mm Hg (14). The underlying etiology of the renal disease (i.e., focal segmental glomerulosclerosis, chronic interstitial nephritis, amyloidosis, etc.), based on results from the previously mentioned studies, determines the immediate and long-term management of renal parenchymal disease. The aggressive treatment and control of BP can slow the progression of renal function loss, especially using ACE inhibitors or ARBs as specific additions to the regimen (61). A significant opportunity exists to improve the treatment of hypertension in CKD by the increased use of ACE inhibitors and ARBs (62). In diabetics, tight control of blood sugar also can slow the loss of renal function. For patients who do progress to ESRD, renal replacement therapies, including hemodialysis or peritoneal dialysis, are available, together with renal transplantation for selected patients.

## Renovascular Disease

The clinical clues for renovascular disease that may be responsible for renovascular hypertension include:

- Abrupt onset of hypertension
- Age younger than 30 years or older than 55 years
- Accelerated or malignant hypertension (grade 3 or 4 retinopathy)
- Hypertension refractory to a triple-drug regimen
- Hypertension and diffuse vascular disease (carotid, coronary, peripheral vascular)
- Systolic/diastolic epigastric bruit
- Hypertension and unexplained renal insufficiency
- Renal insufficiency induced by ACE inhibitor therapy
- Severe hypertension and recurrent "flash" pulmonary edema (59,63,64)

A number of specialized diagnostic tests have been used to screen patients suspected of having renovascular disease. The duplex Doppler ultrasonography, spiral CT angiography, and magnetic resonsonance angiography (MRA) are replacing traditional screening tests (i.e., IVP, plasma renin activity, captopril renogram). Renal arteriography remains the gold standard for diagnosing renal artery stenosis. Renovascular disease can be effectively diagnosed with an acceptable specificity and sensitivity using most forms of newer diagnosis tests (Table 51.8)

Uncontrolled BP and progressive compromise in renal function are the primary indicators for intervention. For younger patients with fibromuscular dysplasia (medial fibroplasia, intimal fibroplasia, periarterial hyperplasia), percutaneous transluminal renal angioplasty is the mainstay of therapy, with surgical revascularization considered a secondary indication. Successful angioplasty results in a reduction of both the disease and hypertension (65). For older patients with atherosclerotic ischemic nephropathy, percutaneous transluminal renal angioplasty plus stenting or surgical revascularization is the usual option. Angioplasty and stent placement in patients with atherosclerotic renal arterial disease will not improve BP management if residual renal function is <40%.

## TABLE 51.8

### SPECIFICITY AND SENSITIVITY OF SCREENING TESTS FOR RENOVASCULAR HYPERTENSION

| Test | Sensitivity (%) | Specificity (%) |
|---|---|---|
| Magnetic resonance angiography (MRA) | 100 | 96 |
| Duplex Doppler ultrasonography | 69 to 96 | 86 to 90 |
| Spiral computed tomography angiography | 98 | 94 |
| IVP | ~75 | ~85 |
| Captopril renogram | 41 to 93 | 95 |
| Captopril stimulated PRA | 75 | 89 |

## Thyroid and Parathyroid Disorders

Thyroid dysfunction, together with renovascular hypertension, represents the most common form of reversible secondary hypertension observed in hypertensive individuals older than 60 years (66,67). Thyrotoxic patients have hyperdynamic hypertension and high cardiac output, seen predominantly as an elevated SBP. Conversely, hypothyroid patients have a high prevalence of elevated DBP, and this can be a valuable clue in the elderly, in whom primary diastolic hypertension is rare. Most patients with primary hyperparathyroidism are asymptomatic, and the clinical diagnosis should be strongly suspected by the finding of hypercalcemia. The side effects of hypercalcemia, such as polyuria, polydipsia, renal calculi, peptic ulcer disease, and hypertension, may offer diagnostic clues. Multiple endocrine neoplasia syndromes are the exception to the above, and the finding of a thyroid nodule, thyroid mass, or cervical lymphadenopathy should suggest the possibility of a medullary thyroid carcinoma.

Additional screening studies may include the assessment of thyroid-stimulating hormone level, serum thyroid hormone level, and serum calcitonin level for thyroid disease. For hyperparathyroidism, serum calcium, serum phosphorus, and serum parathyroid hormone level should be assessed.

For diagnosis and localization, the decreased thyroid-stimulating hormone and increased free thyroxine index should be assessed in the hyperthyroid patient. Increased thyroid-stimulating hormone, decreased free thyroxine index, presence of medullary thyroid carcinoma, and increased calcitonin should be assessed in the hypothyroid patient. Hypercalcemia, hypophosphatemia, and increased parathyroid hormone level should be assessed in the hyperparathyroid patient.

## HYPERTENSIVE EMERGENCIES AND URGENCIES

Hypertensive emergencies are those occasional situations that require immediate BP reduction (not necessarily to normal) to prevent or limit target organ damage. Examples include hypertensive encephalopathy, intracranial hemorrhage, acute pulmonary edema, or a dissecting aortic aneurysm (68). Hypertensive urgencies are those situations in which the reduction of BP over several to 24 hours is desirable. Examples include patients with upper levels of stage III hypertension and those with progressive target organ complications, but no acute deterioration in target organ disease. Elevated BP alone, in the absence of symptoms or new or progressive target organ damage, rarely requires emergency therapy. A number of effective agents are available for the management of hypertensive emergencies and urgencies (Table 51.9).

## TABLE 51.9

### DRUGS FOR THE MANAGEMENT OF HYPERTENSIVE EMERGENCIES AND URGENCIES

| Agent | Dose | Onset/Duration of Action (after discontinuation) | Precautions |
|---|---|---|---|
| Parenteral Vasodilators | | | |
| Sodium nitroprusside | 0.25(10.0 µg/kg/min as i.v. infusion[a]; maximal dose for 10 min only | Immediate/2–3 min after infusion | Nausea, vomiting, muscle twitching; with prolonged use may cause thiocyanate intoxication, methemoglobinemia acidosis, cyanide poisoning; bags, bottles, and delivery sets must be light-resistant |
| Fenoldopam mesylate | 0.1–0.3 mg/kg/min as i.v. infusion | <5 min/30 min | Headache, tachycardia, flushing, local phlebitis |
| Glyceryl trinitrate | 5–100 µg as i.v. infusion[a] | 2–5 min/5–10 min | Headache, tachycardia, vomiting, flushing, methemoglobinemia; requires special delivery system due to drug binding to polyvinyl chloride tubing |
| Nicardipine | 5–15 mg/h i.v. infusion | 1–5 min/15–30 min, but may exceed 12 h after prolonged infusion | Tachycardia, nausea, vomiting, headache, increased intracranial pressure; Hypotension, may be protracted after prolonged infusions |
| Verapamil | 5–10 mg i.v.; can follow with infusion of 3–25 mg/h | 1–5 min/30–60 min | First-, second-, third-degree heart block, concomitant digitalis or beta blockers, bradycardia |
| Diazoxide | 50–150 mg as i.v. bolus, repeated, or 15–30 mg/min by i.v. infusion | 2–5 min/3–12 h | Hypotension, tachycardia, aggravation of angina pectoris, nausea and vomiting, hyperglycemia with repeated injections |
| Hydralazine | 10–20 mg as i.v. bolus or 10–40 mg i.m., repeat every 4–6 h | 10 min i.v./>1 h i.v. 20–30 min i.m./4–6 h i.m. | Tachycardia, headache, vomiting, aggravation of angina pectoris |
| Enalaprilat | 0.625–1.250 mg every 6 h i.v. | 15–60 min/12–24 h | Renal failure in patients with bilateral renal artery stenosis, hypotension |
| Parenteral Adrenergic Inhibitors | | | |
| Labetalol | 20–80 mg as i.v. bolus every 10 min; 2 mg/min as i.v. infusion | 5–10 min/2–6 h | Bronchoconstriction, heart block, orthostatic hypotension |
| Esmolol | 500 mg/kg/bolus injection i.v. or 25–100 (g/kg/min by infusion; may rebolus after 5 min or increase infusion rate to 300 mg/kg/min | 1–5 min/15–30 min | Greater than first-degree heart block, congestive heart failure, asthma |
| Methyldopate | 250–500 mg as i.v. infusion every 6 h | 30–60 min/4–6 h | Drowsiness |
| Phentolamine | 5–15 mg as i.v. bolus | 1–2 min/10–30 min | Tachycardia, orthostatic hypotension |
| Oral Agents | | | |
| Captopril | 25 mg p.o., repeat as needed SL, 25 mg | 15–30 min/6–8 h SL 15–30 min/2–6 h | Hypotension, renal failure in bilateral renal artery stenosis |
| Clonidine | 0.1–0.2 mg p.o., repeat hourly as required to total dose of 0.6 mg | 30–60 min/8–16 h | Hypotension, drowsiness, dry mouth |
| Labetalol | 200–400 mg p.o., repeat every 2–3 h | 30 min to 2 h/2–12 h | Bronchoconstriction, heart block, orthostatic hypotension |
| Prazosin | 1–2 mg p.o.; repeat hourly, as needed | 1–2 h/8–12 h | Syncope (first dose), palpitations, tachycardia, orthostatic hypotension |

[a] Requires special delivery system.

Hypertensive emergencies during pregnancy warrant careful drug selection and hemodynamic monitoring to avoid any increase in fetal risk. Whereas hydralazine, methyldopa and magnesium sulfate are traditional therapeutic agents in pregnancy, labetalol has been used more recently. Bolus injections may achieve therapeutic BP lowering goals sooner than continuous infusion. Consideration for timely delivery to the infant will often help with BP control.

Most hypertensive urgencies represent patients who are noncompliant with therapy or who are inadequately treated for essential hypertension. In most cases, an immediate resumption of medication with appropriate outpatient follow-up represents adequate therapy.

The use of fast-acting nifedipine in hypertensive urgencies has been discouraged by the U.S. Food and Drug Administration (FDA). A number of reported serious adverse effects and the inability to control the rate or degree of decline in BP make this agent unacceptable (69,70). The routine use of sublingual or oral nifedipine in patients with chronic hypertension, when BPs increase beyond a predetermined level, is also considered unacceptable.

## REFERENCES

1. Oparil S, Zaman MA, Calhoun DA. Pathogenesis of hypertension. *Ann Intern Med* 2003;139:761–776.
2. Hajjar I, Kotchen TA. Trends in prevalence, awareness, treatment, and control of hypertension in the United States, 1988–2000. *JAMA* 2003;290:199–206.
3. Abbott KC, Bakris GL. What have we learned from the current trials? *Med Clin North Am* 2004;88:189–207.
4. Chobanian AV, Bakris GL, Black HR, et al. The Seventh Report of the Joint National Committee on Prevention, Detection, Evaluation, and Treatment of High Blood Pressure: The JNC 7 Report. *JAMA* 2003;289:2560–2571.
5. Chobanian AV, Bakris GL, Black HR, et al. Seventh report of the Joint National Committee on Prevention, Detection, Evaluation, and Treatment of High Blood Pressure. *Hypertension* 2003;42:1206–1252.
6. Joint National Committee. The sixth report of the committee on the Prevention, Detection, Evaluation and Treatment of High Blood Pressure (JNC-VI). *Arch Intern Med* 1997;157:2413–2446.
7. Major outcomes in high-risk hypertensive patients randomized to angiotensin-converting enzyme inhibitor or calcium channel blocker vs. diuretic: The Antihypertensive and Lipid-Lowering Treatment to Prevent Heart Attack Trial (ALLHAT). *JAMA* 2002;288:2981–2997.
8. Brenner BM, Cooper ME, de Zeeuw D, et al. Effects of losartan on renal and cardiovascular outcomes in patients with type 2 diabetes and nephropathy. *N Engl J Med* 2001;345:861–869.
9. Parving HH, Lehnert H, Brochner-Mortensen J, et al. The effect of irbesartan on the development of diabetic nephropathy in patients with type 2 diabetes. *N Engl J Med* 2001;345:870–878.
10. Wright JT, Jr., Bakris G, Greene T, et al. Effect of blood pressure lowering and antihypertensive drug class on progression of hypertensive kidney disease: results from the AASK trial. *JAMA* 2002;288:2421–2431.
11. Psaty BM, Lumley T, Furberg CD, et al. Health outcomes associated with various antihypertensive therapies used as first-line agents: a network meta-analysis. *JAMA* 2003;289:2534–2544.
12. Hjalmarson A, Waagstein F. The role of beta-blockers in the treatment of cardiomyopathy and ischaemic heart failure. [Review]. *Drugs* 1994;47 Suppl 4:31–39;discussion 39.
13. Eichhorn EJ. The paradox of beta-adrenergic blockade for the management of congestive heart failure. *Am J Med* 1992;92:527–538.
14. Bakris GL, Weir MR, Shanifar S, et al. Effects of blood pressure level on progression of diabetic nephropathy: results from the RENAAL study. *Arch Intern Med* 2003;163:1555–1565.
15. Hornig B, Landmesser U, Kohler C, et al. Comparative effect of ace inhibition and angiotensin II type 1 receptor antagonism on bioavailability of nitric oxide in patients with coronary artery disease: role of superoxide dismutase. *Circulation* 2001;103: 799–805.
16. Thomas MC, Cooper ME, Shahinfar S, et al. Dialysis delayed is death prevented: a clinical perspective on the RENAAL study. *Kidney Int* 2003;63:1577–1579.
17. Lewington S, Clarke R, Qizilbash N, et al. Age-specific relevance of usual blood pressure to vascular mortality: a meta-analysis of individual data for one million adults in 61 prospective studies. *Lancet* 2002;360:1903–1913.
18. Clausen P, Jensen JS, Jensen G, et al. Elevated urinary albumin excretion is associated with impaired arterial dilatory capacity in clinically healthy subjects. *Circulation* 2001;103:1869–1874.
19. Bakris GL. Maximizing cardiorenal benefit in the management of hypertension: achieving blood pressure goals. *J Clin Hypertens* (*Greenwich*) 1999;1:141–147.
20. Bakris GL, Weir MR, Study of Hypertension and the Efficacy of Lotrel in Diabetes (SHIELD) Investigators. Achieving goal blood pressure in patients with type 2 diabetes: conventional versus fixed-dose combination approaches. *J Clin Hypertens* (*Greenwich*) 2003;5:202–209.
21. Forette F, Lechowski L, Rigaud AS, et al. Does the benefit of antihypertensive treatment outweigh the risk in very elderly hypertensive patients? *J Hypertens* 2000;18:S9–S12.
22. Voko Z, Bots ML, Hofman A, et al. J-shaped relation between blood pressure and stroke in treated hypertensives. *Hypertension* 1999;34:1181–1185.
23. Koren MJ, Devereux RB, Casale PN, et al. Relation of left ventricular mass and geometry to morbidity and mortality in uncomplicated essential hypertension. *Ann Intern Med* 1991;114: 345–352.
24. Liao Y, Cooper RS, McGee DL, et al. The relative effects of left ventricular hypertrophy, coronary artery disease, and ventricular dysfunction on survival among black adults. *JAMA* 1995;273:1592–1597.
25. Gueyffier F, Boutitie F, Boissel JP, et al. Effect of antihypertensive drug treatment on cardiovascular outcomes in women and men. A meta-analysis of individual patient data from randomized, controlled trials. The INDANA Investigators. *Ann Intern Med* 1997;126:761–767.
26. Cicila GT. Strategy for uncovering complex determinants of hypertension using animal models. *Curr Hypertens Rep* 2000;2:217–226.
27. Hunt SC, et al. In: King RA, Roubenoff R, Motulsky AG, eds. *The Genetic Basis of Common Diseases*. New York: Oxford Press, 2002.
28. Cusi D, Barlassina C, Azzani T, et al. Polymorphisms of alpha-adducin and salt sensitivity in patients with essential hypertension. *Lancet* 1997;349:1353–1357.
29. Hunt SC, Geleijnse JM, Wu LL, et al. Enhanced blood pressure response to mild sodium reduction in subjects with the 235T variant of the angiotensinogen gene. *Am J Hypertens* 1999;12:460–466.
30. Turner ST, Schwartz GL, Chapman AB, et al. C825T polymorphism of the G protein beta(3)-subunit and antihypertensive response to a thiazide diuretic. *Hypertension* 2001;37:739–743.
31. Lifton RP. Molecular genetics of human blood pressure variation. *Science* 1996;272:676–680.
32. Luft FC. Present status of genetic mechanisms in hypertension. *Med Clin North Am* 2004;88:1–18, vii.
33. Black HR. The paradigm has shifted, to systolic blood pressure [editorial; comment]. *Hypertension* 1999;34:386–387.
34. Swales JD. Systolic vs. diastolic blood pressure: paradigm shift or cycle? *J Hum Hypertens* 2000;14:477–479.
35. Beevers DG. Epidemiological, pathophysiological and clinical significance of systolic, diastolic and pulse pressure. *J Hum Hypertens* 2004;18:531–533.
36. Franklin SS, Khan SA, Wong ND, Larson MG, Levy D. Is pulse pressure useful in predicting risk for coronary heart disease? The Framingham Heart Study. *Circulation* 1999;100:354–360.

37. Turner ST, Bielak LF, Narayana AK, et al. Ambulatory blood pressure and coronary artery calcification in middle-aged and younger adults. *Am J Hypertens* 2002;15:518–524.

38. Staessen JA, Gasowski J, Wang JG, et al. Risks of untreated and treated isolated systolic hypertension in the elderly: meta-analysis of outcome trials. *Lancet* 2000;355:865–872.

39. Vaccarino V, Berkman LF, Krumholz HM. Long-term outcome of myocardial infarction in women and men: a population perspective. *Am J Epidemiol* 2000;152:965–973.

40. Mitchell GF, Moye LA, Braunwald E, et al. Sphygmomanometrically determined pulse pressure is a powerful independent predictor of recurrent events after myocardial infarction in patients with impaired left ventricular function. SAVE investigators. Survival and Ventricular Enlargement. *Circulation* 1997;96:4254–4260.

41. Franklin SS, Larson MG, Khan SA, et al. Does the relation of blood pressure to coronary heart disease risk change with aging? The Framingham Heart Study. *Circulation* 2001;103:1245–1249.

42. Clement DL, De Buyzere ML, De Bacquer DA, et al. Prognostic value of ambulatory blood-pressure recordings in patients with treated hypertension. *N Engl J Med* 2003;348:2407–2415.

43. Kaplan NM, Izzo JL. Refractory hypertension. In: Izzo JL, Black HR, eds. *Hypertension Primer*. Dallas: American Heart Association, 2003;382–384.

44. Yakovlevitch M, Black HR. Resistant hypertension in a tertiary care clinic. *Arch Intern Med* 1991;151:1786–1792.

45. Taler SJ, Textor SC, Augustine JE. Resistant hypertension: comparing hemodynamic management to specialist care. *Hypertension* 2002;39:982–988.

46. Nieto FJ, Young TB, Lind BK, et al. Association of sleep-disordered breathing, sleep apnea, and hypertension in a large community-based study. Sleep Heart Health Study. *JAMA* 2000;283:1829–1836.

47. Pepperell JC, Ramdassingh-Dow S, Crosthwaite N, et al. Ambulatory blood pressure after therapeutic and subtherapeutic nasal continuous positive airway pressure for obstructive sleep apnoea: a randomised parallel trial. *Lancet* 2002;359:204–210.

48. Serfas D, Borow KM. Coarctation of the aorta: Anatomy, pathophysiology, and natural history. *J Cardiovasc Med* 1983;8:575–581.

49. Rocchini AP. Coarctation of the aorta. In: Izzo JL, Jr., Black HR, eds. *Hypertension Primer*. Dallas: American Heart Association, 1999;146–147.

50. Biglieri EG, Irony I, Kater CE. Identification and implications of new types of mineralocorticoid hypertension. *J Steroid Biochem* 1989;32:199–204.

51. Montori VM, Young WF, Jr. Use of plasma aldosterone concentration-to-plasma renin activity ratio as a screening test for primary aldosteronism. A systematic review of the literature. *Endocrinol Metab Clin North Am* 2002;31:619–632, xi.

52. Mulatero P, Rabbia F, Milan A, et al. Drug effects on aldosterone/plasma renin activity ratio in primary aldosteronism. *Hypertension* 2002;40:897–902.

53. Sigurjonsdottir HA, Manhem K, Axelson M, et al. Subjects with essential hypertension are more sensitive to the inhibition of 11 beta-HSD by liquorice. *J Hum Hypertens* 2003;17:125–131.

54. Blachley JD, Knochel JP. Tobacco chewer's hypokalemia: licorice revisited. *N Engl J Med* 1980;302:784–785.

55. Stormer FC, Reistad R, Alexander J. Glycyrrhizic acid in liquorice—evaluation of health hazard. *Food Chem Toxicol* 1993; 31:303–312.

56. Kaye TB, Crapo L. The Cushing syndrome: an update on diagnostic tests. *Ann Intern Med* 1990;112:434–444.

57. Bravo EL. Pheochromocytoma. *Cardiol Rev* 2002;10:44–50.

58. Nativ O, Grant CS, Sheps SG, et al. The clinical significance of nuclear DNA ploidy pattern in 184 patients with pheochromocytoma. *Cancer* 1992;69:2683–2687.

59. National High Blood Pressure Education Program (NHBPEP) Working Group. 1995 Update of the Working Group Reports on Chronic Renal Failure and Renovascular Hypertension. *Arch Intern Med* 1996;156:1938–1947.

60. Moore MA, Porush JG. Hypertension and renal insufficiency: recognition and management. *Am Fam Phys* 1992;45:1248–1256.

61. Bakris GL, Williams M, Dworkin L, et al. Preserving renal function in adults with hypertension and diabetes: a consensus approach. National Kidney Foundation Hypertension and Diabetes Executive Committees Working Group. *Am J Kidney Dis* 2000;36:646–661.

62. Giverhaug T, Falck A, Eriksen BO. Effectiveness of antihypertensive treatment in chronic renal failure: to what extent and with which drugs do patients treated by nephrologists achieve the recommended blood pressure? *J Hum Hypertens* 2004;18:649–654.

63. Mann SJ, Pickering TG. Detection of renovascular hypertension. State of the art: 1992. *Ann Intern Med* 1992;117:845–853.

64. Conlon PJ, O'Riordan E, Kalra PA. New insights into the epidemiologic and clinical manifestations of atherosclerotic renovascular disease. *Am J Kidney Dis* 2000;35:573–587.

65. Slovut DP, Olin JW. Fibromuscular dysplasia. *N Engl J Med* 2004; 350:1862–1871.

66. Richards AM, Espiner EA, Nicholls MG, et al. Hormone, calcium and blood pressure relationships in primary hyperparathyroidism [published erratum appears in *J Hypertens* 1988 Nov;6(11):ii]. *J Hypertens* 1988;6:747–752.

67. Streeten DH, Anderson GH, Jr., Howland T, et al. Effects of thyroid function on blood pressure. Recognition of hypothyroid hypertension. *Hypertension* 1988;11:78–83.

68. Vidt DG. Management of hypertensive urgencies and emergencies. In: Izzo JL, Jr., Black HR, eds. *Hypertension Primer: The Essentials of High Blood Pressure*. Dallas: American Heart Association, 1999; 437–440.

69. Furberg CD, Psaty BM, Meyer JV. Nifedipine. Dose-related increase in mortality in patients with coronary heart disease. *Circulation* 1995;92:1326–1331.

70. Grossman E, Messerli FH, Grodzicki T, Kowey P. Should a moratorium be placed on sublingual nifedipine capsules given for hypertensive emergencies and pseudoemergencies? *JAMA* 1996;276:1328–1331.

# Critical Fluid and Electrolytic Abnormalities in Clinical Practice

**52**

*Marc A. Pohl*

An understanding of fluid and electrolyte abnormalities in clinical practice requires an appreciation of certain pertinent facts:

- The normal distribution of the body fluid compartments and perturbations in the distribution of these compartments
- Recognition of clinical conditions that either contract or expand the individual body fluid compartments
- Differentiation between disturbances of sodium balance and disturbances in water balance
- Identification of the causes of increased or decreased concentrations of sodium and potassium

This chapter discusses the normal and abnormal distribution of the body fluid compartments, clinical conditions associated with sodium excess or depletion, hypokalemia, hyperkalemia, hyponatremia, hypernatremia, and an approach to polyuria.

## DISTRIBUTION OF THE BODY FLUID COMPARTMENTS

Total body water (TBW) is approximately 50% to 70% of total body weight. It is generally assumed that females have more fat (hence, less water) than males, and most textbooks indicate that TBW is approximately 60% of body weight for men and 50% of body weight for women. The TBW is subdivided into two major compartments: the intracellular fluid (ICF) compartment and the extracellular fluid (ECF) compartment. The ICF compartment accounts for approximately two-thirds of TBW and the ECF compartment for approximately one-third of TBW. Accordingly, the ICF compartment is approximately 40% of body weight and the ECF compartment approximately 20% of body weight. The ECF compartment is further divided into two subcompartments: the interstitial fluid volume compartment and the plasma volume compartment. The plasma volume compartment accounts for approximately one-fourth of the ECF compartment and therefore represents 5% of body weight. This normal distribution of the body fluid compartments is depicted in Figure 52.1. The trans-cellular fluid compartment is a minor subdivision of the ECF compartment and includes small volumes such as aqueous humor, cerebral spinal fluid, and synovial fluid.

## SODIUM

Approximately 3,500 mEq of sodium is present in the body of a 70-kg man. Approximately one fifth of this total body sodium is chemically bound in bone and thought to be metabolically unavailable for exchange among the body fluid compartments. The remainder of the total body sodium, approximately 40 mEq/kg of body weight, is biologically active. Most of the total body exchangeable sodium (approximately 2,000 to 2,500 mEq) resides in the ECF compartment, at a concentration of approximately 135 to 145 mEq/L. Thus, sodium is principally a cation of the ECF compartment.

A relatively small amount of sodium is present within cells (i.e., allocated to the ICF compartment), approximately 5 to 10 mEq/L of intracellular water (in muscle). The great discrepancy between the ECF sodium concentration (135 to 145 mEq/L) and the ICF sodium concentration (5 to 10 mEq/L) does not result from an absolute impermeability of cell membranes to sodium. Rather, sodium is continuously diffusing into cells from the ECF and is continuously being extruded to maintain its low intracellular concentration. This extrusion of sodium ions from within the cells to the ECF compartment appears to be a major transport activity of cells. Because this process requires that sodium be transported out of the cell against both an electrical and a chemical concentration gradient, work must be performed in maintaining the ECF position of sodium. The energy for this process derives from the metabolism within cells and is important in preserving cell volume. Impaired cellular metabolism disrupts the active extrusion of sodium from cells, allowing sodium to continually leak into the cell from the ECF, thereby increasing sodium accumulation within the cells. In this setting, chloride also accumulates in the cell, and as a net gain of intracellular solute occurs, cellular swelling ensues. This cellular swelling may have important consequences in clinical

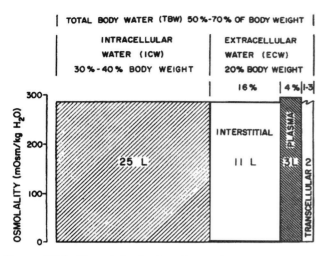

**Figure 52.1** Normal distribution of water between intracellular fluid and extracellular fluid compartments.

conditions of ischemia to kidney tissue cells, heart muscle cells, and brain cells.

## Sodium Balance

The normal daily nutritional sodium requirement is met by the average daily diet and is generally in the range of 75 to 250 mEq/day. This variance in daily sodium intake is conditioned by dietary habit and taste in seasoning one's food. Although a small loss of sodium in the form of sweat and desquamated epithelium (12 to 20 mEq/day) occurs in normal people, for all practical purposes, the urinary sodium excretion is a reflection of the daily dietary sodium intake. Thus, in the steady state, there is no normal value for urinary sodium excretion because the urinary sodium excretion varies directly with the dietary intake of sodium. This concept of sodium balance also holds true for patients receiving chronic diuretic therapy, wherein the 24-hour urinary sodium excretion reflects the dietary sodium intake. A clinical application of sodium balance is the use of the 24-hour urinary sodium excretion in a hypertensive patient who appears to be refractory to antihypertensive drug treatment; such patients frequently ingest large amounts of salt in the diet (and often deny it). Measuring the 24-hour urinary sodium excretion in these patients, whether they are taking diuretics or not, allows the physician to estimate dietary sodium intake accurately.

Because sodium is the major ion in the ECF compartment, the ECF volume is a function of the sodium content in this compartment. External sodium balance is the most important regulator of the ECF volume and hence of the plasma volume. Deficits in total body sodium are clinically reflected by a reduction in the ECF volume, which, if critical enough, leads to serious hemodynamic compromise. Clinical conditions producing ECF volume contraction include gastrointestinal fluid losses (e.g., diarrhea,

malfunctioning ileostomy) and excessive diuresis from diuretic usage. Excesses in total body sodium content (sodium excess states) are manifested by an expansion of the ECF compartment, often producing congestion of the central circulation or edema.

Sodium excess states are common in clinical medicine. They may present clinically as an expansion of the interstitial fluid volume compartment, or edema. Increases in the ECF volume compartment may be present with or without a measurable increase in the plasma volume compartment. Primary aldosteronism, oliguric acute renal failure, severe chronic renal failure of any cause, and acute glomerulonephritis are examples of sodium excess states having increased ECF volume and an increase in measured plasma volume. Patients with congestive heart failure, nephrotic syndrome, and decompensated liver disease with ascites are examples of sodium excess states with increased ECF volume, but these patients may have normal, expanded, or contracted plasma volumes. These patients have decreased effective plasma volume (decreased effective arterial blood volume). Other clinical examples of increased ECF volume with decreased or ineffective arterial blood volume include patients with hypothyroidism, preeclampsia, arteriovenous fistulas, and salt and water retention associated with hydralazine and minoxidil therapy. These are all examples of sodium excess states.

### Serum Sodium Concentration

The serum sodium concentration is the ratio of the amount of sodium in milliequivalents to body water in liters. The serum sodium concentration is regulated primarily by water balance, not by the total amount of sodium in the body. A low serum sodium concentration (hyponatremia) may be present with deficits in total body sodium (e.g., gastrointestinal fluid losses) or in sodium excess states (e.g., edematous conditions such as ascites and congestive heart failure). A high serum sodium concentration (hypernatremia) may be present with total body sodium deficits (e.g., osmotic diuresis from tube feedings or uncontrolled diabetes mellitus) or with excess total body sodium (e.g., primary aldosteronism).

## POTASSIUM

The body of a 70-kg man contains approximately 3,200 mEq of potassium, or approximately 45 to 50 mEq/kg of body weight. In women, because of a smaller body cell mass in proportion to body weight, the normal potassium content is approximately 35 to 40 mEq/kg, or approximately 2,300 to 2,500 mEq of total body potassium. Only a small amount of total body potassium is present in the ECF volume compartment (approximately 70 mEq), at a concentration of 3.5 to 5.0 mEq/L. Most of the total body potassium resides within the cells, where this intracellular potassium forms the major cation of intracellular water, at a concentration of approximately 150 mEq/L. Most of the total body potassium resides within muscle cells. Total body potassium declines with age as body cell mass diminishes. The normal daily dietary potassium requirements are met by an average diet. Daily potassium intake in food is generally in the range of 40 to 100 mEq, almost all of which is excreted in the urine, with a small component excreted in the stool. Accordingly, 24-hour urinary potassium excretion reflects the dietary potassium intake.

The plasma potassium concentration is not a reliable index for estimating total body potassium. Indeed, the serum potassium concentration may be drastically elevated in the presence of marked total body potassium deficits. Several factors affect the distribution of potassium between the ICF and the ECF volume compartments, including ECF pH, ECF osmolality, drugs (e.g., succinylcholine), and cellular catabolic rate or cellular necrosis. Patients with severe hyperglycemia may have concomitant hyperkalemia attributable to the *solvent drag phenomenon*. Metabolic acidosis, with a resulting decrease in blood pH (acidemia), is commonly associated with an elevated serum potassium concentration, reflecting a redistribution of potassium from the ICF to the ECF volume compartment, rather than an increase in total body potassium content. Conversely, metabolic alkalosis with an increase in blood pH (alkalemia) is often associated with a low serum potassium concentration, again due to a redistribution of potassium between the ECF and ICF volume compartments. Thus, acidosis is usually associated with hyperkalemia, and alkalosis is usually associated with hypokalemia, and in neither situation is the serum potassium concentration a reflection of the body's potassium content. Conversely, most patients with metabolic acidosis have moderate deficits of total body potassium, and patients with significant metabolic alkalosis have moderate to large total body potassium deficits. A more extensive listing of causes of hyperkalemia is given in Table 52.1.

Concentrations of the serum potassium of more than 7 mEq/L are extremely dangerous, and values of 9 to 12 mEq/L are usually fatal, the cause of death being cardiac arrhythmia or arrest. Hence, severe hyperkalemia is always a medical emergency. The electrocardiogram is frequently, but not always, useful in assessing the magnitude of hyperkalemia: For patients with elevated serum potassium levels in the range of 6.5 to 7.5 mEq/L, electrocardiography typically demonstrates tall, peaked, or tented T waves. Serum potassium levels in the range of 7.5 to 8.0 mEq/L may be associated with loss of T waves or widening of electrocardiographic wave complexes. For patients with even more severe hyperkalemia (e.g., serum potassium of more than 8.0 mEq/L), electrocardiography demonstrates biphasic electrocardiographic wave complexes, idioventricular rhythm, and terminal sign wave patterns. Treatment options for hyperkalemia are summarized in Table 52.2.

### TABLE 52.1
### CAUSES OF HYPERKALEMIA

| Normal Total Body K$^+$ | Excessive Total Body K$^+$ |
|---|---|
| Pseudohyperkalemia | Excessive intake |
| Hemolysis of drawn blood | K$^+$ penicillin (1.7 mEq/10$^6$ U) |
| | Salt substitutes (10–14 mEq/g) |
| Tourniquet-induced ischemia | Stored blood |
| | Low-salt diet is K$^+$ rich |
| High leukocyte count ($>5 \cdot 10^5$ mm$^3$) | Defects in renin-aldosterone-renal axis |
| High platelet count ($>7.5 \cdot 10^5$ mm$^3$) | Renin-substrate deficiency |
| | |
| Redistributional | Liver failure |
| Acidosis (inorganic $>$organic) | Glucocorticoid deficiency |
| | Hyporeninemia |
| Hormonal | Aging |
| Insulin deficiency | Extracellular fluid expansion |
| α-Adrenergic agonists | Diabetes mellitus |
| β-Adrenergic blockers | Interstitial nephritis |
| Aldosterone deficiency | Hydronephrosis |
| | Drugs and toxins |
| | Nonsteroidal anti-inflammatory drugs |
| Tissue necrosis | |
| Familial periodic paralysis | β-Blockers |
| | α-Agonists |
| Drugs and toxins | Lead |
| Digitalis poisoning | Converting enzyme inhibitor |
| Succinylcholine | Captopril, lisinopril |
| Arginine, lysine | Aldosterone synthetic defect |
| Tromethamine | Generalized adrenal failure |
| Hyperosmolality (in diabetic patients) | Specific synthetic defect |
| | Idiopathic |
| | Drugs: heparin, spironolactone |
| | Enzyme deficiencies |
| | Renal aldosterone resistance |
| | Oliguria, low urinary sodium |
| | Interstitial nephritis (sickle cell, systemic lupus erythematosus) |
| | Drugs: spironolactone |
| | Hydronephrosis |
| | Amyloidosis |
| | Gordon's syndrome |

K$^+$, potassium.

Deficits in total body potassium are often observed in conjunction with a reduced serum potassium concentration (hypokalemia). The normal range for serum potassium in most laboratories is from 3.5 to 5.0 mEq/L. Thus, a serum potassium concentration of less than 3.5 mEq/L is generally regarded as hypokalemic. The more common causes of hypokalemia with a reduction in total body potassium content are due to losses of potassium from the gastrointestinal tract and diarrhea. Occasionally, a very low dietary potassium intake (e.g., anorexia nervosa) may cause significant hypokalemia. Renal losses of potassium, with consequent

## TABLE 52.2
### TREATMENT OF SEVERE OR MODERATE HYPERKALEMIA

| Treatment | Onset | Duration |
|---|---|---|
| Calcium infusion | 5 min | 1–2 h |
| Glucose and insulin | 15–30 min | 1–4 h |
| Sodium bicarbonate | 15–60 min | 1–4 h |
| Hypertonic saline | 30–60 min | 2–6 h |
| Cation exchange resins | | |
|   Rectal | 30–90 min | Indefinite (repeat) |
|   Oral | 2–12 h | Indefinite (repeat) |
|   Dialysis | 2–8 h | Indefinite (repeat) |

## TABLE 52.4
### ESTABLISHING THE CAUSE OF HYPOKALEMIA

| Serum K+ (mEq/L) | Urinary K+ (mEq/24 h) | Cause |
|---|---|---|
| ≤3.0 | >30 | Renal |
| ≤3.0 | <20 | Extrarenal |

$K^+$, potassium.

hypokalemia, are typically seen in patients taking diuretics and in patients with renal tubular acidosis, mineralocorticoid excess, and hyperadrenocorticism. A more complete listing of the causes of hypokalemia is given in Table 52.3.

The symptoms of hypokalemia include muscular fatigue, hypotonicity of muscles, paralysis, and, occasionally, apnea in the case of severe hypokalemia affecting the muscles of respiration. Cardiac manifestations of hypokalemia include ectopic atrial, nodal, and ventricular beats, as well as tachyarrhythmias. Confusion and agitation may be observed with hypokalemia. Electrocardiography commonly shows diagnostic patterns of hypokalemia when the serum potassium decreases to less than 2.5 mEq/L; these electrocardiographic changes include wide T waves with flattening or inversion of the T wave, prolonged Q-T interval, and prominent U waves.

Because most causes of hypokalemia are due to gastrointestinal potassium losses, low dietary potassium intake, and renal potassium losses, pinpointing the reason

for hypokalemia may be simplified by measuring the 24-hour urinary potassium excretion in conjunction with a simultaneous serum potassium value (Table 52.4). Classifying the cause of hypokalemia as either renal or extrarenal guides the differential diagnosis of hypokalemia.

Hypokalemia is not infrequently associated with hypertensive disorders. These hypokalemic/hypertensive conditions may be categorized as being associated with either elevated or depressed plasma renin activity. Renovascular hypertension, malignant hypertension, renin-secreting tumors, and hypertension in association with oral contraceptives are examples of hypokalemia with hypertension and elevated plasma renin activity. Diuretic therapy in patients with essential hypertension also may present with hypokalemia and elevated plasma renin levels. Hypokalemic hypertensive patients with depressed plasma renin activity include patients with primary aldosteronism due to adrenal adenomas or bilateral adrenal hyperplasia, cases of licorice abuse, and deoxycorticosterone acetate or corticosterone excess states.

In nearly all clinical conditions associated with hypokalemia and total body potassium deficits, the potassium replacement should be in the form of potassium chloride because in most of these clinical situations, hypokalemia and total body potassium deficit occur in conjunction with metabolic alkalosis, and the administration of chloride is necessary to correct metabolic alkalosis.

## CHLORIDE

In a 70-kg man, the total body chloride is approximately 2,000 mEq. Although some chloride is contained within the ICF volume compartment, most of the body chloride resides in the ECF volume compartment, at a concentration of 95 to 105 mEq/L. Changes in chloride ion concentration in the plasma generally move in the same direction as the concentration of sodium in the plasma. Thus, hypochloremia (a reduced plasma chloride concentration) is usually seen in conjunction with hyponatremia (e.g., chloride loss from the gastrointestinal tract, as a result of diuretic usage with urinary loss of chloride, and sometimes after administration of adrenal steroids). Hyperchloremia (an increased plasma chloride concentration) is usually seen in combination with hypernatremia,

## TABLE 52.3
### CAUSES OF HYPOKALEMIA

Gastrointestinal losses
  Vomiting, nasogastric suction, intestinal fistulas
  Diarrhea
  Villous adenoma
  Laxative abuse
Low dietary potassium intake (anorexia nervosa)
Hypomagnesemia
Tumors
  Primary aldosteronism
  Cushing's syndrome
  Insulinoma
  Renal losses
  Secondary aldosteronism (cirrhosis, congestive heart failure, accelerated hypertension)
  Alkalosis—metabolic or respiratory
  Diuretics
  Renal tubular acidosis
Familial periodic paralysis

normal anion gap metabolic acidoses (e.g., ureterosigmoidostomies, renal tubular acidosis, diarrhea, mild to moderate chronic renal failure), and iatrogenically, with the excessive administration of ammonium chloride or hydrochloric acid.

## BICARBONATE

The bicarbonate ($HCO_3^-$) concentration of body fluids is usually reported as total serum carbon dioxide or carbon dioxide combining power. Virtually all total carbon dioxide is dissolved $HCO_3^-$. Clinically important fluid and electrolyte disturbances include those clinical conditions associated with either a decrease in ECF $HCO_3^-$ concentration (e.g., diarrhea, renal failure) or an increase in ECF $HCO_3^-$ concentration (e.g., vomiting, diuretic usage). Detailed discussions of abnormalities of the plasma $HCO_3^-$ concentration usually occur in the context of describing clinical acid–base disorders, which are reviewed in detail in Chapter 53.

## RELATIONSHIP OF PLASMA SODIUM CONCENTRATION TO PLASMA OSMOLALITY

Plasma or serum sodium concentration and plasma or serum osmolality are frequently measured in clinical practice. The plasma osmolality (mOsm/kg) depicts the osmotically active particles in the body fluids relative to the amount of water surrounding those particles. As discussed earlier, the osmolality across all the body fluid compartments is essentially the same, approximately 280 to 290 mOsm/kg. The relationship of the plasma sodium concentration to the plasma osmolality is depicted in the following equations:

$$P_{osm} = [2\ P_{Na}] + [glucose/18] + [BUN/2.8]$$
$$\text{Effective } P_{osm} = 2\ P_{Na}$$

where $P_{osm}$ is the plasma osmolality, $P_{Na}$ is the plasma sodium concentration, and BUN is the blood urea nitrogen concentration. In patients with normal values for plasma sugar and BUN, the effective estimated plasma osmolality is essentially twice the plasma (or serum) sodium concentration.

In the setting of severe hyperglycemia (e.g., plasma glucose 900 mg/dL), assuming an elevated BUN of 30 mg/dL and assuming a sodium concentration of 132 mEq/L, the calculated plasma osmolality would be approximately 324 mOsm/kg. If the plasma osmolality were actually measured in the laboratory in this example of hyperglycemia, the measured and calculated plasma osmolalities would be similar. Conversely, if an osmotically active particle (not measured by routine laboratory tests—e.g., mannitol) were to reside in the ECF volume compartment, the measured plasma osmolality would be substantially higher than the osmolality calculated by the formula above. This discrepancy between measured and calculated osmolality is known as the *osmolal gap*. Clinical conditions characterized by a wide osmolal gap (*measured* greater than *calculated* plasma osmolality) include hypermannitolemia, ethylene glycol intoxication, and methanol intoxication. A wide osmolal gap in the setting of severe metabolic acidosis should alert the physician to the likelihood of ethylene glycol or methanol intoxication.

## PERTURBATIONS IN THE DISTRIBUTION OF THE BODY FLUID COMPARTMENTS

As depicted in Figure 52.1, the body fluid compartments are divided into the ECF and ICF compartments. Note that the osmolality of the body fluid compartments is the same across all body fluids, approximately 280 mOsm/kg. Sodium is the major ion in the ECF volume compartment and the major contributor to the osmolality of the ECF. Potassium is the major cation in the ICF compartment, and with its companion anions, phosphate, and proteins, contributes to the osmolality of the ICF. Other osmotically active particles, known as *osmolytes*, reside primarily in the ICF; the major intracellular osmolytes are glutamate, glutamine, taurine, and myoinositol. Other organic osmolytes are glycine, alanine, lycine, and betaine. These osmolytes play an important role in the maintenance of cell volume.

*Hypertonic* states are common in clinical medicine and are characterized by the concentration (i.e., increased osmolality) of the body fluids and a contraction of the ICF compartment. Hyperglycemia, mannitol infusions, and the administration of hypertonic saline are clinical examples of hypertonic states. In these situations, the osmolality of the ECF is acutely increased and water moves out of the ICF (across the semipermeable membrane separating the cells from the ECF) into the ECF compartment. Hyperosmolality of the body fluids ensues, with initial expansion of the ECF and contraction of the ICF. The symptoms of body fluid hypertonicity with associated cell shrinkage include irritability, restlessness, stupor, muscle twitching, hyperreflexia, spasticity, and, possibly, coma and death. The osmotic demyelinization syndrome that occurs with a too rapid correction of chronic hyponatremia is a clinical example of this pathophysiology. *Hypotonic* states are characterized by dilution of the body fluids (i.e., decreased osmolality), with expansion of the body fluid compartments. Acute water intoxication is an example of a hypotonic state. The clinical consequences of acute hypotonic states include cell swelling; if the brain cells swell too much, cerebral edema and seizures ensue. The effects of administering hypertonic saline, water, and isotonic saline are summarized in Table 52.5.

## TABLE 52.5

**OSMOTIC AND VOLUME EFFECTS WITH ADDITION OF SODIUM CHLORIDE, WATER, OR ISOTONIC SALINE**

| | Hypertonic Sodium Chloride | Water | Isotonic Saline |
|---|---|---|---|
| Plasma osmolality | ↑ | ↓ | 0 |
| Plasma sodium | ↑ | ↓ | 0 |
| Extracellular fluid volume | ↑ | ↑ | ↑ |
| Urine sodium | ↑ | ↑ | ↑ |
| Intracellular fluid volume | ↓ | ↑ | 0 |

↓, decrease; ↑, increase.
(Adapted with permission from Rose BD. *Clinical Physiology of Acid–Base and Electrolyte Disorders*, 4th ed. New York: McGraw-Hill, 1994:224.)

## TABLE 52.6

**VOLUME CONTRACTION VERSUS DEHYDRATION**

| Loss of 1 L Saline | Type of Change | Loss of 1 L Water |
|---|---|---|
| −150 mEq | Change in sodium content | 0 |
| −1,000 mL | Change in total body water | −1,000 mL |
| 0 | Change in plasma osmolality | +2.5% (7.5 mOsm/L) |
| −1,000 mL | Change in extracellular fluid volume | −333 mL |
| −250 mL | Change in plasma volume | −83 mL |

## DEHYDRATION VERSUS VOLUME CONTRACTION

Physicians frequently apply the term *dehydration* to any situation wherein a reduction occurs in the amount of fluid in the body. The previous discussion of the body fluid compartments and appreciating the clinical consequences (described in Table 52.5), however, should draw attention to the difference between loss of water and loss of salt and water from the body fluids. When one loses water from the body (dehydration), the amount of water lost is in proportion to the distribution of that water across all the body fluid compartments—that is, when 1 L of water is lost from the body, such as in profuse sweating, one-third of that water loss comes from the ECF volume compartment, and two-thirds come from the ICF volume compartment. When one loses 1 L of salt and water from the body, as in small intestinal and biliary fluid losses, the patient has essentially lost ECF volume because the concentration of sodium in these gastrointestinal fluids is reasonably close to the concentration of sodium in the ECF volume compartment. Thus, the threat to the central circulation in terms of maintaining blood pressure is formidable when large volumes of salt and water are being lost from the body, in comparison with losses of pure water. Loss of water from the body should be referred to as *dehydration*. Loss of salt and water from the body should be termed *ECF volume contraction* or *volume contraction*.

These concepts are highlighted in Table 52.6, which describes the change in milliliters in the body fluid compartments consequent to the loss of 1 L of normal saline, versus the loss of 1 L of water. Greater losses (e.g., 3 to 4 L) of salt and water would produce reductions in ECF volume and plasma volume, with obvious compromise of the circulation. In treating patients who have undergone body fluid compartment loss from one or more body fluid

compartments, it is crucial to recognize the difference between dehydration and volume contraction: Normal saline, not dextrose 5% concentration in water ($D_5W$), is the treatment for ECF volume contraction. Fluid resuscitation for patients who are truly dehydrated should consist primarily of hypotonic fluids (e.g., $D_5W$ or $D_5W$ with normal saline).

## HYPONATREMIA

The range of the serum sodium concentration in most clinical laboratories is 135 to 145 mEq/L. Hyponatremia is present when the serum sodium concentration decreases to less than 135 mEq/L. Although total body sodium balance determines the ECF volume, sodium balance per se does not determine the serum sodium concentration. Indeed, a decrease in the serum sodium concentration (hyponatremia) can exist in the face of either an excess or deficit of total body sodium. Patients with cirrhosis and ascites are typically hyponatremic, despite an obvious excess of total body sodium. Patients with profound diarrhea or excessive gastrointestinal fluid losses are often hyponatremic in the face of total body sodium deficit.

Aberrations in the serum sodium concentration usually reflect abnormalities in water balance. For this discussion, hyponatremia indicates a positive water balance (water intake exceeds water excretion). This situation develops when the kidneys fail to excrete water normally, in conjunction with continued water intake: A positive water balance ensues, with dilution of the body fluids. With this concept at hand, nearly all types of hyponatremia are dilutional, rendering the term *dilutional hyponatremia* of little differential diagnostic value.

In the normal subject, hyponatremia is prevented by the renal excretion of water excess. The physiologic requirements for this elimination of excess water are the following:

- Ability of the hypothalamic osmoregulatory machinery in the brain to inhibit vasopressin [antidiuretic hormone

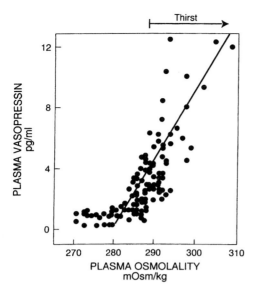

**Figure 52.2** Effect of plasma osmolality on plasma antidiuretic hormone and thirst. (Reproduced with permission from Robertson GL, Aycinena P. Neurogenic disorders of osmoregulation. *Am J Med* 1982;72:339.)

(ADH)] secretion in response to hypoosmolality of the plasma

■ Normal intrinsic renal diluting mechanisms

The relationship between plasma osmolality and plasma ADH is depicted in Figure 52.2. In normal individuals, plasma ADH levels are virtually undetectable when the plasma osmolality falls below 280 mOsm/kg. In most clinical conditions associated with hyponatremia and reduced plasma osmolality (e.g., plasma osmolality of 260 mOsm/kg), however, plasma ADH levels are elevated, thus promoting the retention of water in the collecting tubules of the kidneys and thereby contributing to a persistent reduction in the plasma sodium concentration. The reason for this increase in ADH despite reduced plasma osmolality is the volume stimulus for ADH release—that is, an actual or perceived reduction (decreased effective arterial blood volume) in plasma volume or a tumor producing ADH independent of the plasma osmolality. Normal intrinsic renal diluting mechanisms include (i) adequate delivery of salt-containing fluid to the distal diluting sites of the nephron; (ii) intact salt transport at the diluting sites in the nephron; and (iii) impermeability of the distal nephron to water in the absence of ADH. In most clinical conditions featuring hyponatremia, these normal intrinsic renal diluting mechanisms are impaired such that the urine is not adequately diluted (urine osmolality is elevated). This results in decreased water excretion and contributes to positive water balance and hyponatremia. Because hyponatremia is prevented in normal subjects by the excretion of water excess (for the reasons described previously), the critical pathophysiologic question to ask is "Why is the excess water not excreted?" If patients with congestive heart failure

(frequently hyponatremic) were able to excrete water normally, they would not become hyponatremic. Thus, hyponatremia is a disorder of urinary dilution.

## Approach to the Diagnosis of Hyponatremic Syndromes

Excluding causes of pseudohyponatremia, such as hyperlipidemia and hyperproteinemia, is the first step in evaluating the hyponatremic patient. In these two conditions, although the serum sodium concentration may be factitiously low, the sodium concentration of plasma water is normal. With severe hyperlipidemia, the serum will appear lactescent; factitious hyponatremia in conjunction with severe hyperproteinemia is usually observed when the plasma protein concentration is in excess of 12 to 15 g/dL. In these two conditions, the plasma sodium concentration is low, but the plasma osmolality is normal.

Hyperglycemia and hypermannitolemia, sometimes categorized as examples of pseudohyponatremia, really produce true hyponatremia. In these situations, water moves from the ICF to the ECF compartment, resulting in a reduction of the serum sodium concentration. In contrast to hyperlipidemia and hyperproteinemia, the low serum sodium concentration associated with hyperglycemia or hypermannitolemia is a true reflection of the ECF sodium concentration. In these latter two conditions, the serum or plasma sodium concentration is low and the plasma osmolality may be normal or elevated because of the excess sugar or mannitol in the plasma. In other situations of true hyponatremia (to be discussed), the serum osmolality and the serum sodium concentration are both depressed.

After excluding factitious hyponatremia, hyperglycemia, and hypermannitolemia, it is worthwhile to consider several causes of hyponatremia related to drugs such as morphine, barbiturates, anesthesia, clofibrate, cyclophosphamide, vincristine, oxytocin, and chlorpropamide. Endocrine disorders, such as adrenal insufficiency, hypopituitarism, and myxedema, may be associated with hyponatremia and also should be excluded. Acute water intoxication in an individual with normal renal function is an extremely rare entity and would be expected to occur only when maximal renal water output (approximately 22 L/day) is exceeded by an unusually large water intake (e.g., psychogenic polydipsia). Most clinical situations of acute water intoxication develop in patients with chronic renal failure and a marked reduction of glomerular filtration rate because these patients have an inability to maximally dilute their urine and are more susceptible to developing severe hyponatremia after receiving an acute water load (e.g., hypotonic intravenous solutions, psychogenic polydipsia).

With the previously mentioned clinical situations eliminated, a useful approach to the patient with hyponatremia attempts to place the hyponatremic patient into one of three broad categories, based on the history and physical examination:

I. Hyponatremia with hypovolemia (inadequate circulation)
   A. With renal salt retention (urinary sodium concentration of less than 10 to 15 mEq/L)
      1. Gastrointestinal losses
      2. Profuse sweating
   B. With urinary sodium wasting (urinary sodium of more than 20 mEq/L)
      1. Adrenal insufficiency
      2. Diuretics
      3. Renal salt wasting as in chronic renal failure or distal renal tubular acidosis
II. Hyponatremia with edema (urinary sodium concentration usually of less than 10 mEq/L)
   A. Congestive heart failure
   B. Hepatic cirrhosis with ascites
   C. Nephrotic syndrome
III. Hyponatremia without evidence of hypovolemia or edema
   A. Syndrome of inappropriate secretion of ADH (SIADH)
   B. Reset osmostat
   C. Drugs (as mentioned previously)

The physical examination easily differentiates patients in category I from patients in category II, and patients who are euvolemic (category III) can usually be differentiated, clinically, from those patients who are either hypovolemic (category I) or edematous (category II). Table 52.7 summarizes a more complete diagnostic approach to hyponatremia.

## TABLE 52.7

### DIAGNOSTIC APPROACH TO HYPONATREMIA

**Step 1. Measure serum osmolality**

| Normal (280–285 mOsm) | Low (<280 mOsm) | Elevated (>285 mOsm) |
|---|---|---|
| Step 1A. Measure blood sugar, lipids, protein | ↓ | Step 1B. Measure blood sugar |
| *Isotonic hyponatremia* | ↓ | *Hypertonic hyponatremia* |
| 1. Pseudohyponatremia | ↓ | 1. Hyperglycemia |
| Hyperlipidemia | | 2. Hypertonic infusions |
| Hyperproteinemia | | Glucose |
| 2. Isotonic infusions | ↓ | Mannitol |
| Glucose | | Glycine |
| Mannitol | | |
| Glycine | | |

**Step 2. Clinically assess the extracellular fluid volume**

| Tachycardia, hypotension, poor skin turgor | | | | | Edema | | | | | Normal pulse, blood pressure, skin turgor, no edema | | | | |
|---|---|---|---|---|---|---|---|---|---|---|---|---|---|---|
| **Hypovolemic hypotonic hyponatremia** | | | | | **Hypervolemic hypotonic hyponatremia** | | | | | **Isovolemic hypotonic hyponatremia** | | | | |
| *Causes* | *BUN/ Cr* | *Uric Acid* | *Urinary Osm* | *Na* | *Causes* | *BUN/ Cr* | *Uric Acid* | *Urinary Osm* | *Na* | *Causes* | *BUN/ Cr* | *Uric Acid* | *Urinary Osm* | *Na* |
| GI losses | ↑↑/↑ | ↑ | ↑↑ | ↓↓ | CHF | ↑↑/↑ | ↑ | ↓ | ↓ | Water intoxication | ↓/↓ | ↓ | ↑(↓) | ↓ |
| Skin losses | ↑↑/↑ | ↑ | ↑↑ | ↓↓ | Liver damage | ↑↑/↑ | ↑ | ↑ | ↓ | Renal failure | ↑↑/↑↑ | ↑ | ISO | ↑ |
| Lung losses | ↑↑/↑ | ↑ | ↑↑ | ↓↓ | Nephrosis | ↑↑/↑ (↑↑↑/↑↑) ↑ | | ↑ (ISO ↓↑) ↓ | | K+ loss | ↑/↑ (N) | ↑ | ↑ | ↓ |
| Third-space | ↑↑/↑ | ↑ | ↑↑ | ↓↓ | | | | | | SIADH | ↓/↓ | ↓↓ | ↑ | ↑ |
| Renal losses | | | | | | | | | | Reset osmo stat | N | N | V | V |
| Diuretics | ↑↑/↑ | ↑ | ISO | ↑ | | | | | | | | | | |
| Renal damage | ↑↑/↑↑ | ↑ | ISO | ↑ | | | | | | | | | | |
| Partial urinary tract obstruction | ↑↑/↑ | ↑ | ISO (↓) | ↑ | | | | | | | | | | |
| Adrenal insufficiency | ↑↑ | ↑ | ↑ | ↑ | | | | | | | | | | |

BUN/Cr, blood urea nitrogen/creatinine; CHF, congestive heart failure; GI, gastrointestinal; ISO, isotonic; K+, potassium; N, normal; Na, sodium; Osm, osmolality; SIADH, syndrome of inappropriate secretion of antidiuretic hormone; V, variable.
Note: Arrows indicate direction of change. Single and double arrows define the magnitude of change.
(Reproduced with permission from Narins RG, Jones ER, Stom MC, et al. Diagnostic strategies in disorders of fluid, electrolyte and acid-base homeostasis. *Am J Med* 1982;72:496–519.)

## Syndrome of Inappropriate Antidiuretic Hormone

Any discussion of hyponatremia would be incomplete without some comment about the syndrome of SIADH. This relatively rare condition is characterized by:

- Hyponatremia with corresponding hypoosmolality of the serum and ECFs
- Continued renal excretion of sodium
- Absence of clinical evidence of fluid volume depletion or edema
- Normal renal function
- Normal adrenal and thyroid function
- Osmolality of the urine greater than that appropriate for the concomitant osmolality of the plasma, or urine that is less than maximally dilute

Most patients with SIADH have a low or low/normal serum uric acid level.

Disorders in which there is a syndrome probably resulting from inappropriate secretion or aberrant production of ADH (SIADH) include malignant tumors such as carcinoma of the lung, duodenum, and pancreas; central nervous system tuberculosis, purulent bacterial meningitis, acute intermittent porphyria, and subdural hemorrhage; pulmonary disorders, such as tuberculosis, pulmonary abscess, aspergillosis, and viral and bacterial pneumonias; and, finally, idiopathic SIADH. In patients appearing to have idiopathic SIADH, usually a specific underlying cause surfaces eventually.

In treating patients with SIADH, water restriction is critically important. With acute hyponatremia due to SIADH, hypertonic saline, salt tablets, or loop diuretics may be required. The long-term ambulatory management of patients with SIADH has become easier with the use of demeclocycline in dosages from 600 to 900 mg/day. Caution is warranted in using demeclocycline in patients with severe hypoalbuminemia because acute tubular necrosis may occur.

## Treatment of Hyponatremia

As a general principle, the treatment for hyponatremia depends on the underlying cause:

- If there is contracted ECF volume, the depleted volume should be replenished with sodium and water, usually in the form of normal saline.
- If an edematous state exists, water should be restricted; in most circumstances, both salt and water should be restricted. If congestive heart failure is the reason for the hyponatremia, water restriction, loop diuretics, and cardiotonic measures, such as the use of an angiotensin-converting enzyme (ACE) inhibitor, should alleviate the hyponatremia, especially if cardiac function improves.
- If SIADH is diagnosed, water should be restricted in conjunction with additional treatment recommendations for SIADH as discussed above.

For patients with hypoadrenalism, hypopituitarism, or hypothyroidism, appropriate hormone replacement therapy is required. Patients with adrenal insufficiency who are acutely hyponatremic and volume-contracted will initially require the administration of normal saline.

In treating hyponatremia, the physician also must consider the severity of the hyponatremia and the rate of correction of the condition. For patients with moderate hyponatremia (e.g., serum sodium concentration of less than 125 to 135 mEq/L), one should discontinue the responsible factor (e.g., drug or diuretic), treat the underlying condition (e.g., heart failure), and restrict fluids to allow correction of the hyponatremia through losses of excess water via the skin and mucous membranes and, it is hoped, an increase in renal water excretion. If severe, life-threatening hyponatremia is present (serum sodium concentration of less than 110 to 115 mEq/L) and especially if obtundation, coma, or seizures exist, (i) enough sodium chloride should be given to increase the serum sodium concentration to approximately 120 mEq/L; (ii) isotonic saline or 3% sodium chloride should be administered; (iii) a diuretic should be administered and urinary electrolyte losses replaced; and (iv) free water should be restricted.

In recent years, much discussion has been generated about the speed (rate) of correction of hyponatremia, the osmotic demyelinization syndrome, and central pontine myelinosis. Several points should be emphasized regarding the rate of correction for severe hyponatremia; severe acute hyponatremia (i.e., hyponatremia developing over 24 to 48 hours) may be associated with considerable morbidity, including seizures, coma, irreversible neurologic abnormalities, and death. This is most likely to occur with water administration to postoperative patients or in patients with thiazide-induced hyponatremia. Rapid initial treatment is both safe (because the cerebral adaptation is not complete) and may be lifesaving. The plasma sodium concentration should be increased by 1.5 to 2.0 mEq/L per hour for the first 4 to 6 hours, but by no more than 20 mEq/L per day. For patients with known chronic hyponatremia (i.e., hyponatremia known to be present for more than 48 to 72 hours) or for patients with hyponatremia of unknown duration, overly rapid correction may lead to central pontine myelinolysis, particularly if plasma sodium is increased by more than 25 mEq/L per day, to above 140 mEq/L. Plasma sodium concentration should be increased in asymptomatic chronic hyponatremic patients at a maximum rate of 0.5 mEq/L per hour. Too rapid correction is most likely to occur with hypertonic saline or after correction of hypovolemia with isotonic saline.

# HYPERNATREMIA

*Hypernatremia* is defined as a serum sodium concentration of more than 145 mEq/L. Hypernatremia may exist in the presence of a decrease or increase in total body sodium.

Almost always, hypernatremia is a sign of relative or absolute water deficiency. Because normal osmoregulation and thirst closely fix body fluid osmolality between 280 and 290 mOsm/kg (serum sodium concentration of 135 to 145 mEq/L), hyperosmolality of the body fluids indicates a deficiency of water. The serum sodium concentration is rarely increased by administration of excess sodium per se, unless an usually large amount of sodium salt is given erroneously.

Hypernatremia is prevented in normal people by the thirst mechanism (Fig. 52.2). A slight increase in plasma osmolality stimulates thirst (at a plasma osmolality of approximately 290 mOsm/kg), which, in turn, increases water intake voluntarily. Obviously, this chain of events does not take place if a person is comatose, does not have access to water, cannot communicate thirst, or if not appropriately administered by paramedical personnel. If the thirst mechanism remains intact and water is available, the osmolality of the body fluids is protected, but at the expense of polydipsia and polyuria. Hospitalized patients avoid hyperosmolality of the body fluids from hypernatremia so long as adequate water or dilute intravenous fluids are provided.

The clinical circumstances associated with hypernatremia are:

- Unconscious or confused patients who receive insufficient fluids
- Osmotic diuresis
- Uncontrolled diabetes mellitus
- Tube feedings
- Loss of both thirst and neurohypophyseal function (rare)
- Water-wasting conditions (if not enough water provided)
- True central diabetes insipidus

- Nephrogenic diabetes insipidus (e.g., congenital or lithium toxicity)
- In infants, especially given sodium chloride–containing fluids
- Rapid infusion of hypertonic saline or sodium bicarbonate (unusual)
- Hyperaldosteronism or Cushing's syndrome
- Seizures, excessive exercise, rhabdomyolysis
- Osmotic diarrhea

## Treatment

The mainstay of treatment for hypernatremia is to provide sufficient water. A reduction of solute intake (e.g., moderate dietary protein restriction) decreases obligatory water losses. For patients with central diabetes insipidus, the most physiologic treatment is to administer exogenous vasopressin (ADH), which can be given subcutaneously or intramuscularly or in the form of a lysine-vasopressin nasal spray. Most patients with central diabetes insipidus use desmopressin. Thiazide diuretics in conjunction with a low-salt diet and chlorpropamide are additional nonvasopressin treatment maneuvers that may decrease urine volume in patients with central diabetes insipidus. Thiazides, by producing mild ECF volume contraction, may induce less renal water excretion; and chlorpropamide (125 to 500 mg daily) enhances the action of circulating ADH. Polyuric patients with nephrogenic diabetes insipidus usually do not respond to desmopressin or chlorpropamide. Inducing mild volume contraction with a thiazide diuretic and a low-salt diet, in conjunction with a low-protein diet, may decrease urine volume in these patients. When this condition is due to lithium toxicity, amiloride may be

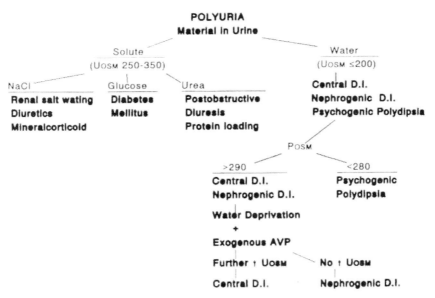

**Figure 52.3** Schematic diagram of polyuria. AVP, arginine vasopressin; D.I., diabetes insipidus; NaCl, sodium chloride; $U_{OSM}$, urine osmolality.

used. Nonsteroidal anti-inflammatory drugs (NSAIDs) may decrease urine volume in patients with congenital nephrogenic diabetes insipidus or lithium toxicity.

## APPROACH TO POLYURIA

Polyuria (daily urine volume of more than 3 to 4 L) is a relatively common patient complaint. The high urine volume may be driven by excessive fluid intake (oral or intravenous infusion of hypotonic solutions) or may be consequent to a solute diuresis. If the urine is remarkably dilute (i.e., urine osmolality of less than 250 mOsm/kg), a water diuresis is present and attributable to either diabetes insipidus or psychogenic polydipsia. If the urinary osmolality is greater than 300 mOsm/kg, a solute diuresis is the likely basis for the polyuria. A schematic approach to polyuria is given in Figure 52.3. Note that when a water diuresis is diagnosed (urine osmolality of less than 200 to 250 mOsm/kg), the next diagnostic step is to obtain a plasma osmolality; if in the setting of a water diuresis the plasma osmolality is less than 280 mOsm/kg, psychogenic polydipsia is likely. If the plasma osmolality is more than 290 mOsm/kg, diabetes insipidus is the explanation for the water diuresis.

## REVIEW EXERCISES

### QUESTIONS

**1.** An internal medical resident ingests 300 mEq of sodium in his diet daily (a "fast-food freak"). His 24-hour urinary sodium excretion, in the chronic steady state, can be expected to be which of the following?
a) 10 mEq/day
b) 100 mEq/day
c) 280 mEq/day
d) 450 mEq/day

**2.** A 70-kg man has profound diarrhea and loses 5 kg in weight. His identical twin (same height and weight) sweats off 5 kg in weight hiking in the desert. Answer true or false to each of the following statements.
a) The man with diarrhea has more evidence of arterial volume contraction than the desert hiker.
b) The man with diarrhea has a lower blood pressure than the desert hiker (both started with identical blood pressures).
c) The optimal treatment of the man with diarrhea is with $D_5W$.
d) The optimal treatment of the desert hiker is with $D_5W$.

**3.** A 52-year-old man with a 20-year history of cigarette smoking is admitted to the hospital because of cough

and weakness. On admission, his serum electrolytes reveal a serum sodium concentration of 112 mEq/L, potassium of 4.5 mEq/L, chloride of 80 mEq/L, and $HCO_3^-$ of 26 mEq/L. The BUN was 8 mg/dL, serum creatinine 0.8 mg/dL, and serum uric acid 3.0 mg/dL. These data are most consistent with which of the following?
a) Addison's disease
b) Congestive heart failure
c) Cirrhosis with ascites
d) SIADH

**4.** Which one of the following applies best to the pathophysiology of patients with hyponatremia?
a) An inability to concentrate the urine
b) An inability to maximally dilute the urine
c) Congestive heart failure
d) SIADH
e) ECF volume contraction

**5.** A 47-year-old man presents to the emergency room with a serum sodium concentration of 115 mEq/L. Physical examination reveals a supine blood pressure of 120/80 mm Hg and a standing blood pressure of 90/60 mm Hg. The skin turgor is diminished. Which one of the following is the best treatment for this man's hyponatremia?
a) Restriction of free water
b) Restriction of salt and water
c) Administration of normal saline
d) Treatment of the hyponatremia with demeclocycline

**6.** A 57-year-old man with a history of chronic congestive heart failure and a 20-year history of cigarette smoking is admitted with a serum sodium concentration of 120 mEq/L. The serum osmolality is 255 mOsm/kg (normal 280 to 300). The urine osmolality is 460 mOsm/kg. These determinations of serum and urine osmolality are most consistent with which one of the following?
a) Congestive heart failure
b) SIADH
c) Cirrhosis and ascites
d) Severe salt and water depletion
e) All of the above

**7.** You are called to the surgical intensive care unit to see a 65-year-old white man with known type II diabetes mellitus, who is oliguric 24 hours after an abdominal aortic aneurysm resection. Electrolytes reveal a serum sodium concentration of 110 mEq/L, potassium of 5.0 mEq/L, chloride of 75 mEq/L, and $HCO_3^-$ of 20 mEq/L; blood sugar is 200 mg/dL, BUN 45 mg/dL, and plasma osmolality 410 mOsm/kg. Answer true or false to the following statements.
a) The measured plasma osmolality is internally consistent with the other reported laboratory test results.
b) The calculated osmolality is approximately 250 mOsm/kg.

c) The discrepancy between the calculated osmolality and the measured plasma osmolality (osmolal gap) could be due to mannitol.

d) If excess mannitol is present in the plasma of this patient, his ICF volume is contracted and his ECF volume is expanded.

## ANSWERS

### 1. c.
In the steady state, the 24-hour urine sodium excretion reflects the dietary sodium intake, and vice versa. The ingestion of 300 mEq of sodium in the diet daily should result in a 24-hour urine sodium excretion of approximately 300 mEq. Of the possible answers for this question, 280 mEq/day is the closest to the amount of sodium ingested in the diet.

### 2. a, true; b, true; c, false; d, true.
The 70-kg male with profuse diarrhea is losing salt and water. The identical twin who sweats off 5 kg in weight is losing essentially water. This water loss comes from TBW—that is, it is lost proportionately to the distribution of water throughout the body fluid compartments. Because the hemodynamic consequences of body fluid losses are greatest when these losses come from the plasma volume or blood volume compartments, the patient with diarrhea loses a substantially larger amount of fluid from his plasma volume than does his identical twin. The man with diarrhea would have more clinical evidence of arterial volume contraction than would the desert hiker and would obviously have a lower blood pressure and more tachycardia than would the desert hiker. Because the man with diarrhea has lost both salt and water from the body, appropriate treatment is normal saline (not $D_5W$). Treatment of the desert hiker with $D_5W$ is appropriate because he has lost primarily water from the body. More profuse water losses, particularly if accompanied by orthostatic hypotension or orthostatic tachycardia, should be treated initially with normal saline to reverse the compromised arterial volume, followed by appropriate administration of $D_5W$.

### 3. d.
The hyponatremia and normal renal function (normal BUN and serum creatinine) in conjunction with a low serum uric acid level all suggest SIADH. The long history of cigarette smoking and cough suggest the possibility of a lung cancer, well known to be associated with SIADH. No evidence of congestive heart failure or cirrhosis with ascites is described on the physical examination. Although the values for sodium, chloride, and potassium concentration are consistent with adrenal insufficiency, one would expect hyponatremia of this magnitude due to adrenal insufficiency to have clinical and biochemical evidence of ECF volume contraction—that is, a higher

BUN, possibly a higher serum creatinine level (depending on the patient's muscle mass), and a higher serum uric acid level.

### 4. b.
Patients with hyponatremia become hyponatremic (unless they have pseudohyponatremia) because of an inability to dilute the urine. Patients with congestive heart failure, SIADH, and ECF volume contraction may all demonstrate hyponatremia, and these three conditions share the pathophysiologic abnormality of an inability to maximally dilute the urine.

### 5. c.
This patient has obvious physical findings of ECF volume contraction (orthostatic hypotension and diminished skin turgor). The proper treatment is to administer ECF (i.e., normal saline). Restriction of salt and water is obviously inappropriate for a patient who requires volume expansion. Although hyponatremic, the restriction of free water would only aggravate the hemodynamic abnormalities present. Consideration of demeclocycline should be reserved for patients with evidence of chronic SIADH, a condition that cannot be diagnosed in the setting of obvious ECF volume contraction.

### 6. e.
This patient has hyponatremia and hypoosmolality of the serum, with evidence of ADH production (i.e., osmolality 460 mOsm/kg). Patients with congestive heart failure, SIADH, ascites, and severe salt and water depletion all may develop hyponatremia with an inability to dilute the urine. ADH levels are increased in all of these clinical situations, contributing to an increase in the urine osmolality. The serum and urine osmolality values given are consistent with all the diagnostic possibilities listed.

### 7. a, false; b, true; c, true; d, true.
The calculated osmolality ($2 \cdot$ serum $[Na^+]$) + (glucose/18) + (BUN/3) is 250 mOsm/kg. The measured osmolality of 410 mOsm/kg reported from the chemistry laboratory is significantly greater than the calculated osmolality. Thus, the measured plasma osmolality (410 mOsm/kg) is not internally consistent with the osmolality calculated on the basis of the measured serum sodium concentration, blood sugar, and BUN. The discrepancy between the calculated and measured osmolalities suggests that some other osmotically active particle is residing in the plasma of this patient. This could be mannitol, particularly because some patients receive intraoperative mannitol during resection of abdominal aortic aneurysm. Assuming that mannitol is present in the plasma of this patient, he qualifies for the label of *hypertonic state*—the osmolality of the body fluids is increased (410 mOsm/kg), and because the mannitol resides entirely in the ECF compartment, water

would come out of the cells, resulting in cell shrinkage. This fluid shift would result in ICF volume contraction and ECF volume expansion.

## SUGGESTED READINGS

Anderson RJ, Chung HM, Kluge R, et al. Hyponatremia: a prospective analysis of its epidemiology and the pathogenetic role of vasopressin. *Ann Intern Med* 1985;102:164–168.

Arieff AI, Llach F, Massry SG. Neurological manifestations and morbidity of hyponatremia: correlation with brain water and electrolytes. *Medicine* 1976;55:121–129.

Ashraf N, Locksley R, Arieff AI. Thiazide-induced hyponatremia associated with death or neurologic damage in outpatients. *Am J Med* 1981;70:1163–1168.

Bartter F, Schwartz WB. The syndrome of inappropriate secretion of antidiuretic hormone. *Am J Med* 1967;42:790.

Berl T. Treating hyponatremia—damned if we do and damned if we don't. *Kidney Int* 1990;37:1006–1018.

Berl T, Anderson RJ, McDonald KM, et al. Clinical disorders of water metabolism. *Kidney Int* 1976;10:117–132.

Carrilho F, Bosoh J, Arroyo V, et al. Renal failure associated with demeclocycline in cirrhosis. *Ann Intern Med* 1977;87:195–197.

DeFronzo RA, Thier SO. Pathophysiologic approach to hyponatremia. *Arch Intern Med* 1980;140:897.

Fichman MT, Vorherr H, Kleeman CP, et al. Diuretic-induced hyponatremia. *Ann Intern Med* 1971;75:853.

Forrest JN Jr, Cox M, Hong C, et al. Superiority of demeclocycline over lithium in the treatment of chronic syndrome of inappropriate secretion of antidiuretic hormone. *N Engl J Med* 1978;298:173–177.

Gullans SR, Verbalis JG. Control of brain volume during hyperosmolar and hypoosmolar conditions. *Ann Rev Med* 1993; 44:289–301.

Hantman O, Rosier B, Zohlman R, et al. Rapid correction of hyponatremia in the syndrome of inappropriate secretion of antidiuretic hormone. *Ann Intern Med* 1973;78:870–875.

Harrington JT, Cohen JJ. Clinical disorders of urine concentration and dilution. *Arch Intern Med* 1973;131:810.

Leaf A. The clinical and physiologic significance of the serum sodium concentration (part 1). *N Engl J Med* 1962;267:24–30.

Leaf A. The clinical and physiologic significance of the serum sodium concentration (part 2). *N Engl J Med* 1962;267:77–83.

Leaf A, Cotran R. *Renal pathophysiology.* New York: Oxford University Press, 1976.

Lee WH, Packer M. Prognostic importance of serum sodium concentration and its modification by converting-enzyme inhibition in patients with severe chronic heart failure. *Circulation* 1986;73: 257–267.

Mange K, Matsuura D, Cizman B, et al. Language guiding therapy: the case of dehydration versus volume depletion. *Ann Intern Med* 1997;127:848–853.

Narins RG, Jones ER, Stom MC, et al. Diagnostic strategies in disorders of fluid, electrolyte and acid–base homeostasis. *Am J Med* 1982;72:496–519.

*Potassium in Clinical Medicine.* Searle & Co. Monograph. Cypress, CA: Medcom Inc., 1973.

Robertson GL, Aycinena P. Neurogenic disorders of osmoregulation. *Am J Med* 1982;72:339–353.

Rose BD. *Clinical Physiology of Acid–Base and Electrolyte Disorders,* 4th ed. New York: McGraw-Hill, 1994:224.

Schrier RW. Pathogenesis of sodium and water retention, high-output and low-output cardiac failure, nephrotic syndrome, cirrhosis, and pregnancy. *N Engl J Med* 1988;319:1065–1072, 1127–1134.

Schrier RW, ed. *Renal and Electrolyte Disorders,* 4th ed. Philadelphia: Lippincott–Raven, 1997.

*Sea Within Us, The.* Searle & Co. Monograph. New York: Science and Medicine Publishing, 1975.

Sterns RH. Severe symptomatic hyponatremia: treatment and outcome. A study of 64 cases. *Ann Intern Med* 1987;107:656–664.

Valtin H, Schafer JA. *Renal Function: Mechanisms Preserving Fluid and Solute Balance in Health,* 3rd ed. Boston: Little, Brown, 1995.

# Acid–Base Disorders

# 53

*Julia Breyer-Lewis*

The acidity of body fluids is expressed in terms of the hydrogen ion concentration ($[H^+]$). The $[H^+]$ is normally 40 nEq/L and usually is expressed in terms of pH, which is the negative log of the $[H^+]$. Figure 53.1 shows the relationship between the pH measured in a patient's blood and the $[H^+]$, the two most commonly used units for specifying the level of acidity. Figure 53.1 shows several important points:

- The pH and the $[H^+]$ are inversely related. As the $[H^+]$ increases, pH decreases.
- A normal pH of 7.4 corresponds to a normal $[H^+]$ of 40 nEq/L.
- A reasonably accurate estimate of proton concentration can be made from pH by exploiting the nearly linear

relationship between pH and the $[H^+]$ between pH 7.0 and 7.5. In this pH range, the $[H^+]$ changes by 1 nEq/L for each 0.01 U change in pH.

To illustrate the pH to $[H^+]$ relationship, given that a normal pH of 7.4 corresponds to a proton concentration of 40 nEq/L, if a patient's pH is 7.2, the proton concentration equals 60 nEq/L:

Change in pH = 0.2 units

Change in $[H^+]$ = (0.2 ÷ 0.01) nEq/L = 20 nEq/L

Therefore,

$[H^+]$ at 7.2 = (40 + 20) nEq/L = 60 nEq/L

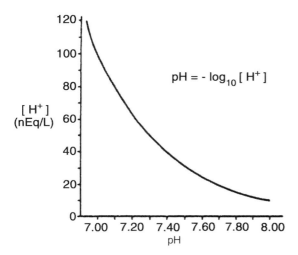

**Figure 53.1** Relationship between pH and hydrogen ion concentration ([$H^+$]), the two most commonly used units for specifying the level of acidity. (Reproduced with permission from Cohen JJ, Kassirer JP. Acid–base chemistry and buffering. In: Kassirer JP, ed. *Acid/Base*. Boston: Little, Brown, 1980;5.)

Estimating the [$H^+$] is important when performing calculations with acid–base data. Another method that relates pH to [$H^+$] compensates for the true curvilinear relationship between pH and [$H^+$]. Although slightly more complex than the preceding technique for estimating [$H^+$], this method is more accurate and works over a broader pH range. This method begins at the point at which pH = 7.40 and [$H^+$] = 40 nEq/L and proceeds as follows:

- To calculate the [$H^+$] for each 0.1 pH decrement, sequentially multiply 40 nEq/L by 1.25.
- To calculate the [$H^+$] for each 0.1 pH increment, sequentially multiply 40 nEq/L by 0.8.

This relationship appears in Table 53.1.

As serum pH falls below 7.36, a patient is said to be *acidemic*. Conversely, as the pH rises above 7.44, a patient is said to be *alkalemic*. Acidemia and alkalemia are descriptions of the patient's actual blood pH. *Acidosis* and *alkalosis* are descriptions of pathophysiologic processes that, if unopposed, may lead to acidemia and alkalemia. In acidosis, the plasma bicarbonate ($HCO_3^-$) concentration may be below normal, whereas in alkalosis the plasma $HCO_3^-$ concentration may be above normal. For example, if a patient is vomiting, he or she will have a high $HCO_3^-$ (32 mEq/L), and thus an alkalosis, but if, at the same time, the patient has respiratory failure and a high carbon dioxide pressure ($P_{CO_2}$) (e.g., 75 mm Hg), arterial pH actually may be in the acidemic range (e.g., pH 7.25).

## ACID–BASE TERMINOLOGY

The principal terms in acid–base disorders are defined as:

- *Acidemia*, an increase in [$H^+$] and a decrease in arterial pH

- *Alkalemia*, a decrease in [$H^+$] and an increase in arterial pH
- *Acidosis*, a process that acidifies body fluids (i.e., lowers plasma $HCO_3^-$) and, if unopposed, leads to a fall in pH and acidemia
- *Alkalosis*, a process that alkalinizes body fluids (i.e., raises plasma $HCO_3^-$) and, if unopposed, leads to an increase in pH and an alkalemia

## THE BODY'S BUFFERS

Despite continuous acid production, the body maintains arterial pH within the narrow range of 7.35 to 7.45. Approximately 15 mol or 15,000 mEq of $CO_2$ are generated each day by tissue metabolism and are carried by hemoglobin (Hgb)-generated $HCO_3^-$ or Hgb-bound carbamino groups to the lung for excretion as $CO_2$. Also, approximately 70 mEq/d or 1 mEq/kg per day of a patient's body weight is generated as nonvolatile acids (mostly phosphoric and sulfuric acids) and excreted by the kidneys.

Daily acid production can be summarized as:

- 12,000 to 15,000 mEq/day of volatile acids are produced and excreted by the lungs as $CO_2$.
- 1 mEq/kg/d of nonvolatile acids are produced and excreted by the kidneys.
- The pH of body fluids is determined by the acid produced, the buffering capacity, and the ability of the lungs and kidneys to excrete the load.

**TABLE 53.1**

**RELATIONSHIP BETWEEN PH AND [$H^+$]**

| pH | [$H^+$] |
|---|---|
| 7.80 | 16 |
| 7.75 | 18 |
| 7.70 | 20 |
| 7.65 | 22 |
| 7.60 | 25 |
| 7.55 | 28 |
| 7.50 | 32 |
| 7.45 | 35 |
| 7.40 | 40 |
| 7.35 | 45 |
| 7.30 | 50 |
| 7.25 | 56 |
| 7.20 | 63 |
| 7.15 | 71 |
| 7.10 | 79 |
| 7.05 | 89 |
| 7.00 | 100 |
| 6.95 | 112 |
| 6.90 | 126 |
| 6.85 | 141 |
| 6.80 | 159 |

(Reproduced with permission from Cohen JJ, Kassirer JP. Acid–base chemistry and buffering. In: Kassirer JP, ed. *Acid/Base*. Boston: Little Brown and Company, 1980;5.)

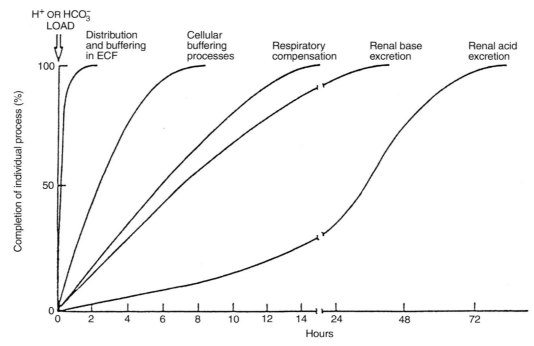

**Figure 53.2** Time course for completion of acid–base compensatory mechanisms. ECF, extracellular fluid; $H^+$, hydrogen ion concentration. (Reproduced with permission from Cogan MG, Rector FC, Seldin DW. Acid–base disorders in the kidney. In: Brenner BM, Rector FC, eds. *The Kidney.* Philadelphia: WB Saunders, 1981; 841–907.)

The latter is a clinically relevant fact. If a patient has renal failure and no longer can excrete the acid that is normally produced, the amount of $HCO_3^-$ needed to buffer the daily acid produced is 1 mEq/kg. If the patient requires more $HCO_3^-$ therapy than 1 mEq/kg to maintain the serum $HCO_3^-$ at any given level, another process, in addition to renal failure, is likely to be contributing to the acidosis.

If an extra base or acid load is introduced, the body reacts with a complex system, composed of buffering and the activation of compensatory mechanisms. As shown in Figure 53.2, if an acid or base load is added, the first defense is extracellular buffering, followed by the intracellular and, more important, skeletal buffering. (The skeleton represents an enormous reservoir of alkaline salts.) As compensation develops, the respiratory system modulates the $CO_2$ tension and, lastly, the kidneys modulate the plasma $HCO_3^-$ concentration.

Clinical acid–base chemistry is really the chemistry of the body's buffers. Simply stated, a *buffer* is a substance that can either absorb or donate protons to a solution. The most important buffer components in the extracellular fluid at physiologically relevant pH are Hgb, plasma proteins, and $HCO_3^-$. The principal buffering system for noncarbonic acid in the extracellular fluid is the $HCO_3^-$ buffering system. Because all buffers behave as though they are in functional contact with a common pool of $[H^+]$, the determination of one buffer pair reflects the states of all other buffer pairs and also of the arterial pH. This relationship, termed the *isohydric principle*, shows that any alteration of

the $[H^+]$ results in parallel changes in the ratio of each buffer pair within any fluid compartment:

$$HA = H^+ + A^-$$

$$K_a = \frac{[H^+][A^-]}{[HA]}$$

$$[H^+] = \frac{K_1 H_2 CO_3}{HCO_3^-} = \frac{K_2 H_2 PO_4^-}{HPO_4} = \frac{KHgbH^+}{Hgb}$$

Clinically, when we assess a patient's acid–base status, we evaluate the carbonic acid $HCO_3^-$ system because it can be measured easily. The most abundant extracellular buffer is $HCO_3^-$. Metabolically produced $CO_2$ is buffered in the red blood cells and provides the substrate for acid secretion in the kidney.

The $P_{CO_2}$-$HCO_3^-$ buffer system is reflected in the following formulas:

$$CO_2 \text{ gas} \rightarrow CO_2 \text{ (dissolved)} + H_2O \leftrightarrow H_2CO_3 + HCO_3^-$$

$$H^+ = \frac{KH_2CO_3}{HCO_3^-}$$

$$pH = pK_a + \frac{(\log[HCO_{3^-}])}{H_2CO_3}$$

$$[H_2CO_3^-] \sim 0.03 \, (P_{CO_2}) \text{ (solubility coefficient)}$$

The chemical species comprising this buffer system are interrelated:

- Dissolved $CO_2$ is reversibly hydrated to $H_2CO_3$ in a slow reaction.

- Carbonic acid is, therefore, a volatile acid because it is in equilibrium with the gaseous $CO_2$.
- Carbonic acid dissociates spontaneously into $[H^+]$ and $HCO_3^-$.
- This equilibrium reaction can be expressed in terms of the Henderson-Hasselbalch equation because the pH equals the $pK_a$ plus the log of the $HCO_3^-$ concentration over the carbonic acid concentration.

Carbonic acid is present in blood in such small quantities that it cannot be measured, but because carbonic acid is in equilibrium with the $CO_2$ in solution and the dissolved $CO_2$ depends on the $PCO_2$ in the arterial blood, the carbonic acid term of the equation can be replaced by the term $PCO_2$ multiplied by the solubility coefficient (0.03). The Henderson-Hasselbalch equation follows:

$$pH = pK_a + \frac{\log[HCO_3^-]}{(0.03)PCO_2} = \frac{kidney}{lung} = \frac{metabolic}{respiratory}$$

$$7.4 = 6.1 + \frac{\log[24]}{(0.03)(40)}$$

Thus, the pH (i.e., the $[H^+]$ of the blood) is determined by the ratio of the serum $HCO_3^-$ concentration to the partial pressure of $CO_2$ in the arterial blood. The $HCO_3^-$ concentration is regulated by the kidney. Metabolic processes, such as metabolic acidosis and metabolic alkalosis, affect primarily the $HCO_3^-$ concentration of the blood. The $PCO_2$ is regulated by the lung, and respiratory acidosis and alkalosis are reflected in primary changes in the $PCO_2$.

The Henderson-Hasselbalch equation can be rearranged and simplified to form the following equation:

$$[H^+] = \frac{24 \times PCO_2}{[HCO_3^-]}$$

As noted previously, the $[H^+]$ is calculated from the pH, given that a pH of 7.4 equals an $[H^+]$ of 40 nEq/L and that there is a linear relationship between pH and $[H^+]$ between a pH of 7.1 and 7.5. Also noted, for every 0.01 change in pH, a 1 nEq/L change in the $[H^+]$ concentration occurs. The advantage of using this simplified equation is that it facilitates the calculation of one unknown parameter from two known parameters. For example, if the plasma $HCO_3^-$ concentration and the pH are known, the $PCO_2$ can be calculated. Also, this equation allows the validity of simultaneous laboratory measurements of pH, $HCO_3^-$ concentration, and $PCO_2$ to be checked. When the reported $HCO_{3-}$ concentration and $PCO_2$ are entered into the right side of the equation, the equation should solve to equal the $[H^+]$ predicted by the arterial pH. If it does not, one of the reported values is wrong. (Many an intern has racked her brain trying to analyze a patient's acid–base problem without checking to see whether the numbers are consistent using this equation.)

## SIMPLE ACID–BASE DISORDERS

Clinical disorders of acid–base equilibrium are classified according to which of the two variables, $PCO_2$ or $HCO_3^-$ concentration, is directly affected by the primary pathologic process:

- Clinical disorders initiated by a primary change in the $HCO_3^-$ are referred to as *metabolic disorders*.
- Clinical disorders initiated by a change in the $PCO_2$ are referred to as *respiratory disorders*.
- Decreases in the plasma $HCO_3^-$ result in metabolic acidosis, whereas increases in the plasma $HCO_3^-$ result in metabolic alkalosis.
- *Hypercapnia*, an increase in the $PCO_2$, results in a respiratory acidosis; *hypocapnia* results in a respiratory alkalosis.

In each of the four primary disturbances shown in Table 53.2, the initiating process not only alters the acid–base equilibrium directly, but it also sets in motion secondary compensatory responses that change the other member of the $PCO_2$-$HCO_3^-$ pair:

- In metabolic acidosis, the primary disturbance is a decrease in the $HCO_3^-$ level; the body, in an attempt to return the pH or $[H^+]$ to normal, induces a fall in $PCO_2$

### TABLE 53.2
### THE FOUR PRIMARY ACID–BASE DISTURBANCES

| Type of Disturbance | Primary Alteration | Compensatory Response | Mechanism of Compensatory Response |
|---|---|---|---|
| Metabolic acidosis | Decrease in plasma $[HCO_3^-]$ | Decrease in $PaCO_2$ | Hyperventilation |
| Metabolic alkalosis | Increase in plasma $[HCO_3^-]$ | Increase in $PaCO_2$ | Hypoventilation |
| Respiratory acidosis | Increase in $PaCO_2$ | Increase in plasma $[HCO_3^-]$ | Increased $HCO_3^-$ reabsorption by the kidney |
| Respiratory alkalosis | Decrease in $PaCO_2$ | Decrease in plasma $[HCO_3^-]$ | Decreased $HCO_3^-$ reabsorption by the kidney |

(by means of hyperventilation), so that the ratio approaches normal.

- In metabolic alkalosis, the primary increase in $HCO_3^-$ is compensated for by a decrease in ventilation and an increase in $Pco_2$.
- In respiratory acidosis, the compensatory response is an increase in the serum $HCO_3^-$ level caused by decreased renal excretion of $HCO_3^-$ and increased renal net acid excretion.
- In respiratory alkalosis, the primary decrease in $Pco_2$ is compensated by increased renal excretion of $HCO_3^-$ and a resultant fall in serum $HCO_3^-$.

By remembering the basic principles relating $Pco_2$ and $HCO_3^-$ to pH or $[H^+]$, and that the body's goal is to maintain a nearly normal pH, all these clinical compensatory responses can be predicted. If only one of these primary processes is present, the patient has a simple acid–base disturbance with an appropriate compensatory response. Conversely, if two or more primary abnormalities are present, the patient is said to have a mixed acid–base disorder. For example, a patient may have a heart attack, become hypotensive, underperfuse his or her organs, and develop a metabolic acidosis as a result of the accumulation of lactic acid, but this patient also may have pneumonia, respiratory failure, and a respiratory acidosis. This patient is said to have a mixed acid–base disorder with two primary processes.

## COMPENSATORY RESPONSES

The role of compensatory processes can be summarized as:

- These processes may return the ratio of $HCO_3^-$ to $Pco_2$ back toward normal and thus help normalize the arterial pH.
- Compensation, with one exception (primary respiratory alkalosis), never returns the pH fully back to normal.
- Compensatory responses require normally functioning lungs and kidneys and take time to occur.
- The lack of compensation in an appropriate interval defines the presence of a second primary disorder.
- The compensatory response creates a second laboratory abnormality.
- The appropriate degree of compensation can be predicted.

Compensatory processes may return the ratio of the $HCO_3^-$ and the $Pco_2$ back toward normal and thus help to normalize the arterial pH, but the compensatory response never returns the pH completely to normal. For example, if a patient has a metabolic acidosis, and thus a low serum $HCO_3^-$, the compensatory response of a decrease in the $Pco_2$ raises the arterial pH. The patient is still acidemic, however; that is, the arterial pH remains below 7.38. The primary process can be determined by looking at the arter-

ial blood gas levels and deciding whether the $HCO_3^-$ or the $Pco_2$ has moved in the right direction to lead to that change in pH. In our example of simple metabolic acidosis, the patient is acidemic because the fall in the $HCO_3^-$ (the primary process) produces the fall in pH. Although the compensatory fall in $Pco_2$ increases the pH, it does not return it to normal and is clearly a secondary event. One exception to this rule is chronic respiratory alkalosis for more than 2 weeks: The compensatory fall in $HCO_3^-$ may return the pH to normal. The primary disorder in this setting must be determined by history.

Compensatory responses require normally functioning kidneys and lungs. A patient with significant renal failure cannot develop full metabolic compensation to a primary respiratory disorder. Similarly, a patient on a ventilator whose respiratory rate is mechanically controlled cannot develop a compensatory respiratory response. Compensatory responses take up to 12 to 24 hours to develop fully. Thus, it cannot be said that a patient has failed to compensate if he or she has not yet had time to do so. If an appropriate amount of time has passed and an adequate compensatory response has not developed, this failure defines the presence of a second primary disorder. A clinical example of this situation could be the patient with diabetic ketoacidosis and severe metabolic acidosis who is obtunded. If the arterial blood gas shows a pH of 7.10, $Pco_2$ of 30, and an $HCO_3^-$ concentration of 9 mEq/L, one can conclude that the respiratory compensation, although present, is incomplete. Thus, the patient has a mixed acid–base disorder consisting of metabolic and respiratory acidosis.

Finally, the limits of appropriate metabolic compensation (change in $HCO_3^-$) for any given degree of primary respiratory acidosis or alkalosis, and the limits of respiratory compensation (change in $Pco_2$) for a given degree of primary metabolic acidosis or alkalosis, have been defined. A $Pco_2$ that lies outside these limits in a patient with a primary metabolic disorder defines a coexistent respiratory disorder. Similarly, an $HCO_3^-$ that lies outside the expected limits of compensation in a patient with a primary respiratory disorder defines a coexistent metabolic disorder. Nomograms such as that shown in Figure 53.3 (which shows 95% confidence limits of compensations for primary "simple" acid–base disturbances) plot the $HCO_3^-$, pH, and $Pco_2$ values expected in primary acid–base disorders. Points within the star-like figure are consistent with, but not diagnostic of, a simple acid–base disorder with a single primary disorder and appropriate compensation. Mixed acid–base disorders that include more than one primary acid–base abnormality have values that fall within the star-like figure between two or three contributing acid–base disorders. It should be noted that values falling outside the star-like figure generally predict a mixed disorder, but values that fall within the star-like figure, although usually representing simple disorders, can result from coincidental mixed disturbances. The mild alkalemia

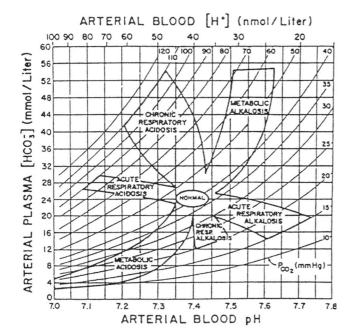

**Figure 53.3** Acid–base nomogram. To predict the pH change with changes in the [$HCO_3^-$] or in the $P_{CO_2}$, trace along the diagonal lines for changes in [$HCO_3^-$] with constant $P_{CO_2}$; trace along the horizontal lines for changes in $P_{CO_2}$ with constant [$HCO_3^-$]. (Reproduced with permission from Cogan MG, Rector FC Jr., Seldin DW, et al. Acid–base disorders. In: Brenner BM, Rector FC, eds. *The Kidney*. Philadelphia: WB Saunders, 1981;860.)

shown in the area of pure chronic respiratory acidosis and the nearly consistent hypercapnia with metabolic alkalosis are still somewhat controversial.

One need not rely exclusively on nomograms. Rather, the degree of compensation and its appropriateness can be calculated using equations that predict the expected degree of compensation (Table 53.3). The most useful, and most often used, equation is the expected respiratory compensation in metabolic acidosis. Note that the degree of compensation in respiratory acidosis and alkalosis varies depending on whether the primary process is acute or chronic.

## PRIMARY ACID–BASE DISORDERS

### Metabolic Acidosis

A summary of the key information concerning metabolic acidosis includes:

- Definition: Begins with fall in serum $HCO_3^-$ due to accumulation of nonvolatile acids
- Primary defect: A fall in $HCO_3^-$; accumulation of metabolic acids is caused by:
  - Excess acid production that overwhelms renal capacity for excretion (e.g., diabetic ketoacidosis)
  - Loss of alkali, leaving unneutralized acid behind (e.g., diarrhea)

- Renal excretory failure: normal total acid production in the face of poor renal function (e.g., chronic renal failure of any cause)
- Compensatory change
- Tissues and red blood cells act to increase serum $HCO_3^-$ by exchanging intracellular $Na^+$ and $K^+$ for extracellular $H^+$, raising serum $HCO_3^-$ and $K^+$
- Pulmonary ventilation increases. A fall in $P_{CO_2}$ brings pH back toward normal

Before the causes of metabolic acidosis can be discussed further, the anion gap (AG) must be reviewed. Total serum anions include chloride and $HCO_3^-$ (routinely measured on the SMA-6), as well as the unmeasured anions. Total anions equal the total cations in blood, which include sodium and unmeasured cations. The unmeasured anions in healthy persons exceed the unmeasured cations, a difference called the *anion gap*, which can be estimated by subtracting the sum of the chloride and $HCO_3^-$ concentrations from the sodium concentration, as shown in the following equations:

$$UA^- + Cl^- + HCO_3^- = Na^+ + UC^+$$
$$UA - UC = AG = Na^+ - (Cl^- + HCO_3^-) = 12$$

In a healthy state, the value is approximately 12. The AG can be increased because of a decrease in unmeasured cations, an increase in unmeasured anions, or laboratory error in the measurement of $Na^+$, $Cl^-$, or $HCO_3^-$ (Table 53.4).

Metabolic acidosis is frequently associated with an increased AG. In fact, metabolic acidoses are categorized clinically by the presence or absence of an abnormally

### TABLE 53.3

**EXPECTED COMPENSATORY CHANGES IN SIMPLE ACID–BASE DISORDERS**

| Primary Disorder | Compensatory Change[a] | |
|---|---|---|
| | **Acute (24 h)** | **Chronic (23 days)** |
| Metabolic acidosis | $P_{CO_2}$ = 1.5 [$HCO_3^-$] + 8 ± 2<br>$P_{CO_2}$ = last 2 digits of the pH | Same |
| Metabolic alkalosis | $P_{CO_2}$ = 40 + 0.6 ($\Delta$[$HCO_3^-$]) | Same |
| Respiratory acidosis | ↑ $\Delta$[$HCO_3^-$] = $\Delta$[$HCO_3^-$]/10 | ↑ $\Delta$[$HCO_3^-$] = 3.5 × $\Delta P_{CO_2}$/10 |
| Respiratory alkalosis | ↓ $\Delta$[$HCO_3^-$] = 2 × $\Delta P_{CO_2}$/10 | ↓ $\Delta$[$HCO_3^-$] = 5 × $\Delta P_{CO_2}$/10 |

[a] Note that some equations give the answers in terms of the change in the plasma measurement (e.g., $\Delta$[$HCO_3$], $\Delta P_{CO_2}$), whereas other equations give the absolute value of the measurement (e.g., $P_{CO_2}$). (Adapted with permission from Narins RG, Emmett M. Simple and mixed acid–based disorders: a practical approach. *Medicine* 1980;59:161–187.)

## TABLE 53.4
### CAUSES OF ANION GAP CHANGES

| Causes of Decreased Anion Gap | Causes of Increased Anion Gap |
| --- | --- |
| Increased unmeasured cation<br>  Increased concentration of normally present cation:<br>    hyperkalemia, hypercalcemia, hypermagnesemia<br>  Retention of abnormal cation: 1 γ-globulin, tromethamine (TRIS)<br>    buffer, lithium<br>Decreased unmeasured anion hypoalbuminemia<br>Laboratory error<br>  Systemic error: hyponatremia due to viscous serum,<br>    hyperchloremia in bromide intoxication<br>  Random error: falsely decreased serum sodium, or falsely<br>    increased serum chloride or $HCO_3^-$ | Decreased unmeasured cation<br>  Hypokalemia, hypocalcemia, hypomagnesemia<br>Increased unmeasured anion<br>  Organic anions: lactate, ketone acids<br>  Inorganic anions: phosphate, sulfate<br>  Proteins: hyperalbuminemia (transient)<br>  Exogenous anions: salicylate, formate, nitrate, penicillin,<br>    carbenicillin, and so forth<br>  Incompletely identified: anion accumulation in paraldehyde,<br>    ethylene glycol, methanol, and salicylate poisoning, uremia,<br>    hyperosmolar hyperglycemic nonketotic coma<br>Laboratory error<br>  Falsely increased serum sodium<br>  Falsely increased serum chloride or $HCO_3^-$ |

elevated AG. In a high-AG acidosis, the proton that titrates $HCO_3^-$ is accompanied by an unmeasured anion, resulting in the accumulation of that anion in the blood and a high-AG acidosis (Fig. 53.4). If the anion accompanying the proton is chloride, the patient has a metabolic acidosis with a normal AG because the fall in $HCO_3^-$ is matched by an increase in chloride. This is, by definition, a hyperchloremic acidosis. For example, a patient can have a loss of $HCO_3^-$ in the stool, with an increase in chloride secondary to volume depletion. The result is a normal AG acidosis or hyperchloremic acidosis. Clinically, the AG should be calculated for every patient each time a set of electrolytes is drawn (Fig. 53.5).

The causes of high-AG metabolic acidosis include:

- Ketoacidosis
- Lactic acidosis
- Uremia
- Salicylate toxicity
- Ethylene glycol toxicity
- Methanol toxicity
- Paraldehyde toxicity
- Massive rhabdomyolysis

If a patient has an elevated AG, lactic acidosis and ketoacidosis are the most common causes. The serum levels

of these organic anions can be measured. Intoxications with aspirin, antifreeze, methanol, or paraldehyde also can cause an AG acidosis and should be considered (Fig. 53.6), especially in an unconscious patient. (As noted, the "normal" AG is approximately 12.) When a patient has an increased AG, most anions that account for this gap are associated with a single proton. In an uncomplicated high-AG acidosis,

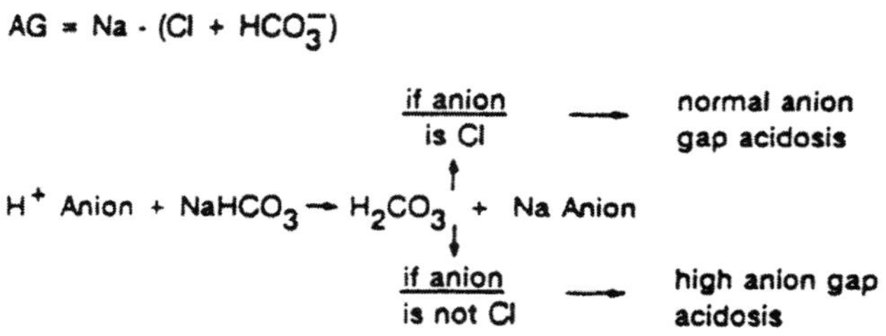

$$AG = Na - (Cl + HCO_3^-)$$

$$H^+ Anion + NaHCO_3 \rightarrow H_2CO_3 + Na\ Anion$$

if anion is Cl → normal anion gap acidosis

if anion is not Cl → high anion gap acidosis

**Figure 53.4** Anion gap in metabolic acidosis.

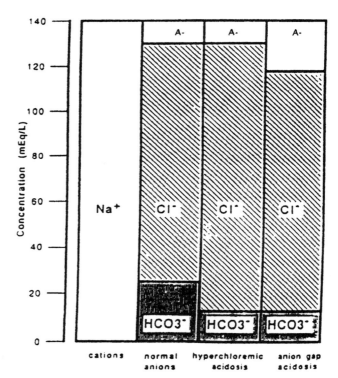

**Figure 53.5** The anion gap. (Reproduced with permission from Breyer MD, Jacobson HR. Approach to the patient with metabolic acidosis or metabolic alkalosis. In: Kelley W, ed. *Textbook of Internal Medicine.* Philadelphia: WB Saunders, 1989;923.)

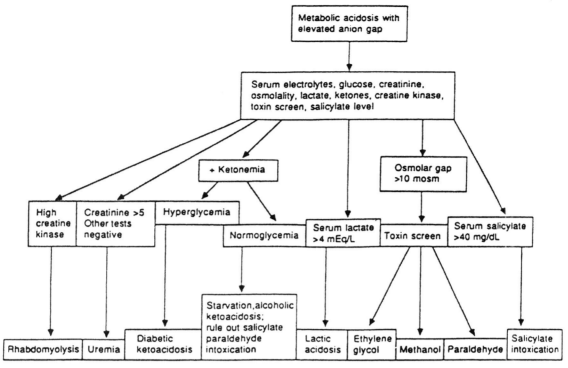

**Figure 53.6** Diagnostic algorithm for metabolic acidosis with elevated anion gap. (Reproduced with permission from Breyer MD, Jacobson HR. Approach to the patient with metabolic acidosis or metabolic alkalosis. In: Kelley WN, ed. *Textbook of Internal Medicine*. Philadelphia: WB Saunders, 1989;926.)

for every 1 mmol rise in the AG, a concomitant fall of 1 mmol should occur in the $HCO_3^-$ concentration. The difference between the patient's AG and a "normal" AG is called the *delta AG* ($\Delta AG$). The $\Delta AG$ and $\Delta HCO_3^-$ are calculated by the following formulas:

$$\Delta AG = \text{observed } AG - \text{upper normal } AG$$
$$\Delta HCO_3^- = \text{lower normal } HCO_3^- - \text{observed } HCO_3^-$$

For example, a patient with an AG of 20 has a $\Delta AG = 20 - 12 = 8$. The eight unmeasured anions would account for a decrease in the serum $HCO_3^-$ concentration of 8 mmol. Any significant deviation from this rule implies the existence of a mixed acid–base disorder. When the fall in $HCO_3^-$ ($\Delta HCO_3^-$) is greater than the rise in AG ($\Delta AG$) ($\Delta HCO_3^-$ >$\Delta AG$), two possible situations exist if laboratory error is excluded. Most commonly, either a mixed high-AG and normal-AG acidosis is present, or a mixed high-AG acidosis and "chronic" respiratory alkalosis with a compensating hyperchloremic acidosis is present. Conversely, when the AG is greater than the $\Delta HCO_3^-$ ($\Delta AG$ >$\Delta HCO_3^-$), a mixed high-AG acidosis and primary metabolic alkalosis almost always is present.

The presence of a hyperchloremic or normal AG acidosis suggests a completely different set of diagnoses, including renal tubular acidosis, diarrhea, ileal conduits, and HCl ingestions (Table 53.5). The diagnostic algorithm appears in Figure 53.7.

In patients with a hyperchloremic metabolic acidosis, the urine AG can be used to distinguish whether the cause of the acidosis is a renal tubular defect or other causes, such as diarrhea. The urine AG is calculated as follows:

$$AG = (\text{urine Na}^+ + \text{urine K}^+) - (\text{urine Cl}^-)$$

**TABLE 53.5**

**CAUSES OF HYPERCHLOREMIC METABOLIC ACIDOSIS**

Hypokalemic
   Proximal renal tubular acidosis, drug induced: acetazolamide, coumarin, mafenide (Sulfamylon)
   Distal renal tubular acidosis
   Posthypocapnea
   Diarrhea
   Ureterosigmoidostomy/ileal loop
   Pancreatic fistula/biliary drainage
   Correction phase of diabetic ketoacidosis
Hyperkalemic/normokalemic
   Type: i.v. renal tubular acidosis, interstitial nephritis, hypoaldosteronism, hydronephrosis
   Hydrochloric acid ingestions/infusions: hyperalimentation, cholestyramine, $CaCl_2$, $NH_4Cl$
   Dilutional acidosis

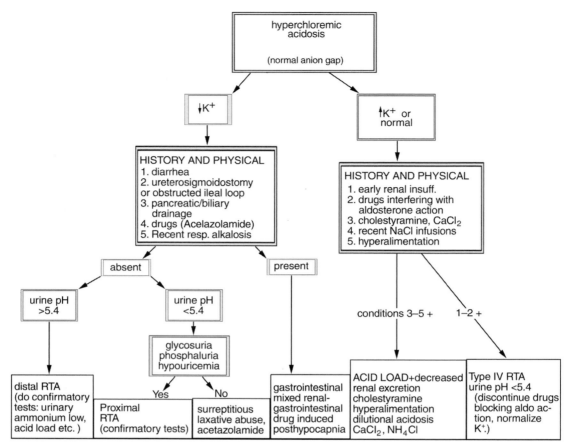

**Figure 53.7** Diagnostic algorithm for hyperchloremic metabolic acidosis. RTA, renal tubular acidosis.

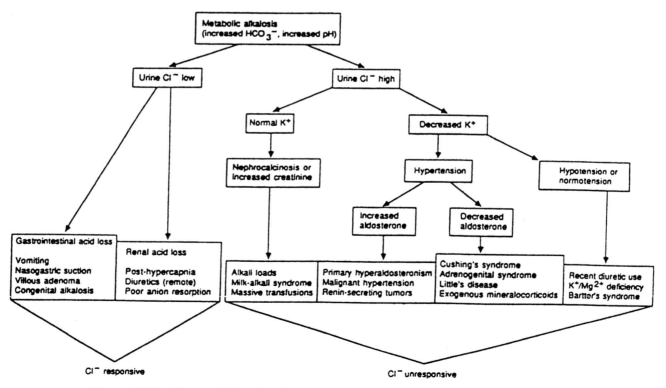

**Figure 53.8** Diagnostic algorithm for metabolic alkalosis. (Reproduced with permission from Breyer MD, Jacobson HR. Approach to the patient with metabolic acidosis or metabolic alkalosis. In: Kelley WN, ed. *Textbook of Internal Medicine*. Philadelphia: WB Saunders, 1989;932.)

Because ammonium is excreted in the urine along with chloride, this index can be used to estimate the concentration of ammonium in the urine in a patient with hyperchloremic metabolic acidosis. A negative urine AG ($Cl^-$ > $Na^+$ + $K^+$) suggests the appropriate excretion of ammonium in the urine with $Cl^-$ and the presence of gastrointestinal loss of $HCO_3^-$. A positive urine AG ($Cl^-$ < $Na^+$ + $K^+$) suggests the presence of a renal tubular acidosis with a distal acidification defect and inadequate ammonium excretion in the urine.

## Metabolic Alkalosis

A summary of the key information concerning metabolic alkalosis includes:

- Definition: A rise in the concentration of serum $HCO_3^-$
- Primary defect: a rise in serum $HCO_3^-$, with two requirements:
  - New $HCO_3^-$ must be added to the blood from renal or extrarenal sources (the process of generation)
  - Kidney must increase its net resorptive capacity to maintain the higher level of serum [$HCO_3^-$] (the stimuli that increase renal $HCO_3^-$ resorption are high $P_{CO_2}$, extracellular fluid contraction, Cl depletion, steroid excess, and $K^+$ depletion)
  - Compensatory change
  - Tissues and red blood cells act to lower serum $HCO_3^-$ by exchanging intracellular $H^+$ for extracellular $K^+$ and $Na^+$, lowering both serum $HCO_3^-$ and $K^+$
  - Alkalosis tends to cause hypoventilation and elevation of $P_{CO_2}$. Compensation for alkalosis is more erratic than for acidosis; generally, $P_{CO_2}$ rarely is greater than 55 mg Hg

The causes of metabolic alkalosis can be divided into those associated with a high urinary excretion of chloride and those associated with a low excretion of chloride and, therefore, responsive to saline administration (Table 53.6 and Fig. 53.8).

## Respiratory Acidosis

A summary of the key information concerning respiratory acidosis includes:

- Definition: Decreases pulmonary clearance of $CO_2$
- Primary defect: Increases $P_{CO_2}$
- Compensatory change: In acute syndromes, tissues and red blood cells generate $HCO_3^-$ by taking up $H^+$ in exchange for $Na^+$ and $K^+$. This acts to increase serum $HCO_3^-$ and $K^+$. In chronic syndromes, renal $HCO_3^-$ synthesis further augments serum $HCO_3^-$.
- Acute respiratory acidosis: Duration of less than 24 hours; no time for renal compensation. Tissue and red blood cells elevate serum $HCO_3^-$ above 4 mEq/L, even with high $P_{CO_2}$. It is rare to see serum $HCO_3^-$ above 31 mEq/L in acute respiratory acidosis.
- Chronic respiratory acidosis: Duration of more than 24 hours; serum $HCO_3^-$ rises further as a result of

**TABLE 53.7**
**CAUSES OF RESPIRATORY ACIDOSIS**

Acute
  Airway obstruction: aspiration of foreign body or vomitus, laryngospasm, generalized bronchospasm, obstructive sleep apnea
  Respiratory center depression: general anesthesia, sedative overdosage, cerebral trauma or infarction, central sleep apnea
  Circulatory catastrophes: cardiac arrest, severe pulmonary edema
  Neuromuscular defects: high cervical cordotomy, botulism, tetanus, Guillain-Barré syndrome, crisis in myasthenia gravis, familial hypokalemic periodic paralysis, hypokalemic myopathy, drugs of toxic agents (e.g., curare, succinylcholine, aminoglycosides, organophosphorus)
  Restrictive defects: pneumothorax, hemothorax, flail chest, severe pneumonitis, infant respiratory distress syndrome (hyaline membrane disease), adult respiratory distress syndrome
  Mechanical ventilators

Chronic
  Airway obstruction: chronic obstructive lung disease (bronchitis, emphysema)
  Respiratory center depression: chronic sedative depression, primary alveolar hypoventilation (Ondine's curse), obesity hypoventilation syndrome (pickwickian syndrome), brain tumor, bulbar poliomyelitis
  Neuromuscular defects: poliomyelitis, multiple sclerosis, muscular dystrophy, amyotrophic lateral sclerosis, diaphragmatic paralysis, myxedema, myopathic disease (e.g., polymyositis, acid maltase deficiency)
  Restrictive defects: kyphoscoliosis, spinal arthritis, fibrothorax, hydrothorax interstitial fibrosis, decreased diaphragmatic movement (e.g., ascites), prolonged pneumonitis, obesity

(Reproduced with permission from Cohen JJ, Kassirer JP. Acid–base chemistry and buffering. In: Kassirer JP, ed. *Acid/Base*. Boston: Little, Brown, 1980;325.)

**TABLE 53.6**
**URINARY CHLORIDE CONCENTRATION IN METABOLIC ALKALOSIS**

| Less than 20 mEq/L | Greater than 30 mEq/L |
| --- | --- |
| Vomiting | Primary hyperaldosteronism |
| Nasogastric suction | Cushing's syndrome: adrenal, ectopic adrenocorticotropic hormone, pituitary |
| Chloride wasting diarrhea | Exogenous steroid: licorice, glucocorticoid, carbenoxalone |
| Colonic villous adenoma | Adrenal 11- or 17-hydroxylase defects |
| Diuretic therapy (remote ingestion) | Liddle's syndrome |
| Posthypercapnia | Bartter's syndrome |
| Poorly reabsorbed anions | $K^+$ and $Mg^{2+}$ deficiency |
| Glucose refeeding | Milk-alkali syndrome |

## TABLE 53.8
### CAUSES OF RESPIRATORY ALKALOSIS

Hypoxia
Decreased inspired oxygen tension
Ventilation–perfusion inequality
Hypotension
Severe anemia
Central nervous system mediated
Voluntary hyperventilation
Neurologic disease: cerebrovascular accident (infarction, hemorrhage), infection (encephalitis, meningitis), trauma, tumor
Pharmacologic and hormonal stimulation: salicylates, dinitrophenol, nicotine, xanthines, pressor hormones, pregnancy
Hepatic failure
Gram-negative septicemia
Postmetabolic acidosis
Anxiety hyperventilation syndrome
Heat exposure
Pulmonary disease
Interstitial lung disease
Pneumonia
Pulmonary embolism
Pulmonary edema
Mechanical overventilation

(Reproduced with permission from Cohen JJ, Kassirer JP. Acid–base chemistry and buffering. In: Kassirer JP, ed. *Acid/Base*. Boston: Little, Brown, 1980;361.)

## TABLE 53.10
### DISORDERS OF SERUM CHLORIDE CONCENTRATION

Hyperchloremia
Proportionate increase in chloride and sodium
Dehydration
Disproportionate increase in chloride compared with sodium
Hyperchloremic metabolic acidosis
Renal compensation for primary respiratory alkalosis
Hypochloremia
Proportionate decrease in chloride and sodium
Overhydration
Disproportionate decrease in chloride compared with sodium
Metabolic alkalosis
Renal compensation for primary respiratory acidosis

## TABLE 53.9
### SYNDROMES COMMONLY ASSOCIATED WITH MIXED ACID–BASE DISORDERS

| Clinical Syndrome | Metabolic Alkalosis | Metabolic Acidosis | Respiratory Alkalosis | Respiratory Acidosis |
|---|---|---|---|---|
| Cardiopulmonary arrest | t | + | t | + |
| Severe pulmonary edema | | + | | + |
| Ethylene glycol + pulmonary edema | | + | | + |
| Methanol + hypoventilation | | + | | + |
| Severe hypophosphatemia | | + | | + |
| Recent alcohol binge | V | + | + | |
| Sepsis | | + | + | |
| Severe liver failure | V/d | + | + | |
| Salicylate intoxication | | + | + | |
| Pregnancy | V | | + | |
| Renal failure | V | + | | |
| Diabetic ketoacidosis | V | + | | |
| Chronic obstructive pulmonary disease | d | | | + |
| Severe hypokalemia | + | | | + |
| Critically ill patients | V/d | + | + | + |

+, syndrome is present; d, diuretics; t, treatment-induced; V, vomiting.
Note: Above are some clinical syndromes in which mixed acid–base disturbances are commonly seen. If metabolic alkalosis from vomiting or diuretics is frequently seen in these disorders, this is denoted by "V" or "d."
(Adapted with permission from Cohen JJ, Kassirer JP. Clinical evaluation of acid–base disorders. In: Cohen JJ, Kassirer JP, ed. *Acid/Base*. Boston: Little, Brown, 1982;405.)

## TABLE 53.11

### REPRESENTATIVE EXAMPLES OF MIXED ACID–BASE DISORDERS

| Type of Mixed Disorder | Example No. | Illustrative | | Laboratory | | | Profile | | Clinical Circumstance |
|---|---|---|---|---|---|---|---|---|---|
| | | pH | Paco2 (mm Hg) | HCO$_3$ | Na+ | mEq/L K+ | Cl | Anion Gap[a] | |
| Metabolic acidosis and respiratory acidosis | 1 | 7.10 | 50 | 15 | 140 | 5.0 | 102 | 23 | Renal failure and hypercapnic respiratory failure |
| | 2 | 6.99 | 34 | 8 | 141 | 6.0 | 105 | 28 | Cardiopulmonary arrest |
| Metabolic alkalosis and respiratory alkalosis | 3 | 7.69 | 30 | 35 | 134 | 4.0 | 84 | 15 | Hepatic failure and nasogastric suction |
| | 4 | 7.60 | 40 | 38 | 131 | 3.6 | 77 | 16 | Congestive heart failure and diuretics |
| Metabolic alkalosis and respiratory acidosis | 5 | 7.44 | 55 | 36 | 135 | 3.8 | 84 | 15 | COPD and diuretics |
| | 6 | 7.45 | 48 | 32 | 133 | 4.2 | 85 | 16 | Adult respiratory distress syndrome and acetate-rich total parenteral nutrition |
| Metabolic acidosis and respiratory alkalosis | 7 | 7.44 | 12 | 8 | 136 | 5.5 | 106 | 22 | Renal failure and Gram-negative septicemia |
| | 8 | 7.40 | 15 | 9 | 138 | 4.1 | 110 | 19 | Salicylate intoxication |
| Metabolic acidosis and metabolic alkalosis | 9 | 7.43 | 39 | 25 | 132 | 3.7 | 84 | 23 | Alcoholic liver disease and diuretics |
| | 10 | 7.37 | 35 | 20 | 138 | 4.0 | 93 | 25 | Diabetic ketoacidosis after NaHCO$_3$ therapy |
| Respiratory acidosis | 11 | 7.54 | 41 | 34 | 140 | 3.8 | 93 | 13 | COPD under mechanical ventilation |
| | 12 | 7.68 | 28 | 32 | 137 | 3.5 | 91 | 14 | COPD under mechanical ventilation |
| Respiratory acidosis, metabolic acidosis, and metabolic alkalosis | 13 | 7.38 | 57 | 33 | 134 | 4.7 | 77 | 24 | COPD, diuretics, and shock |
| Respiratory alkalosis, metabolic acidosis, and metabolic alkalosis | 14 | 7.43 | 25 | 16 | 135 | 3.2 | 97 | 22 | Congestive heart failure, diuretics, and shock |
| Hyperchloremic and high anion gap metabolic acidosis | 15 | 7.12 | 16 | 5 | 137 | 3.6 | 114 | 18 | Diabetic ketoacidosis with adequate salt and water balance |
| Acute or chronic respiratory acidosis | 16 | 7.22 | 80 | 32 | 141 | 4.3 | 99 | 10 | COPD and therapy with O$_2$- rich mixtures |
| Acute or chronic respiratory alkalosis | 17 | 7.54 | 12 | 10 | 132 | 3.2 | 107 | 15 | Alcoholic liver disease and cerebral bleeding |
| Acute or chronic respiratory acidosis and metabolic acidosis | 18 | 7.09 | 65 | 19 | 136 | 3.3 | 105 | 12 | COPD and diarrhea |
| Mixed high anion gap metabolic acidosis and respiratory acidosis | 19 | 7.18 | 44 | 16 | 133 | 5.7 | 100 | 17 | Hepatic, renal, and pulmonary failure |
| Mixed high anion gap metabolic acidosis and metabolic alkalosis | 20 | 7.36 | 31 | 17 | 132 | 4.0 | 89 | 26 | Alcoholic liver disease, vomiting, and lactic acidosis |
| | 21 | 7.40 | 40 | 24 | 143 | 5.5 | 95 | 24 | Diabetic ketoacidosis and lactic acidosis after HCO$_3^-$ therapy |

COPD, chronic obstructive pulmonary disease.
[a] Anion gap is calculated as [Na$^+$] ([Cl] + [HCO$_3$]).

compensatory $HCO_3^-$ synthesis. The elevated $P_{CO_2}$ stimulates renal tubular $H^+$ secretion and ammonia production. More acid is excreted; more $HCO_3^-$ is synthesized and returned to the blood. The high $P_{CO_2}$ also allows the kidney to reclaim new $HCO_3^-$ when filtered at glomerulus. Chloride excreted with $NH_4^+$ acts to lower serum chloride.

The causes of respiratory acidosis are summarized in Table 53.7.

## Respiratory Alkalosis

A summary of the key information concerning respiratory alkalosis includes:

- Definition: Increased pulmonary clearance of $CO_2$
- Primary defect: Fall in $P_{CO_2}$
- Compensatory change: Acute respiratory alkalosis; duration of less than 24 hours. No renal compensation acutely. By exchanging intracellular $H^+$ for extracellular $Na^+$ and $K^+$, tissue and red blood cells act to lower $HCO_3^-$, which rarely falls below 15 mEq/L, and $K^+$. Metabolic acid production (lactate) increases slightly.
- Chronic respiratory alkalosis: Chronic alkalosis impairs the kidney's ability to excrete acid. Retained acid further lowers serum $HCO_3^-$, resulting in more complete compensation. Duration longer than 2 weeks is associated with alkalemia. Greater duration may elicit normal pH. Only acid–base disturbance compensation in which pH may return to normal.

The causes of respiratory alkalosis are listed in Table 53.8. Table 53.9 contains common clinical situations in which more than one primary acid–base problem presents (i.e., a mixed disorder).

A few clues may be helpful in assessing the presence of a mixed acid–base disturbance:

- Normal pH (with the exception of respiratory alkalosis): With the sole exception of chronic respiratory alkalosis, a normal pH value in the setting of an abnormal $P_{CO_2}$ or $HCO_3^-$ concentration signifies a mixed disturbance; compensation rarely corrects the pH to normal. The more severe the primary disorder, the less effective the compensatory mechanism at returning the pH to normal.
- $P_{CO_2}$ + $HCO_3^-$ deviating in opposite directions: The $P_{CO_2}$ and serum $HCO_3^-$ concentration always deviate in the same direction in simple acid–base disorders. If they deviate in opposite directions, a mixed abnormality is present.
- A pH change in the opposite direction for a known primary disorder: A pH change in the opposite direction to that predicted for a known primary disorder signifies a mixed disturbance.

The chloride and potassium concentrations also can provide clues to the underlying acid–base disorder. If the chloride concentration changes in proportion to sodium, it reflects a change in hydration (Table 53.10). If chloride changes in excess of serum sodium, however, the cause is an acid–base disorder, with hyperchloremia suggesting an acidosis and hypochloremia suggesting an alkalosis. Similarly, in a general sense, hyperkalemia is associated with acidosis and hypokalemia is associated with alkalosis.

The approach to the patient with acid–base disorder is summarized as follows:

- Take a careful history: vomiting, diabetes, diarrhea, ingestion of toxin, and sepsis.
- Perform a thorough physical examination: fever, signs of volume depletion, respiratory rate and pattern, blood pressure.
- Determine electrolytes: $Na^+$, $K^+$, $Cl^-$, $HCO_3^-$.
- Calculate the AG.
  - Note that $\Delta AG = \Delta HCO_3^-$ in a simple disorder.
- Check the internal consistencies of arterial blood gases.
- Look for clues of mixed disorder (Table 53.11).
- Check nonelectrolyte laboratory results: creatinine (renal failure), glucose (diabetes), hematocrit (volume depletion), ketones, and lactate.

## SUGGESTED READINGS

Adams SL. Alcoholic ketoacidosis. *Emerg Med Clin North Am* 1990;4: 749–760.

Adrogue HJ, Wilson H, Boyd AE, et al. Plasma acid–base patterns in diabetic ketoacidosis. *N Engl J Med* 1982;307:1603–1610.

Brimioulle S, Kahn RJ. Effects of metabolic alkalosis on pulmonary gas exchange. *Am Rev Respir Dis* 1990;141:1185–1189.

Cooper DJ, Walley KR, Wiggs BR, et al. Bicarbonate does not improve hemodynamics in critically ill patients who have lactic acidosis. *Ann Intern Med* 1990;112:492–498.

Emmett M, Seldin DW. Clinical syndromes of metabolic acidosis and metabolic alkalosis. In: Seldin DW, Giebisch G, eds. *The Kidney: Physiology and Pathophysiology.* New York: Raven Press, 1985: 1567–1639.

Fulop M. Serum potassium in lactic acidosis and ketoacidosis. *N Engl J Med* 1979;300:1087–1089.

Gabow PA, Kaehny WD, Fennessey PV, et al. Diagnostic importance of an increased serum anion gap. *N Engl J Med* 1980;303:854–858.

Hood VL, Tannen RL. Lactic acidosis. *Kidney* 1989;22:1–6.

Jacobson HR, Seldin DW. On the generation, maintenance, and correction of metabolic alkalosis. *Am J Physiol* 1983;245: F425–432.

McLaughlin ML, Kassirer JP. Rational treatment of acid–base disorders. *Drugs* 1990;39:841–855.

Mecher C, Rackow EC, Astiz ME, et al. Unaccounted for anion in metabolic acidosis during severe sepsis in humans. *Crit Care Med* 1991;19:705–711.

Narins RG, Cohen JJ. Bicarbonate therapy for organic acidosis: the case for its continued use. *Ann Intern Med* 1987;106:615–618.

Narins RG, Emmett M. Simple and mixed acid–base disorders: a practical approach. *Medicine* 1980;59:161–186.

Rodriguez-Soriano J, Vallo A. Renal tubular acidosis. *Pediatr Nephrol* 1990;4:268–275.

Rothstein M, Obialo C, Hruska KA. Renal tubular acidosis. *Endocrinol Metab Clin North Am* 1990;19:869–887.

Wilson RF, Binkley LE, Sabo FM, et al. Electrolyte and acid–base changes with massive blood transfusions. *Am Surg* 1992;58:535–545.

Wrenn K. The delta (D) gap: an approach to mixed acid–base disorders. *Ann Emerg Med* 1990;19:1310–1313.

# BOARD SIMULATION: Nephrology and Hypertension

**54**

*Richard A. Fatica*

## QUESTIONS

**1.** A 26-year old man presents with complaints of edema of the lower extremities for the past week. He has been using a COX-2 selective NSAID mg per day for 1 month for a shoulder injury.

He is found to have a blood pressure of 130/90 mm Hg, and 3+ lower extremity edema.

His laboratory values show 10.8 g of urinary protein in 24 hours, no hematuria, and serum creatinine level of 0.9 mg/dL. Urinalysis was normal 6 months previously.

The most likely disorder causing this clinical picture is:
a) Human immunodeficiency virus (HIV) nephropathy
b) Focal segmental glomerulosclerosis
c) Acute tubular necrosis
d) Minimal change glomerulonephritis

**2.** A 26-year-old man presents with hematuria (i.e., tea-colored urine), arthralgias, and a heart murmur. The patient was recently discharged from military service, and he developed an upper respiratory infection 10 days ago.

The results of the physical examination are a swollen and tender right wrist and left elbow, prominent cervical/submandibular nodes, 2/6 systolic ejection murmur, and 2+ edema.

A urinalysis shows the following values: a specific gravity of 1.013; glucose, 0; pH, 6.0; protein, 3+; and 20 RBC/HPF; 3 to 5 RBC casts; and 5 to 10 white blood cells/HPF.

Serology studies reveal a low plasma C3 level; creatinine, 2.2 mg/dL, glucose, 51 mg/dL; increased rheumatoid factor level; FeNa, 71%; and positive cryoglobulins.

The most likely cause for this clinical scenario is:
a) Membranous glomerulonephritis
b) Wegener's granulomatosis
c) Poststreptococcal glomerulonephritis
d) Acute tubular necrosis
e) Fanconi's syndrome

**3.** A 36-year-old woman with recurrent kidney stones presents for further evaluation. Her first kidney stone was approximately 15 years ago; since then, she notes that she has passed approximately 50 stones. She has a strong family history of kidney stones in her father and brother, but no kidney failure. No stone has been recovered for analysis. On advice, she has been restricting her calcium intake for the past few years.

Her laboratory studies reveal the following values:

| Component | Reference Range | Value |
|---|---|---|
| Creatinine | 0.7–1.4 mg/dL | 0.8 mg/dL |
| Sodium | 135–146 mmol/L | 138 mmol/L |
| $CO_2$ | 24–32 mmol/L | 20 mmol/L |
| Calcium | 8.5–10.5 mg/dL | 10.6 mg/dL |
| PTH | 10–60 pg/mL | 66 pg/mL |
| Phosphorous | 2.5–4.5 mg/dL | 2.8 mg/dL |
| **24–hour urine:** | | |
| Calcium | 100–300 mg/24hr | 401.7 mg |
| Citrate | 320–940 mg/24hr | 704 mg |
| Oxalate | 10–50 mg/24hr | 91 mg |
| Sodium | 40–220 mmol/24hr | 315 mmol |
| Uric acid | 250–750 mg/24hr | 1,010.4 mg |
| Volume | | 4,141 cc |

Which of the following is an inhibitor of calcium stone formation?
a) High urinary calcium concentration
b) High urinary citrate concentration
c) High urinary sodium concentration
d) High dietary protein intake
e) High dietary oxalate intake

**4.** Renal manifestations of HIV infection include which of the following?
a) Hyponatremia
b) Tubuloreticular inclusions
c) Focal segmental glomerular sclerosis
d) Acute tubular necrosis
e) All the above

**5.** A 65-year-old man with BPH presents for follow up 5 days into treatment of urinary tract infection with trimethoprim-sulfamethoxazole. He has resolved symptoms, temperature 37.5 C, the remainder of the physical examination is normal. Laboratory work shows the resulting values:

| 2 Weeks Prior | Current |
|---|---|
| BUN 12 mg/dL | 12 mg/dL |
| Creatinine 1.4 mg/dL | 2.0 mg/dL |

**Urinalysis:**
Specific gravity 1.010
Heme negative
Protein negative
Leukocyte esterase negative
No casts

In this patient, the most likely reason for the creatinine increase to 2.0 mg/dL is:
a) Acute interstitial nephritis
b) Acute pyelonephritis
c) Obstructive uropathy
d) Reduced creatinine excretion
e) Acute tubular necrosis

**6.** A 60-year-old man presents to the office with weakness and fatigue of 4 months duration. He has no significant past medical history. His blood pressure is 140/92; conjunctival and mucosal pallor is present. Lower leg edema of 1+ is present.

His laboratory values are a Hgb level of 9 g/dL; 24-hour urine, 5 gm protein/24 hr; and serum creatinine 2.2 mg/dL (1.0 mg/dL one year ago). Protein electrophoresis shows monoclonal spike in γ-region

The patient undergoes a kidney biopsy, which demonstrates diffuse glomerular mesangial expansion with an amorphous hyaline material, glomerular capillary wall thickening, and arteriolar thickening. The congo red stain is positive.

Electron microscopy shows 10 nm fibrils located in the mesangium and glomerular basement membrane.

Which of the following urinalyses would most likely correspond to this patient's disease?
a) pH 5; heme neg; protein neg; SSA 3+
b) pH 5; heme neg; protein 3+; SSA neg
c) pH 5; heme neg; protein 3+; SSA 3+
d) pH 5; heme pos; protein neg; SSA 3+
e) pH 5; heme pos; protein 3+; SSA neg

**7.** A 28-year-old woman with an 18-year history of diabetes mellitus is seen at 12 weeks gestation during her first pregnancy. She is taking enalapril 5 mg per day for hypertension and diabetic nephropathy. Her blood pressure is 160/100. The remainder of the examination is normal.

Laboratory studies reveal a Hgb level of 12 g/dL; Hgb A1C 10%; Cr 0.8 mg/dL; BUN 10 mg/dL; U/A 1+ gluc, 3+ protein; and 24-hour protein excretion 1.2 gm.

Which of the following would you advise?
a) Increase enalapril to 10 mg per day.
b) Continue enalapril and add hydrochlorothiazide 12.5mg per day.

c) Continue enalapril and add α-methyldopa 250 mg twice a day.
d) Replace enalapril with α-methyldopa 250 mg twice a day.
e) Continue enalapril and add amlodipine 5 mg per day.

**8.** A 68-year-old woman with a 20-year history of hypertension presents to you for follow-up after hospital discharge. She was admitted after presenting to the emergency department with headache, at which time her blood pressure was 200/70. Her creatinine was 1.6 mg/dL (stable for 3 years); an ultrasonogram of her kidneys revealed 12 cm kidneys bilaterally. A renal artery duplex was suggestive of renal arterial atherosclerotic disease.

She underwent renal artery angiography, which revealed 55% stenosis on left, and 35% stenosis on right, with a markedly atheromatous aorta.

Her laboratory results are as follow:

| | |
|---|---|
| TSH | 1.5 mU/mL |
| Plasma renin activity | 0.5 mg/L/H |
| Plasma aldosterone | 10 ng/dL |
| Urine dipstick protein | 1+ |
| Urinary protein: creatinine | 0.6 |
| Sodium | 140 mEq/L |
| Potassium | 4.2 mEq/L |
| Carbon dioxide | 26 mEq/L |
| Creatinine | 1.6 mg/dL |

What is the most likely cause of this patient's hypertension?
a) Essential hypertension
b) Primary hyperaldosteronism
c) Glucocorticoid remediable hyperaldosteronism
d) Renal arterial stenosis
e) Pheochromocytoma

**9.** Pick the correct statement concerning fractional excretion of sodium (FeNa):
a) A FeNa is most useful at normal glomerular filtration rates.
b) A FeNa is always greater than 1% in acute tubular necrosis.
c) A normal FeNa is greater than 1%.
d) A FeNa has the most validity when oliguria is present.

**10.** A 45-year-old alcoholic man is brought to the emergency department in a comatose state. His weight is 70 kg, and his urine output is 175mL/hr.

His laboratory data show the following values:

| | |
|---|---|
| Na | 168 mEq/dL |
| K | 4 mEq/dL |
| Cl | 130 mEq/dL |
| $CO_2$ | 25 mEq/dL |
| Plasma osmolality | 350 mOsm/L |
| Urine osmolality | 80 mOsm/L |

What is the approximate water deficit (in L)?
a) 8

**b)** 6

**c)** 7

**d)** 10

**11.** A 55-year-old woman with a 10-year history of idiopathic pulmonary fibrosis is seen in consult for hyponatremia. She presented in pulmonary edema to the emergency department, and underwent aortic valve repair 3 days ago for severe aortic stenosis. At the time of surgery, her serum sodium was 125 mEq/L. Following the surgery, she received intravenous furosemide (Lasix) for leg swelling. On the third day postoperatively, her serum sodium is noted to be 118 mEq/L. She is asymptomatic. The physical examination shows a seated BP of 110/80, pulse 100; standing BP 90/60, pulse 120. Lungs are clear, and no edema of the legs is present. One year ago, her serum sodium was 130 mEq/L.

Additional laboratory studies reveal:

| | |
|---|---|
| Urea nitrogen | 22 mg/dL |
| Creatinine | 0.9 mg/dL |
| Sodium | 118 mEq/L |
| Potassium | 3.9 mEq/L |
| Chloride | 96 mEq/L |
| Bicarbonate | 28 mEq/L |
| Uric acid | 4 mg/dL |
| Urine osmolality | 280 mOsm |

Which of the following is most likely responsible for this patient's hyponatremia?

**a)** Decrease in antidiuretic hormone (ADH) secondary to hypoosmolality

**b)** Increase in ADH secondary to volume depletion

**c)** Increase in ADH secondary to hypokalemia

**d)** Decrease in aldosterone secondary to hyponatremia

**e)** Increase in aldosterone secondary to free-water retention.

**12.** A 45-year-old woman with peptic ulcer disease reports 6 days of nausea and vomiting. On physical examination, here BP is found to be 100/60 without postural change, the skin turgor is decreased, and the neck veins are flat. Her laboratory values are:

| | |
|---|---|
| Sodium | 140 mEq/L |
| Potassium | 2.2 mEq/L |
| Chloride | 86 mEq/L |
| Bicarbonate | 42 mEq/L |
| Urea nitrogen | 80 mg/dL |
| Creatinine | 1.9 mg/dL |
| Urine pH | 5.0 |
| Urine sodium | 2 mEq/L |
| Urine potassium | 21 mEq/L |
| Urine chloride | 3 mEq/L |
| Arterial pH | 7.53 |
| Arterial $P_{CO_2}$ | 53 mmHg |

The most appropriate therapeutic option is

**a)** Administer oral ammonium chloride.

**b)** Administer oral carbonic anhydrase inhibitor.

**c)** Administer intravenous hydrochloric acid solution.

**d)** Administer intravenous 0.9% NaCl solution.

**e)** Administer intravenous D5W solution.

**13.** A 35-year-old patient presents for evaluation of spontaneous bone fracture. She recently had a bone densitometry evaluation that revealed osteopenia.

She has undergone normal growth and development. She has no children. She gives a history of recurrent kidney stones in her father, but she has no history of stones. Her physical examination is unrevealing.

Her laboratory values are:

| | |
|---|---|
| Sodium | 140 mEq/L |
| Potassium | 3.2 mEq/L |
| Chloride | 114 mEq/L |
| Bicarbonate | 16 mEq/L |
| Creatinine | 0.7 mg/dL |
| Calcium | 9.0 mg/dL |
| Urine sodium | 20 mmol/dL |
| Urine pH | 7.0 |

You provide the patient with potassium citrate therapy, and she returns 4 weeks later. At that time, her urine pH is 7.5, and her plasma bicarbonate is 18 mEq/L.

The most likely diagnosis is

**a)** Primary hyperaldosteronism

**b)** Secondary hyperparathyroidism

**c)** D-lactic acidosis

**d)** Bartter's syndrome

**e)** Renal tubular acidosis

**14.** A 75-year-old woman is seen for a preoperative physical examination. She has been followed for 6 years for chronic kidney disease, not yet requiring dialysis. Her most recent creatinine value was 3.0 mg/dL, stable over 6 months. She has been complaining of feeling tired and cold. Her medications are ramipril 10 mg per day, calcium carbonate 1,300 mg with meals, and aspirin 81 mg per day. Her physical examination reveals a blood pressure level of 130/70, pulse 90, mucosal pallor, and no evidence of volume overload. Her laboratory studies reveal a Hgb level of 7.5 g/dL; Hct, 23 mg/dL; MCV, 66; and reticulocyte count, 0.5.

What is the next most appropriate step?

**a)** Oral iron therapy

**b)** Bone marrow biopsy

**c)** Initiate dialysis

**d)** Erythropoietin therapy

**e)** Colonoscopy

**15.** A 30-year-old man is seen with right foot pain. He has a history of congenital reflux, and he received a live donor renal transplant (from his father) at age 20. His medications include prednisone 7.5 mg per day, imuran 100 mg per day, and cyclosporine 125 mg twice a day. On examination, he has an erythematous and tender first metatarsal phalangeal (MTP) joint on the right foot.

He has tophi on the elbow and hands. His creatinine has been stable at 2.0 mg/dL. Arthrocentesis and crystal analysis reveal monosodium urate crystals.

Which of the following would be best appropriate therapy for his gout?
a) Indomethacin
b) Allopurinol
c) Colchicine
d) Ibuprofen
e) Probenecid

## ANSWERS AND DISCUSSION

### 1. d.

Nonsteroidal anti-inflammatory drug (NSAID) use, both nonselective and COX-II selective inhibitors, has been associated with several renal manifestations, including salt and water retention (edema), hyperkalemia, hypertension, acute renal failure, and proteinuria. Acute hemodynamic alterations can result in renal failure. The effect on the renal vasculature is to reduce the renal blood flow by inhibiting the prostaglandin-dependent afferent arteriolar vasodilation in susceptible kidneys. Proteinuria results from a renal glomerular epithelial cell injury that is histopathologically identified as a minimal change lesion, with effacement of the foot processes.

Whereas, as in minimal change disease, focal sclerosis, and HIV nephropathy are causes of nephritic-range proteinuria (>3.5 g/day), they are not typically seen as caused by NSAID exposure. Acute tubular necrosis may be seen as a severe example of the hemodynamic insult secondary to NSAIDs, but it is not associated with heavy proteinuria.

### 2. c.

The diagnosis of poststreptococcal glomerulonephritis should be entertained on the basis of patient history, urinary findings, and hypocomplementemia (i.e., low plasma C3 level). The antistreptolysin titer is elevated in about 75% of patients with pharyngitis. The low plasma C3 level occurs during the first week, and elevated rheumatoid factor titers and circulating cryoglobulins can be found in most patients. Membranous glomerulonephritis, Wegener's granulomatosis, acute tubular necrosis, and Fanconi's syndrome are not associated with low plasma C3 levels. Other entities associated with low C3 level, with or without a low C4 level, include membranoproliferative glomerulonephritis, cryoglobulinemia, systemic lupus erythematosus, subacute bacterial endocarditis, acute poststreptococcal glomerulonephritis, hemolytic uremic syndrome, thrombotic thrombocytopenic purpura, severe malnutrition, and hepatic failure.

### 3. b.

High concentrations of urinary citrate are protective against the formation of calcium-based kidney stones. It is thought that the urinary citrate can complex with calcium and form soluble complexes. A very low urinary citrate is seen in chronic metabolic acidosis, as with renal tubular acidosis or hyperparathyroidism. Hypercalciuria is a risk for calcium-based stone formation, and high urinary sodium levels are a risk for hypercalciuria. High protein intake can be a risk for higher calcium and salt intake, as well as increased urinary uric acid concentrations. High dietary oxalate can lead to hyperoxaluria; oxalate in the urine complexes with calcium to form calcium oxalate stones.

### 4. e.

Of patients infected with HIV, 60% have low serum sodium levels because of volume depletion and dilute fluid replacement. The syndrome of inappropriate antidiuretic hormone (SIADH) can be seen in patients with pulmonary and intracranial diseases, including pneumocystosis, toxoplasmosis, and tuberculosis. Endothelial tubuloreticular inclusion bodies are a marker of HIV infection, and histologically, HIV may demonstrate findings similar to those of focal segmental glomerular sclerosis (FSG) (i.e., diffuse epithelial cell changes and prominent collapse of the glomerular tuft). Acute tubular necrosis in HIV infection can occur in patients with hypovolemia, shock, sepsis, and in those who are receiving nephrotoxic drugs. Drug-induced acute interstitial nephritis can be seen along with interstitial edema from malnutrition, proteinuria, and hypoalbuminemia. Hemolytic uremic syndrome also may be seen in patients with HIV.

### 5. d.

Trimethoprim and other organic cations, such as cimetidine, competitively inhibit the creatinine secretion in the renal tubule. This phenomenon is sometimes used to more accurately reflect the true glomerular filtration rate (GFR; cimetidine preload before creatinine clearance determination).

Although acute interstitial nephritis occurs after TMP/SMX exposure, it is less commonly seen without other systemic allergic symptoms such as rash and fever.

TMP/SMX has not been associated with acute tubular necrosis (ATN), as have aminoglycosides or amphotericin B.

### 6. c.

The urinary dipstick is a pH-sensitive colorometric assay that is used to detect albumin. Because of its negative charge, the presence of albumin in the urine in high enough quantities reacts with the reagent strip. In contrast, sulfosalicylic acid will react with all protein in the urine to form a white precipitate. The SSA test is commonly performed when there is a suspicion of nonalbumin protein, such as light chains. It will, however, precipitate all protein, including albumin, so that in states with heavy albuminuria, both the dipstick and the SSA should be positive.

Amyloidosis, as defined by the pathology report of this kidney biopsy, usually presents with heavy albuminuria, due to the glomerular involvement in the disease. It is not usually manifest with high amounts of hematuria.

### 7. d.

Angiotensin-converting enzyme (ACE) inhibitors are known to be associated with fetal developmental abnormalities in the second and third trimesters. This is likely due to the ability of the ACE-I to cross the placenta. Angiotensin II is thought to be important in the regulation of placental blood flow and normal fetal growth. The teratogenic effects are renal tubular dysplasia, oligohydramnios, limb contractures and craniofacial deformities (oligohydramnios), fetal death, neonatal anuria and renal failure, pulmonary hypoplasia, and prolonged neonatal hypotension.

### 8. a.

This patient, although having marked atherosclerosis, does not appear to have the necessary critical lesion (>75% luminal narrowing) for renovascular hypertension secondary to renal artery stenosis. The duplex ultrasound, in the hands of experienced operators, has a very high sensitivity and specificity for the detection and accurate grading of renal artery lesions. Primary aldosteronism and glucocorticoid remediable aldosteronism are forms of secondary hypertension with abnormal salt and water retention and kaliuresis causing hypokalemia. They are commonly seen with a metabolic alkalosis as well. This patient's potassium concentration is normal, and she does not have a metabolic alkalosis. The plasma renin activity-to-aldosterone ratio has been used as a screening tool for the presence of primary aldosteronism, however there is much dispute on where to set the ratio for best sensitivity and specificity. The duration of her disease, as well as no evidence of a secondary cause, reinforce that this patient most likely has essential hypertension.

### 9. d.

The fractional excretion of sodium (FeNa) is the percentage of filtered sodium that is excreted in the urine. In normal subjects, the FeNa is usually less than 1%. It has the highest predictive power when the subject is oliguric or has a markedly compromised GFR. In that state, it is not physiologic to excrete a sodium concentration that is less than 1%; therefore, if a FeNa of less than 1% is seen, avid sodium conservation is present. Certain causes of acute tubular necrosis may be associated with a FeNa of less than 1%, such as radiocontrast-induced injury or concomitant hypoperfusion. At normal GFRs, and in balance, the FeNa represents normal sodium intake.

### 10. a.

The water deficit is described by the equation:

$$
\begin{aligned}
\text{water deficit (L)} \\
&= 0.6 \times \text{weight (kg)} \times [(\text{serum Na}/140) - 1] \\
&= 0.6 \times 70\text{kg} \times [(168 \text{ mEq/dL}/140 \text{ mEq/dL}) - 1] \\
&= 42\text{kg} \times (1.2 - 1) \\
&= 8.4 \text{ kg} \\
&= 8.4 \text{ L}
\end{aligned}
$$

### 11. b.

Osmoregulation is accomplished in the body by the regulation of water excretion and water intake. ADH is released in response to increases in plasma osmolality, usually reflected by an increase in measured plasma sodium concentration. Thirst is generated as well, resulting in increased water intake if there is free access to water. In the presence of ADH, the distal tubule and collecting ducts become permeable to water, resulting in reabsorption. Effective circulating volume refers to fluid that is effectively perfusing tissues. Regardless of whether true volume depletion or a concomitant edematous state exists (nephrosis, cirrhosis, congestive heart failure), the effect on water excretion is to increase ADH release by unloading carotid sinus baroreceptors and augmenting sodium, therefore causing water reabsorption.

### 12. d.

This patient has a metabolic alkalosis, manifest with an increase in serum bicarbonate concentration, as well as increased plasma pH. This is an example of a chloride-responsive metabolic alkalosis, in which the urinary chloride is less than 25mEq/L. This is commonly seen in association with vomiting or nasogastric suction, late diuretic effect, factitious diarrhea, or low chloride intake. High urinary chloride levels (>40mEq/L) are seen in mineralocorticoid excess states or early diuretic use. Restoring the extracellular volume, specifically using a chloride-containing salt, is the treatment of choice because chloride depletion has been linked to increased bicarbonate generation. Ammonium chloride can lead to a significant accumulation of HCL and ammonia in the liver and should not be used; intravenous HCL may be used in chloride-unresponsive states but is rarely needed. A carbonic anhydrase inhibitor, such as acetazolamide, can be used for chloride resistant alkaloses in volume overload states.

### 13. e.

This patient has a proximal renal tubular acidosis (type 2 RTA), in which the primary defect is a reduction in the set-point for bicarbonate reabsorption in the proximal tubule. If the plasma bicarbonate is at or below that set-point threshold, the urinary pH may be appropriately low with respect to the metabolic acidosis. Only when the patient receives alkali therapy does the plasma bicarbonate exceed the reabsorptive threshold; excess bicarbonate appears in the urine and increases the urinary pH. In a distal, or type 1 RTA, the urinary pH should always be higher than expected for the given metabolic acidosis. Primary hyperaldosteronism and Bartter's syndrome are associated with a metabolic alkalosis and hypokalemia; secondary hyperparathyroidism is seen in patients with decreased GFR; D-lactic acidosis causes typical neurologic manifestations and is usually seen in patients with a history of intestinal resection or bypass.

**14. e.**

The anemia associated with kidney disease is a normocytic normochromic anemia, and the initiation of a workup for anemia begins when the hemoglobin is 80% of normal value for the patients' reference population. Microcytosis may reflect iron deficiency, aluminum excess, or certain hemoglobinopathies; macrocytosis may be associated with vitamin $B_{12}$ or folate deficiency. Iron deficiency should prompt the search for iron (blood) loss; in this patient, colonoscopy is the best choice. Oral iron therapy without excluding a source of blood loss could potentially result in the failure to diagnose a serious condition. The patient does not have an indication to start dialytic therapy. A bone marrow biopsy can sometimes be helpful if more than one cell line is being affected. Erythropoeitin is initiated when other causes of anemia have been excluded, and the anemia is attributed to chronic kidney disease. The effective treatment of the anemia of chronic kidney disease (CKD) improves survival, decreases morbidity, and increases quality of life.

**15. c.**

The best choice for therapy for this acute gouty arthritis in a transplant recipient who has had a prior gouty attack is colchicine. Rarely, even low doses may induce the abrupt or insidious onset of a myoneuropathy, probably due to a decreased clearance of colchicine resulting from the simultaneous administration of calcineurin inhibitors (cyclosporine or tacrolimus). In this setting, myalgias, paresthesias, or weakness may be the first and only sign of colchicine toxicity. NSAIDs are a potential concern because the inhibition of renal prostaglandin synthesis may lead to a further reduction in GFR. Allopurinol generally should generally be avoided in patients treated with azathioprine. Allopurinol interferes with the metabolism of 6-mercaptopurine, the active metabolite of azathioprine, and severe bone marrow toxicity may result. Probenecid should not be used with renal insufficiency. Another commonly used and effective option is a steroid pulse. Treatment commonly begins following an arthrocentesis that demonstrates typical gout crystals.

## SUGGESTED READINGS

### Question 1

Clive DM. Renal transplant-associated hyperuricemia and gout. *J Am Soc Nephrol* 2000;11(5):974–979.

Morales E, Mucksavage JJ. Cyclooxygenase-2 inhibitor-associated acute renal failure: case report with rofecoxib and review of the literature. *Pharmacotherapy* 2002;22(10):1317–1321.

Matzke GR. Nonrenal toxicities of acetaminophen, aspirin, and nonsteroidal anti-inflammatory agents. *Am J Kidney Dis* 1996;28(1 Suppl 1):S63–70.

### Question 2

Baldwin DS, Gluck MC, Schact RG, Gallo G. The long-term course of poststreptococcal glomerulonephritis. *Ann Intern Med* 1974;80:342–358.

Hebert LA, Cosio FG, Neff JC. Diagnostic significance of hypocomplementemia. *Kidney Int* 1991;39:811–821.

Madaio MP, Harrington JT. Current concepts. The diagnosis of acute glomerulonephritis. *N Engl J Med* 1983;309;1299–1302.

Roth KS, Foreman JW, Segal S. The Fanconi syndrome and mechanisms of tubular transport dysfunction. *Kidney Int* 1981;20:705–716.

### Question 3

Coe FL, Parks JH, Asplin JR. Pathogenesis and treatment of kidney stones. *N Engl J Med* 1992;327:1141–1152.

Preminger GM. Renal calculi: pathogenesis, diagnosis and medical therapy. *Semin Nephrol* 1992;12:200–216.

### Question 4

Berns JS, Cohen RM, Stumacher RJ, Rudnick MR. Renal aspects of therapy for human immunodeficiency virus and associated opportunistic infection. *J Am Soc Nephrol* 1991;1:1061–1081.

Humphreys MH. Human immunodeficiency virus associated nephritis. *Kidney Int* 1995;48:311–320.

Masharani U, Schambelan M. The endocrine complications of acquired immunodeficiency syndrome. *Adv Intern Med* 1993;38:323–336.

Rao TK. Clinical features of human immunodeficiency virus associated nephropathy. *Kidney Int* 1991;35(Suppl):S13–S18.

Seney FD Jr., Burns DK, Silva FG. Acquired immunodeficiency syndrome and the kidney. *Am J Kidney Dis* 1990;16:1–13.

### Question 5

Shemesh O, Golbetz H, Kriss JP, Myers BD. Limitations of creatinine as a filtration marker in glomerulopathic patients. *Kidney Int* 1985;28:830–838.

Hilbrands LB, Artz M, Wetzels JF, Koene RA. Cimetidine improves the reliability of creatinine as a marker of glomerular filtration. *Kidney Int* 1991;40:1171–1176 .

### Question 6

Markowitz GS. Dysproteinemia and the kidney. *Adv Anat Pathol* 2004;11(1):49–63.

Gertz MA, Lacy MQ, Dispenzieri A. Immunoglobulin light chain amyloidosis and the kidney. *Kidney Int* 2002;61(1):1–9.

### Question 7

Shotan A, Widerhorn J, Hurst A, Elkayam U. Risks of angiotensin-converting enzyme inhibition during pregnancy: experimental and clinical evidence, potential mechanisms, and recommendations for use. *Am J Med* 1994;96:451–456.

Hou S. Pregnancy in chronic renal insufficiency and end-stage renal disease. *Am J Kidney Dis* 1999;33:235–252.

## Question 8

Onusko E. Diagnosing secondary hypertension. *Am Fam Phys* 2003 1; 67(1):67–74.

Olin JW, Piedmonte MR, Young JR, et al. The utility of duplex ultrasound scanning of the renal arteries for diagnosing significant renal artery stenosis. *Ann Intern Med* 1995 1;122(11):833–838.

Textor SC. Pathophysiology of renovascular hypertension. *Urol Clin North Am* 1984;11(3):373–381.

## Question 9

Steiner RW. Interpreting the fractional excretion of sodium. *Am J Med* 1984;77(4):699–702.

Rose, BD. *Pathophysiology of Renal Disease*, 5th ed. New York: McGraw-Hill, 2001; 408–409.

## Question 10

Rose, BD, Post, TW. *Clinical Physiology of Acid-Base and Electrolyte Disorders*, 5th ed. New York: McGraw-Hill, 2001; 285–296.

## Question 11

Rose, BD, Post, TW. *Clinical Physiology of Acid-Base and Electrolyte Disorders*, 5th ed. New York: McGraw-Hill, 2001; 700–701.

## Question 12

Rose, BD, Post, TW. *Clinical Physiology of Acid-Base and Electrolyte Disorders*, 5th ed. New York: McGraw-Hill, 2001; 551–577.

## Question 13

Rose, BD, Post, TW. *Clinical Physiology of Acid-Base and Electrolyte Disorders*, 5th ed. New York: McGraw-Hill, 2001; 578–646.

## Question 14

Delano BG. Improvements in quality of life following treatment with r-HuEPO in anemic hemodialysis patients. *Am J Kidney Dis* 1989; 14(2 Suppl 1):14–18.

National Kidney Foundation. *K/DOQI Clinical Practice Guidelines for Chronic Kidney Disease: Executive Summary*. New York: National Kidney Foundation, 2002; 51–54.

# Gastroenterology

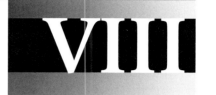

# Liver Disorders

**William D. Carey**

## 55

The recognition of common and uncommon hepatobiliary disorders is a challenge for physicians and surgeons of all specialties. Rote memory will not do. A system of organizing our thoughts will go a long way toward making this task manageable. Perhaps the place to begin is a consideration of laboratory tests and how they help to distinguish liver and biliary tract disorders of various etiologies.

## SERUM-BASED LIVER TESTS

Readily available tests provide information about the state of the liver, but few are absolutely pathognomonic. Instead, a context-based pattern recognition often is required of the clinician. The first pattern distinction is to determine whether the abnormalities are more suggestive of cholestatic or liver cell injury. *Cholestatic liver disease* refers to impairment of hepatic excretion into the biliary system. This type of blockage may occur at any level. In drug-induced cholestasis (e.g., chlorpromazine), the defect is at the level of the bile canaliculus (i.e., intrahepatic cholestasis). In cancer of the bile duct (cholangiocarcinoma), the defect is in the large (macroscopically visible) biliary system. In both kinds of blockage, the same pattern is present in serum-based liver function tests. The alkaline phosphatase and γ-glutamyl transpeptidase (GGTP) are elevated to a much greater degree than that of the transaminases [transferases; serum glutamic-oxaloacetic transaminase (SGOT) or aspartate transaminase (AST), serum glutamate-pyruvic transaminase (SGPT) or alanine transaminase (ALT)]. The bilirubin level may or may not be elevated, depending on the extent and duration of obstruction. If the prothrombin time is elevated in cholestatic liver disease, the abnormality usually reverses upon the parenteral administration of vitamin K.

Special mention must be made of those situations in which an elevation of GGTP is present with a normal bilirubin and normal liver enzymes, including alkaline phosphatase. Current opinion suggests this problem does not, by itself, call for additional testing. If additional clinically relevant issues point to possible liver disease (e.g., alcohol intake, obesity, and so forth), then relevant tests directed by these facts should be considered. In other words, an elevation of GGTP is a frequent finding of little clinical consequence.

When liver disease primarily affects hepatocytes, as in viral hepatitis, alcoholic hepatitis, and many drug-induced problems, a pattern of *liver cell injury* is seen. The transaminases [transferases; SGOT (AST) and SGPT (ALT)] are elevated predominantly. If the hepatocellular process is severe enough to produce an elevation of the prothrombin time, it will not be corrected by parenteral vitamin K. Most often, patients with hepatocyte-centered liver injury do not complain of pruritus, nor do they have xanthelasma or prominent elevations of serum cholesterol.

In fact, most liver and bile duct injuries produce elevations in both the cholestatic and hepatitic tests, and so the predominant elevation must be identified. For example, a tenfold elevation of ALT with a twofold elevation of alkaline phosphatase would indicate a hepatocellular process; the converse would indicate a bile duct disease.

Jaundice first becomes evident clinically when the bilirubin is elevated, usually to a range of 4 mg/dL or greater. Lesser elevations usually are not discernible by examination of the sclera and skin. The inherited disorders of bilirubin metabolism should only be considered if other serum-based liver tests are normal. Among these bilirubin metabolism disorders, only Gilbert's syndrome is common; it must be differentiated from true liver disease to avoid expensive, invasive, and unnecessary evaluations for liver disease. In a patient with suspected Gilbert's syndrome, only two tests are needed. First, the amount of bilirubin present as conjugated and unconjugated direct portions is essential. *Conjugated bilirubin* is measured as direct-reacting bilirubin, and *unconjugated bilirubin* is measured as indirectly reacting bilirubin. In Gilbert's syndrome, 90% or more of the bilirubin is indirect-reacting. Because hemolysis also results in elevations of indirect-reacting bilirubin, a reticulocyte count helps to exclude a compensated hemolytic anemia as a cause for the elevated indirectly-reacting bilirubin. Table 55.1 identifies the key aspects of syndromes that cause an isolated elevation of bilirubin levels.

## HEPATOCELLULAR DISEASES

### Fatty Liver

Fatty liver is one of the most common causes of mild to moderate parenchymal liver test elevations. Benign

**TABLE 55.1**

**ELEVATED BILIRUBIN WITH NORMAL LIVER TEST RESULTS**

| Condition | Defect | Hints | Sequelae |
|---|---|---|---|
| Unconjugated hyperbilirubinemia | | | |
| Gilbert's syndrome | Multiple; hepatic uptake of bilirubin defective; bilirubin usually 1.3–3.0 mg/dL, rarely higher | Common; usually apparent in late adolescence or early adulthood<br>Fasting increases bilirubin further; phenobarbital lowers bilirubin | None |
| Hemolysis | Increased production of (unconjugated) bilirubin by destruction of red blood cells; bilirubin >8 mg% rules out hemolysis as sole abnormality | Low hemoglobin (occasionally normal if hemolysis is compensated) | Those of underlying disease |
| Crigler-Najjar syndrome | Diminished or absent ability of liver to conjugate bilirubin | Present at birth or soon after so will not present as a mystery in an adult; usually high bilirubin (may be >20 mg/dL), kernicterus brain damage usual | Severely debilitating neurologic effects from kernicterus |
| Conjugated hyperbilirubinemia | | | |
| Dubin-Johnson syndrome | Both indirect and direct reacting bilirubin are present | The liver has a black appearance due to pigment deposition; oral cholecystogram does not visualize, raising specter of biliary disease as cause | None |
| Rotor's syndrome | Same as above | Liver not pigmented; otherwise just like Dubin-Johnson syndrome | None |

accumulations of fat may be seen in up to 75% of obese persons and also may be seen in the nonobese, especially in diabetic persons. Certain drugs (e.g., corticosteroids, estrogens, tamoxifen, amiodarone) may cause fatty liver. Fat also may accumulate in Wilson's disease, starvation states, jejunoileal bypass, and in those who consume even moderate amounts of alcohol. Those with elevated serum triglycerides are also at risk. This form of fatty liver is benign, nonprogressive, and requires no specific treatment. A more virulent form of fatty liver, steatohepatitis, often emerges in the same at-risk population, and the clinical distinction of those with benign fat and those with steatohepatitis is impossible without a liver biopsy. The histologic features of steatohepatitis, in addition to fat accumulation, are a polymorphonuclear inflammatory response that includes the destruction of hepatocytes and the presence of Mallory bodies (identical to those in alcoholic hyaline). Steatohepatitis may progress to cirrhosis in 10% to 50% (1). Fatty liver or steatohepatitis (termed *nonalcoholic steatohepatitis*) in patients who do not drink alcohol should be suspected in patients with mild to moderate transaminase elevations and whose serologic studies for viral hepatitis, iron overload, and autoimmune disorders are negative. Additional inference regarding the presence of fatty liver can be obtained from hepatic ultrasound (diffusely echogenic) and computed tomography (CT) scan (low attenuation compared with spleen and hepatic vasculature). Magnetic resonance imaging (MRI) also may provide information, but cost considerations and its lack of additional utility discourage its use for this condition.

Neither blood tests nor scans are able to distinguish benign fatty liver from steatohepatitis, at least before cirrhotic changes become apparent. Liver biopsy is the best method to assess the presence and relative amount of fat and is required to establish a diagnosis of steatohepatitis. Considering the great frequency of fatty liver and the paucity of therapeutic options, a presumptive diagnosis and empiric treatment often is preferable to the cost and risks involved with liver biopsy. Weight loss in obese patients, the control of elevated triglycerides and diabetes, and the avoidance of alcohol are recommended. Reversal of jejunoileal bypass may be necessary to prevent progressive liver failure. For those with steatohepatitis, ursodiol has been shown in limited studies to result in improved liver enzymes and liver histology (2). More data are needed before advocating the routine use of this agent in patients with fatty liver.

## Alcohol

In the United States, alcohol is the most common cause of liver cirrhosis. The consumption of large quantities of alcohol over a long period is required before cirrhosis occurs. Steatohepatitis is considered a precursor lesion in many patients. A reasonable correlation exists between the per capita consumption of alcohol and the prevalence of cirrhosis (3). Women are more susceptible to the hepatic effects of alcohol (4). It is estimated that 80 g of alcohol per day in men and 60 g per day in women, over the course of approximately 10 to 12 years, is required before cirrhosis develops.

Alcohol appears to exert its toxic effect on the liver through the formation of toxic metabolites, induction of enzymes that produce free radicals, and immunologic mechanisms that are activated by free radicals. The parallel and simultaneous enzymatic degradation of alcohol by alcohol dehydrogenase, the microsomal ethanol-oxidizing system within the endoplasmic reticulum, and catalases all convert ethanol to acetaldehyde. This intermediate is toxic; it is rendered nontoxic by a subsequent metabolism to acetate by aldehyde dehydrogenase (5). Chronic alcohol ingestion induces the microsomal ethanol-oxidizing system enzyme family, which includes cytochrome P450 2E. This enzyme produces hydroxyethyl free radicals that bind to cellular proteins and render some of them immunogenic. Antibodies produced in response to this action may injure the liver further (6).

A wide spectrum of liver disease is produced by alcohol. Early on, alcohol ingestion results in the accumulation of fat within hepatocytes (fatty liver). Alcoholic steatohepatitis (described previously) produces a clinical syndrome of alcoholic hepatitis. Fibrosis, especially around the central veins, may herald the beginning of the cirrhotic process. When fully developed, Laennec's cirrhosis is present. Hepatitis C appears to hasten the development of cirrhosis in alcoholic persons.

The diagnosis of alcoholic liver disease often is obvious but may be obscure in the well-nourished person who minimizes or denies alcohol ingestion. Cutaneous spider telangiectasias are frequently present. Other stigmata of acute or chronic liver disease may be present, such as jaundice, ascites, edema, encephalopathy, dilated abdominal veins, parotid enlargement, and gynecomastia. Blood tests frequently show only modest elevations of the SGOT (AST), almost always less than 400 IU. The SGPT (ALT) is characteristically normal or only slightly elevated; thus, the SGOT-to-SGPT ratio is usually greater than 2. Other abnormal tests often reveal macrocytosis (the $B_{12}$ level is almost invariably elevated, and the folate level may be depressed if the patient has consumed a diet deficient in folate), and the γ-globulin levels are frequently elevated. A liver biopsy is usually not necessary in these cases.

The treatment of severe alcoholic hepatitis is largely supportive. Abstinence, multiple vitamins, and fluids are required. In severely ill hospitalized patients, enteral feeding for several weeks produces a better outcome compared with the use of a standard oral diet. Improved survival, Child's score, liver tests, and a lower incidence of encephalopathy have been described (7). The use of corticosteroids remains controversial more than 20 years after they were first studied in this condition. Several studies, however, suggest that steroids improve survival for patients with severe alcoholic hepatitis without gastrointestinal bleeding (8,9). The definition of severity requires an evaluation of the bilirubin level and the prothrombin time (pro time). The so-called *discriminant function value* identifies a group of patients at substantial risk of dying from alcoholic hepatitis.

Discriminant function:

$$4.6 \text{ (pro time} - \text{control [in seconds])} + \text{(serum bilirubin [mg/dL])} = 32$$

When severely ill patients with a discriminant function score of 32 or higher (without gastrointestinal hemorrhage) are given 40 mg of prednisone daily for 28 days, survival is nearly twice as likely. Nutritional therapy appears to benefit patients with moderate malnutrition but not those with severe malnutrition and alcoholic hepatitis. Oxandrolone also may benefit those in whom adequate nutrition can be given (10). Insufficient evidence is available to recommend propylthiouracil or colchicine in alcoholic liver disease (11,12). The treatment of established alcoholic cirrhosis is discussed later.

## Viral Hepatitis

Hepatitis may be caused by myriad viruses. Not all are common and some, especially the herpesviruses, occur in distinctive clinical settings (e.g., the immunocompromised patient). Those in which the hepatocyte appears to be the major locus of infection (hepatatrophic viruses) are shown in Figure 55.1. Most hepatatrophic viruses also infect other organs, thus providing a potential reservoir for recurrence, for example, after liver transplantation. In addition, the extrahepatic manifestations of viral hepatitis may be significant and, from time to time, overshadow the hepatic manifestations. Table 55.2 identifies the important extrahepatic manifestations of hepatitis.

### Hepatitis A

Hepatitis A is spread through fecal-oral contamination. The virus usually is not identified in the serum, where it is present only transiently. It is shed in the stool; usually, shedding (and therefore infectivity) has ceased by the time the index case becomes clinically ill. The affected person

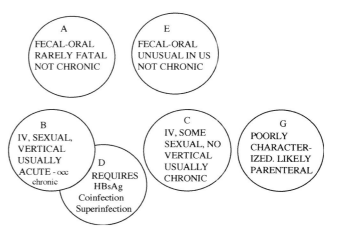

**Figure 55.1** Important hepatatrophic viruses. HBsAg, hepatitis B surface antigen; occ, occasionally; US, United States.

**TABLE 55.2**
**EXTRAHEPATIC FEATURES OF VIRAL HEPATITIS**

| Hepatitis B | Hepatitis C | Unclassified Hepatitis (Non-A, Non-B, Non-C) |
|---|---|---|
| Serum sickness–like illness | Leukocytoclastic vasculitis | Aplastic anemia |
| Polyarteritis nodosa | Porphyria cutanea tarda | |
| Glomerulonephritis (usually membranous) | Glomerulonephritis (usually membranoproliferative) | |
| | Cryoglobulinemia | |
| | Autoimmune thyroiditis | |
| | Sicca syndrome | |
| | Non-Hodgkin's B-cell lymphoma | |

(Reproduced with permission from Brown KE, Tisdale J, Barrett K, et al. Hepatitis-associated aplastic anemia. *N Engl J Med* 1997;336:1059–1064.)

frequently is not jaundiced (*anicteric*). The vast majority of cases resolve within a few days to weeks. Fewer than 1% result in massive hepatic necrosis and death. The diagnosis can be made by demonstration of antihepatitis A antibodies of the immunoglobulin M (IgM) class. Immunoglobulin G (IgG) antibodies denote prior, not acute, infection. No chronic form of hepatitis A or carrier state exists.

Immune globulin provides protection against hepatitis A. Formerly, preexposure prophylaxis was recommended for international travels to endemic regions, but currently such persons are advised to receive active immunization (see discussion later in this section). Postexposure prophylaxis with immune globulin is recommended for (i) household and sexual contacts, (ii) in daycare centers (if children in diapers attend) but not to elementary or secondary school contacts unless an outbreak (more than a single case) has been identified, (iii) within institutions to contacts only, and (iv) in hospitals only if an outbreak occurs. Immune globulin is not recommended for coworkers in offices or factories. Restaurant-exposed persons also may get immune globulin unless the contact was more than 2 weeks previous, in which case no vaccine is recommended. Postexposure prophylaxis is not needed for persons who have been immunized.

In March 1995, the U.S. Food and Drug Administration (FDA) approved an inactivated hepatitis A vaccine (Havrix). This vaccine is safe and highly immunogenic, at least for those with a normal immune system, and it is likely to provide long-lasting immunity. A protective antibody response to this vaccine is apparent within 2 weeks (13). Seroconversion rates approaching 100% are seen 1 month after primary vaccination [1,440 enzyme-linked immunosorbent assay (ELISA) units in adults and two doses of 360 ELISA units in children] (14). A booster dose given 6 to 12 months later is recommended. It seems likely that, in time, this agent will become part of the normal immunization panel for all youngsters, but for the present it is only recommended for (i) those at high risk, such as travelers to endemic areas; (ii) military personnel; (iii) people living in or relocating to areas highly endemic

for hepatitis A; (iv) residents in a community experiencing an outbreak of hepatitis A; (v) institutionalized children and adults; and (vi) children in daycare centers. Limited data suggest that acute hepatitis A may be particularly devastating to those with chronic liver disease (15). For this reason, hepatitis A vaccination is recommended for all susceptible persons with chronic liver disease.

### Hepatitis B

Viral hepatitis B affects more than 300 million people throughout the world. It is spread by three important routes: parenteral, venereal, and through "vertical transmission." In the United States, parenteral and venereal spread is most common, whereas worldwide, vertical transmission (from mother to offspring) is most common. Clinically, most cases are mild and self-limited. Outcomes for those infected as adults are indicated in Figure 55.2. Chronic disease occurs in a minority of adults infected with hepatitis B virus (HBV). The situation is quite different in children. More than 90% of neonates infected with HBV develop chronic infection. Diagnosis is made easier by the many antigen-antibody systems that have been identified in HBV infections. Distinct genotypes of hepatitis B have been described. It is not yet clear if these genotypes have different biologic behavior

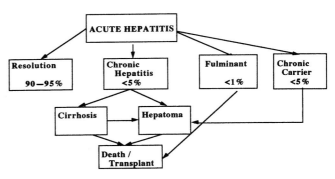

**Figure 55.2** The courses of hepatitis B.

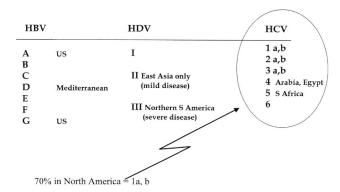

**Figure 55.3** Viral hepatitis genotypes. HBV, hepatitis B virus; HCV, hepatitis C virus; HDV, hepatitis D virus; US, United States.

and respond differently to treatment. Figure 55.3 provides information on the genotypes for hepatitis B, D, and C.

The sequence of antigens and antibodies emergence is available in standard textbooks. A few clinical situations are described:

■ Acute hepatitis B: Early in the disease, the hepatitis B surface antigen (HBsAg) is present, and possibly hepatitis B e antigen (HBeAg), but no antibodies. If the patient comes to medical attention a little later, both the HBsAg and the HBeAg may have disappeared. The HBsAg will have been replaced by IgM class antihepatitis B core (HB$_c$). The disappearance of HBeAg usually is followed by the emergence of anti-e.

■ Remote resolved infection: These patients have antihepatitis B surface (HBS) and anti-HB$_c$ in the serum. Many years later, the waxing and waning antibody titers may yield inconstant results for these assays.

■ Chronic hepatitis B: Found either with disease such as chronic active hepatitis or disease-free (chronic carrier), this disease has HBsAg and anti-HB$_c$ but no anti-HBS. Hepatitis B carriers have normal liver enzymes and normal liver histology. Elevated liver enzymes and positive HBsAg and anti-HB$_c$ usually denote the presence of chronic hepatitis.

■ Successful immunization status: The patient has anti-HBS only.

Acute hepatitis B requires only supportive treatment, preferably out of the hospital. Corticosteroids have no established place in the management of either acute or chronic viral hepatitis. Rarely, hepatitis B results in massive hepatic necrosis and should be treated as such (see Acute Liver Failure, later in this chapter). It may take 6 months or longer before acute hepatitis B resolves.

Interferon-α is useful in many cases of chronic hepatitis B and has received FDA approval for this indication. Five million units of interferon-α, given daily for 16 weeks, or 10 million units given three times per week seem equally effective. The goal of therapy is to convert the HBeAg-positive patient to HBeAg negative, which usually is accom-panied by improved transaminases and improved histology. Interestingly, the elimination of HBeAg often is preceded by a major flare of hepatitis, which can be worrisome and even dangerous to the patient with decompensated cirrhosis. The loss of HBeAg usually implies markedly diminished viral replication, although the HBsAg remains positive. Approximately 35% to 40% of patients have a response to treatment. Treatment successes are durable; few relapses occur in hepatitis B patients. The long-term outlook for those who clear HBeAg positivity with interferon therapy is remarkably improved. Even those with well-compensated cirrhosis appear to benefit from treatment with interferon, if clearance of HBeAg occurs. Such patients have improved aminotransferase levels, experience fewer cirrhotic complications, and live longer than those who do not receive interferon treatment (16). The successful treatment of hepatitis B with interferon reduces the likelihood of subsequent hepatoma (17).

Who should be treated with interferon? The HBsAg carrier (normal liver enzymes) probably requires no treatment because the outcome of this form of hepatitis B seems benign (18). Chinese persons, homosexual patients, and those with long-duration disease (i.e., >2 years) do not respond well to treatment. If coinfection with human immunodeficiency virus (HIV) is present, interferon is of unproven value. Those with decompensated cirrhosis tolerate interferon therapy poorly and may have significant worsening of disease while receiving the drug. Those who have none of these features should be considered for therapy if they have had disease for at least 1 year and if they are HBeAg positive (19).

Nucleoside analogs are active against hepatitis B, and this has created a new opportunity to improve the successful management of hepatitis B. Nucleoside analogs inhibit viral DNA polymerase. Many patients achieve effective blood levels after oral dosing and are relatively free of severe adverse effects; these agents are much less costly than interferon. Most attention has been given to oral lamivudine, which is approved by the FDA for use in hepatitis B (20). It is remarkably free of side effects, although pancreatitis has been observed in pediatric HIV–infected patients receiving this drug. Resistant strains have emerged, caused by mutations in the YMDD locus of the reverse transcriptase of the DNA polymerase gene, but some evidence suggests that, even when this occurs, clinical deterioration is not inevitable. Patients given a dose of 100 mg daily for 1 year had a 72% likelihood of normalization of transaminases and a 16% likelihood of conversion from HBeAg positive to negative. They also had a 56% likelihood of improved histology scores (all results were statistically superior to those given placebo) (21). The limitations of lamivudine include the need for indefinite therapy. Available evidence suggests a rapid reemergence of active viral replication when the drug is stopped. Also, viral mutations (emergence of genotypic mutations in the YMDD locus) occur in approximately 14% of treated patients in the first year. It is too soon

**TABLE 55.3**

**RECOMMENDED DOSES OF HEPATITIS B VACCINE[a]**

| | Recombivax Hepatitis B Dose | | Engerix-B Dose | |
|---|---|---|---|---|
| | (μg) | (mL) | (μg) | (mL) |
| Infants of HBsAg-negative mothers and children <11 years of age | 2.5 | 0.25 | 10 | 0.5 |
| Infants of HBsAg-positive mothers; prevention of perinatal infection | 5.0 | 0.5 | 10 | 0.5 |
| Children and adolescents 11–19 years of age | 5.0 | 0.5 | 20 | 1.0 |
| Adults >19 years of age | 10.0 | 1.0 | 20 | 1.0 |
| Dialysis patients and other immunosuppressed persons | 40.0 | 1.0[a] | 40 | 2.0 |

HBsAg, hepatitis B serum antigen.
*Note:* Usual schedule is three doses, at 0, 1, and 6 months; Engerix-B has been licensed for a four-dose schedule, at 0, 1, 2, and 12 months.
[a] Special high-concentration vaccine is available.

to know whether the long-term administration of lamivudine will alter the natural history of hepatitis B; clinical studies currently are in progress. Patients eligible for either interferon or lamivudine should be offered interferon as first-line treatment because durable responses after a relatively short course of treatment may make additional long-term treatment unnecessary.

Prophylaxis against hepatitis B is possible for most. In April 1991, the Centers for Disease Control and Prevention (CDC) endorsed universal hepatitis B immunization for young children in the United States. This strategy was adopted because of the manifest failure of the former policy of targeting immunization to high-risk groups. Universal immunization will greatly diminish hepatitis B and D in this country within one generation. The CDC guidelines were published in *Morbidity and Mortality Weekly Report* in 1991. Immunization can be started after birth, just before the infant leaves the hospital, and repeated in 1 to 2 months and again at 6 to 18 months of age. Alternatively, the first injection can be given at 1 to 2 months of age, repeated at 4 months, and finally repeated at 6 to 18 months. The hepatitis B vaccine can be given concomitantly with diphtheria, tetanus, and pertussis; *Haemophilus influenzae* type b conjugate; measles-mumps-rubella; and oral polio vaccine. Some children will escape immunization, and a "catch-up" program for adolescents (at age 13 years) is recommended. Dosages for immunoprophylaxis are indicated in Table 55.3. Recommendations for postexposure prophylaxis are indicated in Table 55.4.

## Hepatitis D

Hepatitis D (delta virus), discovered in Italy in 1977, is seen throughout the world. It is more prevalent in other countries than in the United States. Because hepatitis D is a defective RNA virus that can exist only in the presence of hepatitis B, it appears to be a virus infecting a virus. Evidence of delta hepatitis is not found unless the patient is HBsAg positive. The diagnosis of delta hepatitis can be made by detecting hepatitis D antigen in the serum. Two forms of infection may occur. When hepatitis B and delta coinfect the liver simultaneously, the illness produced is more severe than usual hepatitis B. A biphasic peak of SGPT may occur. Fulminant disease may occur, although the patient usually recovers. When delta hepatitis superinfects a liver infected with hepatitis B, a severe, sometimes fatal, disease flare-up occurs. Chronic delta hepatitis may respond to high-dose interferon. Nine million units three times weekly for 48 weeks results in normalization of transaminases in

**TABLE 55.4**

**MANAGEMENT AFTER EXPOSURE TO HEPATITIS B**

| Type of Exposure | Immunoprophylaxis |
|---|---|
| Perinatal | Vaccination HBIG |
| Sexual: acute infection | HBIG ± vaccination |
| Sexual: chronic carrier | Vaccination |
| Household contact: chronic carrier | Vaccination |
| Household contact: acute case | None, unless known exposure |
| Household case: acute, known exposure | HBIG ± vaccination |
| Infant (<12 mo): acute case primary caregiver | HBIG = vaccination |
| Inadvertent: percutaneous/ permucosal | Vaccination ± HBIG |

HBIG, hyperimmune globulin; vaccination, Recombivax HB or Engerix-B.

71% of cases, and most responders lose evidence of circulating hepatitis D virus RNA activity. Although more likely to recrudesce than hepatitis B, approximately half of treated patients continue to have normal transaminases 6 months after treatment is stopped. Despite normal enzymes, many have a reemergence of hepatitis D virus RNA activity once treatment is stopped (22).

### Hepatitis C

Hepatitis C virus (HCV), an RNA virus with similarities to flaviviruses, from which they are, however, distinct, chronically infects 2.7 million Americans; it is estimated that cirrhosis will develop in 20% of those infected (23). Risk factors (Table 55.5) for hepatitis C include blood transfusions before 1992, illicit intravenous drug use, and healthcare workers in contact with blood and blood products. The risk of contracting hepatitis C after a blood transfusion in the United States has diminished from approximately 1 in 10 in the 1980s to a current estimate of 1 case per 100,000 U of blood. A small risk is assumed by sexual partners and household contacts of affected persons. The risk for hemodialysis patients is independent of blood transfusions and is related instead to the total duration of dialysis treatment. Intranasal cocaine use has been recognized as a risk factor. In 40% of infected persons, none of these risks appears to be present. Low socioeconomic status has been invoked to explain this large group with acute hepatitis C without apparent conventional risks. Without further definition, this category appears to serve as a surrogate for a specific risk or risks yet to be identified. The transmission of HCV from mother to infant (vertical transmission) occurs in approximately 6% of mothers whose serum is positive to HCV RNA. The risk seems proportionate to the titer of circulating virus in the mother (24).

Approximately 5% of medical personnel suffering accidental needlestick injuries from needles contaminated with blood from HCV-positive persons develop acute hepatitis C, which is usually subclinical or self-limited and transient (25). No specific postexposure action can be taken to reduce the likelihood of infection in the healthcare worker. Recommendations, therefore, are not entirely comforting to the exposed person. Nevertheless, the CDC, in collaboration with the Hospital Infection Control Practices Advisory Committee, recommends the following policies:

- For the source, baseline testing for antibody to hepatitis C (anti-HCV)
- For the person exposed to an anti-HCV–positive source, baseline and follow-up (e.g., 6-month) testing for anti-HCV and serum alanine aminotransferase activity
- Confirmation by supplemental anti-HCV testing of all anti-HCV results by enzyme immunoassay. Supplemental testing is often recombinant immunoblot antibody testing, but it could be the determination of HCV through the detection of HCV RNA using polymerase chain reaction (PCR)
- Recommendation against postexposure administration of immune globulin or antiviral agents, such as interferons
- Education of healthcare workers about the risk for and prevention of blood-borne infections (26)

### Clinical Course

Hepatitis C has an incubation period of 14 days to 6 months. Acute infection produces a mild undistinguished illness in most persons. It is much more likely than hepatitis B to become chronic (85%) (27). Recent evidence indicates that resolution with permanent elimination of viremia occurs in a small minority of cases (12%), although in another 12%, persistently normal transaminases were present despite viremia. More than three-fourths of patients developed chronic liver disease (28). It is not yet determined what to call those with normal transaminases and persistent anti-HCV or viremia. In a sense, these appear to represent chronic carriers. Yet, unlike those with normal ALT values and positive HBsAg (chronic B carriers), liver biopsies in those with normal ALT values and positive anti-HCV often show chronic hepatitis. The patient with normal ALTs and hepatitis C may have mild to moderate portal hepatic inflammation, although in a few patients, a normal biopsy is seen (29).

Over the course of several decades, hepatitis C may cause cirrhosis, which sometimes decompensates. Increasing evidence suggests that alcoholic liver disease in the presence of hepatitis C results in higher mean aminotransferase levels and mean histologic activity and progression to advanced cirrhosis (30). Daily alcohol consumption, even in low amounts (<50 g/day), has been shown to have an additive effect in the risk of symptomatic cirrhosis, and high alcohol intakes (>125 g daily) have a multiplicative effect (31). Hepatitis C is increasingly recognized as a risk factor for hepatoma. Notwithstanding these observations, Seeff and colleagues described 568 patients who acquired transfusion-associated non-A, non-B hepatitis between 1967 and 1980. After a mean follow-up of 18 years, the mortality was no higher for those who developed non-A, non-B hepatitis than for control patients (51% in each group). The cause of death, however, was more likely due to cirrhosis in the patients who had acquired non-A, non-B hepatitis (32).

**TABLE 55.5**

**TRANSMISSION OF HEPATITIS C VIRUS**

Shared blood
   Intravenous drug abuse
   Blood transfusion before 1992
   Body piercing
   Tattoo
Intrafamilial
Sexual transmission
Intranasal cocaine
Unknown

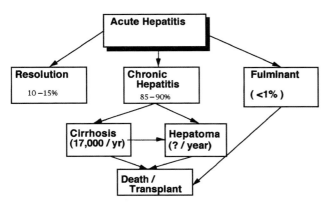

**Figure 55.4**   Hepatitis C.

<table>
<tr><td colspan="3">**TABLE 55.6**</td></tr>
<tr><td colspan="3">**INTERPRETATION OF HEPATITIS C TEST RESULTS**</td></tr>
</table>

| Anti-Hepatitis C Virus | Hepatitis C Virus RNA (Polymerase Chain Reaction) | Interpretation |
|---|---|---|
| Negative | Negative | No infection |
| Positive | Positive | Infection present |
| Negative | Positive | Infection present: early infection or immunocompromised host |
| Positive | Negative | Several possibilities: Resolved infection False-positive antibody Passively acquired antibody Chronic infection, low-level viremia |

- Genotype 1 predominates in North America
- Genotypes 2 and 3 are more amenable to treatment than 1 and 4
- Six months of treatment suffices for genotypes 2 and 3; 12 months for genotypes 1 and 4

### Treatment

The goals of therapy are multiple: reduction in symptoms; improvement in liver tests and liver histology; prevention of development of cirrhosis or cirrhotic decompensation; and reduction in risk for the development of hepatoma. Whether viral eradication is required to achieve each of these goals remains unproven. Certain lifestyle modifications should take precedence over attempts at viral elimination. Complete alcohol abstinence is thought by most to be essential, as is the cessation of illicit drug use and other high-risk behaviors.

Antiviral treatment usually uses multiple drugs, including interferon. Table 55.7 identifies these regimens. Several features are correlated with a relatively good or poor outcome following treatment. These features are compared in Table 55.8. Most patients, of course, have a mixture of favorable and unfavorable traits, which makes precise estimates of response difficult.

Several extrahepatic manifestations of hepatitis C may overshadow hepatic involvement. The glomerular protein leak in membranoproliferative glomerulonephritis may improve if the hepatitis C is treated successfully using interferon (33). As discussed later, some believe that type 2 autoimmune chronic active hepatitis may be triggered by HCV. Porphyria cutanea tarda (PCT), as a result of reduced activity of the enzyme uroporphyrinogen decarboxylase, may be either inherited as an autosomal dominant trait or acquired. Hepatic dysfunction is nearly always seen in PCT, and anti-HCV antibodies are present in four of five patients with acquired PCT, but not in patients with familial PCT (34). Figure 55.4 indicates the many clinical paths this infection can take.

### Diagnosis

Suspicion of hepatitis C relies on the right epidemiologic background, as described previously, and the presence of otherwise unexplained liver test abnormalities. Laboratory testing confirms the diagnosis. ELISA detects anti-C antibodies. This test is quite sensitive, but false-positive results occasionally occur. Confirmatory antibody tests based on recombinant immunoblot antibody testing are widely used. A confirmation of a positive ELISA anti-HCV should be sought in any case, especially if treatment with interferon is being contemplated. The direct measurement of virologic activity is readily available, although not FDA approved. The detection of HCV RNA using PCR represents a powerful new clinical tool. Table 55.6 provides an easy interpretative guide to the tests most often used to detect hepatitis C.

Based on the nucleotide sequence of HCV, several distinct genotypes of HCV are recognized (Fig. 55.3). Great geographic diversity exists with respect to the dominant genotype seen. It has been speculated that different genotypes might influence the severity of disease. Increasing evidence suggests that certain genotypes (especially type 1b) are more likely to produce chronic active hepatitis and cirrhosis (35). Chronic hepatitis C may progress to cirrhosis even with only a modest elevation of transaminases. Currently, the most important observations about HCV genotypes are:

<table>
<tr><td colspan="1">**TABLE 55.7**</td></tr>
<tr><td colspan="1">**HEPATITIS C TREATMENT**</td></tr>
</table>

Drugs used
  Interferon monotherapy
  Interferon + ribavirin
  Pegylated interferon
  Pegylated interferon + ribavirin

## TABLE 55.8

**INTERFERON PREPARATIONS, DOSAGES, AND RECOMMENDED TREATMENT SCHEDULES FOR CHRONIC HEPATITIS C**

| Product | Manufacturer | Dose (Given Subcutaneously) | Duration (Yr) |
|---|---|---|---|
| Interferon alfacon-1 (Infergen) | Amgen | 9 µg three times weekly; 15 µg three times weekly for treatment failures | 1[a] |
| Interferon α-2A (Roferon) | Roche | 3 million units three times weekly | 1[a] |
| Interferon α-2B (Intron A) | Schering | 3 million units three times weekly | 1[a] |
| Interferon α-2B plus ribavirin | Schering | Interferon, 3 million units three times weekly; ribavirin, 1,000 mg; daily (use 1,200 mg daily if weight >65 kg) | 1[b] |

[a] Continue treatment for 1 year only if hepatitis C virus RNA polymerase chain reaction test is negative after 12 weeks of treatment.
[b] Continue treatment for 1 year only if hepatitis C virus RNA test is negative after 6 months of treatment.

By convention, hepatitis C patients are divided into three categories:

- Treatment naïve (never treated)
- Treatment relapser (relapse during or after interferon therapy)
- Treatment nonresponder (no virologic clearance)

Treatment-naïve patients and treatment relapsers have a much higher likelihood of response to therapy than those who have failed a previous course of interferon.

The current primary endpoint of antiviral therapeutic trials is viral elimination that persists for at least 6 months after therapy is ended (sustained virologic response). The absence of circulating virus 6 months after stopping treatment correlates well with absence of virus for the next several years (36). Long-term follow-up in those successfully treated with interferon is encouraging. Those who sustain a durable response (negative serum HCV RNA 6 months after the cessation of therapy) are highly likely to remain HCV RNA negative for up to 13 years, and possibly forever (37). The risk of subsequent hepatoma development appears to be favorably influenced by interferon therapy, both for sustained responders and for responders and relapsers (38).

Landmark publications comparing monotherapy (interferon) with a combination of interferon and ribavirin indicate a substantial benefit from two-drug therapy in those who can tolerate it (39,40). Pegylated interferons (interferon bound to polyethylene glycol) provide for once a week dosing. Pegylated interferon α-2a and pegylated interferon α-2b are superior to interferon in producing sustained virologic responses (41,42). Tables 55.9 and 55.10 indicate the expected likelihood of sustained virologic response using

## TABLE 55.9

**EXPECTED (SUSTAINED VIROLOGIC) RESPONSE RATE IN INTERFERON-NAÏVE PATIENTS WITH HEPATITIS C**

| | Interferon Alone Duration (wk) | | Interferon and Ribavirin Duration (wk) | |
|---|---|---|---|---|
| | 24 | 48 | 24 | 48 |
| All patients | 6% | 13–19% | 31–35% | 35–43% |
| Genotype 2 or 3 | — | 33% | 64% | 64% |
| Best risk[a] | — | 33% | 55% | 80% |
| Worst risk[b] | — | 0% | 8% | 20% |

[a] Best risk = women younger than 40 years, with hepatitis C virus genotype 2 or 3, and viral load <2 million.
[b] Worst risk = men older than 40 years, genotype 1, 4, or 5; septal fibrosis or more; and viral load >2 million.
(Reproduced with permission from Poynard T, Marcellin P, Lee SS, et al. Randomised trial of interferon a2b plus ribavirin for 48 weeks or for 24 weeks versus interferon a2b plus placebo for 48 weeks for treatment of chronic infection with hepatitis C. *Lancet* 1998;352:1426–1437; and McHutchinson JG, Gordon SC, Schiff ER, et al. Interferon α 2b alone or in combination with ribavirin as initial treatment of chronic C hepatitis. *N Engl J Med* 1998;339:1485–1492.)

## TABLE 55.10

### EXPECTED SUSTAINED VIROLOGIC RESPONSE RATE IN INTERFERON-RELAPSER PATIENTS WITH HEPATITIS C RE-TREATED

|  | Interferon Alone (Duration 24 wk) | Interferon and Ribavirin (Duration 24 wk) | Interferon Alone (Duration 48 wk) |
|---|---|---|---|
| All patients | 5% | 49% | 50% |
| Best risk[a] | 18% | 100% | — |
| Worst risk[b] | 0% | 25% | — |

[a] Best risk = genotype other than type 1, and viral load <2 million.
[b] Worst risk = genotype 1 and viral load >2 million.
(Reproduced with permission from Davis GL, Esteban-Mur R, Rustigi V, et al. Interferon alfa-2b alone or in combination with ribavirin for the treatment of relapse of chronic hepatitis C. *N Engl J Med* 1998;339: 1493–1499; and Heathcote EJ, Keefe EB, Lee SS, et al. Retreatment of chronic hepatitis C with consensus interferon. *Hepatology* 1998;27:1136–1143.)

currently available therapies. These results only apply to treatment-naïve patients. The therapy with the best reported outcome—a combination of pegylated interferon and ribavirin—is not yet approved by the FDA. Two studies demonstrate that those who achieve an initial response to interferon and then relapse are good candidates for re-treatment. Forty-eight weeks on consensus interferon results in a 50% sustained response rate (43). Alternatively, the combination of interferon and ribavirin for 24 weeks results in a comparable rate of durable virologic response (44). Expected responses to various treatments are presented in Table 55.11.

The large group of treatment nonresponders is probably best left untreated for now, except in research protocols.

The side effects of hepatitis C antiviral therapy are myriad. Interferons frequently (>50%) induce flu-like symptoms consisting of one or more of the following: headache, fatigue and asthenia, myalgias, fevers, and rigors. Less often seen (13% to 20%) are gastrointestinal symptoms such as anorexia, nausea, and diarrhea. Psychiatric symptoms, either insomnia or depression, may be seen, as well as respiratory symptoms, dermatologic problems, and the

flare-up of putative autoimmune and inflammatory diseases such as psoriasis, inflammatory bowel disease, and so forth. Thyroid abnormalities, both hypothyroidism and hyperthyroidism, are frequent enough that most recommend a thyroid-stimulating hormone test before treatment and 3 months after interferon has been started.

When ribavirin is added to interferon therapy, additional important side effects must be borne in mind. Ribavirin is teratogenic in experimental animals. It is mandatory that effective birth control be in place for both men and women receiving ribavirin, both during and for several months after the cessation of therapy. If pregnancy is a possibility, women should have a negative pregnancy test before starting therapy. Ribavirin accumulates in red blood cells and produces hemolysis (average hemoglobin drop in the first month, 2 g/dL), which may be brisk, resulting in hemoglobin values of <10 g/dL in 10%. This may have dire consequences in patients with ischemic heart disease. Close monitoring of hemoglobin levels early in the course of therapy is mandatory.

The patient with normal ALTs and hepatitis C may have mild to moderate portal hepatic inflammation, although in a few a normal biopsy is seen (29). The poor virologic response rate (6%) to interferon therapy in such individuals, together with the low likelihood of progressive disease, indicates that this group should be spared antiviral therapy for now (45). We do not currently biopsy or treat individuals with hepatitis C with persistently normal ALT levels. HIV-coinfected patients pose a challenge, especially in light of the long life expectancy of those with well-maintained CD4 counts. As yet, we lack convincing evidence that it is helpful to attempt to eradicate hepatitis C in this group.

### Chronic Hepatitis

Chronic hepatitis is a syndrome that may have a number of specific possible etiologies. It is characterized by a sustained elevation of the transaminases and certain histologic features within the liver (e.g., piecemeal necrosis, bridging). To

## TABLE 55.11

### STRATIFICATION OF HEPATITIS C VIRUS TREATMENT CANDIDATES

| Optimal | Questionable |
|---|---|
| Female | Active drug/alcohol use |
| Young | Decompensated cirrhosis |
| Nonobese | Comorbidity |
| Low viral count | Failed previous treatment |
| No severe fibrosis/cirrhosis | Human immunodeficiency virus coinfected |
| Genotype 2 or 3 | Immunocompromised |
| Treatment naïve | Normal liver tests |

*Note:* Most candidates are in neither group.

satisfy the term *chronic*, liver disease must have been present for at least 6 months. Drugs, viruses, and autoimmune liver diseases all can lead to chronic active hepatitis. An idiopathic chronic active hepatitis also exists, in which neither viruses nor drugs can be identified, but autoimmune markers are negative. This subtype of chronic active hepatitis behaves clinically like the autoimmune variant and is just as responsive to corticosteroid therapy. α-Methyldopa, nitrofurantoins, isoniazid, dantrolene, and, rarely, propylthiouracil are drugs that are particularly likely to produce chronic active hepatitis.

### Autoimmune Chronic Hepatitis

Autoimmune chronic hepatitis is one of many liver diseases that produce a prominent elevation of transaminases (transferases) and a histologic response within the liver termed *chronic hepatitis*. Autoimmune type hepatitis predominates in women. Transaminases are markedly elevated; progression to cirrhosis and death within just a few months or years is to be anticipated unless treatment is given. Fatigue, malaise, change in menstruation patterns (often amenorrhea), and prominent extrahepatic effects, such as arthritis and arthralgias, may be present, in which case confusion with rheumatoid arthritis or systemic lupus erythematosus (SLE) may occur. A number of autoantibodies are present, including antinuclear antibody, rheumatoid factor, lupus erythematosus cell phenomena, and false biologic tests for syphilis. The globulin fraction of protein often is elevated markedly. The smooth muscle antibody test is present in up to 75% of patients and is a hallmark of the disease, although it also may be present (usually in low titer) in other diseases.

Several additional autoantibodies have been described, which has allowed the subdivision of autoimmune chronic hepatitis based on the types of autoantibodies present (Table 55.12). Such classification schemes are of little practical importance currently, except to highlight that many patients with autoimmune chronic hepatitis test negative for antinuclear antibody and smooth muscle antibody and thus might be thought to have other disorders.

Liver-kidney microsomal antibodies (anti-LKM) have, in some studies, been linked to hepatitis C infection. Some have claimed that hepatitis C triggers this form of disease. More recent studies cast doubt on this putative association (46). Anti-LKM type 2 affects primarily children and tends to be more severe.

The major histocompatability complex affects autoimmune chronic active hepatitis. Human leukocyte antigens (HLA) A1, B8, and DR3 occur more frequently in younger patients with severe disease activity. Such patients are also more likely to relapse after treatment and require liver transplantation. HLA-DR4 also is associated with autoimmune chronic hepatitis and usually is seen in adult women with higher than usual transaminases; these women are more likely to have additional organs affected by autoimmune diseases and are more likely to respond to corticosteroid therapy (47). These observations do not imply that HLA typing is needed in the evaluation and management of chronic active hepatitis in clinical practice.

The treatment of severe cases (transaminase values 7 to 10 times the upper limit of normal) through the use of prednisone is highly effective in controlling disease and is lifesaving. Azathioprine is frequently added to allow a reduction of the prednisone dose to more acceptable levels. Ordinarily, treatment is given for 6 to 12 months before any attempt is made to wean. Retreatment is frequently necessary, and close follow-up is mandatory to identify recrudescence of disease activity after therapy is stopped. Many patients require lifelong treatment to maintain control.

It is important to distinguish autoimmune chronic hepatitis from hepatitis C. As noted, some patients with the former condition test positive for anti-HCV, especially through ELISA testing. Some patients with chronic C hepatitis have autoantibodies in the serum, usually in low titer. The importance of making the distinction is more than academic because the treatment of autoimmune chronic active hepatitis with interferon may make the disease much worse. If substantial doubt about the diagnosis remains after careful evaluation, a trial of treatment with corticosteroids should precede the administration of interferon. Confusion should be present infrequently if the differences between these entities are borne in mind.

## CHOLESTATIC LIVER DISEASES

Two important causes of cholestatic liver disease are primary biliary cirrhosis (PBC) and primary sclerosing cholangitis (PSC). Whereas a superficial resemblance exists between these disorders, the clinical presentations are usually quite different, and laboratory tests show different patterns (Table 55.13). Autoantibodies are much more likely in PBC.

**TABLE 55.12**

**CLASSIFICATION OF AUTOIMMUNE HEPATITIS BY TYPE OF AUTOANTIBODY**

| Disease | Antinuclear Antibodies | LKM | Soluble Liver Antigens | Smooth Muscle Antibodies |
|---|---|---|---|---|
| Classic (type 1) Autoimmune | + | − | − | + |
| Anti-LKM1 | − | +(1) | − | − |
| Anti-LKM2 | − | +(2) | − | − |
| Soluble liver antigens | − | − | + | ± |
| Smooth muscle antibodies | − | − | − | + |

LKM, liver-kidney microsomal antibodies.

**TABLE 55.13**

**CLINICAL COMPARISON OF CHOLESTATIC DISEASES: PRIMARY BILIARY CIRRHOSIS VERSUS PRIMARY SCLEROSING CHOLANGITIS**

| Marker | Primary Biliary Cirrhosis (n = 258) | Primary Sclerosing Cholangitis (n = 70) |
|---|---|---|
| Immunoglobulin M (mg/dL) | 620 | 70 |
| Antimitochondrial antibodies | 96% | 4% |
| Smooth muscle antibody | 66% | 9% |
| Rheumatoid factor | 70% | 2% |
| Inflammatory bowel disease | 0.04% | 70% |

*Note:* Not helpful: alanine transaminase, alkaline phosphate, bilirubin, albumin, γ-globulin prothrombin time, urine, and hepatic copper.
(Reproduced with permission from Dickson ER, American Association for the Study of Liver Diseases, 1991 course.)

**TABLE 55.14**

**ACQUIRED VANISHING BILE DUCT SYNDROMES**

| Major Differential | Also Consider | To Be Complete |
|---|---|---|
| Primary biliary cirrhosis | Liver allograft rejection | Histiocytosis X |
| Primary sclerosing cholangitis | Graft-versus-host | Mucoviscidosis |
| Autoimmune cholangiopathy? | Hepatic sarcoidosis | Septicemia |
| Idiopathic adulthood ductopenia? | Immunodeficiency and viral | |
| | Drug-induced and toxic | |

(Reproduced with permission from Desmet VJ. Vanishing bile duct disorders. In: Boyer JL, Ockner RK, eds. *Progress in Liver Diseases*, vol X. Philadelphia: WB Saunders, 1992;89.)

## Primary Biliary Cirrhosis

A disease of the interlobular bile ducts, PBC is a chronic disease that is most likely to afflict women older than 30 years. PBC represents a prototypical cholestatic liver disease. Its etiology is poorly understood, but it shares many features with other diseases characterized as autoimmune. Prominent among these are the presence of autoantibodies and the tendency of the disease to involve multiple organs, especially the thyroid, and to exist within Sjögren's syndrome, Raynaud's syndrome, and occasionally CREST syndrome (i.e., *c*alcinosis, *R*aynaud's phenomenon, *e*sophageal dysfunction, *s*clerodactyly, *t*elangiectasia). A regular feature is the presence of antimitochondrial antibodies, discussed later. Th-1 class CD4+ T cells predominate in the inflammatory reaction (48). Most cases are discovered when blood testing done for other reasons reveals abnormal liver test results. Others are discovered during the evaluation of symptoms common in PBC, especially fatigue, pruritus, and skin xanthoma. Metabolic bone disease, especially osteoporosis, is common. The progressive insult to interlobular bile ducts produces a characteristic evolution of bile duct damage, eventuating in the disappearance of most interlobular bile ducts. Thus, it is one of a number of acquired diseases that have been classified as *vanishing bile duct* disorders (Table 55.14) (49).

Immune cholangitis (sometimes termed *autoimmune cholangiopathy* or *autoimmune cholangitis*) appears to represent a trivial variant of PBC—it comprises cases of PBC in which the antimitochondrial antibody is negative. Idiopathic adulthood ductopenia probably refers to this same entity (50). No evidence has been found for a different etiology, clinical course, or response to therapy (51). A more difficult diagnostic problem is the patient with laboratory and histologic evidence of both parenchymal disease (markedly elevated transaminases and inflammatory infiltrate in the hepatic parenchyma) and cholestatic disease (high alkaline phosphatase and significant bile duct injury). These patients have features of both autoimmune chronic active hepatitis and PBC and represent an overlap syndrome (52). These persons often respond dramatically to corticosteroids.

### Natural History

PBC requires 10 to 20 years to display its natural evolution. Among asymptomatic patients, only 50% develop symptomatic disease over 10 years of observation (53). Not surprisingly, the histologic pattern progresses as the disease does (Table 55.15). Some studies have demonstrated a lack of excess mortality, even after 11 years in asymptomatic patients, although the experience of others suggests excess mortality beginning after 4 or 5 years in this group (54,55). Even among initially symptomatic patients, the 4-year survival exceeds 90%. This long disease duration is important in judging the results of clinical therapeutic trials. The Child-Pugh score is an excellent way to predict survival in patients with PBC (Fig. 55.5).

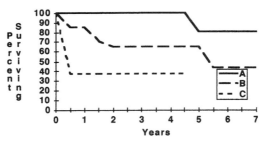

**Figure 55.5** Survival probability in primary biliary cirrhosis using Child-Pugh score at presentation. Pairwise comparison: A versus B, *p* = 0.14; A versus C, *p* < 0.001; B versus C, *p* = 0.005.

**TABLE 55.15**

## HISTOLOGIC STAGES OF PRIMARY BILIARY CIRRHOSIS

| Stage | Key Finding | Additional Findings |
|-------|-------------|---------------------|
| 1 | Mononuclear inflammatory cells around bile ductule in portal areas; some can be seen infiltrating the basement membrane; referred to as *florid duct lesion* | Inflammation in entire portal area, sometimes spilling out into parenchyma; granulomas variably found |
| 2 | Bile duct proliferation | Features of earlier stage may be present |
| 3 | Fibrosis but not cirrhosis; bile ducts may be difficult to identify | Features of earlier stages may be present |
| 4 | Cirrhosis; marked diminution in number of bile ducts; inflammation minimal | Features of earlier stages may be present |

Much has been made of disease-specific predictive scores that claim to be more accurate in predicting outcome. One has won widespread acceptance in clinical research circles (56). Some have found this scoring system awkward to use in clinical practice. We have found that the Child-Pugh score is a simpler yet excellent tool for predicting the likelihood of survival in PBC. The Child's B patient with PBC is reaching the end stage of disease and should be considered for liver transplantation when appropriate. Newer tests, such as soluble intercellular adhesion molecule 1, type III procollagen aminoterminal peptide, and hyaluronic acid levels, appear to correlate with the stage of disease, but are not routinely available and have not been extensively validated (57,58).

### Laboratory Findings

The level of alkaline phosphatase is irrelevant in defining the severity of disease or the extent of liver injury, a point of some importance when judging the effects of therapy discussed later. In early stage disease, tests of liver synthetic function are normal, including serum albumin and prothrombin time. Also normal is the serum bilirubin. When these tests are deranged, late-stage disease (i.e., cirrhosis) is present.

Autoantibodies are a nearly universal feature of PBC. The antimitochondrial autoantibody is seen most regularly (usually with titers >160) and is present in more than 90% of cases. Mitochondria are surrounded by an inner and outer membrane (Fig. 55.6). Multiple antigens are expressed by these membranes; at least 9 (M1 to M9) have been characterized. The presence of antibody directed against the M2 antigen (expressed by the inner membrane) is highly specific for PBC, whereas antibodies against M4 are frequently seen in the chronic active hepatitis overlap syndrome. Evidence suggests that the mitochondrial oxodehydrogenase enzymes are targeted by these antibodies (59). Even though antigens also are expressed by mitochondria from cells in nonhepatic organs, some investigators believe that antibodies to mitochondrial antigens are responsible

for the bile duct injury in PBC. Factors in favor of this association include:

- The highly directed response of the autoantibody
- The absence of such antibodies in other obstructive biliary tract disorders
- The characteristic constellation of T cells and immune complexes seen around the involved bile duct
- The similarity of the lesion of PBC with graft-versus-host disease

This topic has been reviewed (60,61). Other possibly important factors include the aberrant expression of class II major histocompatibility complex and the activation of the complement system (62).

### Diagnostic Workup When Primary Biliary Cirrhosis Is Suspected

The diagnosis of PBC is usually straightforward. A middle-aged woman with elevated cholestatic liver enzymes who is taking no medication, has no pain, and has no previous biliary tract surgery and no signs or symptoms of inflammatory bowel disease needs little diagnostic testing. An

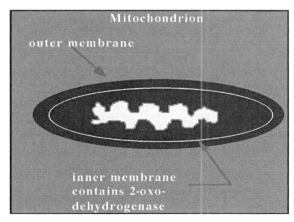

**Figure 55.6** Antimitochondrial antibody in primary biliary cirrhosis is directed against mitochondrial inner membrane.

antimitochondrial antibody in high titer all but establishes the diagnosis in such patients. Most often, an ultrasound examination (or other noninvasive imaging procedure such as a CT scan) of the liver and biliary tract is done, although in an otherwise straightforward case, the value of these tests is minimal.

A liver biopsy is valuable both in confirming the diagnosis and in establishing the stage of disease. The liver biopsy in PBC is highly characteristic. It should not be surprising that the features vary, depending on the stage of disease at which the biopsy was obtained. The most commonly used pathology staging scale used in the United States over the past 15 years was developed by Ludwig and colleagues (63). When considering only biopsy features, a number of conditions may be confused with PBC, but in clinical practice, confusion should not be frequent. Only the PBC–chronic active hepatitis overlap syndrome is likely to create difficulty for the experienced histopathologist. PSC may bear a superficial resemblance to PBC clinically, biochemically, and histologically, but most often the pathology is sufficiently distinguished that confusion is reduced rather than increased by reviewing the histologic features.

If any reason to suspect PSC is present, cholangiography must be done. When in doubt, the biliary anatomy should be defined, however. Cholangiography usually is necessary when any element of pain or previous or current biliary stone disease is present, and if any signs or symptoms of inflammatory bowel disease are evident. Men with apparent PBC, and most patients in whom the antimitochondrial antibody is negative, require cholangiography to exclude PSC.

The extrahepatic manifestations of PBC require attention and occasionally may overshadow the hepatic disease. Some features can be traced to the malabsorption of fat-soluble vitamins, although most patients with PBC have normal serum levels of vitamin A, 25-hydroxy vitamin D, 1,25-dihydroxy vitamin D, prothrombin, and vitamin E levels (64).

Premature osteoporosis and, occasionally in late-stage disease, osteomalacia may be seen. Bone pain, compression spine fractures, and other pathologic bone fractures may be the consequence of PBC-related osteoporosis and occur in up to 20% of affected persons. Malabsorption of vitamin D is one cause, although, as mentioned, only a minority of patients have documented low levels of 25-OH vitamin D. Hepatic biotransformation to 1,25-dihydroxy vitamin D appears to be intact in PBC patients (65). Despite (usually) normal absorption and biotransformation, bone biopsies in PBC show decreased osteoblastic and increased osteoclastic activity (66). Most discouraging is the observation of continued rapid bone loss in PBC patients given adequate replacement with calcium and vitamin D (67).

### Treatment

The treatment for PBC may be divided into *supportive* and *specific* regimens. Surprisingly, few controlled clinical trials

---

**TABLE 55.16**

**SUPPORTIVE THERAPY IN PRIMARY BILIARY CIRRHOSIS**

Bone disease prevention
  Calcium
  Vitamin D
  Hormone replacement therapy in postmenopausal women
  ? Bisphosphonates
Pruritus
  Level 1: Skin lubrication
  Level 2: Antihistamines (e.g., Benadryl)
    Cholestyramine
  Level 3: Rifampin
    Opioid antagonists (nalmefene, naloxone)?
Night blindness
  Vitamin A
Diarrhea (malabsorption)
  Level 1: Low-fat diet
    Vitamin supplements (A, D, E, K)
  Level 2: Medium-chain triglyceride oil

---

have been done to establish the use of most supportive therapy (Table 55.16). It is possible to overburden with polypharmacy a patient with a disease that is causing no difficulty. Treatment should be tailored to the patient; most require little supportive therapy. Short-term studies support the regular use of calcium and vitamin D as a means of improving vertebral bone density (68,69). One retrospective study suggests that hormone replacement therapy in postmenopausal women with PBC had resulted in lower rates of osteoporosis than in women who did not receive hormone replacement therapy (70). Drugs that have an antiresorptive effect (e.g., calcitonin) appear not to be of value in preventing bone disease; newer drugs with a similar mode of action, such as bisphosphonates, require further study in this regard. A small 2-year study comparing the cyclic use of a bisphosphonate (400 mg etidronate orally for 2 weeks followed by a 13-week "rest") and sodium fluoride (50 mg/day) in women with PBC indicated the possible benefit of bisphosphonate administration. Etidronate-treated women had essentially no change in bone densitometry in the lumbar spine, compared with a modest loss in density seen in those who received fluoride. New spontaneous bone fractures were seen only in the fluoride-treated group. These promising results must be confirmed and expanded (71).

Pruritus is frequent in PBC and may be severe and debilitating. The cause is incompletely understood. Early studies incriminated an accumulation of bile acids in the skin; further research has cast considerable doubt on skin bile acids as an important cause of pruritus. Many treatments are available; none is ideal. Endogenous opiate agonists (e.g., enkephalins) accumulate in cholestatic syndromes, and some investigators have wondered whether pruritus is caused by increased opiate agonist availability at opiate receptor sites in the brain (72). In less severe cases, simple measures such as skin lubrication sometimes augmented by the use of antihistamines suffice; this may be particularly valuable at bedtime. More severe cases do not respond to antihistamines, however, and cholestyramine, an anion-exchange resin, is generally effective. Its putative mechanism of action is the binding of bile (which contains the pruritogenic substance). It must be taken at a suitable interval from other medications because binding of medication to the resin will result in decreased absorption.

Rifampin has many complex effects on hepatocytes, the including induction of microsomal enzyme activity and stimulation of hepatic bile acid synthesis. Ghent and Carruthers gave rifampin to eight patients with PBC in a placebo-controlled crossover study. Mean pruritus scores decreased significantly while the patients were on rifampin but not on placebo. They observed no beneficial effect on liver tests (73). In a similar study of 22 patients given 10 mg/kg daily, not only did pruritus improve, but so, too, did mean levels of ALT, AST, alkaline phosphatase, GGTP, bile acids, and aminopyrine (in breath test) (74). The dosage used in this study was somewhat higher than that used by Ghent and Carruthers, which may account for the beneficial effect on liver tests that was not seen in the earlier study. In another short-term (1-week) crossover study, rifampin was effective in relieving pruritus (75). Some of these patients were entered into a longer open-label study lasting 18 months. One patient developed an allergic reaction (rash, eosinophilia, facial edema) and was dropped from the study. Of 18 patients treated, 17 sustained complete relief and one partial relief of itching. Although the mean alkaline phosphatase level decreased from 1,246 to 863, this difference was not statistically significant. Compared with phenobarbitone in a 14-day crossover study of 22 patients, 19 had relief of itching using rifampin compared with eight using phenobarbitone (74). Other studies support an antipruritic effect of this agent. The relevance of these findings to the pruritus in PSC is likely but has not been proved.

No therapy is known to reverse PBC in the native liver. A great deal of interest has been shown in drugs that appear to have some biologic effect against some of the more obvious manifestations of the disease. Colchicine (76), prednisolone (77), ursodiol, cyclosporine (78,79), and tacrolimus (FK506) all have been shown to have some activity. Methotrexate has its champions, but controlled clinical trials have demonstrated a lack of efficacy. Preliminary studies indicate, moreover, that methotrexate, when used in conjunction with ursodiol, appears to provide no advantage (80). Because of its toxicity, the use of this agent for PBC outside of research protocols should be considered with exceptional care. Liver transplantation is available as salvage for patients with advanced stages of PBC. Ursodiol and liver transplantation are the most widely embraced therapies at this time.

Ursodiol has a number of properties that may lead to a beneficial effect in PBC. It affords a cell membrane–stabilizing effect and also may have mild immunomodulating properties. A reduced expression of major histocompatability complex class I molecules is seen on hepatocyte membranes in the presence of ursodiol (81). The first report of the beneficial effect of ursodiol in PBC indicated that this agent improved liver tests and symptoms (82). Ursodiol has been given to hundreds of patients with PBC in randomized placebo-controlled trials (83–87).

The most consistent findings of studies of ursodiol in PBC are those that show an effect on the serum levels used as markers for disease presence (but not severity). Ursodiol regularly reduces the levels of alkaline phosphatase, ALT, and GGTP. It also has an effect on serum bilirubin level and serum albumin, which more closely reflect disease stage. Some, although not all, studies demonstrated a beneficial effect on liver histology. These beneficial effects are easiest to demonstrate in stage 1 and stage 2 disease.

Insufficient numbers of patients have had follow-up of sufficient duration to allow definitive conclusions to be drawn about the most vital question: Does ursodiol prolong life? It requires a minimum of 10 years of study to derive a scientifically sound answer to this core question. In the meantime, the results of shorter studies (2 to 4 years) are available to provide a tentative answer. Some data suggest that ursodiol arrests the clinical course of PBC. Treatment failure is seen less often in ursodiol-treated patients than in controls, although the definitions of treatment failure often seem arbitrary and not clinically useful. It has been more difficult to demonstrate that ursodiol prolongs life or reduces the need for liver transplantation. When the results from three multicenter trials using comparable doses of ursodiol (13 to 15 mg/kg daily) are combined (553 evaluable patients), a benefit of ursodiol on survival of 31% was apparent after up to 4 years of therapy, which also may decrease the manifestations of portal hypertension. Patients who received active treatment also had marked improvement in serum markers of disease. No improvement was seen in metabolic bone disease or fatigue, and a variable effect on pruritus was observed (88). The beneficial effects were observed even in stage 3 and 4 disease.

Until long-term data are available, interval recommendations are reasonable. For patients with precirrhotic PBC, ursodiol therapy (13 to 15 mg/kg daily) is offered. Some would extend that recommendation even to those with well-compensated cirrhosis. Therapy is lifelong. Side effects rarely limit the use of ursodiol. A few develop diarrhea, and occasionally a patient has worsening of pruritus.

Of course, the PBC patient with advanced cirrhosis may develop features of decompensation (ascites, gastrointestinal bleeding, portosystemic encephalopathy). These are handled in the same manner as with other causes of cirrhosis, which are discussed later. Liver transplantation for advanced PBC is highly successful. Although controlled clinical trials comparing liver transplantation and medical therapy have not been performed, survival comparisons of transplantation with the "natural history" have been estimated using the Cox regression model. An apparent advantage of liver transplantation is apparent as early as 6 months after surgery, and this survival benefit is maintained for at least 5 years (89). The outcome of liver transplantation is better than for many other diseases. The disease affecting the native liver has been shown to recur in many diseases for which liver transplantation is performed. Indeed, some evidence has shown that PBC may recur in approximately 10% of transplant recipients. This area is controversial because the histology of rejection shares some features of PBC. In our transplant program, 30 patients received a graft because of PBC; many have had a recurrence of antimitochondrial antibody, but only one has had a clinical course and serial liver histology consistent with recurrent PBC. In the remainder, recognizable PBC has not emerged. Whether this freedom from recurrence reflects the effects of immunosuppression or other factors is unknown.

The timing of referral for transplantation is always difficult because of the complex interplay of disease progression and the long interval between the approval for transplantation and the operation, which frequently exceeds 1 year. Child's B patients with PBC are significantly more likely to die than Child's A, and Child's C patients are more likely to die than either A or B patients. Once a patient with PBC falls into the Child's B range, liver transplantation should be given serious consideration.

## Primary Sclerosing Cholangitis

PSC is a chronic hepatobiliary disease of unknown cause that is characterized by diffuse or multifocal fibrosing inflammatory changes in the bile ducts. It is seen most often in association with inflammatory bowel disease. Some have suggested a common pathogenesis (90,91). Patients with PSC have circulating immune complexes (92,93). An increase in the T-cell helper-to-suppressor ratio has been shown (94). The increased autoreactivity of T lymphocytes after activation in the autologous mixed lymphocyte reaction also occurs (95). All these observations suggest the role of a disordered immune system in the pathogenesis of PSC.

PSC is characterized by disease progression and excessive mortality. Although some investigators suggested that PSC is a relatively indolent disorder (96), most experiences with this disorder are considerably less benign (97). It is apparent that, regardless of liver stage or clinical status, the disease is progressive (98). Our experience indicates a 9-year survival of 49%. In one therapeutic trial, 80% of patients showed evidence of disease progression (as assessed by the development of ascites, esophageal varices, increase in bilirubin, progression of histologic stage, referral for liver transplantation, or death within a 3-year study period) (99).

Diagnosis requires cholangiography, although a strong inferential case can be made clinically, especially in those patients with inflammatory bowel disease and a markedly elevated alkaline phosphatase level. The cholangiogram reveals a ratty, irregular biliary tree produced by the fibrosing process. Between the narrowed segments, the biliary tree may be either normal in caliber or even dilated. The process most often is diffuse, but sometimes it is limited to the intrahepatic or extrahepatic biliary tree. The most important differential diagnosis in the cholangiogram is between PSC and cholangiocarcinoma. The more limited the extent of the biliary abnormality, the more concern exists that cancer is present. So many variations and permutations are possible that certain differentiation is often not possible. Cholangiocarcinoma, although usually focal, may be diffuse. Moreover, cholangiocarcinoma may complicate sclerosing cholangitis, usually in patients older than 60 years. Men are more commonly afflicted. Patients present most often with signs or symptoms or laboratory abnormalities suggesting complete or partial biliary tract obstruction.

There is no proven therapy for PSC. Hope that ursodiol may modulate the liver damage in PSC in a manner analogous to its effect in PBC has not been born out (100). Important differences in biliary bile acid composition in these disorders may, in part, explain ursodiol's lack of effect in PSC. Virtually no lithocholate was seen in the serum of patients with PSC before or after treatment with ursodiol, and no change in the urinary lithocholate levels was seen after treatment (101).

Liver transplantation for PSC with or without inflammatory bowel disease may be lifesaving. The PSC patient with cirrhotic complications can anticipate a 1- and 3-year survival rate after liver transplantation of 90% and 89%, respectively (102). Timing is crucial, particularly in light of the long waiting period required for a donor organ. As in PBC, once a PSC patient is classified as Child's B, it is time to consider referral to a transplant center.

## INHERITED LIVER DISEASES

The three liver diseases to be considered here are Wilson's disease, hemochromatosis, and $\alpha_1$-antitrypsin (A1AT) deficiency. In particular, persons with the first two disorders must be identified because of the potential for life-saving treatment. Genetic counseling and the screening of family members is also important. Wilson's disease may present with either brain or liver disease or occasionally both. It is a disease of abnormal copper metabolism, inherited as autosomal recessive, and it should be suspected in any young person with chronic or severe acute liver disease. It is rare for Wilson's disease to manifest for the first time after the age of 40 years. The serum ceruloplasmin is depressed in 95% of persons, which is helpful because ceruloplasmin is an acutephase reactant and therefore is elevated in most forms of liver disease. A low-normal or clearly low ceruloplasmin level in the setting of liver disease should be considered Wilson's disease until proven otherwise. Other causes for a low level include the healthy heterozygote state and fulminant or end-stage liver disease. Kayser-Fleischer rings (brown pigmented rings around the edge of the cornea) should be present if neurologic signs and symptoms are observed, but these may be absent if only the liver is involved. A slit-lamp examination is required to see all but the most florid Kayser-Fleischer rings. In questionable cases, a liver biopsy with quantitative copper determination usually clarifies the diagnosis. Hepatic copper values greater than 250 μg/g are virtually diagnostic of untreated Wilson's disease. Lesser degrees of hepatic copper elevation may be seen in chronic hepatitis and in chronic cholestatic liver diseases (such as PBC) (103). Copper-chelating drugs are used to treat Wilson's disease. The drug of first choice is D-penicillamine, but trientine may be used if D-penicillamine is poorly tolerated. Oral zinc therapy competes with copper absorption and may be used for maintenance therapy in the decoppered patients (104,105).

*Hereditary hemochromatosis* (genetic hemochromatosis, idiopathic hemochromatosis), a heterogeneous group of disorders, is characterized by excessive iron deposition in many organs, including, importantly, the liver. Other targets for excess iron include the pancreas (diabetes may result), heart (conduction disturbances, heart failure), joints (arthritis), gonads (impotence), and skin (darkening). The constellation of bronze skin, diabetes, heart disease, and liver disease describes the fully developed case. To prevent end-organ damage, this disease should be suspected in any patient with chronic liver disease, especially those who manifest injury in one or more other organ systems. Iron may accumulate due to genetic predisposition or to chronic iron overload, such as occurs in the multiply transfused patient and chronic anemias (e.g., thalassemia), and it is associated with certain conditions such as PCT.

Hereditary hemochromatosis, a relatively common disorder inherited as an autosomal recessive trait carried on the short arm of chromosome 6 in close association to the HLA-A3 locus, results in a failure of feedback inhibition of intestinal iron absorption. The most common form is inherited as an autosomal recessive trait. The homozygous presence of either of two different genes may result in iron accumulation. It has been estimated that as many as 1 in 250 white persons carries both genes necessary for expression of the disease, an estimate that appears to overstate the frequency with which it is recognized clinically. The precise genetic defect for many cases of hereditary hemochromatosis has been identified, and a clinically important laboratory diagnostic test (hemochromatosis DNA polymerase chain reaction) has revolutionized our approach to identifying those affected. The so-called *HFE* gene is located on chromosome 6, near the locus for the *HLA-A* gene. Two mutations have been described (106). Most (69% to 100%) cases of clinically typical hereditary hemochromatosis have a missense mutation (C282Y) that causes cysteine to be substituted for tyrosine at the 282 amino acid protein product of the gene. Another mutation

### TABLE 55.17

## HEMOCHROMATOSIS DNA-BASED DIAGNOSTIC TESTING

| Test Finding | Result | Iron Overload |
| --- | --- | --- |
| C282Y | Homozygote | High association |
| H63D | Homozygote | Mild association |
| C282Y/H63D | Compound heterozygote | Moderate association |
| C282Y | Heterozygote | No association |
| H63D | Heterozygote | No association |

on the *HFE* gene at the H63D locus, which results in the substitution of aspartic acid for histidine at position 63, may be present in those with hereditary hemochromatosis. The presence of homozygous H63D may result in iron overload, but the clinical expression (rate and frequency) appears less than when homozygote C282Y defect is present. Finally, a compound heterozygote (one gene containing C282Y and the other H63D) also may result in iron overload. Table 55.17 provides a guide to the interpretation of hemochromatosis genetic testing.

A laboratory diagnosis of hemochromatosis is important (107). The diagnosis should be suspected in the following situations:

- Any adult with liver disease, especially men
- Transferrin saturation of 55% or higher
- Ferritin elevations (≤200 μg/L in premenopausal women; ≤300 μg/L in men and postmenopausal women)

Confirmation of the diagnosis requires a demonstration of increased hepatic iron by liver biopsy. The value of the biopsy is twofold: It provides information about the degree of fibrosis and cirrhosis present, which is vital in predicting the risk of subsequent development of hepatoma, and it provides an assessment of iron stores. The quantitative assessment of hepatic iron is considered superior to semi-quantitative staining of liver specimens (108). The hepatic iron index is calculated as follows:

$$\text{Hepatic iron index} = \text{hepatic iron concentration (μmol/g dry weight)} \mid \text{patient's age in years}$$

A hepatic iron index level below 2.0 is normal; values greater than 2.0 are seen in hemochromatosis. Interest has been rekindled in assessing hepatic iron through the evaluation of iron stains of liver biopsy material, and this is a satisfactory alternative to quantitative iron determination (109). Bone marrow iron stores are not adequate to assess total body iron stores; indeed, cases of hemochromatosis with absent stainable bone marrow iron have been reported. The treatment of idiopathic hemochromatosis requires phlebotomy on a weekly basis until iron deficiency is depleted, with maintenance phlebotomies every 1 to 3 months thereafter (110).

The physician who makes the diagnosis of hemochromatosis in a patient has a responsibility to inform the patient that the disease is inherited and to urge that patient to ensure that all siblings and offspring are informed and screened. Those older than 25 years should be screened because the likelihood of demonstrating excess iron in children and young adults, even in the presence of homozygosity, is low. Of course, genetic testing for C282Y and H63D can be done at any age.

In the event that cirrhosis is present, the patient with hemochromatosis must be in a regular surveillance program for hepatoma. Annual α-fetoprotein determinations and ultrasound examinations are suggested. Some would argue that twice yearly testing should be done, and others would doubt the value of any screening.

## α₁-Antitrypsin Deficiency

Often, α₁-antitrypsin (A1AT) deficiency presents in childhood with prominent pulmonary disease or, less often, with pediatric liver disease. Some cases do not manifest until adulthood. Unexplained liver dysfunction or complications of cirrhosis may be due to A1AT deficiency. Liver test abnormalities are nonspecific. Occasionally, decompensated cirrhosis is the presentation. Many different genetic forms exist, and the protease inhibitor test most often is used to differentiate these. The normal protease inhibitor type is MM. Those with a double Z allele (protease inhibitor ZZ) are most likely to suffer from the disease. Controversy surrounds the association of a single Z allele (e.g., protease inhibitor MZ) and liver disease. Current published evidence and a review of the Cleveland Clinic material suggest that the isolated presence of a single Z allele poses an increased risk for cirrhosis and liver failure (111). No definitive treatment is available for this disease; liver transplantation should be considered if the stigmata of end-stage cirrhosis develop.

## CIRRHOSIS

The outcome for cirrhotic patients depends on the degree of functional impairment in the liver and the amount of decompensation present. Originally developed to predict survival after portacaval shunt surgery, the Child-Pugh classification (Table 55.18) has been useful in predicting survival in the untreated cirrhotic patient. Only five features (all easily measurable) are needed.

Cirrhosis may produce no symptoms or signs. When cirrhosis becomes decompensated, it manifests as one or more of the following:

- Ascites and edema
- Gastrointestinal bleeding
- Encephalopathy

**TABLE 55.18**

**PUGH-MODIFIED CHILD-TURCOTTE CLASSIFICATIONS**

|  | A (1 Point) | B (2 Points) | C (3 Points) |
|---|---|---|---|
| Bilirubin | <2 mg/dL | 2–3 mg/dL | >3 mg/dL |
| Albumin | >3.5 g/dL | 2.8–3.5 g/dL | <2.8 g/dL |
| Ascites | None | Easily controlled | Poorly controlled |
| Neurologic | No PSE | Mild PSE | Refractory PSE |
| International normalized ratio | <1.7 | 1.7–2.3 | >2.3 |

PSE, portosystemic encephalopathy.
*Note:* For each of five items, a score of 1, 2, or 3 is assigned. The total score is the sum of these items. Child's A = 57; B = 810; C = 11 or more.

Ascites occurs because the kidney behaves as if it were receiving an inadequate blood flow. Low urine volume and urine sodium concentration (often 10 mEq/L) and an activated renin-angiotensin-aldosterone (RAA) system are typical, resulting in sodium and water retention. When the imbalance between sodium intake and excretion goes on long enough, expansion of the intravascular and then extravascular space occurs, which eventually causes edema and or ascites. Atrial natriuretic factor (ANF) often is elevated in patients with cirrhotic ascites. Such elevations probably serve to protect against further volume expansion in early cirrhosis (112). A complete understanding of sodium retention in cirrhosis has been elusive, but the pathophysiology has been investigated extensively.

## Sodium Retention

The vascular, hemodynamic, and humoral characteristics in the cirrhotic patient are dynamic, with fairly subtle early changes and more explicit and numerous abnormalities in decompensated cirrhosis. In a study of 12 cirrhotic patients with diuretic-resistant tense ascites, all had normal or nearly normal serum creatinine (0.85 mg/dL ± 0.2). At the same time, they were mildly hyponatremic (135 mEq/L ± 4). Yet all had avid sodium retention (urine [Na$^+$] 5 mEq/L), and urine volume was only 445 mL/24 hours (113). It is clear that urinary sodium excretion is impaired. Yet this study, like most others, takes a "snapshot" late in the course of a long disease process. If we wish to know more about the evolution of the renal defect in cirrhosis, we need to look at the patient, or an experimental animal, much earlier. A direct correlation exists between renal sodium retention and liver function, as measured by the clearance of antipyrine, caffeine, and chocolate, but no relationship is apparent between sodium retention and degree of portosystemic shunting (114).

Levy has done some of the most elegant experiments in a dog model of cirrhosis and ascites (115). Using dimethylnitrosamine to create cirrhosis, he studied the blood volume, renal, humoral, and autonomic nervous system changes over time. Before dimethylnitrosamine, not surprisingly, urinary sodium excretion matched sodium intake (i.e., homeostasis was demonstrated). As cirrhosis developed and portal pressure began to rise, but well before ascites formed, progressive impairment of renal sodium excretion resulted in a positive sodium balance and increased intravascular volume. In humans with alcoholic cirrhosis, plasma volume was expanded whether or not ascites was present. A positive correlation was found between plasma volume and wedged hepatic venous pressure (a reflection of portal pressure) (116). Splanchnic plasma volume did not contract during the formation of ascites, nor did it expand when ascites was mobilized (117). Thus, in both humans and experimental animals with cirrhosis, plasma volume is expanded. The signal initiating inappropriate sodium retention remains elusive, but most investigators believe that arterial underfilling from cirrhosis activates a yet unidentified intrahepatic low-pressure baroreceptor and signals the kidney to conserve sodium.

## Renin-Angiotensin-Aldosterone

In healthy humans, the volume, distribution, and composition of extracellular fluid vary within a narrow range. Among the neurohumoral regulators of renal sodium handling, the RAA system plays an important role. In cirrhosis, the equilibrium of this feedback loop is frequently severely disturbed. In cirrhotic preascitic rats, early abnormalities can be detected. For example, urinary aldosterone levels rise before ascites forms, and these levels are temporally related to sodium retention (118). In other animal experiments, however, sodium retention predated the activation of the RAA system. In humans with cirrhosis, a good correlation exists between plasma aldosterone levels and urinary sodium excretion, except that the system appears "downregulated" in cirrhotics with ascites. For any given level of aldosterone, cirrhotic patients with ascites excrete less sodium than either cirrhotic patients without ascites or healthy subjects (119). The inhibition of the RAA system by drugs has had a mixed result in increasing natriuresis in cirrhotic ascites. This area of study has not been easy, because drugs that affect the RAA system often have independent effects on the vascular system and renal glomerular blood flow. The greatest support for an important role for the RAA system is the effectiveness of the aldosterone-blocking agent, spironolactone, in cirrhotic ascites. In such a setting, this agent is superior to furosemide in producing natriuresis (120). Nevertheless, other drugs that interfere with the RAA system (e.g., captopril, saralasin, β-blockers) do not seem to be effective agents in cirrhosis, although captopril added to diuretic therapy may be effective in some patients with refractory ascites (121). In summary,

the RAA system plays an important but not an exclusive role in the perpetuation of renal sodium retention once it is activated, probably through other factors. The central role in aldosterone antagonism using spironolactone in the treatment of ascites is well accepted.

## Other Perturbations

Sympathetic nervous system abnormalities are the rule in cirrhotic patients and appear to play a role in the renal response to this condition. The circulating levels of norepinephrine, the principal neurotransmitter of the adrenergic nervous system, are taken as a measure of sympathetic discharge. Levels are higher in patients with more advanced cirrhosis and higher still in the hepatorenal syndrome (122). Adrenergic blockade with agents such as clonidine does result in reduced norepinephrine levels; however, as noted, its effect in reducing perfusing pressure overshadows any beneficial effect of norepinephrine, and enhanced sodium excretion does not occur. It is possible that the observed increases in sympathetic activity seen in cirrhosis represent a defense against other changes, rather than important pathophysiologic events. ANF, a cardiac hormone with powerful vasodilator and natriuretic properties, is often elevated in patients with cirrhotic ascites. Such elevations probably serve to protect against further volume expansion in early cirrhosis (112). This suggests that either ANF is elevated as a normal response to sodium retention or that a blunted renal response to ANF is present in cirrhosis. Like the sympathetic nervous system, the exact importance of ANF in the pathogenesis of ascites remains obscure (123).

## Clinical Features

### Ascitic Fluid Analysis

Cirrhotic ascites is similar to serum, except it contains less protein. The serum albumin–ascitic fluid albumin gradient is usually more than 1:1. This ratio is calculated by subtracting the albumin concentration of ascites from that of serum (albumin ser minus albumin asc). Cardiac ascites will have a similarly high gradient. Low gradients (<1.1) suggest a noncirrhotic (and a noncardiac) cause for ascites, such as malignancy or infection. This test is considered a routine part of the evaluation of ascitic fluid and has largely replaced the exudate–transudate distinction that was based on a consideration of total protein concentration in the ascitic fluid (124). Although ascites is usually not a threat, it becomes so when infection occurs. Spontaneous bacterial peritonitis (SBP) usually is the result of aerobic gut-derived bacteria or *Streptococcus pneumoniae* (Table 55.19). It usually is not polymicrobial, and anerobes are distinctly unusual. In SBP, the ascitic fluid cell count almost always reveals a polymorphonuclear count of greater than $250/mm^3$. Interestingly, infected ascites usually maintains an albumen gradient of greater than one. Cultures are most likely to be

## TABLE 55.19

### TYPICAL ORGANISMS THAT CAUSE SPONTANEOUS BACTERIAL PERITONITIS

| Gram-Negative | Percent | Gram-Positive | Percent |
|---|---|---|---|
| *Escherichia coli* | 37.0 | Pneumococcus | 12.0 |
| *Klebsiella pneumoniae* | 17.0 | *Streptococcus viridans* | 8.5 |
| *Enterobacter* | 6.4 | γ-Hemolytic streptococcus | 4.3 |
| Other | 5.0 | Enterococcus | 3.2 |
| Other group D streptococci | 1.1 | Other | 5.0 |

positive if 10 mL of fluid is poured into a blood culture bottle at the patient's bedside.

The treatment of infected ascites requires systemic antibiotics. Because the kidney of a cirrhotic patient is particularly susceptible to toxicity from aminoglycosides, the use of these agents plus ampicillin has generally given way to the use of a third-generation cephalosporin such as cefotaxime. Five days of treatment are adequate in most cases (125). Costs are an increasingly important part of medical decision making. The dosage of cefotaxime needed to control infection is lower in cirrhotic patients, in part because of decreased hepatic metabolism. Two grams every 12 hours, instead of every 6 hours, results in satisfactory peak and trough levels and controls infection (126). Important endpoints of the treatment of SBP with cefotaxime are infection resolution and mortality. The pretreatment predictors of treatment failure are (127):

- Higher levels of band neutrophils in peripheral blood
- Hospital acquisition of SBP
- Higher blood urea nitrogen
- Higher ALT

Pretreatment predictors of in-hospital mortality are:

- High blood urea nitrogen
- High ALT
- Hospital acquisition of SBP
- Older age
- Child-Pugh score
- Ileus

The prevention of SBP is possible. Both primary prevention (for those with no history of SBP) and secondary prevention studies are available. Quinolone antibiotics are effective, although they are poorly absorbed from the gastrointestinal tract (128–130). They are effective in reducing bacterial counts in the gut and the urinary tract, two reservoirs for organisms commonly seen in SBP. For the typical cirrhotic patient with ascites, norfloxacin, 400 mg twice daily, is a simple and effective regimen. The reports of a rapid emergence of resistant organisms have not translated

(yet) into a reduced effectiveness in using this strategy to reduce episodes of SBP in cirrhotic patients with ascites (131). Other agents also appear to be effective in SBP prophylaxis. Sulfamethoxazole-trimethoprim (800 mg/160 mg) (one double-strength tablet Monday through Friday) reduced by 87% the number of episodes of SBP over a median 90-day follow-up period (132). The 12-month cost of this regimen in the Veteran's Administration Hospital system is $31 per year, compared with $590 per year for norfloxacin.

When should antibiotic prophylaxis be given to cirrhotic patients with ascites? Based on available evidence for those particularly at risk, it seems prudent to consider prophylaxis for those with one or more of the following risk factors:

- Previous history of SBP
- Ascitic fluid protein concentration below 1 g/dL
- Serum bilirubin greater than 3 mg/dL
- Renal dysfunction with elevated serum creatinine
- Hospitalized cirrhotic patients likely to undergo invasive procedures

### Treatment of Cirrhotic Ascites

Bed rest is unquestionably helpful in controlling ascites, but seldom is this treatment practical, except in the sickest patients. The effect of posture on renal sodium handling has been elucidated: In an upright posture, the renin-angiotensin system is activated, sympathetic tone increased, and glomerular filtration decreased (133). The mainstay of treatment for ascites is dietary sodium restriction. A 2-g sodium diet is often prescribed. When this is insufficient, diuretics are used. Spironolactone is the agent of first choice. An initial dose of 50 mg twice daily is often selected. Dose escalation up to 400 mg daily is possible. In men, painful gynecomastia frequently prevents such a high dose. Proximal tubule or loop diuretics then are added, most frequently a thiazide or furosemide. Diuretics have frequent side effects that regularly cause intravascular volume depletion, electrolyte abnormalities, and a reduction in renal function. These problems are particularly likely to occur if more than 500 to 1,000 mL/24 hours of excess fluid is mobilized.

Paracentesis represents an increasingly popular method of controlling large amounts of ascites and is perhaps the most physiologic treatment, given the central role of volume expansion in cirrhotic ascites. The removal of large volumes (even total paracentesis) appears safer than diuretic therapy (134). The patient so treated is simultaneously begun on a salt-restricted diet and diuretics to minimize the reaccumulation of ascites and to reduce the need for repeated paracentesis. Many hepatology units provide intravenous albumin infusions (e.g., 6 g/L of ascites removed), but the value of this expensive replacement therapy has not been established unequivocally. Whereas transient changes are seen in cardiac output, pulmonary wedge pressure, and central venous pressure, along with activation of the renin-angiotensin system when ascites is removed without providing intravenous colloid, the clinical relevance of these observations remains speculative (135). One drawback of repeated large-volume removal is protein depletion. Although not much of a clinical problem, the reduction in ascitic fluid opsonic activity raises the theoretic problem of susceptibility to infection; this was not borne out, however, in a carefully controlled clinical trial designed to compare the relative risks of large-volume paracentesis compared with diuretic therapy for cirrhotic ascites (136).

Peritoneovenous shunting for refractory ascites has been used for 20 years, with mixed results. There seems to be variable success in keeping these shunts patent over an extended period. When they remain patent, rapid natriuresis is observed. Infection, disseminated intravascular coagulation, and clotting are problems described with these shunts. Approximately 50% are occluded within 24 months of placement (137). Consistent with high early patency rates followed by failures, when peritoneovenous shunting was compared with large-volume paracentesis, early and total rehospitalizations were fewer in the shunted group; total time in the hospital during follow-up, total complication rates, and survival rates were similar in both groups.

Early studies using percutaneous transjugular intrahepatic portosystemic shunts (TIPS) suggested that they represent an effective way to manage refractory ascites (138). A reduction in ascites and a reduced need for diuretics or paracentesis have been demonstrated, as have an increase in fractional sodium excretion and decreased plasma renin, aldosterone, and norepinephrine (139). It appears that the size of the shunt created is more critical for ascites control than for bleeding control. Portosystemic encephalopathy may occur, usually within the first 3 months. Clinical manifestations often recede, even when the TIPS remain patent and the arterial ammonia levels remain elevated, suggesting a role of cerebral adaptation (140).

After a few months, TIPS tend to occlude in many patients and require repeated balloon angioplasty to restore patency and function. We consider TIPS for refractory ascites as a bridge to liver transplantation. Hospitalized Child's C cirrhotic patients whose refractory ascites is treated using TIPS do not survive hospitalization unless they undergo transplantation. Longer-term studies are needed before deciding that this is a satisfactory long-term treatment.

The 1- and 3-year survival rates after the first development of ascites are 50% and 20%, respectively (141). These rates compare unfavorably with survival after transplantation. Accordingly, the emergence of conspicuous ascites should at least prompt an inquiry into whether or not liver transplantation should be undertaken in that patient.

*Hepatic hydrothorax* is the accumulation of pleural effusions, most often right sided, in the setting of cirrhotic

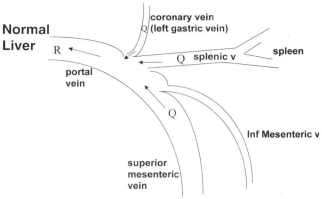

**Pressure is directly proportional to Resistance X Flow**
**Pressure drop across liver (portal vein - hepatic vein) < 5 mm Hg**

**Figure 55.7** Pressure in the normal liver. Q, volume of blood flow; R, resistance.

ascites. Often, ascites becomes less of a problem as fluid accumulates within the pleural space. Defects within the diaphragm are most often the culprit. Symptomatic hepatic hydrothorax represents a difficult management problem that often occurs toward the latest stages of cirrhosis. Treatment through salt restriction and diuretics or large-volume paracentesis is seldom successful. Repeated thoracentesis is usually poorly tolerated because of the required frequency. Both pleurodesis and TIPS have been used, with variable results (142). Most patients with this complication die of end-stage liver failure within a few months unless they undergo transplantation.

## Portal Hypertensive Bleeding

Gastrointestinal bleeding occurs frequently in patients with portal hypertension. A detailed practice guideline has been published (143). The pathogenesis of cirrhotic hypertension is complex. Figure 55.7 indicates the major vessels of interest in portal hypertension, and Figure 55.8 shows the major pertubations. In humans, portal pressure is measured somewhat indirectly because the portal vein is not

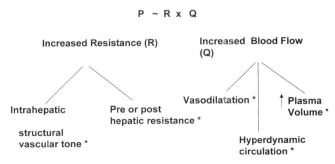

**Figure 55.8** Factors contributing to increased portal pressure. *, potentially reversible.

readily accessible for cannulation. The wedge pressure in the hepatic vein is measured, and from this measurement is subtracted the free hepatic vein pressure (or the inferior vena cava pressure); the result is termed the *portal-hepatic vein gradient*. The normal pressure is less than 5 mm Hg. Bleeding from portal hypertension is not seen until the portal-hepatic vein gradient is greater than 12 mm Hg.

### Primary Prevention

Most often, brisk or massive portal hypertensive bleeding is due to ruptured esophageal or gastric varices. More recently, a diffuse mucosal abnormality termed *portal hypertensive gastropathy* was described as a frequent cause of hemorrhage. The mortality for first variceal bleeds is approximately 20% for Child's A and 60% or higher for Child's C patients. Because of the often disastrous outcome from variceal hemorrhage, therapy administered to the cirrhotic patient with large varices that have never bled has been studied extensively. Currently, two classes of agents appear effective in preventing the first hemorrhage: non-cardioselective β-blockers, especially propranolol, nadolol, and timolol; and long-acting nitrates. β-Blockers have been extensively studied and are reasonably well tolerated and moderately effective in reducing episodes of first hemorrhage (144). Isosorbide mononitrate appears to be as effective in preventing first variceal hemorrhage. One report, however, found a higher incidence of (nonbleeding) deaths in patients older than 50 years receiving isosorbide mononitrate, compared with those who received propranolol (145). The significance of this possible heightened death rate is uncertain. Endoscopic band ligation is an effective alternative to β-blocker therapy for primary prevention (146,147).

### Management of Acute Hemorrhage

A patient with acutely bleeding varices represents a medical emergency and should be admitted to the hospital and monitored closely. At the same time that fluid resuscitation is being carried out, a control of bleeding is attempted by simultaneously initiating pharmacotherapy (Table 55.20) and organizing an upper intestinal endoscopy for a direct endoscopic attack on the bleeding source. Octreotide is easier to use than vasopressin and is virtually devoid of significant hemodynamic side effects. It is more effective than vasopressin and is the pharmacologic agent of first choice (148). When vasopressin is used, the dosage is limited by the occurrence of significant ischemia of other organs, such as the heart, gut, or kidneys. Bradyarrhythmias may occur. The concomitant use of nitroglycerin (usually as a patch or sublingually) has allowed higher doses of vasopressin. Approximately 60% to 75% of bleeding variceal episodes can be controlled by using these agents.

The use of balloons attached to tubes (Sengstaken Blakemore, Minnesota, or Linton) is also effective. Studies suggest that 85% to 90% of initial control of bleeding varices occurs. A high incidence of early rebleeding once the balloons are deflated or removed occurs, so additional therapy must be planned for most of these patients. Balloon tamponade in our unit is reserved for those in whom pharmacologic therapy (octreotide, vasopressin) has failed to control bleeding.

Endoscopic therapy has been used frequently for the control of the acute bleeding episode. A series of sessions directed at the elimination of esophageal varices is required. Endoscopic sclerotherapy or band ligation is appropriate for the control of bleeding from esophageal varices, but not for bleeding from either gastric varices or

## TABLE 55.20
### PHARMACOLOGIC STRATEGIES TO CONTROL ACUTE VARICEAL HEMORRHAGE

| Option | Agent | Adjunctive Therapy | Concomitant Endoscopic Control |
|---|---|---|---|
| A | Octreotide, 50 μg i.v. bolus then 50 μg/h i.v. | No | Yes |
| B | Vasopressin, 20 IU in 100 mL D5W over 20 min; then 0.1 IU to 0.4 IU/min | No | Yes |
| C | Per option B, except infusion rates up to 0.8 IU/min allowed | NTG infusion 40 μg/min and increase by 40 μg/min every 15 min if systolic blood pressure >100 mm Hg. Maximum infusion 400 μg/min or NTG transdermal patch (10 mg over 24 h) or NTG 0.6 mg SL every 30 min over 6 h. | Yes |

D5W, dextrose 5% in water; NTG, nitroglycerin.

portal hypertensive gastropathy. Studies indicate that elastic banding of esophageal varices may be more efficient than injection techniques; fewer sessions are needed, and less bleeding occurs (149).

Where emergency endoscopic services are readily available, the endoscopic control of variceal bleeding is most often used. Adjunctive pharmacotherapy is administered as soon as major variceal hemorrhage is suspected, in preparation for endoscopic control. Octreotide is often given as an intravenous bolus of 50 μg, followed by an infusion of 50 μg/hour. The infusion is continued for up to 5 days. One study suggested that prolonging treatment with octreotide for 15 days (100 μg subcutaneously three times daily), combined with either β-blocker therapy or endoscopic sclerotherapy, significantly reduces rebleeding rates during the first 42 days after the index bleed (150). Rebleeding rates at 6 weeks were lowest (18%) in those who received 15 days of octreotide plus sclerotherapy and highest (82%) in those who received placebo and sclerotherapy.

In the few studies comparing the effectiveness and complication rates of endoscopic and pharmacologic treatment, the results support either approach. A meta-analysis of such studies suggested equivalent efficacy in controlling bleeding and a lower incidence of side effects using drug therapy compared with endoscopic sclerotherapy (151). Rebleeding rates after the cessation of infusion therapy appear higher, however, than that after sclerotherapy, and the cost may be higher as well. Thus, the debate continues. The importance of this issue to the clinician rests in the observation that both forms of treatment are acceptable, and that lack of availability of endoscopic services need not be considered evidence of less than state-of-the-art care. In most centers, these treatment options are both available, and most experts recommend initiating pharmacotherapy and endoscopic therapy simultaneously.

### Secondary Prevention

After acute bleeding is controlled, attention moves to a long-term strategy to prevent additional bleeds (secondary prevention). The most frequent therapy has been a series of endoscopic sessions to obliterate varices.

The endoscopic treatment of esophageal varices with band ligation appears superior to injection sclerotherapy. Rebleeding rates are lower, varices are obliterated in fewer sessions, and mortality may also be less (152). The optimal strategy to prevent bleeding recurrence appears to be with pharmacotherapy plus repetitive band ligation sessions. Nadolol in addition to ligation reduced recurrent hemorrhage from 47% to 21% over 21 months. In this study, those who received nadolol plus ligation therapy also received sucralfate (153). One report suggests that nadolol combined with isosorbide mononitrate is more effective at reducing rebleeding than endoscopic ligation (154).

If bleeding becomes recalcitrant, consideration is given to salvage therapy. Shunt surgery, either central or distal, is considered if the patient is a good surgical risk (Child-Pugh A

or B+). A radiologically placed TIPS is used in poorer risk patients or as salvage therapy for the acutely bleeding patient not responsive to other therapy. TIPS was first introduced as a temporizing measure, as a bridge to liver transplantation.

This procedure is performed by invasive radiologists. By puncturing the jugular vein and traversing the superior and inferior vena cava, the hepatic vein is cannulated. A needle is passed through the cannula, and the hepatic vein is punctured. A communication is established between the hepatic vein and the (hypertensive) portal vein. With the fistulous tract established, portal pressure falls. To keep the fistula open, a stent is placed across the track. Preliminary data suggest that bleeding may be controlled in as many as 90% of patients, and ascites in 70%. Controlled trials are currently under way. This procedure should be considered in cases in which endoscopic therapy is ineffective. The enthusiasm for this treatment almost surely will be modified as the results of clinical trials become available (155,156). Three prospective studies comparing TIPS with endoscopic sclerotherapy have been reported. In two of these studies, TIPS was more effective in reducing subsequent hemorrhage. In one study only, the mortality for those receiving TIPS was higher. In two of three studies, the incidence of worsened portosystemic encephalopathy was higher in those treated using TIPS (157). Until the literature becomes clearer, most will rely first on endoscopic (or pharmacologic) treatment to prevent recurrent hemorrhage, reserving TIPS for patients who fail to respond to or are unlikely to comply with an endoscopic or pharmacologic program. Figure 55.9 is a useful algorithm for portal hypertensive bleeding. Table 55.21 indicates current first- and second-line treatment for primary prevention, acute hemorrhage, and secondary prevention.

## Hepatic Encephalopathy

*Hepatic encephalopathy* is chronic liver disease caused by those toxins present in the splanchnic circulation (absorbed from the gastrointestinal tract) being shunted around the liver into the systemic circulation, where they gain access to

### TABLE 55.21

**VARICEAL HEMORRHAGE MANAGEMENT**

|  | First Choice | Second Choice |
|---|---|---|
| Primary prevention | β-blocker[a] + IMN | Band ligation |
| Active bleed | Octreotide/SMN + band ligation | Vasopressin, TIPS, or balloon tamponade |
| Secondary prevention | Band ligation + β-blocker + IMN | TIPS or shunt |

IMN, isosorbide mononitrate; SMN, somatostatin; TIPS, transjugular intrahepatic portosystemic shunt.
[a] β-blocker = noncardioselective (e.g., nadolol, propranolol, timolol).

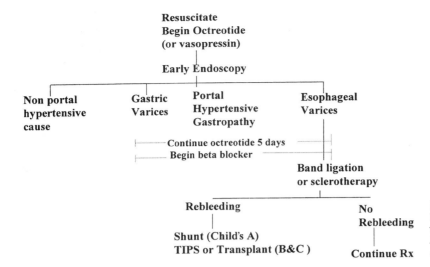

**Figure 55.9** Algorithm for management of bleeding cirrhotics. TIPS, transjugular intrahepatic portosystemic shunt. (Reproduced with permission from American College of Gastroenterology, http://www .acg.gi.org/physicianforum/pated/var_alg2.html.)

the central nervous system and exert their deleterious effect. Ammonia, fatty acids, mercaptans, aromatic amino acids, γ-aminobutyric acid (GABA), and endogenous benzodiazepines are all candidate neurotoxins (158,159). The central nervous system of cirrhotic patients is much more sensitive to hypnotics, sedatives, and narcotics, all of which may precipitate coma in these patients. The artificial creation of shunts (either surgical or through TIPS) may precipitate hepatic encephalopathy. In acute liver failure, other mechanisms are operative as well, including the loss of liver function and cerebral edema. Encephalopathy is graded according to severity (Table 55.22).

The treatment of hepatic encephalopathy in cirrhotic patients depends, in part, on the severity. Dietary protein restriction is used in all stages and may be all that is necessary in stage 0 through II encephalopathy. Pharmacotherapy includes lactulose, neomycin, and metronidazole. The use of flumazenil is discussed later in this section. Lactulose has been shown to improve the results of psychometric testing in stage 0 encephalopathy, but the clinical use may be less apparent (160). We do not routinely use lactulose for very early stage encephalopathy.

Blood in the gut lumen from gastrointestinal bleeding is particularly neurotoxic in cirrhotic patients. Bowel cleansing and reduction or elimination of dietary protein are treatment mainstays. Neomycin, both orally and as enemas, decreases the gut flora that produce many of the toxins. Lactulose acts both as a cathartic and as an ammonia trap (lactulose is fermented, producing acids that favor the equilibrium of $NH_3 + H^+$ $NH_4$). Ammonium is not absorbed across the gut membrane. Newer data suggest that the mechanism of action of lactulose is multifaceted. Probable actions include (i) a direct effect on ammonia production related to changes in bacterial selection; (ii) changes in bacterial protein synthesis and degradation; and (iii) a decrease in the 3- to 6-carbon short-chain fatty acids, with a corresponding increase in the nontoxic short chain acetate (161). Because of reports that endogenous benzodiazepines may play a role in hepatic encephalopathy, the use of a specific benzodiazepine antagonist, such as flumazenil, seems logical. Only a minority of patients with grade III and IV coma appear to achieve a clinical response to flumazenil (162). This agent should be considered a second-line agent for hepatic encephalopathy. Careful

### TABLE 55.22

**GRADING OF HEPATIC ENCEPHALOPATHY**

| Stage | Clinical | Neurologic | Electroencephalography |
|-------|----------|------------|------------------------|
| 0 | Subtle personality changes (apparent only to family or sophisticated neuropsychiatric testing) | Alert; no asterixis | Normal |
| 1 | Definite personality changes; alteration of sleep pattern | Asterixis present | Delta waves present |
| 2 | Sleepy; abnormal behavior | Asterixis present | Delta waves present |
| 3 | Somnolent but arousable | Asterixis present | Delta waves present |
| 4 | Comatose (may respond to painful stimuli) | Asterixis absent | Delta waves present |

attention to drugs that might provoke encephalopathy is important.

## LIVER DISEASE IN PREGNANCY

The pregnant woman with liver disease requires special consideration and knowledge of some liver conditions unique to pregnancy. Liver disease in pregnancy is uncommon but often is serious. Table 55.23 presents some key data about liver diseases associated with pregnancy. An excellent review is available (163).

*Acute fatty liver of pregnancy* most often presents dramatically with signs and symptoms of acute liver failure between weeks 30 and 38 of gestation (164). Vomiting, jaundice, and encephalopathy are frequent. Laboratory tests reveal hyperbilirubinemia (usually <15 mg/dL) and moderately elevated ALT and AST values (usually <1,000). The alkaline phosphatase may be modestly elevated, and evidence of liver synthetic failure as measured by prolonged prothrombin times is frequent; ammonia levels may rise. Leukocytosis is prominent. Because of the rarity of the condition and the frequency with which it may be mimicked by other liver disorders, for example, viral hepatitis, a liver biopsy is recommended. Histologic findings of preserved liver architecture, foamy cytoplasm, and microvesicular fat are diagnostic. Therapy should not be delayed. Prompt delivery of the infant is the treatment. In the event liver failure advances despite delivery, liver transplantation may be required.

*H*emolysis, *e*levated *l*iver enzymes, *l*ow *p*latelets (the HELLP syndrome) is part of the spectrum of preeclampsia–eclampsia (165). Most patients, therefore, have arterial hypertension and frequently other features, such as edema, excessive weight gain, and sometimes renal abnormalities. Nausea, vomiting, and upper abdominal pain are frequent in HELLP. Laboratory values in HELLP include features of microangiopathic hemolytic anemia, elevated bilirubin and lactic dehydrogenase levels, and platelet counts below

100,000. Transaminases are usually only slightly elevated. The complications of HELLP are many, including organ damage as a consequence of microangiopathy and progression of eclampsia. Particularly feared complications include hepatic hematomas and hepatic rupture, a surgical emergency. Treatment is directed toward reducing blood pressure, correcting the coagulopathy, and assessing for liver hemorrhage. For mature fetuses over 35 weeks' gestation, immediate delivery is recommended.

Intrahepatic cholestasis of pregnancy poses little risk to the mother but is associated with excessive fetal death either in utero or because of prematurity. The disorder most often presents in the third trimester as pruritus, but occasionally it may be seen much earlier in pregnancy. In fewer than 10% of patients is jaundice seen. Abnormal laboratory tests include AST and ALT elevations, in addition to a slight elevation of bilirubin levels. Tests usually associated with cholestasis (e.g., GGTP, alkaline phosphatase, 5' nucleotidase) are not more elevated in this disorder than in normal pregnancies. The serum bile acid levels, however, are markedly elevated and serve as a useful marker for this complication. Treatment consists of antihistamines to relieve pruritus. Other agents of possible benefit in this disorder are ursodiol (166), 10-day pulse therapy using dexamethasone (167), and possibly S-adenosyl-L-methionine (168). An excellent review is available (169).

## ACUTE LIVER FAILURE

Acute liver failure is a syndrome characterized by the rapid onset of severe liver dysfunction in a patient who has no prior history of liver disease. Jaundice, coagulopathy, and encephalopathy are the major clinical manifestations. Acute liver failure occurs because of either massive or submassive hepatic necrosis. In the former, the disease runs its course within 8 weeks of onset; in the latter, up to 26 weeks may elapse. An improvement in mortality has accompanied an improved understanding of the nature of complications for

**TABLE 55.23**

**LIVER SYNDROMES SEEN IN PREGNANCY**

| Disease | Trimester | Signs/Symptoms | Outcome | Recurrence |
|---|---|---|---|---|
| Acute fatty liver of pregnancy | 3 | Malaise, nausea, vomiting, abdominal pain, jaundice, portosystemic encephalopathy may occur | Mortality 10–25% for mother and infant; treatment, immediate delivery | Rare |
| HELLP syndrome | 3 | *H*emolysis, *e*levated *l*iver enzymes, *l*ow *p*latelets | Mortality for mother 5%; for infant 10–60% | Rare |
| Intrahepatic cholestasis | 3 | Pruritus, increased alanine transaminase/aspartate transaminase, bilirubin seldom exceeds 5 mg% | Benign course; treat symptomatically | Common |
| Hepatic rupture | 3 | Toxemia usually present; sudden abdominal catastrophe | Mortality >50% for mother and fetus | Rare |

**TABLE 55.24**

### DIAGNOSIS OF ACUTE LIVER FAILURE IN 61 PATIENTS

| Diagnosis | Percent | Survival Rate (%) |
|---|---|---|
| Non-A, non-B hepatitis | 28 | 24 |
| Acetaminophen | 25 | 67 |
| Hepatitis B | 16 | 10 |
| Drug reaction | 10 | 17 |
| Ischemic hepatitis | 8 | 40 |
| Delta hepatitis | 5 | 67 |
| Wilson's disease | 3 | 0 |
| Hepatitis A | 2 | 0 |
| Reye's syndrome | 2 | 0 |
| *Amanita* mushroom | 2 | 0 |

(Reproduced with permission from Donaldson BW, Gopinath R, Wanless IR, et al. The role of transjugular biopsy in fulminant liver failure: relationship to other prognostic indicators. *Hepatology* 1993;18:1370–1376.)

some but not all causes of acute liver failure. With intensive supportive measures, survival rates for established acute liver failure range from 10% to 25% for most causes. Liver transplantation appears to improve survival rates to 50% to 85%. Early transfer to a center with expertise in the management of this syndrome, particularly in a center that offers liver transplantation, is necessary for optimal salvage.

Common causes for acute liver failure are severe viral hepatitis [A, B (sometimes complicated by delta virus), or C], drug intoxication (especially acetaminophen taken in a suicide attempt), and, occasionally, mushroom poisoning (usually *Amanita* species). Table 55.24 indicates the etiology of acute liver failure in one North American liver unit. Other possible causes include ischemia, acute Budd-Chiari, Wilson's disease, and fatty liver of pregnancy. Some drugs that may precipitate acute liver failure are noted in Table 55.25.

The basis for acetaminophen liver injury is particularly well understood. Ninety percent or more of the drug is metabolized to form nontoxic glucuronide or sulfate conjugates, which are excreted in bile. A small percentage of acetaminophen metabolism occurs by means of an alternative pathway that uses cytochrome P450 IIE. Drug metabolized through this pathway produces a toxic metabolite, *N*-acetyl-*p*-benzoquinoneimine, which is rapidly transformed to form mercapturic acid metabolites of acetaminophen, a reaction that requires glutathione. When normal pharmacologic doses of acetaminophen are consumed, glutathione stores are adequate and *N*-acetyl-*p*-benzoquinoneimine does not accumulate. Glutathione can be depleted easily by large amounts of acetaminophen, however. *N*-acetyl-*p*-benzoquinoneimine accumulates and causes cell death by covalently binding to intracellular proteins. Chronic alcoholism and certain medications increase cytochrome P450 enzyme levels and so make acetaminophen toxic at a daily dose much lower than those usually considered toxic.

Early recognition of the patient with acetaminophen overdose leads to treatment that may prevent liver injury. *N*-acetylcysteine administered within 10 hours of ingestion is highly effective in preventing hepatic necrosis (170,171). More recent evidence suggests that, although later administration may not prevent hepatic necrosis, better outcome ensues when *N*-acetylcysteine is given up to 36 hours after ingestion (172). Acetaminophen blood levels may assist in the management of such cases by defining patients particularly at risk for hepatic necrosis. Blood levels below 200 mg/L 4 hours after ingestion (or 100 mg/L after 8 hours or 50 mg/L at 12 hours) are unlikely to be associated with hepatic damage and may not require specific protective treatment. Nomograms relating plasma acetaminophen levels to the risk of hepatic damage are available (173). Despite remarkable hepatic dysfunction caused by massive doses of acetaminophen, recovery is the rule. In one large liver failure referral center, only 110 (20%) of 548 patients transferred with signs of severe hepatic impairment from acetaminophen died, and 44 (8%) received liver transplants (174).

**TABLE 55.25**

### DRUGS THAT MAY CAUSE ACUTE LIVER FAILURE

| Common | Infrequent | Rare | Synergistic Toxicity |
|---|---|---|---|
| Acetaminophen overdose | Isoniazid | Carbamazepine | Alcohol/acetaminophen |
| | Valproate | Ofloxacin | Trimethoprim-sulfamethoxazole |
| | Halothane | Ketoconazole | Rifampin/isoniazid |
| | Phenytoin | Lisinopril | Acetaminophen/isoniazid |
| | Propylthiouracil | Labetalol | |
| | Amiodarone | Etoposide (VP-16) | |
| | Disulfiram | Imipramine | |
| | Dapsone | Interferon-α | |
| | | Flutamide | |

(Reproduced with permission from Lee WM. Acute liver failure. *N Engl J Med* 1993;329:1862–1870.)

## Selected Management Issues in Acute Liver Failure

Problems posed by established acute liver failure include:

- Sepsis
- Coagulopathy
- Renal failure
- Encephalopathy
- Acute cerebral edema
- Metabolic disorders

Sepsis is likely to develop, in part because the acute liver failure patient is immunocompromised. A report of selective gut decontamination in a group of patients with acute liver failure suggests that the incidence of enterobacterial infections can be nearly eliminated. Forty-seven percent of patients developed infection with enterobacteria (*Escherichia coli*, *Klebsiella* spp., *Proteus* spp., *Enterobacter serratia*) before the introduction of selective gut decontamination, whereas only 3% developed such infections when given selective decontamination. Norfloxacin, 400 mg every 24 hours and nystatin 1,000,000 units every 6 hours, was the regimen most often used. The incidence of other Gram-negative and Gram-positive infections was not decreased. The effect on mortality was hard to compare directly because patients treated before selective decontamination was used also were treated in an era when transplantation was never used.

In patients who survive for more than a few days, invasive fungal infections (typically *Candida* or *Aspergillus*) may occur in up to one-third. These infections are difficult to diagnose antemortem. Common sources include indwelling vascular catheters and pulmonary reservoirs. A patient who appears to improve but then relapses may have developed invasive fungal infection. Those with renal insufficiency are at particularly high risk. An unexplained temperature elevation (or one that persists after all identified bacterial infections are being treated appropriately), particularly if the white blood cell count is elevated, should raise the index of suspicion for a fungal coinfection. Our approach in all patients with acute liver failure is to administer norfloxacin and nystatin (Mycostatin) to achieve selective gut decontamination, even in the absence of established infection. Frequent chest radiographs and culture for bacteria and fungi are done. The threshold to begin broad-spectrum antibiotics is quite low. In a patient who does not respond, a further search for fungal infection is considered on a case-by-case basis.

The patient with acute liver failure has some degree of hepatic encephalopathy. The differential diagnosis of neurologic deterioration in a liver failure patient includes cerebral edema, hypoglycemia, infection, and intracerebral bleeding. Encephalopathy in acute liver failure has, at least in part, a different basis from that occurring in the cirrhotic patient, and neither lactulose nor neomycin improves encephalopathy from acute liver failure. More recent studies indicate an association between the level of ammonia in experimental acute liver failure and decreases in brain function, suggesting that ammonia is of key importance in the encephalopathy that develops after both acute and chronic liver injury.

Acute cerebral edema frequently produces tonsillar herniation and death through brainstem compression. The pathophysiology of cerebral edema is poorly understood. A combination of cytotoxic and vasogenic mechanisms are probably responsible for impaired neuronal $Na^+/K^+$ adenosine triphosphatase activity, a disrupted blood–brain barrier, and the accumulation of osmotically active amino acids in the brain cells. The frequency of cerebral edema occurring in fulminant hepatic failure may be as high as 85%.

A recognition of significant cerebral edema is difficult on clinical grounds. Headache, projectile vomiting, bradycardia, and papilledema usually are absent. Other noninvasive measures, such as CT scanning, are relatively insensitive in identifying this rapidly progressive complication. In one center in which the routine placement of an epidural pressure transducer was placed in 15 patients with fulminant hepatic failure, elevated intracranial pressure (>15 mm Hg) was identified in 11 (73%). Routine CT scans showed evidence of effacement or flattening of cortical sulci, a reduction in size, a narrowing or obliteration of the cerebral ventricles or cisterns, or the presence of generalized decreased attenuation of the hemispheres in only 27% of cases in which increased intracranial pressure had been identified by pressure measurement.

Measures useful in lowering the intracranial pressure include elevation of the head of the bed by 30 degrees, hyperventilation of the intubated patient to a $PCO_2$ of 30 mm Hg, mannitol administration, and barbiturate-induced coma. If mannitol is required, it is given in a bolus of 0.5 to 1.0 g/kg to keep the serum osmolality in the range of 310 to 320 mOsm/L. Mannitol cannot be used in oliguric patients who do not exhibit a diuretic response to mannitol. Barbiturate coma lowers intracranial pressure by causing cerebral vasoconstriction and by decreasing both cerebral oxygen demand and neuronal metabolic activity. Corticosteroids, such as dexamethasone, are uniformly unhelpful in preventing or treating the cerebral edema seen in acute liver failure.

The identification of early indicators of prognosis in acute liver failure is essential. Late occurring clinical or laboratory features are not helpful in planning therapy or deciding on liver transplantation. More helpful indicators are those easily monitored aspects of a case at the outset (Table 55.26). The etiology of the acute liver failure is the most powerful in predicting outcome. Those whose acute liver failure is due to hepatitis A, for example, have a 45% survival rate. Acetaminophen-induced liver failure, hepatitis B, and idiosyncratic drug reactions have a survival rate of 34%, 23%, and 14%, respectively. The worst prognosis is from non-A, non-B–induced acute liver failure; a meager 9% survive. Age is also an important determinant of survival, especially for acute liver failure caused by factors other than acetaminophen. Patients under the age of 10 years or older than 40 years are particularly likely to do poorly.

**TABLE 55.26**

## FEATURES ASSOCIATED WITH POOR PROGNOSIS IN ACUTE LIVER FAILURE

| Acetaminophen | Other Causes |
|---|---|
| pH <7.30 | Prothrombin time INR >6.5 |
| or | or |
| (a) Prothrombin time INR >6.5 and | Any three of the following: |
| (b) Creatinine >3.4 mg/dL and | (a) Age <10 or >40 yr |
| (c) Portosystemic encephalopathy grade III or IV | (b) Etiology non-A, non-B, halothane, drug reaction |
| | (c) Jaundice preceded portosystemic encephalopathy >7 days |
| | (d) Prothrombin time INR >3.5 |
| | (e) Bilirubin >17.6 mg/dL |

INR, international normalized ratio.
(Reproduced with permission from O'Grady JG, Alexander GJM, Haylar KM, et al. Early indicators of prognosis in fulminant hepatic failure. *Gastroenterology* 1989;97:439–445.)

The grade of encephalopathy on admission plays a role in the early prediction of outcome, although the relationship is complicated and apparently paradoxical. For example, in liver failure not caused by acetaminophen, survival was lowest (12%) in those admitted with grade 0 to II compared with those with grade III through IV coma (20% survival). Finally, the duration of jaundice before encephalopathy plays a prognostic role. When this interval is 7 days or less, the survival rate is 34%, but when it is longer than 7 days, this rate is only 7%. For acetaminophen-induced acute liver failure, an initial arterial blood pH less than 7.30 also was associated with a poorer outcome. An excellent review is available (175).

Key points in the management of acute liver failure are summarized in Table 55.27. Survival rates for emergency liver transplantation for acute liver failure range from

**TABLE 55.27**

## MANAGEMENT OF THE ACUTE LIVER FAILURE PATIENT

Transfer to intensive care unit if stage III or IV coma develops
Obtain emergent computed tomographic scan of the head
Stat neurosurgery consult for evaluation and placement of intracranial pressure monitor
Treat cerebral edema aggressively
Elective endotracheal intubation in stage III coma to protect airway
Frequent surveillance cultures
Selective gut decontamination protocol; norfloxacin, Mycostatin, and oral antibiotic paste while intubated
Low threshold to empirical use of antibiotics if infection suspected
Dialysis support either for fluid removal or hemodialysis
Swan-Ganz catheter placement for hemodynamic monitoring and resuscitation
Gastrointestinal bleeding prophylaxis with histamine blocker ± sucralfate

50% to 85%. For patients with conditions other than acetaminophen-induced hepatic necrosis, no variable at the time of admission other than cause (Wilson's disease did best; idiosyncratic drug reaction did worst) predicted survival after transplantation. Considering changing variables during hospitalization, serum creatinine is the only factor that emerges from stepwise logistic regression analysis as predicting outcome (176).

# PRIMARY LIVER CANCER (HEPATOMA AND CHOLANGIOCARCINOMA)

## Hepatoma

Substantial variation occurs in the geographic and racial incidence of hepatocellular carcinoma (hepatoma). Etiology varies in high- and low-incidence regions. In high-incidence regions (Africa, south of the Sahara; Taiwan; Southeast China; and other parts of the Far East), the age-adjusted incidence is greater than 20 per 100,000 per year. In North America, hepatoma is much less common, between 3 and 5 cases per 100,000 per year. In high-incidence areas, the age of onset is young in Africa but much older (sixth decade) in the Far East. In low-incidence areas, older onset is the rule. Men are affected more commonly than women (4:1 to 8:1 in high-incidence areas, but only 2.5:1 in low-incidence areas). Malignant hepatic tumors produce one or more of the following:

- Upper abdominal discomfort or pain
- Palpable or visible mass
- Cachexia
- Intractable ascites

Because many malignant tumors occur in the setting of advanced cirrhosis, confusion with the effects of cirrhosis may lead to diagnostic delay. It is not infrequent that hepatoma is diagnosed only at necropsy in a patient who had a rapid downhill course attributed to decompensated cirrhosis.

Strong epidemiologic evidence incriminates environmental factors in the pathogenesis of hepatoma, especially (i) hepatitis B and C infection, (ii) aflatoxins, and (iii) cirrhosis. At least 80% of cases of hepatoma worldwide are associated with evidence of persistent hepatitis B infection. HBV carriers run a higher risk of developing this cancer. This association is particularly relevant in regions of high tumor incidence, but it is also found in the United States. Patients without evidence of current infection usually have evidence of remote infection. The presence of hepatitis B as measured by HBV DNA has been shown in hepatomas from persons without HBsAg positivity (6). Hepatitis B infection precedes the development of hepatoma by many years (often many decades). Evidence from Japan indicates that hepatitis C may be more powerfully associated with hepatoma formation. In a group of 251 patients with chronic hepatitis B or C, followed up prospectively with ultrasound and α-fetoprotein, more than twice as high a percentage (10.4% versus 3.9%) of hepatitis C patients developed hepatoma over a period of 11 years (177).

Aflatoxins are metabolites of the ubiquitous fungus *Aspergillus flavus*. Aflatoxin B1 is a potent hepatic carcinogen. The contamination of foodstuffs, particularly stored nuts and grain, has been demonstrated in many tropical and subtropical areas where hepatoma is prominent. The urinary excretion of aflatoxin has been demonstrated in high-incidence regions in China. Aflatoxins, either alone or together with hepatitis B infection, almost certainly contribute to the hepatoma incidence in high-incidence areas but not to hepatoma as seen in the United States.

Cirrhosis stands out as a risk factor in the United States, and alcohol abuse is the most common cause. It seems likely that alcohol per se is not a cause of hepatoma, but it causes the cirrhosis that sets the stage for hepatoma risk. In some U.S. studies, nearly all cases of hepatoma were related to alcoholic cirrhosis. Evidence suggests that, even in patients with alcoholic liver disease, hepatitis B or C plays a role, at least as a cocarcinogen (178). Experts predict a sharp upsurge in hepatoma in the United States as persons who acquired hepatitis C during young adulthood continue to age.

Hemochromatosis, A1AT deficiency, and PBC also carry a heightened hepatoma risk. Miscellaneous causes of hepatoma include sex-steroid ingestion, particularly androgenic steroids, which is of increasing concern among young athletes, some of whom take androgenic steroids to increase muscle mass and athletic performance.

Radiologic investigations play a major role in the diagnosis of hepatoma. Isotopic scans show lesions 3 cm or larger. CT scans can detect lesions of approximately 2 cm. Ultrasonography can distinguish somewhat smaller lesions. CT, particularly dynamic scanning, can detect and define hepatomas with an improved degree of precision (2-cm lesions), and MRI is also helpful. α-Fetoprotein is a fetal protein whose synthesis is repressed after birth. It is positive in many with persons with hepatoma. This test has been used in screening, and when it is unusually high (e.g., >200 ng/mL), may confer reasonable certainty on the nature of a focal liver lesion even without biopsy.

Symptomatic hepatoma carries a grave prognosis. Small asymptomatic lesions may remain so for several years; once symptoms develop, however, life expectancy is only a few months. Chemotherapy has added little to the quantity or quality of life for those with hepatoma. Treatment options for hepatomas remain few. Percutaneous injection of ethanol for small (<2 cm) solitary hepatomas seems to be as effective as surgical resection (179). This may be done safely even when the neoplasm is located on the surface of the liver (180). Intratumor alcohol injections may extend life expectancy when the lesions are small. Chemotherapy has limited success. Doxorubicin (Adriamycin) is the single agent with the most activity against hepatomas, but it increases life expectancy little. Combination chemotherapy

has been disappointing. Recombinant interferon (50 million units three times weekly) showed a weak activity (median survival 14.0 weeks compared with 7.5 weeks for untreated patients) in Chinese patients (181). Liver transplantation is appropriate only for small asymptomatic hepatomas and for the rare fibrolamellar variant.

## Cholangiocarcinoma

Cholangiocarcinomas derive from bile duct epithelium and may be distal (near or at the terminus of the common bile duct in the duodenum), middle, or proximal (within the liver parenchyma). When the tumor occurs at the bifurcation of the right and left hepatic duct systems, this tumor is referred to as a *Klatskin's tumor*. In the United States, cholangiocarcinoma is seen more frequently than hepatoma. The pathogenesis of cholangiocarcinoma is not clear. Sclerosing cholangitis, with which cholangiocarcinoma may be confused, is said to predispose to bile duct cancer. Cholangiocarcinoma is not associated with cirrhosis or hepatitis B or exposure to mycotoxins.

The disease usually occurs in patients older than the age of 60 years and is rare before age 40. Men are more commonly affected. Patients present most often with signs or symptoms or laboratory abnormalities suggesting complete or partial biliary tract obstruction. The disease is highly suspected after a cholangiogram (endoscopic retrograde cholangiopancreatography or transhepatic cholangiogram) shows the lesion. As noted, cases of diffuse cholangiocarcinoma may be hard to distinguish from sclerosing cholangitis radiologically. Indeed, cancer may develop in sclerosing cholangitis. Brush cytologic material may be obtained during the diagnostic study. Positive results may be seen in as many as 60% of patients after up to three brushings. The high false-negative rate, however, is disappointing.

Treatment is usually palliative. Surgical removal is not usually possible except for a few lesions located in the distal biliary tree. Cholangiocarcinoma that obstructs high in the biliary tree (e.g., at the bifurcation) may be difficult for the surgeon to bypass, although the surgical placement of stents across the lesion may be possible. Either radiologic or endoscopically placed stents usually are favored for these lesions. For lesions in the common bile duct, both surgery and endoscopically placed stents are technically possible and have a high success rate.

## LIVER TRANSPLANTATION

For the past 6 years, a 35% mean annual growth has occurred of patients officially listed as waiting for liver transplantation. The growth in liver transplant operations has been much slower (7% per year). It is estimated that nearly 25,000 patients will be waiting for only 5,300 donor organs (182). Patients selected for liver transplantation usually have common problems related to end-stage cirrhosis (or to fulminant liver failure). Twenty-nine percent of patients seen in the Cleveland Clinic Hepatology Clinic have hepatitis C, and 4% have hepatitis B. Of the hepatomas seen, 26% are associated with hepatitis C and 37% with hepatitis B. In some centers, hepatitis C is the leading disease causing the end-stage liver disease that requires transplantation (183). Some have predicted that a wave of end-stage liver disease resulting from hepatitis C will emerge over the next decade, as the epidemic of high-risk behavior that created a high prevalence of hepatitis C endures long enough for the natural history of C-virus infection to play out. Current selection criteria for liver transplantation candidacy are broad, and contraindications are few and diminishing each year. In general, patients are selected for liver transplantation candidacy if one or more of the following apply: (i) end-stage liver disease with a life expectancy of less than a year; (ii) quality of life judged sufficiently poor that the risks appear justified; or (iii) a liver-based metabolic disease with lethal implications. Those sentinel events in the evolution of cirrhosis that indicate a high likelihood of mortality without transplantation include:

- Child-Pugh score 7 or higher
- Appearance of ascites
- SBP
- Hepatic hydrothorax
- Hepatorenal syndrome

Portal hypertensive bleeding also carries with it a risk of increased mortality, but in the otherwise well-compensated cirrhotic (Child-Pugh <8), this problem is dealt with best by using measures other than liver transplantation. Age per se is usually not considered a contraindication to liver transplantation, although the chances of a disqualifying coexistent disease goes up with age. Acute liver failure patients are suitable for liver transplantation. It is often logistically difficult, however, to obtain a suitable donor organ in the short "window of opportunity" available in such patients. A consensus conference determination of reasonable minimal criteria for liver transplantation is available (184).

Liver allocation policies of United Network for Organ Sharing currently determine minimal eligibility requirements for liver transplantation. An elaborate liver allocation system is currently in place to attempt, insofar as possible, to make the process of allocation of scarce resources as equitable as possible. Five categories of liver disease are recognized for adults:

- *Status 1* is the highest priority for obtaining a donor organ. These patients have fulminant liver failure with a life expectancy without transplantation of less than 7 days. To qualify, a patient must have been without preexisting liver disease (exception, acute decompensated Wilson's disease). In addition, this group includes transplanted patients who have primary nonfunction of the graft and those with hepatic artery thrombosis within a week of transplantation.

- *Status 2A* patients have liver disease requiring an intensive care unit due to chronic liver failure, with a life expectancy without liver transplantation of less than 7 days. Such patients must have a Child-Pugh score (Table 55.18) of at least 10 points and meet additional criteria: unresponsive variceal hemorrhage, hepatorenal syndrome, refractory ascites (or hepatic hydrothorax), and stage III or IV encephalopathy (Table 55.23).

- *Status 2B* is advanced liver disease, a Child-Pugh score of 10 or higher, and one or more of the following: variceal hemorrhage unresponsive to therapy, hepatorenal syndrome, SBP, refractory ascites, or hepatic hydrothorax. These patients do not need to be hospitalized.

- *Status 3* is the lowest priority. A patient may have advanced liver disease and a Child-Pugh score of 7 or higher. Such patients are usually managed as outpatients.

- *Status 4* is temporarily inactive (not eligible to receive a transplant or not in need of a transplant).

Additional details and updated information about changes in United Network for Organ Sharing policies and bylaws can be obtained on the United Network for Organ Sharing Web site at http://www.unos.org.

Alcoholic liver disease is no longer considered a contraindication to liver transplantation, particularly in those in whom sufficient personal or family support resources are available to make resumption of alcohol intake less likely (185). Patients with cholangiocarcinoma do extremely poorly and are not candidates for liver transplantation in most centers. Hepatomas, particularly if small and incidental or fibrolamellar, may have acceptable outcomes, but many question the use of scarce resources for a group who, on average, fare much more poorly after liver transplantation than those with nonmalignant disease. Patients with hepatitis B frequently have disease recurrence in the transplanted organ, sometimes with disastrous consequences (186). Interferon given after liver transplantation does not appear to prevent recurrence and may provoke increased rates of rejection (187). More recent evidence suggests that hepatitis B recurrence may be delayed, and possibly prevented, by the regular posttransplantation administration of hyperimmune B globulin to sustain serum anti-HBs titers at a protective level (188). The use of nucleoside analogs has been discussed herein (viral hepatitis B); these agents also are being explored as tools to reduce the incidence and impact of post–liver transplant hepatitis B recurrence.

A certain aura of inevitability persists about the recurrence of hepatitis C after transplantation (189). This infection is usually better tolerated than recurrent hepatitis B (190,191). Serious hepatic infections are sometimes seen, and fibrosing cholestatic hepatitis has been described (192). Despite reinfection, many centers report 1- and 3-year survival rates, similar to those for other conditions for which transplantation is done. One concern is the possibility that the time horizon has been too short. Evidence suggests a much high rate of fibrosis, with some estimates that cirrhosis may develop, on average, within 7 years after transplantation. No strategy has been shown to be of unequivocal value in moderating the outcome of recurrent hepatitis C, although a pilot study suggests the combination of interferon and ribavirin is helpful (193).

Transplantation for hemochromatosis is associated with a higher than expected mortality and a high incidence of cardiac problems, infection, and immunologic problems, including susceptibility to infection, immunoblastic lymphoma, and cancers. Whether or not iron accumulates in the transplanted liver remains controversial (194).

## Living Related Donors

In many parts of the world, the use of cadaveric organs for transplantation is not possible because of religious or cultural taboos. A viable liver transplantation program can still be effected through the use of living related donors. It has long been recognized in animals and humans that major hepatic resection is well tolerated. In the donor, the remaining liver regenerates, so that within 2 months, total liver volume is approximately what it had been before resection. Liver segments transplanted into the recipient undergo similar regeneration.

Donor selection must proceed with care. Attention to medical and ethical aspects is mandatory. Many programs specify the donor be between 20 and 45 years of age and in excellent health, without evidence of liver disease, and ABO compatible with the potential recipient. Liver mass must be estimated, most often with CT scan or MRI. The graft-mass/recipient body weight ratio should be 1% or higher. The donor liver must be free of significant steatosis.

The donor operation consists of a left or right partial hepatectomy. A left hemihepatectomy is technically easier and often results in a liver mass of 300 to 500 g. This may be sufficient for a small recipient. More often, a right hemihepatectomy is required, which yields 800 to 900 g of liver.

The results of adult living related donor liver transplantation are comparable with cadaveric transplants. Rare donor deaths have been reported.

## Cost of Liver Transplantation

The true costs of transplantation are difficult to determine. Charges, on the other hand, are often a matter of public record. In the United States, considerable regional variation in charges occurs. The U.S. Agency for Health Care Policy and Research records that, in 1996, the average charge for 3,157 liver transplants was $195,409, with mean length of stay 28 days. These charges are not inclusive. The patient successfully transplanted faces years of additional drug therapy and monitoring, with ensuing additional costs. One estimate of charges for transplant evaluation, organ procurement, transplantation, hospital charges, physician charges, and first-year follow-up totals $314,500. Liver transplantation is a costly undertaking.

## REFERENCES

1. Bacon BR, Farahvash MJ, Janney CG, et al. Nonalcoholic steatohepatitis: an expanded clinical entity. *Gastroenterology* 1994;107: 1103–1109.
2. Laurin J, Lindor KD, Crippin JS, et al. Ursodeoxycholic acid or clofibrate in the treatment of non–alcohol induced steatohepatitis: a pilot study. *Hepatology* 96;23:1464–1467.
3. Savolainen VT, Penitlia A, Karhumen PJ. Delayed increase in liver cirrhosis mortality and frequency of alcoholic liver cirrhosis following an increased and redistribution of alcohol consumption in Finland. *Alcohol Clin Exp Res* 1992;16:661–664.
4. Tuyns A, Pequignot G. Greater risk of ascitic cirrhosis in females in relation to alcohol consumption. *Int J Epidemiol* 1983;13:53–57.
5. Lieber CS. Mechanisms of ethanol-induced hepatic injury. *Pharmacol Ther* 1990;46:1–41.
6. Albano E, Clot P, Morimoto M, et al. Role of cytochrome P4502E1-dependent formation of hydroxyethyl free radical in the development of liver damage in rats intragastrically fed with ethanol. *Hepatology* 1996;23:155–163.
7. Kearns PJ, Young H, Garcia G, et al. Accelerated improvement of alcoholic liver disease with enteral nutrition. *Gastroenterology* 1992;102:200–205.
8. Ramond M-J, Poynard T, Rueff B, et al. A randomized trial of prednisolone in patients with severe alcoholic hepatitis. *N Engl J Med* 1992;326:507–512.
9. Imperiale TF, McCullough AJ. Do corticosteroids reduce mortality from alcoholic hepatitis? A meta-analysis of the randomized trials. *Ann Intern Med* 1990;113:299–307.
10. Mendenhall CL, Moritz TE, Roselle GA, et al. A study of oral nutritional support with oxandrolone in malnourished patients with alcoholic hepatitis. *Hepatology* 1993;17:564–576.
11. Orrego H, Blake JE, Blendis LM, et al. Long term treatment of alcoholic liver disease with propylthiouracil. Part 2. *J Hepatol* 1994;20:343–349.
12. Akriviadis EA, Steindel H, Pinto PC, et al. Failure of colchicine to improve short-term survival in patients with alcoholic hepatitis. *Gastroenterology* 1990;99:811–818.
13. DeFraites RF, Feighner BH, Binn LN, et al. Immunization of U.S. soldiers with a two dose primary series of inactivated hepatitis A vaccine. *J Infect Dis* 1995;171[Suppl]:S61–S69.
14. Clemens R, Safary A, Hepburn A, et al. Clinical experience with an inactivated hepatitis A vaccine. *J Infect Dis* 1995;171[Suppl]: S44–S49.
15. Vento S, Garofano T, Renzini C, et al. Fulminant hepatitis associated with hepatitis A virus superinfection in patients with chronic hepatitis C. *N Engl J Med* 1998;338:286–290.
16. Fattovich G, Giustina G, Realdi G, et al. Long-term outcome of hepatitis B e antigen-positive patients with compensated cirrhosis treated with interferon α. *Hepatology* 1997;26:1338–1342.
17. Lin S-M, Sheen I-E, Chien R-N, et al. Long-term beneficial effects of interferon therapy in patients with chronic hepatitis B infection. *Hepatology* 1999;29:971–975.
18. de Franchis R, Meucci G, Vecchi M, et al. The natural history of asymptomatic hepatitis B surface antigen carriers. *Ann Intern Med* 1993;118:191–194.
19. Hoofnagle JH, Di Bisceglie AM. The treatment of chronic viral hepatitis. *N Engl J Med* 1997;336:347–356.
20. Dienstag JL, Perillo RP, Schiff ER, et al. A preliminary trial of lamivudine for chronic hepatitis B infection. *N Engl J Med* 1995; 333:1657–1661.
21. Lai C-L, Chien R-N, Leung NWY, et al. A one-year trial of lamivudine for chronic hepatitis B. *N Engl J Med* 1998;339:61–68.
22. Farci P, Mandas A, Coiani A, et al. Treatment of chronic hepatitis D with interferon α 2a. *N Engl J Med* 1994;330:88–94.
23. National Institutes of Health Consensus Development Conference Panel statement: management of hepatitis C. *Hepatology* 1997; 26[Suppl 1]:2S–10S.
24. Ohto H, Terazawa S, Sasaki N, et al. Transmission of hepatitis C virus from mothers to infants. *N Engl J Med* 1994;330:744–750.
25. Mitsui T, Iwano K, Masuko K, et al. Hepatitis C virus infection in medical personnel after needlestick accident. *Hepatology* 1992;16: 1109–1114.

26. Recommendation for follow-up of health care workers after occupational exposure to hepatitis C virus. *Morb Mortal Wkly Rep* 1997;46:603–606.

27. Alter MJ, Margolis HS, Krawczynski K, et al. The natural history of community-acquired hepatitis C in the United States. *N Engl J Med* 1992;327:1899–1905.

28. Barrera JM, Bruguera M, Ercilla G, et al. Persistent hepatitis C viremia after acute self-limiting posttransfusion hepatitis C. *Hepatology* 1995;21:639–644.

29. Naito M, Hayashi N, Hagiwara H, et al. Serum hepatitis C virus: quantity and histological features of hepatitis C virus carriers with persistently normal ALT levels. *Hepatology* 1994;19:871–875.

30. Fong T-L, Kanel GC, Conrad A, et al. Clinical significance of concomitant hepatitis C infection in patients with alcoholic liver disease. *Hepatology* 1994;19:554–557.

31. Corrao G, Arico S. Independent and combined action of hepatitis C virus infection and alcohol consumption on the risk of symptomatic liver cirrhosis. *Hepatology* 1998;27:914–919.

32. Seeff LB, Buskell-Bales Z, Wright EC, et al. Long-term mortality after transfusion-associated non A, non B hepatitis. *N Engl J Med* 1992;327:1906–1911.

33. Johnson RJ, Gretch DR, Yamabe H, et al. Membranoproliferative glomerulonephritis associated with hepatitis C virus infection. *N Engl J Med* 1993;328:465–470.

34. Herrero C, Vicente A, Bruguera M, et al. Is hepatitis C virus infection a trigger of porphyria cutanea tarda? *Lancet* 1993;341:788–789.

35. Feray C, Gigou M, Samuel D, et al. Influence of the genotype of hepatitis C virus on the severity of recurrent liver disease after liver transplantation. *Gastroenterology* 1995;108:1088–1096.

36. Reichard O, Glaumann H, Fryden A, et al. Two year biochemical, virological and histological follow-up in patients with chronic hepatitis C responding in a sustained fashion to interferon α 2b treatment. *Hepatology* 1995;21:918–922.

37. Lau DT-Y, Ghany MG, Park Y, et al. 10-year follow-up after interferon therapy for chronic hepatitis C. *Hepatology* 1998;28:1121–1127.

38. Kasahara A, Hayashi N, Mochizuki K, et al. Risk factors for hepatocellular carcinoma and its incidence after interferon treatment in patients with chronic hepatitis C. *Hepatology* 1998;27:1394–1402.

39. Poynard T, Marcellin P, Lee SS, et al. Randomised trial of interferon a2b plus ribavirin for 48 weeks or for 24 weeks versus interferon a2b plus placebo for 48 weeks for treatment of chronic infection with hepatitis C. *Lancet* 1998;352:1426–1432.

40. McHutchison JG, Gordon SC, Schiff ER, et al. Interferon α-2b alone or in combination with ribavirin as initial treatment for chronic C hepatitis. *N Engl J Med* 1998;339:1485–1492.

41. Zeuzem S, Feinman V, Rasenack J, et al. Peginterferon α 2a in patients with chronic hepatitis C. *N Engl J Med* 2000;343:1666–1672.

42. Lindsay KL, Trep C, Heintges T, et al. Randomized double blind trial comparing pegylated interferon α 2b to interferon α 2b as initial treatment for chronic hepatitis C. *Hepatology* 2001;34:395–403.

43. Heathcote EJ, Keefe EB, Lee SS, et al. Retreatment of chronic hepatitis C with consensus interferon. *Hepatology* 1998;27:1136–1143.

44. Davis GL, Esteban-Mur R, Rustigi V, et al. Interferon α-2 b alone or in combination with ribavirin for the treatment of relapse of chronic hepatitis C. *N Engl J Med* 1998;339:1493–1499.

45. Sangiovanni A, Morales R, Spinzi GC, et al. Interferon α treatment of HCV RNA carriers with persistently normal transaminase levels: a pilot randomized controlled study. *Hepatology* 1998;27:853–856.

46. Czaja A, Manns MP, Homburger HA. Frequency and significance of antibodies to liver/kidney microsome type 1 in adults with chronic active hepatitis. *Gastroenterology* 1992;103:1290–1295.

47. Czaja A, Carpenter HA, Santrach PJ, et al. Significance of HLA DR4 in type 1 autoimmune hepatitis. *Gastroenterology* 1993;105:1502–1507.

48. Harada K, Van de Water J, Leung PSC, et al. In situ nucleic acid hybridization of cytokines in primary biliary cirrhosis. *Hepatology* 1997;25:791–796.

49. Desmet VJ. Vanishing bile duct disorders. In: Boyer JL, Ockner RK, eds. *Progress in Liver Diseases*, vol X. Philadelphia: WB Saunders, 1992:89.

50. Ludwig J, Weisner RH, La Russo, et al. Idiopathic adulthood ductopenia: a cause of chronic cholestatic liver disease and biliary cirrhosis. *J Hepatol* 1988;7:193–199.

51. Invernizzi P, Crosignani A, Battezzati PM, et al. Comparison of clinical features and clinical course of antimitochondrial antibody-positive and-negative primary biliary cirrhosis. *Hepatology* 1997;25:1090–1095.

52. Geubel AP, Baggenstoss AH, Summerskill WHJ. Response to treatment can differentiate chronic active liver disease with cholangitic features from the primary biliary cirrhosis syndrome. *Gastroenterology* 1976;71:444–449.

53. Long RG, Scheuer PJ, Sherlock S. Presentation and course of asymptomatic primary biliary cirrhosis. *Gastroenterology* 1977;72:1204–1207.

54. Roll J, Boyer JL, Barry D, et al. The prognostic importance of clinical and histologic features in asymptomatic and symptomatic primary biliary cirrhosis. *N Engl J Med* 1983;308:1–7.

55. Balasubramaniam K, Grambsch PM, Wiesner RH, et al. Diminished survival in asymptomatic primary biliary cirrhosis. *Gastroenterology* 1990;98:1567–1571.

56. Dickson ER Grambsch PM, Flemin TR, et al. Prognosis in primary biliary cirrhosis: model for decision-making. *Hepatology* 1989;10:1–7.

57. Lim AG, Jazrawl RP, Ahmed HA, et al. Soluble intercellular adhesion molecule 1 in primary biliary cirrhosis: relationship with disease stage, immune activity, and cholestasis. *Hepatology* 1994;20:882–887.

58. Poupon RE, Balkau B, Guechoy J, et al. Predictive factors in ursodeoxycholic acid-treated patients with primary biliary cirrhosis: role of serum markers of connective tissue. *Hepatology* 1994;19:635–640.

59. Martinez OM, Villanueva JC, Gershwin ME, et al. Cytokine patterns and cytotoxic mediators in primary biliary cirrhosis. *Hepatology* 1995;21:113–119.

60. Gershwin ME, Coppel RL, Mackay IR. Primary biliary cirrhosis and mitochondrial autoantigens—insights from molecular biology. *Hepatology* 1988;8:147–151.

61. Neuberger J, Thomson R. PBC and AMA—What is the connection? *Hepatology* 1999;29:271–276.

62. Mehal W, Gregory WL, Lo Y-M D, et al. Defining the immunogenetic susceptibility to primary biliary cirrhosis. *Hepatology* 1994;20:1213–1219.

63. Ludwig J, Dickson ER, McDonald GS, et al. Staging of chronic non-suppurative destructive cholangitis (syndrome of primary biliary cirrhosis). *Virchows Arch* 1978;379:103–112.

64. Kaplan M, Elta G, Furie B, et al. Fat soluble vitamin nutriture in primary biliary cirrhosis. *Gastroenterology* 1988;95:787–792.

65. Herlong SF, Recker RR, Maddrey WC, et al. Bone disease in primary biliary cirrhosis: histologic features and response to 25 hydroxy vitamin D. *Gastroenterology* 1982;82:103–108.

66. Hodgson SF, Dickson ER, Wahner HW, et al. Bone loss and reduced osteoblast function in primary biliary cirrhosis. *Ann Intern Med* 1985;103:855–860.

67. Eastell R, Dickson R, Hodgson SF, et al. Rates of vertebral bone loss before and after liver transplantation in women with primary biliary cirrhosis. *Hepatology* 1991;14:296–300.

68. Camisasca M, Crosignani A, Battezzati PM, et al. Parenteral calcitonin for metabolic bone disease associated with primary biliary cirrhosis. *Hepatology* 1994;20:633–637.

69. Rosen H. Primary biliary cirrhosis and bone disease [Editorial]. *Hepatology* 1995;21:253–255.

70. Crippin JS, Jorgenson RA, Dickson ER, et al. Hepatic osteodystrophy in primary biliary cirrhosis: effects of medical treatment. *Am J Gastroenterol* 1994;89:47–50.

71. Guanabens N, Pares A, Monegal A, et al. Etidronate versus fluoride for treatment of osteopenia in primary biliary cirrhosis. *Gastroenterology* 1997;113:219–224.

72. Jones E, Bergasa NV. Hypothesis: the pruritus of cholestasis: from bile acids to opiate agonists. *Hepatology* 1990;11:884–887.

73. Ghent CN, Carruthers G. Treatment of pruritus in primary biliary cirrhosis with rifampin. *Gastroenterology* 1988;94:488–493.

74. Bachs L, Elena M, Pares A, et al. Comparison of rifampicin with phenobarbitone for treatment of pruritus in biliary cirrhosis. *Lancet* 1989;1:574–576.

75. Podesta A, Popez P, Terg R, et al. Treatment of pruritus of primary biliary cirrhosis with rifampin. *Dig Dis Sci* 1991;36:216–220.

76. Kaplan M, Alling DW, Zimmerman HJ, et al. A prospective trial of colchicine for primary biliary cirrhosis. *N Engl J Med* 1986; 315:1448–1454.

77. Mitchison HC, Plamer JM, Bassendine MF, et al. A controlled trial of prednisolone treatment in primary biliary cirrhosis: three year results. *J Hepatol* 1992;15:336–344.

78. Wesiner H, Ludwig J, Lindor KD, et al. A controlled clinical trial of cyclosporine in the treatment of primary biliary cirrhosis. *N Engl J Med* 1990;322:1419–1424.

79. Lombard M, Portmann B, Neuberger J, et al. Cyclosporin A treatment in primary biliary cirrhosis: results of a long-term placebo controlled trial. *Gastroenterology* 1993;104:519–526.

80. Lindor KD, Dickson ER, Jorgensen RA, et al. The combination of ursodeoxycholic acid and methotrexate for patients with primary biliary cirrhosis: the results of a pilot study. *Hepatology* 1995;22:1158–1162.

81. Calmus Y, Gane P, Rouger P, et al. Hepatic expression of class I and class II major histocompatibility complex molecules in primary biliary cirrhosis: effect of ursodeoxycholic acid. *Hepatology* 1990;11:12–15.

82. Poupon R, Chretien Y, Poupon RE, et al. Is ursodeoxycholic acid an effective treatment for primary biliary cirrhosis? *Lancet* 1987;1: 834–836.

83. Poupon RE, Balkau R, Eschwege E, et al. A multicenter controlled trial of ursodeoxycholic acid in primary biliary cirrhosis. *N Engl J Med* 1991;324:1548–1554.

84. Heathcote EJ, Cauch-Dudek K, Walker V, et al. The Canadian multicenter double blind randomized controlled trial of ursodeoxycholic acid in primary biliary cirrhosis. *Hepatology* 1994;19:1149–1156.

85. Poupon RE, Poupon R, Balkus B. Ursodiol for the long term treatment of primary biliary cirrhosis. *N Engl J Med* 1994;330: 1342–1347.

86. Lindor KD, Dickson ER, Baldus WP, et al. Ursodeoxycholic acid in the treatment of primary biliary cirrhosis. *Gastroenterology* 1994;106:1284–1290.

87. Combes B, Carithers R, Maddrey W, et al. A randomized double-blind, placebo controlled trial of ursodeoxycholic acid in primary biliary cirrhosis. *Hepatology* 1995;22:759–766.

88. Poupon RE, Lindor KD, Cauch-Dudek K, et al. Combined analysis of randomized controlled trials of ursodeoxycholic acid in primary biliary cirrhosis. *Gastroenterology* 1997;113:884–890.

89. Markus BH, Dickson ER, Grambsch PM, et al. Efficacy of liver transplantation in patients with primary biliary cirrhosis. *N Engl J Med* 1989;320:1709–1713.

90. Chapman RW, Cattone M, Selby WS, et al. Serum autoantibodies, ulcerative colitis and primary sclerosing cholangitis. *Gut* 1986;27: 86–91.

91. Whiteside TL, Lasky S, Si L, et al. Immunologic analysis of mononuclear cells in liver tissues and blood of patients with primary sclerosing cholangitis. *Hepatology* 1985;5:468–474.

92. Bodenheimer HC, LaRusso NF, Thayer WR, et al. Elevated circulating immune complexes in primary sclerosing cholangitis. *Hepatology* 1983;3:150–154.

93. Minuk GY, Angus M, Brickman CM, et al. Abnormal clearance of immune complexes from the circulation of patients with primary sclerosing cholangitis. *Gastroenterology* 1985;88:166–170.

94. Lindor KD, Wiesner RH, Katzmann JA, et al. Lymphocyte subsets in primary sclerosing cholangitis. *Dig Dis Sci* 1987;32:166–170.

95. Lindor KD, Wiesner RH, LaRusso NF, et al. Enhanced autoreactivity of T-lymphocytes in primary sclerosing cholangitis. *Hepatology* 1987;7:884–888.

96. Helzberg JH, Petersen JM, Boyer JL. Improved survival with primary sclerosing cholangitis. *Gastroenterology* 1987;92:1869–1875.

97. Lebovics E, Palmer M, Woo X, et al. Outcome of primary sclerosing cholangitis. *Arch Intern Med* 1987;147:729–731.

98. LaRusso NF, Wiesner RH, Ludwig J. Is primary sclerosing cholangitis a bad disease? *Gastroenterology* 1987;92:2031–2033.

99. LaRusso NF, Wiesner RH, Ludwig J, et al. Prospective trial of penicillamine in primary sclerosing cholangitis. *Gastroenterology* 1988;95:1036–1042.

100. Lindor K. Ursodiol for primary sclerosing cholangitis. *N Engl J Med* 1997;336:691–695.

101. Batta AK, Arora R, Salen G. Effect of ursodiol (UDCA) on bile acid metabolism in primary sclerosing cholangitis (PSC). *Gastroenterology* 1989;96:A575.

102. Mc Entee G, Wiesner RH, Rosen C, et al. A comparative study of patients. *Transplant Proc* 1991;23:1563–1564.

103. Steindl P, Ferenci P, Dienes HP, et al. Wilson's disease in patients presenting with liver disease: a diagnostic challenge. *Gastroenterology* 1997;113:212–218.

104. Stremmel W, Meyerrose KW, Niederau C, et al. Wilson's disease: clinical presentation, treatment, and survival. *Ann Intern Med* 1991;115:720–726.

105. Ferenci P, Gilliam TC, Gitlin JD, et al. An international symposium on Wilson's and Menke's disease. *Hepatology* 1996;24: 953–958.

106. Feder JN, Gnirke A, Thomas W, et al. A novel MHC class I-like gene is mutated in patients with idiopathic hemochromatosis. *Nat Genet* 1996;13:399–408.

107. Powell LW, George K, McDonnell SM, et al. Diagnosis of hemochromatosis. *Ann Intern Med* 1998;129:925–931.

108. Bassett ML, Halliday JW, Powell LW. Value of hepatic iron measurements in early hemochromatosis and determination of the critical iron level associated with fibrosis. *Hepatology* 1986;6:24–29.

109. Deugnier YM, Turlin B, Powell LW, et al. Differentiation between heterozygotes and homozygotes in genetic hemochromatosis by means of histological hepatic iron index: a study of 192 cases. *Hepatology* 1993;17:30–34.

110. Barton JC, McDonnell SM, Adams PC, et al. Management of hemochromatosis. Hemochromatosis Management Working Group. *Ann Intern Med* 1998;129:932–939.

111. Graziadei IW, Joseph J, Wiesner RH, et al. Increased risk of chronic liver failure in adults with heterozygous α-one-antitrypsin deficiency. *Hepatology* 1998;28:1058–1063.

112. Warner L, Skorecki K, Blendis LM, et al. Atrial natriuretic factor and liver disease. *Hepatology* 1993;17:500–513.

113. Pozzi M, Osculati G, Boari G, et al. Time course of circulatory and humoral effects of rapid total paracentesis in cirrhotic patients with tense ascites. *Gastroenterology* 1994;106:709–719.

114. Rector WG Jr., Lewis F, Robertson AD, et al. Renal sodium retention complicating alcoholic liver disease: relation to portosystemic shunting and liver function. *Hepatology* 1990;12:455–459.

115. Levy M. Sodium retention and ascites formation in dogs with portal cirrhosis. *Am J Physiol* 1977;233(F):572–585.

116. Lieberman FL, Reynolds TB. Plasma volume in cirrhosis of the liver; its relation to portal hypertension, ascites and renal function. *J Clin Lab Invest* 1967;46:1297–1308.

117. Lieberman FL, Ito S, Reynolds TB. Effective plasma volume in cirrhosis with ascites. *J Clin Lab Invest* 1969;48:975–981.

118. Jimenez W, Martinez-Pardo A, Arroyo V, et al. Temporal relationship between hyperaldosteronism, sodium retention, and ascites formation in rats with experimental cirrhosis. *Hepatology* 1985; 238:245–250.

119. Bernardi M, Trevisani F, Santini C, et al. Aldosterone related blood volume expansion in cirrhosis before and during the early phase of ascites formation. *Gut* 1983;24:761–766.

120. Perez-Ayuso RM, Arroyo V, Planas R, et al. Randomized comparative study of efficacy of furosemide versus spironolactone in patients with liver cirrhosis and ascites. *Gastroenterology* 1983; 84:961–968.

121. Van Vliet AA, Hackeng WH, Donker AJM, et al. Efficacy of low dose captopril in addition to furosemide and spironolactone in patients with decompensated liver disease. *J Hepatol* 1992;15:40–47.

122. Henrickson JH, Ring-Larsen H. Hepatorenal disorders: role of the sympathetic nervous system. *Semin Liver Dis* 1994;14:35–43.

123. Wong F, Blendis L. Pathophysiology of sodium retention and ascites formation in cirrhosis: role of atrial natriuretic factor. *Semin Liver Dis* 1994;14:59–70.

124. Runyon BA, Montano AA, Akriviadis EA, et al. The serum-ascites albumin gradient is superior to the exudate-transudate concept in the differential diagnosis of ascites. *Ann Intern Med* 1992;117: 215–220.

125. Runyon BA, McHutchison JG, Antillon MR, et al. Short course versus long course antibiotic treatment of spontaneous bacterial peritonitis: a randomized controlled trial of 100 patients. *Gastroenterology* 1991;100:1737–1742.

126. Rimola A, Salmeron JM, Clemente G, et al. Two different dosages of cefotaxime in the treatment of spontaneous bacterial peritonitis: results of a prospective randomized multicenter study. *Hepatology* 1995;21:674–679.

127. Toledo C, Salmeron J-M, Rimola A, et al. Spontaneous bacterial peritonitis in cirrhosis: predictive factors of infection resolution and survival in patients treated with cefotaxime. *Hepatology* 1993;17:251–257.

128. Rimola A, del Pino JL, Gines P, et al. Partially absorbed quinolones in the prophylaxis of spontaneous bacterial recurrence in cirrhosis. *J Hepatol* 1988;100:72.

129. Gines P, Rimola A, Planas R, et al. Norfloxacin prevents spontaneous bacterial peritonitis recurrence in cirrhosis. *Hepatology* 1990;12:716–724.

130. Soriano G, Guarner C, Teixodo M, et al. Selective intestinal decontamination prevents spontaneous bacterial peritonitis. *Gastroenterology* 1991;100:477–481.

131. Dupeyron C, Manganey S, Sedrati I, et al. Rapid emergence of quinolone resistance in cirrhotic patients treated with norfloxacin to prevent bacterial peritonitis. *Antimicrob Agents Chemother* 1994; 38:340–344.

132. Singh N, Gayowski T, Yu V, et al. Trimethoprim-sulfamethoxazole for the prevention of spontaneous bacterial peritonitis in cirrhosis: a randomized trial. *Ann Intern Med* 1995;122:595–598.

133. Bernardi M, Santini C, Trevisani F, et al. Renal function impairment induced by changes in posture in patients with cirrhosis and ascites. *Gut* 1985;26:629–635.

134. Gines P, Arryo V, Quintero E, et al. Comparison of paracentesis and diuretics in the treatment of cirrhotics with tense ascites. *Gastroenterology* 1987;93:234–241.

135. Pinto PC, Amerian AI, Reynolds TB. Large volume paracentesis in nonedematous patients with tense ascites: its effects on intravascular volume. *Hepatology* 1988;8:207–210.

136. Sola R, Andreu M, Coll S, et al. Spontaneous bacterial paracentesis in cirrhotic patients treated using paracentesis or diuretics: results of a randomized study. *Hepatology* 1995;21: 340–344.

137. Gines P, Arroyo V, Vargas V, et al. Paracentesis with intravenous infusion of albumin as compared with peritoneovenous shunting in cirrhosis with refractory ascites. *N Engl J Med* 1991;325: 829–835.

138. Ochs A, Rossle M, Haag K. The transjugular intrahepatic portosystemic shunt procedure for refractory ascites. *N Engl J Med* 1995;332:1192–1197.

139. Quiroga J, Sangro B, Nunez M, et al. Transjugular intrahepatic porto-systemic shunt in the treatment of refractory ascites: effect on clinical, renal, humoral and hemodynamic parameters. *Hepatology* 1995;21:986–994.

140. Nolte W, Wiltfang J, Schindler C, et al. Portosystemic hepatic encephalopathy after transjugular intrahepatic portosystemic shunts in patients with cirrhosis: clinical, laboratory, psychometric, and electroencephalographic investigations. *Hepatology* 1998; 28:1215–1225.

141. Arroyo V, Epstein M, Gallus G, et al. Refractory ascites in cirrhosis: mechanism and treatment. *Gastroenterol Int* 1989;2: 195–207.

142. Jeffries MA, Kazanjian S, Wilson M, et al. Transjugular intrahepatic portosystemic shunts and liver transplantation in patients with refractory hepatic hydrothorax. *Liver Transplant Surg* 1998; 4:416–423.

143. Grace ND. Diagnosis and treatment of gastrointestinal bleeding secondary to portal hypertension. *Am J Gastroenterol* 1997;92: 1082–1090.

144. Poynard T, Cales P, Pasta L, et al. Multicenter study group. β-adrenergic antagonist drugs in the prevention of gastrointestinal bleeding in patients with cirrhosis and esophageal varices: an analysis of data and prognostic factors from 589 patients from four randomized clinical trials. *N Engl J Med* 1991;324:1532–1538.

145. Angelico M, Carli L, Piat C, et al. Effects of isosorbide 5-mononitrate compared with propranolol on first bleeding

146. Imperiale TF, Chalasni N. A meta-analysis of endoscopic variceal ligation for primary prophylaxis of esophageal variceal hemorrhage. *Hepatology* 2001;33:802–807.

147. Lebrec S. Primary prevention of variceal bleeding. What's new? *Hepatology* 2001;33:1003–1004.

148. Corley DA, Cello JP, Adkisson W, et al. Octreotide for acute esophageal variceal bleeding: a meta-analysis. *Gastroenterology* 2001;120:946–954.

149. Gimson AES, Ramage JK, Panos MZ, et al. Randomised trial of variceal ligation versus injection sclerotherapy for bleeding oesophageal varices. *Lancet* 1994;345:391–394.

150. D'Amico G, Politi F, Morabito A, et al. Octreotide compared with placebo in a treatment strategy for early rebleeding in cirrhosis. A double blind randomized pragmatic trial. *Hepatology* 1998;28: 1206–1214.

151. Avgerinos A, Armonis A, Raptis S. Somatostatin or octreotide versus endoscopic sclerotherapy in acute variceal hemorrhage: a meta-analysis. *J Hepatol* 1995;22:247–251.

152. Laine I, El-Newihi HM, Migikovsky B, et al. Endoscopic ligation compared with sclerotherapy for the treatment of esophageal varices. *Ann Intern Med* 1993;119:1–7.

153. Lo g-H, Lai k-H L, Cheng J-S C, et al. Endoscopic variceal ligation plus nadolol and sucralfate compared with ligation alone for prevention of variceal re-bleeding. A prospective, randomized trial. *Hepatology* 2000;32:461–465.

154. Villanueva C, Minina J, Ortiz J, et al. Endoscopic ligation compared with combined treatment with nadolol and isosorbide mononitrate to prevent recurrent variceal hemorrhage. *N Engl J Med* 2001;345:647–655.

155. Conn HO. Transjugular intrahepatic portal-systemic shunts: the state of the art. *Hepatology* 1993;17:148–158.

156. Rossle M, Haag K, Ochs A, et al. The transjugular intrahepatic portosystemic stent shunt procedure for variceal bleeding. *N Engl J Med* 1994;330:165–171.

157. Conn H. Transjugular intrahepatic portosystemic shunts versus sclerotherapy: a discussion of discordant results. *Ann Intern Med* 1997;126:907–909.

158. Basile AS, Jones EA. Hepatic encephalopathy and the GABA-benzodiazepine receptor-chloride ionophore complex: an update. *J Gastroenterol Hepatol* 1988;3:387–388.

159. Mullen KD, Szauter KM, Kaminsky-Russ K. Endogenous benzodiazepine activity in body fluids of patients with hepatic encephalopathy. *Lancet* 1990;336:81–83.

160. Watanabe A, Sakai T, Sato S, et al. Clinical efficacy of lactulose in cirrhotic patients with and without subclinical hepatic encephalopathy. *Hepatology* 1997;26:1410–1414.

161. Mortensen PB. The effect of orally-administered lactulose on colonic nitrogen metabolism and excretion. *Hepatology* 1992;16: 1350–1356.

162. Barbaro G, Di Lorenzo G, Soldini M, et al. Flumazenil for hepatic encephalopathy grade III and IVa in patients with cirrhosis: an Italian multicenter double-blind, placebo-controlled, crossover study. *Hepatology* 1998;28:374–378.

163. Knox TA, Olans LB. Liver disease in pregnancy. *N Engl J Med* 1996;335:569–576.

164. Reyes H. Acute fatty liver of pregnancy. *Clin Liver Dis* 1999;3: 69–81.

165. Barton JR, Sibai BM. HELLP and the liver diseases of preeclampsia. *Clin Liver Dis* 1999;3:31–48.

166. Palma J, Poupon RE, Ribalta J, et al. Ursodeoxycholic acid in the treatment of cholestasis of pregnancy. *J Hepatol* 1997;27:1022–1028.

167. Hirvioja ML, Tuimala R. The treatment of intrahepatic cholestasis of pregnancy by dexamethasone. *Br J Obstet Gynecol* 1992;99: 109–111.

168. Ribalta J, Reyes H, Gonzalez MC, et al. S-adenosyl-L-methionine in the treatment of patients with intrahepatic cholestasis of pregnancy. *Hepatology* 1991;13:1084–1089.

169. Bacq Y. Intrahepatic cholestasis of pregnancy. *Clin Liver Dis* 1999; 3:1–13.

170. Smilkstein MJ, Knapp GL, Kulig KW, et al. Efficacy of oral acetylcysteine in the treatment of acetaminophen overdose. *N Engl J Med* 1988;319:1557–1562.

171. Keays R, Harrison PM, Wendon JA, et al. Intravenous acetylcysteine in paracetamol induced fulminant hepatic failure. *BMJ* 1991;303:1026–1029.

172. Harrison PM, Keays R, Bray GP, et al. Improved outcome of paracetamol-induced fulminant hepatic failure by late administration of acetylcysteine. *Lancet* 1990;335:1572–1573.

173. Flanagan RJ, Meredith TJ. Use of N-acetylcysteine in clinical toxicology. *Am J Med* 1991;91:131S–139S.

174. Bernal W, Wendon J, Rela M, et al. Use and outcome of liver transplantation in acetaminophen-induced acute liver failure. *Hepatology* 1998;27:1050–1055.

175. Hoofnagle JH, Carithers RL, Shapiro C, et al. Fulminant hepatic failure: summary of a workshop. *Hepatology* 1995;21:240–252.

176. Devlin J, Wendon J, Heaton N, et al. Pretransplantation clinical status and outcome of emergency transplantation for acute liver failure. *Hepatology* 1995;21:1018–1024.

177. Takano S, Yokosuka O, Imazeki F, et al. Incidence of hepatocellular carcinoma in chronic hepatitis B and C: a prospective study of 251 patients. *Hepatology* 1995;21:650–655.

178. Paterlini P, Driss F, Nalpas B, et al. Persistence of hepatitis B and hepatitis C viral genome in primary liver cancers from HBsAg negative patients: a study from a low endemic area. *Hepatology* 1993; 17:20–29.

179. Kotoh K, Sakai H, Sakamoto S, et al. The effect of percutaneous ethanol injection therapy on small solitary hepatocellular carcinoma is comparable to that of hepatectomy. *Am J Gastroenterol* 1994;89:194–198.

180. Shilna S, Tagawa K, Fujino H, et al. Percutaneous ethanol injection therapy for neoplasms located on the surface of the liver. *Am J Radiol* 1990;158:507–509.

181. Lai C-L, Lau J Y-N, Wu P-C, et al. Recombinant interferon α in inoperable hepatocellular carcinoma: a randomized controlled trial. *Hepatology* 1993;17:389–394.

182. United Network for Organ Sharing (http://www.unos.org).

183. Wright TL, Pereira B. Liver transplantation for chronic viral hepatitis. *Liver Transplant Surg* 1995;1:30–42.

184. Lucey MR, Brown KA, Everson GT, et al. Minimal criteria for placement of adults on the liver transplant waiting list. *Liver Transplant Surg* 1997;3:628–637.

185. Sherman D, Williams R. Liver transplantation for alcoholic liver disease. *J Hepatol* 1995;23:474–479.

186. Samuel D, Muller R, Alexander G, et al. Liver transplantation in European patients with the hepatitis B surface antigen. *N Engl J Med* 1993;329:1842–1847.

187. Rakela J, Wooten RS, Batts KP, et al. Failure of interferon to prevent recurrent hepatitis B infection in hepatic allograft. *Mayo Clin Proc* 1989;64:429–432.

188. McGory R, Ishitani M, Oliveira W, et al. Improved outcome of orthotopic liver transplantation for chronic hepatitis B cirrhosis with aggressive passive immunization. *Transplantation* 1996;61: 1358–1364.

189. Wright TL, Donegan E, Hsu HH, et al. Recurrent and acquired hepatitis C viral infection in liver transplant recipients. *Gastroenterology* 1992;103:317–322.

190. Feray C, Gigou M, Samuel D, et al. The course of hepatitis C virus infection after liver transplantation. *Hepatology* 1994;20:1137–1143.

191. Shiffman ML, Contos MJ, Luketicv A, et al. Biochemical and histological evaluation of recurrent hepatitis C following orthotopic liver transplantation. *Transplantation* 1994;57:526–532.

192. Scluger LK, Min A, Wolf DC, et al. Severe recurrent cholestatic hepatitis C following orthotopic liver transplantation. *Gastroenterology* 1994;106:A978.

193. Bizollon T, Palazzo U, Ducerf C, et al. Pilot study of the combination of interferon α and ribavirin as therapy of recurrent hepatitis C after liver transplantation. *Hepatology* 1997;26:500–504.

194. Poulos JE, Bacon BR. Liver transplantation for hereditary hemochromatosis. *Dig Dis Sci* 1996;14:316–322.

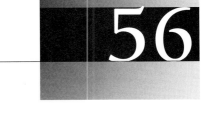

# Pancreatic Diseases

*Darwin L. Conwell*

This chapter addresses the following pancreatic conditions:

- Acute pancreatitis
- Chronic pancreatitis
- Pancreatic adenocarcinoma
- Endocrine neoplasms of the pancreas
- Gastrinoma
- Vasoactive intestinal polypeptide tumor (VIPoma)
- Glucagonoma
- Somatostatinoma

## ACUTE PANCREATITIS

Each year, more than 100,000 persons are admitted to the hospital for pancreatitis in the United States, and approximately 2,000 of them die from severe pancreatitis. Pancreatitis has many causes, an obscure pathogenesis, and few effective treatments. Most cases are mild (75%), but as many as 25% can be severe, with sequelae of systemic organ dysfunction.

### Anatomy and Physiology

The pancreas is a retroperitoneal organ approximately 12 to 20 cm in length and 70 to 120 g in weight. The organ head is apposed to the curvature of the duodenum, and the organ tail extends obliquely, posterior to the stomach, toward the hilum of the spleen. The pancreas has a rich blood supply from branches of the celiac, superior mesenteric, and splenic arteries. Venous drainage of the pancreas enters the hepatic portal system. Both sympathetic and parasympathetic efferent fibers supplied by the vagus and splanchnic nerves innervate the pancreas via the celiac plexuses.

The functional unit of the pancreas is the pancreatic acinus, composed of acinar and ductal cells. Acinar cells have a rich and highly specialized intracellular matrix for the synthesis, storage, and secretion of large amounts of proteins, mainly as digestive enzymes. The ductal cells primarily secrete water and electrolytes.

The three primary phases of postprandial pancreatic secretion include:

- Cephalic
- Gastric
- Intestinal

The cephalic phase is stimulated by the thought, sight, taste, or smell of food via vagal cholinergic innervation. The gastric phase occurs in response to gastric distention, which also is mediated by vagal cholinergic reflexes. The intestinal phase, which is the major phase of postprandial pancreatic secretion, is regulated primarily by the release of secretin and cholecystokinin (CCK). Secretin released into the blood from the duodenum is responsible for bicarbonate and water secretion from pancreatic ductal cells. CCK released into the circulation is primarily responsible for protease enzyme secretion from acinar cells; it also mediates secretin-stimulated electrolyte secretion.

Experimental evidence in rats suggests a feedback inhibition of pancreatic enzyme secretion by intraduodenal pancreatic proteases such as trypsin, chymotrypsin, and elastase. These pancreatic proteases inhibit the release of CCK and thus decrease pancreatic secretion.

## Pathophysiology

The pathophysiology of acute pancreatitis has been extensively studied in experimental models, which reveal a disruption in the normal separation of lysosomal and pancreatic enzymes and the formation of condensing vacuoles. The exposure of pancreatic proenzymes to lysosomal enzymes, such as cathepsin B, activates trypsinogen and leads to the premature activation of other pancreatic enzymes. In turn, this results in pancreatic autodigestion and the potential for profound systemic complications once the activated enzymes leak into the bloodstream.

## Etiology

Acute pancreatitis is caused by gallstones in approximately 45% of patients and by alcohol consumption in approximately 35%. In approximately 10% of cases, it is idiopathic or results from other causes (Table 56.1).

## Clinical Presentation

The typical symptoms of acute pancreatitis include acute abdominal pain, nausea, and vomiting. Patients may also

### TABLE 56.1
### CAUSES OF ACUTE PANCREATITIS

| Cause | Frequency (%) |
|---|---|
| Gallstones | 45 |
| Alcohol | 35 |
| Idiopathic | 10 |
| Other | 10 |
|   Drugs | |
|     Azathioprine | |
|     Thiazide | |
|     Valproic acid | |
|     Didanosine (2',3'-dideoxyinosine) | |
|     Sulfasalazine | |
|     Trimethoprim-sulfamethoxazole | |
|     Pentamidine | |
|     Tetracycline | |
|   Trauma | |
|   Postoperative | |
|   Hyperlipidemia | |
|   Hypercalcemia | |
|   Infectious agents | |
|     Mumps virus | |
|     Coxsackievirus B | |
|     Cytomegalovirus | |
|     *Candida* spp. | |
|     Human immunodeficiency virus | |
|     *Salmonella* spp. | |
|     *Shigella* spp. | |
|     *Escherichia coli* | |
|     *Legionella* spp. | |
|     *Leptospira interrogans* | |
|   Ductal obstruction | |

have reduced bowel sounds secondary to ileus. Jaundice may be evident in the presence of gallstones or compression of the common bile duct by an edematous pancreatic gland. In addition, patients may show evidence of subcutaneous necrosis on skin examination.

Laboratory features may include a transient mild hypoglycemia, hypocalcemia, hyperbilirubinemia, and mild elevations in the serum alanine transaminase and alkaline phosphatase levels. Patients with a bilirubin level greater than 2.5 times the normal value and a serum alanine transaminase twice the normal value are likely to have gallstone pancreatitis.

## Diagnosis

Acute pancreatitis is usually diagnosed on the basis of clinical findings and elevated serum amylase and lipase levels. It is also important to consider other causes of hyperamylasemia in the differential diagnosis; these include small bowel obstruction, perforation, infarction, or perforated duodenal ulcer. When a patient presents with acute pancreatitis, ultrasonography (US) of the right upper quadrant is the imaging modality of choice. This helps to delineate the presence or absence of gallstones and gives some idea of

## TABLE 56.2

### RANSON PROGNOSTIC CRITERIA FOR SEVERITY OF ACUTE PANCREATITIS

At admission
  Age >55 yr
  Leukocyte count >16,000 cells/mm3
  Plasma glucose >200 mg/dL
  Serum lactate dehydrogenase >350 U/L
  Serum aspartate transaminase >250 U/L
During initial 48 h
  Hematocrit decrease of >10%
  Serum urea nitrogen increase of >5 mg/dL
  Serum $Ca^{2+}$ <8 mg/dL
  $PAO_2$ <60 mm Hg
  Base deficit >4 mEq/L
  Fluid sequestration >6 L

the pancreatic morphology. Computed tomography (CT) is only recommended for patients with severe pancreatitis who show no improvement clinically after 72 hours of supportive therapy.

## Prognosis

The degree of elevation in the serum amylase and lipase levels has no prognostic value for determining the severity of pancreatitis. The most accurate method of determining severity within the first 48 hours after hospital admission is well described in the Ranson criteria (Table 56.2). The mortality increases considerably in patients with an increasing number of Ranson criteria. Patients with three or more criteria have severe pancreatitis. The Ranson criteria are no longer valid 48 hours after admission; the Acute Physiology and Chronic Health Evaluation II score is more reliable after this time. Patients with a score of 8 or greater have severe pancreatitis.

Dynamic CT, which is indicated in patients with severe pancreatitis, helps to determine whether necrotizing pancreatitis is present. Uniform enhancement on the scan implies an intact microcirculation and is suggestive of interstitial pancreatitis. Areas of nonenhancement indicate a disruption in pancreatic microcirculation, which is strongly suggestive of pancreatic necrosis. The infection rate in patients with interstitial pancreatitis is approximately 1%, whereas in patients with necrotizing pancreatitis, it is as high as 50%.

## Treatment

The treatment of acute interstitial pancreatitis is usually supportive, using intravenous fluids and analgesia. Patients with severe pancreatitis (i.e., Ranson score of 3 or higher, Acute Physiology and Chronic Health Evaluation score of 8 or higher, or organ dysfunction) require fine-needle aspiration (FNA) of necrotic areas in the pancreas to rule out infection.

These patients also require monitoring in an intensive care unit. Antibiotics do not decrease mortality, but they are strongly recommended. Antibacterial agents with good pancreatic tissue penetration are preferred; these include imipenem/cilastatin sodium (Primaxin) and ciprofloxacin (Cipro). If the Gram's stain of aspirated pancreatic tissue shows evidence of bacterial colonization, surgical debridement is recommended.

Patients with severe pancreatitis can have other systemic complications such as renal failure, acute respiratory distress syndrome, gastrointestinal bleeding, or hypotension. Local pancreatic complications include pancreatic abscess or pseudocyst formation. Pancreatic abscesses are infected primarily with *Escherichia coli* and require both antibiotic therapy and early surgical intervention. Pancreatic pseudocysts occur in approximately 20% of patients with acute pancreatitis and should be drained only if they cause symptoms.

Patients with gallstone pancreatitis who are deteriorating clinically or have evidence of biliary sepsis should undergo emergent endoscopic retrograde cholangiopancreatography (ERCP) for the removal of impacted gallstones. This should be followed by a cholecystectomy.

## CHRONIC PANCREATITIS

### Etiology

The most common cause of chronic pancreatitis—alcohol consumption—accounts for 70% of cases, and approximately 20% of cases are idiopathic. The remaining miscellaneous causes include trauma and prolonged metabolic disturbances (i.e., hypercalcemia, hypertriglyceridemia). Chronic pancreatitis can also be inherited as an autosomal dominant disorder (i.e., hereditary pancreatitis).

The underlying physiology involves a basal hypersecretion of pancreatic proteins with a concomitant decrease of protease inhibitors. This changes the biochemical composition of the pancreatic juice and predisposes patients to the formation of protein plugs and pancreatic stones. The blockage of small ducts results in the premature activation of pancreatic enzymes and the resultant development of acute pancreatitis that causes permanent structural damage to the gland over time.

### Clinical Presentation

The two most common clinical presentations of patients with chronic pancreatitis are abdominal pain and weight loss. The mechanism for abdominal pain is controversial, but it may involve inflammation of the pancreas, increased intrapancreatic pressure, neuroinflammation, or extrapancreatic causes, such as stenoses of the common bile duct and duodenum. Weight loss initially results from a decreased caloric intake because of fear of precipitating abdominal pain. Later, as the pancreatitis advances, pancreatic insufficiency develops, manifested as malabsorption or diabetes mellitus (DM).

## Diagnosis

The diagnosis of chronic pancreatitis is strongly suggested by the history and is confirmed through laboratory tests and imaging studies. The secretin- or CCK-stimulation test, which directly measures pancreatic bicarbonate secretion, has a sensitivity and specificity of approximately 90%. An indirect test of pancreatic function that measures urinary chymotrypsin output, the bentiromide (Chymex) test, has a sensitivity of approximately 85% and a specificity of 90%.

The presence of diffuse calcifications throughout the pancreas on radiography, US, or CT is diagnostic of chronic pancreatitis. Plain film radiography of the abdomen should be the first diagnostic test because it is both simple and inexpensive. US has a sensitivity of 70% and a specificity of 90%. CT increases the sensitivity and specificity by 10% to 30% over those of US alone.

ERCP is the most sensitive and specific diagnostic test for chronic pancreatitis, but it is an expensive procedure with a low but significant rate of complications, notably ERCP-induced pancreatitis. It should be reserved for patients in whom the diagnosis cannot be established clearly or for the evaluation of complications from chronic pancreatitis.

## Treatment

The treatment of chronic pancreatitis is usually supportive and involves control of pain, avoidance of alcohol, and use of adequate analgesics. At present, the mainstay of treatment involves the use of pancreatic enzymes to cause feedback inhibition of pancreatic secretion and thus decreased pancreatic ductal pressure.

Nonenteric-coated enzyme supplementation provides pancreatic protease (i.e., trypsin) to the duodenum in patients with pancreatic insufficiency. Enzyme supplementation decreases the pain of chronic pancreatitis, and enteric-coated preparations that protect lipase from gastric acid destruction help in the treatment of steatorrhea. A histamine $H_2$-receptor antagonist or proton pump inhibitor may be needed to decrease gastric acidity if enteric-coated preparations are not effective in decreasing steatorrhea. It is also important to rule out other causes of steatorrhea in patients whose disease is refractory; these include celiac sprue, Crohn's disease, and bacterial overgrowth.

Surgery is effective in decreasing abdominal pain, producing relief in 60% to 80% of patients. The mortality associated with surgery is 5% or less. A pancreaticojejunostomy is the procedure of choice in most patients.

## Complications

The most common complications in patients with chronic pancreatitis include:

- Pancreatic pseudocysts
- Ascites
- Splenic vein thrombosis

Pancreatic pseudocysts occur in approximately 25% of patients. Asymptomatic pseudocysts can be followed with serial US or CT. Most pseudocysts resolve in time. Large pseudocysts (usually 6 cm or greater) causing symptoms should be drained, either surgically or radiologically.

Patients with pancreatic ascites require ERCP to document the area of duct disruption, and medical treatment with total parenteral nutrition and octreotide (Sandostatin) supplementation has been shown to be effective. Patients who do not respond to medical treatment require surgical intervention.

Splenic vein thrombosis occurs in approximately 4% of patients. These patients are predisposed to gastrointestinal bleeding from gastric varices. The diagnosis is confirmed by celiac angiography, and splenectomy is curative.

# PANCREATIC ADENOCARCINOMA

## Etiology and Risk Factors

The risk factors for developing pancreatic carcinoma include cigarette smoking, a high-fat diet, chronic pancreatitis, hereditary pancreatitis, and industrial exposure to coal tar derivatives. Patients with chronic pancreatitis have a relative risk for pancreatic cancer that increases over time. In addition, hereditary pancreatitis increases the risk for pancreatic cancer fivefold.

## Clinical Presentation

The clinical presentation of pancreatic adenocarcinoma is pain, jaundice, weight loss, or new onset DM. Patients may also have superficial thrombophlebitis, gastrointestinal bleeding, or psychiatric disturbances.

## Diagnosis

The diagnosis usually is established through FNA of a mass seen on US or CT of the abdomen. ERCP has a sensitivity of approximately 90% in patients with negative imaging studies.

## Treatment and Prognosis

Surgery offers the only chance for cure; however, only 10% of patients have resectable tumors. The surgery of choice, a Whipple's procedure in patients with carcinoma at the head of the pancreas, carries a mortality of approximately 2%. Palliative procedures, such as gastrojejunostomy and endoscopic stenting procedures, are undertaken in patients with metastatic disease. Many attempts at radiation therapy and chemotherapy have met with poor results and produced no statistically significant beneficial effect on patient survival. Pancreatic ductal carcinoma has a 5-year survival rate of only 1%.

# ENDOCRINE NEOPLASMS OF THE PANCREAS

Pancreatic endocrine tumors (PETs) originate from the neuroendocrine cell system. PETs are classified as functional if associated with a clinical syndrome that is caused by hormone release. Nonfunctional PETs are those not associated with a clinical syndrome. Pancreatic polypeptide tumors are not associated with a clinical syndrome and are classified as nonfunctional. Histologically, PETs consist of homogenous, small, round cells with uniform nuclei and cytoplasm. The histologic classification fails to describe the growth pattern of the tumor or determine whether it is malignant. Malignancy can be determined only if a patient has evidence of metastatic disease or invasion. The malignant potential of these tumors varies on the basis of histologic type. Most PETs produce multiple hormones. The symptoms caused by these inappropriately released hormones are usually responsible for the initial clinical manifestations. Late in the disease, symptoms caused by the tumor (i.e., abdominal pain) become apparent. PETs may also be part of the multiple endocrine neoplasia type 1 syndrome.

## Gastrinoma

Gastrinomas are found in the pancreas or peripancreatic area in 90% of patients with PET. In 15%, they are located in the duodenal wall.

### Clinical Presentation
Zollinger-Ellison syndrome is characterized by gastric acid hypersecretion, peptic ulceration, and diarrhea. Approximately 25% to 30% of patients with gastrinomas have multiple endocrine neoplasia type 1 syndrome. A serum gastrin concentration greater than 1,000 pg/mL in patients who produce gastric acid is diagnostic of gastrinoma.

### Diagnosis
The diagnosis can be confirmed by the secretin test. An absolute increase in serum gastrin level to greater than 100 pg/mL above baseline confirms the diagnosis. CT or octreotide scanning can localize the tumor.

### Treatment and Prognosis
Patients with Zollinger-Ellison syndrome should be explored surgically for isolated tumors. Patients with multifocal tumors and metastatic disease are not candidates for resection. Omeprazole (Prilosec) minimizes symptoms, and total gastrectomy may be performed in patients who do not respond to medical treatment. Chemotherapy using streptozocin (Zanosar) and fluorouracil (Adrucil) is effective. Approximately 50% of patients with gastrinoma die within 10 years because of metastatic disease.

## Vasoactive Intestinal Polypeptide Tumor

Patients with VIPomas usually present with watery secretory diarrhea and profound hypokalemia. The condition is also commonly called the *Verner-Morrison syndrome*; pancreatic cholera; or watery diarrhea, hypokalemia, and achlorhydria syndrome. The mean age at presentation is 50 years, with a range of 32 to 81 years. There is a female predominance. VIPomas tend to be large and may be detected on CT or US. The diagnosis is established by an elevated serum vasoactive intestinal polypeptide concentration greater than 200 pg/mL and by a pancreatic tumor on imaging studies. Definitive therapy is surgical resection; in many patients, octreotide controls diarrheal symptoms.

## Glucagonoma

Glucagonomas are extremely rare tumors of pancreatic α-cells. The clinical presentation includes DM, necrolytic migratory erythema (a migratory, necrolytic, erythematous rash), stomatitis, glossitis, and weight loss. Most glucagonomas are large at the time of diagnosis, ranging from 0.4 to 35.0 cm in size. Cutaneous lesions are one of the most common and visible manifestations of the disease, occurring in up to 90% of patients. The skin lesions can precede the diagnosis by a mean of 6 to 8 years and are the primary initial clinical manifestation of the disease. Characteristically, the skin lesions start as an erythematous area at the periorofacial or intertriginous areas (e.g., groin, buttocks, thighs, perineum) and then spread laterally. The lesions become raised, blister, and eventually rupture to leave central pigmented areas surrounded by edges that continue to spread, with crusting, well-defined edges. The diagnosis is confirmed by an elevated fasting plasma glucagon level greater than 400 pg/mL in the presence of a characteristic skin rash. Surgical resection is the definitive therapy; symptoms may be controlled using octreotide.

## Somatostatinoma

Somatostatinomas are pancreatic tumor cells that arise from D cells. They are the least common type of PET, and fewer than 50 cases have been reported. The characteristic triad of symptoms includes DM, cholelithiasis, and diarrhea with steatorrhea. The development of DM and gallbladder disease is due to the inhibitory action of somatostatin on insulin release and gallbladder emptying. The diagnosis is established by a somatostatin level greater than 200 pg/mL. No effective treatment is known, but chemotherapy using streptozocin and fluorouracil may have some value.

# REVIEW EXERCISES

## QUESTIONS

**1.** A 76-year-old woman with ERCP-induced pancreatitis continues to have fever (39°C) with a rising white blood cell count on the fourth hospital day. Dynamic CT reveals an area of nonenhancement in the pancreas.

What is the appropriate next step in the treatment of this patient?

**a)** FNA of the pancreas
**b)** Angiography
**c)** Magnetic resonance imaging
**d)** Total parenteral nutrition

**2.** A 21-year-old woman has had recurrent abdominal pain since 3 years of age. She gives a history of similar symptoms in an uncle who died of pancreatic cancer at age 45 years. Kidney-ureter-bladder imaging shows extensive calcification in the upper abdomen.

Which is most likely diagnosis for this patient?

**a)** Celiac sprue
**b)** Zollinger-Ellison syndrome
**c)** Hereditary pancreatitis
**d)** Gastric carcinoma

**3.** A 50-year-old man with DM and a history of intermittent diarrhea is noted to have a small pancreatic mass during laparoscopic cholecystectomy for gallstones.

Which serologic test would you perform?

**a)** Vasoactive intestinal polypeptide
**b)** Calcitonin
**c)** Somatostatin
**d)** Urinary 5-hydroxyindoleacetic acid

**4.** A 35-year-old man presents to the outpatient clinic for evaluation of diarrhea and weight loss. Esophagogastroduodenoscopy performed to obtain a small bowel biopsy sample reveals esophageal erythema with occasional erosions, gastric ulcers, and multiple duodenal ulcerations. The biopsy sample shows blunted or flattened villi.

Which serologic or diagnostic procedure would you perform next?

**a)** ERCP
**b)** Colonoscopy
**c)** Gastrin
**d)** Antigliadin or antiendomysium antibodies

## ANSWERS

**1. a.**
This woman has persistent symptoms suggesting complicated acute pancreatitis. Dynamic CT is indicated to determine whether the blood supply to the pancreas has been compromised and if pancreatic necrosis is present. The presence of necrosis on CT requires prompt evaluation for infection. FNA with Gram's stain has been shown to be most effective at determining the presence or absence of microorganisms.

**2. c.**
This woman has the classic presentation of hereditary pancreatitis: acute bouts of abdominal pain starting in childhood with the eventual development of chronic pancreatitis. Her family history is positive for pancreatitis. Patients with hereditary pancreatitis have a fivefold greater risk for pancreatic cancer than the risk in the average population.

**3. c.**
The classic symptoms of diarrhea, DM, and gallstones raises the suspicion of the rare somatostatinoma tumor. The inhibitory effects of somatostatin cause the clinical manifestations.

**4. c.**
This man has the cardinal features of Zollinger-Ellison syndrome; a serum gastrin level test is indicated. In addition to inflammation and ulceration in the upper gastrointestinal tract, patients with Zollinger-Ellison syndrome may have diarrhea. Zollinger-Ellison syndrome also causes blunting of the small intestinal villi similar to that seen in celiac disease.

## SUGGESTED READINGS

Meko JB, Nortan JA. Endocrine tumors of the pancreas. *Curr Opin Gen Surg* 1994;186–194.

Steer ML, Waxman I, Freedman S. Chronic pancreatitis. *N Engl J Med* 1995;332:1482–1490.

Steinberg W, Tenner S. Acute pancreatitis. *N Engl J Med* 1994;330:1198–1210.

Warshaw AL, Fernandez-del Castillo C. Pancreatic carcinoma. *N Engl J Med* 1992;326:455–465.

# Esophageal Diseases

*Joel E. Richter*

**57**

The esophagus is a relatively simple, tubular organ connecting the oropharynx with the stomach. The pleasures of eating and maintaining adequate nutrition require a normal, healthy esophagus. The esophagus has three major functions:

- To transport ingested material from the oropharynx to the stomach
- To prevent the regurgitation of food and gastric contents from the stomach into the esophagus
- To vent ingested air to reduce abdominal bloating

## ANATOMY AND PHYSIOLOGY

The esophagus can be divided into three functional regions:

- Upper esophageal sphincter (UES)
- Esophageal body
- Lower esophageal sphincter (LES)

### Upper Esophageal Sphincter

The UES consists of striated muscle, which is formed primarily by the horizontal fibers of the cricopharyngeus muscle at the level of vertebrae C5 and C6. Similar to the striated muscles of the oropharynx and upper portion of the esophagus, the UES is innervated, and it receives motor input directly from the brainstem (i.e., nucleus ambiguus) to the motor endplates in the muscles. The UES is tonically closed, and it opens momentarily in response to a swallow (i.e., the first function). The UES also forms a secondary barrier that prevents the aspiration of gastroesophageal contents (i.e., the second function).

### Esophageal Body

The esophageal body consists of an empty tube lined by squamous mucosa, composed of a submucosal layer and two layers of muscles (i.e., the inner circular and outer longitudinal muscles). No serosa overlies the muscle layers. The upper portion of the esophagus is primarily striated muscle, whereas the lower two thirds is predominately smooth muscle.

The nerve network for the esophageal body lies between the muscle layers. The Meissner (submucosal) plexus is between the muscularis mucosae and the circular muscle layer; the Auerback (myenteric) plexus is between the circular and longitudinal muscle layers. Similar to the LES, innervation of the smooth muscles portion of the esophageal body occurs primarily via the vagus nerve, from neurons arising in the dorsal motor nucleus of the brainstem and from nerve endings in the myenteric plexus.

At rest, the esophageal body is quiet, without motor activity. Normal esophageal motor activity is characterized by the orderly progression (peristalsis) of a contraction along the esophagus in coordination with the relaxation and contraction of the UES and LES. Figure 57.1 represents the pressure sequence of a normal, primary peristaltic wave, as measured with esophageal manometry. The single pressure complex that begins in the pharynx progressively opens the UES and moves sequentially down the esophageal body through an opened LES. The food bolus is pushed ahead by this peristaltic wave through the opened LES and into the stomach. These activities are initiated by the voluntary act of swallowing. Perpetuation through the distal esophagus, however, is controlled by the enteric nervous system.

### Lower Esophageal Sphincter

The LES is a high-pressure zone of smooth muscle straddling the diaphragm. It is composed of smooth muscle of the distal esophagus and striated muscle of the crural diaphragm, and it is the major component of the antireflux barrier. At rest, the LES is tonically contracted, which thus prevents the reflux of gastric contents. On swallowing, the LES relaxes and stays relaxed until the peristaltic wave reaches the end of the esophagus and produces sphincter closure. LES relaxation is vagally mediated via preganglionic cholinergic nerves and postganglionic, noncholinergic, nonadrenergic nerves. Candidates for inhibitory neurotransmitters include vasoactive intestinal polypeptide and nitric oxide.

Tonic contractions of the LES predominantly result from intrinsic muscle activity. LES pressure fluctuates greatly over time, even from minute to minute. Much of this fluctuation results from various extraesophageal factors that modulate LES pressure:

- Food ingested during meals (proteins increase and fats decrease LES pressure)

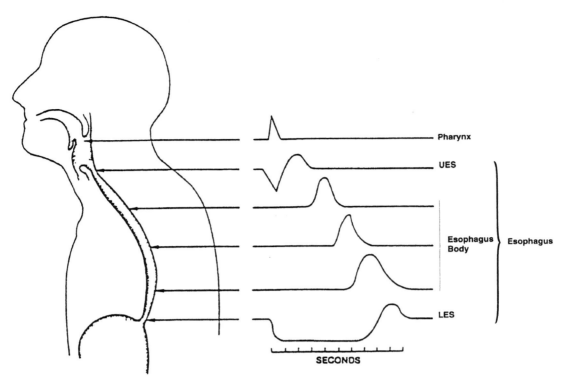

**Figure 57.1** Pressure sequences in swallowing. LES, lower esophageal sphincter; UES, upper esophageal sphincter.

- Cigarette smoking (decreases LES pressure)
- Gastric distention (decreases LES pressure)

Gastric distention is a critical trigger for transient LES relaxation, which is important in venting ingested gases. In response to transient increases in intraabdominal pressure, LES pressure increases to a greater degree than the increases occurring in the abdomen below, which thus prevents gastroesophageal reflux (GER). In addition, many hormones and peptides affect LES pressure. Those that increase LES pressure include:

- Gastrin
- Motilin
- Substance P
- Pancreatic polypeptide

Those that decrease LES pressure include:

- Secretin
- Cholecystokinin
- Glucagon
- Vasoactive intestinal polypeptide

## DIAGNOSTIC PROCEDURES

A thorough patient history and physical examination are critical in evaluating patients with esophageal disorders.

These often identify the appropriate diagnosis and direct further testing (Fig. 57.2).

### Imaging Techniques

The barium esophagram is the single most important test for the diagnosis of structural and motor abnormalities of the esophagus. A proper examination should include videotaping of the oropharyngeal and esophageal portions of swallowing, as well as full-column and air-contrast views of the distended esophagus, to identify mucosal irregularities, masses, and regions of luminal narrowing. A solid bolus, such as a marshmallow or tablet, should be administered to any patient with solid food dysphagia in whom a liquid study has been nondiagnostic. Esophageal peristalsis can be assessed in the prone position, with the patient taking five to ten single swallows of barium; this technique approximates esophageal manometry. To identify GER, the cause and extent of barium reflux should be evaluated by rolling the patient from side to side, having the patient cough, and performing the Valsalva maneuver and the water-siphon test.

Solid food scintigraphy, with the patient upright, best approximates normal food ingestion and bolus transport. This is an excellent technique for measuring the completeness of LES relaxation and esophageal emptying, and it is especially helpful in patients with achalasia.

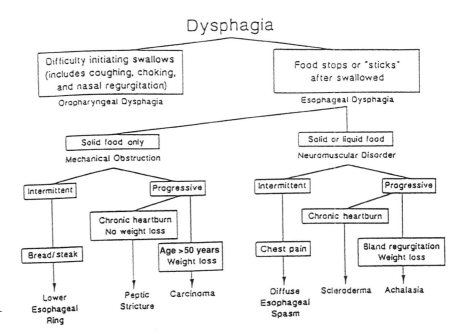

**Figure 57.2**  Diagnostic approach for patients with dysphagia.

A new imaging technique, endoscopic ultrasonography, is useful in diagnosing and staging both benign and malignant esophageal neoplasms. It is superior to computed tomography (CT) in evaluating the depth of tumor infiltration and assessing regional lymph node metastases.

## Esophageal Motility Studies

Manometry is the definitive test for diagnosing esophageal motility disorders because it allows an accurate measurement of sphincter pressures and esophageal pressure waves and more completely evaluates abnormalities of esophageal peristalsis. The test is performed by placing a small catheter into the esophagus and measuring changes in intraluminal pressure simultaneously at multiple sites. Normal values for a broad range of ages have been developed with the use of commercially available equipment.

Esophageal manometry does have limitations, however. It accurately records esophageal pressures, but it does not reliably evaluate other important aspects of esophageal function, including completeness of sphincter relaxation, bolus movement, and esophageal emptying. These can best be evaluated with video-imaging techniques.

## Endoscopy and Mucosal Biopsy

Fiberoptic endoscopy using biopsy and brush cytology is the best method for identifying mucosal abnormalities of the esophagus. The procedure usually is performed on an outpatient basis, with local and sometimes intravenous anesthesia. A small, flexible endoscope, passed orally, permits a thorough evaluation of the esophagus, stomach, and duodenum. Endoscopy is the preferred method for identifying reflux esophagitis, infectious esophagitis, and

neoplasms. Mucosal biopsy is most helpful in identifying Barrett's esophagus, mild esophagitis, neoplasms, and infectious causes of esophagitis.

## Ambulatory Esophageal pH Monitoring

Prolonged ambulatory monitoring of the esophagus for as long as 24 hours is the most reliable means of diagnosing GER. The pH probe is placed transnasally 5 cm above the LES. GER is defined as a decrease in esophageal pH to less than 4. Data are collected in a lightweight box worn on a waist belt, and the information is analyzed by computer. This test usually is performed on an outpatient basis, which allows physiologic activities to be monitored in the supine and upright positions, during wakefulness and sleep, during fasting, and after eating. Recording units have an event marker that can be triggered when symptoms occur. This technique allows the accurate quantitation of acid reflux and permits a correlation between acid reflux and subjective symptoms such as chest pain, cough, heartburn, and wheezing.

## Testing for Esophageal Sensory Mechanisms

Tests assessing esophageal sensory mechanisms are used when the esophagus is suspected of causing atypical symptoms of chest pain. The most commonly used tests include the acid-perfusion Bernstein test for identifying an acid-sensitive esophagus and the edrophonium chloride test for identifying the esophagus as the source of chest pain. Other provocative tests include:

■ Injection of bethanechol chloride, pentagastrin (Peptavlon), or ergonovine maleate (Ergotrate Maleate)

- Infusion of hypertonic solutions
- Esophageal balloon distention

# COMMON ESOPHAGEAL DISEASES

## Gastroesophageal Reflux Disease

GER disease (GERD)—with heartburn as its major symptom—is the most common disorder of the esophagus, the major indication for antacid consumption, and probably the most prevalent condition originating from the gastrointestinal tract. According to a recent Gallup survey, 44% of adults in the United States experience heartburn at least once every month, and 10% complain of weekly symptoms. More than 40% take antacids for their heartburn, but only 25% discuss this complaint with a physician. Pregnant women have the highest prevalence of heartburn, with at least 25% having daily symptoms, usually in the third trimester.

GERD is defined as the sequelae, both clinical and histopathologic, of the chronic movement of gastroduodenal contents into the esophagus. GERD, however, represents a spectrum of disease; for example, it occurs without adverse consequences in many healthy individuals. Episodes of "physiologic" reflux typically are postprandial, short-lived, and asymptomatic, and almost never occur at night. Pathologic reflux leads to inflammatory changes and mucosal injury (i.e., reflux esophagitis) and is usually accompanied by symptoms.

### Pathophysiology

The pathophysiology of GERD reflects a complex interplay of multiple factors (Fig. 57.3). The common denominator for acid reflux is a creation of a common cavity, representing an equilibration of intragastric and intraesophageal pressures. The LES is the major barrier against GER, with a sec-

ondary barrier formed by the crural diaphragm during inspiration, but measurement of a single LES pressure is not very discriminatory. In fact, recent studies determined that transient LES relaxation, occurring with either normal or low LES pressures, is the major mechanism promoting the free reflux of gastric contents. Transient relaxation accounts for nearly all episodes of GER in normal subjects and 65% of episodes in patients with GERD. Other patients experience GER because of very low baseline LES pressures, with either transient increases in intraabdominal pressure (i.e., stress reflux) or spontaneous reflux across an atonic sphincter.

Esophageal acid clearance normally occurs as a two-step process:

- Swallow-induced, peristaltic esophageal contractions rapidly clear fluid volume from the esophagus.
- The small amount of residual acid is neutralized by saliva, which has a pH of 6.4 to 7.8.

A dysfunction of esophageal clearance mechanisms contributes to esophagitis, particularly in patients with severe motility disorders (e.g., scleroderma) or sicca complex.

Both the nature and volume of gastric contents are important. The primary role of acid is indisputable, but its mechanism of mucosal damage involves the action of coexisting pepsin more than direct damage from acid alone. In animal models, bile salts and pancreatic enzymes can produce esophagitis, but their importance in human disease is unknown. Acid hypersecretory states (e.g., Zollinger-Ellison syndrome) may be associated with a high prevalence of esophagitis. Delayed gastric emptying promotes GER but is an important factor in only 10% to 15% of patients with GERD.

The same degree of acid exposure may lead to variable degrees of mucosal damage, which probably relates to individual variations in esophageal mucosal resistance. Factors contributing to mucosal resistance include:

- Mucus
- Bicarbonate ions secreted by submucosal glands
- Stratified squamous cells and their tight junctions
- Mucosal blood flow

The relationship between a sliding hiatal hernia and the development of GERD remains controversial. Most patients with esophagitis have a sliding hiatal hernia, but many patients with hiatal hernias do not have GERD. Recent evidence suggests that a large, nonreducible hernia may interfere with normal esophageal clearance by acting as a fluid trap, thus promoting acid reflux during swallow-induced LES relaxations, particularly in the supine position.

### Clinical Presentation

The symptoms of GERD include:

- Heartburn
- Associated symptoms
- Dysphagia

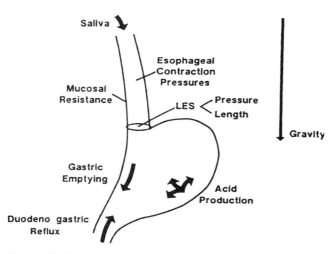

**Figure 57.3** Pathogenesis of gastroesophageal reflux disease. LES, lower esophageal sphincter.

- Odynophagia
- Regurgitation
- Water brash
- Belching

Patients describe their heartburn as a retrosternal burning pain, which may also be noted in the epigastrium, neck, throat, and occasionally the back. Frequently, it occurs post-prandially, and it is exacerbated by lying down or bending over. In patients with heartburn, dysphagia is suggestive of a peptic stricture. Other alternative diagnoses include severe inflammation without stricture, peristaltic dysfunction, and an esophageal cancer arising in a Barrett's esophagus. Odynophagia usually represents ulcerative esophagitis. The effortless regurgitation of acidic fluid, especially postprandi-ally and at night, is highly suggestive of GERD. Water brash is the sudden appearance in the mouth of a slightly sour or salty fluid from the salivary glands in response to intrae-sophageal acid exposure.

GERD may present with extraesophageal symptoms, including:

- Chest pain
- Respiratory complaints
- Ear, nose, and throat problems

In these patients, the clinical symptoms of heartburn or regurgitation may be mild or even absent. Recent studies indicate that GERD may be the major cause of noncardiac chest pain in as many as 50% of patients. Chronic cough, recurrent aspiration pneumonia, and pulmonary fibrosis may relate to GERD, and some studies suggest a close association between asthma and GERD, with up to 80% of patients with asthma having evidence of excessive acid reflux on pH testing. Hoarseness, sore throat, halitosis, dental erosions, vocal cord granuloma, and even laryngeal cancer may be caused by the intermittent aspiration of gastric contents.

### Diagnosis
In most patients with classic symptoms of heartburn or regurgitation, the history is sufficiently typical to permit a trial of therapy without diagnostic tests. The following situations should lead to early investigation:

- Esophageal symptoms that do not respond to medical therapy
- Dysphagia and atypical presentations of suspected GERD
- Possible complications of GERD
- Consideration of antireflux surgery

Tests for GERD evaluate different variables in the disease spectrum; these variables include:

- Potential for reflux
- Hiatal hernia
- Esophageal damage
- Abnormal reflux
- Acid sensitivity

Specific tests include:

- Barium esophagography
- Endoscopy
- Mucosal biopsy
- Manometry
- Acid-perfusion Bernstein test
- 24-hour pH with symptom correlation

There is no single best selection of tests. These tests must be applied selectively, based on the information desired.

All patients with persistent symptoms of GER or with frequent relapses after histamine $H_2$-receptor antagonist therapy should have endoscopy to identify possible esophagitis or other complications of GERD. Patients with esophagitis and complications should undergo biopsy to exclude associated malignancies and Barrett's esophagus. One must remember, however, that most patients with GERD have no evidence of esophagitis at endoscopy.

Barium esophagography should be the first diagnostic procedure in most patients with dysphagia. Optimally administered, double-contrast barium esophagography detects erosive and ulcerative esophagitis in approximately 90% of patients. The radiologic detection of mild (i.e, nonerosive) esophagitis, however, is unreliable. Barium esophagography is also the preferred method for identifying hiatal hernia, and it is good for identifying GER fluoroscopically, particularly when provocative maneuvers are done.

Prolonged esophageal pH monitoring is helpful in patients with atypical presentations or difficult treatment problems, and it has essentially replaced the acid-perfusion Bernstein test. The most common indications for pH monitoring include:

- Noncardiac chest pain
- Suspected pulmonary or ear, nose, and throat presentations of GERD
- Intractable reflux symptoms associated with a negative workup

In addition, prolonged pH monitoring should be conducted before antireflux surgery if there is any question about the diagnosis. A pH evaluation is the single best test for diagnosing GERD, with a sensitivity of 85% and a specificity of greater than 95%.

Manometry of LES pressure is not considered to be a sensitive diagnostic test because fewer than 25% to 50% of patients with GERD have a low resting LES pressure (less than 10 mm Hg). Manometry is reserved for patients in whom another diagnosis (e.g., achalasia) is suspected, and it is mandatory before antireflux surgery to ensure adequate esophageal pump function.

### Treatment
The rationale for GERD therapy depends on a careful definition of specific aims (Table 57.1). In patients without esophagitis, the goal is simply to relieve the acid-related

## TABLE 57.1

### GENERAL APPROACH TO THE TREATMENT OF GASTROESOPHAGEAL REFLUX DISEASE

| | Symptoms without Esophagitis | Mild Esophagitis | Severe Esophagitis or Intractable Symptoms |
|---|---|---|---|
| Acute | Lifestyle changes<br>Medications p.r.n.<br>   H$_2$-receptor antagonists<br>   Antacids<br>   Alginic acid<br>   Prokinetics | Lifestyle changes<br>Daily to scheduled<br>  medications<br>H$_2$-receptor antagonists | Lifestyle changes<br>Daily to scheduled<br>  medications<br>Proton pump inhibitors |
| Maintenance | Medications p.r.n. as above | H$_2$-receptor antagonists | Proton pump inhibitors<br>Antireflux surgery |

p.r.n., as needed.

symptoms; in patients with esophagitis, the ultimate goal also is to heal esophagitis while preventing further complications, such as strictures and Barrett's metaplasia. These goals are set against a complex background, however. GERD is a chronic condition, and patients with esophagitis generally experience relapse when medical therapy is stopped.

### Lifestyle Modifications

Lifestyle changes are the cornerstone of effective antireflux treatment in all patients; these are summarized in Table 57.2.

### Antacids and Alginic Acid

Antacids and alginic acid are useful for treating mild, infrequent reflux symptoms, especially those brought on by lifestyle indiscretions. They are not effective in healing esophagitis, however. Antacids work primarily by neutralizing acid, albeit for relatively short periods. Therefore, patients need to take these agents frequently, usually 20 to 30 minutes after meals and at bedtime. Aluminum hydroxide antacids containing alginic acid form a highly viscous solution that floats on the surface of the gastric pool and acts as a mechanical barrier. Recent studies confirm that

## TABLE 57.2

### LIFESTYLE MODIFICATIONS FOR PATIENTS WITH GASTROESOPHAGEAL REFLUX DISEASE

| Decrease LES Pressure | Improve Acid Clearance | Avoid Direct Esophageal Irritants | Decrease Gastric Distention |
|---|---|---|---|
| Avoid certain foods | Elevate head of bed | Avoid citrus, spicy, or tomato-based products | Avoid large meals |
| Fats | Maintain upright position after meals | | Take evening meals several hours before retiring; lose weight |
| Chocolate | | Avoid medications causing pill-induced esophagitis | |
| Coffee | | | |
| Carminatives | | | |
| Avoid certain medications | | | |
| Theophylline | | | |
| Progesterone | | | |
| Antidepressants | | | |
| Nitrates | | | |
| Calcium channel blockers | | | |

LES, lower esophageal sphincter.

alginic acid tablets (Gaviscon) effectively prevent acid reflux in the upright position.

### Prokinetic Drugs

Bethanechol and metoclopramide (Reglan) are prokinetic drugs that effectively relieve symptoms of heartburn, but their efficacy in treating esophagitis is equivocal. Bethanechol, 25 mg, or metoclopramide, 10 mg, is taken 30 minutes before meals and at bedtime. Side effects are common in both young and elderly patients.

The prokinetic drug cisapride (Propulsid) is more effective than placebo and equal to $H_2$-receptor antagonists in controlling the symptoms of GER and healing mild esophagitis. Cisapride acts by promoting release of acetylcholine at the myenteric plexus, which thereby increases LES pressure, improves peristalsis amplitude, and accelerates gastric emptying. At a dose of 10 mg taken 30 minutes before meals and at bedtime, cisapride has minimal side effects, with abdominal cramps, borborygmi, and diarrhea being the most common. Cisapride has been removed from the market because of an association with dangerous cardiac arrhythmias and death, usually due to toxic blood levels resulting from drug interactions with macrolide antibiotics, antifungal agents, and antiviral drugs.

### $H_2$-Receptor Antagonists

The use of $H_2$-receptor antagonists achieved the first real breakthrough in the treatment of GERD, and it continues to be the backbone of therapy for mild reflux esophagitis. Despite advertising to the contrary, all $H_2$-receptor antagonists (i.e., cimetidine, ranitidine, famotidine, and nizatidine), when properly dosed, are equally effective at improving symptoms of reflux and healing mild to moderate GERD. These agents are usually given once or preferably twice daily. Recent data on patterns of acid exposure show that most acid reflux occurs during the early evening hours after dinner and that it decreases markedly during the sleeping hours. Therefore, it may be preferable to take an $H_2$-receptor antagonist 30 minutes after the evening meal rather than at bedtime. Heartburn can be significantly decreased by $H_2$-receptor antagonists and esophagitis healed in approximately 60% of patients after up to 12 weeks of treatment. Healing rates differ in individual trials, however, depending primarily on the degree of esophagitis before therapy. Mild esophagitis heals in 75% to 90% of patients, whereas moderate to severe esophagitis heals in only 40% to 50% of patients. Studies also suggest that $H_2$-receptor antagonists are effective in preventing a relapse of GERD in patients with reflux symptoms and mild esophagitis. The $H_2$-receptor antagonists are available over the counter at lower doses. Their efficacy is similar to that of antacids, although the duration of symptom relief may be longer. The over-the-counter preparations are best used for prophylaxis before refluxogenic activities (i.e., large meals, exercise, etc.).

### Proton Pump Inhibitors

Omeprazole (Prilosec), lansoprazole (Prevacid), rabeprazole (Aciphex), and pantoprazole (Protonix) are potent, long-acting inhibitors of both basal and stimulated acid secretion. They act by selective, noncompetitive inhibition of the $H^+/K^+$ adenosine triphosphatase pump on parietal cells. Proton pump inhibitors (PPIs) completely abolish reflux symptoms in most patients with severe GERD, usually within 1 to 2 weeks; complete healing of esophagitis occurs after 8 weeks in 80% of patients. PPIs are superior to $H_2$-receptor antagonists, but efficacy is similar across these four drugs. The newest PPI, however, esomeprazole magnesium trihydrate (Nexium), is a purified form of omeprazole and results in superior healing of esophagitis at 4 and 8 weeks. Pantoprazole is the only available intravenous PPI.

Side effects are minimal with short-term use, but the long-term safety of these drugs is not yet established past 15 years of continuous use. PPIs cause profound hypoacidity that stimulates gastrin release, which in turn promotes the proliferation of enterochromaffin-like cells in the gastric fundus. In the rat model, the prolonged use of omeprazole causes gastric carcinoids; however, such carcinoids have not been reported to date in humans treated for uncomplicated reflux or ulcer disease. The FDA has recently approved over-the-counter omeprazole (Prilosec) for 2-week use for frequent heartburn. If symptoms persist, then a physician should be seen. This class of drugs is most effective in patients with severe reflux symptoms and severe esophagitis, as well as in maintenance therapy to prevent relapse of esophagitis.

### Antireflux Surgery

Antireflux surgery, performed either by open or laparoscopic techniques, attempts to maintain a segment of the tubular esophagus below the diaphragm and usually includes wrapping the stomach around the distal esophagus to produce increased LES pressure. Long-term relief of symptoms occurs in approximately 80% of patients followed for up to 20 years. The preservation of esophageal function, as confirmed with esophageal testing before surgery, is critical for successful antireflux surgery, as is performance of the operation by a skillful surgeon. Indications for antireflux surgery include:

- Severe GERD in younger patients who would otherwise require lifelong medical therapy
- Recurrent, difficult-to-dilate strictures
- Nonhealing ulcers
- Severe bleeding from esophagitis
- Aspiration symptoms from related GERD

### Complications of GERD

#### Peptic Strictures

Peptic strictures represent the end stage of ongoing reflux, mucosal damage, healing, and secondary fibrosis. Patients with strictures present with slowly progressive dysphagia for solids, usually without much weight loss. Radiographically, peptic strictures are commonly found in the lower esophagus and are characterized by smooth-walled, tapered, circumferential narrowings. In all patients, the benign nature of the stricture must be confirmed through endoscopy and biopsy.

Therapy for peptic strictures consists of a careful review of dietary and medication habits, aggressive antireflux therapy, and bougienage. Patients should chew their food well, take fluids liberally, and avoid potentially damaging pills, such as aspirin, nonsteroidal anti-inflammatory drugs (NSAIDs), and potassium chloride. Aggressive acid suppression, particularly with PPIs, may reduce the need for subsequent dilations. Dilating (i.e., stretching) the narrowed distal esophagus with blunt bougies passed either freely or over a guidewire can markedly relieve symptoms of dysphagia.

### Barrett's Esophagus

Barrett's esophagus secondary to severe esophagitis produces a unique reparative process in which the original squamous epithelial lining is replaced by metaplastic columnar epithelium. The prevalence of Barrett's esophagus varies depending on the population being studied. Patients with symptomatic GERD have a prevalence rate of 5% to 12%, whereas those with esophagitis, scleroderma, or peptic strictures may have higher rates (11% to 44%). The diagnosis is best made with endoscopy and confirmed with biopsy. Barrett's epithelium may comprise three types of mucosa, but only the specialized columnar epithelium has malignant potential.

Therapy is no different from that for any other form of esophagitis. The major concerns are the increased prevalence and incidence of esophageal adenocarcinoma. The prevalence rate is estimated at 10%, which is thirty- to fortyfold greater than in the general population. The incidence rates are quite variable, however, ranging from 1 in 46 to 1 in 441 patient-years of follow-up. As with colonic adenomas, over time, the columnar lining of the esophagus may evolve through increasing degrees of dysplasia to cancer. For this reason, endoscopic surveillance is recommended in patients with Barrett's esophagus to detect high-grade dysplasia or early cancer, so that curative surgical resection can be performed.

## OTHER INFLAMMATORY DISORDERS OF THE ESOPHAGUS

Other disorders of the esophagus are usually acute in onset and characterized clinically by odynophagia and dysphagia. An algorithm for evaluating patients with odynophagia is shown in Figure 57.4.

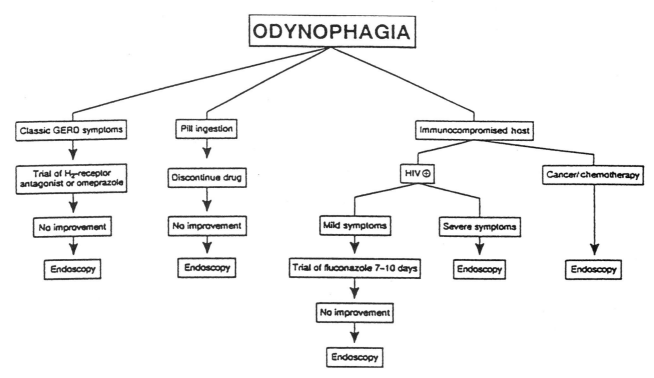

**Figure 57.4** Diagnostic approach for patients with odynophagia. GERO, gastroestophageal reflux disease; HIV⊕, human immunodeficiency virus-positive. (From Wilcox CM, Karowe NW. Esophageal infection: etiology, diagnosis, and management. *Gastroenterologist* 1994;2:188–206, with permission.)

## Infectious Esophagitis

Infections of the esophagus are rare in the general population. When present, however, they should prompt a search for an underlying immune abnormality. Esophageal infection is seen primarily in three groups of immunocompromised patients:

- Patients infected with the human immunodeficiency virus (HIV)
- Patients with cancer and granulocytopenia after chemotherapy
- Organ transplantation patients receiving immunosuppressive therapy

Other predisposing conditions include:

- Malignancy
- Alcoholism
- Diabetes mellitus
- Therapy with corticosteroids or other immunosuppressive agents

The most common causes of infectious esophagitis are:

- *Candida* species
- Herpes simplex virus
- Cytomegalovirus

Candidal esophagitis is most commonly seen in patients who are infected with HIV or have granulocytopenic cancer. Viral esophagitis predominates in patients who received bone marrow transplants. Both candidal and viral esophagitis are encountered after solid organ transplantation. Other less common causes of infectious esophagitis include:

- *Histoplasma* organisms
- *Mycobacterium tuberculosis*
- *Mycobacterium avium*-intracellulare complex
- *Cryptosporidium* species
- *Pneumocystis carinii*
- Epstein-Barr virus
- HIV
- Gram-negative and Gram-positive bacteria

Mixed infections are present in approximately 30% of patients, and esophageal infections should be suspected in immunocompromised patients presenting with odynophagia, dysphagia, or chest pain. Oral thrush is commonly sought, but its presence does not preclude infections with organisms besides *Candida*. In addition, its absence does not preclude *Candida*. Double-contrast barium esophagography has neither high sensitivity nor specificity for infectious esophagitis. Endoscopy with brush cytology, biopsy, and culture is the best initial diagnostic test.

Candidiasis is recognized by discrete, 3- to 5-mm, raised yellowish plaques or confluent cheesy exudates. The diagnosis is most easily established by brushing the plaques, smearing the material on a clear glass slide, allowing it to dry, and then applying 10% potassium hydroxide. The specimen is examined for the typical branched hyphae and budding yeast. Fungal cultures and the histologic examination of biopsy specimens are also helpful. The treatment of candidal esophagitis is determined by the severity of the infection and the nature of the underlying immune defect (Table 57.3).

Herpetic esophagitis is characterized by clear vesicles early in its course. Because these vesicles are short lived, however, the usual finding is discrete, small, superficial

## TABLE 57.3
### TREATMENT FOR COMMON ESOPHAGEAL INFECTIONS

| Infection | Treatment |
| --- | --- |
| *Candida* | |
| Minimal compromise (i.e., diabetes, steroids) | Nystatin, 1–3 million U q.i.d.; or clotrimazole, 100 mg t.i.d. |
| Acquired immunodeficiency syndrome | Ketoconazole, 200–400 mg daily; or fluconazole, 100 mg daily |
| Failure of above | Amphotericin B, 0.3–56.4 mg/kg/day |
| Herpes simplex virus | |
| Immunocompetent patient | Supportive care |
| | Analgesics |
| | Topical anesthetics |
| Immunocompromised patient | |
| Mild cases | Acyclovir, 200–400 mg p.o. 5 times daily |
| More severe cases | Acyclovir, 15 mg/kg/day i.v. |
| Cytomegalovirus | Ganciclovir, 5 mg/kg i.v. every 12 h; or foscarnet, 60 mg/kg/day i.v. every 8 h |
| Human immunodeficiency virus | Prednisone, 40 mg daily |

(Modified with permission from Wilcox CM, Karowe NW. Esophageal infection: etiology, diagnosis, and management. *Gastroenterologist* 1994;2:188–206.)

ulcers with a punched-out appearance and raised yellow edges. The intervening mucosa often appears normal. Brushings and biopsy specimens show cytologic changes that may be suggestive of herpetic infection (i.e., Cowdry type A inclusions).

Cytomegalovirus esophagitis appears as an extensive area of mucosal injury with inflammatory exudate and ulcerations. The ulcers are very deep, progress in size, and occasionally perforate. Biopsy specimens, brush cytologic examination, or viral culture may show evidence of cytomegalovirus. Esophageal ulcerations have been described in patients who undergo HIV seroconversion. These patients present with a syndrome characterized by fever, myalgia, maculopapular rash, and odynophagia. Endoscopy shows multiple discrete esophageal ulcerations, and the electron microscopy of tissue shows retroviral organisms, which thus indicates HIV as the direct cause.

### Pill-Induced Esophagitis

More than 50% of cases of pill-induced esophagitis result from tetracycline hydrochloride or tetracycline derivatives, particularly doxycycline. Other commonly prescribed medications causing esophageal injury include:

- Slow-release potassium chloride
- Iron sulfate
- Quinidine sulfate
- Alendronate sodium (i.e., Fosamax)
- NSAIDs

A common factor among these patients is a history of improper pill ingestions. In nearly 50% of reported cases, patients took little or no fluid while swallowing their pills, or took their pills just before bedtime. Patients with pill-induced esophageal injury generally complain of odynophagia and retrosternal burning; only a minority report that pills get stuck in the chest. Endoscopy, which is the first investigative study, usually reveals discrete ulcers at the aortic arch or distal esophagus.

Pill-induced esophagitis improves after withdrawal of the offending medication. Symptomatic resolution and endoscopic healing are usually evident after 3 days to 6 weeks. In addition to drug discontinuation, other therapies include palliation of odynophagia with viscous lidocaine, prevention of acid reflux, and assurance of adequate nutrition. Rarely, strictures requiring dilation develop. To prevent further pill-induced esophageal injuries, patients should be encouraged to ingest all pills with 8 oz of water while standing or sitting upright, and they should be discouraged from taking pills just before bedtime.

## ESOPHAGEAL MOTILITY DISORDERS

Functional disturbances of the esophagus may result from either neurologic or muscular disorders and may involve the striated muscle, smooth muscle, or both muscle segments. The most common motility abnormalities involved the distal smooth muscle.

### Achalasia

Achalasia is characterized by a double defect in esophageal function. The LES does not relax appropriately and thus offers resistance to the flow of liquids and solids from the esophagus into the stomach. In addition, peristaltic muscle movement is lost in the lower two-thirds (i.e., smooth muscle portion) of the esophagus. Achalasia usually develops between 25 and 60 years of age, and men and women are affected equally. The cause is unknown, but the two most popular theories suggest that achalasia is secondary to an infection or a degenerative disease of neurons. In South America, infection with the protozoan *Trypanosoma cruzi* produces ganglion damage and an achalasia-like syndrome with megaesophagus, but this is rarely seen in the United States.

#### Pathophysiology

Abnormalities in both muscle and nerves can be detected in patients with achalasia, but a neural lesion is thought to be of primary importance. Three major neuroanatomic changes are described:

- Loss of ganglion cell within the Auerbach plexus
- Degeneration of the vagus nerve
- Qualitative and quantitative changes in the dorsal motor nucleus of the vagus

Selective damage occurs to inhibitory neurons, with marked reduction in the levels of vasoactive intestinal polypeptide and nitric oxide receptors, which can account for the observed motility disturbances. Further evidence of denervation is the exaggerated contractions in the LES and esophageal body that are observed when these patients are given methacholine; this response indicates denervation hypersensitivity.

#### Clinical Presentation

Nearly all patients with achalasia have dysphagia for solids, and most also have dysphagia for liquids. The onset is gradual, and most have symptoms for an average of 2 years before the diagnosis is made. Postural changes, such as throwing the shoulders back, lifting the neck, and performing a rapid Valsalva maneuver, help improve esophageal emptying. Fullness in the chest and regurgitation of undigested, nonacidic food are also seen in many patients. Undigested food may be regurgitated postprandially or at night, with the regurgitation causing choking, cough, and aspiration pneumonia. Chest pain occurs in some patients and is more common in younger patients with earlier disease. Surprisingly, heartburn sometimes is described, presumably because of the fermentation of intraesophageal contents. Weight loss is very common and usually increases with disease duration.

## Diagnosis

In a patient with suspected achalasia, the first diagnostic test is a barium esophagram. Early in the course of disease, the esophagus may appear normal in diameter but has a loss of normal peristalsis. As the disease progresses, the esophagus becomes more dilated and tortuous, with retained food and presence of air-fluid levels. The distal esophagus is characterized by a smooth, symmetric, tapering, bird-beak appearance. Clues to the diagnosis may also be found on chest radiographs; these include:

- Widened mediastinum
- Thoracic air-fluid level
- Absence of the gastric air bubble

The diagnosis of achalasia is confirmed through esophageal manometry (Table 57.4). Characteristic manometric features include:

- Absence of peristalsis in the distal smooth muscle esophagus
- Incomplete or abnormal LES relaxation
- Elevated LES pressure
- Elevated intraesophageal pressure relative to gastric pressure

All patients with achalasia should undergo upper gastrointestinal endoscopy to differentiate primary achalasia from pseudoachalasia, which is usually secondary to an adenocarcinoma.

## Treatment

The goal of therapy in patients with achalasia is to diminish the high residual LES pressure after swallowing. If esophageal emptying is improved, esophageal stasis and its consequences are reduced. Peristalsis rarely returns, but patients feel as if swallowing is nearly normal. Three treatments are available:

- Pharmacologic therapy
- Pneumatic dilation
- Surgical myotomy

### Pharmacologic Therapy

Smooth muscle relaxants, including sublingual isosorbide dinitrate, or a calcium antagonist, such as nifedipine, can be used prophylactically with meals or as necessary for pain or dysphagia. These medications provide variable relief of symptoms, but their effectiveness tends to decrease with time. Botulinim toxin injection into the LES during endoscopy has been shown to improve symptoms for 3 months to 1 year. It may be preferred treatment in the elderly or subjects with severe comorbid illnesses who are not good candidates for more definitive treatments.

### Pneumatic Dilation

Pneumatic dilation involves placing a balloon across the LES and then inflating it to a pressure adequate to tear the muscle fibers of the sphincter. Good to excellent results occur in 50% to 90% of patients. The procedure can be performed on an outpatient basis, recovery is rapid, and discomfort is short lived. Approximately 30% of patients may require subsequent dilations, however, and perforation is a major complication, reported in approximately 2.5% of patients and usually requiring surgical repair.

### Surgical Myotomy

Heller myotomy involves incising the circular muscle of the LES and the more distal esophagus down to the mucosa and allowing the muscle to protrude through the incision. Myotomy produces good to excellent results in 60% to 90% of patients, and the operative mortality rate is low. To prevent postoperative GER, many surgeons now add a loose antireflux operation to the myotomy. Laparoscopic and thoracoscopic techniques for esophageal myotomy have

## TABLE 57.4

### MANOMETRIC CHARACTERISTICS OF ESOPHAGEAL MOTILITY DISORDERS

| | Achalasia | Spastic Motor Disorder | | | Scleroderma |
| | | DES | Nutcracker | Hypertensive LES | |
|---|---|---|---|---|---|
| Striated muscle/UES | Normal | Normal | Normal | Normal | Normal |
| Smooth muscle | Aperistalsis | Intermittent peristalsis | Normal peristalsis | Normal peristalsis | Low-amplitude peristalsis or aperistalsis |
| | | Simultaneous, repetitive High amplitude Long duration Spontaneous | High amplitude | | |
| LES | Abnormal relaxation High pressure | Occasional LES dysfunction | Normal | High pressure Normal relaxation | Low or no pressure |

DES, diffuse esophageal spasm; LES, lower esophageal sphincter; UES, upper esophageal sphincter.

replaced the open procedure, which was usually done through the left chest and had a longer hospitalization and recovery period.

## Spastic Motility Disorders

Spastic manometric patterns differ from those of achalasia by the following characteristics:

- Normal peristalsis intermittently interrupted by simultaneous contractions
- High-amplitude or long-duration waves
- Dysfunction of the LES

Confusion has arisen, however, concerning whether these manometric abnormalities represent separate, distinct entities or variations of diffuse esophageal spasm (Table 57.4). The similarities among these disorders in presentation, natural history, and treatment suggest that these syndromes frequently overlap and that they should be designated as spastic motility disorders of the esophagus.

### Pathophysiology

The cause and pathogenesis of these disorders is unknown, and no specific, characteristic pathologic lesion is present. Spastic motility abnormalities are commonly associate with other medical conditions, particularly GER. Central nervous system processing could produce some of these manometric abnormalities. Psychologically stressful interviews, loud noises, or difficult mental tasks can produce simultaneous waves and increase contraction amplitudes in the distal esophagus of both normal persons and patients with spastic motility disorders. These patients also appear to have both a motor and sensory component to their spastic disorder. Acid instillation may stimulate sensitive neural receptors, thus producing esophageal pain at low distention volumes without the accompaniment of noticeable motor changes.

### Clinical Presentation

Spastic disorders of the esophagus generally develop during middle age and occur more commonly in women. Dysphagia and chest pain are the cardinal symptoms; most patients present with both. Dysphagia for liquids and solids is present in 30% to 60% of patients. The symptom is intermittent, however, and it varies daily from mild to very severe, although usually it is not progressive or severe enough to interfere with eating or produce weight loss. Intermittent anterior chest pain, sometimes mimicking that of angina pectoris, is reported by most patients. Episodes of pain last from minutes to hours and may require narcotics or nitroglycerin, which further confuses the distinction between esophageal and cardiac pain. Many patients also have symptoms compatible with that of irritable bowel syndrome, and accompanying urinary and sexual dysfunction may be present in women.

### Diagnosis

Spastic motility disorders are best defined using esophageal manometry. A patient's chief symptom is an important factor in identifying the prevalence and type of motility disorder. In patients with diffuse esophageal spasm, the barium esophagram may reveal severe, lumen-obliterating tertiary contractions that trap barium and delay transit and thereby produce a to-and-fro movement of the bolus. Other spastic motility disorders frequently yield a normal barium esophagram. Endoscopy may be done, but its major role is to identify possible structural lesions or rule out reflux esophagitis. Provocative tests, such as the edrophonium chloride and balloon distention tests, may be able to provoke chest pain. Ambulatory 24-hour pH monitoring is useful to identify associated GERD, which is present in 20% to 50% of these patients.

### Treatment

Many patients respond favorably to confident reassurance that their chest pain has an esophageal origin and is not coming from the heart. GER should be identified and aggressively treated; otherwise, no single drug has a proved efficacy in the treatment of spastic esophageal motility disorders. Smooth muscle relaxants, such as long-acting nitrates, calcium channel blockers, and anticholinergics, may decrease high-amplitude contractions, but they do not relieve chest pain consistently. Antidepressant medications may reduce the amount of discomfort experienced (as well as the patient's reaction to pain), but the esophageal motility abnormality does not change. Botulinim toxin injections into the lower esophagus may help chest pain and dysphagia. Passive dilation of the esophagus has no value; however, pneumatic dilation helps some patients with diffuse esophageal spasm or hypertensive LES who complain of severe dysphagia and have documented delays in esophageal emptying. In rare cases, a long surgical myotomy may help the patient. Aggressive interventions must be used cautiously, however, because symptoms may not be relieved.

## SCLERODERMA

Esophageal involvement is seen in 70% to 80% of patients with scleroderma, and more than 90% have associated Raynaud's phenomenon. Esophageal involvement is seen in patients with either progressive systemic sclerosis or CREST syndrome (calcinosis, Raynaud's phenomenon, esophageal involvement, sclerodactyly, and telangiectasia). The pathophysiology involves an abnormality in muscle excitation and responsiveness resulting from muscle atrophy and decreased cholinergic excitation.

The classic manometric features of advanced scleroderma include (Table 57.4):

- Low LES pressure

- Peristaltic dysfunction of the smooth muscle portion of the esophagus, characterized by low-amplitude contractions or aperistalsis
- Preserved function of the striated esophagus and oropharynx

Because of these manometric abnormalities, patients may have dysphagia and severe GERD. Surprisingly, dysphagia for solids and liquids is reported by fewer than 50% of patients with scleroderma. More severe dysphagia is suggestive of esophagitis, often with an associated stricture. Esophagitis is present in most patients.

The treatment of scleroderma centers around GER and its complications. Patients should chew their food well and drink plenty of fluids. GERD should be identified and aggressively treated using $H_2$-receptor antagonists or PPIs. Strictures respond to frequent dilations. In severe cases, antireflux surgery may be warranted.

## ESOPHAGEAL TUMORS

More than 90% of esophageal tumors are malignant. Squamous cell carcinoma, which is primarily a disease of African American men, remains the most common malignant tumor of the esophagus. Associated risk factors are the excessive use of tobacco and alcohol. Conversely, adenocarcinoma, seen mainly in white men, is a recognized complication of Barrett's esophagus resulting from chronic GER. Recently, a striking five- to sixfold increase has occurred in the incidence of adenocarcinoma of the esophagus, which has changed the ratio of squamous cell carcinoma cases to adenocarcinoma cases from 90% to 10%, to 60% to 40%.

Other types of malignant tumors of the esophagus are rare and include lymphoma and melanoma. Common benign tumors of the esophagus include:

- Leiomyoma
- Lipoma
- Granular cell tumor
- Squamous cell papilloma
- Esophageal cyst

## MISCELLANEOUS ESOPHAGEAL DISORDERS

### Esophageal Diverticula

An esophageal diverticulum is an outpouching of one or more layers of the esophageal wall. It occurs in three main areas:

- Immediately above the UES (i.e., Zenker diverticulum)
- Near the midpoint of the esophagus (i.e., traction diverticulum)
- Immediately about the LES (i.e., epiphrenic diverticulum)

Zenker diverticulum occurs in older patients, who complain of cervical dysphagia, gurgling in the throat, halitosis, regurgitation of foul food, and sometimes a neck mass. It was originally believed to relate to discoordination of UES relaxation, but recent studies show that the sphincter opens incompletely because of reduced muscle compliance. To compensate for this decreased cross-sectional area, the hypopharyngeal bolus pressure increases, which leads to dysphagia and diverticulum formation. Traction diverticula usually are asymptomatic. They are believed to occur secondary either to external inflammatory processes (e.g., tuberculosis) or to a localized segmental motility disorder. Epiphrenic diverticula are invariably associated with esophageal motility disorders, especially achalasia.

Diverticula are best diagnosed with barium esophagography; endoscopy is rarely required. The treatment of symptomatic diverticula requires surgery.

## Esophageal Tears and Perforations

Esophageal tears and perforations can result from the following:

- Prolonged and violent vomiting after a meal or alcoholic binge
- Instrumentation of the esophagus
- Ingestion of foods containing bones or sharp foreign objects

A mucosal tear at the gastroesophageal junction is known as a Mallory-Weiss tear. It can be asymptomatic or associated with significant upper gastrointestinal bleeding. In contrast, spontaneous esophageal rupture (i.e., Boerhaave syndrome) is a rare, life-threatening condition characterized by a full-thickness tear of the esophageal wall. Patients with Boerhaave syndrome present with:

- Severe substernal epigastric pain
- Dysphagia
- Odynophagia
- Dyspepsia

Findings include hypotension, fever, tachycardia, and subcutaneous emphysema. Radiographs frequently reveal pleural effusion, parenchymal infiltrates, pneumothorax, pneumomediastinum, and mediastinal widening.

The diagnosis is confirmed with a barium esophagram obtained with the use of a water-soluble contrast agent (e.g., meglumine diatrizoate). On confirmation, a nasogastric tube should be placed to provide continuous suction, and the patient should be given broad-spectrum antibiotics. Small, self-contained leaks can be treated successfully with conservative management, but larger tears require immediate surgery.

## Rings and Webs

The lower esophageal (Schatzki) ring, located at the squamocolumnar junction, is the most common source of intermittent dysphagia for solids. Rings are usually found in patients older than 50 years, and rarely in those younger than 30 years. The origin of the lower esophageal ring is unknown, but recent studies suggest that it is a complication of GERD. The diagnosis is made with the following:

- Barium swallow examination in the prone position
- Valsalva maneuver
- Having the patient swallow a marshmallow or tablet to bring out the ring

  Treatment includes:

- Simple reassurance with guidance for adjustment of eating habits
- Dilation of the ring with a blunt bougie
- Therapy for associated GERD

Webs are membranous narrowings covered entirely by squamous mucosa. They may occur anywhere along the esophagus but are found primarily in the upper 2 to 4 cm. Some webs are congenital; others are associated with iron deficiency anemia (i.e., Paterson-Kelly or Plummer-Vinson's syndrome). Most webs are asymptomatic and are discovered as incidental radiologic findings. Symptomatic patients are usually women reporting dysphagia for solids rather than liquids. The diagnosis is made using the lateral view of the barium esophagram. Treatment with bougienage often is successful.

## REVIEW EXERCISES

### QUESTIONS

**1.** Which of the following are the components of the LES?
a) Distal esophageal smooth muscle
b) Distal esophageal striated muscle
c) Crural portion of the diaphragm
d) a and c

**2.** A patient reports intermittent dysphagia for solid foods only, and especially for bread and meat. What is the cause?
a) Lower esophageal (Schatzki) ring
b) Esophageal cancer
c) Zenker diverticulum
d) Achalasia

**3.** Which is the most effective medication for relieving heartburn symptoms and healing esophagitis?
a) Antacids
b) Cisapride
c) $H_2$-receptor antagonists
d) PPIs

**4.** Achalasia is usually *not* characterized by which of the following symptoms?

a) Dysphagia for solids and liquids
b) Dysphagia for solids only
c) Bland regurgitation
d) Heartburn

**5.** Which pill is most commonly associated with esophagitis?
a) NSAIDs
b) Quinidine
c) Doxycycline
d) Slow-release potassium

**6.** Which of these diseases has been associated with GERD?
a) Noncardiac chest pain
b) Asthma
c) Dental erosion
d) Laryngeal cancer
e) All of the above

**7.** Which statement is not true about Barrett's esophagus?
a) It results from long-standing acid.
b) The diagnosis is made by endoscopy.
c) The prevalence rate of developing adenocarcinoma is approximately 10%.
d) Endoscopic surveillance is recommended for healthy patients with Barrett's esophagus.

**8.** The best treatment for achalasia in a healthy patient is:
a) Botulinim toxin injection
b) Pneumatic dilation
c) Heller myotomy with fundoplication
d) Either b or c

### ANSWERS

**1. d.**
The LES has two components. Basal pressure is generated by the distal esophageal smooth muscle. The increased sphincter pressure that occurs during inspiration is generated by the crural diaphragm. This augmentation prevents GER upon deep inspiration efforts.

**2. a.**
A lower esophageal ring presents classically with dysphagia for solids and no weight loss. With esophageal cancer, progressive dysphagia and weight loss is present. Achalasia presents with dysphagia for solids and liquids, and regurgitation of nonacidic, undigested food and saliva. Zenker diverticulum is marked by cervical dysplasia, bland regurgitation, and halitosis.

**3. d.**
PPIs decrease acid secretion by at least 80%, thus inhibiting both nocturnal and meal-stimulated acid secretion. They are the most effective medications for relieving the symptoms of reflux and for healing esophagitis. Antacids, which only neutralize acid in the stomach, are best for intermittent relief of mild heart-

burn. Cisapride, which improves LES pressure, esophageal clearance, and gastric emptying, is most effective for relieving mild to moderate symptoms, usually without esophagitis. $H_2$-receptor blockers best inhibit acid secretion at night, and they are best for mild to moderate heartburn associated with mild esophagitis.

### 4. b.

Dysphagia for solids suggests an anatomic (i.e., structural) rather than a functional (i.e., motility) disorder.

### 5. c.

All these medications are associated with pill-induced esophagitis. The most frequent culprit, however, is doxycycline because it is a widely used antibiotic. Classically, young adults taking doxycycline for acne present with dysphagia and odynophagia because they take their medication either with a minimal amount of water or immediately before bedtime.

### 6. e.

More than 50% of patients with noncardiac chest pain have GERD. Extraesophageal presentations of GERD include damage to the lungs (i.e., asthma) and oropharynx (e.g., hoarseness, vocal cord granulomas, dental erosions, laryngeal cancer) secondary to high acid reflux.

### 7. b

The diagnosis of achalasia is *suspected* by endoscopy and confirmed by biopsies showing the presence of specialized columnar mucosa with goblet cells.

### 8. d.

Either pneumatic dilation or Heller myotomy offers long-term relief for dysphagia/regurgitation in patients with achalasia. Botulinim toxin treatments give short-term relief and are best for elderly patients or those with important comorbid illnesses.

## SUGGESTED READINGS

Baehr PH, McDonald GB. Esophageal infections: risks factors, presentation, diagnosis and treatment. *Gastroenterology* 1994;106:509–532.

Baron TH, Richter JE. The use of esophageal function tests. *Adv Intern Med* 1993;38:3661–3686.

Biot WJ, Devesa SS, Kneller RW, et al. Rising incidence of adenocarcinoma of the esophagus and gastric cardia. *JAMA* 1991;265:1287–1289.

Clouse RE. Spastic disorders of the esophagus. *Gastroenterologist* 1997;5:112–127.

DeVault KR, Castell DO. Updated guidelines for the diagnosis and treatment of gastroesophageal reflux disease. *Am J Gastroenterol* 1999;94:1434–1442.

Kim-Deobold J, Kozarek RA. Esophageal perforation: an 8-year review of a multispecialty clinic's experience. *Am J Gastroenterol* 1992;87:1112–1119.

Lagergren J, Bergstrom R, Lindgren A, et al. Symptomatic gastroesophageal reflux as a risk factor for esophageal adenocarcinoma. *N Engl J Med* 1999;340:825–831.

Marks RD, Richter JE. Peptic strictures of the esophagus. *Am J Gastroenterol* 1993;88:1160–1173.

Richter JE. Extraesophageal presentations of gastroesophageal reflux disease. *Semin Gastrointest Dis* 1997;8:75–89.

Sloan S, Rademaker AW, Kahrilas PJ. Determinants of gastroesophageal junction incompetence: hiatal hernia, lower esophageal sphincter, or both? *Ann Intern Med* 1992;117:977–982.

Spechler SJ, Goyal RK. The columnar-lined esophagus, intestinal metaplasia and Norman Barrett. *Gastroenterology* 1996;110:614–621.

Spechler SJ, Lee E, Ahnen D, et al. Long-term outcome of medical and surgical therapies of GERD. Follow-up of a randomized controlled trial. *JAMA* 2001;285:2331–2338.

Vaezi MF, Richter JE. Current therapies for achalasia: comparison and efficacy. *J Clin Gastroenterol* 1998;27:21–35.

Vigneri S, Termini R, Leandro G, et al. A comparison of five maintenance therapies for reflux esophagitis. *N Engl J Med* 1995;333:1106–1110.

# Peptic Ulcer Disease

# 58

*Gary W. Falk   David S. Lever*

Peptic ulcer disease (gastric ulcer and duodenal ulcer) is a common clinical problem. The lifetime prevalence of peptic ulcer disease is approximately 5% to 10%. The most important risk factors are infection with *Helicobacter pylori* and ingestion of a nonsteroidal anti-inflammatory drug (NSAID). However, *H. pylori*-negative, NSAID-negative ulcer disease has become more common in recent years. The unopposed hypergastrinemia of Zollinger-Ellison syndrome is a rare cause of peptic ulcer disease. A number of "myth" factors clearly are not associated with the development of ulcers: personality, occupation, alcohol consumption, and diet. Emotional stress alone is not believed to cause ulcers in most patients. Some recent evidence from earthquake victims in Japan, however, suggests that stress may trigger or exacerbate gastric ulcers.

## GASTRODUODENAL MUCOSAL SECRETION AND PROTECTIVE FACTORS

The formation of ulcers requires acid and peptic activity in gastric secretions. Acid secretion occurs in the parietal cells located in the oxyntic glands of the fundus and body of the stomach (Fig. 58.1). These cells may be stimulated to secrete acid by three different pathways. The *neurocrine pathway* involves the vagal release of acetylcholine, the *paracrine pathway* is mediated by the release of histamine from mast cells and enterochromaffinlike cells in the stomach, and the *endocrine pathway* is mediated by the release of gastrin from antral G cells. Each of these transmitters has a specific receptor located on the basolateral surface of the parietal cell. The stimulation of these receptors leads to activation of intracellular second-messenger systems: gastrin and acetylcholine promote the accumulation of intracellular calcium, whereas histamine causes a stimulatory G protein to activate adenylate cyclase, which in turn generates cyclic adenosine monophosphate (cAMP). These intracellular messengers then activate protein kinases, which activate the proton pump—the $H^+/K^+$ adenosine triphosphatase enzyme, located at the apical surface of the parietal cell—to secrete hydrogen ions in exchange for potassium ions. Prostaglandins and somatostatin inhibit parietal cell function by binding to receptors that act through inhibitory G proteins to inhibit adenylate cyclase. Somatostatin also inhibits gastrin release. Acid is necessary to convert pepsinogen, secreted from gastric chief cells, into pepsin, a proteolytic enzyme

that is inactive at a pH greater than 4. Parietal cells also secrete intrinsic factor, a glycoprotein important in vitamin $B_{12}$ absorption.

Under normal circumstances, gastroduodenal surface epithelial cells resist injury by several protective mechanisms. First, these cells secrete mucins, phospholipids, and bicarbonate to create a pH gradient in the mucous layer between the acidic gastric lumen and the cell surface. Second, the surface cells resist back-diffusion of acid by intrinsic mechanisms of cellular integrity. Finally, prostaglandins enhance mucosal protection by increasing mucus secretion, increasing bicarbonate production, maintaining mucosal blood flow, and enhancing the resistance of epithelial cells to injury.

## PATHOPHYSIOLOGY

Peptic ulcer disease is the end result of an imbalance between aggressive and defensive factors in the gastroduodenal mucosa. *H. pylori*, NSAIDs, and acid-secretory abnormalities are the major factors that disrupt this equilibrium. Although acid peptic injury is necessary for ulcers to form, acid secretion is normal in almost all patients with gastric ulcers and increased in approximately one-third of patients with duodenal ulcers. Zollinger-Ellison syndrome accounts for 0.1% of patients who present with peptic ulcer disease. Gastric ulcers tend to occur in areas of non–acid producing cells, such as the antrum, or in areas of atrophic gastritis. A defect in bicarbonate production, and, hence, acid neutralization in the duodenal bulb, also is seen in patients with

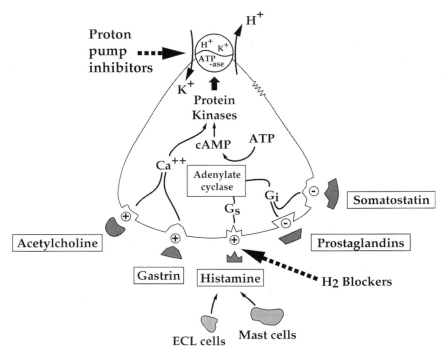

**Figure 58.1** Acid secretion by the parietal cell. Each transmitter has a specific receptor located on the basolateral surface of the parietal cell. Stimulation of these receptors leads to activation of intracellular second-messenger systems: Gastrin and acetylcholine promote accumulation of intracellular calcium, and histamine causes a stimulatory G protein (Gs) to activate adenylate cyclase, which in turn generates cyclic adenosine monophosphate (cAMP). These intracellular messengers then activate protein kinases that activate the proton pump [i.e., the $H^+/K^{+-}$ adenosine triphosphatase (ATPase) enzyme], which is located at the apical surface of the parietal cell, to secrete hydrogen ions in exchange for potassium ions. Prostaglandins and somatostatin inhibit parietal cell function by binding to receptors that act through inhibitory G proteins (Gi) to inhibit adenylate cyclase. Arrows indicate sites of action of various drugs that inhibit acid secretion. ATP, adenosine triphosphate; ECL, enterochromaffin-like cells.

duodenal ulcer disease. This abnormality resolves with eradication of *H. pylori*, if it is present.

## *Helicobacter pylori*

*H. pylori* is a Gram-negative, curved, flagellated rod found only in gastric epithelium or in gastric metaplastic epithelium. *H. pylori* infection causes chronic active gastritis in all infected patients and used to be found in the overwhelming majority of patients with duodenal and gastric ulcers. Recent data suggest, however, that *H. pylori* infection rates for duodenal ulcer patients in the United States are approximately 73%, far lower than previous estimates of 95%. Furthermore, only a minority of patients infected with *H. pylori*, approximately 15% to 20%, develop peptic ulcer disease. A clear age-related prevalence of *H. pylori* infection is seen in healthy subjects, increasing from 10% in those under age 30 to 60% in subjects older than 60 years in the Western world. The majority are infected early in life, although the mode of transmission remains unknown. *H. pylori* colonization in the United States is more common in minorities, immigrants, and the elderly. The prevalence of *H. pylori* infection in the West is declining and is likely to continue to do so. Similar trends are now encountered in formerly high-prevalence regions of the world such as Japan, where the prevalence decreased from 73% in 1974 to 39% in 1999. In contrast, infection is far more common in the developing world, where more than 80% of the population is infected by age 20. Infection with *H. pylori* typically is lifelong unless treated.

*H. pylori* is a noninvasive organism that colonizes the mucous layer overlying gastric epithelium. Factors important in the organism's ability to colonize the stomach include its flagellae, which facilitate locomotion; its ability to adhere to the mucous layer; and its production of urease. Urease increases juxtamucosal pH, which creates a more hospitable microclimate than that of the acidic stomach. Colonization causes acute and chronic inflammation, with the accumulation of neutrophils, plasma cells, T cells, and macrophages accompanied by varying degrees of epithelial cell injury, all of which resolves after treatment.

The ultimate clinical outcome of infection depends on a complex interplay between virulence factors of the organism, the host response, environmental factors, and age at the time of infection. It is now clear that many different strains of *H. pylori* exist, each with different virulence factors. Two such virulence factors are the *vacA* and *cagA* genes. The *vacA* gene encodes a vacuolating cytotoxin that directly damages epithelial cells and is more common in patients with peptic ulcer disease. A strong association exists between the production of the vacuolating cytotoxin and the presence of the *cagA* gene, both of which are more common in patients with peptic ulcer disease.

Acute infection results in short-lived acid hyposecretion that then resolves despite the persistence of the organism. Chronic infection increases the basal gastrin, the gastrin

response to a meal, basal acid output, and gastrin-stimulated acid output. The regulation of antral G cells may be altered by abnormalities in the ability of adjacent somatostatin-producing D cells to shut down gastrin release. All these abnormalities resolve after eradication of the organism. Gastric ulcers may develop in the setting of intense gastritis associated with infection by certain strains of *H. pylori*. The development of duodenal ulcers is more complex and probably involves enhanced gastric acid secretion caused by the dysregulation of somatostatin and gastrin: Gastrin release is increased, whereas the inhibitory influence of somatostatin is diminished. This results in gastric metaplasia in the duodenum, with subsequent *H. pylori* colonization. Duodenal bicarbonate production is also inhibited by *H. pylori* infection. Atrophic gastritis is another end result of infection that may increase the risk of gastric cancer. Finally, the mucosal lymphocytic response to *H. pylori* infection may lead to a monoclonal B-cell proliferation in mucosa-associated lymphoid tissue (MALT) lymphoma.

## Nonsteroidal Anti-inflammatory Drugs

NSAIDs are among the most widely used classes of drugs in the world. A clear relationship exists between the ingestion of NSAIDs and injury to the gastrointestinal tract. Two types of mucosal injury are caused by NSAIDs. The first form develops after acute ingestion and involves direct topical injury to mucosal cells. The acute ingestion of aspirin enhances mucosal permeability by lowering the mucosal potential difference and enhancing the back-diffusion of hydrogen ions. Hyperemia, subepithelial hemorrhage, and superficial erosions are seen endoscopically, although these lesions are typically asymptomatic. Microscopically, a "reactive" pattern of injury is characterized by little or no increase in inflammatory cells. With longer-term NSAID use, these lesions disappear and frank ulceration may develop. Chronic NSAID ingestion inhibits cyclooxygenase (COX), which results in the inhibition of gastroduodenal mucosal prostaglandin synthesis, and, hence, a decrease in mucus and bicarbonate production, mucosal blood flow, epithelial proliferation, and mucosal resistance to injury. Two COX isoenzymes are involved in prostaglandin synthesis. COX-1 is expressed constitutively and is necessary for gastric cytoprotective functions, whereas COX-2 is induced only at sites of tissue inflammation. New NSAIDs that selectively inhibit COX-2 have far less gastrointestinal toxicity.

The use of NSAIDs clearly predisposes patients to ulcers, both duodenal and gastric, as well as to complications of ulcer disease, including hemorrhage, perforation, and obstruction. The risk for gastric ulcers is somewhat greater than that for duodenal ulcers. Endoscopically apparent ulceration occurs in approximately 40% of long-term NSAID users, the majority of whom are asymptomatic. Only approximately 15% of NSAID users have

## TABLE 58.1

### RISK FACTORS FOR DEVELOPMENT OF NSAID-INDUCED ULCERS AND COMPLICATIONS

Age >60 yr
Prior peptic ulcer disease or ulcer bleed
High dosage or use of more than one NSAID
Concurrent use of NSAID and corticosteroids
Concurrent use of NSAID and anticoagulants
Serious systemic disorder

NSAID, nonsteroidal anti-inflammatory drug.

## TABLE 58.2

### ETIOLOGY OF PEPTIC ULCER DISEASE

*Helicobacter pylori*–positive
*H. pylori*–negative
False-negative *H. pylori* test result
Serologic testing in low-prevalence region
Recent use of antibiotics or bismuth
Concurrent use of proton pump inhibitors (PPIs) with urea breath
   test or urease test
Atrophic gastritis
Nonsteroidal anti-inflammatory drug use
Zollinger-Ellison syndrome
Crohn's disease
Idiopathic peptic ulcer disease

clinical manifestations of ulcer disease, however, and serious complications are encountered in approximately 2% each year. NSAID-induced ulceration occurs with all nonselective NSAIDs, including low-dose aspirin, although certain compounds, such as salsalate, nabumetone (Relafen), and etodolac (Lodine), may be associated with a decreased risk of ulceration. The administration of COX-2–selective agents, such as celecoxib (Celebrex), results in lower rates of endoscopic ulcers, symptomatic ulcers, and complications, such as bleeding, perforation, or obstruction, than do conventional nonselective NSAIDs. In fact, the ulcer risk with these agents is no greater than with placebo. Risk factors for NSAID-induced ulceration and complications are shown in Table 58.1. In addition, underlying cardiovascular and cerebrovascular disease may be a risk factor for bleeding peptic ulcer disease as well. Mixed findings have emerged regarding susceptibility to ulcer formation in those taking NSAIDS who are also *H. pylori* positive. A recent meta-analysis suggested that peptic ulcer disease is significantly more common in NSAID takers who are *H. pylori* positive, thus indicating a possible synergy of both types of damage to the gastroduodenal mucosa.

### Peptic Ulcer Disease

*H. pylori* infection is on the decline in the Western world. Because of this decline, the entity of *H. pylori*–negative peptic ulcer disease is becoming more common. In patients with peptic ulcer disease and negative test results for *H. pylori* infection, a number of different diagnoses must be considered (Table 58.2). Many of these patients are acetyl salicylic acid (ASA) or NSAID users, often using over-the-counter medications. Some have a false-negative test result for *H. pylori* because of concurrent proton pump inhibitor (PPI) use. Others may have Zollinger-Ellison syndrome. In rare cases, Crohn's disease may present as gastroduodenal ulceration. This can be diagnosed by the finding of granulomas on biopsy or evidence of Crohn's disease in the small bowel.

If all the previously mentioned entities are excluded, then individuals are said to have idiopathic peptic ulcer disease. This newly described entity is characterized by elevated serum gastrin levels, increased gastric acid output, and abnormally rapid gastroduodenal emptying. The treatment of this entity may be more difficult than the treatment of routine peptic ulcer disease.

## CLINICAL PRESENTATION

Dyspepsia, the classic symptom of peptic ulcer disease, is defined as a pain centered in the upper abdomen or discomfort characterized by fullness, bloating, distention, or nausea. Symptoms may be chronic, recurrent, or of new onset. Dyspepsia is a common clinical problem and may be seen in 25% to 40% of adults. Only 15% to 25% of patients with dyspepsia are found to have a gastric or duodenal ulcer. Up to 60% of patients have no definite diagnosis and are classified as having functional dyspepsia, a condition most likely related to an abnormal perception of events in the stomach caused by afferent visceral hypersensitivity. Other causes of dyspepsia include gastroesophageal reflux disease (GERD) and gastric cancer (Table 58.3). Ulcers may also be asymptomatic, especially in patients ingesting NSAIDs. Patients may present with complications of ulcer disease; hemorrhage may develop in 20%, perforation in 5%, and gastric outlet obstruction in 2%.

## TABLE 58.3

### DIFFERENTIAL DIAGNOSIS OF DYSPEPSIA

| Condition | Frequency (%) |
|---|---|
| Peptic ulcer disease | 15–25 |
| Gastroesophageal reflux disease | 5–15 |
| Functional dyspepsia | 60 |
| Gastric cancer | <2 |

# DIAGNOSIS

## General Approaches

Several possible diagnostic approaches are possible in the patient with dyspepsia: (i) instituting a short trial of empiric antisecretory therapy, (ii) performing immediate endoscopy, and (iii) conducting noninvasive testing for *H. pylori* infection followed by antibiotic treatment of patients with positive test results.

Immediate endoscopic evaluation without a trial of empiric therapy is indicated for individuals with obvious systemic symptoms, such as weight loss, bleeding, nausea, and vomiting, as well as individuals older than 45 to 50 years with new-onset dyspepsia in whom gastric neoplasia is a consideration (Table 58.4). If a gastric ulcer is found at endoscopy, multiple biopsies and brush cytologic examination are required to exclude a malignancy. Endoscopy is also indicated in patients who fail to respond to empiric therapy. Barium radiography has no role in the evaluation of dyspepsia due to its poor sensitivity and specificity.

Initial noninvasive testing for *H. pylori*, followed by antimicrobial therapy in patients with positive test results, is a reasonable approach for patients under the age of 45 years with uncomplicated dyspepsia. The rationale for this is that ulcer disease, if present, will heal and future ulcer diathesis is eliminated. A decision to empirically treat patients with dyspepsia with antibiotics for presumed *H. pylori* infection without proof of infection is not supported by any model to date, however, and should never be done. The indiscriminate use of antimicrobial therapy also may be associated with illnesses related to alteration of normal human flora, increased resistance of *H. pylori* and

other bacteria that are not a target of therapy, and a host of adverse effects, such as *Clostridium difficile* colitis.

Empiric antisecretory therapy with omeprazole is more effective than placebo for the treatment of symptoms of nonulcer dyspepsia, despite an appreciable response to placebo. As the risk of *H. pylori*–induced ulcer disease declines, and because most cases of dyspepsia are not ulcer related, the test and treat approach for *H. pylori* infection likely will become less successful. As the proportion of *H. pylori*–negative ulcers rise, a modest cost advantage may be seen in the use of empiric antisecretory therapy over the test and treat approach for *H. pylori* in patients with uninvestigated dyspepsia.

## Diagnostic Tests for *Helicobacter pylori*

*H. pylori* testing is essential in patients with peptic ulcer disease. A negative test result will focus the subsequent diagnostic evaluation on other causes of peptic ulcer disease, such as NSAID consumption or gastrinoma. An initial negative test result in patients with newly diagnosed peptic ulcer disease should be confirmed by a second test, however, given the importance of diagnosing *H. pylori* infection. Furthermore, a negative test result precludes the use of antimicrobial therapy. Diagnostic tests for the detection of *H. pylori* infection are subdivided into nonendoscopic and endoscopic techniques (Table 58.5). The decline in the prevalence of *H. pylori* in the Western world has resulted in a paradigm shift in testing strategies for *H. pylori* infection. Enzyme-linked immunosorbent assay serologic (ELISA) tests, formerly the cornerstone of *H. pylori* testing, are no longer recommended because of the poor performance characteristics of these tests: sensitivity of 85% and specificity of 79%. The sensitivity (71%) and specificity (88%) of office-based blood and serologic testing is also suboptimal, which makes these tests contraindicated as well. Furthermore, serologic test results may remain positive for

**TABLE 58.4**

**DIAGNOSTIC APPROACHES FOR PATIENTS WITH DYSPEPSIA**

Immediate endoscopy *mandatory*
  Alarm signs
  Weight loss
  Anorexia
  Nausea or vomiting
  Evidence of bleeding (anemia, melena)
  Age >45–50 years with new-onset dyspepsia
  Gastric ulcer or lesion suspicious for cancer on barium radiographs
Immediate endoscopy optional
  Young patients
  Short duration of symptoms
  Absence of alarm signs
  Nonsteroidal anti-inflammatory drug use
  Noninvasive *Helicobacter pylori* testing in patients without alarm signs
  Positive test results antimicrobial treatment
  Negative test results antisecretory treatment

**TABLE 58.5**

**DIAGNOSTIC TESTS FOR *HELICOBACTER PYLORI***

Nonendoscopic
  Antibody tests (no longer recommended)
    Qualitative (serum or whole blood)
    Quantitative (enzyme-linked immunosorbent assay)
  Urease tests
    Carbon 13 urea breath test
    Carbon 14 urea breath test
    Carbon 13 urea blood test
  Fecal antigen test
Endoscopic
  Rapid urease test
  Histologic examination
  Culture

up to 3 years after bacterial eradication, which limits the role of such testing in the documentation of eradication. Currently, the only role for serologic testing is in populations with a high background prevalence (>60%).

In the breath test using urea labeled with carbon 13 or carbon 14, *H. pylori* urease splits off labeled carbon dioxide, which may be detected in the breath of the patient. The urea breath tests are more accurate than serologic tests and are now the noninvasive test of choice for diagnosing *H. pylori* infection and documenting successful *H. pylori* eradication after antibiotic therapy. Patients should not receive PPIs for at least 14 days before the administration of breath tests to avoid false-negative results.

The stool antigen test is emerging as a noninvasive, inexpensive alternative to the urea breath test. In this test, an enzymatic immunoassay detects the presence of *H. pylori* in stool specimens. This technique has excellent sensitivity (93%) and specificity (94%) for the initial diagnosis of *H. pylori* infection. The sensitivity of the test is decreased by the recent use of antibiotics, bismuth, or PPIs. (Because of this, the role of this test in posttreatment evaluation is still evolving.) Recent evidence shows, however, that stool antigen testing can be performed seven days after the completion of treatment to identify those patients in whom the eradication of *H. pylori* is unsuccessful. Stool antigen testing 7 or more days after the completion of eradication therapy identified patients with persistent infection in about 95% of cases. A negative stool test 7 days after treatment correctly identified clearance in 90% of cases. The advantages include the ability for prompt testing after treatment, and earlier retreatment for *H. pylori* positivity, especially in those who are at risk for ulcer rebleeding.

If endoscopy is performed, the diagnosis is made by the rapid urease test or histologic examination. In the rapid urease test, mucosal biopsies are directly inoculated into a urea-containing medium with a pH-sensitive indicator that changes color when ammonia is metabolized from urea by the urease of the organism. Recent treatment with antibiotics or PPIs decreases the yield of both these biopsy tests.

The guidelines for posttreatment testing have changed in recent years. Posttreatment testing is mandatory in patients with complicated peptic ulcer disease (i.e., bleeding, perforation, or obstruction) or MALT lymphoma, or after resection of early gastric cancer. It also should be performed in all patients with newly diagnosed ulcer disease and in patients concerned about persistent infection. (Because antibiotic treatment suppresses the organism even if it is not eradicated, testing to confirm cure should only be done 4 weeks after the completion of therapy.)

## TREATMENT OF PEPTIC ULCER DISEASE

### Initial Treatment

A number of treatment options are available for the healing of peptic ulcers. Antacids are highly effective agents for healing ulcers and controlling symptoms. From a practical perspective, however, the inconvenient dosing frequency and adverse effects of therapy limit the use of antacids to symptom control only. Antacids neutralize acid that is already secreted. This increases intragastric pH, which also inactivates pepsin. The greatest buffering capacity is achieved when antacids are given 1 hour after eating.

Histamine $H_2$-receptor antagonists remain a mainstay of ulcer therapy. Acid secretion is decreased by the competitive and selective inhibition of the histamine $H_2$-receptor of the parietal cell. Four different histamine $H_2$-receptor antagonists are available: cimetidine, ranitidine, famotidine, and nizatidine. All these compounds act by the same mechanism, but all have different relative potencies for inhibiting gastric acid secretion. Cimetidine is the least potent, whereas famotidine is the most potent. As a consequence of gastric acid secretion inhibition, gastric pH rises, and pepsin activity decreases. This class of drugs is uniformly safe and well tolerated, although the risk of adverse effects is slightly increased with cimetidine because it binds to cytochrome P450 and hence drug interactions are increased. Histamine $H_2$-receptor antagonists heal 90% to 95% of duodenal ulcers and 88% of gastric ulcers in 8 weeks. Given as a single full dose at bedtime, each of the available compounds (cimetidine 800 mg, ranitidine 300 mg, famotidine 40 mg, nizatidine 300 mg) has a comparable efficacy for ulcer healing (Table 58.6).

The PPIs bind irreversibly to the $H^+/K^+$–adenosine triphosphatase enzyme of the gastric parietal cell. This blocks the final step of gastric acid secretion in response to any type of stimulation and results in the long-lasting inhibition of gastric acid secretion. For gastric secretory activity to be restored, new enzyme must be resynthesized, which normally takes 2 to 5 days. The PPIs are all remarkably well tolerated. Adverse effects are uncommon and are typically no more common than those experienced with placebo. The PPIs achieve duodenal ulcer healing rates at 4 weeks (90% to 100%) that typically are seen at 8 weeks with $H_2$-receptor antagonists. In addition to accelerating duodenal ulcer healing, the PPIs typically relieve symptoms more rapidly than histamine $H_2$-receptor antagonists. In contrast to the dramatic acceleration of duodenal ulcer healing using PPIs, gastric ulcer healing is essentially comparable to that achieved with histamine $H_2$-receptor antagonists at 8 weeks. The dosing and duration of therapy of the PPIs for peptic ulcer disease is shown in Table 58.6. Little information is currently available for the newest proton pump inhibitor, esomeprazole, when used alone in the treatment of active peptic ulcer disease. It has been shown to be effective when used in combination with antibiotics for the treatment of *H. pylori*.

Sucralfate is a complex salt of sucrose sulfate and aluminum hydroxide that is as effective as $H_2$-receptor antagonists in the treatment of duodenal ulcer disease. It is insoluble in water, and in the acid milieu of the stomach,

**TABLE 58.6**
## ANTISECRETORY THERAPY FOR PEPTIC ULCER DISEASE

| Agent | Duodenal Ulcer | | Gastric Ulcer | |
|---|---|---|---|---|
| | Dose (mg) | Duration (wk) | Dose (mg) | Duration (wk) |
| H₂-receptor antagonists | | | | |
| Cimetidine | 800 | 8 | 800 | 8 |
| Ranitidine | 300 | 8 | 300 | 8 |
| Famotidine | 40 | 8 | 40 | 8 |
| Nizatidine | 300 | 8 | 300 | 8 |
| Proton pump inhibitors | | | | |
| Omeprazole | 20 | 4 | 40 | 8 |
| Lansoprazole | 15 | 4 | 30 | 8 |
| Rabeprazole | 20 | 4 | 20 | 8 |
| Pantoprazole | 40 | 4 | 40 | 8 |

sucralfate is broken down into sucrose sulfate and an aluminum salt. There, it becomes a gel-like substance that binds to both defective and normal mucosa in the stomach and the duodenum. Sucralfate has little or no effect on acid secretion and acts through several different mucosa-protective mechanisms. It binds to mucosal surfaces and acts as a physical barrier to the diffusion of acid, pepsin, and bile acids. The drug is well tolerated, with few adverse effects. The evidence for efficacy in gastric ulcer disease is less compelling. The correct dosage is 1 g q.i.d. This dosing requirement makes it less convenient than other agents for treating peptic ulcer disease, and for this reason it is rarely used today.

## Treatment of *Helicobacter pylori* Infection

The eradication of *H. pylori* accelerates the rate of duodenal and gastric ulcer healing to a point at which it approximates the rate obtained with omeprazole at 4 weeks. The eradication of *H. pylori* essentially cures both duodenal and gastric ulcers and should be attempted in all patients with current or past documented peptic ulcer disease and evidence of infection.

The treatment of *H. pylori* infection is confusing, however, requires multiple drugs, and remains suboptimal. Despite the in vitro sensitivity of the organism to a variety of antibiotics, the in vivo activity of these same drugs against *H. pylori* is disappointing. For this reason, eradication of the organism is difficult. Combinations of two antibiotics plus a PPI are used to maximize the chance of eradication. The efficacy of these regimens is typically approximately 90%. In over 30 trials involving over 3,900 patients, it has been shown that eradication therapy is superior to ulcer healing drugs when treating duodenal ulcers in patients who are *H. pylori*–positive. No significant differences between the two different treatment regimens were identified in *H. pylori*–positive gastric ulcer patients.

Current treatment regimens for *H. pylori* infection are shown in Table 58.7. A reasonable approach is to use either a metronidazole- or clarithromycin-based triple therapy regimen as first-line therapy. Should that fail, then second-line therapy uses the antimicrobial not used, with quadruple therapy reserved as a third-line option.

Factors such as duration of therapy, compliance, and antibiotic resistance, especially to clarithromycin and metronidazole, influence treatment efficacy. Compliance is essential for treatment success. In the United States, resistance to metronidazole is approximately 35% and to clarithromycin 11%. The problem of antibiotic resistance is increasing and in the future may require antimicrobial sensitivity testing before therapy. Given the resistance problems with both clarithromycin and metronidazole, it is recommended that the use of these two agents together in the initial treatment of *H. pylori* infection be avoided.

**TABLE 58.7**
## PREFERRED THERAPIES FOR *HELICOBACTER PYLORI* INFECTION

Twice-daily proton pump inhibitor (PPI)[a]
  PPI
  Plus two of the following three agents
    Amoxicillin, 1 g
    Clarithryomycin, 500 mg
    Metronidazole, 500 mg
Quadruple therapy
  PPI twice daily[b]
  Tetracycline, 500 mg q.i.d.
  Metronidazole, 500 mg t.i.d.
  Bismuth subsalicylate or subcitrate q.i.d.

[a] Esomeprazole may be given as 40 mg once daily with any regimen.
[b] 14-Day therapy superior to 7-day therapy.
(Modified with permission from Graham DY. Therapy of *Helicobacter pylori*: current status and issues. *Gastroenterology* 2000;118:S2–S8.)

## Treatment and Prophylaxis of Ulceration Induced by Nonsteroidal Anti-Inflammatory Drugs

For patients who develop ulcers while ingesting NSAIDs, therapy should be stopped, if possible, and the patient placed on conventional doses of H$_2$-receptor antagonists or PPIs. H. pylori infection should be sought and treated if present. For patients who need continued NSAID therapy, the dosage should be reduced as much as possible. Small ulcers (5 mm or less) in the stomach or duodenum will heal with coadministration of histamine H$_2$-receptor antagonists, whereas larger ulcers require the coadministration of a PPI for healing (Table 58.8).

Given the fact that prophylactic medications are expensive and NSAID use is common, ulcer prophylaxis should be considered only in high-risk individuals. These include (i) those older than 60 years, (ii) those with a prior history of peptic ulcer disease or ulcer bleed, (iii) those concurrently taking anticoagulants or corticosteroids, and (iv) those taking high dosages of NSAIDS. It is important to remember that even low-dose aspirin used for cardiac prophylaxis is a risk factor for bleeding from peptic ulcer disease. There are two options for ulcer prevention: (i) the coadministration of agents that protect the gastroduodenal mucosa, or (ii) the use of COX-2–selective agents.

Misoprostol is a prostaglandin E1 analog that is effective for the prophylaxis of NSAID-induced ulcers in patients. It decreases the incidence of serious gastrointestinal complications such as bleeding, perforation, and gastric outlet obstruction. It acts by prostaglandin-dependent pathways to decrease gastric acid secretion and enhance mucosal defenses. Misoprostol, at a dosage of 200 μg three times a day or four times a day is effective for the prevention of duodenal and gastric ulcers. Adverse effects with misoprostol are common, however, especially diarrhea and abdominal cramps, and these limit its use. A fixed combi-

### TABLE 58.8
### STRATEGY FOR PROPHYLAXIS OF NSAID-INDUCED ULCERS

Discontinue NSAIDs.
If NSAIDs are necessary, use lowest dose possible.
Consider prophylactic therapy for populations at risk:
    Age >60 yr
    Prior peptic ulcer disease
    Prior peptic ulcer bleeding
    Concurrent use of corticosteroids
    Concurrent use of anticoagulants
    High NSAID dosage or use of multiple NSAIDs
If prophylaxis is indicated:
    Omeprazole, 20 mg q.d.
    Misoprostol, 200 μg t.i.d to q.i.d.
    Famotidine, 40 mg b.i.d.

NSAID, nonsteroidal anti-inflammatory drug.

nation of the NSAID diclofenac sodium and misoprostol (Arthrotec) is also available. Use of this compound results in lower rates of ulcer formation than with placebo.

Recent data suggest that omeprazole at a dosage of 20 mg daily is more effective than either histamine H$_2$-receptor antagonists or misoprostol for the prevention of NSAID-induced ulcers. Furthermore, omeprazole is typically better tolerated than misoprostol. High-dose famotidine 40 mg two times a day is more effective than placebo in preventing both duodenal and gastric ulcers in patients receiving long-term NSAID therapy. The cost of such a regimen, however, is considerably higher than that of once-a-day omeprazole. The conventional dosages of famotidine and the other histamine H$_2$-receptor antagonists are effective only for the prophylaxis of duodenal ulcers, not for the prophylaxis of gastric ulcers.

The use of COX-2 agents is a reasonable treatment strategy to consider for high-risk patients, instead of coadministration of a PPI or misoprostol. Celecoxib is as effective as diclofenac plus omeprazole in preventing recurrent bleeding in H. pylori–negative rheumatoid and osteoarthritis patients who initially presented with ulcer bleeding while taking NSAIDs. Low-risk patients, however, may do just as well using nonselective NSAIDs without prophylaxis.

## Interactions between Nonsteroidal Anti-Inflammatory Drugs and Helicobacter pylori: Treatment Implications

The frequency of H. pylori infection and NSAID ingestion both increase with age. Some data suggest that H. pylori increases, has no effect on, and decreases the risk of bleeding in patients taking NSAIDs, including aspirin. In a landmark study by Chan et al., patients with a history of peptic ulcer disease bleeding who were infected with H. pylori and were taking aspirin or other NSAIDs were randomly assigned to receive H. pylori eradication therapy or treatment with omeprazole 20 mg daily for 6 months. The investigators found that, among patients taking low-dose aspirin for cardiac prophylaxis, eradication therapy was equivalent to omeprazole treatment for the prevention of recurrent bleeding, whereas omeprazole therapy was superior to eradication therapy among patients taking other NSAIDs. Therefore, patients with a prior history of peptic ulcer disease or its complications should be tested for H. pylori and treated, if necessary, before NSAID therapy is commenced.

## Treatment of Nonhealing Ulcers

Approximately 10% of ulcers fail to heal after standard acid-suppression therapy (i.e., 8 weeks of histamine H$_2$-receptor antagonists or 4 weeks of PPIs for duodenal ulcers; 12 weeks of H$_2$-receptor antagonists or 8 weeks of PPIs for gastric ulcers). Persistence of symptoms and macroscopically apparent ulceration are not necessarily correlated.

Factors to be considered when ulcers fail to heal are noncompliance, cigarette smoking, NSAID ingestion, acid hypersecretion, Zollinger-Ellison syndrome, idiopathic acid hypersecretion, cancer (gastric ulcers), and *H. pylori* infection. Each of these issues should be addressed before additional therapy is instituted. Infection with *H. pylori* and the surreptitious use of NSAIDs have emerged as the two leading causes of refractory peptic ulcers. A determination of salicylate levels and platelet aggregation studies may be useful in these patients.

Switching from one H$_2$-blocker to another has no advantages. Omeprazole at a dose of 40 mg or other PPIs administered at comparable doses heal almost all peptic ulcer disease refractory to conventional dosages of therapy. The eradication of *H. pylori*, if present, should be attempted in these patients.

## Maintenance Therapy

Maintenance therapy with a long-term low dose (i.e., half strength) of any H$_2$-blocker is an obsolete concept. Before the role of *H. pylori* in peptic ulcer disease was determined, the ulcer relapse rate was reduced to between 10% to 30% at 1 year using this strategy. Today, maintenance therapy is indicated only for a small subset of patients with chronic peptic ulcer disease. Patients with *H. pylori*–positive peptic ulcer disease should be placed on maintenance therapy if eradication is unsuccessful. Patients with *H. pylori*–negative peptic ulcer disease should be placed on maintenance therapy if they have three or more relapses each year or a history of ulcer complications, such as bleeding or perforation, and multiple other medical problems.

## *Helicobacter pylori* and Functional Dyspepsia: Treatment Implications

The role of *H. pylori* in functional dyspepsia has been the subject of intense study. Trials assessing the treatment of *H. pylori* infection in patients with functional dyspepsia indicate that 20% to 25% of these patients experience symptom resolution with effective antibiotic therapy. A recent meta-analysis of randomized, controlled trials of therapy for *H. pylori* in these patients, however, provided little if any support for the use of *H. pylori* eradication therapy in patients with functional dyspepsia. For this reason, routine treatment of *H. pylori* infection in patients with functional dyspepsia should be avoided at present. This disorder more likely relates to an abnormal perception of events in the gut resulting from abnormal visceral afferent hypersensitivity.

## *HELICOBACTER PYLORI* AND GASTRIC NEOPLASIA

Infection with *H. pylori* is an important risk factor for the development of distal gastric cancer, which is the second leading cause of death from cancer worldwide. Some 40% to 60% of tumors of the gastric body or antrum are associated with *H. pylori* infection. The incidence of gastric cancer in the United States is decreasing, however, and it is estimated that only 1% of infected Americans ever develop cancer. Mass screening for *H. pylori* in middle-aged U.S. adults is not indicated at present.

*H. pylori* infection also is associated with gastric MALT lymphoma, which is a low-grade, B-cell subtype of non-Hodgkin's lymphoma of the stomach. Clinical presentation is nonspecific and is related to the size and location of the tumor(s) in the stomach. Diagnosis is based on the characteristic histologic appearance of destructive lymphoepithelial lesions. Endoscopic ultrasonography is useful in predicting a response to therapy; an excellent response is seen if the tumor is limited to the mucosa or submucosa. The eradication of *H. pylori* may cure up to 70% of individuals with MALT-type lymphoma, especially those with superficial disease.

## COMPLICATIONS OF PEPTIC ULCER DISEASE

### Bleeding Peptic Ulcers

Fifteen percent to 20% of patients with peptic ulcer disease develop bleeding, and bleeding ulcer is the most common cause of upper gastrointestinal bleeding. Although bleeding ceases spontaneously in 80% of cases, the mortality of bleeding ulcers is approximately 10%. The major risk factor for bleeding ulcers is consumption of NSAIDs. Patients with bleeding ulcers present with hematemesis, melena, or hematochezia, often without antecedent pain. Clinical predictors for an adverse outcome are shown in Table 58.9.

All patients with upper gastrointestinal bleeding should undergo early upper endoscopy, which allows for both therapeutic intervention and determination of the presence of predictors for rebleeding. Rebleeding rates without endoscopic treatment are approximately 3% for clean-based

**TABLE 58.9**

**CLINICAL PREDICTORS OF AN ADVERSE OUTCOME IN BLEEDING PEPTIC ULCERS**

Hemodynamic instability at presentation
Hematemesis
Hematochezia
Age >60 years
Ongoing transfusion requirements >6 U for a single bleed
Severe comorbid medical or surgical illnesses
Inpatient hemorrhage
Rebleeding from same lesion while hospitalized

(Adapted with permission from Jensen DM. Endoscopic diagnosis and treatment of bleeding peptic ulcers. *Clin Perspect Gastroenterol* 1999; 2(2):73–84.)

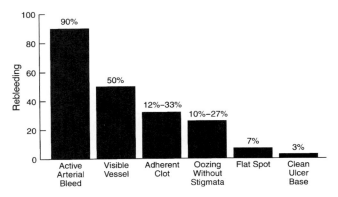

**Figure 58.2**  Natural history of ulcer hemorrhage without endoscopic intervention. [Adapted with permission from Jensen DM. Endoscopic diagnosis and treatment of bleeding peptic ulcers. *Clin Perspect Gastroenterol* 1999;2(2):73–84.]

ulcers, 7% for ulcers with flat spots, 12% to 33% for adherent clots, 50% for nonbleeding visible vessels, and 90% for active arterial spurting from an ulcer (Fig. 58.2). Patients with large ulcers of more than 1 to 2 cm also have higher rebleeding rates and mortality. Endoscopic therapy using techniques such as bipolar or thermal coagulation combined with the injection with epinephrine decreases subsequent rebleeding and clearly improves the outcome in patients with bleeding ulcers by also decreasing mortality, length of hospital stay, number of blood transfusions required, and need for emergency surgery. Because most rebleeding occurs within 3 days of initial presentation, patients with active bleeding or stigmata of hemorrhage, such as pigmented spots in an ulcer crater or clot, can typically be discharged within 3 days if they are stable (Table 58.10). Given the excellent prognosis for patients with clean-based ulcers, discharge within 24 hours of presentation is also reasonable.

Acid-suppression therapy using PPIs decreases rebleeding after the endoscopic treatment of bleeding peptic ulcers. The rationale for aggressive acid suppression is multifactorial:

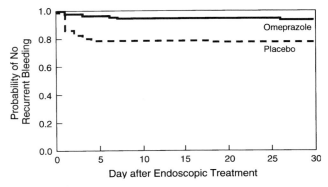

**Figure 58.3**  Probability of no recurrent bleeding within 30 days after endoscopic treatment of bleeding peptic ulcers: effect of initial treatment with intravenous omeprazole versus placebo. (Reproduced with permission from Lau JY, Sung JJ, Lee KK, et al. Effect of intravenous omeprazole on recurrent bleeding after endoscopic treatment of bleeding peptic ulcers. *N Engl J Med* 2000;343:310–316.)

### TABLE 58.10

### IMPLICATIONS OF STIGMATA OF RECENT HEMORRHAGE ON TREATMENT OF BLEEDING PEPTIC ULCERS

| Endoscopic Finding | Endoscopic Therapy | Management |
|---|---|---|
| Clean base | No | Regular diet<br>Discharge within 24 h |
| Flat spot | No | Regular diet<br>Discharge within 24 h |
| Oozing without stigmata | Yes | PPI intravenously then orally[a]<br>Regular diet<br>Observation for 24–48 h after treatment |
| Adherent clot | Yes | PPI intravenously then orally[a]<br>Regular diet<br>Observation for 48 h after treatment |
| Visible vessel | Yes | PPI intravenously then orally[a]<br>Regular diet<br>Observation for 48 h after treatment |
| Active arterial bleeding | Yes | PPI intravenously then orally[a]<br>Liquid diet<br>Observation for 72 h after treatment |

PPI, proton pump inhibitor.
[a] Intravenous PPI should be the equivalent of omeprazole, 80-mg bolus, followed by continuous infusion of 8 mg/hour. Oral PPI therapy should be the equivalent of omeprazole, 40 mg b.i.d. for 3 days, followed by standard-dose PPI or H2-receptor antagonist therapy for ulcer healing.
[Adapted with permission from Jensen DM. Endoscopic diagnosis and treatment of bleeding peptic ulcers. *Clin Perspect Gastroenterol* 1999; 2(2):73–84.]

(i) blood clots are unstable at a low pH, and (ii) pepsin, which requires a pH of less than 4, can lyse blood clots. At a pH level of 6, platelet aggregation and pepsin inactivation are optimized. In a landmark study, Lau et al. found that intravenous omeprazole (80 mg bolus followed by 8 mg/ hour) given for 72 hours was more effective than placebo administration in decreasing rebleeding after endoscopic therapy in patients with actively bleeding ulcers or nonbleeding visible vessels (Fig. 58.3). Parenteral omeprazole is not available in the United States, but pantoprazole is. Intravenous pantoprazole is currently used off label and is administered with an initial 80 mg bolus followed by a continuous infusion of 8 mg/hour. This method for treating bleeding ulcers also has been shown to be cost effective when compared with placebo. High-dose omeprazole (40 mg two times a day) also may be useful in the management of bleeding peptic ulcers if endoscopic therapy is not used. Practically speaking, patients with bleeding peptic ulcers should be treated with high-dose PPI therapy (the equivalent of omeprazole 40 mg two times a day) as soon as oral medications are permitted or with parenteral PPI therapy for 3 days, followed by conventional-dose PPI or histamine $H_2$-receptor antagonist therapy for ulcer healing.

Approximately 20% of patients rebleed after initial endoscopic therapy, especially if ulcers are large and deep. Endoscopic retreatment is effective in approximately 75% of patients; it clearly reduces the need for surgery without increasing the risk of death in these patients and should be offered before alternative modalities are considered. Those in whom retreatment is unsuccessful are then candidates for surgical intervention or, if they are deemed too high a surgical risk, for angiographic treatment using either intraarterial vasopressin or embolization techniques.

Patients with bleeding peptic ulcers who are infected with *H. pylori* have a marked decrease in rebleeding after *H. pylori* eradication, whereas failure to cure the infection results in a rebleeding rate of approximately 33% at 1 year. Therefore, all patients with bleeding peptic ulcers should have their *H. pylori* status determined. Antibiotic therapy should be given to patients who are infected; for these patients, a cure of their infection should be confirmed using the urea breath test. Failure to cure *H. pylori* infection mandates long-term, even indefinite, maintenance therapy with half-dose histamine $H_2$-receptor antagonists.

### Gastric Outlet Obstruction

Gastric outlet obstruction is typically due to either pyloric channel or duodenal ulceration and may be seen in the setting of acute ulceration in which edema, spasm, or inflammation causes gastric outlet obstruction or as a sequela of chronic ulceration with scarring and fibrosis. Patients present with symptoms of early satiety, bloating, nausea, vomiting, and weight loss. Endoscopy is the diagnostic test of choice for gastric outlet obstruction; it should be performed only after adequate gastric decompression and lavage of retained gastric contents. Malignancy accounts for approximately 50% of cases of gastric outlet obstruction and should be excluded with adequate biopsy and cytology samples. Malignancy should be suspected especially in patients older than 55 years with no history of peptic ulcer disease. The treatment of gastric outlet obstruction is aimed at correcting any underlying electrolyte abnormalities resulting from persistent vomiting, in conjunction with nasogastric decompression for 3 to 5 days. During that time, a histamine $H_2$-receptor antagonist or PPI should be administered parenterally as well. Adequacy of response may be assessed empirically with a trial of refeeding. In those patients who respond, the underlying cause of ulcer disease (*H. pylori* infection or NSAID use or both) should be treated appropriately, in conjunction with continued antisecretory therapy. For patients failing to respond, treatment options include endoscopic balloon dilation or surgery.

### Perforation

Peptic ulcer perforation occurs when an ulcer penetrates the full thickness of the stomach or duodenum. This then leads to peritonitis, which if untreated, results in sepsis and death. Perforation can occur with either duodenal or gastric ulcers but is a far less common complication than bleeding. Patients present with the sudden onset of severe abdominal pain beginning in the epigastrium and radiating throughout the entire abdomen. Physical examination demonstrates peritoneal findings, including abdominal pain, rebound tenderness, and board-like rigidity. The clinical suspicion of perforation may be confirmed in most but not all cases by demonstrating pneumoperitoneum with either an upright chest radiograph or upright and supine abdominal radiographs. In less clear-cut cases, computed tomography (CT) or a upper gastrointestinal study using water-soluble contrast may be helpful. Perforation requires surgical intervention. A perforated duodenal ulcer is typically repaired with an omental patch, whereas a perforated gastric ulcer requires either an omental patch or resection.

## ZOLLINGER-ELLISON SYNDROME

Zollinger-Ellison syndrome is characterized by a marked hypersecretion of acid due to high circulating levels of gastrin caused by the presence of a gastrin-secreting tumor. It accounts for less than 1% of cases of peptic ulcer disease. Approximately 80% of gastrinomas are sporadic, whereas the other 20% are associated with multiple endocrine neoplasia syndrome type 1 (MEN1). MEN1 is an autosomal dominant condition. The *MEN1* gene is located on chromosome 11, which may allow for genetic testing for this disorder in the future. It is typically associated with hyperparathyroidism and pituitary tumors.

Zollinger-Ellison syndrome should be suspected in patients with recurrent peptic ulcer disease in the absence of *H. pylori* infection or NSAID consumption. Up to 50% of patients may have diarrhea, whereas others also may have symptoms of gastroesophageal reflux and its complications. The diagnosis of Zollinger-Ellison syndrome is made when a high fasting gastrin concentration of more than 1,000 pg/mL is present in the setting of gastric acid hypersecretion (more than 15 mEq/hour if no gastric surgery, more than 5 mEq/hour if prior gastric surgery). Gastrinomas are a relatively uncommon cause of hypergastrinemia, however. The most common causes of hypergastrinemia are *H. pylori* infection and hypochlorhydria related either to decreased intraluminal acid in the setting of atrophic gastritis or to antisecretory therapy. Other causes of hypergastrinemia include retained gastric antrum (after ulcer surgery), idiopathic G-cell hyperfunction, chronic gastric outlet obstruction, and chronic renal failure. Therefore, acid hypersecretion, as documented by gastric acid analysis, is necessary for the diagnosis of Zollinger-Ellison syndrome. The secretin stimulation test has limited value due to false-negative and false-positive results of up to 10%. The single best imaging test for gastrinomas is somatostatin receptor scintigraphy, which is superior to ultrasonography, CT, magnetic resonance imaging (MRI), and angiography for tumor localization. Endoscopic ultrasonography is also superior to conventional imaging techniques. Should either of these studies give negative results in the setting of a suspected gastrinoma, then MRI is the best alternative imaging technique.

Surgical therapy is the preferred management of sporadic Zollinger-Ellison syndrome. The tumors are often found in the "gastrinoma triangle" demarcated by the common bile duct, the junction of the second and third portions of the duodenum, and the body of the pancreas, but these tumors also have been found in the heart, bile duct, liver, ovary, kidney, and mesentery. All patients with sporadic gastrinomas without evidence of liver metastases should undergo exploration with the intent of removal of local and regional disease, even if preoperative imaging tests yield negative results. Multiple pancreatic or duodenal tumors are the classic finding in gastrinomas that occur as part of the MEN1 syndrome, and the role of surgery in these patients is less clear-cut, although some recommend surgery if a lesion larger than 3 cm is identified with preoperative imaging techniques. Studies clearly show that surgical extirpation of these tumors decreases the chance of metastatic spread to the liver, which is the primary determinant of survival. PPIs are the agents of choice to control acid secretion in these patients. Omeprazole or lansoprazole should be commenced at an initial dosage of 60 mg daily, and the dosage should then be titrated to a basal acid output of less than 10 mEq/hour at 24 hours after the last dose of the drug. If more than 120 mg of a PPI is required, then the dose should be split to twice-daily administration. Long-term therapy with PPIs uniformly results in the continued inhibition of acid secretion, good symptom control, complete healing of any mucosal lesions, and lack of adverse effects. The treatment of Zollinger-Ellison syndrome using proton pump inhibitors does not result in further elevation of gastrin levels.

## STRESS-RELATED MUCOSAL DAMAGE

Stress-related mucosal damage develops in most critically ill patients, and overt upper gastrointestinal bleeding may occur in as many as 15% of untreated patients. Stress-related mucosal injury is caused by mucosal ischemia, which impairs mucosal resistance to acid back-diffusion and the presence of acid. Hyperemia of the mucosa evolves into erosions and then to frank ulceration in the stomach and duodenum. Critical illnesses associated with a risk of stress-related mucosal injury include:

- Burns
- Trauma
- Central nervous system injury
- Prolonged hypotension
- Sepsis
- Respiratory failure
- Hepatic failure
- Multiorgan failure

The mortality rate of patients who progress to bleeding is increased; however, the incidence of major bleeding in critically ill patients has decreased recently. The reason for this is uncertain and cannot necessarily be attributed to the widespread use of prophylactic therapy.

Several prophylactic treatment strategies are effective in preventing upper gastrointestinal bleeding in critically ill patients. Meta-analysis suggests that prophylaxis using antiulcer regimens reduces overt and clinically important gastrointestinal bleeding in critically ill patients. The administration of antacids every 2 hours neutralizes gastric acid but has the disadvantages of inconvenience and increased nursing time, and produces diarrhea. The use of sucralfate requires the placement of a nasogastric tube, and a dosage of 1 g every 4 hours was once thought to decrease the risk of late-onset nosocomial pneumonia. Recent data, however, suggest that no difference exists in the rate of ventilator-associated pneumonia with this agent and with $H_2$-receptor antagonists. $H_2$-receptor antagonists, given either as a continuous infusion or by bolus injection every 12 hours (in the case of more potent agents such as famotidine), are safe and convenient and should be titrated to produce an intragastric pH of higher than 4 to minimize the activity of pepsin. Fewer side effects are encountered with ranitidine and famotidine than with cimetidine. Recent studies suggest that the administration of $H_2$-receptor antagonists results in a significantly lower rate of clinically important bleeding than the administration of sucralfate.

Should all patients in the intensive care unit (ICU) receive prophylaxis, especially in this era of cost constraints? The answer is no. A large multicenter Canadian study involving 2,252 medical and surgical ICU patients identified coagulopathy and respiratory failure requiring mechanical ventilation for 48 hours or longer as the only risk factors for clinically significant bleeding in the ICU. Only 1.5% of all patients had clinically significant bleeding in this large study. Therefore, patients with coagulopathy or mechanical ventilation should continue to receive prophylaxis. Other patients who should receive targeted prophylaxis include those with central nervous system trauma, burns, organ transplantation, or a history of peptic ulcer disease with or without bleeding. Admission to the ICU does not automatically warrant prophylaxis for stress gastropathy.

## REVIEW EXERCISES

### QUESTIONS

**1.** The most common outcome of infection with *H. pylori* is
a) Peptic ulcer disease
b) Functional dyspepsia
c) Asymptomatic chronic active gastritis

**d)** Gastric adenocarcinoma

**e)** Gastric MALT lymphoma

**2.** A 55-year-old previously healthy man sees you, complaining of chronic intermittent epigastric discomfort. Some nausea is present, but no vomiting, melena, or weight loss. No prior history of peptic ulcer disease is reported. The single best diagnostic approach would be

**a)** Immediate upper gastrointestinal barium radiography

**b)** Immediate upper endoscopy

**c)** Serologic test for *H. pylori* and treatment if results are positive

**d)** Empiric antimicrobial treatment of *H. pylori*

**e)** Empiric antisecretory therapy with upper endoscopy if there is no response in 2 weeks

**3.** A 55-year-old woman with a prior endoscopically documented duodenal ulcer is currently taking ranitidine nightly. She is asymptomatic and has never been treated for *H. pylori*. Your approach would be to

**a)** Continue ranitidine therapy as the patient is asymptomatic.

**b)** Schedule the patient for upper endoscopy.

**c)** Institute empiric antibiotic therapy for *H. pylori*.

**d)** Order a urea breath test for *H. pylori* followed by antibiotic therapy if test results are positive.

**e)** Perform serologic testing for *H. pylori* followed by antibiotic therapy if test results are positive.

**4.** All the following are true about omeprazole therapy in patients using NSAIDs except which?

**a)** Decreases the risk of developing a gastric ulcer

**b)** Decreases the risk of developing a duodenal ulcer

**c)** Should be used in all patients receiving NSAIDs

**d)** Is uniformly well tolerated by patients

**5.** A 75-year-old retired steelworker with a history of chronic NSAID use for debilitating osteoarthritis presents with complaints of midepigastric pain for the past 2 months. He also has been taking low-dose aspirin for cardioprohylaxis since his MI 2 years ago, and he has a remote history of a bleeding ulcer. His Hb is 10. On endoscopy he is found to have multiple antral ulcers and a duodenal bulb ulcer. What further management is the least appropriate?

**a)** Switch to a COX-2 and ASA.

**b)** Test and treat for *H. pylori*.

**c)** Maintain NSAID and ASA doses and prescribe a PPI.

**d)** Maintain ASA, switch to a COX-2–selective inhibitor, and begin a PPI.

**6.** The following are true regarding high-dose intravenous omeprazole therapy for treatment of bleeding ulcers used adjunctively to endoscopic hemostasis:

**a)** It is a cost effective treatment.

**b)** It substantially decreases the risk of recurrent bleeding.

**c)** It should be used to treat all ulcers that have recently bled.

**d)** It decreases the need for endoscopic retreatment and blood transfusions.

**e)** It decreases the length of hospital stay.

## ANSWERS

**1. c.**
The overwhelming majority of individuals infected with *H. pylori* have asymptomatic chronic active gastritis. Peptic ulcer disease develops in approximately 20%, but very few ever develop gastric adenocarcinoma or MALT lymphoma. *H. pylori* infection does not appear to be an important factor in functional dyspepsia.

**2. b.**
Patients with new-onset dyspepsia warrant immediate diagnostic evaluation with upper endoscopy if they are older than 45 to 50 years because the risk of gastric cancer increases gradually after this age. The presence at any age of alarm signs such as hematemesis, melena, anemia, nausea, vomiting, and weight loss also warrants immediate endoscopy. The poor performance characteristics of barium radiography makes this an inappropriate study to perform at present. A test-and-treat method is warranted as a cost-effective approach for a young patient with new-onset dyspepsia, but serologic tests are no longer warranted. No justification ever exists for treating anybody for *H. pylori* without proof of infection.

**3. d.**
The treatment of *H. pylori* infection is warranted in any patient with documented present or past peptic ulcer disease. The most appropriate diagnostic approach is to perform a urea breath test or a stool antigen test in previously untreated patients. Serologic tests are no longer accurate enough to be an appropriate diagnostic test for *H. pylori*, except in high-prevalence regions. Any patient with a history of ulcers should undergo determination of *H. pylori* status and then receive treatment if it is present. This approach obviates the need for continued antisecretory therapy. Given the lack of symptoms and the prior endoscopic documentation, there is no need for endoscopy for this patient.

**4. c.**
Omeprazole is a well-tolerated antisecretory agent that is effective in decreasing the risk of developing NSAID-induced ulcers. Because NSAID use is so widespread, however, the economic consequences of universal prophylaxis are prohibitive. Therefore, prophylaxis is warranted only in high-risk patients, such as those who are older than age 60 years, have had prior peptic ulcer disease or ulcer bleed, are taking a high dosage of or more than one NSAID, use corticosteroids or anticoagulants concurrently with an NSAID, or have a serious systemic disorder.

### 5. a.

Any patient with a remote history of ulcer disease followed by a recurrent ulcer should be tested for *H. pylori*. At least 80% of gastric ulcers and 90% of duodenal ulcers will heal with continued NSAID use if accompanied by a PPI. Substituting a COX-2 for a nonselective NSAID and maintaining ASA results in the same risk of GI complications as treating with a nonselective NSAID. Patients who are debilitated, require ASA, and are at significant risk for upper GI ulcer complications also should be treated with a PPI, even if they are switched to a COX-2 selective inhibitor.

### 6. c.

Although treatment using intravenous omeprazole is very effective in preventing rebleeding when administered after endoscopic therapy, its use should be limited to ulcers that are actively bleeding, contain a visible blood vessel, and possibly an adherent clot. It is expensive to use and should be saved for ulcers with the highest chance of rebleeding. Despite the positive benefits listed, no significant evidence suggests that its use decreases mortality.

## SUGGESTED READINGS

American Gastroenterological Association medical position statement: evaluation of dyspepsia. *Gastroenterology* 1998;114:579–581.

Blaser MJ. In a world of black and white, *Helicobacter pylori* is gray. *Ann Intern Med* 1999;130:695–697.

Bombardier C, Laine L, Reicin A, et al. Comparison of upper gastrointestinal toxicity of rofecoxib and naproxen in patients with rheumatoid arthritis. *N Engl J Med* 2000;343:1520–1528.

Chan FK, Chung S, Suen BY, et al. Preventing recurrent upper gastrointestinal bleeding in patients with *Helicobacter pylori* infection who are taking low-dose aspirin or naproxen. *N Engl J Med* 2001;344:967–973.

Chan FKL, Hung LCT, et al. Celecoxib versus diclofenac and omeprazole in reducing the risk of recurrent ulcer bleeding in patients with arthritis. *N Engl J Med* 2002;347:2104–2110.

Ciociola AA, McSorley DJ, Turner K, et al. *Helicobacter pylori* infection rates in duodenal ulcer patients in the United States may be lower than previously estimated. *Am J Gastroenterol* 1999;94:1834–1840.

Cook DJ, Fuller HD, Guyatt GH, et al. Risk factors for gastrointestinal bleeding in critically ill patients. *N Engl J Med* 1994;330:377–381.

Cook DJ, Guyatt GH, Marshall J, et al. A comparison of sucralfate and ranitidine for the prevention of upper gastrointestinal bleeding in patients requiring mechanical ventilation. *N Engl J Med* 1998;338:791–797.

Cook DJ, Guyatt GH, Salena BJ, et al. Endoscopic therapy for acute nonvariceal upper gastrointestinal hemorrhage: a meta-analysis. *Gastroenterology* 1992;102:139–148.

Cook DJ, Reeve BK, Guyatt GH, et al. Stress ulcer prophylaxis in critically ill patients. Resolving discordant meta-analysis. *JAMA* 1996; 275:308–314.

De Boer WA, Tytgat GN. Treatment of *Helicobacter pylori* infection. *BMJ* 2000;320:31–34.

Feldman M, Burton ME. Histamine$_2$-receptor antagonists. Standard therapy for acid-peptic disease. *N Engl J Med* 1990;323: 1672–1680,1749–1755.

Feldman M, McMahon AT. Do cyclooxygenase-2 inhibitors provide benefits similar to those of traditional nonsteroidal anti-inflammatory drugs, with less gastrointestinal toxicity? *Ann Intern Med* 2000;132:134–143.

Gibril F, Reynolds JC, Doppman JL, et al. Somatostatin receptor scintigraphy: its sensitivity compared with that of other imaging methods in detecting primary and metastatic gastrinomas. *Ann Intern Med* 1996;125:26–34.

Graham DY. Therapy of *Helicobacter pylori*: current status and issues. *Gastroenterology* 2000;118:S2–S8.

Graham DY, Lew GM, Klein PD, et al. Effect of treatment of *Helicobacter pylori* infection on the long-term recurrence of gastric or duodenal ulcer. *Ann Intern Med* 1992;116:705–708.

Graham DY. NSAIDs, *Helicobacter Pylori*, and Pandora's Box. *N Engl J Med* 2002; 347:2162-2164.

Hansson LE, Engstrand L, Nyren O, et al. *Helicobacter pylori* infection: independent risk indicator of gastric adenocarcinoma. *Gastroenterology* 1993;105:1098–1103.

Hansson LE, Nyren O, Hsing AW, et al. The risk of stomach cancer in patients with gastric or duodenal ulcer disease. *N Engl J Med* 1996;335:242–249.

Hawkey CJ. Nonsteroidal anti-inflammatory drug gastropathy. *Gastroenterology* 2000;119:521–535.

Hawkey CJ, Karrasch JA, Szczepanski L, et al. Omeprazole compared with misoprostol for ulcers associated with nonsteroidal anti-inflammatory drugs. *N Engl J Med* 1998;338:727–734.

Heaney A, Collins JS, Watson RG, et al. A prospective randomised trial of a "test and treat" policy versus endoscopy based management in young *Helicobacter pylori* positive patients with ulcer-like dyspepsia, referred to a hospital clinic. *Gut* 1999;45:186–190.

Hirschowitz BI. Zollinger-Ellison syndrome: pathogenesis, diagnosis, and management. *Am J Gastroenterol* 1997;92:44S–48S.

Howden CW, Hunt RH. Guidelines for the management of *Helicobacter pylori* infection. *Am J Gastroenterol* 1998;93:2330–2338.

Huang, JQ et al. Role of *Helicobacter pylori* infection and non-steroidal anti-inflammatory drugs in peptic-ulcer disease: a meta-analysis. *The Lancet* 2002;359:14-22.

Jensen DM. Endoscopic diagnosis and treatment of bleeding peptic ulcers. *Clin Perspect Gastroenterol* 1999;2(2):73–84.

Khuroo MS, Yattoo GN, Javid G, et al. A comparison of omeprazole and placebo for bleeding peptic ulcer. *N Engl J Med* 1997;336: 1054–1058.

Laine L, Schoenfeld P, Fennerty MB. Therapy for *Helicobacter pylori* in patients with nonulcer dyspepsia. *Ann Intern Med* 2001;134:361–369.

Laine L, Peterson WL. Bleeding peptic ulcer. *N Engl J Med* 1994;331: 717–727.

Lanas A, Bajador E, Serrano P, et al. Nitrovasodilators, low-dose aspirin, other nonsteroidal anti-inflammatory drugs and the risk of gastrointestinal bleeding. *N Engl J Med* 2000;343:834–839.

Lanas AI, Remacha B, Esteva F, et al. Risk factors associated with refractory peptic ulcers. *Gastroenterology* 1995;109:1124–1133.

Lanza FL. A guideline for the treatment and prevention of NSAID-induced ulcers. *Am J Gastroenterol* 1998;11:2037–2046.

Lassen AT, Pedersen FM, Bytzer P, et al. *Helicobacter pylori* test and eradicate versus prompt endoscopy of dyspeptic patients: a randomised trial. *Lancet* 2000;356:455–460.

Lau JY, Sung JJ, Lam YH, et al. Endoscopic retreatment compared with surgery in patients with recurrent bleeding after initial endoscopic control of bleeding ulcers. *N Engl J Med* 1999;340:751–756.

Lau JY, Sung JJ, Lee KK, et al. Effect of intravenous omeprazole on recurrent bleeding after endoscopic treatment of bleeding peptic ulcers. *N Engl J Med* 2000;343:310–316.

Maton PN. Omeprazole. *N Engl J Med* 1991;324:965–975.

McColl KE. H. pylori-negative ulcer disease. *J Gastroenterol* 2000; 35[Suppl XII]:47–50.

McGowan CC, Cover TL, Blaser MJ. *Helicobacter pylori* and gastric acid: biological and therapeutic implications. *Gastroenterology* 1996;110: 926–938.

Norton JA, Fraker DL, Alexander HR, et al. Surgery to cure Zollinger-Ellison syndrome. *N Engl J Med* 1999;341:635–644.

Parsonnet J, Friedman GD, Vandersteen DP, et al. *Helicobacter pylori* infection and the risk of gastric carcinoma. *N Engl J Med* 1991; 325:1127–1131.

Parsonnet J, Hansen S, Rodriguez L, et al. *Helicobacter pylori* infection and gastric lymphoma. *N Engl J Med* 1994;330:1267–1271.

Peek RM, Blaser MJ. Pathophysiology of *Helicobacter pylori*–induced gastritis and peptic ulcer disease. *Am J Med* 1997;102:200–207.

Peterson WL, Fendrick AM, Cave DR. *Helicobacter pylori*–related disease. Guidelines for testing and treatment. *Arch Intern Med* 2000; 160:1285–1291.

Pounder, Roy E, *Helicobacter pylori* and NSAIDS—the end of the debate? *The Lancet* 2002; 359:3–4.

Raskin JB, White RH, Jackson JE, et al. Misoprostol dosage in the prevention of nonsteroidal anti-inflammatory drug-induced gastric and duodenal ulcers: a comparison of three regimens. *Ann Intern Med* 1995;123:344–350.

Silverstein FE, Faich G, Goldstein JL, et al. Gastrointestinal toxicity with celecoxib vs. nonsteroidal anti-inflammatory drugs for osteoarthritis and rheumatoid arthritis. The CLASS study: a randomized controlled trial. *JAMA* 2000;284:1247–1255.

Silverstein FE, Graham DY, Senior JR, et al. Misoprostol reduces serious gastrointestinal complications in patients with rheumatoid arthritis receiving nonsteroidal anti-inflammatory drugs. *Ann Intern Med* 1995;123:241–249.

Soll AH. Medical treatment of peptic ulcer disease. Practice guidelines. *JAMA* 1996;275:622–629.

Steinbach G, Ford R, Glober G, et al. Antibiotic treatment of gastric lymphoma of mucosa-associated lymphoid tissue. An uncontrolled trial. *Ann Intern Med* 1999;131:88–95.

Sung JJY, Chan FKL, et al. The effect of endoscopic therapy in patients receiving omeprazole for bleeding ulcers with nonbleeding visible vessels or adherent clots. *Ann Intern Med* 2003;139:237–243.

Taha AS, Hudson N, Hawkey CJ, et al. Famotidine for the prevention of gastric and duodenal ulcers caused by nonsteroidal anti-inflammatory drugs. *N Engl J Med* 1996;334:1435–1439.

Talley NJ, Lauritsen K. The potential role of acid suppression in functional dyspepsia: The BOND, OPERA, PILOT and ENCORE studies. *Gut* 2002;50(Suppl):iv36–iv41.

Talley NJ, Silverstein MD, Agreus L, et al. AGA technical review: evaluation of dyspepsia. *Gastroenterology* 1998;114:582–595.

Tytgat GN. *Helicobacter pylori*: past, present, and future. *J Gastroenterol Hepatol* 2000;15:G30–G33.

Vaira D, Vakil N. Blood, urine, stool, breath, money, and *Helicobacter pylori*. *Gut* 2001;48:287–289.

Vaira D, Vakil N. The stool antigen test for detection of *Helicobacter pylori* after eradication therapy. *Ann of Intern Med* 2002;136:4: 280–287.

Veldhuyzen van Zanten SJ. Can the age limit for endoscopy be increased in dyspepsia patients who do not have alarm symptoms? *Am J Gastroenterol* 1999;94:9–11.

Wolf MM, Lichtenstein DR, Singh G. Gastrointestinal toxicity of nonsteroidal anti-inflammatory drugs. *N Engl J Med* 1999;340:1888–1898.

Wolf MM, Soll AH. The physiology of gastric acid secretion. *N Engl J Med* 1988;319:1707–1715.

Yeomans ND, Tulassay Z, Juhasz L, et al. A comparison of omeprazole with ranitidine for ulcers associated with nonsteroidal anti-inflammatory drugs. *N Engl J Med* 1998;338:719–726.

# Colorectal Carcinoma

## *Carol A. Burke*

Colorectal cancer is the third most common cancer and cause of cancer deaths in the United States. As shown in Table 59.1, both men and women face a lifetime risk of 1 in 18 for the development of invasive colorectal cancer. Each year approximately 147,000 new cases of colorectal cancer are diagnosed and 57,000 deaths occur (1). The survival benefit from early detection of colorectal carcinoma through the fecal occult blood test (FOBT) and sigmoidoscopy has been proven; however, fewer than 50% of eligible Americans have undergone screening. More than 45% of patients diagnosed with colorectal cancer present with stage III and stage IV disease, which carry a 5-year survival rate of 50% and 7%, respectively.

## ETIOLOGY

In nearly all cases, colorectal carcinoma arises from an adenomatous polyp. Only 2% of adenomas progress to cancer, however. Observational studies suggest that the adenoma-to-carcinoma sequence takes approximately 10 years

(2). The indirect evidence supporting the adenoma-to-carcinoma sequence includes:

- Anatomic distribution and patient demographics are similar for both adenoma and colorectal cancer.
- Risk of dysplasia or cancer increases with increasing polyp size and villous architecture, and in most cases cancer is associated with the presence of adenomatous polyps.
- Progressive genetic alterations have been found as adenomas progress to cancer.
- Colonoscopic polypectomy has been associated with a diminished incidence of cancer.

## RISK FACTORS

Colorectal carcinogenesis results from complex interactions between genetic susceptibility and environmental factors. Epidemiologic studies implicate dietary variables (e.g., high fat, particularly from red meat, excess alcohol ingestion, and low fiber) as cofactors in the development of polyps and colorectal cancer. Other environmental risk factors include obesity and smoking. The risk of adenomatous polyps and

**TABLE 59.1**

**PERCENTAGE OF U.S. POPULATION DIAGNOSED WITH INVASIVE COLORECTAL CANCER**

|  | Birth–39 Yr | 40–59 Yr | 60–79 Yr | Lifetime Risk |
|---|---|---|---|---|
| Men | 0.06 (1 in 1,678) | 0.86 (1 in 116) | 3.94 (1 in 25) | 5.88 (1 in 17) |
| Women | 0.06 (1 in 1,651) | 0.67 (1 in 150) | 3.05 (1 in 33) | 5.49 (1 in 18) |

(Data reprinted with permission from Jemal A, Tiwani R, Murray T, et al. Cancer statistics, 2004. *CA Cancer J Clin* 2004;54:24.)

cancer is low before age 40, but it increases with age to a peak in the seventh and eighth decades of life. A sex or race predilection does not appear to exist, except among African Americans, who have higher colorectal cancer incidence and mortality rates. Approximately 70% of newly diagnosed colorectal cancers arise in patients without known risk factors. In approximately 30% of patients with colorectal cancer, risk factors have been identified (Table 59.2).

A personal history of adenomatous polyps or colorectal cancer increases the risk for metachronous colorectal cancer. First-degree relatives of patients with colorectal cancer have a two- to threefold increased risk for colorectal cancer and adenomatous polyps (3,4). Recent work has proven that the first-degree family members of patients with adenomatous polyps also have an increased risk of colorectal cancer, particularly when the adenoma is diagnosed before age 60 (5,6).

Patients with the highest risk of colorectal cancer are those who have germline abnormalities in critical genes that control critical cellular function, as in the hereditary colorectal cancer syndromes. *Familial adenomatous polyposis* (FAP) is an autosomal dominant disease with nearly 100% penetrance. Germline mutations of the tumor-suppressor gene *APC*, on the long arm of chromosome 5, are detected in up to 90% of FAP patients. *APC* mutations result in the development of hundreds to thousands of colonic adenomas by the second decade of life. Colon cancer develops in all FAP patients by 40 years of age if prophylactic colectomy is not performed. Upper gastrointestinal adenomas are common in this population, and periampullary cancer is the second leading cause of cancer deaths in this group.

**TABLE 59.2**

**RISK FACTORS FOR COLORECTAL CANCER**

Personal history of adenomas or colorectal cancer
First-degree relative <60 yr with adenoma or colorectal cancer, or
    two first-degree relatives of any age with colorectal cancer
Inherited colorectal cancer syndromes
    Hereditary nonpolyposis colorectal cancer
    Familial adenomatous polyposis
Ulcerative colitis and Crohn's disease

*Gardner syndrome* is a phenotypic variant of FAP. In addition to colonic polyposis, Gardner syndrome may manifest with benign soft tissue tumors, osteomas, supernumerary teeth, desmoid tumors, and congenital hypertrophy of the retinal pigment epithelium.

Recent studies have identified another genetic cause for multiple colonic adenomas. *MYH*, on chromosome 19, is a base-excision-repair gene. Bi-allelic germline mutations in *MYH* have been found to be present in 7.5% of individuals with FAP and no detectable *APC* mutation (7). It also results in a recessive pattern of inheritance to multiple colorectal adenomas and probably an increased risk of colorectal cancer. Bi-allelic *MYH* mutations are found in 3.9% of individuals with multiple (3 to 100) lifetime adenomas and in 29% of those with 15 to 100 adenomas.

*Hereditary nonpolyposis colon cancer* (HNPCC) is an autosomal dominant disease with nearly complete penetrance. Colon cancer occurs in up to 80% of those affected, usually at a young age, and is often right-sided. Mutations in at least four genes, called *mismatch repair genes*, result in carcinogenesis in HNPCC. Alterations in the mismatch repair genes prevent the adequate repair of DNA. Germline mutations in one of four mismatch repair genes can be identified in 50% of patients with HNPCC. The diagnosis of HNPCC is made in families that satisfy the Amsterdam criteria:

- Three or more relatives with colorectal cancer, with one being a first-degree relative of the other two
- At least two successive generations affected
- One cancer diagnosed before age 50

HNPCC families may have extracolonic cancers, which include other gastrointestinal tumors and urologic and gynecologic malignancies. The risk of endometrial carcinoma has been reported to be as high as 60% in women in HNPCC kindreds (8). Therefore, aggressive gynecologic screening for endometrial cancer is recommended.

The chronic inflammatory colitides, *ulcerative colitis* and *Crohn's disease*, are associated with a high risk of colorectal cancer. The proximal extent of colonic involvement and the duration of disease (not activity) stratify the level of risk. Risk is highest in patients with pancolitis and negligible in patients with proctitis. After a decade of disease, the cancer risk increases yearly by 1% to 2%.

**TABLE 59.3**

**GENETIC ALTERATIONS IN COLORECTAL TUMORIGENESIS**

| Oncogenes | Tumor-Suppressor Genes | Mismatch Repair Genes | Base Excision Genes |
|-----------|------------------------|-----------------------|---------------------|
| 12p (k-ras) | 5q (APC) | 2p (MSH2) | 19 (MYH) |
|  | 17p (p53) | 3p (MLH1) |  |
|  | 18q (DCC) | 2 (PMS1) |  |
|  |  | 7 (PMS2) |  |

## PATHOGENESIS

Colorectal tumorigenesis results from multiple acquired genetic alterations within tumor tissue. These alterations, in turn, promote malignant transformation (i.e., the development of oncogenes) or loss in the inhibition of cellular proliferation (i.e., the development of tumor-suppressor genes) (9). Mutations in DNA repair (i.e., mismatch repair) genes are implicated in carcinogenesis in patients with HNPCC and in approximately 20% of patients with sporadic colorectal cancer (Table 59.3).

## CLINICAL PRESENTATION

Colon polyps and early colon cancer are asymptomatic until they are advanced. Gastrointestinal blood loss is the most common sign and may include a positive FOBT result, iron deficiency anemia, or hematochezia. When tumors are advanced, unexplained anorexia, weight loss, or symptoms from obstruction or local invasion, such as a change in bowel habits, abdominal pain, or obstruction may occur.

## DIAGNOSIS

The diagnosis of colorectal polyps and cancer is made most often during a colonic evaluation performed for gastrointestinal symptoms, screening, or surveillance.

**TABLE 59.4**

**CLASSIFICATION OF COLORECTAL POLYPS**

| Neoplastic | Non-neoplastic |
|------------|----------------|
| Adenomatous | Hyperplastic |
| Tubular | Hamartomatous |
| Tubulovillous | Lymphoid aggregate |
| Villous | Inflammatory |

**TABLE 59.5**

**ADENOMA SIZE, HISTOLOGY, AND CANCER RISK**

| Histology | Percentage with Invasive Cancer | | |
|-----------|-------|-------|-------|
|  | <1 cm | 12 cm | >2 cm |
| Tubular adenoma | 1 | 10 | 35 |
| Tubulovillous adenoma | 4 | 7 | 46 |
| Villous adenoma | 10 | 10 | 53 |

(Adapted with permission from Muto T, Bussey HJR, Marson BC. The evolution of cancer of the colon and rectum. *Cancer* 1975;36:2251–2270.)

## Pathology

*Polyp* is an inexact term that indicates a protuberance of tissue into the colonic lumen. A variety of polyps can be found in the colon. The only polyp that can become an adenocarcinoma is an adenomatous polyp (Table 59.4). Adenomas account for approximately two of every three colonic polyps. Both the size and the degree of villous features are predictive of the risk of malignancy within the polyp (Table 59.5) (10).

Hyperplastic polyps are the second most common type of polyp, accounting for 10% to 30% of colonic polyps. Hyperplastic polyps are most often found in the rectosigmoid and have no clinical significance. Hyperplastic polyps and adenomas are indistinguishable at endoscopy, however. Therefore, all polyps detected in the colon and rectum should be removed and sent for histologic analysis.

## Screening

Various methods are available for colorectal cancer screening, and the cost effectiveness of these modalities is under study (11) (Table 59.6). Any positive finding detected by any of the screening tests warrants colonoscopy.

**TABLE 59.6**

**COST, SENSITIVITY, AND SPECIFICITY OF SCREENING TESTS FOR COLORECTAL CANCER**

| | Cost Per Test ($) | Sensitivity (%) | Specificity (%) |
|--|-------------------|-----------------|-----------------|
| Fecal occult blood test | 10–20 | 26–92 | 90–98 |
| Flexible sigmoidoscopy | 150–500 | 90 | 98 |
| Air-contrast barium enema | 300–500 | 60–80 | 98 |
| Colonoscopy | 1,000–1,500 | 75–95 | 100 |

### Fecal Occult Blood Test

The FOBT is the most widely studied screening method. Because large polyps and cancers intermittently bleed, FOBT can be an effective screening tool. The peroxidase activity of hemoglobin can be detected by a color change when it catalyzes the oxidation of guaiac through a peroxide reagent. Compliance rates are low, however, possibly because of both the need to follow a special diet (i.e., meat-free, high-residue diet without vegetables having peroxidase activity, such as turnips and horseradish) for at least 24 hours before specimen collection and the need to obtain three separate stool specimens collected at least 1 day apart. A positive finding on one or more samples on an FOBT is a positive test result.

A randomized trial of screening FOBT involving 46,551 volunteers found a 33% decrease in the mortality rate from colorectal cancer in a group that underwent annual screening (12). This reduced mortality rate was accompanied by a shift to detection of earlier-stage cancer. Overall compliance was low, however, with only 46% of volunteers completing all the screenings. Slide rehydration increased the sensitivity from 81% to 90%, but it decreased the specificity from 98% to 90% and the positive predictive value from 5.6% to 2.2%. In addition, the incidence of colorectal cancer was reduced by 20% in the annual screening group probably because of the use of colonoscopy and polypectomy (13).

### Sigmoidoscopy

Sigmoidoscopic screening allows a portion of the colorectal mucosa to be visualized directly and a diagnostic biopsy to be performed at the time of examination. Both the sensitivity and the specificity is high for the detection of polyps and cancer in the segment of the bowel examined. Unfortunately, however, nearly 40% of polyps and cancers are beyond the limits of detection of the longest (i.e., 60 cm) flexible sigmoidoscope. The detection of adenomas on flexible sigmoidoscopy is considered a positive test result and warrants colonoscopy with polypectomy.

Opinions vary regarding the need for colonoscopy for patients in whom a single tubular adenoma smaller than 1 cm is found on flexible sigmoidoscopy; however, the prevalence of proximal neoplasms in such patients may be substantial enough (7% to 9%) to warrant screening colonoscopy (14).

The results of several case-control studies show a reduction in deaths from colorectal cancer in patients who undergo predominantly rigid sigmoidoscopic examinations. The reported reduction in mortality varies from between 59% and 80%. The most well-known study reviewed the use of sigmoidoscopic screening in 261 patients who died from cancer of the distal colon or rectum, comparing these patients with 868 controls (15). Screening reduced the rectosigmoid cancer mortality rate by 60%, and the protective effect of sigmoidoscopy was noted to last for up to 10 years. This reduction in mortality may have resulted from earlier detection of cancer and removal of premalignant polyps.

### Fecal Occult Blood Testing and Sigmoidoscopy

In one controlled trial, 12,479 people underwent annual screening with rigid sigmoidoscopy or rigid sigmoidoscopy combined with FOBT (16). A reduction in the colorectal cancer mortality rate, detection of earlier-stage cancer, and longer survival were seen in patients undergoing both FOBT and rigid sigmoidoscopy.

### Barium Enema Testing

Barium enema testing has the advantage of imaging the entire colon. Recent evidence, however, suggests that it is inaccurate for the detection of polyps and early cancers, and suboptimal for colorectal cancer screening or surveillance. In a prospective study comparing the use of double-contrast barium enema examination and colonoscopy, the miss rate of barium enema testing for polyps larger than 1 cm was 52% (17).

If barium enema testing is the only option for screening or surveillance, it should be coupled with flexible sigmoidoscopy. The use of flexible sigmoidoscopy allows the visualization of the rectosigmoid, which is not well visualized on barium enema examination because of the overlapping loops of bowel. Lesions detected on barium enema testing warrant colonoscopic evaluation.

### Colonoscopy

Colonoscopy is the only technique with both diagnostic and therapeutic applications. It is considered the gold standard for the detection of colonic neoplasms, and it can be completed in more than 95% of examinations. No published studies have investigated the effectiveness of colonoscopic screening in the prevention of colorectal cancer. In one cohort study of 1,418 patients who underwent colonoscopy and polypectomy, a lower-than-expected incidence of colorectal cancer was observed (18).

### Recommendations

Consortium, multisociety guidelines for colorectal cancer screening were updated in 2003 (19). Recommendations for average-risk patients, for whom screening begins at age 50, include the following:

■ Annual FOBT plus flexible sigmoidoscopy every 5 years, or
■ Colonoscopy every 10 years, or
■ Double-contrast barium enema test every 5 to 10 years

Patients with a greater-than-average risk of colorectal cancer should undergo colonoscopic surveillance individualized according to the risk of cancer, which involves the following factors.

#### Surveillance

**History of Adenomatous Polyps.** Once adenomatous polyps are removed, the next colonoscopy should occur in 3 to 5 years depending on the family history, and the size, number, and pathology of the polyps (20,21).

Patients who have "advanced" (identified by being >1 cm, or with histology containing villous features or severe dysplasia) or multiple adenomas (≥3) should have their first follow-up colonoscopy in 3 years. Patients who have 1 or 2 small, <1 cm, tubular adenomas should have their first follow-up colonoscopy at 5 years. The surveillance interval is individualized for individuals with large (i.e., more than 2 cm) sessile polyps, numerous adenomas, adenomas removed piecemeal, or adenomas with malignancy and favorable prognostic features; this period may be as short as 3 to 6 months.

If the first follow-up colonoscopy is normal, or only 1 or 2 small (<1 cm) tubular adenomas are found, the next colonoscopy can be in 5 years. After one negative result, the interval can be lengthened to 5 to 10 years, depending on the aforementioned risk factors.

*History of Colorectal Cancer.* In patients who undergo curative surgical intervention for colorectal cancer and have a normal preoperative colonoscopy, the subsequent surveillance examination should occur at 3 years and, if results are negative at that time, every 5 years thereafter.

*Familial Adenomatous Polyposis.* Patients with FAP should receive genetic counseling and be offered genetic testing. Beginning at puberty, gene carriers or those with indeterminate status should undergo yearly flexible sigmoidoscopy.

*Hereditary Nonpolyposis Colon Cancer.* Patients with HNPCC should receive genetic counseling and be offered genetic testing. Colonoscopy should be performed every 1 to 2 years beginning at age 25 (or at an age 10 years younger than the age at which cancer occurred in the relative who developed colon cancer at the youngest age). After age 40, surveillance examinations should be conducted yearly. Annual transvaginal ultrasonography and endometrial biopsy should be considered in women older than 25 years.

*Ulcerative or Crohn's Colitis.* Generally, colonoscopy with biopsies for dysplasia is performed every 1 to 2 years after 8 years of pancolitic disease. Patients with disease involving the left colon should begin surveillance after 12 to 15 years of disease.

*Family History of Colon Cancer or Adenomatous Polyps.* In an individual with two first-degree relatives who developed colon cancer at any age, or with a first degree-relative diagnosed with adenomatous polyps or colorectal cancer before age 60, a colonoscopy every 5 years beginning at age 40 (or at an age 10 years younger than the age at which the relative developed cancer) is appropriate. Individuals with one first-degree, or two second-degree relatives older than age 60 with colorectal neoplasia should undergo colonoscopy every 10 years, beginning at age 40.

**TABLE 59.7**

**COMPARISON OF DUKES AND TNM STAGING SYSTEMS**

| Dukes | Stage | TNM | | | 5-Yr Survival (%) |
|---|---|---|---|---|---|
| A | I | T1 or T2 | N0 | M0 | 90 |
| B1 | II | T3 | N0 | M0 | 75 |
| B2 | | T4 | N0 | M0 | |
| C | III | Any T | N1–N3 | M0 | 35–60 |
| D | IV | Any T | Any N | M1 | <10 |

| Primary tumor (T) | |
|---|---|
| Tis | Carcinoma in situ |
| T1 | Tumor invades submucosa |
| T2 | Tumor invades muscularis propria |
| T3 | Tumor invades through muscularis propria |
| T4 | Tumor invades serosa, nodes, and adjacent organs |

| Metastases (M) | |
|---|---|
| M0 | No distant metastases |
| M1 | Distant metastases |

| Regional nodes (N) | |
|---|---|
| N0 | Negative nodes |
| N1 | 1–3 positive nodes |
| N2 | >3 positive nodes |
| N3 | Positive nodes on vascular trunk |

TNM, tumor-node-metastasis.

## TREATMENT

The curability and chance of recurrence of colorectal cancer, and survival after it, are determined on the basis of the disease stage. For most early-stage tumors (i.e., Dukes stages A and B; Table 59.7), surgery alone is curative. For more advanced disease, surgery and adjuvant chemotherapy are recommended to prevent recurrence and prolong survival.

### Adjuvant Treatment

Studies over the last 10 years have proven the benefit of adjuvant therapy in decreasing cancer recurrence and prolonging survival in subgroups of patients with colon cancer (22). In the current view, patients with Dukes stage C colon cancer should receive adjuvant therapy with fluorouracil (5-FU; Adrucil) and leucovorin calcium (Wellcovorin). Patients with Dukes stage B2 disease should be encouraged to participate in ongoing trials because adjuvant therapy has no proven survival benefit for these patients (23). The combination of postoperative radiation and 5-FU significantly reduces the rates of recurrence, cancer-related deaths, and overall mortality in patients with stage II or stage III rectal cancer, compared with radiation therapy alone (24).

### Hepatic Metastases

The prognosis for patients with hepatic metastases is poor, with virtually no survivors at 3 years. A multi-institutional study reviewing hepatic resection as treatment for colorectal cancer metastases found a 5-year survival rate of 33% and a disease-free survival rate of 21% (25). Favorable prognostic factors included a resection margin greater than 1 cm and two or fewer metastases smaller than 8 cm.

## PREVENTION

Chemoprevention is one of the most exciting potential preventive measures against colorectal cancer. The high consumption of fruits and vegetables is consistently associated with a lower risk of colorectal cancer. The mechanism by which fiber may prevent cancer is unknown, but a small randomized, double-blind, placebo-controlled study identified a statistically significant reduction in fecal bile acid concentrations among patients receiving a wheat-bran fiber and calcium supplement (26). Results of epidemiologic studies show that diets high in carotenoid vegetables, cruciferous vegetables, garlic, and tofu (or soybeans) are associated with decreased prevalence of adenoma (27). Nonsteroidal anti-inflammatory drugs (NSAIDs), particularly aspirin, substantially reduce the risk of colorectal cancer by anywhere from 4% to 60%. In two large, prospective double-blind studies, regular aspirin use in dosages similar to those taken for cardioprotection was associated with decreased risk of recurrent colorectal adenomas (28,29). The U.S. Food and Drug Administration has approved the use of the cyclooxygenase 2–selective NSAID celecoxib as an adjunct to promote the regression of adenomas, in addition to the usual surveillance and polypectomy, in patients with FAP. This approval was based on a 6-month trial, which found a 28% reduction in colorectal adenomas in patients with FAP (30). A recent randomized, double-blind, placebo-controlled study detected a significant decrease in the recurrence of adenomas in patients taking 1,200 mg of calcium (31).

## CONCLUSION

Colorectal cancer is one of the leading causes of cancer and death from carcinoma in the United States. Increasing awareness regarding the preventable nature of this disease, along with the widespread use of screening, should favorably affect the incidence of colorectal cancer. Colorectal cancer screening and polyp removal can save lives, and the most exciting area of future research is the primary prevention of adenomas and colorectal cancer through chemoprevention.

## REVIEW EXERCISES

### QUESTIONS

For the cases in Questions 1 through 4, choose the appropriate recommendation from the lettered list (each may be used more than once):

**1.** A single 3-mm rectal adenoma is found on flexible sigmoidoscopy in a 32-year-old woman.

**2.** A 62-year-old man with an 18-year history of pancolitis just underwent colonoscopy.

**3.** A 54-year-old woman has a lifelong history of irritable bowel syndrome.

**4.** A 68-year-old African American man recently underwent removal of an 8 mm villous adenoma.
a) Colonoscopy and polypectomy
b) Yearly FOBT and flexible sigmoidoscopy every 5 years
c) Colonoscopy at age 40 years
d) Colonoscopy in 5 years
e) Colonoscopy in 3 years
f) Colonoscopy in 1 year

**5.** A 71 year-old white man underwent complete colonoscopy with removal of 2 polyps. One was a 7-mm tubulovillous adenoma with severe dysplasia, the other was a 3-mm tubular adenoma.
  What is the best recommendation in this case?
a) Repeat colonoscopy in 3 to 6 months.
b) Repeat colonoscopy in 1 year.
c) Repeat colonoscopy in 3 years.
d) Repeat colonoscopy in 5 years.

For Questions 6 through 10, indicate whether the statement about colorectal cancer and polyps is true or false.

**6.** A 70-year-old man who underwent curative resection of Dukes stage A colon cancer found on a surveillance colonoscopy can wait 3 years until the next examination.
a) True
b) False

**7.** A 53-year-old woman with breast cancer is at increased risk of colorectal cancer and should undergo colonoscopy every 5 years.
a) True
b) False

**8.** A 34-year-old man who has a 52-year-old brother with colon cancer, a sister with endometrial cancer, and a father who died of colon cancer at age 58 should undergo colonoscopy at age 50.
a) True
b) False

**9.** All patients with a T3 N1 M0 colon cancer should be offered adjuvant therapy with leucovorin and 5-FU.
a) True
b) False

**10.** A patient with FAP has a 50% chance of transmitting the disease to his or her children.
a) True
b) False

**11.** A 62-year-old woman arrives in your office with recent-onset abdominal pain and a change in bowel habit. She has no family history of cancer and is otherwise in good health. Physical examination reveals some tenderness in the suprapubic area but is otherwise normal. FOBT reveals one of six smears to be positive.

Which of the following options is most appropriate?

a) Repeat the FOBT.
b) Schedule a colonoscopy.
c) Order a flexible sigmoidoscopy and, if results are negative, do no further evaluation.
d) Reassure the patient that she has symptoms of irritable bowel syndrome and treat with fiber.

12. A 42-year-old man with FAP has two children, ages 12 and 14. He is interested in knowing if his children have FAP. No *APC* mutation was found on his genetic testing, however. What would be the appropriate management of this family?

a) Recommend flexible sigmoidoscopy when the children begin to show symptoms of colonic disease.
b) Offer *MYH* testing to the man.
c) Advise him that he cannot pass FAP on to his children because he has no detectable *APC* mutation.

## ANSWERS

### 1. a.
Until further studies are performed, all patients with an adenoma detected by flexible sigmoidoscopy should undergo a full colonoscopy to detect synchronous, more proximal neoplasms, as well as polypectomy of all detected polyps.

### 2. f.
All patients with ulcerative pancolitis who have had the diagnosis for more than 8 years are at increased risk of colorectal dysplasia and cancer. Yearly colonoscopy with four-quadrant biopsy every 10 cm to detect dysplasia is indicated.

### 3. b.
Patients with irritable bowel syndrome and no risk factors are at average risk for colorectal cancer. Although colonoscopy is the preferred screening strategy, the best answer here is flexible sigmoidoscopy every 5 years and annual FOBT, which is an appropriate screening method for patients at average risk.

### 4. d.
The postpolypectomy surveillance interval is 5 years in patients with fewer than three tubular adenomas smaller than 1 cm detected on colonoscopy. New data has shown that those individuals are not at high risk of having numerous, large, or advanced adenomas on their subsequent colonoscopy.

### 5. e.
The individuals at higher risk of having recurrent neoplasia on the first postpolypectomy examination are those who had more than two, large (>1 cm), or histologically

advanced (villous features or severe dysplasia) adenomas. This group of individuals is recommended to have their follow-up colonoscopy in 3 years.

### 6. a.
True. A 3-year surveillance interval is recommended after colorectal cancer surgery with curative intent. If this patient did not have a perioperative colonoscopy, a colonoscopy should be done within 1 year of surgery.

### 7. b.
False. A personal history of breast cancer is not associated with an increased risk of colorectal carcinoma. Factors that increase the risk of colorectal cancer include a personal or family history of colorectal neoplasia, the inherited colon cancer syndromes, and the chronic colitides, such as ulcerative and Crohn's colitis.

### 8. b.
False. This patient's family history should suggest HNPCC to the clinician. Although the Amsterdam criteria are not met, the strong family history (in two first-degree relatives) of early onset colorectal cancer (occurring before age 60 years) necessitates colonoscopic surveillance beginning at age 40 years, or 10 years earlier than the age at which cancer was diagnosed in the relative in whom cancer occurred at the youngest age.

### 9. a.
True. The clinician should be familiar with the Dukes and tumor-node-metastasis (TNM) cancer staging systems. Adjuvant therapy is recommended only for patients with nodal disease (Dukes C or TNM stage III) colorectal cancer. No benefit was seen in earlier-stage disease.

### 10. a.
True. As in all dominantly inherited diseases, such as FAP and HNPCC, 50% of the offspring are at risk of inheriting the mutation.

### 11. b.
Any patient with symptoms of colorectal cancer should have a complete colonic evaluation. A positive FOBT result includes a positive finding in any of six sample windows; retesting should not be performed.

### 12. b.
It is not appropriate to wait for colonic symptoms in individuals "at risk" of FAP. Surveillance should begin at the time of puberty and colectomy should be performed before bleeding, pain, or cancer develops. About 10% of individuals with FAP are *APC*-negative but still have a 50% chance of passing an FAP disease–causing mutation on to their children. It has recently been discovered that bi-allelic germline mutations in *MYH* account for up to 7.5% of *APC*-negative FAP patients. *MYH* testing should be offered to any patient with multiple adenomas or those with classic FAP but who are *APC*-negative.

## REFERENCES

1. Jemal A, Tiwani R, Murray T, et al. Cancer statistics, 2004. *CA Cancer J Clin* 2004;54:8–29.
2. Morson BC. The evolution of colorectal carcinomas. *Clin Radiol* 1984;35:425–431.
3. St. John DJ, McDermott F, Hopper J, et al. Cancer risk in relatives of patients with common colorectal cancer. *Ann Intern Med* 1993;118:785–790.
4. Bazzoli F, Fossi S, Sottili S, et al. The risk of adenomatous polyps in asymptomatic first-degree relatives of persons with colon cancer. *Gastroenterology* 1995;109:783–788.
5. Winawer S, Zauber A, Gerdes H, et al. Risk of colorectal cancer in the families of patients with adenomatous polyps. *N Engl J Med* 1996;334:82–97.
6. Ahsan H, Neugut A, Garbowski G, et al. Family history of colorectal adenomatous polyps and increased risk for colorectal cancer. *Ann Intern Med* 1998;128:900–905.
7. Sieber O, Lipton L, Crabtree M, et al. Multiple colorectal adenomas, classic adenomatous polyposis, and germ-line mutations in *MYH*. *N Engl J Med* 2003;348;791–798.
8. Brown GJ, St. John DJ, Macrae FA, et al. Cancer risk in young women at risk of hereditary nonpolyposis colorectal cancer: implications for gynecologic surveillance. *Gynecol Oncol* 2001;80:346–349.
9. Vogelstein B, Fearon E, Hamilton S, et al. Genetic alterations during colorectal-tumor development. *N Engl J Med* 1988;319:525–532.
10. Day DW, Morson BC. Pathology of adenomas in the pathogenesis of colorectal cancer. In: Morson BC, ed. *Major Problems in Pathology*. Philadelphia: WB Saunders, 1978;43–57.
11. Lieberman DA. Cost-effectiveness model for colon cancer screening. *Gastroenterology* 1995;109:1781–1790.
12. Mandel JS, Bond JH, Church TR, et al. Reducing mortality from colorectal cancer by screening for fecal occult blood. Minnesota Colon Cancer Control Study. *N Engl J Med* 1993;328:1365–1371.
13. Mandel JS, Church TR, Bond JH, et al. The effect of fecal occult-blood screening on the incidence of colorectal cancer. *N Engl J Med* 2000;343:1603–1607.
14. Lieberman D, Weiss D, Bond J, et al. Use of colonoscopy to screen asymptomatic adults for colorectal cancer. *N Engl J Med* 2000;343:162–168.
15. Selby JV, Friedman GD, Quesenberry CO, et al. Case-control study of screening sigmoidoscopy and mortality from colorectal cancer. *N Engl J Med* 1992;326:653–657.
16. Winawer SJ, Flehinger BJ, Schottenfeld D, et al. Screening for colorectal cancer with fecal occult blood testing and sigmoidoscopy. *J Natl Cancer Inst* 1993;85:1311–1318.
17. Winawer SJ, Stewart ET, Zauber AG, et al. A comparison of colonoscopy and double-contrast barium enema for surveillance after polypectomy. *N Engl J Med* 2000;342(24):1766–1772.
18. Winawer SJ, Zauber AG, Ho MN, et al. Prevention of colorectal cancer by colonoscopic polypectomy. *N Engl J Med* 1993;329:1977–1981.
19. Winawer S, Fletcher R, Rex D, et al. Colorectal cancer screening and surveillance: clinical guidelines and rationale—Update based on new evidence. *Gastroenterology* 2003;124(2):544–560.
20. Bond JH. Polyp guideline: diagnosis, treatment, and surveillance for patients with colorectal polyps. Practice Parameters Committee of the American College of Gastroenterology. *Am J Gastroenterol* 2000;95:3053–3063.
21. Atkin WS, Morson BC, Cuzick J. Long-term risk of colorectal cancer after excision of rectosigmoid adenomas. *N Engl J Med* 1992;326(10):658–662.
22. Engstrom PF, Benson AB III, Cohen A, et al. NCCN colorectal cancer practice guidelines. The National Comprehensive Cancer Network. *Oncology* 1996;10:140–175.
23. Moertel CG, Fleming TR, Macdonald JS. Intergroup study of fluorouracil plus levamisole as adjuvant therapy for stage II/Dukes' stage B2 colon cancer. *J Clin Oncol* 1995;13: 2935–2943.
24. Krook J, Moertel C, Gunderson L, et al. Effective surgical adjuvant therapy for high-risk rectal carcinoma. *N Engl J Med* 1991;324:709–715.
25. Hughes KS, Simon R, Songhorabodi S, et al. Resection of the liver for colorectal carcinoma metastasis: a multi-institutional study of indications for resection. *Surgery* 1990;103: 278–288.
26. Alberts DS, Ritenbaugh C, Story JA, et al. Randomized, double-blinded, placebo-controlled study of effect of wheat bran fiber and calcium on fecal bile acids in patients with resected adenomatous colon polyps. *J Natl Cancer Inst* 1996; 88:81–92.
27. Witte JS, Longnecker MP, Bird C, et al. Relations of vegetable, fruit, and grain consumption to colorectal adenomatous polyps. *Am J Epidemiol* 1996;144:1015–1025.
28. Baron JA, Cole BF, Sandler RS, et al. A randomized trial of aspirin to prevent colorectal adenomas. *N Engl J Med* 2003;348:891–899.
29. Sandler R, Halabi S, Baron J, et al. A randomized trial of aspirin to prevent colorectal adenomas in patients with previous colorectal cancer. *N Engl J Med* 2003;348:883–890.
30. Steinbach G, Lynch PM, Phillips RK, et al. The effect of celecoxib, a cyclooxygenase-2 inhibitor, in familial adenomatous polyposis. *N Engl J Med* 2000;342:1946–1952.
31. Baron JA, Beach M, Mandel JS, et al. Calcium supplements for the prevention of colorectal adenomas. *N Engl J Med* 1999;340:101–107.

## SUGGESTED READINGS

Bond JH. Polyp guideline: diagnosis, treatment, and surveillance for patients with colorectal polyps. Practice Parameters Committee of the American College of Gastroenterology. *Am J Gastroenterol* 2000; 95:3053–3063.

Engstrom P, Benson A, Cohen A, et al. NCCN colorectal cancer practice guidelines. The National Comprehensive Cancer Network. *Oncology* 1996;10:140–175.

Krook J, Moertel C, Gunderson L, et al. Effective surgical adjuvant therapy for high-risk rectal carcinoma. *N Engl J Med* 1991;324: 709–715.

Mandel JS, Bond JH, Church TR, et al. Reducing mortality from colorectal cancer by screening for fecal occult blood. Minnesota Colon Cancer Control Study. *N Engl J Med* 1993;328:1365–1371.

Selby JV, Friedman GD, Quesenberry CO, et al. A case-control study of screening sigmoidoscopy and mortality from colorectal cancer. *N Engl J Med* 1992;326:653–657.

Vogelstein B, Fearon E, Hamilton S, et al. Genetic alterations during colorectal-tumor development. *N Engl J Med* 1988; 319:525–532.

# Inflammatory Bowel Disease

# 60

## Aaron Brzezinski

The term *inflammatory bowel disease* (IBD) applies commonly to two diseases of the gastrointestinal system, namely, Crohn's disease and ulcerative colitis. These are chronic diseases of unknown etiology, and their hallmark is uncontrolled inflammation. IBD is a systemic disorder in that patients frequently have extraintestinal manifestations. A greater understanding of the immunologic abnormalities has resulted in more specific treatments, but therapy is still aimed at limiting morbidity, controlling symptoms, and decreasing mortality. Recent information supports the existence of a genetic predisposition for IBD in some families.

## ETIOLOGY

The cause of IBD remains elusive. The gastrointestinal tract is not only an absorptive organ but also has a major immune function. It is normally in a "controlled state of inflammation." In patients with IBD this balance is lost, and there appears to be a failure to downregulate once the inflammatory process begins. It is believed that in a susceptible individual, an environmental trigger may affect the immune system. The end result is pathologic inflammation, which leads to ulceration and altered remodeling that causes fibrosis and stricture formation.

## EPIDEMIOLOGY

The incidence of ulcerative colitis has remained stable, at 2 to 15 per 100,000 population, whereas the incidence of Crohn's disease is increasing, with current estimates as high as 7 per 100,000. The combined prevalence in the Western world is 150 to 200 cases per 100,000. Great geographic variation exists in the incidence of these diseases, with a direct relation between levels of sanitation and incidence of IBD. IBD is more prevalent in northern Europe and the northern parts of North America (i.e., the northern United States and Canada) than in the southern regions. In Third World countries, where infectious gastroenteritis is common, IBD is uncommon.

A slight female preponderance is observed, and the age at presentation has a bimodal distribution, with the larger peak occurring between ages 15 and 25 and a second, lower peak after the sixth decade of life. Both diseases can occur in children, but ulcerative colitis is more common in this population.

## RISK FACTORS

All populations are at risk, but Whites are more commonly affected. The risk for Ashkenazi Jews in Europe and in the United States is two- to fourfold higher for ulcerative colitis and six- to eightfold higher for Crohn's disease than in the general population in those same areas. Ashkenazi Jews in Israel, however, have a lower risk of IBD than those in Europe or the United States, which suggests a role for an environmental factor as a trigger for the disease.

An interesting association also exists between cigarette smoking and IBD. A larger-than-expected number of patients with Crohn's disease are cigarette smokers, whereas a lower-than-expected number of patients with ulcerative colitis are cigarette smokers.

## PATHOGENESIS

The cause of IBD remains unknown. A genetic predisposition to the disease exists, and there are as-yet-unknown environmental or infectious agents that trigger the disease. Whereas in 75% to 90% of patients no family history of IBD is present, 10% to 25% have a first-degree relative with the disease. IBD inheritance does not follow a mendelian pattern. Ten percent to 25% of patients have a first-degree relative with IBD, and the lifetime risk of IBD among first-degree relatives of patients is 3 to 20 times higher than in the rest of the population; namely, 9% for offspring and siblings, and 3.5% for parents. When a family history of IBD is present, patients usually present with the disease at an earlier age. In many families, a disease concordance for Crohn's disease also exists. The concordance rate among monozygotic twins is approximately 85% for Crohn's disease but not for ulcerative colitis.

A susceptibility locus for Crohn's disease has been mapped to chromosome 16, and it is referred to as *IBD1*. The most compelling evidence for a genetic role in Crohn's disease comes from the description of three mutations within the *NOD2* gene, which is located on chromosome 16 and is involved in apoptosis and antigen recognition. Such mutations have been reported in three studies, and the frequency in patients with a positive family history is 15% to 20%, compared with approximately 10% in controls.

The gastrointestinal system is in a constant state of controlled inflammation because it is continuously exposed to luminal antigens. Therefore, it seems logical that these antigens can trigger an abnormal inflammatory response. The antigens may be dietary, infectious, or environmental. To date, however, no specific antigens have been identified, although many have been proposed, including *Mycobacterium paratuberculosis* and proteins from bacterial cell-wall membranes. It is possible that the trigger antigen or antigens are the normal intestinal microflora. In animal models of IBD, the disease is not manifested as long as the animal is in a germ-free environment.

Whatever the trigger or triggers may be, the mucosal activation of macrophages leads to increased release of proinflammatory cytokines (i.e., interleukin-1, tumor necrosis factor-α, interleukin-6, interleukin-8), which in turn results in cell destruction through different mechanisms (including clonal expansion of natural killer cells and cytotoxic T cells), B-cell proliferation (with increased production of mucosal immunoglobulin G), and increased production of thromboxane $A_2$, leukotriene B, and platelet-activating factor (i.e., proinflammatory mediators that amplify the inflammatory response by recruiting and activating neutrophils).

# ULCERATIVE COLITIS

## Clinical Features

The presenting symptoms of ulcerative colitis depend on both the extent and severity of the disease. Patients with ulcerative colitis usually present with nonbloody diarrhea that rapidly progresses to bloody diarrhea. At presentation, the disease is limited to the rectum in 30% of patients and to the rectum and sigmoid colon in more than 50% of patients. It is for this reason that the initial presentation in most patients is mild to moderate disease, and at least 90% achieve remission with medical treatment. Fewer than 10% of patients present with a severe or fulminant attack, and these patients are likely to need surgery at presentation. The mortality rate from the initial attack is less than 0.5%.

## Diagnosis

The diagnosis of ulcerative colitis relies on the clinical picture, stool testing, endoscopic appearance, and histologic findings. To provide optimal medical treatment and establish the prognosis, it is important to determine the extent of disease. Histology is the most sensitive way of establishing disease extent, and colonoscopy with biopsies is indicated for patients in whom ulcerative colitis is suspected. In patients with severe or fulminant presentation, a limited

examination is sufficient because the rectum is always affected and the risk of significant complications precludes a more extensive examination. Biopsies are also useful in screening patients for dysplasia because those with extensive and long-standing disease have an increased risk of colorectal cancer. Colonoscopy is not necessary to assess patient response to medical treatment or for the routine follow-up of patients with ulcerative colitis. For determining the extent of the disease, colonoscopy without biopsy is less sensitive, and radiology is the least sensitive diagnostic modality. In fact, both these modalities underestimate the true extent of disease.

### Stool Analysis

Stool studies to exclude infectious causes that mimic ulcerative colitis are mandatory at time of presentation and are frequently ordered when patients experience exacerbations of disease. The most common infectious agents that mimic IBD include *Salmonella* species, *Shigella* species, *Campylobacter* species, *Clostridium difficile*, *Yersinia* species, and *Escherichia coli* O157:H7. In endemic areas, stool examination for *Entamoeba histolytica* is indicated because the use of corticosteroids in patients infected with this agent has disastrous results. In patients who are immunosuppressed (through chemotherapy, posttransplantation therapy, or acquired immunodeficiency syndrome), other infectious agents, such as cytomegalovirus, *Mycobacterium avium* complex, *Neisseria gonorrhoeae*, and chlamydia, should be excluded.

### Endoscopy

Patients with untreated ulcerative colitis always have rectal involvement. The earliest endoscopic findings in patients with ulcerative colitis are blurring of the blood vessels and hyperemia. In patients with more severe inflammation, the mucosa becomes granular and friable, and finally, with severe ulcerative colitis, the mucosa is ulcerated, and frequently blood, mucus, and pus are found in the lumen. The mucosa is diffusely involved in a continuous pattern. In chronic disease, the colon becomes tubular in appearance, and pseudopolyps may be present. A sharp demarcation between diseased and healthy mucosa may also be seen (Fig. 60.1).

### Radiology

In patients with severe or fulminant colitis, intestinal perforation or pneumatosis coli should be excluded by plain films of the abdomen before endoscopy is performed. Double-contrast barium enema testing is safe in patients with mild or moderately severe ulcerative colitis, but this modality underestimates the extent of disease and does not allow concurrent histologic sampling; therefore, it is rarely used. In patients with long-standing ulcerative colitis, the haustral folds are lost, and the colon is shortened and narrow ("stem-pipe colon"). Pseudopolyps can be visualized easily at double-contrast barium enema testing.

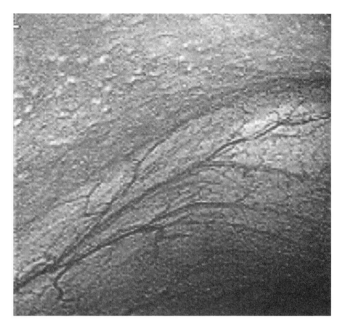

**Figure 60.1**  Line of demarcation in ulcerative colitis. (See Color Fig. 60.1.)

In addition, strictures can be diagnosed by contrast barium enema examination. Patients with strictures should undergo colonoscopy with biopsy and brush cytologic study to rule out dysplasia or cancer.

### Histology

The inflammatory changes in ulcerative colitis are primarily confined to the mucosa. The main findings are an increased number of neutrophils, lymphocytes, plasma cells, and macrophages; and cryptitis with crypt abscesses and goblet cell depletion. In patients with chronic disease, architectural distortion occurs, with crypt atrophy and shortened glands that lose their normal "test-tube array" appearance.

### Severity

Truelove and Witts proposed a classification of severity based on symptoms and laboratory tests (Table 60.1). Such a classification is useful to determine prognosis and establish treatment. Since its initial description, few modifications have been made except for the addition of endoscopic criteria. Such classifications are used most commonly in clinical trials. For the clinician, disease severity can be assessed by history and physical examination. An ambulatory patient seen in the office who does not have significant systemic symptoms has mild disease, whereas the patient who has tachycardia, is febrile, and has abdominal pain and tenderness has severe disease.

### Differential Features

See the later section Differential Features of Ulcerative Colitis and Crohn's Disease.

## Treatment

Patients with mild or moderate disease do not require hospitalization and are treated with 5-aminosalicylic drugs. Patients with severe disease are best treated with corticosteroids. Patients with fulminant disease or toxic megacolon require hospitalization and, frequently, emergency surgery. (See the section Treatment of Inflammatory Bowel Disease.)

## Prognosis

Most patients with ulcerative colitis have intermittent attacks, with remissions lasting from a few weeks to many

## TABLE 60.1
### SEVERITY CRITERIA FOR ULCERATIVE COLITIS, MODIFIED

| Criteria | Mild | Severe[a] | Fulminant |
|---|---|---|---|
| Stool frequency | <4/day | >6/day | >10/day or, at times, no bowel movements |
| Blood in stool | Small amounts | Macroscopic with all bowel movements | Continuous |
| Temperature | No fever | >37.8°C on 2 of 4 days | >37.8°C |
| Heart rate | Normal | >90 | >90 |
| Hemoglobin | Normal | <75% of normal (12 g/dL) | Transfusion requiring |
| Erythrocyte sedimentation rate | <30 mm/h | >30 mm/h | >30 mm/h |
| Radiography | Normal | Thumbprinting | Edematous, dilated |
| Clinical signs | Normal or mild tenderness | Abdominal tenderness | Abdominal distention, absent bowel sounds, tenderness |

[a] Moderate: between mild and severe.
(Modified with permission from Truelove SC, Witts LJ. Cortisone in ulcerative colitis. *BMJ* 1955;1:1041–1048.)

years. Ten percent to 15% of patients have a chronic, continuous course, and 5% to 10% present with a severe attack that requires urgent colectomy. The course and prognosis are largely determined by the extent of the disease. In 70% of patients presenting with proctitis, the disease remains confined to the rectum; in the other 30%, the disease extends proximally as patients are followed for up to 30 years. The risk that colectomy will eventually be required is proportional to the extent of disease and is significantly greater in patients with pancolitis. The rate of colectomy is as high as 30% during the first year of disease in those patients with pancolitis at presentation. After the first year, however, the colectomy rate for all patients with ulcerative colitis, regardless of extent, is 1% per year.

Patients with ulcerative colitis have an increased risk of colorectal cancer. This risk depends on the duration and extent of disease, regardless of clinical activity. The risk is further increased in patients with a family history of colorectal cancer and in patients with primary sclerosing cholangitis (PSC). The risk of colorectal cancer increases after 7 years in patients with pancolitis, and it has been estimated to increase by 1% per year after 15 or 20 years. In patients with left-sided ulcerative colitis, the risk of colorectal cancer is increased, but there is no agreement on how high this risk actually is. Patients with proctitis have no increased risk and do not require screening that differs from that used in the general population.

Colorectal cancer in patients with ulcerative colitis is usually, but not always, preceded by dysplasia. For this reason, patients who have pancolitis for more than 7 years are advised to undergo surveillance colonoscopies with biopsies. There is no universal agreement as to which colonoscopic schedule is best, but a common recommendation is to begin screening colonoscopies with multiple biopsies 7 years after the onset of symptoms. Four-quadrant biopsy samples are obtained at 10-cm intervals, and extra biopsy samples are taken from suspicious areas, such as strictures or masses. Dysplastic changes can be found in areas remote from where a cancer might be; therefore, the entire colon should be screened. If no dysplasia is found, colonoscopy is repeated at 1- to 3-year intervals. If high-grade dysplasia is found and confirmed by a second experienced pathologist, colectomy is recommended. For low-grade dysplasia, debate continues regarding the best recommendation. Some pathologists and gastroenterologists treat dysplasia, whether low- or high-grade, as precancerous and advise colectomy. Others recommend repeat colonoscopies and biopsies every 6 months in patients with low-grade dysplasia either until there is no dysplasia (in which case patients return to yearly screening) or colectomy (if high-grade dysplasia is found). Because of sampling error, however, dysplasia may be missed using this approach. The author views dysplasia—whether low- or high-grade—as premalignant and advises colectomy.

# CROHN'S DISEASE

Crohn's disease is a heterogeneous disease that has different clinical presentations, which are determined by the site of involvement and the type of disease (inflammatory, stricturing, or fistulizing). It can affect any segment of the gastrointestinal system, but the most common types are ileocolitic disease (50% of patients), small bowel involvement alone (30%), and colonic involvement alone (20%). Esophageal and gastroduodenal involvement occurs in 0.5% to 4.0% of patients. Most patients with gastroduodenal involvement also have evidence of Crohn's disease elsewhere in the gastrointestinal tract. Clinically, Crohn's disease can be inflammatory, stenotic, fistulizing, or mixed. The signs, symptoms, and treatment depend on the site of involvement and disease behavior.

## Clinical Presentation

Patients with ileocolitis usually present with nonbloody diarrhea, crampy abdominal pain (usually worse after meals), weight loss, and low-grade fever. The onset is usually subacute, but it can be acute and confused with acute appendicitis. On examination, patients are pale, bowel sounds can be decreased, and tenderness to palpation is present in the right lower quadrant of the abdomen, where a palpable mass may be present. More than 90% of patients with ileocecal disease eventually require surgery. The most common indications for surgery are internal fistulas, abscess, or obstruction.

The terminal ileum is the most common site of involvement in the small bowel. Disease can be diffuse, however, involving the jejunum and the ileum, or only the jejunum. Patients with diffuse disease present with diarrhea, abdominal pain consistent with intermittent and incomplete small bowel obstruction, and weight loss. Patients tend to be older at presentation, and the most common indication for surgery is obstruction. Patients with jejunal involvement have malabsorption and steatorrhea.

Patients with Crohn's disease of the colon usually have inflammatory disease and present with diarrhea and hematochezia. Obstruction may occur because of strictures, and fistulas both to and from the colon generally are found. In patients who require surgery, differentiating Crohn's colitis from ulcerative colitis is of primary importance. In 10% of patients, however, a specific diagnosis cannot be established; such patients are classified as having "indeterminate colitis." Approximately 50% of patients with Crohn's colitis require surgery, and the most common indications in this group are perianal disease and obstruction. Perianal disease occurs in 30% of patients with Crohn's disease, and approximately 10% of female patients with Crohn's colitis develop rectovaginal fistulas.

Gastroduodenal Crohn's disease may be difficult to distinguish from peptic ulcer disease and erosions caused by nonsteroidal anti-inflammatory drugs (NSAIDs). Patients usually present with nausea, vomiting, and abdominal pain that improve with use of antacids.

Gastrocolic fistulas can develop, and these usually originate from the colon rather than the stomach. Patients with gastrocolic fistulas present with diarrhea and malabsorption or with feculent emesis. Gastric outlet obstruction occurs in approximately 30% of patients in this group and is the most common indication for surgery.

Rectal and perianal involvement occurs in 10% to 30% of patients, and it is usually manifested by perianal abscess or fistulas. Rectal and perianal disease can occur without colonic involvement and, at times, before evidence of Crohn's disease is present elsewhere in the gastrointestinal tract. Not infrequently symptoms from perianal disease are the main problem in these patients.

The risk of colorectal cancer also is increased in patients with extensive Crohn's disease of the colon. There are no current guidelines for surveillance in these patients, and it is adequate to follow guidelines similar to those for patients with ulcerative colitis.

## Diagnosis

The diagnosis of Crohn's disease is based on clinical, laboratory, radiologic, endoscopic, and histologic criteria. The clinical presentation (described earlier) depends on the site of involvement and disease behavior. Physical examination may be normal or may reveal pallor, muscle wasting, palpable right lower quadrant mass, or evidence of perianal disease such as skin tags, fissures, or fistulas.

### Laboratory Testing

Most often, laboratory testing confirms the clinical suspicion and helps to rule out conditions that mimic Crohn's disease, such as infectious or parasitic enteritis or colitis. The abnormalities found on laboratory examinations reflect the inflammatory and chronic nature of Crohn's disease. Patients frequently are anemic and have leukocytosis, thrombocytosis, and an elevated erythrocyte sedimentation rate. Perinuclear antinuclear cytoplasmic antibodies are found in only 10% of patients with Crohn's disease, compared with more than 70% of patients with ulcerative colitis.

### Radiology

Contrast studies play a major role in the diagnosis of ileitis and gastroduodenal Crohn's disease. In gastroduodenal Crohn's disease, antral narrowing and duodenal strictures occur. The small intestine is well visualized using a small-bowel series, and a dedicated small-bowel series provides better mucosal detail than an upper gastrointestinal series with small-bowel follow-through. Small-bowel enema testing is indicated in only a small group of patients. The findings on radiographs include mucosal ulceration, loop separation, strictures, fistulas, and cobblestoning. For those patients in whom an abscess is suspected, computed tomography (CT) is useful because it not only confirms the

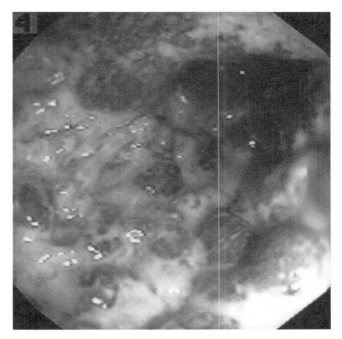

**Figure 60.2**  Severe Crohn's disease. (See Color Fig. 60.2.)

presence of an abscess but also provides guidance for percutaneous drainage.

### Endoscopy

Colonoscopy and esophagogastroduodenoscopy allow the direct visualization of the mucosa as well as mucosal sampling for histologic analysis (Fig. 60.2). Because Crohn's disease is discontinuous, areas of abnormal mucosa with normal intervening mucosa, referred to as *skip lesions*, are visualized at endoscopy. Patients with Crohn's disease may have rectal sparing. Patients may have multiple ulcers in the colon of different sizes, shapes, and depths. Aphthoid ulcers are considered to be pathognomonic of Crohn's disease. Aphthoid ulcers are 3- to 5-mm in size and have a surrounding red halo. Cobblestoning frequently is seen. Fistulas are a feature of Crohn's disease but not of ulcerative colitis.

## Differential Features of Ulcerative Colitis and Crohn's Disease

Distinguishing ulcerative colitis from Crohn's disease can be difficult, especially in patients with fulminant colitis or in patients who have only colonic disease (Table 60.2). Histopathologic examination can be useful in making this distinction. The histologic findings seen in Crohn's disease, but not in ulcerative colitis, are aphthous ulcers, noncaseating granulomas, microscopic skip lesions, and transmural involvement. A number of autoantibodies have been described in patients with IBD. Patients with ulcerative colitis are more likely to have positive test results for perinuclear antineutrophil cytoplasmic antibodies, and patients with Crohn's disease are more likely to test positive

**TABLE 60.2**

**DIFFERENTIAL FEATURES OF ULCERATIVE COLITIS AND CROHN'S DISEASE**

| Features | Ulcerative Colitis | Crohn's Disease |
|---|---|---|
| **Clinical** | | |
| Rectal bleeding | Usual | Sometimes |
| Abdominal mass | Absent | Often |
| Perianal disease | Extremely rare | 30% |
| Upper gastrointestinal symptoms | Unrelated | Frequent |
| Malnutrition | Rare, mild | Frequent, moderate to severe |
| **Endoscopic and radiologic** | | |
| Rectal involvement | Present | Variable |
| Continuous disease | Always | Rare |
| Discrete linear ulcers | Rare | Frequent |
| Aphthoid ulcers | Absent | Common |
| Cobblestoning | Absent | Common |
| Skip areas | Absent | Common |
| Small bowel disease | Absent[a] | Common |
| Fistulas | Absent | Common |
| **Pathologic** | | |
| Aphthous ulcers | Absent | Common |
| Noncaseating granulomas | Absent | 10–30% |
| Crypt abscess | Common | Frequent |
| Transmural involvement | Absent | Present |
| Microscopic skip lesions | Absent | Frequent |

[a] Except backwash ileitis.

for anti–*Sacharomyces cerevisiae* antibodies. The sensitivity of using one or both antibodies to distinguish ulcerative colitis from Crohn's disease is 44% to 60% and the specificity is 86% to 90%, respectively.

The principal differential diagnoses for IBD are infectious enteritis or colitis, ischemia, radiation enteritis, lymphoma, Behçet disease, endometriosis, diverticulitis, and enteropathy or colopathy induced by NSAIDs. A careful history, physical examination, and laboratory tests are critical to exclude conditions that mimic IBD.

## EXTRAINTESTINAL MANIFESTATIONS

To date, more than 100 extraintestinal manifestations of IBD have been described. Some parallel the disease activity; others follow an independent course. Extraintestinal manifestations occur more frequently in patients with colonic disease. Complications that parallel disease activity include:

- Peripheral arthritis
- Erythema nodosum
- Pyoderma gangrenosum
- Keratoconjunctivitis
- Episcleritis
- Hypercoagulability

Extraintestinal manifestations that run an independent course include:

- Ankylosing spondylitis, which more commonly occurs in patients with ulcerative colitis who are positive for HLA-B27
- Sacroiliitis
- Anterior uveitis

### Arthritis

The arthritis of IBD is usually nonerosive, mono- or pauci-articular, asymmetric, and migratory. No synovial destruction is present, and large joints are more commonly affected. Peripheral arthritis is more common in female patients and correlates with disease activity. Axial arthritis is associated with the presence of HLA-B27 and does not correlate with disease activity.

### Skin and Eye Disorders

Erythema nodosum occurs in approximately 3% of patients with IBD. It is characterized by the presence of tender subcutaneous nodules that generally occur along the shins. The area affected is erythematous and exquisitely sensitive to touch.

Pyoderma gangrenosum is characterized by the presence of an ulcerating lesion that becomes purulent and necrotic, and, when it heals, leaves a scar. Commonly found at sites of minimal trauma, these lesions occur in both ulcerative colitis and Crohn's disease. Treatment frequently involves immunosuppressive therapy.

The ocular manifestations of IBD include iritis, keratoconjunctivitis, episcleritis, and uveitis. Patients with uveitis generally test positive for HLA-B27. Frequent symptoms include blurred vision, photophobia, and a painful eye. Some ocular manifestations are medical emergencies because if they are not treated properly, they can lead to blindness. Such patients should be referred to an ophthalmologist.

### Liver Disease

Cholestatic liver disease is the most common manifestation of hepatic involvement in patients with IBD. It occurs in 5% of patients, and it does not parallel disease activity. PSC occurs in 1% to 5% of patients with ulcerative colitis and rarely in patients with Crohn's colitis. The course of PSC is independent of disease activity, and PSC can appear either before the diagnosis of ulcerative colitis or present years after colectomy for ulcerative colitis. In most patients, early diagnosis depends on the detection of biochemical abnormalities, such as an elevated alkaline phosphatase level. The levels of alkaline phosphatase can fluctuate, however, and can even return to normal in patients with established PSC. During the late stages of disease, PSC can be complicated by cholangiocarcinoma.

## TREATMENT OF INFLAMMATORY BOWEL DISEASE

The goals of medical treatment in IBD are to improve symptoms, decrease complications, decrease the need for surgical intervention, and improve the patient's quality of life. Treatment can be divided into two phases: therapy for the acute attack, and maintenance of remission.

### Pharmacologic Treatment

Medications used to treat patients with IBD include:

- 5-aminosalicylic acid (5-ASA)
- Antibiotics
- Corticosteroids
- Immunosuppressive medications
- Biologic medications

#### 5-Aminosalicylic Acid
The 5-ASA drugs (Table 60.3) are anti-inflammatory agents that act at the mucosal level and decrease inflammation,

possibly by inhibiting the formation of both prostaglandin and leukotriene metabolites. The 5-ASA medications also are effective in maintaining remission in patients with ulcerative colitis and, to a lesser degree, in those with Crohn's disease. As mentioned, ulcerative colitis is characterized by periods of activity and periods of quiescence. With the continuous use of 5-ASA, remission can be prolonged in a significant number of patients with ulcerative colitis.

It is important to remember that the therapeutic effect of 5-ASA is local, at the mucosal level, and not systemic. For the medication to be effective, it must be delivered to the site of disease. If a preparation that releases 5-ASA in the colon is given to patients with small bowel disease only, no therapeutic effect is observed. Given orally, 5-ASA is rapidly absorbed in the proximal small bowel, acetylated by the liver, and excreted in the urine. To prevent proximal absorption and allow the 5-ASA to exert its anti-inflammatory effect at the site of inflammation, different delivery methods are available, including the following:

- Creating a larger molecule by binding it to a carrier or another 5-ASA via an azo-bond
- Coating 5-ASA with a pH-sensitive resin
- Using delayed-release preparations

Other 5-ASA preparations currently used are in the form of suppositories and enemas. Suppositories effectively

## TABLE 60.3
### AMINOSALICYLIC ACID FORMULATIONS

| Formulation | FDA Indication | Common Use | Dosage |
|---|---|---|---|
| Azo-compounds | Mild to moderate ulcerative colitis | Same | Acute disease: 4–8 g daily |
| Sulfasalazine (Azulfidine) | Maintenance of remission of ulcerative colitis | Crohn's colitis, mild | Maintenance: 2–4 g daily |
| Olsalazine sodium (Dipentum) | Maintenance of remission of ulcerative colitis in patients intolerant of sulfasalazine | Same<br>Induce remission in mild to moderate ulcerative colitis in patients allergic to or intolerant of sulfasalazine | 500 mg daily p.o. b.i.d. with meals |
| Balsalazide disodium (Colazal) | Mild to moderate ulcerative colitis | 12-Week treatment | 2.25 g t.i.d. |
| pH-sensitive preparations | Mildly to moderately active ulcerative colitis | Same | FDA approved: 1.2–2.4 g daily |
| Mesalamine, polymer-coated (Asacol) | Maintenance of remission in ulcerative colitis | Active mild to moderate Crohn's colitis<br>Maintenance of remission in Crohn's colitis (debatable) | Common use: 2.4–4.8 g daily<br>Higher dosage for active Crohn's disease: 2.4–4.8 g daily for maintenance of remission |
| Delayed-release preparations | Induction of remission in patients with active mild to moderate ulcerative colitis | Mild to moderate Crohn's ileitis or ileocolitis | Active disease: 4 g daily |
| Mesalamine, ethylcellulose-coated (Pentasa) | | Maintenance of remission in Crohn's disease | Maintenance of remission: 3–4 g daily |

FDA, U.S. Food and Drug Administration.

induce remission in patients with ulcerative proctitis; the recommended dosage is 500 mg twice a day for 4 to 6 weeks. Enemas effectively induce remission in patients with proctosigmoiditis; the recommended dosage is 4 g in 60 mL of liquid at bedtime for 4 to 6 weeks. Both suppositories and enemas can maintain remission in patients with ulcerative proctitis or proctosigmoiditis. In patients with more extensive disease and symptoms of proctitis, a combined treatment using oral and topical medications is recommended.

### Azo-Bond Compounds

Sulfasalazine, which is a 5-ASA molecule bound to sulfapyridine by an azo-bond, was the first 5-ASA preparation found to be effective in the treatment of IBD. Sulfapyridine serves as a carrier and has no therapeutic effect. The azo-bond is split by an azo-reductase that is produced by colonic bacteria. Therefore, the main therapeutic use of sulfasalazine is in patients with colonic involvement, whether it is ulcerative colitis or Crohn's colitis. Sulfasalazine effectively induces remission in patients with mild or moderate disease, but patients with severe disease should be treated with corticosteroids.

A therapeutic effect from sulfasalazine is seen in 60% to 80% of patients with mild or moderate ulcerative colitis. The therapeutic dosage is 4 to 6 g daily, divided into four doses. To improve tolerance, the drug is started at a low dose (e.g., 500 mg three or four times a day), and then the dose is gradually increased. Thirty percent of patients are either allergic to or intolerant of sulfapyridine, and they require discontinuation of sulfasalazine therapy. The most common side effects include headache, nausea, anorexia, oligospermia, and dyspepsia; less common side effects include skin rash, pruritus, urticaria, and hemolytic anemia. Rarely, patients can develop life-threatening reactions, such as aplastic anemia or anaphylactic reactions. Because sulfapyridine decreases folic acid absorption by competitive inhibition, patients receiving sulfasalazine should take supplemental folic acid (0.4 to 1.0 mg per day).

Intolerance and allergy to sulfasalazine is usually due to the sulfapyridine moiety, rather than the 5-ASA. A 5-ASA compound that does not contain sulfapyridine can be used in patients who are intolerant of sulfasalazine or allergic to sulfa. Olsalazine sodium (Dipentum) is 5-ASA that is bound by an azo-bond to another molecule of 5-ASA. It is safe for patients who are allergic to sulfa. The azo-bond in olsalazine also is split by azo-reductase from colonic bacteria, so the site of action is colonic as well. Unfortunately, however, as many as 17% of patients taking olsalazine develop secretory diarrhea; this side effect can be minimized by giving the olsalazine with meals.

### pH-Sensitive Preparations

The only pH-sensitive preparation available in the United States is Asacol, which is 5-ASA coated with a methacrylic acid copolymer B (called Eudragit-S) that dissolves at pH 7.0 (i.e., the pH in the distal ileum and the colon). Its main use, therefore, is for patients with colonic disease. The recommended dosage in patients with active mild or moderate ulcerative colitis or Crohn's colitis is 2.4 g per 24 hours in three or four divided doses. Tolerance is good, and larger doses (i.e., 4.8 to 6.0 g per 24 hours) produce better results. Asacol is well tolerated, and very few patients develop diarrhea.

### Delayed-Release Preparations

The only delayed-release preparation currently available is Pentasa, which is an ethylcellulose-coated mesalamine preparation that releases 5-ASA throughout the small intestine and the colon. Pentasa is approved by the U.S. Food and Drug Administration (FDA) for use in patients with ulcerative colitis. In clinical trials, it has effectively induced remission in patients with mild or moderate symptoms of inflammatory Crohn's disease of the small intestine, with or without colonic involvement. Like all 5-ASA medications, the higher the dosage, the more effective it is. The recommended dosage is 4 g per 24 hours in four divided doses.

### *Antibiotics*

Primary treatment with antibiotics is indicated only in patients with Crohn's disease. Controlled data are available for metronidazole and ciprofloxacin. Metronidazole is particularly effective in patients with Crohn's colitis or perianal disease. The most common side effects leading to discontinuation of metronidazole are gastrointestinal intolerance and peripheral neuropathy. Long-term metronidazole use during pregnancy is contraindicated because of the risk of cleft palate; in addition, all patients should be warned of its potential interaction with disulfiram (Antabuse). For those patients who do not tolerate metronidazole, ciprofloxacin is used with similar results. In controlled studies, ciprofloxacin was as effective as mesalazine in inducing remission, and the benefit lasted 6 to 9 months. Combination treatment using metronidazole and ciprofloxacin is very effective. Other antibiotics, such as clarithromycin, trimethoprim-sulfamethoxazole, or tetracyclines, can be tried in patients intolerant of or allergic to metronidazole and ciprofloxacin.

### *Corticosteroids*

Corticosteroids play a major role in the medical treatment of IBD. Their use is indicated in patients with moderate or severe ulcerative colitis or Crohn's disease and in those who fail to respond to 5-ASA or antibiotics. Corticosteroids effectively induce remission, but they are not indicated for maintaining remission. In adult patients with ulcerative colitis or Crohn's disease, 40 to 60 mg of oral prednisolone or prednisone per day is recommended; for pediatric patients, a starting dosage of 1 mg per kilogram per day is recommended. The administration of oral corticosteroids is tapered off slowly (i.e., 5 to 10 mg every 5 to 7 days) once remission is achieved. Initial response occurs in 60% to 80% of patients; however, at least 20% do not improve and another 20% become steroid dependent. If remission or significant improvement is not achieved in 7 to 14 days using oral corticosteroids, patients should be admitted to the hospital and treated with either intravenous steroids or other agents.

Patients with more severe ulcerative colitis are best treated in a hospital with intravenous corticosteroids. Hydrocortisone and methylprednisolone are equally effective. Hydrocortisone usually is prescribed at a dosage of 300 mg per 24 hours. Controlled data are not available, but intravenous hydrocortisone may be more effective when given by continuous infusion rather than by an intravenous bolus every 8 hours. If the patient fails to respond in 5 to 7 days, surgery or other medical treatments should be considered. Adrenocorticotropic hormone is rarely used because it does not offer a significant advantage over other corticosteroids.

Budesonide is a very potent anti-inflammatory steroid that has a high first-pass metabolism in the liver. Because of this, it has less systemic side effects, although some adrenal axis suppression still occurs. It is available in a formulation that releases the drug in the distal ileum, and at 9 mg per day its effectiveness in inducing remission is similar to that of prednisone. In a maintenance trial, it was not effective in maintaining remission.

Corticosteroid enemas are useful in patients with ulcerative proctosigmoiditis, and budesonide is as effective as conventional corticosteroids and has fewer short-term and long-term side effects. Neither corticosteroid enemas nor budesonide is as effective as topical 5-ASA, however. Budesonide enemas are not yet available for clinical use in the United States.

The many side effects of corticosteroids, which are the major factors limiting their use in patients with IBD, include osteoporosis, moon facies, buffalo hump, striae, posterior subcapsular cataracts, aseptic necrosis of bone, glaucoma, immunosuppression, hyperglycemia, acne, mood swings, insomnia, weight gain, and adrenal insufficiency. Arrest of growth occurs in children, but this can be lessened by administering corticosteroids on alternate days rather than daily. Patients should be informed about the potential risks of corticosteroids and the need for glucocorticoid supplementation in case of surgery for up to 1 year after corticosteroid cessation. Patients also should be warned about the severe risks of sudden discontinuation of corticosteroids.

### Biologic Agents

Patients with Crohn's disease have elevated levels of tumor necrosis factor-$\alpha$ (TNF$\alpha$) in the colon, blood, and feces. Because TNF$\alpha$ is a proinflammatory cytokine, it seems logical that blocking its action would have beneficial effects in these patients. Infliximab is a TNF$\alpha$ chimeric antibody that is approved by the FDA as treatment for Crohn's disease. The main uses are in patients with mild or moderate inflammatory Crohn's disease that does not respond to conventional medical treatment and in patients with fistulizing disease. In 70% of patients with inflammatory disease, a response is seen, and in patients with fistulous disease, decreased drainage is seen in 70% of patients and temporary closure is seen in 50% of patients. The medication is administered intravenously. Infliximab is well tolerated, highly effective in inducing remission and, in long-term trials, has been effective as a steroid-sparing drug. Two problems are the need to administer the drug intravenously and the cost of infusion. The most significant side effect to date is the reactivation of tuberculosis, which usually presents with extrapulmonary manifestations. Patients should be given a purified protein derivative (tuberculin) test before infliximab administration. Approximately 2% of patients have side effects that require discontinuation of the drug.

### Immunosuppressive Drugs

The main indications for the use of immunosuppressive drugs in patients with IBD are refractory disease, steroid-dependent disease, and unhealed fistulas. Substantial patient experience exists with 6-mercaptopurine (6-MP) and azathioprine, an S-substituted form of 6-MP. Experience with cyclosporine and with methotrexate sodium is more limited. The exact mechanism by which immunosuppressive drugs reduce symptoms in patients with IBD is unclear, but improvement may result from the blocking of lymphocyte proliferation and activation, as well as through an effect on humoral responsiveness.

The therapeutic benefit of 6-MP and azathioprine is slow in onset. Response is seen 2 to 3 months after initiation of the drug, and therapeutic benefits have been observed even as late as 12 months after the initiation of treatment. These medications allow a reduction or discontinuation of steroid therapy in 60% to 80% of patients who are steroid dependent, improve symptoms in approximately 70% of patients with refractory disease, and promote fistula healing in approximately 60% of patients. In patients with ulcerative colitis, benefit is observed in 50% to 75% of patients. Given that surgery is seen as "curative" in ulcerative colitis, the role of these medications in treating these patients is less clear. The main side effects of 6-MP and azathioprine are pancreatitis (3%), allergic-type reactions (2%), bone marrow suppression (2%), and, with long-term use, cervical cancer. The clinical effectiveness and toxicity are at least in part related to some of the metabolites of these medications. The metabolites are 6-thioguanine, 6- methylmercaptopurine, and 6-thiouric acid. The metabolite 6-thioguanine is associated with clinical response and bone marrow toxicity; 6-methylmercaptopurine is associated with liver toxicity. The relative accumulation of these metabolites depends on genetic polymorphism of the enzymes that participate in the metabolism of these drugs.

Controversy has arisen regarding the risk of lymphoma in IBD patients who are taking 6-MP or azathioprine.

Given that the benefits outweigh the risk, the current practice is to start these medications early in the course of the disease. A randomized trial involving a pediatric population compared treatment with prednisone alone to treatment with prednisone plus 6-MP in children in whom IBD was recently diagnosed. The addition of 6-MP was found to significantly decrease the need for prednisone and to improve maintenance of remission over the 18-month duration of the trial. Patients receiving these drugs are more susceptible to infections, and it is important for them to understand the need for routine blood tests while on these medications.

Cyclosporine is a potent immunosuppressant that frequently is used to prevent rejection in patients undergoing organ transplantation. Cyclosporine does not maintain remission in patients with IBD, and its use may be restricted to those patients with severe ulcerative colitis who do not respond to intravenous corticosteroids and would like to avoid surgery. Because of significant side effects, this medication should be used only by experienced physicians, and preferably in tertiary-care centers. The most common side effects include nephrotoxicity, seizures, paresthesia, hypertrichosis, hypertension, and infections.

Information on the use of methotrexate to treat IBD is limited, but an intramuscular dose of 25 mg once a week is useful for inducing remission in patients with Crohn's disease. Patients receiving methotrexate also should receive folic acid, 1 mg per day, for the duration of treatment, which usually is 16 weeks. Methotrexate also is used to maintain remission. In patients who respond to this regimen, the dose of methotrexate is decreased to 15 mg by intramuscular injection once a week. The most serious toxicities are hypersensitivity pneumonitis, teratogenicity, hepatotoxicity, and bone marrow suppression. Patients should be strongly advised against drinking alcohol, and women with childbearing potential should practice adequate contraception. The risk of hepatotoxicity is greater in patients who are obese and in those who consume alcohol.

### Alternative Treatments

Fish oil is an inhibitor of the activity of leukotriene and other proinflammatory cytokines. It has successfully been used as primary therapy or adjuvant treatment with corticosteroids in patients with ulcerative colitis and Crohn's disease. The main limitations to its use are that, with consumption of the recommended daily dose of 15 to 18 capsules containing 0.18 g eicosapentaenoic acid per capsule, patients experience dyspeptic symptoms and develop a fishy odor.

Transdermal nicotine has been used in patients with refractory ulcerative colitis. It is more effective in ex-smokers. The dosage is 15 to 24 mg per 24 hours. Patients who have never smoked cigarettes have poor tolerance and response to this agent. Transdermal nicotine is not effective in maintaining remission.

Recently, probiotics have been used effectively in patients with ulcerative colitis and pouchitis. The preliminary data are very encouraging, but further information is still needed.

### Surgery

Between one-third and one-half of patients with IBD require surgery. Patients with ulcerative colitis and extensive Crohn's colitis require surgery because of failure to respond to medical treatment, hemorrhage, toxic dilatation, perforation, strictures causing obstruction, and dysplasia or cancer. The type of surgery performed in patients with Crohn's disease differs from that used in patients with ulcerative colitis. Depending on the indication, patients with Crohn's disease may undergo segmental resection or stricturoplasty. Patients with ulcerative colitis should undergo subtotal colectomy, regardless of disease extent. The creation of a pelvic pouch from the terminal ileum and anal anastomosis allow permanent ileostomy to be avoided, but the complication of pouchitis occurs in 5% to 10% of patients.

Recurrence is frequent in patients with Crohn's disease. Approximately 50% require additional surgery within 5 to 10 years of the previous surgery. The recurrence rate, as determined by endoscopy and histological examination, is almost 100% at 1 year, but the symptomatic recurrence rate is lower. Symptomatic recurrence can be delayed in some patients by using 5-ASA, metronidazole, 6-MP, or azathioprine postoperatively, but these medications cannot be recommended for all patients, and their use should be individualized.

## SYSTEMIC COMPLICATIONS

Systemic complications are more common in patients with Crohn's disease than in ulcerative colitis. The most common systemic complications are weight loss, malabsorption, urinary stones, gallstones, thrombotic and embolic events, sepsis, and amyloidosis. Many of the systemic complications in patients with Crohn's disease relate to the involvement of the small intestine and depend on the extent of disease. Weight loss is common. The main cause is decreased oral intake, either because of anorexia or because of postprandial symptoms. Malabsorption, which also is frequent, results from extensive mucosal involvement, which leads to decreased absorptive surface area or protein-losing enteropathy, or from the presence of fistulous tracts that bypass the small bowel. Patients with malabsorption also can present with steatorrhea owing to bile salt depletion.

Gallstones and kidney stones are complications that relate primarily to alterations of small-bowel pathophysiology; these alterations lead to the excess absorption of oxalate and the abnormal recirculation and loss of bile salts. Vitamin $B_{12}$ is selectively absorbed in the distal 100 cm of the terminal ileum; if this segment is diseased or removed surgically, patients develop vitamin $B_{12}$ malabsorption, with subsequent vitamin $B_{12}$ deficiency. In such patients, the optimal route for supplementation is parenteral. Likewise, hydroxy bile acids are absorbed in the distal 100 cm of the terminal ileum. Thus, when *less* than 100 cm is diseased or surgically removed, the malabsorbed hydroxy bile acids enter the colon and cause a secretory diarrhea; these patients respond to oral cholestyramine, which binds bile salts. Conversely, when *more* than 100 cm of terminal ileum is surgically removed, patients deplete their bile salt pool and develop malabsorption and steatorrhea. Patients with steatorrhea malabsorb lipid-soluble vitamins and calcium. Such patients respond to a low-fat diet that is supplemented by medium-chain triglycerides, which do not require bile salts for absorption.

Another complication that leads to malabsorption in patients with Crohn's disease is small-bowel bacterial overgrowth. Bacterial overgrowth results from strictures or fistulas, or it can occur after surgery because of resection of the ileocecal valve and ileocolic anastomosis.

Colorectal cancer and sepsis are the leading causes of mortality in patients with Crohn's disease. Hypercoagulability, which leads to thrombotic and embolic phenomena in patients with IBD, is the third leading cause of disease-related mortality in patients with IBD. Thromboembolism occurs in 1% to 6% of IBD patients, and 25% of these patients die during the first event. Some of the conditions that lead to thromboembolic events in these patients include activated protein C resistance (related to a mutation in factor V Leiden) and hyperhomocysteinemia; these disorders occur with greater frequency in patients with IBD than in the general population. Other abnormalities that have been described include decreased antithrombin III, thrombocytosis, leukocytosis, and abnormal fibrinolysis. Amyloidosis, particularly renal, was a frequent complication in the past, but it is rarely seen now. Other rare extraintestinal complications of IBD include pancreatitis, immune-mediated neutropenia, and immune-mediated thrombocytopenia.

## REVIEW EXERCISES

### QUESTIONS

A 30-year-old White woman presents to your office because of diarrhea and tender nodules on her legs. Three years before this episode, she was on vacation in Mexico and on return home developed bloody diarrhea. She was treated with ciprofloxacin, 750 mg two times a day for 7 days, and the diarrhea resolved. A year later, she had a similar episode, which was diagnosed as irritable bowel syndrome. Two months ago, she discontinued cigarette smoking after an episode of shortness of breath and sharp chest pain that lasted 1 week. Four weeks before consultation, she developed four red "lumps" on

her legs that were extremely painful to touch. She was started on ibuprofen (Advil), and 2 weeks later developed bloody diarrhea. She has predefecational cramps that are followed by small, loose bowel movements and, at times, bloody mucus. On two occasions, she has had nocturnal bowel movements.

She has no systemic symptoms. Her past medical history is unremarkable. She takes ibuprofen for menstrual cramps and is taking birth control pills.

On examination, she is in no distress, with a heart rate of 84, respiratory rate of 16, and a temperature of 37.6°C. Examination of the abdomen reveals normal bowels sounds; the abdomen is soft but tender to palpation in the left lower quadrant. Rectal examination reveals soft stool with bloody mucus. On the shins, she has four quarter-sized brown nodules.

1. Your initial impression is
a) Irritable bowel syndrome
b) Infectious diarrhea
c) Ulcerative colitis
d) Crohn's colitis
e) Collagenous colitis

2. The best diagnostic test is
a) Complete blood cell count/differential
b) Stool test for *C. difficile*
c) Flexible sigmoidoscopy with biopsies
d) Air-contrast barium enema
e) Small bowel series

3. Your recommendation is
a) Admission to hospital
b) Metronidazole (Flagyl) 500 mg orally three times a day for 1 week
c) Fiber and an anticholinergic agent
d) Prednisone 40 mg orally once a day
e) 5-ASA enemas at bedtime

4. A 34-year-old patient with a 12-year history of ulcerative colitis comes with her husband for advice regarding pregnancy and medical treatment. When she was 22 years old, she developed bloody diarrhea. The initial presentation was severe and was treated with prednisone. She was able to wean off prednisone and has remained on sulfasalazine since then. She has mild flare-ups in the spring every year, which are controlled by increasing the dosage of sulfasalazine to 4 g per day from a maintenance dose of 2 g per day. She is otherwise healthy and takes a multivitamin daily. She does not take any other medications.

Your recommendation is
a) Discontinue sulfasalazine because of the risk of kernicterus and start 5-ASA.
b) Discontinue sulfasalazine and do not institute treatment unless she has an exacerbation.

c) Continue sulfasalazine at the present dosage.

d) Add folic acid 1 mg orally once a day.

e) Discontinue sulfasalazine postpartum to decrease the risk of kernicterus.

## ANSWERS

### 1. c.
The patient has new onset ulcerative colitis, which is mild.

### 2. c.
Her symptoms are those of distal ulcerative colitis. This can be confirmed by sigmoidoscopy and biopsy.

### 3. e.
The best initial treatment is a topical 5-ASA product.

### 4. d.
All 5-ASA compounds are safe during pregnancy and lactation, and they should be continued to decrease the risk of a flare-up, with potentially disastrous consequences. Although sulfasalazine contains sulfapyridine, and all sulfas have the potential for inducing kernicterus, this is a theoretical concern; kernicterus has yet to be reported in association with sulfasalazine (Azulfidine). Folic acid should be added, because sulfasalazine interferes with folic acid absorption and because it decreases the risk of spina bifida.

## SUGGESTED READINGS

Aslan A, Triadafilopoulos G. Fish oil fatty acid supplementation in active ulcerative colitis: a double-blind, placebo-controlled, crossover study. *Am J Gastroenterol* 1992;87:432–437.

Bar-Meir S, Chowers Y, Lavy A, et al. Budesonide versus prednisone in the treatment of active Crohn's disease. *Gastroenterology* 1998; 115(4):835–840.

Belluzzi A, Brignola C, Campieri M, et al. Effect of an enteric-coated fish oil preparation on relapses in Crohn's disease. *N Engl J Med* 1996;334:1557–1560.

Brzezinkski A. Medical treatment of Crohn's disease. *Clin Colon Rectal Surg* 2001;14:167–173.

Brzezinski A, Rankin GB, Seidner DL, et al. Use of old and new oral 5-aminosalicylic acid formulations in inflammatory bowel disease. *Cleve Clin J Med* 1995;62:317–323.

Cho J. The Nod2 gene in Crohn's disease: implications for future research into the genetics and immunology of Crohn's disease. *Inflamm Bowel Dis* 2001;7(3):271–275.

Connell WR, Kamm MA, Dickson M, et al. Long-term neoplasia risk after azathioprine treatment in inflammatory bowel disease. *Lancet* 1994;343:1249–1252.

D'Haens GR, Lashner BA, Hanauer SB. Pericholangitis and sclerosing cholangitis are risk factors for dysplasia and cancer in ulcerative colitis. *Am J Gastroenterol* 1993;88:1174–1178.

Ekbom A, Helmick C, Zack M, et al. Increased risk of large bowel cancer in Crohn's disease with colonic involvement. *Lancet* 1990; 336:357–359.

Ekbom A, Helmick CG, Zack M, et al. Survival and causes of death in patients with inflammatory bowel disease. A population-based study. *Gastroenterology* 1992;103:954–960.

Farmer RG, Easley KA, Rankin GB. Clinical patterns, natural history, and progression of ulcerative colitis: a long-term follow up of 1,116 patients. *Dig Dis Sci* 1993;38:1137–1146.

Farmer RG, Whelan G, Fazio VW. Long-term follow-up of patients with Crohn's disease: relationship between clinical pattern and prognosis. *Gastroenterology* 1985;88:1818–1825.

Feagan BG, Fedorak RN, Irvine EJ, et al. A comparison of methotrexate with placebo for the maintenance of remission in Crohn's disease. North American Crohn's Study Group Investigators. *N Engl J Med* 2000;342:1627–1632.

Feagan BG, Rochon J, Fedorak RN, et al. Methotrexate for the treatment of Crohn's disease. *N Engl J Med* 1995;332:292–297.

Fockens P, Tytgat GNJ. Role of endoscopy in follow-up of inflammatory bowel disease. *Endoscopy* 1992;24:582–584.

Gendre JP, May JY, Florent C, et al. Oral mesalamine (Pentasa) as maintenance treatment in Crohn's disease: a multicenter placebo-controlled study. *Gastroenterology* 1993;104:435–439.

Gillen CD, Walmsley RS, Prior P, et al. Ulcerative colitis and Crohn's disease: a comparison of the colorectal cancer risk in extensive colitis. *Gut* 1994;35:1590–1592.

Gionchetti P, Rizzello F, Venturi A, et al. Oral bacteriotherapy as maintenance treatment in patients with chronic pouchitis: a double-blind, placebo-controlled trial. *Gastroenterology* 2000;119(2):305–309.

Greenberg GR, Feagan BG, Martin F, et al. Oral budesonide for active Crohn's disease. *N Engl J Med* 1994;331:836–841.

Greenstein AJ, Lachman P, Sachar DB, et al. Perforating and non-perforating indications for repeated operations in Crohn's disease: evidence for two clinical forms. *Gut* 1988;29:588–592.

Gumaste V, Sachar DB, Greenstein AJ. Benign and malignant colorectal strictures in ulcerative colitis. *Gut* 1992;33:938–941.

Kirsner JB. Problems in the differentiation of ulcerative colitis and Crohn's disease of the colon: the need for repeated diagnostic evaluation. *Gastroenterology* 1975;68:187–191.

Lashner BA. Recommendations for colorectal cancer surveillance in ulcerative colitis: a review of research from a single university-based surveillance program. *Am J Gastroenterol* 1992;87:168–175.

Lashner BA. Risk factors for small bowel cancer in Crohn's disease. *Dig Dis Sci* 1992;37:1179–1184.

Lashner BA, Provencher KS, Seidner DL, et al. The effect of folic acid supplementation on the risk for cancer or dysplasia in ulcerative colitis. *Gastroenterology* 1997;112:29–32.

Lashner BA, Shaheen NJ, Hanauer SB, et al. Passive smoking is associated with an increased risk of developing inflammatory bowel disease in children. *Am J Gastroenterol* 1993;88:356–359.

Lashner BA, Turner BC, Bostwick DG, et al. Dysplasia and cancer complicating strictures in ulcerative colitis. *Dig Dis Sci* 1990;35:349–352.

Lewis JD, Schwartz JS, Lichtenstein GR. Azathioprine for maintenance of remission in Crohn's disease: benefits outweigh the risk of lymphoma. *Gastroenterology* 2000;118(6):1018–1024.

Liebman HA, Kashani N, Sutherland D, et al. The Factor V Leiden mutation increases the risk of venous thrombosis in patients with inflammatory bowel disease. *Gastroenterology* 1998;115(4):830–834.

Lock MR, Farmer RG, Fazio VW, et al. Recurrence and reoperation for Crohn's disease: the role of disease location in prognosis. *N Engl J Med* 1981;304:1586–1588.

Malchow H, Ewe K, Brandes JW, et al. European Cooperative Crohn's Disease Study: results of drug treatment. *Gastroenterology* 1984;86:249–266.

Markowitz J, Grancher K, Kohn N, et al. A multicenter trial of 6-mercaptopurine and prednisone in children with newly diagnosed Crohn's disease. *Gastroenterology* 2000;119:895–902.

Michener WM, Caulfield M, Wyllie R, et al. Management of inflammatory bowel disease: 30 years of observation. *Cleve Clin J Med* 1990;37:685–691.

Orholm M, Munkholm P, Langholz E, et al. Familial occurrence of inflammatory bowel disease. *N Engl J Med* 1991;324:84–88.

Papi C, Luchetti R, Gili L, et al. Budesonide in the treatment of Crohn's disease: a meta-analysis. *Aliment Pharmacol Ther* 2000;14:1419–1428.

Peeters M, Nevens H, Baert F, et al. Familial aggregation in Crohn's disease: increased age-adjusted risk and concordance in clinical characteristics. *Gastroenterology* 1996;111:597–603.

Pennington L, Hamilton SR, Bayless TM, et al. Surgical management of Crohn's disease: influence of disease at margin of resection. *Ann Surg* 1980;192:311–318.

Persson PG, Ahlbom A, Hellers G. Inflammatory bowel disease and tobacco smoke: a case-control study. *Gut* 1990;31:1377–1381.

Petras RE, Mir-Madjlessi SH, Farmer RG. Crohn's disease and intestinal carcinoma: a report of 11 cases with emphasis on associated epithelial dysplasia. *Gastroenterology* 1987;93:1307–1314.

Prantera C, Pallone F, Brunetti G, et al. The Italian IBD Study Group. Oral 5-aminosalicylic acid (Asacol) in the maintenance treatment of Crohn's disease. *Gastroenterology* 1992;103:363–368.

Present DH, Korelitz BI, Wisch N, et al. Treatment of Crohn's disease with 6-mercaptopurine. A long-term, randomized, double-blind study. *N Engl J Med* 1980;302:981–987.

Present DH, Rutgeerts P, Targan S, et al. Infliximab for the treatment of fistulas in patients with Crohn's disease. *N Engl J Med* 1999;340: 1398–1405.

Reiser JR, Waye JD, Janowitz HD, et al. Adenocarcinoma in strictures of ulcerative colitis without antecedent dysplasia by colonoscopy. *Am J Gastroenterol* 1994;89:119–122.

Riddell RH, Goldman H, Ransofhoff DF, et al. Dysplasia in inflammatory bowel disease: standardized classification with provisional clinical implications. *Hum Pathol* 1983;14:931–968.

Rutgeerts P, Lofberg R, Malchow H, et al. A comparison of budesonide with prednisolone for active Crohn's disease. *N Engl J Med* 1994; 331:842–845.

Sachar DB, Andrews H, Farmer RG, et al. Proposed classification of patient subgroups in Crohn's disease. Working Team Report 4. *Gastroenterol Int* 1992;3:141–154.

Sandborn WJ, Tremaine W, Offord KP, et al. A randomized double-blinded placebo-controlled trial of transdermal nicotine for mild to moderately active ulcerative colitis. *Ann Intern Med* 1997; 126(5):364–371.

Silverstein MD, Lashner BA, Hanauer SB, et al. Cigarette smoking in Crohn's disease. *Am J Gastroenterol* 1989;84:31–33.

Steinhart AH, Hemphill DJ, Greenberg GR. Sulfasalazine and mesalazine for the maintenance therapy of Crohn's disease: a meta-analysis. *Am J Gastroenterol* 1994 Dec;89(12):2116–2124.

Sutherland LR, Ramcharan S, Bryant H, et al. Effect of cigarette smoking on recurrence of Crohn's disease. *Gastroenterology* 1990;98: 1123–1128.

Targan SR, Hanauer SB, van Deventer SJH, et al. A short term study of chimeric monoclonal antibody cA2 to tumor necrosis factor a for Crohn's disease. *N Engl J Med* 1997;337:1029–1035.

Thomas GA, Rhodes J, Mani V, et al. Transdermal nicotine as maintenance therapy for ulcerative colitis. *N Engl J Med* 1995;332: 988–992.

Truelove SC, Witts LJ. Cortisone in ulcerative colitis. *BMJ* 1955;1: 1041–1048.

Turunen U, Farkkila M, Hakala K, et al. Long-term treatment of ulcerative colitis with ciprofloxacin: a prospective, double-blind, placebo-controlled study. *Gastroenterology* 1998;115:1072–1078.

Woolrich AJ, DaSilva MD, Korelitz BI. Surveillance in the routine management of ulcerative colitis: the predictive value of low-grade dysplasia. *Gastroenterology* 1992;103:431–438.

# Diarrhea and Malabsorption

## 61

*Edy E. Soffer    John A. Dumot*

## DIARRHEA

Diarrhea is best defined by increased stool weight, essentially as the result of increased water content. For most individuals eating a Western-type diet, diarrhea implies a 24-hour stool output in excess of 200 g. A more practical definition is abnormal looseness of the stools, which is usually associated with increased stool weight and frequency of bowel movements.

Approximately 8 to 9 L of fluid enter the intestine daily; 1 to 2 L represent food and liquid intake, and the rest is from endogenous sources such as salivary, gastric, pancreatic, biliary, and intestinal secretions. After small-bowel absorption, only 1 to 2 L are presented to the colon; most of it is absorbed as it passes through the colon, leaving a stool output of up to 100 to 200 g daily.

## Mechanisms of Diarrhea

Water is absorbed passively in the gut, dependent on osmotic gradient. Consequently, diarrhea is due to an excess of osmotically active substances in the stool, which results in the decreased absorption of nutrients and electrolytes or excess secretion of any combination of electrolytes, water, or nutrients. Four mechanisms of diarrhea are present: osmotic, secretory, altered motility, and exudative.

### Osmotic Diarrhea

Osmotic diarrhea results from the presence of a poorly absorbable solute that causes excessive water output. The presence of the poorly absorbable solute exerts an osmotic pressure effect across the intestinal mucosa. Because the diarrhea is caused by the solute, it tends to stop during fasting. Additionally, a stool "osmotic gap" occurs. Normally, stool osmolality can be accounted for by normal concentrations of stool electrolytes. A reasonable estimate of the stool osmolality can be made by adding the serum concentration of sodium and potassium and by multiplying by 2 for the associated anions. If a nonabsorbable solute is present in the fecal fluid, the concentrations of stool electrolytes are lower. Therefore, adding stool sodium and potassium concentrations and multiplying by 2 (for their associated anions) will result in a stool osmolality value that is lower than the serum osmolality. Because of technical problems associated with measuring total fecal osmolality, one can use the electrolyte estimate method and compare it to the expected serum osmolality, which should be 290 mOsm.

For example, in using stool electrolyte concentrations to estimate the stool osmolality, if stool sodium $[Na^+]$ is 100 mmoles and stool potassium $[K^+]$ is 5 mmoles, then the expected stool osmolality would be:

$$(100 + 5) \times 2 = 210 \text{ mOsm}$$

In a study in which diarrhea was induced in normal volunteers using different agents, it was observed that in secretory diarrhea, the osmotic gap was always less than 50 mOsm, whereas in all forms of osmotic diarrhea, the gap was always considerably higher than 50 mOsm.

To calculate the osmotic gap, consider that estimated serum osmolality is usually 290 mOsm. Thus,

$$290 \text{ mOsm} - \text{calculated stool osmolality} = \text{gap}$$

Using the above example:

$$290 - 210 = 80 \text{ mOsm}$$

which is greater than 50. Thus, unaccounted osmotically agents or unabsorbable solutes account for the "gap." A fecal fluid with a pH level of less than 5.6 helps distinguish diarrhea due to malabsorption of a sugar such as lactulose.

The causes of osmotic diarrhea include:

- Disaccharidase deficiency, such as lactose intolerance
- Malabsorption of osmotically active nutrients
- Poorly absorbed sugars, such as lactulose, sorbitol, and mannitol
- Laxatives containing magnesium, sodium citrate, and sodium phosphate
- Antacids containing magnesium

### Secretory Diarrhea

In secretory diarrhea, an abnormal ion transport occurs across intestinal epithelial cells, the result of the active secretion of ions. In this case, no osmotic gap occurs, and because the diarrhea is not related to the intestinal content, it typically will not cease with fasting. The most striking example of secretory diarrhea is bacterial toxin–associated diarrhea, as occurs in cholera.

The causes of secretory diarrhea include:

- Infections, such as cholera
- Mucosal inflammation, such as celiac sprue or collagenous colitis
- Stimulant laxatives, such as phenolphthalein, senna, and docusate sodium
- Hormonal causes, such as vasoactive intestinal peptide-producing tumor, carcinoid tumor, and hyperthyroidism

### Altered Motility

Motility disturbances of the gastrointestinal (GI) tract can result in decreased absorption. Any anatomic disruption, such as gastrectomy or vagotomy, could produce diarrhea.

Proving motility as the sole cause of diarrhea is very difficult, however. Dysmotility-induced diarrhea often is a diagnosis of exclusion. A consequence of reduced intestinal motility may be bacterial overgrowth, which would aggravate the diarrhea and cause fat malabsorption.

The causes of diarrhea due to altered motility include:

- Irritable bowel syndrome
- Postsurgical (vagotomy, cholecystectomy, gastrectomy)
- Hyperthyroidism

### Exudative Diarrhea

Extensive injury of the small bowel or colon mucosa may result in fluid and protein loss into the intestinal lumen and ensuing diarrhea. Exudation is rarely the only mechanism accounting for the diarrhea.

The causes of exudative diarrhea include:

- Inflammatory bowel disease (IBD)
- Invasive bacterial infections (*Shigella, Salmonella*)

It is important to keep in mind that more than one mechanism may exist. For example, in infectious and inflammatory conditions, both malabsorption (leading to osmotic diarrhea) and active secretion may coexist.

## Evaluation of Diarrhea

### History and Physical Examination

Conducting a careful interview can provide valuable clues that will aid in choosing the most appropriate and cost-effective investigations. Of particular usefulness is the duration of diarrhea. Acute diarrhea is usually infectious in origin and, for the most part, resolves with or without intervention. Chronic diarrhea, defined as lasting more than 4 weeks, is unlikely to be infectious. The presence of blood is also a useful clue, suggesting infections by invasive organisms, inflammation, ischemia, or neoplasm. Large-volume diarrhea suggests small-bowel or proximal colonic disease, whereas small, frequent stools associated with urgency suggest left colon or rectal disease. All current and recent medications should be reviewed, specifically new medications, antibiotics, antacids, and alcohol abuse. Nutritional supplements should be reviewed, including the intake of "sugar-free" foods (containing nonabsorbed carbohydrates), fat substitutes, milk products or shellfish, or the heavy intake of fruits, fruit juices, or caffeine. The social history should include travel, source of drinking water (treated city water or well water), the consumption of raw milk, exposure to farm animals that may spread *Salmonella* or *Brucella*, and sexual orientation. Familial occurrence of celiac disease, IBD, or multiple endocrine neoplasia syndromes also should be checked.

Physical examination in acute diarrhea is helpful in determining the severity of disease and hydration status. In chronic diarrhea, findings such as oral ulcers and pyoderma gangrenosum suggest IBD; dermatitis herpetiformis is associated with celiac disease, and lymphadenopathy with lymphoma.

Further evaluation by laboratory tests and the appropriate selection of tests depend to a great extent on the duration and severity of diarrhea and the presence of blood, overt or occult, in the stool.

### Acute Diarrhea

Acute diarrhea is defined as lasting less than 4 weeks; it is commonly caused by infectious organisms or toxins. It is usually self-limited and, in the absence of blood in the stool, remains mostly undiagnosed. If a patient is seen early in the course of illness and has no systemic symptoms or blood in the stool, and if diarrhea is mild, then observation and follow-up are most appropriate. Otherwise, and particularly in the presence of blood, stool should be sent for evaluation for infectious organisms and treatment instituted when appropriate. If organisms are not identified, sigmoidoscopy should be performed and biopsies obtained. Further investigations will depend on the results of sigmoidoscopy (e.g., if IBD is suspected), severity of diarrhea, immune status of the host, and presence of systemic toxicity.

Traveler's diarrhea is the most common affliction of a highly mobile population. Food-borne illness is the most common cause. Watery diarrhea 5 to 15 days after arrival, with a range 3 to 31 days, is common. *Escherichia coli* is the leading cause and is responsible for more cases than all other infectious agents combined. *Campylobacter* infections are responsible for more than *Shigella* and *Salmonella* combined. Other infectious agents include *Vibrio parahemolyticus*, rotavirus, Norwalk virus, adenovirus, coxsackievirus, *Clostridium difficile*, *Clostridium perfringes*, *Bacillus cereus*, *Staphylococcus aureus*, *Entamoeba histolytica*, *Vibrio cholerae*. Other organisms make up the remaining cases.

Treatment includes the replacement of fluid loss and the administration of loperamide or diphenoxylate (which should be discontinued after 2 days, or immediately in the presence of blood, mucous, or fever). Bismuth subsalicylate 30 ml eight times a day can shorten the course of traveler's diarrhea and also may be used for prevention at 2.4 gm/day. Short-course broad spectrum antibiotics using fluoroquinolone or trimethoprin-sulfamethoxazole plus loperamide have been the standard for severe cases, but data remain unconvincing and theoretical risks do exist for selecting out invasive or resistant organisms. Rifaximin (Xifaxan) 200 mg three times a day, for 3 days, recently has been approved for traveler's diarrhea. Its use is indicated in patients 12 years or older for diarrhea caused by noninvasive strains of *E. coli*.

A general algorithm for the evaluation of acute diarrhea is shown in Figure 61.1.

### Chronic Diarrhea

Clinicians have many tests at their disposal for evaluating a patient with chronic diarrhea, and proper judgment should be used in the choice of the most appropriate tests. The duration of diarrhea, evidence of systemic involvement, nutritional deficiencies, and previous investigations should guide the evaluation. Unlike acute diarrhea, chronic diarrhea of infectious etiology is uncommon. Weight loss and evidence of nutritional deficiencies suggest malabsorption caused by small-bowel or pancreatic pathology, the latter implicated by a history of excessive alcohol intake or abdominal pain. Chronic bloody diarrhea suggests IBD, particularly ulcerative colitis. Chronic diarrhea with no evidence of nutritional or metabolic deficiency suggests lactose intolerance (common); irritable bowel syndrome, particularly when associated with abdominal pain (common); microscopic colitis (particularly in elderly women); fecal incontinence; or surreptitious laxative abuse. Colon cancer should always be excluded. In the absence of nutritional deficiencies, large-volume diarrhea with features of a secretory process usually prompts a search for hormone-producing tumors, but these are rarely found. A general algorithm for the approach to chronic diarrhea is illustrated in Figure 61.2.

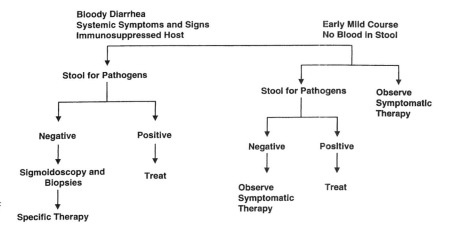

**Figure 61.1** Algorithm for the evaluation of acute diarrhea.

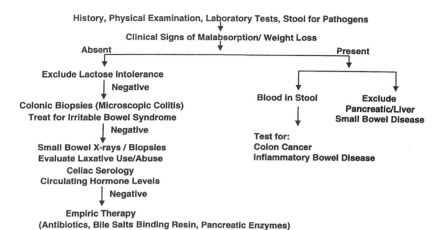

History, Physical Examination, Laboratory Tests, Stool for Pathogens

Clinical Signs of Malabsorption/ Weight Loss

**Absent**             **Present**

**Exclude Lactose Intolerance**
Negative

**Colonic Biopsies (Microscopic Colitis)**
**Treat for Irritable Bowel Syndrome**
Negative

**Small Bowel X-rays / Biopsies**
**Evaluate Laxative Use/Abuse**
**Celiac Serology**
**Circulating Hormone Levels**
Negative

**Empiric Therapy**
**(Antibiotics, Bile Salts Binding Resin, Pancreatic Enzymes)**

**Blood in Stool**

**Test for:**
**Colon Cancer**
**Inflammatory Bowel Disease**

**Exclude**
**Pancreatic/Liver**
**Small Bowel Disease**

**Figure 61.2** Algorithm for the approach to chronic diarrhea.

## Treatment

When possible, therapy is directed toward the underlying etiology. When no specific therapy is available or no cause is found, it is appropriate to give empiric therapy (e.g., an antibiotic for possible bacterial overgrowth or Giardia, or cholestyramine for bile acid malabsorption) or nonspecific therapy with constipating agents, such as loperamide (Imodium), diphenoxylate/atropine sulfate (Lomotil), or, in more severe cases, codeine, paregoric, or a trial of long-acting somatostatin analog.

## MALABSORPTION

The main purpose of the GI tract is to digest and absorb major nutrients (fat, carbohydrates, and protein), essential micronutrients (vitamins and trace elements), water, and electrolytes. Digestion involves both the mechanical and biochemical breakdown of food. Mechanical breakdown is achieved by mastication and gastric trituration, and its biochemical counterpart by a complex enzymatic process that depends on gastric, pancreatic, and biliary secretions; this process is completed by enzymes located at the brush border of enterocytes. The final products are then absorbed through the intestinal brush border. The controlled release of food from the stomach, its normal progression through the intestine, and adequate intestinal surface area are important factors. The term *malabsorption* is used in reference to all aspects of the impaired assimilation of nutrients.

Most food components can be absorbed throughout the length of the small intestine, whereas some can be absorbed only at specific segments (e.g., vitamin $B_{12}$ and bile acids in the terminal ileum). The primary absorptive function of the colon is the salvage of water and electrolytes. Malabsorption results from abnormal digestion, abnormal absorption, or both. The digestive process starts in the stomach, with acid and pepsin, and continues in the upper small bowel, with bile and pancreatic enzymes such as lipase, amylase, and trypsin. As a result, fats are broken down to fatty acids and

monoglycerides, proteins to amino acids and peptides, and carbohydrates into monosaccharides and disaccharides. Further breakdown of these nutrients takes place at the brush border of the intestinal mucosal cells by disaccharidases and oligopeptidases, with final absorption across the large surface area of the small intestine. The products of absorption reach the circulation either through the mesenteric vasculature or through lymphatics.

Of all the nutrients ingested, lipids require the most complex digestive process before being absorbed. Lipolysis starts in the stomach and is completed in the jejunum by pancreatic lipase. This results in the formation of free fatty acids and glycerol. Bile salts manufactured in the liver are necessary to facilitate absorption through micellar formation. Bile salts are then reabsorbed in the terminal ileum to be used over and over again (enterohepatic circulation). Therefore, fat malabsorption can occur because of gastrectomy, pancreatic insufficiency, advanced liver disease, biliary obstruction, or absent or markedly diseased ileum. Bile salt action also can be impaired by deconjugation, which occurs in the presence of bacterial overgrowth.

The causes of malabsorption include:

- Defect in intraluminal phase: pancreatic insufficiency, bile salt deficiency, bacterial overgrowth
- Mucosal defect: disaccharidase deficiency, celiac sprue, Whipple's disease, Crohn's disease, abetalipoproteinemia
- Infections: Giardiasis, tropical sprue
- Lymphatic obstruction: intestinal lymphangiectasia, lymphoma
- Multiple mechanisms: gastrectomy, Crohn's disease, ileal resection
- Drugs: neomycin, laxatives, cholestyramine

## Clinical Presentation

The symptoms of malabsorption are multiple. Diarrhea is almost universally present. Stools are often described as bulky and sticky. Floating stools do not necessarily indicate malabsorption. Abdominal pain is mild unless an inflammatory etiology (IBD) or pancreatic disease is present. Weight loss can be mild or advanced, depending on the severity of malabsorption. Malabsorption may lead to multiple manifestations due to various nutritional deficiencies, such as anemia due to iron, vitamin $B_{12}$, or folic acid deficiency; hypocalcemia; and a bleeding tendency due to vitamin K deficiency, among others.

The past history can provide important clues. A surgical history should be taken, with particular attention to the exact site and extent of any organ resection. A history of alcohol or previous attacks of abdominal pain may lead to the diagnosis of chronic pancreatitis. A drug history must be taken, along with a travel history and inquiry about sexual practices.

## Laboratory Testing

When malabsorption is suspected, blood tests usually include a measurement of albumin, carotene, cholesterol, calcium, and folic acid levels, and a measure of prothrombin time. These data are helpful in assessing the severity of malabsorption but do not aid in the differential diagnosis. Many other tests are available in diagnosing malabsorption; the more clinically useful tests are discussed in the following sections.

### Fecal Fat Analysis

The simplest way to detect stool fat is to perform a Sudan stain on a stool smear. This test has limited sensitivity because of the stain's affinity for dietary triglyceride and its lipolytic products only, but it has the advantage of simplicity and low cost. A more sensitive test for steatorrhea is the quantitative measurement of fat in the stool. Stool is collected for 3 consecutive days and analyzed for fat content while the patient is eating a diet containing 80 to 100 g of fat daily. Normal fat excretion should not exceed 6 g daily. The test is cumbersome and does not identify the cause of fat malabsorption, but it yields an accurate quantification of stool fat excretion.

### Tests of Pancreatic Exocrine Function

Intubation studies of the duodenum near the ampulla of Vater provide the best index of pancreatic function. After stimulation of the pancreas, duodenal contents are aspirated and analyzed for bicarbonate and enzyme output. These tests are invasive and time consuming, however, and are therefore not suitable for screening. Pancreatic calcifications seen on abdominal radiographs or computed tomography (CT) indicate the presence of chronic pancreatitis in late stages but usually are not present early on. Abnormal ductal anatomy can be demonstrated by endoscopic retrograde cholangiopancreatography (ERCP), but this test is invasive and has side effects. Magnetic resonance image (MRI) technology may substitute ERCP in the future.

**TABLE 61.1**

## SMALL-BOWEL BIOPSY IN DIAGNOSING MALABSORPTION

| Often Diagnostic | Abnormal But Not Diagnostic |
|---|---|
| Whipple's disease | Celiac sprue |
| Amyloidosis | Systemic sclerosis |
| Eosinophilic enteritis | Radiation enteritis |
| Lymphangiectasia | Bacterial overgrowth syndrome |
| Primary intestinal lymphoma | Tropical sprue |
| Giardiasis | Crohn's disease |
| Abetalipoproteinemia | |
| Agammaglobulinemia | |
| Mastocytosis | |

### Small-Intestine Biopsy

Small-intestine mucosal biopsy is a key diagnostic test in diseases that affect the cellular phase of absorption. In some diseases, the histologic features are diagnostic, whereas in others the findings are suggestive. Endoscopic biopsies from the duodenum and jejunum have replaced biopsies obtained by specially designed per-oral capsules. Several biopsy samples should be taken from the distal duodenum to increase the diagnostic yield.

The use of small-bowel biopsy specimens in malabsorption is categorized in Table 61.1.

### D-Xylose Absorption Test

D-Xylose is a five-carbon monosaccharide that, when given in a large dose, can cross the intestinal mucosa largely by passive diffusion. The test is performed by having a patient ingest 25 g of D-xylose; urine is collected for the next 5 hours. Healthy individuals excrete more than 4.5 g of D-xylose in 5 hours. The test reflects the permeability and surface area of the mucosa and serves as an indicator of mucosal integrity. False-positive abnormally low results may occur in the presence of poor renal function, large amounts of edema, or ascites. Abnormal results may also be seen in the presence of bacterial overgrowth, but these may normalize after treatment with antibiotics. Many institutions have abandoned this test, and it remains only of historical importance.

### Radiographic Studies

Barium studies of the small bowel in malabsorption usually are nonspecific. They are helpful in the presence of distinct anatomic changes, however, such as small bowel diverticulosis, lymphoma, Crohn's disease, strictures, and enteric fistulas.

### Schilling Test

The absorption of vitamin $B_{12}$ requires several steps. First, it binds to salivary R protein. In the duodenum, pancreatic proteases hydrolyze the R protein, allowing the vitamin to bind with the intrinsic factor secreted by gastric parietal cells. The vitamin $B_{12}$–intrinsic factor complex is then absorbed by specific receptors found on enterocytes in the distal ileum. Consequently, the malabsorption of vitamin $B_{12}$ can occur because of a lack of intrinsic factor (pernicious anemia or gastric resection), pancreatic insufficiency, bacterial overgrowth, or ileal resection or disease. The Schilling test helps identify the cause of vitamin $B_{12}$ deficiency. The test consists of several phases:

- Phase 1: After 1 mg of vitamin $B_{12}$ is injected to saturate the hepatic storage, the patient ingests radiolabeled vitamin, and urine is collected for measurement of radioactivity.
- Phase 2: If malabsorption is diagnosed, the test is repeated while the patient is given vitamin $B_{12}$ and intrinsic factor. If malabsorption is corrected, pernicious anemia is diagnosed.
- Phase 3: If malabsorption is still present, and the test remains abnormal in spite of treatment with antibiotics, an ileal disease is diagnosed.

### Breath Tests

Breath tests rely on the principle that the bacterial degradation of luminal compounds releases gases that can be measured in the breath. In disaccharidase deficiency, the oral ingestion of specific carbohydrates (e.g., lactose) will result in colonic fermentation due to malabsorption in the small bowel, with increased hydrogen in the breath. In the presence of bacterial overgrowth, orally ingested glucose will be fermented in the small bowel, instead of being absorbed, thus resulting in increased breath hydrogen. The measurement of radioactive carbon in the breath ($^{14}C$) has been used in tests devised to measure malabsorption of fat and bile acids, as well as for bacterial overgrowth ($^{14}C$-xylose). The radioactive tests are cumbersome, and their use in clinical practice is limited.

## Approach to Suspected Malabsorption

Because of the large number of available diagnostic tests, a rational use of these tests is necessary when a patient with suspected malabsorption is being evaluated (Fig. 61.3). The best screening test for steatorrhea is the 72-hour fecal fat analysis. The test is cumbersome and difficult to obtain in practice, however. Alternatively, test selection may depend on the clinical presentation. The presence of cholestatic hepatobiliary disease is usually quite obvious clinically. When weight loss, nutritional deficiencies, and diarrhea are present, a qualitative stool analysis may be done to establish steatorrhea.

The absence of a history of excessive alcohol intake, previous episodes of pancreatitis, or abdominal pain makes the presence of chronic pancreatitis unlikely. A urinary D-xylose test or a small bowel biopsy then may be performed to determine whether mucosal disease is present. If these tests are normal, then enzyme tests can be done, along with abdominal radiography, to look for pancreatic disease. If tests are nonrevealing, or the D-xylose test is abnormal in the presence of a normal mucosal biopsy, a hydrogen breath test can be done and small bowel films obtained to test for bacterial overgrowth. When abdominal pain suggestive of a pancreatic origin is present, ultrasound, CT of the abdomen, or ERCP may be performed first to exclude chronic pancreatitis or pancreatic cancer.

When diarrhea is associated with cramps and flatulence with minimal or no weight loss and no nutritional deficiencies, the possibility of carbohydrate malabsorption, particularly lactose intolerance, should be entertained.

## Treatment

The treatment of malabsorption depends on the underlying condition. It consists of dietary manipulations in celiac sprue, antibiotic therapy in bacterial overgrowth, enzyme supplementation in pancreatic insufficiency, surgery for

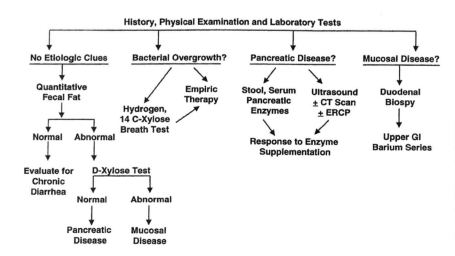

**Figure 61.3** Evaluation of a patient with suspected malabsorption. CT, computed tomography; ERCP, endoscopic retrograde cholangiopancreatography; GI, gastrointestinal. (Adapted with permission from Riley SA, Marsh MN. Maldigestion and malabsorption. In: Feldman M, Sleisenger MH, Scharschmidt BF, et al., eds. *Sleisenger & Fordtran's Gastrointestinal and Liver Disease: Pathophysiology, Diagnosis, Management*, 6th ed. Philadelphia: WB Saunders, 1998;1501–1522.)

small bowel obstruction, or parenteral nutrition when treatment options have failed to maintain an adequate nutritional status. Empiric treatment using pancreatic enzyme supplementation or an antibiotic for suspected bacterial overgrowth or Giardia is occasionally given when the etiology remains unclear.

# CELIAC SPRUE

Celiac sprue, also known as *nontropical sprue* or *gluten-sensitive enteropathy*, is characterized by intestinal mucosal injury resulting from an immunologic intolerance to gluten in genetically predisposed individuals. The prevalence of the disease among relatives of patients with celiac sprue is approximately 10%. Celiac sprue is strong associated with human leukocyte antigen class II molecules, in particular HLA-DQ2 and HLA-DQ8. The disease is induced by exposure to the storage proteins found in grain plants, such as wheat (which contains gliadin), barley, rye, and oats, and their products. The exposure initiates a cellular immune response that results in mucosal damage, particularly in the proximal intestine. Recent investigations suggest that an enzyme, tissue transglutaminase, may be the autoantigen of celiac sprue.

## Clinical Presentation

Celiac disease may present with the classic constellation of symptoms and signs of a malabsorption syndrome. Conversely, the presentation may be atypical, with nonspecific GI symptoms such as bloating, chronic diarrhea without steatorrhea, flatulence, lactose intolerance, or deficiency of a single micronutrient, such as iron-deficiency anemia. Up to 50% of celiac patients do not have diarrhea. Non-GI complaints, such as depression, fatigue, and arthralgia, and manifestations such as osteoporosis or osteomalacia, may predominate. Several diseases are associated with a higher incidence of celiac disease; these include dermatitis herpetiformis, type I diabetes mellitus, autoimmune thyroid disease, and selective immunoglobulin A deficiency.

## Diagnosis

Although celiac disease is part of the differential diagnosis of every malabsorption syndrome, a high index of suspicion should be kept in mind for patients with atypical presentations. Intestinal biopsy is the most valuable test in establishing the diagnosis of celiac sprue. A spectrum of pathologic changes occur, ranging from normal villous architecture with an increase in mucosal lymphocytes and plasma cells (infiltrative lesion) to partial or total villous atrophy. Although abnormal findings on intestinal biopsy are nonspecific, they are highly suggestive, particularly because most other conditions that can mimic celiac dis-

ease, such as Crohn's disease, lymphoma, tropical sprue, graft-versus-host disease, or immune deficiency, may be distinguished on clinical grounds. A clinical response to a gluten-free diet in the presence of an abnormal biopsy should establish the diagnosis and preclude the need, in adults, to document healing by repeat biopsies. Serologic blood tests are helpful for screening patients and the asymptomatic relatives of celiac sprue patients. The panel used in our lab includes a total immunoglobulin A (IgA) level, endomysial IgA, gliadin IgG and IgA, and transglutaminase IgA levels. In patients with low total IgA levels, normal antibody levels are unreliable; these patients should usually undergo small-bowel biopsy. The proper management of patients with serological evidence of celiac disease and normal biopsies is unknown.

## Treatment

A strict, lifelong adherence to a gluten-free diet is the only treatment for celiac disease. Specific nutritional supplementation should be provided to correct deficiencies, particularly of iron, vitamins, and calcium. Clinical response may be seen within a few weeks. Patients should be followed to ensure adequate response and proper adherence to diet. Long-term prognosis is excellent for patients who adhere to a gluten-free diet, although a slight increase in the incidence of malignancies may be present, particularly lymphoma.

# BACTERIAL OVERGROWTH SYNDROME

The proximal small bowel normally contains only a small number of bacteria, fewer than a thousand per milliliter of fluid, with no anaerobic *Bacteroides* organisms and few coliforms. An overgrowth of bacteria can result in diarrhea and malabsorption through several mechanisms:

- Deconjugation of bile salts leading to impaired micelle formation and fat malabsorption
- Patchy injury to enterocytes on the intestinal mucosal surface
- Direct use of nutrients, such as uptake of vitamin $B_{12}$, by Gram-negative organisms
- Secretion of water and electrolytes, secondary to by-products of bacterial metabolism, such as hydroxylated bile acids and organic acids

## Associated Conditions

The most important factor in maintaining the relative sterility of the upper gut is a normal motor function, with other factors being gastric acid and intestinal immunoglobulins. Consequently, conditions that impair these functions can result in bacterial overgrowth. GI stasis may be caused by a motility disorder (scleroderma, intestinal pseudo-obstruction, diabetes) or anatomic impairment (blind loops, obstruction, and diverticulosis). Achlorhydria, pancreatic insufficiency, and immunodeficiency syndromes are also associated with bacterial overgrowth.

## Diagnosis

The direct culture of a jejunal aspirate is the most definitive diagnostic test, but it is invasive and uncomfortable. The $^{14}$C-xylose breath test is the most appropriate test, whereas the glucose breath hydrogen test is the simplest, although not as sensitive or specific. An empiric therapeutic trial of an antibiotic is an acceptable alternative.

## Treatment

When appropriate, specific therapy should be provided, such as surgery for intestinal obstruction. More commonly, patients are treated with an antibiotic effective against aerobic and anaerobic enteric organisms. Tetracycline, trimethoprim-sulfamethoxazole, and metronidazole in combination with a cephalosporin are suitable agents. A single course of therapy for 7 to 10 days may be therapeutic for months. In other patients, intermittent therapy (1 week out of every 4) or even continuous therapy for 1 or 2 months may be needed.

## LYMPHOCYTIC OR COLLAGENOUS COLITIS

This is a relatively common disease or spectrum of diseases, which is characterized by chronic diarrhea and mucosal abnormalities consisting of infiltration of the lamina propria and epithelium with lymphocytes, increased subepithelial collagen plate (in collagenous colitis), or both. The endoscopic and radiological appearance of the colon is normal. The mean age at presentation is in the sixth decade, with a female predominance. An association with autoimmune disorders and celiac sprue has been noted. Typically, patients exhibit no biochemical deficiencies, and the diagnosis can be made only through random biopsies from the colon.

No specific treatment is available for this entity, although sulfasalazine (Azulfidine), mesalamine (Asacol, Pentasa), and local (budesonide) and systemic steroids have been reported to provide relief. In a recent study involving a small number of patients, high-dose bismuth subsalicylate resolved diarrhea and colitis in most patients. Symptomatic therapy using antidiarrheal agents may be the treatment of choice.

## DIARRHEA IN ACQUIRED IMMUNODEFICIENCY SYNDROME

In up to two-thirds of patients with acquired immunodeficiency syndrome (AIDS), diarrhea develops during the course of their disease. An increasing array of infectious and noninfectious etiologies is recognized as causing diarrhea in this population. These include pathogens found in immunocompetent hosts, those related to sexually transmitted organisms, and organisms associated with the immunocompromised host, as well as noninfectious causes. Stool analysis is the most productive investigation, followed by colonoscopy. Upper endoscopy may be done if the workup for small-bowel pathogens is negative.

The causes of diarrhea in patients with acquired immunodeficiency syndrome include:

- Infections
- Organisms affecting immunocompetent hosts: *Salmonella, Shigella, Clostridium difficile, Giardia lamblia, Entamoeba histolytica*
- Sexually transmitted pathogens: *Neisseria gonorrhoeae, Chlamydia trachomatis, Treponema pallidum*
- Organisms affecting immunocompromised hosts: *Mycobacterium avium*-intracellulare, Cytomegalovirus, *Cryptosporidium*, Microsporidia
- Malignancy: Kaposi's sarcoma, Non-Hodgkin's lymphoma
- AIDS enteropathy

## REVIEW EXERCISES

### QUESTIONS

**1.** A 68-year-old woman reports diarrhea and occasional fecal incontinence. She is otherwise healthy; her appetite is good and her weight stable. Which of the following helps you decide whether her diarrhea is significant?
a) Passage of liquid stools
b) Frequent passage of stools
c) Presence of large bowel movements
d) 24-Hour stool weight greater than 250 g
e) The history of fecal incontinence

**2.** Which of the following features can help distinguish osmotic from secretory diarrhea?
a) Secretory diarrhea decreases or disappears with fasting.
b) There is usually no osmotic gap in secretory diarrhea.
c) Osmotic diarrhea is often accompanied by bleeding.
d) Stool weight is higher in osmotic diarrhea due to the nonabsorbable solutes.

**3.** A 52-year-old man presents with a 2-year history of diarrhea and weight loss. No bleeding is present. He admits to heavy alcohol intake in the past but has been without alcohol for several years. His diabetes is well-controlled with insulin. He underwent cholecystectomy 6 years ago. Laboratory tests are normal, except for mild anemia, and radiographs of the small bowel are reported as normal. Which should be the next test?
a) ERCP
b) Small bowel biopsy

**c)** 72-Hour stool collection for volume and fat
**d)** Glucose hydrogen breath test
**e)** Colonoscopy with biopsy

**4.** A 59-year-old African American woman presents with a 6-year history of diarrhea and occasional abdominal pain. Laboratory and stool tests are normal. Which of the following would you proceed with?
**a)** Upper GI endoscopy and biopsy
**b)** Treatment with an anticholinergic
**c)** Colonoscopy and random biopsies
**d)** Hydrogen breath test or lactose free diet for lactose intolerance

**5.** A 55-year-old woman with diarrhea is found to have lymphocytic colitis. She has iron deficiency anemia, and the diarrhea is difficult to control. Which would you proceed with?
**a)** Iron supplementation
**b)** Antigliadin antibody
**c)** Small bowel radiograph
**d)** 72-Hour stool collection for fat
**e)** Upper GI endoscopy and small-bowel biopsy

**6.** A 29-year-old woman seeks medical advice because of chronic low back pain. Tests showed osteoporosis and iron deficiency anemia. She is a mother of two children and complains of heavy menstrual bleeding. Sigmoidoscopy was normal. You would proceed with which of the following?
**a)** Colonoscopy
**b)** Empiric treatment with iron preparation
**c)** Referral to a gynecologist
**d)** Upper endoscopy and small-bowel biopsy

## ANSWERS

**1. e.**
The history of fecal incontinence should always be considered significant and evaluated. In a patient with fecal incontinence who is otherwise healthy, the involuntary loss of stool can be perceived as diarrhea. Although liquid stools are usually associated with increased weight, stool weight remains the only objective way of assessing the degree of diarrhea so answer d is also considered an acceptable answer, but not the best answer.

**2. b.**
Because secretory diarrhea is associated either with the active secretion of electrolytes and water or impaired absorption, no increase in osmotic gap occurs in this condition. Secretory diarrhea is usually not affected by food intake. Osmotic diarrhea is not accompanied by bleeding. Stool volumes may be high in either osmotic or secretory diarrhea. The nonabsorbable solutes in osmotic diarrhea does not cause the stool weight to rise.

**3. c.**
This man has several potential reasons for diarrhea: (i) alcohol intake, which raises the possibility of pancreatic insufficiency; (ii) diabetes, which can lead to bacterial overgrowth or autonomic impairment (diabetic diarrhea); and (iii) cholecystectomy. Given the weight loss (suggestive of malabsorption), a 72-hour collection would be helpful in determining whether steatorrhea is present; this result would be highly suggestive of pancreatic insufficiency or possibly bacterial overgrowth. Although ERCP and invasive tests can provide evidence of chronic pancreatitis, it does not necessarily indicate the presence of pancreatic insufficiency. A colonoscopy would be reasonable in this man, but it would not help determine the presence of steatorrhea, which is likely in this patient.

**4. d.**
Given the history of chronic diarrhea with no evidence of laboratory abnormalities or any suggestion of systemic abnormalities, lactose intolerance is likely, particularly in an African American person. The test is simple and noninvasive, and response to a lactose-free diet will confirm the diagnosis with no need for further testing.

**5. e.**
Lymphocytic colitis is usually not associated with anemia. Because the diarrhea is difficult to control and the patient also has iron deficiency anemia, the possibility of celiac disease should be kept in mind. An upper GI endoscopy and small-bowel biopsy to exclude celiac, as well as other upper GI sources for anemia, would be the most appropriate way to proceed.

**6. d.**
Although heavy blood losses during menses can cause anemia in an otherwise healthy young woman, the presence of osteoporosis suggests the presence of a different problem. Colonoscopy is unlikely to provide an answer in the absence of symptoms related to the colon and in the presence of normal sigmoidoscopy. Malabsorption is highly suspected, and the small-bowel biopsy showed celiac disease. Celiac disease can present with symptoms related to malabsorption in the absence of diarrhea and occasionally only with iron deficiency anemia.

## SUGGESTED READINGS

Achkar E, Carey WD, Petras R, et al. Comparison of suction capsule and endoscopic biopsy of small bowel mucosa. *Gastrointest Endosc* 1988;32:278–286.
Afzalpurkar RG, Schiller LR, Little KH, et al. The self-limited nature of chronic idiopathic diarrhea. *N Engl J Med* 1992;327:1849–1852.
Clinical conference: hormonal diarrhea due to pancreatic tumor. *Gastroenterology* 1980;79:571–582.
Corazza GR, Menozzi MG, Strocchi A, et al. The diagnosis of small bowel bacterial overgrowth: reliability of jejunal culture and inadequacy of breath hydrogen testing. *Gastroenterology* 1990;98:302–309.

Craig RM, Atkinson AJ Jr. D-Xylose testing: a review. *Gastroenterology* 1988;95:223–231.

Cummings JH, Sladen GE, James OF, et al. Laxative-induced diarrhoea: a continuing clinical problem. *BMJ* 1974;1:537–541.

Dieterich W, Ehnis T, Bauer M, et al. Identification of tissue transglutaminase as the autoantigen of celiac disease. *Nat Med* 1997;3: 797–801.

DiMagno EP, Go VL, Summerskill WHJ. Relations between pancreatic enzyme outputs and malabsorption in severe pancreatic insufficiency. *N Engl J Med* 1973;288:813–815.

Eherer AJ, Fordtran JS. Fecal osmotic gap and pH in experimental diarrhea of various causes. *Gastroenterology* 1992;103:545–551.

Fine KD, Lee EL. Efficacy of open-label bismuth subsalicylate for the treatment of microscopic colitis. *Gastroenterology* 1998;114:29–36.

Fine KD, Schiller LR. AGA technical review on the evaluation and management of chronic diarrhea. *Gastroenterology* 1999;116: 1464–1486.

Goggins M, Kelleher D. Celiac disease and other nutrient-related injuries to the gastrointestinal tract. *Am J Gastroenterol* 1994; 89[Suppl]:S2–S17.

Grohmann GS, Glass RI, Pereira HG, et al. Enteric viruses and diarrhea in HIV-infected patients. *N Engl J Med* 1993;329:14–20.

Hofmann AF. Bile acid malabsorption caused by ileal resection. *Arch Intern Med* 1972;130:597–605.

Jessurun J, Yardley JH, Lee EL, et al. Microscopic and collagenous colitis: different names for the same condition? *Gastroenterology* 1986;91: 1583–1584.

Khouri MR, Huang G, Shiau YF. Sudan stain of fecal fat: new insight into an old test. *Gastroenterology* 1989;96:421–427.

Kotler DP, Orenstein JM. Chronic diarrhea and malabsorption associated with enteropathogenic bacterial infection in a patient with AIDS. *Ann Intern Med* 1993;119:127–128.

Matteoni C, Wang N, Goldblum J, et al. Celiac disease is highly prevalent in lymphocytic colitis. *J Clin Gastroenterol* 2001;32:225–227.

Mills LR, Schuman BM, Thompson WO. Lymphocytic colitis: a definable clinical and histological diagnosis. *Dig Dis Sci* 1993;38: 1147–1151.

Phillips S, Donaldson L, Geisler K, et al. Stool composition in factitial diarrhea: a 6-year experience with stool analysis. *Ann Intern Med* 1995;123:97–100.

Saslow SB, Camilleri M. Diabetic diarrhea. *Semin Gastrointest Dis* 1995;6:187–193.

Shamir R. Advances in celiac disease. *Gastroenterol Clin North Am* 2003;32:931–947.

Simon D, Brandt LJ. Diarrhea in patients with the acquired immunodeficiency syndrome. *Gastroenterology* 1993;105:1236–1242.

Smith P, Lane HC, Gill VJ, et al. Intestinal infections in patients with the acquired immunodeficiency syndrome (AIDS): etiology and response to therapy. *Ann Intern Med* 1988;108:328–333.

Trier JS. Diagnosis of celiac sprue. *Gastroenterology* 1998;115:211–216.

Wilcox CM, Schwartz DA, Cotsonis G, et al. Chronic unexplained diarrhea in human immunodeficiency virus infection: determination of the best diagnostic approach. *Gastroenterology* 1996;110: 30–37.

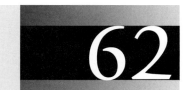

# BOARD SIMULATION:
# Gastroenterology

*John J. Vargo, II*

For the following clinical vignettes, please indicate the most appropriate therapy. The answers may be used once, multiple times, or not at all.

## QUESTIONS

**1.** *Clostridium difficile* colitis in an 86-year-old woman who presents with diarrhea 6 weeks after completing antibiotic therapy for a community-acquired pneumonia. The patient is afebrile, the abdominal examination is normal, and the serum albumin is 4.0 g/dL.

**2.** Chronic active hepatitis C in a patient with tense ascites, a serum albumin of 2.4 g/dL, a platelet count of 36,000 μL, and an international normalized ratio of 2.0.

**3.** A 56 year-old woman with collagenous colitis.

**4.** A 36-year-old healthcare worker with chronic active hepatitis C. The physical examination is normal, and the patient is otherwise healthy.

**a)** Lamivudine, 100 mg/day

**b)** No therapy

**c)** Interferon-α, 3 million units three times per week, and ribavirin, 1,000 mg/day

**d)** Bismuth subsalicylate, eight tablets per day

**e)** Metronidazole, 250 mg four times per day for 10 days

**f)** Interferon-α, 3 million units three times per week

**g)** Vancomycin, 125 mg four times per day for 10 days

**5.** A 43-year-old man with chronic hepatitis C and compensated cirrhosis undergoes a screening endoscopy for sequelae of portal hypertension. The endoscopy reveals large nonbleeding variceal columns in the distal esophagus with red color signs. Which of the following interventions would be most appropriate?

**a)** Repeat the surveillance endoscopy in 1 year.

**b)** Initiate therapy with octreotide, 0.1 mg subcutaneously twice per day.

**c)** Recommend a transjugular intrahepatic portosystemic shunt placement.

**d)** Refer the patient for consideration of a distal splenorenal shunt.

**e)** Begin therapy with a β-blocker with the goal of reducing the basal pulse rate by 25%.

**6.** A 62-year-old woman presents to your office with a 2-month history of midepigastric abdominal pain, anorexia, and a 5-pound weight loss. The discomfort is transiently relieved with antacids. The past medical history is notable for diabetes mellitus, which has been under good control, and osteoarthritis. Medications include oral ibuprofen, 400 mg two times a day, and daily oral glyburide, 5 mg. The physical examination is notable for mild midepigastric tenderness without organomegaly or masses. The stool sample is weakly guaiac positive. The next step in the patient's evaluation should be which of the following?

**a)** Discontinue ibuprofen and initiate a cyclooxygenase-2 selective antagonist. If no improvement, consider endoscopy.

**b)** Perform upper endoscopy.

**c)** Initiate antireflux measures, including a proton pump inhibitor (PPI). If no improvement, consider increasing the PPI to twice daily frequency after 2 weeks of therapy.

**d)** Obtain a serology for *Helicobacter pylori* and, if positive, treat with metronidazole, 500 mg two times a day; omeprazole 20 mg two times a day; and clarithromycin, 250 mg two times a day for 14 days. If there is no improvement, consider endoscopy.

**e)** Obtain a solid-phase gastric emptying study.

Questions 7–11: For the following statements, please choose the most appropriate answer.

**7.** HLA-B27 seronegative arthropathy

**8.** Skip areas of involvement on colonoscopy

**9.** Treatment with a chimeric monoclonal antibody to tumor necrosis factor (TNF) indicated in moderately to severely active disease

**10.** Erythema nodosum

**11.** 5-Aminosalicylic acid enemas useful in the treatment of mild proctitis

**a)** Crohn's disease

**b)** Ulcerative colitis

**c)** a and b

**d)** Neither a nor b

**12.** A 62-year-old woman comes to your office for advice regarding surveillance for colonic polyps. She underwent a colonoscopy 10 years ago, during which three adenomas were removed from the rectum and sigmoid colon. She has no symptoms attributable to a gastrointestinal disorder. The physical examination is normal. The most appropriate management of this patient would be which of the following?

**a)** Perform flexible sigmoidoscopy; if polyps identified, schedule for colonoscopy.

**b)** Schedule for computed tomography (CT) colography; if polyps identified, perform "same-day" colonoscopy.

**c)** Perform double-contrast barium enema; if polyps identified, schedule colonoscopy.

**d)** Schedule colonoscopy.

**13.** A 32-year-old man comes to your office requesting an opinion regarding colorectal cancer screening. The patient's brother was diagnosed at the age of 45 with colon cancer. A sister, aged 62, was recently diagnosed with adenomatous polyps. The patient has not experienced any change in bowel habits and the physical examination, including fecal occult blood testing, is unremarkable. The most appropriate step in the management of this patient would be which of the following?

**a)** Initiate a program of annual fecal occult blood testing and sigmoidoscopy every 5 years now instead of waiting until the patient reaches 50 years of age.

**b)** Schedule a colonoscopy when the patient is 50 and repeat every 10 years.

**c)** Screen the patient and all first-degree relatives for the presence of the *k-ras* oncogene, and perform a colonoscopy in those patients who are positive for this test.

**d)** Begin a screening program with a colonoscopy at the age of 35 and repeat the examination every 5 years.

**e)** Perform a flexible sigmoidoscopy now; if normal, the patient's risk for colorectal neoplasia can now be considered average, and he can then be enrolled in a screening program beginning at the age of 50.

Questions 14–17 are based on endoscopic photographs obtained during screening flexible sigmoidoscopy.

**14.** A 52-year-old man presents to your office with episodes of scant hematochezia and alteration in bowel habits of 4 months' duration (Fig. 62.1). His family medical history is notable for a history of Crohn's disease in a sibling. Which statement regarding the diagnosis and management of the patient is true?

**a)** Therapy with steroid enemas should be instituted. If no response occurs in 2 weeks, oral steroids should be considered, and further evaluation, consisting of a colonoscopy and small bowel series, should be obtained.

**b)** Stool samples should be obtained for *Salmonella* and *Shigella*. Empiric therapy with oral ciprofloxacin, 500 mg two times a day, should be started.

**c)** Biopsies for viral culture, including cytomegalovirus, should be obtained.

**d)** Biopsies of the lesion should be obtained and referral to a colorectal surgeon should be arranged.

**15.** A 52-year-old asymptomatic woman presents for routine screening. A retroflexed view in the rectum reveals the image shown in Figure 62.2. The appropriate

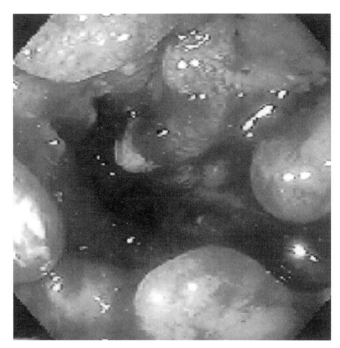

**Figure 62.1** Endoscopic photograph for the patient described in Question 14. (See Color Fig. 62.1.)

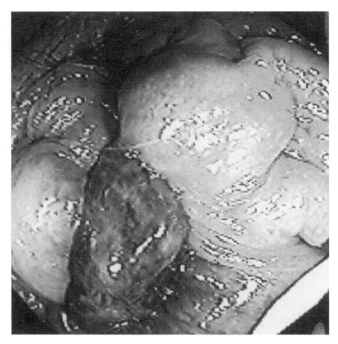

**Figure 62.3** Endoscopic photograph for the patient described in Question 16. (See Color Fig. 62.3.)

management in this case would include which of the following?

a) Obtain a biopsy; if adenomatous tissue is identified, refer for a colonoscopy with polypectomy.

b) No further evaluation is necessary.

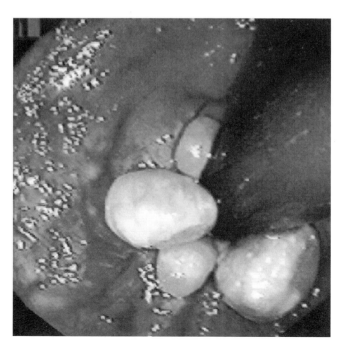

**Figure 62.2** Retroflexed view in the rectum of the patient described in Question 15. (See Color Fig. 62.2.)

c) Start therapy with a fiber supplement.

d) Refer to a colorectal surgeon for banding.

**16.** A 63-year-old man presents with scant hematochezia and pruritus ani (Fig. 62.3). He is otherwise healthy and has experienced an increasing frequency of the symptoms. Which of the following would be the most appropriate management?

a) Refer to a gastroenterologist for the evaluation of possible portal hypertension.

b) Counsel the patient on the deleterious side effects associated with the chronic use of stimulant laxatives.

c) Refer to a colorectal surgeon for banding.

d) This vascular tumor is commonly seen in immunocompromised patients; a human immunodeficiency virus serology should be obtained.

**17.** A 73-year-old woman presents for a screening flexible sigmoidoscopy (Fig. 62.4). Her laboratory values reveal the presence of thrombocytopenia and hypoalbuminemia. The most appropriate management would be which of the following?

a) Evaluate for a hypercoagulable state.

b) Obtain a hepatitis serology and refer to a gastroenterologist.

c) The finding is a normal variant; no further evaluation is necessary.

d) Obtain an obstetrical history with a particular emphasis on traumatic, breech, or forceps deliveries.

Questions 18–22: For the following questions, please choose the most appropriate diagnostic test.

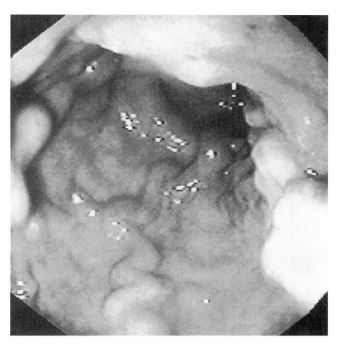

**Figure 62.4** Photograph from screening flexible sigmoidoscopy performed on the patient described in Question 17. (See Color Fig. 62.4.)

**18.** A 64-year-old woman presents with significant dysphagia to both liquids and solids. Which is the most appropriate diagnostic test?
**a)** Esophageal manometry
**b)** 24-Hour pH probe
**c)** Upper endoscopy
**d)** Barium swallow
**e)** Scintigraphy for gastroesophageal reflux

**19.** An 86-year-old man recently suffered a stroke and now is noted to cough and choke when eating. A chest radiograph reveals a right middle lobe infiltrate.
**a)** Esophageal manometry
**b)** Barium esophagram
**c)** Upper endoscopy
**d)** 24-Hour pH probe
**e)** Bernstein test

**20.** A 46-year-old woman presents with crescendo history of episodic right upper quadrant pain, nausea, and vomiting. Ultrasonography of the gallbladder and biliary tree reveals cholelithiasis and a hyperechoic focus, with posterior shadowing in a mildly dilated common bile duct. A liver profile reveals the following laboratory values: alanine aminotransferase, 200 U/L, aspartate aminotransferase, 260 U/L, alkaline phosphatase, 450 U/L, and total bilirubin, 4.8 mg/dL.
The next appropriate intervention would be which of the following?
**a)** Magnetic resonance cholangiography
**b)** Endoscopic retrograde cholangiography

**c)** Computed tomography of the liver with a serum α-fetoprotein level
**d)** Endoscopic ultrasonography

**21.** A 32-year-old man is admitted to the emergency room for the evaluation of painless melena. He recently suffered a knee injury and has been treated with an over-the-counter nonsteroidal anti-inflammatory agent for 1 year. The past medical history is unremarkable, and he takes no other medications. The physical examination reveals a blood pressure of 110/62 and a pulse rate of 62, without orthostatic changes. No stigmata of chronic liver disease is present, and the remainder of the examination, with the exception of melena on rectal examination, is unremarkable. Laboratory values reveal a white blood count of 7,100/μL; hemoglobin 14.1 g/dL; hematocrit 45%; a platelet count of 225,000/μL, international normalized ratio 1.0; a blood urea nitrogen (BUN) level of 46 mg/dL; and a creatinine level of 1.2 mg/dL.
An endoscopy reveals a clean-based antral ulcer. In addition to discontinuation of the nonsteroidal anti-inflammatory agent, which of the following would be an appropriate course of action?
**a)** Admit the patient for 48 hours to ensure that no further bleeding occurs, and begin therapy with an intravenous $H_2$ blocker.
**b)** Discharge the patient, begin therapy with a PPI, obtain an *H. pylori* serology, and repeat the endoscopy in 8 weeks to ensure ulcer healing.
**c)** Admit the patient, perform a colonoscopy to ensure that no right-sided colonic lesion is present that also could lead to melena.
**d)** Discharge the patient, begin therapy with a PPI, obtain an *H. pylori* serology, and perform an upper endoscopy in 48 hours to ensure that no rebleeding has occurred that might require endoscopic therapy.

**22.** Every condition below is associated with a low gradient (i.e., serum-ascites albumin gradient of less than 1.1 g/dL), *except*
**a)** Peritoneal carcinomatosis
**b)** Tuberculous peritonitis
**c)** Nephrotic syndrome
**d)** Budd-Chiari syndrome
**e)** Pancreatic ascites

**23.** A 36-year-old man presents with a 6-month history of intermittent solid food dysphagia. No history of liquid dysphagia or weight loss is present. A barium swallow is obtained (Fig. 62.5). Which statement about the radiographic finding is true?
**a)** The lesion is seen in association with tylosis and iron deficiency.
**b)** The patient is at increased risk for adenocarcinoma of the cardia.
**c)** Treatment should consist of upper endoscopy with esophageal dilatation.

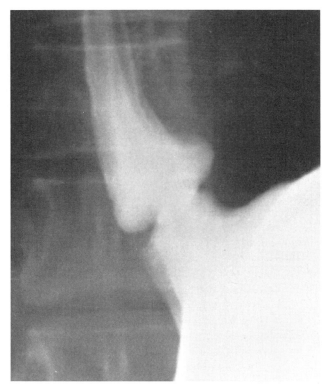

**Figure 62.5** Barium radiographic finding for the patient described in Question 23.

**d)** A trial of a smooth muscle relaxant, such as nifedipine, should be tried before endoscopy.

**e)** Esophageal manometry should be performed.

Questions 24–26: Please provide the most appropriate answer for the following statements.

**24.** A risk factor for the development of pancreatic cancer.

**25.** Associated with pseudocyst formation.

**26.** Hypercalcemia and hypertriglyceridemia are important etiologic factors.
**a)** Acute pancreatitis
**b)** Chronic pancreatitis
**c)** Both a and b
**d)** Neither a nor b

Questions 27–30: For the following clinical vignettes, please choose the correct answer.

**27.** Clinical features after ingestion include anemia, thrombocytopenia, and renal failure.

**28.** Nausea and vomiting occur 6 hours after ingestion of fried rice.

**29.** Diarrhea, vomiting, and mesenteric adenitis occur; it is occasionally mistaken for acute appendicitis.

**30.** A febrile prodrome occurs followed by abdominal pain and diarrhea.

**a)** *Escherichia coli* O157:H7
**b)** *Yersinia enterocolitica*
**c)** *Campylobacter jejuni*
**d)** *Bacillus cereus*

Bonus Question: A 46-year-old man is admitted to the intensive care unit with hypotension and hematemesis. After stabilization, an emergent upper endoscopy is performed, revealing an actively bleeding duodenal ulcer. The ulcer is successfully treated using injections of epinephrine and the application of a heater probe. The next appropriate measure would be which of the following?
**a)** Initiation of an infusion of an $H_2$-receptor antagonist
**b)** Treatment with sucralfate slurry
**c)** Initiation of a high-dose PPI infusion
**d)** Both b and c
**e)** Both a and b

## ANSWERS

**1. e.**
Metronidazole is much less expensive than vancomycin and is quite effective. Vancomycin should be reserved for severely ill patients, those who have not responded to or cannot tolerate metronidazole, pregnant women, or children younger than age 10 years.

**2. b.**
The patient clearly exhibits decompensated cirrhosis. The use of antiviral therapy in such a case could potentially lead to a further decompensation in the cirrhosis and possibly death.

**3. d.**
Bismuth subsalicylate can lead to a 92% clinical response rate and histologic improvement in 75% of patients treated. To date, it is the only therapy that may change the course of the disease.

**4. c.**
The combination of interferon-α and ribavirin is superior to therapy with interferon-α alone in terms of sustained response 24 weeks posttreatment, higher initial response, fewer relapses, and improved liver histology.

**5. e.**
The patient exhibits two endoscopic findings that are associated with an increased risk of variceal hemorrhage: large size of the variceal columns and the presence of red color signs. Mortality from the first episode of variceal bleeding can approach 50%. β-Blockade has been shown to be a cost-effective prophylaxis in patients with high-risk esophageal varices.

**6. b.**
The patient exhibits three alarm signs that would indicate the need for an immediate endoscopy: weight loss, anorexia, and age older than 50 years.

**7. c.**
HLA-B27 seronegative spondyloarthropathies, such as ankylosing spondylitis and sacroiliitis, can occur in both types of inflammatory bowel disease. The disease activity of the seronegative spondyloarthropathies is independent of the intestinal disease activity.

**8. a.**
Crohn's disease has the propensity to have skipped areas of involvement. In contrast, ulcerative colitis always exhibits continuous involvement.

**9. a.**
At present, treatment with a chimeric monoclonal antibody to TNF is indicated only in patients with Crohn's disease who have moderately to severely active disease or fistulizing disease.

**10. c.**
Erythema nodosum can be seen in both Crohn's disease and ulcerative colitis; its activity often parallels that of the intestinal disease activity.

**11. c.**
5-Aminosalicylic acid enemas are useful in the treatment of mild proctitis stemming from Crohn's disease or ulcerative colitis.

**12. d.**
Flexible sigmoidoscopy is not indicated for surveillance in patients with a history of colorectal polyps. In fact, new data suggest that it is inferior to colonoscopy in the detection of proximal neoplasia in average-risk patients who are undergoing screening. Colonoscopy has been found to be superior to double-contrast barium enema as surveillance examination. CT colography is a developing technology that has not replaced colonoscopy as a screening or surveillance tool at this point.

**13. d.**
The patient has a first-degree relative with colon cancer diagnosed before age 60 years. A colonoscopy beginning at an age 10 years younger than that of the relative at the time of the diagnosis of cancer and repeated every 5 years is appropriate.

**14. d.**
The endoscopic photograph shows a circumferential, ulcerated mass in the sigmoid colon that should be considered a malignancy until proved otherwise. Both cytomegalovirus and infections with enteroinvasive bacteria, such as *Salmonella*, can cause ulcerations but will not produce a mass.

**15. b.**
The retroflexed view in the rectum reveals hypertrophied anal papillae, which is a benign, asymptomatic condition. Hypertrophied anal papillae are differentiated from polyps by their white color and the fact that they origi-

nate at or below the dentate line. These should never be biopsied, as this will precipitate pain.

**16. c.**
These are prolapsed internal hemorrhoids. Given the symptomatic nature of the hemorrhoids, referral for definitive treatment such as banding is appropriate.

**17. b.**
Rectal varices are occasionally seen in patients with portal hypertension. They frequently appear as blue, serpiginous columns and can sometimes be the source of serious blood loss. The patient's history of thrombocytopenia and hypoalbuminemia is also suggestive of cirrhosis.

**18. a.**
The patient has dysphagia to both solids and liquids, which is an important clinical indicator of a possible motility disorder, such as achalasia. Esophageal manometry is therefore the test of choice.

**19. b.**
The patient's symptoms suggest oropharyngeal dysphagia secondary to a recent stroke and complicated by an aspiration pneumonia. A videoesophagogram (i.e., a videotaped version of a barium swallow) can be used to assess suspected cases of oropharyngeal dysphagia. Typically, laryngeal penetration of the barium and sometimes frank aspiration can be observed.

**20. b.**
The presence of a hyperechoic focus with posterior shadowing in a dilated common bile duct is highly suggestive of choledocholithiasis. Because the level of clinical suspicion is so high, other noninvasive modalities for studying the biliary tree are not indicated. An endoscopic retrograde cholangiopancreatography should be performed to remove the common bile duct stones before cholecystectomy.

**21. b.**
The patient is hemodynamically stable, is otherwise healthy, and exhibits endoscopic findings of a clean-based ulcer, which has a low risk of rebleeding (5% or less). Therapy with a PPI has been associated with increased rates of healing within the first 2 weeks after diagnosis. Obtaining an *H. pylori* serology will ensure that another important factor in the patient's ulcer formation will be addressed.

**22. d.**
The etiologies of a low serum-ascites albumin gradient include choices a, b, and e, as well as systemic lupus erythematosus, bile ascites, and as a result of bowel infarction or obstruction.

**23. c.**
The barium radiograph reveals a lower esophageal ring, or Schatzki's ring. This is a thin, symmetric ring in the distal esophagus that typically presents with intermittent

solid food dysphagia. Treatment is esophageal dilatation. The etiology of a Schatzki's ring is thought to be gastroesophageal reflux.

**24. b.**

Definite risk factors for chronic pancreatitis include age older than 60 years, male gender, cigarette smoking, chronic pancreatitis, and nonpolyposis cancer syndrome.

**25. c.**

Although more common in acute pancreatitis, both conditions can be associated with the development of pseudocyst formation.

**26. c.**

Metabolic conditions, along with ethanol use, pancreas divisum, and hereditary pancreatitis are important etiologic factors for both acute and chronic pancreatitis.

**27. a.**

Most *E. coli* O157:H7 infections have occurred after eating inadequately prepared beef. Young children and the elderly are at the highest risk of death from the infection.

**28. d.**

*B. cereus* produces a heat-stable toxin that results in nausea and vomiting. Another presentation is that of diarrhea 12 hours after ingesting contaminated food; this presentation is caused by an enterotoxin.

**29. b.**

*Y. enterocolitica* is usually transmitted by incompletely cooked pork or contaminated dairy products.

**30. c.**

Both *C. jejuni* and *Campylobacter coli* can be transmitted by eating incompletely cooked poultry or by drinking raw milk. Typically, a febrile prodrome with headache and vomiting is followed by abdominal pain and bloody diarrhea.

Bonus Question. The correct answer is c.

A recent randomized, placebo-controlled trial found that a continuous high-dose infusion of omeprazole led to a reduction in rebleeding from 22.5% to 6.7%. A meta-analysis found that $H_2$-receptor antagonist infusion therapy reduced bleeding and the need for surgery only in patients with gastric ulcers. Another problem with $H_2$-receptor antagonist therapy is the development of tolerance.

## SUGGESTED READINGS

### Question 1

Kelly CP, Pothoulakis C, LaMont JT. *Clostridium difficile* colitis. *N Engl J Med* 1994;330:257–262.

### Question 2

Management of Hepatitis C. *NIH Consensus Statement* 1997;15(3): 1–4.

### Question 3

Fine KD, Lee EL. Efficacy of open-label bismuth subsalicylate for the treatment of microscopic colitis. *Gastroenterology* 1998;114: 29–36.

### Question 4

McHutchison JG, Gordon SC, Schiff ER, et al. Interferon-α-2b alone or in combination with ribavirin as initial therapy for chronic hepatitis C. *N Engl J Med* 1998;339:1485–1492.

### Question 5

Teran JC, Imperiale TF, Mullen KD, et al. Primary prophylaxis of variceal bleeding in cirrhosis: a cost-effectiveness analysis. *Gastroenterology* 1997;112:473–482.

The North Italian Endoscopic Club for the Study and Treatment of Esophageal Varices. Prediction of the first variceal hemorrhage in patients with cirrhosis of the liver and esophageal varices. *N Engl J Med* 1988;319:983–989.

### Question 6

Bennett JC, Plum F, eds. *Cecil Textbook of Medicine*, 20th ed. Philadelphia: Saunders, 1996;667.

Graham DY, Rabeneck L. Patients, payers, and paradigm shifts: what to do about *Helicobacter pylori*? *Am J Gastroenterol* 1996;91: 188–191.

Health and Public Policy Committee, American College of Gastroenterology. Endoscopy in the evaluation of dyspepsia. *Ann Intern Med* 1985;102:242–249.

### Questions 7–11

Bennett JC, Plum F, eds. *Cecil Textbook of Medicine*, 20th ed. Philadelphia: Saunders, 1996; 707–715.

Targan SR, Hanauer SB, van Deventer SJ, et al. A short-term study of chimeric monoclonal antibody cA2 to tumor necrosis factor alpha for Crohn's disease. *N Engl J Med* 1997;337:1029–1035.

### Question 12

Lieberman DA, Weiss DG, Bond JH, et al. Use of colonoscopy to screen asymptomatic adults for colorectal cancer. *N Engl J Med* 2000;343:162–168.

Winawer SJ, Stewart ET, Zauber AG, et al. A comparison of colonoscopy and double-contrast barium enema for surveillance after polypectomy. *N Engl J Med* 2000;342:1766–1772.

### Question 13

Winawer SJ, Fletcher R, Miller L, et al. Colorectal cancer screening: clinical guidelines and rationale. *Gastroenterology* 1997;112: 594–642.

### Questions 14–17

Sivak MV. *Gastroenterologic Endoscopy*, 2nd ed. Philadelphia: WB Saunders, 1999.

### Question 18

Bennett JC, Plum F, eds. *Cecil Textbook of Medicine*, 20th ed. Philadelphia: Saunders, 1996;654–655.

### Question 19

Bennett JC, Plum F, eds. *Cecil Textbook of Medicine*, 20th ed. Philadelphia: Saunders, 1996;650–659.

### Question 20

Bennett JC, Plum F, eds. *Cecil Textbook of Medicine*, 20th ed. Philadelphia: Saunders, 1996;630–635.

### Question 21

Bennett JC, Plum F, eds. *Cecil Textbook of Medicine*, 20th ed. Philadelphia: Saunders, 1996;667–669.
Graham DY. The relationship between nonsteroidal anti-inflammatory drug use and peptic ulcer disease. *Gastroenterol Clin North Am* 1990;19:171.

### Question 22

Bennett JC, Plum F, eds. *Cecil Textbook of Medicine*, 20th ed. Philadelphia: Saunders, 1996;745.

### Question 23

Bennett JC, Plum F, eds. *Cecil Textbook of Medicine*, 20th ed. Philadelphia: Saunders, 1996;658.

### Questions 24–26

Bennett JC, Plum F, eds. *Cecil Textbook of Medicine*, 20th ed. Philadelphia: Saunders, 1996;729–736.

### Questions 27–30

Bennett JC, Plum F, eds. *Cecil Textbook of Medicine*, 20th ed. Philadelphia: Saunders, 1996;738–739.

### Bonus Question

Collins R, Langman M. Treatment with histamine $H_2$ antagonists in acute upper gastrointestinal hemorrhage. *N Engl J Med* 1985;313: 660–666.
Lau JYW, Sung JJY, Lee KKC, et al. Effect of intravenous omeprazole on recurrent bleeding after endoscopic treatment of bleeding peptic ulcers. *N Engl J Med* 2000;343;310–316.
Merki HS, Wilder-Smith CH. Do continuous infusions of omeprazole and ranitidine retain their effect after prolonged dosing? *Gastroenterology* 1994;106:60–64.

# Cardiology

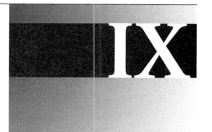

# Coronary Artery Disease

*Richard A. Grimm    Thomas H. Marwick*

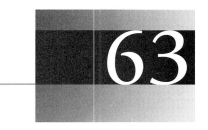

The diagnostic approach to the evaluation of patients with coronary artery disease (CAD) is in the midst of a significant overhaul. Although exercise stress testing has traditionally been the method of choice in determining the functional severity of coronary stenoses and prognosis, several other methods are vying for position as the testing methods most adept at characterizing plaque burden, vulnerable plaque and, hence, prognosis. These include electron beam tomography, magnetic resonance imaging (MRI), intravascular ultrasound, and serum markers of inflammation (i.e., C-reactive protein). Because of the preliminary nature of data regarding the efficacy of these tests, and the present lack of outcome information, it would be premature to include a discussion of these methods with this review. The more conventional approach is therefore discussed, while recognizing that exercise stress testing will likely be only one of several diagnostic modalities used in a more thorough and comprehensive evaluation of CAD patients in the very near future.

## DEFINING "SIGNIFICANT" CORONARY ARTERY DISEASE

In patients with coronary stenoses, the flow of blood is preserved at rest until the lumen diameter is reduced by 90% to 95%, at which time rest pain occurs. Patients with milder lesions develop ischemia during stress when, despite dilation of the distal coronary vasculature, coronary flow becomes restricted by the stenosis. This usually occurs with stenoses of greater than 50% and almost always with lesions of greater than 70% of the artery diameter. In the 50% range, flow reduction is modulated by collateral flow, location and length of stenoses, relation to bends and bifurcations, and other variables. Thus, the gold standard of CAD diagnosis is stenoses of greater than 50% diameter (some centers use >70%) at coronary angiography.

There certainly are a number of problems with this criterion, including a poor correlation between the severity of stenosis and reduction of flow and the interobserver variability in subjective interpretation. Nonetheless, a reference standard is needed, and this is the best that is currently available.

## STATISTICAL APPROACH TO ASSESSING STRESS TESTS

No noninvasive test used for the diagnosis of CAD is perfect. The aim of testing is to inform the ordering physician about the likelihood of disease being present as well as its severity and prognosis. Not every patient with a positive test proceeds to coronary angiography; therefore, the separation of "diagnostic" and "prognostic" testing is artificial. The functional data permit a judgment to be made regarding whether the cost, risk, and discomfort of coronary angiography will be worthwhile.

Several values are used to measure the ability of noninvasive tests to predict the presence of significant coronary stenoses. These include sensitivity, specificity, accuracy, and both positive and negative predictive value. Sensitivity and specificity are the most widely used because they depend less on disease prevalence than do the other variables. The definitions of statistical terms relating to accuracy are:

- Sensitivity = true positives/all patients with CAD
- Specificity = true negatives/all patients without CAD
- Predictive value of positive test = true positives/all positive tests
- Predictive value of negative test = true negatives/all negative tests
- Accuracy = all correct results/all patients

## CLINICAL EVALUATION

Regardless of a patient's clinical status, stress testing is not appropriate for the diagnosis or exclusion of CAD. Applying Bayes' theorem, the posttest probability of disease depends not only on the accuracy of the test but also on the pretest probability of CAD, which may be defined on the basis of age, gender, and symptom status (Table 63.1). The relationship among accuracy, pretest probability, and posttest probability is summarized in Figure 63.1, which shows that patients with a very low (<20%) or very high (>80%) pretest probability of disease will remain in these categories, regardless of test results and accuracy. Thus, in patients with a high or low probability of disease, the usefulness of noninvasive testing for diagnostic

## TABLE 63.1
### DIAGNOSIS OF MYOCARDIAL ISCHEMIA: PRETEST PROBABILITY IN MEN

| Age (Yr) | Asymptomatic | Nonanginal | Atypical | Typical (%) |
|---|---|---|---|---|
| 30–39 | 2 | 5 | 22 | 70 |
| 40–49 | 6 | 14 | 46 | 87 |
| 50–59 | 10 | 22 | 59 | 92 |
| 60–69 | 12 | 28 | 67 | 94 |

## TABLE 63.2
### NONINVASIVE DIAGNOSIS OF ISCHEMIA

| Stress Techniques | Diagnostic Tests |
|---|---|
| Exercise | Electrocardiography only |
|   Bicycle | |
|   Treadmill | |
| Pharmacologic | Perfusion |
|   Adenosine | Thallium-201 |
|   Dipyridamole | Tc-MIBI |
|   Dobutamine | Other technetium-99m |
| Pacing + other | Function |
|   (e.g., cold pressor) | |
| | Two-dimensional echocardiography |
| | Nuclear left ventriculography |
| | New approaches |
| | Positron emission tomography |
| | Magnetic resonance imaging |
| | Fast computerized tomography |

Tc-MIBI, technetium-99m methoxyisobutylisonitrile perfusion imaging.

purposes is limited. These tests may, however, provide useful prognostic data (e.g., exercise capacity, site and extent of ischemia, severity of left ventricular dysfunction), which may influence treatment. (The following sections assume that appropriate decisions about investigation are made on clinical grounds, even though in clinical practice, these "rules" are constantly broken.)

## DIAGNOSTIC TESTS

In the detection of ischemia, a bewildering number of combinations of stress-testing methodologies and electrocardiography (ECG) or imaging techniques is available (Table 63.2). No single test is optimal for the diagnosis of CAD in the population as a whole, but the two major determinants of appropriate testing are interpretability of the stress ECG and ability of the patient to exercise maximally. Patients who can exercise maximally should do so because exercise testing provides useful functional and prognostic information, independent of whether ischemia is detected. If the ECG is nondiagnostic (discussed later), an imaging test should be performed, and this should be planned for all patients who undergo pharmacologic stress because of an inability to exercise. The latter groups (nondiagnostic ECGs) now constitute the majority of tests performed in most tertiary centers (Fig. 63.2).

### Exercise Electrocardiography

#### Indications for Exercise Electrocardiography
Patients should undergo exercise ECG if they can exercise maximally and have an interpretable ST segment. In contrast to the expense of imaging tests (which can exceed $1,000), exercise ECG is "low-tech" and relatively inexpensive. It is difficult to obtain current, specific cost and charge data at most institutions, but the multiples between different tests change little. Table 63.3 lists these multiples for costs, reimbursements, and charges involved with the common diagnostic methodologies.

Despite the potential cost savings of a given methodology, we must consider its effectiveness as well. The exclusive use of standard exercise ECG would have clear disadvantages in relation to accuracy. Only approximately one-third of patients exercise maximally and have an interpretable stress ECG, and among these patients, equivocal results (e.g.,

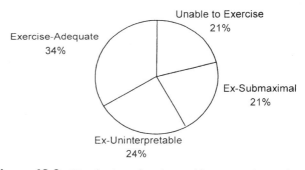

**Figure 63.2** Distribution of patients able to exercise and with interpretable electrocardiography among patients attending a hospital exercise laboratory. Ex-Submaximal, patients who are able to exercise but are unable to increase their heart rate to 85% of the age predicted maximum; Ex-Uninterpretable, uninterpretable electrocardiography because of resting electrocardiography changes.

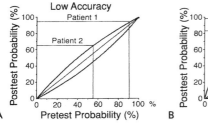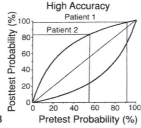

**Figure 63.1** Relation of pretest and posttest probability with tests of **(A)** low accuracy and **(B)** high accuracy.

## TABLE 63.3

**COSTS, REIMBURSEMENTS, AND CHARGES FOR COMMON DIAGNOSTIC METHODOLOGIES AS A MULTIPLE OF THE COST FOR AN EXERCISE STRESS ELECTROCARDIOGRAPHY**

| | Charges | Reimbursement (Medicare) | Cost |
|---|---|---|---|
| Exercise electrocardiography | 2.5 | 0.4 | 1.0 |
| Exercise thallium-201 imaging | 13.3 | 3.2 | 5.1 |
| Exercise echocardiography | 7.7 | 1.6 | 1.4 |
| Coronary angiography | 31.8 | 9.1 | 13.4 |

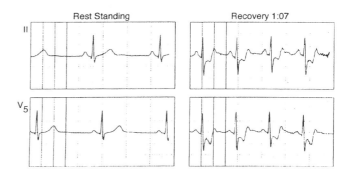

**Figure 63.3** Exercise-induced ST-segment depression consistent with myocardial ischemia.

borderline ST-segment changes without angina) nevertheless may necessitate the performance of a stress-imaging test.

The indications for exercise ECG tests, in addition to those used for the diagnosis of CAD, are:

- Diagnostic evaluation of chest pain
- Physiologic significance of known CAD
- Prognosis of CAD (especially after myocardial infarction)
- Evaluation of therapy (e.g., drug, percutaneous transluminal coronary angioplasty, coronary artery bypass graft)
- Screening for CAD in "at-risk" individuals
- Evaluation of arrhythmias, pacing
- Heart failure (especially evaluation of treatment)
- Estimation of functional capacity
- Follow-up of patients with congenital and valvular diseases

Provided that the contraindications are observed, exercise ECG testing is quite safe, with a recorded serious-event rate of 1:1,000 or lower. Contraindications to exercise ECG are:

- Acutely unstable coronary syndromes*
- Symptomatic, severe aortic stenosis*
- Uncontrolled heart failure
- Uncontrolled serious cardiac dysrhythmias*
- Severe hypertension
- Recent pulmonary embolism
- Serious acute noncardiac disorder
- Inability to cooperate

### Performing Exercise Electrocardiography

Exercise ECG testing simply involves the performance of a standardized exercise protocol while the patient undergoes ECG monitoring for evidence of ischemia. The endpoints of testing are:

- Patient request/exhaustion

_____
* Lesser degrees of these problems, especially after treatment, may benefit from exercise testing.

- Severe angina, marked ST-segment depression (>3 mm) or elevation (>2 mm)
- Fall of systolic blood pressure below resting despite more work
- Poor perfusion, central nervous system symptoms
- Serious arrhythmias
- Hypertension (>280/115 mm Hg)

Note that attaining the "maximum" pulse rate is not an indication to stop in most instances.

A test is identified as being "positive" by a horizontal or downsloping ST-segment depression of greater than 0.1 mV (Fig. 63.3). Upsloping depression is accepted if it occurs 0.06 or 0.08 sec after the J point, but this is less specific than the other changes. Unless it occurs in leads with Q waves, ST-segment elevation is a reliable sign of transmural ischemia. The presence of angina, exercise capacity, hemodynamic response, and rhythm during testing are useful adjunctive results. These data have been combined into various global exercise scores, but these have not been widely accepted.

### Accuracy of Exercise Electrocardiography

The results of studies having minimal referral bias have shown that both the sensitivity and specificity of standard exercise ECG are in the mid 70% range (Table 63.4). The

## TABLE 63.4

**EXERCISE ELECTROCARDIOGRAPHY: SENSITIVITY AND SPECIFICITY**

| Study | Sensitivity [n (%)] | Specificity [n (%)] |
|---|---|---|
| Sketch (*JAMA* 1980) | 40/59 (68) | 39/48 (81) |
| Melin (*Circulation* 1981) | 73/99 (74) | 43/61 (70) |
| Patterson (*Am J Cardiol* 1982) | 27/50 (54) | 35/46 (76) |
| Weintraub (*Am J Cardiol* 1984) | 73/101 (72) | 37/46 (80) |
| Hung (*Am Heart J* 1985) | 99/117 (85) | 34/54 (63) |
| Combined male patients | 312/426 (73) | 188/255 (74) |
| Hung (*J Am Coll Cardiol* 1984) | 20/28 (71) | 38/64 (59) |
| Melin (*Circulation* 1985) | 27/44 (61) | 72/91 (79) |
| Combined female patients | 47/72 (65) | 110/155 (71) |

accuracy is somewhat lower in female subjects, but the reasons for this are not well understood.

The selection of exercise ECG testing must be made with the knowledge that this technique is less accurate than stress-imaging approaches. Equivocal results such as a negative test response in a high-probability patient may occur, thus requiring a stress-imaging test or angiography to be performed to clarify the matter.

In patients who are unable to exercise, the ECG component of either dipyridamole or dobutamine stress is insensitive for the identification of myocardial ischemia. Consequently, if either dipyridamole or dobutamine is selected as a stressor in these patients, a stress-imaging technique should be performed as well.

## Stress-Imaging Techniques

### Indications for Stress Imaging
Stress imaging typically is used in patients with nondiagnostic ST segments. This includes patients with the following conditions:

- Left bundle branch block
- Left ventricular hypertrophy with strain
- Digitalis therapy
- Resting ST-segment changes, Wolff-Parkinson-White syndrome

Stress imaging also is used in patients who require pharmacologic stress because of their inability to exercise maximally, such as those with the following conditions:

- Peripheral vascular disease
- Orthopedic problems (e.g., back, legs)
- Chronic respiratory disease
- Cerebrovascular disease
- Medications, poor motivation
- Poor physical capacity

To these patients, one also might add those with normal resting ST segments in whom exercise ECG may be unreliable, such as women and patients with left ventricular hypertrophy.

### Performing Stress Imaging
Standard nuclear methodologies comprise stress ventriculography and myocardial perfusion imaging. Ventriculography has a poor specificity and is intrinsically insensitive for the identification of segmental ischemic dysfunction. It may have some value in combination with technetium-99m methoxyisobutylisonitrile (MIBI) perfusion imaging for the exclusion of false-positive perfusion defects resulting from soft-tissue attenuation. Otherwise, however, it has been superseded by other methodologies for the diagnosis of CAD.

The widespread application of single-photon emission computerized tomography (SPECT) to myocardial perfusion imaging has enhanced our ability to localize CAD and

to appreciate its extent. Thallium is innately unfavorable for imaging because of its low-energy photon emission, which leads to tissue attenuation and scatter; unfavorable radiation dosimetry, which also contributes to low photon counts; and long half-life, which precludes a true resting scan and leads to ambiguity regarding the presence of infarction and ischemia. These constraints are not shared by technetium-99m, however, which has been attached to various isonitriles, the most widespread of which is MIBI. The benefits of MIBI include:

- Better image quality
- A small increment of accuracy, particularly in the posterior territories of the heart, which are the most poorly visualized areas using thallium-201 imaging
- Ability to perform ventriculography simultaneously with perfusion measurements
- Absence of redistribution, thus allowing the injection of this tracer at one time and imaging at a later time, which is useful in the emergency room or during acute intervention

Recent work has combined the benefits of thallium-201 (i.e., assessment of viability, lesser expense) with those of MIBI (i.e., absence of washout, high-quality images), thus producing a dual-isotope approach that enhances the performance speed of nuclear scintigraphic studies. The benefits of using MIBI in this approach, however, are obtained at a significant increase in cost.

Positron emission tomography (PET) is a sophisticated imaging technique that may be used to examine myocardial perfusion using the tracers $^{13}$N-ammonia, $^{15}$O-water, or rubidium-82. This technology provides accurate measurements of myocardial perfusion, but further development of PET for diagnostic purposes has been inhibited by its cost. Whether the expense of PET is justified on the basis of better prognostic assessment or the prevention of a substantial number of unnecessary catheterizations remains unresolved.

Stress echocardiography involves a comparison of regional function at rest, as well as both during and after stress, to identify myocardial ischemia. Usually, this process is facilitated by a side-by-side display of digitized images in a cine-loop format. Its accuracy, however, depends on the ability of the observer to identify often-subtle changes in regional function. The clinical interpretation of all stress-imaging approaches involves some degree of subjectivity, but a trained observer is especially important during stress echocardiography.

### Accuracy of Stress Imaging
Tomographic myocardial perfusion imaging (i.e., SPECT) offers a greater sensitivity for CAD than planar approaches, but this may occur at the cost of lower specificity (Table 63.5). To an extent, this may reflect referral bias. Perfusion scintigraphy has a particularly low specificity in those subgroups of patients with left ventricular hypertrophy and left

## TABLE 63.5

**EXERCISE THALLIUM SINGLE-PHOTON EMISSION COMPUTED TOMOGRAPHY DIAGNOSIS OF CORONARY ARTERY DISEASE: SENSITIVITY AND SPECIFICITY**

| | Sensitivity (%) | | Specificity (%) | MI (in CAD) (%) |
| --- | --- | --- | --- | --- |
| | Overall | No MI | | |
| Tamaki (n = 104) | 96 | 96 | 91 | 39 |
| DePasquale (n = 210) | 95 | 92 | 74 | 26 |
| Iskandrian (n = 461) | 82 | 78 | 60 | 18 |
| Maddahi (n = 183) | 95 | 90 | 56 | 47 |
| Mahmarian and Verani (n = 360) | 87 | 79 | 87 | 33 |
| Van Train (n = 262) | 94 | 90 | 43 | 40 |
| Total | 90 | 85 | 70 | 31 |

CAD, coronary artery disease; MI, myocardial infarction.

bundle branch block. Thus, whereas perfusion scintigraphy has the benefit of much experience with its use, recent concerns have focused on its cost as well as on its false-positive rate. It remains an excellent choice, however, in patients with previous infarction and at centers without a major commitment to high-quality stress echocardiography.

The accuracy of PET for the diagnosis of CAD is greater than 90%, although many of the studies have been small and included an unacceptable number of patients with previous myocardial infarction (Table 63.6). Comparisons of cardiac PET with SPECT have shown a benefit to PET in terms of accuracy, which mirrors the underlying benefits of PET regarding accurate localization of tracer, ability to obtain high counts (and therefore excellent image quality), and capacity to perform attenuation correction. Clinically, these benefits include a better ability to resolve moderate (i.e., 50% to 70% diameter) coronary stenosis, a reduction of false-positive results because of soft tissue attenuation artifacts, and the ability to accurately diagnose CAD involving the posterior parts of the heart (reflecting the benefits of

attenuation correction, reduction of scatter, and higher counts). Both the cost and availability of PET, however, mandate a selective and sparing use of this technology. For diagnostic purposes, its high specificity is attractive in patients with a lower probability of CAD, and its high diagnostic accuracy is attractive in patients for whom angiography is inappropriate. It also may be useful for studying patients who otherwise are difficult to image (e.g., obese patients). Nonetheless, the major value of PET relates to evaluating the physiologic significance of known coronary lesions, as well as investigating issues of myocardial viability.

The sensitivity and specificity of exercise echocardiography for the identification of CAD are approximately 85% each (Table 63.7). As with other noninvasive tests, however, these values vary among studies relative to the mix of patients, and particularly relative to the prevalence of multivessel disease and previous infarction, which augment the recorded sensitivity of all stress-imaging tests. Two particular problems for stress echocardiography are the identification of multivessel disease in patients without previous infarction

## TABLE 63.6

**ACCURACY OF POSITRON EMISSION TOMOGRAPHY FOR DETECTION OF CORONARY ARTERY DISEASE**

| Study | Tracer | MI (%) | Sensitivity [n (%)] | Specificity [n (%)] |
| --- | --- | --- | --- | --- |
| Schelbert (1982) | Nitrogen-13 | ? | 31/32 (97) | 13/13 (100)[a] |
| Yonekura (1987) | Nitrogen-13 | 43 | 37/38 (97) | 13/14 (93)[a] |
| Tamaki (1988) | Nitrogen-13 | 74 | 47/48 (98) | 3/3 (100)[a] |
| Go (1990) | Rubidium-82 | 47 | 142/152 (93) | 39/50 (78) |
| Stewart (1991) | Rubidium-82 | 42 | 50/60 (83) | 19/21 (90) |

MI, myocardial infarction.
[a] Including healthy volunteers.

## TABLE 63.7

**DIGITAL EXERCISE ECHOCARDIOGRAPHY: SENSITIVITY AND SPECIFICITY**

| Study | Sensitivity [n (%)] | Specificity [n (%)] |
| --- | --- | --- |
| Armstrong (*J Am Coll Cardiol* 1987) | 40/51 (78) | 19/22 (86) |
| Ryan (*J Am Coll Cardiol* 1988) | 31/40 (78) | 24/24 (100) |
| Crouse (*Am J Cardiol* 1991) | 170/175 (97) | 34/53 (64) |
| Marwick (*J Am Coll Cardiol* 1992) | 96/114 (84) | 31/36 (86) |
| Quinones (*Circulation* 1992) | 64/86 (74) | 21/26 (81) |
| Hecht (*J Am Coll Cardiol* 1993) | 127/137 (93) | 37/46 (80) |
| Ryan (*J Am Soc Echocardiogr* 1993) | 192/211 (91) | 76/98 (78) |
| Combined | 720/814 (88) | 242/305 (79) |

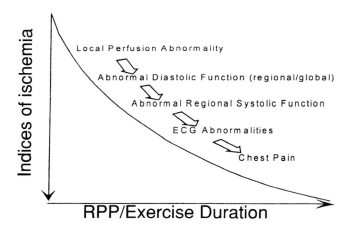

**Figure 63.4** The "ischemic cascade," during which less-sensitive tests become positive at higher workloads. ECG, electrocardiography; RPP, rate-pressure product.

and the detection of ischemia in the setting of resting wall motion abnormalities. Currently, stress echocardiography has the disadvantage of involving subjective interpretation. It has advantages, however, in relation to cost, safety, and patient convenience. In addition, it may be the test of choice for patients with left ventricular hypertrophy and, possibly, those with left bundle branch block.

### Comparative Studies

The sensitivity of stress imaging exceeds that of exercise ECG. This result can be readily anticipated from an appreciation of the "ischemic cascade" (Fig. 63.4).

The overall accuracy of stress echocardiography is comparable to that of nuclear scintigraphy. Scintigraphy has a slightly higher sensitivity, however, and echocardiography has a higher specificity. The strengths of stress echocardiography are its speed, cost, accuracy in patients with left ventricular hypertrophy or left bundle branch block, and ability to acquisition data on resting left ventricular function, valves, and pericardium. Scintigraphy is more sensitive for single-vessel disease, is better for recognizing multivessel disease, and may be better for distinguishing ischemia and infarction. It also is more quantitative, although both techniques require both technical and interpretive expertise.

The decision between echocardiography and nuclear testing is made predominantly on the basis of local expertise and availability. This is particularly true for stress echocardiography, which undoubtedly is the most demanding of the techniques.

### Evaluation of Patients Unable to Exercise

As discussed, pharmacologic stress ECG (without imaging) is not a good option in patients who are unable to exercise. Because myocardial perfusion scintigraphy essentially depends on the evaluation of differences in regional hyperemia, coronary vasodilators (e.g., dipyridamole, adeno-

sine) are the optimal pharmacologic stressors for this test. For echocardiography, dobutamine is a better stressor than coronary vasodilators, which rarely cause ischemia in a functional sense.

Exercise and pharmacologic stress-imaging tests have comparable accuracy. The additional data provided by exercise, however, including its correlation of stress with daily life, exercise capacity, and ST-segment and rhythm evaluation, all favor the use of exercise whenever a patient can exercise maximally.

## PROGNOSIS

In clinical practice, diagnosis rarely is separate from prognostic assessment. In addition, further investigations rarely are determined by the prediction of CAD alone, but on the basis of an assessment of the severity and, hence, the implications of the diagnosis for each individual.

The outcome of patients with CAD is determined by their left ventricular function, amount of jeopardized myocardium, exercise capacity, and noncardiac factors such as age and diabetes. Because functional testing provides most of these data, it is not surprising that its predictive power exceeds that of coronary angiography, which only supplies anatomic data. At exercise testing, exercise capacity, hypotension, and dysrhythmias predict outcome more so than ST-segment changes. At imaging, the extent of ischemic or all abnormal myocardium is the strongest predictor of outcome.

## CONCLUSION

Recent advances in stress testing have enhanced our ability to identify CAD through noninvasive means. Over the last decade, SPECT, stress echocardiography, and PET have become accepted clinical tools, and some initial data suggest their specific usefulness in individual situations. Nonetheless, the standard exercise ECG stress test remains the backbone of functional testing for CAD. Indeed, the challenge of the next few years will be to incorporate these new techniques into the cost-effective treatment of patients with suspected CAD.

### REVIEW EXERCISES

#### QUESTIONS

1. A 56-year-old woman with arthritis has atypical pain but a normal ECG. Which is the best diagnostic option?
a) Stress (exercise or dobutamine) ECG
b) Coronary angiography
c) Exercise echocardiography
d) Dipyridamole thallium imaging
e) None of the above

**2.** A 28-year-old woman presents with left-sided pain at rest and exercise. Which the best diagnostic option?
a) Exercise ECG
b) Coronary angiography
c) Exercise echocardiography
d) Exercise thallium imaging
e) None of the above

**3.** A 68-year-old man presents with central retrosternal pain at exercise. Which is the best diagnostic option?
a) Exercise ECG
b) Coronary angiography
c) Exercise echocardiography
d) Exercise thallium imaging
e) None of the above

**4.** A 48-year-old man with hypertensive left ventricular hypertrophy complains of atypical chest pain. Which is the best diagnostic option?
a) Exercise ECG
b) Coronary angiography
c) Exercise echocardiography
d) Dipyridamole thallium imaging
e) None of the above

**5.** Problems may occur with exercise thallium imaging, except in patients with which of the following?
a) Left bundle branch block
b) Left ventricular hypertrophy
c) Female gender
d) Obesity, posterior circulation disease
e) Left anterior descending (LAD) CAD

**6.** A 52-year-old woman has an uninterpretable ECG and atypical pain. What is the least expensive option?
a) Exercise thallium imaging
b) Coronary angiography
c) Exercise echocardiography
d) Dipyridamole PET imaging
e) None of the above

**7.** A 52-year-old man needs a femoropopliteal bypass. What would you recommend first for risk stratification?
a) Exercise ECG
b) Coronary angiography
c) Dobutamine echocardiography
d) Dipyridamole thallium imaging
e) Clinical evaluation

**8.** The following probably constitute significant CAD, *except*
a) Proximal LAD stenosis of 80%
b) LAD stenosis of 60% with angina
c) Right coronary artery stenosis of 50%
d) Left circumflex coronary artery stenosis of 50% with positive exercise ECG

**9.** Which of the following patients has the greatest probability of CAD?

a) A 48-year-old woman with atypical chest pain
b) A 25-year-old man with typical angina
c) A 45-year-old man with atypical chest pain
d) A 70-year-old man with atypical chest pain

**10.** In what proportion of patients is an exercise ECG adequate for the diagnosis of CAD?
a) Most (approximately 80%)
b) Majority (approximately 60%)
c) Minority (approximately 40%)
d) Few (approximately 10%)

**11.** What is the accuracy of exercise ECG for the diagnosis of CAD?
a) Sensitivity 85%, specificity 85%
b) Sensitivity 85%, specificity 65%
c) Sensitivity 75%, specificity 75%
d) Sensitivity 75%, specificity 95%

**12.** In a patient with intermediate pretest CAD probability, which of the following tests is least sensitive?
a) Stress echocardiography
b) Exercise thallium SPECT
c) Exercise ECG
d) Exercise nuclear ventriculography

**13.** In a middle-aged woman with atypical pain, which of the following tests is most accurate?
a) Exercise ECG
b) Exercise thallium SPECT
c) PET
d) Exercise nuclear ventriculography

**14.** In a patient with hypertensive left ventricular hypertrophy and atypical pain, which of the following tests is most accurate?
a) Exercise ECG
b) Exercise thallium SPECT
c) PET
d) Exercise echocardiography

## ANSWERS

**1. d.**
Because this 56-year-old woman has arthritis, an exercise stress will likely result in the patient being unable to exercise maximally or unable to exercise at all. Because the patient is a woman with atypical pain, she has an intermediate pretest probability and is therefore a good candidate for a stress-imaging study. Proceeding directly to coronary angiography with such a relatively low pretest probability would potentially subject the patient to an unnecessary invasive test.

**2. e.**
This patient has a very low pretest probability for having CAD (approximately 4%) because of her age, gender, and the atypical nature of the pain. Because of this low pretest probability, the accuracy of a given test will not

significantly affect the posttest probability of disease. Only in those patients with an intermediate pretest likelihood of disease will the accuracy of the test have a significant effect on posttest probability. Therefore, none of the choices provides the best diagnostic option because the best option likely includes the consideration of a noncardiac etiology for the pain.

### 3. b.
This patient has a high pretest probability of disease, and therefore coronary angiography would provide information on the site, severity, and extent of the disease. Although an exercise electrocardiographic study, as well as an imaging study with echocardiography or thallium perfusion imaging, would be useful in risk-stratifying such a patient, the definitive diagnosis in detecting disease in patient populations with such a high pretest probability would be attained using coronary angiography.

### 4. c.
An exercise ECG stress test is likely to be nondiagnostic in patients with left ventricular hypertrophy. Because of the resting secondary ST-T wave repolarization changes characteristic of left ventricular hypertrophy, a false-positive result is likely and may therefore inappropriately lead to further testing. A coronary angiogram would lead to undue risk from an invasive procedure, particularly in a 48-year-old man with atypical pain. A dipyridamole thallium study is also limited by the potential of falsely positive perfusion defects; these are likely secondary to subendocardial ischemia due to the abnormal coronary flow reserve seen in hypertrophied hearts, despite the presence of normal epicardial vessels. Exercise echocardiography has been demonstrated to be more specific in this patient population because the basis for this test is an assessment of left ventricular function rather than perfusion, which can be affected by abnormalities in coronary flow reserve.

### 5. e.
Abnormalities may be seen on thallium SPECT imaging in patients with left bundle branch block secondary to abnormalities in septal conduction. Additionally, patients with left ventricular hypertrophy also may manifest false-positive findings on thallium SPECT imaging, likely related to coronary flow reserve related abnormalities, which are characteristic of this patient population. Attenuation defects may be seen in the female population as a result of breast tissue, which may manifest as falsely positive defects, particularly in the LAD territory. Nuclear perfusion imaging, and specifically thallium SPECT imaging, may be limited in obese patients, with potentially false-positive abnormalities arising in the segments served by the posterior circulation and related to the relatively low-energy emissions typical of the thallium-201 radioisotope and its relative inability to penetrate large masses of soft tissue. Therefore, the best answer in this case is

LAD disease because this is a patient population that can be identified with a high degree of sensitivity using nuclear SPECT perfusion imaging.

### 6. c.
Although highly accurate for the diagnosis of CAD, both exercise thallium imaging and dipyridamole PET imaging are relatively expensive and would therefore not qualify as the least expensive option. In addition to being very expensive, a coronary angiogram would subject the patient to an undue relative risk, especially given the relatively low pretest probability of disease (approximately 30%) in this particular patient. An exercise echocardiogram would provide the advantage of both a highly accurate diagnostic imaging study as well as a cost benefit of roughly only 1.5 times the cost of an exercise ECG examination.

### 7. e.
The question specifically requests a recommendation for an initial assessment of risk stratification in this 52-year-old man requiring femoral popliteal bypass surgery. The initial risk stratification should therefore include a clinical examination that initially is directed at determining the presence of angina pectoris, age older than 70 years, history of prior heart failure, history of prior myocardial infarction, or the presence of diabetes mellitus. Only when one or more of the above-noted risk factors can be identified should one proceed to a stress-imaging examination. If none of the above risk factors is identified, this patient would have a very low perioperative risk of a cardiac event (approximately 3%, based on the data of Eagle et al.).

### 8. c.
Significant CAD typically is considered to be present with lesions of greater than 50% or 70% of the artery diameter. Coronary stenoses in the 50% range may or may not be functionally significant in terms of a reduction in coronary flow because flow reduction is modulated by collateral vessels, location, and length of stenoses, and is related to bends and bifurcations, and other variables. Coronary artery stenoses of greater than 90% have been demonstrated to restrict flow at rest without the provocation of stress. Therefore, in this question, answer a, a proximal LAD stenosis of 80%, is almost certainly considered significant disease, and a LAD stenosis of 60% in the presence of typical angina pectoris also quite likely represents significant, flow-limiting coronary disease. Finally, a left circumflex coronary stenosis of 50% with the presence of positive exercise ECG changes is likely to represent significant CAD, yet a right coronary stenosis of 50% in the absence of a functional test that is positive for ischemia or the presence of concomitant symptoms may or may not represent the presence of significant stenosis.

**9. d.**

Based on the Diamond and Forester estimate of pretest probability of disease, which is based on age, gender, and symptoms of chest pain, a 70-year-old man with atypical chest pain is likely to have a pretest probability of disease approximating 70%. Of note, the 25-year-old man with typical angina would also have a significant but slightly lower pretest probability of disease. A 45-year-old man with atypical chest pain would have a pretest probability of approximately 46%, whereas a woman of similar age with atypical symptoms would have a dramatically lower pretest probability of disease, estimated to be approximately 13% and reflecting the delayed onset of disease among the female population, likely related to the protective effect of estrogen.

**10. c.**

Exercise stress ECG testing is of benefit and useful in a patient who is able to maximally exercise and who has a normal resting ECG. Studies have demonstrated that a significant proportion of subjects presenting for an evaluation of coronary disease are either unable to exercise (or cannot exercise maximally) or have uninterpretable electrocardiograms at rest. For this reason, a minority of patients meet both criteria, namely, a normal resting ECG and the ability to maximally exercise.

**11. c.**

More recent investigations that have evaluated the accuracy of exercise ECG have attempted to limit selection bias; these investigations have demonstrated sensitivities and specificities in the 75% range. The sensitivity and specificity of the test in the female population is somewhat lower, at 65% and 71%, respectively.

**12. c.**

The reported sensitivities of stress echocardiography, exercise thallium SPECT imaging, and exercise nuclear ventriculography are approximately 85%, 90%, and 80%, respectively. The reported sensitivity of approximately 75% for exercise ECG make this the least sensitive test of those listed.

**13. c.**

In this middle-aged woman with atypical chest pain, an exercise ECG test is subject to falsely positive result because ST-T wave abnormalities are relatively common in the female population for reasons that are as yet not well understood. Exercise thallium SPECT imaging, although a more sensitive test, is limited by its reported specificity, in large part related to breast attenuation, obesity, and artifacts in the posterior circulation. Exercise nuclear ventriculography is a relatively poorly sensitive study for the detection of CAD. PET imaging, on the other hand, is both highly sensitive as well as highly specific and is particularly good in the female population because attenuation artifacts are largely eliminated, primarily related to the high-energy radioisotopes that are used for this imaging procedure.

**14. d.**

In this patient with left ventricular hypertrophy and atypical chest pain, the least accurate test would be exercise ECG testing because of the presence of uninterpretable secondary ST segment repolarization abnormalities commonly seen on the baseline electrocardiogram in patients with left ventricular hypertrophy. Of note, recent data suggest that, even in patients without resting electrocardiographic abnormalities but with evidence for left ventricular hypertrophy, the propensity for false-positive stress ECG abnormalities is significant. It is suspected that abnormalities in coronary flow reserve, with resultant subendocardial ischemia in the absence of epicardial vessel disease, is responsible for these false-positive perfusion abnormalities noted on SPECT and myocardial PET nuclear perfusion imaging.

## SUGGESTED READINGS

Armstrong WF, O'Donnell J, Ryan T, et al. Effect of prior myocardial infarction and extent and location of coronary disease on accuracy of exercise echocardiography. *J Am Coll Cardiol* 1987;10(3):531–538.

Berman DS, Kiat HS, van Train KF, et al. Myocardial perfusion imaging with technetium-99m-sestamibi: comparative analysis of available imaging protocols. *J Nucl Med* 1994;35:681–688.

Crouse LJ, Harbrecht JJ, Vacek JL, et al. Exercise echocardiography as a screening test for coronary artery disease and correlation with coronary arteriography. *Am J Cardiol* 1991; 67(15):1213–1218.

DePasquale EE, Nody AC, DePuey EG, et al. Quantitative rotational thallium-201 tomography for identifying and localizing coronary artery disease. *Circulation* 1988;77(2):316–327.

Detrano R, Froelicher VF. Exercise testing: uses and limitations considering recent studies. *Prog Cardiovasc Dis* 1988;31:173–204.

Diamond GA, Forrester JS. Analysis of probability as an aid in the clinical diagnosis of coronary artery disease. *N Engl J Med* 1979;300: 1350–1358.

Fletcher GF, Balady G, Froelicher VF, et al. AHA Medical/Scientific Statement. Exercise standards. A statement for healthcare professionals from the AHA. *Circulation* 1995;91:580–615.

Gibbons RJ, Balady GJ, Beasley JW, et al. Guidelines for exercise testing. A report of the ACC/AHA task force on assessment of cardiovascular procedures. *Circulation* 1997;96:345–354.

Go RT, Marwick TH, MacIntyre WJ, et al. A prospective comparison of rubidium-82 PET and thallium-201 SPECT myocardial perfusion imaging utilizing a single dypyridamole stress in the diagnosis of coronary artery disease. *J Nucl Med* 1990;31(12):1899–1905.

Hecht HS, DeBord L, Shaw R, et al. Digital supine bicycle stress echocardiography: a new technique for evaluating coronary artery disease. *J Am Coll Cardiol* 1993;21(4):950–956.

Hung J, Chaitman BR, Lam J, et al. Noninvasive diagnostic test choices for the evaluation of coronary artery disease in women: a multivariate comparison of cardiac fluoroscopy, exercise, electrocardiography, and exercise thallium myocardial perfusion scintigraphy. *J Am Coll Cardiol* 1984;4(1):8–16.

Hung J, Chaitman BR, Lam J, et al. A logistic regression analysis of multiple noninvasive tests for the prediction of the presence and extent of coronary artery disease in men. *Am Heart J* 1985;110(2):460–469.

Iskandrian AS, Verani MS, Heo J. Pharmacologic stress testing: mechanism of action, hemodynamic responses, and results in detection of coronary artery disease. *J Nucl Cardiol* 1994;1(1):94–111.

Kahn JK, McGhie I, Akers MS, et al. Quantitative rotational tomography with 201Tl and 99mTc-methoxyisobutylisonitrile. A direct comparison in normal individuals and patients with coronary artery disease. *Circulation* 1989;79:1282–1290.

Maddahi J, Schelbert H, Brunken R, et al. Role of thallium-201 and PET imaging in evaluation of myocardial viability and management of patients with coronary artery disease and left ventricular dysfunction. *J Nucl Med* 1994;35(4):707–715.

Mahmarian JJ, Verani MS. Exercise thallium-201 perfusion scintigraphy in the assessment of coronary artery disease. *Am J Cardiol* 1991;67:2D–11D.

Marwick TH, Nemec JJ, Pashkow FJ, et al. Accuracy and limitations of exercise echocardiography in a routine clinical setting. *J Am Coll Cardiol* 1992;19(1):74–81.

Marwick T, Willemart B, D'Hondt AM, et al. Selection of the optimal nonexercise stress for the evaluation of ischemic regional myocardial dysfunction and malperfusion: comparison of dobutamine and adenosine using echocardiography and Tc-99m MIBI single photon emission computed tomography. *Circulation* 1993;87: 345–354.

Melin JA, Piret LJ, Vanbutsele RJ, et al. Diagnostic value of exercise electrocardiography and thallium myocardial scintigraphy in patients without previous myocardial infarction: a Bayesian approach. *Circulation* 1981;63(5):1019–1024.

Melin JA, Wijns W, Vanbutsele RJ, et al. Alternative diagnostic strategies for coronary artery disease in women: demonstration of the usefulness and efficiency of probability analysis. *Circulation* 1985; 71(3):535–542.

Patterson RE, Horowitz SF, Eng C, et al. Can exercise electrocardiography and thallium-201 myocardial imaging exclude the diagnosis of coronary artery disease? Bayesian analysis of the clinical limits of exclusion and indications for coronary angiography. *Am J Cardiol* 1982;49(5):1127–1135.

Picano E, Lattanzi F, Orlandini A, et al. Stress echocardiography and the human factor: the importance of being expert. *J Am Coll Cardiol* 1991;17:666–669.

Pryor DB, Shaw L, McCants CB, et al. Value of the history and physical in identifying patients at increased risk for CAD. *Ann Intern Med* 1993;118:81–90.

Quinones MA, Verani MS, Haichin RM, et al. Exercise echocardiography versus 201Tl single-photon emission computed tomography in evaluation of coronary artery disease. Analysis of 292 patients. *Circulation* 1992;85(3):1026–1031.

Ryan T, Segar DS, Sawada SG, et al. Detection of coronary artery disease with upright bicycle exercise echocardiography. *J Am Soc Echocardiogr* 1993;6(2):186–197.

Ryan T, Vasey CG, Presti CF, et al. Exercise echocardiography: detection of coronary artery disease in patients with normal left ventricular wall motion at rest. *J Am Coll Cardiol* 1988;11(5):993–999.

Schelbert HR, Wisenberg G, Phelps ME, et al. Noninvasive assessment of coronary stenoses by myocardial imaging during pharmacologic coronary vasodilation. VI. Detection of coronary artery disease in human beings with intravenous N-13 ammonia and positron computed tomography. *Am J Cardiol* 1982;49(5):1197–1207.

Sketch MH, Mohiuddin SM, Nair CK, et al. Automated and nomographic analysis of exercise tests. *JAMA* 1980;243:1052–1055.

Stewart RE, Schwaiger M, Molina E, et al. Comparison of rubidium-82 positron emission tomography and thallium-201 SPECT imaging for detection of coronary artery disease. *Am J Cardiol* 1991;67(16): 1303–1310.

Tamaki N, Yonekura Y, Senda M, et al. Value and limitation of stress thallium-201 single photon emission computed tomography: comparison with nitrogen-13 ammonia positron tomography. *J Nucl Med* 1988;29(7):1181–1188.

Van Train KF, Maddahi J, Berman DS, et al. Quantitative analysis of tomographic stress thallium-201 myocardial scintigrams: a multicenter trial. *J Nucl Med* 1990;31(7):1168–1179.

Weintraub WS, Madeira SW Jr., Bodenheimer MM, et al. Critical analysis of the application of Bayes' theorem to sequential testing in the noninvasive diagnosis of coronary artery disease. *Am J Cardiol* 1984;54(1):43–49.

Yonekura Y, Tamaki N, Senda M, et al. Detection of coronary artery disease with 13N-ammonia and high-resolution positron-emission computed tomography. *Am Heart J* 1987;113(3):645–654.

# Clinical Electrocardiography: A Visual Board Review

**64**

*Donald A. Underwood*   *Curtis M. Rimmerman*

It has been almost 100 years since Einthoven published his initial observations related to clinical electrocardiography (ECG). From that beginning, the technique has developed over the years into a very important clinical tool for the acute and chronic evaluation and treatment of patients. It is often the first information gathered, after the history and physical examination, for patients who present with chest pain syndromes, syncope, and abrupt changes in their respiratory status. It is the pivotal piece of information in the modern treatment of acute coronary artery syndromes. It is the gate through which patients must pass to be considered for thrombolytic treatments. As isolated information, the ECG has value, but it is always important to remember that it is just one clinical tool, and its greatest impact is when placed in the context of the individual patient who presents with any of a number of symptoms or histories. Mastery of ECG evolves over many years of clinical experience. In fact, it is never truly mastered. Skills with observation and integration continue to be refined, and even the most senior electrocardiographer finds new variations and clinical relationships related to the ECG.

This type of review cannot "teach" ECG. Instead, this review is intended to remind you of clinical situations that you have experienced in which the ECG may have had importance and cement those memories into your basic fund of clinical knowledge. Figures 64.1 through 64.67 are not examples of rare or unusual conditions, nor are the ECGs at all unusual or unique. They are common tracings that you

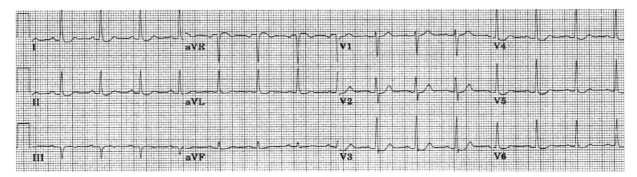

**Figure 64.1**  This patient shows a sinus rhythm. The main abnormality is in the ST segment, which has a scooping depression. Also, the QT interval is relatively short. This is most compatible with digitalis effect, and it is an example of a repolarization change that has an appearance specific enough for a definite diagnosis.

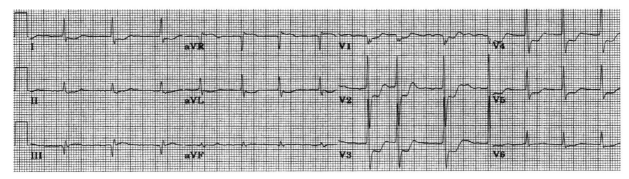

**Figure 64.2**  On this electrocardiograph, atrial fibrillation (an irregularly irregular ventricular response and no definite atrial activity) is present. ST-segment depression also is present in lead I, not inconsistent with digitalis effect. In the mid-precordial leads, however, the ST-segment depression is deeper, horizontal, or downsloping and, although this could be related to digitalis, subendocardial ischemia or infarction must be considered.

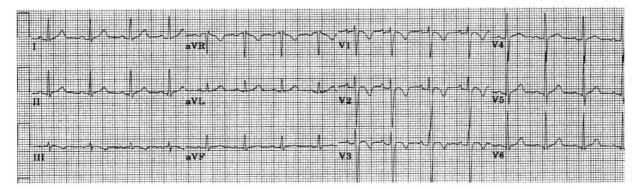

**Figure 64.3**  This electrocardiograph shows a sinus rhythm. Mid-precordial T-wave changes also are present. T-wave changes such as this can be abnormal. This patient, however, is a young girl, aged 7 years, and in this case, the T-wave changes are normal and represent a juvenile pattern. This emphasizes the importance of age, sex, and race notations when interpreting an electrocardiograph.

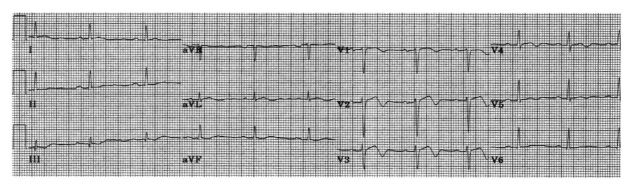

**Figure 64.4** This electrocardiograph also shows T-wave changes. These extend as inversions to lead $V_5$. The T wave in lead $V_6$ is low. This is a nonspecific T-wave abnormality. The electrocardiograph is not normal, but a specific disease process cannot be determined from the electrocardiograph and must be identified through clinical correlation.

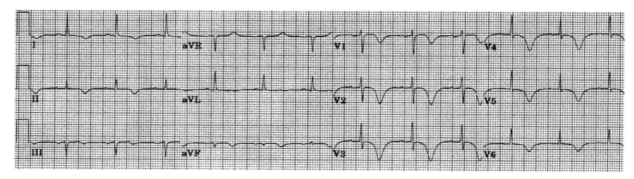

**Figure 64.5** T-wave abnormalities are present on this electrocardiograph. They are generalized and found throughout the electrocardiograph. The T waves are deeply inverted and symmetric. The QT interval is prolonged. This can be seen in coronary disease. Also in the differential diagnosis is significant central nervous system injury, which was the case in this patient.

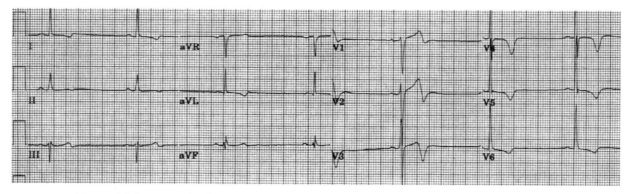

**Figure 64.6** A sinus bradycardia is present on this electrocardiograph. The T-wave changes in the mid-precordium are biphasic and terminally symmetric. This also is a nonspecific T-wave abnormality, but T waves such as this are commonly seen in patients with coronary disease. Sometimes, this appearance can be seen with ventricular hypertrophy, especially hypertrophic cardiomyopathy. Again, clinical correlation is necessary.

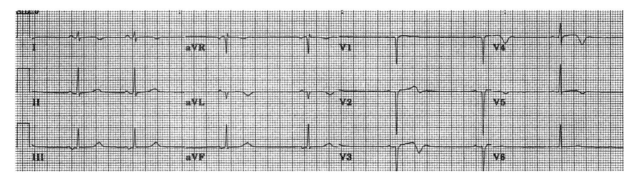

**Figure 64.7**   This electrocardiograph shows T-wave changes with terminal symmetry in the mid-precordium. It also shows poor R-wave progression. This is suggestive of myocardial injury, and although definite Q waves are not present, the combination of T waves of this type with minimal R waves often is seen after myocardial injury with associated wall motion abnormalities on wall motion studies. This electrocardiograph is from a young woman with Ehlers-Danlos syndrome; she had an anterior descending coronary artery dissection and rupture with infarction.

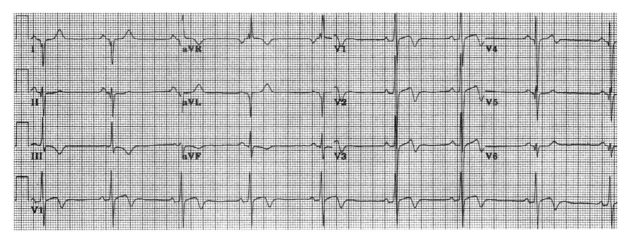

**Figure 64.8**   Terminally symmetric mid-precordial T-wave inversions are present on this electrocardiograph. These are seen in the presence of prominent R waves, even in lead $V_1$. Q waves are present in the lateral leads and, although this could suggest a posterolateral infarct, the narrowness of the Q waves and prominence of the anterior vectors suggest an obstructive hypertrophic cardiomyopathy, which was the case in this patient.

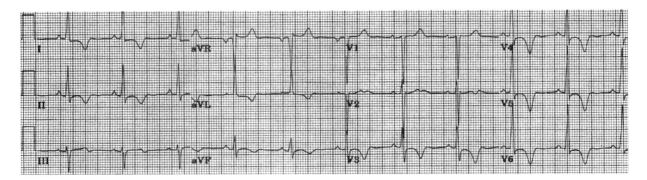

**Figure 64.9**   This patient also shows symmetric T-wave abnormalities, which are found fairly generally throughout the electrocardiograph. Voltage is prominent, and the complexes are broad, raising the possibility of ventricular hypertrophy. This patient also has hypertrophic cardiomyopathy. In this case, the location is toward the apex. This is an example of apical hypertrophy of the heart, which is an idiopathic hypertrophic cardiomyopathy variant.

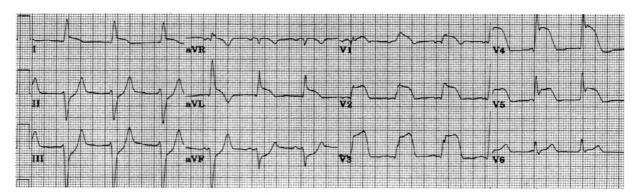

**Figure 64.10**  ST-segment elevation is the hallmark of acute myocardial infarction. That is the case on this electrocardiograph. ST elevations of significance are seen in the anterior and lateral leads. A sinus rhythm is present in the middle portion of the electrocardiograph. To the left and right, however, the complexes are broader, and P waves are absent. This is an example of an accelerated idioventricular rhythm seen in the face of an acute infarct. Accelerated idioventricular rhythm is seen not uncommonly as a reperfusion arrhythmia after thrombolytic therapy for myocardial infarction.

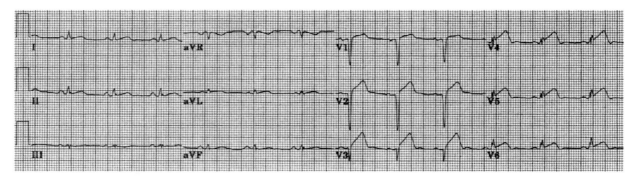

**Figure 64.11**  This is an acute anterior infarct. The ST segments are elevated. The QT intervals are relatively prolonged, and a straightening occurs in the upslope of the ST segments into the T waves. No reciprocal changes are present, which is not an uncommon finding in an acute anterior infarct, unlike inferior and lateral infarcts.

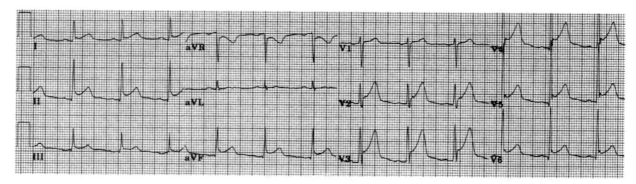

**Figure 64.12**  ST-segment elevation does not always represent acute myocardial infarction. In this case, a definite ST elevation is present. This is seen in all leads except aV$_R$. This is an example of acute pericarditis. Occasionally, PR-segment deviation can be seen, as in this case, in which a PR-segment elevation occurs in lead aV$_R$.

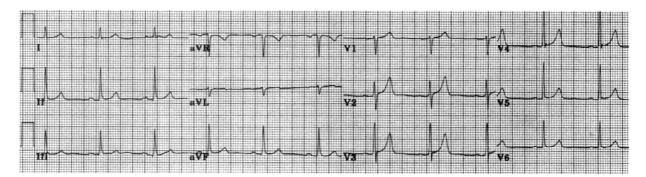

**Figure 64.13**  Regional ST-segment elevation often is due to myocardial infarction, but it is always important to remember early repolarization, which is a normal variant. Here, the J point is distinct, with elevation in lead $V_2$ and especially in lead $V_3$. The QT interval is not prolonged, and the upslope of the T wave is not straightened. This is a normal electrocardiograph with early repolarization.

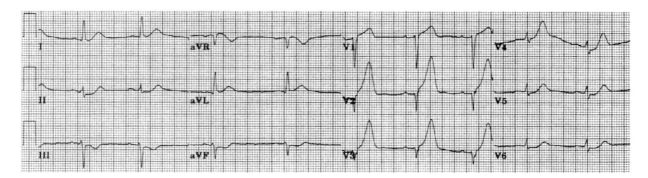

**Figure 64.14**  In this electrocardiograph, the broad, somewhat symmetric T waves are the dominant finding. The QT interval is also prolonged. Minimal ST-segment elevation is present in the mid-precordial leads. This represents the acute phase of an acute myocardial infarction, which often is not seen on the electrocardiograph because it occurs while the patient is in the process of reaching the hospital, and the electrocardiograph has evolved through this picture by the time of arrival.

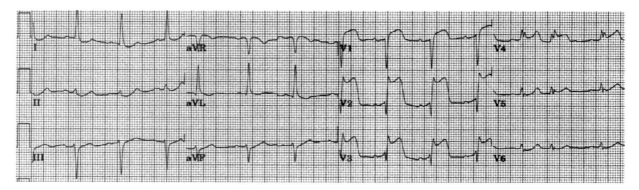

**Figure 64.15**  This is the same patient described in Figure 64.14, 40 minutes later. Very clear ST-segment elevation is seen in the mid-precordial leads, and the diagnosis of acute anteroseptal infarction is clear. In addition, premature atrial contractions are present. Once again, definite reciprocal changes are not seen.

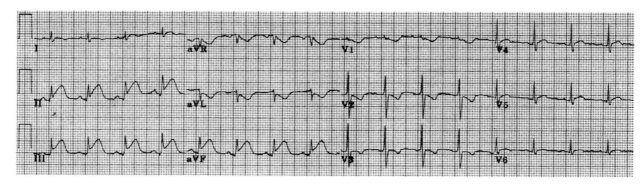

**Figure 64.16** This electrocardiograph shows ST-segment elevation, this time in the inferior leads II, III, and aV$_F$. A reciprocal depression occurs in aV$_L$. This is an acute inferior infarct.

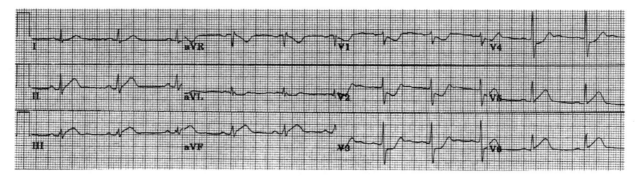

**Figure 64.17** This also is an example of an acute inferior infarction. Some slight ST elevation appears in leads III and aV$_F$, and reciprocal depressions are present in leads V$_1$, V$_2$, and V$_3$. The T waves are broad, and the upslope of the T waves are straightened. These changes also are seen in leads V$_5$ and V$_6$. The differential diagnosis of ST-segment depression in the right precordium that is seen with an acute inferior infarct is (i) simple reciprocal change, (ii) "ischemia at a distance," and (iii) posterior infarction. Posterior infarction is more likely to be the case here, in view of the acute ST-T–wave changes that are seen in leads V$_5$ and V$_6$, in addition to the acute inferior abnormalities.

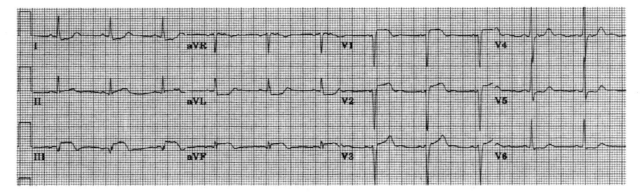

**Figure 64.18** The ST-segment elevation in leads III and aV$_F$ is associated with depressions in leads I and aV$_L$, suggesting acute inferior infarction. In addition, ST-segment elevation is present in leads V$_1$ and V$_2$. Elevations in the right precordial leads in the face of inferior infarct should strongly suggest right ventricular infarct. This can be confirmed with right-sided chest leads, although in this case that would not be necessary because this is a fairly characteristic right ventricular infarct.

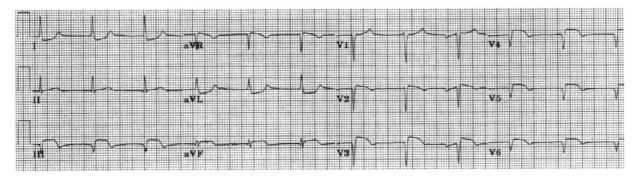

**Figure 64.19** This is the same patient described in Figure 64.18. The frontal plane, which is made up of leads I, II, III, aV$_R$, aV$_L$, and aV$_F$, is in the standard hookup. The precordial leads are right-sided chest leads and show acute ST elevation over the right precordium, especially in leads V$_3$ through V$_6$. These types of ST deviations are seen with an acute RV infarct. This type of right precordial recording is useful in patients in whom elevations in leads V$_1$ and V$_2$ are absent in the face of an acute inferior infarct and a clinical suggestion of right ventricular dysfunction.

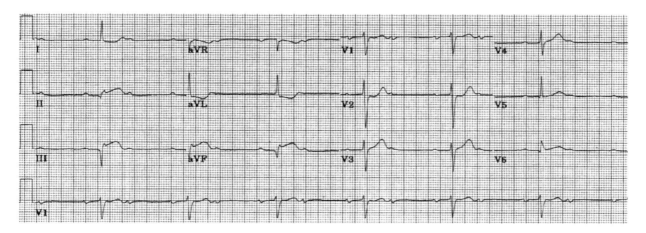

**Figure 64.20** Acute inferior infarctions can be associated with a variety of sinus and atrioventricular node conduction abnormalities. This is an example of one. On this electrocardiograph, an acute inferior infarction pattern is present, with elevation in the inferior leads and reciprocal changes in leads I and aV$_L$. In addition, a 2:1 atrioventricular block can be seen.

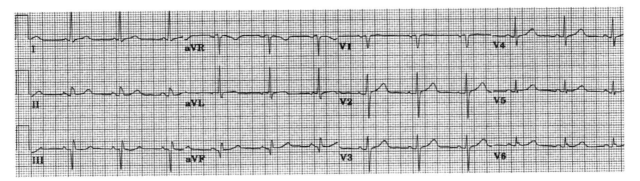

**Figure 64.21** This is an old inferior infarction. Well-developed Q waves are seen in leads III and aV$_F$; aV$_F$ is the key lead. Here, the Q wave is broad, being 0.04 seconds in duration. The ST-segment abnormalities are resolved. T waves are back to normal. This is a well-established (old or remote) infarct.

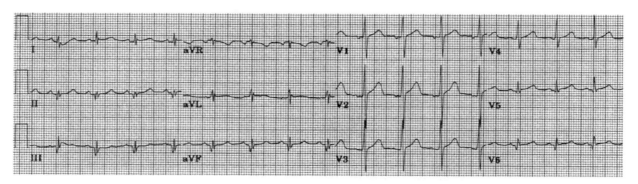

**Figure 64.22** In this electrocardiograph, the inferior directed Q waves are obvious. They are broad and deep relative to the R waves and without question represent an inferior infarct. Lead $V_6$ has a similar Q-wave duration and QR ratio. Of importance, the R waves in lead $V_1$ are prominent, greater, or at least equal to the S wave in that lead, with the T waves being upright. This is an example of an inferoposterior infarct.

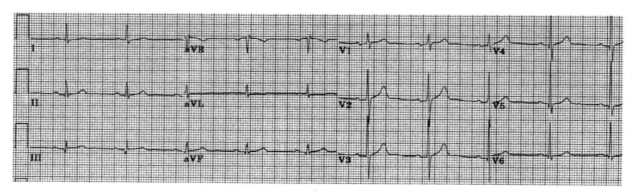

**Figure 64.23** This electrocardiograph shows small inferior Q waves. Those in lead III are prominent, but those in leads II and $aV_F$ are below the diagnostic level. $V_1$, however, shows prominence of the R wave, with an R greater than S and an upright T wave. This is an example of a posterior infarction.

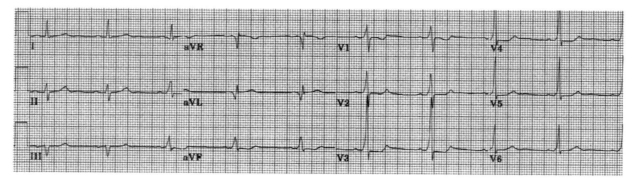

**Figure 64.24** This electrocardiograph, in the right precordial leads, also shows prominence of the R wave, with an upright quality to the T waves. A Q wave is present in $aV_L$, and this could represent an old posterolateral infarction. In looking at leads $V_3$, $V_4$, and $V_5$, however, it can be seen that the PR interval is short, and a delta wave initiates the QRS complexes. This is an example of Wolff-Parkinson-White syndrome or preexcitation with a pseudoinfarct pattern. This tracing actually demonstrates an intermittent preexcitation syndrome because two normal complexes initiate the electrocardiograph.

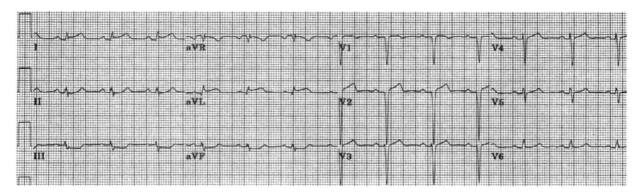

**Figure 64.25**   The ST-segment elevation is slight but definite in this electrocardiograph. It is best seen in lead aV$_L$. Some lesser elevation occurs in lead I, and reciprocal changes are present in the inferior leads, especially leads III and aV$_F$. This is an example of an acute high lateral infarction. The precordial leads are fairly unremarkable, and this type of infarct can evolve as quite a surprise. It results in high enzyme elevations in what seems to be an electrocardiographically limited event. The high lateral wall is relatively electrically silent, and changes in those leads must be respected.

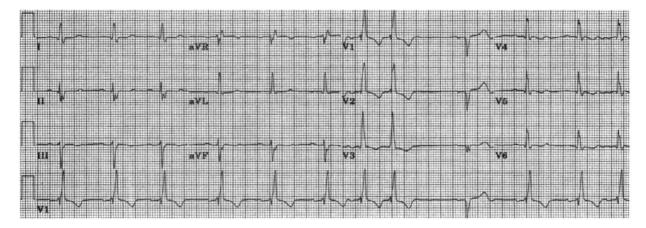

**Figure 64.26**   Electrocardiographs sometimes reveal their secrets in only a few beats. This electrocardiograph shows a right bundle branch block with left axis deviation. In the middle panel, a premature atrial contraction can be seen, and after the compensatory reset, normal intraventricular conduction is permitted to occur. The "normal beat" after the pause shows Q waves that extend from V$_1$ to V$_3$. This is an old anteroseptal infarct uncovered by the premature atrial contraction. Also, this is an example of a rate-dependent right bundle branch block.

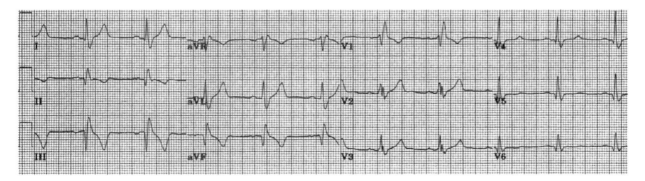

**Figure 64.27**   Right bundle branch block does not obscure the diagnosis of myocardial infarction. Right bundle branch block is defined by a terminal vector that results in a large R′ in lead V$_1$ and a broad terminal S in V$_6$ and often in lead I. Infarcts are defined in the initial portion of the QRS complex, so these diagnoses are not mutually exclusive on the electrocardiograph. This is an example of a right bundle branch block with broad Q waves in the inferior leads of an old inferior infarct. Some lateral involvement with the Q waves is also probable in leads V$_5$ and V$_6$.

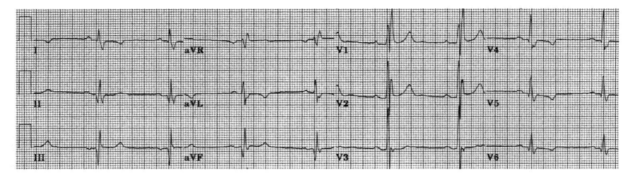

**Figure 64.28** This electrocardiograph, which is similar to the previous tracing, has some important differences. It is a right bundle branch block and an old inferior infarction. Usually, with a right bundle branch block, T-wave inversions are present in the right precordial leads. In this case, the T wave is upright, suggesting a primary T-wave abnormality and supporting the diagnosis of inferior and posterior infarction in the face of a right bundle branch block. Ordinarily, right bundle branch block prevents the diagnosis of posterior infarction, but in this case, the initial vector is prominent, and the T wave is upright in $V_1$, representing inferoposterior infarct.

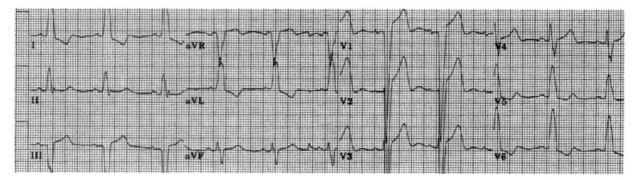

**Figure 64.29** This is a left bundle branch block. The complexes are greater than 120 msec, no Q waves are present in leads I or $V_6$ (which would represent normal septal depolarization), and no secondary repolarization changes are present in the lateral leads. Based on the QRS complex, other diagnoses should not be made in the face of a left bundle branch block.

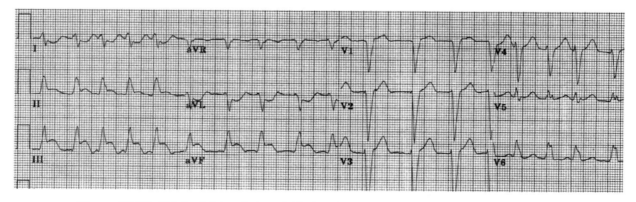

**Figure 64.30** This is a left bundle branch block with ST elevation in the inferior leads and depressions in leads $aV_L$ and I. These are probably reciprocal. This is an example of an acute inferior infarct in the face of a left bundle branch block. The infarct is defined by the ST-segment deviations, which are primary repolarization defects that are not appropriate for a left bundle branch block.

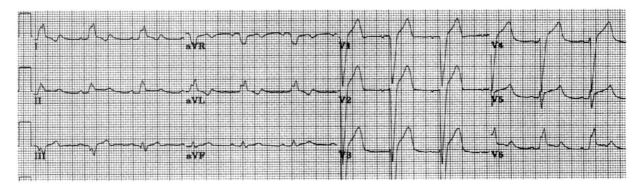

**Figure 64.31**   This electrocardiograph also shows a left bundle branch block. Widespread ST-segment elevations are present. These are primary repolarization findings. The diffuse nature suggests pericarditis. This tracing and that shown in Figure 64.30 are examples of electrocardiographic diagnoses of left bundle branch block based on repolarization changes and not on the basic QRS complexes.

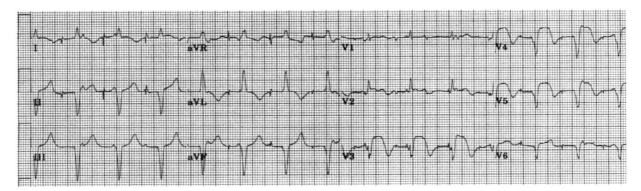

**Figure 64.32**   This is a variation on the primary repolarization story. This is an atrioventricular sequential pacemaker in which the primary ST-T–wave changes are compatible with an acute anterior infarction. The infarct diagnosis is based not on the paced ventricular complexes, but instead on the primary nature of the ST-T–wave changes.

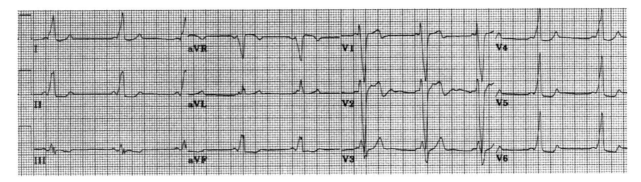

**Figure 64.33**   The gross appearance of this electrocardiograph suggests left bundle branch block. It is, however, preexcitation, with a short PR interval and a delta wave giving a pseudo–left bundle branch block appearance. Wolff-Parkinson-White syndrome can mimic almost anything, as seen in the pseudoposterolateral infarct in Figure 64.24. One should always be aware of short PR intervals and delta waves.

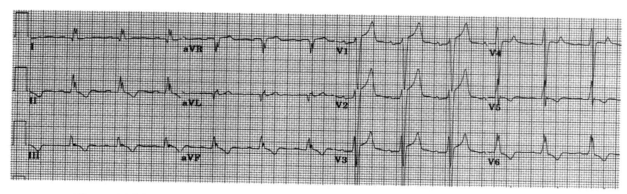

**Figure 64.34** This electrocardiograph has a wide complex that in V₆ has an appearance suggesting left bundle branch block. Q waves, however, are present in lead I. A left bundle branch block is defined by the absence of septal Q waves, and this electrocardiograph is more properly interpreted as an intraventricular conduction defect. A lateral infarct is also possible, also based on the Q waves in leads aV₁ and I.

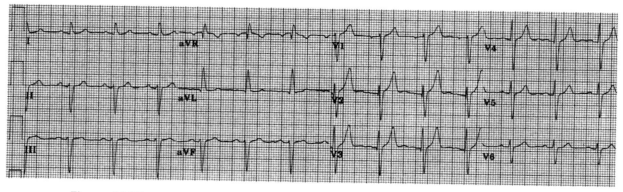

**Figure 64.35** On this electrocardiograph, the dominant finding is marked left axis deviation. This is associated with small Q waves in leads I and aV₁. The total complex is not broad. This, therefore, is an example of an anterior hemiblock. The presence of small Q waves in the right precordial leads is part of the hemiblock pattern and not a sign of myocardial infarction, which would be suggested in the absence of left axis deviation.

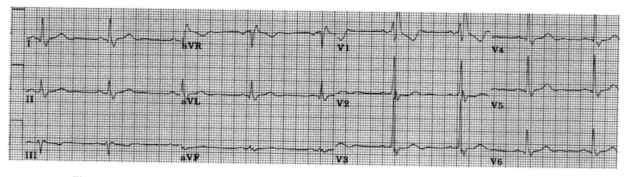

**Figure 64.36** This is an example of a right bundle branch block. Right bundle branch block is defined by a broadening of the QRS complex by a terminal vector. The vector is wide and positive in lead V₁. It is wide and negative in lead V₆. This vector is produced by right ventricular depolarization, unopposed by left ventricular forces. Usually, with a right bundle branch block ST-segment and T-wave changes are present in the right precordial leads, secondary to the conducting defect.

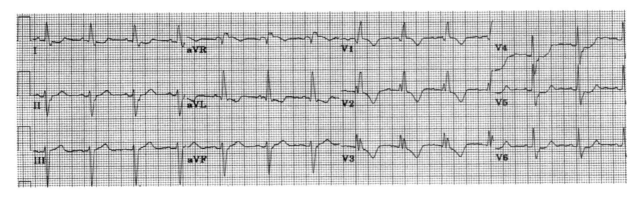

**Figure 64.37** This patient's electrocardiograph shows a sinus rhythm with a normal PR interval. A right bundle branch block with a broad R′ is present in lead $V_1$ and a terminal S is present in $V_6$. Marked left axis deviation and small Q waves also are present in leads I and $aV_L$. This is an example of a bifascicular block–right bundle branch block and anterior fascicular block (hemiblock).

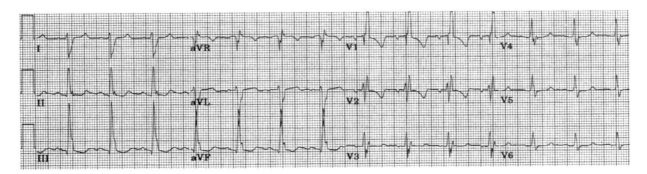

**Figure 64.38** This electrocardiograph shows a sinus rhythm with a normal PR interval. A right bundle branch block and right axis deviation are present. This could be a bifascicular block with right bundle branch block and posterior fascicular block, but posterior fascicular block is a clinical diagnosis. The patient must be examined and right ventricular enlargement excluded before making the diagnosis of posterior fascicular block.

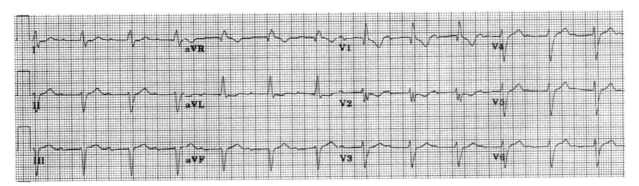

**Figure 64.39** In this electrocardiograph, a right bundle branch block with a broad R′ in $V_1$ and broad terminal S in $V_5$, an anterior hemiblock, and a first-degree atrioventricular block are present. This is, at least, a bifascicular block and certainly could be trifascicular, although that cannot be stated with certainty based on the electrocardiograph alone. Trifascicular block also is a clinical diagnosis.

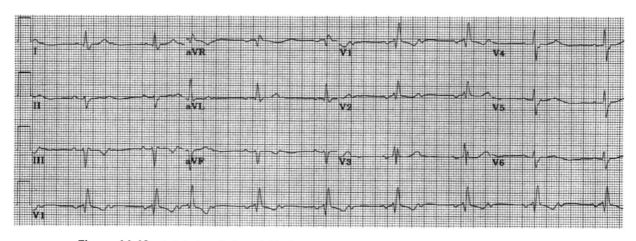

**Figure 64.40** A right bundle branch block and an anterior fascicular block is present in this electrocardiograph. In addition, most of the electrocardiograph shows a 2:1 atrioventricular block. Usually, with conducting system defects and a 2:1 block, the atrioventricular conduction abnormality is Mobitz type II. In this electrocardiograph, however, a Wenckebach sequence is seen at the second and third QRS complexes. The PR interval has a sequential increase, followed by a dropped beat with a 3:2 block. If Wenckebach block is present in one location, it is likely to be the basis of dropped beats elsewhere. This, therefore, is not a trifascicular block.

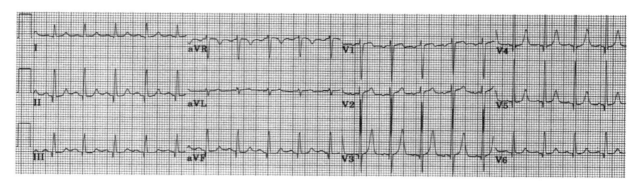

**Figure 64.41** T waves in this electrocardiograph are prominent. The QT interval actually is relatively prolonged, although the presence of tachycardia may make this difficult to assess. Some slight ST-segment elevation is present, especially in lead $V_3$, which represents early repolarization. Although the ST-segment elevation and prominent T waves are seen with myocardial infarction, the narrow symmetry of the T waves here should suggest hyperkalemia.

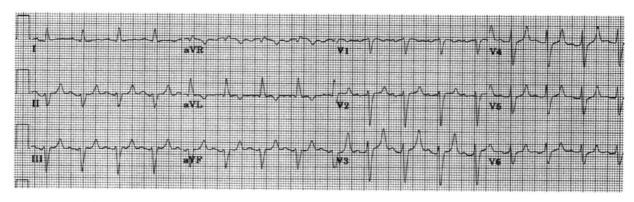

**Figure 64.42** This electrocardiograph also shows prominent, symmetric T waves. It is associated with a broadening of the QRS complex, which is generalized. This is an example of hyperkalemia, but hyperkalemia at a level at which the resting membrane potential has become less negative, activation of the action potential in phase 0 is prolonged, and as a result, intraventricular conduction is prolonged. As hyperkalemia evolves, a broadening of the QRS, producing an intraventricular conduction delay, commonly is seen, as is loss of atrial activity.

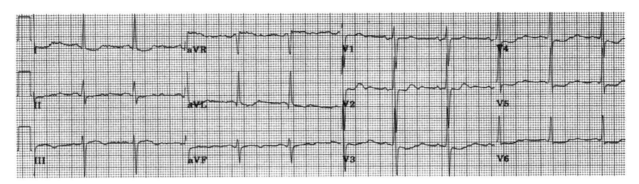

**Figure 64.43**  This is an example of hypokalemia that shows ST-segment depression in the mid-precordium, T waves that are low and broad, U waves that have become prominent with TU fusion, and U waves that are more prominent than the T waves with which they are associated.

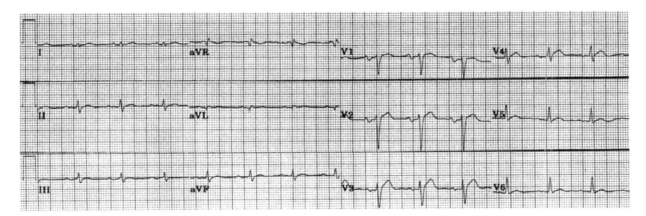

**Figure 64.44**  In this electrocardiograph, the T waves are normal in appearance, but the QT interval is relatively short. This might be passed as a normal electrocardiograph, but it is, in fact, an example of hypercalcemia.

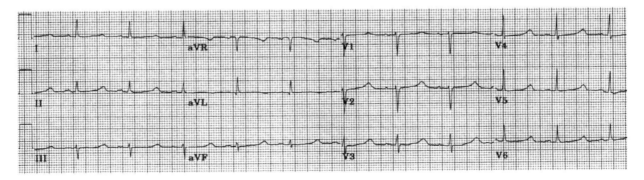

**Figure 64.45**  This electrocardiograph is the opposite of the tracing in Figure 64.44. It shows a prolongation of the QT interval. The T waves, however, have a fairly normal appearance; this is hypocalcemia.

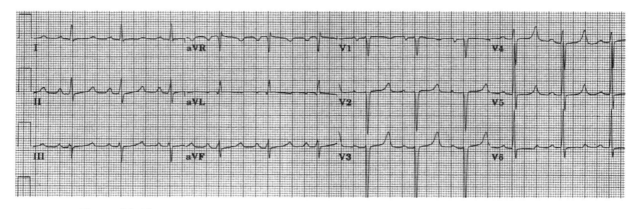

**Figure 64.46**   This is a mixed electrolyte abnormality. The QT interval is prolonged, suggesting hypocalcemia. T waves are symmetric, especially in the mid-precordial leads, compatible with hyperkalemia. This patient has renal insufficiency.

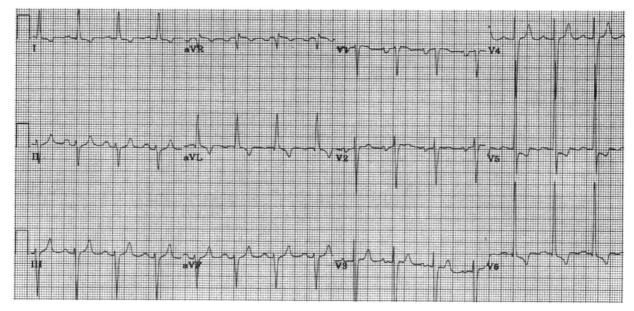

**Figure 64.47**   This is a classic example of left ventricular hypertrophy. The voltage is prominent, with secondary ST-T–wave changes laterally (strain), left axis deviation, prolongation of the QRS complex, and left atrial enlargement. The left atrial enlargement is diagnosed by the presence of the wide P wave, with notching in lead II and a broad terminal negative portion in lead $V_1$.

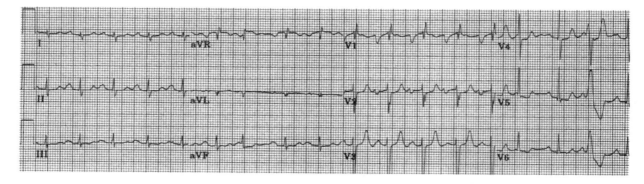

**Figure 64.48**   This patient also has left atrial enlargement with a broad P wave in lead $V_1$ and a broadly negative terminal component of the P wave in lead $V_1$. This is right ventricular hypertrophy, rather than left ventricular hypertrophy. Right ventricular hypertrophy is suggested by the prominent R' in lead $V_1$ with T-wave inversion and right axis deviation. This patient has mitral stenosis. One premature ventricular beat is noted terminally.

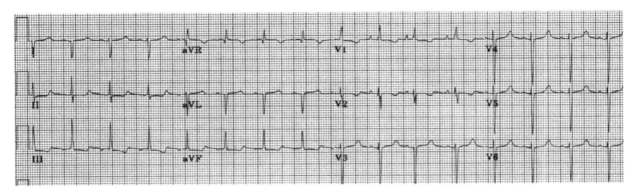

**Figure 64.49** This electrocardiograph shows another example of right ventricular hypertrophy. In this case, a dominant R wave is present, with no S wave and with T-wave inversion in $V_1$. This is a young woman with primary pulmonary hypertension. In addition to the prominent R wave in $V_1$ with T-wave inversion, marked right axis deviation is present, and the S waves are deep relative to the R waves in the lateral leads.

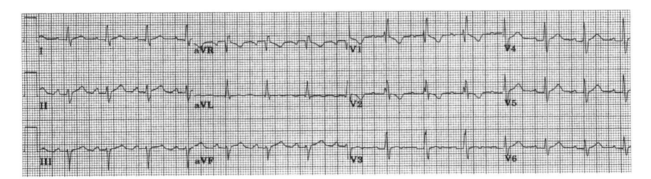

**Figure 64.50** Like the right ventricular hypertrophy depicted in Figure 64.48, this tracing shows an incomplete right bundle branch block with rSR' and R' greater than S, with associated T-wave inversion in lead $V_1$. This pattern of right ventricular hypertrophy can be seen with mitral stenosis and with volume overload states, such as atrial septal defects. An ostium secundum septal defect will have right axis deviation, but an atrial septal defect in which left axis deviation is seen is usually an ostium primum defect. Notching in the P wave raises the possibility of left atrial enlargement. This was a young man with an ostium primum atrial septal defect and right ventricular hypertrophy. He also had a cleft mitral valve and significant mitral insufficiency with left atrial enlargement.

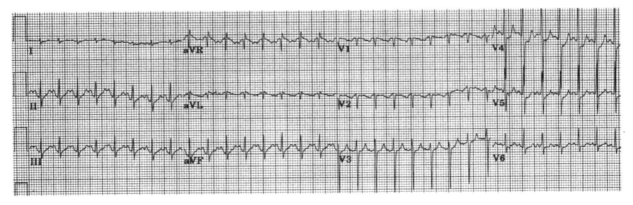

**Figure 64.51** This electrocardiograph shows a significant tachycardia. The differential for narrow complex tachycardia is extensive, but in this case the "dysrhythmia" is sinus tachycardia. This is established by the normal PR interval and the normal vector of the P waves in the frontal plane.

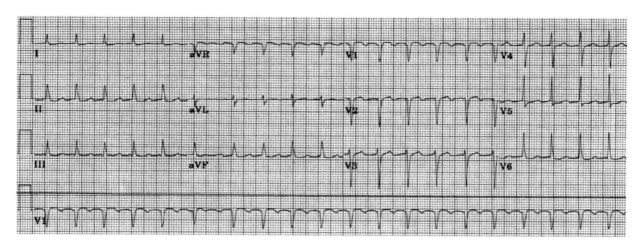

**Figure 64.52** This electrocardiograph also shows a tachycardia. It could be a sinus tachycardia with a first-degree atrioventricular block, but after the sixth beat in the V₁ rhythm strip, a pause occurs. In this interval two discrete atrial waves can be seen, thus establishing this as atrial flutter or atrial tachycardia with largely a 2:1 atrioventricular block.

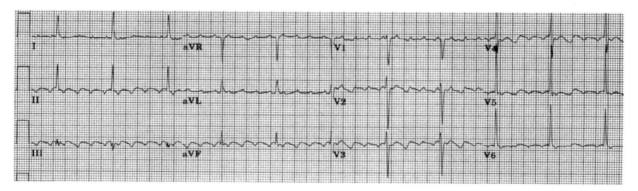

**Figure 64.53** This patient has a more typical atrial flutter. The atrial rate is rapid, at approximately 300 beats per minute. A negative saw-toothed appearance is present in the inferior leads. This is atrial flutter with a controlled ventricular response. This patient is either taking a medication that is slowing atrioventricular conduction or has associated atrioventricular conduction disease.

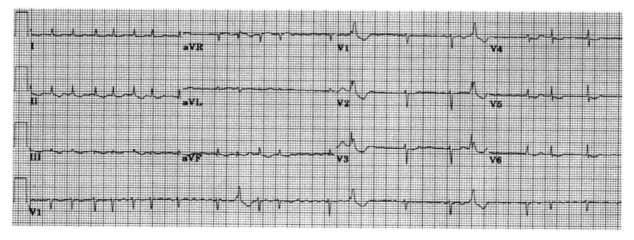

**Figure 64.54** This is an irregularly irregular tachycardia—atrial fibrillation. Occasional wider beats that have a right bundle branch block configuration are present, which is usually seen in aberrantly conducted beats. These are examples of Ashman's phenomenon.

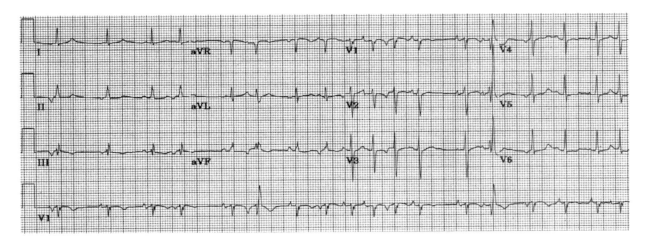

**Figure 64.55** This also is an irregularly irregular narrow complex tachycardia. Fairly distinct atrial waves are present, however, in a chaotic presentation and with a wide variety of forms. This is an example of multifocal atrial tachycardia. The sixth and fourteenth beats have right bundle branch block aberrancy. These also are examples of Ashman's phenomenon. Multifocal atrial tachycardia is usually related to decompensated pulmonary disease. Its treatment is best accomplished through treating the pulmonary problem.

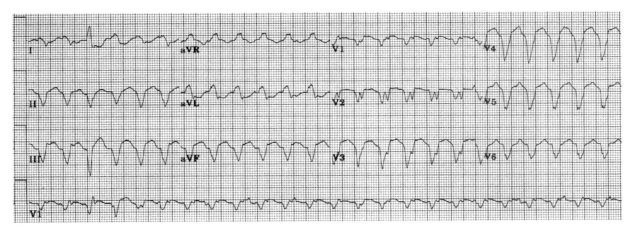

**Figure 64.56** This is an example of wide complex tachycardia—ventricular tachycardia. The key finding is atrioventricular dissociation, which is evident here as P waves that pass through the regular ventricular activity (especially seen in the $V_1$ rhythm strip). Additionally, the third beat is a hybrid or fusion beat. Atrioventricular dissociation has good specificity for ventricular tachycardia, but fusion beats are especially specific. This electrocardiograph also shows the morphologic changes that accompany ventricular tachycardia, in that an anterior negative concordance of voltage is present.

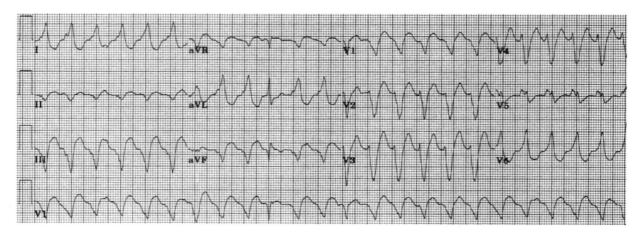

**Figure 64.57** This electrocardiograph also shows a wide complex, regular tachycardia. Atrioventricular dissociation is suggested by the P waves seen on the second complex and after the third complex in lead I. In addition, looking at the V$_1$ rhythm strip, the tenth and thirteenth complexes are narrower and probably represent capture and fusion complexes (highly specific for ventricular tachycardia).

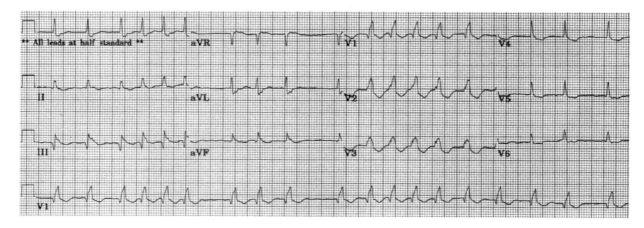

**Figure 64.58** This is a wide complex tachycardia. It has a right bundle branch block-like pattern and is grossly irregular. Although ventricular tachycardia can be subtly irregular, it is never irregular to this degree. This, therefore, is atrial fibrillation with an intraventricular conduction defect, most likely a right bundle branch block.

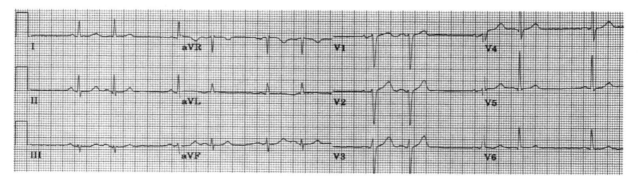

**Figure 64.59** This electrocardiograph shows a group beating with variable RR intervals. The pauses are due to a bigeminal rhythm; in this case, atrial bigeminy. The first P waves in each couplet have normal P vectors. The second P waves in each couplet have a variation. The following pause is not an abnormality; it is merely a delay as the normal mechanism resets itself.

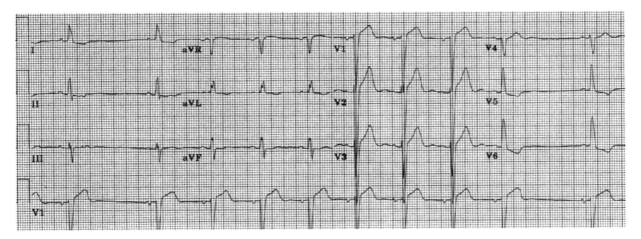

**Figure 64.60** This electrocardiograph shows an incomplete left bundle branch block, with pauses. Here, the T waves preceding the pauses can be seen to have a distorted shoulder and a modified downslope. This is especially evident in the V₁ rhythm strip. This is an example of nonconducted premature atrial contractions. Again, the pauses are not sinister and merely reflect postectopic delay.

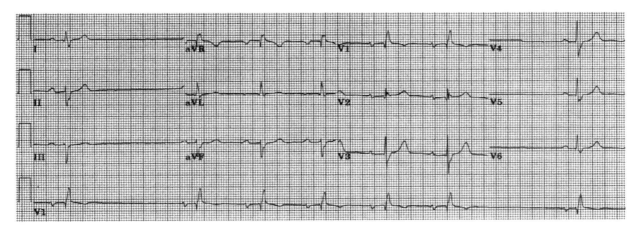

**Figure 64.61** In this electrocardiograph, the obvious problem is the pauses. No obvious premature activity is present that would result in the pause, and as a result, these are either examples of sinus arrest or sinus exit block.

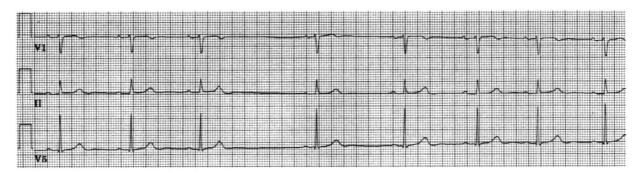

**Figure 64.62** This three-lead rhythm strip shows a prolonged pause. This is an additional example of a nonconducted atrial premature contraction. In the lead II rhythm strip, the T wave of the third beat that precedes the pause can be seen to have a more peaked and notched top, indicating a P wave superimposed on the T wave.

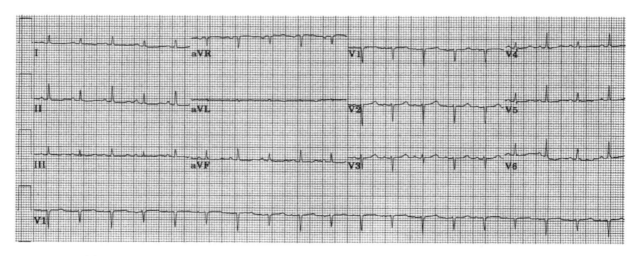

**Figure 64.63**  This electrocardiograph permits a specific clinical diagnosis. A sinus tachycardia is present, voltage is low, and the voltage alternates. This is an example of electrical alternans in a patient with cardiac tamponade.

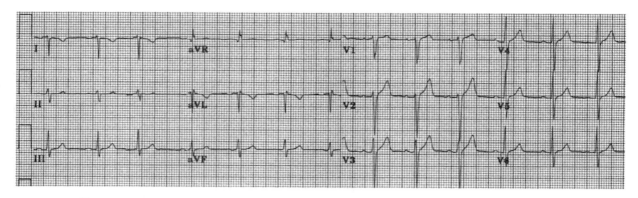

**Figure 64.64**  On this electrocardiograph, a marked right axis deviation appears to be present. Careful inspection of the P waves, however, shows that these are inverted in leads I and aV$_L$. Right axis deviation with P-wave inversion in these leads is usually due to switched arm wires.

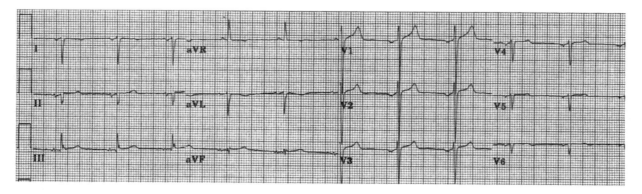

**Figure 64.65**  In this electrocardiograph, the appearance of right axis deviation is present, with an inversion of the P waves in leads I and to some extent aV$_L$. As in Figure 64.64, this could be due to switched arm leads, but in looking at the precordial leads, a drop-off of voltage occurs from right to left. This is an example of dextrocardia (the other cause of inverted P waves in leads I and aV$_L$ with sinus rhythm).

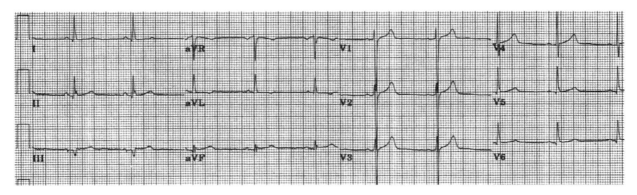

**Figure 64.66**  This is the electrocardiograph from the patient with dextrocardia described in Figure 64.65. Here, the extremity wires have been switched left to right, and the precordial leads have been mounted on the right chest. It produces a fairly normal-looking electrocardiograph.

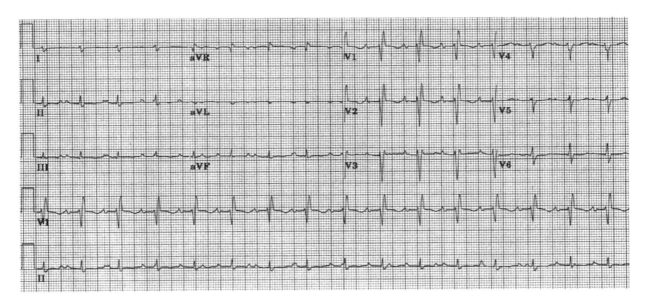

**Figure 64.67**  This is another example in which close scrutiny of the electrocardiograph is important. This is a 12-lead electrocardiograph and a V$_1$ and V$_2$ rhythm strip. In looking at the V$_2$ rhythm strip, a dominant P wave is present, with a PR interval of a little more than 200 msec followed by a QRS complex that has an incomplete right bundle branch block pattern. In addition, an extraneous but regular waveform moves independent of the basic QRS complexes. This is an accessory atrial rhythm and is an example of a cardiac transplantation. In this case, the dissociated atrial rhythm is due to the native sinus and residual atrial tissue. The QRS-related P waves came with the new heart.

have encountered in your patients over years of training, and it is hoped that their review will reinforce important concepts, reassure you about your strengths, and perhaps give some guidance in suggesting additional reading.

## SUGGESTED READINGS

Numerous, excellent texts on electrocardiography are available. It is impossible to list them all, but these are used regularly in clinical practice.

Chou T, Knilans TK. *Electrocardiography in Clinical Practice*, 4th ed. Philadelphia: WB Saunders, 1996.

Fisch C. *Electrocardiography of Arrhythmias*. Philadelphia: Lee & Febiger, 1990.

Lipman BS, Massie E, Kleiger RE. *Clinical Scalar Electrocardiography*, 6th ed. Chicago: Year Book Medical Publishers, 1972. (Out of print.)

Macfarlane P, Lawrie TDV. *Comprehensive Electrocardiography: Theory and Practice in Health and Disease*. New York: Pergamon, 1989.

Marriott HJL. *Practical Electrocardiography*, 7th ed. Baltimore: Williams & Wilkins, 1983.

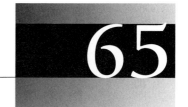

# Valvular Heart Disease

*Brian P. Griffin*

Valvular heart disease remains an important cause of cardiac morbidity, despite a decline in the incidence of rheumatic valvular disease in the developed world. Congenital valvular anomalies (e.g., bicuspid aortic valve, which is seen in approximately 2% of the population) and myxomatous degeneration of valvular tissue (e.g., mitral valve prolapse) are the most common conditions encountered today.

Valvular heart disease may cause problems when the valve becomes stenotic, is regurgitant, or, as frequently occurs, a combined stenotic and regurgitant lesion is present. Multiple valves often are affected either by the primary disease process (e.g., rheumatic fever) or secondarily affected by the pressure or volume effects of another valve lesion. For instance, tricuspid regurgitation commonly is associated with mitral disease because mitral disease increases pulmonary pressures, thus causing the right ventricle to dilate. Right ventricular dilatation causes the tricuspid valve ring or annulus to dilate and, thus, causes the valve to leak.

Stenotic lesions produce problems by reducing cardiac output, particularly during stress, and by increasing the pressure in the chambers proximal to the valve. The heart chambers respond to increased pressure first by hypertrophying and then by dilating. Conversely, regurgitant lesions cause problems by increasing the volume load on the ventricles. For instance, in mitral and aortic regurgitation, the left ventricle dilates to maintain a normal cardiac output. Eventually, with more severe degrees of regurgitation, ventricular dilatation fails to compensate for the regurgitation, and cardiac output falls.

## CLINICAL PRESENTATION

Many patients with valvular heart disease are asymptomatic for years. The onset of symptoms often is insidious, and patients often unwittingly decrease their activities to reduce their symptoms. An acute onset of symptoms may signal valvular disruption (e.g., acute myocardial infarction with papillary muscle rupture or after endocarditis), an acute volume load (e.g., as in pregnancy), or the onset of a tachyarrhythmia (e.g., atrial fibrillation). Symptoms include dyspnea, chest discomfort, syncope, palpitations, embolization, and fatigue.

■ Dyspnea is the most common symptom in valvular heart disease. It usually results from high pulmonary venous pressures, which increase the transudation of fluid into the alveoli and result in diminished gas exchange. It is seen relatively early in mitral stenosis and later in the course of aortic and mitral regurgitation and of aortic stenosis. It is important to determine how limiting the dyspnea is because therapeutic interventions usually are based on the severity of symptoms rather than on the severity of the disease process itself.

■ Chest discomfort may be anginal because of oxygen supply and demand mismatch (e.g., aortic or mitral stenosis) or nonanginal (e.g., mitral valve prolapse).

■ Syncope usually results from an inability to increase cardiac output during peripheral vasodilatation (e.g., with exercise). It is seen in conditions that severely limit cardiac output (e.g., aortic stenosis, mitral stenosis with pulmonary hypertension).

- Palpitations result from an arrhythmia (e.g., atrial fibrillation in mitral disease).
- Embolic events may occur when material on abnormal valves (e.g., calcium) embolizes. An important cause of embolization is endocarditis, and another important cause of embolization is thrombus formation in the left atrium accompanying mitral valve disease.
- Fatigue is common in all forms of valvular heart disease, particularly those associated with low cardiac output (e.g., mitral or aortic stenosis).

## DIAGNOSIS

### Physical Examination

The physical examination is critical to the evaluation of patients with valvular heart disease. It is important to examine thoroughly all aspects of the cardiovascular system. These aspects include:

- Pulse. The pulse is best palpated at the carotid artery. The rhythm, rate, and character (e.g., slow upstroke in aortic stenosis, collapsing in aortic regurgitation) should be assessed.
- Venous pressure. Venous pressure height and wave pattern should be assessed. Valvular disease is characterized by large A waves in pulmonary hypertension and pulmonary stenosis, and large V waves in tricuspid regurgitation.
- Blood pressure. A narrow pulse pressure (i.e., difference between systolic and diastolic blood pressure) is present in aortic stenosis; wide pulse pressure with low diastolic pressure is present in aortic regurgitation.
- Facies. Cyanotic facies often is marked peripherally in low output disorders; mitral facies (i.e., purplish red cheeks) is noted in mitral stenosis.

### Heart Examination

#### Palpation

The patient should be palpated for cardiomegaly and the position of the apex beat, as well as for the following:

- Thrills. Thrills occur with significant valvular lesions and result from turbulent blood flow at the site of the valve lesion. They can be systolic or diastolic in timing, and they are most common with aortic stenosis, ventricular septal defect, and pulmonic stenosis. Diastolic thrills are less common, but they occur with mitral stenosis and aortic regurgitation.
- Character of apex beat. Tapping is less sustained than normal in mitral stenosis and is more sustained than normal or heaving in left ventricular hypertrophy.

- Right ventricular heave. Right ventricular heave is felt along the left sternal border in right ventricular hypertrophy.
- Other sounds. The second heart sound often is palpable in pulmonary hypertension, and $S_3$ and $S_4$ may be palpable as well.

#### Auscultation

The patient should be auscultated for the following:

- First heart sound. The first heart sound is loud in mitral and tricuspid stenosis and soft in mitral regurgitation. Later, with calcification of a stenosed mitral valve, the first heart sound again becomes softer.
- Second heart sound. The second heart sound has a loud pulmonary component in pulmonary hypertension and a soft aortic component in severe aortic stenosis.
- Third heart sound. The third heart sound is a low-pitched, filling sound best heard with the bell of a stethoscope. It is common during severe mitral regurgitation and left ventricular dilatation and may be physiologic in young people.
- Fourth heart sound. The fourth heart sound is the atrial filling sound. It is heard during conditions with left ventricular hypertrophy (e.g., aortic stenosis).
- Opening snap. The opening snap is heard at the lower left sternal border during mitral stenosis. The opening snap follows $S_2$. The shorter the time interval between $S_2$ and the opening snap, the more severe the mitral stenosis.
- Ejection sounds. Early systolic sounds at the base of the heart are heard in congenitally abnormal but mobile valves (e.g., bicuspid aortic valve).
- Mid-systolic clicks. Systolic sounds are heard with myxomatous mitral valve prolapse because of tensing of the redundant leaflets.

Murmurs should be assessed in terms of timing, location, intensity, and provocative maneuvers. Timing involves:

- Systolic
- Ejection (peaking in mid-systole), as in aortic stenosis, pulmonic stenosis, hypertrophic cardiomyopathy
- Pansystolic (heard throughout systole, may encompass $S_1$ and $S_2$), as in mitral regurgitation, tricuspid regurgitation
- Late systolic, as in mitral valve prolapse, ischemic mitral regurgitation because of papillary muscle dysfunction
- Diastolic
- Early, decrescendo, as in aortic regurgitation, pulmonary regurgitation
- Mid-diastolic, as in mitral stenosis, tricuspid stenosis
- Presystolic (late diastole), as in mitral stenosis in normal sinus rhythm

Location involves:

- Apical, as in mitral murmurs; aortic murmur may radiate to the apex

- Base, as in aortic, pulmonary murmurs
- Sternal border, as in tricuspid murmurs, aortic and pulmonary regurgitation
- Radiation, to axilla with mitral, to neck and apex with aortic

Regarding intensity, the severity of the lesion often relates to the loudness of the murmur in systolic murmurs (e.g., aortic stenosis, mitral regurgitation). The severity of diastolic murmurs relates more to the duration of the murmur than to intensity.

Provocative maneuvers include:

- Respiration. Right-sided lesions are louder with inspiration (i.e., increased flow through the right heart). Left-sided lesions are louder with expiration.
- Valsalva. The Valsalva's maneuver decreases intracardiac volume and reduces the intensity of most murmurs. Exceptions are the murmurs of hypertrophic cardiomyopathy, which become louder, and of mitral valve prolapse, which become longer and louder. A reduction in intracardiac volume accentuates outflow obstruction in hypertrophic cardiomyopathy and prolapse in mitral valve prolapse syndrome.
- Position. With standing, intracardiac volume decreases; therefore, most murmurs decrease in intensity (except those of hypertrophic cardiomyopathy and mitral valve prolapse). Squatting accentuates intracardiac volume. Therefore, most murmurs become louder, but those of mitral valve prolapse and hypertrophic cardiomyopathy usually decrease.

## Studies

### Electrocardiography

During electrocardiography, the clinician should look for atrial fibrillation, left or right atrial enlargement, and signs of left ventricular or right ventricular hypertrophy.

### Chest Radiography

A chest radiograph is useful in detecting cardiac chamber enlargement, pulmonary venous hypertension, and more overt signs of pulmonary congestion.

### Doppler Echocardiography

Echocardiography is the most important test currently used for the diagnosis of valvular heart disease. It can define the specific valves that are affected, type of lesion (i.e., stenosis or regurgitation), and severity of the lesion. Transesophageal echocardiography is especially useful when chest wall images are poor, after a prosthesis has been implanted, and when looking at the left atrium for thrombus.

## Severity of Stenosis

Planimetry using two-dimensional echocardiography can directly measure the area of the valve opening in mitral

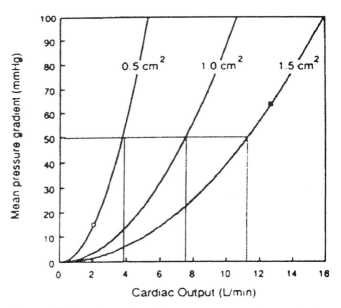

**Figure 65.1**  Relationship of flow to pressure gradient and valve area. A mean pressure gradient of 50 mm Hg across the aortic valve is possible with a valve area of 0.5 to 1.5 cm², depending on the flow (i.e., cardiac output) through the valve.

stenosis. This is the most reliable measurement in mitral stenosis, but it often is technically difficult.

Velocity across the valve as measured by Doppler can be converted to a pressure gradient using the Bernoulli equation:

$$\text{Pressure gradient} = 4 \times \text{velocity}^2$$

Thus, for example, if a peak velocity measured across the aortic valve is 4 m/s, then the peak pressure gradient across the valve is 64 mm Hg.

The pressure gradient depends on the flow across the valve. The higher the flow for any given area, the higher the pressure gradient will be (Fig. 65.1). Therefore, pressure gradients should be interpreted with knowledge of the cardiac output and function.

### Estimation of Valve Area

The continuity equation usually is applied to the aortic valve. Because of the law of conservation of mass-energy, the flow into the valve is equivalent to that leaving the valve. Flow ($F$) is the product of the cross-sectional area ($A$) at a given point and the velocity ($v$) at that point, or

$$F = Av$$

The velocity ($v_p$) and cross-sectional area ($A_p$) below the aortic valve in the left ventricular outflow tract can be measured readily, as can the velocity at the site of maximal narrowing at the aortic valve ($v_d$), which is the highest velocity recorded (Fig. 65.2). The cross-sectional area at the valve itself ($A_d$) can be derived as

$$A_d = A_p v_p / v_d$$

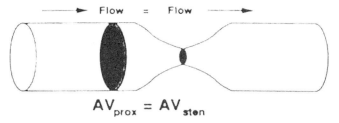

**Figure 65.2**   Flow is the product of area and velocity at a given point, and the continuity equation uses this to calculate the aortic valve area. Flow in the left ventricular outflow tract below the valve can be calculated from the known velocity (*V*) and area (*A*) at this level (*AV*$_{prox}$). The stenotic valve area can be derived from the velocity at this point (*AV*$_{sten}$) as

$$\frac{A_{prox}v_{prox}}{v_{sten}}$$

### Pressure Half-Time

In mitral stenosis, the severity of stenosis inversely relates to the time it takes for the initial pressure to decrease to half its original value. The valve area has been empirically derived as

$$220/\text{Pressure half-time}$$

The shorter the pressure half-time, the less severe the stenosis.

## Assessment of Regurgitant Lesions

The qualitative and quantitative assessment of regurgitant lesion severity is done by using the flow disturbance associated with the regurgitation on color flow mapping. Quantitative assessment uses the determination of flow across the regurgitant valve and across a normal valve. Regurgitant flow is the total flow through the regurgitant valve minus that through the normal valve. The regurgitant fraction equals the regurgitant volume divided by the total volume flow (i.e., forward plus backward).

Newer methods are becoming available to measure regurgitant flow and the size of the regurgitant orifice directly. These use the flow field that is proximal to the regurgitant orifice (proximal convergence).

## Assessment of Effects of Valvular Disease on Ventricular Function

Increasing ventricular size over time in the absence of symptoms is an indication for surgical intervention in patients with mitral and aortic regurgitation. The response of the left ventricle, both in size and function, to exercise stress is increasingly used to assess the effect of valvular regurgitation on contractile function and to help determine optimal timing for surgery.

## Cardiac Catheterization

Cardiac catheterization is less critical today because of reliable, noninvasive measures. It still is used, however, when a discrepancy occurs between clinical findings and noninvasive techniques or to confirm noninvasive findings in selected patients. It also is necessary when coronary disease is suspected or must be excluded (e.g., in patients who need surgery).

With cardiac catheterization, the pressure gradients across the valves can be measured directly rather than simply being derived, as they are with Doppler. The effects of maneuvers, such as exercise, also can be used to determine the severity of a lesion. Valve area is derived empirically using the Gorlin equation from the flow (thermodilution or Fick technique) and the pressure gradient across the valve.

Regurgitation usually is assessed semiquantitatively, by the direct injection of dye into the left ventricle to assess mitral regurgitation or into the aorta to assess aortic regurgitation. The opacification of the chamber receiving the regurgitant flow is then determined.

## TREATMENT

The general principles for treating patients with valvular heart disease are as follows:

1. Assess severity of symptoms.
2. Determine the nature of the valvular lesion and its severity.
3. Assess the effects of the lesion on ventricular function.
4. Assess for other cardiac (or other) pathologies.

Intervention is indicated in the following situations:

- Limiting symptoms with significant stenosis
- Limiting symptoms with significant regurgitation
- Significant left ventricular dysfunction or progressive left ventricular dilatation attributable to the valve lesion in severe mitral or aortic regurgitation or aortic stenosis

Prophylaxis for endocarditis is indicated whenever blood flow is turbulent at a structurally abnormal valve. The benefits of prophylaxis have never been fully established, but it is usual to err on the side of administration. Patients with mild leaks in otherwise normal valves (e.g., physiologic leaks at the mitral, tricuspid, or most commonly, pulmonic valve) have a relatively low risk for endocarditis and probably do not require prophylaxis.

## SPECIFIC VALVE LESIONS

### Mitral Stenosis

Mitral stenosis is twice as common in women as in men. It usually is rheumatic in origin, although congenital mitral stenosis also occurs. The valve becomes fibrosed and tends to calcify with time. The reduction in the size of the mitral valve orifice lowers the cardiac output, and it tends to raise left atrial and pulmonary venous and arterial pressures. In patients with severe mitral stenosis, pulmonary hypertension as high as that of the systemic vasculature may occur. Flow across the mitral valve occurs in diastole and is critically dependent on the heart rate; therefore, the reduction of diastolic filling time caused by increased heart rate worsens the symptoms and can cause acute pulmonary edema. Symptomatic deterioration often results from the onset of atrial fibrillation.

The complications of mitral stenosis may include atrial arrhythmia, atrial fibrillation, and thromboembolism. Left atrial enlargement and atrial fibrillation predispose patients to atrial thrombus and thromboembolism. This may occur in as many as 25% of those who are not anticoagulated, and it often occurs silently.

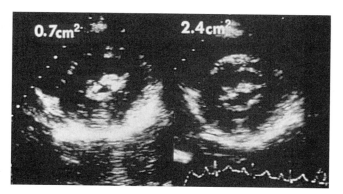

**Figure 65.3** Planimetry of the mitral valve by echocardiography. The mitral valve area increases after balloon valvuloplasty (**right**) compared with baseline (**left**).

### Diagnosis

The symptoms of mitral stenosis are:

- Dyspnea
- Fatigue
- Hemoptysis (from pulmonary venous hypertension)
- Angina; syncope, if there is pulmonary hypertension
- Edema secondary to right heart failure

The signs of mitral stenosis are:

- Tapping apex beat from a loud first heart sound if the valve is pliable
- Diastolic thrill in severe stenosis (classically described as like a purring cat)
- Palpable $P_2$, if there is pulmonary hypertension
- Loud $S_1$, because the valve remains open at the end of diastole and shuts abruptly with the onset of systole; as the valve calcifies, the $S_1$ gets softer
- Opening snap indicates a pliable valve and disappears as the valve calcifies. The opening snap often is heard at the left sternal border rather than at the apex, and with the diaphragm rather than with the bell of the stethoscope
- Diastolic murmur with presystolic accentuation in sinus rhythm, best heard at apex with the bell of the stethoscope and the patient on his left side
- Associated pulmonary hypertension leads to a loud $P_2$, right ventricular heave, tricuspid regurgitation, and pulmonary insufficiency (i.e., Graham-Steel murmur)
- Occasionally, no murmur is heard if flow through the valve is low (e.g., as with severe pulmonary hypertension)

Signs indicating severe stenosis include a long diastolic murmur, a short duration of the interval between $S_2$ and the opening snap (thus indicating high atrial pressure even at the end of systole), and a loud $P_2$.

### Differential Diagnosis

The differential diagnosis of diastolic murmur includes tricuspid stenosis, Austin-Flint murmur of aortic regurgitation (i.e., aortic regurgitant jet hits the mitral valve and prevents full diastolic opening), left atrial myxoma, and cor triatria-

tum. Silent mitral stenosis with pulmonary hypertension simulates primary pulmonary hypertension.

### Studies

Electrocardiography shows left atrial enlargement, right atrial enlargement, right axis, and right ventricular hypertrophy. Chest radiography may show left atrial enlargement, prominence of main pulmonary artery Kerley B lines with edema, and pulmonary hemosiderosis. Doppler echocardiography reveals:

- The appearance of doming of the mitral valve, which has a restricted opening. The opening may be measured directly by planimetry in the short axis (Fig. 65.3), which usually is the most reliable method for assessing severity of the narrowing.
- A pressure gradient across the valve (normal <5 mm Hg) may be as high as 20 mm Hg in those with severe mitral stenosis. The valve area also is derived empirically from the pressure half-time (see Pressure Half-Time, earlier in this chapter).
- A decrease in valve area (normal 4 to 6 $cm^2$) to less than 1 $cm^2$ in patients with critical mitral stenosis.
- A mitral valve score based on thickness, calcification, mobility, and involvement of subvalvular apparatus on transthoracic echocardiography. This score is used to determine the likelihood of success for percutaneous mitral valvuloplasty. The score may vary from 0 to 16. If the score is greater than 8, valvuloplasty will have less chance of success.
- The possible presence of associated lesions such as mitral, aortic, or tricuspid regurgitation.

Stress echocardiography is increasingly used to assess functional capacity and the effects of exercise on valve pressure gradients and pulmonary pressures (as derived from the velocity of tricuspid regurgitation). This is especially useful when patients have severe stenosis but deny symptoms, or when the degree of stenosis apparently is mild but the symptoms are more severe than would be anticipated.

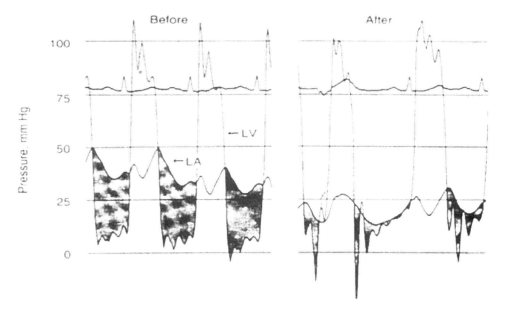

**Figure 65.4**   The mitral valve gradient is the shaded area between the left atrial (LA) and left ventricular (LV) pressure in diastole. (**Left**) The gradient before percutaneous valvuloplasty. (**Right**) The reduced gradient after successful balloon valvuloplasty.

Cardiac catheterization is used to determine the presence of accompanying coronary disease, and it also is useful in confirming the severity of mitral disease. Knowledge regarding the effect of exercise on the mitral pressure gradient may be useful when the severity of the lesion is in doubt. Cardiac catheterization is necessary for percutaneous mitral valvuloplasty (Fig. 65.4).

### Treatment

Survival rates are lower among patients with mitral stenosis in whom symptoms have appeared. Patients increasingly are treated with balloon valvuloplasty, which at 2 years has results similar to those of open mitral commissurotomy regarding symptoms and valve area. Balloon valvuloplasty is feasible if the valve is pliable and relatively uncalcified (as assessed by the echocardiographic splitability score), if no more than mild mitral regurgitation is present (i.e., mitral regurgitation usually increases one grade with the balloon procedure), if no thrombus is present in the left atrium (i.e., a thrombus could be dislodged by wires during valvuloplasty), and if severe tricuspid regurgitation is absent (i.e., severe tricuspid regurgitation often persists after a balloon procedure).

Asymptomatic patients usually can be treated conservatively. Indications for intervention in patients without symptoms include significant pulmonary hypertension, prophylaxis in those undergoing major surgery during which a large volume shift might be encountered, or women of childbearing age with severe stenosis who wish to start a family.

With symptomatic patients, intervention with balloon valvuloplasty or surgery may be considered. Valve replacement is indicated in patients with calcified valves or severe mitral regurgitation.

Patients with mitral stenosis must be monitored closely during pregnancy because the volume load and tachycardia may cause severe, symptomatic deterioration even in those with mild mitral stenosis. The risk of heart failure is greatest during the first trimester and at delivery. Careful monitoring and slowing of the heart rate allows most patients with mitral stenosis to carry their pregnancies to term without intervention. In those with severe, symptomatic deterioration, commissurotomy (preferably with a balloon) is indicated.

With medical treatment, the control of heart rate in patients with atrial fibrillation is important. In older patients who are not considered to be good surgical candidates, rate control and diuretics may effectively reduce symptoms. In younger patients, prophylaxis against rheumatic fever usually is required. Patients with chronic atrial fibrillation and mitral stenosis have a high risk for thromboembolism and should receive anticoagulation.

Surgical treatment consists of open commissurotomy, in which the fused mitral valve leaflets are opened under direct vision by the surgeon or by prosthetic valve insertion.

## Mitral Regurgitation

### Etiology

Primary mitral regurgitation is an abnormality of the valve or apparatus. The causes of primary mitral regurgitation are:

- Rheumatic, more often men than women
- Myxomatous, as in mitral valve prolapse
- Congenital, as in endocardial cushion defects with primum atrial septal defect
- Endocarditis, as in bacterial and marantic infections, Libman-Sacks vegetations in lupus
- Ischemic, as in papillary muscle dysfunction or rupture

Secondary mitral regurgitation results from dilatation of the left ventricle from any cause. This can include ischemia, cardiomyopathy, or aortic valve disease.

### Pathophysiology

When volume load occurs on the left atrium and left ventricle, the left ventricle initially responds by pumping more vigorously and emptying more completely. Subsequently, progressive dilatation occurs, with eventual impairment of left ventricular function. This may be permanent despite valve surgery.

### Diagnosis

Mitral regurgitation often is asymptomatic for many years. Dyspnea and heart failure are the most common symptoms, and right-sided heart failure with hepatic congestion and cachexia also are seen.

No specific pulse findings are present. The jugular venous pressure often is elevated because of right-sided heart failure.

The murmur generally is holosystolic, louder in expiration, best heard at the apex, and radiates to the axilla. A murmur that radiates to the back indicates a posterior-directed jet (e.g., anterior prolapse of the mitral valve). It often is associated with an $S_3$ gallop, which is consistent with severe mitral regurgitation and a dilated left ventricle. $S_1$ usually is soft, and $S_2$ may be loud in patients with pulmonary hypertension.

### Studies

Electrocardiography shows a volume overload pattern and left atrial enlargement. Echocardiography allows the anatomy of the valve and cause of the leak to be delineated precisely. It also is useful in determining the severity of the leak, either semiquantitatively by the size and extent of the regurgitant jet on color Doppler or quantitatively as the regurgitant volume. The leak can be quantified by a new color Doppler technique proximal to the hole through which the leaks occur (i.e., regurgitant orifice). The size of the regurgitant orifice also can be estimated; in patients with severe mitral regurgitation, it usually is greater than 0.3 cm$^2$.

Over time, any change in size of the chambers, particularly the left ventricle, is useful for monitoring the progress of the lesion and determining the need for surgery. The contractile function of the left ventricle is difficult to assess accurately through noninvasive means because the ventricle is volume loaded and ejects much of its blood back into the lower pressure left atrium. Left ventricular function always appears to be better than it really is when using ejection indices such as ejection fraction. An ejection fraction of less than 60% should suggest possible contractile dysfunction in this condition.

Increasingly, left ventricular volume measurements are made to determine the appropriate timing of surgery. We have used the response of the left ventricle to exercise stress

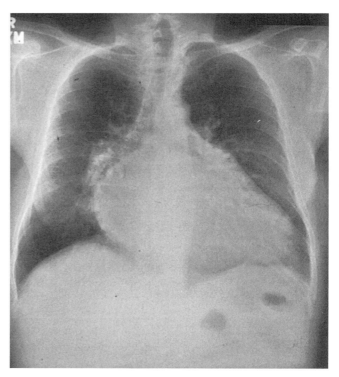

**Figure 65.5**  Chest radiograph of a patient with chronic mitral regurgitation showing left atrial and left ventricular enlargement.

as a means of determining contractile reserve in this condition. A failure of the left ventricle to decrease in size at peak exercise, or of the ejection fraction to increase, is indicative of left ventricular dysfunction, which is often manifest postoperatively.

Chest radiography shows left atrial and left ventricular enlargement as well as congestive changes (Fig. 65.5), and cardiac catheterization can determine the severity of mitral regurgitation (using ventriculography) or the presence of coronary disease. Large V waves in pulmonary wedge tracings also suggest severe mitral regurgitation. A succession of pressure–volume loops, as defined using high-fidelity catheters and by changing the loading conditions, allows myocardial elastance to be measured. This is the best load-independent measure of true contractile function in this condition. It remains a research tool, however, because it is difficult to measure and requires catheterization as well as intravenous pressors and vasodilators for its measurement.

### Treatment

#### Medical Treatment

No treatment is needed for mild regurgitation, but these patients should undergo serial echocardiography. Afterload reduction usually is not indicated in those with primary mitral regurgitation because this has not been shown to postpone surgical intervention. Antibiotic prophylaxis generally is necessary. If congestive heart failure is present, treatment includes diuretics, digoxin, and afterload reduction. In patients with secondary mitral regurgitation, the primary disease should be treated. Vasodilators or afterload reduction should be used in patients with cardiomyopathy.

### Surgical Treatment

Patients with mitral regurgitation eventually develop heart failure. The onset of heart failure is associated with reduced survival rates, as is significant ventricular dysfunction. Mitral regurgitation should be corrected before the signs of left ventricular dysfunction or failure become overt. Indications for surgery, therefore, are severe mitral regurgitation with symptoms of heart failure, dyspnea, evidence of deteriorated left ventricular function, or progressive left ventricular enlargement. In asymptomatic patients, an end-systolic dimension of 2.6 cm/m² is considered to be an indication for surgery. Because patients with mitral regurgitation should have hyperdynamic function, even a low-normal left ventricular ejection fraction (i.e., <60%) should be considered to be a sign of incipient left ventricular dysfunction, and surgery should be recommended accordingly. With exercise, those patients in whom the left ventricular ejection fraction fails to increase, or the end-systolic volume fails to decrease, likely have contractile dysfunction and should be considered for early surgery (Fig. 65.6).

Surgical therapy includes mitral valve repair and mitral valve replacement. Mitral valve repair is the surgical intervention of choice. It is successful in selected patients, especially those with myxomatous valves (i.e., prolapse) or mitral regurgitation from ischemia. It is less likely to be feasible, however, in patients with endocarditis or rheumatic disease. Mitral valve repair has a lower mortality than replacement (i.e., <1%) and allows a better preservation of left ventricular systolic function through the conservation of valve-supporting structures. Freedom from reoperation at 20 years has been reported in >90% of patients who have undergone repair for mitral valve prolapse.

Mitral valve replacement is indicated when repair is not feasible, especially in rheumatic or elderly patients with calcified valves. Replacement has both a higher mortality (i.e., <5%) and morbidity than valve repair.

## Mitral Valve Prolapse

Mitral valve prolapse is a relatively common condition and is associated with myxomatous degeneration of the mitral valve. It occurs in 1% to 2% of the population and is equally prevalent in men and women. An increased amount of acid mucopolysaccharides accumulates in the valve tissue to cause prolapse. Mitral valve prolapse is associated with Marfan's syndrome, but it usually occurs as an isolated entity involving the mitral valve. Occasionally, however, the tricuspid and the aortic valves also are involved. In prolapse, the annulus may be dilated, and elongation of the chordae occurs. The valve leaflets often are redundant, with excess tissue that causes them to prolapse. The degree of abnormality tends to increase with age.

Mitral valve prolapse is associated with a spectrum of abnormality, varying from asymptomatic to severe heart

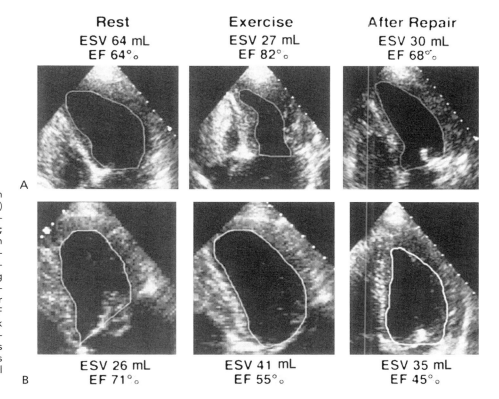

**Figure 65.6** Effects of exercise on left ventricular ejection fraction (LVEF) and end-systolic volume (ESV) in patients (A; *top three panels*) and (B; *bottom three panels*), both of whom have severe mitral regurgitation. In patient A, LVEF increases at peak exercise and ESV decreases, thus indicating preserved left ventricular systolic function. The LVEF remains normal after mitral valve repair. In patient B, LVEF declines and ESV increases at peak exercise, thus indicating latent left ventricular dysfunction, which becomes overt once the volume-loading effects that mask it are removed after mitral valve repair.

Rest
ESV 64 mL
EF 64°%

Exercise
ESV 27 mL
EF 82°%

After Repair
ESV 30 mL
EF 68°%

A

ESV 26 mL
EF 71°%

ESV 41 mL
EF 55°%

ESV 35 mL
EF 45°%

B

failure resulting from mitral regurgitation. Mitral valve prolapse often is a relatively benign condition, especially in women. In many women, prolapse becomes less prominent with age, which may reflect a relative disproportion between the size of the valve leaflets and the ventricle, which is lessened as the ventricle dilates with increasing age. Men, on the other hand, are more prone to the complications of mitral valve prolapse and are at least twice as likely as women to require surgical intervention for mitral regurgitation. Mitral valve prolapse often is associated with ventricular arrhythmia in the form of ectopy and more rarely with sustained ventricular tachycardia and sudden death.

### Diagnosis

Mitral valve prolapse often is asymptomatic at presentation and detected by a mid-systolic click on auscultation. Another presentation is with congestive heart failure from severe mitral regurgitation that results from acute chordal rupture. Patients with prolapse and regurgitation are prone to endocarditis, and they may present as such.

In young women especially, a syndrome of chest pain of nonanginal quality, paresthesia, and arrhythmia (especially ventricular ectopy) is seen. These symptoms have been attributed to autonomic imbalance, but they are as common in matched populations without prolapse as in those with prolapse.

Signs are a mid-systolic click, with or without a systolic apical murmur. The murmur typically occurs after the click in late systole, but in those with more severe prolapse, the murmur may be holosystolic. Clicks may be present even without echocardiographic prolapse. Maneuvers that decrease intracardiac volume accentuate the click and murmur, causing them to begin earlier in systole.

### Studies

Electrocardiography commonly shows inferior T-wave inversion. Mitral valve prolapse is a cause of false-positive stress electrocardiograms.

Echocardiography reveals late systolic prolapse of the posterior leaflet on M mode, as well as thickening and redundancy of the leaflets and chordae. Prolapse of either or both leaflets (posterior is much more common) can be seen on a two-dimensional echocardiogram. It is important to make the diagnosis with the parasternal or apical long-axis views rather than with the apical views. In apical views, apparent prolapse of the mitral leaflets occurs even in normal patients because the mitral annulus is not a flat plane but is saddle shaped. Thus, in this view, the mitral leaflets often appear to be displaced superior to the annular plane. Mitral regurgitation of varying severity may be present as well.

### Treatment

If severe mitral regurgitation is present, surgery is indicated. Reassuring patients of the relatively benign nature of

this condition often is beneficial. Autonomic symptoms and ventricular ectopy often respond to treatment with β-blockade (in small doses).

According to the American Heart Association guidelines, antibiotic prophylaxis is indicated for dental work and selected procedures if both a click and a murmur are present, but such prophylaxis usually is not required for a click alone.

## Aortic Stenosis

Aortic stenosis is increasingly common. Approximately 2% of the population has a bicuspid aortic valve, and 80% of cases occur in male subjects. Aortic stenosis may occur at, above, or below the valve.

### Etiology

The causes of aortic (valvular) stenosis are congenital (bicuspid, occasionally unicuspid), rheumatic, or degenerative (valvular calcification). Bicuspid valves are familial and occur in approximately 10% of first-degree relatives. Degenerative aortic valve disease has been shown to have histologic characteristics similar to that of to atherosclerosis. The progression of stenosis is promoted by hyperlipidemia, and lipid-lowering agents may slow the rate of progression. Subaortic (nonvalvular) stenosis occurs because of a congenital membrane that is seen below the aortic valve, in the left ventricular outflow tract. Hypertrophic cardiomyopathy is a dynamic obstruction of the left ventricular outflow tract as the left ventricle contracts. Supravalvular aortic stenosis is associated with hypercalcemia.

### Pathophysiology

The obstruction of the aortic valve initially leads to increased left ventricular hypertrophy and then to left ventricular dilatation and failure. The normal aortic valve opens from 3 to 4 $cm^2$. The valve area is greater than 1.5 $cm^2$ in patients with mild aortic stenosis, 1.0 to 1.5 $cm^2$ in those with moderate stenosis, and less than 1 $cm^2$ in those with severe stenosis. Critical aortic stenosis is present when the valve area is less than 0.75 $cm^2$. A normalization of the valve area, as based on the body surface area, often is useful. A valve area of less than 0.5 $cm^2/m^2$ is considered to be critical stenosis.

The pressure gradient across the valve also is used to indicate the severity of aortic stenosis, but this depends on the flow. In patients with normal heart function and without significant aortic regurgitation, a mean gradient of 50 mm Hg by Doppler or a peak-to-peak gradient of 50 mm Hg at cardiac catheterization is consistent with severe aortic stenosis. In patients with heart failure, flow may be reduced, thus giving a small gradient across the aortic valve and underestimating the degree of stenosis. Aortic regurgitation increases the flow across the valve and, in turn, the gradient for any degree of stenosis. It generally is best to measure the valve area rather than rely on the pressure gradient alone.

### Diagnosis

The symptoms of aortic stenosis are:

- Angina in patients without coronary disease because of mismatch between the blood supply and demand, especially of the subendocardium of the hypertrophied heart
- Dyspnea because of increased pulmonary capillary pressure
- Syncope caused by an inability of the heart to increase output with systemic vasodilatation, thus leading to decreased cerebral perfusion; arrhythmia also can cause syncope or sudden death in these patients

The signs of aortic stenosis are:

- Pulse is anacrotic (i.e., pulsus parvus et tardus), with slow delayed upstroke. This is the most reliable physical sign of significant aortic stenosis.
- Pulse usually is best examined at the carotid artery.
- Systolic thrill often is felt in patients with critical aortic stenosis.
- In young people with mobile valves, an ejection click may be heard.
- A harsh ejection systolic murmur over the aortic area, radiating to the neck, usually with a soft $S_2$ and $S_4$, is heard. The murmur often radiates to the apex as well.

### Studies

Electrocardiography reveals left atrial enlargement and left ventricular hypertrophy. Doppler echocardiography reveals a thickened, abnormal valve, and this study can define the severity of the lesion with the pressure gradient and valve area. Cardiac catheterization is used to assess the valve area and pressure gradient, but it usually is not indicated if Doppler gradients appear to be reliable and the patient is under 40 years of age and does not have angina.

### Treatment

Survival rates are lower among patients in whom symptoms have appeared. Once left ventricular dysfunction or congestive heart failure occurs, the 2-year survival rate is low.

Asymptomatic patients with severe aortic stenosis, except for young patients with severe congenital aortic stenosis, have a relatively low risk of death. In studies, patients who died suddenly with aortic stenosis usually had the onset of symptoms before death. In older patients, especially those with calcific aortic stenosis, the asymptomatic interval in severe aortic stenosis usually is relatively short (typically 2 to 3 years).

Therefore, patients with symptoms of syncope, angina, or dyspnea and severe aortic stenosis should be considered for surgery. No treatment usually is indicated in patients without symptoms, except in those with severe stenosis and resultant left ventricular dysfunction or in those with

severe aortic stenosis and pressure gradients of greater than 100 mm Hg; these patients may have an increased risk of sudden death. Patients with asymptomatic, severe aortic stenosis must be monitored closely using serial echocardiography at 6-month intervals (at least) and must be alerted to report their symptoms. In older patients with calcific aortic stenosis, elective surgery may be considered, even among those who are asymptomatic, given the high likelihood of its being necessary anyway. Asymptomatic patients with severe aortic stenosis should avoid heavy exertion, and young patients with aortic stenosis should refrain from competitive sports.

In young patients with fused commissures, aortic valvotomy provides good palliation for years. Often, this treatment results in significant aortic regurgitation, but it also obviates a prosthesis while growth is still occurring. Prosthetic valve replacement may be either mechanical or bioprosthetic. Biologic valves should be avoided in young patients because early degeneration is common. The mortality typically is from 2% to 3%, although it is lower in young patients.

Homograft implantation using cadaveric human valves has good intermediate-term results, but the long-term results are not known. This procedure does not require long-term anticoagulation. Aortic valve repair is possible at some centers in selected patients with congenitally bicuspid valves.

The Ross procedure involves the autotransplantation of the native pulmonic valve to the aortic position and a pulmonary homograft to the pulmonary position. This is indicated in adolescent patients because the autograft grows with the patient. The procedure, however, is technically complex.

Balloon valvuloplasty accomplished with percutaneous dilatation of the aortic valve is feasible in patients with congenital stenosis and even calcific stenosis. Results are better in younger patients. In older patients, it is used as a palliative procedure in those who cannot withstand surgery, and most often as a bridge to surgery. Short-term hemodynamic results are reasonable, and early restenosis (<6 months) is the rule. Survival rates are not affected in those patients who cannot undergo valve replacement. Morbidity and mortality, however, are substantial (i.e., 5%). This procedure is not an alternative to surgery in older patients.

## Aortic Regurgitation

### Etiology

The causes of aortic regurgitation include:

- Congenital anomaly (e.g., bicuspid valve, aortic valve prolapse)
- Rheumatic disease
- Diseases of the aorta, such as aortic root aneurysm because of Marfan's syndrome or aortic dissection

involving the ascending aorta; the mechanism of aortic regurgitation usually involves dilatation of the aortic root with poor coaptation of leaflets

- Aortitis caused by connective tissue disease or syphilis
- Endocarditis
- Degeneration (an area of leaflet coaptation becomes friable with aging)

Aortic regurgitation is rarely, if ever, caused by ischemic heart disease

### Pathophysiology

Aortic regurgitation causes volume overload of the left ventricle, which dilates to compensate for the volume load. Left ventricular dilatation is well tolerated for a long time, but, eventually, it leads to impaired systolic function and heart failure. The pressure gradient between the aorta and left ventricle is greatest at aortic valve closure and decreases progressively throughout diastole, thus giving rise to the decrescendo nature of the aortic regurgitation murmur.

### Diagnosis

Aortic regurgitation often is asymptomatic for years. If it is acute, such as in dissection or endocarditis, it may give rise to congestive symptoms that are poorly tolerated. Chest pain of an anginal nature also may be reported.

The signs of aortic regurgitation are:

- High-volume pulse with rapid falloff as blood leaks back into the left ventricle (i.e., collapsing or Corrigan's water-hammer pulse). Increased capillary pulsation also is seen (i.e., Quincke's pulse) at the nail bed, where alternate flushing and pallor of the skin is seen when light pressure is applied to the nail tip. Other signs of severe aortic regurgitation are pistol-shot femoral artery pulses and Duroziez's sign (i.e., a to-and-fro murmur over the femoral artery when it is lightly compressed with a stethoscope).
- The pulse pressure is widened, with a high systolic and a low diastolic pressure.
- Prominent pulsation of the carotid arteries is seen.
- The apex beat is hyperdynamic, and a diastolic thrill may be felt on occasion.
- The murmur of valvular aortic regurgitation is decrescendo and is heard over the aortic area and along the left sternal border. The murmur is best heard during expiration, with the patient leaning forward. When aortic regurgitation results from aortic root dilatation, the murmur frequently is heard at the right rather than the left sternal border.
- Aortic regurgitation usually is associated with an ejection systolic murmur, even in patients without clinically significant stenosis. The ejection murmur reflects increased flow across the aortic valve.
- $S_3$ and $S_4$ may be heard.
- During severe aortic regurgitation, the jet may impinge on

the opening of the anterior mitral valve leaflet and cause a mid-diastolic murmur (i.e., Austin-Flint murmur).

### Studies

Electrocardiography reveals diastolic volume overload and left ventricular hypertrophy. Doppler echocardiography can quantify and determine the mechanism of the aortic regurgitation. Serial echocardiography is used to follow left ventricular size and function over time. The chest radiography shows cardiomegaly and a prominent aorta.

Cardiac catheterization aortography is used to determine semiquantitatively the severity of aortic regurgitation. It currently is the gold standard for assessing such severity.

### Treatment

Acute, severe aortic regurgitation needs urgent surgical treatment. Afterload reduction using sodium nitroprusside can stabilize the patient while he or she is waiting for surgery. Intraaortic balloon counterpulsation increases the severity of aortic regurgitation by increasing the diastolic pressure in the aorta, and it should not be used to treat this condition.

Chronic aortic regurgitation is well tolerated for many years. Valve surgery is indicated once symptoms occur or left ventricular dysfunction manifests. After left ventricular dysfunction is present for more than 1 year, it may not normalize, even after aortic valve replacement. Sudden death is more likely once left ventricular size is greatly increased; therefore, a careful follow-up of patients with significant regurgitation is required.

Echocardiography is used to follow both the size and function of the left ventricle. Even in asymptomatic patients, surgery should be considered if the left ventricle end-systolic dimension is greater than 5 cm because surgical intervention in patients with large ventricles is associated with poor outcome. Surgery may be considered at smaller end-diastolic and end-systolic dimensions if the left ventricular enlargement is rapidly progressive or left ventricular function is declining. In asymptomatic patients with left ventricular dilatation, afterload reduction using nifedipine delays the need for surgery. Valve surgical options are similar to those for aortic stenosis, except that aortic valve repair is more likely to be possible in patients with aortic regurgitation, as compared with those with aortic stenosis.

## Tricuspid Stenosis

Tricuspid stenosis is less common than mitral stenosis. Tricuspid stenosis occurs in 5% to 10% of patients with severe mitral stenosis. Carcinoid is an additional rare cause.

Tricuspid stenosis leads to elevated right atrial pressure. In turn, this leads to peripheral edema, ascites, and low cardiac output.

## Diagnosis

Isolated tricuspid stenosis is rare, but it may lead to low cardiac output and peripheral edema. The signs include a jugular pressure with a large A wave if the patient is in normal sinus rhythm. Elevated jugular venous pressure is present as well. Auscultation reveals a diastolic murmur similar to that of mitral stenosis, except that it is best heard during inspiration and over the left sternal margin and xiphoid.

## Studies

Electrocardiography shows right atrial enlargement. Doppler echocardiography is used to measure the gradient across the tricuspid valve.

## Treatment

Right-sided symptoms should be treated with diuretics first. Balloon valvuloplasty is feasible in suitable candidates, and surgical treatment should be considered in patients undergoing mitral surgery, if the mean tricuspid gradient is greater than 4 or 5 mm Hg. If surgical repair is unsuccessful, prosthetic replacement usually is performed using a tissue valve (because of the increased risk of thrombosis with mechanical prostheses at this position).

## Tricuspid Regurgitation

Tricuspid regurgitation may be either primary or secondary. Primary tricuspid regurgitation usually results from rheumatic disease. Other causes include carcinoid, congenital abnormalities (e.g., Ebstein's anomaly), right ventricular ischemia or infarction, tricuspid valve prolapse, trauma, or endocarditis.

   Secondary tricuspid regurgitation results from conditions that cause pulmonary hypertension, with resultant right ventricle dilatation and dilatation of the tricuspid annulus. Tricuspid regurgitation leads to reduced cardiac output, with peripheral edema as well as hepatic and gastrointestinal congestion.

## Diagnosis

Tricuspid regurgitation causes symptoms of low cardiac output (e.g., fatigue) or right-sided failure (e.g., anorexia) from passive congestion of the liver and gastrointestinal tract. The signs include large V waves in the jugular venous pulse. Auscultation reveals a pansystolic murmur, which is heard best during inspiration at the left sternal border and subxiphoid area.

## Studies

Electrocardiography reveals right atrial enlargement and right ventricular hypertrophy. Doppler echocardiography can be used to determine both the severity of the regurgitation and its cause.

## Treatment

Isolated, severe tricuspid regurgitation may not require any treatment apart from diuretics. Surgical repair or replacement might be considered in patients with congestive symptoms that are refractory to medical treatment. In patients with secondary tricuspid regurgitation, the primary condition should be treated. In those with tricuspid regurgitation secondary to mitral or aortic valve disease, however, tricuspid annuloplasty should be considered at the time of surgery for the primary condition.

## Diet Drugs and Valve Disease

Certain anorexigenic drugs, either alone or in combination, have been associated with a valvulopathy. Drugs involved include phentermine, fenfluramine, and dexfenfluramine. The valvulopathy occurs mainly at the mitral and aortic valves and has similarities to rheumatic disease, carcinoid syndrome, and ergot valve disease. The pathophysiology of the valve lesion currently is unknown, although serotonin has been implicated, given the similarity to carcinoid syndrome. The predominant hemodynamic abnormality is regurgitation rather than stenosis. Valvulopathy consists of thickening and restriction of the valve leaflets and supporting structures. A minority of patients taking the drugs develop valvulopathy, although some patients have required surgical repair or replacement of the affected valves. The longer the duration of treatment with these anorexigenic agents, the more likely is a valvulopathy to develop. Improvement in the valvulopathy after cessation of the anorexigenic agents has been reported. Patients who have taken anorexigenic drugs should undergo physical examination of the heart, and echocardiography is recommended if any clinical suspicion of valve disease emerges.

## REVIEW EXERCISES

### QUESTIONS

   **1.** The most common cause of mitral regurgitation in the United States today is
a) Rheumatic disease
b) Myxomatous disease (prolapse)
c) Endocarditis
d) Hypertension
e) None of the above

   **2.** Which of the following is untrue about mitral stenosis?
a) It is more common in men.
b) It is usually rheumatic in origin.
c) It is associated with a diastolic murmur.
d) A presystolic murmur is heard in mitral stenosis in those in sinus rhythm.
e) The duration of the diastolic murmur predicts severity of the stenosis.

3. All the following are indications for surgery in severe mitral regurgitation, *except*
a) Shortness of breath on exertion
b) Left ventricular ejection fraction 45%
c) Dilated left ventricle (end-systolic dimension 5 cm)
d) Frequent ventricular ectopy
e) Recurrent atrial fibrillation

4. Consider the following hemodynamic data: left atrial pressure, 25 mm Hg; left ventricular pressure, 120/10 mm Hg; aortic pressure, 120/80 mm Hg; and cardiac index, 1.9 L/min/m². These are most consistent with which valvular lesion?
a) Mitral stenosis
b) Mitral regurgitation
c) Aortic stenosis
d) Aortic regurgitation
e) None of the above

5. Recognized complications of isolated mitral stenosis include all of the following, *except*
a) Atrial fibrillation
b) Pulmonary hypertension
c) Atrial thrombus
d) Right heart failure
e) Left ventricular enlargement

6. The following statements concerning surgical correction of mitral regurgitation are correct, *except*
a) Repair is most likely to be possible in rheumatic valves.
b) Repair has a lower complication rate than prosthetic replacement.
c) Left ventricular function declines more after prosthetic replacement than with repair.
d) Surgery is indicated in severe mitral regurgitation with symptomatic deterioration.
e) Men are more likely to require surgical correction of regurgitation than women.

7. Common symptoms of aortic stenosis include all of the following, *except*
a) Dyspnea
b) Syncope
c) Ankle edema
d) Angina
e) Fatigue

8. The most reliable physical finding in predicting severe aortic stenosis is
a) Loudness of the murmur
b) Absent first heart sound
c) Loud second heart sound
d) Delayed carotid upstroke
e) Left ventricular heave

9. Surgical intervention is indicated in severe aortic stenosis for all of the following, *except*
a) Recent exercise-induced syncope

b) Left ventricular ejection fraction of 45% with normal coronary vessels
c) Shortness of breath on walking two blocks
d) Associated significant aortic regurgitation
e) Exertional chest pain usually relieved by rest

10. Consider the following hemodynamic data: left atrial pressure, 15 mm Hg; left ventricular pressure, 220/15 mm Hg; aorta pressure, 100/60 mm Hg; and cardiac index, 1.9 L/min/m². These are most consistent with which valvular lesion?
a) Tricuspid stenosis
b) Mitral stenosis
c) Aortic stenosis
d) Aortic regurgitation
e) Tricuspid regurgitation

11. Indications for surgical treatment in severe aortic regurgitation include the following, *except*
a) Left ventricular ejection fraction 53%
b) Increasing left ventricular size on sequential echo (left ventricular end-systolic dimension 6 cm)
c) Shortness of breath
d) Aortic root size >6 cm
e) Anginal chest pain

12. A 27-year-old woman has recent onset of shortness of breath going upstairs and a history of palpitations. Physical examination reveals a regular pulse, loud $S_1$, and an apical diastolic murmur. The most likely diagnosis is
a) Aortic stenosis
b) Mitral stenosis
c) Aortic regurgitation
d) Tricuspid stenosis
e) None of the above

## ANSWERS

1. b.
Mitral valve prolapse is the most common cause of mitral regurgitation in the United States today.

2. a.
Mitral stenosis is more common in women than in men.

3. d.
Frequent ventricular ectopy is common and does not necessarily improve with surgery. It is not considered an indication for valve surgery in mitral regurgitation.

4. a.
Mitral stenosis; high left atrial pressure with a pressure gradient across the mitral valve in diastole and a low cardiac output.

5. e.
Isolated mitral stenosis does not cause left ventricular enlargement; left ventricle size is normal or small due to reduced inflow to the left ventricle.

**6. a.**

Mitral valve repair is most likely to be successful in mitral valve prolapse and least likely in rheumatic disease and endocarditis.

**7. b.**

Ankle edema is uncommon in aortic stenosis.

**8. d.**

Delayed carotid upstroke is the most reliable predictor of severe aortic stenosis.

**9. d.**

Aortic regurgitation does not affect the decision regarding surgery in aortic stenosis. Surgery is indicated for symptoms and left ventricular dysfunction.

**10. c.**

Low cardiac output and large pressure gradient between left ventricle and aorta in systole diagnose aortic stenosis.

**11. a.**

Reduced left ventricular ejection fraction, to less than 50%, is considered an indication for surgery.

**12. b.**

Mitral stenosis.

## SUGGESTED READINGS

Bonow RO, Carabello BA, de Leon AC, et al. ACC/AHA Guidelines for the management of patients with valvular heart disease. *Circulation* 1998;98:1949.

Connolly HM, Crary JL, McGoon MD, et al. Valvular heart disease associated with fenfluramine-phentermine. *N Engl J Med* 1997;337:581.

Dajani AS, Taubert KA, Wilson W, et al. Prevention of bacterial endocarditis. Recommendations by the American Heart Association. *JAMA* 1997;277:1794–801.

Durack DT, Lukas AS, Bright DK. New criteria for diagnosis of infective endocarditis: utilization of specific echocardiographic findings. *Am J Med* 1994;96:200–209.

Griffin BP. Valvular heart disease. *Sci Am Med* 2001;11:1–12.

Levine HJ, Gaasch WH. Vasoactive drugs in chronic regurgitant lesions of the mitral and aortic valves. *J Am Coll Cardiol* 1996;28: 1083.

Marso S, Griffin BP, Topol EJ, ed. *Manual of Cardiovascular Medicine.* Philadelphia: Lippincott Williams & Wilkins, 2000.

# Arrhythmias

66

*Mina K. Chung*

Cardiac arrhythmias can be categorized on the basis of mechanisms, rates, and associated risk. When considering rate, tachycardias generally consist of arrhythmias with rates of more than 100 beats/min. Significant bradycardias generally consist of arrhythmias with rates of less than 60 beats/min. The appropriate diagnosis and assessment of the risk associated with arrhythmias is important to their treatment.

## TACHYARRHYTHMIAS

### Mechanisms

The mechanisms underlying cardiac arrhythmias usually are categorized into disorders of impulse formation, impulse conduction, or a combination of both.

#### Disorders of Impulse Formation

##### Automaticity

Automaticity is the property of a cell or fiber to initiate a spontaneous impulse without previous stimulation. Spontaneously discharging cardiac cells that initiate spontaneous action potentials during phase 4 diastolic depolarization result in automaticity. The rate at which the sinus node discharges usually is faster than, and suppresses, the discharge rate of other potential latent or subsidiary automatic pacemaker sites. Normal or abnormal automaticity at the sinus node or other ectopic sites, however, can lead to rates that are faster and can gain control of the cardiac rhythm for one or more cycles. This may manifest if the discharge rate of the sinus node slows or that of the latent pacemaker increases.

***Normal Automaticity.*** Cells that can exhibit spontaneous phase 4 diastolic depolarization are located in the sinus node, atria, atrioventricular junction, and the His-Purkinje system. Normal automaticity generally occurs in normal cells with normal membrane resting potentials. It can be suppressed by overdrive pacing, but generally resumes after the termination of pacing. Subsidiary pacemakers can become dominant in the settings of acidosis, ischemia, sympathetic stimulation, and use of certain drugs. Examples of arrhythmias in this category include sinus tachycardia that is inappropriate to the clinical situation and, possibly, ventricular parasystole.

***Abnormal Automaticity.*** Normal myocardial cells maintain membrane resting potentials at approximately −90 mV, and they depolarize only when stimulated. Abnormal automaticity, however, can occur in cells with reduced maximum diastolic potentials, often at membrane potentials of −50 to −60 mV. The partial depolarization and failure to reach or maintain the normal maximum diastolic potential may induce automatic discharge. Examples of tachycardias that likely result from abnormal automaticity include accelerated junctional rhythm (i.e., nonparoxysmal junctional tachycardia), accelerated idioventricular rhythms, certain atrial tachycardias, some ventricular tachycardias (VTs) in patients without structural heart disease, exercise-induced VT, VT during the first several hours of myocardial infarction (MI), and some VTs in patients with marked electrolyte imbalance.

##### Triggered Activity

Unlike automaticity, which does not require previous stimulation to occur, triggered activity is initiated by oscillations in the membrane potential (i.e., afterdepolarizations) that are induced by preceding action potentials. Afterdepolarizations that occur before full repolarization is completed are called *early afterdepolarizations* (EADs); those that occur after completion of repolarization, during phase 4, are called *delayed afterdepolarizations* (DADs). If afterdepolarizations reach threshold potential, an action potential can be generated, which potentially can trigger another or repetitive afterdepolarization(s).

***Early Afterdepolarizations.*** Occurring during phase 2 or 3 of the action potential, EADs are thought to be responsible for VTs associated with prolonged repolarization, such as long QT syndromes (acquired or congenital) and torsades de pointes (TdP). Rapid rates and magnesium both suppress EADs as well as these arrhythmias. Experimentally, EADs can be produced by hypoxia, cesium, as well as class IA (e.g., quinidine) and III (e.g., sotalol) antiarrhythmic agents.

***Delayed Afterdepolarizations.*** Occurring after repolarization during phase 4, DADs have been demonstrated in Purkinje's fibers as well as in atrial and ventricular fibers exposed to digitalis. Faster rates may augment DADs and are associated with an increase in intracellular calcium

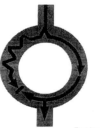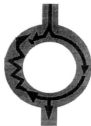

- Pathway of conduction
- Unidirectional block
- Slow conduction

**Figure 66.1** Reentry.

overload. Clinically, DADs have been classically implicated in digitalis toxicity as well as in those tachyarrhythmias associated with catecholamine excess, acidosis, MI, and certain VTs (e.g., verapamil-responsive VT).

### Disorders of Impulse Conduction

Conduction delay or block can produce bradyarrhythmias or tachyarrhythmias. The most common mechanism of tachyarrhythmias is reentry. Classically, reentry requires

- Alternate or separate pathways of conduction as defined by anatomic barriers (e.g., myocardial scar, atrioventricular node, and accessory pathway) or functional properties (e.g., no anatomic boundaries but contiguous fibers with different electrophysiologic properties, such as local differences in refractoriness, excitability, or anisotropic intercellular resistances)
- An area of unidirectional block in one pathway
- An area of conduction in the alternate pathway that is slow enough for the propagating and returning impulse to meet and excite tissue proximal to the block that has recovered (Fig. 66.1)

Reentry is thought to be the mechanism underlying most recurrent paroxysmal tachycardias. These include atrial flutter, atrial fibrillation, atrioventricular nodal reentry, atrioventricular reentry involving accessory pathways (including Wolff-Parkinson-White syndrome), and most VTs associated with ischemic heart disease and previous MI.

## Diagnosis

### Patient History and Physical Examination

A key to diagnosing and appropriately treating patients with arrhythmias is the determination of the underlying, predisposing cardiac substrate. Known structural heart disease, particularly in patients with known coronary artery disease or ischemic or nonischemic cardiomyopathies, can greatly influence both treatment and diagnosis. Patients presenting with wide QRS complex tachycardias and previous MI almost always have VT. Triggering agents (e.g., inotropic or QT-prolonging drugs) or events may be important to longer term treatment and the subsequent

**TABLE 66.1**
**DIFFERENTIAL DIAGNOSIS OF TACHYCARDIAS**

| Regular Rhythm | Irregular Rhythm |
|---|---|
| Narrow QRS complex | |
|   Atrial tachycardia | Atrial fibrillation |
|     Sinus tachycardia | Atrial flutter, variable AV block |
|     Sinus node reentry | Multifocal atrial tachycardia |
|     Ectopic atrial tachycardia | |
|   Atrial flutter, fixed AV block | |
|   AV nodal reentrant tachycardia | |
|   Orthodromic AV reentry | |
| Wide QRS complex | |
|   Ventricular tachycardia | Ventricular tachycardia |
|   Supraventricular tachycardia | Atrial fibrillation with |
|     Preexisting BBB |   Preexisting BBB |
|     Functional BBB |   Functional BBB |
|     Preexcitation |   Preexcitation |
|       Antidromic AV reentry | Torsades de pointes |
|       Bystander accessory pathway | |

AV, atrioventricular; BBB, bundle branch block.

prevention of arrhythmias. In addition to hemodynamic status and the evidence of underlying valvular or ventricular dysfunction, helpful physical findings include evidence of atrioventricular dissociation (i.e., cannon A waves in the jugular venous pulse) and termination or slowing with vagal maneuvers (e.g., carotid sinus massage, Valsalva's maneuver, cough, cold-water immersion) or adenosine.

### Differential Diagnosis

Tachyarrhythmias can be classified into wide versus narrow QRS complex and regular versus irregular tachycardia (Table 66.1). An electrocardiographic (ECG) evaluation of tachycardias should begin by assessing the rate, regularity, and QRS complex width. Narrow QRS complex tachycardias, which are defined as tachycardias with a QRS complex width of less than 120 ms, implies ventricular activation over the rapidly conducting His-Purkinje system, which in turn suggests a supraventricular tachycardia (SVT; a tachycardia requiring atrial or atrioventricular junctional tissue for initiation or maintenance). Irregularity of the ventricular rate during an SVT suggests atrial fibrillation, atrial flutter with variable block, or multifocal atrial tachycardia. A wide QRS complex tachycardia may result from VT or SVT and is discussed later.

### Narrow QRS Complex Tachycardias

ECG evaluation of narrow QRS complex tachycardias should include assessment of:

- Rate
- Regularity
- QRS complex width
- Atrial activation pattern and relationship to the QRS complex (RP/PR relationship, morphology of the P wave)

- QRS complex morphology
- Effect of bundle branch block (BBB) aberration (if present)
- Mode of initiation
- Effect of vagal maneuvers and drugs

SVTs may be classified as:

- Sinus node tachycardias
  - □ Inappropriate sinus tachycardia
  - □ Sinus node reentry
- Atrial tachycardias
  - □ Automatic
  - □ Reentrant
- Atrial flutter
- Atrial fibrillation
- Multifocal atrial tachycardia
- Junctional tachycardias
  - □ Nonparoxysmal
  - □ Automatic
- Atrioventricular nodal reentry
  - □ Typical
  - □ Atypical
- Atrioventricular reciprocating tachycardia and other SVTs associated with accessory pathways

In narrow QRS complex tachycardias, the relationship of the QRS complex and P waves can be important in establishing the diagnosis. Figure 66.2 shows the QRS complex and P-wave relationships and configurations commonly seen in patients with various SVTs, and these conditions are discussed further in later sections on specific arrhythmias.

In typical atrioventricular nodal reentrant tachycardia (AVNRT), which is characterized by near simultaneous atrial and ventricular activation, the P wave is buried in the QRS complex, and it either is not visible or is detected at the end of the QRS complex (within 80 ms) in 94% of cases. In 2% of cases, the P wave barely precedes the QRS complex and can be diagnostic. Atypical AVNRT occurs in 4% of cases and is characterized by a long RP interval and a short PR interval, with inverted P waves in the inferior (i.e., II, III, $aV_F$) leads. In orthodromic atrioventricular reentrant tachycardia (AVRT) mediated by a retrograde-conducting accessory pathway, the retrograde P wave often can be detected early in the ST segment. Slowly conducting retrograde accessory pathways can have long RP intervals. Atrial tachycardias, sinus tachycardia, and sinoatrial node reentrant tachycardia have long RP and short PR intervals, with the P-wave morphology differing from that of sinus rhythm in ectopic atrial tachycardias, but being similar in sinoatrial node reentrant tachycardia or sinus tachycardia.

Thus, close examination of the PR and RP intervals can be helpful. The differential diagnosis of short RP (i.e., RP interval shorter than the PR interval) and long RP (i.e., RP interval longer than the PR interval) SVTs is shown in Figure 66.3. Short RP narrow complex tachycardias most likely result from AVNRT or orthodromic AVRT mediated by a retrograde-conducting accessory pathway; atrial tachycardia is a much less likely cause. Long RP narrow complex tachycardias result from atrial (or sinus) tachycardias, atypical AVNRT, or orthodromic AVRT mediated by a slow-retrograde-conducting accessory pathway.

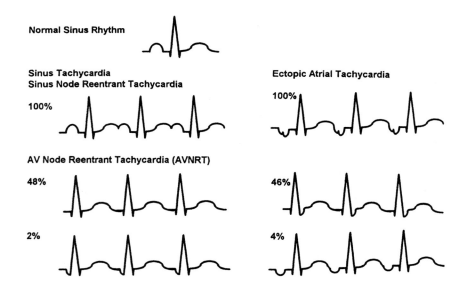

**Figure 66.2** Relationships and configurations of QRS and P waves in supraventricular tachycardia. AV, atrioventricular. (Adapted with permission from Josephson ME. *Clinical Cardiac Electrophysiology: Techniques and Interpretation*, 2nd ed. Malvern, PA: Lea & Febiger, 1993;269.)

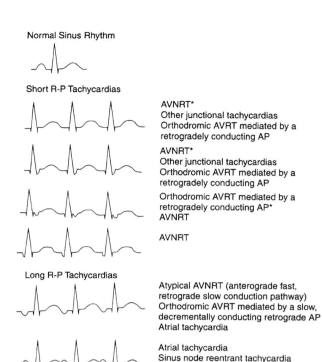

Normal Sinus Rhythm

Short R-P Tachycardias

AVNRT*
Other junctional tachycardias
Orthodromic AVRT mediated by a
retrogradely conducting AP

AVNRT*
Other junctional tachycardias
Orthodromic AVRT mediated by a
retrogradely conducting AP

Orthodromic AVRT mediated by a
retrogradely conducting AP*
AVNRT

AVNRT

Long R-P Tachycardias

Atypical AVNRT (anterograde fast,
retrograde slow conduction pathway)
Orthodromic AVRT mediated by a slow,
decrementally conducting retrograde AP
Atrial tachycardia

Atrial tachycardia
Sinus node reentrant tachycardia
Sinus tachycardia

**Figure 66.3** Differential diagnosis of supraventricular tachycardias by RP/PR relationships and P-wave configurations. *, most common; AP, accessory pathway; AVNRT, atrioventricular nodal reentrant tachycardia; AVRT, atrioventricular reentrant tachycardia. (Adapted with permission from Josephson ME. *Clinical Cardiac Electrophysiology: Techniques and Interpretation*, 2nd ed. Malvern, PA: Lea & Febiger, 1993;270.)

### Wide QRS Complex Tachycardia

Wide complex tachycardia (WCT) has a QRS duration of 120 ms or longer, with a ventricular rate of 100 beats/min or more.

### Differential Diagnosis

The differential diagnosis of WCT includes:

- VT
- SVT
  - SVT with preexisting BBB or intraventricular conduction defect
  - SVT with aberrant His-Purkinje system conduction (i.e., functional BBB)
  - Ashman's phenomenon after long-short RR interval
  - Rate-related, acceleration-dependent BBB
  - Maintenance of functional BBB by transseptal concealed conduction (i.e., linking)
  - SVT with antegrade conduction via an accessory pathway
    - Antidromic SVT with antegrade conduction via an accessory pathway
    - Atrial fibrillation/flutter/tachycardia with antegrade conduction via an accessory pathway
    - AVNRT with antegrade conduction down a bystander accessory pathway
  - SVT with slowed conduction because of electrolyte or metabolic imbalance or an antiarrhythmic drug

The diagnosis of WCT often can be established on the basis of clinical presentation, physical examination, ECG findings, and provocative maneuvers. As a general rule, however, treat as a VT when in doubt, particularly in patients with structural heart disease.

### Clinical Presentation

In multiple studies, VT was the correct diagnosis in more than 80% of patients presenting with WCT. VT is more likely to occur in older patients, but age alone is not a useful marker. In very young patients (<20 years), SVT is a more frequent cause of WCT. VT can occur in younger patients with structurally normal hearts, but this is uncommon. Hemodynamic instability is a poor discriminating factor because hemodynamic stability depends on rate, ventricular function, cardiac disease, and concomitant pharmacologic therapy. A history of structural heart disease, particularly of coronary artery disease with previous MI, is important. In patients with a history of MI, 98% of WCTs result from VT; a history of MI and symptoms of tachycardia starting only after the MI strongly favor VT.

### Physical Examination

Rate and blood pressure are not useful in determining the cause of WCTs. The finding of atrioventricular dissociation, however, strongly favors VT. This is because approximately two-thirds of patients with VT have atrioventricular dissociation at electrophysiology study, and atrioventricular dissociation is rare in SVT. An asynchronous contraction of the atria and ventricles can cause cannon A waves in the jugular venous pulsation, wide split heart sounds, variable $S_1$, and variability in blood pressure resulting from changes in stroke volume with atrioventricular dissociation.

### Provocative Maneuvers

Vagal maneuvers can depress sinus node automaticity and slow atrioventricular nodal conduction. A gradual slowing of the rate of the WCT suggests sinus tachycardia. A termination of the rhythm suggests reentry involving the atrioventricular node or sinus node (e.g., sinoatrial node reentrant tachycardia, AVNRT, AVRT). Transient block with reinitiation suggests atrial tachycardia, atrial fibrillation, or atrial flutter. VT rarely is affected by vagal maneuvers.

It is important that intravenous verapamil not be used to treat WCT because hemodynamic collapse and death have been reported, regardless of the cause of the WCT. Adenosine has a much shorter duration of action (i.e., seconds) and is delivered intravenously as a 6- to 12-mg rapid bolus. Like vagal maneuvers, adenosine can terminate supraventricular arrhythmias resulting from reentry involving the atrioventricular or sinus node, or it can allow the demonstration of atrial flutter waves, atrial tachycardia, or atrial fibrillation. Some uncommon forms of VT in structurally normal hearts can be terminated by vagal maneuvers or adenosine.

### Electrocardiographic Findings

In patients with preexisting complete BBB, the QRS complex is wide, and a comparison with previous ECGs can be helpful. The QRS complex may be wide in any supraventricular rhythm, however, if functional aberrancy occurs. Patients receiving antiarrhythmic drugs, particularly class IC agents, may develop rate-related aberrancy. Preexcitation via an anterograde-conducting accessory pathway (i.e., Wolff-Parkinson-White syndrome) also causes a wide QRS complex. The ECG should be analyzed, with specific attention paid to the atrioventricular relationship, presence of capture or fusion beats, and QRS duration, axis, and morphology.

Fusion beats occur when conducted supraventricular impulses depolarize the ventricle coincident with ventricular depolarization from the VT circuit. A narrower, usually intermediate-width QRS complex results. Narrow beats during WCT strongly favor the diagnosis of VT, but they are not pathognomonic [e.g., premature ventricular contraction (PVC) during SVT with BBB could also result in a narrower QRS complex].

Capture beats represent the conduction of a supraventricular impulse to the ventricle and depolarization before it is depolarized by the VT circuit. It appears as a narrow complex beat with a shorter coupling interval than the tachycardia interval, which indicates that the WCT is VT. Capture beats virtually exclude SVT with aberrancy because they occur after a shorter interval with a narrow QRS complex; aberrancy is more likely to occur with wider QRS complexes after shorter rather than longer intervals.

Atrioventricular dissociation strongly favors the diagnosis of VT, but this feature is not always identifiable on surface ECGs. One-third of VTs may have 1:1 ventriculoatrial

(VA) conduction. Even so, variable retrograde VA conduction, or VA Wenckebach conduction, strongly suggests VT. Rare SVTs may exhibit VA dissociation (e.g., automatic junctional tachycardia with retrograde block). The recording of an atrial electrogram through a right atrial or an esophageal electrode may facilitate assessment.

QRS complex morphology can help to distinguish SVT with aberrancy from VT. QRS concordance in leads $V_1$ through $V_6$ is predictive of VT, but also can be seen in patients with Wolff-Parkinson-White syndrome. Delayed or slowed initial QRS deflection suggests VT. The QRS complex morphology can be classified into a left BBB or a right BBB pattern on the basis of QRS polarity in $V_1$. Right BBB morphology has a predominantly positive QRS deflection, and left BBB morphology a predominantly negative QRS deflection, in $V_1$. In right BBB morphology WCT (Fig. 66.4), a monophasic R, qR, RS, or R greater than r′ pattern in $V_1$ favors VT. In $V_6$ a QS, QR, or monophasic R pattern also favors VT. In contrast, triphasic complexes in $V_1$ or $V_6$ favor SVT. In left BBB morphology WCT (Fig. 66.5), an R in $V_1$ or $V_2$ of 40 ms or greater, notched downstroke on the S wave in $V_1$ or $V_2$, any Q in $V_6$, or more than 60 ms from the QRS onset to the S nadir in $V_1$ or $V_2$ favors VT.

A commonly used four-level algorithm for distinguishing VT from SVT (i.e., the Brugada criteria) is shown in Figure 66.6. This algorithm was prospectively validated for more than 500 WCTs with electrophysiologic diagnoses. It had a high sensitivity (0.987) and specificity (0.965). Using these criteria, if no RS can be identified in any precordial lead, VT is diagnosed. If an RS complex is present and the RS interval is longer than 100 ms, VT is diagnosed. If the RS interval is shorter than 100 ms, evidence of atrioventricular dissociation indicates VT. If none of the first three criteria is met, then morphologic criteria for VT are analyzed in leads $V_1$ or $V_2$, as well as $V_6$. If both leads fulfill the criteria for VT,

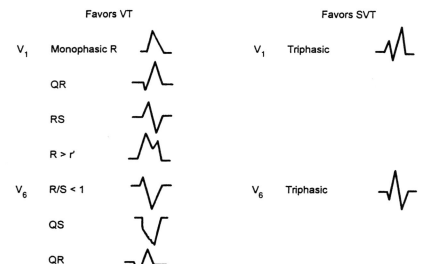

**Favors VT**

$V_1$  Monophasic R

    QR

    RS

    R > r′

$V_6$  R/S < 1

    QS

    QR

    Monophasic R

**Favors SVT**

$V_1$  Triphasic

$V_6$  Triphasic

**Figure 66.4** Right bundle branch block morphologic criteria for distinguishing ventricular tachycardia (VT) from supraventricular tachycardia (SVT). (Adapted with permission from Wellens HJJ, Bar FWHM, Lie KI. The value of the electrocardiogram in the differential diagnosis of a tachycardia with a widened QRS complex. *Am J Med* 1978;64:27–33.)

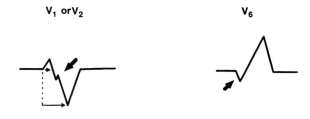

**V₁ orV₂**          **V₆**

1    R in V₁ or V₂ ≥ 40 ms sec.

2    >60 msec from QRS onset to S nadir in V₁ or V₂.

3    Notched downstroke S wave in V₁ or V₂.

4    Any Q in V₆.

**Figure 66.5** Left bundle branch block morphologic criteria for ventricular tachycardia in leads V₁ and V₆. (Adapted with permission from Kindwall KE, Brown J, Josephson ME. Electrocardiographic criteria for ventricular tachycardia in wide complex left bundle branch block morphology tachycardias. *Am J Cardiol* 1988; 61:1279–1283.)

then VT is diagnosed; otherwise, the diagnosis of SVT with aberrancy is made by exclusion of VT.

Other ECG clues include the consistent initiation of WCT by premature atrial contractions, which favors a supraventricular rhythm. The initiation of WCT preceded by constant PP intervals, but a short PR interval (with the QRS complex fused to the P wave), in patients without preexcitation suggests VT. Grossly irregular RR intervals suggest atrial fibrillation. If a rapid, irregular WCT has beat-to-beat variation in the QRS complex duration, Wolff-Parkinson-White syndrome should be suspected. A comparison with previous sinus rhythm ECGs is helpful to determine preexisting preexcitation or baseline BBB/intraventricular conduction defect.

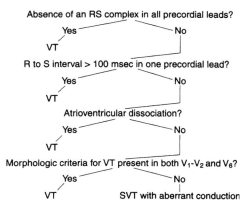

Absence of an RS complex in all precordial leads?

Yes ———————— No

VT

R to S interval > 100 msec in one precordial lead?

Yes ———————— No

VT

Atrioventricular dissociation?

Yes ———————— No

VT

Morphologic criteria for VT present in both V₁-V₂ and V₆?

Yes ———————— No

VT          SVT with aberrant conduction

**Figure 66.6** Brugada criteria for distinguishing ventricular tachycardia (VT) from supraventricular tachycardia (SVT) in tachycardia with widened QRS complexes. (Reprinted with permission from Brugada P, Brugada J, Mont L, et al. A new approach to the differential diagnosis of a regular tachycardia with a wide QRS complex. *Circulation* 1991;83:1649–1659.)

A QRS complex duration of longer than 140 ms with WCT of right BBB morphology, or of longer than 160 ms with left BBB morphology, favors the diagnosis of VT. Most SVTs with aberrancy have QRS complex durations of 140 ms or less, but wide QRS complex durations can be seen with preexcitation and marked baseline intraventricular conduction defects. In addition, 15% to 35% of patients with VT also may have QRS complex durations of 140 ms or less.

QRS axis deviation with a right superior axis (i.e., negative in I, aV_F) suggests VT. Left superior axis (i.e., left axis deviation; negative in aV_F, II; positive in I) in WCT with right BBB morphology suggests VT, but it is not helpful in WCT with left BBB morphology.

### Treatment

For hemodynamically unstable WCT, including pulmonary edema or severe angina, cardioversion should be performed (including 200 J to 300 to 360 J if initially unsuccessful). Sedation should be given before cardioversion if the patient is awake. For hemodynamically stable WCT, a clinical history (including cardiac disease, previous arrhythmias, previous MI, drug use) should be elicited and physical examination performed (including inspection for cannon A waves). A 12-lead ECG and laboratory studies to exclude electrolyte and metabolic abnormalities, ischemia, hypoxia, or drug toxicity should be obtained. If the diagnosis is in doubt, placement of an esophageal lead can be considered. Adenosine, 6 to 12 mg delivered intravenously as a rapid bolus, can be given. Lidocaine or procainamide can be attempted as well, and if the WCT persists, bretylium or intravenous amiodarone can be considered. Cardioversion under anesthesia or overdrive pace termination can be attempted for persistent WCT. If WCT is incessant, consider the possibility of electrolyte abnormalities, digitalis toxicity, acute severe ischemia, reperfusion arrhythmias, proarrhythmia, or TdP. Consideration also should be given to empiric MgSO₄, treatment for acute ischemia or MI, and intravenous amiodarone.

An evaluation after the termination of WCT should include a consideration of electrophysiologic testing to determine the WCT etiology. Subsequent therapy depends on the diagnosis but can include pharmacologic, ablation, or device therapies.

## SPECIFIC SUPRAVENTRICULAR ARRHYTHMIAS

### Atrial Premature Depolarizations

Atrial premature depolarizations can be frequent and occasionally symptomatic. Although not associated with significant risk, they can be associated with underlying cardiovascular or pulmonary disease. Treatment generally includes reassurance, avoidance of precipitating factors (e.g., caffeine, sympathomimetic agents), and occasionally β-blockers or calcium channel blockers.

## Sinus Tachycardia

Sinus tachycardia is defined in an adult as a sinus rate of greater than 100 beats/min. The sinus node is located in the high right atrium and is sensitive to catecholamines and autonomic tone. Therefore, sinus tachycardia may be secondary to many physiologic and pathologic states. It is a normal response to exertion, anxiety, and a variety of stresses, including fever, hypotension, hypovolemia, hyperthyroidism, congestive heart failure, pulmonary embolism, myocardial ischemia or infarction, inflammation, and drugs, such as catecholamines, caffeine, alcohol, or nicotine. Because of the location and automatic properties associated with the sinus node, physiologic sinus tachycardia has normal P-wave morphology (i.e., upright in II, III, and $aV_F$) and exhibits gradual rate acceleration and deceleration that varies with changes in the autonomic tone and volume. Treatment should focus on the cause of sinus tachycardia, avoidance of stimulants, fluid replacement in patients with hypovolemia, fever reduction, and, possibly, β-blockers or calcium channel blockers.

### Inappropriate Sinus Tachycardia

Inappropriate sinus tachycardia, in which otherwise healthy patients have chronic, nonparoxysmal sinus tachycardia without apparent cause or at an inappropriate rate, may result from increased automaticity, increased sympathetic tone, increased sensitivity to catecholamines, decreased vagal tone, or an automatic atrial focus located near the sinus node. Treatment may require β-blockers, calcium channel blockers, digitalis, or sinus node radiofrequency modification or surgical ablation.

### Sinus Node Reentry

Sinus node reentry, which only rarely occurs, may be difficult to distinguish from sinus tachycardia. The onset typically is sudden and paroxysmal, and it often is precipitated by a premature atrial beat, which is important in establishing the diagnosis. The heart rate can vary from 80 to 200 beats/min, but generally is slower than in other SVTs, with an average rate of 130 to 140 beats/min. The rate also can fluctuate with the autonomic tone. P-wave morphology demonstrates a high-to-low atrial activation sequence (i.e., upright in II, III, $aV_F$) that is identical to sinus rhythm in morphology. The PR interval relates to the SVT rate, with a long RP interval and a shorter PR interval. Atrioventricular block can occur (e.g., Wenckebach) without affecting the tachycardia. Vagal maneuvers (e.g., carotid sinus massage, Valsalva's maneuver) or adenosine can slow and terminate the tachycardia. Drugs, such as β-blockers or calcium channel blockers, as well as class I or III antiarrhythmic agents, also have been used successfully. Surgical or radiofrequency catheter ablation occasionally may be indicated.

## Atrial Tachycardias

Tachycardias originating in the atria at sites other than the sinus or atrioventricular node are called atrial, or ectopic atrial, tachycardias. Heart rates generally are regular, ranging from 100 to 250 (generally 150 to 200) beats/min, with a P-wave morphology differing from that in sinus rhythm and isoelectric periods between P waves, thus distinguishing it from atrial flutter or atrial fibrillation. A long RP interval (with a shorter PR interval) that is variable in duration usually is present. Atrioventricular conduction block (i.e., spontaneous Wenckebach second-degree atrioventricular block or atrioventricular block induced by carotid sinus massage, other vagal maneuvers, or adenosine) typically does not terminate the tachycardia. A positive or biphasic P wave in aVL suggests a right atrial origin. A positive P wave in $V_1$ suggests a left atrial focus. At physical examination, rapid A waves in the jugular venous pulse may be evident.

Atrial tachycardia can occur paroxysmally in short, nonsustained runs or in longer, sustained runs, and they occasionally may be incessant, potentially leading to a tachycardia-mediated cardiomyopathy. It often is associated with significant structural heart disease, pulmonary disease, hyperthyroidism, or digitalis intoxication. Three mechanisms of atrial tachycardias have been described: abnormal automaticity, reentry, and triggered activity. In general, and depending on the clinical situation, treatment in patients not receiving digitalis may include atrioventricular node-blocking agents (e.g., calcium channel blockers, β-blockers, digitalis); class IA, IC, or III antiarrhythmic agents; or surgical or radiofrequency catheter ablation.

### Atrial Tachycardia with Block Resulting from Digitalis Toxicity

In digitalis toxicity, the concomitant impairment of atrioventricular conduction can cause atrial tachycardia with block, and triggered activity (i.e., DAD) is believed to be the mechanism responsible for the atrial tachycardia. This may occur in patients with atrial fibrillation or flutter, but it can be distinguished by isoelectric periods between P waves. Treatment includes cessation of digitalis, administration of potassium (if the potassium level is not already elevated) and, depending on the ventricular rate and presence of other digitalis-toxic arrhythmias, potentially a β-blocker, lidocaine, or phenytoin.

### Automatic Atrial Tachycardia

Automatic atrial tachycardia generally is characterized by a warm-up phenomenon, in which the heart rate gradually accelerates after initiation. Usually, it can be overdrive suppressed, but not terminated, through pacing. Automatic atrial tachycardia can occur in all age groups and can be seen in association with MI, lung disease, alcohol ingestion, and metabolic abnormalities.

### Reentrant Atrial Tachycardia

Reentrant atrial tachycardia can result from anatomic abnormalities, including surgical scars or atriotomy incisions. It can be initiated by premature atrial stimuli that induce conduction delay or block, usually can be terminated through atrial pacing, and not uncommonly is associated with atrial flutter.

### Multifocal Atrial Tachycardia

Multifocal atrial tachycardia is characterized by a heart rate of greater than 100 beats/min, multiple (more than three) P-wave morphologies, and variable PP, PR, and RR intervals. The multiple P-wave morphologies result from multiple depolarizing foci in the atria. The irregularly irregular ventricular rate can mimic atrial fibrillation, and a differentiation from "coarse" atrial fibrillation can be made by isoelectric periods between P waves. Multifocal atrial tachycardia predominantly occurs in patients who are elderly or critically ill with advanced chronic pulmonary disease. Other commonly associated conditions include pneumonia, infection or sepsis, postoperative states, lung cancer, pulmonary embolism, cor pulmonale, congestive heart failure, hypertensive heart disease, and other acute cardiac or pulmonary processes. Rarely, digoxin toxicity, hypokalemia, and hypomagnesemia may be associated. Multifocal atrial tachycardia also may progress to atrial fibrillation. In critically ill patients, it is associated with a high hospital mortality. Treatment is directed toward the underlying disease, which often is pulmonary. Antiarrhythmic agents often are ineffective, and β-blockers can be effective but often are contraindicated in patients with severe bronchospastic disease. Verapamil, amiodarone, and potassium, as well as magnesium replacement, have been helpful. The mechanism underlying multifocal atrial tachycardia may be enhanced automaticity or triggered activity.

## Atrial Flutter

The incidence of atrial flutter is lower than that of atrial fibrillation, and two general categories of atrial flutter have been described. The typical (i.e., type I) form is caused by macroreentry in the right atrium. Atrial depolarization in this reentrant circuit typically propagates in the counterclockwise direction, craniocaudally down the free wall, through a corridor of functionally slow-conducting tissue in the posterolateral to posteromedial right atrium, and caudal cranially up the atrial septum. This pattern of atrial activation inscribes the typical sawtooth flutter waves on the surface ECG that typically are negative in the inferior leads (i.e., II, III, $aV_F$). Clockwise propagation along the posterior corridor also can occur, producing positive flutter waves in the inferior leads. The atrial rate usually is 250 to 350 beats/min, but this may be slowed by class IA, IC, and III antiarrhythmic drugs. Type I atrial flutter often can be terminated through atrial pacing. It also can be cured, with a success rate of 75% to 90%, by radiofrequency catheter ablation, in which the application of radiofrequency energy produces a line of conduction block across the posterior corridor.

Atypical (i.e., type II) atrial flutter has an atrial rate that usually is 250 to 400 beats/min and may not be influenced or terminated through atrial pacing. Atrial flutter/tachycardias due to reentrant circuits around areas of atrial scars or prior incisions may have slower rates, depending on the size of the macroreentrant pathway and atrial conduction times. In type II atrial flutter, the right atrial posterior corridor, as described in type I atrial flutter, is generally not a critical component of the reentrant circuit, with other right or left atrial pathways of conduction participating in the arrhythmia.

In untreated patients with type I atrial flutter, the atrial rate usually is 300 beats/min, with 2:1 atrioventricular conduction and a ventricular rate of 150 beats/min. Slower rates may occur with treatment (e.g., atrioventricular node-blocking agents) or atrioventricular nodal disease. The ventricular response often occurs with 2:1, 4:1, alternating 2:1/4:1, or variable conduction patterns. Thus, the ventricular rate may be constant or variable and irregular. Occasionally, 1:1 atrioventricular conduction can be seen in patients with preexcitation syndromes (e.g., Wolff-Parkinson-White syndrome), with hyperthyroidism, or in children, and this can be a medical emergency. Slowing of the atrial rate, as occurs with the administration of antiarrhythmic agents, also may result in 1:1 atrioventricular conduction. Vagal maneuvers or adenosine can help to establish the diagnosis by blocking the ventricular response and enhancing appreciation of the flutter waves. Esophageal or intracardiac atrial electrogram recordings can help in patients for whom the diagnosis remains unclear.

Paroxysmal atrial flutter can occur in patients without structural heart disease, but chronic, persistent atrial flutter most often occurs in patients with underlying heart disease. Conditions associated with atrial flutter include coronary artery disease, rheumatic heart disease, cardiomyopathy, hypertensive heart disease, pulmonary disease with or without cor pulmonale, hyperthyroidism, alcohol ingestion, pericarditis, acute MI, pulmonary embolism, septal defects, congenital heart disease, after surgical repair of congenital defects or valve disease, and other causes of atrial dilatation. In patients treated with class IC antiarrhythmic drugs that can significantly slow conduction, a recurrence of atrial arrhythmias often occurs in the form of type I atrial flutter and tachycardia because significant slowing of conduction can facilitate reentry along the typical atrial flutter posterior corridor circuit.

The treatment of atrial flutter commonly involves controlling the ventricular response with agents such as verapamil, diltiazem, β-blockers, or digoxin. Synchronized direct current (DC) cardioversion is effective and may require only low energies (i.e., 25 to 100 J). Rapid atrial overdrive pacing may terminate type I atrial flutter. Antiarrhythmic agents (i.e., class IA, IC, III) have been used successfully, but because the facilitation of atrioventricular conduction may occur during the use of class IA agents with vagolytic activity or class I or III agents that slow the atrial rate enough to allow 1:1 conduction, concomitant negative dromotropic (i.e., atrioventricular nodal slowing) agents may be required. The long-term prevention of atrial flutter has been difficult with medical treatment. As noted, however, type I atrial flutter can be cured, with a success rate of 75% to 90%, using radiofrequency catheter ablation, in which the application of radiofrequency energy produces a line of conduction block across the posterior corridor. Atypical atrial flutters also may be approached with catheter ablation methods and advanced mapping techniques, although with success rates that are lower than those for type I atrial flutter. Radiofrequency ablation also has been used successfully as adjunctive therapy in patients on antiarrhythmic agents to cure the atrial flutter that can be facilitated by these agents.

## Atrial Fibrillation

Atrial fibrillation is the most common sustained tachyarrhythmia. During atrial fibrillation, an electrical activation of the atria occurs in rapid, multiple waves of depolarization, with continuously changing, wandering pathways. Intraatrial activation can be recorded as irregular, rapid depolarizations, often at rates exceeding 300 to 400 beats/min. Mechanically, this pattern of rapid, disordered atrial activation results in a loss of coordinated atrial contraction. Irregular electrical inputs to the atrioventricular node lead to irregular ventricular rates. Focally initiating atrial fibrillation has been recognized as a more common cause of atrial fibrillation than previously appreciated, particularly in lone atrial fibrillation that occurs in the absence of structural heart disease. These fibrillations most frequently arise from the ostia of the pulmonary veins and potentially can be catheter ablated to achieve long-term cure, even in patients with structural heart disease.

On the surface ECG, atrial fibrillation is characterized by an absence of discrete P waves, the presence of irregular fibrillatory waves, or both, and an irregularly irregular ventricular response. Complete BBB or aberrancy (e.g., Ashman's phenomenon) can mimic VT. At physical examination, the pulse is irregularly irregular, variable stroke volumes may produce pulse deficits, and the jugular venous waveform lacks A waves.

The incidence of atrial fibrillation increases with age. The most common underlying cardiovascular diseases associated with atrial fibrillation are hypertension and ischemic heart disease. Age, valvular disease, congestive heart failure, hypertension, and diabetes mellitus are independent risk factors for atrial fibrillation. Other associated conditions include rheumatic heart disease (especially mitral valve disease), nonrheumatic valvular disease, cardiomyopathies, congenital heart disease, pulmonary embolism, thyrotoxico-

| TABLE 66.2 | | |
| --- | --- | --- |
| **AMERICAN COLLEGE OF CHEST PHYSICIANS GUIDELINES FOR ANTITHROMBOTIC THERAPY FOR ATRIAL FIBRILLATION** | | |
| **Risk Factors** | **No.** | **Recommendation** |
| High[a] | 1 | Warfarin[b] |
| Moderate[c] | >1 | Warfarin[b] |
| | 1 | Warfarin[b] or aspirin[d] |
| None | 0 | Aspirin[d] |

[a] Prior transient ischemic attack, systemic embolus or stroke, hypertension, poor left ventricular function, rheumatic mitral valve disease, or prosthetic heart valve, age >75 years.
[b] Warfarin target international normalized ratio: 2.5 (range, 2.0–3.0).
[c] Age 65–75 years, diabetes mellitus, coronary artery disease with preserved left ventricular systolic function.
[d] Aspirin, 325 mg/day.
(Reproduced with permission from Albers GW, Dalen JE, Laupacis A, et al. Antithrombotic therapy in atrial fibrillation. *Chest* 2001;119: [Suppl]194S–206S.)

sis, chronic lung disease, sick sinus syndrome and degenerative conduction system disease, Wolff-Parkinson-White syndrome, pericarditis, neoplastic disease, postoperative states, and normal hearts affected by high adrenergic states, alcohol, stress, drugs (especially sympathomimetics), excessive caffeine, hypoxia, hypokalemia, hypoglycemia, or systemic infection.

One of the most important clinical consequences of atrial fibrillation is its association with thromboembolic events and stroke. Recommended guidelines for antithrombotic therapy are listed in Tables 66.2 and 66.3.

### Acute Treatment

The acute treatment of atrial fibrillation that is symptomatic with an increased heart rate should include the consideration of urgent cardioversion if the patient is hemodynamically unstable (e.g., hypotensive) or has evidence of ischemia or pulmonary edema. For moderate to severe symptoms, acute control of the ventricular rate usually can be achieved using intravenous β-blockers, verapamil, diltiazem, or digoxin (Table 66.4). Digoxin can be used safely in patients with heart failure, but it has a delayed peak onset of heart rate–lowering effect, a narrow therapeutic window, and is less effective in the rate control of paroxysmal atrial fibrillation or rapid rates during hyperadrenergic states when the vagal tone is low (such as in the intensive care unit) because of increased sympathetic tone. Pharmacologic or electrical cardioversion, the use of antiarrhythmic agents, and anticoagulation should be considered. Pharmacologic conversion can be attempted intravenously, using procainamide, ibutilide, or amiodarone, or orally, using class I or III antiarrhythmic agents (Table 66.5). If the duration of atrial fibrillation is more than 48 hours, anticoagulation using warfarin for 3 weeks versus transesophageal echocar-

## TABLE 66.3
### GUIDELINES FOR ELECTRICAL CARDIOVERSION

Anticoagulation (e.g., warfarin PT/international normalized ratio 2.0–3.0) should be given for 3 wks before elective cardioversion of patients who have been in atrial fibrillation for >48 h and continued until normal sinus rhythm has been maintained for 4 wks. In some circumstances, a transesophageal protocol may be substituted for conventional therapy but adjusted-dose warfarin continued until sinus rhythm has been maintained at least 4 wks.

Consideration should be given to treating patients in atrial flutter in the same manner as patients in atrial fibrillation.

Long-term anticoagulation beyond the 4 wk after cardioversion should be considered if cardiomyopathy, history of previous embolism, mitral valve disease, or other indications for long-term anticoagulation also exist, as listed previously.

Heparin anticoagulation followed by oral anticoagulation may be indicated for patients requiring emergency cardioversion for hemodynamic instability. For atrial fibrillation <48 h, risk of embolism after cardioversion appears low, but pericardioversion anticoagulation is recommended.

Note: Many of these patients were excluded from the multicenter trials on atrial fibrillation. There is an increased risk of bleeding that correlates with the level of anticoagulation (i.e., international normalized ratio >4). A marked decrease in efficacy is noted at international normalized ratio <2.

Contraindications to anticoagulation include hemorrhagic tendencies, recent intracranial hemorrhage or neurosurgery, recent major hemorrhage or trauma, and uncontrolled diastolic hypertension with blood pressure >105 mm Hg. Other critical considerations include patients at risk of falling, alcohol abuse, drug interactions, poor compliance or follow-up, and concomitant use of nonsteroidal anti-inflammatory drugs.

(Adapted with permission from Albers G, Dalen J, Laupacis A, et al. Antithrombotic therapy in atrial fibrillation. *Chest* 2001;119[Suppl]: 194S–206S.)

diographically guided cardioversion using anticoagulation should be considered (Table 66.3). For shorter durations of atrial fibrillation (i.e., <48 hours), anticoagulation still should be considered if the patient has underlying heart disease or risk factors for thromboembolism. Anticoagulation also should be considered for the pericardioversion period.

### Long-Term Treatment

The long-term treatment of atrial fibrillation should include evaluation for underlying structural heart disease, risk factors, and, potentially, other precipitating arrhythmias. Anticoagulation using warfarin or aspirin should be considered (Table 66.2). Control of the ventricular rate using β-blockers, calcium channel blockers, or digoxin also may be required (Table 66.4). In addition, restoring and maintaining sinus rhythm through cardioversion, maintenance antiarrhythmic therapy, or both can be considered. The Atrial Fibrillation Follow-up Investigation of Rhythm Management (AFFIRM) study, a large randomized trial of rate- vs. rhythm-control strategies for atrial

fibrillation, showed no significant survival benefit for either approach, although a trend toward better survival was observed in the rate control arm. Nevertheless, for first-onset atrial fibrillation, or continued symptoms despite rate control, a rhythm control strategy still may be of some benefit. Available primary antiarrhythmic agents that may effectively maintain sinus rhythm include class IA (i.e., quinidine, procainamide, disopyramide), class IC (i.e., flecainide, propafenone), class IA/B/C (i.e., moricizine), and class III (i.e., sotalol, amiodarone, dofetilide) antiarrhythmic drugs (Table 66.5). Nonpharmacologic approaches for refractory patients include catheter ablation directed toward electrical isolation of the antrums of the pulmonary vein ostia. Permanent pacemaker implantation may be helpful for symptomatic bradyarrhythmias, or tachycardia-bradycardia syndrome, and include the use of mode-switching, dual-chamber devices for paroxysmal atrial fibrillation. Implantable defibrillators with programmable atrial therapies may be useful for some patients but are limited by discomfort from shocks. Complete atrioventricular junction ablation or atrioventricular junction modification through the implantation of a rate-responsive, permanent pacemaker has produced symptomatic benefit, particularly in patients with difficult-to-control ventricular rates. The *maze procedure* is an operation that was designed to cure atrial fibrillation by dividing the atria into mazelike corridors and blind alleys, which limit the development of reentry by limiting the available path length. Much of the success of this procedure likely has been due to surgically created pulmonary vein isolation.

## Junctional Tachycardias

Abnormal junctional tachycardias can be divided into nonreentrant and reentrant tachycardias.

### Nonparoxysmal Junctional Tachycardia

Nonparoxysmal atrioventricular junctional tachycardia is characterized by gradual onset and termination, and it likely results from accelerated automatic discharge in or near the bundle of His. In this form of accelerated junctional rhythm, atrioventricular junctional tissue may exhibit faster discharge rates or usurp the dominant pacemaker status during sinus slowing. Heart rate generally ranges from 70 to 130 beats/min, but it can be faster. Nonparoxysmal atrioventricular junctional tachycardia occasionally occurs in patients with underlying heart disease, such as acute MI, myocarditis, after open heart surgery (particularly valve procedures), or with digitalis intoxication. It also can occur in otherwise healthy, asymptomatic individuals. In infants or children, it is associated with a high mortality. Incessant tachycardia may lead to a tachycardia-mediated cardiomyopathy. Treatment generally is supportive and directed toward the underlying disease.

**TABLE 66.4**

**MEDICAL TREATMENT FOR VENTRICULAR RATE CONTROL IN SUPRAVENTRICULAR ARRHYTHMIAS, INCLUDING ATRIAL FIBRILLATION**

| Agent | Loading Dose | Maintenance Dose | Side Effects/Toxicity | Comments |
|---|---|---|---|---|
| Digoxin | 0.25–0.50 mg i.v., then 0.25 mg i.v. every 4–6 h to 1 mg in the first 24 h | 0.125–0.250 mg p.o. or i.v. every day | Anorexia, nausea, AV block, ventricular arrhythmias; accumulates in renal failure | Used in congestive heart failure, vagotonic effects on the AV node, delayed onset of action, narrow therapeutic window, less effective in paroxysmal atrial fibrillation or high adrenergic states |
| Class II (β-blockers) | — | — | Bronchospasm, congestive heart failure, decreased blood pressure | Effective in heart rate control even with exercise, rapid onsets of action |
| Propranolol | 1 mg i.v. every 2–5 min to 0.1–0.2 mg/kg | 10–80 mg p.o. t.i.d. to q.i.d. | — | — |
| Metoprolol | 5 mg i.v. every 5 min to 15 mg | 25–100 mg p.o. b.i.d. | — | — |
| Esmolol | 500 μg/kg i.v. over 1 min | 50 μg/kg i.v. for 4 h, repeat load as needed and increase maintenance to 20–50 μg/kg/min every 5–10 min as needed | — | Esmolol short-acting |
| Class IV (calcium channel blockers) | — | — | Decreased blood pressure, congestive heart failure | Rapid onset, can be used safely in chronic obstructive pulmonary disease and diabetes mellitus |
| Verapamil | 2.5–10.0 mg i.v. over 2 min | 5–10 mg i.v. every 30–60 min or 40–160 mg p.o. t.i.d. | Increased digoxin level | — |
| Diltiazem | 0.25 mg/kg over 2 h, repeat as needed every 15 min at 0.35 mg/kg | 5–15 mg/h i.v. or 30–90 mg p.o. q.i.d. | — | — |
| Class III | | | | |
| Sotalol | — | 80–240 mg p.o. b.i.d. | Bradycardia, congestive heart failure, bronchospasm, decreased blood pressure, increased QT, torsades de pointes, proarrhythmia | — |
| Amiodarone | 600–1,600 mg/day, divided | 100–400 mg p.o. daily | Bradycardia, pulmonary, thyroid, liver, skin, gastrointestinal, ophthalmologic | Drug interactions |
| Adenosine | 6–18 mg i.v. rapid bolus | — | Transient sinus bradycardia, sinus arrest, AV block, flushing, chest discomfort, bronchospasm; may precipitate atrial fibrillation by shortening of atrial refractoriness | Not effective in controlling ventricular rate in atrial fibrillation flutter, but may be useful diagnostically; can terminate reentrant paroxysmal supraventricular tachycardias using the AV node |

AV, atrioventricular.

## TABLE 66.5

### CLASS I AND III ANTIARRHYTHMIC AGENTS

| Antiarrhythmic Drug | Dose | Side Effects/Comments |
|---|---|---|
| **Class IA** | | Increased QT, proarrhythmia/TdP, potential increased AV node conduction can be seen with all three |
| Quinidine | 200–400 mg p.o. t.i.d. to b.i.d. | Diarrhea, nausea, increased digoxin levels |
| Procainamide | 10–15 mg/kg i.v. at 50 mg/min or 500–1,000 mg p.o. every 6 h (sustained release) | Decreased blood pressure, congestive heart failure, drug-induced lupus; metabolite N-acetylprocainamide (class III) can accumulate in renal failure |
| Disopyramide | 100–300 mg p.o. t.i.d. | Anticholinergic effects (e.g., urinary retention, dry eyes/mouth), congestive heart failure |
| **Class IB** | | |
| Lidocaine | 50–100 mg i.v. (0.5–1.5 mg/kg) bolus, infusion of 1–4 mg/min, and rebolus in 5–15 min | Reduce dosage in congestive heart failure, elderly, hepatic dysfunction, bradycardia, hypotension, CNS side effects (tremors, seizures, altered mental status) |
| Mexiletine | 150–300 mg p.o. every 8 h | Gastrointestinal side effects (nausea, vomiting) common, may be minimized by dosing with meals; CNS effects (tremor, dizziness, nervousness) |
| Tocainide | 400–600 mg p.o. every 8 h | Gastrointestinal side effects (nausea, vomiting), CNS less common (dizziness, vertigo, nervousness); rare but potentially life-threatening agranulocytosis and pulmonary fibrosis |
| Phenytoin | 100 mg p.o. every 8 h; loading up to 1 g in divided doses; or 20–50 mg/min i.v. to maximum 1 g | Rarely used as an antiarrhythmic agent outside of digitalis toxicity; CNS side effects common; dermatologic reactions |
| **Class IC** | | Proarrhythmia |
| Flecainide | 50–200 mg p.o. b.i.d. | Visual disturbance, dizziness, congestive heart failure, avoid in coronary artery disease or left ventricular dysfunction |
| Propafenone | 150–300 mg p.o. t.i.d. | Congestive heart failure, ? avoid in coronary artery disease/left ventricular dysfunction |
| **Class IA/B/C** | | |
| Moricizine | 200–300 mg p.o. t.i.d. | Proarrhythmia, dizziness, gastrointestinal/nausea, headache, caution in coronary artery disease/left ventricular dysfunction |
| **Class III** | | |
| Sotalol | 80–240 mg p.o. b.i.d. | Congestive heart failure, bronchospasm, bradycardia, increased QT, proarrhythmia/TdP; renally excreted |
| Bretylium | 5–10 mg/kg i.v. bolus; 1–2 mg/min i.v. infusion | Hypotension; transient increased arrhythmias possible due to initial norepinephrine release; reduce dose in renal failure |
| Amiodarone | 600–1,600 mg/day loading in divided doses p.o., 100–400 mg p.o. daily maintenance; i.v. available | Pulmonary toxicity, bradycardia, hyperthyroidism or hypothyroidism, hepatic toxicity, gastrointestinal (nausea, constipation), neurologic, dermatologic, and ophthalmologic side effects, drug interactions |
| Ibutilide | 1.0 mg i.v. over 10 min, may repeat in 10 min | Monitor for QT prolongation, TdP |
| Dofetilide | 125–500 μg p.o. every 12 h; initial dose: CrCl (mL/min) >60: 500 μg b.i.d.; 40–60: 250 μg b.i.d.; 20–40: 125 μg b.i.d. | In-hospital initiation mandated; exclude if CrCl <20 mL/min; monitor for QT prolongation, proarrhythmia/TdP; headache, muscle cramps |

AV, atrioventricular; CNS, central nervous system; TdP, torsades de pointes.

Standard treatment for digitalis toxicity may be required. β-Blockers and class IA, IC, and III antiarrhythmic agents have been used, as has radiofrequency catheter ablation.

### Atrioventricular Nodal Reentrant Tachycardia

The most common form of paroxysmal reentrant SVT is AVNRT, which accounts for 60% to 70% of patients with paroxysmal SVT. Reentry occurs within the atrioventricular node and perinodal tissue, and at least two functional pathways of conduction can be demonstrated within the atrioventricular node in patients with AVNRT (Fig. 66.7). Typically, one (fast) pathway conducts rapidly, with a relatively long refractory period. A second (slow) pathway conducts more slowly, and usually with a shorter refractory

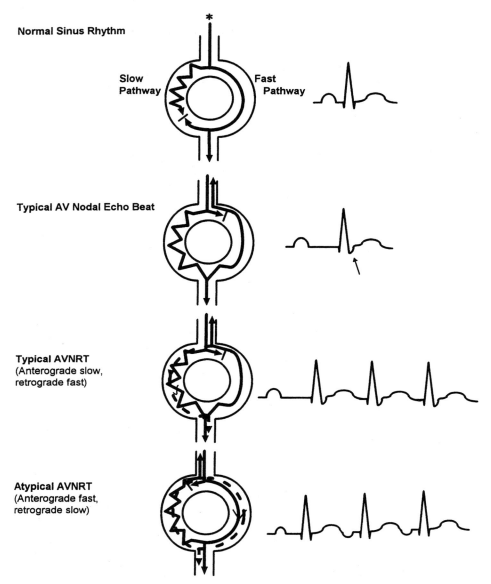

**Normal Sinus Rhythm**

Slow Pathway

Fast Pathway

**Typical AV Nodal Echo Beat**

**Typical AVNRT**
(Anterograde slow, retrograde fast)

**Atypical AVNRT**
(Anterograde fast, retrograde slow)

**Figure 66.7**  Atrioventricular nodal reentrant tachycardia (AVNRT).

period. During sinus rhythm, conduction generally occurs over the fast pathway. A premature atrial depolarization that blocks conduction in the fast pathway because of the longer refractory period, however, still may conduct over the slow pathway. If conduction through this pathway is slow enough that the fast-pathway refractory period ends and the impulse can travel retrogradely back to the atrium, then atrioventricular node reentry can occur. In common, or typical, AVNRT, anterograde conduction occurs via the slow pathway and retrograde conduction via the fast pathway. Rapid retrograde activation of the atrium via the fast pathway occurs nearly simultaneously with the ventricular activation, and it usually causes the P wave to be simultaneous with, or buried within, the QRS complex. In 5% to 10% of patients with AVNRT, atypical or uncommon AVNRT occurs, in which anterograde conduction takes place via the fast pathway and retrograde conduction via

the slow pathway. This causes retrograde P waves that usually are negative in the inferior leads (i.e., II, III, aV$_F$) and are separated from the QRS complex, with an RP interval that is longer than the PR interval (i.e., a mechanism of long RP tachycardia).

Clinically, AVNRT commonly occurs in patients with no structural heart disease, and 70% of patients are women. It may occur at any age, but most patients present during the fourth or fifth decade of life. Symptoms may include palpitations, lightheadedness, near syncope, weakness, dyspnea, chest pain, rarely syncope, and frequently neck pounding with prominent A waves that can be seen on the jugular pulse, representing atrial contraction against a closed tricuspid valve.

Electrocardiographically, the rate of AVNRT usually is 150 to 200 beats/min, although rates as high as 250 beats/min can occur. The initiation of typical AVNRT usually occurs with a premature atrial contraction that is followed by a long PR interval, thus indicating blocked conduction in the fast pathway and conduction down the slow pathway. Because atrial and ventricular activation occur simultaneously during the tachycardia, P waves generally are buried in the QRS complex. A pseudo r′ in $V_1$ may be seen during typical AVNRT. A longer RP interval indicates retrograde conduction via a slower retrograde pathway.

### Treatment

Vagal maneuvers (e.g., carotid sinus massage, Valsalva's maneuver) may slow or terminate the tachycardia. Adenosine, 6 to 12 mg administered as a rapid intravenous bolus, is the initial drug of choice. Termination of a narrow complex tachycardia by vagal maneuvers or adenosine can be helpful diagnostically by suggesting that the atrioventricular node may be a component of the circuit (in contrast to atrial tachycardias, in which atrioventricular block can be produced with continued tachycardia). β-blockers, verapamil, or diltiazem also can be successful. The long-term use of these agents or of class IA, IC, or III antiarrhythmic drugs can be successful, but radiofrequency catheter ablation, particularly of the slow atrioventricular nodal pathway, has become the standard therapy for cure of AVNRT, having success rates that can exceed 95% and less than a 1% risk of inducing complete atrioventricular block or the need for a permanent pacemaker.

## Supraventricular Tachycardia Mediated by Accessory Pathways

Accessory pathways are bands of excitable conducting tissue that connect the atrium and the ventricle, thus bypassing either all or part of the normal atrioventricular conduction system. Preexcitation syndromes are disorders in which anterograde ventricular or retrograde atrial activation occurs, either in part or totally, through anomalous pathways distinct from the normal conduction system. Anterograde conduction (i.e., from atrium to ventricle) via an accessory pathway during sinus rhythm causes manifest ventricular preexcitation (i.e., Wolff-Parkinson-White syndrome). This results in wide QRS complexes because the accessory pathway inserts into the ventricular myocardium, with activation occurring from myocyte to myocyte rather than via the faster conducting His-Purkinje system. On ECG, a short PR interval and a delta wave (i.e., initial slurring of the QRS complex) usually are seen. Approximately 1 to 3 per 1,000 ECGs show ventricular preexcitation. Accessory pathways that conduct only in the retrograde direction are called *concealed* (i.e., no ventricular preexcitation or delta wave seen on surface ECG), yet these still may participate in SVT. Typical accessory pathways conduct rapidly and nondecrementally. Variant accessory pathways include those with slow, decremental conduction and connections from the atrium to the distal atrioventricular node, the atrium to the His bundle, and the atrium to the right bundle, distal Purkinje network, or apex via a duplicate atrioventricular node/His bundle–like connection (i.e., Mahaim fiber). Congenital abnormalities associated with accessory pathways include Ebstein's anomaly, coarctation of the aorta, hypertrophic cardiomyopathy, ventricular septal defects, and D-transposition of the great arteries.

### Atrioventricular Reentrant Tachycardia

During AVRT, the accessory pathway, as well as the atria and ventricles, are essential parts of the circuit (Fig. 66.8). In orthodromic AVRT, anterograde conduction occurs via the atrioventricular node and retrograde conduction via the accessory pathway. In antidromic AVRT, anterograde conduction occurs via an accessory pathway and retrograde conduction via the atrioventricular node or a second accessory pathway. Other accessory pathway–associated tachycardias include atrial fibrillation, atrial flutter, atrial tachycardia, or AVNRT, with conduction via a bystander accessory pathway, in which the accessory pathway is not integral to the tachycardia but conducts to the ventricle. Slowly conducting, concealed accessory pathways, which usually are located in the posteroseptal region, can mediate near incessant orthodromic SVT, with retrograde, slow conduction via the accessory pathway (i.e., permanent form of junctional reciprocating tachycardia); these can present as a tachycardia-mediated cardiomyopathy. The most common tachycardias associated with accessory pathways are discussed in the following sections; their treatment is summarized in Table 66.6.

### Orthodromic Atrioventricular Reentrant Tachycardia

Orthodromic AVRT is the most common SVT in patients with accessory pathways, occurring in 90% of those who are symptomatic. Anterograde conduction occurs via the atrioventricular node and His-Purkinje system, inscribing a narrow QRS complex (with no preexcitation) on the surface ECG, unless BBB aberrancy occurs. Because retrograde conduction occurs via the accessory pathway, patients with either manifest or concealed accessory pathways can experience orthodromic AVRT. The heart rate of the tachycardia usually is 150 to 250 beats/min, and the tachycardia usually initiates with an atrial or ventricular premature depolarization. Because the atria and ventricles are requisite parts of the circuit, a 1:1 relationship must be present. The demonstration of atrioventricular dissociation or intermittent atrioventricular block during SVT excludes AVRT as a diagnosis. The P wave commonly is visualized in the early part of the ST segment, with a constant RP interval despite the tachycardia rate. Spontaneous or induced BBB during orthodromic AVRT that slows the tachycardia rate indicates the participation of an accessory pathway ipsilateral to the side of the BBB (Fig. 66.9). For example, during orthodromic AVRT using a left free wall

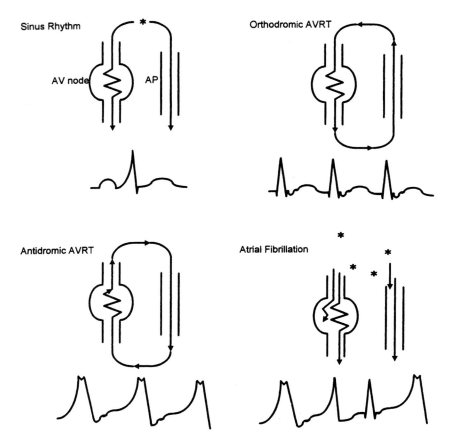

**Figure 66.8** Tachycardias associated with accessory pathways (APs). AVRT, atrioventricular reentrant tachycardia.

accessory pathway as the retrograde limb, the production of block in the left bundle forces ventricular activation to occur via the right bundle, thus requiring conduction through a longer ventricular myocardial path back up to the accessory pathway and slowing the tachycardia cycle length.

Short-term treatment of the two common, regular, narrow complex tachycardias (i.e., orthodromic AVRT and AVNRT) is similar because the atrioventricular node is an integral part of the circuit in the anterograde direction. To terminate the tachycardia, vagal maneuvers or adenosine are the first options of choice, followed by intravenous β-blockers, verapamil, or diltiazem. Adenosine can shorten atrial refractory periods but occasionally may precipitate atrial fibrillation with a rapid ventricular response. In patients with very rapid SVT and hemodynamic impairment, DC cardioversion is the initial treatment of choice. Longer term treatment may include β-blockers, verapamil, diltiazem, digoxin, or class IA, IC, or III antiarrhythmic drugs. Radiofrequency catheter ablation, however, can be curative and have high success rates; in many patients, it can be considered as a first-line or early therapeutic option.

### Antidromic Atrioventricular Reentrant Tachycardia
Antidromic AVRT is uncommon, occurring in less than 5% to 10% of patients with Wolff-Parkinson-White syndrome.

The anterograde limb of the circuit is an accessory pathway. In 33% to 60% of patients with antidromic AVRT, however, multiple accessory pathways are present, and the retrograde limb may be via either the atrioventricular node or another accessory pathway. Because ventricular activation occurs via an accessory pathway, the QRS complex is wide, bizarre, and preexcited. Mahaim fibers, which are accessory pathways with decremental conduction properties that connect the atrium to the distal right bundle branch or apex via a duplicate atrioventricular node/His bundle-like connection, also can mediate a form of antidromic AVRT with left BBB morphology. In antidromic AVRT, if the atrioventricular node makes up the retrograde limb, then vagal maneuvers or adenosine may terminate the tachycardia, but these measures will not be effective if both limbs are accessory pathways. In the short-term, treatment may require DC cardioversion or procainamide.

### Atrial Fibrillation and Wolff-Parkinson-White Syndrome
In patients with manifest accessory pathways having a short refractory period, rapid conduction to the ventricles during atrial fibrillation via the accessory pathway can provoke ventricular fibrillation. The shortest preexcited RR interval during atrial fibrillation gives an indication of the refractory period of the accessory pathway. Short

## TABLE 66.6

**MANAGEMENT OF PREEXCITATION SYNDROMES**

Initial evaluation
  Determine presence or absence of symptoms
  Characterize symptoms, including frequency and severity
  Determine previous treatment regimens and effectiveness
  Document specific arrhythmias present during symptoms
  Determine presence of concomitant heart disease
Acute treatment of arrhythmias associated with preexcitation syndromes
  Orthodromic SVT
    Vagal maneuvers (e.g., Valsalva's, carotid sinus massage)
    Adenosine i.v. (6–12 mg rapid bolus)
    Verapamil i.v. (5–10 mg), β-blocker, or diltiazem
    Procainamide i.v. (1 g over 20–30 min)
    Cardioversion
  Antidromic SVT (retrograde conduction may occur via a second AP or the AV node)
    Procainamide i.v.
    Cardioversion
  Atrial fibrillation (digoxin and verapamil may accelerate ventricular rate and should not be used)
    Procainamide i.v.
    Cardioversion
Long-term treatment of patients with preexcitation syndromes
  Pharmacologic management
    Concealed AP
      Digoxin/verapamil/beta blocker
      Class IC: flecainide/propafenone
      Class IA: disopyramide/quinidine/procainamide
      Class III: sotalol/amiodarone
    Manifest AP
      Class IC: flecainide/propafenone
      Class IA: disopyramide/quinidine/procainamide
      Class III: sotalol/amiodarone
  Indications for nonpharmacologic management
    Life-threatening ventricular rate during atrial fibrillation/ flutter
    SVT refractory to medical therapy
    Intolerance to medical therapy
      Alternate first-line therapy in patients with symptomatic arrhythmias, high-risk occupations, or preference for nonpharmacologic treatment
  Nonpharmacologic approaches
    Radiofrequency catheter ablation
    Surgical ablation (rarely required)
  Indications for electrophysiology studies
    Delineation of the mechanism of arrhythmias
    Localization/mapping of pathways for ablation
    Assess efficacy of antiarrhythmic agents
    Assessment of the refractory periods of the AP as an indicator of the risk of sudden death

AP, accessory pathway; AV, atrioventricular; SVT, supraventricular tachycardia.

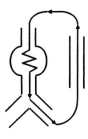 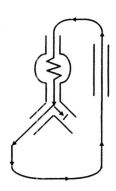

Orthodromic AVRT    Orthodromic AVRT with ipsilateral BBB

**Figure 66.9** Orthodromic atrioventricular reentrant tachycardia (AVRT) with bundle branch block (BBB) ipsilateral to the accessory pathway.

## SPECIFIC VENTRICULAR ARRHYTHMIAS

VT is defined as three or more consecutive ventricular beats at a rate of 100 beats/min or more. Nonsustained VT is defined as VT lasting three or more beats under 30 seconds in duration and that does not require intervention for termination. Sustained VT is VT lasting 30 seconds or more or requiring intervention for termination. QRS complex morphology may be either monomorphic (i.e., uniform) or polymorphic (i.e., variable). The usual heart rate of VT ranges from 100 to 280 beats/min. VT is wide because of the slower rate of conduction through ventricular tissue, compared with that through Purkinje's fibers. Hemodynamic stability depends on the rate, underlying cardiac disease, ventricular function, and concomitant pharmacologic treatment. VA dissociation occurs in 60% to 70% of these patients, but it may be evident on surface ECGs only in one-third of patients.

### Premature Ventricular Depolarizations

Isolated premature ventricular depolarizations are not associated with significant risk in patients without structural heart disease, but frequent or complex premature ventricular complexes can be markers for a potential increased risk in those with structural heart disease. The treatment of isolated, symptomatic premature complexes generally includes an assessment of risk in the presence of structural heart disease or risk factors, avoidance of precipitating factors (e.g., caffeine, sympathomimetic agents), and reassurance, with the administration of occasional β-blockers or (rarely) other antiarrhythmic agents for persistently symptomatic patients. An electrophysiology study, using mapping and catheter ablation of focally originating premature ventricular complexes or tachycardias, also has been performed for frequent and refractory symptoms.

refractory periods (<250 ms) are associated with an increased risk of sudden death. Verapamil can increase the ventricular rate during atrial fibrillation; intravenous verapamil may precipitate ventricular fibrillation and should not be given. The treatment of choice is procainamide or DC cardioversion.

## Sustained Ventricular Tachycardia or Fibrillation: Aborted Sudden Cardiac Death

The patient who survives hemodynamically compromising sustained ventricular arrhythmias or aborted sudden cardiac death in the absence of reversible causes or acute MI faces a high recurrence rate. The implantation of cardioverter-defibrillator (ICD) is usually indicated. Randomized studies, such as the Antiarrhythmics versus Implantable Defibrillator (AVID) trial, have demonstrated the superiority of ICDs over medical therapies using antiarrhythmic drugs in these high-risk patients.

## Ventricular Tachyarrhythmias after Myocardial Infarction

Premature ventricular complexes, nonsustained or sustained VT, ventricular fibrillation, and polymorphic VT can occur during the acute phases of ischemia and infarction. Coronary reperfusion has been associated with accelerated idioventricular rhythms and ventricular tachyarrhythmias. Nonsustained or sustained VT, which often results from reentry, can occur late after MI.

Use of lidocaine as prophylaxis for ventricular fibrillation in patients with suspected acute MI has been controversial. Prophylactic lidocaine may produce a small decrease in the incidence of ventricular fibrillation. It has not been shown to improve the mortality, however, and significant side effects can occur. Potential adverse effects include asystole, bradyarrhythmias, neurologic symptoms, seizures, respiratory arrest, nausea, and vomiting. Current data suggest that the routine use of prophylactic lidocaine in patients with suspected acute MI should be avoided when facilities and personnel for prompt resuscitation are available, but when defibrillation is unavailable, prophylactic lidocaine might be beneficial.

The short-term treatment of ventricular arrhythmias after MI depends on the hemodynamic status of the patient and presence of ongoing or recurrent ischemia (as well as other precipitating factors). The long-term prognosis depends on the timing of these arrhythmias in relation to the acute infarction as well as to the degree of ventricular dysfunction. Asymptomatic premature ventricular complexes or nonsustained VTs generally do not require short-term therapy, but they may be associated with an increased mortality when they are frequent or complex, detected late in the course of MI, or associated with left ventricular dysfunction. Accelerated idioventricular rhythms have been associated with coronary reperfusion, but they have not been specific or highly sensitive as predictors of reperfusion and generally do not require specific short-term therapy. Early VT and sustained fibrillation are associated with an increased in-hospital mortality. Among hospital survivors, however, it may not signify a worsened long-term prognosis. Short-term therapy may require DC counter-shock, antiarrhythmic therapy, correction of electrolyte and metabolic imbalances, or assessment and treatment of associated recurrent or ongoing ischemia.

Long-term treatment requires an assessment of prognostic significance. Sustained ventricular arrhythmias after the acute phase of MI are associated with a high rate of recurrence, and ICD implantation is usually indicated. Patients with prior MI and LVEF ≤30% also should be considered for ICD implantation because the Multicenter Automatic Defibrillator Implantation Trial II (MADIT-2) demonstrated a survival benefit from ICDs in this group of patients without a requirement of nonsustained VT or EP testing. MADIT-2 enrolled patients at least 1 month after MI and 3 months after revascularization. Patients with nonsustained VT and LVEF ≤40% after MI should be considered for electrophysiology study, with the implantation of an ICD if the study induces sustained VT or reproducible ventricular fibrillation, because some trials (e.g., MADIT I and Multicenter Unsustained Tachycardia Trial [MUSTT]) have demonstrated that mortality is reduced in these high-risk patients through ICD implantation. Frequent or complex ventricular arrhythmias occurring after the acute phase of MI (i.e., the first 48 to 72 hours) are more frequent in patients with significant myocardial dysfunction and also are an independent prognostic factor. The empiric suppression of PVCs or nonsustained VT using antiarrhythmic agents, with the possible exception of amiodarone, however, is associated with the potential for an increased mortality. β-Blockers and angiotensin-converting enzyme (ACE) inhibitors, which also have been associated with improved survival rates in many studies, should be routinely advocated in the absence of contraindications.

## Ventricular Arrhythmias Associated with Nonischemic Cardiomyopathy

VT or fibrillation associated with nonischemic cardiomyopathy may result from reentry, triggered activity, or increased automaticity. A form of macroreentry caused by bundle branch reentry is more common in patients with nonischemic dilated cardiomyopathy and preexisting His-Purkinje system disease, as can be manifested by an intraventricular conduction delay in sinus rhythm, most commonly of the left BBB type. Bundle branch reentrant VT most commonly presents as a rapid VT of left BBB morphology, although rare right BBB morphologies have been described. This arrhythmia potentially can be cured by selective radiofrequency ablation of one of the bundle branches (most commonly the right).

The presence of nonsustained VT in patients with nonischemic cardiomyopathy has been associated with an increased risk of mortality. The roles of prophylactic ICD implantation and empiric amiodarone in heart failure patients were subjects of recent large multicenter trials. The Defibrillators in Non-Ischemic Cardiomyopathy Treatment

Evaluation (DEFINITE) randomized patients with nonischemic cardiomyopathy and LVEF ≤35% and PVCs or NSVT to single-chamber ICD implantation or standard medical therapy. A reduction in all-cause mortality that did not reach statistical significance (p = 0.08) and a significant reduction in sudden death from arrhythmia was reported in the ICD group. The Sudden Cardiac Death in Heart Failure Trial [SCDHeFT] randomized nonischemic and ischemic cardiomyopathy patients with NYHA functional class II or III heart failure symptoms and LVEF ≤ 35% to ICD implantation, amiodarone, or placebo. No significant survival benefit was recently reported in the amiodarone group, compared to placebo, but ICD implantation resulted in a significant reduction in mortality.

## Arrhythmogenic Right Ventricular Dysplasia

Arrhythmogenic right ventricular dysplasia (ARVD) results from a cardiomyopathy, possibly familial in some patients (e.g., chromosome 14), that predominantly involves the right ventricle with hypokinetic and thinned areas that often have fatty infiltration. ARVD can cause ventricular arrhythmias in patients with an apparently normal left ventricle. VTs associated with ARVD generally have a left BBB morphology and may result from reentry. Pharmacologic therapies using antiarrhythmic drugs, surgery, ICD therapy, and radiofrequency ablation have been used as treatments of ventricular arrhythmias in patients with ARVD.

## Ventricular Tachycardias in Patients with Structurally Normal Hearts

Syndromes of repetitive, monomorphic, nonsustained, or sustained VT and paroxysmal VTs can present in patients with structurally normal hearts.

Outflow tract VT (arising from the right or left ventricular outflow tract or aortic cusp) can present with symptomatic, minimally symptomatic, or asymptomatic frequent, repetitive, or paroxysmal nonsustained or sustained VT, or with frequent symptomatic PVCs. It may be precipitated by stress, exercise, or high catecholamine states. Vagal maneuvers or adenosine may terminate the tachycardia. The PVCs or VT are monomorphic and characterized by left BBB morphology with an inferior axis (i.e., positive QRS in aV$_F$, II, and III). The VT often is associated with a gradual onset (i.e., warm-up) and offset, may not be inducible with programmed ventricular extrastimulation (i.e., at electrophysiology study), but may occur during rapid pacing or infusion of isoproterenol. The mechanism may result from triggered activity or increased automaticity. Radiofrequency catheter ablation has been effective in abolishing the right ventricular outflow tract focus. Left ventricular outflow tract or aortic cusp sites have also been targets for ablation. Treatment also may include β-blockers, calcium channel blockers, and type I or III antiarrhythmic agents.

Idiopathic left ventricular or fascicular tachycardia may present as a paroxysmal VT and usually can be induced through programmed ventricular extrastimulation, rapid pacing, isoproterenol, or exercise. It is characterized by right BBB morphology, usually with left superior axis (i.e., left-axis deviation; negative in II and aV$_F$), and it usually arises in the left inferoposterior septum through a mechanism believed to result from fascicular reentry or triggered activity. It may be terminated or suppressed by verapamil or diltiazem, and it has been successfully treated using radiofrequency catheter ablation, usually at sites where the VT is preceded by a fascicular potential.

## Torsades de Pointes

A form of polymorphic VT associated with prolonged QT intervals, TdP is a potentially life-threatening condition that can occur as a complication of several medications or in association with congenital long QT syndromes. The heart rate ranges from 150 to 250 beats/min, with twisting of the QRS complexes around the baseline. QT prolongation and QTU abnormalities are characteristic but may be present only in beats preceding TdP. TdP typically is rate dependent, and sinus bradycardia, bradycardia resulting from atrioventricular block, or abrupt prolongation of the RR interval (e.g., with a pause after a premature complex) can trigger its onset. It usually initiates with "long-short" coupled intervals, which may occur because of a PVC on the previous, long QT–associated T wave. A pause followed by a subsequent sinus or supraventricular beat and another PVC with a short coupling interval then may initiate TdP.

Acquired or congenital forms of long QT syndromes can predispose an individual to TdP. Congenital syndromes include the Romano-Ward syndrome (i.e., autosomal dominant) and Jervell and Lange-Nielsen syndrome (i.e., double dominant, associated with deafness). Linkage studies have revealed multiple separate loci (including on chromosomes 3, 4, 7, 11, and 21) that cause abnormalities in potassium (K$^+$) or sodium (Na$^+$) channels. The acquired long QT syndromes, many of which are associated with drugs that can prolong repolarization, are more commonly encountered. Long QT syndromes identified thus far with their respective genetic and ion channel defects are summarized in Table 66.7.

Drugs or conditions associated with TdP include:

- Antiarrhythmic drugs that prolong QT interval
  - Quinidine
  - Procainamide (including its metabolite *N*-acetylprocainamide)
  - Disopyramide
  - Sotalol
  - Amiodarone
  - Ibutilide
  - Dofetilide

**TABLE 66.7**

**LONG QT SYNDROMES**

| | Chromosome | Clinical Characteristics | Gene | Ion Current Change | Frequency |
|---|---|---|---|---|---|
| LQT1 | 11 | Events during exercise, swimming; broad T wave | KvLQT1 | ↓IKs α subunit | 45% |
| LQT2 | 7 | Events during auditory stimuli, startle, emotion; notched or low T wave | HERG | ↓IKr α subunit | 45% |
| LQT3 | 3 | Events during sleep; bradycardia; long flat ST | SCN5A | ↑INa | 10% |
| LQT4 | 4 | | Ankyrin | unknown | rare |
| LQT5 | 21 | | minK | ↓IKs β subunit | rare |
| LQT6 | 21 | | MiRP1 | ↓IKr α subunit | rare |
| LQT7 | 17 | Andersen's syndrome: intermittent muscle weakness; ventricular ectopy | KCNJ2 | ↓IKir2.1 | rare |
| JLN1 | 11 | Deafness; autosomal recessive | KvLQT1 | ↓IKs | rare |
| JLN2 | 21 | Deafness, autosomal recessive | minK | ↓IKs | rare |

□ Bepridil
□ Tedisimil
■ Tricyclic antidepressants
■ Phenothiazines
■ Nonsedating antihistamines
  □ Terfenadine
  □ Astemisole
■ Antibiotics
  □ Erythromycin
  □ Pentamidine
  □ Trimethoprim-sulfamethoxazole
  □ Ampicillin
  □ Ketoconazole
  □ Itraconazole
  □ Spiramycin
■ Other QT-prolonging drugs
  □ Probucol
  □ Ketanserin
  □ Cisapride
■ Organophosphates
■ Electrolyte abnormalities
  □ Hypokalemia
  □ Hypomagnesemia
  □ Hypocalcemia (uncommon)
■ Bradyarrhythmias
■ Hypothyroidism
■ Liquid protein and other diets, anorexia
■ Central nervous system abnormalities, particularly affecting sympathetic outflow
  □ Subarachnoid hemorrhage
  □ Brainstem, cervical cord lesions

Treatment includes the avoidance of offending agents and may require an acceleration of the heart rate, which can be accomplished through either pharmacologic agents (e.g., isoproterenol) or pacing, and intravenous magnesium. Lidocaine, mexiletine, or phenytoin can be tried as well.

# PHARMACOLOGIC THERAPY FOR TACHYARRHYTHMIAS

The most commonly accepted classification of antiarrhythmic drugs is the Vaughan-Williams classification (Harrison's modification). All drug classifications possess shortcomings, and specific agents may block more than one ion channel with effects that are characteristic of multiple classes. This scheme, however, has proved useful. Class I antiarrhythmic drugs block $Na^+$ channels, thereby decreasing action potential upstroke velocity (i.e., phase 0) and slowing conduction. Class I drugs are further divided into three subdivisions. Class IA agents, which prolong repolarization or action-potential duration, have a moderate effect on conduction slowing and the depression of phase 0. Class IB drugs have little effect on conduction and phase 0 in normal tissue, but they exhibit moderate effects in abnormal tissue. In addition, they show either no effect or a shortening of repolarization/action potential duration. Class IC agents have a marked effect on conduction slowing and phase 0, with mild or no effects on repolarization or action potential duration. Class II contains the β-adrenergic blocking agents, and class III potassium channel–blocking agents prolong repolarization/action potential duration. Class IV contains calcium channel blockers. Tables 66.4 and 66.5 list commonly used antiarrhythmic agents and their suggested dosages.

# BRADYARRHYTHMIAS

## Sinus Node Dysfunction

Sinus node dysfunction includes a range of abnormalities, including sinus bradyarrhythmias (e.g., sinus pauses, sinus bradycardias, chronotropic incompetence, sinus arrest, sinoatrial exit block), sick sinus syndrome, and tachycardia–bradycardia syndrome (e.g., paroxysmal or persistent atrial tachyarrhythmias with periods of bradyarrhythmia). Other forms of sinus node dysfunction that cause tachycardias (e.g., sinus tachycardia, inappropriate sinus tachycardia, sinus node reentry) were discussed previously.

### Sinus Bradycardia

Sinus bradycardia, which generally is defined as sinus rates of less than 60 beats/min, is common in young, healthy adults (especially in athletes), with normal rates during sleep falling to as low as 35 to 50 beats/min. It usually is benign, but it can be associated with diseases, such as hypothyroidism, vagal stimulation, increased intracranial pressure, MI, and drugs, such as β-blockers (including those used for glaucoma), calcium channel blockers, amiodarone, clonidine, lithium, and parasympathomimetic drugs. Treatment often is unnecessary if the patient is asymptomatic. Patients with chronic bradycardia or chronotropic incompetence and symptoms of congestive heart failure or low cardiac output, however, may benefit from permanent pacing.

### Sinus Pauses or Sinus Arrest

Sinus pauses or arrest may result from degenerative changes of the sinus node, acute MI, excessive vagal tone or stimuli, digitalis toxicity, sleep apnea, or stroke. Symptomatic or very long pauses may require permanent pacing.

### Sinoatrial Exit Block

Sinoatrial exit block results from a block in conduction from the sinus node to the atria. It usually appears as the absence of a P wave, with the sinus pause duration being a multiple of the basic PP interval (i.e., type II). In type I (Wenckebach pattern) sinoatrial exit block, the PP interval shortens before the pause, and the pause is less than two PP intervals. Sinoatrial exit block usually is transient but may be caused by drugs, vagal stimulation, or degenerative disease of the sinus node and atrium. Therapy for symptomatic sinoatrial exit block involves the avoidance of precipitating factors and, potentially, pacing for persistent symptoms.

### Sick Sinus Syndrome

Sick sinus syndrome includes a variety of sinus nodal disorders, such as inappropriate sinus bradycardia; sinus pauses, arrest, or sinoatrial exit block; combinations of sinoatrial and atrioventricular conduction abnormalities; and tachycardia-bradycardia syndrome, in which periods of rapid atrial tachyarrhythmias, as well as periods of slow atrial and ventricular rates, occur. Treatment depends on the basic rhythm disturbance. Drug therapy for rapid atrial arrhythmias may aggravate the bradyarrhythmias, and permanent pacing may be required.

## Hypersensitive Carotid Sinus Syndrome

Carotid sinus hypersensitivity can produce sinus arrest or atrioventricular block that leads to syncope, and it may be demonstrable with carotid sinus massage. Two types of responses are noted. Through carotid sinus massage, a cardioinhibitory component, with pauses of longer than 3 seconds, or a vasodepressor component, with a decrease in systolic blood pressure, may be provoked. Symptomatic patients may require pacemaker implantation to treat the cardioinhibitory component. Continued symptoms caused by vasodepressor reactions, even after pacemaker implantation, may require further treatment, including support stockings, high-sodium diets, or sodium-retaining drugs.

## Atrioventricular Dissociation

Atrioventricular dissociation refers to an independent depolarization of the atria and ventricles. It may be caused by

- Physiologic interference resulting from a slowing of the dominant pacemaker (e.g., sinus node) and the escape of a subsidiary or latent pacemaker (e.g., junctional or ventricular escape)
- Physiologic interference resulting from the acceleration of a latent pacemaker that usurps control of the ventricle (e.g., accelerated junctional tachycardia or VT)
- Atrioventricular block preventing the propagation of the atrial impulse from reaching the ventricles, thus allowing a subsidiary pacemaker (e.g., junctional or ventricular escape) to control the ventricles

Note that patients with complete atrioventricular block have atrioventricular dissociation and, generally, a ventricular rate that is slower than the atrial rate. Patients with atrioventricular dissociation, however, may have complete atrioventricular block or dissociation resulting from physiologic interference, with the latter typically having an atrial rate that is slower than the ventricular rate.

## Atrioventricular Block

Atrioventricular block occurs when the atrial impulse either is not conducted to the ventricle or is conducted with delay at a time when the atrioventricular junction is not refractory. It is classified on the basis of severity into three types.

In first-degree atrioventricular block, conduction is prolonged (PR interval >200 ms), but all impulses are conducted. The conduction delay may occur in the atrioventricular node, the His-Purkinje system, or both. If the QRS complex is narrow and normal, the atrioventricular delay usually occurs in the atrioventricular node.

In second-degree atrioventricular block, an intermittent block in conduction occurs. In Mobitz type I (i.e., Wenckebach) second-degree atrioventricular block, a progressive prolongation of the PR interval occurs before the block in conduction. In the usual Wenckebach periodicity (Fig. 66.10), the PR interval gradually increases, but with a decreasing increment, thus leading to a gradual shortening

## TABLE 66.8
### INDICATIONS FOR PERMANENT PACEMAKERS

| Disorder | Class of Indication | Indication |
|---|---|---|
| SND | I | 1. SND with documented symptomatic bradycardia, including as a consequence of necessary long-term drug therapy<br>2. Symptomatic chronotropic incompetence |
| | II | 1. SND with heart rates <40 beats/min, no clear associations between symptoms and bradycardia<br>2. Syncope of unexplained origin with major SND found at electrophysiologic testing<br>3. In minimally symptomatic patients, chronic heart rate <40 beats/min while awake |
| | III | 1. No symptoms<br>2. Symptoms clearly documented as not associated with slow heart rate<br>3. Symptomatic bradycardia due to nonessential drug therapy |
| Acquired AVB | I | 1. Advanced 2nd- or 3rd-degree AVB at any anatomic level associated with:<br>  a. Bradycardia with symptoms (including heart failure) presumed due to AVB<br>  b. Arrhythmias and other medical conditions needing drugs that result in symptomatic bradycardia<br>  c. Periods of asystole ≥ 3.0 secs or escape rate <40 bpm in awake, asymptomatic patients<br>  d. AV junction ablation<br>  e. Postoperative AVB not expected to resolve<br>  f. Neuromuscular diseases (e.g. myotonic muscular dystrophy, Kearns-Sayre syndrome, Erb's limb-girdle dystrophy, peroneal muscular atrophy) with AVB, with or without symptoms, as progression of AVB may be unpredictable<br>2. 2nd degree AVB at any level with symptomatic bradycardia<br>3. 2nd degree AVB type II with a wide QRS |
| | II | 1. Asymptomatic 3rd-degree AVB with average awake ventricular rates of ≥40 bpm, especially if LV dysfunction or cardiomegaly is present<br>2. Asymptomatic 2nd-degree AVB type II with narrow QRS<br>3. Asymptomatic type I 2nd-degree AVB at intra- or infra-His levels found at electrophysiology study<br>4. 1st- or 2nd-degree AVB with symptoms similar to those of pacemaker syndrome<br>5. Marked 1st-degree (>0.30 s) in LV dysfunction and congestive heart failure in which shorter AV interval results in hemodynamic improvement<br>6. Neuromuscular diseases with any degree of AVB (including 1st degree), as progression of AVB may be unpredictable |
| | III | 1. Asymptomatic 1st-degree AVB<br>2. Asymptomatic 2nd-degree AVB type I at the AV node level<br>3. AVB expected to resolve and unlikely to recur (e.g., drug toxicity, Lyme disease, hypoxia in sleep apnea syndrome in absence of symptoms) |
| AV block associated with myocardial infarction | I | 1. Persistent advanced 2nd-degree with bilateral BBB or 3rd-degree AVB with block in the His-Purkinje system<br><br><br>2. Transient advanced (2nd or 3rd degree) infranodal AVB and associated BBB<br>3. Persistent and symptomatic 2nd- or 3rd-degree AVB |
| | II | Persistent 2nd- or 3rd-degree AVB at the AV node level |
| | III | 1. Transient AVB in the absence of intraventricular conduction defects or in the presence of isolated left anterior fascicular block<br>2. Acquired left anterior fascicular block without AVB<br>3. Persistent 1st-degree AVB with BBB that is old or age indeterminate |
| Bifascicular or trifascicular block | I | 1. Intermittent 3rd-degree AVB<br>2. 2nd-degree type II AVB<br>3. Alternating BBB |

(continued)

**TABLE 66.8**

## INDICATIONS FOR PERMANENT PACEMAKERS (*Continued*)

| Disorder | Class of Indication | Indication |
|---|---|---|
| | II | 1. Syncope not demonstrated to b due to AVB when other likely causes, including ventricular tachycardia, have been excluded<br>2. HV interval ≥100 ms or nonphysiologic pacing-induced infra-His block found at electrophysiologic study<br>3. Neuromuscular diseases with any degree of fascicular block with or without symptoms, as progression of AV conduction disease may be unpredictable |
| | III | Asymptomatic fascicular block or fascicular block with associated 1st-degree AV node block |
| Neurocardiogenic syncope or carotid sinus hypersensitivity | I | Recurrent syncope provoked by carotid sinus stimulation; pauses of >3 sec induced by minimal carotid sinus pressure |
| | II | 1. Recurrent syncope without clear provocative events and with a hypersensitive cardioinhibitory response<br>2. Significantly symptomatic and recurrent neurocardiogenic syncope associated with bradycardia documented spontaneously or at tilt-table testing<br>3. Neurally medicated syncope with significant bradycardia reproduced by head upright tilt with or without provocative maneuvers |
| | III | 1. Hyperactive cardioinhibitory response to carotid sinus stimulation that is asymptomatic or minimally/vaguely symptomatic<br>2. Recurrent syncope, lightheadedness or dizziness in the absence of a hyperactive cardioinhibitory response<br>3. Situational vasovagal syncope in which avoidance behavior is effective |
| Cardiomyopathy | I | None |
| | II | 1. Medically refractory, symptomatic hypertrophic obstructive cardiomyopathy with significant resting or provoked LV outflow tract obstruction<br>2. Biventricular pacing in medically refractory, symptomatic NYHA class III or IV patients with idiopathic or ischemic cardiomyopathy, QRS interval ≥ 130 ms, LV end-diastolic diameter ≥ 55 mm, and LVEF ≤ 35%.<br>3. Symptomatic drug-refractory dilated cardiomyopathy with prolonged PR interval when acute hemodynamic studies have demonstrated hemodynamic benefit of pacing |
| | III | 1. Asymptomatic or medically controlled patients with hypertrophic obstructive cardiomyopathy or dilated cardiomyopathy<br>2. Symptomatic patients without LV outflow tract obstruction<br>3. Symptomatic ischemic cardiomyopathy when ischemia is amenable to intervention |

SND, sinus node dysfunction; AVB, atrioventricular block; BBB, bundle branch block; LV, left ventricular; LVEF, left ventricular ejection fraction.
[Modified and adapted with permission from Gregoratos G, Abrams J, Epstein AE, et al. ACC/AHA/NASPE 2002 Guideline Update for Implantation of Cardiac Pacemakers and Antiarrhythmia Devices: Summary Article: A Report of the American College of Cardiology/American Heart Association Task Force on Practice Guidelines (ACC/AHA/NASPE Committee to Update the 1998 Pacemaker Guidelines) *Circulation* 2002;106:2145–2161.]

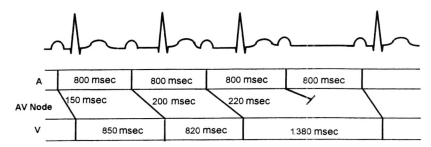

**Figure 66.10**  Second-degree atrioventricular (AV) block Mobitz type I (Wenckebach) periodicity.

of the RR intervals. The longest PR interval usually precedes the block, and the shortest PR interval usually occurs after the block, thereby resulting in the long RR interval of the blocked impulse being shorter than twice the basic PP interval. Variants of this pattern are not uncommon. In Mobitz type II second-degree atrioventricular block, PR intervals before the block are constant, and sudden blocks in P-wave conduction occur. Advanced or high-degree atrioventricular block refers to a block of two or more consecutive impulses. In Mobitz type I block, the level of the block is almost always at the atrioventricular node. Rarely, type I Wenckebach periodicity in the His-Purkinje system may be seen in patients with BBB. In contrast, Mobitz type II block is almost always at the level of the His-Purkinje system and has a higher risk of progressing to complete atrioventricular block.

In third-degree (i.e., complete) atrioventricular block, no impulses are conducted from the atria to the ventricles. The level of the block can occur at the atrioventricular node (usually congenital), His bundle, or in the His-Purkinje system (usually acquired). Escape beats that are junctional at rates of 40 to 60 beats/min generally occur with congenital complete atrioventricular block. Escape beats that are ventricular in origin often are slow, ranging from 30 to 40 beats/min.

## Indications for Permanent Pacing

Conditions for which permanent pacing is or is not indicated are outlined in Table 66.8, based on a three-part classification of indications:

- Class I: conditions for which evidence and/or general agreement exists that permanent pacemakers should be implanted
- Class II: conditions for which pacemakers frequently are used but for which conflicting evidence and/or disagreement exists regarding their usefulness or efficacy.
- Class III: conditions for which general agreement exists that pacemakers are unnecessary

## Indications for Temporary Pacing

In general, temporary pacing is indicated for patients with medically refractory, symptomatic bradyarrhythmias without contraindications to pacing. In the absence of acute MI, particularly while awaiting the implantation of a permanent pacemaker (if indicated), temporary pacing can be warranted for patients with medically refractory, symptomatic or hemodynamically compromising sinus node

bradyarrhythmias, second- or third-degree atrioventricular block, or third-degree atrioventricular block with a wide QRS complex escape rhythm or a ventricular rate of less than 50 beats/min. In the presence of acute MI, temporary pacing is indicated for:

- Third-degree atrioventricular block
- Second-degree atrioventricular block
  - Mobitz II with anterior MI
  - Mobitz II with inferior MI and wide QRS complex or recurrent block with narrow QRS complex
- Mobitz I with marked bradycardia and symptoms
- Atrioventricular block associated with marked bradycardia and symptoms (e.g., hypotension, heart failure, low cardiac output)
- BBB
  - New bifascicular block
  - Alternating BBB
  - New BBB with anterior MI
  - Bilateral BBB of indeterminate age with anterior or indeterminate MI
  - Bilateral BBB with first-degree atrioventricular block

## SUGGESTED READINGS

Albers GW, Dalen JE, Laupacis A, et al. Antithrombotic therapy in atrial fibrillation. *Chest* 2001;119[Suppl 1]:194S–206S.

Antiarrhythmics Versus Implantable Defibrillators (AVID) Investigators. A comparison of antiarrhythmic-drug therapy with implantable defibrillators in patients resuscitated from near-fatal ventricular arrhythmias. *N Engl J Med* 1997;337:1576–1583.

Atrial Fibrillation Follow-Up Investigation of Rhythm Management (AFFIRM) Investigators. A comparison of rate control and rhythm control in patients with atrial fibrillation. *N Engl J Med* 2002; 347:1825–1833.

Brugada P, Brugada J, Mont L, et al. A new approach to the differential diagnosis of a regular tachycardia with a wide QRS complex. *Circulation* 1991;83:1649–1659.

Fuster V, Ryden LE, Asinger RW, et al. ACC/AHA/ESC Guidelines for the Management of Patients with Atrial Fibrillation: Executive Summary. A Report of the American College of Cardiology/ American Heart Association Task Force on Practice Guidelines and the European Society of Cardiology Committee for Practice Guidelines and Policy Conferences (Committee to Develop Guidelines for the Management of Patients With Atrial Fibrillation) Developed in Collaboration with the North American Society of Pacing and Electrophysiology. *Circulation* 2001;104:2118–2150.

Gregoratos G, Abrams J, Epstein AE, et al. ACC/AHA/NASPE 2002 Guideline Update for Implantation of Cardiac Pacemakers and Antiarrhythmia Devices: Summary Article: A Report of the American College of Cardiology/ American Heart Association Task Force on Practice Guidelines (ACC/AHA/NASPE Committee to Update the 1998 Pacemaker Guidelines). *Circulation* 2002;106:2145–2161.

Moss AJ, Zareba W, Hall WJ, et al., for the Multicenter Automatic Defibrillator Implantation Trial II Investigators. Prophylactic implantation of a defibrillator in patients with myocardial infarction and reduced ejection fraction. *N Engl J Med* 2002;346:877–883.

# Adult Congenital Heart Disease

### Douglas S. Moodie

**67**

Adult congenital heart disease will become increasingly important over the next 20 years. Children who have undergone corrective or palliative operations during infancy and childhood are surviving well into adulthood, and cardiologists who care for these children now are faced with young or middle-aged adults who require a lifetime of follow-up. In addition, many patients first present with their congenital heart lesions as adults. These patients represent an increasingly important area in adult cardiovascular disease, as evidenced by numerous publications on this topic (1–9).

Treating adults with congenital heart disease is difficult because physicians involved in such care generally have not been trained to deal with the issues involved. Many pediatric cardiologists stop following their patients after 20 years of age, turning them over to adult cardiologists. Adult cardiology programs generally have not concentrated on the problems of adults with congenital heart disease, focusing mainly on acquired heart disease. Thus, adult patients with congenital heart disease who had surgery as children or initially present as adults encounter physicians who are somewhat ill-equipped to address their problems.

Where these patients should receive care can be problematic as well. It is difficult for adults to obtain care in the setting where most pediatric cardiologists practice (i.e., children's hospitals). The special needs of adults with congenital heart disease also are not always evident in adult institutions, which primarily are equipped to deal with acquired coronary or valvular heart disease. Thus, it is increasingly important for pediatric and adult cardiologists to work closely together, and for a "new breed" of congenital cardiologists to appear. These cardiologists most likely will come from pediatric cardiology settings, but they also must feel comfortable dealing with adult congenital heart disease. At the Cleveland Clinic, all patients with congenital cardiac disease are followed by the pediatric cardiologist from infancy to late adulthood. Board-certified internists who are advanced fellows in cardiology rotate on the congenital cardiology service. These fellows manage those complications and problems, seen in adult medicine, that are unfamiliar to pediatric cardiologists. A cardiologist who is trained in specific congenital lesions, however, manages the major cardiac problems.

It is important that cardiologists caring for adults with congenital cardiac disease know how individuals present as adults. Current studies (10,11) have dealt primarily with infants and children followed into adulthood. This chapter concentrates on experience at my institution with adults who presented with their defects as adults. The congenital lesions we have encountered most commonly in adults are atrial septal defect (ASD), ventricular septal defect (VSD), patent ductus arteriosus (PDA), coarctation of the aorta, tetralogy of Fallot, pulmonary stenosis (PS), corrected transposition of the great arteries, and Ebstein's anomaly.

## ATRIAL SEPTAL DEFECT

If congenitally bicuspid aortic valve and mitral valve prolapse are excluded, ASD is the most common form of congenital heart disease in adults, constituting approximately 22% to 25% of these patients (1). Some 65% to 75% of all ASDs are of the ostium secundum type, 15% to 20% are of the ostium primum type (i.e., partial atrioventricular canal), and 5% to 10% are the sinus venosus type (Fig. 67.1), which is associated with partial anomalous pulmonary venous connection of the right upper pulmonary veins. ASDs account for 7% to 11% of all cardiac defects in general. The female-to-male ratio is approximately 2:1.

In young adults, the dominant shunt is left to right because the left atrial pressure exceeds the right atrial pressure during the major portion of the cardiac cycle. Immediately after atrial systole, the right atrial pressure briefly may exceed that of the left, and blood may shunt right to left. Despite the marked increase in pulmonary blood flow (i.e., as high as three to four times the systemic blood flow), pulmonary artery pressure almost always is normal until later in adult life, and although pulmonary arteries may have medial hypertrophy and intimal proliferation, pulmonary vascular changes greater than grade II are rare even in middle-aged adults.

Between 1956 and 1981, 295 patients (219 women and 76 men) with ASD were seen at the Cleveland Clinic who eventually underwent surgical closure. Patients ranged in age from 19 to 70 years, with a mean age of 40 years.

### Clinical Presentation

The most common presenting symptoms were shortness of breath (51%) and easy fatigability (43%). Forty-three percent also reported palpitations, 12% experienced atrial

Atrial Septal Defect

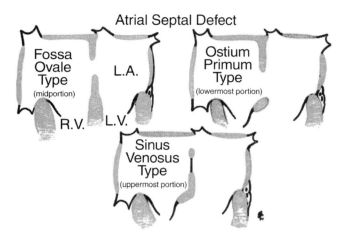

**Figure 67.1**  Diagrammatic representation of the three forms of atrial septal defect demonstrating a secundum, primum, and sinus venosus type defect. LA, left atrium; LV, left ventricle; RV, right ventricle. (Reproduced with permission from the American College of Cardiology.)

fibrillation, and 15% were asymptomatic. Eleven percent reported one or more episodes of heart failure, 4% had cyanosis, and 3% had suffered a stroke.

Seventy-six patients were New York Heart Association (NYHA) functional class I, 179 were class II, 34 were class III, and six were class IV. Twenty-nine percent of patients were taking digoxin, and 18% were on diuretics. Six percent were taking antiarrhythmics, and 9% were on other medications. A positive family history for ASD was present in 27% of patients. A heart murmur was detected in 97%, and a fixed, split $S_2$ was noted in 54%.

### Radiographic Features

Chest radiography demonstrated cardiomegaly in 71% of patients. Fifty-one percent had mildly increased vascularity, 38% were normal, 11% had moderately increased vascularity, and 1% had greatly increased vascularity.

### Electrocardiographic Features

Electrocardiography revealed sinus rhythm in 92% of patients. Right ventricular hypertrophy was present in 52%, atrial fibrillation in 7%, and complete heart block in 1%. The mean QRS axis was 82 degrees, with a range of 0 to 160 degrees; the mean P axis was 72 degrees with a range of 30 to 150 degrees. Right ventricular hypertrophy correlated strongly with pulmonary artery pressure but did not correlate with age. Preoperative atrial fibrillation correlated with both increasing pulmonary artery pressure and age.

### Cardiac Catheterization

Cardiac catheterization was performed on 290 patients. The systolic pulmonary artery pressures varied from 13 to 146 mm Hg, with a mean pressure of 40 mm Hg. Left atrial pressures ranged from 2 to 28 mm Hg, with a mean of 8.5 mm Hg, and right atrial pressures were slightly lower, with a mean of 7 mm Hg. The mean pulmonary flow to systemic flow ratio ($Q_p$:$Q_s$) was 2.8:1, with a range of 1.2 to 10:1. Mean total pulmonary vascular resistance was 3.9 U, with a range of 1.4 to 8.6 U. Mean systemic resistance was 28 U.

Thirteen percent of these patients were noted to have anomalous pulmonary venous connection. Nine percent had coronary artery disease, 5% had PS, and 1% had tricuspid insufficiency and aortic valve disease. Fifteen percent of the patients had pulmonary vascular disease.

Left ventricular function, as assessed by ventriculography, was normal in 96%, mildly impaired in 2%, moderately impaired in 2%, and severely impaired in none. Mitral insufficiency was noted in 7% of the patients, being mild in 5%, moderate in 1%, and severe in 1%. Eighty-six percent of the defects were of the ostium secundum type, and ostium primum and sinus venosus defects were each found in 6% of the patients.

## VENTRICULAR SEPTAL DEFECT

In 1879, Henri Roget wrote, "The congenital defect of the heart compatible with life and perhaps a long one, one of the most frequent which I have encountered . . . is the communication between the two ventricles because of failure of occlusion of the interventricular septum and its upper portion" (12). VSD (Fig. 67.2) is a common anomaly, occurring in

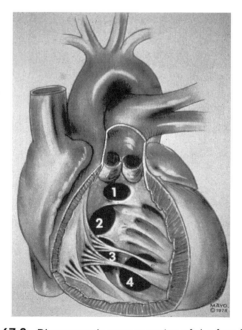

**Figure 67.2**  Diagrammatic representation of the four forms of ventricular septal defect as viewed from the right ventricle. The figure demonstrates that the supracristal and subcristal ventricular septal defects are both subaortic on the left ventricular side. The diagram also shows an atrioventricular canal type ventricular septal defect and a muscular ventricular septal defect. (Reproduced with permission from the American College of Cardiology.)

approximately 10% of adult patients with congenital heart disease (1). Campbell (13) has described the natural history of adults with VSD in his practice: 27% of his patients died by age 20, 53% by age 40, and 69% before age 60.

At our institution, 79 patients (42 men and 37 women) older than 18 years with isolated VSD were seen between 1951 and 1981. These patients ranged in age from 18 to 59 years, with a mean age of 34 years. Twelve patients had surgical closure soon after presentation, whereas 67 were treated medically.

## Clinical Presentation

The medical group consisted of 67 patients (33 men and 34 women) who ranged in age from 18 to 59 years at presentation, with a mean age of 33 years. At the time of diagnosis, 42 of these patients were in NYHA functional class I, 15 in class II, eight in class III, and two in class IV. Only 29% were taking medication, with digitalis and diuretics being most common. The most common symptoms among these patients are listed in Table 67.1.

Almost all patients had a holosystolic murmur of VSD audible along the left sternal border. Seventy-four percent were grade 2 to 4 out of 6, and 51% had a palpable thrill. The physical findings among these patients are summarized in Table 67.2.

Chest radiography showed cardiomegaly in 32% of the patients. The pulmonary vascularity was increased in 28%.

The initial electrocardiogram revealed a variety of rhythm patterns. Normal sinus rhythm was the most common, occurring in 58 of the 67 patients (Table 67.3).

## Cardiac Catheterization

Forty-six patients had cardiac catheterization; however, only 38% of these patients had sufficient data available to calculate the pulmonary artery resistance. The results of these catheterizations are listed in Table 67.4. After the initial evaluation, 8 patients were placed on medication, and 58 required no treatment.

## Course

The medical group was followed from between 1 month and 24 years, with a mean follow-up of 9 years. Patient age at follow-up ranged from 24 to 74 years, with a mean age of 42 years. At follow-up, 51 patients were alive, and 15 had expired. Only one patient had bacterial endocarditis and succumbed. The most common causes of death among these patients are listed in Table 67.5. Of the catheterization data available for the medically followed patients who died, 73% had a systolic pulmonary artery pressure of greater than 50 mm Hg (Table 67.6).

Fifteen patients continued to have symptoms, including palpitations, atypical chest pain, dysrhythmias, shortness of breath, angina, and fatigability. Fourteen patients were maintained on medication. At follow-up, 42 patients were NYHA functional class I, eight were class II, and two were class III. Only one patient was severely restricted in physical activity, and 32 patients continued to work. Excluding

### TABLE 67.1

**ADULT VENTRICULAR SEPTAL DEFECT (MEDICAL GROUP): SYMPTOMS IN 87 PATIENTS**

| Symptom | Patients [n (%)] |
| --- | --- |
| Dyspnea | 19 (28) |
| Exercise intolerance | 16 (24) |
| Shortness of breath | 15 (22) |
| Edema | 13 (19) |
| Hypertension | 3 (4) |
| Fever | 2 (3) |
| None | 23 (34) |

### TABLE 67.2

**ADULT VENTRICULAR SEPTAL DEFECT (MEDICAL GROUP): PHYSICAL FINDINGS IN 67 PATIENTS**

| Finding | Patients [n (%)] |
| --- | --- |
| Systolic murmur | 66 (99) |
| Split $S_2$ | 57 (85) |
| Normal pulmonary component | 38 (57) |
| Increased pulmonary component | 22 (33) |
| Systolic thrill | 34 (51) |
| Cyanosis | 11 (16) |
| Clubbing | 6 (9) |
| $S_3$ | 10 (15) |
| Right ventricular lift | 7 (10) |
| Hepatomegaly | 5 (7) |
| Systolic click | 2 (3) |
| $S_4$ | 1 (1) |

### TABLE 67.3

**ADULT VENTRICULAR SEPTAL DEFECT (MEDICAL GROUP): ELECTROCARDIOGRAPHIC FINDINGS IN 67 PATIENTS**

| Finding | Patients [n (%)] |
| --- | --- |
| Sinus rhythm | 58 (87) |
| Sinus bradycardia | 6 (9) |
| Sinus tachycardia | 2 (3) |
| Supraventricular tachycardia | 1 (1) |
| First-degree atrioventricular block | 4 (6) |
| Premature ventricular contractions | 2 (3) |
| Right ventricular hypertrophy | 16 (24) |
| Left ventricular hypertrophy | 2 (3) |
| Biventricular hypertrophy | 3 (4) |

### TABLE 67.4

**ADULT VENTRICULAR SEPTAL DEFECT (MEDICAL GROUP): CARDIAC CATHETERIZATION FINDINGS IN 46 PATIENTS**

| Finding | Mean | Patients (n) |
|---|---|---|
| Femoral artery pressure (mm Hg) | | |
| Systolic | 127 ± 24 | 45 |
| Diastolic | 79 ± 14 | 45 |
| Femoral artery saturation (%) | 92 ± 6 | 31 |
| Mixed venous saturation (%) | 69 ± 16 | 29 |
| Pulmonary artery saturation (%) | 78 ± 8 | 37 |
| Left ventricular pressure (mm Hg) | | |
| Systolic | 128 ± 24 | 42 |
| Diastolic | 12 ± 6 | 42 |
| Right ventricular pressure (mm Hg) | | |
| Systolic | 53 ± 44 | 43 |
| Diastolic | 8 ± 6 | 43 |
| Pulmonary artery pressure (mm Hg) | | |
| Systolic | 50 ± 42 | 43 |
| Diastolic | 23 ± 24 | 43 |
| Cardiac index (L/min/m$^2$) | 3.2 ± 1.2 | 26 |
| Pulmonary index (L/min/m$^2$) | 5.0 ± 5.5 | 25 |
| $Q_p/Q_s$ | 1.6 ± 1.4 | 26 |
| Pulmonary resistance (U) | 10.3 ± 13.8 | 26 |
| Pulmonary arteriolar resistance (U) | 6.4 ± 13.7 | 11 |
| Systemic resistance (U) | 35.8 ± 16.2 | 24 |
| Left-to-right shunt (%) | 30 ± 23 | 20 |

$Q_p$, pulmonary flow; $Q_s$, systemic flow.

those patients who died, only three deteriorated, with the remainder either stable or improved.

Patients who were class I at presentation had a better survival rate than the more symptomatic patients. Survival at 10 years was 90% for class I patients and 58% for others. Cardiomegaly at initial presentation significantly reduced

### TABLE 67.5

**ADULT VENTRICULAR SEPTAL DEFECT (MEDICAL GROUP): CAUSE OF DEATH IN 15 PATIENTS**

| Cause | (%) |
|---|---|
| Heart failure | 45 |
| Myocardial infarct | 45 |
| Sudden death | 31 |
| Pulmonary embolus | 29 |
| Renal failure | 37 |
| Noncardiac, other | 42 |
| Heart failure and endocarditis | 42 |
| Cerebrovascular accident | 43 |
| Major hemorrhagic complications and pulmonary hypertension | 43 |

### TABLE 67.6

**ADULT VENTRICULAR SEPTAL DEFECT (MEDICAL GROUP): PULMONARY ARTERY PRESSURE IN PATIENTS WHO DIED**

| Patient | Pulmonary Systolic Pressure (mm Hg) | Pulmonary Diastolic Pressure (mm Hg) |
|---|---|---|
| 1 | 122 | 58 |
| 2 | 96 | 52 |
| 3 | 88 | 50 |
| 4 | 98 | 54 |
| 5 | 48 | 4 |
| 6 | 38 | 15 |
| 7 | 30 | 12 |
| 8 | 173 | 80 |
| 9 | 100 | 55 |
| 10 | 115 | 70 |
| 11 | 118 | 72 |

the chance for survival. The 10-year survival rates were 90% for patients without cardiomegaly and 50% for those with elevated pulmonary artery pressure ($p < 0.001$) in the medical group.

## PATENT DUCTUS ARTERIOSUS

Between 1951 and 1984, we evaluated 117 patients with the diagnosis of isolated PDA (Fig. 67.3). These patients ranged in age from 18 to 81 years, with a mean age of

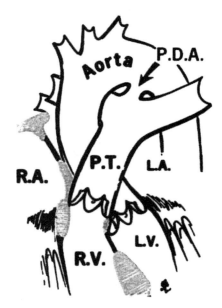

**Figure 67.3** Diagrammatic representation of a patent ductus arteriosus (PDA). LA, left atrium; LV, left ventricle; PT, pulmonary trunk; RA, right atrium; RV, right ventricle. (Reproduced with permission from the American College of Cardiology.)

36 years. There were 95 women and 22 men. Follow-up was obtained for 114 of these patients.

Thirty-three patients received no therapy, and 12 received medical therapy alone. Sixty-eight patients underwent surgical closure of the PDA. All patients were classified functionally at the initial diagnosis. Fifty-seven were in NYHA functional class I, 51 in class II, seven in class III, and two in class IV. No significant difference existed between the surgical and nonsurgical groups in terms of functional class.

## Clinical Presentation

Symptoms at diagnosis were comparable in the two groups (Table 67.7). Thirty-seven of the 117 patients presented with exercise intolerance, and 29% complained of dyspnea. Cyanosis was more frequent in the nonsurgical group. Thirty-seven patients were asymptomatic at initial presentation.

Ninety-seven percent of these patients presented with a systolic murmur, which generally was grade 2 to 4 in intensity. It was best heard at the left upper sternal border in most patients. The intensity of the murmur was comparable in both groups. A continuous murmur was heard in 61%, and four patients presented with no heart murmur. Only 38% of the nonsurgical patients presented with a diastolic murmur, whereas 71% of the surgical patients had a diastolic murmur, which ranged in intensity from grade 2 to 4 ($p < 0.0001$). The pulmonary component of $S_2$ was heard with equal intensity in the nonsurgical and surgical groups. The frequency of a systolic thrill or $S_3$ was not different between the two groups.

No difference was observed between the surgical and nonsurgical groups in terms of the type or amount of medications taken at initial presentation. Eighty-nine patients were taking no medication. Endocarditis was seen in three of the patients preoperatively.

## Radiographic Features

Sixteen patients demonstrated calcification of the ductus, either at chest radiography or surgery. In the surgical group, 11 patients had calcification; their ages ranged from 28 to 70 years, with a mean age of 49 years. In the nonsurgical group, five patients had calcification; their mean age of 61 years was somewhat greater.

Cardiomegaly was found in 46% of the patients. Sixteen patients demonstrated increased pulmonary vascularity.

## Electrocardiographic Features

The electrocardiogram revealed normal sinus rhythm in 95% of patients. In the nonsurgical group, 13 patients demonstrated right ventricular hypertrophy, and five demonstrated left ventricular hypertrophy. In the surgical group, ten patients had evidence of right ventricular hypertrophy, and 13 had evidence of left ventricular hypertrophy.

## COARCTATION OF THE AORTA

Between 1952 and 1970, 69 adult patients (49 men and 20 women) underwent surgical correction for coarctation of the aorta (Fig. 67.4) and were evaluated preoperatively. Their ages ranged from 18 to 50 years, with a mean age of 30.5 years.

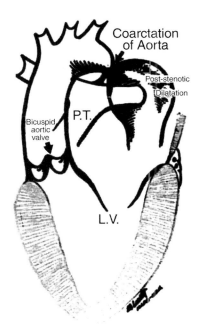

**Figure 67.4** Diagrammatic representation of a classical isolated coarctation of the aorta. The figure represents prestenotic and poststenotic dilatation of the descending aorta and a bicuspid aortic valve. LV, left ventricle; PT, pulmonary trunk. (Reproduced with permission from the American College of Cardiology.)

## TABLE 67.7

### ADULT PATENT DUCTUS ARTERIOSUS: SYMPTOMS IN 117 PATIENTS

| Symptom | Nonsurgically Treated [n (%)] | Surgically Treated [n (%)] |
|---|---|---|
| Patients | 45 (100) | 72 (100) |
| Asymptomatic | 19 (42) | 18 (25) |
| Symptomatic | 25 (58) | 54 (75) |
| Exercise intolerance | 11 (24) | 26 (38) |
| Dyspnea | 11 (24) | 23 (32) |
| Cyanosis | 9 (20) | 0 (0) |
| Peripheral edema | 5 (11) | 4 (5) |
| Clubbing | 3 (7) | 0 (0) |

(Reprinted with permission from Fisher RC, Moodie DS, Sterba R, et al. Patent ductus arteriosus in adults long-term follow-up: nonsurgical versus surgical treatment. *J Am Acad Cardiol* 1986;8:281–284.)

## Clinical Presentation

Fifty-eight percent (40 of 69) of these patients were asymptomatic. Twenty-three percent (16 of 69) had exercise intolerance, and 17% (12 of 69) complained of claudication. Ten percent experienced dyspnea and had angina, and one patient was cyanotic. Ninety percent (62 of 69) were hypertensive, and 44% (30 of 69) had a heart murmur. Ten percent had already experienced bacterial endocarditis, 4% had a myocardial infarction, and 1% had aortic dissection. Five patients had suffered a stroke.

As mentioned, 62 of these patients had hypertension, and 21 were on antihypertensive medication or diuretics. The mean blood pressure in this group was 152/86 mm Hg, with systolic blood pressure ranging from 100 to 260 mm Hg and diastolic from 40 to 148 mm Hg. Femoral pulses were absent in 18%, normal in 2%, and diminished in 80%.

## TETRALOGY OF FALLOT

Tetralogy of Fallot (Fig. 67.5) was the most common form of cyanotic congenital heart disease. It is estimated that without surgical intervention, only approximately 10% of these patients survive beyond 21 years of age (14–16). Several studies have addressed the adult with tetralogy of Fallot (17–21).

Between 1951 and 1981, we saw 13 patients older than 18 years needing total intracardiac repair of tetralogy of Fallot. These 13 patients included eight men and five women. Three had no previous palliation. Of the ten who had undergone previous palliation, six had a Potts anastomosis, three had a Blalock shunt, and one patient had an aortopulmonary artery graft. Patient age at palliation ranged from 5 months to 19 years, and time from palliation to total repair ranged from 2 to 80 years, with a mean time of

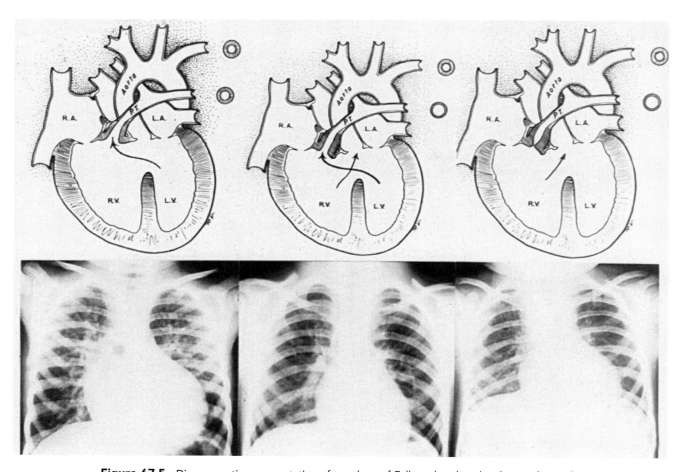

**Figure 67.5** Diagrammatic representation of tetralogy of Fallot related to the chest radiograph. The left-hand panel shows a pink tetralogy of Fallot with mild right ventricular outflow tract obstruction and a left-to-right shunt. The radiograph demonstrates a cardiomegaly with increased vascularity. The mid-panel represents bidirectional shunting at the ventricular level. The heart on radiography is smaller and the vascularity somewhat reduced. The right-hand panel represents classic tetralogy of Fallot with a right-to-left shunt at the ventricular level and severe right ventricular outflow tract obstruction. The radiograph shows a boot-shaped heart with decreased vascularity. LA, left atrium; LV, left ventricle; PT, pulmonary trunk; RA, right atrium; RV, right ventricle. (Reproduced with permission from the American College of Cardiology.)

20 years. Patient age at total intracardiac repair ranged from 18 to 42 years, with a mean age of 30 years.

## Clinical Presentation

Cyanosis and dyspnea on exertion were the most common symptoms before total repair. Other, less frequent findings were fatigue, restricted activity, hemoptysis, pneumonia, headache, syncope, and endocarditis. On the NYHA functional classification, one patient was class I, one was class II, ten were class III, and one was class IV.

Cyanosis was present in 11 patients, and clubbing was present in ten. No patient had heart failure, but all had a systolic murmur. Other findings were as noted in Table 67.8.

## Radiographic Features

Cardiomegaly was present in five patients. Seven patients had evidence of right ventricular enlargement, whereas two had evidence of left ventricular enlargement. Decreased pulmonary vascularity was apparent in only one patient.

## Electrocardiographic Features

All patients had normal sinus rhythm. Eleven had evidence of right ventricular hypertrophy, and nine showed right-axis deviation. Three patients had complete right bundle branch block. One patient had first-degree atrioventricular block.

## Cardiac Catheterization

Hemodynamic data were obtained in 11 of these patients (Table 67.9). Right ventricular systolic pressure ranged from 70 to 130 mm Hg, and right ventricular outflow tract

### TABLE 67.9

**ADULT TETRALOGY OF FALLOT: HEMODYNAMIC DATA**

| Patient No. | Right Ventricular Systolic Pressure (mm Hg) | Right Ventricular Outflow Tract Gradient (mm Hg) | Pulmonary Artery Pressure (mm Hg) |
|---|---|---|---|
| 1 | 82 | 57 | 25/15 |
| 2 | — | — | — |
| 3 | 130 | — | — |
| 4 | 130 | 112 | 18[a] |
| 5 | 110 | — | — |
| 6 | 115 | 90 | 25/15 |
| 7 | 110 | 85 | 25/20 |
| 8 | 115 | —[b] | 85/65 |
| 9 | 120 | 100 | 20[a] |
| 10 | 95 | 75 | 20[a] |
| 11 | — | — | — |
| 12 | 70 | 50 | 20/15 |
| 13 | 125 | 85 | 40/25 |

—, not obtained.
[a] Systolic.
[b] Previous Potts shunt.
(Reprinted with permission from Kreindel M, Moodie DS, Sterba R, et al. Total repair of tetralogy of Fallot in the adult: The Cleveland Clinic experience, 1951–1981. *Cleve Clin Q* 1985;fall:376.)

gradients were measured in nine patients. These gradients ranged from 50 to 112 mm Hg. In addition, pulmonary artery pressures were measured in ten patients. Systolic pressure ranged from 18 to 85 mm Hg, and diastolic pressure ranged from 15 to 65 mm Hg.

# PULMONARY STENOSIS

Between 1951 and 1981, we saw 68 patients older than 20 years of age with PS. Thirty-seven of these patients had PS with associated defects, and 31 had isolated PS. Of those patients with associated defects, 19 had a VSD, ten an ASD, four aortic insufficiency, three mitral valve prolapse, two mitral insufficiency, two corrected transposition of the great arteries, two univentricular heart, two congenital coronary anomalies, two isolated dextrocardia, and one patient each with PDA, supravalvular PS, aortic stenosis, tricuspid stenosis, bicuspid aortic valve, subvalvular PS, double-outlet right ventricle, and double-outlet left ventricle.

Of the 31 patients with isolated PS, 13 were men and 18 were women. These patients ranged in age from 18 to 51 years. Sixty-five percent were on no medication. Only one patient had hepatomegaly.

## Clinical Presentation

Of the 31 patients with isolated PS, 13 had shortness of breath, 11 exercise intolerance, seven dyspnea on exertion,

### TABLE 67.8

**ADULT TETRALOGY OF FALLOT: PHYSICAL FINDINGS IN 13 PATIENTS**

| Finding | Patients [n (%)] |
|---|---|
| Cyanosis | 11 (85) |
| Clubbing | 10 (77) |
| Right ventricular lift | 9 (64) |
| Systolic thrill | 5 (39) |
| Systolic click | 3 (22) |
| Single $S_2$ | 8 (62) |
| Diminished pulmonary component | 4 (31) |
| $S_4$ | 1 (7) |
| Systolic murmur | 13 (100) |
| Continuous murmur | 4 (29) |
| Diastolic murmur | 0 (0) |

(Reprinted with permission from Kreindel M, Moodie DS, Sterba R, et al. Total repair of tetralogy of Fallot in the adult: The Cleveland Clinic experience, 1951–1981. *Cleve Clin Q* 1985;fall:375–381.)

three tachypnea or edema, and one each hypertension and cyanosis. Five patients were in NYHA functional class I, 16 in class II, and ten in class III or IV.

All patients had systolic murmurs. Twelve had at least a grade 3 systolic murmur, and 21 had systolic murmurs ranging in severity from grade 3 to 5. No patients had a diastolic murmur.

Four had a right ventricular lift and 12 a systolic thrill. The $S_2$ could be appreciably auscultated as split in 23 patients. $S_4$ was heard in five patients and $S_3$ in four patients.

## Radiographic Features

Heart size was normal in 28 patients, and five patients had cardiomegaly. Vascularity was normal in 28, increased in two, and decreased in one.

## Electrocardiographic Features

Electrocardiography showed sinus rhythm in all patients. One had sinus bradycardia, and two had first-degree atrioventricular block. Fifteen showed right ventricular hypertrophy. Sixteen demonstrated no hypertrophy of either the right or left ventricle.

## CORRECTED TRANSPOSITION OF THE GREAT ARTERIES

Congenitally corrected transposition (Fig. 67.6) of the great arteries is an unusual cardiac malformation in which normal hemodynamic pathways are not altered by the anatomic abnormalities. The entity originally was described by Von Rokitansky in 1875 (22), and in most patients, it is accompanied by associated anomalies that dictate the symptomatology and considerably affect the prognosis. We use this term to refer to patients with ventricular inversion and to those in whom the aorta is anterior and to the left of the pulmonary artery.

We reviewed patient records from 1960 to 1986, which revealed 18 patients with corrected transposition. These patients ranged in age from 10 to 67 years at initial assessment. Fifteen patients were older than 20 years at initial assessment, and three patients younger than 20 years were included because their follow-up extended well into adulthood.

## Clinical Presentation

Seventeen of these patients had associated cardiac lesions. The most common lesions were left atrioventricular valve insufficiency (11 patients), VSD (seven patients), ASD (four patients), and PS (three patients).

Six patients were NYHA functional class I, six class II, five class III, and one class IV. Patients presenting with class III or IV had hemodynamically significant associated lesions, which may have accounted for their poor clinical status, and one of these patients had a cardiomyopathic systemic ventricle.

## Electrocardiographic Features

Fifteen patients were in sinus rhythm, and three had permanent pacemakers inserted for complete heart block. In two patients, the complete heart block was congenital, and in one, it occurred after closure of a VSD.

## Course

Our data suggest that the morphologic right ventricle can function for a long time as the systemic ventricle, even in patients with associated lesions that pose a significant

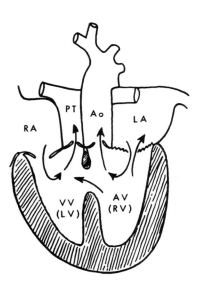

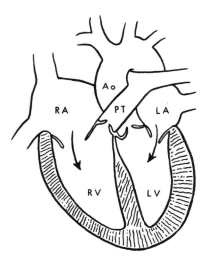

**Figure 67.6** Diagrammatic representation of corrected transposition showing that the right atrium (RA) sits above a morphologic left ventricle (LV) connected by a morphologic mitral valve. Pulmonary venous return is to a morphologic left atrium (LA) that sits above a morphologic tricuspid valve connected to a systemic morphologic right ventricle (RV). The aorta (Ao) is anterior and to the left of the pulmonary artery. AV, arterial ventricle; PT, pulmonary trunk; VV, venous ventricle.

CORRECTED TRANSPOSITION

NORMAL

hemodynamic load. Using radionuclide angiographic techniques, Benson et al. (23) provided data that suggested a normal response to exercise in the morphologic right ventricle in adolescent patients with isolated corrected transposition of the great arteries. Clearly, the associated lesions may determine the long-term outlook for these patients.

## EBSTEIN'S ANOMALY

Between 1950 and 1985, we saw 22 patients with Ebstein's anomaly (Fig. 67.7). These patients ranged in age from 15 to 58 years.

### Clinical Presentation

Seventeen of these patients had easy fatigability and dyspnea on exertion, and five had palpitations and shortness of breath. Two patients presented with heart failure, and two patients were asymptomatic. No family history of Ebstein's anomaly was present in these patients, but four siblings in these families had either an ASD or a VSD.

On physical examination, six patients were cyanotic. Eighteen had a widely split and a questionable fixed $S_2$. All patients had a systolic heart murmur that was grade 2 to 4 in intensity, and two patients had a diastolic murmur. Ebstein's anomaly has been called "the great masquerader," in that it may manifest with different presentations, but 19 of our 22 patients had cardiomegaly.

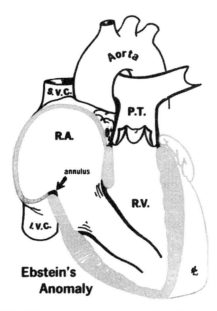

**Figure 67.7** Diagrammatic representation showing the downward displacement and elongated leaflets of the tricuspid valve in a patient with Ebstein's anomaly. IVC, inferior vena cava; PT, pulmonary trunk; RA, right atrium; RV, right ventricle; SVC, superior vena cava.

### Electrocardiographic Features

Electrocardiography demonstrated complete or incomplete right bundle branch block in 16 patients. Right atrial enlargement was present in four patients and first-degree atrioventricular block in three. One patient had Wolff-Parkinson-White syndrome.

Five patients had atrial fibrillation, with three before and two after cardiac surgery. Two patients had complete heart block after surgery and required a permanent pacemaker. Two patients had paroxysmal supraventricular tachycardia, and four had unifocal premature ventricular contractions. The single patient with Wolff-Parkinson-White syndrome eventually underwent surgical ablation.

### Cardiac Catheterization

Cardiac catheterization was performed on all 22 patients. Twelve demonstrated at least a moderate ASD, eight severe tricuspid insufficiency, four mitral insufficiency and mitral valve prolapse, two tricuspid stenosis, and one each PS and VSD. In a single patient, the diagnosis was missed at cardiac catheterization but confirmed at surgery. No deaths occurred during the catheterizations in these patients. Two patients sustained ventricular tachycardia in the catheterization laboratory and required cardioversion.

### Course

Follow-up for these patients extended for 2 to 25 years. Eight of the 22 patients died, with two of these deaths occurring after cardiac surgery.

In those patients treated nonsurgically, one died suddenly at age 24 during competitive athletics. Another patient died of a stroke at age 57, and two patients died of heart failure, one at age 45 and one at age 48.

Fourteen of these patients are alive. Six who underwent surgery are NYHA functional class I, and eight who were treated medically are currently class II. One patient had four miscarriages, with increasing shortness of breath during pregnancy. Another patient had three pregnancies with no difficulties. Three patients underwent one pregnancy each without difficulty, and one patient had four pregnancies with slight shortness of breath and normal deliveries.

## REVIEW EXERCISES

### QUESTIONS

**1.** A 48-year-old woman appears in the emergency room with sudden onset of atrial fibrillation. She is acyanotic and hemodynamically stable but has a systolic murmur at the left upper sternal border radiating to the back, a widely fixed split second heart sound, and a diastolic

flow rumble along the right lower sternal border. The most likely diagnosis is
a) VSD
b) ASD
c) PS
d) Aortic stenosis

**2.** A 28-year-old professional baseball player was noted to have an unusual murmur on his sports physical before the season began. The doctor thought he heard a continuous murmur at the left upper sternal border associated with a slightly widened pulse pressure and brisk to abounding pulses. The most likely diagnosis is
a) VSD
b) ASD
c) Coarctation of the aorta
d) PDA

**3.** A 27-year-old man is noted to have a systolic blood pressure of 170/100 mm Hg. He has a prominent aortic ejection click and murmurs heard over the ribs on both sides anteriorly and over the back posteriorly. In addition, no pulses are palpable in the lower extremities, and he complains of mild claudication with exertion. The most likely diagnosis is
a) ASD
b) Aortic stenosis
c) Coarctation of the aorta
d) VSD

**4.** A 48-year-old man was known in his county as the "blue boy of the county." He has always been cyanotic, clubbed, and physically restricted. His hematocrit was 68%, with a hemoglobin level of 24 g. He has never undergone surgery, and his oxygen saturation on room air is 62%. Cardiac catheterization demonstrates a large VSD, overriding aorta, and severe calcification of the entire right ventricular outflow tract with small pulmonary arteries bilaterally. The diagnosis in this patient is
a) Double-outlet right ventricle
b) Truncus arteriosus
c) Tetralogy of Fallot
d) Atrioventricular canal

**5.** A 40-year-old man presents to your office with the murmur of mitral regurgitation. He has been known to have a complete heart block since childhood and is now somewhat fatigued and short of breath. You noticed that on his chest radiograph he has a completely straight left heart border. The most likely diagnosis in this patient is
a) VSD
b) Rheumatic mitral regurgitation
c) Corrected transposition of the great vessels
d) PDA

**6.** A 26-year-old man has been known to have Wolf-Parkinson-White syndrome with episodes of supraventricular tachycardia. You order a chest radiograph and are surprised at the significant cardiomegaly, with what appears to be marked right atrial enlargement. The patient also has a murmur of tricuspid regurgitation. The most likely diagnosis is
a) ASD
b) VSD
c) Tricuspid stenosis
d) Ebstein's anomaly

## ANSWERS

**1. b.**
ASD commonly presents in the adult, and the first symptom may be the sudden onset of atrial fibrillation. At least 12% to 15% of adult patients have atrial fibrillation preoperatively. Physical findings that demonstrate this as an ASD are the murmur of increased pulmonary blood flow at the left upper sternal border radiating to the back, the pathognomonic finding of a fixed split second heart sound, and the diastolic flow rumble along the right mid-right lower sternal border (functional tricuspid stenosis), which suggests that this patient has a large left-to-right shunt at atrial level. Adult patients with ASD tend to have large defects that raise the question of whether somewhat smaller defects in childhood actually get stretched and become larger defects in adults with significant left-to-right shunts. ASDs are also more common in women, with a female-to-male ratio of 2 to 3:1.

**2. d.**
Many adult patients with patent ductus are asymptomatic, depending on the size of the left-to-right shunt and the size of the ductus. Frequently, the condition is discovered by the unusual quality of a continuous murmur at the left upper sternal border that can sound like an innocent venous hum. Because a patent ductus is an aortopulmonary runoff, however, the pulse pressure frequently is widened, and the pulses are brisk to bounding. Today, most lesions of ductus can be closed in the catheterization laboratory without surgery.

**3. c.**
Adult patients with coarctation almost always present with systolic hypertension, and one may occasionally see diastolic hypertension as well. A bicuspid aortic valve is noted in 60% to 80% of patients with coarctation; therefore, one may hear an aortic ejection click. These patients frequently have collateral murmurs from intercostal arteries heard over the anterior and posterior chest as well as increased collateral from the thyrocervical trunk. The pulses in the lower extremity tend to be absent. If the coarct is severe enough, the individuals may complain of claudication

with exercise. The approach to correction in adult patients is surgery, with resection and reanastomosis.

### 4. c.

Tetralogy of Fallot is the most common form of cyanotic congenital heart disease in adolescents and adults. The hallmark of tetralogy is severe valvular and subvalvular PS associated with a large VSD. Patients shunt right to left at the ventricular level; therefore, they are cyanotic and clubbed. In addition, they are polycythemic; once their hematocrit gets above 65%, they are at risk for stroke or spontaneous cerebral hemorrhage. The approach to tetralogy is surgical, with relief of the right ventricular outflow tract obstruction and closure of the VSD.

### 5. c.

Patients with corrected transposition frequently present as adults. Although a morphologic right atrium is connected to a morphologic left ventricle via the mitral valve, the blood flows from that ventricle to the pulmonary artery. It returns then to a morphologic left atrium, which crosses a tricuspid valve into a morphologic right ventricle that pumps blood out the aorta, and the aorta is anterior and to the left. Patients with this condition frequently present in adulthood because the blood is flowing from inverted ventricles, but out the appropriate arteries. Patients with corrected transposition, however, are either born with complete heart block, or develop heart block at a rate of 1% per year. In addition, they have ventricular septal defect and pulmonary stenosis. The chest radiograph shows a completely straight left heart border because of the anterior and leftward position of the aorta. They also frequently have an Ebstein's malformation of the left AV valve (tricuspid valve), and that valve is frequently regurgitant.

### 6. d.

Ebstein's anomaly is the only congenital cardiac defect commonly associated with preexcitation syndromes like Wolf-Parkinson-White syndrome. Patients frequently have significant tricuspid regurgitation with a markedly dilated right atrium. Ebstein's patients are prone to all rhythm disorders, including both atrial and ventricular arrhythmias, and they have a significant incidence of sudden death.

## REFERENCES

1. Fuster V, Bradenburg RO, McGoon DC, et al. Clinical approach management of congenital heart disease in the adolescent and adult. *Cardiovasc Clin North Am* 1980;10:161–197.
2. Kusumoto M, Amemiya K. Congenital heart disease in patients over 40 years old who have not undergone cardiac surgery. *Jpn Circ J* 1981;45:243–248.
3. Abinader EG, Oliven M. Congenital heart disease in the middle aged and elderly. *J Ir Med Assoc* 1980;73:201–205.
4. Danielson GK, McGoon DC. Surgical therapy and results. In: Roberts WC, ed. *Adult Congenital Heart Disease*. Philadelphia: FA Davis, 1987;543–560.
5. Nicks R, Halliday EJ. Surgery for congenital heart disease in adults. *Med J Aust* 1971;5:424–428.
6. Gonzalez-Lavin L, Neirotti R, Ross JK, et al. Surgical correction of congenital malformation of the heart and great vessels in patients over 20 years of age. *Mich Med* 1975;74:9–12.
7. Bekoe S, Magovern GJ, Liebler GA, et al. Congenital heart disease in adults. Surgical management. *Arch Surg* 1975; 110:960–964.
8. Fetzer JA. Congenital heart disease in the adult. *J Alpha Omega Alpha* 1973;72:1150–1155.
9. Shibuya M. The natural history of adult congenital heart disease. *Jpn Circ J* 1972;36:832.
10. Roberts WC. Congenital heart disease in adults. In: Brest A, ed. *Cardiovascular Clinics*. Philadelphia: FA Davis, 1987.
11. Roberts WC. *Adult Congenital Heart Disease*. Philadelphia: FA Davis, 1987.
12. Perloff JK. *The Clinical Recognition of Congenital Heart Disease*. Philadelphia: WB Saunders, 1978:396.
13. Campbell M. Natural history of ventricular septal defect. *Br Heart J* 1971;33:246–257.
14. Freisinger GC, Bahnson HT. Tetralogy of Fallot. Report of a case with total correction at 54 years of age. *Am Heart J* 1966;71:107–111.
15. Holladay WE, Witham AC. The tetralogy of Fallot. *Arch Intern Med* 1957;100:400–414.
16. Higgins CB, Mulder DC. Tetralogy of Fallot in the adult. *Am J Cardiol* 1972;29:837–846.
17. Abraham KA, Cherian G, Rao VD, et al. Tetralogy of Fallot in adults. A report on 147 patients. *Am J Med* 1979;66: 811–816.
18. Garson AJ, Nihill MR, McNamara DG, et al. Status of the adult and adolescent after repair of tetralogy of Fallot. *Circulation* 1979;59:1232–1240.
19. Garson AJ, McNamara DG, Cooley DA. Tetralogy of Fallot in adults. *Cardiovasc Clin* 1979;10:341–364.
20. Beach PM, Bowman FO, Kaiser GA, et al. Total correction of tetralogy of Fallot in adolescents and adults. *Circulation* 1971;5[Suppl I]:37–44.
21. Abraham KA, Cherian G, Sukumar IP, et al. Hemodynamics in adult tetralogy of Fallot. *Indian Heart J* 1979;31:88–91.
22. Von Rokitansky D. *Die Defecte der Scheidewonde Meczens*. Vienna: W Braumuller, 1875;81.
23. Benson LN, Burns R, Schwaiger M, et al. Radionuclide angiographic evaluation of ventricular function isolated congenitally corrected transposition of the great vessels. *Am J Cardiol* 1986;48:319–324.

# Acute Coronary Syndromes

**68**

*Hani Jneid    Curtis M. Rimmerman    A. Michael Lincoff*

Acute coronary syndromes represent a spectrum of ischemic heart events that share a common pathophysiology and encompass the following entities:

- Unstable angina
- Non–ST elevation myocardial infarction (MI)
- ST-elevation MI

Some also include sudden cardiac death, defined as an unexpected cardiac death occurring within 1 hour of chest discomfort onset.

## EPIDEMIOLOGY

Acute coronary syndromes account for 2 million annual visits to the emergency department among a total of 4 to 5 million visits for chest pain. Almost 900,000 people suffer an acute MI in the United States each year. Of these, approximately 25% die, with 50% of these deaths occurring in the prehospital setting before effective treatment can be given. Invariably, these prehospital deaths are arrhythmogenic in origin. To minimize out-of-hospital mortality, a multidisciplinary approach should be implemented including patient education, rapid patient evaluation and triage, prompt initiation of reperfusion therapy, and ready access to public external defibrillators for witnessed out-of-hospital ventricular dysrhythmias. Successful early infarct-related coronary artery reperfusion reduces both the infarct size and the incidence of subsequent complications, including congestive heart failure, arrhythmia, and death.

## PATHOPHYSIOLOGY

An acute coronary syndrome is caused by an unstable atheromatous plaque that fissures (mostly in women) or ruptures (mostly in men) (1) in an epicardial coronary artery; this leads to the formation of a superimposed platelet and fibrin thrombus. The unstable plaque and the superimposed thrombus result in the rapid interruption of regional myocardial blood flow, causing acute myocyte ischemia and infarction in the absence of prompt reperfusion.

Unstable plaques associated with acute coronary syndromes are most often lipid-rich, atheromatous lesions with a thin fibrous cap and high macrophage infiltration, whereas stable plaques causing chronic stable angina generally possess a thick fibrous cap, less lipid core, and less inflammatory burden.

Most fissured and ruptured coronary artery unstable plaques leading to acute coronary syndromes are not flow-limiting (70% of these plaques possess less than a 50% angiographic stenosis).

Unstable plaques do not occur in isolation in the coronary arteries of patients with an acute coronary syndrome: Up to 40% of patients with an acute MI had multiple complex plaques with angiographic features of instability (thrombus, ulceration, etc.) (2). This is in line with the accumulating evidence demonstrating the diffuse nature of coronary artery inflammation rather than its being confined to the culprit lesion (3).

## CLINICAL PRESENTATION

The classic symptoms of an acute coronary syndrome include chest discomfort, pain, or heaviness. Associated symptoms include dyspnea, palpitations, light-headedness, nausea, vomiting, and diaphoresis. Symptoms develop mostly in the central or left chest area, with radiation to the jaw, neck, shoulders, back, and arms, but almost never below the waist. The discomfort is usually not highly localized, does not vary with position or inspiration (as is pleuropericarditic pain), and is not reproducible by palpation (as is costochondritis).

Usually, if the duration of unstable angina symptoms extends beyond 20 minutes, an MI documentable by positive cardiac enzymes transpires secondary to irreversible myocyte necrosis. Fleeting chest pain of few seconds' duration is unlikely to represent a cardiac origin.

Most chest discomfort episodes representing an unstable coronary syndrome occur at rest or with minimal activity, although strenuous activity is well known to trigger acute ischemic events, especially among patients who exercise infrequently. Circadian variation in acute coronary syndrome onset is well described, with a peak occurrence in the morning, believed secondary to an increase in catecholamines and platelet aggregability (4).

The differential diagnosis of chest pain may include other life-threatening conditions. Aortic dissection and pulmonary embolism are important to consider and differentiate in a

## TABLE 68.1

### DIFFERENTIAL DIAGNOSIS OF NONISCHEMIC CHEST PAIN

Chest pain from other cardiovascular causes
Pericarditis
Dissection of the aorta
Pulmonary embolism/infarction
Chest pain from gastrointestinal causes
Esophageal reflux
Esophageal spasm
Esophageal rupture
Gallstone colic
Peptic ulcer disease
Chest pain from other causes
Tietze's syndrome (pain associated with tender swelling of the
 costochondral joints)
Chest wall pain
Spontaneous pneumothorax
Herpes zoster
Mondor's disease (phlebitis of the veins in the left breast region)

timely manner. Benign conditions also merit consideration (Table 68.1). Aortic dissection is abrupt in onset, perceived as "ripping" chest, interscapular, or back pain. These qualities distinguish it from chest pain of ischemic origin, in which the discomfort is less severe and intensifies gradually. Patients with an acute aortic dissection often have a history of hypertension (often severe) and manifest pulse deficits and a widened mediastinum on the chest radiograph.

Pulmonary embolism is characterized by pleuritic chest pain that worsens while in a supine position, accompanied by dyspnea, tachycardia, tachypnea, and unexplained hypoxemia. The chest radiograph is typically normal. Frequently, an antecedent history of immobility, previous congestive heart failure, or previous pulmonary embolism is present, thus making the clinical and past medical history diagnostically important.

Chest pain alleviation using nitroglycerin has little diagnostic utility in patients presenting with a chest pain syndrome. In a study of 223 patients presenting to the emergency room with chest pain, their response to nitroglycerin was equally present in both patients with cardiac and noncardiac chest pain (88 vs. 92%, p = 0.50) (5). In addition, patients with esophageal spasm are known to exhibit relief secondary to the smooth muscle relaxation associated with nitrate therapy.

## DIAGNOSIS

### Physical Examination

During an acute coronary syndrome, patients often appear to be restless and are unable to assume a comfortable position. Diaphoresis and skin pallor often are visible, and the pulse is regular and rapid. Premature systoles also are common. The blood pressure response varies, including:

- Hypertension (in the setting of increased adrenergic stimulation)
- Normal blood pressure
- Hypotension (particularly in patients with larger infarctions and superimposed left ventricular failure)

The jugular venous pulse usually is normal, unless a right ventricular infarct is present. Rales may be present on pulmonary examination, reflecting a larger, left-sided infarction and a component of heart failure. Cardiac examination frequently demonstrates an $S_4$ gallop, and a dyskinetic cardiac apex may be palpable precordially, particularly during an anterolateral infarction. A third heart sound may be either preexisting or new, with a newly discovered third heart sound reflecting a more extensive MI. Newly audible systolic murmurs, which are reflective of transient or persistent mitral regurgitation, commonly are detected during the periinfarction period.

The combined findings of a carefully obtained patient history and physical examination strongly suggest the diagnosis of an acute coronary syndrome in most patients. Additional essential studies include electrocardiography (ECG) and serum analysis of cardiac enzyme levels.

## Electrocardiography

### Diagnostic Findings

The diagnosis of acute ST-elevation MI can be made on the basis of ECG criteria, including ST-segment elevation of greater than 1 mm in at least two contiguous leads. Reciprocal ST-segment depression is an associated and helpful finding that makes the possibility of acute pericarditis mimicking acute infarction less likely. Electrocardiographically, ST-segment elevation is thought to represent acute myocardial injury, whereas Q-wave formation is most appropriately labeled as infarction, and Q waves in the setting of ST-segment elevation are best labeled as acute infarction. In the absence of ST-segment elevation, Q waves represent an MI of indeterminate age. Unlike right bundle branch block, left bundle branch block obscures Q waves and interferes with the ability to diagnose Q waves, unless Q waves develop newly in the presence of left bundle branch block, in which setting they should be considered pathologic. Premature ventricular complexes with a complete right bundle branch morphology, and, thus, a left ventricular origin, may manifest Q waves. When present, they can be a useful diagnostic adjunct for the presence of coronary artery disease. Tall and peaked T waves have been noted in the early phases of acute MI and represent hyperacute T waves.

Common ECG findings of unstable angina and non–ST-elevation MI include ST-segment depression and T-wave inversion.

An ECG also provides an estimate of infarction size, particularly if the ECG demonstrates ST-segment elevation in leads $V_2$ through $V_6$, I, and $aV_L$, which collectively indicate an extensive anterolateral MI. Infarction involving the left circumflex coronary artery, which most commonly is reflected in leads $V_5$, $V_6$, I, and $aV_L$, is frequently "silent" on ECG.

The ECG is an indispensable adjunct to the patient history and physical examination, but it may sometimes provide inconclusive information despite a transpiring acute coronary syndrome. In the Thrombolysis in Myocardial Infarction (TIMI) III trial, with 1,473 patients enrolled having unstable angina or non–ST-segment-elevation MI, 9% of the patients demonstrated no ischemic ECG changes (6).

### ST-Segment Elevation and Q Waves

Traditionally, MIs have been classified as Q-wave MI or non–Q-wave MI, based on the presence or absence of ECG Q waves in patients with a myocardial enzyme release consistent with acute MI. It is not possible to ascertain whether a Q-wave infarction truly is transmural and a non–Q-wave infarction nontransmural. Significant overlap occurs, and it is best to limit oneself to an ECG description. The development of Q waves depends to some extent on the speed and completeness of spontaneous or therapeutic coronary reperfusion. Patients with Q-wave infarcts tend to suffer larger infarctions and have less prominent coronary collaterals, lower associated ejection fractions, and higher peak cardiac enzyme levels. In-hospital mortality is greater among patients with Q-wave infarctions, which likely is secondary to their larger size. Importantly, postinfarction ischemia is more common in those patients with non–Q-wave infarctions, as is reinfarction. The 3-year mortality is similar for both groups.

With the advent of reperfusion therapy for acute MIs, a more important distinction at presentation is based on the presence or absence of ST-segment elevation. With ST-segment elevation MI, acute coronary angiography typically demonstrates an occlusive thrombus in more than 80% of patients, compared with only 10% to 20% of patients without ST-segment elevation. Fibrinolytic therapy has been recommended for those patients with ST-segment elevation MIs (or new bundle branch block) presenting within 12 hours of symptoms (7). Thus, the identification of ST-segment elevation on the ECG represents the key decision point in the acute management of these patients.

### Laboratory Studies

With the discovery and clinical introduction of the highly sensitive cardiac troponins, clinicians can detect minimal degrees of myocardial necrosis (of <1 g) (8). The diagnosis of an acute MI can be made either histopathologically or by the rise of cardiac markers along with any one of the following four criteria:

■ Ischemic symptoms
■ ECG evidence of myocardial ischemia
■ New Q waves on the ECG
■ Direct visualization of a freshly occlusive coronary thrombus on coronary angiography

Serial testing of serum cardiac enzyme levels should be performed routinely in those patients with a suspected acute coronary syndrome. Also, successful reperfusion, whether spontaneous, pharmacologic, or mechanical, results in a higher and earlier peak of enzyme levels secondary to a "washout" phenomenon, which serves as a useful bedside clinical indicator of reperfusion success.

### Troponins T and I

These serum markers are components of the cardiac myocyte contractile apparatus and are highly specific for a cardiac origin. They also possess a greater sensitivity for the detection of acute myocardial injury when they are offered in a rapid assay form (8,9). Troponins start to rise by 3 hours from chest pain onset and last longer in the circulation (7 to 14 days) than creatine kinase (CK), reducing their value for reinfarction detection, in which setting CK-MB are the markers of choice (Fig. 68.1). Troponin levels should be interpreted with caution in the presence of renal failure (10,11). These markers are being used increasingly in patients with acute onset chest discomfort syndromes of uncertain etiology to expediently assess for serum evidence of acute myocardial injury. This permits prompt patient triage, including the more appropriate use of intravenous thrombolytic therapy and urgent cardiac catheterization.

Patients with elevated troponins but a normal CK-MB tend to have worsened outcomes compared with patients with ischemic symptoms and no elevation in serum markers (unstable angina patients) (12,13). In a study comparing patients on hospital admission with an acute chest discomfort syndrome, a low CK-MB (<7.0 ng/mL) and an elevated troponin T (>0.1 ng/mL) versus a low troponin T

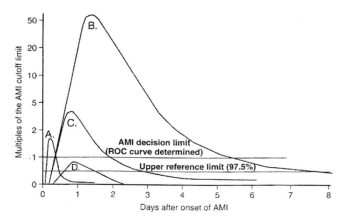

**Figure 68.1** Typical plasma profiles for various biomarkers after acute, ischemic myocardial infarction (AMI). Peak A, early release of myoglobin or creatine kinase (CK)-MB isoforms after AMI; peak B, cardiac troponin after AMI; peak C, CK-MB after AMI; peak D, cardiac troponin after unstable angina. ROC, receiver operating characteristic. (Reproduced with permission from Wu AH, Apple AS, Gibler WB, et al. Recommendations for the use of cardiac markers in coronary artery disease. *Clin Chem* 1999;45:1104–1121.)

(<0.1 ng/mL) demonstrated a threefold 30-day mortality increase (12.3% vs. 4.1%) in the patient subset with elevated troponin T (13). This has substantiated the adverse prognostic importance of detected myocardial damage, irrespective of its extent.

### Creatine Kinase

The measurement of the CK-MB isoenzyme level continues to be a useful laboratory test for the diagnosis of acute MI. CK-MB isoenzyme level comes second to troponins in specificity for diagnosing MI. Initial elevations can be detected 4 hours after acute injury. Mean peak levels occur at approximately 24 hours and return to baseline within 48 to 72 hours. Levels should be obtained at initial presentation, 8 to 12 hours, and 16 to 24 hours after the onset of chest discomfort (Fig. 68.1).

### Nonspecific Markers

The elevation of levels in white blood cell count, serum myoglobin, lactate dehydrogenase (LDH) and its isoenzymes (mainly LDH1), and aspartate aminotransferase represent nonspecific biochemical markers for the detection of MI. Myoglobin is one of the earliest cardiac markers to rise (1 to 4 hours) and may be of certain value, especially in an emergency room setting. Levels of LDH exceed the normal range 24 to 48 hours after the acute event and peak at approximately 78 to 96 hours (Fig. 68.1). Fractionation of total LDH is important because LDH1 is cardiac in origin. This test is best reserved for patients in whom the suspicion for recent MI is high but the CK level has normalized. Its use has been replaced by the use of the troponin assays.

Although markers of myocardial necrosis are helpful in the diagnosis of myocardial infarction, other emerging markers have important prognostic value. Myeloperoxidase (a marker of leukocyte activation) and brain natriuretic peptide (BNP, a marker of neurohormonal activation) predict future cardiovascular events in patients presenting to the emergency room with chest pain and in patients with an acute coronary syndrome (including mortality), respectively (14–16).

High-sensitivity C-reactive protein (hs-CRP), a nonspecific marker of inflammation, stands as an independent prognostic marker for recurrent events after an acute coronary syndrome, including death, MI, and restenosis after percutaneous coronary interventions (17,18). It is especially important, however, in the primary prevention setting in subjects with intermediate risk for cardiovascular events (10% to 20% risk within 10 years).

## TREATMENT

All patients with an acute coronary syndrome warrant hospitalization and telemetry monitoring. Those who develop an acute MI or manifest persistent ischemic symptoms should be observed in the intensive care unit.

## Oxygen

The routine administration of oxygen during the first few hours of an acute coronary syndrome is recommended. Higher dose mask oxygen or endotracheal intubation may be necessary as well, particularly in those patients with concomitant congestive heart failure.

## Reperfusion Therapy

The mainstay of therapy for acute ST-segment elevation MI is immediate reperfusion therapy, based on the observation that myocardial necrosis occurs as a wavefront over 4 to 6 hours post–coronary artery occlusion. The operative paradigm is that early reperfusion arrests this wavefront, salvages myocardium, preserves left ventricular function, and reduces mortality. Many large-scale placebo-controlled trials have demonstrated that therapy with fibrinolytic (thrombolytic) agents during the first 6 hours after onset of symptoms reduces short-term (4 to 5 week) mortality by 25% to 35% among patients with acute MI (19–22). Primary angioplasty or stenting is a viable alternative to pharmacologic reperfusion, with evidence of greater efficacy than fibrinolytic agents when performed at expert centers (23–26).

A recent meta-analysis of 23 trials, including 7,739 patients with acute ST-elevation MI, confirmed the superiority of primary angioplasty/stenting over thrombolytic therapy, independent of the fibrinolytic agent used (27).

## Fibrinolytic (Thrombolytic) Therapy

Indications for fibrinolytic therapy in those patients with acute MI include ST-segment elevation in two or more contiguous leads or new (or presumably new) bundle branch block, with ischemic symptoms of less than 12 hours in duration. Clinical benefit is noted to be greater in larger (i.e., anterior) infarctions, in diabetic patients, and in patients with previous infarctions. A clear relationship exists between the magnitude of beneficial treatment effect and time to therapy, with the greatest patient benefit in those patients with a short period (ideally <1 hour) between symptom onset and thrombolytic therapy administration. The value of thrombolytics 12 to 24 hours after symptom onset is less clear. Patients with ongoing chest discomfort and ST-segment elevation likely will benefit. In TIMI IIIB, patients with non–Q-wave MIs had higher reinfarction rates when treated with thrombolysis compared with placebo (6). Fibrinolytics should not be given to patients with ST-segment depression because evidence points to increased morbidity in this setting (6,28).

Four fibrinolytic agents are currently approved in the United States for the treatment of acute MI. The first of these, streptokinase, is a nonfibrin-specific agent. Of the available agents, streptokinase produces the lowest rate of acute infarct vessel recanalization. Better rates of patency are achieved using the second- and third-generation agents alteplase, reteplase, and tenecteplase. These latter agents vary with regard to circulating half-life and fibrin specificity. Mortality rates in patients receiving alteplase, reteplase, and tenecteplase therapy are lower than that with streptokinase. Tenecteplase, a mutant of alteplase with higher fibrin specificity and one of the newest fibrinolytics approved, has shown efficacy similar to alteplase (29), but it offers the advantage of a single and rapid bolus infusion over 5 seconds (as opposed to reteplase, which is administered as two boluses 30 minutes apart).

The principal limitation of fibrinolytic therapy is bleeding, most notably intracranial hemorrhage. Rates of intracranial hemorrhage after thrombolysis have risen recently to approximately 0.9%. Risk factors for intracranial hemorrhage include female gender, advanced age, low body weight, concurrent warfarin therapy, excessive heparinization, and use of fibrinolytic agents other than streptokinase.

Absolute contraindications for fibrinolytic administration reflect bleeding risk and include:

- Intracranial neoplasm or arteriovenous malformation
- Active internal bleeding (excluding menses)
- Cerebrovascular accident within the prior year or any prior intracranial hemorrhage
- Suspected aortic dissection

Relative contraindications for thrombolytic administration include:

- Blood pressure above 180/110 mm Hg on presentation
- History of cerebrovascular accident more than 1 year prior
- History of chronic, severe hypertension
- Anticoagulant therapy with international normalized (INR) ratio greater than 2.0
- Active peptic ulcer
- Pregnancy
- Recent trauma or internal bleeding (within 2 to 4 weeks)
- Noncompressible vascular puncture within the prior 24 hours
- Cardiopulmonary resuscitation
- Recent major surgery

## Mechanical Reperfusion

Because only 29% to 54% of patients treated with fibrinolytics achieved complete reperfusion (TIMI III flow) (30), primary angioplasty (percutaneous transluminal coronary angioplasty [PTCA]) has been advocated as an attractive alternative to thrombolytic therapy. Smaller randomized trials have, in aggregate, shown that primary PTCA is associated with a lower mortality and reduced rates of intracranial hemorrhage when compared with fibrinolytic therapy. Primary PTCA also may be applied to patients for whom fibrinolysis is relatively or absolutely contraindicated. In the high-risk subset of patients with acute MI presenting with cardiogenic shock, primary angioplasty is clearly the preferred modality of therapy (except in the subset of elderly

patients >75 years of age) (31). Limitations of primary angioplasty include the requirement for specialized facilities with skilled and experienced personnel. Moreover, as with fibrinolysis, the greatest clinical benefit is clearly derived if direct angioplasty is performed within a timely period (60 to 90 minutes) from hospital presentation. In broad clinical practice, differences in outcome among patients receiving thrombolytic agents compared with primary angioplasty have not been as marked as in the clinical trials, likely reflecting practical difficulties in providing rapid access to the facilities and expertise required to conduct primary angioplasty. Thus, primary angioplasty is the preferred means of reperfusion compared with fibrinolytic therapy in settings in which it can be applied with expertise, within optimal door-to-balloon time (i.e., within 60 to 90 minutes of the patient's presentation). This short time window has been recently challenged, however, by studies demonstrating the superiority of a strategy of transporting patients with ST-elevation MI to invasive centers for mechanical revascularization compared with on-site thrombolysis, even at the expense of a more prolonged door-to-balloon time (32,33).

PTCA may also be indicated on a rescue basis in those patients who have evidence of continued myocardial ischemia and failed reperfusion after administration of thrombolytic agents. One small randomized trial demonstrated a reduction in the incidence of death and heart failure among patients with anterior infarctions who received rescue angioplasty (34). The routine application of angioplasty immediately or early after successful thrombolysis confers no demonstrable clinical benefit and may be associated with increased risks of bleeding and reinfarction.

## Coronary Stenting

Coronary stents are commonplace as an adjunct to coronary angioplasty to percutaneously restore coronary blood flow during an acute MI. Stents help prevent elastic recoil in the coronary arteries after balloon inflation and reduce the restenosis rate at 6 months up to 44% in some studies (35). The regular use of intravenous glycoprotein IIb/IIIa inhibitors in combination with stents during a coronary intervention reduces the rate of embolization to the distal coronary microcirculation and the rise of troponin postintervention, translating into a reduction in myocardial events. When administered with provisional glycoprotein IIb/IIIa inhibitors, bivalirudin (a direct thrombin inhibitor) demonstrated a similar efficacy to a combination of heparin and glycoprotein IIb/IIIa in reducing periprocedural ischemia and lower periprocedural bleeding rates (36). The demonstration of the clinical superiority of prolonged clopidogrel therapy (for 12 months) after percutaneous coronary interventions beyond the 1-month standard treatment was another major advance in interventional cardiology (37).

A new era in the management of acute coronary syndrome has emerged with the development of drug-eluting stents. These stents, coated with biological agents (such as rapamycin or paclitaxel) that inhibit smooth muscle cell proliferation and consequently neointimal hyperplasia, reduce restenosis rates to a single-digit number (38,39).

Stents have not been shown to reduce mortality or enhance myocardial salvage relative to balloon angioplasty.

## PHARMACOLOGIC THERAPY

### Antiplatelet Therapy

The prompt administration of 160 to 325 mg of aspirin (chewed) is indicated for all patients presenting with acute coronary syndromes, and daily use of aspirin should be continued indefinitely thereafter. The Second Interventional Study of Infarct Survival examined the efficacy of aspirin and demonstrated a reduction of 23% in the 35-day mortality (Fig. 68.2). Additionally, aspirin reduces the incidence of coronary reocclusion and recurrent myocardial ischemia. In the absence of acute ischemic symptoms, 81 mg of aspirin daily is as effective and has less gastroenterologic toxicity than larger doses of aspirin (40).

Data from the Clopidogrel in Unstable Angina to Prevent Recurrent Ischemic Events trial demonstrated a 20% additional reduction in the composite endpoint of cardiovascular death, MI, and stroke in patients with unstable angina and non–ST-segment elevation MI randomized to dual antiplatelet therapy with aspirin and clopidogrel compared with aspirin alone (41). That benefit was evident as early as 2 hours after the acute event and persisted for the total follow-up period of 12 months.

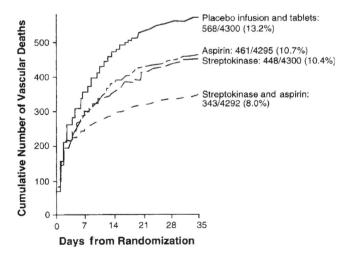

**Figure 68.2** Cumulative vascular mortality for days 0 to 35 in the Second Interventional Study of Infarct Survival. [Reproduced with permission from ISIS-2 (Second Interventional Study of Infarct Survival) Collaborative Group. Randomized trial of intravenous streptokinase or aspirin, both or neither, among 17,187 cases of suspected acute myocardial infarction: ISIS-2. *Lancet* 1988;2: 349–360.]

### Heparin

After the administration of streptokinase, heparin does not reduce ischemic events and does increase hemorrhage rates. Unless indicated for other reasons, such as the prevention or treatment of mural thrombus or deep vein thrombosis, heparin therefore is not recommended in the immediate period after treatment with streptokinase. For the fibrin-specific agents (alteplase, reteplase, and tenecteplase), heparin has been associated with improved reperfusion rates, although hemorrhage rates are also increased. It is recommended that heparin be administered for 1 to 3 days after the administration of fibrin-specific thrombolytic agents, to those patients with an acute MI, targeted to an optimal activated partial thromboplastin time of 55 to 75 seconds. Unfractionated heparin is used routinely in the catheterization laboratory among patients undergoing primary angioplasty or stent implantation. Unlike unfractionated heparin, low-molecular-weight heparin (LMWH) offers the advantages of reduced protein binding, subcutaneous dosing, reduced platelet activation, reduced monitoring requirements, and a reduced incidence of heparin-induced thrombocytopenia. Enoxaparin is the only LMWH that showed superiority to unfractionated heparin in two large, blinded, randomized studies. In the ESSENCE study, enrolling 3,171 patients with unstable angina and non–ST-elevation MI, fewer patients randomized to enoxaparin reached the primary combined endpoint of death, MI, and recurrent angina at 14 days compared with those assigned to unfractionated heparin (16.6% vs. 19.8%) (42). The TIMI IIB results confirmed the enoxaparin superiority over unfractionated heparin in unstable angina and non–ST-elevation MI patients, with a 12% relative reduction in the primary combined endpoint of death, MI, and urgent revascularization at day 43 (43). The enoxaparin superiority over unfractionated heparin was maintained at 1-year follow-up (44).

### Platelet Glycoprotein IIb/IIIa Receptor Antagonists

Each platelet contains thousands of glycoprotein IIb/IIIa receptors on its surface; these receptors undergo conformational changes on platelet activation, enabling them to bind fibrinogen dimers and cross-link platelets. Glycoprotein IIb/IIIa inhibitors effectively block the final common pathway of platelet aggregation and thus represent the most potent antiplatelet therapy available.

Abciximab, a chimeric human-murine monoclonal antibody with a high affinity to the glycoprotein IIb/IIIa receptor and a long physiologic half-life of 12 hours, is the pharmacologic agent of choice as an adjunct in patients undergoing percutaneous coronary interventions (45–47). Data from the Global Use of Strategies to Open Occluded Coronary Arteries in Acute Coronary Syndromes IV trial showed no benefit of this agent in those patients presenting with acute coronary syndromes and not undergoing early revascularization (48).

The small molecules, eptifibatide (a synthetic peptide inhibitor) and tirofiban (a nonpeptide mimetic), have shorter half-lives (90 to 120 minutes). They are the agents of choice in those patients with unstable angina and non–ST-elevation MI.

Abciximab remains the standard of care in percutaneous coronary intervention, after it showed superiority to tirofiban in a head-to-head comparative trial (the Do Tirofiban and ReoPro Give Similar Efficacy trial) in patients presenting with an acute coronary syndrome and subsequently undergoing percutaneous coronary intervention (49).

The role of glycoprotein IIb/IIIa blockade as an adjunct to fibrinolytic therapy is currently under investigation. The Global Use of Strategies to Open Occluded Coronary Arteries in Acute Coronary Syndromes V study compared the use of the fibrinolytic reteplase with the combination of half-dose reteplase plus abciximab. Although it did not show a statistical difference in the 30-day mortality primary endpoint between the two regimens, a promising lesser reinfarction rate (a prespecified secondary endpoint) was noted for the combination regimen, but at the expense of higher nonintracranial bleeding rate (50).

## β-Blockers

β-Blockers are appropriately administered to patients within the first 12 hours of an acute coronary syndrome and should be continued daily thereafter. By lowering the heart rate, blood pressure, and consequently myocardial oxygen demand, β-blockers reduce the rates of cardiac rupture and ventricular fibrillation, relieve pain, and reduce infarct size. Patients with heart failure, hypotension (blood pressure <90 mm Hg), bradycardia (heart rate <60), or advanced heart block should be excluded. A common protocol is to initiate intravenous metoprolol in three separate 5-mg boluses 5 minutes apart, subsequently beginning oral metoprolol therapy (50 mg every 6 hours), provided the patient is hemodynamically stable (51).

## Angiotensin-Converting Enzyme Inhibitors

Early in the course of an acute MI, administration of an angiotensin-converting enzyme (ACE) inhibitor reduces mortality (52). The greatest benefit occurs in those patients with anterior infarctions and heart failure. Therapy with ACE inhibitors should be started promptly (i.e., within 24 hours of presentation), but immediate intravenous therapy is unnecessary and may be detrimental (53). If left ventricular systolic function remains normal, the discontinuation of ACE inhibitors 4 to 6 weeks after initiation is appropriate. If the left ventricular ejection fraction is reduced to approximately 35% to 40%, ACE inhibitors should be continued indefinitely.

Data from the Heart Outcomes Prevention Evaluation Study extended the use of the ACE inhibitor ramipril to all patients at risk for cardiovascular events, who were devoid of heart failure or left ventricular dysfunction. It showed a 22% reduction in cardiovascular events with a once daily oral dose of ramipril (10 mg) at a mean of 5 years of follow-up in patients with vascular disease or in diabetics with one additional cardiac risk factor (54). Whether these benefits of ramipril represent a class effect of all ACE inhibitors or a unique property belonging to ramipril (known to have high tissue penetrance) remains a matter of unresolved debate.

## Nitroglycerin

Nitroglycerin reduces both right and left ventricular preload, produces peripheral vasodilation, and reduces ventricular afterload, thereby lowering myocardial oxygen requirements and work. In addition, it has direct vasodilator effects on the coronary arteries. The routine administration of nitroglycerin has not been associated with reduced mortality in randomized trials and may even be detrimental in those patients with right ventricular infarction or intravascular volume depletion. Similarly, long-term nitrate administration to patients after an acute coronary syndrome is not clearly beneficial. Nitroglycerin does remain helpful in those patients with persistent ischemia, hypertension, or congestive heart failure during the initial 24 to 48 hours after an acute coronary syndrome. After 48 hours, continued use is appropriate in the settings of recurrent ischemia and persistent heart failure.

## Calcium Channel Blockers

Calcium channel blockers are used most appropriately in the setting of acute infarction when ischemia or atrial arrhythmias persist and there is a contraindication to the administration of β-blockers. Calcium channel blockers have not been shown to reduce the mortality after acute MI, and in some patient subgroups, these agents may even increase the mortality (55).

## Analgesia

Ongoing chest discomfort causes increased sympathetic output, and, therefore, an increase in the heart rate and blood pressure. This ultimately increases myocardial oxygen consumption. Prompt administration of an intravenous analgesic (e.g., morphine sulfate) is therefore recommended. Morphine sulfate also reduces ventricular preload and helps relieve dyspnea. It is therefore of special importance in acute MI patients with the complication of left-sided heart failure. Acute right ventricular infarction is a preload-sensitive state, in which setting nitroglycerin and morphine should be used with extreme caution.

## Hydroxymethylglutaryl–Coenzyme A Reductase Inhibitors

The Scandinavian Simvastatin Survival Study (4S) demonstrated a 30% mortality reduction in patients with coronary artery disease randomized to simvastatin compared with placebo and was the first secondary prevention trial to prove a survival benefit of hydroxymethylglutaryl–coenzyme A (HMG-CoA) reductase inhibitors (56). Other trials using various HMG-CoA reductase inhibitors showed benefit in both primary (57,58) and secondary prevention (56,59,60). The Myocardial Ischemia Reduction with Aggressive Cholesterol Lowering trial, a study of unstable angina and non–Q-wave MI patients, demonstrated a significant benefit using early (within 24 to 96 hours) and aggressive (80 mg) atorvastatin therapy compared with placebo in reducing recurrent ischemic events in the first 16 weeks. This immediate intensive lipid-lowering strategy was safe and well tolerated (61). A strategy of aggressive lipid lowering therapy (atorvastatin 80 mg daily) after an ACS to a median LDL of 62 mg/dl was superior to that of routine lipid lowering (pravastatin 40 mg daily) to a median LDL of 95 mg/dl, with an additional 16% reduction in hard cardiovascular events within 2 years of therapy (62). The benefits of aggressive lipid lowering therapy were supported by another study of 502 patients randomized to atorvastatin 80 mg versus pravastatin 40 mg daily. The intensive lipid-lowering arm showed less progression in atheroma burden (and even mild regression) on serial coronary intravascular ultrasound procedures 18 months apart compared with the routine lipid-lowering therapy (63).

The above data therefore support the utility of early and aggressive use of HMG-CoA reductase inhibitors (statins) after an acute coronary syndrome. Statins are known to exert their benefits through lipid lowering and nonlipid effects (so called pleiotropic effects), such as anti-inflammatory and antithrombotic effects.

As new lipid-modifying agents emerge therapy is directed increasingly at the HDL cholesterol component. In a pilot study of 47 patients with an acute coronary syndrome, 5 weekly treatments with an intravenous experimental therapy, recombinant ApoA-I Milano/phospholipid complexes (ApoA-I Milano is a variant of apolipoprotein A-I), demonstrated significant regression in coronary atherosclerosis, as measured by serial intravascular ultrasound (64).

## HEMODYNAMIC MONITORING

The placement of a Swan-Ganz catheter and continuous measurement of right-sided cardiac pressures are indicated in select circumstances. These include severe or progressive congestive heart failure, cardiogenic shock, and suspected mechanical complications of acute infarction (e.g., papillary muscle rupture, ventricular septal defect, pericardial tamponade).

Patients with severe congestive heart failure, cardiogenic shock, or both often require intravenous inotropes as well as ventricular preload- and afterload-reducing agents, best administered and dosed with full knowledge of the cardiac-filling pressures. This allows the differentiation in critically ill patients of inadequate left ventricular volumes and an underfilled left ventricle versus a volume replete state with extensive left ventricular systolic impairment. The routine uncomplicated acute MI, regardless of its location, is not an indication for right-sided heart catheter monitoring.

## INTRAAORTIC BALLOON COUNTERPULSATION

Intraaortic balloon counterpulsation is reserved for critically ill patients. Subgroups in which this therapy is indicated include patients with the following conditions:

- Persistent cardiogenic shock despite pharmacologic therapy as a bridge to coronary revascularization
- Refractory arrhythmias resulting in hemodynamic instability
- Refractory post-MI angina despite maximal antianginal therapy
- Acute mechanical complications of MI (e.g., ventricular septal defect, papillary muscle rupture)
- High-risk percutaneous revascularization (unprotected left main disease, left ventricular dysfunction, target vessel supplying >40% territory, or severe congestive heart failure)

Contraindications to intraaortic balloon counterpulsation include aortic dissection, aortic aneurysms, peripheral arterial disease, descending aortic and peripheral vascular grafts, and moderate to severe aortic regurgitation.

## COMPLICATIONS OF ACUTE MYOCARDIAL INFARCTION

### Arrhythmias

With the widespread use of fibrinolytics and primary interventions, arrhythmias are observed less frequently in the presence of an acute MI. Arrhythmias are more common in patients with the following conditions:

- Anterior MI
- Large MI
- MI complicated by congestive heart failure
- Hypotension and hypoperfusion
- Older age
- Post-MI patients with ongoing myocardial ischemia

### Atrial Fibrillation

Atrial fibrillation is the most common sustained arrhythmia in this setting, occurring in approximately 10% of

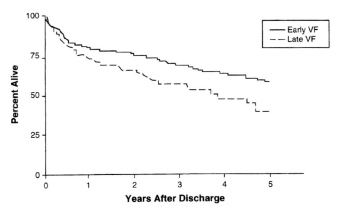

patients with acute MI. If hemodynamic compromise develops during an episode of atrial fibrillation, prompt electrical cardioversion is indicated. If the patient is not clinically compromised, the initial cautious use of intravenous β-blockade is useful in slowing the ventricular response and attenuating superimposed ischemia. If atrial fibrillation persists, intravenous heparin should be initiated and antiarrhythmic therapy should be considered.

## Ventricular Arrhythmias

Often fatal, ventricular arrhythmias commonly occur during an acute infarction. It is important to distinguish early ventricular fibrillation, which occurs within the first few hours of infarction, from late ventricular fibrillation, which occurs more than 48 hours after infarction (Fig. 68.3). Early ventricular fibrillation suggests a higher immediate mortality that can reach 20%. The out-of-hospital mortality is far greater in those patients experiencing late ventricular fibrillation because this is often associated with larger infarctions, greater left ventricular systolic dysfunction, and congestive heart failure (51).

The use of routine in-hospital intravenous lidocaine administration during an acute infarction has been abandoned (65). Lidocaine reduces the incidence of primary in-hospital ventricular fibrillation but does not exert a favorable effect on mortality (66). On the other hand, lidocaine appears to have a negative effect on mortality (67,68), which likely is related to increased episodes of bradycardia and asystole.

The early administration of intravenous β-blockade followed by oral doses exerts a favorable impact on ventricular fibrillation frequency and should be administered routinely to patients with acute infarction devoid of advanced heart block, significant hypotension, or cardiogenic shock. In addition, close monitoring of electrolyte levels, specifically potassium and magnesium levels, is important in

arrhythmia prevention. The treatment of ventricular fibrillation requires prompt, unsynchronized electric shock, followed by pharmaceutical therapy, as outlined in the advanced cardiac life support protocol.

Ventricular tachycardia is classified as either nonsustained (<30 seconds) or sustained (>30 seconds). Nonsustained, nonhemodynamically compromising ventricular tachycardia does not require specific treatment other than attenuation of persistent ischemia, normalization of electrolyte levels, and β-blockade. Hemodynamically compromising sustained ventricular tachycardia requires electric shock. Hemodynamically noncompromising sustained ventricular tachycardia can be treated with pharmacologic agents, including intravenous lidocaine or procainamide. In addition, intravenous amiodarone also is indicated for sustained ventricular tachycardia and is highly effective. Drug-refractory sustained ventricular tachycardia in the setting of acute MI is best treated using β-blockade, intravenous amiodarone, balloon pump insertion, and urgent revascularization.

## Bradyarrhythmias

Sinus bradycardia is another frequent complication of acute MI, especially in those patients with inferior infarctions and reperfusion of the right coronary artery (the Bezold-Jarisch reflex). Heart block occurs in approximately 10% of patients with acute infarction, and new left or right bundle branch block also can develop. Patients with heart block or bundle branch block have a greater in-hospital mortality, most likely related to the greater size of their presenting infarctions. Atropine is an effective treatment for bradycardia associated with hypotension or ischemia. It also is effective as prompt treatment for ventricular asystole or symptomatic atrioventricular (AV) block.

Temporary pacing is an effective bridge therapy for symptomatic bradycardia and heart block during an acute MI. It can be performed by the transcutaneous or transvenous route. The transcutaneous mode is safer, especially in the setting of thrombolytic therapy. The transvenous mode is best used in those patients with a high likelihood of proceeding to advanced heart block. Indications for temporary pacing include:

- Symptomatic bradycardia unresponsive to drug therapy
- Mobitz type II AV block
- Third-degree heart block
- New bilateral bundle branch block
- Newly acquired left bundle branch block
- New right bundle branch block or left bundle branch block and first-degree AV block

Relatively few patients with acute infarction require permanent pacemakers. Rhythm disturbances that indicate a need for permanent pacing are persistent second-degree AV block in the His-Purkinje system, complete heart block, and symptomatic AV block.

**Figure 68.3** Kaplan-Meier survival curves. VF, ventricular fibrillation. (Reproduced with permission from Jensen GVH, Torp-Pedersen C, Kober L, et al. Prognosis of late versus early ventricular fibrillation in acute myocardial infarction. *Am J Cardiol* 1990;66:10.)

## Mechanical Complications

### Acute Mitral Regurgitation

Acute mitral regurgitation, which usually occurs 2 to 7 days after an acute MI, is mostly associated with an inferior MI. It commonly results from a partially ruptured posteromedial papillary muscle because of its single blood supply (from the posterior descending coronary artery), as opposed to the dual supply of the anterolateral papillary muscle (from both the left anterior descending and the left circumflex coronary arteries). It should be suspected on physical examination when a new holosystolic murmur develops, and it is best confirmed using two-dimensional echocardiography and color Doppler analysis. It is an indication for prompt surgical repair, with an overall mortality from 40% to 90%.

### Ventricular Septal Defect

Similar to acute mitral regurgitation, a ventricular septal defect occurs 3 to 5 days after an acute infarction. A new murmur almost always is audible, occurring in approximately two-thirds of cases in the setting of an anterior infarction. This defect also can be diagnosed echocardiographically. The mortality without surgery is greater than 90%.

### Ventricular Free Wall Rupture

Ventricular free wall rupture occurs approximately 3 to 6 days after an acute infarction and without any clear predilection for infarction location. The mortality approaches 100%. The incidence is thought to be reduced in those patients receiving thrombolytic therapy and prompt β-blockade at initial presentation by reducing infarct size and left ventricular systolic wall tension.

## CONCLUSION

Prompt treatment of acute coronary syndromes is essential. All MI patients and high-risk unstable angina patients should be placed in coronary intensive care units, where experienced personnel can provide close monitoring and promptly attend to any complications. Aspirin is a first-line treatment. Unless contraindications exist, patients with ECG and clinical criteria for an acute ST-elevation MI should receive either intravenous fibrinolytic therapy or be transported promptly to the catheterization laboratory for primary percutaneous coronary intervention. Early invasive strategy is becoming the standard of care for unstable angina non–Q-wave MIs. Glycoprotein IIb/IIIa inhibitors are indicated in high-risk patients presenting with unstable angina or a non–Q-wave MI (tirofiban and eptifibatide) and are useful adjuncts to stenting in angioplasty procedures (abciximab). Clopidogrel has been shown to have an incremental benefit over aspirin alone in acute coronary syndromes, and the combination may become the standard of care in such patients.

Pharmaceutical agents that should be administered concomitantly if no contraindications exist include:

- Aspirin
- β-blockers
- ACE inhibitors
- Intravenous nitroglycerin
- Heparin (unfractionated or low molecular weight)

The prognosis depends on the following factors:

- Age
- Infarction size and location
- Hemodynamic stability
- Intervening congestive heart failure
- Arrhythmia development

With the improvement in medical and interventional therapies and the emergence of a solid body of evidence-based coronary care, a significant decrease in case-fatality rate is presently observed in acute MIs. Knowing that many of the medical therapies are underused (69,70), however, and that subgroups of patients including minorities and women (71) remain undertreated, considerable room for improvement still exists.

## REVIEW EXERCISES

### QUESTIONS

**1.** Which of the following statements *does not* pertain to the anatomy and pathology of acute MI?
**a)** Even during an acute MI, angiography remains safe.
**b)** More than 85% of infarct-related arteries are totally occluded during the acute infarction phase.
**c)** The incidence of totally occluded infarct vessels is reduced after MI secondary to spontaneous thrombolysis.
**d)** Most patients who die from an acute infarction have a critical obstruction in one coronary artery.

**2.** Which of the following statements concerning risk stratification after an acute MI is false?
**a)** Women possess an improved post-MI prognosis compared with that of men.
**b)** The single most important determinant of both short- and long-term survival is the residual left ventricular systolic function.
**c)** Silent ischemia as detected by Holter monitoring has a similar prognosis to that of symptomatic ischemia after MI.
**d)** Diabetes mellitus contributes to an increased postinfarction risk.

**3.** The following items are features of non–Q-wave MI, *except*
**a)** The residual coronary artery stenosis generally is severe.

**b)** Prominent collaterals serve the infarct-related artery.
**c)** A greater likelihood of a previous MI exists.
**d)** Recurrent infarction is less likely compared with a Q-wave infarction.

**4.** The following statements regarding thrombolytic therapy are true, *except*
**a)** An improved mortality has been shown in patients with inferior infarction after thrombolytic administration.
**b)** The earlier the thrombolytic treatment, the greater the impact on survival.
**c)** Preservation of left ventricular function depends on early thrombolytic administration.
**d)** Cardiopulmonary resuscitation is an absolute contraindication for thrombolytic therapy.

**5.** Indications for a temporary pacemaker in patients with acute MI include the following, *except*
**a)** New left anterior fascicular and right bundle branch block
**b)** New second-degree Mobitz I AV block
**c)** New left bundle branch block
**d)** Complete heart block

**6.** True statements concerning the ECG findings during an acute MI include the following, *except*
**a)** Sinus tachycardia is frequently present.
**b)** An accelerated idioventricular rhythm postthrombolytic therapy warrants urgent electric cardioversion.
**c)** Atrial dysrhythmias such as atrial fibrillation are commonly observed.
**d)** The development of complete heart block portends a worse prognosis.

**7.** In a patient presenting with an acute chest discomfort syndrome and an ECG demonstrating an extensive anterolateral myocardial injury pattern, appropriate treatment measures include the following, *except*
**a)** The prophylactic placement of an intraaortic balloon pump to attenuate the degree of myocardial injury given the large MI
**b)** Intravenous thrombolytic therapy
**c)** Intravenous β-blocker administration in the absence of advanced heart failure and hemodynamic compromise
**d)** An urgent cardiac catheterization with the goal of percutaneous coronary angioplasty and possible coronary stent placement

## ANSWERS

**1. d.**
During an acute MI, angiography remains safe and, with angioplasty, often is the appropriate treatment. Of importance, most infarct-related arteries are occluded during the acute infarction phase. This is reduced after infarction secondary to spontaneous thrombolysis. Most patients who die of an acute infarction have advanced coronary atherosclerosis involving more than one coronary artery.

**2. a.**
Important adverse prognostic predictors after an MI include the extent of left ventricular systolic dysfunction and coexistent morbidity, including diabetes mellitus. Silent ischemia, as detected at Holter monitoring, portends a worse prognosis, as does female gender.

**3. d.**
Non–Q-wave infarctions are characterized by the residual, high-grade coronary stenosis, prominent collaterals, and greater likelihood of previous MI. The total creatine phosphokinase level is less, but the reinfarction rate is higher compared with that in patients with Q-wave infarctions.

**4. d.**
Thrombolytic therapy is most beneficial within the early phases of an acute MI. Reduced morbidity and mortality are shown for all infarcts, including inferior infarctions. Enhanced left ventricular systolic function is noted with earlier thrombolytic administration. Cardiopulmonary resuscitation remains a relative, not an absolute, contraindication to thrombolytic therapy.

**5. b.**
Indications for temporary pacing during an acute MI include new-onset bifascicular block, second-degree Mobitz II AV block, and complete heart block. First-degree AV block and Mobitz I Wenckebach second-degree AV block require careful observation but not temporary pacing.

**6. b.**
In the presence of an acute MI, increased sympathetic tone often is reflected in the form of sinus tachycardia. Atrial arrythmias frequently are demonstrated in part related to atrial ischemia, increased circulating catecholamines, acutely elevated intracardiac pressures, and cardiac chamber dilatation. Advanced forms of heart block are associated with larger infarctions, which portend a worse prognosis. Accelerated idioventricular rhythms frequently manifest after successful reperfusion during the acute myocardial injury phase, rarely require treatment other than careful observation, and represent a noninvasive marker of successful coronary blood flow restoration.

**7. a.**
In the presence of an acute chest discomfort syndrome and an ECG demonstrating acute myocardial injury, the restoration of coronary artery blood flow in the most expedient manner results in reduced morbidity and mortality. This can be achieved by administering intravenous

thrombolytic therapy or proceeding directly with heart catheterization and a catheter-based coronary intervention. β-blockers reduce myocardial oxygen demand, attenuate myocardial ischemia, and limit the size of an infarction. β-blockers should be administered to all acute MI patients in the absence of a hemodynamic contraindication. In the presence of cardiogenic shock, drug-refractory congestive heart failure, and recurrent life-threatening cardiac dysrhythmias believed to be ischemia-mediated, the placement of an intraaortic balloon pump in the peri-MI period can achieve a positive clinical benefit. The routine use of an intraaortic balloon pump is not indicated and may subject the patient to excess morbidity secondary to vascular injury, cholesterol and systemic embolization, and infection, all without a tangible benefit. The use of an intraaortic balloon pump is an individualized decision for each acute MI patient.

## REFERENCES

1. Patel VB, Topol EJ. The pathogenesis and spectrum of acute coronary syndromes: from plaque formation to thrombosis. *Cleve Clin J Med* 1999;66:561–571.
2. Goldstein JA, Demetriou D, Grines CL, et al. Multiple complex coronary plaques in patients with acute myocardial infarction. *N Engl J Med* 2000;343(13):915–922.
3. Buffoon A, Biasucci LM, Liuzzo G, et al. Widespread coronary inflammation in unstable angina. *N Engl J Med* 2002;347(1):5–12.
4. Muller JE, Abela GS, Nesto RW, et al. Triggers, acute risk factors and vulnerable plaques: the lexicon of a new frontier. *J Am Coll Cardiol* 1994;23:809–813.
5. Shry EA, Dacus J, Van De Graaff E, et al. Usefulness of the response to sublingual nitroglycerin as a predictor of ischemic chest pain in the emergency department. *Am J Cardiol.* 2002;90(11):1264–1266.
6. The TIMI IIIB Investigators. Effects of tissue plasminogen activator and a comparison of early invasive and conservative strategies in unstable angina and non-Q-wave myocardial infarction: results from the TIMI IIIB Trial. *Circulation* 1994;89:1545–1556.
7. Lee TH. Guidelines: diagnosis and management of acute myocardial infarction. In: Braunwald E, Zipes DP, Libby P, eds. *Heart disease: A Textbook of Cardiovascular Medicine*, 6th ed. Philadelphia, WB Saunders, 2001;1219–1231.
8. Alpert JS, Antman E, Apple F, et al. Myocardial infarction redefined—a consensus document of the Joint European Society of Cardiology/American College of Cardiology Committee for the Redefinition of Myocardial Infarction. *J Am Coll Cardiol* 2000;36:959–969.
9. Hamm CW, Goldmann BU, Heeschen C, et al. Emergency room triage of patients with acute chest pain by means of rapid testing for cardiac troponin T or troponin I. *N Engl J Med* 1997;337:1648–1653.
10. Musso P, Cox I, Vidano E, et al. Cardiac troponin elevations in chronic renal failure: prevalence and clinical significance. *Clin Biochem* 1999;32:125–130.
11. Van Lente F, McErlean ES, DeLuca SA, et al. Ability of troponins to predict adverse outcomes in patients with renal insufficiency and suspected acute coronary syndromes: a case-matched study. *J Am Coll Cardiol* 1999;33:471–478.
12. Antman EM, Tanasijevic MJ, Thompson B, et al. Cardiac-specific troponin I levels to predict the risk of mortality in patients with acute coronary syndromes. *N Engl J Med* 1996;335:1342–1349.
13. Ohman EM, Armstrong PW, Christenson RH, et al. Cardiac troponin T levels for risk stratification in acute myocardial infarction. *N Engl J Med* 1996;335:1333–1341.
14. Brennan ML, Penn MS, Van Lente F, et al. Prognostic value of myeloperoxidase in patients with chest pain. *N Engl J Med* 2003;349(17):1595–1604.
15. de Lemos JA, Morrow DA, Bentley JH, et al. The prognostic value of B-type natriuretic peptide in patients with acute coronary syndromes. *N Engl J Med* 2001;345(14):1014–1021.
16. Omland T, Persson A, Ng L, et al. N-terminal pro-B-type natriuretic peptide and long-term mortality in acute coronary syndromes. *Circulation* 2002;106(23):2913–2918.
17. Danesh J, Wheeler JG, Hirschfield GM, et al. C-reactive protein and other circulating markers of inflammation in the prediction of coronary heart disease. *N Engl J Med* 2004;350(14):1387–1397.
18. Pearson TA, Mensah GA, Alexander RW, et al. Markers of inflammation and cardiovascular disease: application to clinical and public health practice: a statement for healthcare professionals from the Centers for Disease Control and Prevention and the American Heart Association. *Circulation* 2003;107(3):499–511.
19. Gruppo Italiano per lo Studio della Streptochinasi nell'Infarto Miocardico (GISSI). Effectiveness of intravenous thrombolytic treatment in acute myocardial infarction. *Lancet* 1986;1:397–401.
20. ISIS-2 (Second Interventional Study of Infarct Survival) Collaborative Group. Randomized trial of intravenous streptokinase or aspirin, both or neither, among 17,187 cases of suspected acute myocardial infarction: ISIS-2. *Lancet* 1988;2:349–360.
21. AIMS (APSAC Intervention Mortality Trial) Trial Study Group. Effects of intravenous APSAC on mortality after acute myocardial infarction: preliminary report of a placebo-controlled clinical trial. *Lancet* 1988;1:545–549.
22. Wilcox RG, Von der Lippe G, Olsson CG, et al. for the ASSET (Anglo-Scandinavian Study of Early Thrombosis) Study Group. Trial of tissue plasminogen activator for mortality reduction in acute myocardial infarction (ASSET). *Lancet* 1988;2:525–530.
23. The Global Use of Strategies to Open Occluded Coronary Arteries in Acute Coronary Syndromes (GUSTO IIb) Angioplasty Substudy Investigators. A clinical trial comparing primary coronary angioplasty with tissue plasminogen activator for acute myocardial infarction. *N Engl J Med* 1997;336:1621–1628.
24. Grines CL. Should thrombolysis or primary angioplasty be the treatment of choice for acute myocardial infarction? Primary angioplasty—the strategy of choice. *N Engl J Med* 1996;335:1313–1316.
25. Weaver WD, Simes RJ, Betriu A, et al. Comparison of primary coronary angioplasty and intravenous thrombolytic therapy for acute myocardial infarction: a quantitative review. *JAMA* 1997;278:2093–2098.
26. Grines CL, Cox DA, Stone GW, et al. Coronary angioplasty with or without stent implantation for acute myocardial infarction. *N Engl J Med* 1999;341:1949–1956.
27. Keeley EC, Boura JA, Grines CL. Primary angioplasty versus intravenous thrombolytic therapy for acute myocardial infarction: a quantitative review of 23 randomised trials. *Lancet* 2003;361(9351):13–20.
28. Fibrinolytic Therapy Trialists (FTT) Collaborative Group. Indications for fibrinolytic therapy in suspected acute myocardial infarction: collaborative overview of early mortality and major morbidity results from all randomized trials of more than 1,000 patients. *Lancet* 1994;343:311–322.
29. Assessment of the Safety and Efficacy of a New Thrombolytic (ASSENT-2) Investigators. Single-bolus tenecteplase compared with front-loaded alteplase in acute myocardial infarction. The ASSENT-2 double-blind randomized trial. *Lancet* 1999;354:716–722.
30. The GUSTO Angiographic Investigators. The effects of tissue plasminogen activator, streptokinase, or both, on coronary artery patency, ventricular function, and survival after acute myocardial infarction. *N Engl J Med* 1993;329:1615–1622.
31. Hochman JS, Sleeper LA, Webb JG, et al. Early revascularization in acute myocardial infarction complicated by cardiogenic shock. *N Engl J Med* 1999;341:625–634.
32. Andersen HR, Nielsen TT, Rasmussen K, et al. A comparison of coronary angioplasty with fibrinolytic therapy in acute myocardial infarction. *N Engl J Med* 2003;349(8):733–742.
33. Widimsky P, Budesinsky T, Vorac D, et al. Long distance transport for primary angioplasty vs. immediate thrombolysis in acute myocardial infarction. Final results of the randomized national multicentre trial—PRAGUE-2. *Eur Heart J* 2003;24(1):94–104.

34. Ellis SG, Ribeiro-da Silva E, Heyndrickx G, et al. Randomized comparison of rescue angioplasty with conservative management of patients with early failure of thrombolysis for acute anterior myocardial infarction. *Circulation* 1994;90:2280–2284.

35. Raimund E, Haude M, Hans W. Coronary-artery stenting compared with balloon angioplasty for restenosis after initial balloon angioplasty. *N Engl J Med* 1998;339:1672–1678.

36. Lincoff AM, Bittl JA, Harrington RA, et al. Bivalirudin and provisional glycoprotein IIb/IIIa blockade compared with heparin and planned glycoprotein IIb/IIIa blockade during percutaneous coronary intervention: REPLACE-2 randomized trial. *JAMA* 2003; 289(7):853–863.

37. Steinhubl SR, Berger PB, Mann JT 3rd, et al. Early and sustained dual oral antiplatelet therapy following percutaneous coronary intervention: a randomized controlled trial. *JAMA* 2002;288(19): 2411–2420.

38. Morice MC, Serruys PW, Sousa JE, et al. A randomized comparison of a sirolimus-eluting stent with a standard stent for coronary revascularization. *N Engl J Med* 2002;346(23):1773–1780.

39. Stone GW, Ellis SG, Cox DA, et al. A polymer-based, paclitaxel-eluting stent in patients with coronary artery disease. *N Engl J Med* 2004;350(3):221–231.

40. Jneid H, Bhatt DL. Advances in antiplatelet therapy. *Expert Opin Emerg Drugs* 2003;8(2):349–363.

41. Yusuf S, Zhao F, Mehta SR, et al. Effects of clopidogrel in addition to aspirin in patients with acute coronary syndromes without ST-segment elevation. *N Engl J Med* 2001;345(7):494–502.

42. Cohen M, Demers C, Gurfinkel EP, et al. A comparison of low-molecular-weight heparin with unfractionated heparin for unstable coronary artery disease. Efficacy and Safety of Subcutaneous Enoxaparin in Non-Q-Wave Coronary Events Study Group. *N Engl J Med* 1997;337:447–452.

43. Antman EM, McCabe CH, Gurfinkel EP, et al. Enoxaparin prevents death and cardiac ischemic events in unstable angina/non-Q-wave myocardial infarction (TIMI) 11B trial. *Circulation* 1999;100: 1593–1601.

44. Antman EM, McCabe C, Gurfinkel E, et al. Treatment benefit of enoxaparin in unstable angina/non-Q-wave myocardial infarction is maintained at one-year follow up in TIMI 11B. *Circulation* 1999; 100[Suppl 1]:I-497.

45. EPIC Investigators. Use of a monoclonal antibody directed against the platelet glycoprotein IIb/IIIa receptor in high- risk coronary angioplasty. *N Engl J Med* 1994;330:956–961.

46. EPILOG Investigators. Platelet glycoprotein IIb/IIIa blockade with abciximab with low-dose heparin during percutaneous coronary revascularization. *N Engl J Med* 1997;336:1689–1696.

47. EPISTENT Investigators. Randomized placebo-controlled and balloon-angioplasty controlled trial to assess safety of coronary stenting with use of platelet glycoprotein IIb/IIIa blockade. *Lancet* 1998;352:87–92.

48. The GUSTO IV-ACS Investigators. Effect of glycoprotein IIb/IIIa receptor blocker abciximab on outcome in patients with acute coronary syndromes without early coronary revascularisation: the GUSTO IV-ACS randomised trial. *Lancet* 2001;357:1915–1924.

49. Topol EJ, Moliterno DJ, Herrmann HC, et al. Comparison of two platelet glycoprotein IIb/IIIa inhibitors, tirofiban and abciximab, for the prevention of ischemic events with percutaneous coronary revascularization. *N Engl J Med* 2001;344:1888–1894.

50. The GUSTO V Investigators. Reperfusion therapy for acute myocardial infarction with fibrinolytic therapy or combination reduced fibrinolytic therapy and platelet glycoprotein IIb/IIIa inhibition: the GUSTO V randomised trial. *Lancet* 2001;357:1905–1914.

51. Antman EM, Braunwald E. Acute myocardial infarction. In: Braunwald E, Zipes DP, Libby P, eds. *Heart Disease: A Textbook of Cardiovascular Medicine*, 6th ed. Philadelphia: WB Saunders, 2001;1114–1231.

52. Latini R, Tognoni G, Maggioni AP, et al. Clinical effects of early angiotensin-converting enzyme inhibitor treatment for acute myocardial infarction are similar in the presence and absence of aspirin: systematic overview of individual data from 96,712 randomized patients. *J Am Coll Cardiol* 2000;35:1801–1807.

53. Sigurdsson A, Swedberg L. Left ventricular remodeling, neurohormonal activation and early treatment with enalapril (CONSENSUS II) following myocardial infarction. *Eur Heart J* 1994;15[Suppl B]:14.

54. The Heart Outcomes Prevention Evaluation Study Investigators. Effects of an angiotensin-converting–enzyme inhibitor, ramipril, on cardiovascular events in high-risk patients. *N Engl J Med* 2000; 342:145–153.

55. Alexander RW, Pratt CM, Ryan TJ, et al. Diagnosis and management of patients with acute myocardial infarction. In: Fuster V, Alexander RW, O'Rourke R, et al, eds. *Hurst's The Heart*, 10th ed. New York: McGraw-Hill, 2001;1275–1359.

56. Scandinavian Simvastatin Survival Study Group. Randomized trial of cholesterol lowering in 4,444 patients with coronary heart disease. *Lancet* 1994;344:1383–1389.

57. Downs JR, Clearfield M, Weis S, et al. Primary prevention trial of acute coronary events with lovastatin in men and women with average cholesterol levels. Results of AFCAPS/ TexCAPS. *JAMA* 1998;279:1615–1622.

58. Shepherd J, Cobbe SM, Ford I, et al. Prevention of coronary heart disease with pravastatin in men with hypercholesterolemia. *N Engl J Med* 1995;333:1301–1307.

59. Sacks FM, Pfeffer MA, Moye LA, et al. The effect of pravastatin on coronary events after myocardial infarction in patients with average cholesterol levels. *N Engl J Med* 1996;335:1001–1009.

60. The Long-Term Intervention with Pravastatin in Ischemic Disease (LIPID) Study Group. Prevention of cardiovascular events and death with pravastatin in patients with coronary heart disease and a broad range of initial cholesterol levels. *N Engl J Med* 1998;339: 1349–1357.

61. Schwartz GC, Olsson AG, Ezekowitz MD, et al. Effects of atorvastatin on early recurrent ischemic events in acute coronary syndromes: the MIRACL study: a randomized controlled trial. *JAMA* 2001;285:1711–1718.

62. Cannon CP, Braunwald E, McCabe CH, et al. Intensive versus moderate lipid lowering with statins after acute coronary syndromes. *N Engl J Med* 2004;350(15):1495–1504.

63. Nissen SE, Tuzcu EM, Schoenhagen P, et al. Effect of intensive compared with moderate lipid-lowering therapy on progression of coronary atherosclerosis: a randomized controlled trial. *JAMA* 2004;291(9):1071–1080.

64. Nissen SE, Tsunoda T, Tuzcu EM, et al. Effect of recombinant ApoA-I Milano on coronary atherosclerosis in patients with acute coronary syndromes: a randomized controlled trial. *JAMA* 2003; 290(17):2292–2300.

65. Tan HL, Lie KI. Prophylactic lidocaine use in acute myocardial infarction revisited in the thrombolytic era. *Am Heart J* 1999;137: 770–773.

66. Alexander JH, Granger GB, Sadowski Z, et al. Prophylactic lidocaine use in acute myocardial infarction: incidence and outcomes from two international trials. The GUSTO-I and GUSTO-IIb Investigators. *Am Heart J* 1999;137:799–805.

67. MacMahon S, Collins R, Peto R, et al. Effects of prophylactic lidocaine in suspected acute myocardial infarction: an overview of results from the randomized, controlled trials. *JAMA* 1988;260: 1910–1916.

68. Archbold RA, Sayer JW, Ray J, et al. Frequency and prognostic implications of conduction defects in acute myocardial infarction since the introduction of thrombolytic therapy. *Eur Heart J* 1998; 19:893–898.

69. Goldberg RJ, Gurwitz JH. Disseminating the results of clinical trials to community-based practitioners: is anyone listening? *Am Heart J* 1999;137:4–7.

70. McCormik D, Gurwitz JH, Lessard D, et al. Use of aspirin, β-blockers, and lipid-lowering medications before recurrent acute myocardial infarction: missed opportunities for prevention? *Arch Intern Med* 1999;159:561–567.

71. Jneid H, Thacker HL. Coronary artery disease in women: different, often undertreated. *Cleve Clin J Med* 2001;68:441–448.

## SUGGESTED READINGS

Braunwald E, Antman EM, Beasley JW, et al. ACC/AHA guideline update for the management of patients with unstable angina and non-ST-segment elevation myocardial infarction—2002: summary article: a report of the American College of Cardiology/ American Heart Association Task Force on Practice Guidelines

(Committee on the Management of Patients With Unstable Angina). *Circulation* 2002;106(14):1893–1900.

DeWood MA, Spona J, Notske R, et al. Prevalence of total coronary occlusion during the early hours of transmural myocardial infarction. *N Engl J Med* 1980;303:897–902.

ISIS-2 (Second Interventional Study of Infarct Survival) Collaborative Group. Randomized trial of intravenous streptokinase or aspirin, both or neither, among 17,187 cases of suspected acute myocardial infarction: ISIS-2. *Lancet* 1988;2:349–360.

Kleiman NS, White HD, Ohman EM, et al. Mortality within 24 hours of thrombolysis from myocardial infarction: the importance of early reperfusion. *Circulation* 1994;90:2658–2665.

Ryan TJ, Anderson JL, Antman EM, et al. ACC/AHA guidelines for the management of patients with acute myocardial infarction: a report of the ACC/AHA Task Force on Practice Guidelines (Committee on Management of Acute Myocardial Infarction). *J Am Coll Cardiol* 1996;28:1328–1428.

Ryan TJ, Antman EM, Brooks NH, et al. ACC/AHA revised guidelines for the management of patients with acute myocardial infarction. *J Am Coll Cardiol* 1999;34:890–911.

TIMI 3-B Investigators. Effects of tissue plasminogen activator and a comparison of early invasive and conservative strategies in unstable angina and non Q-wave myocardial infarction: results of the TIMI-3B trial. *Circulation* 1994;89:1545–1556.

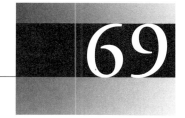

# Hyperlipidemia Update

*Dennis L. Sprecher*

Perhaps the most significant advance in the concept of cholesterol reduction and coronary disease is the association between cholesterol reduction and reduction in cardiac events (1). The angiographic rate of regression with cholesterol reduction is extremely small, albeit statistically significant, whereas the reduction in event rate in these angiographic studies is often well above 50%. It is thought that the cholesterol reduction alters the organization of the plaque so that rupture and consequent myocardial infarction (MI) is less likely. This pathway otherwise depends on a weakening of the shoulders of the plaque, perhaps due to collagen breakdown, as well as subsequent thrombogenicity of the lipid core. Cholesterol lowering is thought to reduce inflammation around the plaque borders and enrich the area with collagen. In the Cholesterol and Recurrent Events (CARE) trial (2) and Air Force/Texas Coronary Atherosclerosis Prevention Study (AFCAPS) trials (3), it was found that pravastatin (Pravachol) and lovastatin (Mevacor) treatment, respectively, resulted in a reduction of C-reactive protein, a marker of inflammation. Such lowering is not statin–dose dependent (4) and is thought to represent a class effect (5). Herein lies a considerable restructuring of thought. The progressive stenoses of a vessel leading to hemodynamic compromise are not as relevant in predicting a future infarct as the integrity of the plaque because cardiac events often are the result of lesions that demonstrate less than 50% stenosis. Such lesser lesions make up the bulk of plaque in a coronary artery. Therefore, the lack of hemodynamically significant stenoses may not reduce, and certainly does not exclude, the probability of a new cardiac event. Cholesterol lowering reduces the incidence of MI. According to large clinical trials, specifically Scandinavian Simvastatin Survival Study

(4S) (6), West of Scotland Coronary Prevention Study (WOSCOPS) (7), CARE (8), Long-Term Intervention with Pravastatin in Ischaemic Disease (LIPID) (9), AFCAPS (3), and most recently the Heart Protection Study (HPS) (10), the time to plaque stabilization, if it is to occur, is between 6 months and 2 years of continuous treatment in the stable, nonacute setting. Statin therapy initiated during the acute setting may influence subsequent outcomes more rapidly [as per the Pravastatin or Atorvastatin Evaluation and Infection-Thrombolysis (PROVE-IT) study].

## RECENT CLINICAL TRIALS

A further follow-up of previous trials, as well as numerous new trials indicating a reduction of cardiac events with a reduction in cholesterol serum levels have been published or presented. The 4S study (6) evaluated more than 4,000 individuals who had cardiac disease and were randomized to simvastatin, a hydroxymethylglutaryl–coenzyme A (HMG-CoA) reductase inhibitor, or placebo. A reduction in the percentage of death and nonfatal MI, and a reduction in overall mortality was noted. This was the first cholesterol-lowering study to definitely indicate the reduction in cardiac mortality (>40%) and total mortality (30%). The 8-year follow-up data suggest a continuing divergence of the survival curves, even though many placebo patients went on simvastatin at the end of the original 6-year study (11). Total mortality remained at 30% reduction after 8 years (15.8% placebo versus 11.4% treatment group, p = 0.0001). Further, as noted during the trial (12), 8-year data indicate a cardiac event rate benefit depending on the percent reduction in low-density lipoprotein (LDL) levels (a 44% to 70% reduction leads to an 18.2% reduction in event rate, 34% to 44% reduction to 13.8%, and less than 34% reduction of LDL to 10.6% event rate). In a potentially parallel fashion, utilizing intravascular ultrasound (IVUS), statin therapy demonstrated a direct relation between percent change in plaque volume and percent LDLc, promoting the overall relevance of LDLc to CV risk (13). The WOSCOPS primary prevention trial (7) indicated the benefit of use of pravastatin versus placebo, demonstrating an approximately 30% reduction in the combined endpoint of death and nonfatal MI, with some strong suggestive trends in the arena of mortality. The higher the risk, the more the absolute benefit of cholesterol lowering. Further, there was some suggestion of attenuation of event rate benefits after LDL levels were lowered beyond 20%. This has been supported by Fager and Olov (14), who also suggest an attenuation of benefit as the LDL level is lowered. This is countered by the more linear relationship found in the Lipid Research Clinics data (15,16) and associated meta-analyses (17), the 4S data cited previously, and the further benefit noted in the post–coronary artery bypass graft trial in saphenous vein grafts (18). In the Reversal of Atherosclerosis with Aggressive Lipid Lowering (REVERSAL) trial, percent plaque volume was correlated down to at least a 50% reduction in LDLc levels (13).

The CARE study tested pravastatin (Pravachol) in patients who had coronary artery disease (CAD) but whose LDLc level was within a more normal level (115 to 175 mg/dL). Again, the numbers were comparable with other research data, suggesting that even at LDL values as low as 127 to 130 mg/dL, a benefit was derived from the further reduction of the LDLc value. Results from the CARE trial (and LIPID trial) data analyses revealed no benefit of Pravachol over 5 years in subjects with baseline LDL values of less than 125 mg/dL. The Harvard Atherosclerosis Reversibility Project, an angiographic study, indicated no benefit in CAD lesions with LDL cholesterol (LDLc) levels below 140 mg/dL, over a 2.5-year period (19,20). In some contrast, the Lipoprotein and Coronary Atherosclerosis study using fluvastatin suggested similar angiographic benefits with LDLc values between 115 to 130 mg/dL as with LDLc values above 150 mg/dL. Saphenous vein grafts also are protected through LDL lowering in the lower ranges. In the post–coronary artery bypass graft trial, using lovastatin, LDL was lowered from a baseline mean of 155 to 135 mg/dL (modest treatment), and the outcome was compared with a lowering to 95 mg/dL (aggressive treatment). Benefit was observed angiographically and through a reduction in repeat procedures (29%) (21). Seven-year follow-up reveals continued benefits (22). Although coumadin was not found to be of value in the initial trial, coumadin began to contribute to outcomes (22) during the sixth and seventh years. The 4S and WOSCOPS (as well as pre-statin primary and secondary studies) included subjects with high isolated LDLc levels (17).

Two further trials have been reported that incorporate subjects with more modest to moderate LDL values. First, 6,605 healthy men and women (15%) were studied in AFCAPS (3) (average age, 58 years), with mean LDL of 150 mg/dL and high-density lipoprotein (HDL) levels of 37 mg/dL, treated with lovastatin, placebo, or both for approximately 5 years. A 25% reduction in LDL was associated with a 35% reduction in fatal and non-fatal MI, with too few events occurring to determine mortality. Women appeared to derive a benefit equal to that for men. Criteria used for the treatment of AFCAPS patients were not consistent with current National Cholesterol Education Program (NCEP) guidelines; the application of these more aggressive approaches would add another 6 to 8 million people to the NCEP inclusion algorithm.

LIPID (9) is the one of the largest secondary prevention trials (9,014 men and women). LIPID was performed in Australia and New Zealand over the course of 5 years, with characteristics similar to the CARE study. Average LDL values were approximately equal to 150 mg/dL. Pravastatin reduced LDL by 25% and resulted in a 23% reduction in fatal and non-fatal MI. Further, total mortality and coronary mortality decreased by 23% and 24%, respectively. Here again, patients who presented with baseline LDL values less than 125 mg/dL did not appear to enjoy benefits from LDLc lowering. In distinct contrast to these two studies, the dramatic outcomes realized in the HPS (10) suggests that those with LDL cholesterol below 100 mg/dL continued to appreciate cardiovascular benefits comparable to those above this value. This may be due to the larger number of subjects with such low values, or the higher risk characterized by recruitment to the HPS, or some aspect (s) of the particular agent used.

The HPS, the largest study yet in the lipid field (10), included 20,000 people with a total cholesterol level of >135 mg/dL who were suspected of high vascular event risk over the ensuing 5 years (history of current coronary artery disease, vascular disease, diabetes mellitus, or hypertension). The participants were randomized to placebo or simvastatin 40 mg (n = 10,269) by local practitioners. All-cause death was reduced from 14.7% to 12.9% over the 5 years of the trial (12% reduction, p = 0.0003). Both a significant 18% reduction in coronary death rate and an approximate 25% reduction in each of three outcomes—non-fatal MI or coronary death, nonfatal or fatal stroke, and coronary and noncoronary revascularization—was observed. The results were noted regardless of gender, age, presence of diabetes, medication status (e.g., ASA and ACE inhibitor), and most important, regardless of baseline LDLc. The considerable 30% cross-over deployment of statin to the placebo group potentially led to an underestimate of the real value of simvastatin in this intent-to-treat analysis.

The baseline cholesterol level may have some relevance toward reduction in risk. The CARE study (utilizing pravastatin) recommends a progression of enhanced benefit from a LDLc level less than 125 to greater than 150 mg/dL.

Although it has been suggested that the percentage reduction in LDLc is more relevant to angiographic change than average LDLc levels during the study (23), it has been recommended that both factors are relevant (24). Recent studies have reinforced the value of LDLc percentage reduction, whereas on-trial levels must be reevaluated.

It is noteworthy that among 5,800 high-risk, elderly subjects (>70 years of age), followed for 3.5 years, pravastatin reduced cardiovascular events but did not alter overall death, nor influence stroke rates (25). A further correlation between the same percent reduction in LDLc for two statins (atorvastatin and pravastatin) versus the percentage reduction in plaque volume through IVUS suggested an advantage for atorvastatin, thus recommending a statin-specific benefit (13) beyond LDLc lowering alone. A recent meta-analysis of trials over the last 2 years (26) suggests that atorvastatin may provide more potent vascular benefits, particularly more stroke protection, than pravastatin. Whether specific statins have unique attributes remains controversial, however.

## HIGH-DENSITY LIPOPROTEIN AND TRIGLYCERIDE VALUES

A meta-analysis by Hokanson and Austin (27) indicates that triglyceride values are predictive of CAD even after an adjustment for high density lipoprotein cholesterol (HDLc) values. This is consistent with data from the Framingham Heart Study. The data are weak on modifying HDL or triglyceride plasma levels to effect cardiovascular protection, compared with that supporting LDL reduction.

In the Veterans Affairs High-Density Lipoprotein Intervention Trial (28), more than 2,500 men with HDL levels of less than 40 mg/dL, LDL levels of less than 140 mg/dL, and triglyceride levels of less than 300 mg/dL were divided into gemfibrozil and placebo groups. Over 5 years, a 6% increase in HDL levels, 24% decrease in triglyceride levels, and an increase of 3% in LDL levels resulted in a 24% decrease in cardiovascular events. This is the first major trial to suggest a cardiovascular value in reducing triglyceride levels and increasing HDL-implicating intermediate particles. The HDLc level was found to directly correlate with benefits in this trial, although triglyceride-rich particles are suggested as relevant in a small substudy (29). Insulin-resistant subjects (based on fasting glucose and insulin levels) enjoyed the greatest benefit or risk reduction from gemfibrozil therapy, despite demonstrating the least HDLc level elevation (30). Lipid changes, particularly HDLc, explained no more than one-third of the benefits. This dichotomy suggests that the HDLc level is not fully informative about fibrate-related protective attributes, a position also suggested by the Bezafibrate Infarction Trial (31), in which a positive result was observed only in those with baseline triglyceride values above 200 mg/dL (39.5% endpoint reduction, p = 0.02). Otherwise, in the total of 3,090 patients with CAD, a 22%

decrease in triglyceride levels, 12% increase in the HDLc level, and a 5% decrease in the LDL level resulted in a nonsignificant reduction in cardiac events (9% decrease, p = 0.27). The results of two outcomes studies, the Stockholm Ischemic Heart Disease Secondary Prevention Study (32) and the Helsinki Heart Study (33), are consistent with changes in the levels of either HDL or triglyceride effecting a benefit in cardiovascular protection. The actual decrease in triglyceride values in the Helsinki trial, however, did not correspond to a reduction in coronary events, in contrast to the results observed in Stockholm, in which triglyceride level reduction was associated.

Six angiographic trials, the National Heart, Lung, and Blood Institute type II trial (resin) (34); the Familial Atherosclerosis Trial (FATS; niacin and resin versus lovastatin and resin) trial (35); the Lopid Coronary Angiography Trial (LOCAT; gemfibrozil) (36); the Bezafibrate Coronary Atherosclerosis Intervention Trial (BECAIT) (37); the HDL-Atherosclerosis Treatment Study (HATS; simvastatin versus simvastatin and niacin) (38); and the Diabetes Atherosclerosis Intervention Study (DAIS) (23) are consistent with the benefits of altering the levels of HDLc, triglycerides, or both. The LOCAT trial in patients with isolated low HDL levels (mean, 31 mg/dL) demonstrated angiographic benefit in the treatment arm.

The BECAIT trial (37) further showed bezafibrate improves dyslipidemia, lowers plasma fibrinogen, and slows atherosclerosis, and reduces coronary events over the course of 5 years in young survivors (<45 year) of MI. The most recent DAIS trial (23), where HDLc levels were increased by 6%, indicated the angiographic value of fenofibrate in type II subjects. Furthermore, the 4S, WOSCOPS, and post–coronary artery bypass graft substudies indicate a loss of any predictive value for triglyceride levels and much of the value related to baseline HDL levels after substantial LDL level lowering (37). HDL level elevations during 4S added to the benefits observed with LDL level lowering. Change in HDL, apolipoprotein AI (ApoA1), and apolipoprotein B (ApoB) levels were an excellent univariate predictors in AFCAPS, with a change in ApoB/ApoA1 levels possibly being the best lipid-related predictors (39). In subjects with low HDLc levels, the combination of simvastatin and niacin resulted in dramatic benefits (70% reduction in events) over that of placebo, with clear additive benefit for the combination therapy. The author theorized that a HDLc level elevation of 31% and a LDLc level reduction of 42% (each translating into a 1% change per 1% risk reduction), results in the about 70% reduction in events observed. True angiographic regression was noted, rather than a simple delay or lack of progression.

A very novel direct infusion of recombinant apoA-I Milano/phospholipid complex (HDL-like particles) weekly over 5 weeks after an acute cardiac event demonstrated IVUS-based plaque-volume improvement benefits consistent with direct HDL particle vascular influence (40). It is believed that an enhanced apoAI-to-HDL ratio presence in the serum space is associated with cardiovascular improvement, whether through enhanced production (41), direct infusion, or reduced catabolism (42). The complex metabolic pattern of HDL cholesterol transit (43), however, the variability in HDL-subfraction activity and HDL's high integration with the VLDL:LDL; apoB pathway currently complicates the on-trial explanations of HDL benefit. Fibrates and niacin do appear to initiate an improvement in CV endpoints, at least in part, via their association with HDLc level-elevation, as measured using a simple HDLc serum evaluation.

## ASSOCIATION WITH HIGH-DENSITY LIPOPROTEIN/TRIGLYCERIDE MODIFICATION

Forty percent to 50% of subjects who present with both high triglyceride and low HDL levels are obese, and close to 50% of their family members also have HDL and triglyceride level abnormalities (44,45). Triglyceride elevation abnormalities are highly related to the "dense LDL" familial phenotypes associated with CAD. These abnormalities, no doubt, are part of a spectrum of many familial disorders that present with a cluster of risk-associated factors, specifically low HDL and high triglyceride levels, obesity, high blood pressure, glucose intolerance, insulin resistance, or all these factors. This clustering was previously reported by Reaven (46). More recently reviewed, Superko (47) has noted that statins are particularly successful angiographically when the patient expresses dense LDL. Triglyceride values, although not accurate in defining the LDL phenotype, suggest a progressively enhanced dense phenotype when levels of more than 200 mg/dL are present, and a progressively less dense phenotype as triglyceride levels drop below 150 mg/dL.

Two large hypertension trials, in which many of the subjects would meet the definition for metabolic syndrome (i.e., the above clustering of dense LDL–related risk factors), were evaluated for response to statin therapy. The Anglo-Scandinavian Cardiac Outcomes Trial (ASCOT) included a 10 mg atorvastatin dose administered to 10,000 of the overall 19,000 hypertensive subjects; this resulted in a 36% drop in events during the interim of the study (48). This result led to prematurely stopping the study 3.3 years after initiation. This runs counter to the results in the Antihypertensive and Lipid-Lowering treatment to prevent Heart Attack Trial (ALLHAT) study (n = 10,000), where 40 mg of pravastatin therapy provided to approximately 5,000 subjects above age 55 (mean age 66 years), with a moderate baseline LDLc of 146 mg/dL (with 4 to 8 years of follow-up), revealed no obvious benefit. Modest LDLc lowering in the treated group and some LDL reduction in the usual-care group led to a 17% LDLc difference at the trial's end. Recent analysis suggests that the disorder results between the ASCOT and ALLHAT trials may relate to inadequate study power to show an effect of therapy (49).

## MODIFIED LOW-DENSITY LIPOPROTEIN

Considerable animal data suggest that the oxidation of LDL is associated with the development of vascular disease. Human data are still minimal. One study using probucol, which is a significant antioxidant, was unsuccessful in reducing femoral artery disease (50), yet valuable in reducing restenosis after percutaneous transluminal coronary angioplasty (51). The use of vitamin E in epidemiologic analyses has revealed a positive correlation with reduced cardiac outcomes and some reduction in events in post-MI subjects (Cambridge Heart Antioxidant Study). Two large clinical trials, however, the Gruppo Italiano Per lo Studio Della Streptokinase Nell'Infarto Miocardio and the Heart Outcomes Prevention Evaluation, both revealed a lack of value for vitamin E administration in secondary prevention. The most recent HPS again indicated a lack of benefit in the use of antioxidant vitamins (600 mg vitamin E, 250 mg vitamin C, and 20 mg β-carotene) (10). The standard use of vitamin E for cardiovascular protection is not routinely recommended (52,53). Free radical, modified arachidonic acid results in isoprostane synthesis, which is noted to be increased in hypercholesterolemic patients (54). This may be a helpful, although expensive, marker for oxidant stress (55). Other more effective and less expensive markers are becoming available.

## TREATMENT GUIDELINES

The adult treatment panel guidelines for cholesterol control have gone through three iterations. The most recent nuances to these guidelines include a coronary heart disease equivalent (i.e., diabetes and global risk scores >2% per year) (23), the maintenance of HDLc values below 40 mg/dL, and the targeting of non-HDLc levels when triglyceride serum values are found to be greater than 200 mg/dL. The LDL goals are equivalent, based on the findings of the Cholesterol Lowering Atherosclerosis Study of Blackenhorn (56), as well as on the meta-analyses of data discussed earlier. As suggested by Cleeman, who reviewed the NCEP guidelines, no new LDL cutpoint changes were incorporated for the Adult Treatment Panel III (ATPIII), although subtle modifications may be made over time (57). The most recent guidelines are summarized in Figure 69.1 and also are available online at www.nhlbi.nih.gov/guidelines/cholesterol/index.htm.

Risk factor modification data on women has been significantly supplemented from data from the HPS, in which one-fourth of the participants were women. Currently, the data from 4S, CARE, LIPID, AFCAPS, and HPS indicate cholesterol reduction through statin use is at least as beneficial in women as in men, based on point estimates and/or clear significantly proven advantage. The treatment for women in the lipid arena should parallel that for men, a fact which belies the apparent undertreatment of women and their own inaccurate perception that heart disease is

# How to determine the goal LDL level and whether to start drug therapy

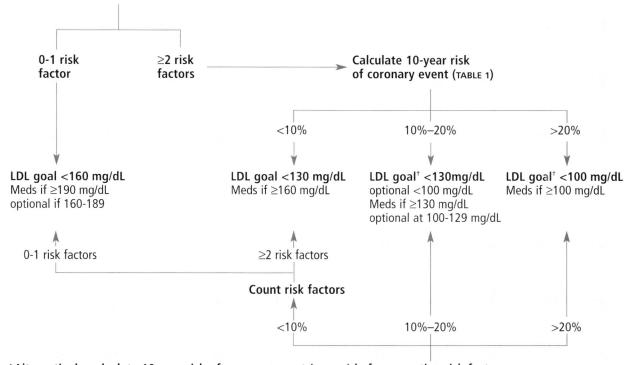

**If any**
- Coronary artery disease
- Peripheral vascular disease
- Abdominal aortic aneurysm
- Symptomatic carotid disease
- Diabetes mellitus

**LDL goal <100mg/dL**
(<70mg/dL optional in acute coronary syndrome or cardiovascular disease with other risk factors)
Meds if ≥100 mg/dL

**If none of the above, count risk factors***
- Hypertension (blood pressure ≥140/90 mm Hg or taking meds)
- Cigarette smoking
- HDL <40 mg/dL (subtract 1 risk factor if HDL is ≥60)
- Age ≥40 years (men) or ≥55 years (women)
- Family history of coronary artery disease (before age 55 in a male first-degree relative or before age 65 in a female first-degree relative)

**0-1 risk factor**

**≥2 risk factors**

**Calculate 10-year risk of coronary event (TABLE 1)**

<10%          10%–20%          >20%

**LDL goal <160 mg/dL**
Meds if ≥190 mg/dL
optional if 160-189

**LDL goal <130 mg/dL**
Meds if ≥160 mg/dL

**LDL goal[†] <130mg/dL**
optional <100 mg/dL
Meds if ≥130 mg/dL
optional at 100-129 mg/dL

**LDL goal[†] <100 mg/dL**
Meds if ≥100 mg/dL

0-1 risk factors

≥2 risk factors

**Count risk factors**

<10%          10%–20%          >20%

*Alternatively, calculate 10-year risk of coronary event (TABLE 1) before counting risk factors

**If LDL goal is reached, treat secondary targets**

**Triglycerides.** If triglyceride level is ≥200 mg/dL, calculate non-HDL level (total cholesterol minus HDL); goal is 30 mg/dL higher than the LDL goal

**Metabolic syndrome.** If three or more of the following are present, treat with weight reduction, increased physical activity, antihypertensive treatment (if blood pressure is elevated), aspirin (if coronary disease is present), and therapy to reduce triglycerides and raise HDL levels
- Waist >40 inches (men) or >35 inches (women)
- Triglyceride level ≥150 mg/dL
- HDL level <40 mg/dL (men) or <50 mg/dL (women)
- Blood pressure ≥130/85 mm Hg
- Glucose level ≥110 mg/dL

[†]For high and moderate risk patients requiring drug therapy, clinicians should seek to lower LDL levels 30% to 40%

CCF
©2004

**Figure 69.1**  Proposed algorithm for starting drug therapy.

not a primary risk issue. Targeted therapeutic recommendations for women have been published (58), but also are more fully available online at http://atvb.ahajournals.org/cgi/content/full/24/3/e29.

The baseline cardiac event rate is substantially higher in CAD patients compared with asymptomatic subjects. Risk reduction has a more statistically significant effect in this CAD population. Although it is clear that cholesterol reduction is effective for both primary and secondary prevention, the decision to treat cholesterol elevation may ultimately be an economic one. The guidelines for internists, as published by the American College of Physicians (59), defines "high-risk" at a fairly elevated threshold, a set point considerably above that established by the NCEP. The global risk score is a continuum that can be dichotomized to select a community-wide level of health improvement, as well as a level of fiscal exposure. The NCEP has established that a below-1% risk of cardiac events per year over the ensuing 10 years is little reason to provide expensive cholesterol level modifying drugs, but levels above the 1% risk baseline are worthy of receiving medical intervention, based on specific risk determinants. An above-2% risk is clearly worthy of drug therapy to prevent the inevitable high cost of support during and after an actual event. It is very likely, however, that compliance deficiencies with pharmaceutical agents such as statins will limit their economic impact. This deficiency will, unfortunately, also seriously erode the expected lipid alterations and, in turn, place a ceiling on their potential cardiovascular benefit (60).

Currently, the NCEP guidelines (ATPIII) (61) recommend treatment for LDLc first—including diet modification (which incorporates fiber as well as plant-sterol enriched margarines) followed by drugs—prior to initiating any therapeutic efforts directed toward triglyceride or HDLc values. Therapeutic lifestyle changes (TLC) are recommended if triglyceride values are above 150 mg/dL, and possible medication if above 200 mg/dL. Weight loss, reduction in fat and simple sugar intake, reduction in alcohol use, and control of diabetes are strongly suggested. With triglycerides levels of more than 400 mg/dL, and general environmental issues implemented, drugs are recommended if:

- Familial CAD is present,
- The patient has CAD,
- At least two significant risk factors are present, or
- All three

Niacin is the first choice, with fibric acid derivatives such as gemfibrozil or fenofibrate as second choice. Subjects with triglyceride levels of more than 1,000 mg/dL can develop pancreatitis. In this scenario, weight loss and the use of either niacin or fibric acid derivative [gemfibrozil (Lopid) or fenofibrate (Tricor)] is recommended.

An attractive addition to the guidelines, although admittedly a complexity, is the calculation of non–HDL cholesterol values. This value (Total cholesterol − HDLc value), equates to the overall apoB-related burden, including LDL and other intermediate lipid forms. In subjects who present with triglyceride values greater than 200 mg/dL, and who have properly controlled their LDLc (through drugs or diet), the guidelines recommend that the non-HDLc value be calculated. If levels are 30 mg/dL or more above that of the concurrent LDLc goal (e.g., if the LDLc goal is 130 mg/dL, a non-HDLc goal of above or equal to 160 mg/dL would prompt therapy), then recommendations for reducing high triglyceride levels should be implemented (e.g., diet and possibly drugs). The finding of low HDLc in the setting of high risk (>2% per year) over the next 10 years, prompts, first, LDL control and subsequently the progressive addition of therapeutic lifestyle changes, fibric acid derivatives, niacin and/or some contribution with a statin to ultimately control this dyslipidemia.

## DRUG THERAPY

HMG-CoA reductase inhibitors, called *statin* agents, are the current major therapeutic approach toward pharmacologic cholesterol lowering. Those available are fairly equal in their convenience of use and side-effect profiles. Simvastatin is approximately twice as potent, milligram per milligram, as pravastatin and lovastatin, and perhaps three times as potent as other drugs, including fluvastatin, which is the least expensive at the lower dose levels. Atorvastatin was approved in January 1997 (62,63). It can lower LDLc up to 60%. It is more potent and more efficacious in LDLc lowering than simvastatin, but does not appear to have comparable HDLc-elevating effects (64). The half-life is uniquely prolonged (14 hours) and its effect is maximal in 2 to 3 weeks, rather than in the less than 2 weeks achieved with other statins. Cerivastatin (Baychol) was released in January 1998 (65), but after 1 or 2 years of general use, it was demonstrated to result in a marked increase in rhabdomyolysis (particularly in combination with gemfibrozil) leading to death. It was consequently removed from the market. Recently, rosuvastatin (Crestor) was introduced; it achieves about 8% more cholesterol-lowering power than atorvastatin and some enhanced HDLc-raising characteristics. Renal concerns limit the dose to 40 mg (rather than the original 80 mg daily) and continued concern at this dose has prompted the European regulatory agencies to recommend specialist involvement at the 40 mg dose. These two recent statin safety issues have fueled concerns about the safety of chronic pharmaceutical therapy for preventive care and have widened the interest in nonsystemic agents for lipid modification, for monotherapy but also for combination therapy with a statin. Ezetimibe introduces a further 18% LDLc level reduction when administered concurrently with a statin (41). It also can permit lower dosing of a statin if goals are achieved (10 mg atorvastatin plus ezetimibe = 80 mg atorvastatin for LDLc lowering). The ease of use and safety profile of ezetimibe has decreased, but not eradicated, the use of other more traditional intestinally directed agents. A potent combination of bile acid–absorbing resin and statin agents has provided LDLc level lowering above 50%. A low-dose combination of both a statin and resin (i.e., between 10 and 20 mg/day of statin, and 4 and 8 g/day of resin) provides approximately a 10% improvement in cholesterol lowering above statin alone, with minimal side effects. These various agents are particularly appropriate for isolated LDL elevation. Resins can produce GI symptoms (e.g., bloating), however, are often constipating, and can produce an elevation in triglyceride values, particularly at the higher dosing. Resins are usually avoided when triglyceride levels exceed 200 mg/dL. Because of the major side effects of the statin agents, liver enzyme (serum glutamic-oxaloacetic transaminase and serum glutamic-pyruvic transaminase) and creatine phosphokinase serum levels must be followed. The latter measurement is not required by the U.S. Food and Drug Administration (FDA), but a baseline value is recommended, with follow-up values assessed every year unless symptoms of myositis are observed.

Subjects with abnormalities not only in LDL levels but also in triglyceride and HDL levels often are encountered more frequently than are patients with isolated LDLc level elevations, especially among CAD patients. In this group of patients, niacin and the fibric acid derivatives (e.g., gemfibrozil) are candidate drugs. Niacin, however, particularly predisposes or produces glucose intolerance in those subjects who are already diabetic. The most notable side effect is flushing, making niacin often not well tolerated. A newer drug, Niaspan (niacin extended-release formula) is a once per day formulation, dosed at 1,000 to 2,500 mg. Its benefits are commensurate with regular niacins, with fewer side effects; it is still undergoing safety testing. Fibric acid derivatives, including gemfibrozil, fenofibrate, and clofibrate, produce a moderate reduction in LDLc levels of approximately 15%, but produce excellent triglyceride level lowering and moderate HDL level elevation. Fenofibrate (66) is a classic European fibrate providing an LDL level lowering effect of greater than 20%, which is more potent than gemfibrozil. The combination of statin and gemfibrozil still poses some minor enhanced risk for muscle damage and liver toxicity.

The combination of niacin and statin also is used (excluding diabetics) to treat mixed hyperlipidemia. A newer combination agent (Nicostatin or Advicor, i.e., Niaspan and lovastatin) has produced marked lipid-altering results, with reductions of LDLc and triglyceride levels by 45% and 42%, respectively, while concurrently raising HDLc levels by 41% (67). Cholesterol ester transfer protein-inhibitors, which block the transfer of cholesterol ester from HDL to very low density lipoprotein (VLDL), improve HDL serum residence times, a step postulated to enhance direct reverse cholesterol transport and possibly improve anti-inflammatory influences on the vessel wall (68,69). Whether the resulting increase of HDLc levels by over 50% changes vessel wall atherosclerosis is not known, but the results of ongoing testing are awaited (70). Other new lipid-profile altering agents under development have been reviewed (71).

On the average, statins reduce triglyceride values by more than 20% when triglyceride levels are greater than 250 mg/dL, 10% when triglyceride levels are 150 to 250 mg/dL, and have no effect when triglyceride levels are less than 150 mg/dL. Further, the ratio of triglyceride-to-LDL percent reduction is 1.2%, 0.5%, and 0%, respectively, at the previously mentioned cutpoints. No differences in these relationships are noted among the statins (72). Thus, if the triglyceride value is above 250 mg/dL, every 1% reduction in LDL is matched by an equivalent 1% reduction in triglyceride values, regardless of the statin used.

## Statin Therapy in Acute Coronary Syndromes

It is hypothesized that the acute or near-term benefits of statins occur through an influence on endothelium-dependent flow (73), consistent with changes shortly after LDL apheresis (74), along with statin-dependent decreases in thrombus formation (75).

The Myocardial Ischemia Reduction with Aggressive Cholesterol Lowering Study (MIRACL) (76) provided 80 mg of atorvastatin or placebo to 3,806 individuals within 96 hours of an acute coronary syndrome; this regimen resulted in a 16% decrease in a combined cardiovascular endpoint after 4 months. Lowering the LDLc level from 124 to 72 mg/dL (a 40% decrease) was unrelated to the outcomes, suggesting nontraditional benefits from the statin agent. A small study (n = 350), Atorvastatin versus Revascularization Treatments, randomized relatively asymptomatic patients to percutaneous transluminal coronary angioplasty with medical therapy or to atorvastatin; this study revealed fewer subsequent events (13.4% versus 20.9%) in the statin arm over 1.5 years. These results are countered by the Sibrafiban versus Aspirin to Yield Maximum Protection from Ischemic Heart Events Post-Acute Coronary Syndrome (SYMPHONY) study of 12,000 subjects with acute coronary syndromes. In the SYMPHONY study, statins (evaluated post-hoc from a database) did not reveal a benefit at any time up to one year, or for any event.

In the PROVE-IT TIMI-22 study encompassing nearly 4,162 subjects, a statin (atorvastatin or pravastatin) was administered within 7 days of an acute coronary event (69% with stents), with a high percentage of patients receiving concomitant medications (aspirin, ACE inhibitors) (77). Atorvastatin revealed a 16% reduction of major cardiovascular endpoints compared to pravastatin therapy, a finding suggested within the first 30 days post-event. Smaller studies have suggested similar outcomes, with benefits both in-hospital and after discharge. Large observational data studies in the United States and Sweden of lipid lowering on discharge in subjects with acute coronary syndromes have suggested profound benefits in the reduction in mortality within the first year of therapy after the event (78,79).

The ATPIII guidelines recommend statins at discharge for all acute coronary syndrome patients with LDL values above 130 mg/dL, with an option of beginning with values above 100 mg/dL. We have expressed the view that perhaps all acute coronary syndrome patients should be discharged with a statin agent (80), regardless of their LDLc values, although some controversy remains.

## Diabetes

Based on 4S (11) and WOSCOPS (81–84) data, statins may be the drugs of choice in mixed hyperlipidemias, particularly in diabetics (21,82,83). A clearance of lipid remnants may be successfully accomplished through the upregulation of the ApoB/E receptors, which is the mode of action for statins. Among the 5,963 people with diabetes in the HPS, a 25% reduction in events (equivalent to those without diabetes) was observed. This was comparable again when evaluating those with baseline LDLc levels below and above 100 mg/dL. The Collaborative Atorvastatin Diabetes Study (CARDS) suggested benefits derived from atorvastatin therapy for vascular events. Although the percent risk reduction is comparable in patients with diabetes and nondiabetics, the absolute risk in diabetes mellitus is very high, thus translating into more benefits versus the costs of therapy. For this reason, the American Diabetes Association (ADA) recently augmented its current diabetes guidelines to recommend LDLc level lowering in the diabetic patient if levels are above 130 mg/dL, with a target value of less than 100 mg/dL, and (more recently) a 30% reduction in LDLc regardless of the baseline LDLc value.

## Vasoregulation

Within 3 months of cholesterol reduction, alterations in vasoregulation occur, and some data suggest improvements within a much shorter period (74,84). Positron emission tomography (PET) studies in chronic angina patients, and outcome studies in unstable angina patients, are ongoing.

## Stroke

More recent data have strongly indicated the benefit of statin therapy in the reduction of stroke, despite a meta-analysis done in 1993 (pre-statins) that suggested otherwise. Three separate meta-analyses, published in 1997 and 1998 (85–87), suggest that statin therapy achieving an LDL level reduction of 25% to 35% results in a 20% to 30% reduction in the development of stroke over the approximate 5 years of these studies. It does not appear that the benefit is directly correlated with LDL reduction. Furthermore, the results of several reports, including the LIPID trial, have found statin therapy to decrease carotid intimal medial thickness (88). Recently, as part of the CARDS trial, atorvastatin was provided to diabetics and showed a clear benefit in stroke reduction (10).

## Cardiac Transplant

Over 60% of heart transplant recipients are observed to have hypercholesterolemia (89). Because vascular disease is a major cause of ultimate transplantation failure, and cholesterol reduction in congestive heart disease patients has been profoundly successful, serious efforts at cholesterol lowering have been made within the transplantation population. At present, pravastatin and simvastatin are the only pharmaceutical agents that have demonstrated a benefit in reducing rejection after human cardiac transplantation and decreasing the level of vasculopathy (50,90,91).

## Human Immunodeficiency Virus

Lipodystrophy (a redistribution of body fat), high triglyceride and low HDL levels, and some insulin resistance have been noted in human immunodeficiency virus (HIV) patients using protease inhibitors (92,93). In addition, premature CAD has been reported in these patients. One study using gemfibrozil and atorvastatin in an HIV-infected population has been reported (94), and a full lipid algorithm has been developed for the optimal management of dyslipidemia in this population (95). The dramatic increase in life expectancy using protease inhibitors prompts further attention to preventive issues.

## REVIEW EXERCISES

### QUESTIONS

**1.** Which of the lipoprotein particles is composed primarily of cholesterol?
a) LDL
b) HDL
c) VLDL
d) None of the above

**2.** LDL is derived from which of the following?
a) Intraplasmic processing from very low density lipoprotein
b) Chylomicron remnant
c) Direct hepatic synthesis
d) Both a and c

**3.** If a person has high cholesterol and heart disease or high cholesterol, multiple risk factors, and at least moderate risk, it is important to reduce the cholesterol value to
a) Produce a reduction in the plaque size and therefore an increase in lumen diameter
b) Reduce the incidence of plaque rupture and thereby reduce the incidence of cardiac events

c) Improve the cholesterol to HDL ratio

d) Achieve at least a 30% to 40% reduction in LDLc, according to the NCEP guidelines

**4.** A 55-year-old man has no known CAD and is totally asymptomatic. He does not smoke, and his systolic blood pressure is less than 120 mm Hg. His father had heart disease before the age of 65 years. His total cholesterol level is 240 mg/dL; triglyceride 96 mg/dL; and HDLc 39 mg/dL. What is the best treatment regimen for his cholesterol control?

a) He should be placed on an HMG-CoA reductase inhibitor because his LDLc is above 190 mg/dL.

b) He should be placed on an HMG-CoA reductase inhibitor because his LDLc is above 160 mg/dL, and he has a high risk.

c) Statin therapy is recommended because his LDLc is above 130 mg/dL, and his risk is moderate.

d) Patients without CAD should not be treated for hypercholesterolemia.

**5.** A 48-year-old man who suffered an MI and had bypass surgery to place grafts in three of his vessels 3 years ago presents to your office. A check of his lipid profile indicated an LDLc level of 150 mg/dL, HDLc level of 45 mg/dL, and triglyceride level of 110 mg/dL. Other risk factors are well controlled. The recommended treatment for his cholesterol is

a) Initiate diet modification therapy for 6 months, and then, if values have not reduced to below 100 mg/dL for LDLc, initiate medication.

b) Begin an HMG-CoA reductase inhibitor to bring the LDLc below 70 mg/dL.

c) Simultaneously initiate diet modification and an HMG-CoA reductase inhibitor to bring the LDLc below 100 mg/dL.

d) Use gemfibrozil in combination with an HMG- CoA reductase inhibitor to both decrease the LDL below 100 mg/dL and increase HDLc.

**6.** The patient, a man 30 years of age, felt great, without any known coronary heart disease and no other risk factors. His nonfasting lipid levels were total cholesterol 200 mg/dL and HDLc 40 mg/dL. Dr. Lipid said, "You're OK. Come back in 5 years and have it rechecked." What do you think of this advice?

a) Good

b) Bad

**7.** A new food label was introduced in 1994. It includes

a) The total percentage of calories from fat in each serving

b) The number of grams of saturated fat in the entire package

c) Total calories, number of calories from fat, and total fat in grams in a defined serving

d) Whether the product is indeed healthy for you

**8.** A man was placed on an HMG-CoA reductase inhibitor. When he returns to your office for a 6-week follow-up, you should check

a) Renal function

b) Renal, liver, and thyroid function tests

c) Liver function tests

d) Liver function tests, creatine phosphokinase, and ophthalmoscopic examination

## ANSWERS

**1. a.**

While each of the particles houses some cholesterol, HDL has more protein, and VLDL is predominantly fat. LDL is over 50% cholesterol.

**2. d.**

**3. b and d.**

In the new amendment, it is suggested that, in those who have moderate or high risk and in whom lipid lowering therapy is contemplated, at least a 30% reduction in the LDLc level should be targeted. Furthermore, although it was once thought that cholesterol reduction would markedly enhance the luminal size of the vessel, we now know that its major benefit is reducing the number of events, and/ or plaque rupture.

**4. c.**

This man has two risk factors (age and low HDLc), with a calculated LDLc of 182 mg/dL [240 − (96/5 + 39)]. Note that family history in male first-degree relatives is positive when age of onset is less than 55 years (not 65). Adding up the global risk score (Age 8; TC 4; HDLc 2) gives 14 points, or a 16% risk over 10 years, thus representing a moderate risk. Therefore, statin therapy is recommended because his LDLc level is higher than 130 mg/dL, and his risk is moderate.

**5. b.**

For stable coronary disease, the current LDL goal level is <100 mg/dL. If such a subject had uncontrolled risk factors, including such items as metabolic syndrome, it is recommended that the LDLc level be brought down to below 70 mg/dL. Alternatively, if the subject came to have a more unstable condition (e.g., acute coronary syndrome), then the lower target is put into effect. In addition, in subjects at high risk, drug and therapeutic lifestyle changes are instituted concurrently. Finally, both the HDL and triglyceride values for this subject are within normal range. In cases where HDL and/or triglyceride levels are abnormal, it is suggested that fibrate or niacin therapy be seriously considered.

**6. b.**

Technically, the answer is b. In healthy, low-risk adults, age 20 and above, the major lipid fractions should be tested once every 5 years. In nonfasting samples, only triglyceride and HDLc levels are measured. If the HDLc level is ≥40 mg/dL and triglyceride level is <200 mg/dL, the subject can return in 5 years. Because the triglyceride value is 200 mg/dL, the next visit should be within 2 years of the current date. Usually this translates into a 1-year return visit.

**7. c.**

**8. c.**

## REFERENCES

1. Brown B, Zhao X-Q, Sacco D, et al. Lipid lowering and plaque regression. New insights into prevention of plaque disruption and clinical events in coronary disease. *Circulation* 1993;87:1781–1791.
2. Ridker PM, Rifai N, Pfeffer MA, et al. Long–term effects of pravastatin on plasma concentration of C–reactive protein. The Cholesterol and Recurrent Events (CARE) Investigators. *Circulation* 1999;100:230–235.
3. Downs J, Clearfield M, Weis S, et al. Primary prevention of acute coronary events with lovastatin in men and women with average cholesterol levels. *JAMA* 2004;1998(279):1615–1622.
4. Ridker P, Rifai N, Pitman Lowenthal S. Rapid reduction in C-reactive protein with cerivastatin among 785 patients with primary hypercholesterolemia. *Circulation* 2001; (103):1191–1193.
5. Jialal I, Stein D, Balis D, et al. Effect of hydroxymethyl glutaryl coenzyme a reductase inhibitor therapy on high sensitive C-reactive protein levels. *Circulation* 2001;103:1933–1935.
6. Scandinavian Simvastatin Survival Study Group. Randomised trial of cholesterol lowering in 4,444 patients with coronary artery disease: the Scandinavian Simvastatin Survival Study (4S). *Lancet* 1994;344:1383–1389.
7. Shepherd J, Cobbe SM, Ford I, et al. Prevention of coronary heart disease with pravastatin in men with hypercholesterolemia. West of Scotland Coronary Prevention Study Group. *N Engl J Med* 1995;333:1301–1307.
8. Sacks F, Pfeffer M, Moye L, et al. The effect of pravastatin on coronary events after myocardial infarction in patients with average cholesterol levels. *N Engl J Med* 1996;335:1001–1009.
9. The Long-Term Intervention with Pravastatin in Ischaemic Disease (LIPID) Study Group. Prevention of cardiovascular events and death with pravastatin in patients with coronary heart disease and a broad range of initial cholesterol levels. *N Engl J Med* 1998;339:1349–1357.
10. Heart Protection Study Collaborative Group. MRC/BHF Heart Protection Study of cholesterol lowering with simvastatin in 20536 high-risk individuals: a randomised placebo-controlled trial. *Lancet* 2002;360:7–22.
11. Pedersen TR, Olsson AG, Faergeman O, et al. Lipoprotein changes and reduction in the incidence of major coronary heart disease events in the Scandinavian Simvastatin Survival Study (4S). *Circulation* 1998;97:1453–1460.
12. Pedersen T, Kjekshus J, Olsson A, et al. 4S results support AHA guideline to reduce LDL cholesterol to less than 100 mg/dL in patients with CHD. *Circulation* 1997;96[Suppl I](I–717).
13. Nissen SE, Tuzcu EM, Schoenhagen P, et al. Effect of intensive compared with moderate lipid-lowering therapy on progression of coronary atherosclerosis: a randomized controlled trial. *JAMA* 2004;291:1071–1080.
14. Fager G, Olov W. Cholesterol reduction and clinical benefit: are there limits to our expectations? *Arterioscler Thromb Vasc Biol* 1997;17:3527–3533.
15. Lipid Research Clinics Program. The Lipid Research Clinics Coronary Primary Prevention Trial results. II. The relationship of reduction in incidence of coronary heart disease to cholesterol lowering. *JAMA* 1984;251:365–374.
16. Levy RI, Brensike JF, Epstein SE, et al. The influence of changes in lipid values induced by cholestyramine and diet on progression of coronary artery disease: results of the NHLBI Type II Coronary Intervention Study. *Circulation* 1984;69:325.
17. Law M, Wald N, Thompson S. By how much and how quickly does reduction in serum cholesterol concentration lower risk of ischaemic heart disease? *BMJ* 1994;308:367–372.
18. Effect of fenofibrate on progression of coronary–artery disease in type 2 diabetes: the Diabetes Atherosclerosis Intervention Study, a randomized study. *Lancet* 2001;357:905–910.
19. Sacks F, Pasternak R, Gibson C, et al. Effect on coronary atherosclerosis of decrease in plasma cholesterol concentrations in normocholesterolemic patients. Harvard Atherosclerosis Reversibility Project (HARP) Group. *Lancet* 1994;344:1182–1186.
20. Sacks F, Gibson C, Rosner B, et al. The influence of pretreatment low density lipoprotein cholesterol concentrations on the effect of hypocholesterolemic therapy on coronary atherosclerosis in angiographic trials. Harvard Atherosclerosis Reversibility Project Research Group (Review). *Am J Cardiol* 1995;76:78C–85C.
21. The Post Coronary Artery Bypass Graft Trial Investigators. The effect of aggressive lowering of low-density lipoprotein cholesterol levels and low-dose anticoagulation on obstructive changes in saphenous-vein coronary artery bypass grafts. *N Engl J Med* 1997;336:153–162.
22. Knatterud GL, Rosenberg Y, Campeau L, et al. Long-term effects on clinical outcomes of aggressive lowering of low-density lipoprotein cholesterol levels and low-dose anticoagulation in the post coronary artery bypass graft trial. Post CABG Investigators. *Circulation* 2000;102:157–165.
23. Thompson G, Hollyer J, Walters D. Percentage change rather than plasma level of LDL-cholesterol determines therapeutic response in coronary heart disease. *Curr Opin Lipidol* 1995;6:386–388.
24. Watts GF, Burke V. Lipid-lowering trials in the primary and secondary prevention of coronary heart disease: new evidence, implications and outstanding issues. *Curr Opin Lipidol* 1996;7:341–355.
25. Shepherd S, Blauw G, Murphy M, et al. Pravastatin in elderly individuals at risk of vascular disease (PROSPER): a randomised controlled trial. *Lancet* 2002;360:1623–1630.
26. Cheung B, Lauder I, Lau C, et al. Meta-analysis of large randomized controlled trials to evaluate the impact of statins on cardiovascular outcomes. *B Jr Clin Pharmacol* 2004;57:640–651.
27. Hokanson J, Austin M. Plasma triglyceride level is a risk factor for cardiovascular disease independent of high-density lipoprotein cholesterol level: a meta-analysis of population-based prospective studies. *J Cardiovasc Risk* 1996;3:213–219.
28. Rubins HB, Robins SJ, Collins D, et al. Gemfibrozil for the secondary prevention of coronary heart disease in men with low levels of high-density lipoprotein cholesterol. Veterans Affairs High-Density Lipoprotein Cholesterol Intervention Trial Study Group. *N Engl J Med* 1999;341:410–418.
29. Elam M, Schaefer E, NcNamara J, et al. Fasting and postprandial remnant–like particles (RLP) as predictors of cardiovascular events in the VA-HDL Intervention Trial (VA-HIT). *Circulation* 1998;100:I–470.
30. Robins SJ, Rubins HB, Faas FH, et al. Insulin resistance and cardiovascular events with low HDL cholesterol: the Veterans Affairs HDL Intervention Trial (VA-HIT). *Diabetes Care* 2003;26(5):1513–1517.
31. Secondary prevention by raising HDL cholesterol and reducing triglycerides in patients with coronary artery disease: the Bezafibrate Infarction Prevention (BIP) study. *Circulation* 2000;102:21–27.
32. Carlson LA, Rosenhamer G. Reduction of mortality in the Stockholm Ischaemic Heart Disease Secondary Prevention Study by combined treatment with clofibrate and nicotinic acid. *Acta Med Scand* 1998;223:405–418.
33. Manninen V, Tenkanen L, Koskinen P, et al. Joint effects of serum triglycerides and LDL cholesterol and HDL cholesterol concentrations on coronary heart disease risk in the Helsinki Heart Study—implications for treatment. *Circulation* 1992;85:37–45.
34. Brensike JF, Levy RI, Kelsey SF, et al. Effects of therapy with cholestyramine on progression of coronary arteriosclerosis: results of the NHLBI Type II Intervention Study. *Circulation* 1984; 69:313.
35. Brown G, Albers JJ, Fisher LD, et al. Regression of coronary artery disease as a result of intensive lipid–lowering therapy in men with high levels of apolipoprotein B. *N Engl J Med* 1990;323:1289–1298.

36. Frick M, Syvanne M, Niemminen M, et al. Prevention of the angiographic progression of coronary and vein-graft atherosclerosis by gemfibrozil after coronary bypass surgery in men with low levels of HDL cholesterol. *Circulation* 1997;96:2137–2143.

37. Ericsson C, Hamsten A, Nilsson J, et al. Angiographic assessment of effects of bezefibrate on progression of coronary artery disease in young male postinfarction patients. *Circulation* 1996;96:2137–2143.

38. Brown BG, Zhao XQ, Chait A, et al. Simvastatin and Niacin, antioxidants vitamins, or the combination for the prevention of coronary disease. *N Engl J Med* 2001;345(22):1583–1592.

39. Gotto AM Jr, Whitney E, Stein EA, et al. Relation between baseline and on-treatment lipid parameters and first acute major coronary events in the Air Force/Texas Coronary Atherosclerosis Prevention Study (AFCAPS/TexCAPS). *Circulation* 2000;101:477–484.

40. Nissen SE, Tsunoda T, Tuzcu EM, et al. Effect of recombinant ApoA-I Milano on coronary atherosclerosis in patients with acute coronary syndromes: a randomized controlled trial. *JAMA* 2003; 290:2292–2300.

41. Saku K, Gartside PS, Hynd BA, et al. Mechanism of action of gemfibrozil on lipoprotein metabolism. *J Clin Invest* 1995;75:1702–1712.

42. Jin FY, Kamanna VS, Kashyap ML. Niacin decreases removal of high-density lipoprotein Apolipoprotein A-I but not cholesterol ester by Hep G2 cells : Implication for reverse cholesterol transport. *Arterioscler Thromb Vasc Biol* 1997;17:2020–2028.

43. Tall A, Costet P, Wang N. Regulation and mechanisms of macrophage cholesterol efflux. *J Clin Invest* 2002;110:899–904.

44. Sprecher DL, Feigelson HS, Laskarzewski PM. The low HDL cholesterol/high triglyceride trait. *Arterioscler Thromb* 1993;13: 495–504.

45. Sprecher DL, Hein MJ, Laskarzewski PM. Conjoint high triglycerides and low HDL-cholesterol across generations: analysis of proband hypertriglyceridemia and lipid/lipoprotein disorders in first-degree family members. *Circulation* 1994;90:1177–1184.

46. Reaven GM. The role of insulin resistance and hyperinsulinemia in coronary heart disease. *Metabolism* 1992;41:16–19.

47. Superko H. What can we learn about dense low density lipoprotein and lipoprotein particles from clinical trials? *Curr Opin Lipidol* 1996;7:363–368.

48. Lindholm L, Samuelsson O. What are the odds at ASCOT today? *Lancet* 2003;361(9364):1144–1145.

49. Hennekens CH. The ALLHAT–LLT and ASCOT–LLA Trials: are the discrepancies more apparent than real? *Curr Atheroscler Rep* 2004; 6(1):9–11.

50. Walldius G, Erikson U, Olsson A, et al. The effect of probucol on femoral atherosclerosis: the Probucol Quantitative Regression Swedish Trial (PQRST). *Am J Cardiol* 1994;74:875–883.

51. Tardif J, Cote G, Lesperance J, et al. Probucol and multivitamins in the prevention of restenosis after coronary angioplasty. *N Engl J Med* 1997;337(365):372.

52. Anderson T, Meredith I, Yeung A, et al. The effect of cholesterol-lowering and antioxidant therapy on endothelium-dependent coronary vasomotion. *N Engl J Med* 1995;332:488–493.

53. Witztum JL. To E or not to E—how do we tell? [editorial;comment]. *Circulation* 1998;98:2785–2787.

54. Reilly MP, Pratico D, Delanty N, et al. Increased formation of distinct F2 isoprostanes in hypercholesterolemia. *Circulation* 1998; 98:2822–2828.

55. Zhang R, Brennan ML, Fu X, et al. Association between myeloperoxidase levels and risk of coronary artery disease. *JAMA* 2001; 286(17):2136–2142.

56. Blankenhorn DH, Nessim SA, Johnson RL, et al. Beneficial effects of combined colestipol-niacin therapy on coronary atherosclerosis and coronary venous bypass grafts. *JAMA* 1987;257:3233–3240.

57. Cleeman J, Lenfant C. The National Cholesterol Education Program. *JAMA* 1998;280:2099–2104.

58. Mosca L, for the expert panel/writing group. Summary of the American Heart Association's evidence based–guidelines for cardiovascular disease prevention in women. *Arterioscler Thromb Vasc Biol* 2004;24:394–396.

59. American College of Physicians. Guidelines for using serum cholesterol, high density lipoprotein cholesterol, and triglyceride levels as screening tests for preventing coronary heart disease in adults. *Ann Intern Med* 1996;124:515–517.

60. Frolkis JP, Pearce GL, Nambi V, et al. Statins do not meet expectations for LDL-cholesterol lowering when used in clinical practice. *Am J Med* 2002;113:625–629.

61. Executive Summary of the third report of the National Cholesterol Education Program (NCEP) Expert Panel on Detection, Evaluation, and Treatment of High Blood Cholesterol in Adults (Adult Treatment Panel III). *JAMA* 2001;285(2486):2497.

62. Austin MA, King MC, Vranizan KM, et al. Low-density lipoprotein subclass patterns and risk of myocardial infarction. *JAMA* 1990; 82:495–506.

63. Nawrocki J, Weiss S, Davidson M, et al. Reduction of LDL cholesterol by 25% to 60% in patients with primary hypercholesterolemia by atorvastatin, a new HMG-CoA reductase inhibitor. *Arterioscler Thromb Vasc Biol* 1995;15:678–682.

64. Davidson MH, Ose L, Frohlich J, et al. Differential effects of simvastatin and atorvastatin on high-density lipoprotein cholesterol and apolipoprotein A-I are consistent across hypercholesterolemic patient subgroups. *Clin Cardiol* 2003;26(11):509–514.

65. Stein E, Sprecher D, Allenby K, et al. Cerivastatin, a new potent synthetic HMG Co-A reductase inhibitor: effect of 0.2 mg daily in subjects with primary hypercholesterolemia. *J Cardiovasc Pharmacol Ther* 1997;2:7–16.

66. Steinmetz A, Schwartz T, Hehnke U, et al. Multicenter comparison of micronized fenofibrate and simvastatin in patients with primary type IIA or IIB hyperlipoproteinemia. *J Cardiovasc Pharmacol* 1996;27:563–570.

67. Moon YS, Kashyap ML. Niacin extended-release/lovastatin: combination therapy for lipid disorders. *Expert Opin Pharmacother* 2002;3(12):1763–1771.

68. Clark RW, Sutfin TA, Ruggeri BA. Raising high-density lipoprotein in humans through inhibition of cholesteryl ester transfer protein: an initial multidose study of torcetrapib. *Arterioscler Thromb Vasc Biol* 2004;24:490–497.

69. Brousseau EM, Schaefer EJ, Wolfe ML, et al. Effects of an inhibitor of cholesteryl ester transfer protein on HDL cholesterol. *N Engl J Med* 2004;350:1505–1515.

70. Brewer HB. High–density lipoproteins: a new potential therapeutic target for the prevention of cardiovascular disease. *Arterioscler Thromb Vasc Biol* 2004;24:387–391.

71. Bays H, Stein EA. Pharmacotherapy for dyslipidaemia—current therapies and future agents. *Expert Opin Pharmacother* 2003;4(11): 1901–1938.

72. Stein EA, Lane M, Laskarzewski P. Comparison of statins in hypertriglyceridemia. *Am J Cardiol* 1998;81:66B–69B.

73. Dupuis J, Tardif JC, Cernacek P, et al. Cholesterol reduction rapidly improves endothelial function after acute coronary syndromes. The RECIFE (Reduction of Cholesterol in Ischemia and Function of the Endothelium) trial. *Circulation* 1999;99:3227–3233.

74. Tamai O, Matsuoka H, Itabe H, et al. Single LDL apheresis improves endothelium-dependent vasodilation in hypercholesterolemic humans. *Circulation* 1997;1997:76–82.

75. Dangas G, Badimonn JJ, Smith DA, et al. Pravastatin therapy in hyperlipidemia: effects on thrombus formation and the systemic hemostatic profile. *J Am Coll Cardiol* 1999;33:1294–1304.

76. Schwartz GG, Olsson AG, Ezekowitz MD, et al. Effects of atorvastatin on early recurrent ischemic events in acute coronary syndromes: an observational study. *Lancet* 2001;285:1711–1718.

77. Cannon C, Braunwald E, McCabe C, et al. Intensive versus moderate lipid lowering with statins after acute coronary syndromes. *N Engl J Med* 2004;350:1495–1504.

78. Aronow HD, Topol EJ, Roe MT, et al. Effect of lipid lowering therapy on early mortality after acute coronary syndromes: an observational study. *Lancet* 2001;357:1063–1068.

79. Stenestrand U, Wallentin L. For the Swedish register of Cardiac Intensive Care (RISKS–HIA). Early statin treatment following acute myocardial infarction and 1–year survival. *JAMA* 2001;285: 430–436.

80. Acevedo M, Sprecher DL, Lauer MS, et al. Routine statin treatment after acute coronary syndromes? *Am Heart J* 2002;143(6): 940–942.

81. Influence of pravastatin and plasma lipids on clinical events in the West of Scotland Coronary Prevention Study (WOSCOPS). *Circulation* 1998;97:1440–1445.

82. Pyorala K, Pedersen TR, Kjekshus J, et al. Cholesterol lowering with simvastatin improves prognosis of diabetic patients with coronary heart disease. A subgroup analysis of the Scandinavian Simvastatin Survival Study (4S). *Diabetes Care* 1997;20:614–620.

83. Pfeffer M, Sacks F, Lemuel A, et al. Cholesterol and recurrent events: a secondary prevention trial for normolipidemic patients. *Am J Cardiol* 1995;76:98C–106C.

84. Treasure C, Klein J, Weintraub W, et al. Beneficial effects of cholesterol-lowering therapy on the coronary endothelium in patients with coronary artery disease. *N Engl J Med* 1995;332: 481–487.

85. Crouse J, Byington R, Hoen H, et al. Reductase inhibitor monotherapy and stroke prevention. *Arch Intern Med* 1997;157: 1305–1310.

86. Hebert P, Gaziano J, Chan K, et al. Cholesterol lowering with statin drugs, risks of stroke, and total mortality. *JAMA* 1997;278: 313–321.

87. Bucher H, Griffith L, Guyatt G. Effect of HMGcoA reductase inhibitors on stroke. *Ann Intern Med* 1998;128:89–95.

88. MacMahon S, Sharpe N, Gamble G, et al. Effects of 4 years with pravastatin on carotid atherosclerosis in patients with coronary heart disease: final results from the LIPID Study Research Group. *Circulation* 1996;94[Suppl]:I–539.

89. Miller L, Schlant R, Kobashigawa J, et al. 24th Bethesda Conference: Cardiac transplantation. Task Force 5: complications. *J Am Coll Cardiol* 1993;22:41–54.

90. Kobashigawa J, Katznelson W Laks H, et al. Effects of pravastatin on outcomes after cardiac transplantation. *N Engl J Med* 1995; 333:621–627.

91. Wenke K, Meiser B, Thiery J, et al. Simvastatin reduces graft vessel disease and mortality after heart transplantation: a four-year randomized trial. *Circulation* 1997;96:1398–1402.

92. Laurence J. Vascular complications associated with use of HIV protease inhibitors [letter; comment]. *Lancet* 1998;351:1960.

93. Carr A, Samaras K, Chisholm DJ, et al. Pathogenesis of HIV-1–protease inhibitor–associated peripheral lipodystrophy, hyperlipidaemia, and insulin resistance. *Lancet* 1998;351(1881):1883.

94. Henry K, Melroe H, Huebesch J, et al. Atorvastatin and gemfibrozil for protease–inhibitor related lipid abnormalities [letter]. *Lancet* 1998;352:1031–1032.

95. Dube MP, Stein JH, Aberg JA. Clinical Infectious Disease, 2003;37(5):613–627.

# Heart Failure

**70**

*Robert E. Hobbs*

Heart failure is a complex clinical syndrome characterized by structural, functional, and biological alterations leading to impaired cardiac function and circulatory congestion. In this syndrome, impaired cardiac function is inadequate to meet the metabolic needs of the body, resulting in decreased perfusion of organs and tissues as well as fluid retention. Half the cases of heart failure result from systolic dysfunction, in which the contractility of the left ventricle is impaired. An equal number of cases involve impaired relaxation of the ventricles during diastole (i.e., diastolic failure or heart failure with preserved systolic function).

## ETIOLOGY

The most common cause of heart failure in the United States is end-stage coronary artery disease (CAD), accounting for more than half of the cases. Other causes include cardiomyopathies, hypertensive heart disease, valvular heart disease, and congenital heart disease.

Heart failure may be characterized in several ways: acute versus chronic, systolic versus diastolic, left- versus right-sided, forward versus backward, low- versus high-output. *Acute heart failure* refers to a rapid decompensation leading to dyspnea, acute pulmonary edema, or fluid retention. *Chronic heart failure* refers to prolonged impairment due to dyspnea, effort intolerance, and fluid retention. Chronic heart failure with acute exacerbations is the most common clinical presentation. *Systolic heart failure* refers to contractile impairment manifested by low left ventricular ejection fraction (LVEF). *Diastolic heart failure* occurs in the setting of preserved LVEF and is associated with abnormal left ventricular relaxation and filling, left ventricular hypertrophy, and elevated intracardiac pressures. Diastolic heart failure occurs with hypertensive heart disease, CAD, hypertrophic cardiomyopathy, restrictive cardiomyopathy, and aortic valve disease with or without valve replacement. Left-sided failure is manifested by effort intolerance and dyspnea. Right-sided failure is characterized by fluid retention, edema, and ascites. The causes of right-sided failure include left-sided failure, mitral stenosis, pulmonary hypertension (primary or secondary), cor pulmonale from chronic obstructive pulmonary disease, pulmonic valve disease, tricuspid valve disease, right ventricular infarction, and arrhythmogenic right ventricular dysplasia. Low cardiac output failure is common, but high-output failure is rare. The causes of high-output heart failure include thyrotoxicosis, arteriovenous fistula, pregnancy, Paget's disease, anemia, and beriberi.

## EPIDEMIOLOGY

Heart failure affects 1% to 2% of the population (approximately 5 million Americans), with 550,000 new cases diagnosed each year. It is the only cardiovascular disease that is increasing in prevalence. During the last decade, hospitalizations for heart failure have increased 159% and now account for 1 million hospital admissions each year. The prevalence of heart failure increases with age and approaches 10 cases per 1,000 population after age 65. Seventy-five percent of patients have antecedent hypertension. Heart failure is the leading DRG diagnosis in the Medicare population, accounting for 20% of all hospitalizations. It the largest expense for the Center for Medicare and Medicaid Services (CMS), accounting for at least $38 billion in healthcare expenditures annually. Heart failure has the highest readmission rate of any medical condition, with half the patients readmitted for cardiac decompensation within 6 months. Heart failure is more common in men than in women until late in life. It is estimated that 10% of the population older than age 75 has experienced heart failure.

The annual mortality for heart failure exceeds that of most malignancies, approaching 20% for all cases. The high annual mortality gives rise to a 70% all-cause mortality rate at 5 years. Sudden death occurs in half these patients and is six to nine times more common than in the general population. Heart failure deaths have increased 35% during the last decade, whereas mortality from myocardial infarction (MI) has declined. The prognosis of heart failure is related to a number of factors: exercise impairment, low LVEF, elevated neurohormones [B-type natriuretic peptide (BNP), norepinephrine, etc.], cachexia, wide QRS complex, elevated serum creatinine, hyponatremia, and hypocholesterolemia The most important prognostic indicator is exercise tolerance.

## PATHOPHYSIOLOGY

Factors contributing to the syndrome of heart failure include structural cardiac abnormalities, hemodynamic derangements, and neurohormonal activation. Hemodynamic derangements characteristic of heart failure are low cardiac output and high intracardiac pressures. Low cardiac output accounts for fatigue and exercise intolerance, whereas high intracardiac pressures lead to exertional dyspnea and peripheral edema. Heart failure patients have poor exercise capacity because of low cardiac output and an exercise-induced pulmonary hypertension. Hemodynamic abnormalities contribute to symptoms, whereas neurohumoral abnormalities lead to the progression to heart failure. Neurohormonal abnormalities consist of sympathetic nervous system activation, renin-angiotensin-aldosterone stimulation, release of vasopressin, elevation of endothelin, activation of proinflammatory cytokines, and secretion of natriuretic peptides. In general, neurohormonal abnormal-

ities lead to vasoconstriction, sodium and water retention, and cardiovascular growth and remodeling. Although the immediate neurohormonal actions are beneficial, long-term effects are deleterious. Neurohormones are elevated in heart failure and correlate with severity and prognosis. Baroreceptor dysfunction contributes to sympathetic nervous system activation and inhibits the parasympathetic nervous system. Circulating catecholamines cause resting tachycardia, arrhythmias, myocyte toxicity, β-receptor dysfunction, and renin-angiotensin stimulation.

The renin-angiotensin system is activated when renin is released from the juxtaglomerular apparatus of the kidney by a variety of stimuli. Renin acts as a substrate for the conversion of angiotensinogen to angiotensin I. After passage through the circulation, angiotensin I is converted to angiotensin II. Angiotensin II is a potent vasoconstrictor that stimulates thirst, releases aldosterone, and promotes sodium and water retention. It is a growth factor that may lead to progressive cardiac deterioration. Vasopressin is released from the hypothalamus secondary to baroreceptor or osmotic stimuli, and it causes vasoconstriction as well as sodium and water retention. The actions of the sympathetic nervous system, renin-angiotensin system, and vasopressin are balanced by the natriuretic peptides. These hormones are released from the cardiac myocytes and exert their physiologic actions on the vasculature and kidneys. The physiologic effects of natriuretic peptides include vasodilation, sodium and water excretion, vasodilation, and neurohormonal modulation. Endothelin is derived from a variety of sources from within the cardiovascular system. It is both a vasoconstrictor and a growth factor. The proinflammatory cytokine, tumor necrosis factor, is released from macrophages and may cause cardiac cachexia, exercise intolerance, and apoptosis in the failing heart. As a consequence of myocardial injury, the heart undergoes remodeling to compensate for low stroke volume. Remodeling consists of hypertrophy, dilatation, and spherical reshaping of the left ventricular chamber, which leads to increased wall stress, mitral regurgitation, and decreased inotropic reserve. In chronic heart failure, the skeletal muscles undergo biochemical and physiologic deterioration. These abnormalities account for some of the exercise intolerance seen in these patients.

## HEART FAILURE WITH PRESERVED SYSTOLIC FUNCTION (DIASTOLIC FAILURE)

Systolic dysfunction is characterized by impaired contractility, whereas diastolic dysfunction is characterized by impaired relaxation. In patients with diastolic dysfunction, the LVEF is normal, but the ventricular filling is impaired (i.e., "stiff-heart syndrome"). The left ventricle often is hypertrophied, left ventricular cavity size is small, and overall heart size is not grossly enlarged. Diastolic dysfunction occurs with hypertensive heart disease, ischemic heart disease, hypertrophic cardiomyopathy, restrictive cardiomyopathy (including infiltrative diseases), and aortic valve disease. Echocardiography is the most important test for assessing LVEF and diastolic filling patterns. Hemodynamically, diastolic dysfunction is characterized by elevated intracardiac pressures. Treatment is directed at the underlying cause. Therapeutic goals include relieving congestion, improving relaxation, decreasing hypertrophy, and reducing ischemia.

## Clinical Presentation

The symptoms of congestive heart failure (CHF) are caused by low cardiac output or high intracardiac pressures. The general manifestations of heart failure include breathlessness, fatigue, effort intolerance, and fluid retention. Respiratory symptoms are common: dyspnea, orthopnea, paroxysmal nocturnal dyspnea, cough, wheezing, or respiratory distress. Abdominal manifestations are indicative of right-sided heart failure: weight gain, fluid retention, bloating, early satiety, anorexia, weight loss, right upper-quadrant pain, nausea, and vomiting. The degree of functional impairment usually is stated in terms of the New York Heart Association (NYHA) Classification:

- *Class I* refers to no limitation of physical activity and no dyspnea or fatigue with ordinary physical activities.
- *Class II* indicates mild limitation of physical activity and dyspnea or fatigue occurring with ordinary physical activities. The patient has no symptoms at rest.
- *Class III* implies marked limitation of activity. Less than ordinary physical activities cause symptoms. The patient is asymptomatic at rest.
- *Class IV* refers to symptoms at rest and with any physical exertion.

## Physical Examination

Patients with severe, acute decompensated CHF and pulmonary edema have respiratory distress, tachypnea, diaphoresis, pallor, cyanosis, cool extremities, jugular venous distension, rales, rapid heart rate, and $S_3$ and $S_4$ gallops. Most patients with chronic heart failure have fluid retention, but are comfortable at rest. Those with end-stage heart failure may have cardiac cachexia and muscle wasting. The blood pressure may be normal, low, or high. The resting heart rate frequently is increased and pulsus alternans, a beat-to-beat variation in the intensity of the pulse, may be present. Jugular venous distension is an important finding in patients with decompensated failure, indicating fluid overload. A prominent V wave is seen with tricuspid regurgitation. The lungs usually are clear in chronic heart failure, but rales indicate decompensated heart failure. Decreased breath sounds and dullness at the lung bases

reflect an underlying pleural effusion. Wheezing may occur because of bronchospasm (*cardiac asthma*). Cheyne-Stokes respirations, a manifestation of central sleep apnea, occur with advanced heart failure. Examination of the heart reveals a diffuse apical impulse that is displaced downward and to the left. A left ventricular heave and occasionally a right ventricular heave may be palpable. If the heart rate is rapid, the first heart sound will be accentuated. The second heart sound may be paradoxically split because of delayed electric activation or mechanical ejection of the left ventricle. A third heart sound is characteristic of left ventricular failure, whereas a fourth heart sound suggests a noncompliant left ventricle. Murmurs of mitral and tricuspid regurgitation are common. Abdominal examination may reveal hepatomegaly, right upper-quadrant tenderness, and ascites. Pressing on the liver may further distend the jugular veins (positive hepatojugular reflux). An examination of the extremities may reveal edema, muscle wasting, or cyanosis.

## Diagnostic Studies

The BNP assay is a useful test for determining whether dyspnea is due to heart failure. Elevated levels of BNP correlate with severity and prognosis of heart failure.

Electrocardiography may reveal normal sinus rhythm or atrial fibrillation. Left ventricular hypertrophy and left bundle branch block are common patterns, and Q waves reflect previous MI. Chest radiography often shows cardiomegaly, increased pulmonary vascularity, redistribution of blood flow to the upper lobes, prominent pulmonary arteries, Kerley-B lines, interstitial and alveolar edema, and pleural effusions.

Echocardiography is the most useful diagnostic test in heart failure. Imaging usually reveals a dilated left ventricle with decreased LVEF. The right ventricle may be normal or dysfunctional. Mitral and tricuspid regurgitation often is detected through Doppler imaging. Pulmonary artery pressures may be estimated indirectly and frequently are elevated. Echocardiography also excludes tamponade or pericardial diseases as possible causes of heart failure. Doppler measurements provide information about diastolic dysfunction.

Metabolic stress testing using respiratory gas measurement provides an objective assessment of functional capacity. Normal middle-aged adults achieve a peak oxygen consumption of 25 mL/kg per minute or greater. Values of less than 14 mL/kg per minute indicate severe functional impairment.

Cardiac catheterization provides hemodynamic data that help to guide therapy. Coronary angiography is the most accurate means of diagnosing CAD. The status of the cardiac valves and left ventricle also may be assessed by catheterization. Although right ventricular endomyocardial biopsy is no longer performed routinely in heart failure patients, myocardial tissue diagnosis may be helpful in assessing patients with giant cell myocarditis, restrictive cardiomyopathy or infiltrative diseases.

## TREATMENT PRINCIPLES

The management of heart failure consists of identifying the underlying cause of heart failure, determining precipitating factors for decompensation, initiating clinically proven therapies, and providing patient education. The etiology of heart failure should be determined: CAD, cardiomyopathy, valvular heart disease, hypertensive heart disease, or congenital heart disease. Precipitating factors for decompensation include excessive salt or fluid intake, noncompliance (with diet, fluids, medications, or follow-up) , arrhythmias, infection, renal failure, ischemia or MI, drugs, pulmonary embolism, anemia, and thyrotoxicosis. Patient education is an important aspect of management because noncompliance is the most frequent causes of rehospitalization. The management of heart failure has changed dramatically during the last 30 years. Initially, bed rest, fluid removal, and oxygen were used for treatment. Later, efforts were directed at increasing contractility and improving hemodynamics. Newer therapies for heart failure attempt to modulate neurohormonal factors. Sympathetic nervous system excess may be modulated through the use of β-blockers and digoxin. The renin-angiotensin system may be inhibited by angiotensin-converting enzyme (ACE) inhibitors or angiotensin II receptor blockers (ARBs) and aldosterone antagonists.

## OUTPATIENT THERAPIES

### Angiotensin-Converting Enzyme Inhibitors

ACE inhibitors are important drugs for treating patients with all levels of heart failure, including those with asymptomatic left ventricular dysfunction. These drugs inhibit the formation of angiotensin II by blocking converting enzyme (ACE). They enhance the action of kinins and augment prostaglandin synthesis. In addition to prolonging survival, ACE inhibitors improve symptoms, hemodynamics, neurohormones, quality of life, and exercise tolerance. The beneficial actions of ACE inhibitors appear to be a class effect. ACE inhibitors should be started at low dose and titrated to target doses to achieve optimal clinical benefit. ACE inhibitors may be limited by side effects, including azotemia, hyperkalemia, cough, angioedema, dysgeusia, and agranulocytosis. ARBs may be substituted for ACE intolerance due to cough or angioedema. The combination of hydralazine and nitrates may be used when ACE inhibitors are not tolerated due to azotemia or hyperkalemia. Hydralazine is an arterial vasodilator that prevents nitrate tachyphylaxis and has antioxidant properties. Nitrates are venous dilators that inhibit cardiovascular growth and remodeling.

### β-Blockers

Numerous studies have shown that β-blockers improve ejection fraction, symptoms, exercise capacity, quality of life, and survival. β-Blockers are as important as ACE inhibitors in the long-term management of heart failure. β-Blockers modulate catecholamine excess, which has numerous adverse effects on the failing heart. β-Blockers improve or prevent remodeling, apoptosis, β-receptor pathway dysfunction, wall stress, myocardial oxygen demand, and arrhythmias. These agents should be started in euvolemic patients at low doses and titrated slowly upward over a period of weeks to target levels. The initiation of a β-blocker decreases adrenergic stimulation of the failing heart and may be associated with a temporary decrease in LVEF, increased left ventricular volume, and worsening hemodynamics. Thus, patients may feel worse initially, but most patients improve clinically after several months of therapy. The risks of β-blocker use in heart failure include hypotension, lightheadedness, fluid retention, worsening heart failure, bradycardia, and heart block.

### Angiotensin Receptor Blockers

ARBs modulate the peripheral effects of angiotensin II by blocking the angiotensin II receptor at the tissue level. Clinical trials have shown that these agents are not superior to ACE inhibitors, but are similar to ACE inhibitors in their beneficial effects. ARBs are better tolerated than ACE inhibitors, although they can cause hypotension, worsening renal function, and hyperkalemia. ARBs are considered second-line drugs for heart failure in patients who are ACE intolerant due to cough or angioedema. ARBs may be added to an ACE inhibitor and a β-blocker for additional morbidity benefit.

### Diuretics

Most patients with heart failure benefit from diuretics. These agents produce rapid symptomatic improvement and control fluid retention. Many diuretics are available; each group or class of diuretic has different sites of action in the kidney, different potencies, and different metabolic effects. Thiazide diuretics may be added to loop diuretics to promote fluid excretion. Diuretics are useful in systolic or diastolic failure and are the key to success when used in conjunction with other drug therapies. These drugs are available at relatively low cost and may be administered once daily. Diuretics may cause electrolyte depletion, overdiuresis, hypotension, and azotemia. They activate neurohormones, and for this reason should not be prescribed as monotherapy for heart failure. It is important to achieve an euvolemic state without overdiuresis; a patient-directed flexible diuretic regimen helps to facilitate this goal.

## Aldosterone Antagonists

Angiotensin II stimulates the release of aldosterone from the adrenal cortex. Aldosterone promotes the sodium and water retention associated with potassium and magnesium loss. It activates the sympathetic nervous system and inhibits parasympathetic outflow. Aldosterone may cause fibrosis of myocardial, vascular, renal, and cerebral tissue as well as cardiac and vascular remodeling. Spironolactone, an aldosterone antagonist, reduces mortality and heart failure hospitalizations in patients with severe heart failure. It has not been studied in patients with mild to moderate heart failure or in patients with asymptomatic left ventricular dysfunction.

Therefore, an aldosterone antagonist is indicated in patients with NYHA functional class III–IV heart failure despite the use of an ACE inhibitor, β-blocker, and diuretic. Hyperkalemia may occur, especially when the serum creatinine level is >2 mg/dL, and an aldosterone antagonist is best avoided in this group of patients. Potassium levels should be determined during the first week of therapy and regularly thereafter. Potassium supplementation may not be necessary when these drugs are administered. Eight percent of men taking spironolactone develop gynecomastia. Eplerenone, a selective aldosterone antagonist, improved survival in patients with MI and left ventricular dysfunction. It is associated with a lower incidence of side effects, especially gynecomastia, compared with spironolactone, but may still cause hyperkalemia in 5% of patients.

## Digoxin

Digoxin, a centrally acting neurohormonal modulating agent, has several direct and indirect actions on the myocardium and conducting system. It exerts its actions through the binding and inhibition of the enzyme sodium-potassium ATPase. In the heart, this leads to increased intracellular calcium, which enhances contractility. In the central nervous system, it reduces sympathetic excess, and within the kidney, it decreases the release of renin. Clinically, digoxin improves exercise capacity, LVEF, and hemodynamics. Although it decreases the frequency of hospitalizations, digoxin has a neutral effect on long-term survival. Digoxin has a relatively low therapeutic–toxic range, and its dose should be decreased in women, the elderly, patients with renal dysfunction, or when combined with amiodarone. Serum digoxin levels should be maintained at <0.9 ng/mL.

## Calcium Channel Blockers

Standard calcium channel blockers should not be used in patients with CHF because these agents depress left ventricular function, activate neurohormones, worsen symptoms, and increase the risk of death. Amlodipine has a neutral effect on cardiac function and may be added to an ACE inhibitor and a β-blocker to treat patients with angina pectoris or hypertension associated with heart failure.

## INPATIENT THERAPIES

### Nitroprusside

Sodium nitroprusside is an intravenous vasodilator that dilates arteries and veins, thereby lowering systemic arterial blood pressure and intracardiac pressures. It is used to treat acute pulmonary edema, decompensated heart failure, or hypertensive emergencies in an intensive care unit with invasive hemodynamic monitoring. Nitroprusside is metabolized to nitric oxide and cyanide by the liver. Nitric oxide activates guanylate cyclase in smooth muscle and epithelial cells, increasing the intracellular concentration of cyclic guanosine-5' monophosphate (cGMP), a second messenger, and resulting in smooth muscle relaxation and vasodilation. The drug is administered by continuous intravenous infusion. Hypotension is a common side effect, mandating frequent blood pressure measurements. It may cause coronary steal syndrome and should be avoided in ischemic syndromes. Prolonged infusions, especially in patients with hepatic or renal dysfunction, have been associated with thiocyanate toxicity.

### Nitroglycerin

Intravenous nitroglycerin is a venous vasodilator at low doses and an arterial vasodilator at high doses. It is biotransformed into nitric oxide, which activates guanylate cyclase, increases cGMP, relaxes smooth muscle cells, and causes vasodilation. Intravenous nitroglycerin lowers intracardiac pressures and improves pulmonary congestion. It relieves myocardial ischemia through coronary artery dilation and increased collateral flow. Its long-term use is limited by tachyphylaxis (loss of effect) occurring within 24 hours as a result of sulfhydryl group depletion. Headache occurs in 20% of patients and hypotension in 5%.

### Nesiritide (B-type Natriuretic Peptide)

Nesiritide, synthetic BNP, is a systemic and pulmonary vasodilator with modest diuretic and natriuretic properties. It is administered in a weight-based intravenous bolus followed by a continuous intravenous infusion in patients with decompensated heart failure. This vasodilator improves heart failure symptoms by lowering intracardiac pressures and increasing cardiac index. Nesiritide has no inotropic properties and no proarrhythmic effects. It is does not require frequent titrations and is not associated with tachyphylaxis.

## Dopamine

Dopamine, an intravenous inotropic agent, is the immediate precursor of norepinephrine. It has distinct physiologic properties (mesenteric vasodilation, positive inotropic effects, and peripheral vasoconstriction) depending on the infusion rate. When used at low doses, dopamine activates dopaminergic receptors in the mesenteric and renal arteries, causing vasodilation. At moderate doses, dopamine stimulates cardiac β-receptors and increases cardiac output. At high doses, it activates peripheral α-receptors, causing vasoconstriction.

## Dobutamine

Dobutamine is a directly acting positive inotropic agent. It is useful for treating hospitalized patients with decompensated heart failure who have hypotension or shock. Routine infusions of dobutamine for decompensated heart failure (without hypotension) are not recommended, and intermittent outpatient dobutamine infusions are discouraged. Continuous home dobutamine may be considered as palliative therapy to improve quality of life and prevent recurrent hospitalizations in patients with end-stage heart failure.

## Milrinone

Milrinone, a phosphodiesterase III inhibitor, is a positive inotropic agent and a vasodilator. It may be used as a primary agent or combined with dobutamine or dopamine. It is more potent as a pulmonary vasodilator than dobutamine, and it is less likely to increase heart rate and myocardial oxygen consumption. It is the preferred inotrope for use in patients treated with β-blockers.

## ELECTRONIC DEVICE THERAPIES

### Defibrillator Therapy

Half of heart failure deaths occur suddenly and without warning. These deaths probably are caused by ventricular tachyarrhythmias or bradyarrhythmias. Sudden death is six to nine times more common in heart failure patients than in the general population. In general, the most important risk factor for sudden cardiac death is the presence of heart failure. Current indications for implantable cardiac defibrillator (ICD) placement include survivors of a cardiac arrest, sustained ventricular tachycardia, inducible ventricular tachycardia, and post-MI with low ejection fraction. The use of defibrillator therapy will likely expand to a larger heart failure population in the future, despite the high costs of therapy.

### Resynchronization Therapy

Conduction abnormalities occur in approximately 50% of heart failure patients, usually left bundle branch block, and are associated with poorer survival. Conduction abnormalities delay the electrical activation of the left ventricle and cause ventricular dyssynchrony (inefficient contractility), prolonged mitral regurgitation, and impaired diastolic filling. Biventricular pacing involves the placement of a right atrial lead, right ventricular lead, and a third pacing lead in a left cardiac vein. Atrial contractility and biventricular contractility are synchronized through echocardiography. Resynchronization therapy improves ventricular contractility, cardiac output, mitral regurgitation, heart failure symptoms, functional class, exercise capacity, and survival. Approximately 75% of patients experience immediate benefit through the use of biventricular pacing, although symptomatic improvement declines with time.

## CARDIAC MECHANICAL SUPPORT

Intraaortic balloon pumping (IABP) temporarily improves hemodynamics in patients with severe heart failure. A balloon pump may increase cardiac output by 20% as a result of improved forward flow and diastolic augmentation. Device complications, such as limb ischemia, bleeding, thrombosis, neurologic injury, and infection, occur at a rate of 10% per day and limit the usefulness of a balloon pump to a period of 1 week.

Left ventricular assist devices (LVADs) currently available include the HeartMate, Novacor, Thoratec, and Abiomed pumps. Small continuous flow devices (DeBakey, Jarvik 2000 Heartmate II, and Cor Aide) are undergoing clinical trials. The major indication for LVAD placement is cardiogenic shock that persists despite inotropes and intraaortic balloon pumping. Patients should be suitable candidates for cardiac transplantation because most of these devices are used as a bridge to cardiac transplantation. Occasionally, LVADs may be implanted as permanent mechanical support or "destination therapy." LVAD support rarely may be used as a "bridge to recovery" after a myocardial insult.

Following LVAD placement, patients are weaned from respiratory and inotropic support. Renal and hepatic dysfunction improve with the normalization of cardiac output. The LVAD allows patients to become physically rehabilitated, making them better candidates for cardiac transplantation. Complications from these devices are frequent and serious. Perioperative bleeding is common, resulting from coagulation abnormalities and liver dysfunction. Most patients receive blood products at the time of device implantation, which may lead to antibody formation against potential organ donors. Infections are the limiting factor to long-term success. Thromboembolic and mechanical complications were more common with earlier devices. Deaths after LVAD implantation usually result from irreversible organ dysfunction, stroke, or infection.

## SURGICAL THERAPIES

### Ventricular Reconstruction

Ventricular reconstruction surgery may be performed in patients with ischemic cardiomyopathy who have evidence of ischemic or hibernating myocardium. The procedure involves a combination of techniques, including coronary artery bypass grafting, mitral and tricuspid valve repair, left ventricular scar or aneurysm resection, left ventricle reconstruction, and epicardial left ventricular pacing lead placement. Postoperatively, the reconstructed elliptically shaped left ventricle becomes a smaller, more efficient pumping chamber. Candidates include patients with CAD, NYHA functional class III or IV symptoms, severe left ventricular dysfunction with scar/aneurysm, hibernating or ischemic myocardium, and mitral and/or tricuspid valvular regurgitation.

### Cardiac Transplantation

Approximately 2,100 heart transplants are performed annually in the United States. This therapy is limited by inadequate numbers of donor hearts and serves only a small fraction of patients with severe heart failure who remain functionally impaired despite medical therapy. The criteria for transplant listing include end-stage heart disease refractory to medical or surgical therapy, disabling symptoms despite maximal medications, and anticipated poor survival. Contraindications include irreversible pulmonary hypertension, other serious illnesses limiting longevity or rehabilitation, drug or alcohol abuse, and medical noncompliance. After transplantation, patients are treated with a multidrug immunosuppressive regimen. Complications often are related to immunosuppression and include infection, rejection, malignancy, and allograft CAD. Other problems occur frequently in the transplant population, including hypertension, renal insufficiency, weight gain, hyperlipidemia, diabetes mellitus, and osteoporosis. Mortality averages 10% to 15% during the first year, and 4% annually thereafter.

## OTHER THERAPIES

### Antiarrhythmic drugs

Antiarrhythmic drug prophylaxis in heart failure is controversial. Amiodarone is the agent of choice for treating atrial fibrillation or ventricular tachycardia, but its use is limited by multiple toxicities. Defibrillator therapy is more effective than amiodarone in preventing sudden death. Amiodarone is not a substitute for β-blocker therapy in heart failure. Dofetilide, a restricted class III antiarrhythmic agent, is effective in maintaining sinus rhythm, but does not improve survival in heart failure.

### Anticoagulation

The routine use of warfarin in heart failure is controversial because the risk of thromboembolic events and hemorrhagic complications from the drug is 1% to 3% annually. Specific indications for warfarin include atrial fibrillation, left ventricular thrombi (especially mobile), left ventricular aneurysms, hypercoagulable states, history of thromboembolism, and patent foramen ovale. Aspirin is indicated in patients with ischemic cardiomyopathy. No evidence supports the routine use of aspirin in patients with normal coronary arteries. At present, the risk–benefit ratio does not justify the routine use of either aspirin or warfarin in heart failure patients as a group.

### Treatment of Sleep Apnea

Sleep-related breathing disorders occur commonly in heart failure. Forty percent of patients have central sleep apnea (Cheyne-Stokes respirations) and 10% have obstructive sleep apnea. Sleep apnea is associated with nocturnal catecholamine surges, hypertension, cardiac arrhythmias, and increased mortality in heart failure. Patients suspected of having sleep apnea should undergo polysomnography. Central sleep apnea improves with the intensification of heart failure therapy and nocturnal oxygen. Persistent central sleep apnea should be treated with continuous positive airway pressure (CPAP) ventilation, whereas overdrive atrial pacing requires further study. Obstructive sleep apnea improves with weight loss and the avoidance of alcohol and sedatives, but not with heart failure therapy. CPAP ventilation is indicated for moderately severe obstructive sleep apnea associated with daytime somnolence. Surgical procedures and mandibular advancement devices have not been studied in heart failure populations.

### Treatment of Anemia

Anemia occurs in 10% to 20% of patients with heart failure. The presence of anemia correlates directly with the severity of heart failure. Anemia is associated with worsening symptoms, impaired exercise tolerance, increased risk of hospitalizations, and poor survival. The causes of anemia in heart failure are multifactorial, with anemia of chronic disease the most common diagnosis. Low cardiac output impairs bone marrow production, whereas renal dysfunction and ACE inhibitors decrease erythropoietin production. Proinflammatory cytokines suppress bone marrow function and inhibit erythropoietin effects. Poor nutrition, gastrointestinal blood loss, and iron deficiency may contribute to low hemoglobin. The treatment of anemia using erythropoietin alone or in combination with iron therapy may improve the natural history of heart failure, quality of life, functional class, and exercise capacity. The threshold level for initiating therapy and the target level of hemoglobin as a therapeutic endpoint are unresolved issues at this time.

## Ultrafiltration

The standard treatment for severe fluid retention from advanced heart failure consists of high-dose intravenous diuretics, or combined loop and thiazide diuretics, or continuous diuretic infusion. Occasionally, diuretic resistance occurs in the setting of cardiorenal syndrome (persistent fluid overload, rising creatinine levels, and hyponatremia). In this setting, ultrafiltration may be utilized to remove water from the blood and extravascular spaces. The balanced diuresis from ultrafiltration maintains plasma volume and avoids hypotension. Ultrafiltration has been shown to relieve pulmonary edema, decrease ascites/edema, correct electrolyte abnormalities, improve hemodynamics, restore diuretic responsiveness, and shorten hospital length of stay.

## Enhanced External Counterpulsation (EECP)

Enhanced external counterpulsation sequentially compresses the lower extremities through the use of inflatable pneumatic cuffs synchronized with the patient's ECG. EECP is similar to a noninvasive intraaortic balloon pump. Hemodynamically, EECP causes diastolic augmentation (increasing coronary blood flow) and systolic unloading (reducing afterload). A typical EECP treatment program consists of 3 to 5 daily 1-hour sessions. EECP improves exercise capacity, quality of life, and cardiac output and decreases angina pectoris. Potential mechanisms of action include an improvement in endothelial function, collateral blood flow, and neurohormone levels. EECP is approved by the U.S. Food and Drug Administration (FDA) as heart failure therapy, although additional results are pending ongoing clinical trials.

## MISCELLANEOUS THERAPIES

Statins are recommended for patients with ischemic cardiomyopathy. Supplements such as coenzyme Q10, carnitine, antioxidants, growth hormone, and thyroid hormone are not recommended. Exercise training, especially cardiac rehabilitation, improves clinical status in heart failure patients. Disease management programs with multidisciplinary staff have been shown to decrease readmissions for cardiac decompensation.

## REVIEW EXERCISES

### QUESTIONS

**1.** Which of the following is not associated with poor prognosis in heart failure?
a) Obesity (Body Mass Index 34)
b) QRS complex 170 msec
c) BNP level 800 pg/mL
d) Serum cholesterol 79 mg/dL
e) Serum sodium 119 mmol/L

**2.** Which statement about angiotensin-II is true?
a) It is a vasodilator.
b) It promotes sodium excretion.
c) It inhibits growth and remodeling.
d) It causes release of aldosterone.
e) It inhibits thirst.

**3.** Heart failure with preserved systolic function is not characteristic of
a) Hypertensive heart disease
b) Ischemic heart disease
c) Hypertrophic cardiomyopathy
d) Restrictive cardiomyopathy
e) Dilated cardiomyopathy

**4.** Which statement about ACE inhibitors is false?
a) They prevent degradation of bradykinin.
b) They cause gynecomastia in 8% of men.
c) They may improve cough due to heart failure.
d) They cause hyperkalemia in some patients.
e) Dysgeusia is a known side effect.

### ANSWERS

**1. a.**
Heart failure is associated with reversed epidemiology. Better prognosis correlates with body mass index, level of blood pressure, and cholesterol level.

**2. d.**
Angiotensin-II is a potent vasoconstrictor that promotes sodium and water retention, releases aldosterone, stimulates thirst, and causes cardiovascular growth and remodeling.

**3. e.**
Dilated cardiomyopathy is characterized by left ventricular enlargement and systolic dysfunction.

**4. b.**
Gynecomastia is a side effect of spironolactone and digoxin.

## SUGGESTED READINGS

Abraham WT, Fisher WG, Smith AL, et al. Cardiac resynchronization in chronic heart failure. *N Engl J Med* 2002;346:1845–1853.

ACC/AHA Task Force on Practice Guidelines. Guidelines for the evaluation and management of heart failure. *Circulation* 1995;92:2764–2784.

Advisory Council to Improve Outcomes Nationwide In Heart Failure (Action HF). Consensus recommendations for heart failure. *Am J Cardiol* 1999;83:1A–38A.

American Heart Association. *Heart Disease and Stroke Statistics–2004 Update.* Dallas: American Heart Association, 2003.

Auricchio A, Ding J, Spinelli JC, et al. Cardiac resynchronization therapy restores optimal atrioventricular mechanical timing in heart failure patients with ventricular conduction delay. *J Am Coll Cardiol* 2002;39:1163–1169.

Bonetti PO, Holmes DR, Lerman A, et al. Enhanced external counterpulsation for ischemic heart disease. *J Am Coll Cardiol* 2003; 41:1918–1925.

Bradley TD, Floras JS. Sleep apnea and heart failure. Part I: Obstructive sleep apnea. *Circulation* 2003;107:1671–1678.

Bradley TD, Floras JS. Sleep apnea and heart failure. Part II: Central sleep apnea. *Circulation* 2003;107:1822–1826.

Brater DC. Diuretic therapy. *N Engl J Med* 1998;339:387–395.

Brophy JM, Joseph L, Rouleau JL. Beta blockers in congestive heart failure: a Bayesian meta-analysis. *Ann Intern Med* 2001;134:550–560.

Brown NJ, Vaughn DE. Angiotensin-converting enzyme inhibitors. *Circulation* 1998;97:1411–1420.

Burnier M. Angiotensin II type 1 receptor blockers. *Circulation* 2001; 103:904–912.

Cohn JN, Tognoni G. A randomized trial of the angiotensin-receptor blocker valsartan in chronic heart failure. *N Engl J Med* 2001;345: 1667–1675.

Felker GM, O'Connor CM. Inotropic therapy for heart failure: An evidence-based approach. *Am Heart J* 2001;142:393–401.

Goldsmith SR. Vasopressin: a therapeutic target in congestive heart failure. *J Cardiac Fail* 1999;5:347–356.

Gomberg-Maitland M, Baran DA, Fuster V. Treatment of congestive heart failure: guidelines for the primary care physician and the heart failure specialist. *Arch Intern Med* 2001;161:342–352.

Granger CB, McMurray JJV, Ostergren J, et al. Effects of candesartan in patients with chronic heart failure and reduced left-ventricular systolic function taking angiotensin-converting-enzyme inhibitors: The CHARM-Alternative Trial. *Lancet* 2003;362:772–776.

Hauptman PJ, Kelly RA. Digitalis. *Circulation* 1999;99:1265–1270.

Heart Failure Society of America. HFSA guidelines for management of patients with heart failure caused by left ventricular systolic dysfunction—pharmacological approaches. *J Cardiac Fail* 1999; 5:357–382.

Herrera-Garza EH, Stetson SJ, Cubillos-Garzon A, et al. Tumor necrosis factor-alpha: a mediator of disease progression in the failing human heart. *Chest* 1999;115:1170–1174.

Hollenberg SM, Kavinsky CJ, Parrillo JE. Cardiogenic shock. *Ann Intern Med* 1999;131:47–59.

Hunt SA, Frazier OH, Myers TJ. Mechanical circulatory support and cardiac transplantation. *Circulation* 1998;97:2079–2090.

Hunt SA, Baker DW, Chin MH, et al. ACC/AHA guidelines for the evaluation and management of chronic heart failure in the adult: executive summary: a report of the American College of Cardiology/American Heart Association Task Force on Practice Guidelines (Committee to Revise the 1995 Guidelines for the Evaluation and Management of Heart Failure). *Circulation* 2001; 104:2996–3007.

Jaski BE, Ha J, Denys BG, et al. Peripherally inserted veno-venous ultrafiltration for rapid treatment of volume overloaded patients. *J Cardiac Fail* 2003;9:227–231.

Jessup M, Brozena S. Heart failure. *N Engl J Med* 2003;348:2007-2018.

Josephson ME, Callans DJ, Buxton AE. The role of the implantable cardioverter—defibrillator for prevention of sudden cardiac death. *Ann Intern Med* 2000;133:901–910.

Leclercq C, Hare JM. Ventricular resynchronization. *Circulation* 2004;109:296–299.

Maisel A. B-type natriuretic peptide levels: a potential novel "white count" for congestive heart failure. *J Cardiac Fail* 2001;7:183–193.

McCarthy PM, Starling RC, Young JB, et al. Left ventricular reduction surgery with mitral valve repair. *J Heart Lung Transplant* 2000;19: S64–S67.

McMurray JJV, Ostergren J, Swedberg K, et al. Effects of candesartan in patients with chronic heart failure and reduced left-ventricular systolic function taking angiotensin-converting-enzyme inhibitors: The CHARM-Added Trial. *Lancet* 2003;362:767–771.

Mills RM, Hobbs RE. Nesiritide in perspective: Evolving approaches to the management of acute decompensated heart failure. *Drugs Today* 2003;39:767–774.

Moss AJ, Zareba W, Hall WJ, et al. Prophylactic implantation of a defibrillator in patients with myocardial infarction and reduced ejection fraction. *N Engl J Med* 2002;346:877–883.

Packer M. The neurohormonal hypothesis: a theory to explain the mechanism of disease progression in heart failure. *J Am Coll Cardiol* 1992;20:248–254.

Packer M, Coats AJS, Fowler MB, et al. Effect of carvedilol on survival in severe chronic heart failure. *N Engl J Med* 2001;344:1651–1658.

Pfeffer MA, Swedberg K, Granger CB, et al. Effects of candesartan on mortality and morbidity in patients with chronic heart failure: The CHARM Overall Programme. *Lancet* 2003;362:759–766.

Pfeffer MA, McMurray JJV, Velazquez EJ, et al. Valsartan, captopril or both in myocardial infarction complicated by heart failure, left ventricular dysfunction, or both. *N Engl J Med* 2003;349:1893–1906.

Pitt B, Zannad F, Remme WJ, et al. The effect of spironolactone on morbidity and mortality in patients with severe heart failure. *N Engl J Med* 1999;341:709–717.

Pitt B, Remme W, Zannad F, et al. Eplerenone, a selective aldosterone blocker, in patients with left ventricular dysfunction after myocardial infarction. *N Engl J Med* 2003;348:1309–1321.

Poole-Wilson PA, Swedberg K, Cleland JG, et al. Comparison of carvedilol and metoprolol on clinical outcomes in patients with chronic heart failure in the Carvedilol or Metoprolol European Trial (COMET): randomised controlled trial. *Lancet* 2003; 362:7–13.

Pitt B, Poole-Wilson PA, Segal R, et al. Effect of losartan compared with captopril on mortality in patients with symptomatic heart failure randomised trial—the Losartan Heart Failure Survival Study ELITE II. *Lancet* 2000;355:1582–1587.

Rathore SS, Wang Y, Krumholz HM, et al. Sex-based differences in the effect of digoxin for the treatment of heart failure. *N Engl J Med* 2002;347:1403–1411.

Rathore SS, Curtis JP, Wang Y, et al. Association of serum digoxin concentration and outcomes in patients with heart failure. *JAMA* 2003;289:871–878.

Remme WJ, Swedberg K. Task Force for the Diagnosis and Treatment of Chronic Heart Failure, European Society of Cardiology. Guidelines for the diagnosis and treatment of chronic heart failure. *Eur Heart J* 2001;22:1527–1560.

Silverberg DS, Wexler D, Iaina A. The importance of anemia and its correction in the management of severe congestive heart failure. *Eur J Heart Fail* 2002;4:681–686.

Suresh D, Lamba S, Abraham WT. New developments in heart failure: role of endothelin and the use of endothelin receptor antagonists. *J Cardiac Fail* 2000;6:359–368.

The Digitalis Investigation Group. The effect of digoxin on mortality and morbidity in patients with heart failure. *N Engl J Med* 1997;336:525–533.

Vasan RS, Benjamin EJ, Levy D. Congestive heart failure with normal LV systolic function: clinical approaches to the diagnosis and treatment of decompensated heart failure. *Arch Intern Med* 1996; 156:146–157.

Yusuf S, Pfeffer MA, Swedberg K, et al. Effects of candesartan in patients with chronic heart failure and preserved left-ventricular ejection fraction: The CHARM-Preserved Trial. *Lancet* 2003;362: 777–781.

# BOARD SIMULATION: Cardiology

*Sasan Ghaffari*

## 71

Questions regarding cardiology constitute the highest percentage of questions on the American Board of Internal Medicine Certification Examination, (~14%) so its significance cannot be overemphasized. The areas covered in this chapter include acute coronary syndromes, valvular heart disease, dysrhythmias such as atrial fibrillation and Wolff-Parkinson-White syndrome, congestive heart failure (CHF), and primary prevention.

## QUESTIONS

**1.** The mechanism of action of acetylsalicylic acid (aspirin) is:
**a)** Adenosine diphosphate-mediated platelet aggregation inhibitor
**b)** Phosphodiesterase inhibitor
**c)** Glycoprotein IIb/IIIa receptor inhibitor
**d)** Cyclo-oxygenase inhibitor
**e)** None of the above

**2.** A 70-year-old man seeks a second opinion regarding frequent episodes of paroxysmal atrial fibrillation that were detected on 48-hour Holter monitor. He is markedly symptomatic, with frequent palpitations and presyncope. Each episode can last from 30 minutes to 2 hours. His past medical history is significant for old anterior wall myocardial infarction (MI), his left ventricular ejection fraction (LVEF) is 20%. His medications include enalapril, digoxin, and warfarin. On physical examination, his blood pressure is 120/80 mmHg and his heart rate is 78/bpm. He appears well compensated and is free of signs of CHF.

Which of the following is the most appropriate antiarrhythmic agent?
**a)** Sotalol
**b)** Amiodarone
**c)** Flecainide
**d)** Disopyramide
**e)** Quinidine

**3.** A 45-year-old man developed an acute anterior wall MI that was treated with primary percutaneous transluminal coronary angioplasty (PTCA). His cardiac catheterization study showed 100% occlusion of the mid-left anterior descending artery; this was successfully opened, with residual narrowing of 10%. His other coronary arteries demonstrated mild atherosclerotic changes. His LVEF is 40%. On admission, his total serum cholesterol level was 230 mg/dL and his LDLc level was 140 mg/dL. He had an uneventful hospital course.

His discharge medications should include all the following, *except*
**a)** Isosorbide dinitrate
**b)** Metoprolol
**c)** Simvastatin
**d)** Captopril
**e)** Aspirin

**4.** The clinical features of constrictive pericarditis include all the following, *except*
**a)** Cardiac surgery is an important etiological factor.
**b)** Commonly misdiagnosed as hepatic cirrhosis.
**c)** Systolic dysfunction is the earliest echocardiographic finding.
**d)** Exertional dyspnea is the most common symptom.
**e)** "Square root" sign is an important finding during simultaneous right and left heart catheterizations.

**5.** An active 32-year-old woman presents with a chief complaint of fatigue and exercise intolerance. She had an uncomplicated pregnancy and delivered her second child 2 months ago. On examination, her blood pressure is 110/80 mm Hg and her heart rate is 86/bpm. Her neck veins are flat, without elevation of jugular venous pressure, and her point of maximal intensity is enlarged and laterally displaced. A 2/6 holosystolic murmur is present at the apex, without $S_3$ gallop. The rest of the examination is unremarkable. Her chest radiograph shows cardiomegaly. An EKG reveals normal sinus rhythm with complete left bundle branch block. Her 2D-echo shows bi-ventricular enlargement with an LVEF of 30% and 2+ mitral regurgitation.

Which of the following agents is first-line therapy?
**a)** Spironolactone
**b)** Prazosin
**c)** Digoxin
**d)** Enalapril
**e)** Carvedilol

**6.** A 27-year-old white woman has had recurrent palpitations for the past 5 years. Her most recent episode was

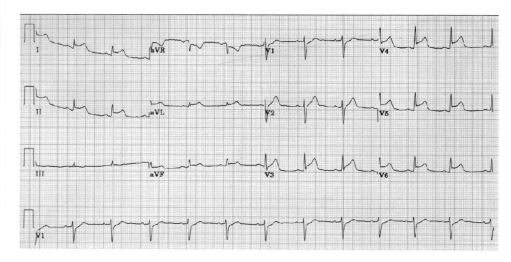

**Figure 71.1** Electrocardiogram for patient in Question 6.

2 days ago; that episode lasted 45 minutes and resulted in near syncope. Her past medical history (PMH) is unremarkable and she takes no medications. Her thyroid stimulating hormone (TSH) level is normal. Her EKG today is shown in Figure 71.1.

The most appropriate recommendation at this time is

a) No treatment, provide reassurance
b) Procainamide
c) Digoxin
d) Verapamil
e) Radiofrequency ablation of accessory pathway

**7.** Based on the National Cholesterol Education Panel guidelines, what is the target goal of lipid management in a diabetic patient with no history of coronary artery disease?

a) Raise high density lipoprotein (HDL) cholesterol levels to >45 mg/dL.
b) Raise HDL cholesterol levels to >55 mg/dL.

c) Lower low density lipoprotein (LDL) cholesterol levels to <130 mg/dL.
d) Lower LDL cholesterol to levels <75 mg/dL.
e) Lower LDL cholesterol to levels <100 mg/dL.

**8.** What is the most likely EKG diagnosis (Fig. 71.2) in this 45-year-old man with acute chest pain syndrome?

a) Acute MI
b) Acute pericarditis
c) Left ventricular aneurysm
d) Early repolarization
e) Hyperkalemia

**9.** A 55-year-old man with multiple cardiac risk factors presents to the emergency department with acute onset of intermittent chest pressure that occurred while he was sitting and watching TV, lasting 6 hours, associated with dyspnea and diaphoresis. Each episode lasted 30 minutes, and there was no relief with Maalox. On physical

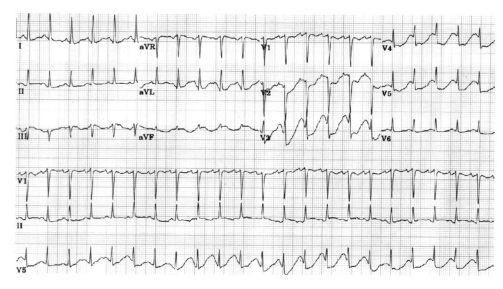

**Figure 71.2** Electrocardiogram for patient in Question 8.

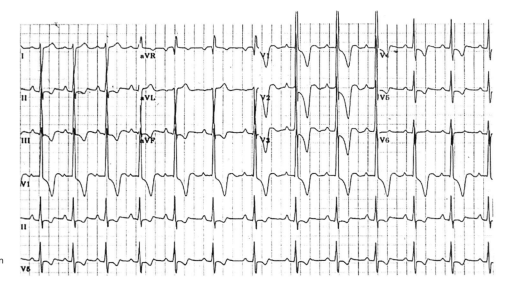

**Figure 71.3** Electrocardiogram for patient in Question 9.

examination, his blood pressure is 150/90 mm Hg, and his heart rate is 130/bpm. His examination is remarkable for tachycardia and no murmurs. He has bi-basilar rales. His creatine phosphokinase (CPK) level is 140 mg/dL, with a CK-MB level of 3 (normal, 0–4), and his troponin T level is 5.6 (normal, 0–0.1). His EKG is shown in Figure 71.3:

The most appropriate combination therapy in this patient is
a) Aspirin, fibrinolysis with tissue plasminogen activator (tPA), heparin, metoprolol, nitroglycerin
b) Aspirin, fibrinolysis with streptokinase, metoprolol, nitroglycerin
c) Aspirin, enoxaparin, nitroglycerin, magnesium
d) Aspirin, enoxaparin, metoprolol, magnesium
e) Aspirin, heparin, tirofiban, metoprolol, nitroglycerin

**10.** A 60-year-old woman presents for preoperative consultation prior to her abdominal aortic aneurysm (AAA; 6 cm) surgery. She is a chronic smoker and has an extensive history of hypertension. She is inactive and has exercise intolerance secondary to her obstructive pulmonary disease. She has no prior cardiac history and reports no angina pectoris. Her medications include theophylline, albuterol inhaler, and hydrochlorothiazide.

On physical examination, her blood pressure is 150/90 mm Hg, and her heart rate is 86/bpm. Her cardiovascular examination is normal, with no evidence of fluid overload or congestion. She has decreased breath sounds with diffuse expiratory wheezes throughout both lung fields and has a palpable pulsatile abdominal mass. Her chest radiograph reveals hyperinflation of both lungs, with flattening of both diaphragms and normal cardiac silhouette. Her EKG shows normal sinus rhythm, with Q waves in inferior leads suggesting remote inferior wall MI.

The most appropriate initial recommendation is
a) Schedule cardiac catheterization
b) Dipyridamole nuclear study
c) Cancel her operation
d) Dobutamine stress echocardiography
e) Proceed with surgery without further work-up

**11.** Indications for surgical intervention during active infective endocarditis include all the following, *except*
a) Systemic emboli
b) Fungal endocarditis
c) CHF and hemodynamic instability
d) Paravalvular invasion and abscess
e) 8 mm tricuspid valve *Staphylococcus aureus* endocarditis

**12.** 35-year-old man is hit in the chest by a baseball and visits the emergency department with pleuritic chest wall pain. He states that when he was a child, his pediatrician heard a heart murmur but he never followed up and has not seen a physician since age 8. He has felt well and takes no medications.

On examination, his blood pressure is 130/40 mm Hg and his heart rate is 90/bpm. He has a left lateral rib cage contusion without deformity. On auscultation, he is found to have a 3/6 diastolic murmur, heard best at the left upper sternal border in a sitting position. His chest radiograph shows incidental cardiomegaly with clear lungs, no infiltrates, and no rib fractures. A 2D-echo reveals dilated left ventricle with mild global systolic dysfunction and an ejection fraction of 45%. He has a bicuspid aortic valve with severe 4+ aortic insufficiency.

What is the most appropriate long-term therapeutic strategy in this asymptomatic patient with severe aortic insufficiency?
a) Watchful waiting and repeat 2D-echo in 6 months
b) Afterload reduction with nifedipine

c) Cardiothoracic surgical consultation for corrective aortic valve surgery

d) Oral furosemide

e) Aortic valve valvuloplasty

**13.** The following statements regarding severe aortic stenosis are all true, *except*

a) Symptoms dictate the timing of aortic valve replacement.

b) As a presenting symptom, angina has a worse prognosis than CHF.

c) Bacterial endocarditis prophylaxis is required.

d) Diagnosis using a cardiac catheter is not mandatory.

e) The incidence of sudden death is very low.

**14.** A 32-year-old Vietnamese nurse requested a routine physical examination and an EKG because of a strong family history of coronary artery disease (CAD). She is asymptomatic. On examination, she appears healthy, with a blood pressure reading of 122/76 mm Hg and a heart rate of 76/bpm. Her cardiac examination is notable for regular rate and rhythm, with normal $S_1$ and widely fixed split $S_2$. She has a 2/6 systolic ejection murmur, heard best at the left upper sternal border, third interspace, and no gallops or diastolic murmurs are present. Her lungs are clear, and she has no evidence of ascites or peripheral edema. No cyanosis or clubbing is present. Her chest radiograph demonstrates enlarged pulmonary arteries with increased vascularity in both lung fields. Her EKG is shown in Figure 71.4.

The most likely diagnosis is

a) Ventricular septal defect

b) Congenital pulmonary stenosis

c) Patent ductus arteriosus

d) Atrial septal defect

e) Mitral stenosis

**15.** The following drugs have all demonstrated a significant reduction in all-cause mortality in patients with CHF, *except*

a) Digoxin

b) Enalapril

c) Metoprolol XL

d) Spironolactone

e) Carvedilol

**16.** All the following clinical markers predict adverse outcome in patients presenting with acute MI, *except*

a) Tachycardia

b) Pulmonary congestion

c) Age >70

d) Systolic blood pressure <90 mm Hg

e) Current cigarette smoker

**17.** Which of the following is true regarding coronary angiography in stable patients after acute ST elevation MI who were successfully treated with fibrinolytic therapy?

a) Predicts reinfarction

b) Predicts mortality

c) Often leads to revascularization and higher income for invasive cardiologists

d) Is a cost-effective risk-stratification strategy

e) Is recommended for all post-MI patients

**18.** A 54-year-old white man with a history of uncontrolled hypertension and end-stage renal disease on hemodialysis develops shortness of breath and hypotension during a dialysis session. His blood pressure is 92/60 mm Hg, his heart rate is 116/bpm, his respiratory rate is 32, his temperature is 37 C. His cardiac examination demonstrated elevated jugular venous pulsation with muffled heart sounds and clear lungs. No ascites or peripheral edema is present.

What would you do next?

a) Echocardiogram (ECHO)

b) Ventilation–perfusion (VQ) scan

c) Measure pulsus paradoxus

d) Obtain blood cultures

e) Perform pericardiocentesis

**19.** A 55-year-old man presents with a 10-hour history of severe chest pressure and is promptly diagnosed with acute inferior wall MI and receives reteplase. His chest pressure and ST segment elevations completely resolve

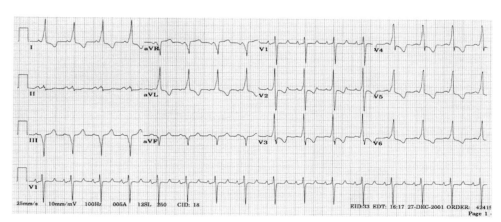

**Figure 71.4** Electrocardiogram tracing for patient in Question 14.

after 40 minutes of thrombolytic administration. He is then placed on a regimen of aspirin, heparin, and metoprolol. On the fourth hospital day, he develops sudden onset dyspnea, diaphoresis, palpitations, and dizziness.

On examination, his respiratory rate is 38 breaths per minute, his blood pressure is 86/60 mm Hg, and his heart rate is 130/bpm. He has an irregularly irregular rhythm with a loud 4/6 holosystolic murmur, heard best at the apex. Pulmonary rales are present two-thirds of the way up both lung fields. The rest of the examination is unremarkable. His EKG demonstrates atrial fibrillation with rapid ventricular response, Q waves inferiorly, and no acute ST segment changes. His chest radiograph is consistent with acute pulmonary edema. Pulmonary artery catheter hemodynamics reveal:

|  | Pressure (mm Hg) | Oxygen Saturation (%) |
|---|---|---|
| Right atrium | 7 | 55 |
| Right ventricle | 50/8 | 57 |
| Pulmonary artery | 50/28 (mean 36) | 58 |
| Mean pulmonary artery wedge | 26 (v wave = 42) | |

What is the most appropriate treatment strategy?
a) Pericardiocentesis
b) Thrombolytic therapy
c) Surgical repair or replacement of mitral valve
d) Angioplasty of left circumflex artery
e) Surgical repair of ventricular septum

**20.** All the following are risk factors for stroke in patients with atrial fibrillation, *except*
a) Hypertension
b) Prior embolic event
c) Ejection fraction <30%
d) Pericardial effusion
e) Mitral stenosis

**21.** A 32-year-old previously healthy woman has experienced four recurrent episodes of transient ischemic attacks (TIAs) with right hemiparesis and dysarthria. She is on no medications. Her physical examination, laboratory evaluation (including coagulation studies), and carotid ultrasound are all within normal limits. Her transesophageal echo (TEE) reveals a patent foramen ovale (PFO).

Which of the following is most likely responsible for her symptoms?
a) Paradoxical emboli
b) Endocarditis
c) Atrial myxoma
d) Atrial dysrhythmias
e) Munchausen syndrome by proxy

**22.** All the following are indications for the placement of a permanent pacemaker, *except*
a) Second-degree atrioventricular block, Mobitz type I
b) Symptomatic third-degree atrioventricular block
c) Carotid artery hypersensitivity syndrome
d) Sinus node dysfunction with angina pectoris
e) Uncontrolled atrial fibrillation with rapid ventricular rate

**23.** Which of the following adult congenital heart diseases is an absolute contraindication to pregnancy?
a) Eisenmenger's syndrome
b) Ebstein's anomaly
c) Rheumatic mitral stenosis
d) Asymptomatic congenital aortic stenosis
e) Atrial septal defect

**24.** What is the treatment of choice in a patient with the EKG tracing in Figure 71.5?
a) Thrombolysis with tissue plasminogen activator
b) Kayexalate
c) Calcium gluconate

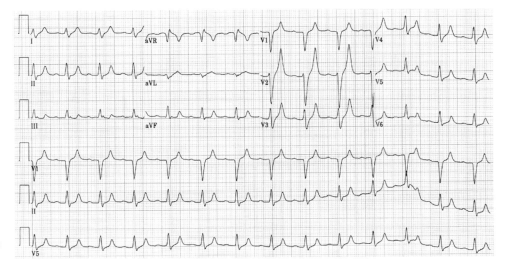

**Figure 71.5** Electrocardiogram for patient in Question 24.

d) Digoxin

e) Amiodarone

**25.** Which of the following conditions results in a paradoxically split $S_2$?

a) Right bundle branch block

b) Left bundle branch block

c) Second-degree atrioventricular block

d) Atrial septal defect

e) Patent ductus arteriosus

**26.** A 46-year-old woman presents with acute inferior wall MI, 3 hours within onset of chest pain, sinus bradycardia of 36 beats per minute, and blood pressure of 92/70 mm Hg. She received aspirin, immediate reteplase (r-PA), and heparin. She complaints of lightheadedness.

Which of the following therapeutic strategies should be implemented next at the bedside?

a) Nitroglycerine

b) Metoprolol

c) Tirofiban

d) Magnesium

e) Atropine and transcutaneous pacing

**27.** A 76-year-old previously healthy, active man accidentally falls and fractures his right hip at the femoral neck. On review of systems, he denies any cardiovascular symptoms, and he has been able to swim 45 minutes three times a week for the past 10 years. His blood pressure is 130/70 mmHg and his heart rate is regular at 70/bpm. Further examination is unremarkable except for right hip swelling and tenderness and immobile right lower extremity. His EKG is normal.

Which of the following would you recommend?

a) Proceed with urgent right hip surgery

b) Adenosine stress sestamibi nuclear scan

c) Cardiac catheterization

d) Proceed with urgent right hip surgery with pulmonary artery catheter hemodynamic monitoring

e) Right lower extremity duplex ultrasound

**28.** Which of the following cardiovascular drugs poses an absolute contraindication to taking sildenafil (Viagra)?

a) Amiodarone

b) Celecoxib

c) Isosorbide dinitrate

d) Nifedipine

e) Enalapril

**29.** A 60-year-old black woman presents with acute ST elevation inferior wall MI and undergoes primary percutaneous coronary intervention with stent to her right coronary artery within 4 hours of the onset of her chest pain. Her left ventricular systolic function is normal, with an ejection fraction of 55%. She has an uncomplicated hospital course. Her PMH is significant for hypertension.

Her discharge medications should include the following, *except*

a) Atorvastatin

b) Isosorbide mononitrate

c) Clopidogrel

d) Metoprolol

e) Ramipril

f) Aspirin

**30.** All the following would be expected to increase the intensity of the murmur of hypertrophic obstructive cardiomyopathy, *except*

a) Valsalva maneuver

b) Amyl nitrite administration

c) Standing position

d) Prompt squatting

e) Postpremature ventricular contraction beat

**31.** All the following meet the major Jones criteria for the diagnosis of acute rheumatic fever, *except*

a) Arthralgia

b) Carditis

c) Erythema marginatum

d) Chorea

e) Subcutaneous nodules

**32.** The most common coexisting congenital anomaly in patients with coarctation of aorta is

a) Cleft mitral valve

b) Bicuspid aortic valve

c) Ebstein's anomaly

d) Ventricular septal defect

e) Patent ductus arteriosus

## ANSWERS AND EXPLANATIONS

**1. d.**

This question is always on the Boards. Both oral and intravenous antiplatelet agents are the main components of therapy in patients who present with acute coronary syndromes. The oral agents, aspirin and clopidogrel, also are used in secondary prevention in patients with atherosclerotic vascular disease, and these agents have shown to decrease vascular events over the long term. Aspirin is the oldest and cheapest agent available, and it has been tested extensively in clinical trials. It has consistently and significantly reduced mortality in patients with acute coronary events. Aspirin irreversibly inhibits the cyclooxygenase enzyme pathway, and it shuts off production of platelet thromboxane $A_2$. Thromboxane $A_2$ is one of many potent mediators of platelet aggregation. The most potent antiplatelet agents are the intravenous glycoprotein IIb/IIIa receptor inhibitors (abciximab, tirofiban, and eptifibatide) that block the final common pathway to platelet aggregation. Ample clinical evidence suggests that these agents reduce the ischemic complications associated with percutaneous coronary interventions.

When added to aspirin and heparin, tirofiban and eptifibatide have been shown to reduce death or MI) in patients with unstable angina or non-ST elevation MI. The thienopyridines (ticlopidine and clopidogrel) exert their antiplatelet effect by inhibiting adenosine phosphate (ADP)–mediated platelet aggregation. An association exists between ticlopidine and thrombocytopenic purpura (TTP) and therefore clopidogrel is more widely used. As a class, these agents increase the risk of bleeding, so platelet levels and function should be monitored closely. Phosphodiesterase inhibitors have vasodilatation properties and minimal or no antiplatelet effect.

## 2. b.
This patient had a previous MI and has depressed left ventricular systolic function. He is symptomatic with his atrial fibrillation and must be treated aggressively. Amiodarone, a Class III antiarrhythmic medication, is a potent agent that exerts its effect broadly on all phases of action potential. It is ideal in this situation, because it has negligible negative inotropic effect. Patients are orally loaded in the hospital and are observed for the development of symptomatic bradycardia and torsade de pointe due to QT prolongation (an uncommon complication). Sotalol, a Class III antiarrhythmic drug is classified as a nonselective β-blocker, and it blocks the potassium channel and prolongs the repolarization phase. It has negative inotropic properties and can induce or exacerbate heart failure. Sotalol should not be prescribed if the ejection fraction is <35%. Flecainide is a Class IC antiarrhythmic agent, and its use is contraindicated in patients with structural heart disease (coronary artery disease, MI, CHF, or undifferentiated cardiomyopathy). Disopyramide is a Class IA antiarrhythmic agent that has profound negative inotropic properties, and its use is contraindicated in patients with depressed left ventricular systolic function. Quinidine is a Class IA agent that has negative inotropic properties. A meta-analysis of several small trials demonstrated excess mortality in patients taking quinidine, and its use has become quite limited. The only other viable option in this patient is dofetilide, a new class III antiarrhythmic therapy that is given to patients with low ejection fraction who have a contraindication to amiodarone.

## 3. a.
All the listed medications and their respective classes have demonstrated a mortality benefit in secondary prevention trials, with the exception of nitrates, isosorbide dinitrate. β-Blockers [Beta Blocker Heart Attack Trial (BHAT)], statins [Scandinavian Simvastatin Survival Study(4S)], ACE-inhibitors [Survival and Ventricular Enlargement (SAVE) study], and aspirin have all shown a significant decrease in mortality and recurrent MI in patients with prior MI when compared with placebo.

## 4. c.
Constrictive pericarditis (CP) is a challenging diagnosis and requires a careful assessment of history, physical examination, imaging modalities, and invasive right and left heart catheterizations before it is confirmed. The most common etiology in the United States is idiopathic or postviral pericarditis; globally, the most common etiology is tuberculosis. With the rise in the number of cardiac surgeries, postoperative CP is emerging as an important etiology. It is a progressive and chronic disorder and shares similar clinical characteristics with hepatic cirrhosis. The most common symptom is dyspnea on exertion followed by peripheral edema and increased abdominal girth. Elevation in jugular venous pressure distinguishes CP from primary liver disease. The earliest echocardiographic findings are changes consistent with diastolic (impaired filling of both right and left ventricles) as opposed to systolic dysfunction. Both atria become enlarged, and the inferior vena cava becomes dilated. For the most part, the left ventricular systolic function is preserved. Chest computed tomography (CT) scans and cardiac magnetic resonance imaging (MRI) can delineate the precise thickness of the pericardium and provide added diagnostic value. The "square root" sign can be seen with simultaneous right and left heart catheterizations and reflects an early diastolic dip with sharp transition to plateau. Elevation and equalization of right and left ventricular diastolic pressures is present.

## 5. d.
The patient's diagnosis is postpartum cardiomyopathy, and she has moderate left ventricular systolic dysfunction and moderate mitral regurgitation. She is clinically well-compensated and has mild limitation in her activities of daily living. The first-line therapy for her is the ACE-inhibitor enalapril. The Studies of Left Ventricular Dysfunction (SOLVD) trial demonstrated a significant reduction in both mortality and rate of hospitalization in both symptomatic and asymptomatic patients with reduced left ventricular systolic function regardless of etiology. Spironolactone has shown a mortality benefit in patients with severe forms of heart failure [New York Heart Association (NYHA) functional classification IV]. Digoxin has a neutral effect on mortality and has shown to reduce the rate of hospitalization for CHF in patients with depressed systolic function. It is not considered first-line therapy, however. Carvedilol, a nonselective β-blocker with α-blocker and antioxidant properties, has been shown in clinical trials to have a mortality benefit in patients with moderate and severe forms of heart failure when compared to placebo. Carvedilol was added to a background regimen of ACE-inhibitor, however, and therefore is not the correct answer.

## 6. e.
One must recognize that the patient's EKG demonstrates Δ-waves and a pseudo-inferior wall MI pattern suggestive of accessory arterioventricular (AV) conduction or Wolf-Parkinson-White (WPW) syndrome. The main symptom of this congenital abnormality is palpitations. The most

feared complication is atrial tachyarrhythmias, with 1:1 AV conduction via the accessory pathway resulting in ventricular fibrillation and sudden death. Thus, nodal blocking agents (digoxin, β-blockers, calcium channel blockers) must *not* be used in patients with WPW and tachycardia. Our patient with presyncope and recurrent palpitations is a very good candidate for electrophysiologic study and radiofrequency ablation of her accessory pathway.

### 7. e.

The Third National Cholesterol Education Program's (NCEP) updated guidelines were published in the *Journal of the American Medical Association* (JAMA) on May 16, 2001. The Adult Treatment Plan III calls for more intensive LDL-lowering therapy and focuses on primary prevention in persons with multiple risk factors. Diabetes is currently considered a coronary heart disease risk equivalent (+ peripheral vascular disease, abdominal aortic aneurysm, carotid artery disease), and the goal of therapy is to lower LDL cholesterol to <100 mg/dL even in the absence of coronary heart disease. Greater emphasis is placed in measuring absolute long-term risk and performing 10-year risk assessment using Framingham scoring. Multiple risk factors estimates (age, gender, total cholesterol level, smoking status, HDL level, systolic blood pressure), which confer a greater than 20% 10-year risk for coronary heart disease, also require a LDL cholesterol reduction to <100 mg/dL. HDL at this time is not the primary target. A small study using recombinant HDL, Apo-Milano, has shown plaque regression using intravascular ultrasound. Larger studies, with longer follow-up times and clinical endpoints, will assess the benefits of HDL elevation; these studies are in the early stages of planning and enrollment. Evidence suggests that the early and prompt initiation of statin therapy (bypass dietary modification) is warranted for secondary prevention to improve compliance and avoid unnecessary delays in effective treatment.

### 8. b.

It its imperative for the clinician to distinguish acute MI from pericarditis electrocardiographically. Acute MI causes localized ST segment elevation that is convex, not concave, with inverted T waves. It is common to see reciprocal ST depressions in the leads without ST elevations. The ST-to-T amplitude ratio in $V_6$ is <0.25. Acute pericarditis, conversely, causes diffuse concave ST segment elevation, with upright T waves. Once the ST segment changes return to baseline in later stages of pericarditis, the T waves become inverted. No reciprocal ST segment depression is noted. PR segment elevation in $aV_R$ and PR segment depression in inferior leads are specific changes seen in pericarditis and not acute MI. Left ventricular aneurysm presents as persistent localized ST segment elevation. Q waves suggest prior infarction. Early repolarization is common in young black Americans and is mainly seen in the precordial leads. Electrocardiographic

changes associated with worsening hyperkalemia include peak-tented T waves >10 mv; prolongation of PR interval, with flattening and eventual disappearance of P waves; widening of QRS, with merging of QRS; and T waves resulting in a sine wave pattern.

### 9. e.

This patient is experiencing a non-ST elevation MI. He has chest pains, marked dynamic ST depressions, and an elevation in troponin T. Fibrinolytic agents are only indicated in the treatment of ST-segment elevation MI. The only exception is isolated 2mm ST depressions in $V_1$–$V_3$ that corresponds to ST elevations in posterior leads $V_7$–$V_9$; this indicates acute posterior infarction. Evidence suggests that fibrinolytic agents cause harm to patients with non-ST elevation MI by inducing a heightened thrombotic state; these agents therefore are contraindicated. Low molecular weight heparins, such as enoxaparin, have a role in the management of this patient, but the key missing ingredients in answers c and d are β-blocking agents and nitrates, respectively. The current guidelines call for a combination of aspirin, standard heparin (or low molecular weight heparin), and potent antiplatelet glycoprotein IIb/IIIa receptor antagonists (tirofiban or eptifibatide) in addition to β-blockers and nitrates. When these glycoprotein IIb/IIIa receptor blockers were added to aspirin and heparin in the Platelet Receptor Inhibition for Ischemic Syndrome Management in Patients Limited to Very Unstable Signs and Symptoms (PRISM-PLUS) and Platelet Glycoprotein IIb/IIIa in Unstable Angina: Receptor Suppression Using Integrilin Therapy (PURSUIT) multi-center placebo-controlled trials, patients showed a significant reduction in the combined rate of death, MI, and recurrent ischemia.

### 10. d.

One of the most common consults for an internist is to provide a preoperative assessment for patients who are scheduled for noncardiac surgery. Our patient is scheduled for AAA repair, which carries a high surgery-specific risk. She has active asthma and an abnormal EKG. Cardiac catheterization is an invasive and aggressive approach and is reserved for symptomatic patients (unstable coronary symptoms or evidence of CHF). A dipyridamole nuclear study is contraindicated due to her active asthma state. Dipyridamole can cause severe bronchospasm and has the potential to induce respiratory failure in asthmatic patients. She needs the operation because the risk of rupture is high and increases with time. She deserves a functional test because a large proportion of patients with AAA harbor atherosclerotic coronary artery disease that requires further risk stratification. Dobutamine stress echocardiography provides valuable information on the status of her left ventricular systolic function and valvular function, and it can determine presence or absence of myocardial ischemia.

Patients with normal dobutamine stress echoes have a very low risk of perioperative MI.

**11. e.**

Remember the mnemonic PPCAFE: *p*rosthetic endocarditis, *p*ersistent bacteremia, *c*ongestive heart failure, *p*erivalvular abscess, *f*ungal endocarditis, and *e*mbolization. *Staphylococcus aureus* has surpassed *Streptococcus viridans* as the most common bacterial cause of acute infective endocarditis. This disorder continues to carry a high (25% to 50%) risk of major morbidity and mortality despite aggressive treatment.

**12. c.**

This patient was initially found to have an incidental heart murmur that led to the diagnosis of severe aortic regurgitation. Although he is asymptomatic, the echocardiographic features—not the presence or lack of symptoms—dictate his course of treatment. He has a reduced ejection fraction with evidence of left ventricular dilatation in a setting of severe 4+ aortic regurgitation. Natural history studies have shown a significant increase in morbidity and mortality in patients whose ejection fraction falls below 50%, with an end-systolic dimension increase of >50 mm. Therefore, watchful waiting is not the right course of action. Research by Rahimtoola et al. (*New England Journal of Medicine* 1994;331:689–694) demonstrated a statistically significant delay in the development of CHF and the need for aortic valve replacement in patients with normal ejection fractions >55% who received nifedipine 20 mg two times a day, as compared with patients who received daily digoxin 0.25 mg. No evidence suggests that this patient is fluid-overloaded, and diuretics do not change the natural history of aortic regurgitation. Aortic valve valvuloplasty has no role in aortic regurgitation.

**13. b.**

As opposed to regurgitant valvular lesions, the management of stenotic valvular lesions is guided by the presence of symptoms. Based on the natural history studies of patients with severe aortic stenosis, angina pectoris has a more favorable prognosis when compared with syncope. Patients who present with CHF have the worst outcome and prognosis if they are medically treated. Bacterial endocarditis prophylaxis is recommended. Echocardiography has superior accuracy when compared with cardiac catheterization and is better able to provide instantaneous maximal peak gradient across the aortic valve. The incidence of sudden cardiac death is very low (~1% per year) and justifies watchful waiting in truly asymptomatic patients.

**14. d.**

This patient has evidence of right-sided volume overload with EKG changes consistent with right ventricular hypertrophy. The fixed split $S_2$ is the key distinguishing feature that is pathognomonic for atrial septal defect.

Ventricular septal defect produces a loud, harsh murmur that is best heard in the mid to lower left sternal border. The murmur of congenital pulmonary stenosis is a loud crescendo/decrescendo systolic ejection murmur that radiates to the left clavicle. Pulmonary stenosis does not cause an increase in pulmonary vascularity. Patent ductus arteriosus is characterized by a continuous systolic/diastolic murmur. Mitral stenosis produces a loud $S_1$, with an opening snap and a diastolic rumble heard best at the apex of the heart.

**15. a.**

Digoxin is the only agent that had a neutral effect in mortality in trials of CHF. The ACE-inhibitors, β-blockers (except bucindolol), and spironolactone all have shown a significant reduction in mortality in randomized double-blind placebo-controlled trials of patients with moderate and severe forms of heart failure (NYHA functional Class II–IV).

**16. e.**

More than 200,000 acute MI patients have been enrolled into various fibrinolytic trials that demonstrated a reduction in mortality. Sinus tachycardia, pulmonary congestion, age >70, systolic blood pressure of <90 mm Hg, and anterior location of MI all have been independent markers of higher mortality. Paradoxically, current smokers with acute MI had a lower mortality rate, most likely due to younger age at presentation.

**17. c.**

Coronary angiography has been shown to be a poor predictor of outcomes in stable patients who present with ST-elevation infarction and receive successful fibrinolytic therapy in a timely manner (<6 hours from onset of chest pain). The stable patient is defined as *not* experiencing postinfarct angina, CHF, or ventricular tachyarrhythmias. In the acute setting, the best predictors of 30-day mortality are advanced age (>70), hypotension (systolic blood pressure < 0 mm Hg), tachycardia (heart rate >100/bpm), prior infarction, anterior location of an infarct, presence of symptoms and signs of CHF, and elevated troponins (T and I). In stable patients, the strategy of submaximal exercise stress test on day 5 post-MI, followed by full exercise treadmill functional test (nuclear or echo) at 6 weeks is quite an acceptable approach. If ischemia is demonstrated, then angiography and revascularization is performed. Of note, no data shows revascularization in stable post-MI patient leads to lower mortality or coronary events. Data does show, however, that the early institution of aspirin, β-blockers, statins, and ACE-inhibitors post-MI leads to a significant reduction in morbidity and mortality and is a highly cost-effective strategy.

**18. c.**

The patient's clinical presentation should elevate the existence of symptomatic pericardial effusion and cardiac tamponade to the top of the differential diagnosis list. In a previously hypertensive patient with end-stage renal disease who acutely becomes hypotensive without obvious blood loss, uremic pericarditis should be considered strongly. The next step is to check for pulsus paradoxus, which is an exaggeration of inspiratory drop in systolic blood pressure (a drop of >10 mm Hg). A 2D echo then is ordered to confirm the diagnosis. (The board members who make up board examination questions place heavy emphasis on physical examination and cost-effective strategy in diagnostic work-ups.)

### 19. c.

The Board definitely will ask you to diagnose and treat all the mechanical complications of acute MI. The mechanical complications associated with acute MI include ventricular septal defect, rupture of free wall of the left ventricle, right ventricular infarction, and papillary muscle rupture with acute mitral regurgitation. The characteristic holosystolic murmur and presence of atrial fibrillation (acute left atrial dilatation) point toward papillary muscle rupture, which is a true cardiac surgical emergency. The triad of right ventricular infarction include hypotension, elevated jugular venous pressure, and clear lung fields on auscultation.

Dressler's syndrome is an autoimmune reaction with resultant pericarditis weeks after MI. The hemodynamics do not demonstrate diastolic equalization and, therefore, cardiac tamponade is excluded and pericardiocentesis is the wrong choice. The EKG failed to show recurrent ST elevation, therefore reinfarction or infarct extension is less likely and a trip to the catheterization laboratory or thrombolysis is not warranted.

### 20. d.

Atrial fibrillation is the most common cardiac dysrhythmia in the general population, and its incidence increases substantially in people older than 70 years. Warfarin anticoagulation is superior to aspirin and is indicated in high-risk patients to prevent embolic strokes. The high-risk category includes patients with long-standing hypertension, low ejection fraction with or without CHF, mitral stenosis, and prior embolic events. Pericardial effusion does not increase the risk of stroke in the setting of atrial fibrillation.

### 21. a.

This young woman has had recurrent neurologic events with essentially negative work-up and cryptogenic TIAs. The most common indication for ordering a TEE is to rule out a cardiac source of emboli. PFO is present in about 25% to 30% of the general population. It is not entirely clear if the presence of PFO is a definite cause, a major contributing factor, or an innocent bystander in this case. Because of the seriousness of recurrent neurologic event(s), most experts will refer the patient for PFO closure, using either a percutaneous or surgical

approach. The clinical findings and absence of vegetations on TEE rule out endocarditis and atrial myxoma. Atrial fibrillation should be in the differential diagnosis. No history of palpitations is present; neither is objective data, such as abnormal EKG or Holter findings; therefore, choice d is wrong.

### 22. a.

In general, documented bradycardia with advanced degrees of heart block symptoms (presyncope, syncope, angina, CHF, extreme fatigue), and symptomatic carotid artery hypersensitivity constitute definite indications for the placement of a permanent pacemaker. A patient with sinus node dysfunction (tachycardia-bradycardia) in need of antianginal medications, such as β-blockers and calcium antagonists, would greatly benefit from a pacemaker. Difficult-to-control atrial fibrillation is another special circumstance in which the ablation of the AV node and placement of a pacemaker can significantly reduce symptoms and improve quality of life.

### 23. a.

The conditions that result in the greatest risk to the mother and/or the fetus include Eisenmenger's syndrome, severe pulmonary hypertension, severe left ventricular outflow obstruction, Marfan's syndrome with enlarged aortic root, and NYHA Class III or IV heart failure. It is commonly advised to terminate pregnancy if any of the above conditions are recognized. The other congenital abnormalities listed pose relative or no contraindication to the continuation of pregnancy.

### 24. c.

This EKG demonstrates the classic findings of hyperkalemia: peaked tented T waves, decreased amplitude P wave, slight ST-segment elevation, and prolongation of QRS. This patient's serum potassium level is 6.4 mEq/L. With a further rise in serum potassium, sine waves will develop, followed by asystole. The acute management of hyperkalemia includes calcium gluconate to stabilize the myocyte membrane, insulin and glucose, and sodium bicarbonate. Kayexalate, either orally or rectally administered, takes time to lower serum potassium and is therefore given to patients with mild to moderate hyperkalemia.

### 25. b.

Left bundle branch causes the depolarization wave to capture the right ventricle first and propagate via the interventricular septum to capture the left ventricle. Therefore, the pulmonary valve $P_2$ will close before the aortic valve $A_2$ does, resulting in a paradoxically split $S_2$. Atrial septal defect results in fixed normal split $S_2$ and is a favorite Board question.

### 26. e.

Nitroglycerin is wrong because of borderline systolic pressure and lack of active chest pain. Metoprolol will exacerbate the patient's bradycardia further, which is her primary problem at this time. There is no role for tirofiban in ST-elevation MI patients who receive a fibrinolytic. If needed, atropine and transcutaneous pacing are highly effective in raising the heart rate and improving marginal hemodynamics.

**27. a.**

Patients with acute hip fractures are at increased risk of major morbidity and mortality if their surgical treatment is delayed. This elderly patient is quite active and is free of any cardiovascular symptoms. His EKG is normal, therefore he is at low risk for perioperative complications (Eagle risk score 1/5, age >70). Delaying his surgery by performing various noninvasive tests can potentially harm him. Cardiac catheterization is not indicated and should not be done.

Concomitant hemodynamic monitoring using a pulmonary artery catheter is performed less and less and is reserved for selected patients with tenuous volume or hemodynamic states and not in this relatively healthy, active individual.

**28. c.**

There is no trick to this question. Currently, three oral medications that inhibit phosphodiesterase 5 (PDE 5) are approved to treat erectile dysfunction: sildenafil (Viagra), vardenafil (Levitra), and tadalafil (Cialis). All these medications are contraindicated in patients who take any form of nitroglycerin. Cases of profound persistent hypotension and death have been reported to the FDA.

**29. b.**

All the medications listed have shown to significantly benefit patients who are status-post MI. Atorvastatin, representing the statin class, has shown in multiple secondary prevention trials to reduce the risk of recurrent MI or death. Clopidogrel is given for a minimum of 1 month (using bare metal stents) and 3 months (using drug-eluting stents), and for up to 1 year post stenting to reduce the risk of in-stent thrombosis, target vessel revascularization, and ischemic complications. Aspirin and metoprolol have been the cornerstone of secondary prevention in reducing recurrent MI or death. Ramipril, representing the ACE-inhibitor class, also is indicated, despite the setting of a normal LVEF. Recent data have demonstrated beneficial effects of ACE-inhibitors in ischemic heart disease patients with normal ejection fraction. One of the proposed mechanisms for ACE-inhibitor benefit is its positive effect on endothelial function.

**30. d.**

Hypertrophic cardiomyopathy results in left ventricular outflow obstruction, and severe forms can cause syncope and sudden death. Any maneuver that reduces preload and therefore left ventricular cavity volume will result in greater systolic anterior motion of the mitral valve and greater left ventricular outflow tract obstruction, and therefore increase the intensity of the systolic murmur. Prompt squatting results in an increase in preload and decrease in the intensity of the systolic murmur.

**31. a.**

Globally, rheumatic fever (RF) is the most common cause of acquired heart disease in children and young adults. Rheumatic valvular heart disease is quite prevalent in the developing world and is a major cause of morbidity and mortality. The clinical manifestations of acute RF follow a group A streptococcal infection of the tonsillo-pharynx after a 3-week latent period. Major Jones criteria for its diagnosis include all listed options, except arthralgia, which is a minor manifestation.

The fifth element is polyarthritis. Rheumatic carditis is a pancarditis affecting the pericardium, myocardium, or the endocardium to varying degrees. A prompt treatment with penicillin antibiotics and anti-inflammatory salicylates is recommended. Cardiac medications, such as diuretics, ACE-inhibitors, or digoxin can be used if left ventricular systolic dysfunction and CHF develop.

**32. b.**

Aortic coarctation is a common congenital defect that consists of a constriction just distal to the left subclavian artery at the site of residual ligamentum arteriosus. A bicuspid aortic valve is the most common coexisting congenital anomaly. A combination of the two poses increased risk to the development of life-threatening aortic dissection. The presence of ventricular septal defect, patent ductus arteriosus, and malformations of mitral valve apparatus, however, are well documented. No association exists between aortic coarctation and Ebstein's anomaly.

# Cardiovascular Emergencies

## 72

*Vidyasagar Kalahasti*    *Samir R. Kapadia*

Cardiovascular emergencies occur from a hemodynamic compromise of the system resulting from mechanical or electrical dysfunction. In this chapter, we focus on understanding the pathophysiology, modes of diagnosis, and appropriate management of those mechanical problems of the cardiovascular system that result in life-threatening emergencies. A prototypical case is presented for each condition and salient features are discussed in a case-based approach.

## CASE 1: CARDIAC TAMPONADE

A 50-year-old man with history of lung cancer presents with shortness of breath and dizziness. On examination his blood pressure is 90/60 mm Hg, pulse rate is 110 beats per minute (bpm), and breath rate is 20 per minute. Jugular venous pressure (JVP) is elevated. Heart sounds are distant. Lung examination reveals normal breath sounds bilaterally. No peripheral edema is present. Cardiac tamponade is suspected.

### Question

1. Which of the following statements is true?
a) Malignancy is the most common cause for pericardial effusion.
b) Pulsus paradoxus is pathognomonic of cardiac tamponade.
c) JVP will increase with inspiration.
d) Tachycardia, hypotension, and increased JVP constitutes Beck's triad for cardiac tamponade.
e) None of the above.

### Answer and Explanation

1. a.
Cardiac tamponade is a clinical syndrome that is characterized by cardiac decompensation due to the compression of cardiac chambers from increased intrapericardial pressure. It is important to recognize that this is a clinical diagnosis. Although imaging modalities help to visualize the compression of different chambers of heart, clinical decompensation must be present for the diagnosis of cardiac tamponade. Hemodynamic compromise is

determined by intrapericardial pressure, volume status, and peripheral vascular tone.

### Etiology

Cardiac tamponade results from increasing intrapericardial pressure caused by increasing pericardial effusions. The intrapericardial pressure increases rapidly even in the presence of a small increase in pericardial fluid if the process is acute (Fig. 72.1). This typically is seen in patients with traumatic effusion and bleeding in the pericardium. Therefore, in acute trauma patients, any effusion is considered serious and warrants immediate attention. Table 72.1 lists common causes of pericardial effusion. Note that the most common cause of pericardial effusion in current practice is malignancy. Tuberculosis is a common cause of effusion in Third World countries. Although autoimmune and infectious diseases are important causes of pericardial effusion, tamponade is not common in these disease processes, because intrapericardial pressure is not greatly elevated by the relatively small effusions that develop slowly in these disease processes.

### Clinical Features

Cardiac tamponade is suspected based on history and physical examination. The symptoms of tamponade are reflective of a low cardiac output state and include dyspnea on exertion, restlessness, dizziness, drowsiness, and fatigue. The physical signs are increased JVP, tachypnea, tachycardia, hypotension, and decreased heart sounds. Low blood pressure, increased JVP, and distant cardiac sounds constitute Beck's triad.

The most characteristic physical sign is pulsus paradoxus, defined as a decline in systolic blood pressure >10 mm Hg upon inspiration (Fig. 72.2). Upon inspiration, some decrease in systolic blood pressure *normally* occurs, due to the decrease in left ventricular stroke volume. In normal breathing, however, the decrease in blood pressure is minimal. In pericardial tamponade, this normal response is exaggerated due to even further decreases in left ventricular (LV) filling, caused by the bowing of the interventricular septum towards the LV during inspiration (Fig. 72.3). It is important to note that patients should be asked to breathe normally while checking for pulsus paradoxus because deep breaths can exaggerate the inspiratory pressure drop.

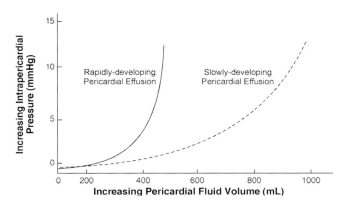

**Figure 72.1** The relationship between pericardial fluid volume and intrapericardial pressure in acute and chronic pericardial effusion.

Pulsus paradoxus is not specific for cardiac tamponade. It is seen in other pericardial diseases, such as in constrictive pericarditis (~50% of patients), or in situations in which marked intrathoracic pressure changes are present, as in emphysema, bronchial asthma, hypovolemic shock, pulmonary embolism, pregnancy, and extreme obesity. Pulsus paradoxus may be absent in severe LV dysfunction, positive pressure breathing, atrial septal defect, localized tamponade in postoperative cardiac surgery patients, and severe aortic regurgitation.

An increase in jugular venous distension during inspiration, which is known as Kussmaul's sign, is seen in constrictive pericarditis. At inspiration, increased intra-abdominal pressure is present, which leads to increased venous return, which in turn leads to an increase in right atrial (RA) pressure. This increase in RA pressure is seen as distended jugular veins. Because the abdominal veins typically are not engorged in cardiac tamponade, this sign is not present in the majority of patients with cardiac tamponade.

**TABLE 72.1**
## CAUSES OF PERICARDIAL EFFUSION

*Malignancy (~30%)*
**Secondary (Metastatic)**
Lung
Breast
Hematological cancers
Adenocarcinoma (ovarian, GI, GU, unknown, thymoma, osteogenic sarcoma, mesothelioma)
**Primary**
Mesothelioma
Sarcoma

*Infectious (~25%)*
Viral (most common):
    Coxsackie, influenza, HIV, hepatitis A, EBV
Bacterial:
    Tuberculosis (4%–7%)
    Sepsis, any organism
    Rickettsiae
    *Mycoplasma pneumoniae*
    Parasitic (hydatid cyst)

*Autoimmune Diseases (~20%)*
Rheumatoid arthritis
Systemic lupus erythematosus (SLE)
Mixed connective tissue disease (MCTD)
Scleroderma

*Postoperative (~5%)*
Postcardiac surgery

*Others (~20%)*
*Metabolic Diseases*
Uremia
Myxedema
*Pleura or Pulmonary Diseases*
*Trauma*
*Iatrogenic*
Pacemaker placement
Extraction of pacemaker leads
Coronary artery perforation
*Radiation Pericarditis*
*Post MI*
<10% in postthrombolytic era

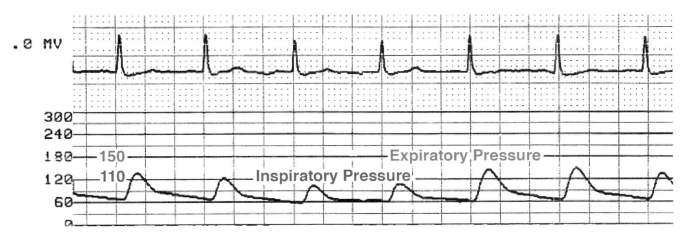

**Figure 72.2** Arterial pressure tracing showing significant decrease in arterial pressure in inspiration and increase in expiration (pulsus paradoxus).

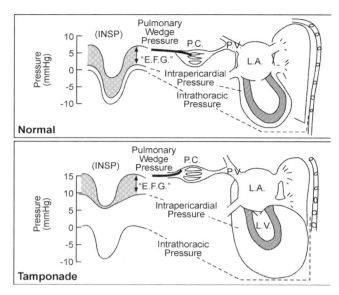

**Normal**

**Tamponade**

**Figure 72.3** Interrelationships between pulmonary capillary wedge pressure, intrathoracic pressure, and intrapericardial pressure during inspiration in normal subject and in patients with cardiac tamponade. Note that the intrapericardial pressure remains elevated in tamponade despite the decrease in intrathoracic pressure. PC, pulmonary capillary; PV, pulmonary veins; LA, left atrium; LV, left ventricle; EFG, effective filling gradient.

## Question

**2.** The patient undergoes further diagnostic testing, including a chest radiograph (CXR), echocardiogram (ECG), and right heart catheterization. Which of the following statements is *not* true?

**a)** "Water bottle heart" on CXR or pulsus alternans on the ECG are suggestive of large pericardial effusion.

**b)** Early diastolic collapse of right ventricular (RV) or RA, increased respiratory variation in mitral inflow, and distended IVC indicate presence of cardiac tamponade.

**c)** Equalization of pressure of RA and left atrial (LA) (the pulmonary capillary wedge pressure; PCWP) is pathognomonic of cardiac tamponade.

**d)** ECG is useful in determining the approach for draining the effusion.

**e)** Cardiac tamponade can occur with a small pericardial effusion.

## Answer and Explanation

**2. c.**

### Diagnosis

An ECG and CXR are performed routinely when a patient presents with symptoms of shortness of breath. In patients with pericardial effusion, the ECG may be normal or may show pulsus alternans in patients with a large effusion (Fig. 72.4). The classic appearance of a large pericardial effusion on a CXR is a "water bottle heart," showing a heart with a small base and enlarged cardiac silhouette that is different from that seen with chamber enlargements (Fig. 72.5). Transthoracic echocardiogram (TTE) is the imaging modality of choice to confirm the diagnosis of cardiac tamponade when it is clinically suspected.

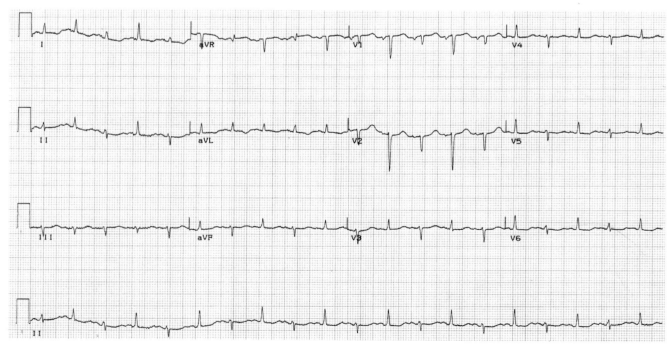

**Figure 72.4** The ECG in a patient with a large pericardial effusion demonstrates a classic electrical alternans pattern.

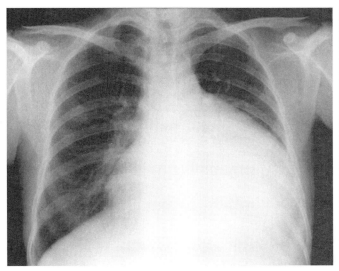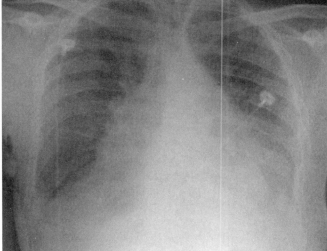

**Figure 72.5** Chest radiographs in patients with large pericardial effusion showing "water bottle heart" and enlarged cardiac silhouette.

The signs of cardiac tamponade on TTE are a collapse of the right atrium and right ventricle in early diastole. Prominent respiratory variation in flows across all cardiac valves is seen in patients with hemodynamic compromise. This is analogous to the change in systolic pressures seen with pulsus paradoxus. A distended inferior vena cava corroborates the clinically observed elevated JVP. Because TTE images are not optimal in postoperative patients with clinical signs of tamponade, transesophageal echocardiography (TEE) may be needed. TEE is very useful to evaluate for hematoma, which is common in postoperative patients.

Hemodynamic pressure measurements can help determine the functional significance of pericardial effusion in difficult cases. The increased intrapericardial pressure is transmitted to all cardiac chambers and, therefore, when the chambers are not actively contracting (diastole), pressures in all chambers are equal and reflect intrapericardial pressure. Although equalization of diastolic pressures [RA, LA (or PCWP), LV and RV] is typical for cardiac tamponade, it can be seen in other diseases affecting the pericardium, such as constrictive pericarditis.

*Treatment*

Volume resuscitation is the most important and useful medical intervention in patients with cardiac tamponade. Diuretics and vasodilators should not be used when tamponade is suspected. The definitive therapy for tamponade is drainage of pericardial fluid. In most situations, percutaneous drainage is the best approach. If the pericardial fluid is loculated and not approachable percutaneously, surgical drainage must be done. In trauma patients, surgical exploration is a must because pericardial hemorrhage is a sign for chamber rupture, and percutaneous drainage is contraindicated. Pericardial fluid can be drained percutaneously using a subcostal, apical, or parasternal approach.

The specific approach depends on the location of the fluid and operator preferences. ECG guidance is extremely helpful for the drainage procedure.

## Key Points

- Cardiac tamponade is a clinical diagnosis.
- Characteristic physical signs are pulsus paradoxus, increased JVP, and low BP.
- TTE is helpful in making the diagnosis of tamponade.
- Volume resuscitation and immediate drainage of the fluid are essential.
- Even a small amount of fluid (typically blood) can lead to tamponade if the accumulation is rapid.

## CASE 2: PAPILLARY MUSCLE RUPTURE

An 80-year-old woman with inferior myocardial infarction (MI) develops severe shortness of breath on day 4 after MI. On exam, she has a systolic murmur. An ECG was performed; it shows severe mitral regurgitation (MR).

## Question

**3.** Which of the following is least likely to be the cause of her MR?
a) Papillary muscle dysfunction
b) Papillary muscle rupture
c) Restricted mitral valve leaflet
d) Myxomatous degeneration of mitral valve
e) All of the above

## Answer and Explanation

**3. d.**

### Etiology

Mitral regurgitation (MR) occurs in almost one-fourth (13% to 45%) of the patients suffering MI. Post-MI MR can result due to various mechanisms. The most common mechanism is the restriction of the posterior mitral leaflet secondary to an akinetic inferior-posterior wall. The akinetic wall pulls the papillary muscle, thus restricting the movement of the posterior leaflet and leading to incomplete coaptation with the anterior leaflet and, finally, MR. The ischemic papillary muscle can cause MR through a similar mechanism. The most serious cause of MR after MI is papillary muscle rupture, which can be rapidly fatal if not recognized and treated immediately. Papillary muscle rupture occurs typically 1 to 7 days after MI. Papillary muscle rupture occurs most commonly after inferior MI because the blood supply of the posteromedial papillary muscle is from a single coronary artery, usually the posterior descending artery branch of the right coronary artery. The anterolateral papillary muscle derives its blood supply from dual coronaries (left anterior descending and left circumflex), making it less vulnerable to ischemic insult.

### Clinical Features

Patients with complete papillary muscle rupture may die of cardiogenic shock from severe acute MR. Patients with a rupture of one of the heads of the papillary muscle may present with sudden onset shortness of breath and hypotension. Interestingly, the MI leading to this complication is usually small in the vast majority of patients.

The signs of papillary muscle rupture include a new holosystolic murmur that is best heard at the apex and radiates to the axilla or to the base of the heart. The mur-mur may be soft and relatively short due to a rapid increase in LA pressure from acute, severe MR in a noncompliant left atrium.

### Diagnosis

An ECG shows evidence of recent inferior or posterior MI and the CXR reveals pulmonary edema. ECG is the diagnostic modality of choice to assess papillary muscle rupture. TEE may be needed to see the details of flail segment and the extent of papillary muscle involvement (Fig. 72.6 and Fig. 72.7). Hemodynamic monitoring with pulmonary artery catheterization shows a large V wave on the PCWP tracing (Fig. 72.8). The large V wave represents the increase in sudden LA pressure from severe MR and a noncompliant small LA that did not have a chance to dilate, as occurs in chronic causes of MR. It is important to note that large V waves also are seen with acute ventricular septal defect (VSD) after MI and therefore are not pathognomonic of acute MR.

### Treatment

Acute MR should be recognized early because 24-hour mortality is as high as 70% without immediate surgical repair. A high index of suspicion is required to diagnose this condition. Medical therapy with vasodilators to decrease afterload can be attempted after recognition of MR, but hypotension may limit the use of such therapy. In patients with hypotension and shock, an intraaortic balloon pump (IABP) should be placed. The IABP decreases afterload, improves coronary blood flow, and augments forward cardiac output. Urgent surgery is needed for the definitive repair of papillary muscle rupture.

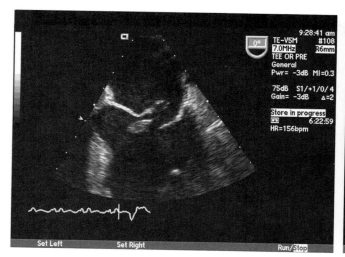
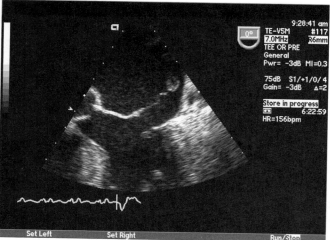

**Figure 72.6**  Transesophageal echocardiogram (TEE) of a patient with a ruptured head of the papillary muscle. The left panel shows a flail anterior mitral valve leaflet attached to the ruptured papillary muscle head in early systole. The right panel shows the flail mitral valve leaflet prolapsing into the left atrium during systole. In this view, the top and bottom chambers are the left atrium and left ventricle, respectively.

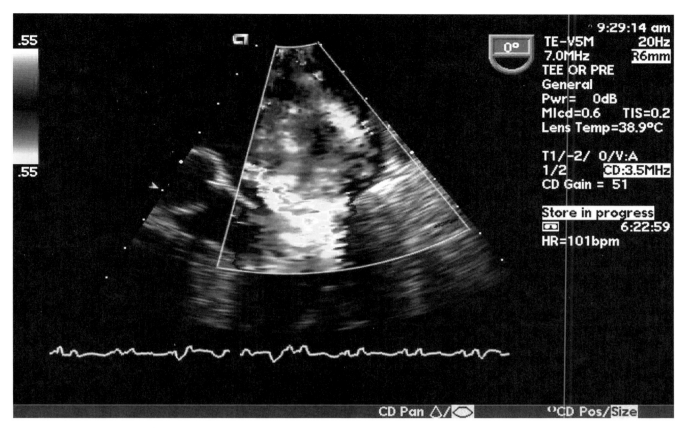

**Figure 72.7** Transesophageal echocardiogram (TEE) showing severe mitral regurgitation by color Doppler secondary to flail anterior mitral valve leaflet from a ruptured papillary muscle.

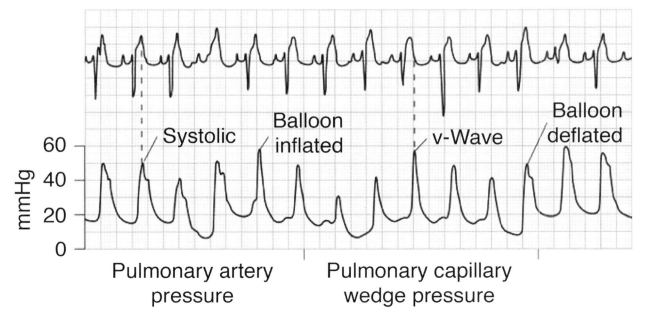

**Figure 72.8** Prominent V waves on PCWP tracing reflective of an increase in LA pressure from severe MR.

## Key Points

- Papillary muscle rupture causing acute MR is more common after inferior MI.
- Acute pulmonary edema is the most common clinical presentation.
- A new holosystolic murmur may be an early clue in papillary muscle rupture.
- ECG is the diagnostic imaging modality of choice.
- Immediate surgical repair can be lifesaving in these patients.

## CASE 3: FREE WALL RUPTURE

An 80-year-old woman presents to the hospital with severe chest pain for 4 hours and is found to have an acute anterior wall MI. She is taken to the cardiac catheterization laboratory emergently and her left anterior descending artery (LAD) is stented. A partial resolution of ST segments is achieved, and final flow in the LAD is TIMI II. She does well for 3 days, then starts having sharp substernal CP.

## Question

4. The likely cause for CP is:
a) Pericarditis
b) Recurrent MI
c) Pulmonary embolism
d) Myocardial rupture
e) All of the above

## Answer and Explanation

4. a.

### Etiology

Left ventricular free wall rupture is a catastrophic complication that can occur after transmural MI. It is seen in 1% to 8% of patients after an acute MI. Free wall rupture accounts for approximately 10% of mortality after MI. This complication is typically encountered 1 to 4 days after MI, although early (within 24 hours) or delayed (3 weeks) presentations have been reported.

Unlike papillary muscle rupture, free wall rupture is seen more frequently with anterior wall MI. Free wall rupture is seen more commonly in elderly woman, with a history of hypertension, and with prior use of steroids and nonsteroidal anti-inflammatory drugs (NSAIDs). It is more common with first MI, late thrombolytic therapy, and large transmural MI involving ≥20% of the myocardium.

### Clinical Features

Patients with acute free wall rupture die suddenly due to electromechanical dissociation. Patients with subacute rupture may present with chest pain and hypotension suggestive of pericarditis and tamponade. The signs of tamponade and a "to and fro" murmur have been described in subacute rupture, although this is uncommon.

### Diagnosis

A high index of clinical suspicion is necessary to make a timely diagnosis. Any patient with a complaint of sharp pain within the first few days after a large anterior MI should have ECG assessment. Intramural hematoma, partial rupture, subacute rupture, or any other mechanical complications of MI should be carefully excluded. Computed tomography (CT) or magnetic resonance imaging (MRI) may have a role in evaluation of some stable patients.

### Treatment

Anticoagulants should be discontinued immediately. Immediate surgical repair is the only treatment option for patient survival. Surgical mortality is high, however, and secondary failure (i.e., dehiscence of the patch) is common because the suturing may be difficult with a recent acute MI.

## Key Points

- Free wall rupture is a catastrophic complication after large transmural MI.
- Free wall rupture is seen more commonly after anterior MI.
- Surgery is a treatment option, but with significant limitations.

## CASE 4: LEFT VENTRICULAR PSEUDOANEURYSM

Left ventricular (LV) rupture contained by pericardial adhesions and thrombus is known as pseudoaneurysm. The pseudoaneurysm has a narrow neck, which is characterized by <50% of the size of the fundus of the aneurysm.

### Clinical Features

The patient typically presents with pleuritic pain. The presentation may be clinically silent and detected only on routine investigations. Alternatively, patients may present with heart failure symptoms and recurrent tachyarrhythmias. Examination may reveal a continuous murmur across the pseudoaneurysm.

### Diagnosis

A CXR may reveal cardiomegaly with an abnormal bulge of the cardiac shadow. The ECG may show persistent ST-segment elevation, as in a true left ventricular aneurysm.

A variety of imaging modalities are used to define the pseudoaneurysm. ECG, cardiac CT, and cardiac MRI are used to confirm the diagnosis (Fig. 72.9).

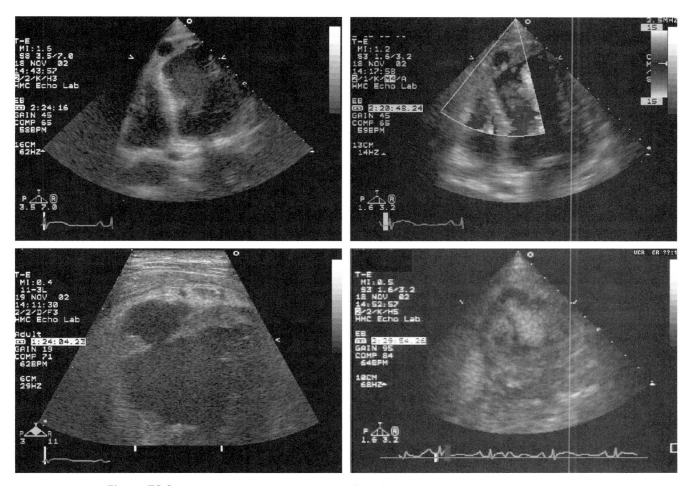

**Figure 72.9** Echocardiographic (ECG) images of a left ventricular pseudoaneurysm. The upper left panel shows an apical pseudoaneurysm and the upper right panel shows flow through the neck of the pseudoaneurysm. The bottom left panel shows the classic appearance of pseudoaneurysm, with a narrow neck. In the bottom right panel, echo contrast is used to delineate the pseudoaneurysm more clearly.

### Treatment

Patients with LV pseudoaneurysm must be referred for definitive surgical repair because of the risk for sudden rupture and death. This is irrespective of the size or symptoms.

### Key Points

- A contained LV free wall rupture is known as pseudoaneurysm.
- Surgical repair is the definitive treatment.

## CASE 5: VENTRICULAR SEPTAL DEFECT

A 79-year-old woman with no history of coronary artery disease presents with an inferior wall MI. The patient develops severe shortness of breath and hypotension. On exam, a loud holosystolic murmur with a thrill is detected. A Swan-Ganz catheter is placed. Oxygen saturation in the right atrium is 50%, and in the pulmonary artery it is 75%. A large V wave was noted on pulmonary capillary wedge tracing.

### Question

5. All the following statements are true, *except*
a) Acute VSD explains the systolic murmur and step up in saturation but not a large V wave.
b) VSD can happen with a relatively small MI.
c) Surgical repair is the best treatment option for this patient.
d) IABP prior to surgery may be helpful to stabilize the patient.
e) Recurrence of VSD after surgical repair is relatively common.

## Answer and Explanation

5. a.

### Etiology

VSD occurs as a result of necrosis of the interventricular septum following a transmural MI. It occurs in up to 2% of acute MI patients and accounts for 1% to 5% of in-hospital deaths. It is usually seen within 3 to 7 days after MI, but can occur as early as 24 hours post-MI. The early presentation is seen after inferior MI and after thrombolytic therapy. The incidence of acute VSD is similar after anterior and inferior MI. The typical patient with VSD is an elderly, hypertensive woman with multivessel disease that presented late after first MI and did not receive revascularization.

Acute VSD is located apically in anterior MI and posterior-basal in inferior MI. The defect may be a through-and-through hole or a serpiginous meshwork of channels. RV involvement is common with posterior-basal defects.

### Clinical Features

Patients with an acute VSD may present insidiously with few symptoms or may present precipitously with pulmonary edema, biventricular failure, and shock. A loud holosystolic murmur, best heard over the lower left sternal border, and associated with a systolic thrill, is present in 50% of patients. The intensity of murmur is inversely related to the defect size.

### Diagnosis

ECG with color-flow Doppler is very useful in the detection of a VSD. Echo is useful in assessing the location and extent of the defect and in the assessment of left and right ventricular function. Doppler flow helps to quantify the magnitude of the left-to-right shunt. Right heart catheterization with oximetry is helpful in the diagnosis of an acute VSD by demonstrating an oxygen step-up between the right atrium and pulmonary artery. The step allows the calculation of the shunt fraction. V waves on a PCWP tracing may be seen in acute VSD due to increased flow in the left atrium from the shunt.

### Treatment

Medical therapy has a minimal role but is helpful in stabilizing the patient prior to surgical treatment. Intravenous vasodilators, such as sodium nitroprusside, are the treatment of choice, because they help to decrease the left-to-right shunt and increase systemic flow. An IABP is helpful to decrease the systemic vascular resistance and therefore decrease left-to-right shunting. Surgical repair is the treatment of choice for all but the smallest VSD and should be performed early. Small VSDs have the best survival and posterior-basal VSDs have the worst prognosis. Percutaneous closure of a VSD using various closure devices has been reported, but this approach still has technical limitations depending on anatomical location and the nature of the defect.

## Key Points

- VSD occurs equally after anterior and inferior MI.
- Clinical presentation can be acute pulmonary edema, biventricular failure, or shock.
- A new holosystolic murmur with thrill is the important physical sign.
- ECG with color and Doppler and right heart catheterization with oxygen step-up are confirmatory tests.
- Surgical correction is the standard treatment, but percutaneous closure is emerging as a treatment option in some of these patients.

## CASE 6: AORTIC DISSECTION

A 40-year-old man presents with acute onset of chest pain radiating to the back, described as sharp and tearing. His blood pressure is 180/100 mm Hg. The cardiac examination is remarkable for tachycardia with normal first and second heart sounds and a soft 3/6 early diastolic murmur at the left lower sternal border. The lungs are clear. Distal pulses are equal bilaterally in both upper and lower extremities. Aortic dissection is suspected.

## Question

6. Which of the following statements is *true* about aortic dissection?
a) Thoracic aortic dissection is less common than abdominal aortic aneurysm rupture.
b) Marfan's syndrome is the most frequent cause of aortic dissection.
c) Blood pressure control is very important in ascending and descending aortic dissection.
d) Surgery is the treatment of choice for descending aortic dissection.
e) None of the above.

## Answer and Explanation

6. c.

### Etiology

Aortic dissection is the most common aortic emergency. The incidence is twice that of ruptured abdominal aortic aneurysm. It is rare in patients <40 years of age. It is seen most commonly between 50 and 70 years. The male-to-female ratio is 2:1. Aortic dissection is seen in patients with hypertension, Marfan's syndrome, Ehlers-Danlos syndrome, Turner's syndrome, giant cell arteritis, bicuspid aortic valve, and in any condition that leads to a medial degeneration of the aortic wall. The other causes for aortic dissection are blunt trauma and iatrogenic trauma, as may occur following cardiac catheterization, IABP placement, and cardiac surgery.

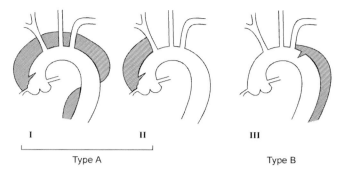

I          II          III

Type A                    Type B

**Figure 72.10**  Stanford and DeBakey classifications of aortic dissection by the anatomic location of intimal tear.

## Pathology

An intimal tear results in blood splitting the aortic media. This leads to a false lumen that can progress in an antegrade or retrograde direction. Aortic rupture can occur back into the lumen or externally into the pericardium or mediastinum. External rupture often results in fatal cardiac tamponade. The most common site of intimal tear is within 2 to 3 cm of the aortic valve. The second most common site is in the descending aorta distal to the left subclavian artery. The dissection can result in an occlusion of the aortic branches, such as the renal, spinal, coronary, or iliac arteries, and result in acute end organ ischemia.

## Classification

Two classifications that use anatomical location for dissection are commonly used, the Stanford classification Type A and B and the DeBakey classification types I, II, and III. (Fig. 72.10).

## Clinical Features

Aortic dissection usually presents with severe chest or back pain that starts upon physical exertion. The pain usually is sudden in onset and described as sharp, tearing, or stabbing. Other less common presentations include heart failure with acute aortic regurgitation or end-organ compromise (acute renal failure, paraplegia, acute limb ischemia, cerebrovascular accident, inferior MI, etc.) or syncope and collapse, in the case of tamponade. Examination may show hypertension or hypotension (depending on presentation), a soft early diastolic murmur of aortic regurgitation, and reduced or absent peripheral pulses.

## Diagnosis

The CXR may show a widened mediastinum. The electrocardiogram may be normal or may show evidence of acute MI if the coronary arteries are involved. The diagnosis can be confirmed through a variety of imaging modalities. The choice of test depends on availability of technology and the stability of the patient. TEE and CT scan are useful in emergency situations. CT scan and MRI are useful in the serial follow-up of chronic dissections.

## Treatment

Aggressive control of blood pressure is important in the initial management of ascending and descending aortic dissection. The primary aim is to reduce blood pressure and the rate of rise of blood pressure (dP/dT). The agents commonly used are intravenous $\alpha$- and $\beta$-blockers (e.g., labetalol) followed by sodium nitroprusside. Ascending aortic dissections require early surgical intervention. Surgery should be coordinated urgently because there occurs an approximately 1% mortality per hour in ascending aortic dissection. Type B dissections typically may be managed medically with aggressive blood pressure control. Percutaneous fenestrations can be considered if there is end-organ compromise from branches coming out of the false lumen. Surgery is reserved for situations in which the threat of aortic rupture is present.

## Key Points

- Aortic dissection is the most common aortic emergency.
- Sharp or tearing chest pain radiating to the back in a hypertensive patient should alert for the possibility of aortic dissection.
- Aggressive blood pressure control is essential in ascending and descending aortic dissection.
- Emergent surgery is needed for the best outcome after ascending aortic dissection.
- Conservative management is preferred for descending aortic dissection.
- Stenting of the aortic dissection is emerging as a promising new therapy for some patients with aortic dissection.

## SUGGESTED READINGS

Braunwald EG, ed. *Heart Disease. A Textbook of Cardiovascular Medicine*, 6th edition. New York: W. B. Saunders Company, 2001.
Shabetai R, ed. *Diseases of the Pericardium*. Cardiology Clinics, Philadelphia: W. B. Saunders, 1990.
Topol EJ, ed. *Textbook of Cardiovascular Medicine*, 2nd edition. Philadelphia: Lippincott Williams & Wilkins, 2002.

# Mock Board Simulation

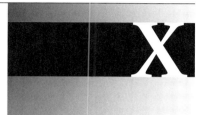

# Mock Board Simulation

**73**

*Amjad Almahameed    Amanda Curnock    Anil K. Jain*
*Vakesh Rajani*

## QUESTIONS

**1.** A 40-year-old woman with cirrhosis awaiting liver transplantation presents to the emergency department with an elevated serum creatinine level (3.0 mg/dL).

    Which of the following would be most supportive of the diagnosis of hepatorenal syndrome?
**a)** Fractional excretion of sodium ($FE_{Na}$) less than 1%
**b)** Normal urine output
**c)** Hypernatremia
**d)** Acute onset of the renal failure
**e)** The patient has primary biliary cirrhosis

**2.** A 55-year-old man undergoing hemodialysis three times a week missed his previous dialysis 2 days ago and presents to the emergency department, concerned about his missed dialysis. He is without specific complaints, except stating that he is several pounds over his dry weight. His vitals signs reveal that he is afebrile at 36.5°C, heart rate is 80/bpm, respiratory rate is 14/min, and blood pressure is 130/80 mm Hg. He has no jugular venous distension. His lungs are clear, and his heart sounds are regular with no $S_3$ gallop or murmur. He has 1+ peripheral edema. His chemistry profile shows $Na^+$ 138 mEq/L, $K^+$ 5.8 mEq/L, $Cl^-$ 104 mEq/L, $HCO_{3-}$ 22 mEq/L, blood urea nitrogen (BUN) 120 mg/dL, creatinine 7.0 mg/dL, and glucose 125 mg/dL. An electrocardiogram (ECG) performed because of hyperkalemia is normal.

    Which of the following is an indication for emergent hemodialysis in this patient?
**a)** Hyperkalemia
**b)** Elevated BUN
**c)** Elevated creatinine
**d)** Metabolic acidosis
**e)** None of the above

**3.** An 88-year-old woman is admitted to the hospital after a fall that resulted in a fractured hip. She previously lived alone and cared for most of her daily needs. She had recently employed a helper to do the weekly shopping and the heavier housework because the arthritis in her knees was limiting her efficiency in performing this heavier work. She had hip surgery yesterday, and today you are asked by the orthopedic surgeon to see her as a medical consult because she is combative and trying to get out of bed. The history and examination are difficult to perform because she fluctuates between falling asleep and shouting that she needs to go to the shops because the cupboards are empty and she has no food. She will listen to you and follow simple commands, but she is easily distracted by the noises of the hospital, is unable to concentrate, and wants to leave the bed to go shopping.

    All the following are true about the most likely cause of her confusion, *except*
**a)** It is a common condition in the hospitalized elderly.
**b)** Common causes include medications.
**c)** The best plan for her safety is to restrain her with soft restraints until the confusion resolves.
**d)** A reduced level of consciousness and inability to focus or sustain concentration are key characteristics.
**e)** Perceptual disturbances such as illusions, hallucinations, and delusions help establish the diagnosis.

**4.** A 60-year-old Asian man is referred to you for evaluation of a heart murmur. He speaks no English and is not accompanied by any family member able to translate. As you wait for the translator to arrive, you are able to communicate sufficiently to obtain permission for a physical examination. His pulse is regular, with a rate of 80/bpm; blood pressure is 100/85 mm Hg. Carotid pulse has a slow upstroke. No jugular venous distension is present. The apex is slightly displaced laterally. A systolic thrill is palpable over the aortic area and carotids. Auscultation reveals a harsh ejection systolic murmur. Valsalva's maneuver does not accentuate the murmur. The second aortic sound is soft.

    With which of the following are these findings most consistent?
**a)** Mitral regurgitation
**b)** Mitral valve prolapse
**c)** Aortic stenosis
**d)** Hypertrophic obstructive cardiomyopathy
**e)** Mitral stenosis

**5.** A 42-year-old man presents with intermittent chest pain. Further history reveals that the character of the pain is typical of angina. He also has had episodes of dyspnea, dizziness, and syncope. He is a nonsmoker and denies illicit drug use. His past medical history is significant for tonsillectomy in childhood. Family history includes the sudden death of his brother at age 33 years of unknown cause. On examination of the cardiovascular system, the pulse is regular, with a rate of 68/bpm, and no jugular venous distension is present. The apical impulse is forceful and displaced laterally. A double apical impulse and a palpable systolic thrill are present. On auscultation of the heart, an $S_4$ and an ejection systolic murmur are heard. ECG shows left ventricular hypertrophy and Q waves in the inferior and lateral precordial leads. Chest radiograph reveals a mild increase in the cardiac silhouette. Echocardiographic findings include left ventricular hypertrophy with asymmetric septal hypertrophy and a small left ventricular cavity.

This murmur may be increased by all of the following, *except*
a) Dopamine
b) Amyl nitrite
c) Diuretics
d) Valsalva's maneuver
e) Handgrip

**6.** Which of the following statements regarding acute tubular necrosis (ATN) is false?
a) If the primary insult can be corrected, most patients with ATN have a renal failure phase of 7 to 21 days followed by increased urine output and then recovery.
b) ATN is the most frequent cause of acute renal failure at tertiary care hospitals.
c) The $FE_{Na}$ is usually greater than 2% in patients with ATN.
d) Because of decreased urine output in ATN, the urine is abnormally concentrated, resulting in a urine osmolality greater than 450 mOsm/kg.
e) The absence of muddy-brown granular and epithelial casts on urine sediment examination does not exclude the diagnosis of ATN.

**7.** A previously healthy 25-year-old man presents to his internist after referral from the emergency department for microhematuria. His vital signs and physical examination are normal. His urine dipstick is positive for both 1+ protein and 3+ hemoglobin (Hgb), and the urine sediment, examined under the microscope, reveals red and white blood cells (WBCs) with granular and red cell casts. On further questioning, he denies a history of cough, hemoptysis, chest pain, sinus infections, or dyspnea. The chemistry profile reveals a BUN level of 40 mg/dL and a creatinine level of 4.0 mg/dL. He is sent for further testing, including a chest radiograph, which is reportedly normal. Anti–glomerular basement membrane (GBM) antibody testing is positive, as is testing for perinuclear pattern anti-neutrophil cytoplasmic antibodies (P-ANCA). A complete blood count (CBC) is normal.

Which of the following statements is false?
a) He has Goodpasture's syndrome.
b) He has anti-GBM antibody disease.
c) He has antibodies directed against myeloperoxidase.
d) He has antibodies directed against a chain of the type IV collagen found in basement membranes.
e) He has a more treatable disease than he would if P-ANCA tests were negative.

**8.** The risk of ovarian cancer increases with all of the following, *except*
a) First-degree relative with ovarian cancer
b) Early menarche
c) Late menopause
d) Nulliparity
e) Use of an oral contraceptive for more than 3 years

**9.** A 48-year-old man presents with his wife, who complains of her husband's snoring. Further history reveals snoring for at least 20 years, with restless sleep observed by the wife. The patient denies any problem sleeping, but on direct questioning, he admits to dry mouth and headaches in the morning and sleepiness throughout the day. He confesses that he almost fell asleep at the wheel of the car several times, but he ascribes this to long hours and overwork. Physical examination reveals a stocky man, somewhat overweight, but the examination is otherwise normal.

Which would be the most appropriate next step?
a) Sedative medication for the patient to ensure that he gets a better night's sleep
b) Sedative medication for the wife so that she can sleep through his snoring
c) Sending the patient for sleep studies
d) Advising a weight loss program and following up in 6 months
e) Advising stopping smoking because doing so has been proven to stop snoring in more than 50% of patients

**10.** All the following statements are true of cystic fibrosis, *except*
a) The disease is autosomal recessive in inheritance.
b) *Pseudomonas* organisms are ultimately isolated from the respiratory secretions of most patients.
c) Sinus disease develops in most patients.
d) A sweat chloride test result of less than 70 mEq/L is highly suggestive of cystic fibrosis.
e) More than 95% of men with cystic fibrosis are infertile.

**11.** A 32-year-old woman presents with double vision. The significant findings on examination include ptosis, diplopia, and facial weakness, causing her to appear to snarl when she attempts to smile. During counting aloud, her speech becomes progressively less distinct and more nasal. Proximal muscle weakness is present, which increases with repetitive movements and improves with rest.

All the following statements are true about this disease, *except*

a) It is more common in women.
b) The most common ages at presentation are the 20s and 30s for women and the 60s for men.
c) Pupils are small and irregular and react to accommodation but not to light.
d) The diagnostic test involves intravenous injection of an anticholinesterase inhibitor.
e) A pathophysiologically similar syndrome that affects proximal muscles but improves with brief exercise is associated with malignancy, most commonly small cell carcinoma of the lung.

**12.** A 55-year-old white man was recently diagnosed with colon cancer. He asks you what the average survival at 5 years is for people with his type of cancer. You obtain the surgical pathology report that indicates that the cancer extends into the perirectal fat. In addition, the report indicates that regional nodes are also involved.

You report to him that the average 5-year survival is

a) 70% to 80%
b) 80% to 90%
c) 60% to 70%
d) 40% to 60%
e) Less than 40%

**13.** You are seated in the hospital cafeteria in the middle of a busy call day when the medical student with whom you are having dinner complains of pruritus and appears flushed. He states that he has felt like this previously, is allergic to peanuts, and thinks that there may have been nuts in the cake that he just ate. He states that he does not feel too bad and that this is nothing like the last time, when he had some difficulty with breathing; he says that he will go lie down in the call room for a while and he should be fine. You assess his airway and breathing, and they are normal.

What would be the most appropriate next step?

a) Let him go and rest; you will go and see a patient who has just arrived and then check on the medical student in an hour or so.
b) Keep him with you so that you can take him to the emergency department if he starts to feel any worse or has any pulmonary symptoms.
c) Take him to the emergency department, and administer 1 mL of 1:10,000 epinephrine intravenously with cardiac monitoring.
d) Take him to the emergency department, recruit assistance from the medical team there, have his airway and cardiopulmonary status assessed and monitored, obtain intravenous access, and administer 0.5 mL of 1:1,000 epinephrine subcutaneously or intramuscularly as soon as possible.
e) Give him an antihistamine that you happen to have in your pocket, and keep him with you so that you can take him to the emergency department if he starts to feel any worse or has any pulmonary symptoms.

**14.** A solitary pulmonary nodule is seen on the chest radiograph of a 60-year-old woman. You request computerized tomography (CT) of the chest.

Which of the following patterns of calcification is compatible with carcinoma as a cause rather than a benign lesion?

a) Popcorn calcification
b) Laminated calcification
c) Central calcification
d) Eccentric calcification
e) Diffuse homogeneous calcification

**15.** A 55-year-old man with a history of polycythemia vera sees his family physician for routine follow-up. A hematocrit (Hct) drawn at the visit is 48%.

Which of the following is most likely?

a) The iron stores in his bone marrow would be increased.
b) He has decreased cerebral blood flow and is at increased risk of thrombotic complications.
c) His bone marrow will be hypocellular, except for hyperplasia of red cell progenitors.
d) An increased level of circulating erythropoietin is present in his plasma.
e) He does not have an increased bleeding tendency due to preservation of platelet function.

**16.** A 30-year-old man, who has been your patient for several years, presents for his regular checkup. He is known to have dextrocardia. He suffers from recurrent sinusitis and for years has had mucopurulent sputum and episodic hemoptysis. He has digital clubbing and bilateral crackles on auscultation of the lungs.

With which of the following conditions are this patient's symptoms most consistent?

a) $\alpha_1$-Antitrypsin deficiency
b) Kartagener's syndrome
c) Young's syndrome
d) Williams-Campbell syndrome
e) Yellow nail syndrome

**17.** A 38-year-old man with a history of hepatitis B virus infection and significant alcohol abuse, who has not seen a physician in 7 years, presents to the emergency department with fever and altered sensorium. On examination, he is febrile, tachycardic, hypotensive, and somnolent. He is markedly jaundiced, with a distended abdomen. Initial blood work reveals a $Na^+$ level of 130 mg/dL, creatinine level of 1.6 mg/dL, Hgb of 10 mg/dL, and platelet count of 90,000/$mm^3$.

Which of the following diagnoses is most consistent with these findings?

a) Splenic sequestration
b) Idiopathic thrombocytopenic purpura
c) Thrombotic thrombocytopenic purpura (TTP)

**d)** Heparin-induced thrombocytopenia

**e)** Systemic lupus erythematosus (SLE)

**18.** A 32-year-old woman is referred to you from her obstetrician. She has had mild hypertension for several years but has been hesitant to start any medications. She is now attempting to have a baby and is concerned that her elevated blood pressure may pose a risk to her baby. She is also concerned that any medications that she takes not be harmful to the fetus. At a preconception visit, her obstetrician recommended consultation with you. She denies any complaints. Her blood pressure during this visit is 160/90 mm Hg, and her heart rate is 85/bpm. She has a normal physical examination. Urinalysis is negative.

You tell her all the following, *except*

**a)** Methyldopa and hydralazine have been shown to be safe to the developing fetus.

**b)** Reducing her blood pressure will reduce the chances of preeclampsia or eclampsia developing.

**c)** Eighty-five percent of hypertensive women have uncomplicated pregnancies.

**d)** Some women with mild hypertension can stop antihypertensive medications in the second trimester.

**e)** Drug treatment would be indicated if hypertensive end-organ damage were found on evaluation.

**19.** A 45-year-old man reports generalized fatigue. Vital signs and physical examination are normal, but an initial CBC reveals a leukocyte count of 7,000/mm$^3$, Hgb of 7 mg/dL, Hct of 20%, and platelet count of 300,000/mm$^3$. The mean cell volume (MCV) is normal. Additional blood work is ordered to diagnose the cause of his anemia.

Which of the following statements is correct?

**a)** In iron deficiency anemia, marrow iron stores are absent, and the serum iron level is low, whereas the erythrocyte porphyrin level is high.

**b)** In iron deficiency anemia, marrow iron stores are absent, and the serum iron, serum ferritin, and erythrocyte porphyrin levels are depressed.

**c)** In anemia of chronic disease, the red blood cells (RBCs) become hypochromic and microcytic.

**d)** The reticulocyte index in both iron deficiency anemia and anemia of chronic disease increases to compensate for the anemia.

**e)** None of the above.

**20.** A 26-year-old man has had recurrent episodes of mild, crampy abdominal pain accompanied by bloody diarrhea over the last year. He has no other significant past medical history and does not smoke or drink alcohol. He has undergone colonoscopy as part of his evaluation. The colon appears to be continuously inflamed from the anal verge to the more proximal colon. Shallow ulcers were noted, and there were no hemorrhoids. Biopsy is consistent with ulcerative colitis. He now presents with a 5-day history of bloody diarrhea and mild abdominal pain with a rather abrupt onset. Stool studies are negative for *Clostridium difficile* or a microbiologic cause of colitis.

All the following are true about this patient's condition, *except*

**a)** Total parenteral nutrition is not effective as primary therapy.

**b)** Sulfasalazine can be effective in maintaining remission, as well as in acute disease.

**c)** If he responds to a corticosteroid, he should be maintained on it indefinitely once in remission.

**d)** Sclerosing cholangitis may be an associated condition.

**e)** Oral anticholinergics for control of symptoms are contraindicated.

**21.** A 50-year-old woman presents for a routine annual examination. She feels well. Past medical history is notable for peptic ulcer disease. Examination reveals a healthy-appearing middle-aged woman. Results of a chemistry panel are as follows:

| | |
|---|---|
| Na$^+$ | 136 mEq/L |
| K$^+$ | 3.9 mEq/L |
| Cl | 102 mEq/L |
| HCO$_3$ | 26 mEq/L |
| BUN | 18 mg/dL |
| Creatinine | 1.0 mg/dL |
| Mg$^{2+}$ | 2.1 mg/dL |
| Ca$^{2+}$ | 11 mg/dL |
| P | 2.0 mg/dL |
| Albumin | 4.0 g/dL |

Her parathyroid hormone level is 90 pg/mL.

All the following statements about the diagnosis are true, *except*

**a)** An increased level of urinary excretion of cyclic adenosine monophosphate is present.

**b)** The majority of patients are symptomatic at presentation.

**c)** This condition occurs in multiple endocrine neoplasia types 1 and 2a.

**d)** Peptic ulceration and pancreatitis may be associated.

**e)** A single abnormal gland is the cause in approximately 80% of patients.

**22.** A 19-year-old man is seen in an urgent care center. He reports dysuria for the last 2 days and admits to two sexual partners in the last 3 weeks. Physical examination reveals an otherwise healthy man with a purulent urethral discharge. A Gram's-stained smear of the discharge reveals intracellular Gram-negative diplococci.

Along with appropriate counseling and serologic testing, which of the following would be the most appropriate treatment?

**a)** Intramuscular dose of a long-acting antimicrobial, such as benzathine penicillin G combined with a 7-day course of doxycycline

b) Single intramuscular dose of ceftriaxone, 125 mg

c) Single oral dose of azithromycin, 2 g

d) Single oral dose of ciprofloxacin, 500 mg

e) Intramuscular dose of cefazolin, 0.5 g, with a 7-day course of doxycycline

**23.** A 64-year-old man schedules an urgent visit for severe pain in his right great toe. The pain was sudden in onset and has prevented him from bearing weight on the right foot. He was recently hospitalized for elective coronary angioplasty and is also known to have moderate renal sufficiency as a result of long-standing diabetes mellitus. His medications consist of aspirin, lisinopril, and glyburide. He does not drink alcohol and is an ex-smoker. Physical examination shows him to be in moderate distress, and the right first metatarsophalangeal joint is inflamed. A polarizing light microscope is used to examine an aspirate from the joint, and needle-shaped crystals with negative birefringence are seen. A Gram's stain of the fluid is negative for bacteria.

What would be the *least* appropriate next step in management?

a) Single intramuscular dose of adrenocorticotropic hormone

b) Intravenous colchicine given through a carefully placed intravenous catheter

c) High dose of indomethacin

d) Allopurinol given orally for at least 2 weeks

e) Stopping aspirin and commencing naproxen

**24.** A 28-year-old woman reports palpitations for the last 6 months. They are accompanied by lightheadedness, chest pressure, and nausea. Initially, they tended to occur only two or three times a day; however, they have now become more frequent, and she has missed work on several occasions and has stopped socializing with friends except at her own home. She has no psychiatric history and does not drink alcohol or abuse drugs. Her caffeine intake is limited. Her family history is notable for maternal hypertension; her father suffered a stroke 7 months ago. The workup reveals no evidence of thyroid disease. Ambulatory ECG monitoring shows that her symptoms are accompanied by sinus tachycardia.

All the following statements about her condition are true, *except*

a) She may benefit from a short-acting benzodiazepine, such as alprazolam.

b) She may benefit from a serotonin reuptake inhibitor, such as paroxetine, in a dose similar to that used for depression.

c) First-degree relatives have an increased incidence of the same condition.

d) Behavioral exposure techniques may be helpful.

e) Patients using alcohol to relax in social situations have a lower incidence of this condition.

**25.** A 69-year-old businessman is assessed for halitosis and a sensation of fullness in his throat. On being questioned, he explains that he is embarrassed by this and has started to avoid social situations. He has also found that he has some difficulty in swallowing that seems to be relieved by bringing up foul-smelling food particles. He has tried over-the-counter famotidine without relief.

Which of the following is the single, most likely diagnosis?

a) Dental abscess

b) Gastroesophageal reflux disease

c) Zenker's diverticulum

d) Globus pharyngeus

e) Progressive systemic sclerosis

**26.** A 17-year-old woman reports aching in the groin area. She is athletic, jogs several miles a day, and is a member of a cheerleading team. She describes an abnormal sensation over the anterolateral thigh. On occasion, she has noticed an "electric jab" type sensation on extending the knee and has curtailed her running. Her past medical history is noncontributory, and she feels well otherwise. You observed her gait to be normal when she entered the office. A normal range of movement is present on examination, and reflexes in the lower extremities are symmetric. Tenderness is not elicited.

What is the most likely diagnosis?

a) Early onset hip arthritis (limited internal rotation)

b) Multiple sclerosis (MS)

c) Lumbar disc herniation (decreased knee reflex, posterior quadriceps weakness)

d) Lateral cutaneous nerve syndrome

e) Trochanteric bursitis

**27.** A 40-year-old man undergoing treatment for lymphoma presents with new-onset vertigo. On further questioning, he also admits to a change in his sense of taste. Along with his prescribed medications, he is also self-medicating with Echinacea. On physical examination, he has a vesicular rash in the right external auditory canal and right-sided facial palsy.

Which is the most likely etiology of his new symptoms?

a) Side effect of herbal medication

b) Disseminated malignancy

c) A virus often identified by Tzanck smear

d) Parvovirus infection

e) A virus often identified by heterophile antibody testing

**28.** A 21-year-old woman is seen in the outpatient department with a 3-month history of watery diarrhea. She has had similar episodes on three prior occasions, with negative stool cultures. Past medical history is notable for knee surgery 2 years ago. Her medications include an oral contraceptive. She has not traveled out of state in the recent past and is a nonsmoker. Examination reveals a slender woman in no acute distress. Office proctoscopy shows black mucosa but an otherwise normal examination.

Which of the following statements is correct?
a) Colonoscopy with multiple biopsies should be the next step in management.
b) Fecal smears should be examined using fluorescent techniques.
c) The patient's condition is highly infectious.
d) The patient's condition could be explained by surreptitious laxative abuse.
e) All first-degree relatives should undergo genetic testing.

**29.** A 41-year-old man reports dull pain over the maxillary areas for the last 10 days and a yellow nasal discharge. He has tried over-the-counter nasal decongestants without relief. Physical examination shows that percussion of the teeth causes pain. You recommend the use of oxymetazoline 0.05% spray and a 10-day course of trimethoprim-sulfamethoxazole. He is seen in routine follow-up 4 months later when he explains that his symptoms did improve for a few days but soon returned. His symptoms are much the same as they were 4 months ago, but he now has a postnasal drip associated with cough.

Which of the following statements relating to this patient's condition is incorrect?
a) Oral amoxicillin for 1 month would be an acceptable next step in management.
b) CT is more sensitive than plain radiography.
c) Up to one-third of patients may respond to treatment with an antihistamine and decongestant preparation.
d) A topical corticosteroid is contraindicated.
e) For patients who do not respond to empiric medical therapy, surgical drainage should be considered.

**30.** A 64-year-old diabetic woman is hospitalized with a diagnosis of myocardial infarction (MI). During the hospitalization, she undergoes coronary angiography and is discharged on the sixth day. You see her in follow-up 8 weeks later, and she explains that she has right-sided shoulder discomfort. She also reports some stiffness in the fingers of her right hand. She explains the pain has come on gradually and is not related to ambulation. Use of the upper extremity on her dominant left side is without pain. She explains that after her hospitalization, she felt low in her mood, and a psychiatrist told her that she was depressed. Physical examination reveals significant reduction in both active and passive range of motion of the right shoulder compared with the left side. Movement of the right shoulder is painful. Tenderness to palpation also is present. Plain radiographs of the shoulder are reported as normal.

Which is the most likely cause of her shoulder pain?
a) Adhesive capsulitis
b) Impingement syndrome
c) Angina
d) Rotator cuff tear
e) Fibromyalgia

**31–35.** From the list below, match the characteristic clinical and laboratory feature with the appropriate vasculitis in questions 31 to 35:
a) Arterial bruits are present, and there are no peripheral pulses.
b) Pulmonary involvement is manifested as asthma.
c) Angiographic evidence of aneurysms is present in the small- and medium-sized arteries of the kidneys.
d) Nonsyphilitic interstitial keratitis is present with vestibuloauditory symptoms.
e) Positive antineutrophil cytoplasmic antibody test is highly specific.

**31.** Wegener's granulomatosis

**32.** Churg-Strauss disease

**33.** Polyarteritis nodosa

**34.** Takayasu's arteritis

**35.** Cogan's syndrome

**36.** A 29-year-old woman is seen in the outpatient department with a dry cough, dyspnea, and headache for 2 weeks. A physician in employee health gave her a 5-day course of clarithromycin without improvement. She had previously been well, except for recurrent sinus infections from which she is presently asymptomatic. She is not taking any medications at the moment, does not smoke, and has not traveled outside the country. Symptoms of fatigue since she returned from a field trip to Arizona 3 weeks ago have caused her to miss several days from work. On examination, a nonspecific maculopapular erythematous rash is noted. A chest radiograph demonstrates a focal upper lobe infiltrate and hilar adenopathy. Biopsy of the rash shows eosinophilic infiltrates.

Which is the most likely cause of this presentation?
a) *Mycoplasma* pneumonia
b) Lyme borreliosis
c) Varicella pneumonia
d) Coccidioidal pneumonia (valley fever)
e) Streptococcal pneumonia

**37.** Which of the following statements regarding hepatitis C is false?
a) In patients with chronic infection with hepatitis C virus, hepatitis A virus immunization is indicated if patients have not previously been exposed.
b) Chronic infection develops in approximately 20% of patients.
c) Cirrhosis develops in 20% of infected patients.
d) Cryoglobulinemia is associated.
e) Of patients with hepatitis C, 30% to 40% have no identifiable risk factors for acquiring the infection.

**38.** A 42-year-old man is found to be anemic on workup for fatigue. He has been taking multivitamins and oral iron supplements for the last 20 years. He is a nonsmoker and seldom drinks alcohol. On direct questioning, he explains that he has frequent bowel movements with stools that are difficult to flush away. Physical examination is notable for a blistering rash at the elbows and knees. On testing, he is found to be anemic, with a mean corpuscular volume (MCV) of 65. Review of his peripheral blood smear demonstrates Howell-Jolly bodies. Endomysial antibody test result is positive, and antinuclear antibody test negative. He is instructed to eat a gluten-free diet, and his symptoms improve.

All the following statements about this patient's condition are true, *except*

a) A positive endomysial antibody test is consistent with the clinical picture.
b) Small bowel biopsy shows periodic acid–Schiff-positive granules in macrophages.
c) Lymphoma is a late complication.
d) Osteomalacia is an association.
e) Response to the gluten-free diet is diagnostic.

**39.** A 27-year-old man, a concert pianist, reports gradually worsening back pain and stiffness for 6 months. He describes the pain as being worst on waking and located in the lumbar and gluteal region. He recalls being awakened by the pain on a number of occasions, and he has arisen and stretched his back to relieve the discomfort. Taking a warm shower helps alleviate the stiffness, and sitting for prolonged periods exacerbates it. The Schrober test demonstrates a separation of 3 cm.

Which of the following is most compatible with this patient's illness?

a) Occupation-related illness
b) The finding of an early diastolic murmur
c) Positive antinuclear antibodies (ANA) test
d) A disease moderately responsive to systemic glucocorticoids
e) Dry mouth and eyes

**40.** A new ultrasound technique is available to screen for ovarian cancer. The sensitivity is said to be 80% and the specificity 95%. The prevalence of ovarian cancer is thought to be 2% in a sample population of adult women.

If the entire sample population undergoes imaging with the new technique, what will be the predictive value of a positive test?

a) 10%
b) 49%
c) 24%
d) 80%
e) 95%

**41.** A 25-year-old woman reports rectal bleeding. She is admitted for further investigation. Physical examination reveals pigmented lesions of the mouth, hands, and feet. Radiologic investigation shows multiple polypoid

tumors of the small bowel, which are also found on endoscopic evaluation of the ascending colon. Biopsy demonstrates findings consistent with hamartomas.

Which of the following statements about this woman's condition is correct?

a) An increased incidence of ovarian sex cord tumors is present in patients with this condition.
b) A high risk of colonic malignancy is present.
c) Total colectomy is absolutely indicated.
d) First-line treatment is a corticosteroid.
e) The inheritance pattern of this condition is autosomal recessive.

**42.** A 28-year-old woman reports not being able to sleep. On questioning, she admits to having lost 8 lb over the last 4 weeks despite an increased appetite. She also feels weak and has noticed difficulty in climbing stairs. Her menstrual cycle has become irregular over the last few months. On examination, she appears restless, and a stare-like gaze is particularly noticeable. Her pulse is 96/bpm, and she appears diaphoretic. Diffuse enlargement of the thyroid gland is present. The dorsa of the legs show thickening of the dermis. Thyroid function tests are reported as follows:

| | |
|---|---|
| Serum thyroid-stimulating hormone | Undetectable |
| Serum T4 | 22 µg/dL |
| Serum T3 | 690 µg/dL |
| Free T4 index | 35 |
| Radioactive iodine uptake | 40% |

Methimazole is started.

Which of the following statements about this patient's condition is false?

a) Once a euthyroid state is achieved, the dose of methimazole can be reduced.
b) Once a euthyroid state is achieved, methimazole can be continued at the original dose and levothyroxine supplementation started.
c) Leukopenia is a potential complication.
d) Hypertrophic pulmonary osteoarthropathy may be seen.
e) Thyroglobulin levels will be low at the time of diagnosis.

**43–47.** Match the following drugs with the mechanism by which they can raise blood pressure in hypertensive patients in questions 43 to 47:

a) Alcohol
b) Prednisone
c) Nonsteroidal antiinflammatory drugs (NSAIDs)
d) Monoamine oxidase inhibitors
e) Cold formulas

**43.** Prevention of metabolism of norepinephrine

**44.** Increased cortisol levels

**45.** Promotion of sodium retention

**46.** Increased peripheral resistance and activation of the sympathetic nervous system

**47.** Iatrogenic Cushing's disease

**48.** Which of the following statements relating to colorectal cancer is false?
a) High-fat diet increases the risk of colorectal cancer.
b) High-fiber diet has a protective effect.
c) Personal history of female genital or breast cancer increases the risk for colorectal cancer.
d) Fecal occult blood testing is highly specific.
e) Hereditary nonpolyposis colon cancer is an autosomal dominant disease.

**49.** A 45-year-old man has recently moved into the area and has been renovating his home. He reports severe pain over the right elbow and back of the upper forearm. Examination reveals pain to pressure over the wrist extensor muscles 1 cm below the lateral epicondyle. Strength is preserved.

Which of the following is the most likely cause of his pain?
a) Tennis elbow
b) Radial nerve entrapment
c) Olecranon bursitis
d) Ruptured biceps tendon
e) Golfer's elbow

**50.** All the following statements about the cough associated with angiotensin-converting enzyme (ACE) inhibitors are true, *except*
a) Dry and hacking
b) More frequent in asthmatics
c) Women affected more often than men
d) Generally occurring on rechallenge
e) Usually beginning within 1 to 2 weeks of institution of therapy

**51.** The following statements about influenza therapy are true, *except*
a) In recommended populations, frequency of immunization is annual because of the changing strains, as well as immunity declining over the year.
b) Concurrent administration of influenza and pneumococcal vaccines is safe and does not affect the effectiveness of either vaccine.
c) In a known outbreak of influenza B in a nursing home, amantadine or rimantadine should be prescribed with the vaccination because these drugs have been shown to reduce the development of influenza B.
d) Amantadine and rimantadine have been shown to be beneficial as prophylaxis in some situations.
e) Vaccination for pregnant women of at least 14 weeks' gestation is indicated because they are at risk for influenza-related complications.

**52.** A 25-year-old man reports a lump and tenderness in the left inguinal region. On examination, he is afebrile with tender left-sided inguinal and femoral lymphadenopathy. No genital ulceration or penile discharge is present.

All the following statements regarding the diagnosis of lymphogranuloma venereum (LGV) are true, *except*
a) The patient may have had a self-limited genital ulcer at the inoculation site.
b) The presentation of unilateral lymphadenopathy is an unusual presentation of LGV.
c) The diagnosis is made by serologic markers after other causes of inguinal lymphadenopathy are excluded.
d) Doxycycline, 100 mg orally twice daily for 3 weeks, is the recommended treatment regimen.
e) The infectious agent that causes LGV is *Chlamydia trachomatis.*

**53–55.** You are considering the options for antianginal medications for a patient with stable angina. Select the major side effect associated with the medications in questions 53 to 55:
a) Constipation
b) Bronchospasm
c) Hypercalcemia
d) Headache
e) Hypertension

**53.** Verapamil

**54.** Nitroglycerin

**55.** Propranolol

**56.** A 30-year-old woman is brought to the emergency department by ambulance after her boyfriend found her in her garage. He says that she may have ingested antifreeze. She is comatose.

Which of the following sets of laboratory studies is most consistent with her diagnosis?
a) $Na^+$ 141 mEq/L, $K^+$ 2.6 mEq/L, $Cl^-$ 115 mEq/L, $HCO_3^-$ 14 mEq/L, creatinine 3.0 mg/dL, arterial pH 7.31, urine pH 6.1
b) $Na^+$ 138 mEq/L, $K^+$ 6.2 mEq/L, $Cl^-$ 107 mEq/L, $HCO_3^-$ 18 mEq/L, creatinine 3.0 mg/dL, arterial pH 7.34, urine pH 5.2
c) $Na^+$ 144 mEq/L, $K^+$ 4.7 mEq/L, $Cl^-$ 100 mEq/L, $HCO_3^-$ 10 mEq/L, creatinine 3.0 mg/dL, arterial pH 7.25, urine pH 5.0
d) $Na^+$ 136 mEq/L, $K^+$ 4.4 mEq/L, $Cl^-$ 108 mEq/L, $HCO_3^-$ 20 mEq/L, creatinine 3.0 mg/dL, arterial pH 7.38, urine pH 5.0
e) $Na^+$ 140 mEq/L, $K^+$ 5.2 mEq/L, $Cl^-$ 105 mEq/L, $HCO_3^-$ 22 mEq/L, creatinine 3.0 mg/dL, arterial pH 7.36, urine pH 5.2

**57–60.** For the clinical scenarios in questions 57 to 60, select the best treatment option:

**57.** A 45-year-old woman recently immigrated from India exhibits a 6-mm reaction on a Mantoux skin test during an immigration physical. She is well and has a normal physical examination and chest radiograph. She denies any history of a bacille Calmette-Guérin vaccination.

What is the best approach?
a) No treatment
b) Isoniazid daily
c) Isoniazid plus rifampin
d) Ethambutol and pyrazinamide

**58.** A 30-year-old man diagnosed with human immunodeficiency virus (HIV) infection 5 years ago shows a 6-mm reaction on the Mantoux skin test. He is well, with a normal physical examination and chest radiograph. A friend recently died while undergoing treatment for multiple drug-resistant tuberculosis.

What is the best approach?
a) No treatment
b) Isoniazid daily
c) Isoniazid plus rifampin
d) Ethambutol and pyrazinamide

**59.** A 27-year-old medical resident 9 months into his training at a rural community hospital shows a 10-mm reaction on the Mantoux skin test. Testing 9 months ago revealed no reaction. He is well, with a normal physical examination and chest radiograph. He does not recall caring for a patient with tuberculosis.

What is the best approach?
a) No treatment
b) Isoniazid daily
c) Isoniazid plus rifampin
d) Ethambutol and pyrazinamide

**60.** A 55-year-old woman who denies any exposure to tuberculosis is found to have a 10-mm reaction on the Mantoux skin test. She was negative at a preemployment physical 2 years ago. She is well, with a normal physical examination and chest radiograph. She is currently living at home with her husband.

What is the best approach?
a) No treatment
b) Isoniazid daily
c) Isoniazid plus rifampin
d) Ethambutol and pyrazinamide

**61.** A 67-year-old man reports "lethargy." History and physical examination suggest no physical disease, but he is not sleeping well, has lost his appetite, is not enjoying his retirement, and is staying in bed for much of the day. He states that his wife has been trying to get him to play golf and bridge with his friends, which he used to enjoy doing, but he feels too lethargic and is not interested in socializing. You are concerned that he may be depressed, and you consider his suicidal risk.

All the following statements about suicide are true, *except*
a) His age puts him in a high-risk group.

b) Women are more likely to attempt suicide and successfully complete it than men.
c) Family history of suicide is a risk factor for suicide.
d) History of recent loss, such as retirement, is a risk factor for suicide.
e) Being single puts one at greater risk of suicide than being divorced.

**62.** Which of the following statements regarding complications of mechanical ventilation in patients with acute respiratory distress syndrome (ARDS) is false?
a) Barotrauma is often a significant direct cause of death in ARDS patients.
b) Tissue breakdown, excessive tidal volumes, and low airway pressures predispose to barotrauma.
c) Although often accompanied by nonspecific findings, nosocomial pneumonia is an important cause of morbidity and mortality in ARDS patients, with a prevalence of approximately 55%.
d) The combination of a corticosteroid and a neuromuscular blocking agent used for paralysis in these patients can lead to a reversible myopathy.
e) Decreased radiolucency at the lung bases and the presence of the deep sulcus sign on a chest radiography are clues to the diagnosis of pneumothorax.

**63.** A 29-year-old woman presents to the emergency department with shortness of breath and palpitations. The triage nurse finds that she has a heart rate of 170/bpm and establishes an intravenous line, starts oxygen therapy, and attaches a cardiac monitor. You assess her airway, breathing, and circulation. Her respiratory rate is 24/min and blood pressure 70/40 mm Hg. She starts to complain of chest tightness.

What should your next step be?
a) Drawing blood for a metabolic profile and cardiac enzymes
b) Synchronized cardioversion
c) Defibrillation
d) Lidocaine
e) Verapamil

**64.** A 55-year-old man with a history of hypertension and renal artery stenosis is brought to the emergency department by his wife because of confusion. His blood pressure is 220/120 mm Hg. Head CT is negative for ischemia or hemorrhage.

Which of the following additional findings would be *least* consistent with malignant hypertension?
a) Retinal hemorrhages and exudates
b) Hematuria
c) Proteinuria
d) Abrupt onset of confusion
e) Bilateral papilledema

**65.** A 35-year-old woman reports dysuria. Other than minor back pain, for which she is taking ibuprofen, she has generally been healthy. Her vital signs and physical examination are normal. A urine dipstick test reveals 2+ leukocyte esterase. Urine is immediately sent to the laboratory for culture and sensitivity. She is told that she has a urinary tract infection and is given a prescription for trimethoprim-sulfamethoxazole. Two days later, the urine culture report indicates no bacterial growth.

In interpreting this report, you consider all the following, *except*

a) Sterile pyuria may occur in the presence of urinary tract infection if this patient had been self-medicating with an antibiotic.

b) Sterile pyuria may be caused by an atypical organism such as *Chlamydia trachomatis, Ureaplasma urealyticum,* or *Mycobacterium tuberculosis.*

c) Obtain further history regarding her analgesic intake and consider chronic interstitial nephritis in the differential.

d) Repeat the urine dipstick, as vaginal leukocytes may have contaminated the original urine sample.

e) You consider all of the above.

66. All the following statements concerning acne vulgaris are true, *except*

a) It is the most common cutaneous disorder in the United States.

b) Inflammation results from the proliferation of the organism *Propionibacterium acnes* within follicles.

c) Typical areas affected include the face, neck, upper back, and upper arms.

d) A topical antibiotic may help eliminate *P. acnes* and thus help suppress the inflammation, but it may produce resistant strains.

e) Tetracyclines are effective only through inhibition of growth of *P. acnes.*

67. A 65-year-old woman presents to the emergency department with hypoxic and hypercapnic respiratory failure. She is intubated and transferred to the intensive care unit (ICU).

Which of the following statements about mechanical ventilation is true?

a) In pressure-cycled ventilation, inspiration ceases when a preset maximum pressure is reached. Volume varies with changes in lung mechanics.

b) In volume-cycled ventilation, inspiration terminates after delivery of a fixed set tidal volume.

c) In assist-control mechanical ventilation, the ventilator senses each inspiratory effort and delivers a fixed tidal volume. A backup rate can be set.

d) In intermittent mandatory ventilation, the ventilator delivers a preset tidal volume at fixed intervals. In addition, patients are allowed to breathe spontaneously and receive a tidal volume relative to their effort.

e) All the above.

68. All the following statements regarding coccidioidomycosis are true, *except*

a) Endemic areas include south central California, southern Arizona, Nevada, and New Mexico.

b) Sixty percent of infections are asymptomatic.

c) Cutaneous manifestations, such as a nonspecific maculopapular or erythematous rash, are seen in 25% of patients, indicate disseminated disease, and portend a poor prognosis.

d) A focal bronchopneumonic infiltrate in a single lobe is the most common finding on chest radiography.

e) Eosinophilia may be seen in up to 25% of patients with coccidioidomycosis.

69. Emergency medical services brings a 55-year-old man with a previous history of coronary artery disease (CAD) and prior MI to the emergency department with severe substernal chest pain radiating to the left shoulder and jaw. Pain has been persistent for approximately 20 minutes. On questioning, he has experienced similar pain intermittently throughout the previous 48 hours. In addition to the pain, he has experienced shortness of breath, diaphoresis, and nausea. His pain improves somewhat after he is given two nitroglycerin tablets sublingually. His vital signs are stable, and his ECG reveals changes consistent with an anterior MI. He is admitted to the coronary ICU. While there, severe systemic hypotension (blood pressure 80/30 mm Hg) and dyspnea develop. He is given vasopressor and inotrope support. A pulmonary artery catheter is placed. The pulmonary artery wedge pressure is 18 mm Hg, and the cardiac index (CI) is calculated to be 2.0 L/min/m².

All the following statements regarding this man's diagnosis are true, *except*

a) It is unusual for cardiogenic shock to develop in this man because in most patients it develops before presentation to the hospital.

b) The hemodynamic measurements obtained for this patient are consistent with those for classic cardiogenic shock.

c) Severe mitral regurgitation from a ruptured chordae tendineae or papillary muscle, cardiac tamponade, or rupture of the intraventricular septum may also lead to cardiogenic shock in the setting of an acute MI.

d) Urgent echocardiography with Doppler flow is indicated and would be helpful in narrowing the differential for this man's hypotension.

e) All the above statements are true.

70. An 87-year-old woman presents for a checkup. She has no complaints and considers herself healthy. On direct questioning, she confesses to falling in her home a couple of weeks ago but states that she was in no way injured. She is taking no medications. She remains in the family home where she raised her seven children and had lived with her husband for 65 years until he died there 5 years ago. Her children live nearby and visit her frequently. You perform a full history and physical examination and assess her with respect to her risk for falls.

All the following are risk factors for falls, *except*
a) Increasing age
b) Female sex
c) A history of falls
d) Arthritis
e) Hypertension

**71.** A 48-year-old man reports drooping of the face and difficulty in speaking for 48 hours. On examination, a paralysis of the upper and lower face is present on the right side. He cannot raise his eyebrows or close his eye tightly. Drooping of the right side of the mouth is present, and the nasolabial fold is smoothed out.

Which of the following is true about the most likely cause of this man's symptoms?
a) This is an upper motor lesion.
b) The most common cause is herpes zoster of the external auditory meatus and geniculate ganglion, called *Ramsay Hunt syndrome.*
c) This is a rare condition occurring in approximately 1 in 10,000 persons in a lifetime.
d) This is permanent in 60% of patients.
e) There may be associated loss of taste sensation from the ipsilateral anterior two thirds of the tongue.

**72.** All the following signs are associated with diffuse toxic goiter (Graves' disease), *except*
a) Lid retraction
b) Ectropion
c) Lid lag
d) Exophthalmos
e) Ophthalmoplegia

**73.** Your patient reports a history of penicillin allergy and requests desensitization.

All the following statements are true, *except*
a) It is important to verify the history because the patient may incorrectly assume that a nonallergic side effect, such as a gastrointestinal side effect, is allergic in origin.
b) Fatal reactions to penicillin skin tests have been reported.
c) Skin testing should not be performed in patients with a high risk for an anaphylactic reaction, unless no alternative drug to a β-lactam is available.
d) Patients with a positive skin test to penicillin are at a fourfold increased risk for an allergic reaction to cephalosporins.
e) Desensitization helps reduce the incidence of Stevens-Johnson syndrome, hemolytic anemia, and serum sickness associated with penicillin.

**74.** A 30-year-old fit man presents with deep vein thrombosis (DVT). He has a history of allergic rhinitis each summer. He has had no recent trauma or surgery and has not traveled in the last 6 months. He is adopted and does not have any medical family history.

What is the most common underlying cause of DVT?
a) Factor V Leiden, activated protein C resistance
b) Protein C deficiency
c) Protein S deficiency
d) Antithrombin III deficiency
e) Dysfibrinogenemia

**75.** Which of the following is not a correctly matched drug and side effect?
a) Enalapril and hyperkalemia
b) Hydrochlorothiazide and hypouricemia
c) Metoprolol and heart block
d) Nifedipine and peripheral edema
e) Prazosin and orthostatic hypotension

**76.** A 42-year-old woman presents with a pruritic erythematous rash around her neck after wearing a new necklace. In the past, she experienced a similar reaction to a cheap pair of earrings.

All the following statements are true, *except*
a) Perfumes and cosmetics can produce the same type of response.
b) Diagnosis can be confirmed with a patch test read in 48 hours.
c) This type of reaction can be caused by topical medications, including antibiotics.
d) Poison ivy produces the same type of response.
e) This is a type II cell-mediated response.

**77.** Occupational exposure is associated with lung cancer in all the following, *except*
a) Asbestos
b) Silica
c) Inorganic arsenic
d) Chromium compounds
e) Polycyclic hydrocarbons (coal by-products)

**78.** A 25-year-old man presents to the emergency department with fever, chills, cough, shortness of breath, and dyspnea on exertion. He is reluctant to give any further history. On examination, he is febrile, tachypneic, tachycardic, and normotensive. He appears to have significant muscle wasting. The physical examination is notable for the presence of oral thrush, poor dentition, normal lung examination, and rapid but regular heart sounds without evidence of murmur. Further laboratory testing and radiologic examinations are done. Meanwhile, a friend mentions that he was diagnosed with HIV infection 9 years ago and last saw his physician 3 months ago.

Which of the following findings or additional history would be *least* supportive of the diagnosis of *Pneumocystis carinii* pneumonia?
a) CD4 count is 600/mm$^3$.
b) He has been on aerosolized pentamidine monthly.
c) Arterial blood gas readings taken while breathing room air are pH 7.43, PCO$_2$ 36 mm Hg, PO$_2$ 64 mm Hg, HCO$_3^-$ 28 mEq/L, and SaO$_2$ 93%.

**d)** Chest plain film reveals a right lower lobe consolidation.

**e)** Lactate dehydrogenase (LDH) level is 550 U/L.

**79.** A 20-year-old man presents with a rash that he has had since he was a teenager. In your opinion, it may be psoriasis.

All the following statements are true of psoriasis, *except*

**a)** Lesions are typically sharply demarcated.

**b)** Salmon-pink lesions with a silvery-white scale are typical.

**c)** Distribution typically involves the elbows, knees, scalp, nails, and intergluteal cleft.

**d)** An increased risk of psoriasis exists if one or both of one's parents have the disease.

**e)** A high incidence of psoriasis is present in Eskimos and North and South American Indians.

**80–82.** The following hemodynamic indices are obtained: CI, systemic vascular resistance (SVR), pulmonary vascular resistance (PVR), mixed venous oxygen saturation ($SvO_2$), and pulmonary artery occlusion pressure (PAOP).

Which of the following diagnoses is most consistent with the parameters in questions 80 to 82?

**80.** CI ↓; SVR ↑; PVR Normal; $SvO_2$ ↓; PAOP ↓

**a)** Neurogenic shock

**b)** Hypovolemic shock

**c)** Cardiogenic shock

**d)** Septic shock

**e)** None of the above

**81.** CI ↑; SVR ↓; PVR Normal; $SvO_2$ Normal ↓; PAOP Normal ↓

**a)** Neurogenic shock

**b)** Hypovolemic shock

**c)** Cardiogenic shock

**d)** Septic shock

**e)** None of the above

**82.** CI ↓; SVR ↑; PVR Normal; $SvO_2$ ↓; PAOP ↑

**a)** Neurogenic shock

**b)** Hypovolemic shock

**c)** Cardiogenic shock

**d)** Septic shock

**e)** None of the above

**83.** A 25-year-old heterosexual man with a single sex partner presents to his primary care physician requesting an HIV test.

Which of the following would be the most correct statement?

**a)** Testing should not be done because he has no risk factors.

**b)** A positive enzyme immunoassay test would need confirmation with a Western blot to lessen the likelihood of a false-positive test result.

**c)** The false-positive and false-negative rates of the enzyme immunoassay and Western blot tests are related to the prevalence of HIV in the population being tested.

**d)** b and c.

**e)** None of the above.

**84.** Which of the following is the leading cause of cancer deaths in the United States?

**a)** Lung cancer

**b)** Breast cancer

**c)** Colorectal cancer

**d)** Prostate cancer

**e)** Ovarian cancer

**85.** Which of the following statements regarding the amniotic fluid embolism syndrome (AFES) is true?

**a)** Disseminated intravascular coagulation with resultant hemorrhage develops in less than 20% of women with AFES.

**b)** Maternal mortality is reported to be approximately 20% with supportive therapy and surpasses pulmonary embolism as a cause of maternal mortality.

**c)** The majority of women diagnosed with AFES die from cardiogenic shock or its complications.

**d)** Noncardiogenic pulmonary edema develops in approximately 70% of patients who survive the first hours of AFES. The resultant damage of the alveolar capillary membrane produces a clinical pattern typical of ARDS.

**e)** None of the above.

**86.** A 28-year-old man presents to the emergency department with a 1-week history of fever, chills, and cough productive of sputum. He is short of breath and has pleuritic left-sided chest pain. On physical examination, he has a respiratory rate of 22/min, blood pressure of 110/78 mm Hg, and a pulse of 98/bpm. Dullness to percussion is present and audible rales in the left base. Sputum and blood cultures reveal *Streptococcus pneumoniae*.

All the following statements concerning pneumococcal pneumonia are true, *except*

**a)** Cigarette smoking is a risk factor.

**b)** HIV infection is a risk factor.

**c)** The risk of pneumococcal sepsis is increased in splenectomized patients.

**d)** If sputum culture is negative, it is unlikely that a concurrent bacteremia is present.

**e)** Bacteremia accompanies pneumococcal pneumonia in 20% to 30% of patients.

**87.** A 76-year-old man admitted to the hospital 2 weeks ago for pneumonia and transferred to the ICU 1 week ago has been deteriorating for the last 3 days, requiring mechanical ventilation with full support and 100% oxygen. He has a history of CAD and chronic obstructive pulmonary disease. Given the poor prognosis, the ICU team meets with his wife.

Which of the following statements is most valid?

a) Instruct the wife that the patient's prognosis is poor and that she will need to make a decision regarding her husband's thoughts on end-of-life issues.

b) Instruct the wife that because there is no "do not resuscitate" order on the chart, even if her husband's physicians believe that cardiopulmonary resuscitation is futile, it will have to be performed in the event of cardiopulmonary arrest.

c) If a durable power of attorney for healthcare is appointed, that person should be making decisions, but only in the absence of the patient's wife.

d) Because the prognosis is poor, the ICU team should be instructed to only run "slow" codes on this patient.

e) Use of pain medications can be construed as a form of physician-assisted suicide because these medications can hasten the patient's death.

88. A 35-year-old woman traveling to Africa in 2 weeks presents to her local physician. She takes no medications and has been healthy.

Which of the following statements is most accurate?

a) Malaria prophylaxis with chloroquine is recommended because travel to sub-Saharan Africa does not increase her chance of chloroquine-resistant *Plasmodium falciparum* exposure.

b) Mefloquine is the drug of choice in most chloroquine-resistance areas and is effective against all strains of *P. falciparum.*

c) Mefloquine should not be prescribed for individuals with cardiac conduction abnormalities because of the association with sinus bradycardia and a prolonged QT interval.

d) If this patient is pregnant and travel cannot be deferred, she should be given doxycycline because chloroquine and mefloquine have been shown to be teratogenic.

e) None of the above.

89. A 65-year-old diabetic woman presents to the hospital with fever. On examination, her temperature is 38.5°C, heart rate 100/bpm, blood pressure 120/70 mm Hg, and respiratory rate 24/min. On physical examination, she does not have a focus for infection. Laboratory studies reveal a WBC count of 12,500 cells/mm³, and urinalysis is positive for leukocyte esterase and nitrites. Urine culture and blood cultures are ordered.

Which of the following terms most accurately describes her present condition?

a) Septic shock

b) Systemic inflammatory response syndrome

c) Sepsis

d) Infection

e) Bacteremia

90. A 32-year-old woman reports increasing shortness of breath. On examination, pulse is regular, and a parasternal heave is noted. On auscultation, a continuous, machinery-type murmur is present, with systolic accentuation that is best heard at the second intercostal space and left sternal border; it is also heard posteriorly. Clubbing and cyanosis of the toes is present, but not of the fingers.

All the following are true of this condition, *except*

a) It is more common in men.

b) Endocarditis prophylaxis should be given before dental procedures.

c) Cyanosis of the lower extremities is associated with the development of Eisenmenger's syndrome.

d) Maternal rubella is associated.

e) It is normal anatomy before birth.

91. A 55-year-old woman reports gradually increasing shortness of breath. On examination, respiratory rate is 24/min, and she appears in mild distress, with difficulty in breathing. Blood pressure is 138/89 mm Hg. Expansion appears to be normal. Percussion is stony-dull in the right base and halfway up the right lung field, with diminished tactile fremitus, vocal resonance, and breath sounds in the same areas. Chest radiograph is consistent with the clinical suspicion of a pleural effusion.

Which of the following statements about pleural effusion is true?

a) An exudative effusion is suggested by pleural fluid lactic dehydrogenase (LDH) more than one-third of the normal upper limit for serum.

b) A transudative pleural effusion is suggested by a ratio of pleural fluid LDH to serum LDH of greater than 0.6.

c) Pulmonary emboli may be associated with both transudates and exudates.

d) The pleural effusion associated with neoplastic disease usually is transudative.

e) In a patient with a parapneumonic effusion, an indication for thoracostomy tube placement is a pleural fluid glucose level greater than 50 mg/dL.

92. Which of the following statements regarding renovascular hypertension is false?

a) Renovascular hypertension is less common in African Americans.

b) Renovascular hypertension should be suspected when an abrupt rise in plasma creatinine levels occur after the institution of an ACE-inhibitor.

c) Patients with moderate to severe hypertension who have recurrent episodes of acute "flash" pulmonary edema should be screened for renovascular hypertension.

d) The gold standard for diagnosing renal artery stenosis is the renal arteriogram.

e) The baseline plasma renin level is elevated in virtually all patients with renovascular hypertension.

**93.** Which of the following features suggests a lower motor neuron lesion rather than an upper motor lesion?
a) Extensor plantar response
b) Hyperreflexia of the tendon reflexes
c) Increased tone (spasticity)
d) Fasciculation
e) Weakness

**94.** A 35-year-old man presents to the emergency department with abdominal cramping, tenesmus, and sudden onset of bloody diarrhea. On examination, he is toxic-appearing with a temperature of 40°C. His blood pressure and respiratory rate are normal. He is slightly tachycardic. He is slightly tender in the right lower quadrant. A presumptive diagnosis is made after examination of the stool for fecal leukocytes and is confirmed by culture of rectal swab.

All the following regarding this diagnosis are true, *except*
a) Stool examination would reveal polymorphonuclear leukocytes on methylene blue stain.
b) Blood cultures would likely reveal the causative organism.
c) In general, antibiotics are not essential in the treatment because this illness is generally self-limited in duration, averaging approximately 7 days.
d) Antibiotic treatment in infected patients can reduce the transmission of this organism to other individuals.
e) The development of bacteremia in this condition is more common in children than adults.

**95.** A 65-year-old man reports back pain. In review of his chart, you note an Hgb level of 10 mg/dL and an elevated total protein. You entertain the diagnosis of multiple myeloma.

Which of the following statements is true?
a) Among neurologic manifestations of myeloma, 5% to 10% of patients have extramedullary plasmacytomas leading to cord compression, although peripheral neuropathy is more common.
b) The anemia is most likely microcytic and hypochromic and occurs in a majority of patients with multiple myeloma.
c) Hypercalcemia is common, occurring in more than 50% of patients with multiple myeloma.
d) The two major causes of renal failure in these patients include cast nephropathy and hypercalcemia.
e) In myeloma kidney, casts accumulate in the loop of Henle. These casts are composed of precipitated monoclonal light chains that interact with Tamm-Horsfall mucoprotein synthesized by the tubular cells in the ascending limb of the loop of Henle.

**96.** All the following statements concerning rhinitis are true, *except*
a) An increased risk of allergic rhinitis exists if there is a family history of allergic rhinitis.

b) Eosinophils can be seen on Wright's-stained nasal secretions.
c) Over-the-counter oral sympathomimetic agents may provide some relief of congestive symptoms, but they can cause elevation of blood pressure and can be dangerous in patients with hypertension or at risk for cardiac events.
d) Nasal sympathomimetic agents are an excellent choice for long-term symptom relief.
e) Hot and spicy foods may produce an episodic rhinitis termed *gustatory rhinitis*, which is a vagally mediated reflex.

**97.** A 56-year-old man asks for advice concerning a nodule seen on a chest radiograph obtained during a physical examination for a new job.

Which of the following statements concerning a solitary pulmonary nodule is true?
a) It is a single, radiologically visible lesion that must be surrounded on all sides by pulmonary parenchyma.
b) The upper limit in size is 2 cm.
c) The type of malignancy most commonly presenting as a solitary pulmonary nodule is small cell carcinoma.
d) It may present with associated pleural effusion.
e) It may present with associated mediastinal lymphadenopathy.

**98.** A 21-year-old woman with a history of sickle cell disease is admitted to the hospital with a pain crisis. This is her sixth admission in the past 4 years. She has been on folate and hydroxyurea therapy as an outpatient. On the day of admission, her temperature is 39°C, blood pressure 130/90 mm Hg, pulse 120/bpm, and respiratory rate 12/min. Her physical examination reveals that she is in moderate distress. Her head, eyes, ears, nose, and throat examination is unremarkable, as are her pulmonary and cardiovascular examinations, except for tachycardia. The abdomen is soft and nontender, with normal bowel sounds. Examination of her extremities does not demonstrate any edema. Initial laboratory tests show a normal chemistry profile. Complete blood count (CBC) shows that her white cell count is 15,000/mm³, Hgb level is 7.5 mg/dL, and Hct is 20%.

Which of the following is *least* appropriate in the initial management of this patient?
a) Continuous intravenous fluids: dextrose water with potassium chloride at 200 mL/h
b) A narcotic analgesic given for adequate pain control
c) Packed RBC transfusion, 2 units, each over 4 hours
d) Cultures of blood and urine, chest radiograph, and careful examination of the skin for a potential source of fever and infection
e) Reticulocyte count

**99.** A 76-year-old man admitted to a general medicine ward for pneumonia is found by a nurse to be unresponsive and without a palpable pulse or spontaneous breathing. As the first physician to the scene, you confirm the absence of pulse and respiration. You then ask the respiratory therapist to establish an airway and begin mask-bag ventilation. Meanwhile, leads are placed for cardiac monitoring. A subclavian central access line had already been placed 2 hours before the arrest. The initial rhythm seen is pulseless electrical activity at 70 complexes per minute. A Doppler ultrasound, operated by the nurse, is unable to detect a blood pressure. Cardiopulmonary resuscitation is initiated.

According to the American Heart Association (AHA) guidelines on the advanced cardiac life support protocol, all the following steps are appropriate in the initial management of this patient, *except*
a) Give epinephrine, 1 mg intravenously.
b) Order a draw of arterial blood for blood gas and chemistry.
c) Begin synchronized direct-current cardioversion.
d) Start intravenous fluid infusion after bolus.
e) Order (but do not wait for) a portable chest radiograph and examine the patient for equal breath sounds bilaterally.

**100.** In the patient from Question 99, the cardiac monitor now reveals a wide complex tachycardia; heart rate is 120/bpm. Blood pressure is now 80/50 mm Hg.

In the interpretation and treatment of this patient's rhythm, which of the following statements is incorrect?
a) If a wide complex tachycardia cannot be differentiated between supraventricular tachycardia (SVT) and ventricular tachycardia (VT), the patient should be treated initially with low-dose verapamil intravenously.
b) The presence of CAD in this patient would make the diagnosis of VT more likely than SVT.
c) The recurrence of a wide complex tachycardia over the past couple of years in the same patient would make it more likely that this is SVT.
d) The observation of cannon "a" waves would make the diagnosis of VT more likely.
e) None of the above.

**101.** A 32-year-old woman presents with slurred speech and ataxia. You have seen her previously with two episodes of blurred vision, 10 and 6 months ago. On examination of her lower extremities, she has increased tone and bilateral spasticity and weakness. Bilateral ankle clonus is present, and the plantar reflexes are extensor. You consider the possibility of MS.

Which of the following statements about MS is true?
a) It is more common in men.
b) The predominant age at presentation is 50 to 65 years.
c) Northern European descent or living in a temperate climate are risk factors for MS.
d) CT and magnetic resonance imaging (MRI) are equally sensitive in the diagnosis of MS.
e) Cerebrospinal fluid examination that suggests the diagnosis of MS includes a normal or slightly low

protein level, a low level of γ-globulin immunoglobulin G (IgG), and negative serology for syphilis.

**102.** All the following statements regarding renal tubular acidosis (RTA) are true, *except*
a) All forms of RTA are characterized by a normal anion gap (hyperchloremic) metabolic acidosis.
b) Proximal (type 2) RTA originates from the inability to reabsorb bicarbonate normally in the proximal tubule and is marked by a urine pH greater than 7.5 and the appearance of filtered bicarbonate during bicarbonate infusion. This is often associated with Fanconi's syndrome.
c) The most common causes of distal (type 1) RTA in adults are autoimmune disorders, such as Sjögren's syndrome and other hyperglobulinemic states.
d) Distal RTA is associated with hyperkalemia, unless decreased tubular sodium reabsorption occurs, in which case hypokalemia is present.
e) Type 4 RTA is due to aldosterone deficiency or resistance of the tubular cells to aldosterone; typically, urinary pH is acidic and serum bicarbonate is greater than 17 mEq/L.

**103.** The following are all risk factors for the development of carcinoma of the bladder, *except*
a) Cyclophosphamide use
b) Family history
c) Tobacco smoke exposure
d) *Schistosoma haematobium* infestation
e) Recurrent stones

**104.** A 65-year-old man with a history of chronic renal insufficiency is now progressing to end-stage renal disease. In preparation for hemodialysis, you counsel him about the possible complications of chronic hemodialysis.

Which of the following do you *not* discuss as a possible complication?
a) Gastrointestinal bleeding
b) Hepatitis
c) Dementia
d) Osteoporosis
e) Cerebrovascular accidents

**105.** A 35-year-old woman who was diagnosed with HIV infection 9 years ago and has been reluctant to start treatment now presents to you for advice. You obtain her CD4 cell count, which is 200/mm$^3$, and her viral load (RNA-polymerase chain reaction), which is 30,000 copies/mL. In addition, a pregnancy test is negative.

Of the following options, which would you recommend as the most appropriate initial therapy for this patient?
a) No treatment, as she does not meet criteria for drug therapy
b) Didanosine, zalcitabine, and indinavir
c) Zidovudine

d) Zidovudine, didanosine, and nevirapine
e) Zidovudine and didanosine

**106.** A 60-year-old man on your inpatient service for 3 days presented with melenic stools. He has been doing well; his Hgb has been stable at 13 mg/dL, and his vital signs also have been stable and normal. He arrived on the Friday of a holiday weekend, and you have been unable to schedule an esophagogastroduodenoscopy until tomorrow. You are paged by his nurse, who reports that he has been restless all afternoon, and now he is demanding and threatening to leave and go home. You immediately go to see the patient, surprised at the behavior described to you by the nurse because he had been very pleasant the previous 3 days. You look at his vital signs chart outside his room. His blood pressure has been rising over the last 24 hours and is now 170/98 mm Hg; on admission it had been 128/76 mm Hg. He has also developed a sinus tachycardia of 118/bpm and a temperature of 37.8°C. When you enter the room, he appears agitated and tremulous and is pacing around the room. On seeing you, he states that he must leave. He appears to be watching something in the room and, on inquiry, states that he is watching the little angels who are flying around the room.

Which of the following is most likely to cause this presentation?
a) Alcohol withdrawal
b) Alcohol intoxication
c) Opiate withdrawal
d) Schizophrenia
e) Personality disorder

**107.** All the following statements about the medication adenosine are true, *except*
a) The AHA subcommittee on advanced cardiac life support protocol recommends adenosine as the initial drug of choice for hemodynamically stable paroxysmal SVT (PSVT).
b) It should be administered as a rapid intravenous push followed by a fluid flush.
c) Patients frequently experience a few seconds of chest discomfort similar to ischemic chest pain.
d) In the treatment of PSVT, the rhythm can recur in up to 50% to 60% of patients.
e) The highest dose recommended for use in PSVT is 6 mg.

**108.** In a confused elderly patient, which feature suggests a diagnosis of delirium rather than dementia?
a) Onset over months to years rather than hours to days
b) Postural tremor, myoclonus, and asterixis
c) Normal rather than slurred speech
d) Impaired recent memory and preserved distant past memory
e) Normal electroencephalogram

**109.** All the following statements regarding aspirin intoxication are true, *except*
a) Toxicity can result with plasma levels of 400 to 500 mg/L.
b) Respiratory alkalosis can occur due to stimulation of the respiratory center by salicylates.
c) A nonanion gap metabolic acidosis develops soon after the respiratory alkalosis.
d) Sodium bicarbonate should be given to alkalinize the plasma.
e) All the above are true.

**110.** A 30-year-old man is evaluated for dyspepsia. His history is remarkable for an 11-lb weight loss in the last month, and he also complains of diarrhea. He denies any NSAID use. On endoscopic examination, duodenal bulb ulceration is noted. Biopsy of the involved area is negative for *Helicobacter pylori*.

What would be the most appropriate next step in managing this patient?
a) Culture of the biopsy specimen for *H. pylori*
b) A 4-week trial of oral famotidine with follow-up endoscopy
c) Breath test for *H. pylori*
d) CT of the abdomen
e) Serum gastrin level

**111.** A 26-year-old woman is undergoing autologous bone marrow transplantation for non-Hodgkin's lymphoma. On the third day of her admission, she is found to have a temperature of 39°C. She feels well, and the examination does not reveal any localizing signs of infection. Laboratory studies show an absolute neutrophil count of 420/mm³.

What would now be the most appropriate management for this patient?
a) Close observation only
b) Blood cultures
c) Blood cultures and empiric treatment with an aminoglycoside and piperacillin
d) Blood cultures and empiric treatment with an aminoglycoside only
e) Blood cultures and empiric treatment with vancomycin and an aminoglycoside

**112.** A 34-year-old woman reports shooting pain between the third and fourth toes of her left foot that has progressively worsened over the past 5 months. The pain occurs with walking and is relieved by stopping and massaging the affected area. On examination, compression of the forefoot causes the patient to wince in pain.

Which of the following is the most accurate statement relating to this patient's condition?
a) Elevating the heel of her shoe will help alleviate her pain.
b) NSAIDs are effective.
c) Men and women are affected in equal numbers.

d) The condition is caused by the compression of interdigital nerves.

e) Surgical treatment is never indicated.

**113.** A 51-year-old man consults you because he is concerned about his risk of cardiovascular disease. His father died at 52 years of age from MI. For exercise, he runs for 30 minutes five times per week. In discussing his diet, you find that he typically eats eggs for breakfast and usually has some sort of fast food for lunch on working days. He does not smoke or drink alcohol and is normotensive on examination. Results of fasting cholesterol and glucose testing are as follows:

| | |
|---|---|
| Total cholesterol | 231 mg/dL |
| Low-density lipoprotein cholesterol | 161 mg/dL |
| High-density lipoprotein cholesterol | 56 mg/dL |
| Triglycerides | 72 mg/dL |
| Glucose | 107 mg/dL |

Liver function tests are normal. He is concerned that he may die of a heart attack and urges you to treat him with "some of the pills" that he has seen advertised.

What would be the most appropriate response?

a) Explain that he should be treated with active diet therapy, and there is no need to start medication at this time.

b) Repeat his laboratory work in 3 to 6 months and discuss the matter further at that time if the lipid profile has not improved.

c) Evaluate for primary and secondary causes of hypercholesterolemia and institute drug therapy.

d) Reassure him, explaining that he is not at increased risk and that he should continue exercising.

e) Suggest that he take a glass of red wine four to five times per week.

**114.** A 52-year-old man reports bilateral ear pain. He describes no change in his hearing or any febrile episodes. His past medical history is notable for a history of episcleritis, and he has stiffness and pain in both upper extremities, which have been bothering him intermittently over the last 6 months. He had some epistaxis after taking ibuprofen for the stiffness and was advised to discontinue it by a pharmacist. On examination, tenderness and swelling of the cartilaginous portion of the ears is present. You have to talk loudly to be understood, and you note that the patient's voice is hoarse.

What is the most appropriate initial management for this patient?

a) Start oral prednisone, 40 mg daily.

b) Prescribe a mild topical corticosteroid to be applied to the ears twice daily.

c) Prescribe a nasal decongestant for 2 weeks.

d) Request ANA studies.

e) Restart ibuprofen.

**115.** You have encouraged a 42-year-old patient to take more exercise. He has recently started to play soccer and now comes to you, complaining of back pain. The pain is worse on standing or bending and eased by sitting or lying down. The pain does not radiate. Pain is not reproducible on straight-leg raising, and neurologic examination is intact.

All the following statements concerning this patient's condition are true, *except*

a) Spinal manipulation can be helpful, if used in the first month of symptoms.

b) Biofeedback has proved to be helpful in reducing recovery time.

c) Controlled physical activity, NSAIDs, and muscle relaxants have a role in the initial management.

d) Bed rest for more than 4 days may lead to debilitation.

e) Lumbosacral strain is the most likely diagnosis.

**116.** A 21-year-old woman reports a thin, malodorous vaginal discharge with vulvar itch. She is sexually active with more than one partner and does not use condoms. She thinks her last menstrual period was 3 weeks ago. Examination of the discharge reveals a pH of 5.0 and a fishy odor on addition of 20% potassium hydroxide solution. The saline wet preparation is significant for squamous cells covered by adherent bacteria.

Which of the following statements relating to this patient is the most accurate?

a) Treatment of choice is oral metronidazole, 2 g.

b) Treatment of choice is oral metronidazole, 500 mg twice daily for 7 days.

c) There is no need for pregnancy testing at this time.

d) There are no findings indicating an increased risk of cervical carcinoma.

e) Treatment with ketoconazole is effective.

**117.** A 46-year-old overweight postal worker has had multiple emergency department visits for chest pain. Cardiac catheterization done 1 month ago was significant for mild atherosclerotic disease. His past medical history is notable for hypercholesterolemia. Exercise stress testing was negative for ischemia. He is worried that he should not continue working and seeks further evaluation.

Which of the following tests would be the most appropriate for this patient?

a) Bernstein test

b) Ambulatory ECG monitoring

c) 24-Hour pH monitoring

d) Endoscopy

e) Esophageal manometry

**118.** A 38-year-old nurse is seen for symptoms consistent with recurrent hypoglycemia. On occasion, she has collapsed at work. Her plasma glucose has been noted as 48 mg/dL on one occasion when she felt faint at work. Her past medical history is notable for irritable bowel syndrome, and her mother is known to be an insulin-requiring diabetic. Fasting laboratory values are as follows:

| | |
|---|---|
| Plasma insulin | 468 μU/mL (normal, 626 μU/mL) |
| C-peptide | 8.0 ng/mL (normal, 1.02.0 ng/mL) |
| Proinsulin to insulin ratio | 15% |

What would be the most appropriate next step in management?
a) Angiography with selective venous sampling for insulin levels
b) Two-phase contrast CT
c) Trial of octreotide and two-phase contrast CT
d) Search for needlestick marks
e) Urinary drug testing

**119.** A 28-year-old male medical assistant is seen in occupational health for preemployment screening. He is asymptomatic, and his physical examination is normal. He undergoes drug screening and is offered a hepatitis immunization. He explains that a physician at his previous place of employment told him that he does not need hepatitis B immunization. You take samples for hepatitis B virus serology and ask him to return in 2 days when you will have the results.

The following results are reported:

| | |
|---|---|
| HbsAg | Negative |
| Anti-HBs | Positive |
| HBc | Negative |
| HbeAg | Negative |
| Anti-Hbe | Negative |

What would be the most accurate advice for this patient?
a) He has a high level of infectivity and should not be employed under federal guidelines.
b) He has low-level infectivity and can be employed as long as universal precautions are followed.
c) He most likely has chronic hepatitis B virus infection and should have liver function testing.
d) All his sexual partners must be advised to undergo testing.
e) None of the above.

**120.** A 59-year-old diabetic man is seen in the outpatient clinic. He reports left-sided ear pain for the last 2 weeks. His wife describes a greenish exudate. His diabetes is well controlled, and he is known to be compliant with your recommendations. His medications include an oral hypoglycemic agent, and he does not have any allergies. However, to help himself get to sleep without discomfort, he has self-medicated with tramadol that was prescribed for his wife. He appears comfortable but is noted to have a temperature of 39.1°C. On examination, the external auditory meatus is exquisitely tender, and you note some friable reddish tissue.

What would be the most appropriate next step in management?

a) Recommend instillation of a suspension of polymyxin B/neomycin/hydrocortisone four times daily for 7 days, with a scheduled return outpatient visit every 7 days until cure is achieved.
b) Prescribe clotrimazole 1% solution, three drops twice daily for 14 days.
c) Prescribe clotrimazole 1% solution, three drops twice daily for 14 days in combination with a topical steroid cream.
d) Prescribe clotrimazole 1% solution applied to a wick left in the ear canal and recommend avoidance of moisture entering the ear canal when he is bathing by use of cotton wool for plugging.
e) Admit him for intravenous antibiotics and possible debridement.

**121.** A 45-year-old woman reports a neck mass. On examination, she is found to have a goiter with a rubbery consistency. A review of systems is positive for weight gain, fatigue, and cold intolerance. High titers of antithyroid peroxidase antibody are present on laboratory studies.

All the following statements about this patient's diagnosis are true, *except*
a) Some patients present with symptoms of hyperthyroidism.
b) The prognosis is poor despite appropriate hormone replacement treatment.
c) A small increased risk of lymphoma exists.
d) An association with autoimmune diseases exists.
e) It is a common cause of hypothyroidism in the United States.

**122.** A 28-year-old visiting student from India is seen in an urgent care facility. He reports that his friend's dog bit his hand 1 hour ago. The dog is apparently in good health. Examination of the affected hand reveals small, superficial puncture wounds. He does not have any allergies. He does not recall any childhood immunizations.

What is the most appropriate management for this patient?
a) Thorough cleansing of the wound with soap and water only
b) Wound irrigation and a 7-day course of antibiotics, with observation of the dog for 10 days
c) Wound irrigation and tetanus and diphtheria toxoid immunization, with destruction of the dog
d) Irrigation, 7 days of antibiotics, tetanus and diphtheria toxoid immunization, tetanus immunoglobulin, and observation of the dog for 10 days, with repeat tetanus and diphtheria immunizations in 1 and 6 months
e) Irrigation, tetanus and diphtheria toxoid immunization, tetanus immunoglobulin, and observation of the dog for 10 days, with repeat tetanus and diphtheria immunizations in 1 and 6 months

**123–127.** Match the following antihypertensive agents with the side effect or contraindication in questions 123 to 127:
a) Lisinopril
b) Metoprolol
c) Minoxidil
d) Hydralazine
e) Nitroprusside

**123.** Severe chronic obstructive pulmonary disease

**124.** Contraindicated during pregnancy

**125.** Lupus-like syndrome

**126.** Hirsutism

**127.** Cyanide toxicity

**128.** A 69-year-old man is seen in the emergency department, complaining of substernal chest pain at rest. He is admitted to the hospital for further evaluation. He is known to have hypercholesterolemia and is a long-time smoker. No other past medical history is noted as being significant. On the morning of the second hospital day, he undergoes cardiac catheterization and is found to have single-vessel CAD. He undergoes what appears to be a successful angioplasty. He is started on aspirin and a β-blocker. On the evening of the second hospital day, he complains of new-onset abdominal pain that is not relieved by morphine administered by the house officer. Physical examination of the abdomen is noted to be normal. His respiratory rate is 24/min. ECG done during the pain is unchanged from his postprocedure tracing.

Which of the following statements about this patient's condition is correct?
a) A thrombolytic should be administered as soon as possible.
b) The pain that he is experiencing could be explained by a condition that would manifest itself on abdominal radiography with the appearance of thumbprinting.
c) The ECG should not have been done, as it is not useful in this context.
d) β-Blockers are contraindicated in this heavy smoker.
e) The normal physical examination rules out bowel pathology as the cause of his abdominal pain.

**129.** A 22-year-old woman, a nurse, has mild discomfort and tearing of her right eye. She is afebrile. On examination, no purulent drainage is present, but there is hyperemia of the conjunctiva. Preauricular adenopathy is also noted.

Which of the following is the most important recommendation?
a) Topical vasoconstrictive drops and cold compress alone
b) Oral tetracycline, 250 mg four times daily for 21 days
c) No specific medication, but a request for her to use thorough hand washing, not to share towels, and to remain away from work until her tearing has settled down
d) Cold compress for symptomatic relief alone
e) Gentamicin solution, one or two drops every 4 hours

**130.** A 56-year-old woman reports urinary incontinence. She explains that she has leakage of urine associated with laughing or making sudden movements. Her past medical history is notable for migraines and two uncomplicated pregnancies. A postvoid residual volume is recorded as 30 mL. Urinalysis is unremarkable.

What would be the most appropriate management at this time?
a) Prompted voiding
b) Intermittent catheter drainage
c) Environmental manipulation
d) Fluid intake modification
e) Pelvic muscle exercises

**131.** All the following statements regarding chronic myelogenous leukemia (CML) are true, *except*
a) It is genetically characterized by the Philadelphia chromosome, a reciprocal translocation between chromosomes 9 and 22, t(9;22).
b) The translocation that accounts for the Philadelphia chromosome is most commonly found in all hematopoietic cell lines but not nonhematopoietic cell lines.
c) The translocation seen in CML is also seen in other myeloproliferative disorders, such as polycythemia vera and idiopathic myelofibrosis.
d) The propensity of CML to progress to acute transformation is approximately 90%, much higher than that seen for other myeloproliferative disorders.
e) Patients often present with a palpable spleen and have an elevated leukocyte count, often higher than 200,000/mm$^3$.

**132.** All the following statements are true, *except*
a) Chronic use of long-acting β-agonists has been associated with loss of potency of bronchodilation and decreased duration of effect.
b) Zafirlukast is an orally administered leukotriene receptor antagonist.
c) Cromolyn is a mast cell stabilizer that has no known serious side effects.
d) Long-term use of high-dose inhaled steroids (>1,000 μg daily) has been associated with cataracts.
e) Oral candidiasis is a side effect associated with inhaled corticosteroids.

**133.** All the following are features of a third (oculomotor) cranial nerve palsy, *except*
a) Loss of taste in the posterior one-third of the tongue
b) Ptosis
c) Dilatation of the pupil
d) Outward and downward deviation of the affected eye
e) Absent pupillary reflexes

**134.** After an appendectomy, a 2-year-old boy has significant bleeding. His parents deny any bleeding tendencies in the family. Results of laboratory studies are as follows:

| | |
|---|---|
| Platelet count | 250,000/mm³ |
| Bleeding time | Less than 4 minutes |
| Prothrombin time (PT) | 12 seconds (same as control) |
| Partial thromboplastin time (PTT) | 28 seconds (same as control) |

Which of the following is the most likely diagnosis for this patient?
a) Thrombasthenia
b) Protein S deficiency
c) Factor XIII deficiency
d) Prekallikrein deficiency
e) Factor XII deficiency

**135.** All the following are common presenting symptoms of depression and *Diagnostic and Statistical Manual of Mental Disorders*, Fourth Edition, criteria for major depression, *except*
a) Fatigue or loss of energy
b) Beliefs of worthlessness or guilt
c) Recurring thoughts of death or suicide
d) Auditory hallucinations
e) Significant weight loss or weight gain

**136.** All the following are true of Horner's syndrome, *except*
a) Ptosis
b) Dilatation of the pupil
c) Anhidrosis
d) Interruption of sympathetic nerve fibers
e) Occasional association with apical bronchogenic carcinoma

**137.** A 45-year-old man was admitted to the ICU 5 days ago for acute respiratory failure.

Which of the following statements about this man's risk of catheter-related infection is *not* true?
a) Peripheral catheters placed in the lower extremity in comparison with those placed in the upper extremity increase the risk of subsequent catheter-related infection.
b) Central venous catheters placed into the internal jugular vein increase the risk, compared with those placed into the subclavian vein.
c) The duration of catheterization has been established as a significant risk factor for catheter-related infection.
d) Heparin-bonded central venous catheters reduce the risk of infections.
e) Catheters placed under emergency conditions are associated with higher rates of infection.

**138.** Which of the following statements regarding the mortality of ICU patients is *not* true?

a) The in-hospital mortality of mechanically ventilated patients presenting with status asthmaticus ranges from 10% to 38%.
b) The in-hospital mortality of mechanically ventilated patients with a history of chronic obstructive pulmonary disease who present with acute respiratory failure ranges from 20% to 60%.
c) Patients with ARDS who present without multiple organ failure have a mortality of approximately 35%.
d) Patients who have systemic inflammatory response syndrome have a mortality of less than 10%, but patients who progress to septic shock have a mortality of greater than 40%.
e) Cancer patients who require mechanical ventilation have an average in-hospital mortality of greater than 70%; however, patients presenting after bone marrow transplantation have only a 50% in-hospital mortality.

**139.** A 78-year-old African American man is brought to the emergency department by his family. He is known to have a mild baseline dementia but still lives alone and has been able to carry out the basic activities of daily living. The family states that over the last 24 hours he has become more confused. He has been unable to tolerate anything to eat or drink for the last 2 days and has been incontinent of very loose feces, with nausea, vomiting, and a low-grade fever. On examination, he appears frail and is oriented to person but not to place or time. Skin turgor is decreased. Lying blood pressure and pulse are 128/68 mm Hg and 80/bpm, and standing readings are 86/50 mm Hg and 118 beats/min. Examination of the respiratory, cardiovascular, and abdominal systems is normal.

Which of the following statements concerning this man's condition is true?
a) You expect a urinary $Na^+$ level less than 25 mEq daily.
b) You expect a urinary $Na^+$ level greater than 25 mEq daily.
c) If the serum $Na^+$ level is greater than 150 mEq/L, vasopressin therapy should be considered.
d) Because of the high risk of seizures in this case, prophylactic phenytoin should be started.
e) You expect a urinary $K^+$ level greater than 20 mEq daily.

**140.** Which of the following statements regarding the diagnosis of minimal change disease (MCD) is incorrect?
a) It accounts for 90% of nephrotic syndrome cases in children younger than 10 years, 50% in older children, and approximately 15% to 25% in adults.
b) On electron microscopy, diffuse fusion of the epithelial cell foot processes is seen.
c) A renal biopsy is necessary in both children and adults to confirm the diagnosis before the start of treatment.

d) Corticosteroids are the mainstay of therapy in MCD.

e) NSAIDs are the most common cause of secondary MCD, and most affected patients concurrently have an acute interstitial nephritis.

**141.** All the following statements about cholesterol screening are true, *except*

a) Cholesterol lowering and, therefore, cholesterol screening are more effective in primary prevention than in secondary prevention.

b) Measuring blood cholesterol levels is widely accepted as a convenient, safe, and inexpensive screening test.

c) Elevated blood cholesterol levels increase the risk for coronary heart disease (CHD).

d) The effects on CHD from lowering cholesterol depend on the magnitude of the cholesterol reduction.

e) In men and women with CHD, cholesterol reduction retards or reverses the progression of atherosclerotic plaques and reduces mortality from CHD.

**142.** A 45-year-old African American woman presents to the emergency department with fever, cough productive of reddish sputum, shortness of breath, and dyspnea on exertion. She was well until approximately 5 days ago. She denies any chest pain, palpitations, abdominal pain, diarrhea, or neurologic symptoms. Her vital signs reveal that she is febrile, normotensive, and tachycardic. On examination, she appears in mild respiratory distress. She has a normal head, eyes, ears, nose, and throat examination. Her neck is supple without any lymphadenopathy. On examination of her lungs, decreased breath sounds and egophony are heard in the left lower base, and dullness to percussion is present in the same region. Cardiovascular, abdominal, and neurologic examinations are unremarkable.

All the following regarding the diagnosis of community-acquired pneumonia in this patient are true, *except*

a) The clinical presentation of an abrupt illness with fever, chills, cough, and pleuritic pain is compatible with *Streptococcus pneumoniae* infection.

b) *S. pneumoniae* is the most common pathogen responsible for community-acquired pneumonia in all age groups.

c) *S. pneumoniae* is acquired through the nasopharynx and is carried asymptomatically by 50% of people at some point in their lives.

d) If this patient has *S. pneumoniae* infection, sputum culture will grow the organism in more than 80% of cases.

e) Mortality of patients with *S. pneumoniae* infection is low, even among ICU patients, who experience a 25% mortality.

**143.** A 40-year-old woman presents to you after reading an article in the newspaper about screening for ovarian cancer. She is concerned because although she comes for annual physical examinations and has her regular pelvic examinations, Pap tests, and all the tests that are recommended to her, nobody has told her that she needs to have screening tests for ovarian cancer. She feels very well and wants to remain so. She has no family history of ovarian cancer, but a friend was recently diagnosed with it. Her history and physical examination reveal nothing that suggests any increased risk of ovarian cancer.

What would be the most appropriate next step for this patient?

a) Call your lawyer in case she has ovarian cancer and you missed it.

b) Test for the tumor marker CA125.

c) Perform transvaginal ultrasonography.

d) Test for the tumor marker CA125, and perform trans-abdominal ultrasound.

e) Explain to her why no screening is indicated.

**144.** According to the revised AHA guidelines for the prevention of endocarditis, in which of the following groups (there may be more than one) would antimicrobial prophylaxis before a dental procedure *not* be recommended?

a) Patients with bioprosthetic and homograft valves

b) Patients with a surgically reconstructed pulmonary conduit

c) Patients with an unrepaired secundum atrial septal defect

d) Patients with previous rheumatic fever without valvular dysfunction

e) Patients diagnosed with mitral valve prolapse with valvular thickening

f) Patients diagnosed with hypertrophic cardiomyopathy

g) Patients with a history of infective endocarditis

**145.** All the following statements concerning asbestos-induced lung disease are true, *except*

a) Most patients are asymptomatic for at least 20 to 30 years.

b) Cough, sputum production, and wheezing are the most common presenting symptoms.

c) ANA and rheumatoid factor may be present.

d) Cigarette exposure increases the risk of lung cancer associated with asbestos exposure.

e) Asbestos exposure increases the risk of lung cancer associated with cigarette smoke exposure.

**146.** A 35-year-old woman presents with "recurrent chest infections." She has a long history of asthma but no other past medical history. She is a nonsmoker. In the past year, she has had several episodes of fever, malaise, and increased sputum production; twice, she had chest radiographs that showed infiltrates consistent with pneumonia. She now has recurrence of her symptoms. Chest radiography shows a parenchymal infiltrate in the left upper lobe and some atelectasis in the right base. Immediate skin test reactivity is positive for *Aspergillus* antigens, and she has serum antibodies to *A. fumigatus*.

All the following statements concerning this woman's condition are true, *except*

a) Proximal bronchiectasis is a feature of this disease.
b) Peripheral blood eosinophilia greater than 55/mm$^3$ is a feature of this disease.
c) Treatment should be an antimicrobial effective against *Aspergillus*.
d) Treatment should be a corticosteroid.
e) Serum IgE concentration greater than 1,000 ng/mL is a feature of this disease.

**147.** A 65-year-old man with a history of CAD and hypertension is admitted for unstable angina. He has been taking ticlopidine since his last angioplasty with stent placement. Vital signs reveal a temperature of 37.5°C, heart rate of 90/bpm, blood pressure of 130/90 mm Hg, and respiratory rate of 12/min. His lungs are clear, and his heart examination reveals a regular rate and rhythm, without an S$_3$ gallop or murmur. He has no peripheral edema. He is started on aspirin, metoprolol, nitroglycerin, heparin, and simvastatin. He is also given haloperidol for the "mental confusion" experienced in the coronary ICU. One day later, a platelet count is obtained, showing 25,000 cells/mm$^3$. His creatinine level is 2.5 mg/dL. Review of medical records from 6 months ago reveals a normal platelet count and creatinine. Heparin is stopped, and a hematology consultation is obtained. The peripheral smear reveals a few fragmented RBCs.

Which of the following diagnoses is most consistent with these findings?

a) Splenic sequestration
b) Idiopathic thrombocytopenic purpura
c) TTP
d) Heparin-induced thrombocytopenia
e) SLE

**148.** A 60-year-old man reports intermittent "indigestion." He rarely visits you; the last time was 5 years ago for a tetanus shot after a dirty cut that he sustained while working in his garden. He describes chest discomfort across the anterior aspect of his chest that lasts 1 to 5 minutes, is squeezing in nature, and is associated with shortness of breath, nausea, and a sense of foreboding. He was completely well until 2 months ago. Initially, the episodes occurred while he was playing tennis or doing heavy garden work; occasionally, they occurred after meals. Last month, he experienced more frequent symptoms brought on by walking upstairs, and today he had one episode at rest.

After further history and physical examination, which of the following is the best plan for this patient?

a) Admit him to the hospital for observation, further diagnosis, and treatment.
b) Arrange for a dobutamine echocardiogram within the next 2 weeks.
c) Arrange for a treadmill stress test within the next 2 days.
d) Prescribe nitroglycerin for sublingual use as needed, and follow up in 1 week or sooner if the discomfort does not resolve after three tablets.
e) Start a trial of an H$_2$-receptor blocker.

**149.** A 46-year-old man with a past history of CAD and diabetes mellitus presents to your office for a routine checkup. He denies angina since undergoing coronary artery bypass graft 3 years ago. His activity is limited by osteoarthritis of the knees and hips. Medications include an ACE inhibitor, a β-blocker, aspirin, digoxin, insulin, and ibuprofen. Routine laboratory studies reveal a K$^+$ level of 5.8 mEq/L.

All the following medications can cause an increase in potassium levels, *except*

a) ACE-inhibitors
b) Insulin
c) β-Blockers
d) Digoxin
e) Ibuprofen

**150.** A 25-year-old woman is noted on preoperative laboratory testing to have an abnormal CBC. She is otherwise well and awaiting a laparoscopy for chronic abdominal pain. Leukocyte count is 5,000/mm$^3$, Hgb level is 12 mg/dL, Hct is 36%, and platelet count is 14,000/mm$^3$; chemistry profile and serum creatinine are normal. On further questioning, she admits to easy bruising and heavy menses. Further testing is done. An antinuclear antibody (ANA) test result is negative.

Which of the following diagnoses is most consistent with these findings?

a) Splenic sequestration
b) Idiopathic thrombocytopenic purpura
c) TTP
d) Heparin-induced thrombocytopenia
e) SLE

**151.** A 39-year-old man presents with a nonproductive cough for 6 to 8 months. He states that the cough is very irritating because he frequently has to speak in public. Six months ago, he saw your colleague who he reports told him that it was a "postviral cough" and gave him an albuterol inhaler, which he used twice a day for 4 months. He discontinued it 2 months ago because it did not help the cough. Further history reveals nasal discharge, frequent throat clearing, and no wheezing or shortness of breath. The cough is worse in the morning but does not wake him from sleep; it is not associated with exercise. On examination, he appears generally well; his respiratory rate is 12/min and pulse is 72/bpm. Nasopharyngeal mucosa has a cobblestone appearance and the presence of secretions is noted. Auscultation of the lung fields is clear with no wheeze. Cardiovascular and abdominal examinations are normal. You observe his inhaler technique, and it is good.

What would be the most appropriate next step in his treatment?

a) Obtain spirometry to investigate for asthma.
b) Recommend restarting the albuterol in addition to an inhaled steroid.
c) Start a trial of an $H_2$ blocker.
d) Reassure him that the cough is probably postviral, and have him return in 3 months if the cough has not resolved.
e) Start a trial of a nasal steroid spray.

**152.** A 45-year-old man undergoing rehabilitation after hip surgery as a result of a motor vehicle accident is noted on a routine CBC to have a platelet count of 55,000/mm$^3$; at hospital discharge 3 weeks ago it was 200,000/mm$^3$. He has been taking a narcotic analgesic and lorazepam, as well as subcutaneous heparin injections, since admission to the rehabilitation center. Heparin has been stopped. Peripheral blood smear is unremarkable, except for thrombocytopenia.

Which of the following diagnoses is most consistent with these findings?

a) Splenic sequestration
b) Idiopathic thrombocytopenic purpura
c) TTP
d) Heparin-induced thrombocytopenia
e) SLE

**153.** A 39-year-old woman presents to the emergency department with shortness of breath and chest pain. She reluctantly confesses to smoking two packs of cigarettes per day, although she had told her primary care doctor that she had stopped smoking. The only medication she is taking is an oral contraceptive. The chest pain is sharp and "catches" when she takes a deep breath. She has no fever, cough, or sputum production. She had a history of DVT approximately 6 months ago, for which she was treated with warfarin for 3 months. Her left calf has remained a little swollen since the incident of DVT. On physical examination, she is breathing uncomfortably and rapidly at a rate of 28/min; pulse is regular at 110/bpm. The trachea is central, percussion is resonant, and breath sounds are normal in all areas. The chest pain is not reproduced on palpation, although it occurs on deep inspiration. You highly suspect that she may have a pulmonary embolus.

All the following statements concerning the diagnosis of pulmonary embolus are true, *except*

a) In this case, a high-probability perfusion scan would indicate a high likelihood of pulmonary embolus.
b) In this case, a low-probability lung scan does not exclude the diagnosis of pulmonary embolus.

c) A raised D-dimer (>500 ng/mL) is highly specific for the diagnosis of pulmonary embolus.
d) Pulmonary angiography is the gold standard.
e) Echocardiography has a low sensitivity.

**154.** Which of the following statements regarding superior vena cava (SVC) syndrome are true?

a) The most common histologic type of lung cancer associated with SVC syndrome is squamous cell carcinoma.
b) The incidence of SVC syndrome in patients with lung cancer is approximately 20%.
c) Patients often experience headache or fullness in the head and dyspnea.
d) a and b.
e) b and c.

**155.** While on call in the hospital, you are walking through a ward when a nurse comes running to you, requesting your help with a patient whose doctor she is unable to locate. The patient is a 62-year-old man who has a heart rate of 38/bpm and is feeling lightheaded and short of breath.

Which of the following statements concerning this situation is true?

a) Atropine, 1 mg intravenously, is an appropriate treatment if the patient is recovering from heart transplantation.
b) High-dose isoproterenol is an appropriate treatment for this bradycardia.
c) Adenosine is a first-line choice of drug therapy.
d) Transcutaneous pacing can be effective treatment, but it is often painful.
e) If the patient is unstable with a falling blood pressure, then synchronized direct-current cardioversion is the appropriate therapy.

**156.** A 55-year-old man presents with confusion and fever. He presented with an acute inferoposterior MI 1 week prior and underwent coronary angioplasty with stent placement to the right coronary artery. He has been receiving aspirin, metoprolol, and clopidogrel since the procedure. On physical examination he is febrile (38.4°C), disoriented to place and time, his heart rate is 85, and his blood pressure is 95/73 mm Hg. The medical resident witnesses a short-lived tonic-clonic seizure while examining the patient. Although his postictal state lasts an hour, no focal neurologic abnormalities are detected on repeated neurologic examinations. A brain CT is unremarkable. Laboratory studies reveal the following:

| | |
|---|---|
| Hct | 24% |
| WBC | 7,100/mm$^3$ |
| Platelets | 11,000/mm$^3$ |
| PT | 12 seconds |
| PTT | 31 seconds |
| BUN | 21 mg/dL |

| | |
|---|---|
| Serum creatinine | 2.9 mg/dL |
| LDH | 900 U/L |
| Direct Coombs' test | Negative |

The next step in the management of this patient at this time is
a) Pulmonary artery catheterization placement for hemodynamic guided management
b) Intravenous fluid resuscitation and positive inotropic agents
c) Broad-spectrum intravenous antibiotics and cerebrospinal fluid analysis
d) Transthoracic echocardiography
e) Peripheral blood smear review

**157–159.** Match the host defense defect with the clinical presentation in questions 157 to 159:
a) Common variable immunodeficiency
b) Selective IgA deficiency
c) Reduced activity of the late components of serum complement pathway: C6, C7, or C8
d) Complement deficiency factors H and I (alternate pathways)
e) Job's syndrome

**157.** A 19-year-old white woman with history of recurrent sinus and lung infections presents with weight loss, anemia, night sweats, and mediastinal lymph node enlargement by chest radiograph.

**158.** Recurrent *Neisseria meningitidis* and *Neisseria gonorrhoeae*

**159.** Recurrent "cold" staphylococcal abscesses, failure to shed primary teeth, eczema, hyperimmunoglobulinemia E, and impaired neutrophil chemotactic responses.

**160–165.** Match the disease with the laboratory findings in questions 160 to 165:

| | Alkaline Phosphatase | Serum Calcium | Serum Parathyroid Hormone | Urine Calcium |
|---|---|---|---|---|
| a) | – | _ or | | |
| b) | | | | – |
| c) | – | – | – | – |
| d) | – | | | or _ |
| e) | – | – | _ or | _ or |
| f) | – | – | – | – |

**160.** Osteoporosis

**161.** Metastatic neoplasm to the bones

**162.** Osteomalacia

**163.** Paget's disease

**164.** Primary hyperparathyroidism

**165.** Vitamin D excess

**166.** A 75-year-old man presents with fatigue and decreased energy. He has lived alone since his wife died 2 years ago. His last physical examination was in 1978, when he changed jobs. He is edentulous, and he cooks for himself. On examination, temperature is 36.5°C, respiratory rate is 18/min, heart rate is 83/bpm, and blood pressure is 142/87 mm Hg. His lung, heart, and abdominal examinations are unremarkable. Perifollicular hyperkeratotic papules containing hemorrhages and purpuric rash are noted on the backs of his thighs. Laboratory tests reveal the following:

| | |
|---|---|
| WBC | 4,239/mm³ (normal differential) |
| Hgb | 9.8 |
| Platelets | 145,000/μL |
| MCV | 101 |
| Blood smear | Hypersegmented neutrophils and macrocytic RBCs |
| BUN | 32 mg/dL |
| Serum creatinine | 1.3 mg/dL |
| ANA | Positive |

The most likely diagnosis is
a) Vitamin A deficiency
b) Vitamin $B_{12}$ deficiency
c) Folic acid deficiency
d) Vitamin C deficiency
e) Lead poisoning

**167.** A 45-year-old woman reports being "off-balance" for the past several weeks. She has sustained several falls and was treated at the local urgent care clinic for skin lacerations and mild bruises. She reports no head injury but states that she consumed five cans of beer and enjoyed two to three martinis with dinner daily for the past 9 years. On review of systems, she complains of chronic abdominal pain. Her past medical history is remarkable for hypertension and weekly marijuana use. On examination, she is mildly delirious, her temperature is 35.4°C, blood pressure is 187/110 mm Hg, and pulse is 78/bpm. She has poor dental hygiene, horizontal nystagmus, diplopia, ataxia, and a distended abdomen. A kidney, ureter, and bladder examination reveals calcifications in the midepigastric area. A brain CT reveals cerebral atrophy without evidence of intracranial bleed or masses. Laboratory tests indicate the following:

| | |
|---|---|
| Hgb | 11.6 g/dL |
| WBC | 8,323 mm³/dL (normal differential) |
| Platelets | 138,000/μL |
| MCV | 107 |

The most likely explanation of her neurologic symptoms is which of the following?
a) Acute alcohol intoxication

b) Cocaine overdose
c) Wernicke's encephalopathy
d) Cerebellar degeneration
e) Korsakoff's psychosis

**168.** An 82-year-old white man with past medical history of hypertension, CAD, cerebrovascular accident, T12 compression fracture, and asthma presents with malaise, anorexia, hip and shoulder pain and stiffness, and an inability to arise from chair, walk, and care for himself. On further questioning, he reports a 3-month history of fatigue, weight loss, and bilateral shoulder and hip stiffness. He recalls feeling relief from his symptoms after self-administration of tapered corticosteroid doses taken during episodes of asthma exacerbation. On examination, he is afebrile, has limited range of motion of the hips and shoulders, and is unable to raise the right arm laterally above 30 degrees. Point tenderness at the sub-acromial bursa is noted. His examination is otherwise unremarkable. A brain CT shows no evidence of intracranial hemorrhage or recent infarct. Laboratory tests indicate the following:

| | |
|---|---|
| Na$^+$ | 135 mEq/dL |
| K$^+$ | 4.1 mEq/dL |
| BUN | 21 mg/dL |
| Creatinine | 1.1 mg/dL |
| HCO$_{3-}$ | 23 mEq/dL |
| WBC | 5,300/mm$^3$ |
| Hgb | 10.0 g/dL |
| Platelets | 389,000/μL |
| Westergren sedimentation rate | 99 mL/hour |
| C-reactive protein | 6.6 |
| Creatine phosphokinase | 241 U/L |

He receives prednisone (20 mg/day) and exhibits dramatic subjective and objective improvement after 24 hours. Ten days after the initiation of prednisone, he has no further complaints, and his Westergren sedimentation rate and C-reactive protein levels have decreased to 22 mm/hour and 0.3, respectively; his Hgb level has increased to 12.3 g/dL.

The most likely cause of this patient's musculoskeletal symptoms is
a) Inflammatory polymyositis
b) Fibromyalgia
c) Pseudoosteoarthritis
d) Inclusion body myositis
e) Polymyalgia rheumatica

**169.** A 79-year-old African American man presents to the office for follow-up of hypertension and hyperkalemia. His past medical history is remarkable for long-standing diabetes mellitus and congestive heart failure. His medications include enalapril (5 mg/day), hydrochlorothiazide (25 mg/day), insulin (70/30, 20 units in a.m. and 14 units in p.m.), digoxin

(1.25 mg/day), metoprolol (25 mg/day), and aspirin (81 mg/day). He reports medical and dietary compliance and denies using any over-the-counter medications. On examination, he is afebrile, heart rate is 74/bpm, and blood pressure is 173/102 mm Hg. His weight is 73 kg and height is 5 ft, 10 in. A nonradiating systolic murmur, best heard at the apex, is auscultated. Abdominal examination reveals no bruits. Trace pitting pedal edema and decreased distal pulses are evident on lower extremity examination. His funduscopic examination reveals grade II arteriolosclerotic retinopathy on the Keith-Wagener-Barker classification scale. Laboratory studies obtained the morning of the visit were as follows:

| | |
|---|---|
| Na$^+$ | 132 mEq/dL |
| K$^+$ | 5.9 mEq/dL |
| BUN | 58 mg/dL |
| Creatinine | 1.8 mg/dL |
| HCO$_{3-}$ | 21 mEq/L |
| Chloride | 115 mEq/L |
| Calcium | 8.4 mg/dL |
| Glucose | Fasting 198 mg/dL |
| Arterial blood gases (room air) | |
| Po$_2$ | 94 mm Hg |
| Pco$_2$ | 41 mm Hg |
| pH | 7.31 |
| O$_2$ saturation | 77% |

His aldosterone and renin activity shows low normal values, which do rise with postural changes and diuretics.

The most likely cause of this patient's abnormalities is
a) Addison's disease
b) Conn's syndrome
c) Secondary aldosteronism
d) Hyporeninemic hypoaldosteronism
e) Iatrogenic Cushing's syndrome

**170–172.** Match the laboratory findings of a 72-hour fast with the most likely underlying cause of fasting hypoglycemia in questions 170 to 172:

| | Insulin | C-Peptide | Urine Drug Screen |
|---|---|---|---|
| a) | – | – | |
| b) | – | – | |
| c) | – | – | Positive |
| d) | – | – | |

**170.** Exogenous insulin use

**171.** Sulfonylurea use

**172.** Insulinoma

**173–179.** For each of the physical auscultatory findings described here, select the most likely diagnosis in questions 173 through 179:
a) Tricuspid regurgitation
b) Austin-Flint murmur

c) Mitral stenosis
d) Aortic valve stenosis
e) Aortic regurgitation
f) Ostium secundum atrial septal defect
g) Hypertrophic obstructive cardiomyopathy
h) Patent ductus arteriosus
i) Mitral prolapse

**173.** A grade 3 harsh systolic ejection murmur begins well after $S_1$. It is best heard in the lower left sternal border and the apex. The murmur becomes louder with Valsalva's maneuver and standing, and diminishes with squatting.

**174.** A grade 2 midsystolic ejection murmur is heard at the base, loudest in the pulmonary area. $S_1$ is normal, but $S_2$ is widely split and is relatively fixed in relation to respiration. A prominent right ventricular cardiac impulse is palpated.

**175.** A low-pitched rumbling murmur is heard throughout diastole. The murmur is best heard with the diaphragm of the stethoscope with the patient in the left lateral recumbent position. An additional sound that occurs shortly after $S_2$ may precede the murmur. The murmur may become louder just before $S_1$.

**176.** A grade 2 mid-diastolic murmur is heard in patients with aortic regurgitation.

**177.** A grade 4 diastolic murmur at the left sternal border begins at $S_2$ and is best heard in the sitting position. It is accentuated when the patient leans forward and exhales.

**178.** A grade 3 blowing holosystolic murmur is heard, loudest at the lower left sternal border, and increasing with inspiration and diminishing with Valsalva's maneuver.

**179.** A grade 3 low-pitched rough murmur, loudest at the base of the heart, reaches a peak in mid-systole. Concordant bruits are heard in the carotid arteries.

**180.** A 63-year-old man with severe chronic obstructive pulmonary disease presents to the emergency department with severe respiratory distress. Arterial blood gas measurement is obtained as follows:

| | Current | 1 Month Ago (Office Visit) |
|---|---|---|
| $Pa_{O2}$ | 51 mmHg | 59 mmHg |
| $Pc_{O2}$ | 73 mmHg | 51 mmHg |
| pH | 7.25 | 7.38 |

He continues to deteriorate despite maximal therapy, and mechanical ventilation is instituted.

Which of the following arterial blood gases values would be most desirable for this patient?

| | $Pa_{O2}$ | $Pa_{CO2}$ | pH | $Fi_{O2}$ | $Sa_{O2}$ |
|---|---|---|---|---|---|
| a) | 91 | 62 | 7.31 | 40% | 94% |
| b) | 55 | 42 | 7.43 | 50% | 86% |
| c) | 65 | 50 | 7.37 | 40% | 93% |
| d) | 65 | 40 | 7.47 | 40% | 93% |

**181.** A 33-year-old 34-week pregnant woman presents with petechial rash and epistaxis. Laboratory tests reveal the following:

| | |
|---|---|
| WBC | 6,000/mm³ (normal differential) |
| Hgb | 14.8 g/dL |
| Platelets | 18,000/μL |
| Chemistry profile | Normal |
| Bone marrow aspirate | Normal with abundant megakaryocytes |

She is started on prednisone (60 mg/day). Four days later, she begins to have contractions, and delivery is expected within the next 12 hours. Repeat CBC reveals a platelet count of 31,000/μL.

Your next step in management is which of the following?
a) Pulse glucocorticoid (Solumedrol, 1 g/day for 3 days)
b) Danazol, orally
c) Continuous platelet transfusion until 6 hours after delivery
d) Emergent plasma exchange
e) Intravenous gamma globulin

**182–187.** For each patient listed, select the most likely set of liver function test findings for questions 182 through 187:

| | Alanine Aminotransferase (ALT) (U/L) | Aspartate Aminotransferase (AST) (U/L) | Alkaline Phosphatase (U/L) | Total Bilirubin (mg/dL) | Albumin (g/dL) | PT/control (seconds) |
|---|---|---|---|---|---|---|
| a) | 994 | 518 | 110 | 2.2 | 4.1 | 11.8/11 |
| b) | 87 | 81 | 902 | 6.1 | 3.1 | 14.8/11 |
| c) | 18,900 | 17,230 | 269 | 7.1 | 3.1 | 20/11 |
| d) | 63 | 273 | 121 | 3.7 | 2.2 | 16/11 |
| e) | 21 | 23 | 70 | 2.6 | 4.1 | 11.2/11 |
| f) | 44 | 46 | 444 | 0.9 | 4.5 | 12.2/11 |

**182.** A 23-year-old man develops mild icterus 48 hours after fasting. His examination is otherwise unremarkable.

**183.** A 28-year-old college student presents with right upper quadrant pain, diarrhea, anorexia, and fever 2 weeks after returning from a trip to Mexico.

**184.** A 55-year-old woman with 10-year history of progressive pruritus develops increasing abdominal girth and dark urine.

**185.** A 51-year-old farmer develops increasing abdominal girth over the preceding month. He presents with fever, abdominal pain, and vomiting. He drinks four to six beers every day and two glasses of wine with dinner.

**186.** A 35-year-old African American woman presents with progressive shortness of breath on exertion. Her chest radiograph reveals hilar lymphadenopathy and interstitial infiltrates. She is found to be anergic on skin testing.

**187.** A 49-year-old woman with history of hepatitis C and bipolar disorder was found unconscious. An empty bottle of acetaminophen was found on the floor.

**188.** A 19-year-old man presents with dysuria and penile discharge for 5 days. He reports having unprotected sexual encounters with multiple prostitutes over the past 3 weeks. On examination, an indurated 2- to 4-cm warm, tender inguinal mass is palpated. An ultrasound examination of the groin suggests that the mass represents enlarged inguinal lymph nodes. A Gram's stain of the discharge shows numerous neutrophils and Gram-negative intracellular diplococci. Rapid plasma reagin is nonreactive, and HIV serology is negative.

The next most appropriate step in management is
a) Give a single dose of ceftriaxone intravenously, 250 mg.
b) Give a single dose of ceftriaxone intravenously, 250 mg, and doxycycline for 7 days.
c) Give a single dose of ceftriaxone orally, 2 g, and doxycycline for 14 days.
d) Give a single dose of ceftriaxone (125 mg intramuscularly) and doxycycline (100 mg two times a day for 7 days), until *Chlamydia trachomatis* serology is back.
e) Await the results of culture and sensitivity testing and counsel him regarding safe sex practices.

**189.** A 53-year-old man with a history of chronic pancreatitis and chronic hepatitis secondary to alcoholism presents to the emergency department complaining of worsening epigastric pain and dizziness. Recently, his chronic pain has been hard to control despite adequate pain medications. On examination, he is afebrile, orthostatic, and has heme-positive stool. Laboratory evaluation reveals the following:

| | |
|---|---|
| Hgb | 5.0 g/dL |
| Platelets | 402,000/µL |
| MCV | 86.4 |
| WBC | 9,800/mm$^3$ |
| PT | 11.2 seconds |
| International normalized ratio | 0.98 |
| PTT | 31.1 seconds |
| Albumin | 3.0 g/dL |
| AST | 81 U/L |
| ALT | 56 U/L |
| Alkaline phosphatase | 377 U/L |
| Bilirubin | 0.8 mg/dL |
| Amylase | 55 U/L |
| Lipase | 12 U/L |

Fresh blood is apparent on gastric lavage, and an urgent esophagogastroduodenoscopy confirms the presence of fresh blood clots in the fundus, with multiple gastric varices and one bleeding varix. The bleeding site is successfully injected with epinephrine. Blood transfusion, octreotide, and propranolol therapy are initiated. The bleeding does not recur, and his hospital course is uncomplicated.

Before discharge, which of the following diagnostic tests is indicated to further explore the cause of this patient's gastric varices?
a) Endoscopic retrograde cholangiopancreatography
b) Percutaneous transhepatic cholangiography
c) Visceral angiography
d) Transjugular hepatic biopsy
e) Radionuclide (hepatobiliary iminodiacetic acid) biliary scan

**190.** A 59-year-old man with a history of hypertension and end-stage renal disease develops refractory hypotension during dialysis. He has missed two dialysis sessions, and his BUN level on presentation is 109 mg/dL. He reports constant chest discomfort, dyspnea on exertion, and easy fatigability over the past week. On examination, he is alert and oriented, heart rate is 112 beats/min and regular, and blood pressure is 88/57 mm Hg. On inspiration, his systolic blood pressure (SBP) falls to 62 mm Hg. His jugular veins are distended and elevated to the jaw angle. Chest radiography shows cardiomegaly and mild interstitial edema, and the ECG reveals diffuse low voltage.

The most appropriate next step in management is which of the following?
a) Start heparin infusion and aim for a prothrombin time (PTT) of 55 to 75 seconds and obtain lung perfusion scan.
b) Start dobutamine and place pulmonary artery catheter to guide management.
c) Infuse 1 L of normal saline followed by dextrose 5% in water and observe.
d) Admit to the telemetry unit and obtain a set of cardiac enzymes.
e) Admit to the ICU and obtain an urgent echocardiogram.

**191–194.** For each patient described with dysphagia, select the most likely diagnosis for questions 191 through 194:

a) Esophageal carcinoma

b) Esophageal web

c) Achalasia

d) Gastroesophageal reflux disease

e) Scleroderma

**191.** A 42-year-old woman with a history of episodes of digital pallor

**192.** A 49-year-old man with recurrent chest pain and negative recent stress test presents with nocturnal cough

**193.** A 56-year-old man with a history of progressive dysphagia and constant retrosternal discomfort over the past 2 months who requests a prescription for a nicotine patch

**194.** A 48-year-old woman with long-standing menorrhagia and glossitis

**195.** A 42-year-old Boy Scouts scoutmaster presents with a painful violet pustule on the dorsum of his right hand that appeared 2 weeks after returning from a fishing trip. A crusted ulcer is seen in the mid portion of the pustule. He denies any constitutional symptoms.

The most likely cause of this infection is

a) *Mycobacterium leprae*

b) *Pseudomonas aeruginosa*

c) *Sporothrix schenckii*

d) *Rickettsia rickettsii*

e) *Mycobacterium marinum*

**196.** Paradoxical splitting of the second heart sound may be heard with which of the following?

a) Right bundle branch block

b) Restrictive cardiomyopathy

c) Pulmonic stenosis

d) Aortic dissection with new diastolic murmur

e) Aortic stenosis

**197.** A 23-year-old man with a history of nephrotic syndrome presents with the acute onset of severe right flank pain, gross hematuria, and left testicular pain. On examination he is afebrile, heart rate is 87/bpm, and blood pressure is 158/94 mm Hg. A left-sided varicocele is palpated and severe left flank tenderness is evident. He has 2+ pitting pedal edema. His medications include prednisone (20 mg/day) and cyclophosphamide (2 mg/kg/day). Laboratory tests reveal the following:

| | **Currently** | **3 Weeks Ago** |
| --- | --- | --- |
| BUN | 76 mg/dL | 34 mg/dL |
| Serum creatinine | 4.3 mg/dL | 1.9 mg/dL |
| Serum albumin | 2.4 g/dL | 3.2 g/dL |
| Serum uric acid | 6.9 mg/dL | 7.1 mg/dL |
| Serum calcium | 7.1 mg/dL | 7.9 mg/dL |
| Urinalysis | | |
| RBC | Too numerous to count | 510/high-power field |
| WBC | 05/high-power field | 03/high-power field |
| Protein | 4+ | 1+ |
| Casts | Occasional granular | Occasional granular |

Renal ultrasound shows an increased size of the left kidney with no collecting system dilatation or nephrolithiasis. The most likely diagnosis is which of the following?

a) Renal cell carcinoma

b) Obstructive uropathy secondary to retroperitoneal hematoma

c) Emphysematous pyelonephritis

d) Perinephric abscess

e) Renal vein thrombosis

**198.** A 21-year-old college student who was found confused and disruptive by the dorm security staff is brought to the emergency department. He states that he has no complaints, is not tired, and is "getting ready to party for 8 more hours." On examination, he is agitated, heart rate is 113/bpm, blood pressure is 155/96 mm Hg, respiratory rate is 19, and temperature is 37.1°C. His pupils are dilated. Heart examination reveals regular tachycardia, and an ECG confirms sinus tachycardia.

A urine drug screen is most likely to be positive for which of the following?

a) Nicotine

b) Cocaine

c) Opiates

d) Amphetamines

e) Hallucinogens

**199.** A 56-year-old diabetic woman presents with new-onset diplopia and headache. On examination, she has left eye ptosis, and her left pupil is dilated and fixed to light. The left eye is deviated laterally and slightly downward.

The etiology of these abnormalities is which of the following?

a) Diabetic third nerve palsy on the left

b) Diabetic sixth nerve palsy on the right

c) Left pontine lacunar infarct

d) Surgical third nerve palsy secondary to aneurysm of the posterior communicating artery

e) Migraine attack

**200–205.** Match the serologic findings with the appropriate patient in questions 200 through 205:

a) HBsAg (+), Anti-HBs (−), Anti-HBc (−)

b) Anti-HBs (+), Anti-HBc (+)

c) Anti-HBs (+), Anti-HBc (−)

d) HBsAg (+), HBeAg (+)

e) HBsAg (−), Anti-HBs (−), Anti-HBc (+)

f) HBsAg (+), Anti-HBe (+)

**200.** Late acute hepatitis B (window phenomenon)

**201.** Recent hepatitis B, highly infectious

**202.** Status postvaccination for hepatitis B

**203.** Early acute hepatitis B

**204.** Previous hepatitis B infection, full recovery

**205.** Acute hepatitis B, noninfectious

## ANSWERS AND DISCUSSION

### 1. a.
In patients with cirrhosis and ascites, the hepatorenal syndrome has been shown to occur in up to 19% of patients at 1 year and 39% at 5 years. Patients who are hyponatremic or hyperreninemic or have preexisting renal insufficiency are at highest risk. Interestingly, patients with primary biliary cirrhosis are relatively protected against the development of the hepatorenal syndrome. The development of hepatorenal syndrome is insidious, often with little (0.1 mg/dL) or no daily rise in creatinine. It can, however, be precipitated by an acute insult, such as gastrointestinal bleeding, infection, or overly rapid diuresis. A very low sodium excretion and oliguria also characterize the hepatorenal syndrome (in the absence of diuretics).

### 2. e.
Indications for emergent hemodialysis should not be based on the value of BUN or creatinine levels. Indications for emergent hemodialysis include symptomatic uremia (including pericarditis, neuropathy, or unexplained alterations in mental status), significant fluid overload, refractory hyperkalemia, or refractory metabolic acidosis. This man is neither symptomatic from uremia nor significantly fluid overloaded. Furthermore, his ECG does not demonstrate changes typically seen with significant hyperkalemia (he may have a baseline $K^+$ of 5.5 mEq/L). His metabolic acidosis is probably also near his baseline. He may need hemodialysis in the very near future, but not emergently.

### 3. c.
Delirium is a common condition in elderly hospitalized patients. Physical restraints are not the best plan in this case. The use of physical restraints has associated morbidity and mortality, and they should be used only when other management possibilities, such as environmental changes or nursing and family support, cannot be established. As well as immediate safety, evaluation and determination of the underlying cause of delirium is important to enable treatment of the underlying cause, and, consequently, the confusion.

### 4. c.
It is important to know the clinical findings associated with all valvular abnormalities. All the signs and symptoms in this case point to aortic stenosis. This is a systolic murmur, which eliminates mitral stenosis. The murmur of hypertrophic obstructive cardiomyopathy is increased with Valsalva's maneuver. Neither mitral regurgitation nor mitral valve prolapse is associated with narrowed pulse pressure or slow upstroke.

### 5. e.
Features of hypertrophic obstructive cardiomyopathy include left ventricular hypertrophy with asymmetric septal hypertrophy, causing a dynamic left ventricular outflow tract pressure gradient and diastolic dysfunction from stiffness of the hypertrophied muscle. Interventions that increase the murmur include those that decrease preload (diuretics, nitrates, Valsalva's maneuver, standing from squatting), decrease afterload (vasodilators, amyl nitrite, ACE-I inhibitor), or increase contractility (digoxin, dopamine, and premature ventricular contractions). Interventions that decrease the murmur include those that increase preload (intravenous fluids, passive leg raising, squatting), increase afterload (handgrip), or decrease contractility (β-blockers, disopyramide, verapamil).

### 6. d.
Renal failure in acute renal failure due to ATN lasts for 7 to 21 days. It is usually followed by a period of diuresis and then recovery back to baseline renal function. Patients with underlying kidney disease may have a prolonged failure phase and may not entirely recover back to baseline. ATN is the most common cause of acute renal failure in hospitalized patients. It has a variety of causes including ischemia and exposure to nephrotoxins, such as aminoglycosides and radiocontrast media. Prerenal azotemia is the second most common cause. The urine sediment is often helpful in distinguishing prerenal azotemia from ATN. In ATN, one may see muddy-brown granular and epithelial casts. However, in nonoliguric ATN, these casts may not be seen. In addition, hyperbilirubinemia can lead by unclear mechanisms to the formation of granular and epithelial casts in the absence of overt tubular disease. The $FE_{Na}$ and urine osmolality are helpful in distinguishing prerenal azotemia from ATN. In prerenal azotemia, the $FE_{Na}$ is usually less than 1%, and the urine osmolality is greater than 500 mOsm/kg. Conversely, in ATN, the $FE_{Na}$ is usually greater than 2%, and the urine osmolality is less than 450 mOsm/kg (often less than 350 mOsm/kg).

### 7. a.
With his positive anti-GBM antibody status, this man has evidence of glomerulonephritis. These antibodies are directed to a target on the NC1 domain of the α3 chain of type IV collagen found in the basement membrane. Goodpasture's syndrome requires the presence of

glomerulonephritis, pulmonary hemorrhage, and anti-GBM antibodies. This man does not have evidence of pulmonary hemorrhage. He also is positive for P-ANCA, which can be seen in 10% to 38% of patients with anti-GBM antibody disease. P-ANCAs are directed against myeloperoxidase. Thus, overlap with Wegener's granulomatosis or a related disease may exist, with occasional evidence of a systemic vasculitis. Treatment for these patients has a more favorable outcome than for P-ANCA–negative individuals.

**8. e.**

An oral contraceptive taken for more than 3 years decreases the risk of ovarian cancer.

**9. c.**

This man's clinical picture suggests obstructive sleep apnea. Patients with unexplained excessive daytime sleepiness deserve further evaluation, and the diagnosis of obstructive sleep apnea requires examining a patient during sleep.

**10. d.**

Sinus disease develops in most patients with cystic fibrosis, with pan-opacification of the paranasal sinuses in 90% to 100% of patients older than 8 months. A sweat chloride test result of greater than 70 mEq/L discriminates cystic fibrosis from other lung diseases. More than 95% of men with cystic fibrosis are infertile, mostly due to incomplete development of the wolffian structures, particularly the vas deferens.

**11. c.**

Myasthenia gravis is the diagnosis suggested by the findings in this woman. The disease is more common in women than men (3:1). Pupillary reactions are always spared in myasthenia gravis. Small, irregular pupils that react to accommodation but not to light are described as Argyll Robertson pupils and are found in patients with neurosyphilis and occasionally in those with diabetes mellitus. The diagnostic test for myasthenia gravis involves intravenous injection of the anticholinesterase inhibitor edrophonium chloride.

**12. d.**

According to Astler and Coller's modification of the Dukes' staging system (Table 73.1), this patient has stage C2 cancer. Penetration into the perirectal fat makes it stage B2, but lymph node involvement makes it stage C2. Furthermore, this staging system is helpful in predicting prognosis, which is directly related to cancer penetration and nodal involvement at the time of resection.

**13. d.**

Anaphylaxis can occur within 5 to 60 minutes after exposure to an allergen. This medical student is at risk of anaphylaxis and death. He needs a controlled and monitored environment. Epinephrine is the drug of choice;

**TABLE 73.1**

**STAGING OF COLORECTAL CANCER**

| Stage | Penetration | 5-Yr Survival (%) |
|---|---|---|
| A | Mucosal, above muscularis propria, no involvement of lymph nodes | 97 |
| B1 | Into muscularis propria but above pericolic fat, no involvement of lymph nodes | 78 |
| B2 | Into pericolic or perirectal fat, no involvement of lymph nodes | 78 |
| C1 | Same penetration as B1 with nodal metastases | 74 |
| C2 | Same penetration as B2 with nodal metastases | 48 |
| D | Distant metastases | 4 |

fatality rates are highest in patients in whom epinephrine administration is delayed. Severe airway edema, severe bronchospasm, or hypotension requires intravenous administration of 0.5 to 1.0 mL of epinephrine. Mild or moderate symptoms without laryngeal edema, bronchospasm, or hypotension should be treated with 0.3 to 0.5 mL of 1:1,000 epinephrine subcutaneously or intramuscularly.

**14. d.**

Eccentric calcification should raise concern of a carcinoma. Popcorn, laminated, central, and diffuse homogenous calcification patterns strongly suggest that the lesion is benign.

**15. b.**

Patients with polycythemia vera who have an Hct greater than 45% usually have decreased cerebral blood flow and an increased thrombotic tendency. The bone marrow is usually hypercellular, with hyperplasia of all bone marrow elements. Iron stores are not increased, and patients actually may be iron deficient due to an increased tendency for gastrointestinal blood loss because of dysfunctional platelets. Finally, a characteristic finding in polycythemia vera is a decreased erythropoietin level due to feedback inhibition (i.e., the proliferation of marrow elements occurs independently of erythropoietin stimulation).

**16. b.**

The pulmonary symptoms and signs are suggestive of bronchiectasis. Kartagener's syndrome consists of dextrocardia, sinusitis, and bronchiectasis. Young's syndrome is defined as obstructive azoospermia; approximately 20% to 30% of patients have bronchiectasis. Early panacinar emphysema, as well as bronchiectasis, may develop in patients with $\alpha_1$-antitrypsin deficiency. Yellow nail syndrome is characterized by the triad of lymphedema, pleural effusion, and yellow discoloration of the nails;

40% of patients have bronchiectasis. Patients with Williams-Campbell syndrome have a deficiency of the bronchial cartilage of medium-sized airways, which dilate and can be complicated by bronchiectasis.

### 17. a.

This man most likely has portal hypertension and ascites. Splenic sequestration of platelets secondary to portal hypertension often leads to a decrease in the platelet count. Alcohol also has a direct cytotoxic effect on megakaryocytes. Furthermore, inadequate thrombopoietin production may be present in the failing liver, also leading to the decreased production of platelets. Nevertheless, the platelet count rarely falls to less than 10,000/mm$^3$.

### 18. b.

Eighty-five percent of women with preexisting mild hypertension do well through pregnancy. Of those taking medication, some may be able to reduce the dose or stop the antihypertensive agent during the second trimester because of the usual drop in blood pressure. Studies have shown that treatment of mild hypertension before and during pregnancy does not reduce the risk for preeclampsia or eclampsia and does not improve maternal or fetal health. Indications for drug treatment usually include a diastolic blood pressure (DBP) of greater than 100 mm Hg or evidence of end-organ damage from the hypertension. Methyldopa and hydralazine have been shown to be safe for the fetus, as opposed to ACE-inhibitors, which have been associated with poor fetal outcome, perhaps related to dysregulation of uteroplacental blood flow.

### 19. a.

In iron deficiency anemia, marrow iron stores are absent and the serum iron and serum ferritin levels are low, whereas the erythrocyte porphyrin level is high. Iron deficiency anemia is characterized by hypochromic, microcytic RBCs in contrast to the normocytic, normochromic RBCs seen in anemia of chronic disease. Finally, the reticulocyte index is a measure of RBC generation of the marrow. In both iron deficiency anemia and anemia of chronic disease, the reticulocyte index is not increased because it is an anemia resulting from RBC loss or destruction.

### 20. c.

This man most likely has ulcerative colitis. Corticosteroids are used in the treatment of ulcerative colitis and Crohn's disease, but controlled trials have shown no benefit in maintaining remission. In patients with a severe exacerbation of colitis, oral intake can promote colonic activity, and intravenous alimentation serves as a component of therapy, although no evidence suggests that it alone is effective as primary therapy. Sulfasalazine is a well-established agent for use in remission, but can also be used in therapy of an acute flare. Drugs such

as codeine, diphenoxylate, or anticholinergics are contraindicated because they can promote colonic dilatation and toxic megacolon.

### 21. b.

The most likely diagnosis is primary hyperparathyroidism. Elevated circulating parathyroid hormone in the presence of elevated calcium is highly suggestive of primary hyperparathyroidism. Serum phosphorus is usually low but can be normal in patients with renal insufficiency. In the majority of cases, the diagnosis is made by routine blood samples when a chemistry panel is ordered. Peptic ulcer disease, pancreatitis, mental status changes, nephrolithiasis, and osteoporosis are all potential presentations.

### 22. c.

This man most likely has gonorrhea. First-generation cephalosporins and long-acting penicillins have no place in the treatment of gonorrhea. Ceftriaxone or ciprofloxacin alone would be inadequate because a high incidence of chlamydial infection is present in patients with gonorrhea. Dual antimicrobial coverage is therefore necessary, and a single dose of azithromycin would be appropriate treatment.

### 23. d.

This question relates to the acute management of gout. Intravenous radiocontrast dye can serve as a precipitant of gouty arthritis. Adrenocorticotropic hormone, 40 U in a single intramuscular injection, can be used in acute gouty arthritis. Intravenous colchicine is frequently given when a good intravenous site can be used; however, it is contraindicated in patients with renal insufficiency, as is high-dose indomethacin. Allopurinol should not be started while signs of acute inflammation are present. Stopping aspirin would not be appropriate because it is being used for prophylaxis against MI.

### 24. e.

Symptoms of panic disorder are characterized by discrete attacks of anxiety associated with a sensation of chest pain, palpitations, or nausea. Patients may have multiple emergency department visits before they are diagnosed. The embarrassment or fear of having panic attacks in public without an easy escape often disrupts social interactions. Alcohol can actually intensify symptoms.

### 25. c.

The symptoms are most likely to be explained by the presence of a Zenker's diverticulum, which is an outpouching of the esophageal wall. This condition usually presents in older individuals complaining of cervical dysphagia, gurgling in the throat, halitosis, and regurgitation of foul food. Regurgitation of old food is unlikely with a dental abscess or gastroesophageal reflux disease. Symptoms of globus pharyngeus do not include dysphagia. Scleroderma of the esophagus can cause gastroesophageal reflux disease, but if dysphagia occurs, it is progressive.

**26. d.**

Entrapment of the lateral cutaneous nerve is characterized by pain, dysesthesia, or hypesthesia at the lateral thigh. Repetitive exercise, particularly extending the hips while doing the splits, could be a factor in this woman. Tight clothing, obesity, and trauma have also been implicated in causing irritation to the lateral cutaneous nerve, particularly in its path adjacent to the anterosuperior iliac spine. Hip arthritis would be expected to demonstrate limited internal rotation. The diagnosis of MS requires documentation of neurologic events over time at different sites of the neuraxis. Normal knee reflexes are less likely with lumbar disc herniation, which can also affect quadriceps strength. Tenderness would be expected on physical examination in trochanteric bursitis.

**27. c.**

Immunocompromised individuals are particularly susceptible to symptomatic herpes zoster, which can result in Ramsay Hunt syndrome. Pain and vesicles appear in the external auditory canal, and there may be loss of taste sensation in the anterior two-thirds of the tongue. The geniculate ganglion of the sensory branch of the facial nerve is involved.

**28. d.**

The appearance of black rectal mucosa is consistent with a diagnosis of melanosis coli, which results from laxative abuse.

**29. d.**

Symptoms of sinusitis of more than 3 months are termed *chronic*. Obstructed sinus drainage is implicated, leading to persistent infection. Diagnosis can be made, based on clinical history, although CT is particularly helpful if there is doubt. Oral amoxicillin for 1 month is appropriate, and an antihistamine/decongestant may help relieve the cough. A topical corticosteroid may actually accelerate resolution of symptoms.

**30. a.**

Adhesive capsulitis is characterized by gradual onset of symptoms, with pain and progressive reduction in active and passive range of motion. Patients often have a recent history of immobilization in a hospital bed. Diabetic patients are known to have an increased risk of capsulitis that is particularly resistant to treatment. Hypothyroidism and Parkinson's disease are also associated. Patients with impingement syndrome usually have good range of motion, and osteoarthritis would be seen on radiography. Examination in rotator cuff tear would show normal passive range of movement. Fibromyalgia is associated with depression, but this patient does not meet other criteria for the diagnosis. The symptoms of tenderness in this patient are not consistent with angina.

**31. e.**

**32. b.**

**33. c.**

**34. a.**

**35. d.**

**36. d.**

The presentation is typical for coccidioidal infection. Coccidioidomycosis is a fungal infection acquired by the inhalation of fungal arthrospores. The disease is endemic in south central California, southern Arizona, Nevada, New Mexico, and parts of Texas. Many cases elude diagnosis because symptoms may be mild and nonspecific. Cutaneous lesions may be present in as many as 25% of patients. Chest radiology most commonly shows a single focal infiltrate. Laboratory studies typically show eosinophilia, and mild elevation of ALT may also be present. A common clue to the diagnosis is nonresolution of symptoms when treatment is directed toward bacterial pneumonia.

**37. b.**

The most common presentation of hepatitis C is a chronic asymptomatic elevation of hepatic transaminases. A state of chronic infection occurs in at least 50% of patients, and in those in whom cirrhosis develops, an increased risk of hepatic malignancy is present.

**38. b.**

This man has a history suggestive of celiac sprue, a gluten-sensitive enteropathy. Iron-deficiency anemia unresponsive to oral supplements often is seen. Dermatitis herpetiformis and Howell-Jolly bodies are clues to the diagnosis. Although a positive endomysial antibody test is not specific, it is sensitive, and the response to the gluten-free diet is virtually diagnostic. If a patient becomes unresponsive to dietary therapy after many years, lymphoma should be a consideration. Periodic acid–Schiff-positive granules on small bowel biopsy are seen in Whipple's disease, not in celiac sprue.

**39. b.**

Insidious onset, morning stiffness, and symptom duration of more than 3 months suggest that the most likely cause of his back pain is inflammatory. Limitation of spinal movement demonstrated by the Schrober test suggests the diagnosis of ankylosing spondylitis. Aortic insufficiency is an association, as are inflammatory bowel disease and iritis. A positive ANA test is not a feature of the illness, although up to 90% of patients carry the HLA-B27 gene. Glucocorticoids have not been found to be helpful in management. Sitting with a poor posture for prolonged periods may be implicated in back pain, as could be suspected in a pianist, but it would not explain morning stiffness. Dry mouth and eyes are features of Sjögren's syndrome.

**40. c.**

Suppose a sample population of 1,000: The reader should construct a $2 \times 2$ table. A prevalence of 2% would mean 20 patients have the disease ($a + c = 20$). The sensitivity is 80%, and of the 20 patients with the disease, 16 would test positive ($a = 20 \times 0.8$). Of the 980 patients without disease, 931 would test negative [$d = 980 \times 0.95$ (specificity)]. This now means 49 patients ($b = 980 - 931$) would test positive despite the absence of disease. The positive predictive value is calculated as $a/(a + b)$.

**41. a.**

This woman most likely has Peutz-Jeghers syndrome of hamartomas and pigmented lesions. This condition is associated with an increased risk of ovarian sex cord tumors. The risk of colonic malignancy is close to that of the general population, and the inheritance pattern is autosomal dominant. Corticosteroids do not play a role in management. Total colectomy is not mandatory.

**42. e.**

This case is typical of a patient with Graves' disease. The symptoms described are those of hyperthyroidism in general. Older patients may have apathy. Ophthalmopathy with exophthalmos and dermatopathy, also termed *pretibial myxedema*, often are seen and are characteristic of Graves' disease. Clubbing may be seen. Treatment is an oral antithyroid agent, and the dose can be lowered when euthyroidism is achieved, or levothyroxine can be added. After 12 to 24 months of treatment, the drug can be discontinued, and up to 50% of patients remain well for an extended time. Thyroglobulin levels are typically low in patients with thyrotoxicosis factitia; levels are usually elevated in Graves' disease.

**43. d.**

**44. a.**

**45. c.**

**46. e.**

**47. b.**

**48. d.**

Fecal occult blood testing has a low specificity and a positive predictive value of approximately 5% for colorectal malignancy.

**49. a.**

Repetitive overuse of the forearm muscles can result in lateral epicondylitis or tennis elbow. The description given is most suggestive of this process. Golfer's elbow is also associated with overuse of the forearm but involves the medial epicondyle. Ruptured biceps tendon results in weakness, and olecranon bursitis most often manifests with posterior elbow pain. Radial nerve entrapment is rare and, therefore, not the most likely cause of pain.

**50. b.**

The cough associated with ACE inhibitors does *not* occur more frequently in asthmatics than in nonasthmatics, although it may be accompanied by bronchospasm.

**51. c.**

Amantadine or rimantadine is effective in the prophylaxis and treatment of influenza A but not influenza B. Amantadine and rimantadine have been shown to be beneficial as prophylaxis when taken daily during the period of highest risk, particularly in the nonimmunized and during institutional outbreaks of influenza A.

**52. b.**

LGV is caused by the L1, L2, and L3 serovars of *C. trachomatis* and is rare in the United States. Unilateral inguinal or femoral lymphadenopathy is the usual presentation in heterosexual men, whereas proctocolitis or fistula or stricture formation (from inflammatory involvement of perirectal or perianal lymphatic tissues) may occur in women or homosexual men. By the time patients seek medical advice, the self-limited genital ulcer at the inoculation site may not be present. Diagnosis is established serologically and by excluding other etiologies for inguinal lymphadenopathy. In addition to aspiration of buboes, 21 days of therapy with twice daily doxycycline is recommended. Alternatively, erythromycin, 500 mg orally four times daily for 21 days, can be used and is the drug of choice for pregnant women. Sex partners of this patient should be examined, and if they have had sexual contact in the last 30 days, they also should be treated.

**53. a.**

**54. d.**

**55. b.**

In the prescription of medications, it is important to consider the side-effect profile as it relates to the patient. Verapamil is associated with peripheral edema. Nitroglycerin is associated with headache, lightheadedness, and flushing due to vasodilation. Propranolol is associated with bronchospasm and consequently is contraindicated in asthma.

**56. c.**

The anion gap is defined as the measured cations minus the measured anions or sodium concentration minus the combination of the chloride and bicarbonate concentrations. Traditionally, the normal range has been between 7 and 13 mEq/L, but because of newer analyzers, the normal range may fall to 3 to 11 mEq/L due to higher reported chloride concentrations.

Ethylene glycol ingestion causes acute renal failure in addition to a metabolic acidosis. In addition, the metabolic acidosis is characterized by a high anion gap; thus, choice c is correct. In choice c, the anion gap is 34 ($144 - 100 - 10$), whereas in choice a, the anion gap is 12 (141 − 115 − 14), and in choice b, it is 13 (138 − 107 − 18). Choice a may refer to a patient with a distal or type I RTA. These patients have hyperchloremic or non–anion gap metabolic acidosis and are unable to lower urinary pH. Choice b may refer to a patient with a type IV RTA. Choice d refers to a patient with a low anion gap, as seen in multiple myeloma due to the positive charge of paraproteins. Finally, choice e may refer to a patient with mild renal insufficiency who has a mild metabolic acidosis with a normal or mildly elevated anion gap and mildly elevated potassium.

**57. a.**

**58. d.**

**59. b.**

**60. b.**
Each individual must be stratified in terms of his or her risk of progressing on to tuberculosis. The benefit of prevention then needs to be weighed with the risk of drug therapy for each patient.

**61. b.**
Suicide among men peaks at age 75 years and among women at 55 years. The predominant age groups for suicide are the elderly (>65 years) and adolescents (15 to 24 years). Women are more likely to attempt suicide (3:1), but men are more likely to complete it (3:1). History of recent loss, such as retirement or bereavement, is a risk factor for suicide. Marital status is important in assessing suicide risk. Single individuals have a higher suicide risk than those who are divorced. Widowed individuals are at higher risk than those who are married.

**62. a.**
ARDS patients who are mechanically ventilated have an ICU course complicated by barotrauma, nosocomial pneumonia, and multiple organ failure. Additional complications include deep vein thromboses, gastrointestinal bleeding, malnutrition, and side effects from sedatives and paralytics. Barotrauma occurs in a minority of ventilated patients (13% in one study), with barotrauma rarely directly causing death. The tissue breakdown seen in ARDS, high airway pressures, and high tidal volumes predisposes to barotrauma. Barotrauma is evidenced by the development of pneumothorax, subcutaneous emphysema, pneumomediastinum, and interstitial emphysema. Increased radiolucency at the lung bases and the presence of the deep sulcus sign on a chest radiograph are clues to barotrauma and pneumothorax. Nosocomial pneumonia is present in 55% of patients with ARDS and is accompanied by nonspecific findings. The combination of a corticosteroid and a neuromuscular blocking agent has been associated with a reversible myopathy that takes several months to resolve.

**63. b.**
This woman has unstable tachycardia with serious signs and symptoms, including hypotension, heart rate greater than 150/bpm, shortness of breath, and chest tightness. According to the AHA, this should be treated with immediate synchronized cardioversion.

**64. d.**
Malignant hypertension is characterized by elevated blood pressure. Retinal involvement may include hemorrhages, exudates, and bilateral papilledema. Malignant nephrosclerosis leads to hematuria, proteinuria, and acute renal failure. Renal injury is due to fibrinoid necrosis in arterioles and capillaries, the same pathology as in hemolytic-uremic syndrome and scleroderma. Neurologic symptoms may be due to intracerebral or subarachnoid bleeding, lacunar infarction, or hypertensive encephalopathy. The encephalopathy seen in malignant hypertension is insidious in onset, unlike the abrupt onset of encephalopathy seen in strokes or hemorrhage.

**65. e.**
True infection without pyuria is rare, but pyuria in the absence of infection does occur. This woman may have had a urinary tract infection that has been partially treated with an antibiotic. In addition, vaginal leukocytes may have contaminated the original urine specimen. Atypical organisms, such as *C. trachomatis*, *U. urealyticum*, or *M. tuberculosis*, may not grow in standard cultures, and thus patients who have symptoms of a urinary tract infection with a negative culture result should be tested for these organisms. Other important causes of sterile pyuria include chronic interstitial nephritis (hence the questioning regarding analgesic use), urothelial tumors, and nephrolithiasis. Nevertheless, the presence of leukocyte esterase and nitrite on urine dipstick has a 95% sensitivity and a 75% specificity for the diagnosis of bacterial urinary tract infection.

**66. e.**
Tetracyclines have direct anti-inflammatory properties, as well as inhibiting growth of *P. acnes*.

**67. e.**
The statements are all true. In volume-cycled ventilation, the ventilator delivers a fixed tidal volume with each breath. The maximum airway pressure varies, depending on stiffness (inverse of compliance) of the lung. Minute ventilation is approximately the set rate multiplied by the tidal volume. Conversely, in pressure-cycled ventilation, the airway pressure is preset with the tidal volume, varying with each breath according to the lung's compliance. Minute ventilation cannot be predicted. In both assist-control and intermittent mandatory ventilation, a backup rate can be set to prevent hypoventilation. In assist-control mode, however, the ventilator delivers a

fixed tidal volume when a spontaneous breath is sensed, whereas in intermittent mandatory mode, a preset tidal volume is delivered at a specified rate. In addition, patients are allowed to trigger a spontaneous breath at a rate and volume that depends on their need. Most often, in this mode, the ventilator-delivered breaths are synchronized to the patient's own, and this is referred to as *synchronized intermittent mandatory ventilation.*

## 68. c.

Coccidioidomycosis is a fungal infection caused by the inhalation of the spore form of *Coccidioides immitis.* In the United States, endemic areas include south central California, southern Arizona, Nevada, New Mexico, and the western half of Texas. Most (60%) of patients are asymptomatic; however, the vast majority of symptomatic patients usually have a self-limited pneumonic process, and a minority progress to disseminated disease. Most symptoms are nonspecific; they include fatigue, nonproductive cough, chest pain, dyspnea, headaches, myalgia, and arthralgia. Cutaneous manifestations, such as a nonspecific maculopapular or erythematous rash, are seen in 25% of patients and do *not* indicate disseminated disease, nor does their presence portend a poor prognosis. On skin biopsy, a nonspecific vasculitic process with variable eosinophilic infiltration is usually seen. A focal bronchopneumonic infiltrate in a single lobe is the most common finding on chest radiography. Occasionally, two or more lobes may be involved. In addition, pleural effusion of clinically insignificant sizes may occur. Laboratory abnormalities include the presence of eosinophilia in 25% of patients and mild elevations of AST and ALT. Diagnosis is made by serologic means. A new enzyme-linked immunosorbent assay has a sensitivity of 98.5% and a specificity of 94.8%. Treatment usually consists of antifungal azoles in mild cases and amphotericin B in severe cases and in patients with concomitant HIV infection.

## 69. a.

Cardiogenic shock, clinically described as severe systemic hypotension, cool extremities, and respiratory distress, occurs in approximately 6% to 7% of patients with acute MI. These patients are often older and of the female gender and have an anterior or large infarction, previous MI, or diabetes mellitus. In the Global Utilization of Streptokinase and t-PA for Occluded Coronary Arteries I trial however, only 0.8% of patients had shock on presentation to the hospital, with shock developing either suddenly (as in this patient) or gradually in the remaining 5.3% after admission. Most cases occur within 24 hours to days afterward, with cases occurring 1 week afterward being rare. Severe left ventricular dysfunction is the most common cause of cardiogenic shock, most commonly from an anterior MI. Right ventricular dysfunction does not usually lead to respiratory distress unless the left ventricle is also involved. Acute mitral regurgitation from ruptured chordae tendineae or papillary muscle, ruptured intraventricular septum, or cardiac tamponade may all lead to cardiogenic shock from mechanical means. As with any patient who is in "shock" (hypoperfusion), other causes and types of shock must be ruled out. Echocardiography (either transthoracic or transesophageal) is essential in the initial evaluation of patients with cardiogenic shock. Not only is left and right ventricular function assessed, but also mechanical complications of MI can be ruled in or out. Finally, the insertion of a balloon-tipped pulmonary artery catheter can confirm the hemodynamic criteria for cardiogenic shock. The American College of Cardiology and the AHA Task Force guidelines define cardiogenic shock as two subsets:

- Pulmonary capillary wedge pressure greater than 15 mm Hg, SBP less than 100 mm Hg, and CI less than 2.5 L/min/m$^2$
- Pulmonary capillary wedge pressure greater than 15 mm Hg, SBP less than 90 mm Hg, and CI less than 2.5 L/min/m$^2$

Subset 2 has a worse prognosis.

## 70. e.

Postural hypotension, rather than hypertension, has been associated with falls. In the elderly, it is important to assess the risk factors for falls and to address them to prevent falls because falls are one of the most common problems that threaten the independence of the elderly and are associated with significant morbidity and mortality.

## 71. e.

These clinical findings are consistent with Bell's palsy, in which there may be associated loss of taste sensation from the ipsilateral anterior two-thirds of the tongue. Clinically, this is a lower motor lesion. In an upper motor lesion of the facial nerve, there would be sparing of the frontalis muscle and an ability to raise his eyebrows. Ramsay Hunt syndrome is a lower seventh cranial nerve lesion associated with herpes zoster of the external auditory meatus and geniculate ganglion, but it is not the most common cause of this facial nerve lesion; the most common cause is idiopathic. This is a common condition occurring in approximately 1 in 60 or 70 persons in a lifetime. Bell's palsy is usually a self-limiting disease; most patients recover in a few weeks.

## 72. b.

Ectropion is not associated with Graves' disease; it is common in the elderly and may be seen in chronic facial nerve palsy.

## 73. e.

Desensitization has no effect on the incidence of Stevens-Johnson syndrome, hemolytic anemia, or serum sickness associated with penicillin because these are all non–IgE-mediated reactions. Fatal reactions to penicillin skin tests have been reported, but they occur in less than 1% of those tested.

### 74. a.
Inherited thrombophilia is associated with a genetically increased risk for venous thromboembolism. Factor V Leiden mutation accounts for 40% to 50% of cases. Protein C, protein S, and antithrombin III deficiencies and dysfibrinogenemia are all causes of inherited thrombophilia, but they are less common.

### 75. b.
Hyperuricemia, not hypouricemia, is a side effect of hydrochlorothiazide.

### 76. e.
Contact dermatitis is a type IV cell-mediated response.

### 77. b.
Silica exposure is associated with the lung disease silicosis but not associated with lung cancer. Silicosis has several different clinical manifestations, including chronic simple nodules or progressive pulmonary fibrosis. The calcification of hilar lymph nodes produces a characteristic "eggshell" pattern. Patients with silicosis are at increased risk for the development of *M. tuberculosis* infections—silicotuberculosis.

### 78. a.
The two most common laboratory abnormalities in HIV patients with *Pneumocystis carinii* pneumonia is a CD4 cell count less than 200/mm$^3$ and an elevated LDH level. Although it is possible, *Pneumocystis carinii* pneumonia is unlikely to develop in patients with CD4 counts greater than 200/mm$^3$.

### 79. e.
A low incidence of psoriasis occurs in Eskimos and a very low incidence occurs in Native Americans.

### 80. b.

### 81. d.

### 82. c.
In hypovolemic and cardiogenic shock, the CI is low, SVR is high, and SvO$_2$ is low, whereas the PAOP is low in hypovolemic shock and high in cardiogenic shock. Finally, in septic shock, an increased CI is present due to a drop in SVR, the SvO$_2$ may be either normal or elevated (reflecting the increased cardiac output), and the PAOP is either normal or depressed.

### 83. d.
This man should be tested because he is requesting it. To diminish the chances of a false-positive result, a Western blot should be performed to confirm a positive enzyme immunoassay. Unlike sensitivity and specificity, the false-positive and false-negative rates are directly related to the prevalence of disease in the population. For example, the higher the prevalence of disease, the higher the false-negative rate will be; the lower the prevalence of disease, the higher the false-positive rate will be.

### 84. a.
Lung cancer is the leading cause of cancer death in the United States.

### 85. e.
AFES occurs in 1 in 20,000 to 30,000 births in the United States and is associated with a 80% to 90% mortality in affected women. It is second only to pulmonary embolism as an aggregate source of maternal mortality. Of patients diagnosed with AFES, 86% die from cardiogenic shock or its complications. Left-sided heart failure is more common than right-sided heart failure. Disseminated intravascular coagulation develops in approximately 40% of patients. Of the patients surviving the first hours, noncardiogenic pulmonary edema develops in 70%. Although damage to the alveolar-capillary membrane occurs, the clinical pattern seen in these survivors is *not* typical of ARDS. In contrast to the protracted course often seen with ARDS, these patients' conditions improve rapidly. Diagnosis and anticipation of the complications of AFES are crucial in affording patients the best chances for survival.

### 86. d.
Sputum culture is negative in approximately 50% of patients with concurrent pneumococcal bacteremia.

### 87. a.
Because this man cannot make decisions about end-of-life issues, the responsibility falls on his wife to make the decision on his behalf. Essentially, she is being asked to decide what he would want done, not what she would want done. In addition, if a durable power of attorney for health care has been appointed, this individual would be the surrogate decision maker, even if the wife were involved in the patient's hospitalization or illness. The individual with the power of attorney must also act on behalf of the patient and not merely project his or her own view. Finally, "slow" codes have no role in the care of a terminally ill patient because there also is no requirement that cardiopulmonary resuscitation be performed in the event that it has been deemed futile. Competent physicians who use standard pain medications in terminally ill patients who suffer from chronic pain are not engaging in physician-assisted suicide.

### 88. c.
Malaria leads to 1 million deaths out of 200 million cases worldwide each year. Of *P. falciparum, P. vivax, P. ovale,* and *P. malariae, P. falciparum* can lead rapidly to coma and death. Travel to sub-Saharan Africa poses the greatest risk for acquisition of *P. falciparum* for American travelers. Strains of *P. falciparum* are becoming more and more resistant to chloroquine; thus, mefloquine is the

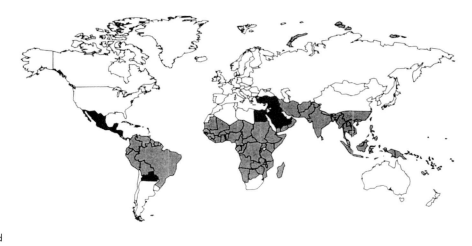

**Figure 73.1** Distribution of malaria and chloroquine-resistant *Plasmodium falciparum*, 1997. (Reproduced with permission from Centers for Disease Control and Prevention (CDC) Web site, http://www.cdc.gov.)

◉ Chloroquine-resistant *P. falciparum*

● Chloroquine-sensitive malaria

chemoprophylactic agent of choice in areas where chloroquine resistance prevails (Fig. 73.1). Adverse effects associated with mefloquine include nausea, dizziness, and vertigo. Mefloquine has been associated with neuropsychiatric effects, including inability to concentrate, bad dreams, paranoid ideation, seizures, and psychosis, as well as cardiac conduction abnormalities leading to sinus bradycardia and a prolonged QT interval. Pregnancy should not be a contraindication to chemoprophylaxis if travel cannot be postponed. Chloroquine is without any established teratogenicity, and mefloquine also seems to be safe. On the other hand, a tetracycline such as doxycycline should not be prescribed because of harmful effects on the fetus (dental discoloration and dysplasia and inhibition of bone growth).

### 89. c.
The American College of Chest Physicians and the Society of Critical Care Medicine have defined this series of terms. This patient meets criteria for having systemic inflammatory response syndrome, as well as clinical evidence of urinary tract infection; thus, the most accurate term for her condition would be *sepsis*. The terms *infection* or *systemic inflammatory response syndrome* would not completely describe her condition. *Infection* is a microbial phenomenon characterized by an inflammatory response to the presence of organisms or to invasion of normally sterile host tissue by these organisms. *Bacteremia* is defined by the presence of viable bacteria in the blood. Systemic inflammatory response syndrome is a widespread inflammatory response defined by the presence of two or more of the following:

- Temperature greater than 38°C or less than 36°C
- Heart rate greater than 90/bpm

- Respiratory rate greater than 20/min or $Paco_2$ less than 32 mm Hg
- WBC count greater than 12,000/mm³ or less than 4,000/mm³ or greater than 10% bandemia

*Sepsis* is the presence of systemic inflammatory response syndrome together with evidence of infection. *Severe sepsis* is the presence of sepsis associated with organ dysfunction, hypotension, or hypoperfusion. *Septic shock* is sepsis with hypotension despite adequate fluid resuscitation and the presence of lactic acidosis, oliguria, or acute mental status changes. *Hypotension* is defined as an SBP of less than 90 mm Hg or a 40 mm Hg or greater decrease from baseline (in the absence of other causes for the decrease).

### 90. a.
Patent ductus arteriosus is more common in women than in men (3:1). It is associated with maternal rubella. Complications include infective endocarditis and Eisenmenger's syndrome. Prophylaxis for endocarditis is indicated, unless treatment by surgical ligation has been performed. Severe pulmonary vascular disease leads to a reversal of flow and shunting of deoxygenated blood to the lower extremities, resulting in differential cyanosis. Once Eisenmenger's syndrome has developed, corrective surgical intervention is no longer an option. The ductus is patent in the fetus but normally closes immediately after birth.

### 91. c.
An exudative effusion is suggested by at least one of the following three criteria, whereas a transudate has none of these criteria:

- Pleural fluid LDH more than two-thirds of the normal upper limit for serum

- A ratio of pleural fluid LDH to serum LDH of greater than 0.6
- A ratio of pleural fluid protein to serum protein of greater than 0.5

The pleural effusion associated with neoplastic disease is usually exudative. Pulmonary emboli are associated with both transudates and exudates. In a patient with a parapneumonic effusion, any of the following is an indication for thoracostomy tube placement:

- Pleural fluid glucose level less than 50 mg/dL
- Presence of gross pus in the pleural space
- Organisms visible on Gram's stain of the pleural fluid
- Pleural fluid pH less than 7.0 and 0.15 units lower than arterial blood pH

### 92. e.

Renovascular hypertension is less common in African Americans. Moderately or severely hypertensive individuals with atherosclerosis, recurrent "flash" pulmonary edema, or asymmetric kidney sizes should be screened. In addition, patients who have a rise in serum creatinine levels after the initiation of an ACE inhibitor should also be screened. The gold standard for diagnosing renal artery stenosis is renal arteriography; however, intravenous pyelography can demonstrate delayed calyceal appearance of contrast and diminished kidney size in the presence of unilateral stenosis. In bilateral stenosis, the differences between the two kidneys may be difficult to see. Other methods for noninvasive screening are available; these include renogram, duplex Doppler ultrasound, magnetic resonance angiography, and spiral CT with angiography. The baseline plasma renin level is elevated in only 50% to 80% of patients with renovascular hypertension, but the administration of an ACE inhibitor can increase the predictive value of obtaining an elevated plasma renin level.

### 93. d.

Fasciculation suggests a lower motor neuron lesion rather than an upper motor lesion. Extensor plantar response, hyperreflexia of the tendon reflexes, and increased tone (spasticity) are all suggestive of an upper motor lesion. Weakness is a feature of both upper and lower motor lesions.

### 94. b.

Acute-onset bloody diarrhea, high fever, and crampy abdominal pain with tenesmus typically characterize *Shigella* gastroenteritis. Initial diagnostic tests may include an examination of stool stained with methylene blue to look for polymorphonuclear leukocytes. Fecal leukocytes may occur in other bacterial diarrheas and are not specific for *Shigella*. The presence of fecal leukocytes suggests a bacterial etiology. Culture of stool or rectal swab can confirm the diagnosis. Blood cultures are rarely helpful, as bacteremia is rare, occurring in approximately

7% of children but few adults. Patients at risk for bacteremia include those who are elderly, HIV-infected, or malnourished or those who have underlying diseases, such as diabetes mellitus. Untreated, shigellosis is highly contagious and is generally a self-limited illness with an average duration of 7 days. The organism can be shed in the stool for up to 6 weeks. For this reason, food handlers, daycare workers and children, and health care workers should be treated along with anyone with bacteremia. Treatment in the United States should start with trimethoprim-sulfamethoxazole. Healthy adults with mild disease alternatively can be treated with norfloxacin. Ampicillin should not be used because of developing resistance. Treatment outside the United States generally consists of a quinolone.

### 95. d.

More than two-thirds of patients with multiple myeloma have a normocytic and normochromic anemia during their illnesses; 50% have rouleaux formation, and only approximately 15% have hypercalcemia. The most common neurologic manifestations are thoracic or lumbosacral radiculopathy, with a cord compression secondary to extramedullary plasmacytomas developing in 5% to 10% of patients. Peripheral neuropathy is rare. The major causes of renal failure in these patients are cast nephropathy and hypercalcemia. In myeloma kidney, casts formed by precipitating monoclonal light chains that interact with the Tamm-Horsfall mucoprotein (synthesized by the tubular cells in the ascending limb of the loop of Henle) accumulate in the distal and collecting tubules.

### 96. d.

Nasal sympathomimetic agents are not to be used for long-term symptom relief. Their use is limited to 2 to 3 days to avoid the development of rhinitis medicamentosa. In rhinitis medicamentosa, rebound nasal congestion occurs after the discontinuation of a strong nasal decongestant, creating a vicious cycle, with the patient restarting the nasal spray to treat the congestion, which is directly caused by the nasal spray itself.

### 97. a.

The definition of a solitary pulmonary nodule is a single radiologically visible lesion that is within and surrounded on all sides by pulmonary parenchyma. It is not associated with potentially related pathology, such as pleural effusion or mediastinal lymphadenopathy. The upper limit of the size of a nodule may be 3 or 4 cm; larger lesions are considered masses. Adenocarcinoma most commonly presents as a solitary pulmonary nodule; small cell carcinoma usually presents as a central endobronchial lesion.

### 98. c.

Packed RBC transfusions are the least appropriate choice for a patient with sickle cell anemia. The reticulocyte count is essential in ruling out the possibility of an aplastic crisis. Cultures of the blood and urine, along with chest radiography, help rule out infection. Pain control and intravenous hydration are the mainstays of therapy for patients with a sickle cell crisis.

## 99. c.
This man is in cardiopulmonary arrest. Specifically, his electrical cardiac activity is pulseless electrical activity. All the choices are appropriate in the initial management of pulseless electrical activity, except synchronized direct-current cardioversion. In addition to pneumothorax, hypoxia, and hypotension, other causes of pulseless electrical activity that must be investigated in the initial management of these patients include cardiac tamponade, hypothermia, massive pulmonary embolism, drug overdose, hyperkalemia, severe acidosis, and massive MI. Atropine may also be given in the event of bradycardia or relative bradycardia.

## 100. a.
In the treatment of wide-complex tachycardia (heart rate greater than 100/bpm, QRS duration 120 ms or more), if one cannot diagnose it as SVT, verapamil, adenosine, or a β-blocker should not be given because they can lead to rapid deterioration in the presence of VT and hypotension. The presence of CAD is a strong predictor of VT rather than SVT. Multiple recurrences of the tachycardia over more than 3 years suggest SVT, and the development of the tachycardia after the recent diagnosis of MI suggests VT. Finally, the observation of cannon "a" waves indicates atrioventricular disassociation and thus VT.

## 101. c.
Northern European descent or living in a temperate climate are risk factors for MS. MS is more common in women. The predominant age at presentation is 16 to 40 years. MRI is more sensitive than CT in the diagnosis of MS. Cerebrospinal fluid examination that suggests the diagnosis of MS includes a normal or slightly *high* protein level (50 to 100 mg/dL), a *high* level of γ-globulin IgG, and negative serology for syphilis.

## 102. d.
All forms of RTA lead to a normal anion gap metabolic acidosis. Fanconi's syndrome is a generalized proximal tubular dysfunction and is most often associated with proximal or type 2 RTA. In Fanconi's syndrome, glucose, phosphate, uric acid, and amino acids also are spilled inappropriately, in addition to bicarbonate. The most common causes of Fanconi's syndrome in adults include the excretion of light chains in multiple myeloma and the use of a carbonic anhydrase inhibitor. Multiple myeloma should be excluded in all patients with a proximal RTA unless another cause is identified. Urinary pH is variable in proximal RTA. Distal RTA results from defects in hydrogen ion secretion: decreased proton pump ($H^+$-adenosine triphosphatase) activity, hydrogen back-leak due to

increased luminal membrane permeability, and reduction of the electrical gradient necessary for proton secretion due to decreased distal tubular sodium reabsorption. Distal RTA often is associated with hyperglobulinemic states. The urinary pH is inappropriately high (>5.5) and often is associated with hypercalciuria due to bone loss from the chronic metabolic acidosis. In addition, hypokalemia often is seen, unless it is caused by decreased tubular sodium reabsorption. In this case, hyperkalemia is seen. Type 4 RTA is due to either aldosterone deficiency or resistance by the tubular cells. The most common cause of aldosterone deficiency in adults is hyporeninemic hypoaldosteronism, seen in mild to moderate renal insufficiency (especially diabetic nephropathy). Finally, aldosterone resistance commonly is seen with potassium-sparing diuretics and chronic tubulointerstitial disease. It is associated with a mild metabolic acidosis due to the suppression of ammonia excretion due to hyperkalemia and an appropriately low urinary pH (<5.3) and serum bicarbonate greater than 17 mEq/L.

## 103. b.
Transitional cell carcinoma of the bladder is more common than either squamous cell carcinoma or adenocarcinoma and has a more favorable prognosis. A risk factor for the squamous subtype includes schistosomal infestations. Other risk factors include aromatic amines present in the products of chemical dyes and cigarette smoke, recurrent stones or infection, and use of cyclophosphamide. Family history is not a risk factor for bladder carcinoma; it is a risk factor for renal cell carcinoma.

## 104. d.
Osteomalacia, not osteoporosis, is a complication of dialysis. In addition to osteomalacia, aluminum toxicity is also associated with dialysis dementia. Hepatitis is a potential complication arising from the increased need for blood product transfusions. Liver failure arising from hepatitis can lead to portal hypertension that can lead to gastrointestinal bleeding. In addition, heparin used during dialysis also can increase the risk of gastrointestinal bleeding. Cerebrovascular accidents and cardiovascular disease are seen with increased frequency in uremic patients, accounting for 50% of deaths of hemodialysis patients.

## 105. d.
The criteria for the initiation of therapy in HIV-infected patients include acute HIV infection or within the first 6 months of seroconversion, symptomatic HIV infection, or asymptomatic infection with a CD4 cell count less than 500/mm$^3$ or viral load (RNA-polymerase chain reaction) greater than 20,000 copies/mL. Recommended initial therapy in these patients includes the combination of two nucleoside reverse transcriptase inhibitors (zidovudine, lamivudine, zalcitabine, or didanosine) and a protease inhibitor (indinavir, saquinavir, ritonavir, or

nelfinavir). Therefore, choice b would be correct, except that the combination of zalcitabine and didanosine should be avoided because of possible toxicity. Alternately, one can use two nucleoside reverse transcriptase inhibitors and a non–nucleoside reverse transcriptase inhibitor (nevirapine, delavirdine, or efavirenz). Therefore, choice d would be the best choice. Combination therapy with two nucleoside reverse transcriptase inhibitors or monotherapy is not recommended. In the case of a pregnant woman, however, in the absence of the indications mentioned previously, monotherapy with zidovudine is indicated in the second and third trimesters to reduce the risk of fetal transmission.

### 106. a.

Restlessness, tachycardia, fever, hypertension, and visual hallucinations after 3 days in the hospital are most suggestive of withdrawal from alcohol. Similar presentations may occur with withdrawal from sedative hypnotics. Withdrawal from either alcohol or sedative hypnotics can cause seizures and may be life threatening. Alcohol intoxication is suggested by slow or slurred speech, confusion, gait disturbance, and nystagmus. Opiate withdrawal may present with agitation, but other features include dilated pupils, rhinorrhea, nausea, cramps, and restlessness. Schizophrenia does disturb thoughts and behavior and may have features of tactile, auditory, and olfactory, as well as visual, hallucinations, but they usually do not present with restlessness, tachycardia, fever, and hypertension. Personality disorder can present with agitated, aggressive, or violent behavior, but usually it is not associated with restlessness, tachycardia, fever, and hypertension.

### 107. e.

The highest dose recommended for use in PSVT is not 6 mg. If 6 mg fails to convert the rhythm after 1 to 2 minutes, a dose of 12 mg should be administered. Adenosine should be administered as a rapid intravenous push followed by a fluid flush because of its very short half-life.

### 108. b.

The differentiation between dementia and delirium is important because of the many reversible underlying causes that require treatment in patients with delirium. Motor signs of postural tremor, myoclonus, and asterixis are suggestive of delirium rather than dementia. Dementia rather than delirium is suggested by onset over months to years rather than hours to days, normal rather than slurred speech, and impaired recent memory and preserved distant past memory. A normal or mildly slow electroencephalogram is found in dementia, whereas in delirium pronounced diffuse slowing is typically seen.

### 109. c.

Aspirin is rapidly converted to salicylic acid in the body. Toxicity is seen in most patients with plasma levels of 400 to 500 mg/L. Therapeutic levels are 200 to 350 mg/L. Fatal overdose can occur with 10 to 30 g in adults. Salicylates directly stimulate the respiratory centers, promoting respiratory alkalosis. In addition, the accumulation of organic acids, including lactic acid and ketoacids, leads to a high anion gap metabolic acidosis. The lactic acidosis may be a response to the respiratory alkalosis. Most patients have either a combined respiratory alkalosis with metabolic acidosis or just a respiratory alkalosis. Finding just metabolic acidosis in these patients is rare. Treatment consists of minimizing absorption of the aspirin with the use of charcoal and preventing accumulation by alkalinizing the plasma with sodium bicarbonate. Urinary alkalinization also may aid in removing of salicylic acid from the body.

### 110. e.

The coexistence of duodenal bulb ulceration with diarrhea is suspicious for Zollinger-Ellison syndrome. This patient also lacks risk factors for *H. pylori* or NSAID use. Histologic evaluation for *H. pylori* is 98% sensitive, and workup with culture and breath test is redundant here. CT can be used to localize a gastrinoma, but the first step would be to evaluate the serum gastrin level.

### 111. c.

This woman has neutropenic fever. Neutropenia is defined as an absolute neutrophil count less than $500/mm^3$. Patients with an absolute neutrophil count less than $500/mm^3$ due to chemotherapy or marrow failure are at high risk for overwhelming bacterial infection. Blood cultures are indicated, and antibiotics should be commenced as soon as possible. Most antibiotic regimens target Gram-negative bacilli. The choice of a β-lactam and an aminoglycoside is appropriate.

### 112. d.

This is a description of Morton's neuroma, a common cause of metatarsalgia. The condition is not caused by a true neuroma, but is due to an interdigital nerve fibrosis caused by irritation. Women are affected approximately five times more often than men, and wearing high-heeled or restrictive shoes aggravates symptoms. Patients should be instructed to wear low-heeled shoes with a wide toe box. Local injection with lidocaine can be helpful in avoiding surgery, which may be necessary.

### 113. c.

This man has two risk factors for CAD: being a man older than 45 years and a significant family history. The National Cholesterol Education Program suggests that with a low-density lipoprotein cholesterol level greater than 160 mg/dL, active drug therapy should be instituted. Although epidemiologic studies suggest that a lowered risk of coronary events is present in those consuming certain types of alcohol, the recommendation that someone who does not otherwise drink starts taking red wine is controversial.

### 114. a.

This man has the typical features of relapsing polychondritis. Disease activity can be suppressed with oral glucocorticoids. NSAIDs, topical steroids, and decongestants are unlikely to affect the disease course. Anemia of chronic disease and an elevated erythrocyte sedimentation rate can be seen. Although rheumatoid factor and ANA may be positive, they do not contribute to the diagnosis in this case.

### 115. b.

The most likely diagnosis is lumbosacral strain. Biofeedback has not been proven to reduce recovery time.

### 116. b.

Bacterial vaginosis is characterized by the appearance of clue cells on a saline wet preparation, as described. The vaginal pH is usually greater than 4.5, and a fishy odor may be present on addition of 20% potassium hydroxide solution. The treatment of choice is metronidazole, 500 mg twice daily for 7 days. Intravaginal clindamycin cream may also be used in the first trimester of pregnancy, when metronidazole is contraindicated. Human papillomavirus has been implicated in the etiology of cervical cancer. Multiple sex partners, smoking, and HIV infection are considered to be risk factors for cervical cancer. Ketoconazole is an antifungal agent and is not effective for bacterial vaginosis.

### 117. a.

This man has chest pain that is unlikely to be of cardiac origin. Reflux disease may mimic cardiac chest pain. A positive Bernstein test would imply that the symptoms are due to reflux and should be treated as such. With convincing evidence that the cause is noncardiac, further evaluation for atherosclerotic disease is redundant. The use of pH monitoring helps establish whether reflux is present, but it may not explain symptoms. Similarly, endoscopy and manometry evaluate for esophagitis and the mechanism of reflux, respectively.

### 118. e.

This woman has a laboratory picture consistent with factitious hypoglycemia. The most likely cause is sulfonylurea abuse. Patients with access to drugs are at higher potential for abuse. An elevated C-peptide level makes surreptitious insulin use an unlikely cause. Angiography and CT may be used to search for an insulinoma. An insulin-producing tumor can cause hypoglycemia; however, the proinsulin-to-insulin ratio is usually greater than 20%. Urinary testing is the most effective way to search for evidence of sulfonylurea intake.

### 119. e.

It is important to be aware of common serologic patterns relating to hepatitis B. This patient is positive only for surface antibody, which is consistent with prior immunization or past exposure. Hepatitis E virus antigen is correlated with high infectivity, and its disappearance (appearance of anti-HBe) in infected patients heralds lower infectivity. Patients with chronic infection would be positive for hepatitis B virus surface antigen.

### 120. e.

Otitis externa is also termed *swimmer's ear*. Maceration of the skin of the external auditory canal is present, and there may be impairment of hearing as debris obstructs the canal. A greenish exudate suggests *Pseudomonas* infection. In uncomplicated cases, debris should be removed and a topical antibiotic applied. If bacterial infection is suspected, an antibacterial steroid solution is appropriate. A fungal infection is treated with clotrimazole solution applied locally for 14 days. Malignant otitis externa is more common in diabetics and is characterized by severe pain and fever. In this situation, there may be rapid spread of infection to local skin and bone, and immediate hospital admission for intravenous antibiotics is indicated.

### 121. b.

This woman almost certainly has Hashimoto's thyroiditis, which is most common in middle-aged women. On histopathologic examination, lymphocytic infiltration of the thyroid gland is present. Antithyroid peroxidase antibodies are invariably present. The disease is associated with a number of other autoimmune disorders, such as chronic active hepatitis, pernicious anemia, and diabetes mellitus. The goitrous form is associated with HLA-DR5 antigen. The prevalence of Hashimoto's thyroiditis is thought to be increasing due to increased iodine intake. A goiter is the usual presentation. High titers of antithyroid peroxidase in pregnant women suggest an increased risk of miscarriage. Elevated thyroid-stimulating hormone is a marker for replacement therapy, and prognosis is usually good. Long-standing disease is associated with an increased risk of lymphoma.

### 122. d.

The appropriate treatment of animal bites before the appearance of local infection is of paramount importance. Appropriate prophylaxis for tetanus is necessary. It is uncertain whether this patient previously received tetanus immunization, and he should therefore receive tetanus immunoglobulin and a primary series of immunizations. Dog bites can cause local infection with multiple organisms and always raise a concern about rabies. Precautions for rabies involve observing the dog for 10 days by quarantine, if necessary. If the dog cannot be observed, then human rabies immune globulin and diploid vaccine should be administered to the patient. Minor abrasions should be cleaned thoroughly and puncture wounds irrigated. Antibiotic use is necessary if bites involve the hand or face, or if there is any sign of infection.

**123. b.**

**124. a.**

**125. d.**

**126. c.**

**127. e.**

It is important to be aware of the potential side effects of antihypertensive agents. The ACE inhibitor class of medications should not be used in pregnancy or in patients with bilateral renal artery stenosis. Hyperkalemia and cough are common, and angioedema and leukopenia are both known to occur. β-Blockers potentially can cause bronchospasm and should be used with caution in patients with pulmonary disease. Other side effects include depression and hypercholesterolemia. β-Blockers should be used with caution in diabetics, as the symptoms of hypoglycemia may be masked. Minoxidil can promote facial hair growth and can worsen anginal symptoms. Intravenous hydralazine has been used in preeclampsia. A lupus-like syndrome has been well documented in some patients taking hydralazine, and it may also induce headaches. A side effect of prolonged nitroprusside use is cyanide toxicity; it is often used in the setting of malignant hypertension.

**128. b.**

This man exhibits a clinical syndrome consistent with mesenteric ischemia.

**129. c.**

This woman has viral conjunctivitis. Preauricular adenopathy is a characteristic feature, but it is not always found. The infection is highly contagious, and patients should be cautioned to use strict hygiene. If the patient is in an occupation that may pose the risk of spread, time off work may be prudent. Symptomatic treatment can be helpful, but hygiene advice takes priority. Oral tetracycline is used in inclusion conjunctivitis to treat chlamydial infection. Gentamicin drops are indicated in chronic bacterial conjunctivitis.

**130. e.**

This postmenopausal woman has stress incontinence. The history shows leakage associated with increased intraabdominal pressure. Instruction in pelvic muscle exercises can be effective, as can bladder training. Prompted voiding, fluid-intake modification, and environmental manipulation are strategies used in functional incontinence. Intermittent catheter drainage can be used in overflow incontinence.

**131. c.**

CML is the only myeloproliferative disorder characterized by the Philadelphia chromosome, a reciprocal translocation between chromosomes 9 and 22. This translocation is commonly found in all hematopoietic cell lines but not in nonhematopoietic cell lines. The

propensity of the myeloproliferative disorders to progress to acute transformation is highest in CML (approximately 90%) and lowest for essential thrombocytopenia (<5%).

**132. a.**

The chronic use of long-acting β-agonists has *not* been associated with loss of potency or decreased duration of effect in bronchodilation.

**133. a.**

Taste sensation in the posterior one-third of the tongue is transmitted via the glossopharyngeal nerve.

**134. c.**

Acquired or inherited factor XIII deficiency frequently leads to significant bleeding. An assay for clot solubility in urea screens for this disorder because the bleeding time, platelet count, PT, and PTT are all normal. PTT is prolonged in patients with factor XII deficiency or prekallikrein deficiency, although no associated increase in bleeding tendency is present. Patients with thrombasthenia do not have normal bleeding times because defective platelet aggregation is present. Finally, patients with protein S deficiency often have a thrombotic rather than bleeding tendency.

**135. d.**

Auditory hallucinations are not common symptoms of depression and are not included among the nine *Diagnostic and Statistical Manual of Mental Disorders*, Fourth Edition criteria, of which at least five are required for the diagnosis of major depression.

**136. b.**

Horner's syndrome is associated with constriction (miosis) rather than dilatation of the pupil.

**137. c.**

The duration of catheter placement has not been firmly established as a risk factor for catheter-related infection. Several studies demonstrated an increased risk with increased duration, whereas others demonstrated no increased risk.

**138. e.**

In general, cancer patients have a mortality of 50%. If they are ventilated, mortality rises to greater than 70%. Furthermore, bone marrow transplantation patients who require mechanical ventilation have a mortality that exceeds 95%.

**139. a.**

This man is hypovolemic from gastrointestinal fluid loss. The serum sodium is likely to be raised and the urinary sodium low (<25 mEq daily) because the kidneys are attempting to retain sodium to compensate for the lost volume. In the same way, potassium is lost in vomiting and diarrhea, and the kidney attempts to compensate for this with a reduced urinary loss of potassium. Vasopressin may be used in the syndrome of central diabetes insipidus, but not in this case. Phenytoin is not indicated in this patient.

### 140. c.

MCD is the most common cause of nephrotic syndrome in children (age <10 years, 90%; older, 50%) but in adults accounts for only 15% to 25%. Immunofluorescence and light microscopy do not show immune complex disease, but electron microscopy reveals diffuse fusion of the epithelial cell foot processes. Corticosteroid therapy is the mainstay of empiric treatment in children without biopsy because of the high frequency of MCD in this nephrotic population. Even in young adults (20 to 30 years), corticosteroids treat both MCD and focal glomerulosclerosis, the second most common cause of nephrotic syndrome. In older adults, other causes (e.g., primary amyloid, membranous nephropathy) of nephrotic syndrome must be ruled out with a renal biopsy before treatment. NSAIDs, ampicillin, rifampin, and interferon all have been reported to cause secondary MCD. MCD may be associated with an underlying hematologic malignancy (Hodgkin's disease and less commonly other lymphomas or leukemias), whereas solid tumors usually produce an immune complex–mediated disease such as membranous nephropathy.

### 141. a.

Smith and colleagues pooled primary and secondary prevention studies, and their meta-analysis shows that the net benefit of cholesterol lowering depends on the underlying risk for death from CHD. The risks for developing and dying of CHD are much lower in primary-prevention settings than in secondary-prevention settings. Hence, cholesterol lowering is more effective in secondary prevention (patients who have had a MI) than in primary prevention. The effects of lowering cholesterol on CHD depend on the magnitude of cholesterol reduction. Each 10% reduction in cholesterol levels is associated with roughly a 20% to 30% reduction in the incidence of CHD.

### 142. d.

*S. pneumoniae* is the most common pathogen associated with community-acquired pneumonia and accounts for up to 66% of bacterial pneumonia in some series in which serologic techniques were used. Nevertheless, the organism is isolated in only 5% to 18% of the cases. In fact, the sputum culture is negative in 50% of patients with bacteremic pneumococcal pneumonia. Fever, chills, cough with rusty-colored sputum, and abrupt-onset pleuritic pain are the symptoms often ascribed to pneumococcal pneumonia. Rales and tubular sounds often are heard over the affected lobe. Most cases are uncomplicated, and even among patients in the ICU, mortality is only 25%. Risk factors for the development of compli-

cations include age, preexistent lung disease, acquired immunodeficiency syndrome or other forms of immunodeficiency, or nosocomial acquisition. Abscesses are usually culture-positive and respond rapidly to drainage. Parapneumonic effusions are associated with concurrent bacteremia with penicillin–nonsusceptible pneumococci. Finally, the most serious complication, bacteremia, occurs in 25% of patients. This complication is increased in splenectomized patients. The use of the sputum Gram's stain and sputum culture in the diagnosis of *S. pneumoniae* infection is debated, but these tests sometimes may aid in choosing the optimal antimicrobial regimen. Penicillin covers the majority of cases, but increasing resistance to penicillin is occurring, thus necessitating use of a cephalosporin or, in some cases with significant resistance, vancomycin.

### 143. e.

No expert group in the United States recommends screening for ovarian cancer in asymptomatic women. A National Institutes of Health consensus conference on ovarian cancer recommends a family history and annual pelvic examination for all women. Screening for CA125 and vaginal ultrasound are recommended only for those with presumed hereditary cancer syndrome.

### 144. c, d.

The AHA 1997 guidelines for the prevention of endocarditis stratify cardiac conditions on the basis of whether prophylaxis is indicated, usually recommended, or not indicated:

- Indicated
  - Prosthetic heart valve
  - History of infective endocarditis
  - Single ventricle states
  - Transposition of the great arteries
  - Tetralogy of Fallot
  - Surgically constructed systemic or pulmonary conduits
- Recommended
  - Acquired valvular dysfunction
  - Hypertrophic cardiomyopathy
  - Mitral valve prolapse with valvular regurgitation, valvular thickening, or both
  - Intracardiac defects that have been repaired within the preceding 6 months or that are associated with significant hemodynamic instability
- Not indicated
  - Physiologic, functional, or innocent heart murmurs
  - Isolated secundum atrial septal defects
  - Surgically repaired atrial septal defects
  - Ventricular septal defect, patent ductus arteriosus, or mitral valve prolapse without associated regurgitation or valvular leaflet thickening
  - Mild or hemodynamically insignificant tricuspid regurgitation

☐ CAD, including previous coronary artery bypass grafting surgery

☐ Intracardiac lesions that have been repaired more than 6 months previously in which there is minimal or no hemodynamic abnormality

☐ Previous rheumatic fever or Kawasaki's disease without valvular dysfunction

☐ Cardiac pacemakers (intravascular and epicardial) and implanted defibrillators

### 145. b.

Dyspnea is the most common presenting symptom of asbestos-induced lung disease. Cough, sputum production, and wheezing are unusual presenting symptoms and, if present, tend to be due to cigarette smoke rather than asbestos exposure. It is true that ANA and rheumatoid factor may be present, as may a raised erythrocyte sedimentation rate, but these are not clinically useful, being nonspecific and not related to disease severity. The risk of lung cancer associated with exposure to both asbestos and cigarette smoke appears to be multiplicative. A 1979 report in the *Annals of the New York Academy of Science* showed that asbestos is associated with a sixfold increase, cigarette smoking with an 11-fold increase, and both cigarette smoke and asbestos exposure with a 59-fold increase in risk of lung cancer.

### 146. c.

Allergic bronchopulmonary aspergillosis is a hypersensitivity reaction in patients with asthma. Colonization with aspergilli occurs, rather than infection, and an antimicrobial is not indicated. Treatment with a corticosteroid is very effective.

### 147. c.

Although this man has been on heparin, abnormal mental status, abnormal renal function, and the presence of fragmented RBCs should raise the suspicion of TTP. In addition, ticlopidine has been associated with TTP.

### 148. a.

It is important to recognize unstable angina, which is defined by one or more of the following:

■ Angina of new onset (<2 months)
■ Frequency of three or more episodes per day
■ Accelerating frequency, severity, duration, or ease of precipitation
■ Angina at rest

Management of all patients with unstable angina is hospital admission for treatment and evaluation.

### 149. b.

β-Blocker and digoxin toxicity can produce hyperkalemia through the redistribution of potassium. ACE inhibitors and NSAIDs, as well as trimethoprim, cyclosporine, and pentamidine, can produce hyperkalemia through renal mechanisms. Insulin, along with β-agonists, causes redistribution and may produce hypokalemia.

### 150. b.

Idiopathic thrombocytopenic purpura in adults normally presents as chronic idiopathic thrombocytopenic purpura, a more indolent form. Patients are more often women (3:1) 20 to 40 years of age and have a history of easy bruising and menometrorrhagia. Because a low platelet count may be seen in SLE, ANA testing and bone marrow biopsies are often required to rule out other causes.

### 151. e.

Chronic cough is defined as a cough persisting for 3 weeks or longer. Postnasal drip, asthma, and gastroesophageal reflux represent approximately 90% of the causes found for chronic cough (and an even higher percentage in nonsmokers with a normal chest radiograph). The approach to such patients should include a detailed history, including a drug history to evaluate for the use of an ACE inhibitor (associated with cough in 3% to 20% patients taking one), and an appropriate physical examination. This man has a history of nasal discharge and frequent throat clearing, and examination revealed nasopharyngeal mucosa with a cobblestone appearance and the presence of secretions, all of which suggest postnasal drip. Hence, a trial of a nasal steroid spray is the most appropriate next step. No clues are suggestive of gastroesophageal reflux, but if there were such clues, a trial of an $H_2$ blocker would have been a possible option. Postviral cough can persist for up to 8 weeks after the acute syndrome but should resolve after 6 months in this case. The diagnosis of asthma is not suggested as the most likely diagnosis here because no nighttime or exercise-related symptoms are present, and 4 months of twice daily albuterol with a good technique had no effect on the symptoms. Therefore, persisting with albuterol and adding an inhaled steroid are not indicated, and at this point, spirometry would not be the best choice.

### 152. d.

This man has been receiving heparin subcutaneously since his surgery. The development of heparin-induced thrombocytopenia may occur from 5 to 10 days after the initiation of therapy. A nonimmunogenic thrombocytopenia (type 1) may occur in 10% to 20% of patients on heparin. It is characterized by a decrease in the platelet count in the initial days of therapy, with a return to normal range with continued therapy, and poses no clinical risk. Immunogenic thrombocytopenia (type 2) may occur in 2% to 3% of patients on heparin; however, it is characterized by a progressive decrease in platelet count, along with an increased risk of both venous and arterial thrombosis. The antigen is thought to be a heparin–platelet factor IV complex in most patients. Treatment is immediate discontinuation of heparin therapy. The diagnosis of heparin-induced thrombocytopenia must be made clinically, although better assays are becoming available to detect the presence of heparin-induced platelet antibodies.

**153. c.**

An elevated D-dimer level (>500 ng/mL) is present in the majority of patients with pulmonary embolus, but raised levels are also found in malignancy and post-surgery. Therefore, a raised D-dimer level is not specific for pulmonary embolus. A D-dimer value less than 200 ng/mL contributes to excluding the diagnosis of pulmonary embolus, with a negative predictive value of 97% when combined with a nondiagnostic lung scan.

**154. c.**

The SVC syndrome occurs in approximately 4% of patients with lung cancer and is most often associated with small cell carcinoma. Patients often experience headache or fullness in the head, along with dyspnea. On examination, patients have facial or upper extremity swelling, plethora, dilatated neck veins, and a prominent venous pattern on the anterior chest.

**155. d.**

Atropine, 1 mg intravenously, is not an appropriate treatment if the patient is recovering from heart transplantation because denervated hearts do not respond to atropine; transcutaneous pacing or catecholamine infusion would be appropriate therapies in that situation. Low-dose isoproterenol may be used with caution after other therapeutic options have failed, but at high doses, it is a Class III drug, has been shown to be harmful, and so is never an appropriate treatment for bradycardia. Adenosine is an appropriate first-line choice of drug therapy for some tachycardias, but not bradycardia. If a patient is unstable with tachycardia and a falling blood pressure, then synchronized direct-current cardioversion is appropriate therapy; however, if a patient with bradycardia is unstable, then transcutaneous pacing is indicated.

**156. e.**

TTP is an acute syndrome that affects myriad systems. The classic pentad of clinical features includes thrombocytopenia, microangiopathic hemolytic anemia, neurologic changes, renal function abnormalities, and fever. Because of the association between ticlopidine use and TTP, clopidogrel, a newer thienopyridine derivative whose mechanism of action and chemical structure are similar to those of ticlopidine, has largely replaced ticlopidine in clinical practice. Several reports showed, however, that TTP also could occur after the initiation of clopidogrel therapy, often within the first 2 weeks of treatment. Although TTP remains an extremely rare complication of clopidogrel, physicians should be aware of the possibility of this potentially life-threatening syndrome when initiating clopidogrel treatment.

**157. a.**

**158. c.**

**159. e.**

Common variable immunodeficiency is a primary immunodeficiency characterized by defective antibody formation. Among populations of European origin, common variable immunodeficiency is the most frequent of the primary specific immunodeficiency diseases. It affects men and women equally. The usual age at presentation is the second or third decade of life. The clinical presentation of common variable immunodeficiency disease is generally that of recurrent pyogenic sinopulmonary infections. Recurrent attacks of herpes simplex are common, and herpes zoster develops in approximately one-fifth of patients. An unusually high incidence of malignant lymphoreticular and gastrointestinal conditions is present in common variable immunodeficiency. A 50-fold increase in gastric carcinoma has been observed. Lymphoma, which seems to be the presenting illness in this patient, is approximately 300 times more frequent in women with common variable immunodeficiency than in affected men.

Deficiencies in both the late and early components of the complement system can lead to increased susceptibility to meningococcal infection. The risk of meningococcal disease for a person with a complement deficiency is estimated to be 0.5% per year. This represents a relative risk of 5,000, as compared with the incidence of meningococcal disease among persons without a complement deficiency.

Job's syndrome is an autosomal recessive disorder characterized by a defective neutrophil chemotactic response, with the development of recurrent cold staphylococcal abscesses and eczema. Patients also have elevated levels of IgE in the serum.

**160. b.**

**161. e.**

**162. a.**

**163. d.**

**164. c.**

**165. f.**

Osteoporosis, the most common bone disease, is characterized by low bone mass and a disruption of the normal bony architecture, which undermines the structural integrity of the bone and leads to skeletal fragility and an increase in fracture risk. The chemistry panel of patients with osteoporosis is nonspecific. The diagnosis of osteoporosis is established by measuring bone mineral density. Ten percent to 20% of cancer patients are hypercalcemic. Hypercalcemia can occur through three major mechanisms in cancer patients: osteolytic metastases, tumor secretion of parathyroid hormone–related protein, and tumor production of calcitriol. Osteomalacia is a disease of decreased bone mineralization. The diagnosis of Paget's disease is usually made incidentally through a routine chemistry screen showing an elevated serum alkaline phosphatase concentration or through a plain radiograph obtained for some other reason. Serum calcium and phosphorus concentrations are normal in most patients with Paget's disease. The diagnosis of primary hyperparathyroidism is made by the demonstration of an inappropriate PTH value in the face of hypercalcemia. The serum phosphorus concentration may be decreased but typically is in the lower range of normal. Approximately 40% of patients with primary hyperparathyroidism are hypercalciuric. Vitamin D excess can cause hypercalcemia by increasing calcium absorption and bone resorption. PTH usually is suppressed by negative feedback of the high calcium levels.

### 166. d.
Although rare in the United States, ascorbic acid deficiency (vitamin C deficiency, scurvy) occurs mostly in severely malnourished individuals, drug and alcohol abusers, or those living in poverty. One group at particularly increased risk comprises adults living alone, most commonly men ("bachelor" or "widower" scurvy) but sometimes women, who have deficient dietary intake because of such factors as poverty, poor access to groceries, dementia, or nutritional ignorance. They mostly prepare their own meals.

The clinical syndrome seen in vitamin C deficiency is due to impaired collagen synthesis. The most distinctive cutaneous finding in scurvy is hemorrhagic skin lesions that usually occur in a perifollicular distribution, especially on the legs, where the hydrostatic pressure is highest. Besides fatigue and decreased exercise tolerance, symptoms of scurvy include ecchymoses, bleeding gums, petechiae, hyperkeratosis, Sjögren's syndrome, arthralgias, and impaired wound healing.

### 167. c.
Wernicke's encephalopathy is caused by thiamine deficiency. Alcoholics are the most commonly affected population in the United States. Patients with significant malnutrition also are at risk. The classic triad is ophthalmoplegia, ataxia, and confusion. Cardiovascular beriberi may coexist. The treatment of choice is parenteral thiamine (50 mg daily until the patient resumes a normal diet, which should begin before starting intravenous glucose infusion). Korsakoff's psychosis is a part of Wernicke's disease and may occur together with the other components of the illness. Cocaine inhibits catecholamine reuptake at adrenergic nerve endings, thus potentiating sympathetic nervous system activity. Tachycardia, hypertension, pyrexia, and mood stimulation are seen in cocaine overdose.

### 168. e.
Although this patient has several medical problems, note that the examiner is interested in the most likely cause of his musculoskeletal problems. Polymyalgia rheumatica

is the leading diagnosis when an elderly patient presents with girdle pain and stiffness, increased acute phase reactants, and anemia, especially when the symptoms improve with systemic glucocorticoids.

Polymyositis is less likely in the absence of elevated creatine phosphokinase and with the presence of muscle pain. Fibromyalgia does not cause the laboratory abnormalities described in this case. Pseudo-osteoarthritis is a condition that describes the progression of calcium pyrophosphate dihydrate crystal deposition disease to joint degeneration. Multiple joints are usually involved, but the most commonly affected joints are the knees, followed by the wrists and metacarpophalangeal joints. Inclusion body myositis is an idiopathic inflammatory myopathy that presents with the insidious onset of weakness over several years. Symmetric proximal lower extremity weakness is usually the first sign. Myalgias are encountered in approximately 40% of cases.

### 169. d.
Hyporeninemic hypoaldosteronism is seen in elderly patients with diabetes mellitus or renal disease. Patients usually have mild renal insufficiency, hyperchloremic metabolic acidosis, and hyperkalemia. Coexisting hypertension and congestive heart failure are common in this patient population. The acidosis is best corrected by treating the hyperkalemia with cation exchange resins and, in the absence of contraindications, mineralocorticoid replacement.

### 170. b.

### 171. c.

### 172. a.
Plasma C-peptide distinguishes endogenous from exogenous hyperinsulinemia. C-peptide is high in patients with insulinomas and sulfonylurea-induced hypoglycemia. Plasma insulin values are high in patients with exogenous insulin administration, whereas plasma C-peptide values are appropriately low.

### 173. g.

### 174. f.

### 175. c.

### 176. b.

### 177. e.

### 178. a.

### 179. d.
Cardiac murmurs and the maneuvers commonly used to characterize them are a popular topic of the Board examination. A full understanding of this topic is highly recommended.

### 180. c.
The goal of mechanical ventilation in patients with chronic obstructive pulmonary disease exacerbation is to

achieve an arterial oxygen tension ($PaO_2$) of 60 mm Hg. Although higher levels increase the risk of oxygen toxicity, they do not increase tissue oxygenation. $PaCO_2$ should be brought as close to the baseline value (i.e., the value recorded when the patient was compensated) but not necessarily normalized. For this patient, choice c meets these criteria.

## 181. e.

The management of idiopathic thrombocytopenic purpura in the early stages of pregnancy is similar to the management of the disease in nonpregnant patients. Prednisone is the drug of choice for patients whose platelet counts are between 30,000 and 50,000/$\mu$L. Although splenectomy remains the most effective treatment for severe idiopathic thrombocytopenic purpura, splenectomy should be reserved for refractory cases that fail medical therapy. Intravenous immunoglobulin is a temporary therapy, especially useful for patients with severe thrombocytopenia who have to undergo urgent surgical procedures or those who go into labor.

## 182. e.

## 183. a.

## 184. b.

## 185. d.

## 186. f.

## 187. c.

Gilbert's syndrome is the most common inherited disorder of bilirubin glucuronidation. Routine laboratory tests are usually normal, except for hyperbilirubinemia. Baseline bilirubin levels are usually less than 3 mg/dL. Certain stressors such as fasting (or receiving a lipid-free diet), febrile illnesses, and physical exertion cause further elevation in serum bilirubin levels, but the level usually stays below 6 mg/dL. The bilirubin level returns to normal 12 to 24 hours after resuming normal diet, removal of the stressor, or both.

Hepatitis A infection is common in areas in which food and water hygiene and sanitation are suboptimal. The incubation period averages 30 days. Patients experience prodromal symptoms including malaise, nausea, vomiting, anorexia, fever, and right upper quadrant pain. Jaundice and hepatomegaly are the most common physical findings in symptomatic patients. Serum aminotransferases are markedly elevated (usually >1,000 IU/dL); serum bilirubin (total and direct) and alkaline phosphatase are also elevated. ALT is commonly higher than AST.

Ninety-five percent of primary biliary cirrhosis patients are women. Although fatigue and pruritus once were the most common presenting symptoms of primary biliary cirrhosis, presently up to half the patients are asymptomatic at diagnosis. Significantly elevated serum alkaline phosphatase is characteristic of primary biliary cirrhosis. The aminotransferases may be normal and, when elevated, they rarely increase more than fivefold above normal. The serum bilirubin concentration becomes elevated in most patients as the disease progresses. Antimitochondrial antibodies are the serologic hallmark of primary biliary cirrhosis.

A disproportionate elevation of serum AST compared with ALT is the most common biochemical abnormality in alcoholic liver disease. Although the absolute values of serum AST and ALT are almost always less than 500 IU/L, the AST to ALT ratio is usually greater than 2.0.

Although hepatic granulomas are present in almost all patients who have sarcoidosis with involvement of their gastrointestinal tract, clinically apparent liver disease is uncommon even in patients who have numerous hepatic granulomas. Mild elevation in alkaline phosphatase and $\gamma$-glutamyltransferase is the usual laboratory finding.

Liver function abnormalities peak from 72 to 96 hours after ingestion in patients with acetaminophen overdose. The plasma ALT and AST levels often exceed 10,000 IU/L. Total bilirubin concentration generally does not exceed 4.0 mg/dL, which is primarily indirect.

## 188. d.

Penile discharge should be treated aggressively, and the physician should look carefully for clinical and laboratory clues for coinfections with sexually transmitted diseases. The Centers for Disease Control and Prevention recommend concomitant chlamydia treatment for cases of presumed or confirmed gonorrheal infection at any site. Choice d represents the preferred recommended therapy.

Conversely, the history of exposure to several prostitutes and presence of inguinal lymph node enlargement in this patient is suspicious for concomitant LGV infection. The diagnosis of LGV is difficult because there is no characteristic clinical presentation. Sexual partners of patients diagnosed with *N. gonorrhoeae* who have had sexual contact with the infected patient within the past 60 days should be evaluated and treated, even if they were asymptomatic.

## 189. c.

Splenic and portal vein thrombosis is a relatively common complication of chronic pancreatitis. In patients with the disorder, studies have estimated a splenic vein thrombosis prevalence rate of between 5% and 24%. In a surgical series, a surprising 10% prevalence of portal or superior mesenteric vein thrombosis has been noted. Besides the fact that many cases are silent, splenic and portal vein thrombosis symptoms in chronic pancreatitis patients may be indistinguishable from the patients' chronic symptoms. Hence, it is not uncommon that many cases go undetected until patients present with complications of portal hypertension. Worsening of the chronic abdominal pain in chronic pancreatitis patients warrants further evaluation to rule out splenic and portal vein thrombosis. Visceral angiography is the diagnostic test of choice for splenic and portal vein thrombosis.

**190. e.**

Pericardial tamponade is a well-recognized complication in patients with chronic renal failure and uremic pericarditis. Pericardial tamponade is a medical emergency. The management of patients suspected of having pericardial tamponade includes aggressive fluid resuscitation and immediate echocardiography by a cardiologist trained to perform pericardiocentesis.

**191. e.**

**192. d.**

**193. a.**

**194. b.**

Raynaud's phenomenon is an early manifestation of scleroderma. Esophageal involvement in scleroderma is present in up to 50% of patients and includes burning pain in the retrosternal region. Gastroesophageal reflux disease and the subsequent esophagitis and esophageal spasm can cause retrosternal chest pain that mimics angina. It is not uncommon for these patients to undergo full cardiac evaluation before the attention is directed to the esophagus. Smoking is a risk factor for esophageal carcinoma. Plummer-Vinson syndrome is a combination of iron-deficiency anemia and a hypopharyngeal web in middle-aged women.

**195. e.**

Swimming pool and fish tank granuloma is caused by *M. marinum*. A small violet nodule or pustule appears at a skin surface exposed to contaminated water. A crusted ulcer or a small abscess evolves thereafter. The incubation period is 1 to 8 weeks after exposure. *M. leprae* is the causative agent of leprosy. The incidence of leprosy in the United States has fallen to an average of 150 cases per year. The incubation period ranges between 3 and 5 years. *P. aeruginosa* bacteremia may be associated with ecthyma gangrenosum, which is characterized by central necrosis surrounded by violaceous ecchymotic areas. Lymphangitic sporotrichosis is the most common manifestation of *Sporothrix schenckii* infection. A painless, red nodule forms at the site of inoculation, followed by several nodules along the lymphatic channels over the next few weeks. *Rickettsia rickettsii* causes Rocky Mountain spotted fever, a tick-borne disease. This is a systemic disease with skin rash that manifests as macules, up to 5 mm in diameter, on the wrists and ankles.

**196. e.**

Because the left ventricular systole may become prolonged in severe aortic stenosis, the aortic valve closure may no longer precede the pulmonic valve closure. This phenomenon causes paradoxical splitting in the second heart sound. Left bundle branch block is another common cause of paradoxical splitting in $S_2$. In right bundle branch block, however, the delayed activation of the right ventricle causes the $S_2$ splitting, which normally occurs during inspiration, to persist during expiration.

**197. e.**

Nephrotic syndrome leads to a reduction in antithrombin III and free protein S levels and an elevation in total protein S and protein C levels. These abnormalities predispose to thrombosis, especially renal vein thrombosis. An abrupt deterioration in renal function or exacerbation of baseline proteinuria and hematuria in a patient with known nephrotic syndrome warrants investigation to rule out renal vein thrombosis.

**198. d.**

The use of amphetamines as drugs of abuse has increased markedly since 1975. This use affects myriad systems, resulting in a wide range of symptoms that may make it a difficult addiction to recognize. The drug is known to cause a massive release of dopamine in the brain, resulting in agitation, anxiety, delirium, hallucinations, and death. In addition, it causes a decrease in *N*-acetylaspartate in the frontal lobes and basal ganglia that may explain the chronic central nervous system side effects, such as lasting psychosis after its use is stopped and choreoathetoid movements. A high index of suspicion is necessary to make an early diagnosis.

**199. d.**

Total palsy of the third nerve causes ptosis, a dilated pupil, and diplopia. Typically, the eye looks down and out. This occurs when all the nerve fibers are affected, which is the case when a circle of Willis aneurysm causes nerve compression and subsequent injury, especially when such an aneurysm ruptures. Most cases of pupil-sparing oculomotor (third cranial nerve) palsy result from microvascular infarction of the nerve. This occurs in patients with long-standing diabetes mellitus and hypertension. Spontaneous recovery over a period of months is the rule.

**200. e.**

**201. d.**

**202. c.**

**203. a.**

**204. b.**

**205. f.**

HBsAg is the first serologic marker detectable in the serum of patients with acute hepatitis B infection. It becomes undetectable 1 to 2 months after the appearance of jaundice. Anti-HBs antibody becomes detectable after HBsAg disappears and remains so indefinitely thereafter. HBcAg is sequestered in the coat of HBsAg and not routinely detected in the serum of hepatitis B–infected patients. Anti-HBc, however, is readily detectable 1 to 2 weeks after the appearance of HBs Ag and before the appearance of anti-HBs. Thus, anti-HBc is used to diagnose acute hepatitis B infection during this gap "window phenomenon" when the HBsAg has disappeared and the anti-HBs has not yet appeared. Anti-HBc thus signifies a current or recent hepatitis B infection. HBeAg occurs transiently early in acute hepatitis B infection, concurrently or shortly after the appearance of HBsAg. HBeAg signifies ongoing viral replication and relative infectivity.

## SUGGESTED READINGS

### Question 1

Arroyo V, Gines P, Gerbes AL, et al. Definition and diagnostic criteria of refractory ascites and hepatorenal syndrome in cirrhosis. International Ascites Club. *Hepatology* 1996;23:164–176.
Better OS. Renal and cardiovascular function in liver disease. *Kidney Int* 1986;29:598–607.
Gines A, Escorsell A, Gines P, et al. Incidence, predictive factors, and prognosis of the hepatorenal syndrome in cirrhosis with ascites. *Gastroenterology* 1993;105:229–236.

### Question 2

Blumberg A, Weidmann P, Shaw S, et al. Effect of various therapeutic approaches on plasma potassium and major regulating factors in terminal renal failure. *Am J Med* 1988;85:507–512.
Conger JD. Interventions in clinical acute renal failure: what are the data? *Am J Kidney Dis* 1995;26:565–576.
Rutsky EA, Rostand SG. Treatment of uremic pericarditis and pericardial effusion. *Am J Kidney Dis* 1987;10:2–8.

### Question 3

Rummans TA, Evans JM, Krahn LE, et al. Delirium in elderly patients: evaluation and management. *Mayo Clin Proc* 1995;70:989–998.

### Question 6

Dixon BS, Anderson RJ. Nonoliguric acute renal failure. *Am J Kidney Dis* 1985;6:71–80.
Liano F, Pascual J. Epidemiology of acute renal failure: a prospective, multicenter, community-based study. Madrid Acute Renal Failure Study Group. *Kidney Int* 1996;50:811–818.
Miller TR, Anderson RJ, Linas SL, et al. Urinary diagnostic indices in acute renal failure: a prospective study. *Ann Intern Med* 1978;89:47–50.
Myers BD, Moran SM. Hemodynamically mediated acute renal failure. *N Engl J Med* 1986;314:97–105.
Nolan CR, Anderson RJ. Hospital-acquired acute renal failure. *J Am Soc Nephrol* 1998;9:710–718.

### Question 7

Hellmark T, Johansson C, Wieslander J. Characterization of anti-GBM antibodies involved in Goodpasture's syndrome. *Kidney Int* 1994;46:823–829.
Hoffman GS, Specks U. Antineutrophil cytoplasmic antibodies. *Arthritis Rheum* 1998;41:1521–1537.
Jayne DR, Marshall PD, Jones SJ, et al. Autoantibodies to GBM and neutrophil cytoplasm in rapidly progressive glomerulonephritis. *Kidney Int* 1990;37:965–970.

Kalluri R, Meyers KM, Mogyorosi A, et al. Goodpasture syndrome involving overlap with Wegener's granulomatosis and anti-glomerular basement membrane disease. *J Am Soc Nephrol* 1997;8:1795–1800.

### Question 8

Whittemore AS, Harris R, Itnyre J. Characteristics relating to ovarian cancer risk: collaborative analysis of 12 U.S. case-control studies. II. Invasive epithelial ovarian cancers in white women. Collaborative Ovarian Cancer Group. *Am J Epidemiol* 1992;136:1184–1203.

### Question 10

Ramsey B, Richardson MA. Impact of sinusitis in cystic fibrosis. *J Allergy Clin Immunol* 1992;90:547–552.

### Question 11

Phillips LH II, Melnick PA. Diagnosis of myasthenia gravis in the 1990s. *Semin Neurol* 1990;10:62–69.
Ryder REJ, Mir MA, Freeman EA. *Myasthenia Gravis. An Aid to the MRCP Short Cases.* Oxford: Blackwell Scientific, 1991:246–247.

### Question 12

Cohen AM, Tremiterra S, Candela F, et al. Prognosis of node-positive colon cancer. *Cancer* 1991;67:1859–1861.
Eisenberg B, Decosse JJ, Harford F, et al. Carcinoma of the colon and rectum: the natural history reviewed in 1,704 patients. *Cancer* 1982;49:1131–1134.

### Question 13

Sampson HA, Mendelson L, Rosen JP. Fatal and near-fatal anaphylactic reactions to food in children and adolescents. *N Engl J Med* 1992;327:380–384.

### Question 14

Lillington GA, Caskey CI. Evaluation and management of solitary and multiple pulmonary nodules. *Clin Chest Med* 1993;14:111–119.

### Question 15

Adamson JW. The myeloproliferative diseases. In: Wilson JD, Braunwald E, Isselbacher KJ, et al., eds. *Harrison's Principles of Internal Medicine,* 12th ed. New York: McGraw-Hill, 1991:1563–1565.
Dickstein JI, Vardiman JW. Hematopathologic findings in the myeloproliferative disorders. *Semin Oncol* 1995;22:355–373.

### Question 17

Girard DE, Kumar KL, McAfee JH. Hematologic effects of acute alcohol abuse. *Hematol Oncol Clin North Am* 1987;1:321–324.
Peck-Radosavljevic M, Zacherl J, Meng YG, et al. Is inadequate thrombopoietin production a major cause of thrombocytopenia in cirrhosis of the liver? *J Hepatol* 1997;27:127–131.

### Question 18

Cunningham FG, Lindheimer MD. Hypertension in pregnancy. *N Engl J Med* 1992;326:927–932.
Redman CW. Controlled trials of antihypertensive drugs in pregnancy. *Am J Kidney Dis* 1991;17:149–153.
Remuzzi G, Ruggenenti P. Prevention and treatment of pregnancy-associated hypertension: what have we learned in the last 10 years? *Am J Kidney Dis* 1991;18:285–305.

Shotan A, Widerhorn J, Hurst A, et al. Risk of angiotensin-converting enzyme inhibition during pregnancy: experimental and clinical evidence, potential mechanisms, and recommendations for use. *Am J Med* 1994;96:451–456.

Sibai BM. Treatment of hypertension in pregnant women. *N Engl J Med* 1996;335:257–265.

Sibai BM, Mabie WC, Shamsa F, et al. A comparison of no medication versus methyldopa or labetalol in chronic hypertension during pregnancy. *Am J Obstet Gynecol* 1990;162:960–966.

## Question 19

Cook JD. Clinical evaluation of iron deficiency. *Semin Hematol* 1982; 19:6–19.

Cook JD, Skikne BS. Iron deficiency: definition and diagnosis. *J Intern Med* 1989;226:349–355.

## Question 20

Kirsner JB, Shorter RG, eds. *Inflammatory Bowel Disease*, 3rd ed. Philadelphia: Lea & Febiger, 1988.

Podolsky DK. Inflammatory bowel disease (1). *N Engl J Med* 1991; 325:928–937.

## Question 21

Silverberg SJ, Bilezikian JP. Evaluation and management of primary hyperparathyroidism. *J Clin Endocrinol Metab* 1996;81:2036–2040.

## Question 22

1998 Guidelines for treatment of sexually transmitted diseases. Centers for Disease Control and Prevention. *MMWR Morb Mortal Wkly Rep* 1998;47(RR-1):1–111.

## Question 23

Pascual E. The diagnosis of gout and CPPD crystal arthropathy. *Br J Rheumatol* 1996;35:306–308.

Terkeltaub RA. What stops a gouty attack? *J Rheumatol* 1992;19:8–10.

## Question 24

Anderson DJ, Noyes R Jr., Crowe RR. A comparison of panic disorder and generalized anxiety disorder. *Am J Psychiatry* 1984;141:572–575.

Lydiard RB, Ballenger JC. Antidepressants in panic disorder and agoraphobia. *J Affect Disord* 1987;13:153–168.

## Question 25

Koch W. Swallowing disorders: diagnosis and therapy. *Med Clin North Am* 1993;77:571–582.

Zenker FA, Von Ziemssen H. Krankheiten des Oesophagus. In: Von Ziemssen H, ed. *Handbuch der Specielen Pathologie und Therapie*. Leipzig: FC Vogel, 1877.

## Question 26

Lieberman JR, Berry DJ, Bono JV, et al. The hip and thigh. In: Snider RK, ed. *Essentials of Musculoskeletal Care*. Rosemont, IL: American Academy of Orthopaedic Surgeons, 1997:265–303.

## Question 27

Locksley RM, Flournoy N, Sullivan KM, et al. Infection with varicella-zoster virus after marrow transplantation. *J Infect Dis* 1985;152:1172–1181.

## Question 28

Donowitz M, Kokke FT, Saidi R. Evaluation of patients with chronic diarrhea. *N Engl J Med* 1995;332:725–729.

Ewe K, Karbach U. Factitious diarrhea. *Clin Gastroenterol* 1986;15:723–740.

## Question 29

Fairbanks DN. Inflammatory diseases of the sinuses: bacteriology and antibiotics. *Otolaryngol Clin North Am* 1993;26:549–559.

## Question 30

Johnson TR. The shoulder. In: Snider RK, ed. *Essentials of Musculoskeletal Care*. Rosemont, IL: American Academy of Orthopaedic Surgeons, 1997:72–121.

Lequesne M, Dang N, Bensasson M, et al. Increased association of diabetes mellitus with capsulitis of the shoulder and shoulder-hand syndrome. *Scand J Rheumatol* 1977;6:53–56.

Pal B, Anderson J, Dick WC, et al. Limitation of joint mobility and shoulder capsulitis in insulin- and non-insulin-dependent diabetes mellitus. *Br J Rheumatol* 1986;25:147–151.

## Question 35

Hunder GG, Arend WP, Block DA, et al. American College of Rheumatology 1990 criteria for the classification of vasculitis: introduction. *Arthritis Rheum* 1990;33:1065–1067.

## Question 36

Galgiani JN. Coccidioidomycosis. *West J Med* 1993;159:153–171.

Stevens DA. Coccidioidomycosis. *N Engl J Med* 1995;332:1077–1082.

## Question 37

Alter MJ, Mast EE. The epidemiology of viral hepatitis in the United States. *Gastroenterol Clin North Am* 1994;23:437–455.

Takahashi M, Yamada G, Miyamoto R, et al. Natural course of chronic hepatitis C. *Am J Gastroenterol* 1993;88:240–243.

## Question 38

Kagnoff M. Celiac disease: a gastrointestinal disease with environmental, genetic, and immunologic components. *Gastroenterol Clin North Am* 1992;21:405–425.

Trier JS. Celiac sprue. *N Engl J Med* 1991;325:1709–1719.

## Question 39

Mau W, Zeidler H, Mau R, et al. Clinical features and prognosis of patients with possible ankylosing spondylitis: results of a 10-year follow-up. *J Rheumatol* 1988;15:1109–1114.

O'Neill TW, King G, Graham IM, et al. Echocardiographic abnormalities in ankylosing spondylitis. *Ann Rheum Dis* 1992;51:652–654.

## Question 40

Goldman L. Quantitative aspects of clinical reasoning. In: Isselbacher KJ, Braunwald E, Wilson JD, et al., eds. *Harrison's Principles of Internal Medicine*, 13th ed. New York: McGraw-Hill, 1994:43–48.

## Question 41

Utsunomiya J, Gocho H, Miyanaga T, et al. Peutz-Jeghers syndrome: its natural course and management. *Johns Hopkins Med J* 1975; 136:71–82.

Young RH, Welch WR, Dickersin GR, et al. Ovarian sex cord tumor with annular tubules: review of 74 cases including 27 with Peutz-Jeghers syndrome and four with adenoma malignum of the cervix. *Cancer* 1982;50:1384–1402.

## Question 42

Singer PA, Cooper DS, Levy EG, et al. Treatment guidelines for patients with hyperthyroidism and hypothyroidism. Standards of Care Committee, American Thyroid Association. *JAMA* 1995;273: 808–812.

Torring O, Tallstedt L, Wallin G, et al. Graves' hyperthyroidism: treatment with antithyroid drugs, surgery, or radioiodine—a prospective, randomized study. Thyroid Study Group. *J Clin Endocinol Metab* 1996;81:2986–2993.

## Question 48

Hardcastle JD, Thomas WM, Chamberlain J, et al. Randomised, controlled trial of faecal occult blood screening for colorectal cancer: results for first 107,349 subjects. *Lancet* 1989;1:1160–1164.

## Question 49

Johnson TR. The elbow and forearm. In: Snider RK, ed. *Essentials of Musculoskeletal Care.* Rosemont, IL: American Academy of Orthopaedic Surgeons, 1997:125–129.

## Question 50

Israili ZH, Hall WD. Cough and angioneurotic edema associated with angiotensin-converting enzyme inhibitor therapy: a review of the literature and pathophysiology. *Ann Intern Med* 1992;117:234–242.

Lunde H, Hedner T, Samuelsson O, et al. Dyspnoea, asthma, and bronchospasm in relation to treatment with angiotensin converting enzyme inhibitors. *BMJ* 1994;308:18–21.

## Question 51

Prevention and control of influenza: recommendations of the Advisory Committee on Immunization Practices (ACIP). Centers for Disease Control and Prevention. *MMWR Morb Mortal Wkly Rep* 1998;47(RR-6):1–26.

## Question 56

Gabow PA. Disorders associated with an altered anion gap. *Kidney Int* 1985;27:472–483.

Gabow PA, Kaehny WD, Fennessey PV, et al. Diagnostic importance of an increased anion gap. *N Engl J Med* 1980;303:854–858.

Winter SD, Pearson R, Gabow PA, et al. The fall of the serum anion gap. *Arch Intern Med* 1990;150:311–313.

## Question 60

Management of persons exposed to multidrug-resistant tuberculosis. *MMWR Morb Mortal Wkly Rep* 1992;41(RR-11):61–71.

Prevention and control of tuberculosis in U.S. communities with at-risk minority populations. Recommendations of the Advisory Council for the Elimination of Tuberculosis. *MMWR Morb Mortal Wkly Rep* 1992;41(RR-5):1–11.

Prevention and treatment of tuberculosis among patients infected with human immunodeficiency virus: principles of therapy and revised recommendations. Centers for Disease Control and Prevention. *MMWR Morb Mortal Wkly Rep* 1998;47(RR-20):1–58.

## Question 61

Currier MB, Olsen EJ. Suicide. In: *Griffith's 5-minute Clinical Consult.* Baltimore: Lippincott Williams & Wilkins, 1999:1030–1031.

## Question 62

Chastre J, Trouillet JL, Vuagnat A, et al. Nosocomial pneumonia in patients with acute respiratory distress syndrome. *Am J Respir Crit Care Med* 1998;157:1165–1172.

Gammon RB, Shin MS, Buchalter SE. Pulmonary barotrauma in mechanical ventilation: patterns and risk factors. *Chest* 1992;102: 568–572.

Gammon RB, Shin MS, Groves RH Jr., et al. Clinical risk factors for pulmonary barotrauma: a multivariate analysis. *Am J Respir Crit Care Med* 1995;152:1235–1240.

Schnapp LM, Chin DP, Szaflarski N, et al. Frequency and importance of barotrauma in 100 patients with acute lung injury. *Crit Care Med* 1995;23:272–278.

## Question 64

Kaplan NM. Management of hypertensive emergencies. *Lancet* 1994; 344:1335–1338.

McGregor E, Isles CG, Jay JL, et al. Retinal changes in malignant hypertension. *BMJ* 1986;292:233–234.

Phillips SJ, Whisnant JP. Hypertension and the brain. The National High Blood Pressure Education Program. *Arch Intern Med* 1992; 152:938–945.

The sixth report of the Joint National Committee on prevention, detection, evaluation, and treatment of high blood pressure. *Arch Intern Med* 1997;157:2413–2446. [Erratum: *Arch Intern Med* 1998; 158:573.]

Strandgaard S, Paulson OB. Cerebral blood flow and its pathophysiology in hypertension. *Am J Hypertens* 1989;2:486–492.

## Question 65

Michel DM, Kelly CJ. Acute interstitial nephritis. *J Am Soc Nephrol* 1998;9:506–515.

Pappas PG. Laboratory in the diagnosis and management of urinary tract infections. *Med Clin North Am* 1991;75:313–325.

Stamm WE, Wagner KF, Amsel R, et al. Causes of the acute urethral syndrome in women. *N Engl J Med* 1980;303:409–415.

## Question 66

Hurwitz S. Acne vulgaris: pathogenesis and management. *Pediatr Rev* 1994;15:47–52.

Kaminer MS, Gilchrest BA. The many faces of acne. *J Am Acad Dermatol* 1995:32:S6–S14.

Webster GF, Toso SM, Hegemann L. Inhibition of a model of *in vitro* granuloma formation by tetracyclines and ciprofloxacin: involvement of protein kinase C. *Arch Dermatol* 1994;130:748–752.

## Question 67

Slutsky AS. Mechanical ventilation. American College of Chest Physicians' Consensus Conference. *Chest* 1993;104:1833–1859. [Erratum: *Chest* 1994;106:656.]

Tobin MJ. Mechanical ventilation. *N Engl J Med* 1994;330:1056–1061.

## Question 68

Drugs for AIDS and associated infections. *Med Lett Drugs Ther* 1995; 37:87.

Martins TB, Jaskowski TD, Mouritsen CL, et al. Comparison of commercially available enzyme immunoassay with traditional serological tests for detection of antibodies to *Coccidioides immitis*. *J Clin Microbiol* 1995;33:940–943.

Sarosi GA, Davies SF. Therapy for fungal infections. *Mayo Clin Proc* 1994;69:1111–1117.

Stevens DA. Coccidioidomycosis. *N Engl J Med* 1995;332:1077–1082.

## Question 69

Califf RM, Bengtson JR. Cardiogenic shock. *N Engl J Med* 1994;330: 1724–1730.

Goldberg RJ, Gore JM, Alpert JS, et al. Cardiogenic shock after myocardial infarction: incidence and mortality from a community wide perspective, 1975 to 1988. *N Engl J Med* 1991;325:1117–1122.

Guidelines for the early management of patients with acute myocardial infarction. A report of the American College of Cardiology/American Heart Association Task Force on Assessment of Diagnostic and Therapeutic Cardiovascular Procedures (Subcommittee to Develop Guidelines for the Early Management of Patients with Acute Myocardial Infarction). *J Am Coll Cardiol* 1990;16:249–292.

Hands ME, Rutherford JD, Muller JE, et al. The in-hospital development of cardiogenic shock after myocardial infarction: incidence, predictors of occurrence, outcome and prognostic factors. *J Am Coll Cardiol* 1989;14:40–46.

Holmes DR Jr., Califf RM, Van de Werf F. Differences in countries' use of resources and clinical outcome for patients with cardiogenic shock after myocardial infarction: results from the GUSTO trial. *Lancet* 1997;349:75–78.

## Question 70

Tinetti ME, Speechley M, Ginter SF, et al. Risk factors for falls among elderly persons living in the community. *N Engl J Med* 1988;319:1701–1707.

## Question 71

Ryder REJ, Mir MA, Freeman EA. *Lower Motor Neurone VIIth Nerve Palsy. An Aid to the MRCP Short Cases.* Oxford: Blackwell Scientific, 1991:192–193.

## Question 73

Lin RY. A perspective on penicillin allergy. *Arch Intern Med* 1992;152:930–937.

## Question 74

Mateo J, Oliver A, Borrell M, et al. Laboratory evaluation and clinical characteristics of 2,132 consecutive unselected patients with venous thromboembolism: results of the Spanish Multicentric Study on Thrombophilia (EMET-Study). *Thromb Haemost* 1997;77:444–451.

Ridker PM, Hennekensch, Lindpainter K, et al. Mutation in the gene coding for coagulation factor V and the risk of myocardial infarction, stroke, and venous thrombosis in apparently healthy men. *N Engl J Med* 1995;332:912–917.

## Question 75

Kostis JB, Shelton B, Gosselin G, et al. Adverse effects of enalapril in the Studies of Left Ventricular Dysfunction (SOLVD). SOLVD Investigators. *Am Heart J* 1996;131:350–355.

Langford HG, Blaufox MD, Borhani NO, et al. Is thiazide-produced uric acid elevation harmful? Analysis of data from the Hypertension Detection and Follow-up Program. *Arch Intern Med* 1987;147:645–649.

Materson BJ, Reda DJ, Cushman WC, et al. Single-drug therapy for hypertension in men: a comparison of six antihypertensive agents with placebo. The Department of Veterans Affairs Cooperative Study Group on Antihypertensive Agents. *N Engl J Med* 1993;328:914–921. [Erratum: *N Engl J Med* 1994;330:1689.]

Oren S, Gossman E, Frohlich ED. Effects of calcium entry blockers on distribution of blood volume. *Am J Hypertens* 1996;9:628–632.

## Question 78

DeLorenzo LJ, Huang CT, Maguire GP, et al. Roentgenographic patterns of *Pneumocystis carinii* pneumonia in 104 patients with AIDS. *Chest* 1987;91:323–327.

Hoover DR, Saah AJ, Bacellar H, et al. Clinical manifestations of AIDS in the era of pneumocystis prophylaxis. Multicenter AIDS Cohort Study. *N Engl J Med* 1993;329:1922–1926.

Jules-Elysee K, Stover DE, Zaman MB, et al. Aerosolized pentamidine: effect on diagnosis and presentation of *Pneumocystis carinii* pneumonia. *Ann Intern Med* 1990;112:750–757.

Stansell JD, Osmond DH, Charlebois E, et al. Predictors of *Pneumocystis carinii* pneumonia in HIV-infected persons. Pulmonary Complications of HIV Infection Study Group. *Am J Respir Crit Care Med* 1997;155:60–66.

Zaman MK, White DA. Serum lactate dehydrogenase levels and *Pneumocystis carinii* pneumonia: diagnostic and prognostic significance. *Am Rev Respir Dis* 1988;137:796–800.

## Question 79

Fitzpatrick TB, Johnson RA, Wolff K, et al., eds. *Psoriasis. Color Atlas and Synopsis of Clinical Dermatology: Common and Serious Diseases*, 3rd ed. New York: McGraw-Hill, 1997:76–95.

## Question 82

Rodgers KG. Cardiovascular shock. *Emerg Med Clin North Am* 1995;13:793–810.

Shoemaker WC. Temporal physiologic patterns of shock and circulatory dysfunction based on early descriptions by invasive and noninvasive monitoring. *New Horiz* 1996;4:300–318.

## Question 83

Public Health Service guidelines for counseling and antibody testing to prevent HIV infection and AIDS. *MMWR Morb Mortal Wkly Rep* 1987;36:509–515.

Recommendations for HIV testing services for inpatients and outpatients in acute-care hospital settings. Centers for Disease Control and Prevention. *MMWR Morb Mortal Wkly Rep* 1993; 42(RR-2):1–6.

Update: serologic testing for HIV-1 antibody—United States, 1988 and 1989. *MMWR Morb Mortal Wkly Rep* 1990;39:380–383.

## Question 85

Clark SL. Amniotic fluid embolism. *Crit Care Clin* 1991;7:877–882.

Dashow EE, Cotterill R, Benedetti TJ, et al. Amniotic fluid embolism. *J Reprod Med* 1989;34:660–666.

## Question 86

Arnow PM, Flaherty JP. Fever of unknown origin. *Lancet* 1997;350:575–580.

Hirschmann JV. Fever of unknown origin in adults. *Clin Infect Dis* 1997;24:291–300.

Knockaert DC, Dujardin KS, Bobbaers HJ. Long-term follow-up of patients with undiagnosed fever of unknown origin. *Arch Intern Med* 1996;156:618–620.

Petersdorf RG. Fever of unknown origin: an old friend revisited. *Arch Intern Med* 1992;152:21–22.

## Question 87

Consensus report on the ethics of foregoing [sic] life-sustaining treatments in the critically ill. Task Force on Ethics of the Society of Critical Care Medicine. *Crit Care Med* 1990;18:1435–1439.

Consensus statement of the Society of Critical Care Medicine's Ethics Committee regarding futile and other possibly inadvisable treatments. *Crit Care Med* 1997;25:887–891.

Guidelines for the appropriate use of do-not-resuscitate orders. Council on Ethical and Judicial Affairs, American Medical Association. *JAMA* 1991;265:1868–1871.

Quill TE, Cassel CK, Meier DE. Care of the hopelessly ill: proposed clinical criteria for physician-assisted suicide. *N Engl J Med* 1992;327:1380–1384.

Schneiderman LJ, Jecker NS, Jonsen AR. Medical futility: response to critiques. *Ann Intern Med* 1996;125:669–674.

## Question 88

Centers for Disease Control and Prevention. http://www.cdc.gov.

Davis TM, Dembo LG, Kaye-Eddie SA, et al. Neurological, cardiovascular and metabolic effects of mefloquine in healthy volunteers: a double-blind, placebo-controlled trial. *Br J Clin Pharmacol* 1996; 42:415–421.

*Health information for international travel, 1996 to 1997.* Atlanta, GA: Department of Health and Human Services, 1997.

## Question 89

American College of Chest Physicians/Society of Critical Care Medicine consensus conference: definitions for sepsis and organ failure and guidelines for the use of innovative therapies in sepsis. *Crit Care Med* 1992;20:864–874.

## Question 90

Ryder REJ, Mir MA, Freeman EA. *Eisenmenger's Syndrome. An Aid to the MRCP Short Cases.* Oxford: Blackwell Scientific, 1991:192–193.

## Question 92

Detection, evaluation, and treatment of renovascular hypertension: final report. Working Group on Renovascular Hypertension. *Arch Intern Med* 1987;147:820–829.

Mann SJ, Pickering TG. Detection of renovascular hypertension: state of the art: 1992. *Ann Intern Med* 1992;117:845–853.

Olin JW, Piedmonte MR, Young JR, et al. The utility of duplex ultrasound scanning of the renal arteries for diagnosing significant renal artery stenosis. *Ann Intern Med* 1995;122:833–838.

Setaro JF, Saddler MC, Chen CC, et al. Simplified captopril renography in diagnosis and treatment of renal artery stenosis. *Hypertension* 1991;18:289–298.

Van de Ven PJ, Beutler JJ, Kaatee R, et al. Angiotensin converting enzyme inhibitor-induced dysfunction in atherosclerotic renovascular disease. *Kidney Int* 1998;53:986–993.

## Question 94

Dupont HL. *Shigella* species. In: Mandell GL, Douglas RG Jr., Bennett JE, eds. *Principles and Practice of Infectious Diseases*, 4th ed. New York: Churchill Livingstone, 1995:203.

Gotuzzo E, Oberhelman RA, Maguina C, et al. Comparison of single-dose treatment with norfloxacin and standard 5-day treatment with trimethoprim-sulfamethoxazole for acute shigellosis in adults. *Antimicrob Agents Chemother* 1989;33:1101–1104.

Struelens MJ, Patte D, Kabir I, et al. Shigella septicemia: prevalence, presentation, risk factors, and outcome. *J Infect Dis* 1985;152: 784–790.

## Question 95

Blade J, Kyle RA. Multiple myeloma in young patients: clinical presentation and treatment approach. *Leuk Lymphoma* 1998;30:493–501.

Cohen DJ, Sherman WH, Osserman EF, et al. Acute renal failure in patients with multiple myeloma. *Am J Med* 1984;76:247–256.

Winearls CG. Acute myeloma kidney. *Kidney Int* 1995;48:1347–1361.

## Question 96

Lundback B. Epidemiology of rhinitis and asthma. *Clin Exp Allergy* 1998;28[Suppl 2]:3–10.

Raphael GD, Raphael MH, Kaliner M. Gustatory rhinitis: a syndrome of food-induced rhinorrhea. *J Allergy Clin Immunol* 1989;83:110–115.

## Question 97

Lillington GA, Caskey CI. Evaluation and management of solitary and multiple pulmonary nodules. *Clin Chest Med* 1993;14:111–119.

Midthun DE, Swensen SJ, Jett JR. Approach to the solitary pulmonary nodule. *Mayo Clin Proc* 1993;68:378–385.

Quoix E, Fraser R, Wolkove N, et al. Small cell lung cancer presenting as a solitary pulmonary nodule. *Cancer* 1990;66:577–582.

## Question 98

Bunn HF. Disorders of hemoglobin. In: Wilson JD, et al., eds. *Harrison's Principles of Internal Medicine*, 12th ed. New York: McGraw-Hill, 1991:1544–1548.

Platt OS, Thorington BD, Brambilla DJ, et al. Pain in sickle cell disease: rates and risk factors. *N Engl J Med* 1991;325:11–16.

## Question 99

Guidelines for cardiopulmonary resuscitation and emergency cardiac care. Emergency Cardiac Care Committee and Subcommittees, American Heart Association. Part III. Adult advanced cardiac life support. *JAMA* 1992;268:2199–2241.

## Question 100

Akhtar M, Shenasa M, Jazayeri M, et al. Wide QRS complex tachycardia: reappraisal of a common clinical problem. *Ann Intern Med* 1988; 109:905–912.

Buxton AE, Marchlinski FE, Doherty JU, et al. Hazards of intravenous verapamil for sustained ventricular tachycardia. *Am J Cardiol* 1987; 59:1107–1110.

Stewart RB, Bardy GH, Greene HL. Wide complex tachycardia: misdiagnosis and outcome after emergency therapy. *Ann Intern Med* 1986;104:766–771.

Tchou P, Young P, Mahmud R, et al. Useful clinical criteria for the diagnosis of ventricular tachycardia. *Am J Med* 1988;84:53–56.

## Question 101

Ryder REJ, Mir MA, Freeman EA. *Multiple Sclerosis. An Aid to the MRCP Short Cases.* Oxford: Blackwell Scientific, 1991:316.

Smith SG. Multiple sclerosis. In: Dambro MR, ed. *Griffith's 5-minute Clinical Consult.* Baltimore: Lippincott Williams & Wilkins, 1999: 700–701.

## Question 102

Gluck SL. Acid-base. *Lancet* 1988;352:474–479.

Rose BD. *Clinical Physiology of Acid-Base and Electrolyte Disorders*, 4th ed. New York: McGraw-Hill, 1994:572–586.

## Question 103

Garnick MB, Brenner BM. Tumors of the urinary tract. In: Wilson JD, Braunwald E, Isselbacher KJ, et al., eds. *Harrison's Principles of Internal Medicine*, 12th ed. New York: McGraw-Hill, 1991:1211–1212.

## Question 104

Delmez JA, Slatopolsky E. Hyperphosphatemia: its consequences and treatment in patients with chronic renal failure. *Am J Kidney Dis* 1992;19:303–317.

Farias MA, McClellan W, Soucie JM, et al. A prospective comparison of methods for determining if cardiovascular disease is a predictor of mortality in dialysis patients. *Am J Kidney Dis* 1994;23:382–388.

Henrich WL. Dialysis considerations in the elderly patient. *Am J Kidney Dis* 1990;16:339–341.

Sherrard DJ, Hercz G, Pei Y, et al. The spectrum of bone disease in end-stage renal failure: an evolving disorder. *Kidney Int* 1993;43: 436–442.

Zuckerman GR, Cornette GL, Clouse RE, et al. Upper gastrointestinal bleeding in patients with chronic renal failure. *Ann Intern Med* 1985;102:588–592.

### Question 105

Carpenter CC, Fischl MA, Hammer SM, et al. Antiretroviral therapy for HIV infection in 1998: updated recommendations of the International AIDS Society–USA Panel. *JAMA* 1998;280:78–86.

Drugs for HIV infection. *Med Lett Drugs Ther* 1997;39:111–116.

Guidelines for the use of antiretroviral agents in HIV-infected adults and adolescents. Department of Health and Human Services and the Henry J. Kaiser Family Foundation. *Ann Intern Med* 1998;128: 1079–1100.

Montaner JS, Reiss P, Cooper D, et al. A randomized, double-blind trial comparing combinations of nevirapine, didanosine, and zidovudine for HIV-infected patients. The INCAS trial. Italy, the Netherlands, Canada and Australia Study. *JAMA* 1998;279:930–937.

### Question 106

Turner RC, Lichstein PR, Peden JG Jr., et al. Alcohol withdrawal syndromes: a review of pathophysiology, clinical presentation and treatment. *J Gen Intern Med* 1989;4:432–444.

### Question 108

Rummans TA, Evans JM, Krahn LE, et al. Delirium in elderly patients: evaluation and management. *Mayo Clin Proc* 1995;70:989–998.

### Question 109

Gabow PA, Anderson RJ, Potts DE, et al. Acid-base disturbances in the salicylate-intoxicated adult. *Arch Intern Med* 1978;138:1481–1484.

Hill JB. Salicylate intoxication. *N Engl J Med* 1973;288:1110–1113.

Prescott LF, Balali-Mood M, Critchley JA, et al. Diuresis or urinary alkalinisation for salicylate poisoning? *BMJ (Clin Res Ed)* 1982; 285:1383–1386.

### Question 110

Deveney CW, Deveney KE. Zollinger-Ellison syndrome (gastrinoma): current diagnosis and treatment. *Surg Clin North Am* 1987;67: 411–422.

### Question 111

Elting LS, Rubenstein EB, Rolston KV, et al. Outcomes of bacteremia in patients with cancer and neutropenia: observations from two decades of epidemiological and clinical trials. *Clin Infect Dis* 1997; 25:247–259.

### Question 112

Wu KK. Morton's interdigital neuroma: a clinical review of its etiology, treatment, and results. *J Ankle Foot Surg* 1996;35:112–119.

### Question 113

Summary of the second report of the National Cholesterol Education Program (NCEP) Expert Panel on Detection, Evaluation, and Treatment of High Blood Cholesterol in Adults. *JAMA* 1993;269: 3015–3023.

### Question 114

Michet CJ. Vasculitis and relapsing polychondritis. *Rheum Dis Clin North Am* 1990;16:441–444.

### Question 115

Bigos S, Bowyer O, Braen G, et al. *Acute low back pain problems in adults: clinical practice guideline.* Rockville, MD: US Department of Health and Human Services, Public Health Service, 1994. Agency for Health Care Policy and Research publication no. 95-0643.

Lahad A, Malter AD, Berg AO, et al. The effectiveness of four interventions for the prevention of low back pain. *JAMA* 1994;272:1286–1291.

### Question 117

Richter JE. Typical and atypical manifestations of gastroesophageal reflux disease: the role of esophageal testing in diagnosis and management. *Gastroenterol Clin North Am* 1996;25:75–102.

### Question 118

Bauman WA, Yalow RS. Hyperinsulinemic hypoglycemia: differential diagnosis by determination of the species of circulating insulin. *JAMA* 1984;252:2730–2734.

Service FJ. Hypoglycemic disorders. *N Engl J Med* 1995;332:1144–1152.

### Question 119

Maddrey WC. Chronic viral hepatitis: diagnosis and management. *Hosp Pract (Off Ed)* 1994;29:117–120.

### Question 120

Bojrab DL, Bruderly T, Abdulrazzak Y. Otitis externa. *Otolaryngol Clin North Am* 1996;29:761–782.

### Question 121

Mariotti S, Caturegli P, Piccolo P, et al. Antithyroid peroxidase autoantibodies in thyroid diseases. *J Clin Endocrinol Metab* 1990;71:661–669.

### Question 122

Dire DJ. Emergency management of dog and cat bite wounds. *Emerg Med Clin North Am* 1992;10:719–736.

Goldstein EJ. Bite wounds and infection. *Clin Infect Dis* 1992;14:633–638.

### Question 128

Schneider TA, Longo WE, Ure T, et al. Mesenteric ischemia: acute arterial syndromes. *Dis Colon Rectum* 1994;37:1163–1174.

Silen W. *Cope's Early Diagnosis of the Acute Abdomen.* Oxford: Oxford University Press, 1990.

### Question 129

Newell FW. *Ophthalmology: Principles and Concepts*, 8th ed. St. Louis: Mosby, 1996.

Schachat AP, Cruess AF. *Ophthalmology.* Baltimore: Williams & Wilkins, 1984.

### Question 130

Fantl JA, Newman DK, Colling J, et al. *Urinary incontinence in adults: acute and chronic management. Urinary Incontinence in Adults Guideline Panel. Clinical practice guideline update.* Rockville, MD: US Department of Health and Human Services, 1996. Agency for Health Care Policy and Research Publication No. 96-0682.

### Question 131

Gaidano G, Guerrasio A, Serra A, et al. Molecular mechanisms of tumor progression in chronic myeloproliferative disorders. *Leukemia* 1994;8:S27–S29.

Najean Y, Rain JD. The very long-term evolution of polycythemia vera: an analysis of 318 patients initially treated by phlebotomy or $^{32}$P between 1969 and 1981. *Semin Hematol* 1997;34:6–16.

Tefferi A, Litzow MR, Noel P, et al. Chronic granulocytic leukemia: recent information on pathogenesis, diagnosis, and disease monitoring. *Mayo Clin Proc* 1997;72:445–452.

## Question 132

Drazen JM, Israel E, Boushey HA, et al. Comparison of regularly scheduled with as-needed use of albuterol in mild asthma. Asthma Clinical Research Network. *N Engl J Med* 1996;335:841–847.

## Question 134

Girolami A, Sartori MT, Simioni P. An updated classification of factor XIII defect. *Br J Haematol* 1991;77:565–566.

Suchman AL, Griner PF. Diagnostic uses of the activated partial thromboplastin time and prothrombin time. *Ann Intern Med* 1986;104:810–816.

## Question 135

American Psychiatric Association. *Diagnostic and Statistical Manual of Mental Disorders*, 4th ed. Primary Care Version (*DSM*-IV-PC). Washington: American Psychiatric Association Press, 1995.

## Question 136

Smith SG. Horner's syndrome. In: Dambro MR, ed. *Griffith's 5 minute Consult*. Baltimore: Lippincott Williams & Wilkins, 1999:502–503.

## Question 137

Appelgren P, Ranjso U, Bindslev L, et al. Surface heparinization of central venous catheters reduces microbial colonization *in vitro* and *in vivo*: results from a prospective, randomized trial. *Crit Care Med* 1996;24:1482–1489.

Cobb DK, High KP, Sawyer RG, et al. A controlled trial of scheduled replacement of central venous and pulmonary-artery catheters. *N Engl J Med* 1992;327:1062–1068.

Eyer S, Brummitt C, Crossley K, et al. Catheter-related sepsis: prospective, randomized study of three different methods of long-term catheter maintenance. *Crit Care Med* 1990;18:1073–1079.

Maki DG, Ringer M. Risk factors for infusion-related phlebitis with small peripheral venous catheters: a randomized, controlled trial. *Ann Intern Med* 1991;114:845–854.

## Question 138

Abel SJ, Finney SJ, Brett SJ, et al. Reduced mortality in association with acute respiratory distress syndrome (ARDS). *Thorax* 1998;53:292–294.

Crawford SW, Petersen FB. Long-term survival from respiratory failure after marrow transplantation for malignancy. *Am Rev Respir Dis* 1992;145:510–514.

Mansel JK, Stogner SW, Petrini MF, et al. Mechanical ventilation in patients with acute severe asthma. *Am J Med* 1990;89:42–48.

Marquette CH, Saulnier F, Leroy O, et al. Long-term prognosis of near-fatal asthma: a 6-year follow-up study of 145 asthmatic patients who underwent mechanical ventilation for a near-fatal attack of asthma. *Am Rev Respir Dis* 1992;146:76–81.

Milberg JA, Davis DR, Steinberg KP, et al. Improved survival of patients with acute respiratory distress syndrome (ARDS): 1983–1993. *JAMA* 1995;273:306–309.

Rangel-Frausto MS, Pittet D, Costigan M, et al. The natural history of the systemic inflammatory response syndrome (SIRS): a prospective study. *JAMA* 1995;273:117–123.

Schapira DV, Studnicki J, Bradham DD, et al. Intensive care, survival, and expense of treating critically ill cancer patients. *JAMA* 1993; 269:783–786.

Weiss SM, Hudson LD. Outcome from respiratory failure: predicting intensive care unit outcome. *Crit Care Clin* 1994;10:197–215.

Westerman DE, Benatar SR, Potgieter PD, et al. Identification of the high-risk asthmatic patient: experience with 39 patients undergoing ventilation for status asthmaticus. *Am J Med* 1979;66:565–572.

## Question 140

Dabbs DJ, Striker LM, Mignon F, et al. Glomerular lesions in lymphomas and leukemias. *Am J Med* 1986;80:63–70.

Nolasco F, Cameron JS, Heywood EF, et al. Adult-onset minimal change nephrotic syndrome: a long-term follow-up. *Kidney Int* 1986;29:1215–1223.

Warren GV, Korbet SM, Schwartz MM, et al. Minimal change glomerulopathy associated with nonsteroidal antiinflammatory drugs. *Am J Kidney Dis* 1989;13:127–130.

## Question 141

Garber AM, Browner WS, Hulley SB. Cholesterol screening in asymptomatic adults, revisited. Part 2. *Ann Intern Med* 1996;124:518–531.

Guidelines for using serum cholesterol, high-density lipoprotein cholesterol, and triglyceride levels as screening tests for preventing coronary heart disease in adults. American College of Physicians. Part 1. *Ann Intern Med* 1996;124:515–517.

Screening for high blood cholesterol and other lipid abnormalities. In: *Guide to Clinical Preventive Services: Report of the U.S. Preventive Services Task Force*, 2nd ed. Baltimore: Williams & Wilkins, 1996: 15–38.

Smith GD, Song F, Sheldon TA. Cholesterol lowering and mortality: the importance of considering initial level of risk. *BMJ* 1993;306: 1367–1373.

Summary of the second report of the National Cholesterol Education Program (NCEP) Expert Panel on Detection, Evaluation, and Treatment of High Blood Cholesterol in Adults. *JAMA* 1993;269: 3015–3023.

## Question 142

Fine MJ, Smith MA, Carson CA, et al. Prognosis and outcome of patients with community-acquired pneumonia: a meta-analysis. *JAMA* 1996;275:134–141.

Potgieter PD, Hammond JM. The intensive care management, mortality and prognostic indicators in severe community-acquired pneumococcal pneumonia. *Intensive Care Med* 1996; 22:1301–1306.

Tuomanen EI, Austrian R, Masure H. Pathogenesis of pneumococcal infection. *N Engl J Med* 1995;332:1280–1284.

## Question 143

NIH consensus conference. Ovarian cancer: screening, treatment, and follow-up. NIH Consensus Development Panel on Ovarian Cancer. *JAMA* 1995;273:491–497.

## Question 144

Dajani AS, Taubert KA, Wilson W, et al. Prevention of bacterial endocarditis: recommendations by the American Heart Association. *JAMA* 1997;277:1794–1801.

Durack DT. Prevention of infective endocarditis. *N Engl J Med* 1995; 332:38–44.

Strom BL, Abrutyn E, Berlin JA, et al. Dental and cardiac risk factors for infective endocarditis: a population-based case-control study. *Ann Intern Med* 1998;129:761–769.

## Question 146

Greenberger PA, Patterson R. Diagnosis and management of allergic bronchopulmonary aspergillosis. *Ann Allergy* 1986;56:444–448.

## Question 147

Bennett CL, Weinberg PD, Rozenberg-Ben-Dror K, et al. Thrombotic thrombocytopenic purpura associated with ticlopidine: a review of 60 cases. *Ann Intern Med* 1998;128:541–544.

George JN, Gilcher RO, Smith JW, et al. Thrombotic thrombocytopenic purpura–hemolytic uremic syndrome: diagnosis and management. *J Clin Apheresis* 1998;13:120–125.

Leavey SF, Weinberg J. Thrombotic thrombocytopenic purpura associated with ticlopidine therapy. *J Am Soc Nephrol* 1997;8:689–693.

## Question 148

Brainwald E, Jones RH, Mark DB, et al. Diagnosing and managing unstable angina. Agency for Health Care Policy and Research. *Circulation* 1994;90:613–622.

## Question 150

George JN, el-Harake MA, Raskob GE. Chronic idiopathic thrombocytopenic purpura. *N Engl J Med* 1994;331:1207–1211.

Stasi R, Stipa E, Masi M, et al. Long-term observation of 208 adults with chronic idiopathic thrombocytopenic purpura. *Am J Med* 1995;98:436–442.

## Question 151

Irwin RS, Curley FJ, French CL. Chronic cough: the spectrum and frequency of causes, key components of the diagnostic evaluation, and outcome of specific therapy. *Am Rev Respir Dis* 1990;141:640–647.

Israili ZH, Hall WD. Cough and angioneurotic edema associated with angiotensin-converting enzyme inhibitor therapy: a review of the literature and pathophysiology. *Ann Intern Med* 1992;117:234–242.

Mello CJ, Irwin RS, Curley FJ. Predictive values of the character, timing, and complications of chronic cough in diagnosing its cause. *Arch Intern Med* 1996;156:997–1003.

Pratter MR, Bartter T, Akers S, et al. An algorithmic approach to chronic cough. *Ann Intern Med* 1993;119:977–983.

## Question 152

Brieger DB, Mak KH, Kottke-Marchant K, et al. Heparin-induced thrombocytopenia. *J Am Coll Cardiol* 1998;31:1449–1459.

Warkentin TE, Levine MN, Hirsh J, et al. Heparin-induced thrombocytopenia in patients treated with low-molecular-weight heparin or unfractionated heparin. *N Engl J Med* 1995;332:1330–1335.

## Question 153

Ginsberg JS, Wells PS, Kearon C, et al. Sensitivity and specificity of a rapid whole-blood assay for D-dimer in the diagnosis of pulmonary embolism. *Ann Intern Med* 1998;129:1006–1111.

## Question 154

Bunn PA Jr. Lung cancer. *Semin Oncol* 1988;15:138.

Midthun DE, Jett JR. Clinical presentation of lung cancer. In: Pass HI, et al., eds. *Lung Cancer: Principles and Practice.* Philadelphia: Lippincott–Raven Publishers, 1996:421.

## Question 155

Austrian R, Gold J. Pneumococcal bacteremia with especial reference to bacteremic pneumococcal pneumonia. *Ann Intern Med* 1964;60:759.

Barrett-Conner E. The non-value of sputum culture in the diagnosis of pneumococcal pneumonia. *Am Rev Respir Dis* 1970;103:845.

## Question 156

Amorosi E, Utmann J. Thrombotic thrombocytopenic purpura: report of 16 cases and review of the literature. *Medicine (Baltimore)* 1966;45:139.

Bennett CL, Connors JM, Carwile JM, et al. Thrombotic thrombocytopenic purpura associated with clopidogrel. *N Engl J Med* 2000;342:1773–1777.

CAPRIE Steering Committee. A randomised, blinded, trial of clopidogrel versus aspirin in patients at risk of ischemic events (CAPRIE). *Lancet* 1996;348:1329–1339.

Connors JM, et al. Clopidogrel associated TTP. *Transfusion* 1999;39[Suppl]:56S–56S.

Soltero ER, et al. Thrombotic thrombocytopenic purpura occurring after exposure to clopidogrel. *Blood* 1999;94[Suppl 1]:78b–78b(abst).

## Questions 157–159

Cunningham-Rundles C, Siegal FP, Cunningham-Rundles S, et al. Incidence of cancer in 98 patients with common varied immunodeficiency. *J Clin Immunol* 1987;7:294–299.

Densen P. Complement deficiencies and meningococcal disease. *Clin Exp Immunol* 1991;86[Suppl 1]:57.

Ellison RT III, Kohler PF, Curd JG, et al. Prevalence of congenital or acquired complement deficiency in patients with sporadic meningococcal disease. *N Engl J Med* 1983;308:913.

Kinlen LJ, Webster AD, Bird AG, et al. Prospective study of cancer in patients with hypogammaglobulinaemia. *Lancet* 1985;1:263–266.

## Questions 160–165

Consensus Development Conference. Consensus development conference: diagnosis, prophylaxis, and treatment of osteoporosis. *Am J Med* 1993;94:646.

Gardsell P, Johnell O, Nilsson BE. The predictive value of forearm bone mineral content measurements in men. *Bone* 1990;11:229–232.

Kanis JA, Melton LJ III, Christiansen C, et al. The diagnosis of osteoporosis. *J Bone Miner Res* 1994;9:1137.

Rosen FS, Cooper MD, Wedgwood RJP. Medical progress: the primary immunodeficiencies. *N Engl J Med* 1995;333:431–440.

Rosol TJ, Capen CC. Mechanisms of cancer-induced hypercalcemia. *Lab Invest* 1992;67:680.

Seymour JF, Gagel RF. Calcitriol: the major humoral mediator of hypercalcemia in Hodgkin's disease and non-Hodgkin's lymphomas. *Blood* 1993;82:1383.

Silverberg SJ, Shane E, Jacobs TP, et al. Nephrolithiasis and bone involvement in primary hyperparathyroidism. *Am J Med* 1990;89:327.

Silverberg SJ, Bilezikian JP. Evaluation and management of primary hyperparathyroidism. *J Clin Endocrinol Metab* 1996;81:2036.

Sneller MC, Strober W, Eisenstein E, et al. NIH conference: new insights into common variable immunodeficiency. *Ann Intern Med* 1993;188:720–730.

Walport MJ. Advances in immunology: complement—first of two parts. *N Engl J Med* 2001;344:1058–1066.

## Question 166

Connelly TJ, Becker A, McDonald JW. Bachelor scurvy. *Int J Dermatol* 1982;21:209–211.

Hirschmann JV, Raugi GJ. Adult scurvy. *J Am Acad Dermatol* 1999;41:895–906.

Hodges RE, Baker EM, Hood J, et al. Experimental scurvy in man. *Am J Clin Nutr* 1969;22:535–548.

Reddy AV, Chan K, Jones JIW, et al. Spontaneous bruising in an elderly woman. *Postgrad Med J* 1998;74:273–275.

Reuler JB, Broudy VC, Cooney TG. Adult scurvy. *JAMA* 1985;253:805–807.

Stewart CP, Guthrie D. *Lind's treatise on scurvy.* Edinburgh: Edinburgh University Press, 1953:113–126.

## Question 167

Lieber CS. Medical disorders of alcoholism. *N Engl J Med* 1995;333: 1058.

Victor M, et al. *The Wernicke-Korsakoff Syndrome and Related Disorders due to alcoholism and Malnutrition.* Philadelphia: Davis, 1989.

## Question 168

Beyenburg S, Zierz S, Jerusalem F. Inclusion body myositis: clinical and histopathological features of 36 patients. *Clin Invest* 1993;71: 351.

Gerster JC, Vischer TL, Fallet GH. Destructive arthropathy in generalized osteoarthritis with articular chondrocalcinosis. *J Rheumatol* 1975;2:265.

Hamilton EBD, Richards AJ. Destructive arthropathy in chondrocalcinosis articularis. *Ann Rheum Dis* 1974;33:196.

Kula RW, Sawchak JA, Sher JH. Inclusion body myositis. *Curr Opin Rheumatol* 1989;1:460.

## Questions 170–172

Service FJ, O'Brien PC, McMahon MM, et al. C-peptide during the prolonged fast in insulinoma. *J Clin Endocrinol Metab* 1993;76:655–659.

## Question 181

George JN, Woolf SH, Raskob GE, et al. Idiopathic thrombocytopenic purpura: a practice guideline developed by explicit methods for the American Society of Hematology. *Blood* 1996;88:3–40.

Moise KJ Jr. Autoimmune thrombocytopenic purpura in pregnancy. *Clin Obstet Gynecol* 1991;34:51–63.

## Questions 182–187

Balasubramaniam K, Grambsch PM, Wiesner RH, et al. Diminished survival in asymptomatic primary biliary cirrhosis. A prospective study. *Gastroenterology* 1990;98:1567–1571.

Gollan JL, Bateman C, Billing BH. Effect of dietary composition on the unconjugated hyperbilirubinaemia of Gilbert's syndrome. *Gut* 1976;17:335–340.

Kaplan MM. Primary biliary cirrhosis. *N Engl J Med* 1996;335:1570–1580.

Lednar WM, Lemon SM, Kirkpatrick JW, et al. Frequency of illness associated with epidemic hepatitis A virus infections in adults. *Am J Epidemiol* 1985;122:226–233.

## Question 197

Llach F. *Renal Vein Thrombosis.* New York: Futura, 1983.

# Index